Essentials of Communication Sciences & Disorders

Paul T. Fogle, Ph.D., CCC-SLP

Private Practice
Sacramento/Elk Grove, California

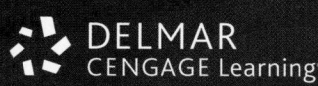
DELMAR
CENGAGE Learning

Australia • Brazil • Japan • Korea • Mexico • Singapore • Spain • United Kingdom • United States

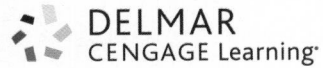
DELMAR
CENGAGE Learning·

**Essentials of Communication Sciences
& Disorders, International Edition**
Paul T. Fogle, Ph.D., CCC-SLP

Vice President, Careers and Computing:
Dave Garza

Director of Learning Solutions:
Matthew Kane

Associate Acquisitions Editor: Tom Stover

Managing Editor: Marah Bellegarde

Senior Product Manager: Laura J. Wood

Editorial Assistant: Anthony Souza

Vice President, Marketing: Jennifer Baker

Marketing Director: Wendy E. Mapstone

Marketing Manager: Matthew Williams

Senior Director, Education Production:
Wendy A. Troeger

Production Manager: Andrew Crouth

Senior Content Project Manager:
Kara A. DiCaterino

Senior Art Director: David Arsenault

Library of Congress Control Number: 2011942788

International Edition:
ISBN-13: 978-1-133-68730-6
ISBN-10: 1-133-68730-X

Cengage Learning International Offices

Asia
www.cengageasia.com
tel: (65) 6410 1200

Australia/New Zealand
www.cengage.com.au
tel: (61) 3 9685 4111

Brazil
www.cengage.com.br
tel: (55) 11 3665 9900

India
www.cengage.co.in
tel: (91) 11 4364 1111

Latin America
www.cengage.com.mx
tel: (52) 55 1500 6000

UK/Europe/Middle East/Africa
www.cengage.co.uk
tel: (44) 0 1264 332 424

**Represented in Canada by
Nelson Education, Ltd.**
www.nelson.com
tel: (416) 752 9100 /
(800) 668 0671

Cengage Learning is a leading provider of customized learning solutions
with office locations around the globe, including Singapore, the United
Kingdom, Australia, Mexico, Brazil, and Japan. Locate your local office at:
www.cengage.com/global

For product information and free companion resources:
www.cengage.com/international

Visit your local office: **www.cengage.com/global**
Visit our corporate website: **www.cengage.com**

Printed in the United States of America
1 2 3 4 5 16 15 14 13 12

Contents

CHAPTER 1

Essentials of Communication and Its Disorders   2

CHAPTER 2

Speech-Language Pathologists and Audiologists   24

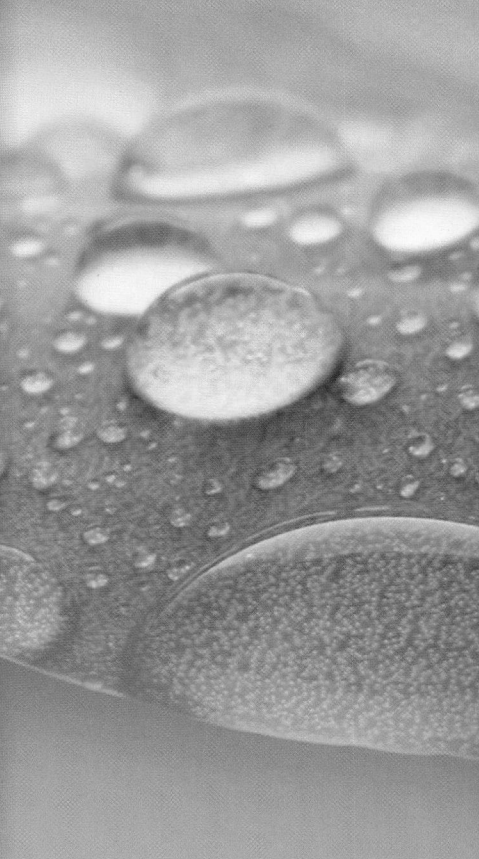

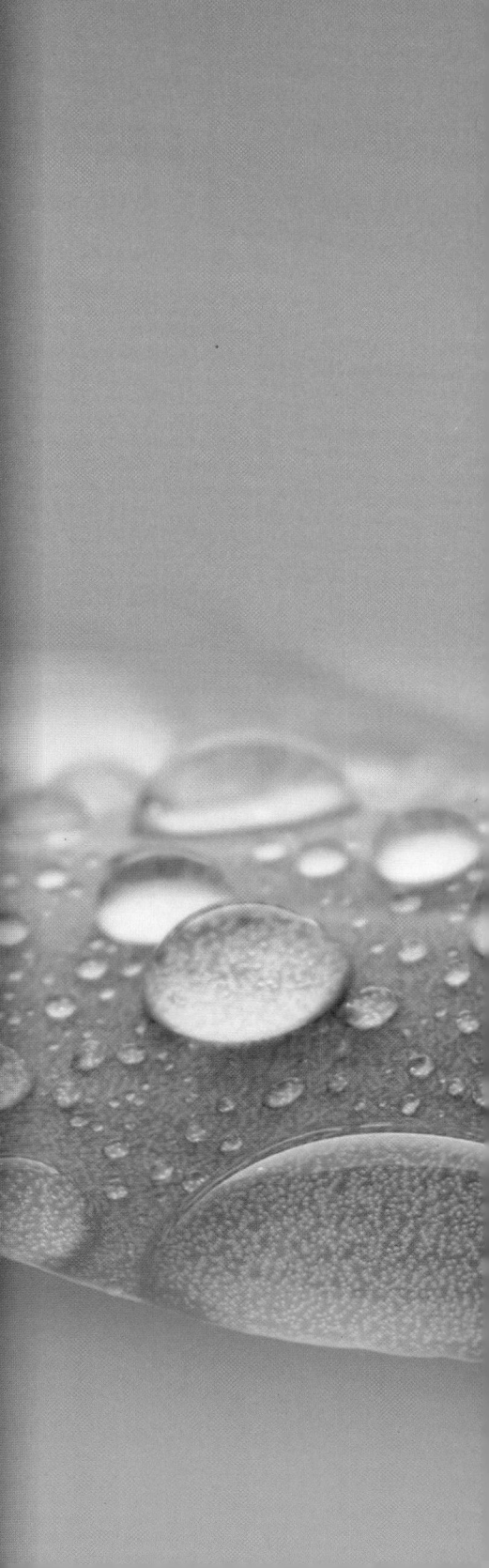

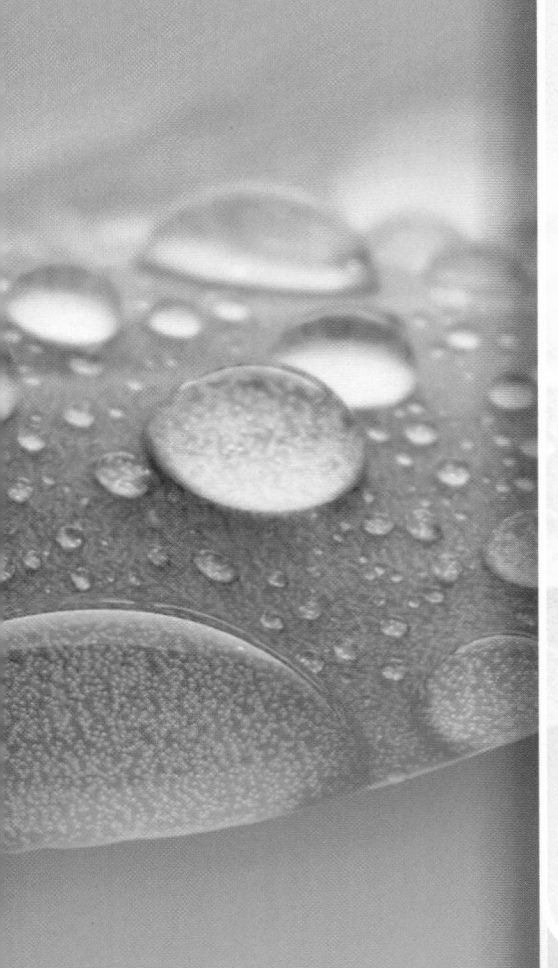

CHAPTER 8

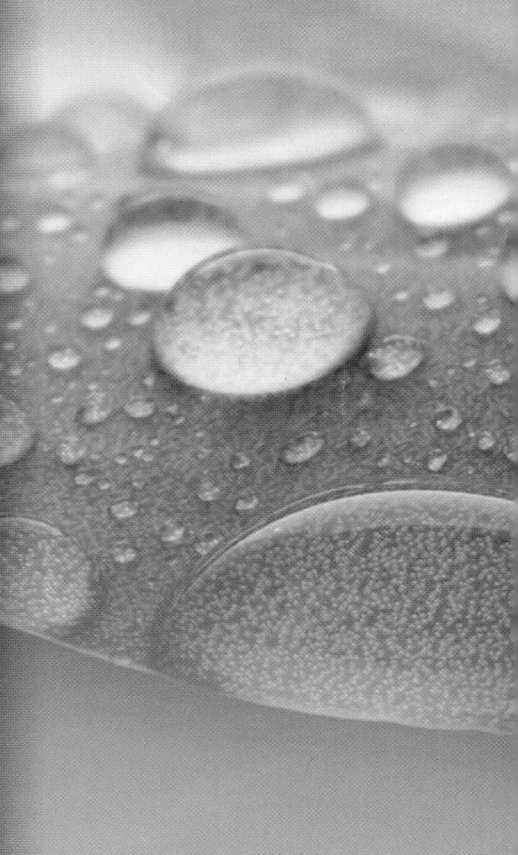

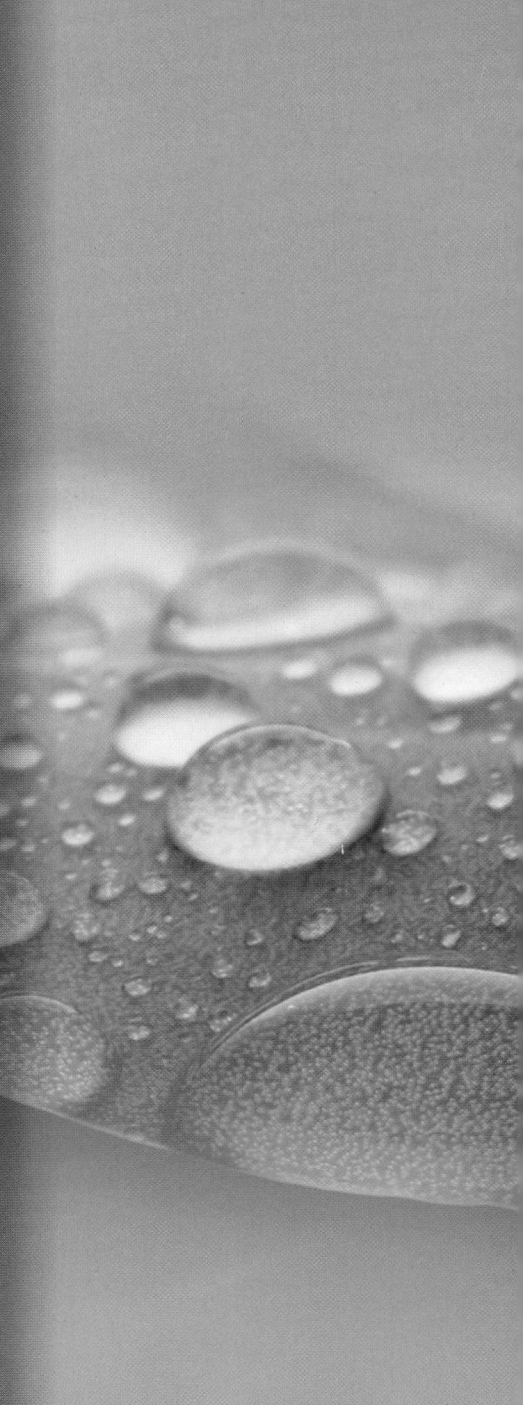

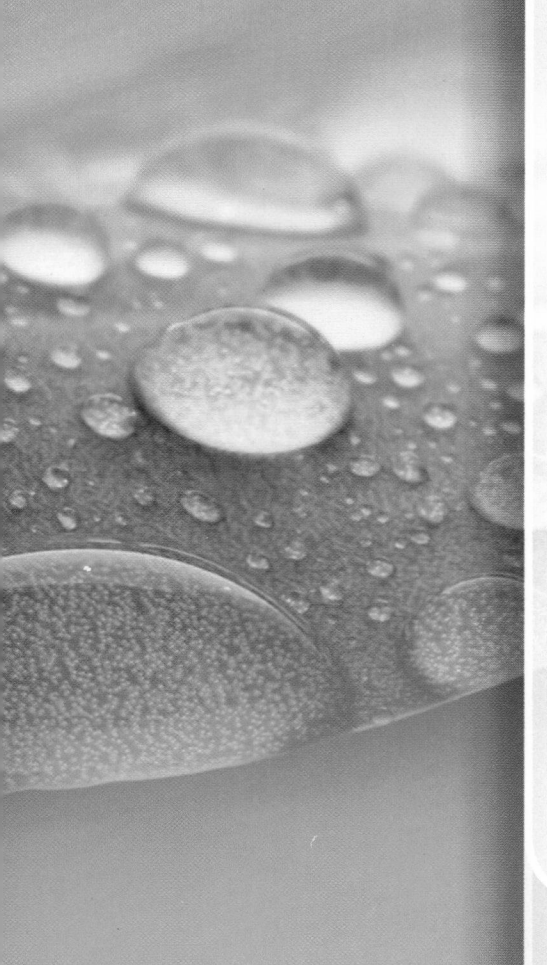

INTRODUCTION

Essentials of Communication Sciences & Disorders is a shorter version of the extensive 920-page *Foundations of Communication Sciences & Disorders* text (Fogle, 2008). Both texts were written for students just beginning their education in speech-language pathology and audiology (communicative disorders). The *Essentials* text focuses on what is considered the vital information beginning students need, whereas the *Foundations* text goes well beyond that level of information. Both texts are based on the skills and knowledge specified in the American Speech-Language-Hearing Association's (ASHA's) 2005 Standards for the Certificate of Clinical Competence (CCC) that address the Knowledge and Skills Acquisition Summary (KASA). Both texts are written in a student-friendly manner so they are both understandable and interesting.

Other Groups of Students

There are other groups of students for whom the *Essentials* text is written—students who take an introductory course in speech-language pathology and audiology who have no intention of going into the major. During the years I have taught the introductory course, students from a wide range of majors have taken the course because someone recommended it, it sounded interesting, or it just worked well into their schedules. Some of these students find the information very interesting and change their majors. For them, the course is serendipitous. These students often bring into their new major valuable perspectives from their past majors, such as premedicine, predentistry, prepharmacy, education, psychology, business, and many others. The professions of speech-language pathology and audiology are all the richer for having students enter who come from other majors. However, for the students who take the introduction to speech-language pathology and audiology course who do not change their major, they and their future professions often benefit from having an understanding of how this course and this book can relate to their work. In addition, students later realize that much of what they learn may help them in their personal lives as parents and possible caregivers to their own parents. As instructors of the introductory course, we know that the information we present relates to life in general and not just to the disciplines of speech-language pathology and audiology.

DESIGN OF THE TEXT

This text was designed for students to enjoy. One of the first things students notice is that all of the illustrations, photos, and figures are in full color. Students also find the writing clear and understandable, with many colorful stories and examples of real-life cases. In other words, we have created an inviting place for students to learn.

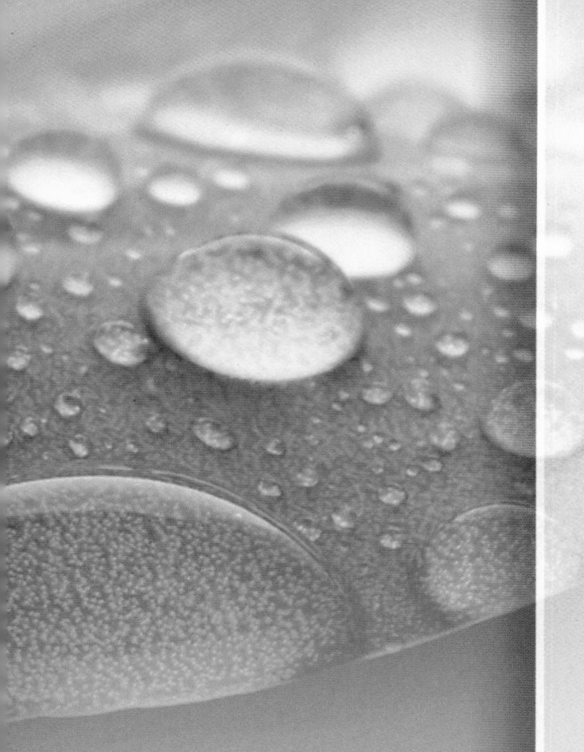

The text presents much of the most recent literature in each chapter. This text also cites literature that is not often cited in introductory texts. There are many references from professional journals outside of speech-language pathology and audiology that are relevant to our professions. These were included to help students understand that there is important information from other professions that relates directly and indirectly to our work.

Essentials of Communication Sciences & Disorders includes literature from numerous foreign journals that are not normally cited by an American author. This was done for several reasons. First, there is a vast amount of literature published in journals around the world that adds important information to our understanding of the many disorders we work with, as well as providing directions for assessment and treatment. Second, this text was written for an international market because speech-language pathology and audiology are practiced in countries around the world. Third, it is important for students to realize that in many countries where they may choose to travel or live and work, they are in a fraternity of speech-language pathologists (SLPs) and audiologists (Auds) with whom they can immediately relate.

CONCEPTUAL APPROACH TO THE TEXT

The conceptual approach to this text is based on several considerations, which may be seen as themes throughout the book. First and foremost, solid, up-to-date information is the foundation of this text. Second, our work is always a team approach, and the most important person on the team is the person with the communication disorder. Third, all of our therapy involves working with the central and peripheral nervous systems. Fourth, people of all ages with communication impairments have emotional and social reactions to their problems. As clinicians, we must work with our clients and patients holistically; we must work with the whole person and not just the disorders that we diagnose and treat. Likewise, the family members of our clients and patients often experience their own emotional and social effects from their loved one's problems. Fifth, there is a joy in being a therapist—a person in a helping profession. As clinicians, we receive much satisfaction from our work. People recognize that we are excited about our work even after doing therapy for many years.

ORGANIZATION AND FEATURES OF THE TEXT

Essentials of Communication Sciences & Disorders was carefully organized for the benefit of students and for ease in teaching. Each chapter begins with learning objectives, a list of key terms, a chapter outline, and an introduction. When an important term is first introduced in the text, it is placed in bold type to highlight it. The term is defined in the margin of the text, and all definitions are compiled in a comprehensive glossary at the back of the book.

Throughout each chapter there are various application questions designed to help students consider how they might use the information they are learning in their personal lives. Most chapters also have case studies and personal clinical stories that are relevant to the material. These features are intended to help paint a vivid picture of the profession, long before students have the opportunity to participate in a clinical practicum.

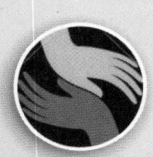

Multicultural considerations are discussed in nearly all chapters as the text material relates specifically to this important area. The multicultural considerations are indicated with a special margin icon, so while the content is part of the main narrative, it can still be easily identified.

Each chapter ends with a Summary that highlights some of the basic concepts discussed. Numerous study questions are provided that are based on Bloom's (1956) taxonomy of educational objectives. That is, three general levels of question difficulty are presented for each chapter: (1) knowledge/comprehension, (2) application, and (3) analysis/synthesis. By answering these questions, students can demonstrate several levels of learning. Each chapter ends with an extensive list of references that students may use to further research the information and concepts presented.

A Word About Words

Many of the terms we use in our profession have Greek or Latin origins, some of which date back 1,000 to 2,000 years. When possible, the end-of-the-book glossary definitions include etymologies of words. Having an understanding of the etymology of words may be helpful in learning the words. Words evolve and meanings change, and the etymology may provide a sense of the history of a word and how it relates to its current use. Also, as with English, the ancient Greek and Latin languages had synonyms for words, and students may find some variability in the terms we use and their etymologies (e.g., in Latin, *aqua* and *lympha* both mean water). Several sources were consulted for definitions of terms and their etymologies, including the *Cambridge International Dictionary of English* (1999), *Mosby's Nursing and Allied Health Dictionary* (2009), Nicolosi, Harryman, and Kresheck's *Terminology of Communication Disorders: Speech-Language-Hearing* (5th ed.) (2004), the *Oxford Dictionary of English Etymology* (1994), *Webster's New Universal Unabridged Dictionary* (2003), and the glossaries of many of the texts that are cited in the various chapters.

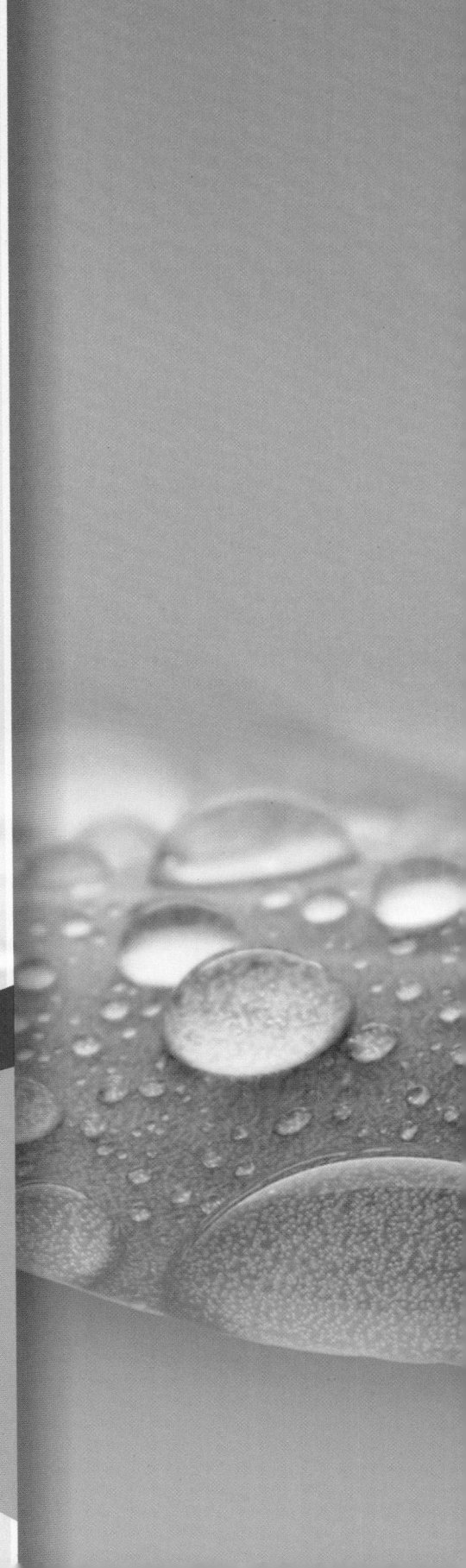

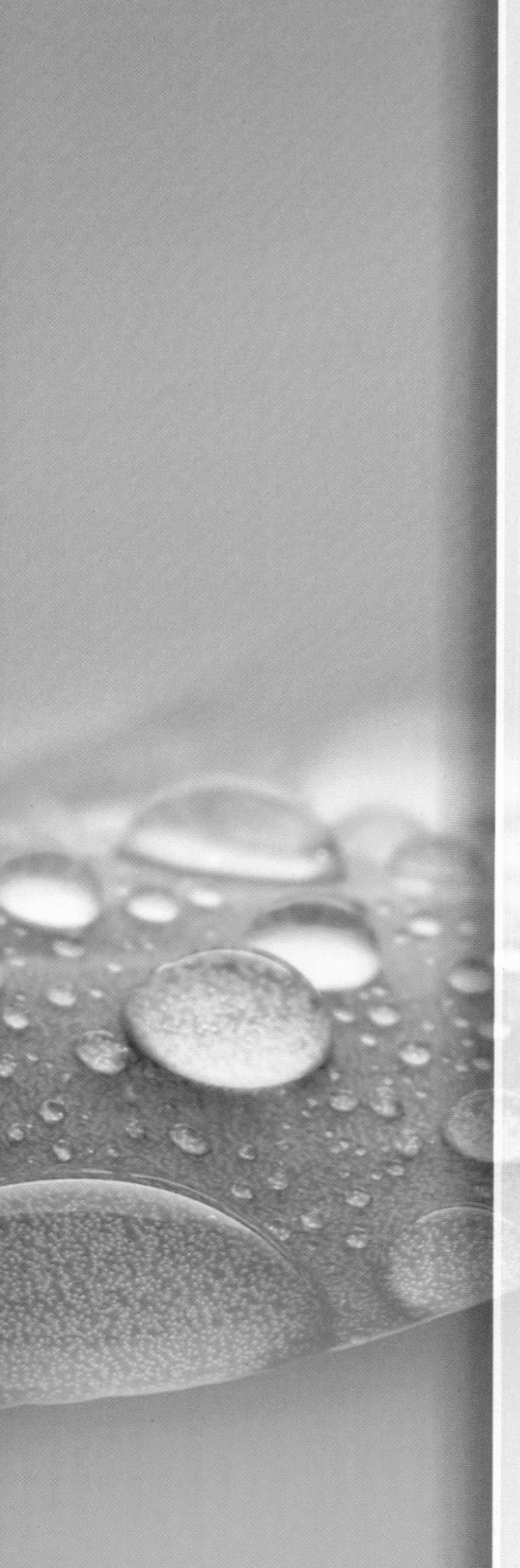

CHAPTERS

Chapter 1: Essentials of Communication and Its Disorders

Chapter 1 introduces the study of human communication and disorders of communication, including communication modalities and classification of communication disorders. It also discusses the concept that there are always emotional and social effects of a communication disorder on the person and the family, and these are discussed further in each chapter on the various disorders.

Chapter 2: Speech-Language Pathologists and Audiologists

A discussion of the professions and the professionals is placed early in the text because students want to know whether these are professions they want to work in and are these the kinds of professionals they want to work with. Some of the topics include the professional organizations, professional ethics, personal qualities (attributes) of effective professionals, the team approach, work settings of SLPs and Auds, and the employment outlook.

Chapter 3: Anatomy and Physiology of Speech and Language

This chapter discusses each of the speech systems (respiratory, phonatory, resonatory, and articulatory) and the essential information about the nervous system that is needed by students in an introductory course on communicative disorders. The numerous illustrations are helpful in understanding both the anatomy and physiology of the structures.

Chapter 4: Speech and Language Development

This chapter begins with theories (perspectives) of speech and language development. The material on speech and language development attempts to provide a sequential but "blended" (i.e., the stages overlap) explanation of how children learn speech and language through early adolescence.

Chapter 5: Articulation and Phonological Disorders in Children

This is one of the longest chapters in the book but it also includes information beyond articulation and phonological disorders.

The material on General American English and Etiologies of Communication Disorders provides foundations from which all other information about children's speech and language disorders can build. Beyond articulation and phonological disorders, there also are discussions about childhood apraxia of speech and dysarthria in children. The ending material in this chapter, as well as in all succeeding chapters, deals with the emotional and social effects of the disorders discussed in the chapter.

Chapter 6: Language Disorders in Children

This chapter begins with essential background information on definitions of language disorders, language disorder vs. language delay, language disorder vs. language difference, prevalence vs. incidence, and severity levels. The discussions of language disorders in this chapter generally follow a chronological sequence, from young children through adolescence. The essential components of a language evaluation are presented and a discussion of operationally defined goals and an outline of a therapy session are included.

Chapter 7: Literacy Disorders in Children

A solid case for literacy disorders being within the scope of practice of SLPs is presented, as well as ASHA guidelines for the roles and responsibilities of SLPs in literacy for children and adolescents. Common problems of children with literacy disorders are discussed and the essentials of assessment and intervention for reading and writing problems are presented.

Chapter 8: Fluency Disorders

This chapter begins with a discussion of normal fluency and defining stuttering, with emphasis on overt and covert behaviors. The essential information about stuttering and theories of its etiology are presented. The rest of the chapter focuses on working with children who stutter and working with adolescents and adults who stutter. The emotional and social effects of stuttering are discussed.

Chapter 9: Voice Disorders in Children and Adults

The various voice disorders are discussed in groupings or classifications relating to functional etiologies and faulty usage, organic etiologies, and neurological etiologies. Both the otolaryngologist's and

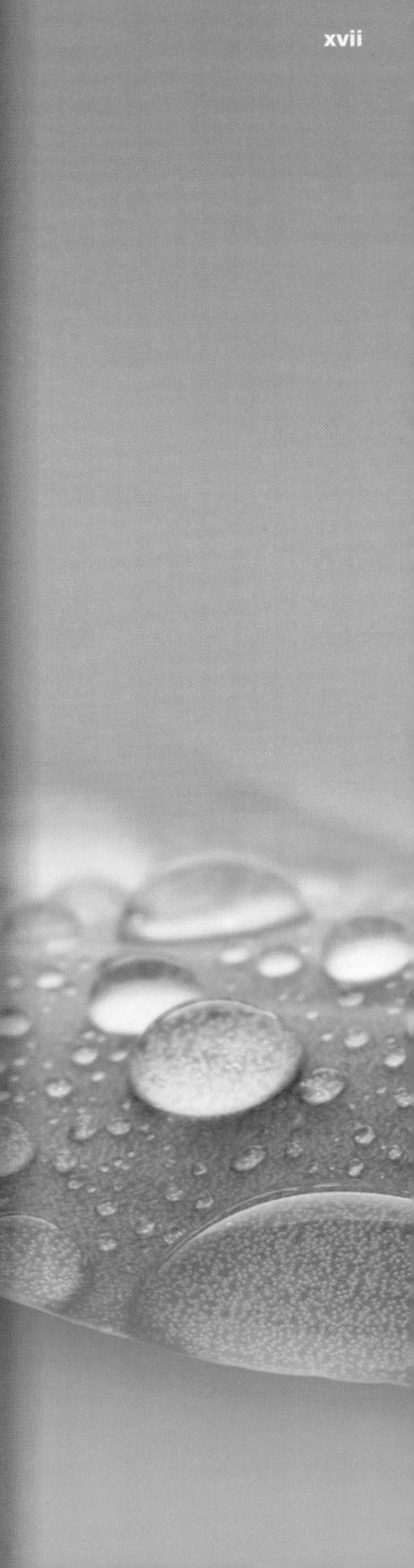

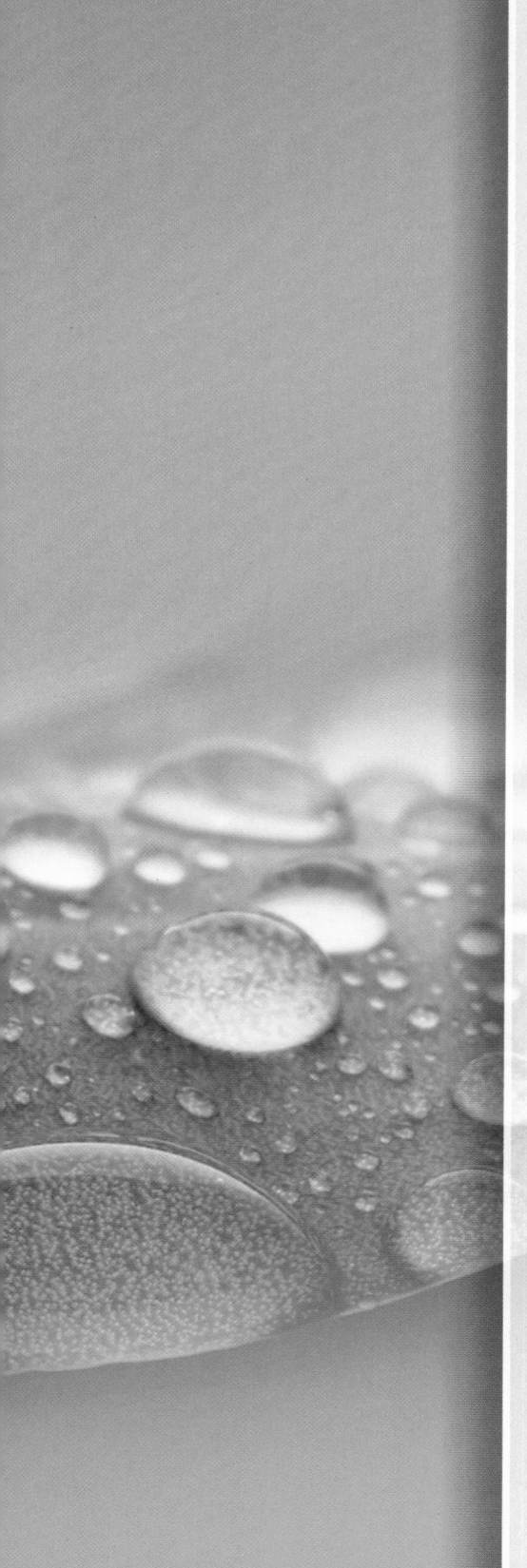

the speech pathologist's assessments are discussed. Three foundational voice therapy approaches are presented: physiologic voice therapy, hygienic voice therapy, and symptomatic voice therapy. Laryngectomy and alaryngeal speech are discussed.

Chapter 10: Cleft Lip and Palate

This chapter presents the primary etiologies of clefts of the lip and palate associated problems with clefts and craniofacial anomalies, including articulation disorders. Surgical management of cleft lip and palate and speech assessment and therapy are discussed. The numerous photographs of real people with clefts enhance the student's understanding of the complexity of these problems.

Chapter 11: Neurological Disorders in Adults

This is a relatively long chapter because the area of neurological disorders in adults is extensive and complex. The essentials of the etiologies of neurological disorders are presented, from strokes to traumatic brain injuries to dementia. The aphasias and cognitive disorders are discussed, and assessment and general principles of therapy for the disorders are included.

Chapter 12: Motor Speech Disorders and Dysphagia/Swallowing Disorders

Apraxia and dysarthria in children were discussed earlier in Chapter 5: Articulation and Phonological Disorders. These disorders, however, are more commonly seen in adults and are discussed in more detail in this chapter. General principles of assessment and therapy for apraxia and dysarthria are presented. SLPs are considered the medical experts in the area of dysphagia/swallowing disorders and this section of the chapter emphasizes the phases of the normal swallow followed by discussions of the various swallowing disorders and their diagnosis and treatment.

Chapter 13: Special Populations with Communication Disorders

This chapter introduces several diverse topics, including intellectual disabilities, autism and pervasive developmental disorders, attention deficit disorders, auditory processing disorders, traumatic brain injury in children, cerebral palsy, and augmentative and alternative communication. There are numerous references that students can use for further information on each of these special populations and their communication disorders.

Chapter 14: Hearing Disorders in Children and Adults

The chapter on hearing disorders is traditionally the last chapter in introductory textbooks; however, its placement does not diminish its importance. This chapter is relatively long but numerous figures that add visual information are included. The chapter begins with discussions of the anatomy and physiology of the ear and central auditory nervous system. These are followed by information on the types and causes of hearing impairments, communication disorders associated with hearing impairments, hearing assessment, and amplification for individuals with hearing impairments. Discussions about aural rehabilitation and the emotional and social effects of hearing impairments end the chapter.

Epilogue

The Epilogue is intended to help students understand that what they have in the book and the introductory course is more than just information about communication disorders, but about the kinds of interesting work speech-language pathologists and audiologists do on a daily basis. The textbook they have and the information they have learned in the course can help them not only in their professional lives but also in their personal lives.

ALSO AVAILABLE

CourseMate to accompany Essentials of Communication Sciences and Disorders

INSTANT ACCESS CODE ISBN-13: 978-1-111-64251-8
PRINTED ACCESS CARD ISBN-13: 978-1-111-64252-5

CourseMate includes:

- an interactive eBook, with highlighting, note taking and search capabilities
- interactive learning tools including:
  - Quizzes
  - Flashcards
  - Animations
  - Games and activities
  - Internet Search Terms
  - and more!
- Engagement Tracker, a first-of-its-kind tool that monitors student engagement in the course.

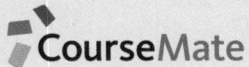 Go to **www.cengagebrain.com** to access these resources, and look for this icon to find resources related to your text.

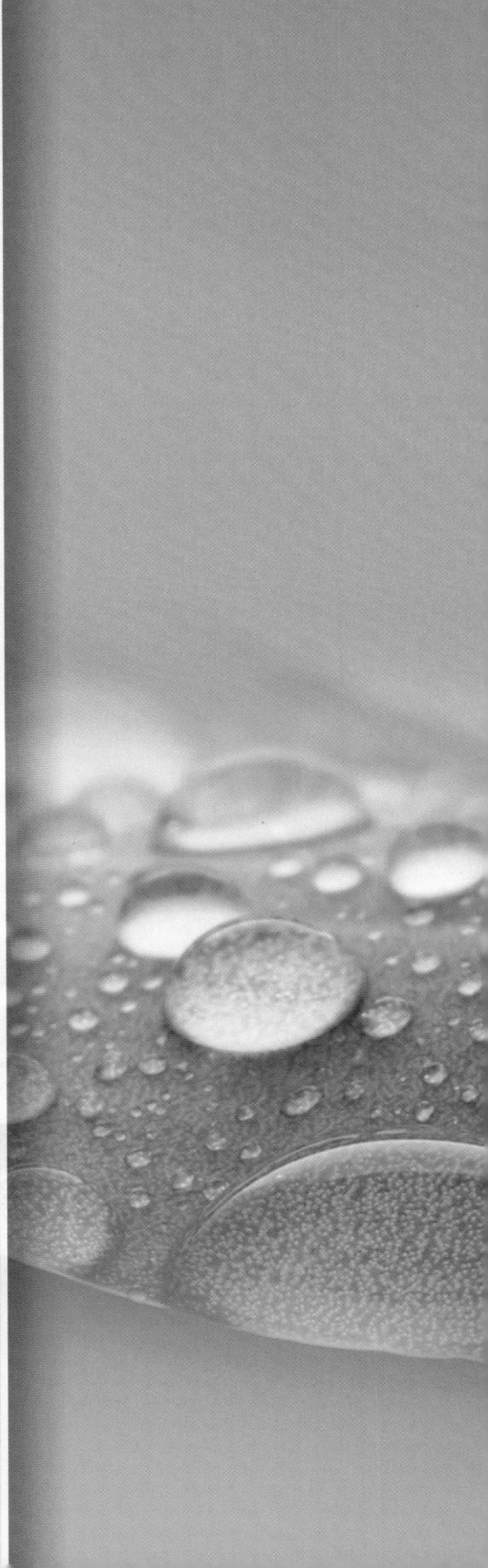

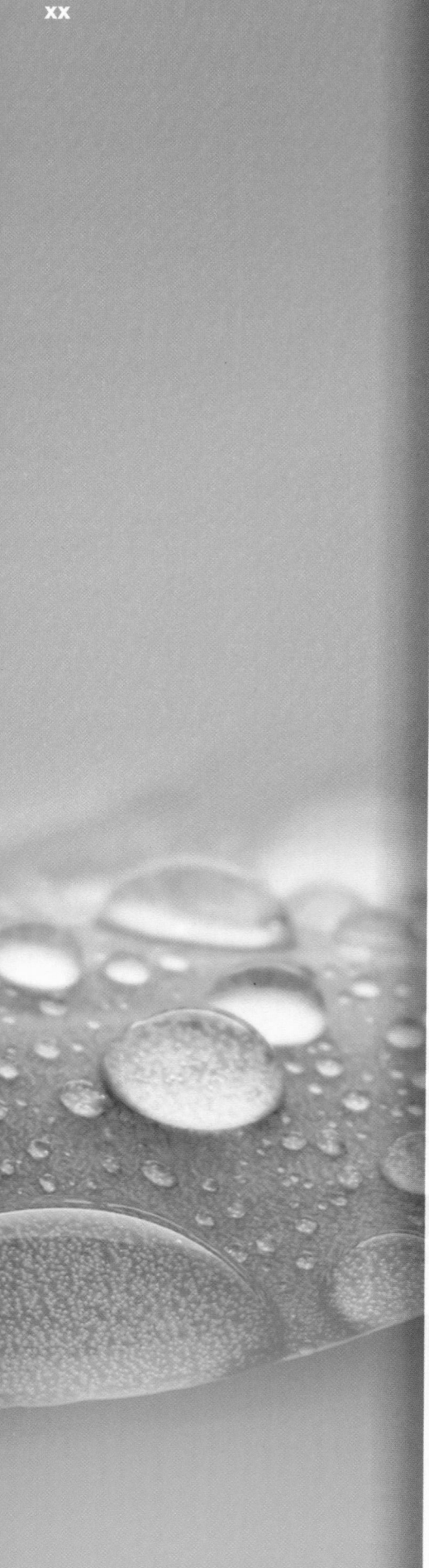

Instructor Companion Website to Accompany Essentials of Communication Sciences and Disorders

ISBN-13: 978-0-840-02255-4

Spend Less Time Planning and More Time Teaching!

With Delmar, Cengage Learning's Instructor Companion Website to Accompany *Essentials of Communication Sciences and Disorders,* preparing for class and evaluating students has never been easier! As an instructor, you will find this tool offers invaluable assistance by giving you access to all of your resources – anywhere and at any time. Features:

- The **Instructor's Manual** contains a course syllabus, teaching tips, and answers to the end of chapter study questions; it is available in Adobe Acrobat PDF® format.
- The **Computerized Testbank** in **ExamView®** makes generating tests and quizzes a snap. With hundreds of questions and different styles to choose from, including multiple choice, true/false, completion, matching, and short answer, you can create customized assessments for your students with the click of a button. Add your own unique questions and print answers for easy class preparation.
- Customizable instructor support slide presentations in **PowerPoint®** format focus on key points for each chapter. Use for in-class lectures or as hand outs for note taking.
- Use the **Image Library** to enhance your instructor support slide presentations, insert art into test questions, or add visuals wherever you need them. These valuable images, which include all artwork form the textbook, are organized by chapter and are easily searchable.
- **Animations** offer enhanced visual aids to help students comprehend important concepts. Animations include The Process of Respiration, The Process of Hearing, The Process of Phonation, and more!

ExamView® is a registered trademark of eInstruction Corp.

PowerPoint® is a registered trademark of the Microsoft Corporation.

To access these resources, contact your sales representative or go to http://login.cengage.com.

ACKNOWLEDGMENTS

This text emphasizes the team approach when working with clients and patients. Likewise, the writing of this book was a team approach with so many people contributing their time, energy,

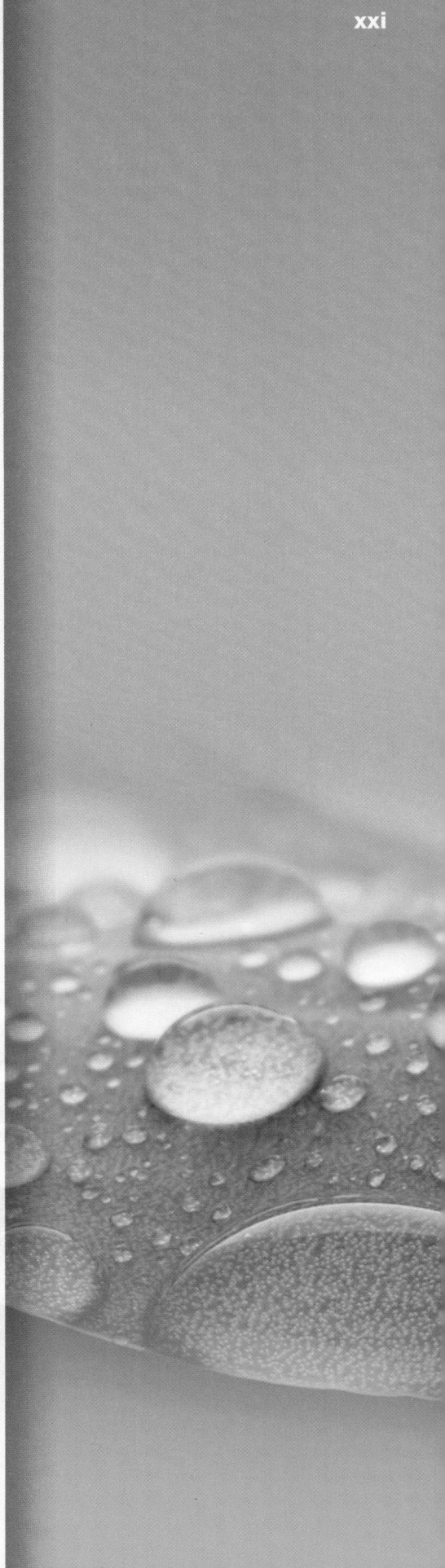

and talents to my education, professional development, and ultimately this writing.

Mr. Rex Fisher, my high school biology and anatomy and physiology teacher, and eventually my friend, introduced me to the fascinating study of life and the human body. These became the foundations of my life's work.

Dr. Joseph and Mrs. Vivian Sheehan inspired my interest in stuttering, trained me well at the Psychology Adult Stuttering Clinic at the University of California, Los Angeles (UCLA), and encouraged me to pursue my doctorate in speech-language pathology.

Dr. Dean Williams, professor and expert in stuttering at the Wendell Johnson Speech and Hearing Center, the University of Iowa, was my mentor and dissertation advisor. His statement to the students in one of his classes remains an inspiration to me: "I hope all of you find someone who helps you become more than what you ever thought you could be." Dr. Williams was that person for me.

Sherry Dickinson, Senior Acquisitions Editor, Delmar Cengage Learning, had the foresight to suggest the need for this text, and Tom Stover, Associate Acquisitions Editor, supported this project.

Laura Wood, Senior Product Manager, Delmar Cengage Learning, provided her expertise and diligence in all steps during the writing, editing, and production of this book. Her insightful comments and dedicated work were essential from the inception to the completion.

Marlene Salas-Provance, Ph.D., MHA, CCC-SLP, contributed significantly to the Multicultural Considerations material throughout this text. Dr. Salas-Provance is the Director of the Graduate Program in Communication Disorders at New Mexico State University; President and CEO of Bilingual Advantage, Inc.; past Coordinator of ASHA Division 14, Communication Disorders and Sciences in Culturally and Linguistically Diverse Populations; past President of the Hispanic Caucus, an ASHA-related professional organization; and is a founding steering committee member and coordinator (2012–2014) of ASHA's Special Interest Group 17, Global Issues in Communication Sciences and Related Disorders. She serves as New Mexico's representative on ASHA's Speech-Language Pathology Advisory Council (2011–2013). She is an ASHA Fellow and a recipient of ASHA's Certificate of Recognition for Special Contributions in Multicultural Affairs.

Barbara Hutchinson, M.A., CCC-SLP, carefully reviewed and edited Chapters 1–7 of this text. Her suggestions were very helpful in strengthening and making clearer each of those chapters.

Rotary International and Rotaplast International Cleft Palate Team provided opportunities for me to travel to Venezuela, Egypt, and India to work with infants, children, and adults with cleft lips and palates, and from those "missions" photographs have been included in this text.

The libraries of Macquarie University, Sydney, Australia; Canterbury University, Christchurch, New Zealand; and the University of Reading, Reading, England, provided excellent facilities for research for the international emphasis of this text.

Tom Stock of Stock Photography provided many of the beautiful photographs of children and adults with communication disorders.

Tiana Pendleton, M.S., CCC-SLP arranged for her patients and colleagues to participate in a photo shoot at St. Peter's Hospital in Albany, New York, and helped ensure the accuracy of each photograph.

Carol Fogle, R.N., my wife of over 40 years, whose love, support, and encouragement for all of my projects has allowed me to contribute to the profession I love. My daughters Heather Brooke Morrison and Heather Lea Fogle are appreciated and loved for being such joys in my life.

Reviewers

Tausha Beardsley, M.A., CCC-SLP
   Clinical Instructor
   Wayne State University
   Detroit, MI

Dana J. Boyd, MS, CCC-SLP
   Clinic Director
   University of Montevallo
   Montevallo, Alabama

Chris Gaskill, PhD, CCC-SLP
   Assistant Professor
   The University of Alabama
   Tuscaloosa, AL

John K. Gould, PhD, CCC-SLP
   Assistant Professor
   Elms College, Division of Communication Sciences
      and Disorders
   Chicopee, Massachusetts

Chip Hahn, MS, AuD, CCC-A/SLP
   Visiting Assistant Professor
   Miami University (OH)
   Oxford, Ohio

Nancy L. Martino, PhD, CCC-SLP
    Xavier University of Louisiana
    New Orleans, LA

Kate Battles Skinker, M.A., CCC-SLP
    Instructor, Director of Undergraduate Program
    University of Maryland
    College Park, Maryland

Suzanne Swift, Ed.D., CCC-SLP
    Chair, Health and Human Services, Associate Professor of CDIS
    Eastern New Mexico University
    Portales, New Mexico

ABOUT THE AUTHOR

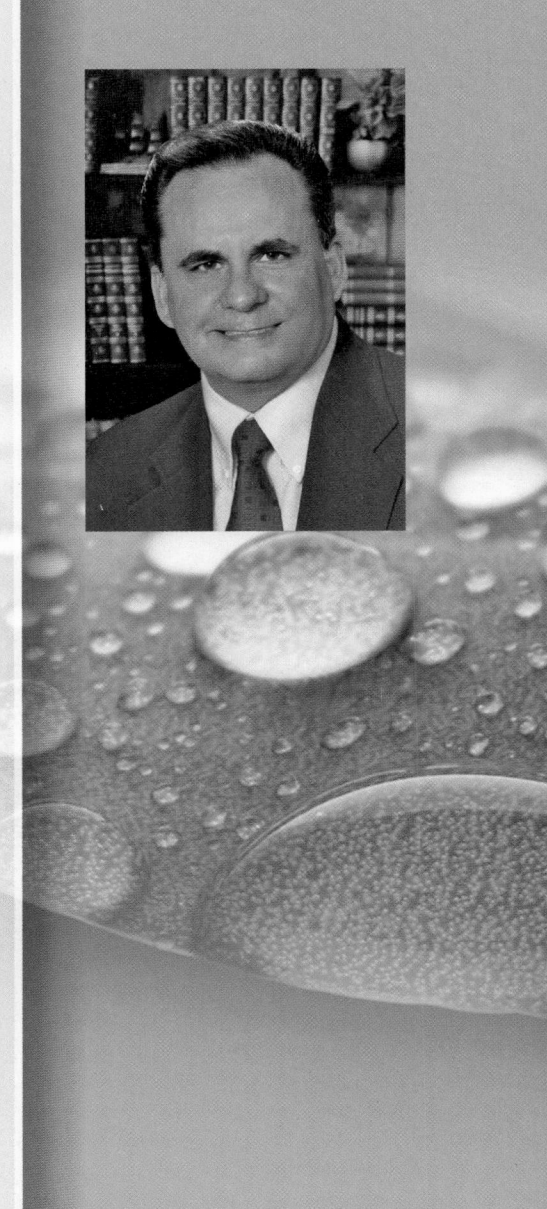

Paul T. Fogle, Ph.D., CCC-SLP, (Fogle is pronounced with a long o, as in FO-GULL) has been studying, training, and working in speech-language pathology for over 40 years. Although he earned all of his degrees in speech-language pathology, he minored in psychology throughout each degree. He earned his Bachelor of Arts in 1970 and his Masters of Arts in 1971, both at California State University, Long Beach. After receiving his M.A., he worked for two years as an Aphasia Classroom Teacher for the Los Angeles County Office of Education and started the first high school aphasia class in California, teaching and working with adolescents who had sustained traumatic brain injuries, strokes, and other neurological impairments. Between 1970 and 1973, Dr. Fogle worked as a therapist at the University of California, Los Angeles (UCLA) Psychology Adult Stuttering Clinic, training under Dr. Joseph Sheehan and Mrs. Vivian Sheehan. Concurrently, he trained on human brain autopsy procedures at Rancho Los Amigos Medical Center in Southern California.

Dr. Fogle earned his doctorate in 1976 from the University of Iowa. He specialized in neurological disorders in adults and children, and stuttering. His dissertation was directed by Dr. Dean Williams and he was awarded membership in Sigma Xi, the Scientific Research Society of North America, for his research. Since receiving his Ph.D. he has taught undergraduate courses on Introduction to Speech-Language Pathology and Audiology, Anatomy and Physiology of Speech and language, Speech Science, and Organic Disorders. At the graduate level he has taught Neurological Disorders in Adults, Motor Speech Disorders, Dysphagia/Swallowing Disorders, Gerontology, Voice Disorders, Cleft Palate and Oral-Facial Anomalies, and

Counseling Skills for Speech-Language Pathologists. Since the early 1990s, he has been training in counseling psychology and family therapy. Most recently he has been receiving education and training in the area of neuropsychology.

Dr. Fogle has worked extensively in hospitals, including Veteran Administration Hospitals, university hospitals, and acute, subacute, and convalescent hospitals. He has maintained a year-round private practice for over 30 years. He has presented numerous seminars, workshops, and short courses on a variety of topics at state, ASHA, international (IALP), and Asia-Pacific Society for the Study of Speech-Language Pathology and Audiology conventions and conferences. Dr. Fogle has presented all-day workshops and seminars in cities around the United States and in countries around the world on counseling skills for speech-language pathologists and audiologists, and on auditory processing disorders and attention deficit disorders. He has been involved with forensic speech-language pathology (court testifying as an expert witness) for over 25 years and has published and presented on this topic. Most recently he has been the speech-language pathologist on Rotaplast (Rotary) International Cleft Palate teams in Venezuela, Egypt, and India.

Dr. Fogle's primary publishing has been textbooks and clinical materials. He is the author of *Foundations of Communication Sciences and Disorders* (Delmar Cengage Learning, 2008) and coauthor of *Counseling Skills for Speech-Language Pathologists and Audiologists* (1st ed. 2004, 2nd ed. 2012, Delmar Cengage Learning), *Ross Information Processing Assessment-Geriatric* (1st ed. 1996, 2nd ed. 2012, Pro-Ed), *The Source for Safety: Cognitive Retraining for Independent Living* (LinguiSystems, 2008), and the *Classic Aphasia Therapy Stimuli* (CATS) (Plural Publishing, 2006). His website is: www.PaulFoglePhD.com and his e-mail address is paulfoglephd@gmail.com.

LETTER TO STUDENTS

Dear Students,

Welcome! Thank you for purchasing this textbook for the beginning of your study about the professions of speech-language pathology and audiology. I hope that you find not only interest in the information but a genuine joy in its learning. If you do, there is a good chance you will find that joy will remain with you throughout your life as you continue to learn about and work in these remarkable professions.

You will find several themes throughout this book that will help you in your learning and work as either a speech-language pathologist or audiologist.

First, our work is always a team approach, and the most important person on the team is the person with the communication disorder because without that person no other team members are needed.

Second, all of our therapy is "brain therapy;" that is, whether we are working with a child or adult with an articulation disorder, language disorder, stuttering problem, neurological disorder, or other disorder, we are working with neurons, axons, dendrites, and synapses within the person's brain to change the muscles that relax and contract for specific behaviors to occur. More subtly, when we are helping people change their attitudes, beliefs, feelings, and reactions toward their communication problems (e.g., stuttering), we are working with the brain.

Third, people of all ages with communication impairments have emotional and social reactions to their problems. A problem may be physical, for example a cleft palate or a hearing loss, but there are always emotional and social effects of the problem. This tells us that, as clinicians we must work with our clients and patients holistically—the whole person and not just the disorders that we diagnose and treat. Likewise, the family members of our clients and patients commonly have their own emotional reactions to their loved one's problems. The therapy we provide one person often has subtle to profound effects on the lives of a constellation of people. If you are going to be a speech-language pathologist or audiologist, you are going to touch countless lives.

Fourth, there is a joy to being a therapist, a person in a helping profession. We give our time, energy, and talents to others, but we receive back more than we give. Yes, you can make a living and support yourself with your profession, but we go into our profession and stay in it not so much because of the financial rewards, but because of the satisfaction we receive knowing that we have helped others have better lives. Ultimately, that becomes our greatest reward.

I hope that you enjoy reading and studying this book as much as I enjoyed writing it for you.

Best Wishes,

Paul T. Fogle, Ph.D., CCC-SLP
www.PaulFoglePhD.com

How to Use *Essentials of Communication Sciences & Disorders*

Application Question

What are your comfort foods? How would you feel if the foods you need or crave for comfort were the very foods you could not have, particularly when you needed them most—when you are sick, anxious, or depressed?

Parentese

Parentese (also called *motherese* and *baby talk*, but more professionally called *child-directed speech*) refers to how parents and other caregivers often talk to infants. Adults using parentese typically (1) use a high-pitched voice with greater pitch variation; (2) use one- and two-syllable words in short, simple sentences; and (3) speak at a slower rate with clearer articulation, sometimes emphasizing every syllable (Berko-Gleason, 2001).

Learning Objectives

Each chapter provides a list of the main concepts to be presented. Read these objectives before reading the chapter to focus your study and then review these objectives as a study tool.

Key Terms

This brief list provides the most important terms from each chapter. Each term is highlighted in the chapter and definitions are included in the margins. You will also find these terms listed in the glossary at the back of the book. These are an excellent tool for review and study.

Chapter Outline

To help you understand the organization of information, a chapter outline has been provided. This prepares you for the information to come and helps show the relationship and order of concepts.

Application Questions

Throughout every chapter application questions give you the chance to think about the material being discussed in terms of your own experiences. Consider these questions as you read the chapter to strengthen your comprehension of information and empathy for your clients and their families.

Sidebars

Throughout the chapters you will find boxes of additional information related to the core concepts under discussion. These boxes provide greater depth about the profession, disorder, or other information in the chapter. These interesting boxes enrich your reading and awareness of the field of communication sciences and disorders.

Personal Story

In these features, the author shares his personal experiences to paint a vivid picture of what it means to be a professional in this field. These stories highlight the clinician's experiences and the challenges and opportunities faced by professional speech-language pathologists and audiologists.

Multicultural Considerations

Rather than confine discussion of multicultural issues to a box or sidebar, these discussions occur as part of the main text to more accurately reflect the reality of professional practice. A special icon appears in the margin next to sections on multicultural issues, allowing you to quickly find this information when you need it.

Case Study

Where appropriate, case histories are included to highlight individual experiences with a particular disorder, as well as the clinician's approach to the case.

Study Questions

Each chapter concludes with study questions that offer three different levels of difficulty: knowledge/comprehension, application, and analysis/synthesis. These questions can be used for self-study or as part of course assignments.

References

A comprehensive listing of key resources used to write the chapter, these references are also ideal if you are looking for additional information on the topics covered in the chapter. Reliable and well respected, the chapter references are a good place to start when preparing for a term paper, report, or research project.

A $40,000 Phone Call — Personal Story

A private client of mine who was in his late 20s was already successful farming orchard crops. John had avoided the telephone all of his life; he even had his wife make the initial phone call to set up the first appointment with me. After several weeks of therapy, John was increasingly working on overcoming his feared situations, especially those involving the telephone. At the beginning of one appointment, he smiled, shook my hand, and thanked me for helping him make $40,000 that week. He told me that for the first time he made a phone call to talk directly to one of his buyers and from that conversation landed an additional $40,000 contract that he had never expected to obtain. Beyond all of the emotional and psychological "costs" of stuttering, for many people their fears and avoidances can be financially costly. ■

Multicultural Considerations

All cultures have their own food preferences and unique ways of preparing foods. In addition, cultures have rituals around food and meals. There may be religious and dietary preference and taboos related to the use of special spices and food preparation practices, when and where meals are served, and even who is present during meals (some cultures have rigid rules as to whether both males and females can be present) (Shoemaker, 1997). Patients in hospitals are presented "institutional food" that the kitchen staff tries to make as nutritious and enjoyable as possible. However, many patients would agree that the food is often rather bland and not always appetizing or appealing.

For patients who are accustomed to "ethnic" foods because of their ethnic and cultural backgrounds, the hospital food presented may be totally foreign to them. A patient with dysphagia may be a visitor to this country or a long-time resident, but has not adopted the food choices and prepar... tion methods of this country. The hospital kitchen staff can-

CASE STUDY — Daddy Wanted to Hear "Daddy"

I was conducting a research study on the speech-sound development of 11-month-old babies with cleft palate. One of the babies produced many glottal stops. The parents were proud of their daughter because she produced this sound to communicate in an expressive manner. It sounded like "uh uh uh." She was a "daddy's girl," and Daddy was happy with the glottal stops but was hurt because the baby had only one recognizable word, "mamma." No matter how hard the father worked with her, she would never say "daddy." When I explained to him that it was physically impossible at this time for her to make a /d/ sound, he was so relieved he just squeezed his little girl and said, "You do love daddy, I knew you did!" In addition, I took the opportunity to tell the parents not to reinforce the glottal stop sounds and taught them how to help th... other speech sounds with...

STUDY QUESTIONS
Knowledge and Comprehension

1. Define voice disorder.
2. Explain hoarseness.
3. What is an otolaryngologist?
4. Why might the interview of a client with a voice disorder be sensitive?
5. What is acute (traumatic) laryngitis, and what are some common causes?

REFERENCES

Alexander-Passe, N, (2010). *Dyslexia and depression: The hidden sorrow.* London South Bank University: London.

ASHA. (2001). *Roles and responsibilities of speech-language pathologists with respect to reading and writing for children and adolescents: Practice guidelines.* Rockville, MD: ASHA.

ASHA. (2009). *National Outcomes Measurement System Fact Sheet: Do SLP services have an impact on students' classroom performance? What teachers think.* Rockville, MD: ASHA.

Catts, H. W., Fey, M. E., Tomblin, J. B., & Zhang, X. (2002). A longitudinal investigation of reading outcomes in children with language

Essentials of Communication Sciences & Disorders

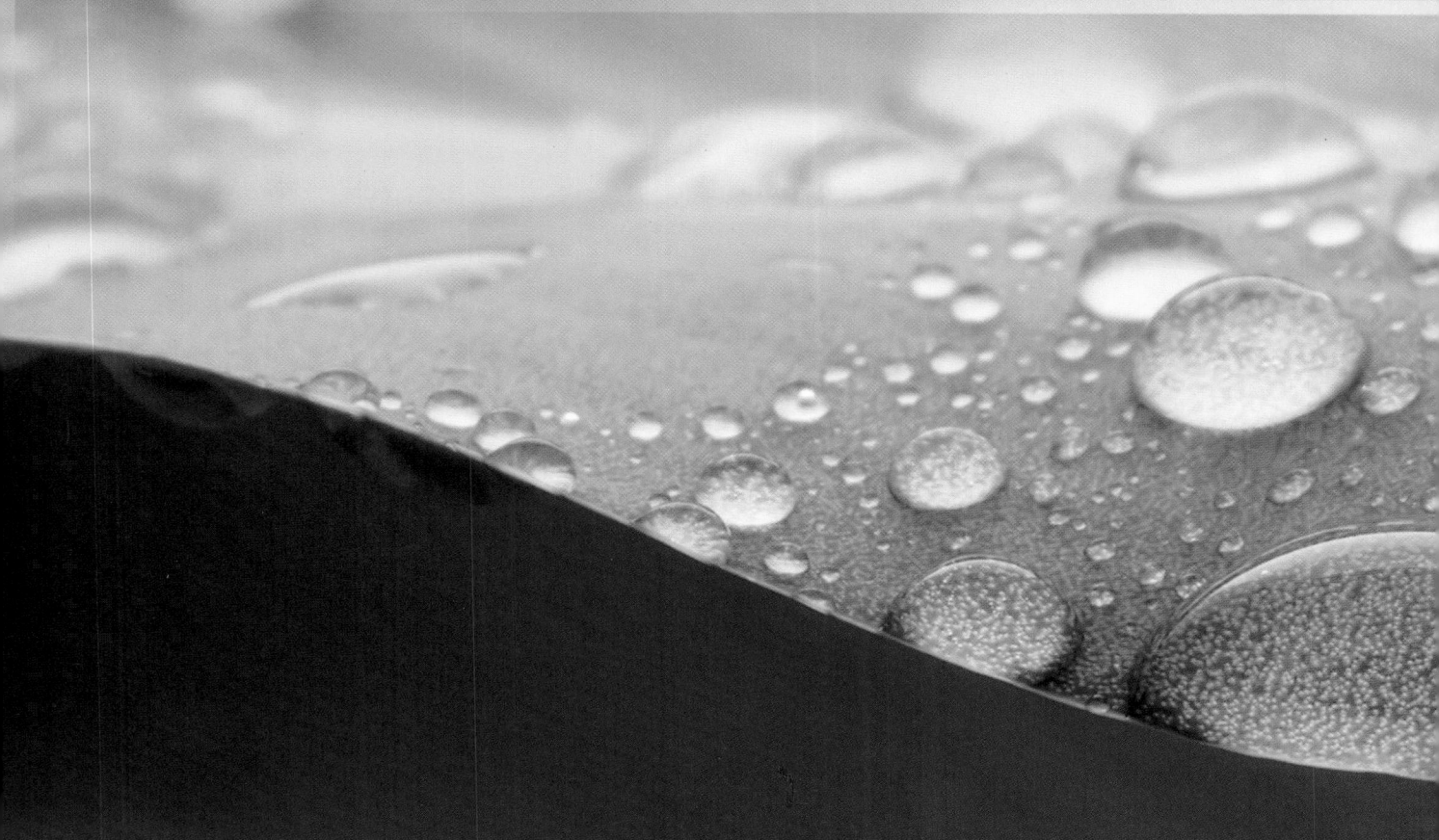

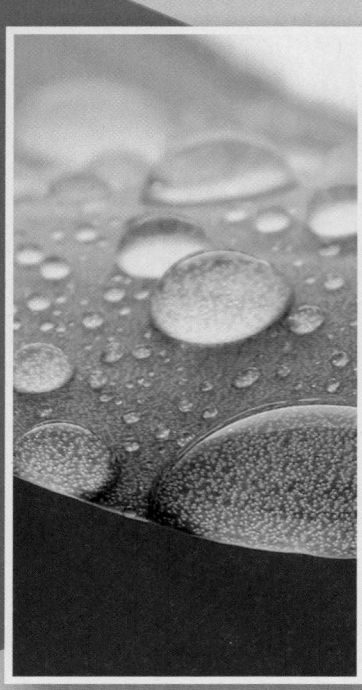

CHAPTER 1
Essentials of Communication and Its Disorders

LEARNING OBJECTIVES

After studying this chapter, you will:

- Know the modalities of communication.
- Be familiar with each of the speech systems.
- Be able to discuss the essentials of oral language: phonology, morphology, syntax, semantics, and pragmatics.
- Understand various classifications of communication disorders.
- Be able to define each of the communication disorders.
- Be aware of the emotional and social effects of communication disorders on the person and the family.

KEY TERMS

acquired disorder

aphasia (dysphasia)

aphonia

articulation disorder

articulator/articulation

audiologist

clinicians

cluttering

cognition

cognitive disorder

communicate

communication (communicative) disorder

conductive hearing loss

congenital disorder

consonant

context

dementia

disability

disorder/impairment

dysphonia

etiology

expressive language

functional disorder

General American English (GAE)

grammar

habilitate/habilitation

handicap

hearing impairment

hoarseness

hypernasal/hypernasality

hyponasal/hyponasality (denasal/denasality)

idiom

KEY TERMS continued

incidence

inner speech

intelligibility

language

language delay

language differences

language disorder

linguistics

modality

morpheme

morphology

motor speech disorder

organic disorder

perception

phoneme

phonological disorder

phonology

pragmatics

prevalence

quality of life

receptive language

rehabilitate/rehabilitation

resonance disorder

semantics

sensorineural hearing loss

sign

speech

speech disorder

speech-language pathologist/ speech pathologist/speech therapist

stuttering (disfluency)

suprasegmentals/paralinguistics/ prosody (prosodic) features

syllable

symptom

syndrome

syntax

traumatic brain injury (TBI)

voice disorder

vowel

World Health Organization (WHO)

CHAPTER OUTLINE

INTRODUCTION

Welcome! You are beginning the study of a basic human need: the need to **communicate**. When two people are interacting, a message is always being communicated, even when neither person is speaking. The old adage still holds true: *We cannot not communicate.* Our ability to communicate is often taken for granted until we have some difficulty communicating or see someone else having difficulty. This text is about the difficulties children and adults of all ages (newborns to end of life) have with **communication disorders**. As **clinicians**, we need to have a solid foundation in the understanding of the **modalities** of communication, that is, the various ways we communicate. Although **speech-language pathologists (SLPs)** and **audiologists (Auds)** focus on the *auditory-verbal* modalities (hearing and speaking), the *nonverbal modalities* (body language and facial expressions) are essential to our understanding what a person is saying and communicating our messages in return.

In a way, good communication is like a dance in which each person takes turns leading and following. The individuals try to stay "in step" with one another, "reading" every nuance of choice of words, tone of voice, *inflections* (variations of pitch during speech), pauses, hesitations, facial expressions, postures, and gestures (i.e., *total communication*) so that there is an easy and enjoyable flow during the conversation. When we meet someone new, it usually does not take long before we decide whether or not we can "dance" well together and whether we even want to try to dance again. We use communication to survive and thrive in our homes, communities, schools, and work places. With a communication disorder, surviving and thriving are much more difficult. Reed (2005) presents the modes we use in communicating (see Figure 1–1). As clinicians, we learn to be increasingly aware of the interactions of these modalities and the effects of subtle to complete breakdowns in these modalities.

THE STUDY OF HUMAN COMMUNICATION

Thirty-thousand-year-old cave paintings of geometric symbols and animals are the earliest forms of communication designed to preserve human experiences. Three-thousand-year-old Egyptian pictographic hieroglyphs were a formal writing system that used symbols for words and letters of the Egyptian alphabet that were carved into stone and later

communicate/ communication

Any means by which individuals relate their wants, needs, thoughts, knowledge, and feelings to another person.

communication (communicative) disorder

Speech, language, voice, resonance, cognitive, or hearing that noticeably deviates from that of other people, calls attention to itself, interferes with communication, or causes distress in both the speaker and the listener; any speech, language, voice, resonance, cognitive, or hearing impairment, disability, or handicap that interferes with a person conveying his wants, needs, thoughts, knowledge, and feelings to another person.

clinicians

Health care professionals, such as physicians, nurses, physical therapists, occupational therapists, speech-language pathologists, audiologists, psychiatrists, or psychologists involved in clinical practice who base their practice on direct observation and treatment of patients and clients.

modality

Any sensory avenue through which information may be received, i.e., auditory, visual, tactile, taste, and olfactory (smell).

speech-language pathologist/speech pathologist/speech therapist

A professional who is specifically educated and trained to identify, evaluate, treat, and prevent speech, language, cognitive, and swallowing disorders.

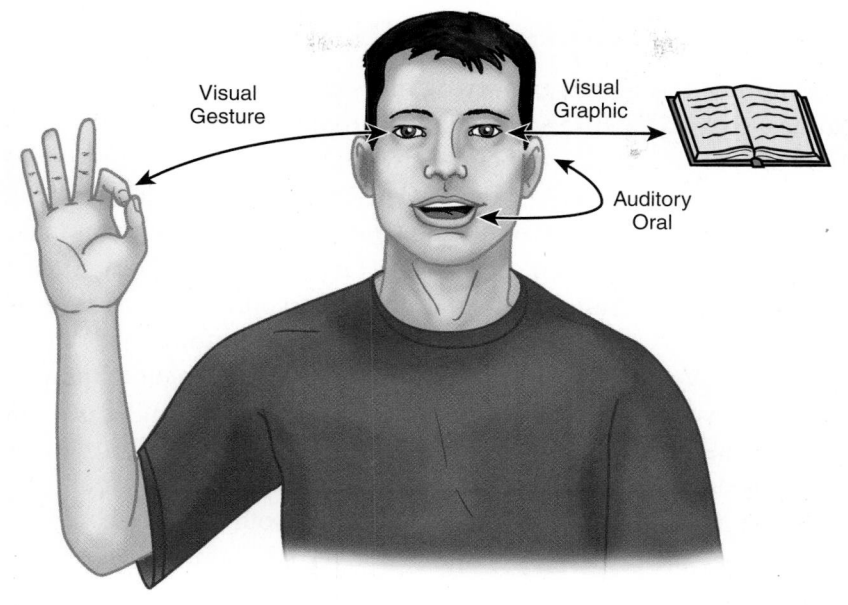

Figure 1–1

Modes of communication.

Source: Adapted from Reed, 2005.

painted on papyrus. The evolution of communication from basic sounds and signs to more sophisticated systems is one of the most important developments in human history. More recently, Wolfgang von Kempelen (1734–1804), a Hungarian author and inventor, described, illustrated, and constructed mechanical devices that could produce speech sounds for words. His devices (see Figure 1–2) were composed of bellows for the lungs, a vibrating reed for the vocal folds, and a leather tube whose shape helped produce different vowel sounds, with constrictions controlled by fingers for generating consonants. To study the production of plosive sounds (e.g., p, b, t, d, k, g), he included movable "lips" and a hinged "tongue" in his device. The device could produce intelligible whole words and short sentences. Von Kempelen may be considered the first speech scientist (Gedeon, 2006).

audiologist

A professional who is specifically educated and trained to identify, evaluate, treat, and prevent hearing disorders, plus select and evaluate hearing aids, and **habilitate** or **rehabilitate** individuals with hearing impairments.

habilitate/habilitation

The process of developing a skill to be able to function within the environment; the initial learning and development of a new skill.

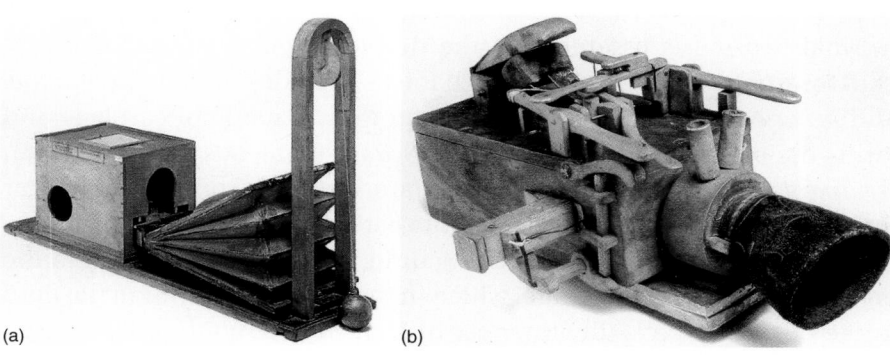

(a)   (b)

Figure 1–2

Von Kempelen's (1791) (a) "lungs" and "voice box" and (b) articulating mouth.

Source: *Science and technology in medicine: An illustrated account based on ninety-nine landmark publications for five centuries*, 2005, pages 138 and 141, "Wolfgang Von Kempelen," Andras Gedeon, Figure 25:4 and 25:8. With kind permission of Springer Science and Business Media.

**rehabilitate/
rehabilitation**

Restoration to normal or to as satisfactory a status as possible of impaired functions and abilities.

inner speech (internal discourse, stream of consciousness)

The nearly constant internal monologue a person has with himself at a conscious or semi-conscious level that involves thinking in words; a conversation with oneself.

speech

The production of oral language using phonemes for communication through the process of respiration, phonation, resonation, and articulation.

language

According to Owens (2012), "a socially shared code or conventional system for representing concepts through the use of arbitrary symbols [sounds and letters] and rule-governed combinations of those symbols [grammar]."

COMMUNICATION MODALITIES

Communication means conveying messages through one or more modalities; that is, listening, speaking, reading, and writing. We normally think of communication as being between two or more people; however, much of what we "hear" every day is us talking to ourselves. We commonly have an internal monologue (**inner speech**) going on inside of our heads that we refer to as *thinking* (Luria, 1961; Vygotsky, 1962). We silently (and sometimes not so silently) talk to ourselves and even argue with ourselves, wrestling with decisions from the mundane (Where am I going to have lunch?) to the profound (What am I going to do with my life?). Our verbal communication is mostly a reflection of our wants, needs, thoughts, feelings, and knowledge (i.e., sharing information).

However, spoken words may communicate only a small portion of a person's total message. SLPs and Auds also need to become skilled in "reading" facial expressions and nonverbal communication as well (Fogle, 2009). Burgoon, Guerrero, & Floyd (2010) reviewed 100 studies on *verbal* (oral) and *nonverbal* (body postures, gestures, eye contact, and facial expressions) communication and, among other points, determined the following:

- Verbal content is more important for factual, abstract, and persuasive communication; nonverbal content is more important for judging emotions and attitudes.
- When verbal and nonverbal channels conflict, adults rely more on nonverbal cues (i.e., people believe what they see more than what they hear).

When we think of communication disorders, we usually think of talking and listening. Most of your education and training in speech-language pathology and audiology will focus on these modalities. However, because communication may involve three different input modalities (auditory, visual, and tactile) and three different output modalities (speaking, gesturing, and writing), SLPs and Auds work with more than just speech and hearing. Any or all of the input and output modalities may be involved in a communication disorder.

Hearing

Normal hearing is essential for the development of normal **speech** and **language**. The hearing mechanism includes the *outer, middle,* and *inner ear* (see Figure 1–3). The outer ear is made of cartilage and forms the *pinna* or *auricle* and the *ear canal* that leads to the eardrum (*tympanic membrane*). Sound waves are directed from the outer ear into the ear canal where they reach the eardrum and cause it to vibrate. The vibration of the eardrum causes three small bones (*ossicles*) in the enclosed middle ear to vibrate, which in turn sets into vibration the fluid in the next chamber—the inner ear or *cochlea*. The fluid in the cochlea stimulates minute structures (*hair cells*) that transmit nerve impulses

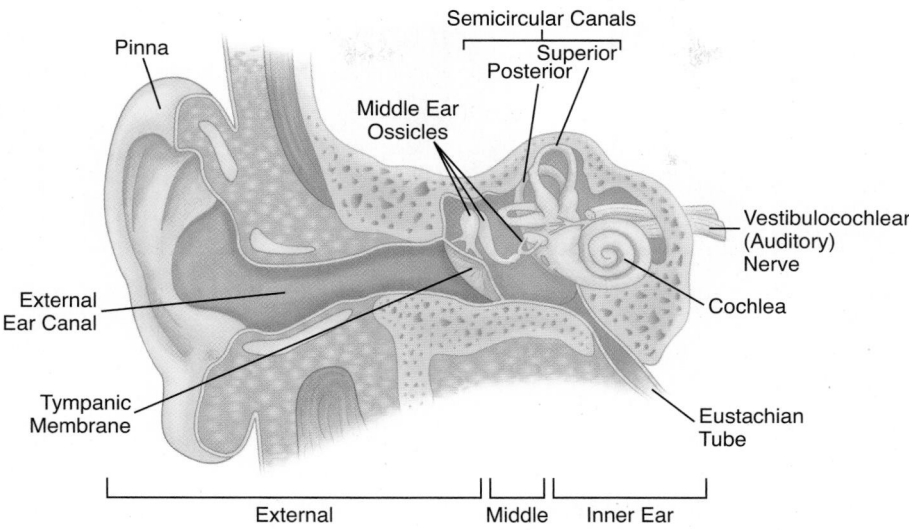

Figure 1-3

The human peripheral auditory system has three divisions: external, middle, and inner ear. The external ear consists of the pinna (or auricle) and the external ear canal (or external auditory meatus). The tympanic membrane (eardrum) closes off the medial end of the external ear canal. The middle ear is an air-filled cavity that contains the three middle-ear ossicles. The middle-ear cavity is connected to the nasopharynx by the Eustachian tube. The inner ear includes the cochlea, vestibule, and three semicircular canals. The cochlea contains the end organ for hearing. The vestibule and three semicircular canals contain the end organs for balance and motion detection, respectively.

© Cengage Learning 2013.

through a nerve to the brain that interprets the sound and its meaning. If speech sounds are not perceived normally by infants and young children, they will not be able to understand the speech of others or hear their own speech to make appropriate adjustments in voice and articulation and develop normal speech and language.

Speech Systems

Speech is the result of several physiological systems interacting and functioning in near perfect timing and harmony (the individual speech systems will be discussed in more detail in Chapter 3). To produce a single sound, the *respiratory system* (lungs, diaphragm, and chest muscles) must have adequate inhalation and controlled exhalation (see Figure 1-4). The *phonatory system* is composed of the *vocal folds* and other muscles inside and outside the *larynx*. The numerous muscles within the larynx that are necessary to close and open the vocal folds must have sufficient strength for the vocal folds to vibrate and create sound. The vocal folds must have the proper tension for subtle changes of loudness, pitch, and quality from instant to instant. But the voice does more than just produce sounds to speak words; it also gives a tone to the voice that can convey the true meaning of the message, which may in some cases be

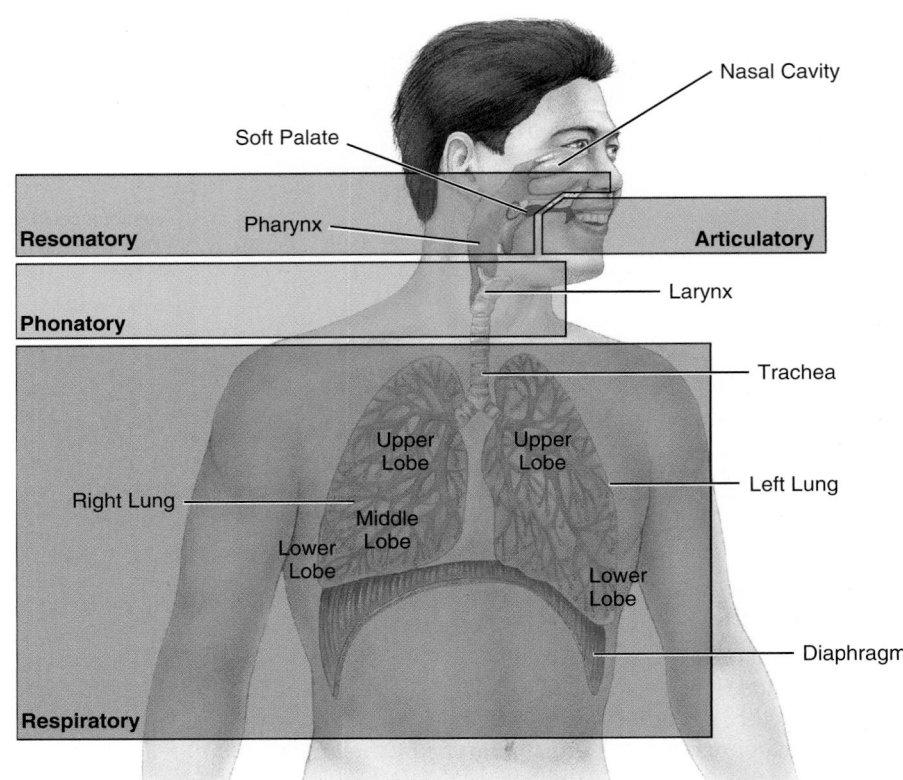

Figure 1-4

The speech systems: respiratory, phonatory, resonatory, and articulatory.

© Cengage Learning 2013.

articulator/articulation

In speech, the mandible, lips, tongue, and soft palate are the articulators; *articulation* refers to the movements of the articulators for speech sound production that involves accuracy in placement, timing, direction of movement, and pressure of the articulators on one another; the totality of motor processes involved in the planning and execution of speech.

intelligible

The degree to which a person's utterances are understood by the average listener; influenced by articulation, rate of speech, fluency, vocal quality, and intensity of voice.

syllable

Either a single **vowel** (V) or a vowel and one or more **consonants** (C); e.g., V+ consonant (VC), VCC, CV, CCV, CVC, etc.

the opposite of what the words mean (as in sarcasm). A simple sigh can convey numerous meanings just by its tone.

The *resonatory system* in the throat, nose, and mouth modifies the sounds produced by the larynx. For example, a tense throat (*pharyngeal region*) can significantly alter the sound produced by the vocal folds. The position of the *soft palate* (the back of the roof of the mouth) determines whether sounds will come through the mouth (soft palate up for *oral sounds* [e.g., p, t, s]) or the sound will come through the nasal passages (soft palate down for *nasal sounds* [e.g., m, n, ng]). The *articulatory system* (**articulators**) includes the *maxilla* (upper jaw), *mandible* (lower jaw), lips, teeth, and tongue. The articulators modify the sounds that enter the *oral cavity* (mouth) into words. Incredibly fast and precise movements of the articulators and their muscles allow us to produce **intelligible** speech.

Oral/Spoken Language

When sounds are organized into **syllables** and words are organized into grammatical sentences, spoken language is generated. As noted previously, language has been defined as "a socially shared code or conventional system for representing concepts through the use of arbitrary symbols [sounds and letters] and rule-governed combinations of those symbols [grammar]" (Owens, 2012). Spoken language is our primary and usually most efficient form of communication. There are approximately

7,000 "living languages" (languages widely used as a primary form of communication by specific groups of people) and an unknown number of dead or extinct languages (Lewis, 2009).

Spoken language gives the listener not only the *content* (the words in the message) but the **suprasegmentals** (also called **paralinguistics** or **prosody [prosodic] features**) that help the listener understand the true intent of the message by using voice inflections for emphasis or deemphasis (e.g., the difference between "I scream" and "ice cream"). Suprasegmentals include *prosody* (rate and rhythm), *intonation* (pitch change within an utterance), and *stress* (combination of pitch, loudness, and duration). Suprasegmentals are important in conveying the emotional aspects of messages, such as happiness, sadness, fear, and surprise. When we cannot see a person's face (e.g., while on the telephone), we usually can still discern the emotions behind the messages based on the suprasegmentals.

Linguistics

Linguistics is the scientific study of language, and *linguists* are individuals who specialize in the study of linguistics. Traditionally, linguists divide language into several components: *phonemes* (sounds), *morphemes* (groups of sounds that form words or parts of words), *syntax* (rules for combining words into sentences), *semantics* (meaning of the language or message), and *pragmatics* (the rules governing the use of language in social situations). *Linguistic competence* is a person's underlying knowledge about the system of rules of a language. Linguistic competence helps us recognize when a sentence is grammatically correct or incorrect.

Phonology

Phonology is the study of speech sounds (**phonemes**) and the rules for using them to make words in a language. The English language has a limited number of phonemes, but an almost limitless variety of sound combinations can be used in words and to make up new words. Each year, hundreds of words are added to our language that must follow phonological rules (see Chapter 4, Speech and Language Development). Consider all of the new words that were created when automobiles first arrived on the scene, or when televisions and computers were invented. Whenever there is a significant technological advancement such as computers, a large number of words are added to our language (e.g., *Google*—the search engine).

For new words to be accepted by the public, certain phonological rules for combining sounds must be followed. For example, a single letter is not used as a new word, nor is a combination of more than two consonants with no **vowels**. A combination of three or more vowels also is not considered to follow English phonological rules. Some foreign languages are difficult for English speakers to learn because their phonologies use consonant and vowel combinations not used in English. Many people

consonant

Speech sounds articulated by either stopping of the outgoing air stream or creating a narrow opening of resistance using the articulators.

suprasegmentals/ paralinguistics/prosody (prosodic) features

Voice inflections used in a language such as stress, intensity, changes in pitch, duration of a sound, and rhythm that help listeners understand the true intent of a message and that convey the emotional aspects of a message, such as happiness, sadness, fear, or surprise.

linguistics

The scientific study of the structure and function of language and the rules that govern language; includes the study of phonemes, morphemes, syntax, semantics, and pragmatics.

phonology

The study of speech sounds and the system of rules underlying sound production and sound combinations in the formation of words.

phoneme

The shortest arbitrary unit of sound in a language that can be recognized as being distinct from other sounds in the language.

vowel

Voiced speech sounds from the unrestricted passage of the air stream through the mouth without audible stoppage or friction.

trying to learn English as a second language find it difficult because the pronunciation of a word may vary considerably depending on the context, and the differences in the pronunciation can significantly change a word's meaning. For example, "He could lead if he got the lead out." "The girl had tears in her eyes because of the tears in her dress." "Since there is no time like the present, he decided to present the present."

Authors of fiction books sometimes create new words by following phonological rules of English; for example, J.R.R. Tolkien, in *The Lord of the Rings* trilogy, created a great number of new words, including *hobbit, glede,* and *Fallohides.* J. K. Rowling, the author of the *Harry Potter* books, also created *quidditch* and *muggle* (*muggle* is now in the *New Oxford English Dictionary*). These words "sound like they could be words," just as any new technical word must follow accepted English phonological rules to eventually become part of our vocabulary (e.g., *byte, megabyte,* and *telecommunication*).

Morphology

Morphology is the study of the way words are formed out of basic units of language—**morphemes**. Morphemes are one or more letters or sounds that may be used as prefixes, such as *un*comfortable; base (root) words, such as *comfort*; or suffixes such as *able*. When a morpheme is able to stand alone, that is, it does not need any other morphemes attached to it to make it a true word, it is called a *free morpheme* (e.g., *horse, culture,* and *accept*). Morphemes that cannot stand alone and must be attached to a free morpheme are referred to as *bound morphemes* (e.g., prefixes such as *pre-, dis-,* and *mis-*; suffixes such as the plural *-s*, the past tense *-d*, and the gerund *-ing*; and base words such as *-celerate-* and *audio-*). Table 1–1 shows how prefixes, base words, and suffixes (morphemes) combine to make whole words.

Syntax

Syntax and morphology are the two major categories of language structure (i.e., **grammar**). Syntax is the study of the rules for acceptable sequences (order) and word combinations in sentences. Various languages

---

morphology

The study of the structure (form) of words.

morpheme

The smallest unit of language having a distinct meaning, for example, a prefix, root word, or suffix.

syntax

Rules that dictate the acceptable sequence and combination of words in a sentence to convey meaning; the study of sentence structure.

grammar

The rules of the use of morphology and syntax in a language.

TABLE 1–1	Examples of Whole Words, Prefixes, Base Words, and Suffixes		
WHOLE WORD	**PREFIX**	**BASE WORD**	**SUFFIX**
miscommunication	mis	communicate	tion
indefensible	in	defense	ible
disorienting	dis	orient	ing

© Cengage Learning 2013.

have different word orders for sentences. In an English declarative sentence, the subject comes before the verb: "David is going to work." However, when the subject (*David*) and the auxiliary or helping verb (*is*) are reversed in order, the sentence becomes a question—"*Is David* going to work?" English syntax has the adjective preceding the noun (e.g., the green room); however, the syntax of Spanish and French has the adjective following the noun (e.g., the room green). Most English sentences flow from subject to verb to objects or complements. Most sentences conform to variations of the following patterns:

Subject/verb/direct object (*The woman took her purse.*)

Subject/verb/indirect object (*The horse ran to the barn.*)

Subject/verb/subject complement (*The man worked hard.*)

Native speakers of a language develop a grammatical intuition by which they can recognize when a sentence is not quite grammatically correct, but they may have some difficulty pinpointing or explaining what is not correct. When people who have learned English as a second language are speaking, they may use some incorrect word order or omit morphemes (e.g., the plural *-s*) that a native speaker of English recognizes and may be a little uncomfortable with, feeling a need to correct the nonnative speaker.

Semantics

Semantics is the study of meaning in language that is conveyed by the words, phrases, and sentences communicated. Semantics may be thought of as the *content expressed* by the speaker and the *content understood* by the listener. Miscommunication occurs when there is a discrepancy between the two.

Social and cultural factors play significant roles in the way we use and understand language. For example, a word's meaning in one region of the United States may be considerably different from its meaning in another region. In many western regions of the United States *dinner* is the evening meal but in many midwestern and southern regions *dinner* is the noon meal and *supper* is the evening meal. Among English-speaking countries, there can be significant differences in the use of words for the same thing. For example, in England a *restroom* is sometimes called a *water closet* and in Australia a *napkin* is a *diaper*. The differences in the semantic use of words and the meanings of words can certainly affect communication, even among people who do not have communication disorders.

Idioms (figures of speech) are a way of expressing a thought by referring to one thing in terms of another (see Figure 1–5). We use countless idioms in our language, most of which when analyzed word by word make little or no sense, although we assume that the listener will automatically know what we mean when we say "I'm all ears," "He has butterflies in his stomach," "She has a heart of gold," and "He put his foot in his mouth."

Application Question

How good is your grammatical intuition; that is, how easily do you automatically detect or recognize grammatical errors in other people's speech? In your own speech?

semantics

The study of meaning in language conveyed by words, phrases, and sentences.

idiom

An expression in the usage of a language that is peculiar to itself either grammatically (e.g., "Zip your lip.") or in having a meaning that cannot be derived from the normal combination of words (e.g., "Keep your eyes on the ball, your shoulder to the wheel, and your nose to the grindstone.").

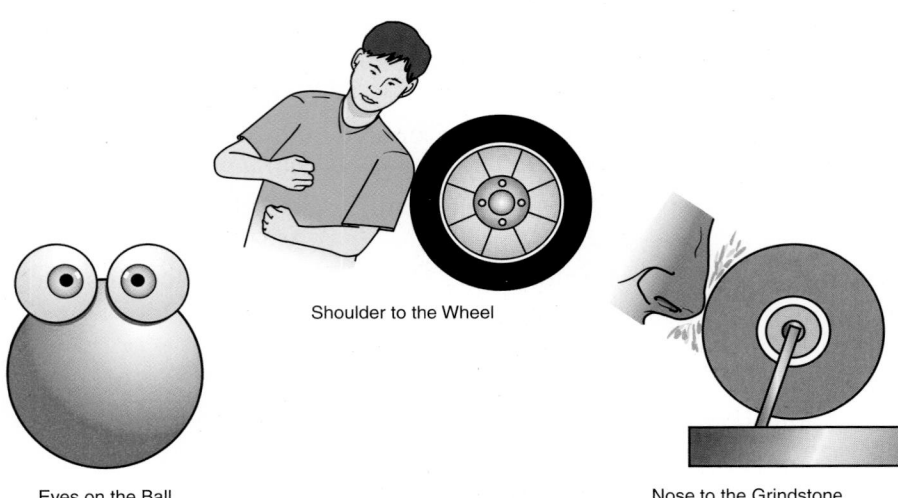

Figure 1–5

How an idiom might look. ("Keep your eyes on the ball, your shoulder to the wheel, and your nose to the grindstone.")

© Cengage Learning 2013.

Eyes on the Ball

Shoulder to the Wheel

Nose to the Grindstone

Pragmatics

Pragmatics are the rules governing the use of language in social situations. Some elements included in pragmatics are the *relationship* of the people talking, the **context** or environment they are in (e.g., social vs. business), and the *intentions* of the communication (e.g., friendliness or hidden agendas). The context in which a message is framed significantly affects its true meaning. Pragmatics places greater emphasis on the functions of language than on the structure of language.

Pragmatics are culturally based or influenced. For example, in some regions of the world, such as the Middle East, an initial business meeting may be devoted to sharing about family and friends, and the business may not be discussed until a later meeting. Also, the beginning of each new business meeting may be devoted to extended casual conversation rather than moving to the task at hand. When businesspeople do not know the cultural traditions of the people they are dealing with, disastrous consequences may result.

pragmatics

The rules governing the use of language in social situations; includes the speaker–listener relationship and intentions and all elements in the environment surrounding the interaction—the context.

context

The circumstances or events that form the environment within which something exists or takes place; also, the words, phrases, or narrative that come before and after a particular word or phrase in speech or a piece of writing that helps to explain its full meaning.

Reading and Writing

Many speech-language pathologists are involved in the area of literacy with children who have reading and writing disabilities, particularly in the public schools. Reading and writing may be more challenging for the brain to process and, therefore, more difficult to develop than auditory-verbal abilities. In a way, we have two languages: listening-speaking (*auditory-verbal* or *aural-oral*) and reading-writing (*visual-graphic*). The auditory-verbal language is developed in the early years of life; however, the reading-writing language does not normally start developing until the early years of schooling. Also, a person may become verbal and be considered a good communicator, but that does not mean he is an equally good reader or writer.

DISORDERS OF COMMUNICATION

When we listen to someone talk, we typically (consciously or subconsciously) pay attention or notice several features. We notice the person's articulation and how clearly and easily we can understand him. We pay attention to the person's voice and whether we think it is appropriate for the person's age and gender, and whether it is relatively smooth and clear. We hear whether a person has a resonance problem and sounds like he is either "talking through his nose" or sounds like he has a "stuffy nose." We listen for the person's language skills and whether good syntax is being used with a reasonably appropriate choice of words. We notice whether the person's speech is relatively fluent or whether he has unusual pauses and hesitations, repetitions of sounds and words, or prolongations of sounds. We also notice whether the person's hearing is adequate when we are talking to him or whether we have to speak louder than normal or repeat ourselves often. We also may notice whether the person seems embarrassed or frustrated with his own communication. In social conversations, when we notice problems in any of these areas we usually try not to let the speaker know that we are aware of them. However, in our professional work as speech-language pathologists and audiologists we need to recognize, analyze, diagnose, and treat a person's communication disorders.

Charles Van Riper's (1978) classic definition of communication disorder is commonly used by SLPs; that is, speech (or language) is disordered when it deviates from that of other people, calls attention to itself, interferes with communication, or causes distress in both the speaker and the listener. However, based on the earlier definition of *communication* (i.e., any means by which individuals relate their wants, needs, thoughts, knowledge, and feelings to another person), a communication disorder, therefore, may be defined as any voice, resonance, articulation, language, cognitive, or hearing impairment that interferes with people relating their wants, needs, thoughts, knowledge, and feelings to another person.

As professionals, SLPs and Auds try to provide objectivity in their definitions of terms and diagnoses of communication disorders. In reality, the subjective feelings of clients and patients and their listeners are what determine how much a communication disorder actually affects an individual. Some individuals have very negative reactions to even minor communication problems, whereas others appear (or try to appear) remarkably tolerant, unconcerned, or unaware of even fairly significant problems. In essence, a communication disorder can affect our **quality of life**, and the task of SLPs and Auds is to help improve the quality of life of our clients, patients, and their families. The term **handicap** is generally avoided because of its negative connotations, with the terms **disability** and **impairment** now more commonly used.

Prevalence refers to the number of individuals diagnosed with a particular disorder at a given time. **Incidence** is the rate at which a disorder appears in the normal population over a period, typically one year.

quality of life

A global concept that involves a person's standard of living, personal freedom, and the opportunity to pursue happiness; a measure of a person's ability to cope successfully with the full range of challenges encountered in daily living; the characterization of health concerns or disease effects on a person's lifestyle and daily functioning.

handicap

Loss or limitation of opportunities to take part in the life of the community on an equal level with others **(World Health Organization [WHO])**; a congenital or acquired physical or intellectual limitation that hinders a person from performing specific tasks.

World Health Organization (WHO)

An agency of the United Nations established in 1948 to further international cooperation in improving health conditions throughout the world.

disability

Any restriction or lack (resulting from an impairment) of ability to perform an activity in the manner or within the range considered normal for a human being (World Health Organization [WHO]); the impairment, loss, or absence of a physical or intellectual function; *physical disability* is any impairment that limits the physical functions of limbs or gross or fine motor abilities; *sensory disability* is impairment of one of the senses (e.g., hearing or vision); *intellectual disability* encompasses intellectual deficits that may appear at any age.

disorder/impairment

Any loss or abnormality of psychological, physiological, or anatomical structure or function that interferes with normal activities (World Health Organization [WHO]).

The prevalence of disorders is more clinically relevant and, therefore, more commonly reported than is the incidence. It is nearly impossible to determine the precise prevalence of communication disorders in the United States or any country, and it is likely that overall estimates are underestimated because not all communication disorders are diagnosed or diagnosed with the same criteria, or systematically reported to calculate their totals. In the United States, approximately 25% of all children between 3–21 years of age receive services from a speech-language pathologist or audiologist at some time. More than 25% of all children with learning or physical disabilities also have one or more communication disorders (e.g., articulation and language, language and literacy, speech, language, and hearing). Males are more likely to have communication disorders at all ages than females (American Speech-Language-Hearing Association [ASHA], 2008a; Catts & Kamhi, 2005; National Dissemination Center for Children with Disabilities, 2010).

CLASSIFICATIONS OF COMMUNICATION DISORDERS

There are numerous approaches to classifications of **speech** and **language disorders**, but in general they are divided into *articulation* (articulation disorders, phonological disorders, and motor speech disorders), *language* (receptive language and expressive language), *fluency* (stuttering and cluttering), *voice* (aphonia and dysphonia), *resonance* (hypernasality and hyponasality), *cognition* (developmental and acquired disorders), *literacy* (reading disorders and writing disorders), and *hearing* (conductive, sensorineural, and mixed losses) (see Figure 1–6). A swallowing disorder is not a communication disorder but is a major area of concern for SLPs, particularly in medical settings. In addition to the term *disorder*, clinicians often use the terms *impairment, disability*, or *problem* as synonyms when discussing clients and patients of all ages.

SLPs and Auds often try to determine *dichotomies* (i.e., either this or that) when classifying disorders. For example, a disorder may be considered *congenital* or *acquired, organic* or *functional*, an *articulation disorder* or *phonological disorder*, a *receptive language disorder* or an *expressive language disorder*, a *child communication disorder* or an *adult communication disorder*, or a *stroke* or *traumatic brain injury (TBI)*. In many cases two or more disorders may occur concurrently (i.e., a *mixed, coexisting*, or *comorbid* disorder), such as a child who has articulation and language disorders or an adult who has both language and **cognitive disorders**.

Congenital disorders are those that are present at birth and are usually considered either hereditary (e.g., some **syndromes**), problems caused during the pregnancy (e.g., maternal drug or alcohol use), or a complication at birth (e.g., fetal *anoxia* [no oxygen] or *hypoxia*

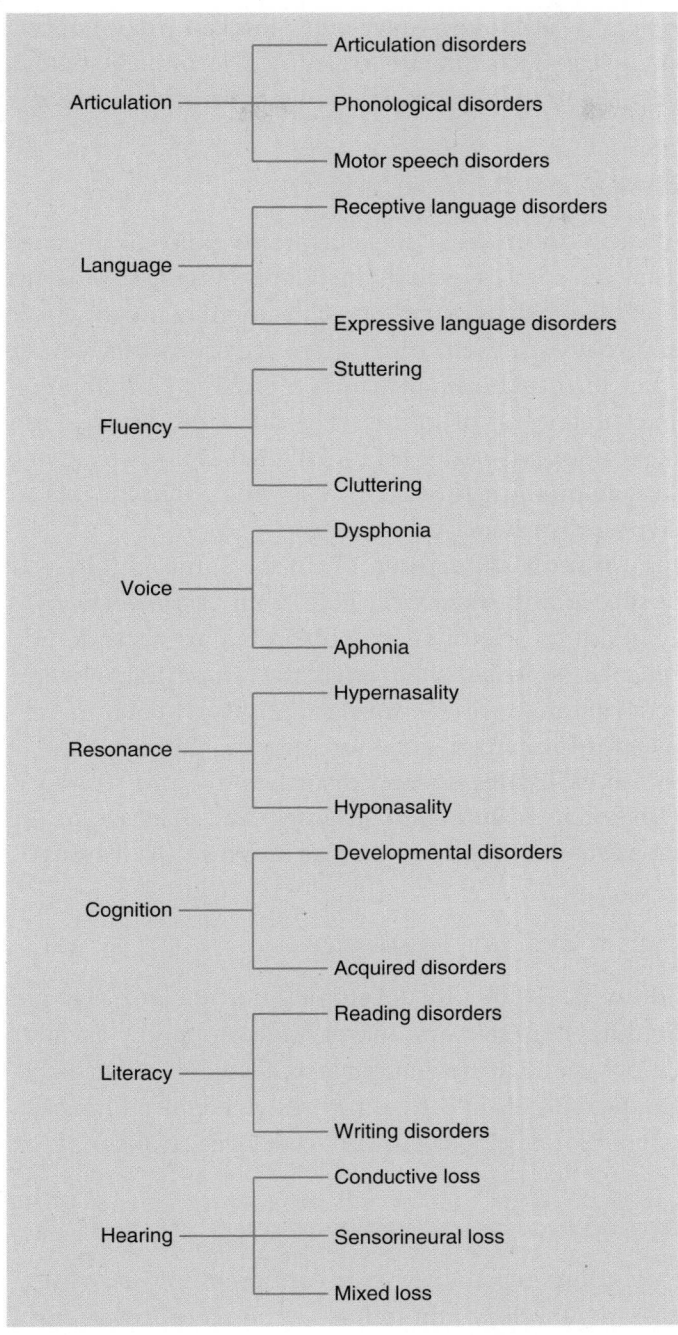

Figure 1–6

Major categories of communication disorders.

© Cengage Learning 2013.

[inadequate oxygen]). **Acquired disorders** are those that begin after an individual has developed normal communication abilities, such as a hearing loss from loud noise exposure, or a speech, language, or cognitive disorder caused by a **traumatic brain injury**.

When considering the **etiology** or cause of a disorder, some clinicians will use the terms **functional disorder** and **organic disorder**. A functional disorder is a problem or impairment that has some behavioral and/or emotional components but no known anatomical, physiological, or neurological basis. An organic disorder has an anatomical, physiological,

symptom

A subjective indication of a disease or change in condition as perceived by the patient or other nonmedical or rehabilitation specialist, such as a family member.

acquired disorder

A disorder that begins after an individual has developed normal communication abilities, such as a hearing loss from loud noise exposure or a speech, language, or cognitive disorder caused by a traumatic brain injury.

traumatic brain injury (TBI) (head trauma, acquired brain injury-ABI)

An acquired injury to the brain caused by an external force that results in partial or total functional disability, including physical, communication, cognitive, and psychosocial impairments.

etiology

The cause of an occurrence (e.g., a medical problem that results in a disorder or disability).

functional disorder

A problem or impairment with no known anatomical, physiological, or neurological basis that may have behavioral or emotional causes or components.

organic disorder

A problem or impairment with a known anatomical, physiological, or neurological basis.

articulation disorder

The incorrect production of speech sounds due to faulty placement, timing, direction, pressure, speed, or integration of the movements of the mandible, lips, tongue, or velum.

phonological disorder

Errors of phonemes that form patterns in which a child simplifies individual sounds or sound combinations.

or neurological basis and may have behavioral and/or emotional components. In many cases it is difficult to clearly determine whether a disorder is purely or primarily a functional disorder or an organic disorder.

Disorders of Articulation

An **articulation disorder** is present when a child cannot correctly *produce* (say) speech sounds used in the child's language. Most articulation disorders are the result of inaccurate placement of the tongue. A **phonological disorder** is present when there are errors of several *phonemes* (sounds) that form patterns in which a child is simplifying individual sounds or combinations of sounds (i.e., the child is unintentionally trying to make the sounds easier for himself to say). Ninety-two percent of SLPs working in public schools report serving children with articulation or phonological disorders (ASHA, 2010).

Motor speech disorders occur in some children (*childhood apraxia of speech* and *dysarthria* [e.g., with *cerebral palsy*]) but more commonly in adults. Motor speech disorders are considered the result of neurological impairments that affect the *motor* (i.e., movement) planning and coordination, or the strength of the articulators for the rapid and complex movements needed for smooth, effortless, and intelligible speech. In adults, motor speech disorders are most often caused by strokes, TBIs, or *neuromuscular diseases* (i.e., diseases of the nervous system that affect the muscles), such as Parkinson's disease.

Disorders of Language

Many children have difficulty developing normal language abilities and these difficulties may become increasingly apparent as the child gets older and more sophisticated language is expected. Adults who have had normal language all of their lives may have acquired language impairments because of neurological disorders such as strokes or head injuries.

Language Disorders in Children

Language disorders in children can vary greatly in how they manifest during language development in both **receptive language** (how well a child understands what he hears) and **expressive language** (how well a child can verbally communicate his messages), with age of a child being a significant factor. Children who have difficulty understanding language commonly have difficulty expressing themselves. Some children are slow to develop language and may be considered to have a **language delay**, but then develop normal language. Parents often refer to these children as "slow talkers" and "late bloomers." Language disorders are associated with more than 75% of children who have learning disabilities (Barnes, Fletcher, & Fuchs, 2007). Some causes of language disorders include hearing loss, traumatic brain injuries, autism, various genetic syndromes, and intellectual disabilities. Most of these children have articulation disorders in conjunction with their language disorders or language delays (ASHA, 2008a). Ninety percent of SLPs working in schools report that they work with children who have language impairments (ASHA, 2010).

Children's culturally and linguistically diverse backgrounds can significantly affect their expressive language. However, expressive language affected by cultural and linguistic diversity is not a disorder—it is a *difference*. **Language differences** are variations in speech and language production that are the result of a person's cultural, linguistic, and social environments. When determining whether a particular child's language is a disorder or a difference, we must consider two norms: **General American English (GAE) (Standard American English [SAE])** and the cultural norms of the child (Hegde, 2007; Paul, 2006). A 1983 American Speech-Language-Hearing Association position paper (p. 24) on social dialects stated "No dialect variety of English is a disorder or a pathological form of speech or language. Each social dialect is considered adequate as a functional and effective variety of English."

Language Disorders in Adults

Impaired language in adulthood may be a continuation of the language problems of a child or adolescent. However, generally we think of language disorders in adults as being acquired because of neurological impairments such as strokes and head injuries. These adults have lived their entire lives, often at very high functioning levels, and then because of medical problems or accidents have communication disorders that they could never have imagined. Damage to the brain's left hemisphere can cause both language impairments (**aphasia**) and motor speech disorders. It is estimated that between 5% to 10% of adults have neurological impairments that result in language disorders (ASHA, 2008c).

Disorders of Fluency

Stuttering (disfluency) is likely the most common problem people think of when they think of a speech disorder. (Note: Most current authorities on stuttering use *dis*fluency rather than *dys*fluency [Bloodstein & Bernstein Ratner, 2008; Guitar, 2006; Manning, 2010; Ramig & Dodge, 2010; Ward, 2006; Yairi & Ambrose, 2005]). Probably most adults have encountered someone who stutters, and the media (including cartoons) have parodied people who stutter countless times. Stuttering is usually heard as repetitions of sounds, syllables, or words; prolongations of sounds; and abnormal stoppages or "silent blocks" while a child or adult is talking. There can be visible tension and struggle behaviors, such as blinking their eyes, looking away just as they begin to stutter, and a variety of facial grimaces and unusual arm, hand, and other body part movements. Stuttering can be one of the most emotionally difficult of all the communication disorders (Bloodstein & Bernstein Ratner, 2008). About 5% of preschool-age children have episodes of disfluency, and in

motor speech disorder

Impaired speech intelligibility that is caused by a neurological impairment that affects the motor (movement) planning or the strength of the articulators needed for rapid, complex movements in smooth, effortless speech.

receptive language/ comprehension/ decoding

What a person understands of what is said.

expressive language/ production/encoding

The words, grammatical structures, and meanings that a person uses verbally.

language delay

An abnormal slowness in developing language skills that may result in incomplete language development.

language differences

Variations in speech and language production that are the result of a person's cultural, linguistic, and social environments.

General American English (GAE)/ Standard American English (SAE)

The speech of native speakers of American English that is typical of the United States and that excludes phonological forms easily recognized as regional dialects (e.g., Northeastern or Southeastern) or limited to particular ethnic or social groups, and that is not identified as a nonnative American accent; the norm of pronunciation by national radio and television broadcasters.

aphasia/dysphasia

An impairment in language processing that may affect any or all input modalities (auditory, visual, and tactile) and any or all output modalities (speaking, writing, and gesturing).

stuttering/disfluency (dysfluency)

A disturbance in the normal flow and time patterning of speech characterized by one of more of the following: repetitions of sounds, syllables, or words; prolongations of sounds; abnormal stoppages or "silent blocks" within or between words; interjections of unnecessary sounds or words; circumlocutions (talking around an intended word); or sounds and words produced with excessive tension.

cluttering

Speech that is abnormally fast with omission of sounds and syllables of words, abnormal patterns of pausing and phrasing, and often spoken in bursts that may be unintelligible; frequently includes abnormalities in syntax, semantics, and pragmatics.

voice disorder

Any deviation of loudness, pitch, or quality of voice that is outside the normal range of a person's age, gender, or geographic cultural background that interferes with communication, draws unfavorable attention to itself, or adversely affects the speaker or listener.

dysphonia

A general term that means a voice disorder, with the person's voice typically sounding rough, raspy, or hoarse.

the general population approximately 1% of school-age children and adults stutter (Yairi & Ambrose, 2005).

Cluttering is considered a fluency disorder that shares some characteristics of stuttering but differs in several important ways. Cluttered speech is abnormally fast with omissions of sounds and syllables so that words sound compressed or *truncated* (reduced in length). A person who clutters has abnormal patterns of pausing and phrasing, and has bursts of speech that may be unintelligible.

Disorders of Voice

A **voice disorder** occurs when the loudness, pitch, or quality (i.e., "smoothness") of a person's voice is outside the normal range for the person's age, gender, or the speaking environment, or the voice is unpleasant to hear. Children and adults can have severe voice disorders that leave them without a functional voice for communicating essential messages. Most voice disorders in children and adults are diagnosed as **dysphonias** in which the person's voice sounds rough, raspy, or **hoarse**. Dysphonia may be caused by laryngitis, masses on the vocal folds (e.g., vocal nodules [cheerleaders nodules]), neurological damage that causes weakness of the vocal folds, or psychological causes, such as tension in the vocal mechanism (*larynx*). **Aphonia** is a complete loss of voice, which is rare, and typically has psychological causes such as emotional stress. Following the complete loss of voice the person may use whispering or writing to communicate and often avoids communication. Voice disorders have been reported to occur in 6% to 23% of children and almost 30% of SLPs report that they serve children or adults with voice disorders (ASHA, 2008a).

Disorders of Resonance

Resonance disorders involve abnormal structures or functioning of the *hard* and *soft palates* (the roof of the mouth, front to back) that cause the voice to be directed into the nasal cavities on oral sounds or not directed into the nasal cavities on nasal sounds (i.e., /m/, /n/, and "ng"). Most resonance disorders in children are the result of cleft palates, with an overall prevalence of about 0.001% to 0.002% of the general population (i.e., 1 to 2 per 1,000 live births) (Peterson-Falzone, Hardin-Jones, & Karnell, 2009). **Hypernasality** is the result of clefts of the hard and soft palates or weakness of the soft palate. In hypernasality, oral consonants and vowels that should exit the mouth pass into the nasal passages where they are *resonated* (i.e., increased vibration and amplification of sounds) and listeners perceive the person's speech as though the person is "talking through his nose." **Hyponasality (denasality)** occurs because of partial or complete obstruction of the nasal passages (e.g., enlarged adenoids), causing the /m/, /n/ and "ng" sounds to not have their normal nasal resonance. Acquired resonance disorders in adults are usually the result of a weak soft palate that is caused by strokes and head injuries.

Disorders of Cognition

Cognition is the act or process of thinking or learning that involves perceiving, memory, reasoning, judgment, and problem solving. Cognitive disorders in children are usually associated with intellectual disabilities. The majority of children who have intellectual disabilities also have mild to profound language delays, with some children never developing functional language skills or the ability to live independently. Relatively intact cognitive abilities are important for development of both speech and language.

Adults may have acquired cognitive disorders, which are usually the result of damage to the right hemisphere or the frontal lobes of the brain. Cognitive disorders affect attention, **perception**, memory, reasoning, judgment, and problem solving (in a word, *thinking*). Mild to moderate TBIs can result in significant cognitive disorders in individuals of all ages, and severe neurological impairments can result in any combination of aphasia, motor speech disorders, and cognitive disorders. Approximately 1% to 2% of children and adults have TBIs that result in long-term disability (Zaloshnja, Miller, Langlois, et al., 2008). Many elderly people develop **dementia**, which is a neurological disorder that is a progressive deterioration of cognitive functioning and personality. Alzheimer's disease is just one form of dementia. It is estimated that approximately 8% to 15% of people between 65 and 70 years of age have some level of dementia; this percent increases significantly every 5 years (Plassman, Langa, Fisher, et al., 2007).

Hearing Impairments

Hearing is the foundation for development of speech and language. **Hearing impairments** can cause numerous speech and language delays and disorders in children that can affect them throughout their lives. Adults may acquire hearing impairments at any age from loud noises, medical problems that affect the ear, or the progressive hearing losses that often come with age. The two primary types of hearing impairments are conductive and sensorineural. A **conductive hearing loss** is a decrease in the loudness of a sound because of poor conduction of sound through the outer or middle ear. In severe conductive hearing losses, the fluid in the *cochlea* (hearing portion of the inner ear) may not be set into motion sufficiently to stimulate the nerves in the cochlea and, therefore, little or no auditory information is sent to the brain. Conductive hearing losses can have numerous causes, including malformations of the outer ear (*pinna*), occlusion of the ear canal from ear wax (*cerumen*), damage to the eardrum (*tympanic membrane*) or the three small bones in the middle ear (*ossicles*), or middle ear infections (*otitis media with effusion*).

hoarseness

A common symptom of dysphonia that is a combination of breathiness and harshness that affects how pleasant and smooth a voice sounds.

aphonia

A complete loss of voice followed by whispering for oral communication that typically has psychological causes such as emotional stress.

resonance disorder

Abnormal modification of the voice by passing through the nasal cavities during production of oral sounds (*hypernasality*) or not passing through the nasal cavities during production of nasal sounds (*hyponasality*).

hypernasal/hypernasality

A resonance disorder that occurs when oral consonants and vowels enter the nasal cavity because of clefts of the hard and soft palates or weakness of the soft palate, causing a person to sound like he is "talking through his nose."

hyponasal/hyponasality (denasal/denasality)

Lack of normal resonance for the three English phonemes, m, n, and ng, resulting from partial or complete obstruction in the nasal tract.

cognition/cognitive processing/cognitive functioning

The act or process of thinking or learning that involves perceiving, memory, abstraction, generalization, reasoning, judgment, and problem solving; closely related to intelligence.

perception/perceive

The process of detecting, discriminating, and recognition of a stimulus.

dementia

A neurological disease that causes intellectual, cognitive, and personality deterioration that is more severe than what would occur through normal aging.

hearing impairment/ hearing loss

Abnormal or reduced function in hearing resulting from an auditory disorder.

conductive hearing loss

A reduction in hearing sensitivity because of a disorder of the outer or middle ear.

sensorineural hearing loss

A reduction of hearing sensitivity produced by disorders of the cochlea and/or the auditory nerve fibers of the vestibulocochlear (VIII cranial) nerve.

In a **sensorineural hearing loss** there is a reduction of hearing sensitivity caused by disorders of the cochlea and/or the auditory nerve fibers of the vestibulocochlear (VIII cranial) nerve. This type of hearing loss typically results in difficulty discriminating speech sounds and, consequently, understanding speech. Infants may be born with sensorineural hearing losses or they may develop losses in childhood because of infections such as measles, mumps, and chicken pox. In older children, adolescents, and young adults, sensorineural hearing losses are often caused by listening to loud music for long periods of time (Thaker & Jongnarangsin, 2007). In older adults sensorineural hearing losses are common with advancing age.

Hearing loss is the most common of all physical impairments. In infants and children, approximately 1 in every 22 newborns in the United States has some kind of hearing problem, and 1 in every 1,000 infants has a severe to profound hearing loss. Of school-age children, 83 out of 1,000 have a significant hearing loss (ASHA, 2008b; National Dissemination Center for Children with Disabilities, 2010). Approximately 4.5% of adults 18 to 44 years of age, 14% of adults 45 to 64 years of age, and 54% of adults 65 years of age and older have some degree of hearing loss (Pleis & Lethbridge-Cejku, 2007).

EMOTIONAL AND SOCIAL EFFECTS OF COMMUNICATION DISORDERS

Communication disorders can have untold emotional and social effects on people of all ages. Many of these effects are likely undocumented and even unacknowledged by the individuals. However, beyond the individuals with the communication disorders are the parents, grandparents, siblings, husbands and wives, and other family members who are bewildered and anguished by their loved one's communication problems. A communication disorder affects a family, not just the person who has it, and it is essential to educate the family about the communication disorder their loved one has (Flasher & Fogle, 2012; Tye Murray, 2012). Each chapter in this text that deals with a disorder has a discussion of the emotional and social effects of that disorder on the person and the family.

As clinicians, we always need to keep in mind the entire person (and the family) with whom we are working, not just the disorder the person has. We need to place considerable importance on developing good, caring, working relationships with clients and their families in order to optimally carry out therapy and provide the necessary family education and training. Good people skills and counseling skills are essential when working with clients of all ages and their families (Flasher & Fogle, 2012).

CHAPTER SUMMARY

Speech-language pathologists and audiologists work with all areas of communication, including hearing, speaking, reading, writing, and nonverbal communication. For speech, we need to consider the various systems involved, including respiration, phonation, resonation, and articulation. We work with all areas of speech and language, including phonology, morphology, syntax, semantics, and pragmatics. Communication disorders may affect articulation, language, fluency, voice, resonance, cognition, and hearing. Communication disorders can have untold emotional and social effects on children, adolescents, and adults, and their families.

STUDY QUESTIONS

Knowledge and Comprehension

1. What are the four speech systems?
2. Explain morphology. In two three-syllable words, indicate each morpheme.
3. What are pragmatics? What are some elements included in pragmatics?
4. What is a communication disorder?
5. What are receptive language and expressive language?

Application

1. When talking with clients and their families, why is it helpful to understand that verbal content is usually more important for factual communication and nonverbal content is more important for judging emotions and attitudes?
2. How do suprasegmentals help us communicate?
3. Discuss the importance of good pragmatics when working with clients and their families.
4. Discuss how being familiar with the major categories of communication disorders could be helpful in your personal life.
5. Discuss the importance of appreciating and understanding the emotional and social effects of language disorders in children.

Analysis/Synthesis

1. What does the sentence, "We cannot not communicate." mean?
2. Explain the differences between speech and language.
3. How are *linguistic competence* and *grammatical intuition* similar and different?
4. Why might determining dichotomies be helpful in diagnosing a speech or language disorder?
5. How might cognitive disorders in children affect their language abilities?

REFERENCES

American Speech-Language-Hearing Association [ASHA]. (1983). Position paper: Social dialects and implications of the position on social dialects. *ASHA, 25*(9), 23–27.

ASHA. (2008a). *Communication facts.* Science and Research Department, Rockville, MD: ASHA.

ASHA. (2008b). *Incidence and prevalence of communication disorders and hearing loss in children in the United States: 2008 edition.* http://www.asha.org. Accessed August 27, 2010.

ASHA. (2008c). *Incidence and prevalence of speech, voice, and language disorders in adults in the United States: 2008 edition.* http://www.asha.org. Accessed August 27, 2010.

ASHA. (2010). *2010 School Survey report: Caseload characteristics.* Rockville, MD: ASHA.

Barnes, M. A., Fletcher, J., & Fuchs, Lynn. (2007). *Learning disabilities: From identification to intervention.* New York, NY: The Guilford Press.

Bloodstein, O., & Bernstein Ratner, N. (2008). *A handbook on stuttering* (6th ed.). Clifton Park, NY: Delmar Cengage Learning.

Burgoon, J. K., Guerrero, L., & Floyd, K. (2010). *Nonverbal communication.* New York, NY: Pearson.

Catts, H. W., & Kamhi, A. G. (2005). *Language and reading disabilities* (2nd ed.). Boston, MA: Allyn & Bacon.

Flasher, L. V., & Fogle, P. T. (2012). *Counseling skills for speech-language pathologists and audiologists* (2nd ed.). Clifton Park, NY: Delmar Cengage Learning.

Fogle, P. T. (2009). *Counseling skills: Recognizing and interpreting nonverbal communication (body language, gestures, and facial expressions),* Gaylord, MI: Northern Speech/National Rehabilitation Services.

Gedeon, A. (2006). *Science and technology in medicine: An illustrated account based on ninety-nine landmark publications from five centuries.* New York, NY: Springer Science.

Guitar, B. (2006). *Stuttering: An integrated approach to its nature and treatment.* Philadelphia, PA: Lippincott Williams & Wilkins.

Hegde, M. N. (2007). *Pocket guide to assessment in speech-language pathology* (3rd ed.). Clifton Park, NY: Delmar Cengage Learning.

Lewis, M. P. (Ed.). 2009. *Ethnologue: Languages of the world* (16th ed.). Dallas, TX: SIL International.

Luria, A. (1961). *The role of speech in the normal and abnormal processes in the child.* Baltimore, MD: Penguin.

Manning, W. H. (2010). *Clinical decision making in fluency disorders* (3rd ed.). Clifton Park, NY: Delmar Cengage Learning.

National Dissemination Center for Children with Disabilities. (2010). *Disability fact sheet.* Washington, DC: NDCCD.

Owens, R. E., Jr. (2012). *Language development: An introduction* (8th ed.) San Antonio, TX: Pearson/Allyn & Bacon.

Paul, R. (2006). *Language disorders from infancy through adolescence: Assessment and intervention* (3rd ed.). St. Louis, MO: Mosby.

Peterson-Falzone, S. J., Hardin-Jones, M. A., & Karnell, M. P. (2009). *Cleft palate speech* (4th ed.). St. Louis, MO: Mosby.

Plassman, B. L., Langa, K. M., Fisher, G. G., Heeringa, S. G., Weir, D. R., Ofstedal, M. B., & Burke, J. R. (2007). Prevalence of dementia in the United States: The aging, demographics, and memory study. *Neuroepidemiology, 29,* 125–132.

Pleis, J. R., & Lethbridge-Cejku, M. (2007). Summary health statistics for U.S. adults: National Health Interview Survey, 2006. National Center for Health Statistics. *Vital Health Statistics, 10*(235), table 11.

Ramig, P. R., & Dodge, D. M. (2010). *The child and adolescent stuttering treatment and activity resource guide* (2nd ed.). Clifton Park, NY: Delmar Cengage Learning.

Reed, V. A. (2005). *An introduction to children with language disorders* (3rd ed.). Boston, MA: Pearson Allyn and Bacon.

Thaker, J., & Jongnarangsin, K. (2007). iPods and pacemakers. *ASHA Leader,* June 19, 5.

Tye Murray, N. (2012). Counseling for adults and children who have hearing loss. In L. Flasher & P. Fogle, *Counseling Skills for Speech-Language Pathologists and Audiologists* (2nd ed.). Clifton Park, NY: Delmar Cengage Learning.

Van Riper, C. (1978). *Speech correction: Principles and methods* (6th ed.). Englewood Cliffs, NJ: Prentice-Hall.

Vygotsky, L. (1962). *Thought and language.* Cambridge, MA: MIT Press.

Ward, D. (2006). *Stuttering and cluttering: Framework for understanding and treatment.* East Sussex, England: Psychology Press.

Yairi, E., & Ambrose, N. G. (2005). *Early childhood stuttering.* Austin, TX: Pro-Ed.

Zaloshnja, E., Miller, T., Langlois, J. A. & Selassie, A. W. (2008). Prevalence of long-term disability from traumatic brain injury in the civilian population of the United States, 2005. *Journal of Head Trauma Rehabilitation, 23*(6), 394–400.

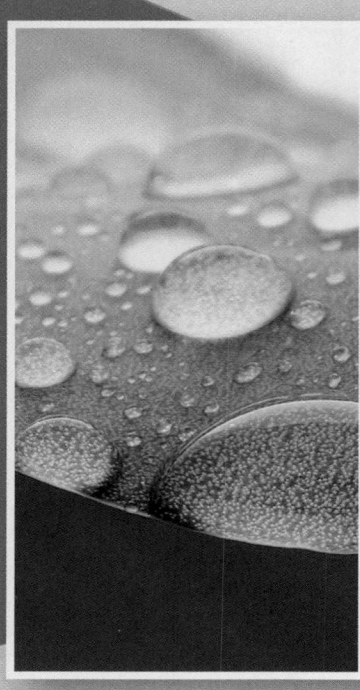

CHAPTER 2
Speech-Language Pathologists and Audiologists

LEARNING OBJECTIVES

After studying this chapter, you will:

- Appreciate that speech-language pathologists and audiologists help many people beyond the clients and patients directly receiving therapy.

- Be aware of numerous personal qualities of effective professionals.

- Recognize that as professionals we are always using a team approach.

- Know the basic educational and clinical experience requirements to become a nationally certified and state-licensed speech-language pathologist or audiologist.

- Be aware of the scope of practice of speech-language pathologists and audiologists.

- Know the variety of work settings in which speech-language pathologists and audiologists practice.

- Understand the employment outlook for speech-language pathologists and audiologists.

- Be aware of the professional organizations that oversee speech-language pathologists and audiologists.

- Be familiar with the National Student Speech-Language-Hearing Association (NSSLHA).

KEY TERMS

CHAPTER OUTLINE

INTRODUCTION

Speech-language pathology and audiology are wonderful professions filled with caring and amiable professionals who serve interesting people with challenging disabilities. Speech-language pathology and audiology are professions that likely will be increasingly fascinating as you study them. It eventually becomes nearly impossible to separate the individual from the profession. The knowledge and skills you learn as a speech-language pathologist or audiologist become an important part of who you are as a person and how you interact and communicate with others.

BEGINNING YOUR STUDY OF SPEECH-LANGUAGE PATHOLOGY AND AUDIOLOGY

This textbook is designed to answer your questions about speech-language pathology and audiology, and it will likely give you a picture of the scope of these professions that is broader than what you imagined. Speech-language pathologists and audiologists learn about and are concerned about people from the moment of conception to their last breaths of life. Every age of infants, children, adolescents, young adults, middle-aged adults, and elderly adults have unique challenges that may affect their speech, language, cognitive, hearing, and swallowing functions. You will learn about many of these challenges through this course and this text. If you decide to major in communication disorders, you will learn about each of the areas introduced in this text in more depth. If, however, you choose to take only this course, you will still learn information that will be invaluable throughout your adult life.

Some clinicians feel that speech-language pathology and audiology are the best majors for preparation for adult life and parenthood. During their education and training students learn about normal and abnormal development of infants and children; how to work with children one-on-one and in small groups of two or three; how to talk with children about what is bothering them and how to talk with parents regarding their concerns about their children; how to motivate children to work hard to improve their communication and academic skills and how to work with children who are fearful of failure and who need special care to learn to trust you and themselves; how to work with adults and elderly people with a variety of neurological problems and the sensitive and sometimes emotional issues that accompany impairment or loss of communication abilities; about the problems of the hearing impaired at all ages and the effects not only on the child with a hearing loss but also the parents and family of the child; and how to be a patient, active listener—a trained listener—which is perhaps the most important interpersonal skill you can develop.

Communication disorders can affect people throughout their life span—for example, children born with hereditary disorders and syndromes, cleft lips and palates, hearing impairments, auditory processing disorders, and cerebral palsy. Adults with acquired communication disorders caused by strokes or traumatic brain injuries may never be able to communicate easily and effectively again, which can prevent returning to work or force them to work at a lower-level (and lower-paying) job.

The person with a communication disorder is, in a way, the tip of an iceberg. A child or adult with a communication disorder affects the family around him, as well as countless other people with whom the child or adult tries to communicate (see Figure 2–1). Therefore, when we help individuals improve their communication abilities we also are helping many other people, both directly and indirectly—most of whom we never meet.

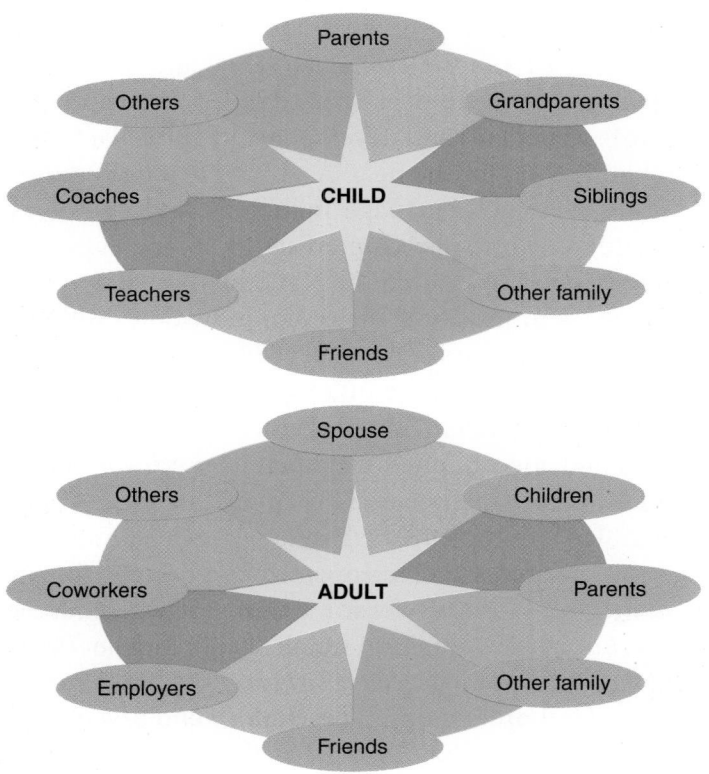

Figure 2–1

Who is really helped?

© Cengage Learning 2013.

Application Question

Have you ever had a "problem" by which other people referred to you (e.g., "Big nose!" "Skinny!" "Fatty!")? How did you feel about being referred to primarily as a problem and secondarily as a person?

Person-First Language

Students and professionals in speech-language pathology and audiology must keep in mind that the problems individuals experience do not define who they are. People are not their problems; problems are something people experience. Therefore, as clinicians and researchers we follow the "client/person first" convention as closely as possible; in other words, we refer to "a boy with an articulation disorder," "a girl with a hearing impairment," "a woman with a voice disorder," and so on. Professionally, we avoid phrases such as "He's an articulation client," "She's hearing impaired," "She's a voice case," and so on, because the wording implies that the person's problem is his or her identity. It is easy to slip into the habit of referring to the problem that the person has rather than to the person who has a problem. We need to learn early and maintain our vigilance to always use person-first language.

A BRIEF HISTORY OF THE PROFESSIONS

The professions of speech-language pathology and audiology are relatively new compared to medicine and education. The common origins of these professions can be traced back to Alexander Graham Bell, whose father and grandfather had been *elocutionists* (individuals who studied formal speaking in pronunciation, grammar, style, and tone) in Edinburgh, Scotland, in the 1860s. A. G. Bell and his father were interested in people who were deaf or hard of hearing (both A. G. Bell's mother and wife were deaf) and developed and applied a formal system of speech rehabilitation for the deaf. A. G. Bell recognized the need for the professions of speech-language pathology and audiology. In the early 1900s, groups with special interests in *speech correction* in the United States were formed within the National Association of Teachers of Speech (NATS), a professional society for individuals with interests in rhetoric, theater, and public speaking. In 1925, the American Academy of Speech Correction (AASC) was unofficially chartered by a group within NATS. The AASC members included physicians, psychologists, professors of English and speech, phonetician, and *speech correctionists*. The AASC eventually evolved to become the American Speech and Hearing Association (ASHA). In the 1970s when language disorders became an essential area of the profession, the organization became the **American Speech-Language-Hearing Association** but retained the abbreviation ASHA (Lubinski, Golper, & Frattali, 2007), Moeller (1975), in her *Speech Pathology & Audiology: Iowa Origins of a Discipline,* discussed the beginnings of our professions in psychology and psychiatry. In 1924, Lee Edward Travis, a doctoral student at the University of Iowa with training in psychology and medicine became "the first individual in the world to be trained by clearly conscious design at the doctoral level for

American Speech-Language-Hearing Association (ASHA)

The professional organization that represents speech-language pathologists and audiologists and sets standards for their education, training, and certification. The organization was formerly called the American Speech and Hearing Association, and retained the ASHA abbreviation.

a definite and specific professional objective of working experimentally and clinically with speech and hearing disorders."

Rehabilitation is a relatively new concept. Even after World War I, when thousands of injured soldiers were released from hospitals, little rehabilitation was provided (certainly, there was no speech therapy or hearing aids for hearing losses caused by acoustic traumas from explosions). If soldiers were medically able to be discharged, they were sent home; how they functioned when they arrived was not the concern of the medical personnel. After World War II, rehabilitation of injured individuals (including those with head injuries) became an important focus of their overall treatment.

Special education and special services for children struggling educationally were not federally mandated and widespread until the 1960s. During that decade and the following decades, important federal legislation was enacted to provide the necessary services to school-age and even preschool children:

- 1965—The *Elementary and Secondary Education Act (Public Law 89-10)* was enacted. This law required states to provide funds so that students with special needs, including the gifted, would be evaluated and appropriately educated.

- 1975—The passage of the *Education of All Handicapped Children Act (Public Law 94-142)* mandated that all school-age children with disabilities must be provided a free and appropriate education in the least restrictive environment. This included providing all related services, such as speech-language therapy, physical therapy, and occupational therapy, for children to maximally benefit from their education.

- 1986—The *Education of the Handicapped Amendments (Public Law 99-457)* provided federal funds to states to develop programs for children with disabilities from birth through 2 years of age, and provisions for Public Law 94-142 were extended to children with disabilities between 3 and 5 years of age.

- 1990—The *Individuals with Disabilities Act (IDEA)* came into being, and the *Americans with Disabilities Act (ADA) (Public Law 101-336)* mandated improved access for individuals with handicaps to buildings and facilities and provided effective communication for people with disabilities, including the use of interpreters, sign language, and **telecommunication devices for the deaf (TDD)**.

The professions of speech-language pathology and audiology have grown as the services they provide have been increasingly valued and funded. From the early years of emphasis on stuttering and articulation disorders grew a profession that touches every communication problem known to science. With the addition of swallowing disorders to our scope of practice, speech-language pathologists can work with disorders of anatomy and physiology that involve the oral, pharyngeal (*pharynx*), laryngeal (*larynx*), and respiratory systems, regardless of a person's communication abilities.

telecommunication devices for the deaf (TDD)

Telephone systems used by those with significant hearing impairments in which a typewritten message is transmitted over telephone lines and is received as a printed message.

PROFESSIONAL ORGANIZATIONS

ASHA is the primary scholarly and professional organization for individuals in the field of communication sciences and disorders in the United States. ASHA considers communication sciences and disorders to be a single discipline with two separate professions: speech-language pathology and audiology. ASHA also establishes the "Scope of Practice in Speech-Language Pathology" and "Scope of Practice in Audiology." These documents are available on the ASHA website at http://www.asha.org. ASHA's Certificates of Clinical Competence (CCC) in Speech-Language Pathology (CCC-SLP) and Audiology (CCC-A) are nationally recognized professional credentials that indicate individuals have met rigorous academic and professional standards, and that they have the knowledge, skills, and expertise to provide high-quality clinical services. SLPs and Auds must engage in ongoing professional development to keep their certification current. In addition to being members of ASHA, many audiologists are also members of the American Audiological Association (referred to as "Triple A"—AAA). AAA is separate from ASHA and has its own national conventions designed to meet the needs of audiologists.

As the need for speech-language pathology and audiology services has increased, membership in ASHA has steadily grown. As of 2010, ASHA had a membership of more than 140,000, including members from countries other than the United States. Speech and hearing associations around the world have their own memberships, for example:

- Speech Pathology Australia
- Royal College of Speech and Language Therapists (Great Britain)
- Canadian Association of Speech-Language Pathology and Audiology
- Israeli Speech, Hearing, and Language Association
- Japanese Association of Speech-Language-Hearing Therapists
- Russian Association of Phoniatricians and Speech Therapists
- Swedish Association of Phoniatrics and Logopedics

Children and adults worldwide experience communication disorders, and perhaps in countries where there is the greatest need (the "developing countries") there are the fewest professionals and resources to provide help.

Student Organizations

Students can join the **National Student Speech-Language-Hearing Association (NSSLHA)** while undergraduates or graduate students (full or part time, national or international). NSSLHA provides students with a closer affiliation to professionals in the discipline, as well as monthly professional publications and other support designed specifically for them (see http://www.nsslha.org).

National Student Speech-Language-Hearing Association (NSSLHA)

The preprofessional association for students interested in the study of communication sciences and disorders.

NSSLHA also has developed an excellent manual for students, titled *Communication Sciences Student Survival Guide* (NSSLHA, 2010), which provides, among other things, information on financing your education and advice (from students' perspectives) about enhancing your education and involvement in the profession throughout your education.

State Associations

Each state has its own state association for speech-language pathologists and audiologists, which provides professional support, public awareness, opportunities for professional growth, and advocates for the professions and the individuals they serve. Both states and ASHA have annual conventions and provide numerous opportunities for continuing education and professional development.

Individual state licensing boards also regulate the practice of speech-language pathology and audiology. State licensing requirements generally follow the requirements for ASHA certification. Most states also have continuing education requirements for licensure renewal. Medicare, Medicaid, and private health insurers generally require a practitioner to be licensed to qualify for reimbursement of clinical services.

PROFESSIONAL ETHICS

In order to be nationally certified professionals, the members must adhere to a code of ethics. Ethics is the process of deciding what is the right thing to do in a moral dilemma (Aiken, 2008). Ethics are standards of conduct that guide our professional behavior. They define acceptable versus unacceptable behaviors and promote high and consistent standards of practice.

The establishment of a code of ethics has been a major function of ASHA since its founding in 1925. For speech-language pathologists and audiologists, ethical practice transcends employment settings, levels of experience, and nature of clientele. Once a speech-language pathologist or audiologist signs the agreement to follow the ASHA Code of Ethics and holds a current Certificate of Clinical Competence, he or she must abide by the ASHA Code regardless of certification held or the location of services provided (Miller, 2007). Failure to abide by the Code of Ethics could result in loss of certification or licensure. Refer to ASHA's website (http://www.asha.org) for a copy of the Code of Ethics.

PERSONAL QUALITIES (ATTRIBUTES) OF EFFECTIVE PROFESSIONALS

Speech-language pathologists and audiologists are professionals. Several personal qualities (attributes) of effective professionals have been identified in the literature (Flasher & Fogle, 2012):

- *Encouraging*—The ability to encourage may be one of the most important qualities of clinicians. Encouragement helps people learn to believe in their potential for improvement.

Personal Story

Elizabeth Smith, M.Ed., CCC-SLP

On an unusual snowy day in Atlanta, Georgia, in March 1983, kindergartner Elizabeth Smith was walking to a friend's nearby house when she stepped on a downed power line that had been hidden under the snow. While she was unconscious, she was rushed to the hospital, and over the next 6 weeks she underwent a series of surgeries that included amputation of both arms at her shoulders and her left leg at the high thigh level. This was followed by physical and occupational rehabilitation for the young girl with triple amputations. She eventually returned to school, and over the next 5 years, with the help of the hospital rehabilitation staff and her schoolteachers, she learned to walk using a prosthetic leg. Although she was fitted with prosthetic arms, she abandoned them because they felt heavy and awkward. Instead, she learned to use her one foot to perform most functions her arms and hands would have done: she learned to eat, type, write, apply makeup, brush her hair, and most everything else people use two arms and hands to do (see Figure 2-2).

Elizabeth said that her hospital stay after the accident inspired her to go into rehabilitation as an adult—as a speech-language pathologist. She said that during her hospital stay as a child, "Rehabilitation was difficult, but I could always communicate." In college, Elizabeth decided that becoming a speech-language pathologist would put all of her interests and talents to good use: verbal skills, interest in science, teaching ability, and talent for interacting with people. In 1999, Elizabeth graduated magna cum laude with a B.A. in speech communication from Georgia State University in Atlanta, followed by a master's degree in communication disorders, which included an internship at a skilled nursing facility (nursing home). Here, she learned even more about overcoming her own clinical challenges on the job, such as working with patients who have feeding and swallowing problems. Her first professional work

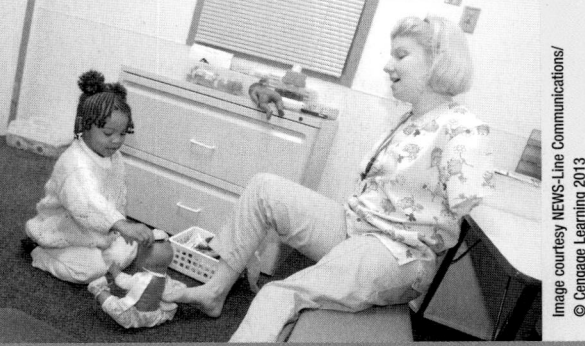

Image courtesy NEWS-Line Communications/
© Cengage Learning 2013

Figure 2-2
Elizabeth Smith on the job.

after completing her master's degree was as a public school speech-language pathologist, but she eventually decided that hospital work in a rehabilitation center for children was her passion. Only a few work-environment accommodations have been made for her, such as lowering the therapy table and having files and materials stored at a comfortable height to make it easier for her to use her foot. Even with its occasional challenges, Elizabeth says of her work, "It is my dream job." ■

- *Emotionally stable*—Most speech-language pathologists and audiologists are at least fairly well-adjusted people.
- *Self-aware*—Self-awareness is related to self-acceptance, self-esteem, and self-realization. Self-awareness is important to maintain our emotional stability.
- *Patient*—One of the hallmark characteristics of speech-language pathologists and audiologists is patience; that is, the ability and willingness to persevere during the often long, slow road of speech and language development or rehabilitation of our clients and patients. It also means not becoming anxious or frustrated about a person's slow rate of improvement and realizing that most people are doing about as well as they can at the moment.
- *Sensitive to others*—Sensitivity requires awareness of others, particularly the sometimes almost unobservable emotional responses to what is being said or what is happening in the person's life.
- *Empathic*—Speech-language pathologists and audiologists attempt to understand the client from the client's point of view; that is, they try to understand what the person is thinking, feeling, and experiencing and communicate this understanding back to the client.

Application Question

Which of the personal qualities do you feel are some of your strongest? Your weakest? How could you strengthen your weakest qualities?

THE TEAM APPROACH

As professionals working with communication disorders, we are members of a team—in all of our work, we take the team approach. We are typically working with other professionals, as well as family members of clients. At minimum, the people on the team are the client and the clinician, with the client always being the most important team member because without the client there would be no need for any other team members. In most cases, the team includes several others, such as family members of the client, the clinician's supervisor or administrator, teachers, and reading specialists in a school setting. Depending on the setting and the needs of the client or patient, physicians, nurses, physical therapists, occupational therapists, respiratory therapists, and other professionals may all be involved directly with helping the person (see Figure 2–3).

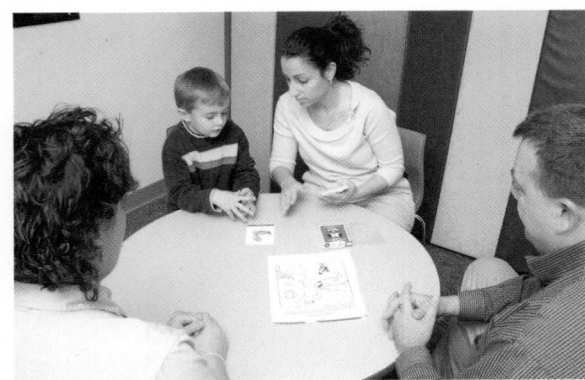

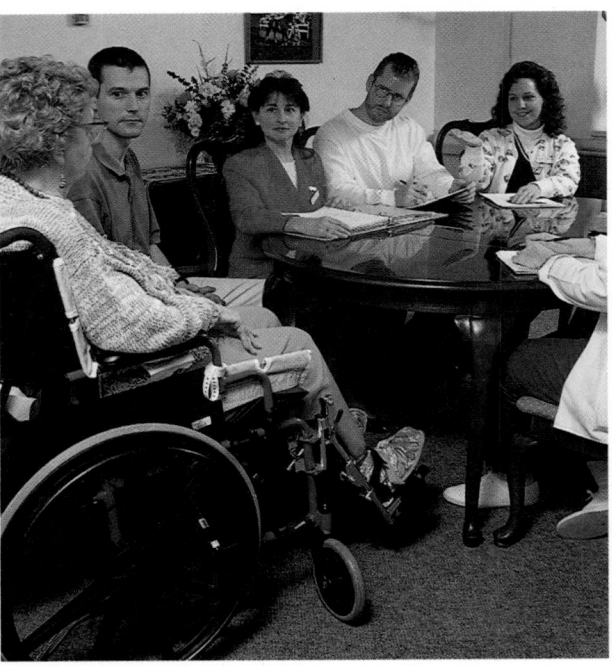

© Cengage Learning 2013

Figure 2-3

The team approach always includes the client/patient, family, and other professionals.

Typical treatment teams for different settings are as follows:

- University clinic: Client, family, student clinician, and supervisor
- School: Child, family, school speech-language pathologist, and classroom teacher
- Hospital: Patient, family, physician, nurse, dietitian, speech-language pathologist , physical therapist, and occupational therapist

Countless other people are indirectly involved with helping clients and patients, including secretarial and administrative staff, custodial and maintenance workers, and kitchen workers. The list of the "behind the scenes" people is long, and if any of these people are not doing their job well it can affect the person we are trying to help. After clinicians have been working for a while, they begin to realize that what makes the "machinery" of the work environment function are the people who are the least acknowledged for their contributions. We as communication specialists need to show our appreciation for all people who are part of the big picture of helping people with communication disorders.

COMMUNICATION DISORDERS PROFESSIONALS

The field of communication (communicative) disorders involves interrelated professionals who begin with earning a bachelor's degree (either a B.A. or a B.S., depending on the institution) in speech-language pathology, communication (communicative) disorders, or speech and hearing sciences (other terms may be used). Students also may earn an undergraduate degree in another major and then begin their education at the graduate level, although they must take a series of undergraduate speech-language pathology and audiology courses to prepare for the more advanced courses in the major. After earning a bachelor's degree, a student needs to attend graduate school and it is at this level that individuals begin to specialize in either speech-language pathology or audiology. The entry-level requirement for speech-language pathologists to work professionally is an M.A. (Master of Arts) or M.S. (Master of Science). The entry-level requirement for audiologists is a doctoral degree, either a Ph.D. (Doctor of Philosophy) or Au.D. (Doctor of Audiology). After receiving a master's degree in speech-language pathology or a doctorate in audiology, passing the national examination, and becoming nationally certified and state licensed (to be discussed later), individuals become independent practitioners. In some countries (e.g., Great Britain, Australia, and New Zealand), a bachelor's degree in speech-language pathology (therapy or logopedics) is a professional degree; however, students begin their education in speech-language pathology in their freshman year of college, and their senior year is roughly equivalent to a graduate year in the United States.

Some individuals in speech-language pathology choose to continue their graduate education after their master's degree by pursuing a Ph.D. or Ed.D. (Doctor of Education). During their doctoral studies, which usually take 3 to 5 years after earning an M.A. or M.S., the individuals continue to specialize in either speech-language pathology or audiology. A few individuals also choose to become *dual certified*, that is, they must meet all educational, training, examination, and professional experience to qualify to be both a certified speech-language pathologist and an audiologist. In all clinical settings for SLPs and Auds, those with Ph.D.s have wide opportunities as teachers and professors, clinicians, and researchers. The following is a brief explanation of the work of speech-language pathologists and audiologists.

The Need for New Ph.D.s

Most men and women who earned Ph.D.s in the 1960s and 1970s in either speech-language pathology or audiology and who became university professors are retiring or have retired. This leaves a significant number of faculty positions in universities around the country struggling to be filled. For individuals with doctoral degrees interested in teaching at a university and doing research, employment prospects are excellent. If students beginning their education and training in speech-language pathology and audiology can look beyond the master's degree and consider pursuing a doctorate, they may find the rewarding (and relatively flexible) career as a university professor to their liking.

Speech-Language Pathologists

The American Speech-Language-Hearing Association has designated our professional title as *speech-language pathologist*; however, many other English-speaking countries prefer to use the designation *speech-language therapist* (e.g., England, Ireland, and New Zealand). What we are called by other professionals, clients, patients, and their family members depends somewhat on the setting in which we are working. For example, in public schools we are more likely to be called speech therapists, speech-language therapists, speech teachers (mostly by children), or speech and hearing specialists. In medical settings, we are commonly referred to by physicians, nurses, and patients as speech therapists or speech pathologists. Rarely is the entire designation *speech-language pathologist* used, perhaps because of the number of sounds and syllables in the complete title. Also, the terms **therapy** and *therapist* are positive terms that suggest helping (e.g., physical therapy, occupational therapy, and respiratory therapy) and include us as regular members of the rehabilitation team. The term *pathology* in the medical field typically connotes diseased tissue, and *pathologist* refers to a physician specializing in the study of diseases.

Outside of university clinics, the term *clinician* is not commonly used. (Interestingly, in textbooks we typically refer to ourselves as *clinicians* rather than *therapists*.) Many universities that train students to become speech-language pathologists refer to their departments as the Department of Communication (or Communicative) Disorders, Department of Communication Sciences and Disorders, or other variations around the term *communication*. However, in many countries around the world students train in a Department of Phoniatrics and Logopedics and become *logopedists*.

The education, coursework, and clinical training of speech-language pathologists are specified by ASHA. The national professional organization specifies coursework and clinical training requirements and standards to help with consistency throughout the country in the quality of new professionals. Upon completion of an M.A. or M.S. in the major, individuals are eligible to take the national *Praxis Examination* administered by the Educational Testing Service (ETS). In addition, to earn ASHA certification, individuals must complete a 36-week **Clinical Fellowship** of full-time work (35 hours per week) or the equivalent part-time experience totaling a minimum of 1,260 hours. After successful completion of all of these requirements, the person becomes a nationally certified speech-language pathologist.

Most states have licensing boards that specify criteria that must be met to be eligible for a state license to work in hospitals and practice independently. States also have credentialing boards that specify education and training criteria to work in public schools. ASHA, as well as most states, requires SLPs to earn **continuing education units (CEUs)** throughout their professional careers to keep abreast of new developments in the field and to maintain their state license or credential. CEUs are essential to the continued professional development of clinicians

---

therapy/treatment

Treatment of any significant condition to prevent, alleviate, or cure it; note: *therapy* and *treatment* are interchangeable.

Clinical Fellowship

A 36-week full-time (35 hours per week) or the equivalent part-time mentored clinical experience totaling a minimum of 1,260 hours begun after all academic coursework and university clinic training are completed; required by ASHA to be eligible for the Certificate of Clinical Competence (CCC).

continuing education units (CEUs)

Additional education or training required by ASHA and most states throughout a professional's career to help the professional remain current in the field.

Application Question

How could attending state and national conferences be valuable to your professional development and career?

and researchers and to strengthening the profession. CEUs are provided in numerous settings, such as national and state conferences and conventions, one- or two-day seminars and workshops provided at the local level, ASHA professional publications, and online coursework in an array of areas. SLPs may continue their formal education at any time by entering one of the many fine doctoral programs throughout the United States. An earned doctorate (Ph.D., Ed.D., or Au.D.) is usually required to be a university professor.

Scope of Practice

The **scope of practice** or work of speech-language pathologists may be described in a few words: we identify, evaluate, diagnose, and help (treat) people with communication and swallowing disorders. The following is a brief description of the primary roles in which speech-language pathologists may be involved when working with clients and patients.

Evaluate Communication and Swallowing Delays and Disorders

When a speech-language pathologist suspects a communication, cognitive, or swallowing problem, a thorough **evaluation** is in order (note: the terms *evaluation* and *assessment* may be used interchangeably). The evaluation generally includes an interview and standardized or *clinician-devised* assessments (i.e., nonstandardized tests designed for specific patients). The purposes of the evaluation are to determine, if possible, the cause of the problem, the nature of the problem, whether it is progressive or static, the characteristics of the problem, what makes it better and what makes it worse, the severity of the problem, treatment goals, and the potential for habilitation or rehabilitation.

Diagnose Communication and Swallowing Delays and Disorders

Making a **diagnosis** means the SLP makes a professional decision and commitment as to the specific diagnostic terms that may be used to represent the client's or patient's communication, cognitive, or swallowing problems. Specific diagnostic terms, with their associated billing codes, are necessary for SLPs to be reimbursed by insurance companies, Medicare, or other third-party payers. A written description of a client's or patient's problems in a formal report is essential, as is *documentation* (reporting) of all therapy goals, rationales, and treatment procedures.

Treat Communication and Swallowing Delays and Disorders

Most speech-language pathologists love doing therapy and developing creative strategies for helping clients and patients. Our best therapy is always based on sound research and theoretical principles with *evidence-based practice* (EBP) as the goal. Evidence-based practice is the integration of (a) clinical expertise, (b) best current evidence, and (c) client/patient perspectives to provide high-quality services reflecting the interests, values, needs, and choices of the individuals we serve.

scope of practice

ASHA's delineation of the general and specific areas in which speech-language pathologists and audiologists may engage with the appropriate and necessary education, training, and experience.

evaluation/assessment

The overall clinical activities designed to understand an individual's communication abilities and disabilities before a treatment program is determined and established. Also called assessment.

diagnosis

The determination of the type and cause of a speech, language, cognitive, swallowing, or hearing disorder based on the signs and symptoms of the client or patient obtained through case history, observations, interviews, formal and informal evaluations, and other methods.

The *art of therapy* involves flexibility and thinking on our feet. It also includes the understanding of when and how to use particular therapy approaches and techniques. No two therapy sessions are the same. Each session has its own uniqueness in the client's responses to the approaches, techniques, materials, and stimuli we present. In addition, the personal interactions and dynamics between the client and the clinician can vary from session to session and sometimes from moment to moment. Our insightfulness into our clients and their problems, our **clinical intuition**, and our counseling skills help make a challenging therapy session into a productive therapy session (Flasher & Fogle, 2012).

Work Settings

Speech-language pathologists work in a variety of work settings, with considerable diversity among clients and patients. The work settings can roughly be divided into educational and medical settings. The largest employer of speech-language pathologists is the public schools, with the legal mandate in the United States to provide services to every child from birth to 21 years of age, and to students who are in adult transition programs who need and qualify for services. Many SLPs also work in infant and early childhood programs funded by local and state agencies. Speech-language pathologists are working with increasingly complex clinical cases, including children with multiple handicaps, most with unidentified etiologies and others that are related to premature birth, mothers who abused substances during pregnancy, and children with HIV or AIDS.

On the other end of the educational spectrum, increasing numbers of speech-language pathologists are being employed by community colleges to provide services to older students and to direct or be involved with programs for people of all ages who have sustained neurological damage. Some speech-language pathologists also provide clinical supervision in university training programs and may do some clinical teaching.

Many SLPs work in medical settings of all types, including **acute care hospitals**, **subacute hospitals**, **convalescent hospitals**, and **inpatient** and **outpatient** clinics. *Home health care* (i.e., therapy in the patient's home) is an increasingly popular employment opportunity for SLPs. Home health care is designed to provide rehabilitation services without the high cost of hospitalization. *Private practice* provides opportunities for SLPs to work with a variety of clients or to specialize in a specific age group or disorder. Private practice also allows speech-language pathologists to have considerable independence and flexibility in their work schedules and allows them to develop their entrepreneurial skills (Fogle, 2001).

Aging presents an increasing number of clinically complex cases with multiple impairments. For example, it is not uncommon to see a patient with a hearing loss, stroke, heart disease, cancer, and visual impairments, along with arthritis and diabetes mellitus. Because speech-language pathologists are good communicators with good to excellent interpersonal skills, they are often advanced into administrative positions

---

clinical intuition

A decision-making process that is used unconsciously by experienced clinicians that is rapid, subtle, and based on the entire context of the situation, but does not follow simple, cause-and-effect logic.

acute care hospital

A hospital where patients are treated for brief but severe episodes of illness, injury, trauma, or during recovery from surgery.

subacute hospital

A level of care needed by patients who do not require acute care but who are medically fragile and require special services, e.g., respiratory therapy, intravenous tube feeding, and complex wound management care.

convalescent hospital/ skilled nursing facility (SNF)/extended care facility/nursing home

A medical facility, such as a skilled nursing facility, extended care facility, or nursing home, that provides extended medical, nursing, or custodial care for individuals over a prolonged period, e.g., during the course of a chronic illness or the rehabilitation phase after an acute illness or injury.

inpatient

A patient who has been admitted to a hospital or other health care facility for at least an overnight stay.

outpatient

A patient who is not hospitalized but is being treated in an office, clinic, or medical facility.

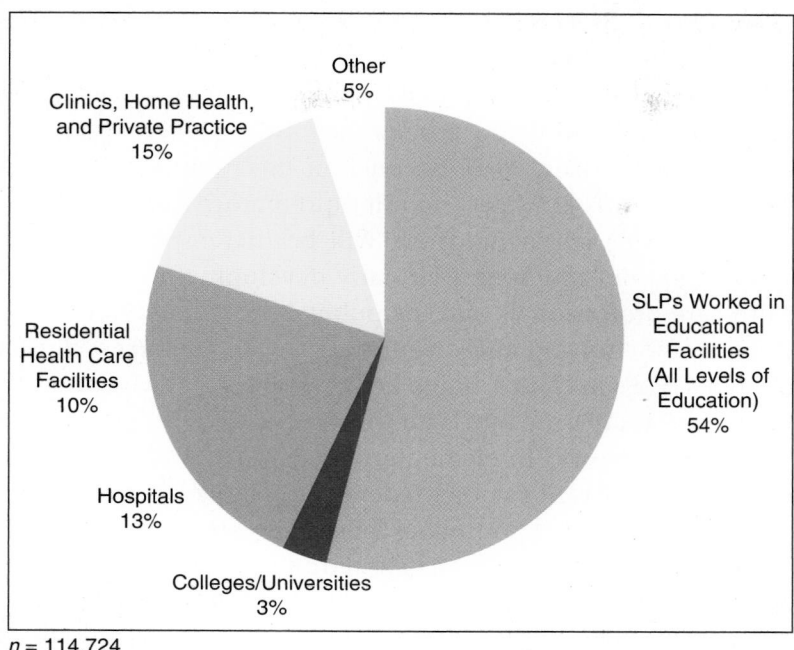

Other
5%

Clinics, Home Health,
and Private Practice
15%

SLPs Worked in
Educational
Facilities
(All Levels of
Education)
54%

Residential
Health Care
Facilities
10%

Hospitals
13%

Colleges/Universities
3%

n = 114,724

Figure 2–4

ASHA-certified speech-language pathologists by primary employment setting.

Source: ASHA Summary Membership and Affiliation Counts, year ending 2010.

in various work settings, which increases their opportunities in a variety of ways (Lubinski, Golper, & Frattali, 2007).

Speech-language pathologists can devote their time to the age groups they most enjoy—for example, early childhood, school-age, adolescence, adult, or elderly. Many SLPs like working in more than one setting. For example, some clinicians work in public schools during the day as their primary job and work in hospitals or their own private practice for a few hours after leaving the school in the afternoon.

Job opportunities in foreign countries are plentiful; all industrialized countries have speech-language pathologists. In addition, military bases worldwide often provide speech-language pathologists for the dependents of service men and women who are being educated in schools on the base. Various military and VA hospitals have speech-language pathologists on staff. Figure 2–4 shows the primary employment settings of speech-language pathologists in 2010.

Application Question

Many people are surprised by our relatively broad scope of practice, the variety of clients and patients SLPs work with, and the array of work settings in which SLPs are employed. Are there any surprises for you?

Employment Outlook

In articles on "The 50 Best Jobs in America" in the November 2009 and 2010 issues of *Money* magazine, speech-language pathology was rated as one of the best, with job satisfaction rated as very high. According to the U.S. Department of Labor's Bureau of Labor Statistics, in its *Occupational Outlook Handbook* (2010), the job outlook is very good for speech-language pathologists. The report projected that between 2010 and 2018 employment of speech-language pathologists is expected to grow by 19%, which is faster than the average for all other occupations. The outlook for a strong job market also exists in Canada, England, Australia, New Zealand, and other English-speaking countries with shortages of SLPs. If you are bilingual, your job market is even broader.

The number of jobs in all types of medical settings will continue to increase for SLPs, partly because of the growing elderly population's susceptibility to strokes. Also, because of the number of premature (i.e., under 5 pounds [2.7 kg]) and micropremature infants (i.e., under 2 pounds [.91 kg]) surviving, there will be increased needs for our services throughout much of their early development and education. As health care professionals and the public become more aware of the importance of identifying and diagnosing speech, language, and hearing problems, SLPs in clinics, home health care, and private practice are expected to see increasing needs for their services.

Anticipated growth in elementary, secondary, and special education enrollments, as well as other federally mandated services, has created more employment opportunities for speech-language pathologists in schools. There will continue to be a long-term shortage of speech-language pathologists in inner cities, rural, and less densely populated areas. Overall, speech-language pathologists will continue to be in great demand in many work settings and most communities in the United States and many other countries. Having a job you enjoy should never be a problem.

Audiologists

Audiologists are professionals who, "by virtue of academic degree, clinical training, and license to practice and/or professional credential, are uniquely qualified to provide a comprehensive array of professional services related to . . . the audiologic identification, assessment, diagnosis, and treatment of persons with impairments of auditory and vestibular function, and to the prevention of impairments associated with them" (American Academy of Audiology, 2004).

ASHA, in conjunction with the *American Academy of Audiology* (AAA), determines the education, coursework, and clinical training of audiologists. Audiologists must earn either a Ph.D. or Au.D., complete a clinical fellowship in audiology, and pass the national (ASHA) examination in audiology. Audiologists need to be licensed, credentialed, or both in their state of employment and must earn CEUs. In some states, in order for audiologists to work with and dispense hearing aids, they must also become licensed hearing instrument specialists.

Scope of Practice

Audiologists evaluate an individual's hearing loss to determine the type and extent of the loss. They further assess the benefits of amplification (e.g., hearing aids) and habilitation or rehabilitation to maximize the person's hearing ability. Many audiologists are able to sell and dispense hearing aids or other amplification devices as part of their practice. Most states have enacted legislation requiring universal screening of newborn infants, which has become an important new area of practice for audiologists. Another area of practice for some audiologists involves testing for balance disorders that may be associated with inner ear problems. As with speech-language pathologists, the scope of practice of audiologists is expanding.

Work Settings

Audiologists work in a variety of settings, including public schools, hospitals, clinics, private practices, and industry. Some audiologists also function as consultants to various agencies and help determine appropriate hearing conservation and protection requirements for state and local government employees, as well as industry standards. Some audiologists work in two or more settings in any one week—for example, private practice, industry, and consulting. Audiologists also teach and supervise in university programs. Even when a university does not offer an audiology program, an audiologist still must provide the basic coursework and training in audiology and aural rehabilitation for the speech-language pathology majors. Figure 2–5 shows the primary employment settings of audiologists in 2010.

Employment Outlook

The 2010 *Occupational Outlook Handbook* from the U.S. Department of Labor's Bureau of Labor Statistics reported that the job outlook is good for audiologists, projecting that between 2010 and 2018 there will be approximately a 25% increase in the need for audiologists. The number of jobs in all types of medical settings will continue to increase for audiologists, partly because of the growing elderly population susceptible to hearing losses. On the other end of the age spectrum, micropremature infants (weight less than 1 pound, 12 ounces [800 grams]) tend to have increased needs for audiological services throughout much of their early

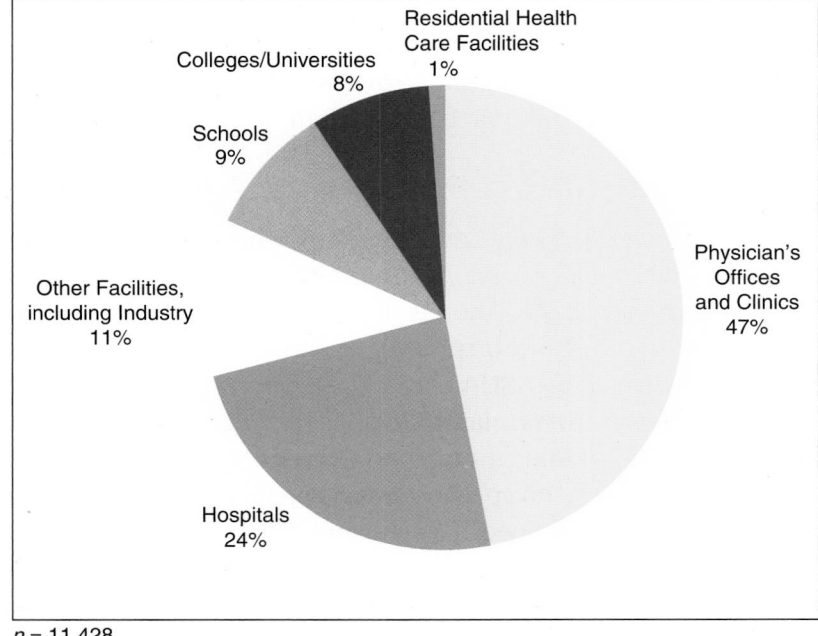

n = 11,428

Figure 2–5

ASHA-certified audiologists by primary employment setting.

Source: ASHA Summary Membership and Affiliation Counts, year ending 2010.

development and education. As health care professionals and the public become more aware of the importance of protecting hearing, identifying and diagnosing hearing problems, and wearing hearing aids as willingly as most people wear contact lenses or eyeglasses, audiologists are expected to see increasing needs for their services.

Audiologists also expect to see employment opportunities in schools grow if enrollment increases in elementary, secondary, and special education classes. The long-term shortage of audiologists in inner cities and less densely populated areas, including rural communities, is likely to continue. Overall, audiologists are and will be needed in many work settings and most communities worldwide.

Speech, Language, and Hearing Scientists

Speech, language, and hearing scientists are a relatively small portion of the professions (less than 5%). They have doctorates and mostly work in universities but also in government agencies, research centers, laboratories, or industry. Some also provide clinical services in either speech-language pathology or audiology. Depending on their specialty (speech, language, or hearing), these scientists usually are involved with *basic research*—that is, investigating the anatomy and physiology of the speech and hearing mechanisms, the physics and acoustics of speech-sound production, or the acquisition and structure of language. In many cases, they generate grants to carry on their research.

Speech, language, and hearing scientists are the skeletal framework of speech-language pathology and audiology because without them the normative data would not be available for clinicians to compare the normal with the abnormal or to understand the scientific rationales for many clinical procedures. The research data collected by scientists are essential to those who provide direct services to clients and patients of all ages. A firm grounding in normal communication processes through courses such as anatomy and physiology, speech science, and hearing science provides the foundation from which clinicians can better understand, diagnose, and treat communication disorders and delays.

Speech-Language Pathology Assistants

speech-language pathology assistant (SLPA)

A support person who performs tasks as prescribed, directed, and supervised by ASHA certified SLPs.

For individuals who do not want to or cannot pursue a B.A. and M.A. in speech-language pathology, ASHA established **speech-language pathology assistants (SLPAs)** as support personnel who, following academic and/or on-the-job training, perform tasks prescribed, directed, and supervised by ASHA certified speech-language pathologists. Individuals may earn an Associate of Arts degree (AA) in speech-language pathology assistant training programs. According to ASHA guidelines and state licensure laws, no speech-language pathologist can employ an SLPA without a certified speech-language pathologist as a supervisor. SLPAs are more commonly employed in school-based programs than in medical settings or clinics. ASHA is the credentialing body that offers a national registration process to ensure basic knowledge and competencies are developed for those wanting to become SLPAs. Many SLPAs eventually choose to pursue a B.A. and M.A. to become state licensed and ASHA certified speech-language pathologists (Moore & Pearson, 2003).

The following is a list of SLPA responsibilities taken from Background Information and Criteria for the Registration of Speech-Language Pathology Assistants (ASHA, October, 2000).

- Assist the SLP with speech-language and hearing screenings (without interpretation).
- Follow documented treatment plans or protocols developed by the supervising SLP.
- Document patient/client performance (e.g., tally data for the SLP to use; prepare charts, records, and graphs) and report this information to the supervising SLP.
- Assist the SLP during assessment of patients/clients.
- Assist with informal documentation as directed by the SLP.
- Assist with duties such as preparing materials and scheduling activities as directed by the SLP.
- Collect data for quality improvement.
- Perform checks and maintenance of equipment.
- Support the SLP in research projects, in-service trainings, and public relations programs.
- Assist with departmental operations (e.g., scheduling, record keeping).
- Exhibit compliance with regulations, reimbursement requirements, and other responsibilities associated with the assistant position.

Audiology Assistants

The American Academy of Audiology has defined the functions of audiology assistants (AAA, 2006).

> An audiology assistant is a person who, after appropriate training and demonstration of competence, performs delegated duties and responsibilities that are directed and supervised by an audiologist. The role of the assistant is to support the audiologist in performing routine tasks and duties so that the audiologist is available for the more complex evaluative, diagnostic, management and treatment services that require the education and training of a licensed audiologist (p. 5).

The duties of an audiology assistant may include equipment maintenance, hearing aid repair, neonatal screening, preparation of patients for electrophysiologic and balance testing, hearing conservation, air-conduction hearing evaluation, assisting the audiologist in testing, record keeping, clinical research, and other tasks after full and complete training and delineation by the supervising audiologist.

The minimal educational background for an audiology assistant is a high school diploma or equivalent, and competency-based training.

Some community colleges and online training programs offer an Associate Degree in Audiology for training of audiology assistants. However, the state licensed audiologist who employs and supervises an assistant must assure that the assistant can perform all duties and responsibilities that are delegated (AAA, 2010).

CHAPTER SUMMARY

You have begun learning about the professions and professionals of speech-language pathology and audiology, and you are in good company. Most countries with speech-language pathologists and audiologists have strong national organizations that help support and regulate the professions. There are excellent job opportunities throughout the United States and in many other countries for both professions. The people who study and work in these professions are interesting and caring people who enjoy helping others. These professionals are team players who interact regularly with colleagues, as well as many other professionals.

STUDY QUESTIONS

Knowledge and Comprehension

1. By helping a child with a communication delay or impairment, whom in the child's life are you also helping?

2. By helping an adult with a communication impairment, whom in the adult's life are you also helping?

3. Why is it important, as students and professionals, to use person-first language?

4. What is the "team approach" and why is it important in the work of speech-language pathologists and audiologists?

5. What is the American Speech-Language-Hearing Association (ASHA)?

6. What is the National Student Speech-Language-Hearing Association (NSSLHA)?

Application

1. Discuss how you might use some of the information you learn in this text and course in your personal life, even if you do not become a speech-language pathologist or audiologist.

2. What are three qualities of effective professionals? How could you apply these to your personal life?

3. How are public laws affecting the work of speech-language pathologists and audiologists?

4. What are some specific things you could do to keep yourself abreast of new developments in the profession?

Analysis/Synthesis

1. What are the similarities and differences between speech-language pathologists and audiologists?

2. Why is it important for a professional organization (e.g., ASHA) to specify the education, coursework, and training of individuals entering a profession?

3. Why might speech-language pathologists be referred to by different titles, depending on the setting in which they work?

REFERENCES

Aiken, T. D. (2008). *Legal and ethical issues in health occupations.* Philadelphia, PA: W. B. Saunders.

American Academy of Audiology. (2004). Audiology: Scope of practice. *Audiology Today, 16*(3), 44–45.

American Academy of Audiology. (2006). Position statement on audiologist's assistants. *Audiology Today, 18*(2), 27–28.

American Academy of Audiology. (2010). Audiology assistant task force report. *Audiology Today, 22*(3), 68–73.

ASHA. (2000). Background information and criteria for the registration of speech-language pathology assistants. Rockville, MD: ASHA.

Bureau of Labor Statistics. (2010). *Occupational outlook handbook, 2004–2005 edition.* Washington, DC: U.S. Department of Labor.

Flasher, L. V., & Fogle, P. T. (2012). *Counseling skills for speech-language pathologists and audiologists* (2nd ed.). Clifton Park, NY: Delmar Cengage Learning.

Fogle, P. T. (2001). Professors in private practice: Rediscovering the joy of therapy. *Advance for Speech-Language Pathologists & Audiologists,* 18–19.

Lubinski, R., Golper, L. A. C., & Frattali, C. (2007). *Professional issues in speech-language pathology and audiology* (3rd ed.). Clifton Park, NY: Delmar Cengage Learning.

Miller, T. D. (2007). Professional ethics. In R. Lubinski, L. Golper, & C. Frattali (Eds.). *Professional issues in speech-language pathology and audiology* (3rd ed.). Clifton Park, NY: Delmar Cengage Learning.

Moeller, D. (1975). *Speech pathology & audiology: Iowa origins of a discipline.* Iowa City, IA: The University of Iowa Press.

Moore, S. M., & Pearson, L. D. (2003). *Competencies and strategies for speech-language pathology assistants.* Clifton Park, NY: Delmar Cengage Learning.

NSSLHA. (2010). *Communication sciences: Student survival guide.* Clifton Park, NY: Delmar Cengage Learning.

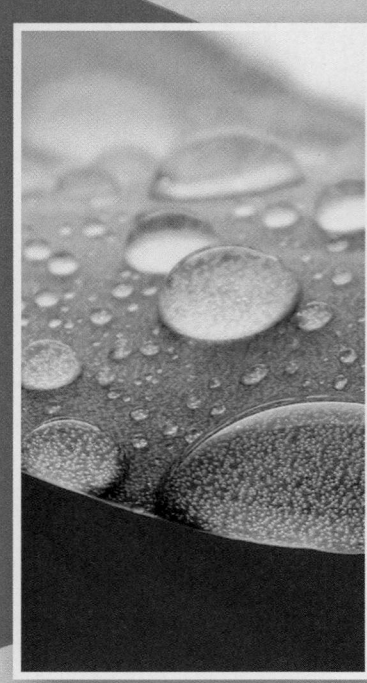

CHAPTER 3
Anatomy and Physiology of Speech and Language

LEARNING OBJECTIVES

After studying this chapter, you will:

- Understand the essentials of the anatomy and physiology of respiration.
- Be able to discuss the contributions of the respiratory system to the production of speech.
- Understand the essentials of the anatomy and physiology of phonation.
- Be able to discuss the contributions of the phonatory system to the production of speech.
- Understand the essentials of the anatomy and physiology of resonation.
- Be able to discuss the contributions of the resonatory system to the production of speech.
- Understand the essentials of the anatomy and physiology of articulation.
- Be able to discuss the contributions of the articulatory system to the production of speech.
- Understand the essentials of the anatomy and physiology of the nervous system.
- Be able to discuss the contributions of the nervous system to speech, language, and cognition.

KEY TERMS

abduct	arytenoid cartilages	brainstem
adduct	auditory	Broca's area
alveolar ridge	comprehension	cartilage
alveolar sacs	axon	central nervous
anoxia	Bernoulli's law	system

KEY TERMS continued

cerebellum
cerebral hemisphere
cortex
cricoid cartilage
decibels (dB)
deciduous teeth
deglutition
dendrite
dentition
diaphragm
epiglottis
executive functions
expiration
   (exhalation)
false vocal folds
   (ventricular folds)
formulate
frequency
hard palate
hertz (Hz)
incisors
inspiration

integrate
intensity
intonation
labia
larynx
malocclusion
mandible
mastication
maxilla
motor
myofunctional
   therapy
neuron
occlusion
open bite
orbicularis oris
peripheral nervous
   system
phonation
process
produce
protrude

range of motion
reflex
resonance
respiration
retract
sensory
soft palate
   (velum)
spinal cord
synapse
thoracic cavity
thyroid cartilage
tongue (lingua,
   glossus)
trachea
true vocal folds
uvula
velopharyngeal
   closure
voice quality

CHAPTER OUTLINE

Introduction
The Respiratory System
   Structures of Respiration
   Muscles of Respiration
   The Respiratory Process
The Phonatory System
   Framework of the Larynx
   The Vocal Folds
The Resonatory System
   Embryological Development of the Upper Lip and Palates
   Hard and Soft Palates
The Articulatory System
   The Skeletal Structures of Articulation
   Facial Muscles
   Tongue
   Dentition
The Nervous System
   The Central Nervous System
   Peripheral Nervous System
Chapter Summary
Study Questions
References

INTRODUCTION

Therapy to improve speech usually focuses on helping children and adults do something different with their articulators (mandible, lips, and tongue) to be more intelligible to their listeners or to have smoother, more fluent speech. However, clinicians need to know and understand the anatomy and physiology of each of the speech systems (respiratory, phonatory, resonatory, and articulatory) and the nervous system to evaluate and treat clients with all types of communication disorders. The foundations of speech are the *anatomy* (structures) and *physiology* (functions and movements) of each of the speech systems. Before any muscle contracts or relaxes in order for each speech system to perform with near perfect timing, the brain must actively decide what will be communicated and how. Most of the processes involved with producing speech are never consciously thought about until we make a speech error or have a communication disorder. Clinicians need to be aware of each speech system (and sometimes specific muscle groups) when working with clients and patients in order to help them make subtle changes so they can better communicate their messages.

THE RESPIRATORY SYSTEM

Other than the beating of our heart, our respiratory system works harder than any other organ in our body. Every minute while sitting quietly, we breathe (one inhalation and one exhalation) about 15 times, or about once every 4 seconds. In 1 hour we breathe about 900 times and in 1 day we breathe more than 20,000 times. To **produce** voice (**phonation**) and speech, humans have learned to control **respiration** by taking quick, short **inspirations (inhalations)** and sustaining the **expirations (exhalations)**. An intricate and interdependent balance exists between respiration and phonation. The first demand of the respiratory system is to supply freshly oxygenated blood to every cell in our bodies and to rid our bodies of the carbon dioxide (CO_2) that is produced when we use up the oxygen (O_2). Producing voice is an *overlaid function* (i.e., not necessary to sustain life) of the respiratory system.

Structures of Respiration

The bones in the chest (*rib cage* and *sternum/breastbone*) provide protection and a framework for the respiratory system. The **thoracic cavity (thorax)** is the upper part of the trunk that contains the principle

produce/production

In speech, to create an utterance (sound, syllable, word, sentence, or longer) that is spontaneous or imitated.

phonation (voice)

The vibration of air passing between the two vocal folds that produces sound that is used for speech.

respiration (ventilation, pulmonary ventilation, breathing)

The movement of air into and out of the lungs that allows for the exchange of oxygen and carbon dioxide.

inspiration (inhalation)

The process of drawing air into the lungs.

expiration (exhalation)

The process of breathing air out of the lungs.

thoracic cavity (thorax, rib cage, chest)

The upper part of the trunk that contains the organs of respiration (lungs) and circulation (heart).

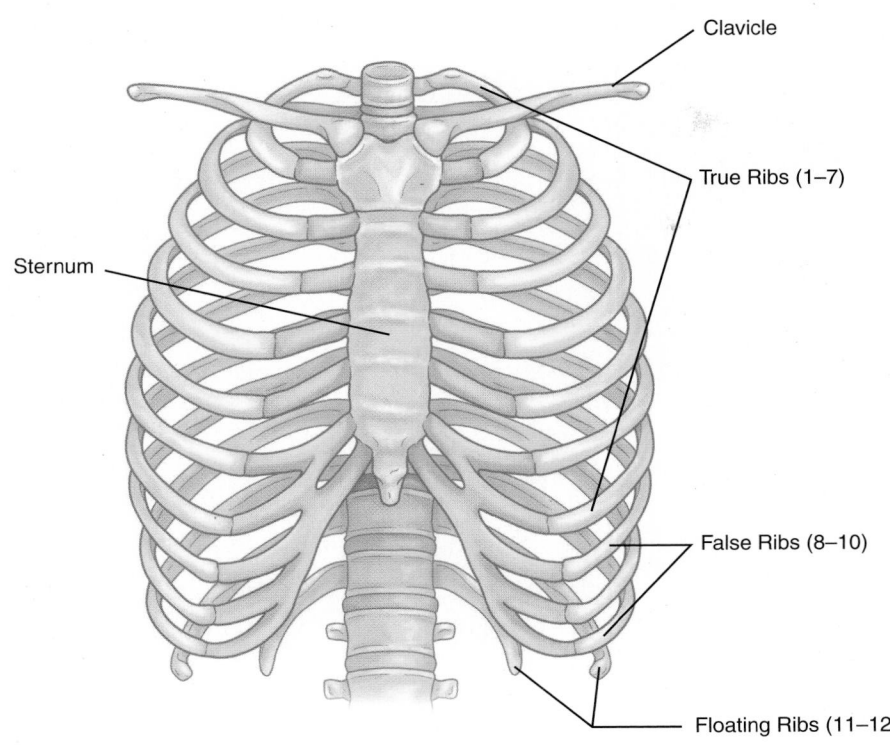

Clavicle

True Ribs (1–7)

Sternum

False Ribs (8–10)

Floating Ribs (11–12)

Figure 3–1

Anterior view of the skeletal framework for respiration.

© Cengage Learning 2013.

organs of respiration (lungs) and circulation (heart). The thorax extends from the *clavicle* (collarbone) and first rib down to the twelfth rib. The ribs attach to the sternum in the center of the chest and the *vertebral (spinal) column* is in the back. The bones of the thoracic cavity (plus the *pelvis*) provide attachments for the many muscles involved in respiration (see Figure 3–1).

During quiet breathing, inspired air enters through the nostrils and flows into the nose and *nasal cavities,* where it is warmed, moistened, and filtered. From the nasal cavities, the air passes through the *larynx* and flows past the open *vocal folds*. The **trachea**, or "windpipe," begins just below the larynx and continues down to where it divides into the lungs. The trachea is a tube about 4 to 5 inches (10 to 13 cm) long and 1 inch (2.5 cm) in diameter and is formed by about 20 rings made of **cartilage** (see Figure 3–2). The bottom of the trachea divides into the *mainstream (primary) bronchi,* which enter into the left and right lungs. The bronchi continue to divide into smaller diameter branches and extend out much like the branches of a tree.

Muscles of Respiration

Twenty-six pairs of muscles are involved in the processes of inspiration and expiration. Most are used during quiet breathing, and additional muscles are used during forced inspiration or expiration. We will only discuss some of the most important muscles involved in respiration.

trachea (windpipe)

The tube that begins just below the larynx and continues down to where it divides into the lungs; carries air down to and up from the lungs.

cartilage

Firm, fibrous, and strong connective tissue that does not contain blood vessels.

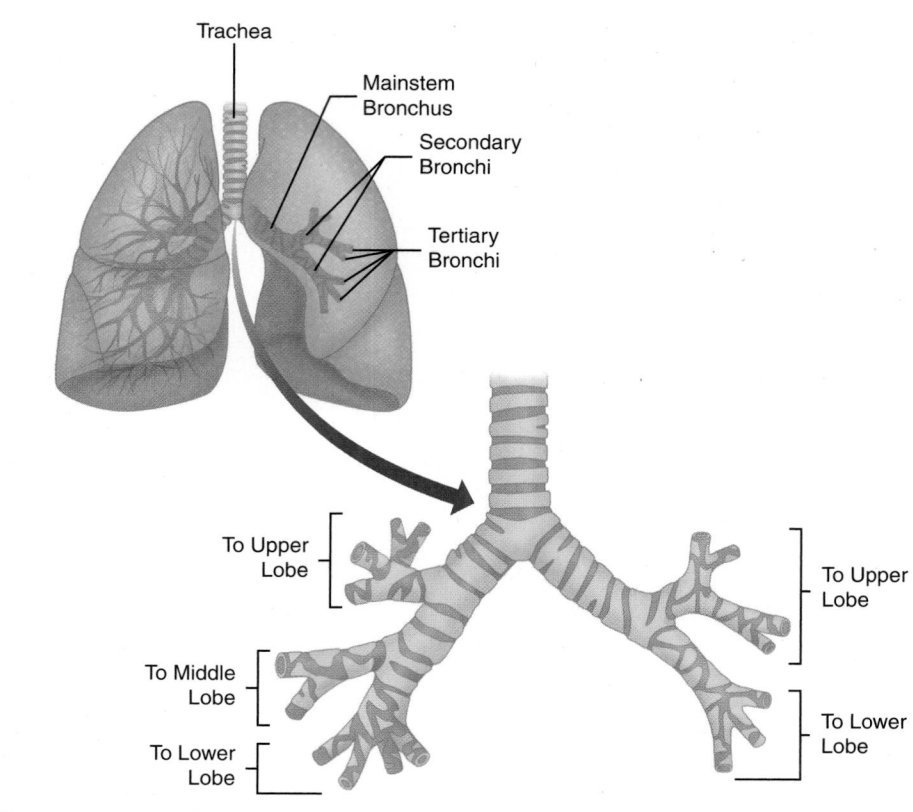

Trachea

Mainstem
Bronchus

Secondary
Bronchi

Tertiary
Bronchi

To Upper
Lobe

To Upper
Lobe

To Middle
Lobe

To Lower
Lobe

To Lower
Lobe

Figure 3-2

Trachea and bronchial tree.

© Cengage Learning 2013.

diaphragm

A large, dome-shaped muscle that separates the thoracic and abdominal cavities and is the main muscle of respiration; during inspiration it moves down to increase the volume in the thoracic cavity, and during expiration it moves up to decrease the volume.

alveolar sacs (alveoli, air sacs)

The spongy tissue of the lungs where gas exchange takes place; walls of alveoli are one cell thick and porous, allowing rapid transfer of fresh O_2 into the capillary bed surrounding the alveoli, and of CO_2 from the capillary bed into the alveoli to be exhaled.

The **diaphragm** is the primary muscle involved with respiration. It is a large, dome-shaped muscle that separates the thoracic and abdominal cavities. During inspiration, it moves down and increases the volume in the thoracic cavity; during expiration, it moves up and decreases the volume. In the thoracic cavity, the volume changes affect the air pressures, which allow air to passively or actively flow into or out of the lungs (see Figure 3–3). Between each rib are muscles that help raise and lower the ribcage during inspiration and expiration (the muscles you eat when eating pork spare ribs). The muscles over the stomach are important in *forced exhalation* when we pull in our stomachs to try to blow out air. When these muscles are well developed they are sometimes called "six-pack abs."

The Respiratory Process

During a single, quiet respiratory cycle, several neurological and physiological processes are occurring. The respiratory center in the brainstem sends messages to the muscles we use for inhalation. The diaphragm contracts and lowers, and the rib cage slightly raises and expands. The volume (space) inside the thoracic cavity increases, which decreases the air pressure inside the lungs. The difference in air pressure between the environmental air and the pressure in the lungs causes air from the outside to flow through the nose, down the trachea, and into the lungs to equalize the pressure (inhalation). The millions of **alveolar sacs** (similar to the holes in a sponge) that make up the lungs are expanded

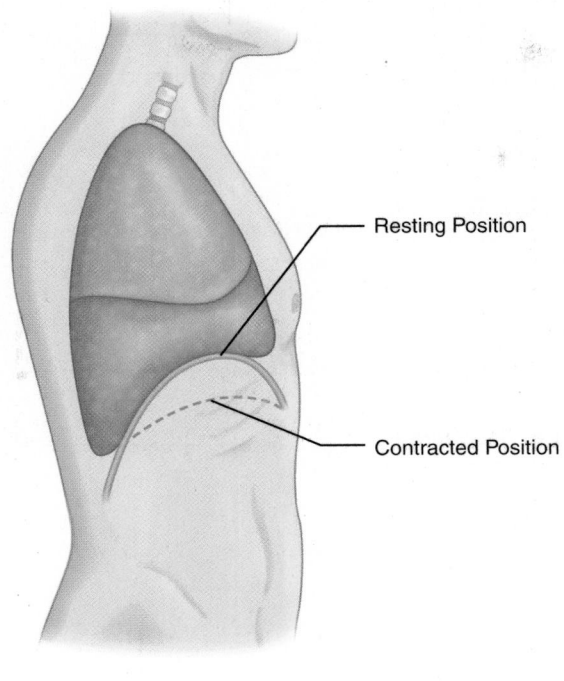

Resting Position

Contracted Position

LATERAL VIEW

Figure 3-3

Lateral-view schematic of the diaphragm showing relative positions during quiet (passive) inspiration and expiration.

© Cengage Learning 2013.

and stretched slightly (much like a balloon that is blown up part way). Because the alveolar sacs cannot remain in a stretched position for long, they begin to relax (deflate), which forces the air back out of the lungs and up the trachea. At the same time, the expanded chest relaxes down, creating more *intrathoracic air pressure* and contributing to the air being forced out of the lungs (exhalation) (Seikel, King, & Drumright, 2010).

THE PHONATORY SYSTEM

The voice is probably one of the speech systems that we most take for granted. The anatomy and physiology of the **larynx** (voice box) are both simple and complex. The simplicity of the anatomy is that the individual structures of the larynx are basically stacked on top of one another; the complexity is that each structure can move in various subtle ways that can alter the loudness, pitch, and quality of the voice. The simplicity of the physiology of the larynx is that the various muscles both inside and outside the larynx can only contract and relax; the complexity is that the precise combinations and amounts of muscle contraction and relaxation can provide the beautiful, pure sounds of opera singers or the grating, strident voices of some people.

Framework of the Larynx

The larynx is located between the top of the trachea and just below the horseshoe-shaped *hyoid bone* that helps support it. Several cartilages make up the larynx, including (1) the circular shaped **cricoid cartilage**

larynx (pl. larynges) (voice box)

Located just above the trachea, the structure that contains cartilages, muscles, and membranes that produce voice by air passing between the vocal folds.

cricoid cartilage

A solid circle of *cartilage* (nonvascular dense supporting connective tissue) shaped like a signet (class) ring located below and behind the thyroid cartilage and on top of the first tracheal ring.

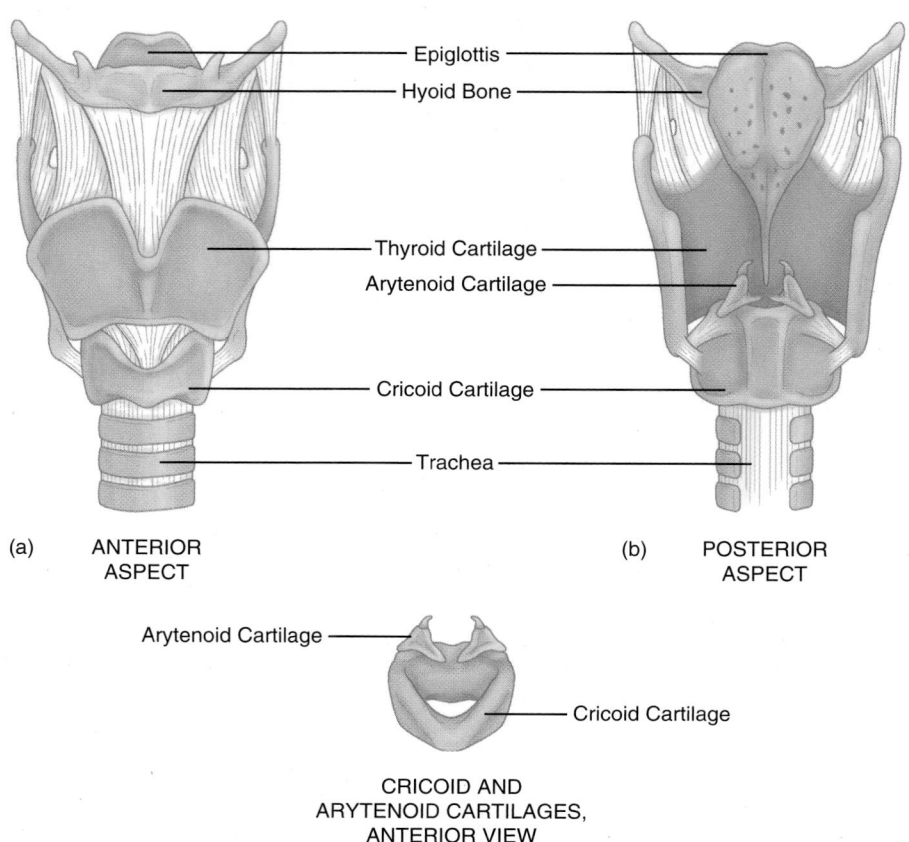

Epiglottis
Hyoid Bone

Thyroid Cartilage
Arytenoid Cartilage

Cricoid Cartilage

Trachea

(a)   ANTERIOR
        ASPECT

(b)   POSTERIOR
        ASPECT

Arytenoid Cartilage

Cricoid Cartilage

CRICOID AND
ARYTENOID CARTILAGES,
ANTERIOR VIEW

Figure 3–4

(a) Anterior and
(b) posterior views
of the larynx.

© Cengage Learning 2013.

thyroid cartilage

The largest of the *laryngeal cartilages* that is the main structure of the larynx and encloses and protects the vocal folds; its *anterior* (front) point is popularly referred to as the "Adam's apple."

arytenoid cartilages

A pair of pyramid-shaped cartilages that sit on top of the posterior edge of the cricoid cartilage and rotate to open and close the vocal folds and pivot back and forth to help change the pitch of the voice.

epiglottis

A large cartilage that is wide at the top and narrow at the bottom that is attached to the anterior edge of the cricoid cartilage and drops over the vocal folds like a lid to prevent food and liquid from entering the trachea and lungs when swallowing.

that sits on top of the first tracheal ring and is below and behind the thyroid cartilage; (2) the large **thyroid cartilage** that is the main structure of the larynx and encloses and protects the vocal folds (its *anterior* [front] point is popularly referred to as the "Adam's apple" [*laryngeal prominence*]); (3) the two pyramid shaped **arytenoid cartilages** that sit on top of the *posterior* (back) portion of the cricoid cartilage and rotate to open and close the vocal folds and pivot back and forth to help change the pitch of the voice; and (4) the **epiglottis**, a large cartilage that is wide at the top and narrow at the bottom (like a leaf or egg that comes to a sharp point) that has an important role protecting the airway during swallowing (see Figure 3–4).

The Vocal Folds

Two pairs of vocal folds, the **true vocal folds** and the **false vocal folds** (**ventricular folds**), stretch across the airway. When talking about the *vocal folds* we are referring to the true vocal folds unless we specifically say *false (ventricular) vocal folds*. (Note: SLPs prefer the term "vocal folds" over "vocal cords" because they are two folds of tissue with attachments on the sides of the thyroid cartilage rather than two "cords" [thick strings] with attachments at either end, although the term *cord* is acceptable in some medical literature.) The true vocal folds are muscles covered with mucous membranes that make them look pearly white (see Figure 3–5).

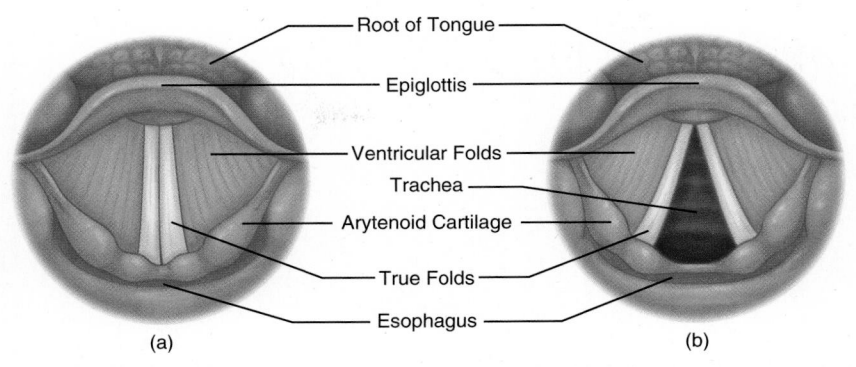

Root of Tongue

Epiglottis

Ventricular Folds

Trachea

Arytenoid Cartilage

True Folds

Esophagus

(a)   (b)

Figure 3-5

Superior view of the vocal folds (a) closed and (b) open.

© Cengage Learning 2013.

The biological function of the vocal folds is to prevent food and liquid from entering the trachea and lungs, and their overlaid function is to produce voice. Each vocal fold is composed of two joined muscles that are covered by a *mucous membrane* (membrane that protects a structure, secretes mucus, and absorbs water, salts, and other materials).

The vocal folds lie in the midline at the level of the laryngeal prominence. When looking down upon the true vocal folds, they have a V shape when open, with the upper point of the V facing anteriorly and the two lower points attaching to the two arytenoid cartilages posteriorly. The space between the open vocal folds is referred to as the *glottis*. Because the trachea below the vocal folds is circular, the shape and position of the vocal folds create a constriction for air passing into or out of the larynx. The false vocal folds lie slightly superior to the true vocal folds inside the thyroid cartilage and are composed of thick mucous membranes with few muscle fibers. They do not vibrate during speech but close tightly during swallowing to prevent material from entering the trachea.

Vocal Fold Vibration

During normal breathing the vocal folds are at rest and partially open (**abducted**), but when we want to phonate the vocal folds must close (**adduct**). (Note: *Abduct* is usually pronounced "A-B-duct," with the "A" and "B" pronounced as the first two letters of the alphabet to prevent confusion between the similar sounding *adduct* and *abduct*.) To produce voice, the vocal folds are told by the brain to close and simultaneously the respiratory system is sent a message to exhale air. As the air coming up the trachea reaches the closed vocal folds *subglottic air pressure* (air pressure below the vocal folds) builds up and blows the vocal folds open in the shape of a football or rugby ball with both the anterior and the posterior points closed. However, because the vocal folds have been told by the brain to stay closed, their elasticity, along with **Bernoulli's law** (a law of physics involving airflow and air pressure) causes them to instantaneously close again, which causes subglottic air pressure to build and then blow them open again. One complete open-close (abduct-adduct) sequence is referred to as a complete *vibratory cycle*. Every time the open phase occurs in the vibratory cycle, a small "puff" of air escapes and travels up to our mouths to be articulated.

true vocal folds

Paired muscles (thyroarytenoid and vocalis) covered with mucous membranes with a pearly white appearance inside the thyroid cartilage at the level of the Adam's apple that open and close extremely rapidly to produce voice; closure during swallowing protects the trachea and lungs from penetration of food and liquid.

false vocal folds

Paired, thick folds of mucous membranes with few muscle fibers that lie just above the true vocal folds in the larynx at the level of the laryngeal prominence (*Adam's apple*); they do not vibrate during speech but close tightly during swallowing to prevent material from entering the trachea.

abduct/abduction

The opening of the vocal folds away from the midline.

adduct/adduction

The closing of the vocal folds toward the midline.

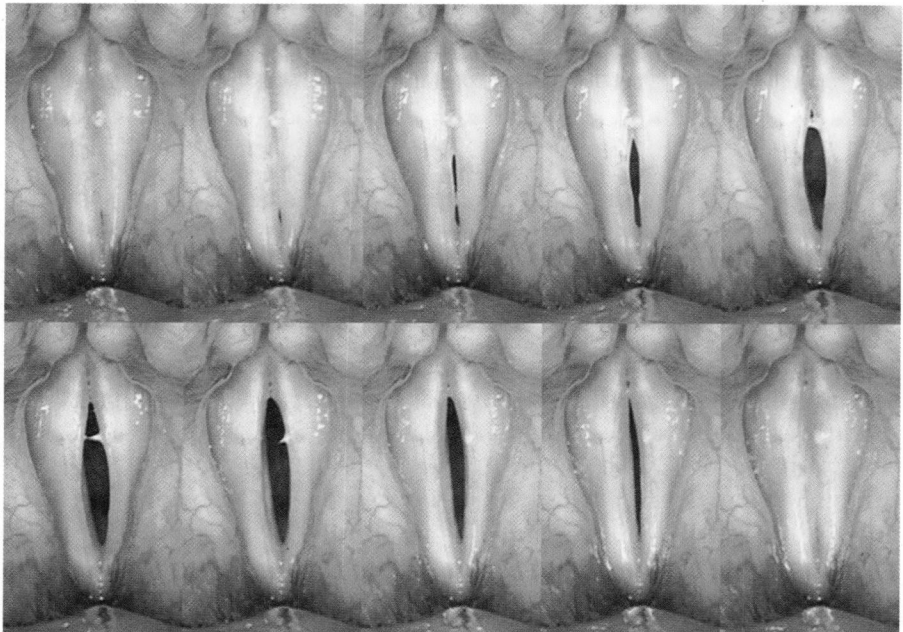

Courtesy of KayPENTAX, Montvale, NJ.

Figure 3-6

Stroboscopic film images of the vocal folds during one complete vibratory cycle.

Bernoulli's law (principle)

A law in physics that states when air flowing through a tube (e.g., trachea) reaches a constriction (e.g., vocal folds) there is an increase in speed of the flow of air that causes decreased pressure on the walls of the constriction that results in a slight negative pressure (i.e., slight vacuum) at the constriction; in voice, this slight negative pressure contributes to the vocal folds closing during vibration; (Daniel Bernoulli, Swiss scientist, 1700–1782).

frequency

In speech, the number of complete cycles (opening, closing) per second that the vocal folds vibrate; *pitch* is the psychological perception of frequency.

hertz (Hz)

The unit of vibration adopted internationally to replace cycles *per second* (CPS).

It is the extremely rapid puffs of air that escape that we perceive as voice (Hixon, Weismer, & Hoit, 2008) (see Figure 3-6).

Frequency, Intensity, and Quality of Voice

Frequency is the number of complete cycles (opening, closing) per second that the vocal folds vibrate per second. *Pitch* is the psychological perception (sensation) of frequency. Frequency is measured in **hertz (Hz)** and a frequency of 100 complete cycles per second (opening-closing) of the vocal folds would be 100 Hz. The rate at which the vocal folds vibrate during normal voicing of the "ah" sound is a person's *fundamental frequency* (f_0). Adult males typically have a fundamental frequency of about 120 Hz and adult females have a fundamental frequency of about 220 Hz.

Intensity, in reference to voice, is the force with which the vocal folds open and close and the amount of air that escapes between the open vocal folds (the puffs of air). *Loudness* is the psychological perception of intensity. Intensity is measured in **decibels (dB)**. A person's average intensity level is related to how loud other people perceive the person (some people are perceived as loud talkers and others as soft spoken). During normal conversation, we use subtle interactions of loudness, pitch, and duration of sounds to give our speech **intonation** (i.e., some variability, "vitality" or "life").

The auditory perceptual judgments of **voice quality** are highly subjective. Generally voice quality is affected by adequate vocal fold closure, efficient timing of closure, and the amount of muscle tone of the folds. Normal voice quality is difficult to describe and may be described more easily by saying what it is *not* rather than what it is. Nicolosi, Harryman, and Kresheck (2004) describe normal voice quality as nontense, nonbreathy, not having extraneous noise, and being easily produced and sustained throughout phonation. However, the voice that is produced at the level of the vocal folds is actually a rather raucous buzzing sound, somewhat like hearing the mouth piece of a saxophone being blown without the rest of the horn to alter the vibration of the reed by adding resonance.

THE RESONATORY SYSTEM

The structures important for normal speech and **resonance** are the facial structures, the articulators, the hard and soft palates, and the pharyngeal region. The anatomy and physiology of these may affect speech intelligibility. When anatomy is abnormal the secondary effect is abnormal physiology. However, it is possible to have intact structures and still have abnormal function resulting in disorders of resonance (e.g., when there is weakness in the muscles of the soft palate).

Embryological Development of the Upper Lip and Palates

The first trimester of pregnancy is crucial in facial and palatal development, with the lips and hard and soft palates forming. The upper and lower lips have formed by 8 weeks gestation and the shape of the upper lip is typically referred to as the "cupid's bow" (see Figure 3–7). Between the 8th and 12th weeks of gestation, the hard and soft palates of the roof of the mouth are formed and fused together, with the fusion occurring in an anterior to posterior direction (see Figure 3–8). We need to keep in mind how very small each of these structures is during the embryological development and the numerous potential influences that may interfere with normal facial and palatal development.

Hard and Soft Palates

The **maxilla** (upper jaw) contains the **hard palate**, which is a thin, bony, shelf-like structure that is covered by mucous tissue and separates the

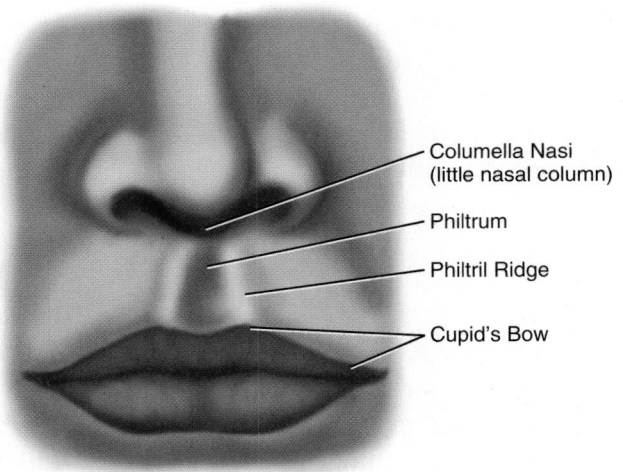

Columella Nasi
(little nasal column)

Philtrum

Philtril Ridge

Cupid's Bow

Figure 3–7

Landmarks of the lips.

© Cengage Learning 2013.

intensity

In reference to voice, the force with which the vocal folds open and close and the amount of air that escapes between the open vocal folds; *loudness* is the psychological perception of intensity.

decibels (dB)

A basic unit of measure of the intensity of sound; it is one-tenth of 1 bel (B); an increase in 1 bel is perceived as a 10-fold increase in loudness.

intonation

Variations in pitch on syllables, words, and phrases that produce *stress* to give emphasis and meaning to utterances.

voice quality

The auditory aspects of the function of the vocal folds that is affected by adequate closure, efficient timing of closure, and the amount of muscle tone of the vocal folds; normal voice quality is a described as nontense, no extraneous noise, nonbreathy, and easily produced and sustained throughout phonation.

resonance

The quality of the voice that results from the vibration of sound in the vocal tract (i.e., spaces and tissues of the pharynx, oral cavity, and nasal cavity).

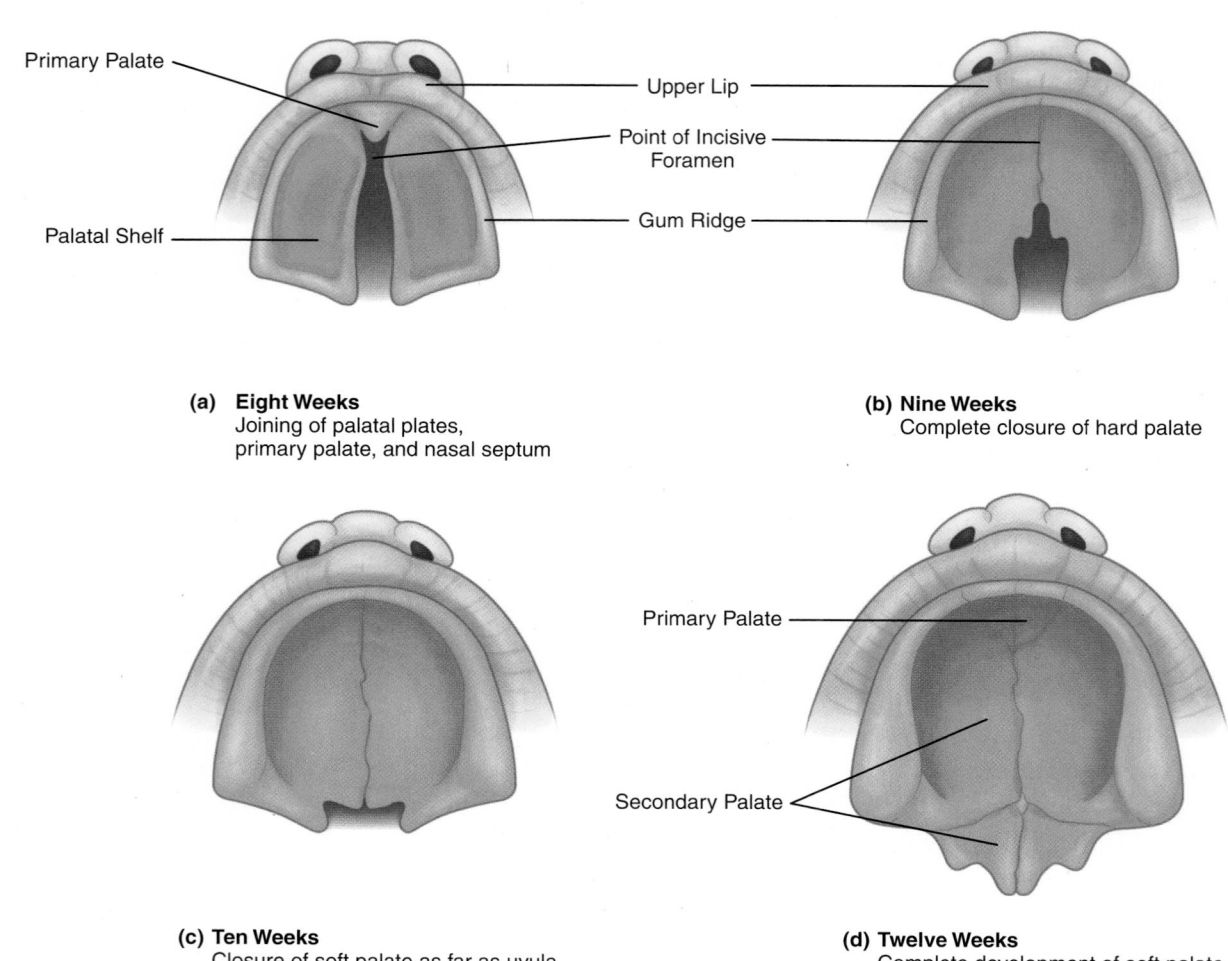

(a) **Eight Weeks**
Joining of palatal plates,
primary palate, and nasal septum

(b) **Nine Weeks**
Complete closure of hard palate

(c) **Ten Weeks**
Closure of soft palate as far as uvula

(d) **Twelve Weeks**
Complete development of soft palate

Figure 3-8

Development of the hard and soft palates looking up toward the roof of the mouth.

© Cengage Learning 2013.

maxilla

The upper jaw that includes the hard palate and contains sockets for the upper teeth; forms much of the midfacial structure.

hard palate

The bony anterior two-thirds of the roof of the mouth that separate the oral cavity from the nasal cavity.

alveolar ridge (alveolar process, dental arch)

The upper portion of the mandible and the lower portion of the maxilla that contain sockets for the roots of the teeth.

oral cavity from the *nasal cavity* (see Figure 3–9). The hard palate is the anterior two-thirds of the roof of the mouth. The ridge surrounding the hard palate on three sides is referred to as the **alveolar ridge**, which is covered by the "gums" (*gingiva*). The anterior portion of the hard palate is the *premaxilla*, which holds the four front teeth. The rest of the hard palate is composed of the *maxillary* and *palatine bones* (two on each side of the midline). Down the center of the hard palate a slight ridge can be felt with the tip of the tongue, which is where the two halves of the hard palate have fused together during the first trimester of gestation. However, wherever there is supposed to be a fusion there is the possibility that fusion may not occur, which can result in a cleft. The hard palate provides points of contact for tongue placement to produce several sounds (e.g., the tongue tip makes contact with the alveolar ridge just behind the top front teeth to produce a /t/ or /d/). The posterior border of the hard palate is the location of the beginning of the **soft palate (velum)**.

The soft palate is the muscular structure that forms the posterior one-third of the roof of the mouth. At the posterior end of the soft palate

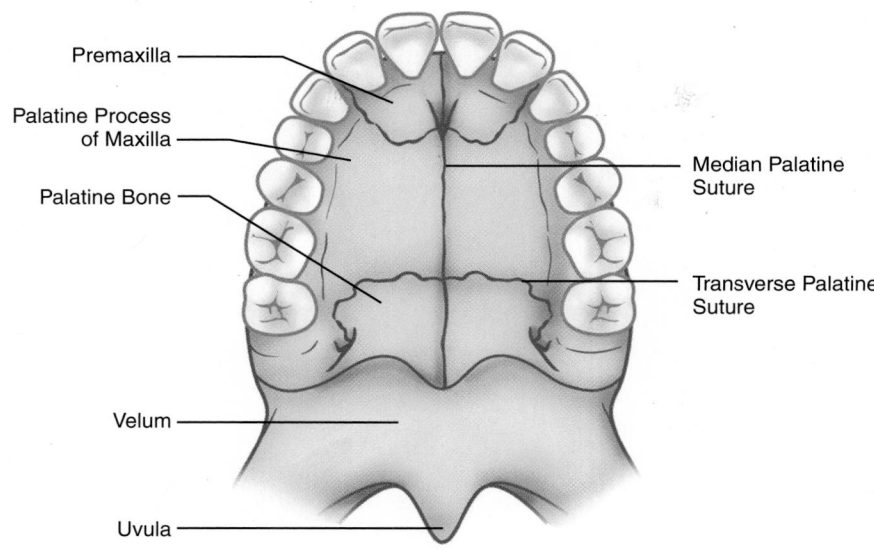

Premaxilla

Palatine Process
of Maxilla

Palatine Bone

Median Palatine
Suture

Transverse Palatine
Suture

Velum

Uvula

Figure 3–9

Bony structures of the hard
palate.

© Cengage Learning 2013.

is the **uvula**, the cone-shaped structure that hangs from the back of the soft palate but does not have any known function. At rest, the soft palate is down and rests near the base of the tongue, which allows an open passageway for breathing through the nose. During speech, the soft palate raises and moves posteriorly (up and back) to make contact with the *posterior pharyngeal wall* (back of the throat) to separate the oral cavity from the nasal cavity for all oral sounds (vowels and consonants) except /m/, /n/, and "ng." Those three sounds are *nasal sounds* and are produced with the soft palate down. The terms *velopharyngeal mechanism* and *velopharyngeal system* refer to the *velum* and the *lateral* and *posterior pharyngeal walls* at the level of the velum (see Figure 3–10). The upward and backward movement of the soft palate to make contact with the posterior pharyngeal wall to close off the coupling of the oral and nasal cavities is referred to as **velopharyngeal closure**.

THE ARTICULATORY SYSTEM

The biological purpose of the mouth is not speech but eating, although most people do more talking than eating. We need to keep in mind that the actions of each articulator are determined by the neurological impulses sent from the brain to tell specific muscles when, how much, and how long to contract or relax. The **sensory** and **motor** systems of the brain are involved in every movement of an articulator. This is noteworthy for both SLPs and Auds because it emphasizes that our therapy to improve articulation (as well as all other aspects of communication) causes changes in neuronal firing and synaptic connections inside the brain.

The Skeletal Structures of Articulation

Numerous bones make up the face and skull, but SLPs are primarily concerned with the maxilla (see above) and **mandible**. The mandible

soft palate (velum)

The muscular tissue in the posterior one-third of the roof of the mouth that separates the oral cavity from the nasal cavity when raised and in contact with the posterior pharyngeal wall.

uvula

The cone- or teardrop-shaped structure that hangs from the back of the soft palate but does not have any known function.

velopharyngeal closure

The upward and backward movement of the soft palate to make contact with the posterior pharyngeal wall to close off the coupling of the oral and nasal cavities.

sensory

Pertaining to sensation or awareness of stimuli that are received in the central nervous system.

motor

Pertaining to motion or movement; nerve cells that initiate and regulate contracting and relaxing of muscle fibers.

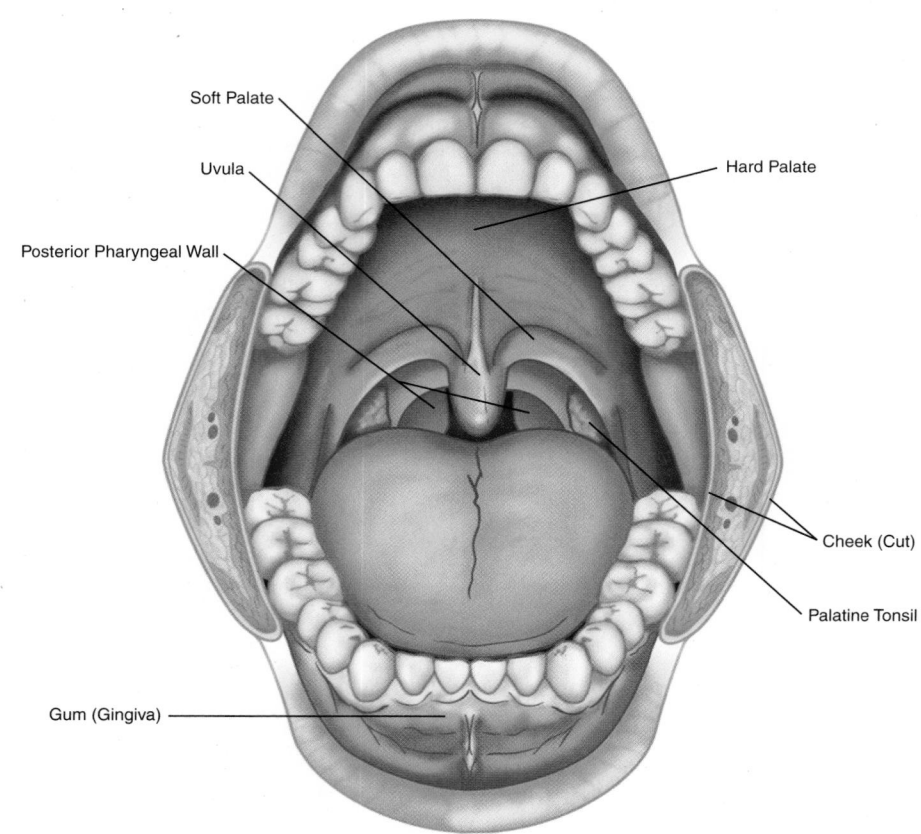

Figure 3-10

Anterior view of the oral cavity.

© Cengage Learning 2013.

---

mandible

The lower jaw that is hinged to the temporal bone for opening and closing and contains sockets for the lower teeth.

is the lower jaw that is hinged to the temporal bones of the skull (*temporomandibular joins—TMJ*) for opening and closing the mouth. Like the maxilla, the mandible's alveolar ridge is covered by *gingiva* ("gums") and contains sockets for the lower teeth. The mandible is normally held in a closed position so that the lips are touching but the teeth are not in contact with the maxillary teeth. During speaking the mandible moves up and down only slightly in the production of many sounds, but a more open mouth position allows more sound to escape, creating a "megaphone" effect and a louder voice.

Facial Muscles

The facial muscles are connected to the numerous bones that make up the front and sides of the skull, including the *frontal bone* (forehead), *temporal bones* (sides of the skull behind and around the ears), *zygomatic bones* (cheek bones), maxilla, and mandible. Although we do not use all of our facial muscles for articulation, we use most of them for communicating our facial expressions, which may either agree or disagree with the words we are articulating.

Lips and Cheeks

labia

Pertaining to the lips.

The biological function of the lips (**labia**) is to hold food and liquid in the oral cavity during chewing, drinking, and swallowing, and the overlaid function is to help with the articulation of some speech sounds. The lips are particularly sensitive to touch so that nothing can enter the mouth (and possibly be swallowed) without a person's awareness. The muscular structure of the lips is the oval-shaped sphincter **orbicularis oris**. The lips are the second most important articulator and have several movements that involve speech: opening, closing, rounding, flattening, **protruding**, and **retracting**. The timing and extent of each of these movements help shape various sounds and allow sounds to exit the mouth.

The *masseter* and *buccinator* muscles make up the bulk of the cheeks, and the inner surfaces of the cheeks are covered with mucous membranes. Biting and chewing are the biological purposes of these muscles, and their overlaid function is to contribute to the production of oral sounds.

Tongue

The three biological functions of the **tongue** (**lingua** or **glossus**) are taste, movement of food in the mouth while chewing (**mastication**), and movement of food and liquid posteriorly for swallowing (**deglutition**). Taste is achieved through the taste buds, which give the tongue its characteristic rough texture. Speech requires the most rapid and complex muscular coordination in the entire body and the tongue is the primary articulator. The slightest movement can modify the air stream to produce the numerous consonants and vowels in our language, as well as the countless different sounds and dialects articulated by speakers of languages around the world (see Figure 3–11).

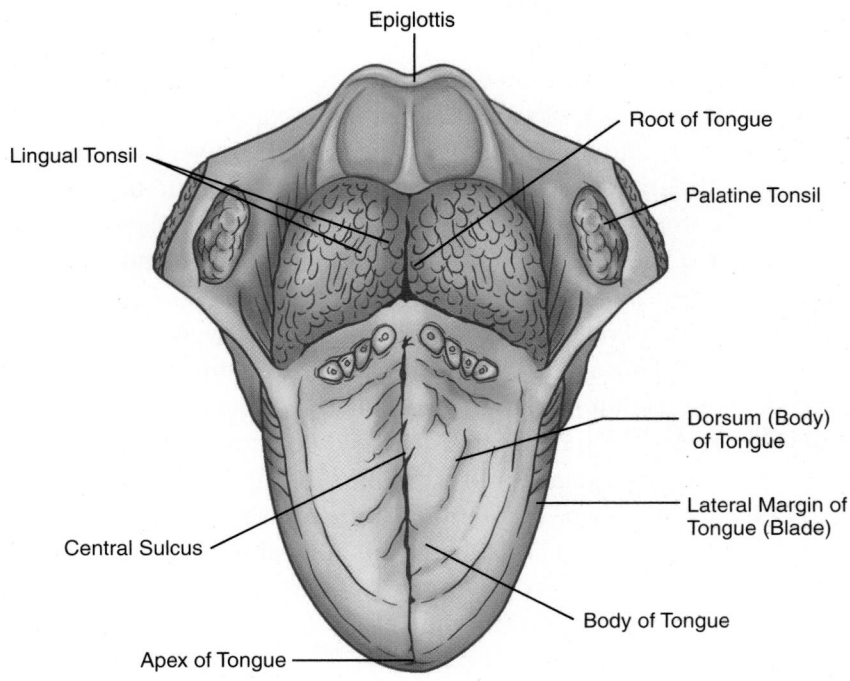

orbicularis oris

The muscle surrounding the opening of the mouth; the muscular structure of the lips.

protrude

In speech, the puckering of the lips forward or the movement of the tongue forward past the lips.

retract

In speech, the pulling back of the lips past their neutral, resting position or the movement of the tongue back into the oral cavity after protrusion or past the neutral, resting position.

tongue (lingua/lingual or glossus/glossal)

The primary articulator, whose movements creates consonants and vowels as well as perform biological functions.

mastication

The act of chewing food in preparation for swallowing and digestion.

deglutition

The act of swallowing.

Figure 3–11

The tongue.

© Cengage Learning 2013.

The tongue is divided in the midline by the *central sulcus* and is made up of eight pairs of muscles on each side. Four of the muscle pairs help *position* (protrude, retract, elevate, depress, lateralize) the tongue in the mouth and four of the muscle pairs help *shape* (round, flatten, groove, hump) the tongue to refine the production of specific sounds. Any significant abnormalities in **range of motion**, strength, coordination, or rate of ability to move, position, or shape the tongue rapidly and precisely may noticeably affect speech intelligibility.

Tongue Thrust

Tongue thrust refers to the habitual pushing of the tongue against the inner surface of the front teeth (**incisors**) or the protrusion of the tongue between the upper and the lower teeth. Although the tongue is not thrust forward forcefully when producing *sibilant sounds* (e.g., /s, z/), the forward movement creates distortions of sibilants (i.e., a *frontal lisp*). Some children have a tongue-resting position with the tongue tip lightly pressing against the frontal incisors, and during swallowing they tend to push the tongue forward against the incisors (sometimes referred to as a *tongue thrust swallow* or *reverse swallow*), which may contribute to misalignment of teeth. Some clinicians take additional training in the area of **myofunctional therapy** to provide intervention for tongue thrust and have had considerable success helping children who have problems in this area. Some orthodontists refer children who have a tongue thrust to an SLP for management before proceeding with placement of appliances (braces).

Dentition

Development of the **dentition** begins in utero when tooth buds are forming. The **deciduous teeth** (primary or "baby teeth") usually begin to erupt between six and nine months of age, with the lower incisors erupting first and the upper incisors after that. Teeth continue to erupt over 18–24 months until all 20 (10 uppers and 10 lowers) are in place. *Shedding* (losing) of the deciduous teeth usually occurs between 6 and 13 years of age, with the front teeth being lost first (first-grade school photographs are often permanent records of the beginning of this process). During the shedding, permanent teeth erupt to replace the deciduous teeth. There are 32 permanent ("adult teeth"), with 16 in the upper dental arch and 16 in the lower dental arch (i.e., four incisors [two central and two lateral], two canines, four premolars, and six molars in each arch).

There are three basic dental **occlusions** (see Figure 3–12). Class I (*neutrocclusion*) is considered the normal relationship in which the upper incisors are slightly forward of the lower incisors and the molars of the upper and lower dental arches are in proper relationship and alignment. In class II **malocclusion** (*overbite*), the upper incisors are considerably anterior of the lower incisors. In class III malocclusion

range of motion/movement (ROM)

For speech, the limits the mandible can open and close, the lips can protrude and retract, and the tongue can protrude, retract, elevate, lower, and move side to side (*lateralize*).

incisors

The four front upper and lower teeth (central and lateral incisors).

myofunctional therapy

Treatment designed to correct a tongue thrust or habitual forward-resting position of the tongue against the front teeth.

dentition

The type, number, and arrangement of teeth in the maxilla and mandible, including the incisors, cuspids (canines), bicuspids (premolars), and molars.

deciduous teeth

The set of 20 teeth that appear during infancy and early childhood (10 uppers, 10 lowers), with the front teeth appearing (erupting) through the gums about 6 months of age; all 20 teeth normally have erupted by 18–24 months. Shedding (losing) the deciduous teeth occurs between 6 and 13 years of age.

occlusion

The process of bringing the upper and lower teeth into contact.

malocclusion

Misalignment of the maxillary teeth with the mandibular teeth.

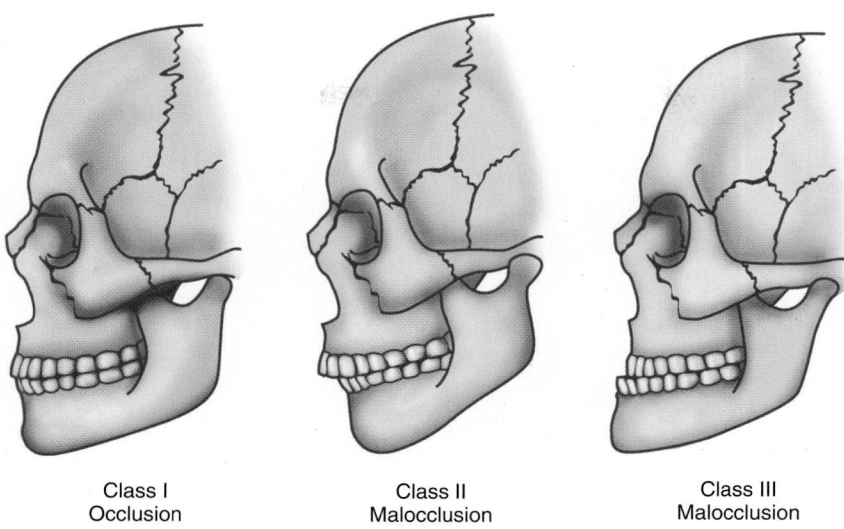

Class I
Occlusion

Class II
Malocclusion

Class III
Malocclusion

Figure 3-12

Types of dental occlusions.

© Cengage Learning 2013.

(*underbite*) the upper incisors rest behind the lower incisors and the mandible juts forward. An **open bite** (not one of the three classes) describes an abnormal vertical space between the anterior maxillary and mandibular teeth that often allows the tongue tip to be seen when a person smiles.

It has long been known that there is not a strong relationship between dentition and articulation of speech because the articulatory mechanism (especially the tongue and lips) is highly adaptable (Bernthal, Bankson, & Flipsen, 2009). People rapidly and automatically make subtle adjustments of their articulators while talking, when chewing gum, or after receiving a local anesthetic at the dentist office. Most pipe smokers learn to articulate clearly with a pipe clenched tightly between their teeth. Although mild dental anomalies usually do not affect articulation of sounds and speech intelligibility, severe dental malocclusions or missing front teeth may contribute to or result in some articulation errors.

THE NERVOUS SYSTEM

The brain is a three-pound glob of matter, the consistency of Jell-O and the color of day-old slush. The brain contains about 100 billion **neurons** (cell bodies) and each neuron has thousands of connections to other neurons, giving us trillions of connections within the brain. Every fleeting thought, emotion, and movement is the result of chemical and electrical activity within our brains. Our brains understand many things, but what the brain does not understand is *how* the brain understands. How does the brain transform sight, sound, touch, taste, and smell into thoughts and emotions? Where in the brain does a thought begin and where does it go from there? What happens when the brain does not do what it is supposed to do? Humans will never fully understand the brain—and perhaps we are never meant to (see Figure 3–13).

open bite

An abnormal vertical space between the anterior maxillary and mandibular teeth that often allows the tongue tip to be seen when a person smiles.

neuron (gray matter)

The basic nerve cell of the nervous system, containing a nucleus within a cell body and extending an axon and multiple dendrites.

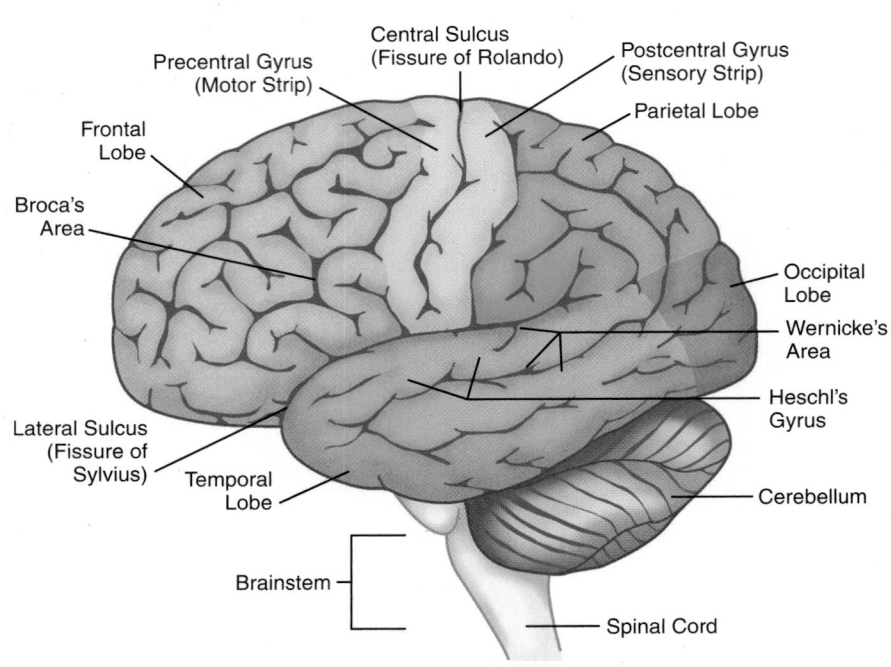

Figure 3-13

The brain, cerebellum, and brainstem.

© Cengage Learning 2013.

---

process/processing

In reference to neurological functioning, the activation of neurons (hundreds to millions at any instant) with their impulses sent through axons and dendrites to other neurons to bring about general and specific cognitive, linguistic, and motor activity.

axon (white matter)

The cellular extension of a neuron that carries impulses away from the cell body.

dendrite (white matter)

A branching extension of a neuron that carries impulses to the cell body.

synapse

The junction at which two neurons communicate with each other.

central nervous system (CNS)

The brain, cerebellum, brainstem, and spinal cord.

Before any of the speech systems are set in motion, the brain must **process** countless bits of information to decide what needs to be communicated and how. The motor and sensory systems then initiate every movement of the structures and muscles that will communicate the message. As SLPs and Auds we need to keep in mind that all of our therapy for hearing, speech, language, cognition, and swallowing disorders involves the brain. That is, whether we are working with a child or adult with a hearing impairment, an articulation disorder, language disorder, stuttering problem, neurological disorder, or any other communication or swallowing disorder, we are working with neurons, **axons**, **dendrites**, and **synapses** within the person's brain to change the way muscles contract and relax for specific behaviors to occur. More subtly, when we are helping people change their attitudes, thoughts, feelings, and reactions toward their communication problems (e.g., stuttering), we are working on new or different neuronal connections within the brain (see Figure 3-14).

The Central Nervous System

The **central nervous system (CNS)** is composed of the brain (*cerebrum*), cerebellum, brainstem, and spinal cord. All incoming and outgoing signals are generated and processed through the CNS. The skull rests on the *atlas*, the top vertebra in the spinal column, named after the mythical figure Atlas who carried the world on his shoulders. Essentially, our brain is our world.

The brain is divided into left and right **cerebral hemispheres** that look grossly the same; however, their functions differ significantly. Each hemisphere has four lobes (*temporal, frontal, parietal*, and *occipital*).

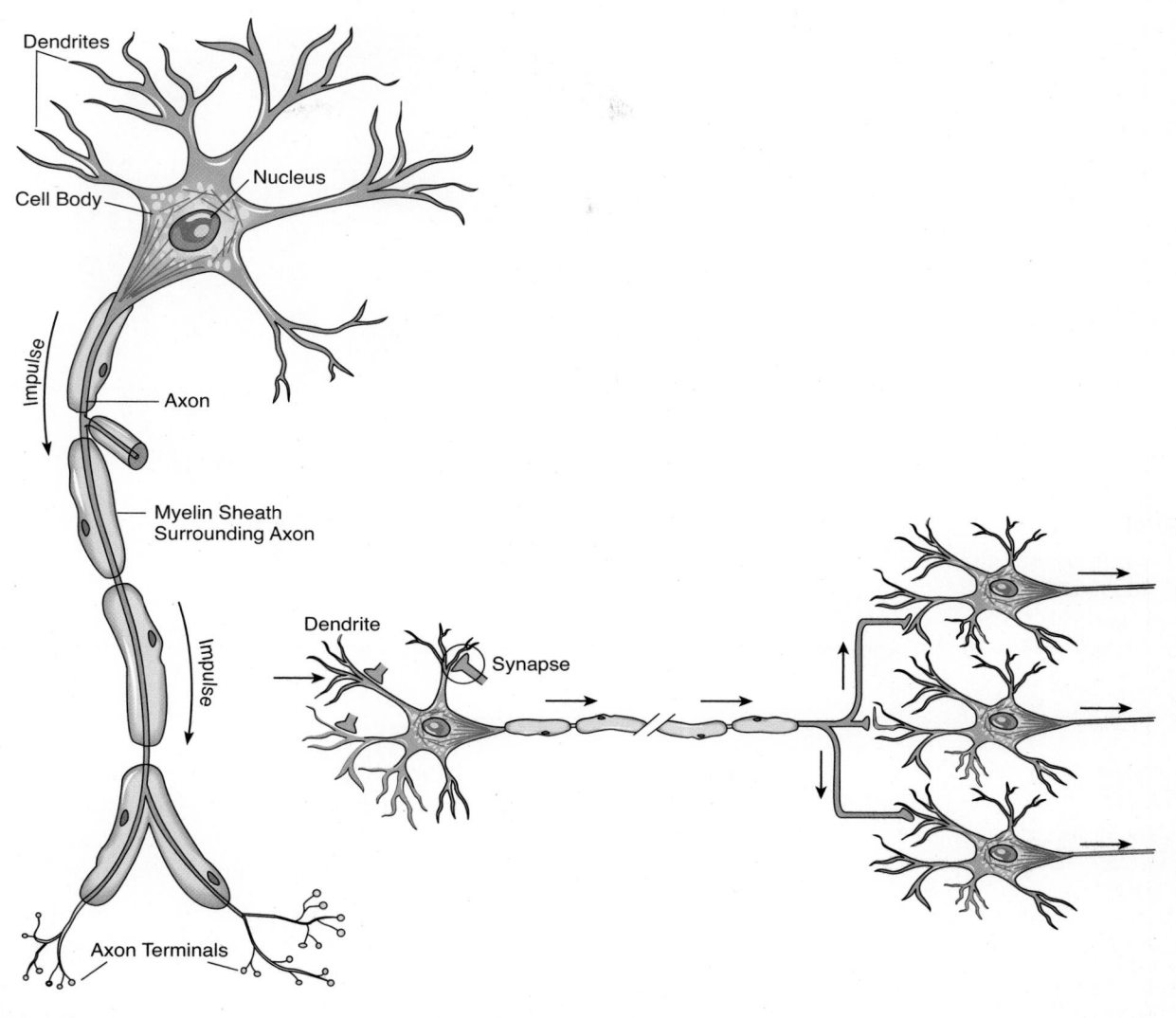

Figure 3–14

Neurons, axons, dendrites, and synapses.

© Cengage Learning 2013.

The left hemisphere is important for receptive and expressive language and speech, for processing rapidly changing information, and for perceiving and analyzing information in a sequential order (e.g., sounds in words and words in sentences). The left hemisphere is commonly referred to as the *dominant hemisphere* for speech, language, and motor functioning. Approximately 95% of right-handed people have dominant left hemispheres and approximately 80% of left-handed people have dominant left hemispheres for speech and language even though their right hemisphere is dominant for motor functioning (Nolte, 2008).

The right hemisphere is particularly important for *attention, orientation* (e.g., self-awareness, where the person is, time of day, etc.),

cerebral hemisphere

Either of the two halves of the brain that contains a frontal lobe, parietal lobe, occipital lobe, and temporal lobe.

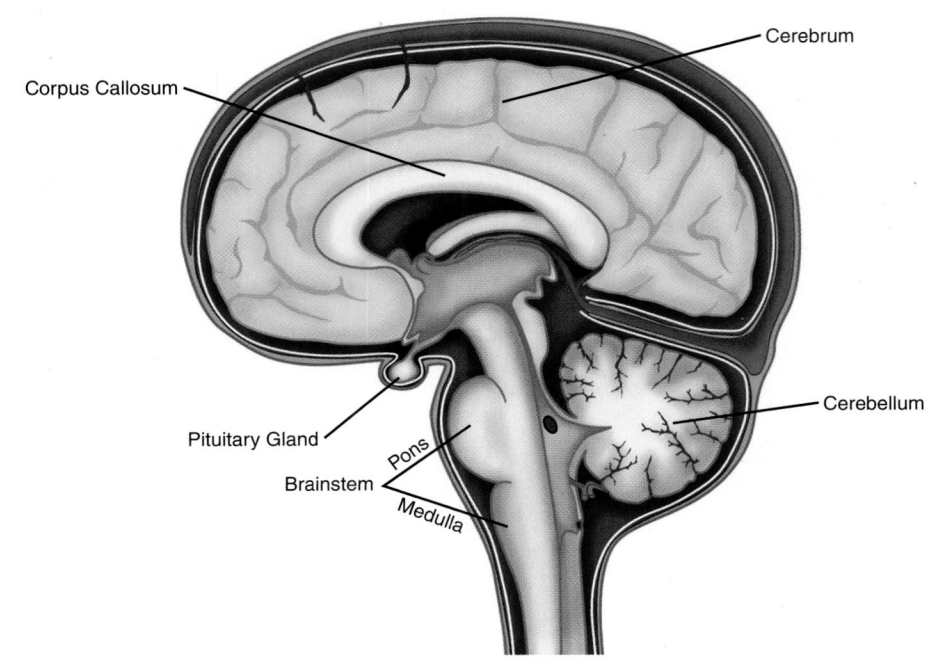

Figure 3–15

Corpus callosum. Midline view of the brain.

© Cengage Learning 2013.

cortex (gray matter)

The outer layer (approximately one-fourth to one-half inch) of brain tissue containing nerve cell bodies (neurons).

emotions, and *cognition* (Ponsford, 2004). The two hemispheres of the brain work together because they are connected by a large band of nerve fibers (*corpus callosum*) in the center of the brain (see Figure 3–15). Both hemispheres are needed to competently and completely analyze information from the various modalities (auditory, visual, tactile, taste, and smell), and to program an appropriate and timely response (Carter, 2009; Gazzaniga, 2004).

Most of the estimated 100 billion neurons in the brain are in the **cortex**—the outer one-fourth to one-half inch of brain tissue. The cell bodies in various areas of the brain have similar structures but diverse functions, which allow different brain areas to have various responsibilities. When the brain is damaged, millions or even billions of neurons, axons, dendrites, and synapses may not function normally or at all (see Figure 3–16).

The brain has a limited capacity to process incoming stimuli; therefore, it must focus its attention on relevant stimuli and ignore or inhibit much of the other stimuli. For example, in a noisy room filled with people we try to attend to one or two people talking while ignoring all other sounds and words that are reaching our ears. Likewise, we try to visually ignore all people and objects in the room that may distract us from the person we are visually focusing on. At the same time, we are ignoring almost everything touching our bodies, from our clothes to jewelry, yet attending to the glass we are holding. Nevertheless, our discussion of language processing focuses on auditory skills, keeping in mind that similar processing may be occurring in other modalities.

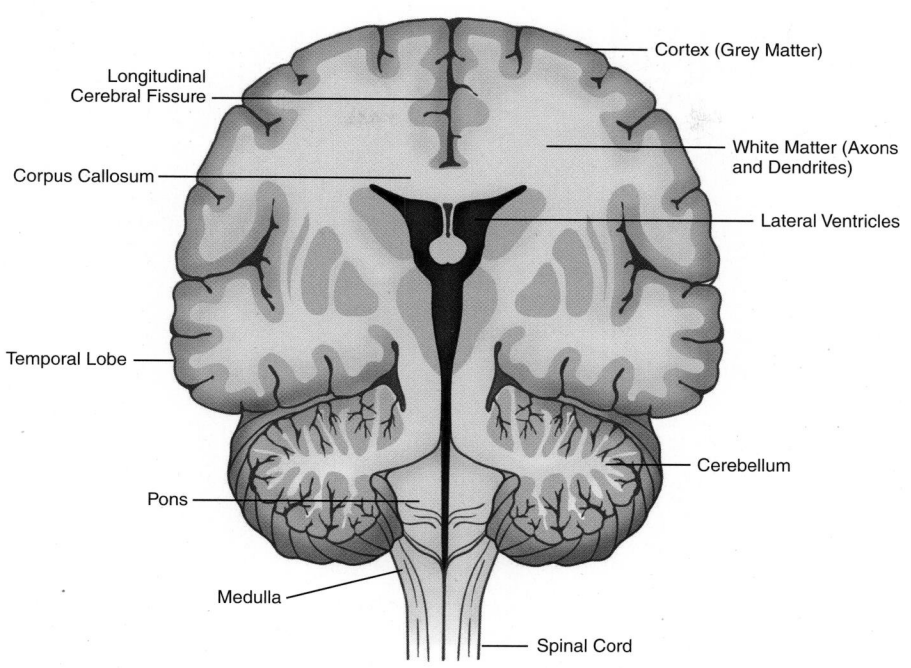

Figure 3-16

Corpus callosum. Cross section of the brain.

© Cengage Learning 2013.

Blood Circulation in the Brain (Cerebrovascular System)

Three arteries supply each hemisphere of the brain (see Figure 3–17). Although the brain weighs only about 3 pounds, it uses 20% to 25% of the blood that is pumped from the heart, depending on the activity level of the brain. This means, for example, that a 150-pound person will use 20% to 25% of his blood every minute for just 2% of his body. When the oxygen-rich blood is prevented from reaching the brain for several seconds (**anoxia**), a person will lose consciousness, and if blood and oxygen cannot reach the brain for just a few minutes, irreversible brain damage will result (e.g., in cases of *near-drowning*). The brain can function normally only with the help of the extensive vascular system supplying it with blood.

Temporal Lobes

The temporal lobes lie behind the frontal lobes, under the parietal lobes, and in front of the occipital lobes. The temporal lobes are essential for *auditory processing* of sounds and language processing. Nerve impulses from the ears are received by the *primary auditory cortex (Heschl's gyrus)* at the top margins of the temporal lobes. The right ear sends impulses to the left hemisphere's primary auditory cortex and the left ear sends impulses to the right hemisphere's primary auditory cortex; however, the information received in the right hemisphere must cross over by way of the corpus callosum to the left hemisphere's temporal lobe for language processing. The primary auditory cortex of both hemispheres perceives sounds as human speech or *environmental* sounds (e.g., animals, telephone ringing, and all other nonhuman sounds)

anoxia

Lack of oxygen in the brain usually caused by asphyxiation (e.g., near-drowning or loss of airway from choking) or inadequate blood circulation (e.g., heart attack) that results in unconsciousness and death of brain tissue.

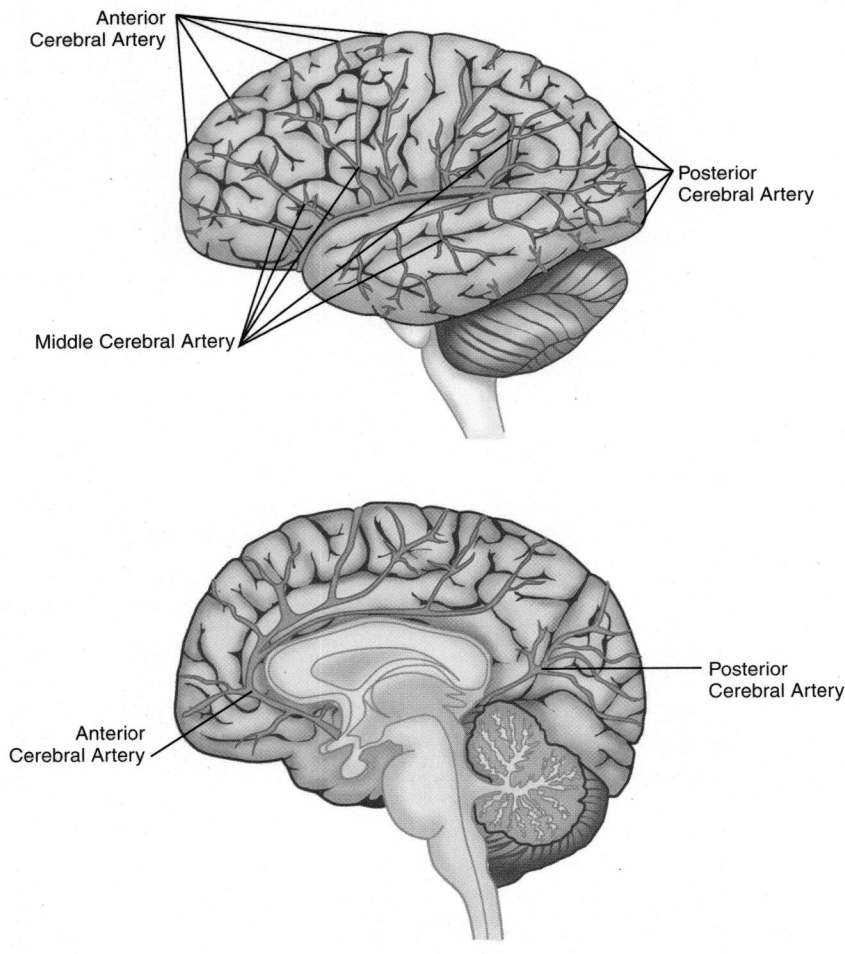

Figure 3-17

The major cerebral arteries (red—middle cerebral artery, blue—anterior cerebral artery, green—posterior cerebral artery).
© Cengage Learning 2013.

auditory comprehension

The ability to understand spoken language at the single word, phrase, simple sentence, complex sentence, paragraph, and conversational speech levels.

but does not interpret their meanings. The auditory information is then sent to an area of the cortex called *Wernicke's area* for interpretation and language processing. Wernicke's area lies just behind the primary auditory cortex but is only in the left temporal lobe in right-handed people, as well as the vast majority of left-handed people (recall the discussion of the dominant hemisphere).

Language Processing

Language processing is a complex phenomenon for the brain that involves not only Wernicke's area in the left hemisphere, but may involve all lobes of the brain at any given instant. SLPs and Auds typically are more concerned about auditory processing than visual or tactile processing. However, when we are in conversation with someone, our brains are processing information from all modalities being stimulated (including in some situations taste and smell, such as when talking about food).

Language processing and **auditory comprehension** involve numerous areas and functions within the brain and occur simultaneously (Bellis, 2002; Geffner & Ross-Swain, 2007). Auditory comprehension begins when meaning is attached to auditory information. However, to comprehend, **integrate**, and **formulate** language, all lobes in both hemispheres of the brain may be involved. Overall, we cannot separate auditory, visual, and tactile processing of information from cognition (Byrnes, 2007). We use language for cognition and we use cognition to comprehend, integrate, and formulate language. When language is impaired, cognition is impaired; when cognition is impaired, language processing is impaired.

Frontal Lobes

The frontal lobes are located behind the forehead and are the largest lobes of the brain. The *prefrontal cortex* (anterior two-thirds of the frontal lobes) is essential for cognition and, along with the right hemisphere of the brain, is involved in a variety of mental activities, including attention, reasoning, judgment, decision making, and problem solving. Our personalities, character, philosophies, religious beliefs, political orientation, and abilities to monitor and regulate our own behaviors, set goals and see them through (**executive functions**) are largely functions of the anterior portions of our frontal lobes (Casey, Gledd, & Thomas, 2000; Sowell, Dells, Stiles, & Jernigan, 2001). We develop our cognitive skills and ability to make thoughtful, wise decisions because of maturity of our brains, learning, and life experiences.

Behind the prefrontal cortex lie the motor areas (*premotor cortex* and *motor cortex*) that generate the impulses for voluntary movement. The left premotor and motor cortex of the brain control the right side of the body, and the right premotor and motor cortex control the left side of the body. The largest portions of the premotor and motor cortex are for movements of the face and hands. **Broca's area** in the premotor cortex of the left hemisphere controls motor movements of the articulators for speech. The motor cortex takes direction from the premotor cortex and is the primary pathway for carrying neural impulses to muscles throughout the body.

Motor Control of Speech

To communicate with Broca's area in the left frontal lobe of the brain, Wernicke's area in the left temporal lobe sends impulses over an axonal pathway (the *arcuate fasciculus*) to Broca's area. Broca's area plans, sequences, coordinates, and initiates the motor movements of the articulators. After this processing, the information is conveyed to the motor cortex in the left and right frontal lobes for execution. Simultaneous feedback by the *sensory cortex* in the left and right parietal lobes allows for fine adjustments of the articulators. Speech is a *sensorimotor* process that involves the parietal lobes for feedback about muscle activity (Kent, 2004; Duffy, 2005). The production of speech is an extraordinarily complex process that involves extensive interaction of different areas of the brain in rapid coordination (see Figure 3–18).

integrate/integration

In neurology, the process of combining information from various input modalities, attaching meaning and interpreting the information, storing (remembering), and making decisions about responding.

formulate/formulation

In language, the choice of words and grammatical structures in the construction of a meaningful verbal expression.

executive functions

A composite of the following activities related to goal completion: anticipation, goal selection, planning, initiation of activity, self-regulation or self-monitoring, and use of feedback to adjust for future responses.

Broca's area

The center for motor speech control (planning, sequencing, coordinating, and initiating) of the articulators located in the lower posterior portion of the left hemisphere's frontal lobe.

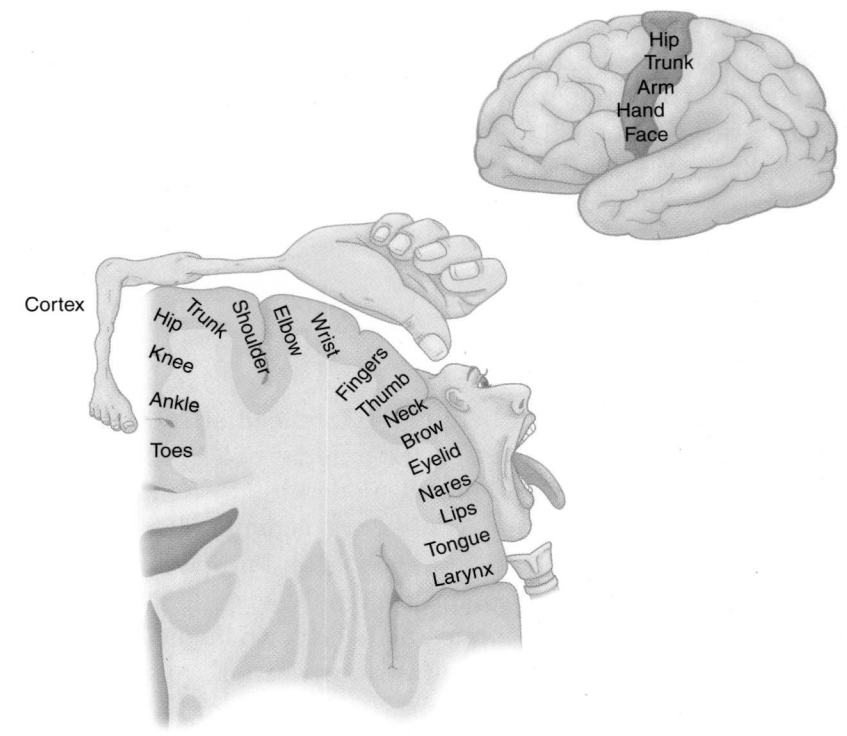

Figure 3-18

Homunculus (L. *homo*, man, + *uncula*, little), representing relative amounts of cortical areas devoted to motor movements.

© Cengage Learning 2013.

Parietal Lobes

The parietal lobes lie just behind the frontal lobes. The left parietal lobe receives sensations from the right side of the body and the right parietal lobe receives sensations from the left side of the body. The anterior portion of the parietal lobes is important in the *tactile* (touch) detection of objects touching the body. The largest portions of the parietal lobes are for sensations of the hands and face, including sensations of taste from the tongue. The remaining areas of the parietal lobes interpret what is detected and integrate bodily sensations such as temperature, touch, pressure, and pain (*somesthetic information*).

Occipital Lobes

The occipital lobes are in the back of the brain and lie posterior and inferior to the parietal lobes. Impulses from the retinas of the eyes travel along the optic nerve to the most posterior areas of the occipital lobes where visual images are received. The visual images are then processed in the *visual association cortex* (the rest of the occipital lobes) to interpret what is seen and enable the cerebrum to use the information. The occipital lobes also are involved with recognizing and interpreting spatial relationships, such as judging distance and seeing things in three dimensions.

Cerebellum, Brainstem, and Spinal Cord

The **cerebellum** lies just below the temporal and occipital lobes and communicates with the brain, brainstem, and spinal cord. The cerebellum is important in coordinating muscle groups for complex motor activity to

cerebellum

The CNS structure largely concerned with the coordination of muscles and the maintenance of balance and body equilibrium.

allow for smooth, accurate movements of the body, limbs, and articulators. The cerebellum is also essential in maintaining balance and equilibrium.

The two components of the **brainstem** (*pons* and *medulla oblongata* [*medulla*]) connect the brain to the spinal cord. All sensory and motor impulses sent to and from the brain pass through the brainstem. Most sensory and motor nerve fibers cross over at the level of the medulla in the brainstem, which is the reason the left hemisphere of the brain controls the right side of the body and the right hemisphere controls the left side of the body. The brainstem controls the face, mouth, and larynx, for the production of speech.

Twelve pairs of *cranial nerves* exit the pons and medulla and course to the mouth, face, neck, and shoulders (see Figure 3–19). The 12 pairs

brainstem

The structure (pons and medulla oblongata [medulla]) that connects the brain to the spinal cord; it is important in sensory and motor functions and contains neurons for the cranial nerves that exit the pons and medulla.

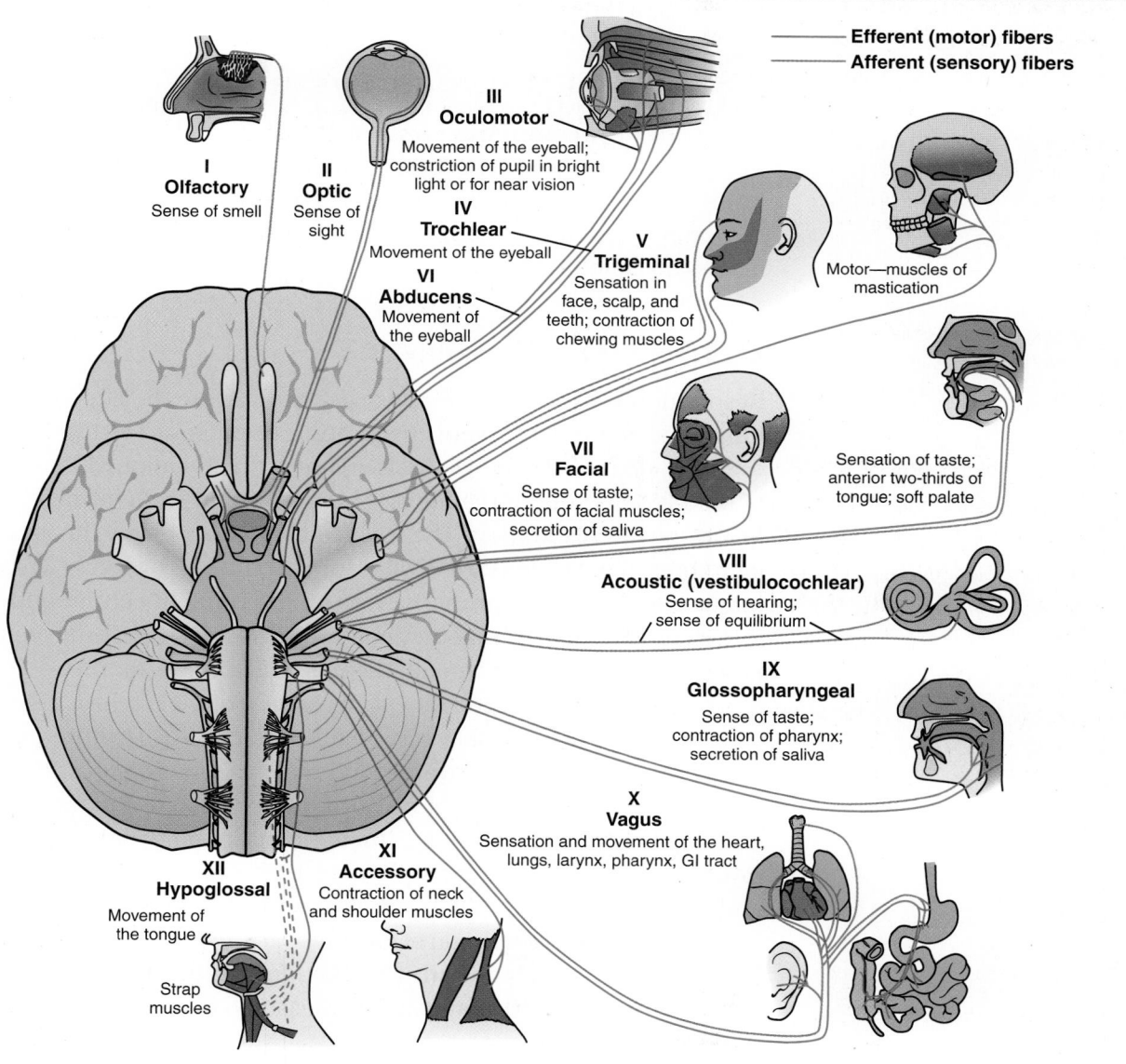

Figure 3–19

Brainstem and cranial nerves coursing to the head and neck.
© Cengage Learning 2013.

of cranial nerves have both motor and sensory pathways for impulses to be sent from the brain to the muscles and for impulses from the muscles to be sent back to the brain. Seven of the cranial nerves are important for speech: *trigeminal* (V) [face and jaws], *facial* (VII) [face and tongue], *vestibulocochlear* or *auditory* (VIII) [hearing and balance], *glossopharyngeal* (IX) [tongue and pharynx], *vagus* (X) [larynx, respiration, heart, gastrointestinal system], *accessory* (XI) [neck and shoulder], and *hypoglossal* (XII) [tongue and neck].

The **spinal cord** is a thick "cord" (approximately the diameter of a finger) of nerve fibers located in the passageway of the vertebral column. The spinal cord *conducts* (sends) sensory and motor impulses of the body to and from the brain and controls many body **reflexes**. Thirty-one pairs of spinal nerves originate from the spinal cord and send branches to innervate every muscle of the body below the face.

Peripheral Nervous System

The **peripheral nervous system (PNS)** is composed of the cranial nerves that exit from the brainstem and the spinal nerves that exit from the spinal cord (see Figure 3–20). The PNS allows the body to communicate sensory information to the brain and the brain to communicate motor information to the body.

CHAPTER SUMMARY

Respiration is the exchange of oxygen and carbon dioxide between the lungs and the environment. Inspiration (inhalation) is the process of drawing air into the lungs, and expiration (exhalation) is the process of breathing air out of the lungs. The diaphragm is the primary muscle involved with respiration. The trachea begins just below the larynx and continues down to where it divides into the lungs. The trachea branches into the left and right primary bronchi; the bronchi continue to divide into smaller branches until they enter the alveolar sacs. The alveolar sacs make up the lung tissue and do the real work of respiration.

The larynx is located at the superior end of the trachea. The thyroid cartilage is what we normally consider the "voice box." The true vocal folds are paired muscle tissue covered with mucous membranes with a pearly white appearance. Closure of the vocal folds helps prevent material from entering the trachea and lungs (their biological purpose), and vibration produces voice (their overlaid function). The vocal folds close (adduct) and open (abduct) to produce voice for one complete vibratory cycle. Pitch is the psychological sensation of the physical property of the frequency of a sound and is measured in hertz (Hz). Loudness is the psychological sensation of the intensity of a sound and is measured in decibels (dB).

The structures important for normal speech and resonance are the facial structures, the articulators, the hard and soft palates, and the pharyngeal region. The first trimester of pregnancy is crucial in facial and palatal development. The maxilla (upper jaw) contains the hard palate

---

spinal cord

A thick "cord" of nerve fibers that passes through the vertebral column that conducts sensory and motor impulses to and from the brain and controls many body reflexes.

reflex

An involuntary response to a sensory input, such as the corneal reflex in which both eyes blink in response to something irritating an eye; the gag reflex, caused by something touching the posterior wall of the pharynx; and the knee jerk (deep tendon) reflex, caused by a sharp tap just below the knee.

peripheral nervous system (PNS)

The cranial nerves that exit the brainstem and the spinal nerves that exit the spinal cord that allow the body to communicate sensory information to the brain and the brain to communicate motor information to the body.

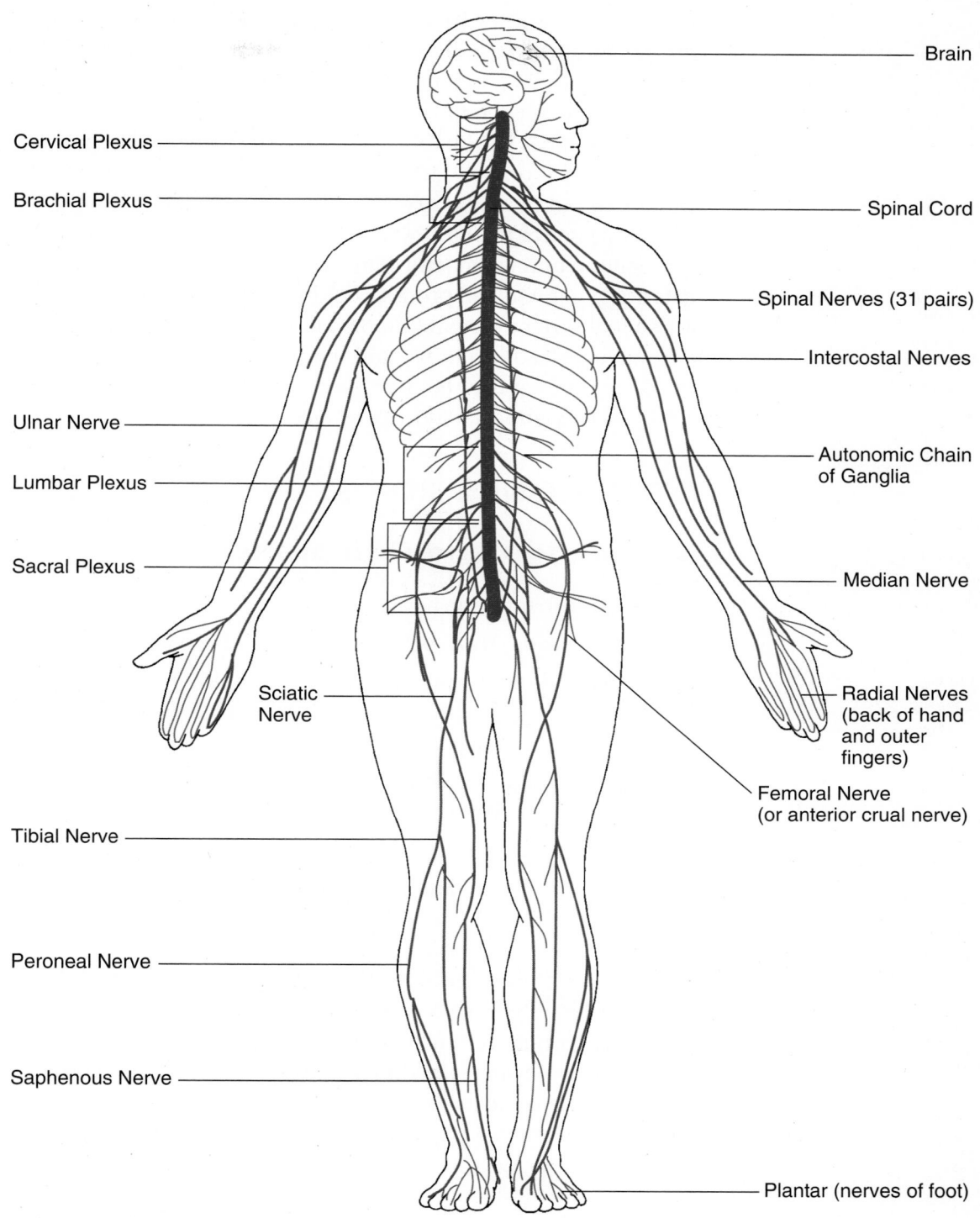

Cervical Plexus

Brachial Plexus

Ulnar Nerve

Lumbar Plexus

Sacral Plexus

Sciatic Nerve

Tibial Nerve

Peroneal Nerve

Saphenous Nerve

Brain

Spinal Cord

Spinal Nerves (31 pairs)

Intercostal Nerves

Autonomic Chain of Ganglia

Median Nerve

Radial Nerves (back of hand and outer fingers)

Femoral Nerve (or anterior crual nerve)

Plantar (nerves of foot)

Figure 3–20

The peripheral nervous system.

© Cengage Learning 2013.

and is the anterior two-thirds of the roof of the mouth. The soft palate is the muscular posterior one-third of the roof of the mouth that separates the oral cavity from the nasal cavity when raised.

The structures important for articulation are the maxilla, mandible, lips, and tongue. The lips and tongue are the two most important articulators. It is the timing and extent of their movements that help shape various sounds and allow sounds to exit the mouth.

The central nervous system is composed of the brain (*cerebrum*), cerebellum, brainstem, and spinal cord. All incoming and outgoing signals are generated and processed through the CNS. The brain is divided into left and right cerebral hemispheres, with each hemisphere having a frontal, parietal, occipital, and temporal lobe. The left hemisphere is the dominant hemisphere for speech and language and the right hemisphere is very important for cognition.

STUDY QUESTIONS

Knowledge and Comprehension

1. Define inspiration and expiration.
2. Describe the true vocal folds and their functions.
3. Explain the anatomical relationship of the hard palate to the soft palate.
4. Why is it important to keep in mind that the physiology of each articulator is determined by the neurological impulses sent from the brain to the muscles?
5. What are the primary functions of the left hemisphere of the brain?

Application

1. How could difficulty inspiring a normal amount of air during a normal breath affect voice?
2. How could you explain respiration and phonation (voice) to an 8-year-old child who has a voice disorder, including some important anatomical (body) terms?
3. How could you explain to an adult client how the soft palate moves during speech?
4. Why could a person have severe speech, voice, and swallowing problems following damage to the brainstem?
5. How could damage to a person's frontal lobes severely affect his quality of life?

Analysis/Synthesis

1. Why is it important to be able to explain in nontechnical terms the processes of respiration and phonation to clients?

2. Why is it important to understand the movement of the soft palate during speech?

3. Discuss the concept that speech requires essentially perfect timing and coordination of muscle contraction and relaxation for precision of articulator movements.

4. Compare and contrast the functions of the left hemisphere with those of the right hemisphere.

5. Why are auditory comprehension and language processing essentially inseparable?

REFERENCES

Bellis, T. (2002). *Assessment and management of central auditory processing disorders in the educational setting: From science to practice* (2nd ed.). Clifton Park, NY: Delmar Cengage Learning.

Bernthal, J. E., Bankson, N. W., & Flipsen, P. (2009). *Articulation and phonological disorders* (6th ed.). Upper Saddle River, NJ: Pearson.

Byrnes, J. P. (2007). *Cognitive development and learning in instructional context* (3rd ed.), Boston, MA: Allyn and Bacon.

Carter, R. (2009). *The human brain book.* London: DK Publishers.

Casey, B., Gledd, J., & Thomas, K. (2000). Structural and functional brain development and its relation to cognitive development. *Biological Psychology, 54,* 241–257.

Duffy, J. R. (2005). *Motor speech disorders: Substrates, differential diagnosis, and management* (2nd ed.). Philadelphia, PA: Elsevier Mosby.

Gazzaniga, M. S. (Ed.). (2004). *The cognitive neurosciences* (3rd ed.). Boston, MA: Massachusetts Institute of Technology.

Geffner, D., & Ross-Swain, D. (2007). *Auditory processing disorders: Assessment, management and treatment.* San Diego, CA: Plural Publishing.

Hixon, T. J., Weismer, G., & Hoit, J. D. (2008). *Clinical speech science: Anatomy, physiology, acoustics, perception.* San Diego, CA: Plural Publishing.

Kent, R. D. (2004). The uniqueness of speech among motor systems. *Clinical Linguistics and Phonetics, 18*(6), 495–505.

Nicolosi, L., Harryman, E., & Kresheck, J. (2004). *Terminology of communication disorders: Speech-language-hearing* (5th ed.). Philadelphia, PA: Lippincott Williams & Wilkins.

Nolte, J. (2008). *The human brain: An introduction to its functional anatomy* (6th ed.). Philadelphia, PA: Elsevier Mosby.

Ponsford, J. (2004). *Cognitive and behavioral rehabilitation: From neurobiology to clinical practice.* New York, NY: Guilford Press.

Seikel, J. A., King, D. W., & Drumright, D. G. (2010). *Anatomy and physiology for speech, language, and hearing* (4th ed.). Clifton Park, NY: Delmar Cengage Learning.

Sowell, E., Dells, D., Stiles, T., & Jernigan, J. (2001). Structural and functional brain development and its relation to cognitive development. *Journal of International Neuropsychological Society, 7,* 312–319.

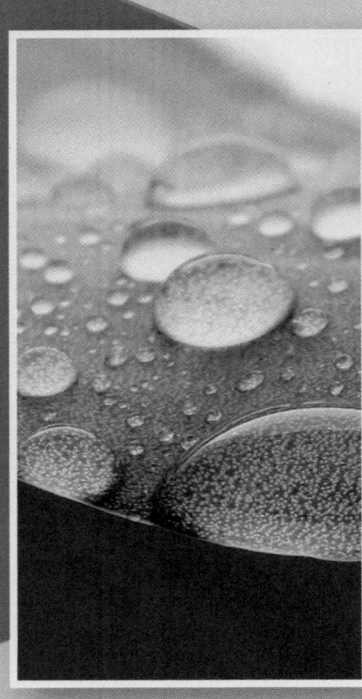

CHAPTER 4
Speech and Language Development

LEARNING OBJECTIVES

After studying this chapter, you will:

- Be able to discuss each of four theories of speech and language development.
- Be able to discuss the four general stages of speech development that children follow in any language or culture.
- Be familiar with multicultural considerations of speech and language development.

KEY TERMS

accent

babbling

behavioral theory

bilingual

blend

code switching

cognitive development

communicative competence

cooing

cultural–linguistic diversity (CLD)

culture

dialect

discourse

echolalia

English as a second language (ESL)

functor (function) words

holophrastic language

inner speech

jargon

language development

lexicon

mean length of utterance (MLU)

multicultural

narrative

nativistic theory

natural processes

neonate

KEY TERMS continued

operant (instrumental)
  conditioning

parallel speech

parentese

phonological processes

prelinguistic (preverbal)
  vocalizations

semantic-cognitive theory

social-pragmatic theory

speech development

standard dialect

stress

telegraphic speech (language)

utterance

vocal play

CHAPTER OUTLINE

Introduction
Theories of Speech and Language Development
  Behavioral Theory
  Nativistic Theory
  Semantic-Cognitive Theory
  Social-Pragmatic Theory
  Cultural and Linguistic Diversity Perspective
Speech Development
  Stage I: Birth–12 Months (Infancy)
  Stage II: 12–24 Months (Toddlerhood)
  Stage III: 2–5 Years (Early Childhood)
  Stage IV: 6–12 Years (Middle Childhood to Early
      Adolescence)
Language Development
  Stage I: Birth–12 Months (Infancy)
  Stage II: 12–24 Months (Toddlerhood)
  Stage III: 2–5 Years (Early Childhood)
  Stage IV: 6–12 Years (Middle Childhood to Early
      Adolescence)
Chapter Summary
Study Questions
References

speech development

The progressive evolving and shaping of individual sounds and syllables that are used as arbitrary symbols and applied in rule-governed combinations to produce words to communicate a person's wants, needs, thoughts, knowledge, and feelings.

language development

The progressive growth of a receptive and expressive communication system for representing concepts using arbitrary symbols (sounds and words) and rule-governed combinations of those symbols (grammar).

behavioral theory (behaviorism)

In reference to speech and language, a perspective of development that asserts that speech and language are behaviors learned through operant conditioning.

operant (instrumental) conditioning

A learning model for changing behavior in which a desired behavior is reinforced immediately after it spontaneously occurs.

INTRODUCTION

Speech and **language development** in infants and children is a complex and intricately interrelated process. For normal communication to develop there must be an integration of anatomy and physiology of the speech systems, neurological development, and sufficient interaction for infants and children to be encouraged and rewarded for communication attempts. Language development involves the development of both receptive language (i.e., what a child understands of what is said) and expressive language (i.e., the words, grammatical structures, and meanings that a child uses verbally) (Owens, 2012).

THEORIES OF SPEECH AND LANGUAGE DEVELOPMENT

Four general theories explain much of speech and language development: behavioral, nativistic, semantic-cognitive, and social-pragmatic. Although not necessarily considered a theory of language development, speech-language pathologists and audiologists need to be aware of cultural and diversity perspectives.

Behavioral Theory

B. F. Skinner is considered the father of modern **behavioral theory**. Behavioral theory may be applied to many aspects of human learning, including speech and language. The behavioral perspective maintains that language is a set of verbal behaviors learned through **operant (instrumental) conditioning**. Operant conditioning is a method of changing behavior in which a desired behavior is reinforced immediately after it spontaneously occurs.

Behaviorists believe that language behaviors are learned by imitation, reinforcement, and successive approximations toward adult language behaviors. They consider language to be determined not by self-discovery or creative experimentation, but by selective reinforcements received from speech and language models (usually parents and other family). Behaviorists focus on the external forces that shape a child's verbal behaviors into language and see the child primarily as a reactor to these forces (Hulit, Howard, & Fahey, 2011).

Two other concepts important in the operant model for speech and language development are *imitation* and *practice*. A young child imitates as best he can the sounds and words he hears his parents say. When a word is said by a child that *approximates* (sounds close to) the word the parents say, they accept and reinforce it. That is, they begin *shaping* the word until the child, through practice, eventually can say the word as the parents do. James (1960, p. 165) provided a well-known illustration of operant conditioning of verbal behavior using selective reinforcement:

> A child says *mama* as his mother starts to pick him up. The mother, who is delighted that the child knows her name, gives him a big hug and kiss and says, *Mama, that's right—I'm mama!* The affectionate physical response from the mother is undoubtedly pleasurable and is likely, therefore, to increase the probability that the child will say *mama* again. In other words, the mother's response to the child's behavior was a reinforcer.

Clinical Application

For decades, clinicians have used a behavioral approach to study children's language by observing, describing, and counting specific language behaviors. This basic *stimulus–response* [S-R] paradigm first teaches children to imitate a sound and then reinforces the production with verbal praise (e.g., "Good job!" and "That was super!"). The children's productions are then shaped into increasingly closer approximations of the target sound, and when they are finally able to produce the sound correctly, the sound is practiced in a variety of sound and word combinations. This same approach is used for language structures and numerous other targets being developed for speech and language.

Parentese

Parentese (also called *motherese* and *baby talk*, but more professionally called *child-directed speech*) refers to how parents and other caregivers often talk to infants. Adults using parentese typically (1) use a high-pitched voice with greater pitch variation; (2) use one- and two-syllable words in short, simple sentences; and (3) speak at a slower rate with clearer articulation, sometimes emphasizing every syllable (Berko-Gleason, 2001).

Application Question

Have you ever used parentese when playing with an infant? How did your speech differ from its normal form? Why do you think this came naturally to you?

Nativistic Theory

The **nativistic theory** emphasizes that the acquisition of language is an innate, physiologically determined, and genetically transmitted phenomenon. That is, a newborn is "prewired" for language acquisition and a linguistic mechanism is activated by exposure to linguistic stimuli (speech and language) (Hulit, Howard, & Fahey, 2011). This theory considers that language is universal and unique among humans and that unless there are severe mental or physical limitations or severe isolation and deprivation, humans will acquire language. The nativistic perspective argues that caregivers (e.g., parents) do not teach children a

nativistic theory

A perspective of language development that emphasizes the acquisition of language as an innate, physiologically determined, and genetically transmitted phenomenon.

progressive understanding of language forms, and that young children are exposed to complex and inconsistent language and are usually not provided feedback about the correctness of their utterances (Pinker, 1984).

Clinical Application

When children do not use certain language structures that are appropriate for their age, they likely have not acquired them through their natural tendency and, therefore, a goal would be to target those language structures in therapy. Helping children learn how to combine words, phrases, and sentences lets them convey their messages to others. Instructing children about how to use language appropriately in different social situations and environments allows them to use appropriate pragmatics when communicating.

Semantic-Cognitive Theory

semantic-cognitive theory

A perspective of language development that emphasizes the interrelationship between language learning and cognition; that is, the meanings conveyed by a child's productions.

The **semantic-cognitive theory** emphasizes the interrelationship between language learning and cognition. Children demonstrate certain cognitive abilities as a corresponding language behavior emerges (Bloom & Lahey, 1978). The semantic meaning that a person wants to communicate determines the words and word order (syntactic form) the person uses—that is, meaning precedes form. For example, children know what they want to communicate (cognition) but do not always use the correct semantics or grammar. Also, children may not know the correct use of a word or understand that a two-word utterance can have many meanings.

Clinical Application

Clinicians use the semantic-cognitive theory by describing children's strategies for acquiring new information (i.e., cognitive skills). For example, the *complexity* of a sentence (the message), the *amount* of information in a sentence, and the *rate* (*c-a-r*) at which a sentence is said may significantly affect a child's understanding of a sentence. A child with delayed or disordered language may benefit from a clinician who is able to adjust one or all of these variables. That is, a clinician may be able to make a sentence simpler (less *complex*), with less information for the child to process (decreased *amount*), and slow the *rate* of speech so the child has a better opportunity to understand a message.

Social-Pragmatic Theory

social-pragmatic theory

A perspective of language development that considers communication as the basic function of language.

The **social-pragmatic theory** considers communication as the basic function of language. This perspective is first seen in infant–caregiver interactions in which the caregiver responds to an infant's sounds and gestures. The prerequisites for the social-pragmatic theory are: (1) the infant must have a caregiver in close proximity to see, hear, or touch;

(2) the caregiver must provide the infant with basic physical needs such as food, warmth, and exploring the environment; (3) the infant must develop an attachment to the caregiver; (4) the infant and caregiver must be able to simultaneously attend to the same objects or actions; and (5) the infant and caregiver engage in *turn-taking* in both verbal and nonverbal behaviors (McLaughlin, 2006). In ideal parent–child communication, all five of these prerequisites are occurring in most interactions. The social-pragmatic perspective emphasizes the importance of the communicative partner's role; the partner's interpretation of what is said defines the results of the speech act.

Clinical Application

Caregivers can facilitate language in a number of ways, including playing social games (e.g., peekaboo) that are stimulating and exciting to infants; taking turns in activities in which the caregiver speaks and expects the infant to respond in some manner; and reading books with young children (see Figure 4–1). Clinicians can assess and treat children's language impairments from a social-communicative and contextual perspective. The therapeutic goal is maximizing communicative competence.

Cultural and Linguistic Diversity Perspective

Regardless of the theory of language acquisition that is followed, children mature within the context of caregivers, whether they are parents, family members, or other individuals within the community.

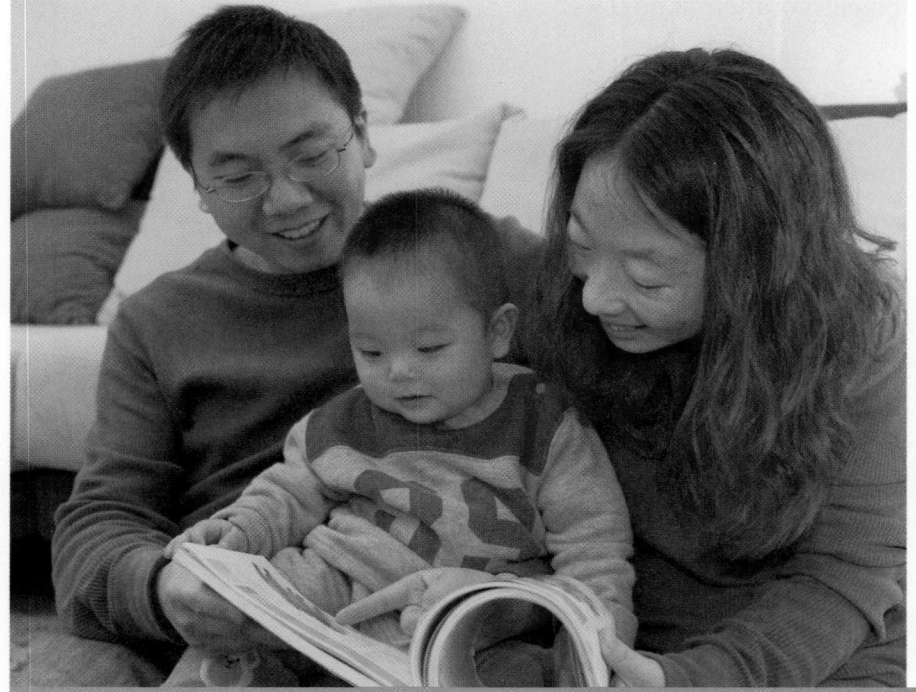

© William Ju/www.shutterstock.com

Figure 4–1

Parents and children reading together is an excellent application of the social-pragmatic perspective.

culture

The philosophies, values, attitudes, perceptions, religious and spiritual beliefs, educational values, language, customs, child-rearing practices, lifestyles, and arts shared by a group of people and passed from one generation to the next.

multicultural

A society characterized by a diversity of cultures, languages, traditions, religions, and values, as well as socioeconomic classes, sexual orientations, and ability levels; ideally, where individuals are respected and valued for their contributions to the whole of that society.

cultural–linguistic diversity (CLD)

A perspective of language development that emphasizes the similarities and differences of the people and the languages spoken around the world, and that stresses how one language or dialect is no better than another.

accent

Usually considered the speech pronunciation and inflections used by nonnative American English speakers (foreign accent).

dialect

A specific form of speech and language used in a geographical region or among a large group of people (*social* or *ethnic dialects*) that differs significantly from the standard of the larger language community in pronunciation, vocabulary, grammar, and idiomatic use of words.

standard dialect

The dialect of a language that is commonly spoken or established by individuals with considerable formal education.

These people provide a communicative environment for the maturing child that is reflective of the range of meanings, values, perceptions, and beliefs of the **cultures** of which they are a part. Like many other countries, the United States is considered **multicultural**. Speech-language pathologists and audiologists must understand and appreciate the **cultural–linguistic diversity (CLD)** of client populations in order to better serve them (Owens, 2012).

Cultural diversity is not determined by the origin of a person's ancestors or color of skin but by numerous other factors, including linguistic background, regional affiliations, educational levels, socio-economic status, and religious beliefs. Any of these factors may influence speech and language development. Many children in America are in families who have recently immigrated to America. These families often continue to speak their native language at home and in their social environments. The children, therefore, typically develop the family's native language as their first language. Many children, however, may be exposed to both English and the family's native language in the home and community and learn to speak English with a distinct **accent**.

There are approximately 1,000 languages in the world spoken by at least 10,000 people (Crystal, 2010). Most of these languages have a variety of forms and **dialects** that vary in phonology, vocabulary, and grammar. One dialect is no better than another within a language. However, the concept of a **standard dialect** within a language is strongly associated with the higher educational levels of the native speakers and is used in educational environments. It is important to consider that standard dialects for the same language may vary significantly among nations. For example, America, England, Australia, New Zealand, and Singapore all use the English language but have significantly different standard dialects for their nations.

ASHA's Position on Dialects of Speech-Language Pathologists

ASHA (1998) provided a position statement and technical report on speech-language pathologists working in school settings who, themselves, have dialectical variations from the local community dialect. ASHA maintains that members may not discriminate against people who speak with a nonstandard dialect in educational programs, employment, or service delivery. However, clinicians must have the necessary diagnostic and clinical skills and be able to model required treatment targets. In addition, the clinician may not have limited English proficiency.

In the United States, the four major ethnic groups are: Hispanics (Latinos), African Americans, Asian and Pacific Island Americans, and Native Americans (American Indians and indigenous Alaskans). Together, these groups represent between 30% and 35% of the nation's approximate 313,000,000 people; however, for individual states, certain ethnic groups significantly exceed the national average. For example, in California slightly more than 50% of the population is now Hispanic (U.S. Bureau of the Census, 2011). All major ethnic groups have broad and specific linguistic and cultural differences that influence their speech and language development (see Battle, 2002, Roseberry-McKibbin, 2008, and ASHA Division 14, *Communication Disorders and Sciences in Culturally and Linguistically Diverse Populations*, for more information on various cultures).

Hispanic (Latino)

Children of immigrants constitute the fastest-growing portion of the child population of the United States and the overall Hispanic population is approximately 15.5% of the population (U.S. Census Bureau, 2011). It is important for clinicians to keep in mind the differences in Spanish morphology and syntax when making decisions about whether a child has a language difference or a language disorder. When a clinician hears a child from a different linguistic and cultural background use morphology and syntax that differs from General American English, it is important to consider whether the child's first language is interfering with his second language (i.e., English). Clinicians who speak Spanish fluently have a distinct advantage working with these children.

English as a Second Language

Native Spanish-speaking parents who are learning **English as a second language (ESL)** (English language learner [ELL]) must decide whether to raise their children as English speakers, Spanish speakers, or **bilinguals**. Families often base their choices about the language their children will learn on fear of discrimination, limited information about the benefits of bilingualism, and other negative sociocultural considerations (Hammer, Miccio, & Wagstaff, 2003). Immigrant parents want their children to succeed; therefore, a common assumption among family members is that they must choose English over their home language, which may for some children result in the loss of the home language. Unfortunately, many educators and professionals (likely including some speech-language pathologists) continue to discourage the use of a child's home or first language and recommend that children focus on learning English to the exclusion of the language of the home. Children who become fluent in both their home language and English can choose to use one language one moment and the other language the next moment (**code switching**), depending on whom they are talking to and what they are talking about.

African American

African Americans comprise almost 13% of the U.S. population and are the largest racial minority in the United States (U.S. Census Bureau, 2011). African American English (AAE) is a systematic, rule-governed,

---

English as a second language (ESL)

Learning English after a child's native (home) language has been established.

bilingual

Children who often speak the parents' native language in the home environment and speak American English in school or other environments.

code switching

An occurrence for bilingual individuals in which sounds, words, semantics, syntactic, or pragmatic elements from one language are included when speaking another language, either automatically or intentionally; also can be expanded to include nonstandard and standard dialects.

phonological, grammatical, syntactic, semantic, and pragmatic system of language (Terrell & Jackson, 2002). AAE is considered a dialect of General American English (GAE) (Seymour & Pearson, 2004). AAE has both verbal and nonverbal aspects, including the use of personal space, body postures and gestures, eye contact, vocal inflections, word choice, and word order. Not all African Americans use AAE and its use is on a continuum that ranges from African Americans who do not use the dialect to those who use most AAE features in all communicative contexts (Wyatt, 2001).

Asian and Pacific Island American

Approximately 3.5% of the U.S. population is Asian and about 1.0% is Native Hawaiian or Pacific Islander (U.S. Census Bureau, 2011). Millions of people from Asian countries (e.g., China, Taiwan, Hong Kong, Japan, Korea, Singapore, Malaysia, Indonesia, India, and Pakistan) and the Pacific Island countries (e.g., Philippines, Guam, Fiji, Samoa, and Hawaii) have immigrated to America over the past 200 years. In addition, since 1975 more than 1 million refugees from Southeast Asia (e.g., Vietnam, Cambodia, Laos, and Thailand) have come to the United States. Asian and Pacific Island countries have diverse and unique languages, cultures, religious beliefs, folk beliefs, worldviews, values, and attitudes toward education and child rearing. Each of these factors, plus the complicated interactions of factors, can profoundly affect the speech-language pathology services we try to provide (Cheng, 2002).

The attitudes of Asian and Pacific Island Americans toward disabilities can be traced in part to folk beliefs, spiritualism, and superstitions. Attitudes range from beliefs that a disability is the result of wrongdoing of an ancestor to an imbalance of inner forces, gods, spirits, or demons. Some cultures believe that a disability is a gift from God, and the person with a disability is then protected and sheltered by the family and community. On the other hand, some cultures view individuals who have obvious disabilities as cursed and ostracize them from society. Treatment of disabilities varies widely among cultures, and Western methods may be counter to Asian religious and cultural beliefs. (For a fascinating and enlightening account of a Hmong child from Laos with cerebral palsy and her parents' struggles with Eastern versus Western medicine and rehabilitation, read Fadiman's 1997 book *The Spirit Catches You and You Fall Down.*)

Native American (American Indians and Indigenous Alaskans)

Native Americans (American Indians and indigenous Alaskans) comprise about 1% of the total U.S. population (U.S. Census Bureau, 2011). Native American societies and cultures vary significantly from one another, as do their languages. Many Native American languages have been lost and some have relatively few speakers (Harrison, 2010). Similar to other ethnic groups, Native Americans have experienced hardships through loss of their ancestral lands, conflicts with mainstream values, and stereo-typing that has resulted in confusion of who they are as a people.

American Indians often bypass professionals and instead choose to use a *medicine man/woman* (a person believed to be able to heal others by making use of supernatural powers) or *shaman* (a spiritual leader who is believed to have special powers such as prophecy and the ability to heal) and healing ceremonies to work through a variety of problems. The *worldviews* (an individual's or group's perception of reality and framework of ideas, beliefs, and attitudes about the world, life, and themselves) of some Native Americans may be considerably different from those of clinicians and may affect understanding of and compliance with therapy (Ryback, Eastin, & Robbins, 2004).

The Influence of Poverty on Language Development

Complicating our work with children from culturally and linguistically diverse backgrounds are the effects of poverty. Many bilingual children in the United States live in low-income families, which increases their risk for language and learning problems, partly because they tend to have limited exposure to both oral and written language (Oller & Pearson, 2002; Rosin, 2006). English language proficiency is an important factor for family economic security and child well-being in at least three ways: (1) limited English language proficiency among both parents and children is associated with poor educational outcomes among children; (2) parents' limited English language proficiency can hamper their ability to communicate effectively with their children and help with their children's English language-related homework; and (3) children for whom English is their second language often have academic and social difficulties in school (Shields & Behrman, 2004; Kindler, 2002).

Children born into poverty are often raised in environments similar to the environments in which their mothers and fathers were raised; that is, with poor nutrition, inadequate stimulation, emotional neglect, and physical danger. There is a culture of poverty, and even children who are born with the potential to develop normal language and communication skills may never realize their potential because of their cultural influences (Kishiyama, Boyce, Jimenez, Perry, & Knight, 2009; Pence & Justice, 2008).

Clinical Application

Clinicians routinely work with children with culturally and linguistically diverse backgrounds to maximize their speech and language development (Roseberry-McKibbin, 2006). In reality, it is not possible for clinicians to have a ready knowledge of each of the hundreds of individual cultures, religious beliefs, folk beliefs, values, and attitudes of the numerous cultures and populations with whom we work. However, it is important for clinicians to become familiar with and develop some functional level of understanding and appreciation of the various cultures of clients and family members with whom they work. As Salas-Provance (2012) emphasizes about working with Native American clients, clinicians need to focus on the people in front of them and not on our expectations of what these people should or should not be. Rapport is achieved by being open, warm, and genuine, and being aware that as clinicians we make mistakes because of our cultural ignorance, and by stating so before mistakes occur. Reading books and other literature on multicultural issues can help clinicians continually expand their multicultural knowledge and understanding (ASHA, 2004).

SPEECH DEVELOPMENT

Child development, including speech development, refers to an increase in complexity—a change from the relatively simple to the more complex and refined. The process involves a sequential progression along an expected continuum that is similar for all children of any culture or language. The rate of development, rather than the sequence, shows great variability among children (Owens, 2012). Speech and language development are intricately interrelated; however, for learning purposes it can be helpful to view them separately.

Speech development may be divided into four stages based on the ages of children and their biological development. Stage I is birth to 12 months; stage II is 12 to 24 months; stage III is 2 to 5 years; and stage IV is 6 to 12 years. Keep in mind that these stages always overlap and that a child emerges into a new stage while merging out of an earlier stage; that is, stages are never discrete (Allen & Marotz, 2007).

Stage I: Birth—12 Months (Infancy)

The foundations for all future speech and language development are built between birth and 6 months of age. From the earliest days of life, newborns absorb information through all of their senses, learning from what they see, hear, touch, taste, and smell. Stage I can be divided into **prelinguistic (preverbal) vocalizations**, birth–6 months and 6–12 months. The months are approximate beginnings and endings for acquisition of both speech and language skills.

Birth–6 Months: Prelinguistic (Preverbal) Vocalizations

Prelinguistic (preverbal) vocalizations are the sounds produced by an infant before the production of true words (e.g., crying, **babbling**, **cooing**, and **echolalia**). The first preverbal vocalization is, ideally, a robust cry at the moment of birth. This cry is important because it begins with a quick and forceful inhalation of air that fills the lungs and closes a valve in the newborn's heart to allow blood to be directed for the first time from the heart to the lungs for oxygenation. The cry is also a **neonate's** first communication—that it is alive and breathing.

prelinguistic (preverbal) vocalizations

The sounds produced by an infant before the production of true words and language (e.g., crying, cooing, babbling, and echolalia).

babbling

The production of a consonant and vowel in the same syllable, either reduplicated *(ba-ba, gaa-gaa)* or nonreduplicated *(baa-da-gi)*, that tends to appear at about 6 or 7 months of age.

cooing

The production of vowel-like sounds (usually /u/ and /oo/ with occasional brief consonant-like sounds similar to /k/ and/g/), usually produced by infants when feeling comfort or pleasure and interacting with a caregiver.

echolalia

An infant's immediate and automatic reproduction or imitation of speech heard from the sounds made by others in the environment; the words infants imitate are not yet meaningful to them.

neonate

A child within the first 28 days after birth.

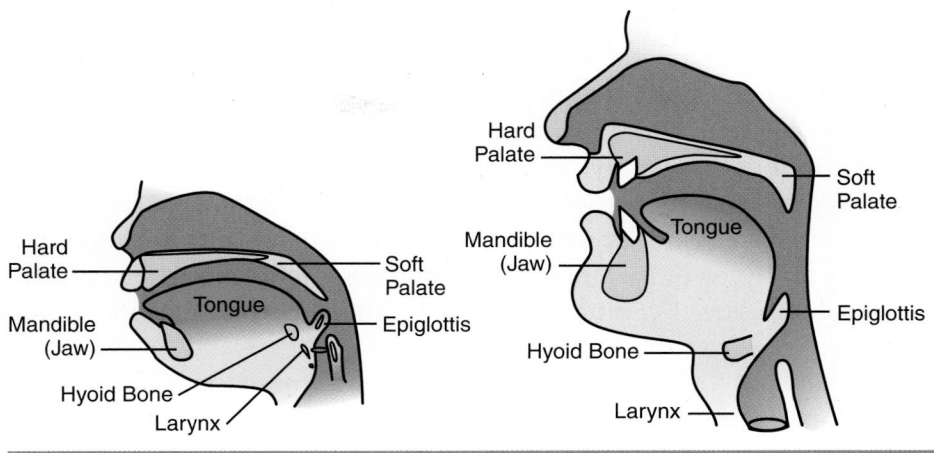

Figure 4–2

Vocal tracts of infants and adults.

© Cengage Learning 2013.

By 2 to 4 months of age infants have begun making cooing and gooing sounds. The consonants infants typically produce are /g/ and /k/, and the vowels are /u/ and /oo/. These sounds are produced in the back of the oral cavity and are easier to produce than other sounds that require more precise movements of the mandible, lips, and tongue in the anterior region of the mouth. The cooing sounds of infants are not intentional forms of communicating with caregivers, although these vocal behaviors usually elicit attention from caregivers followed by closeness, cuddling, and soft, caring speech.

An infant's *vocal tract* (pharyngeal, oral, and nasal cavities) is significantly different from an adult's vocal tract in terms of its size, shape, and location of structures. These differences also play an important role in the sounds an infant can produce (see Figure 4–2). Before about the sixth month of life, an infant does not have control of the movement of the soft palate and, therefore, makes random oral and nasal sounds.

6–12 Months: Prelinguistic (Preverbal) Vocalizations

Between about 6 and 8 months of age infants can produce a variety of vowels and several consonants, although not in a voluntary, intentional manner. They begin to babble and engage in **vocal play** using longer strings of syllables that extend babbling (e.g., *gaga, googoo, baa-da-gi-daa-um-ma*). During vocal play, infants also playfully produce squeals, grunts, screams, growls, and the always entertaining "raspberries." Some children seem to fixate on one particular sound or noise for a few days before moving on to another. If an infant does not babble or begin vocal play by about the eighth month of life, the infant's hearing should be checked by an audiologist. Infants who do not hear well do not receive the enjoyment and motivation of hearing their own babbling and vocal play and, therefore, usually begin decreasing their vocalizations.

After about the sixth month infants have gained some control of the soft palate and can more consistently produce either oral (e.g., *dada*) or nasal (e.g., *mama*) sounds. Over the next several months, an infant's

vocal play

The longer strings of syllables that extend babbling (e.g., *baa-da-gi-daa-um-ma*).

vocal tract begins to more closely resemble the vocal tract of an adult in terms of location and shape of structures, which further changes the acoustic characteristics of the child's sounds. During this time, infants are playing and experimenting with their newly developing ability to make sounds voluntarily. They make sounds when they are happy and are happy when making sounds. They express emotions such as pleasure and displeasure by making different sounds. During the latter part of the first year of life, infants are producing long strings of syllables (consonant–vowel combinations) with different stress and intonation patterns.

Between 8 and 12 months of age, infants are preparing for two major developmental milestones—talking and walking. They are becoming increasingly social and like being the center of attention. Their increasing ability to imitate sounds of adults (*echolalia*) extends their social interactions and helps them develop new skills. During this time the upper and lower front teeth begin to erupt, which also is the time that many mothers wean their infants from nursing and begin feeding them baby (*pureed*) foods. Learning to eat pureed foods may help develop the tongue control that is necessary for developing speech. Better control of the tongue, lips, mandible, and soft palate helps infants develop more precise, rapid, and independent movements needed for articulation.

During this age, infants babble or jabber deliberately to initiate social interaction and shout to attract attention. They babble in sentence-like sequences with inflections as though they are actually talking (sometimes referred to as **jargon**). About 90% of the sounds produced by infants between 11 and 12 months of age are stops (/p, b, t, d, k, g/), nasals (/m, n/), glides (/w, j, h/), and the fricative /s/. It is also during this time that infants begin to say "da-da" and "ma-ma," which parents take as their infant talking to them. Infants are learning that their sounds can control others.

jargon

Strings of syllables produced with stress and intonation that mimic real speech but are not actual words.

Stage II: 12–24 Months (Toddlerhood)

The term *toddlerhood* refers to children learning to stand and walk when they are clumsy and may "toddle" over. We can extend that thought to children's early attempts to speak when they are clumsy with their communicative abilities. Toddlers begin this period of life with the limited abilities of an infant and end with the relatively sophisticated skills of a young child. The first true word emerges about the 12th month of life, and by the 24th month toddlers are typically using two-word sentences to communicate. The ability to stand upright and eventually walk occurs about 12 months of age and allows toddlers to explore their available environments, which significantly expands their world and experiences.

By about 12 months of age, infants express their needs and wants through vocalization and gestures. An infant's first words mark the beginning of a transition from preverbal to verbal communication (Pence-Turnbull & Justice, 2012). The designation of "true" word is not always easy to agree upon. From a parent's point of view, the first time an infant says "mama" or "dada" the infant is using intentional and meaningful speech (true words to the parents). However, a vocalization is considered a true word only if it meets three specific criteria (Locke, 1993):

1. A word must be uttered with a clear intention and purpose. For example, when an infant or toddler is petting a cat and says "kitty," it is a clear intention and purpose that it is in reference to the cat. If a parent tells the child to say "kitty" and the child does, it is considered an imitation or repetition rather than a true word.

2. A true word must be recognizably close to an adult's pronunciation of the word. For example, if a child says "itty-itty" for "kitty-kitty," most adults would recognize the child's word as a good attempt at saying the word correctly. However, if a child uses a consistent but not close approximation (e.g., *ga-ku-me*) for "kitty," it would not be considered a true word.

3. A true word is used consistently by a child in various contexts. For example, if a child only uses *itty* for the family cat but does not use *itty* for other cats, for pictures of cats, or upon hearing a cat's meow, then the use of *itty* would not have a symbolic reference in addition to its specific reference to the family cat.

Phonologically, children's first true words are typically characterized by simple syllables, such as consonant–vowel (CV), vowel–consonant (VC), vowel–consonant–vowel (VCV), or consonant–vowel–consonant–vowel (CVCV) combinations. The sound combinations are usually stops, nasals, and glides—the same combinations used in the late babbling period (/k, g, t, d, p, b, m, n, w, h/). The preferred vowels tend to be /i, a, u/. However, from a speech development perspective, words such as *mommy, daddy, ba* (ball), *ca* (car), *goggy* (doggy), *iddy* (kitty), and *uss* (juice) are more likely to be considered true words than the first productions of *mama* or *dada*. By toddlerhood, children have emerged from prelinguistic vocalizations into linguistic communication. It is important to remember that after toddlers say their first true words, most of their vocalizations continue to be babbling. That is, during vocalizations there is a mixture of true words and babbling, with babbling eventually decreasing and being replaced with true words.

By about 18 months of age children usually can say approximately 50 words that are intelligible to parents and most other people. Even though children may produce a variety of CVC words, the final consonant is still often omitted, with the actual production of the word being a CV combination and the listener "filling in" the final consonant. The final consonant in a CVC word usually begins to emerge around 18 months and is typically the /t/ sound (e.g., *cat*). Three-syllable words are often reduced to two syllables; for example, *banana* (ba-nan-a) becomes *nana*, where the unstressed syllable of the word (e.g., *ba-*) is omitted and the **stressed** syllables *(-nana)* become the child's production of the word.

Between 18 and 24 months of age, children begin to use two-word sentences that are generally intelligible, particularly if the context is

stress

Variations in intensity, frequency, and duration on one syllable more than another in a word, which usually results in the syllable sounding both louder and longer than other syllables in the same word.

known, for example, "More juice," "Daddy go," and "Where mommy?" By 24 months of age, children are more consistently producing a variety of final consonants, including /t, p, k, n/ and sometimes /r/ and /s/. As children are developing intelligible sequences of sounds and words, they are developing the rules for combining phonemes to produce intelligible words that convey information. By 2 years of age, most children are approximately 25–50% intelligible to adults (Locke, 1993).

Stage III: 2–5 Years (Early Childhood)

The differences between a 2-year-old and a 5-year-old child are like night and day. A 2-year-old's speech is usually understandable when the context is known. However, by 5 years of age, most children develop adult-like speech that is approximately 90% intelligible to both familiar and unfamiliar listeners. Although these years are considered early childhood, they may be more specifically classified as early-early childhood (2-year-olds), middle-early childhood (3- and 4-year-olds), and late-early childhood (5-year-olds).

2-Year-Olds (Early-Early Childhood)

Two-year-olds no longer rely on pointing and gestures as primary forms of communication. They use their limited speech and language to communicate their wants, needs, thoughts, and feelings—and they feel strongly about many things. Many of the speech sounds have emerged or are well established and they are usually about 75% intelligible in their two- to three-word sentences. Two-year-olds can use their voice and articulators to produce unstressed syllables in the initial position of words (e.g., they can produce both the unstressed *ba* and the stressed *nana* in the word *banana*). Secord and Donohue (2002), in their *Clinical Assessment of Articulation and Phonology,* used the developmental age norms shown in Table 4–1.

TABLE 4–1 Clinical Assessment of Articulation and Phonology

	STOPS						NASALS			GLIDES		FRICATIVES									AFFRICATES		LIQUIDS		
Age of Mastery*	p	b	t	d	k	g	m	n	ŋ	w	j	h	f	v	s	z	ʃ	ʒ	θ	ð	tʃ	dʒ	l	ɾ	ɚ
75%	2	2	2	2	2	2	2	2	2	2	2	2	3	3	3	3	3	3	6	5	3	3	3	4	3
95%	2	3	3	2	3	3	2	2	4	2	4	2	4	5	5	5	5	6	8	7	5	5	5	6	6

*Age when 75% or 95% of children mastered the sound.
Based on data from Secord and Donohue (2002).

3- and 4-Year-Olds (Middle-Early Childhood)

Vowel development is mostly completed by 3 years of age. Several consonants are considered established by age 3 (e.g., /m, n, p, b, d, k, g, h, f, w/), some of which children have been using since the babbling stage but not in a voluntary, intentionally produced manner. In general, sounds typically acquired by children by the end of 3 years of age are *early developing sounds* and sounds typically acquired after 3 years of age are *later developing sounds* (Bauman-Waengler, 2009). Children this age typically speak in three- to four-word sentences that are approximately 90% intelligible.

Four-year-old children are at least 95% intelligible, even though several sounds and most blends have not yet emerged or fully developed. It is not surprising, however, that children's speech is about as clear and well articulated as the adults' around them. Adult listeners fill in the sounds omitted or mispronounced by children to easily understand their speech. It is interesting, if not somewhat surprising, how easily children learn to understand the often-slurred speech of other children and even adults. Adults say many things for which listeners must fill in the sounds to make complete words and sentences, for example, "g'nai" (Good night) or "djaeet?" (Did you eat?).

5-Year-Olds (Late-Early Childhood)

Most speech sounds have emerged or are fully developed by age 5, although some sounds may not yet be completely and consistently established for some children until age 6 to 8 years of age (e.g., /r, l, s, z, sh, ch, dz, j, v/ "ng", "th", and **blends**) (see Figure 4–3). Many children this age begin to lose their front teeth, which affects the production of some sounds that may be emerging or already acquired (e.g., /s, z/). Speech is at least 95% intelligible even though some consonants and blends are not yet fully developed (e.g., /r, l/, /tr, spl, skw/).

Phonological Processes

Children younger than about 4½ years of age may not have sufficient ability to fully coordinate the movements of the vocal folds, soft palate, and each of the articulators. As a consequence, certain sounds, sound combinations or transitions from one sound to another may be too difficult for them. Young children may, therefore, simplify the production of some words (Williamson, 2010). These simplifications are common in the speech development of children across languages and are called **natural processes** or **phonological processes**. There are three common natural processes: (a) *syllable structure processes* describe changes that affect the structure of the syllable; (b) *substitution processes* for sound modifications in which one sound class (e.g., plosive) is replaced by another; and (c) *assimilatory processes* in which a sound is influenced by a neighboring sound in a word (Bauman-Waengler, 2009).

Five-year-olds are often still confused or have not learned the numerous changes in vowel productions with variations of words (e.g., *nature*

blend (consonant cluster)

A blend or consonant cluster occurs when two or more sounds appear together with no vowel separation (e.g., /tr, sp, bl, str, spl, str, skw/).

natural processes

The processes that are common in the speech development of children across languages.

phonological processes

The simplification of sounds that are difficult for children to produce in an adult manner; phonological processes help explain errors of substitution, omission, and addition that children may use to simplify the production of difficult sounds.

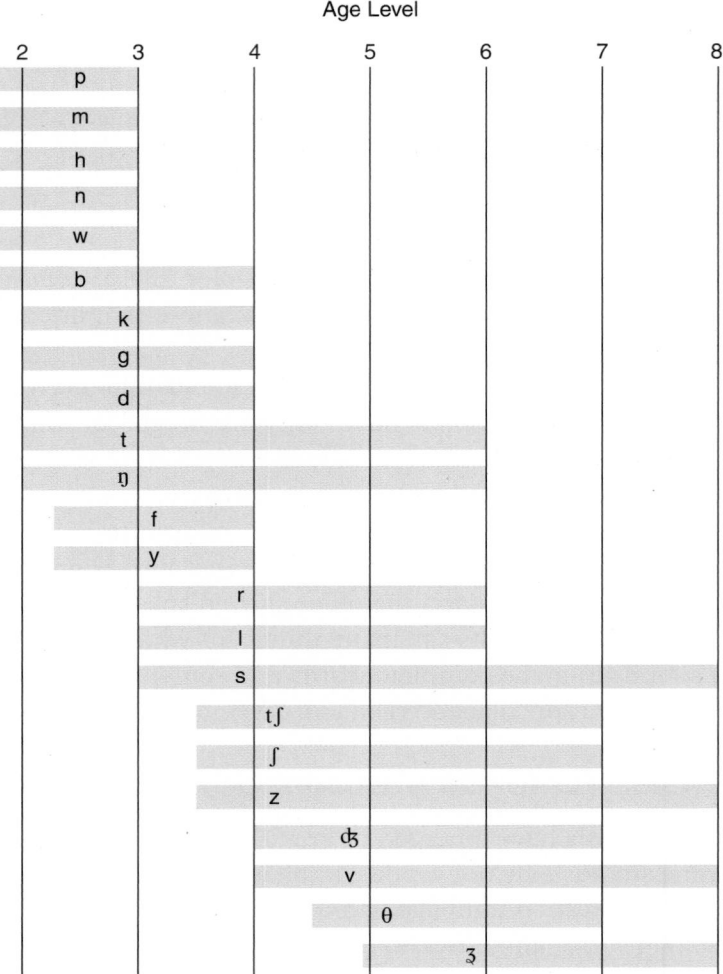

Figure 4–3

Sander's 1972 customary ages of production of English consonants.

Source: Sander, E. K. (1972). When are speech sounds learned? *Journal of Speech and Hearing Disorders, 37,* 62. Copyright 1972 by American Speech-Language-Hearing Association. Reprinted with permission.

versus n*a*tural and expl*a*in versus expl*a*nation). They are able to appropriately place stress on syllables in multisyllabic words (e.g., *happi*ness and *uncomfor*table) and on compound words (e.g., *WHITEhouse,* a noun) versus adjective–noun combinations (e.g., *white HOUSE*).

Stage IV: 6–12 Years (Middle Childhood to Early Adolescence)

When children enter stage IV, they are still very much children but they end as preteens, with the early signs of adolescence developing. At the beginning of stage IV many children have already been in nursery or preschool for a few years and are now entering kindergarten. At the end of this stage, they will be in junior high school.

Most children who are 6, 7, and 8 years of age are 95–100% intelligible, even though some later developing sounds and blends may still not be articulated clearly. Children who are 9, 10, 11, and 12 years old have mastered speech. They communicate easily and freely with people of all ages and adjust their communication to the age of the individual they are talking to; for example, they use early childhood speech with young children, slang and profanity with peers, and mature speech with older adults. This is an important step in pragmatics.

LANGUAGE DEVELOPMENT

For normal communication to develop, there must be an integration of three elements: (1) biological structures and functions must develop within normal limits; (2) cognitive functioning must be sufficient for language skills to emerge and be cultivated; and (3) social interaction (usually with parents or other caregivers) must be sufficient for infants and children to be encouraged and rewarded for communication attempts. As with speech development, language development may be divided into four stages based on the chronological ages of children: Stage I is birth to 12 months (further divided into birth to 6 months and 6 to 12 months); stage II is 12 to 24 months; stage III is 2 to 5 years; and stage IV is 6 to 12 years. Although the ages of the stages are discrete, the developmental levels are not; children merge into the next stage of development.

Stage I: Birth–12 Months (Infancy)

Language development begins in the earliest weeks and months of life. The five senses (sight, hearing, touch, taste, and smell) are the sources of stimuli from the environment that the infant responds to. Every new stimulus helps create new neural pathways and connections in the brain. When the environment is stimulating the language centers of the brain (as well as all other areas of the brain) are "primed" with millions (billions) of connections of neurons and synapses that can eventually be used to form concepts for language.

Sensory and Emotional Deprivation

Infants who have been deprived of sensory stimulation during their early months of life and into toddlerhood have difficulty ever developing normal cognitive–linguistic abilities, as well as emotional and social bonds. In some parts of the world, infant and child sensory deprivation is common. Some orphanages "warehouse" infants and children, keeping them in cribs for years with minimal nourishment and lack of emotional caring and socialization; the only stimulation is primarily self-stimulation. They learn that their whimpering and cries do not bring them attention or comforting.

Some of these infants and children are rescued and adopted by families from other countries. The adoptive parents often feel that all these infants or children need is "a lot of love and they will come around." However, when neural circuits for attachment and loving care are not established during infancy, it is difficult for them to be cultivated later in life for normal emotional and social bonding (attachment) to develop. For more information about development of emotions, read Goleman's (1995) *Emotional Intelligence: Why It Can Matter More Than IQ.*

Birth–6 Months: Prelinguistic (Preverbal) Vocalizations

The primary sensory systems of infants are vision, hearing, taste, and smell. Tactile sensation is less developed, which goes along with their relatively poorly developed motor system. As their first year progresses, they begin integrating their senses by coordinating the use of their hands, mouth, and eyes to explore their own bodies, toys, and surroundings. After visually inspecting objects, they like to put them in their mouths because taste and smell are two of their strongest senses during this time.

The reflexive crying and vegetative grunts and other such sounds may communicate something to parents, but they are often just educated guesses as to what the infant wants or needs. The infant's body and limb movements are generally random without much specific intention, other than to withdraw from an unwanted stimulus or to move toward a wanted stimulus. The cooing and gooing sounds made by infants begin as reflexive and later develop into more intentionally produced sounds. When the sounds become intentionally produced to draw or hold a parent's attention, infants may be using their first verbal expressive language.

6–12 Months: Prelinguistic (Preverbal) Vocalizations

The early months of life created neural pathways that now become knowledge about the environment—the objects and people in it. Infants have an affinity for certain objects, toys, and sounds, as well as the familiar people they see and voices they hear. They also learn how to obtain what they want by whimpering or crying until food or a favorite toy is given to them, or smiling and giggling to keep an adult's attention (all ways of communicating). During the first year of life, infants form attachments (emotional bonds) to people and seek stimulation and comfort from them (Peluso, et al., 2004).

In the latter half of their first year, infants are using their facial expressions and body language to communicate turn-taking (e.g., giving or taking a toy) and parents begin to feel that their child is becoming a true partner in their interactions. Infants this age may be trying to communicate more than what parents and other caregivers think they are because the adults in the environment are not able to consistently and accurately interpret the infants' verbal (jargon) and nonverbal (facial expressions, body and limb movements) messages.

Language Development of Visually Impaired Children

Most students of speech-language pathology probably think more about the effects of a hearing impairment on a child's speech and language development than the effects of a visual impairment. The American Foundation for the Blind recommends the term *blind* be used to refer to individuals with no usable sight. Individuals with even minimal usable vision are referred to as *visually impaired, partially sighted,* or *low visioned.* Congenital blindness is rare compared to visual impairments, and both of these are rare compared to congenital hearing impairments. The following discussion will refer to children who are severely visually impaired or blind.

Application Question

What could you do as a new parent to encourage language development of your infant?

The language development of children who are severely visually impaired or blind is neither delayed nor deviant; rather, an alternative route of language acquisition is followed. Children with severe visual impairments rely on auditory and tactile resources more fully than do children with normal sight. Infants with severe visual impairments cannot make eye contact or use eye gaze to interact with parents, so they must rely on auditory and tactile cues. They need active encouragement to vocalize, which serves as an emotional link to the parents and an important sensory experience for the infant (Perez-Pereira & Conti-Ramsden, 1999).

The onset of meaningful speech occurs slightly later for children with severe visual impairments than for children with normal vision. Children with severe visual impairments tend to have a narrow use of words rather than generalizing or overextending them (e.g., anything round is a ball), as is typical of normally visioned children. Objects that cannot be directly touched are named or requested less often by children who are severely visually impaired. They usually are slower to develop some basic concepts that require vision, such as *clean, dirty, open, shut, in, out, up,* and *down.*

Action words may be used only to refer to things they are doing and not to the actions of others (actions they cannot see). They are slightly delayed in using two- and three-word combinations, but by the end of the third year the average number of morphemes they use in an **utterance** is comparable to sighted children. Visually impaired children tend to echo phrases of others before they can use the syntax voluntarily. They have difficulty understanding and using words such as *here, there, this,* and *that,* although by age 7 they usually have these words mastered (Landau & Gleitman, 1985).

Severely visually impaired children tend to use rising voice intonation to maintain a person's attention and interaction, and sighted children typically use eye contact. Visually impaired children tend to talk louder than necessary because they cannot judge the distance of their listener. They tend to nod their heads less often but smile more often. Some facial expressions may not match their sound and word meanings.

Overall, language development in children who have severe visual impairments or are blind cannot always be judged accurately by comparing them to normally sighted children. However, children with visual impairments may have all of the same phonological, morphological, syntactic, semantic, and pragmatic problems of other children, plus unique developmental differences. Therapeutically, the challenge for speech-language pathologists with these children is that we cannot use the visual modality that we so often rely on, particularly for teaching articulator placement for correct sound production and language therapy.

utterance

A unit of vocal expression preceded and followed by a pause or silence; may be a single sound, word, phrase, or sentence.

Application Question

Have you ever considered what it would be like to work with visually impaired children? Would you consider someday working with this population? What do you imagine some challenges would be working as a clinician with children who have both hearing and visual acuity impairments?

Stage II: 12–24 Months (Toddlerhood)

Toddlerhood allows children to explore their environment more independently because of their increased *ambulatory* (walking) and general motor skills. If something will not come to the toddler, the toddler may be able to go to it. Every new perception and sensation that enters the toddler's brain may be stored for further language development.

Toddlers like to attach words to the new things they are exploring and, therefore, have dramatic increases in receptive and expressive language abilities. Toddlers can understand more than they can express, particularly when spoken to at a moderate rate and with one- or two-syllable words that are in short (three- to five-word) sentences. It is important to understand that the early expressive language of young children is built on what they have experienced and know of their world; that is, children must first experience objects, events, or relationships and understand the words that relate to them before they can use the words meaningfully in expressive language.

Between 12 and 18 months of age children usually have an expressive vocabulary (**lexicon**) of approximately 50 words. They use one word to convey an entire thought; that is, they use one-word sentences (**holophrastic language**) such as "uus" for "I want some juice." The most typical forms of early words are common nouns such as *ball (ba)*, *milk, doggie, mommy, baby,* and *car (ca)*. Toddlers learn to use action words, such as *go, bye-bye,* and *look;* modifiers, such as *red, pretty,* and *hot;* and personal–social words, such as *no, want,* and *please (pweez)*. Between 12 and 26 months normally developing children begin using one-word utterances with a rising inflection to ask yes-or-no questions; for example, they may say "juice?" as in "Am I going to get some juice now?"

By 18 to 24 months of age, children begin to use two-word utterances, which significantly decrease the ambiguity of a child's communication. For example, when a child says "Mommy" there are any number of possible references; however, when the child says "Mommy home," "Mommy go," or "Mommy hurt," the listener has a better idea of the child's meaning. **Communicative competence** increases significantly with two-word utterances. A toddler can more easily communicate requests ("More milk."), negation ("No more!"), and commentary ("Me home!"). Children this age also begin to use grammatical morphemes such as articles (*a, the*), copulas (*is, be*), and auxiliary verbs (*have, can*) to make their utterances longer and more complex.

Brown (1973) investigated the **mean length of utterance (MLU)** of young children's language by counting the number of morphemes (not individual words) they used in single utterances. Brown viewed language as developing in five stages, with an increase of one morpheme per stage (see Table 4–2).

Stage III: 2–5 Years (Early Childhood)

Following toddlerhood, the next few years of life help prepare children cognitively and communicatively for beginning school. Between 2 and 5 years of age, dramatic changes occur in all aspects of children's development. Although these years are considered early childhood, they may

---

lexicon

Refers to all morphemes, including words and parts of words, that a person knows.

holophrastic language

The use of a single word to express a complete thought.

communicative competence

A child's grammatical knowledge of phonology, morphology, syntax, semantics, and pragmatics.

mean length of utterance (MLU)

The average number of morphemes in a young child's individual utterances; generally equivalent to a child's chronological age.

TABLE 4-2	Brown's Stages of Language Development			
STAGES	**CHARACTERIZED BY**	**FEATURES**	**EXAMPLES**
Stage I MLU: 1.0–2.0 Age 12–26 months	First words; semantic roles expressed in simple sentences	Single-word utterances; Combining semantic roles.	Naming significant objects, persons, and events in their daily experiences (*cup, spoon, Mommy, Daddy,* etc.) Agent + Action, Action + Object, Action + Location, Entity + Location, Entity + Attribute, Demonstrative + Attribute.
Stage II MLU: 2.0–2.5 Age 27–30 months	Modulation of meaning	Emerging of grammatical morphemes	Present progressive (*-ing*), prepositions (*in, on*), plural(*-s*), Irregular past (e.g., *ran, ate*), possessive (*-'s*), articles (*a, the*), regular past (*-ed*), third person regular, third person irregular, auxiliary and copula verbs (*is, are, was, were*).
Stage III MLU: 2.5–3.0 Age 31–34 months	Development of sentence form	Noun phrase elaboration and auxiliary development	Noun phrases elaborated in subject and object positions (*Big boy running fast, Billy ate my cookie*). Auxiliary verbs allow more mature interrogatives and negatives.
Stage IV MLU: 3.0–3.75 Age 35–40 months	Emergence of complex sentences	Embedding sentence elements	Object noun phrase complements (*I know you are my friend*); bedded with questions (*I know who is hiding*); relative clauses (*I helped boy who is nice*).
Stage V MLU: 3.75–4.50 Age 41–46 months	Emergence of compound sentences	Conjoining sentences	Conjoining two simple sentences (*I have a book and you have a toy*).

Adapted from *A First Language: The Early Stages* by R. Brown, 1973. Cambridge MA: Harvard University Press. In McLaughlin, 2006.

be more specifically classified as early-early childhood (2-year-olds), middle-early childhood (3- and 4-year-olds), and late-early childhood (5-year-olds).

2-Year-Olds (Early-Early Childhood)

Two-year-olds understand much of what is said to them when spoken in simple, clear sentences. They love being read to, especially if allowed to turn the pages and point to different objects in pictures. Remarkable growth occurs in their abilities to understand what they hear and to communicate their many thoughts and experiences in simple sentences. They understand more than they can express; however, they like to communicate whatever fleeting thoughts they have. By the end of their second year, 2-year-olds have vocabularies of approximately 300 words; nevertheless, their favorite word tends to be "No!" They often have definite opinions about what they like and do not like, what they want and do not want—and what they want, they want *right now.* When they do not get what they want, they may communicate their displeasure with temper tantrums.

3- and 4-Year-Olds (Middle-Early Childhood)

Three-year-old children understand most of what is said to them; if one or two words are not familiar to them, they can usually figure them out from the context. Their receptive vocabularies are growing faster than their expressive vocabularies. Children this age begin to learn that more than one word can mean the same thing (*little, small, tiny*), but they tend to use one word rather than alternative words to express themselves. Children brought up in homes in which parents or other caregivers use a variety of synonyms benefit from the increased language exposure. This is an important reason for parents and caregivers to engage in **parallel speech**—that is, naming, describing, and explaining what the child is experiencing and probably feeling, almost as if the caregiver is the child. For example, "Mommy is turning on the bathroom light now. Now it is really bright in the bathroom. Mommy is turning on the faucet to wash your hands. The water is cold at first but it will warm up and feel good when I'm washing your hands." Parallel speech provides language and concepts for a child when the child does not have the language or concepts for **inner speech**. Parallel speech can help the child's speech, language, and **cognitive development**.

By the end of their third year children may have a 1,000-word vocabulary that they use in their typical 3-word sentences. Sentences used by 3-year-old children often omit the **functor (function) words**, such as articles (*a, the*), conjunctions (*and, but*), determiners (*this, that*), prepositions (*in, on,* etc.), and auxiliary verbs (*have, had*). This omission results in **telegraphic speech (language)**; that is, only the essential nouns, verbs, and adjectives are used. This is also a time when learning grammar and syntactical rules becomes increasingly important to convey meaning (Eisenberg, Guo, & Germezia, 2012). Children learn basic word order to convey simple messages, such as subject/verb/direct object (*"Mommy spill juice."*); subject/verb/indirect object (*"Girl go home."*); and subject/verb/subject complement (*"Boy run fast."*). Later they learn that when the subject and the auxiliary or helping verb are reversed in order, the sentence is changed into a question (*"Is the boy running fast?"*).

Three- and four-year-old children have developed several *grammatical morphemes,* such as *-ing* (eating), *-s* (shoes), *-'s* (baby's), *-ed* (jumped), and others. They begin using **narratives** for relating events and making up stories, but often without including the essential *who, what, when, where,* and *how* information, leaving listeners uncertain or confused. **Discourse** becomes part of 4-year-olds' communication abilities, with children relating long and intertwined stories.

Conversations demonstrate an organizational structure based on such elements as *initiation of topics*, *turn-taking*, and *topic maintenance* (staying on a topic) and *repairs* (rewording or restating an utterance that was not understood); that is, good pragmatics. Normal conversation adheres to the *cooperation principles* (Grice, 1975). That is, each participant must (1) include an appropriate *quantity* of information that is (2) of adequate *quality* and truthfulness, is (3) *relevant* to the established topic, and is (4) delivered in a *manner* that is clear and understandable. Through interactions with adults, young children learn these conversation or cooperation principles, and some become adept with conversation, also contributing to pragmatic skills.

discourse

An extended verbal exchange on a topic (i.e., a conversation or long narrative).

5-Year-Olds (Late-Early Childhood)

Five-year-olds have the foundations of language from which all other language development is built. Children this age have learned to use functor words and grammatical morphemes, but still most of their sentences are declarative sentence forms or basic questions. Children begin refining and using more adult sentence structure that can better communicate the increasing subtleties of their messages. Children primarily use the contracted forms of many words (*can't, won't, don't, wouldn't, shouldn't, couldn't,* etc.) but have not learned the uncontracted forms (*cannot, will not,* etc.). It is sometimes surprising to clinicians that even children who do not have language development problems do not know the uncontracted forms and need to be taught the words.

Stage IV: 6–12 Years (Middle Childhood to Early Adolescence)

6-, 7-, and 8-Year-Olds

Middle childhood is a continual evolution of more complex and elaborate forms of language use. Children are increasingly using compound and complex sentences, passive sentences, and a variety of morphemes that may be used with *root* (base) words. Language is their tool for learning, and when they have language problems, they have learning problems.

9- and 10-Year-Olds

Nine- and 10-year-old children continue to develop increased language complexity as well as social and pragmatic skills. During these years, children gradually develop more awareness and insight into the effects of their language on others. Children are now "reading between the lines" of what others say. They often do not take statements at face value but increasingly interpret them from a personal perspective, asking, "What do you mean by *that*?" to even the most innocuous statements or questions, particularly from parents.

By the preteen years children ideally have developed their receptive and expressive language abilities to prepare them for high school and more advanced education if they choose. Their communication abilities will likely determine much of their educational success, social success, and future employment success. Speech and language are learned to communicate our wants, needs, thoughts, knowledge, and feelings with increasing accuracy and ease.

11- and 12-Year-Olds

During early adolescence children continue to develop language. However, as language demands at school are increasing in areas of both comprehension and expression, children who have borderline skills have increasing problems with academics and interactions with others. Adolescence is a peak period for learning and using *figurative language*, including idioms, metaphors and similes, and verbal humor that is often based on ambiguities and double meanings (being able to take a word or statement more than one way). Slang and jargon (which seem to be the foundation of many teenagers' social communication) are based primarily on figurative language. Competence in figurative language is important (if not essential) for peer acceptance and the social lives of teenagers.

CHAPTER SUMMARY

From the earliest days of life newborns absorb information through all of their senses. Speech development allows children to begin communicating with caregivers about their wants, needs, and feelings. The first 6 months of life lay the foundations for speech and language development. Speech development continues well after the beginning of the early school years. Language development is a long and complex process that all children must go through to develop communication skills in whatever native language they learn. The stages of language development are predictable, but each child has an individual rate of development. By knowing the language expectations of the various stages, parents and clinicians may have impressions of a child's development and whether it is at or near what is expected for the child's chronological age.

STUDY QUESTIONS

Knowledge and Comprehension

1. What is babbling and at what age does it normally begin?
2. What are three criteria for an infant's vocalization to be considered a true word?
3. By what age are most children using adult-like speech?
4. What three elements must be integrated to develop normal communication?
5. What is the *mean length of utterance*?

Application

1. How could knowing the age ranges and sequence of speech and language development help clinicians determine whether a child is developing speech and language at a normal rate?

2. Why should parents be concerned and what should they do if their infant does not begin to babble within the normal age range?

3. What can parents and other caregivers do regularly that can help children's speech and language development?

4. What could be the effects of a child not having a stimulating language environment?

5. Discuss the importance of children developing the ability to communicate their wants, needs, thoughts, information, and feelings to other children and to adults.

Analysis/Synthesis

1. How could knowing various theories of speech and language development help you understand a child's speech and language problems?

2. What is the relationship between speech development and language development?

3. Discuss the possible effects of an infant's severe hearing impairment on the development of speech and language.

4. Discuss the importance of a child developing narrative and discourse language abilities.

5. Discuss the cooperation principles and their importance in a child's language development.

REFERENCES

Allen, K. E., & Marotz, L. R. (2007). *Developmental profiles: Pre-birth through twelve*. Belmont, CA: Wadsworth Cengage Learning.

American Speech-Language-Hearing Association. (2004). Knowledge and skills needed by speech-language pathologists and audiologists to provide culturally and linguistically appropriate services. *The ASHA Leader, 24 (Supplement)*.

Battle, D. (2002). *Communication disorders in multicultural populations* (3rd ed.). Boston, MA: Butterworth-Heinemann.

Bauman-Waengler, J. (2009). *Introduction to phonetics and phonology: From concepts to transcription*. Boston, MA: Pearson.

Berko-Gleason, J. (Ed.). (2001). *The development of language* (5th ed.). Boston, MA: Allyn and Bacon.

Bloom, L., & Lahey, M. (1978). *Language development and language disorders*. New York, NY: John Wiley.

Brown, R. (1973). *A first language: The early stages.* Cambridge, MA: Harvard University Press.

Cheng, L. (2002). Asian and Pacific American cultures. In D. E. Battle (Ed.). *Communication disorders in multicultural populations* (3rd ed.). Boston, MA: Butterworth-Heinemann.

Crystal, D. (2010). *The Cambridge encyclopedia of language* (3rd ed.). Cambridge, MA: Cambridge University Press.

Eisenberg, S. L., Guo, L., & Germezia, M. (2012). *How grammatical are 3-year-olds? Language, Speech, and Hearing Services in the Schools, 43,* 36–52.

Fadiman, A. (1997). *The Spirit Catches You and You Fall Down.* New York, NY: Farrar, Straus and Giroux.

Goleman, D. (1995). *Emotional intelligence: Why it can matter more than IQ.* New York, NY: Bantam Books.

Grice, H. P. (1975). Logic and conversation. In P. Cole & J. Morgan (Eds.), *Syntax and semantics: Speech acts.* New York, NY: Academic Press.

Hammer, C., Miccio, A. W., & Wagstaff, D. (2003). Home literacy experiences and their relationship to bilingual preschoolers' developing English literacy abilities: An initial investigation. *Language, Speech, and Hearing Services in Schools, 34,* 20–30.

Harrison, K . D. (2010). *The last speakers: The quest to save the world's most endangered languages.* Washington, D.C.: National Geographic Society.

Hulit, L. M., Howard, M. R., & Fahey, K. R. (2011). *Born to talk: An introduction to speech and language development* (5th ed.). Boston, MA: Allyn and Bacon.

James, S. (1960). *Normal language acquisition.* Boston, MA: Little Brown.

Kindler, A. (2002). *Survey of the states' limited English proficient students and available educational programs and services.* Washington, DC: National Clearinghouse for English Language.

Kishiyama, M. M., Boyce, W. T., Jimenez, A. M., Perry, L. M., & Knight, R. T. (2009). Socioeconomic disparities affect prefrontal function in children. *Journal of Cognitive Neuroscience, 21*(6), 1106–1115.

Landau, B. & Gleitman, L. R. (1985). *Language and experience: Evidence from the blind child.* Cambridge, MA: Harvard University Press.

Locke, J. L. (1993). *The child's path to spoken language.* Cambridge, MA: Harvard University Press.

McLaughlin, S. F. (2006). *Introduction to language development* (2nd ed.). Clifton Park, NY: Delmar Cengage Learning.

Oller, D. K., & Pearson, B. (2002). Assessing the effects of bilingualism: A background. In D. K. Oller & R. Eilers (Eds.), *Language and literacy in bilingual children.* Clevedon, England: Multilingual Matters.

Owens, R. E., Jr. (2012). *Language development: An introduction* (8th ed.). San Antonio, TX: Pearson/Allyn & Bacon.

Peluso, P. R., Peluso, J. P., Kern, R. M., White, J. A. (2004). *A comparison of attachment theory and individual psychology: A review of the literature. Journal of Counseling and Development, 83*(2), 139–145.

Pence-Turnbull, K. L., & Justice, L. M. (2012). *Language development from theory to practice* (2nd ed.). Upper Saddle River, NJ: Pearson Prentice Hall.

Perez-Pereira, M., & Conti-Ramsden, G. (1999). *Language development and social interactions in blind children*. Hove, England: Psychology Press.

Pinker, S. (1984). *Language, learnability, and language development*. Cambridge, MA: Harvard University Press.

Roseberry-McKibbin, C. (2006). *Language disorders in children: A multicultural and case perspective*. Boston, MA: Allyn and Bacon.

Roseberry-McKibbin, C. (2008). *Multicultural students with special language needs: Practical strategies for assessment and intervention* (3rd ed.). Oceanside, CA: Academic Communication Associates.

Rosin, P. (2006). Literacy intervention in culturally and linguistically diverse worlds: The Linking Language and Literacy Project. In L. M. Justice (Ed.). *Clinical approaches to emergent literacy intervention*. San Diego, CA: Plural Publishing.

Ryback, C., Eastin, C. L., & Robbins, I. (2004). Native American healing practices and counseling. *Journal of Humanistic Counseling, Education, and Development, 43*(1), 25–33.

Salas-Provance, M. (2012). Counseling in a multicultural society: Implications for the field of communicative disorders. In L. V. Flasher & P. T. Fogle, *Counseling skills for speech-language pathologists and audiologists*. Clifton Park, NY: Delmar Cengage Learning.

Sander, E. K. (1972). When are speech sounds learned? *Journal of Speech and Language Disorders, 37*, 62.

Secord, W. A., & Donohue, J. S. (2002). *Clinical assessment of articulation and phonology*. Greenville, SC: Super Duper.

Seymour, H. N., & Pearson, B. (2004). Evaluating language variation: Distinguishing dialect and development from disorder. *Seminars in Speech and Language, 25*(1), 18–26.

Shields, M. K., & Behrman, R. E. (2004). Children of immigrant families: Analysis and recommendations. *The Future of Children, 14*(2), 4–15.

Terrell, S. L., & Jackson, R. S. (2002). African Americans in the Americas. In D. E. Battle (Ed.), *Communication disorders in multicultural populations* (3rd ed.). Boston, MA: Butterworth-Heinemann.

U.S. Census Bureau. (2011). *Statistical abstract of the United States: 2012* (130th ed.). Washington, DC: U.S. Census Bureau.

Willamson, G. (2010). *Phonological processes: Natural ways of simplifying speech production*. London, England: Speech Therapy Information and Resources.

Wyatt, T. A. (2001). *The role of the family, community, and school in children's acquisition and maintenance of African American English: Sociocultural and historical contexts of African American English*. Amsterdam, Netherlands/Philadelphia, PA: John Benjamin Publishing.

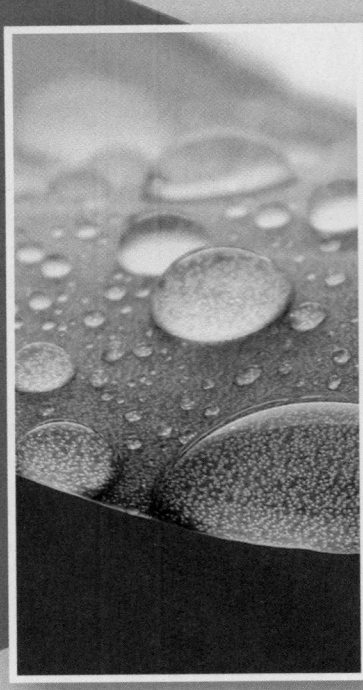

CHAPTER 5
Articulation and Phonological Disorders in Children

LEARNING OBJECTIVES

After studying this chapter, you will:

- Be able to discuss vowels and consonants and how they are produced.
- Be able to discuss the etiologies of articulation and phonological disorders.
- Understand the essentials of articulation disorders.
- Understand the essentials of phonological disorders.
- Understand the essentials of childhood motor speech disorders.
- Be able to discuss the assessment of articulation and phonology.
- Be able to discuss the general principles of therapy for articulation and phonological disorders.
- Be familiar with multicultural considerations of children with articulation and phonological disorders.
- Appreciate the emotional and social effects of articulation and phonological disorders on children.

KEY TERMS

addition
allophone
anoxia
auditory
    discrimination
    training
    (ear training)
bilabial
cerebral palsy

childhood apraxia
    of speech (CAS)
cognate
diadochokinetic
    (diadochokinesis,
    diadochols)
diphthong
distinctive feature
distortion

dysarthria
failure to thrive
frenum/frenulum
fricative
functional
gavage feeding
generalization
glide

KEY TERMS continued

hypertonicity

hypotonicity

idiopathic

infantile hypoxia

International
   Phonetic
   Alphabet (IPA)

labiodental

letter

linguadental
   (interdental)

linguapalatal

linguavelar

low birth weight

manner

multifactorial

nasal

nasogastric (NG) tube

omission

organic

perinatal

perseverate/
   perseveration

phonetics

place

positive
   reinforcement
   (positive
   feedback,
   reward)

premature

sensorimotor

sibilant

significant

social reinforcer

spontaneous
   (connected,
   running) speech
   sample

stimulability

stop

substitution

symmetry
   (symmetrical)

voice

INTRODUCTION

Articulation and phonological disorders are the most common communication disorders of children. As defined previously, an articulation disorder is an incorrect production of speech sounds because of faulty placement, timing, direction, pressure, speed, or integration of the movements of the mandible, lips, tongue, or soft palate. A phonological disorder is defined as errors of several phonemes that form patterns or clusters and are the result of a child simplifying speech sounds and sound combinations that are used by normal speaking adults. Articulation and phonological disorders may occur as isolated problems or as part of other delays or disorders, including language disorders, developmental delays, neurological disorders such as cerebral palsy or brain injuries, and *orofacial* (oral-facial) anomalies such as cleft lip and cleft palate. However, before articulation and phonological disorders can be discussed, it will be helpful to have more of an understanding of General American English (GAE) speech sounds, followed by some causes of articulation and phonological disorders.

GENERAL AMERICAN ENGLISH

American English has as its foundation British English; however, the glossary of this book provides many Latin and Greek derivatives of our professional terminology, and some can be traced back hundreds to thousands of years. General American English or "American English" speech is spoken by millions of people throughout the United States and is considered not to have a regional dialect associated with it. This is the speech normally used by radio and television broadcasters, and when used a person is less likely to be asked, "Where are you from?" General American English is considered the speech of most people in the western regions of the United States (Edwards, 2003).

Speech-language pathologists, audiologists, linguists, and phoneticians make a distinction between a **letter** and a phoneme. A letter is an arbitrary written or printed symbol or character representing a speech sound. A phoneme is the shortest arbitrary unit of sound in a language that can be recognized as being distinct from other sounds in the language. In the English language there are 26 letters but 45 speech sounds (phonemes) because as the language developed, sounds were added after the 26-letter alphabet was established. Other languages may have significantly more or fewer letters in their alphabets and more or fewer phonemes.

The "name" of a letter may not have any resemblance to the sound associated with the letter. For example, we have the letter "h," which we pronounce as "eytch," but the sound is made by opening the vocal folds

letter

An arbitrary written or printed symbol or character representing a speech sound.

and forcing air through with no vibration (as in whispering), while holding the mandible in a slightly open position and with the articulators not creating any restriction of the air. Also, the alphabet has the letter "c," but the sound of the letter is either /s/ or /k/, as in *city* or *cup*. The many variations of spellings of the same sound cause confusion for children learning to spell (e.g., the sound /f/ may be spelled *f* [*for*], *ff* [*off*], *ph* [phone], or *gh* [*rough*]).

In the study of phonology, SLPs use **phonetics** to describe the individual sounds in a language and use the **International Phonetic Alphabet (IPA)** transcription symbols in an attempt to identify specific sounds for any language or dialect (see Table 5–1). The IPA includes 25 consonants (compared to 21 letters in the alphabet), 15 vowels (compared to 5 in the alphabet), and 5 **diphthongs** (not represented by single letters in the alphabet), giving a total of 45 phonemes (compared to 26 letters) (Small, 2012). (Note: Phoneticians do not necessarily agree on the precise number of consonant and vowel phonemes.) However, although a single phonetic symbol may be used for a phoneme, in reality there are slight variations in the way different people produce individual phonemes, and there can be variations of a phoneme depending on whether it is in the *initial, middle (medial)*, or *final* position of a word, or what sounds precede or follow an individual phoneme. These slight variations in individual phonemes are referred to as **allophones**.

Vowels

Vowels, as defined in Chapter 1, are voiced speech sounds from the unrestricted passage of the air stream through the mouth without audible stoppage or friction. Vowels can be described by the placement of the tongue during their production. The *vowel quadrilateral diagram* is a four-sided figure (usually shown as a trapezoid) that represents tongue positions and movements. The corners are labeled *high front, high back, low front*, and *low back*. Figure 5–1 shows a vowel quadrilateral with key words representing the sound of each vowel (note: there can be some variation of vowels in words depending on dialects and accents). You can experiment with producing different vowels by keeping the mandible slightly open and the lips in a neutral position, and then slowly moving the tongue forward and backward, raising and lowering it, and flattening and then humping it up in back. Then keeping the tongue in a neutral position and the mandible slightly open, slowly protrude and retract the lips while voicing.

Consonants

As defined in Chapter 1, consonants are speech sounds articulated by either stopping of the outgoing air stream or creating a narrow opening of resistance using the articulators. Consonants are commonly described by their **distinctive features**; that is, the smallest individual differences required to differentiate one phoneme from another. The three

phonetics

The study of speech-sound production and the special symbols that represent speech sounds.

International Phonetic Alphabet (IPA)

Specially devised signs and symbols designed to represent the individual speech sounds of all languages.

diphthong

A combination of two vowels in which one vowel glides continuously into the second vowel; in American English: /eɪ/, /aɪ/, /oʊ/, and /aʊ/.

allophone

Slight variation in the way different people produce individual phonemes that can be affected by the initial, middle, or final position of a word, or what sounds precede or follow an individual phoneme.

distinctive feature

The smallest individual differences required to differentiate one phoneme from another in a language.

TABLE 5-1 International Phonetic Alphabet Symbols

CONSONANTS		VOWELS	
SYMBOL	**COMMONLY HEARD IN**	**SYMBOL**	**COMMONLY HEARD IN**
p	pick	i	eat
b	book	I	it
t	take	ɛ	egg
d	day	æ	apple
k	cat	ʌ	oven
g	get	ə (schwa)	among
f	fish	a	father*
v	vase	ɔ	father*
θ	think	ɑ	hop
ð	that	o	ocean
s	sit	u	use
z	zoo	ʊ	foot
ʃ š	shoe	ɜ	girl*
ʒʹ ž	measure	ɝ	bird*
h	home		

		ENGLISH DIPHTHONGS	
ʧ č	chip	**SYMBOL**	**COMMONLY HEARD IN**
ʤ ǰ	job		
m	moon	eɪ	ate
n	no	aɪ	I'm
ŋ	ring	oʊ	oats
j y	yes	aʊ	ouch
w	week	ɔɪ	oil
(r)	red	u	use
l	lake		
ʌ*	what		

*May be regional or individual pronunciations.
Based on Tables 2–1 and 2–2 in Yavas, M. (1998). *Phonology development and disorders.* Clifton Park, NY: Delmar Cengage Learning.

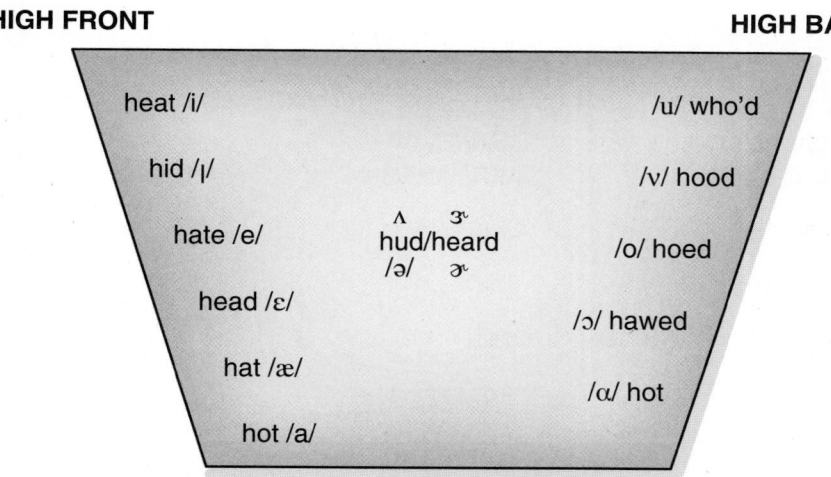

HIGH FRONT

heat /i/

hid /ɪ/

hate /e/

head /ɛ/

hat /æ/

hot /a/

LOW FRONT

HIGH BACK

/u/ who'd

/ʊ/ hood

ʌ ɝ
hud/heard
/ə/ ɚ

/o/ hoed

/ɔ/ hawed

/ɑ/ hot

LOW BACK

Figure 5–1

Vowel quadrilateral with key words and phonetic symbols.

© Cengage Learning 2013.

major distinctive features are place, manner, and voice (see Table 5–2). Speech sounds may be **voiced**, with the vocal folds vibrating (e.g., /b, d, g, z, v/ and all vowels), or *unvoiced,* with no vocal fold vibration (e.g., /p, t, k, s, f/). When sounds are articulated in the same place and differ only in being voiced or unvoiced, they are referred to as **cognates** (e.g., /b-p, t-d, k-g, s-z, f-v/). Table 5–2 shows the classification of consonants by place, manner, and voice.

    Place refers to the location in the mouth where two articulators come together (constrict) to produce specific sounds. Places may include the lips, teeth, alveolar ridge, tongue, and hard and soft palates. The place where articulator constriction occurs is used to classify consonants:

- *Bilabial* consonants are produced when there is contact between the two lips (/p, b, m/) or the two lips *approximate* (/w/).
- *Labiodental* sounds are produced with the upper incisor teeth in contact with the lower lip (/f, v/).
- *Linguadental* consonants are produced when the tongue tip is placed between the upper and the lower incisor teeth (i.e., *lingua-dental* voiced and unvoiced /th/).
- *Alveolar* consonants are produced when the tip of the tongue (*apex*) is in contact with the alveolar ridge of the maxilla, just behind the upper incisor teeth (i.e., *lingua [tongue]-alveolar* /t, d, s, z, n, l/). This point of contact produces more sounds than any other; however, it is the pressure of the tongue tip against the alveolar ridge and the length of time the tongue tip and alveolar ridge are in contact that allow us to produce the various sounds.
- *Palatal* consonants are produced when the blade or body of the tongue is near the hard palate (i.e., *linguapalatal* /ʃ/ [sh], /ʧ/ [ch], /ʤ/, /j/, and /r/).
- *Velar* consonants are produced by the back of the tongue (root) approaching the soft palate (velum) (i.e., *linguavelar* /k/, /g/, and /ŋ/).

voice

The distinctive feature that refers to a sound produced either with the vocal folds vibrating (*voiced*) or not vibrating (*unvoiced*).

cognate

Two sounds that differ only in voicing (e.g., /p/ - /b/).

place

The location in the mouth where two articulators come together (make contact or near contact to constrict the air) to produce specific sounds; places may include the lips, teeth, alveolar ridge, tongue, and hard and soft palates.

TABLE 5-2   Classification of Consonants by Distinctive Features: Place, Manner, and Voice

PLACE OF ARTICULATION	PHONETIC SYMBOL AND KEY WORD	MANNER OF ARTICULATION	VOICE
Bilabial	/p/ (pay)	Stop	−
	/b/ (bay)	Stop	+
	/m/ (may)	Nasal	+
Labial	/ʍ/ (which)	Glide (semivowel)	−
	/w/ (witch)	Glide (semivowel)	+
Labiodental	/f/ (fan)	Fricative	−
	/v/ (van)	Fricative	+
Linguadental	/θ/ (thin)	Fricative	−
(interdental)	/ð/ (this)	Fricative	+
Lingua-alveolar	/t/ (two)	Stop	−
	/d/ (do)	Stop	+
	/s/ (sue)	Fricative	−
	/z/ (zoo)	Fricative	+
	/n/ (new)	Nasal	+
	/l/ (Lou)	Lateral	+
Linguapalatal	/ʃ/ (shoe)	Fricative	−
	/ʒ/ (rouge)	Fricative	+
	/tʃ/ (chin)	Affricative	−
	/dʒ/ (gin)	Affricative	+
	/j/ (you)	Glide (semivowel)	+
	/r/ (rue)	Rhotic	+
Linguavelar	/k/ (back)	Stop	−
	/g/ (bag)	Stop	+
	/ŋ/ (bang)	Nasal	+
Glottal (laryngeal)	/h/ (who)	Fricative	−
	—	Stop	+ (−)

Source: Gelfer, M. P. (1996). *Survey of communication disorders: A social and behavioral perspective.* New York: McGraw-Hill. Reproduced with permission of the McGraw-Hill Companies.

- The *glottal* consonant is produced at the level of the vocal folds by having the vocal folds in an open position and briefly exhaling air (/h/).

Manner is the way in which the air stream is modified as a result of the interaction of the articulators (Bauman-Waengler, 2012). One manner of articulation, *stop-plosives*, consists of consonants that are produced when a complete occlusion between two articulators occurs, for example, /p/, /b/, /t/, /d/, /k/, and /g/. Another manner is **fricatives**, which are produced when air is forced through a narrow constriction between two articulators, such as /f/ and /v/. **Sibilants** are a subcategory of fricative and are produced with a hissing noise, such as /s/, /z/, /ʃ/ [sh], and /ʒ/. *Affricates* are produced as a stop-plosive that releases into a fricative /tʃ/ and /dʒ/. Nasals are produced by lowering the velum so the air passes into the nasal passages resulting in /m/, /n/, or /ŋ/. *Approximates* are produced when the articulators are near one another but do not close enough to cause friction, such as /w/, /j/, /r/, and /l/.

The lips are important in producing several sounds, especially the **bilabial** (two lips) **stops** /p/ and /b/, where both lips touch and then release for sound to escape; the **nasal** sound /m/, where the lips are closed and the sound passes behind the soft palate and through the nasal passage; the bilabial **glide (semivowel)** /w/, where the lips are rounded and slightly protruded then relaxed; and the **labiodental fricatives** /f/ and /v/, where the upper front teeth are in contact with the lower lip (compare to other fricatives: e.g., /θ/ [th], /ð/ [th], and /s/, /z/).

In English, the tongue is particularly important when producing the **linguadental (interdental)** voiced and unvoiced /th/ sounds, where the tongue tip is placed lightly between the top and the bottom front teeth; the lingua-alveolar voiced and unvoiced /d/ and /t/ sounds, where the tongue tip makes contact with the alveolar ridge just behind the upper front teeth; the **linguapalatal** /ʃ/ [sh] and /tʃ/ [ch] sounds, where the top center of the tongue is near the hard palate; and the **linguavelar** /k/ and /g/ consonants, where the back of the tongue moves near the soft palate.

Blends (consonant clusters)

Blends (consonant clusters) are combinations of two or three consonants where each consonant can be heard. There are four major categories of consonant blends: *l*-blends (e.g., <u>bl</u>ack, <u>cl</u>ean, <u>fl</u>at), *r*-blends (e.g., <u>br</u>own, <u>cr</u>edit, <u>dr</u>eam), *s*-blends (e.g., <u>st</u>ate, <u>sm</u>ooth, <u>sp</u>in, <u>sw</u>im, <u>scr</u>am, <u>squ</u>are, <u>spl</u>ash, <u>spr</u>ing, <u>str</u>aw), and middle/end blends (*pa<u>st</u>ure, ex<u>pl</u>ain, fo<u>ld</u>, mi<u>lk</u>*). (Note: When two consonants are together but one is silent, it is not considered a blend [e.g., half], or when two consonants are combined to form one sound it is not considered a blend [e.g., children].) Blends are typically later developing sounds for children.

Figure 5–2 shows the relationship between the articulators and their corresponding places of articulation for consonants. Figure 5–3 illustrates the general places of articulation for the primary consonants in American English.

---

manner

The way in which the air stream is modified as a result of the interaction of the articulators; direction of airflow (e.g., oral or nasal sounds), or the degree of narrowing of the vocal tract by the articulators in the various places.

fricative

A sound formed by forcing the air stream through a narrow opening between articulators (tongue-teeth /θ/, /ð/ [th]; lips /f/, /v/; tongue-alveolar ridge /s/, /z/, and tongue-hard palate /ʃ/).

sibilant

A fricative sound whose production is accompanied by a "hissing" sound (/s/, /z/, /ʃ/ [sh], and /ʒ/).

bilabial

Referring to the two lips or bilabial sounds, /p/ and /b/.

stop

A sound made by building up air pressure in the mouth and then suddenly releasing it; the airflow can be blocked momentarily by pressing the lips together (bilabial—/p, b/) or by pressing the tongue against either the gums (lingua-alveolar—/t, d/) or the soft palate (linguavelar—/k, g/).

nasal

A sound resulting from the closing of the oral cavity, preventing air from escaping through the mouth, with a lowered position of the soft palate and a free passage of air through the nose (/m/, /n/, and /ŋ/ [ng]).

glide (semivowel)

A type of consonant that has a gradual (gliding) change in an articulator (lips or tongue) position and a relative long production of sound; /w/, /j/.

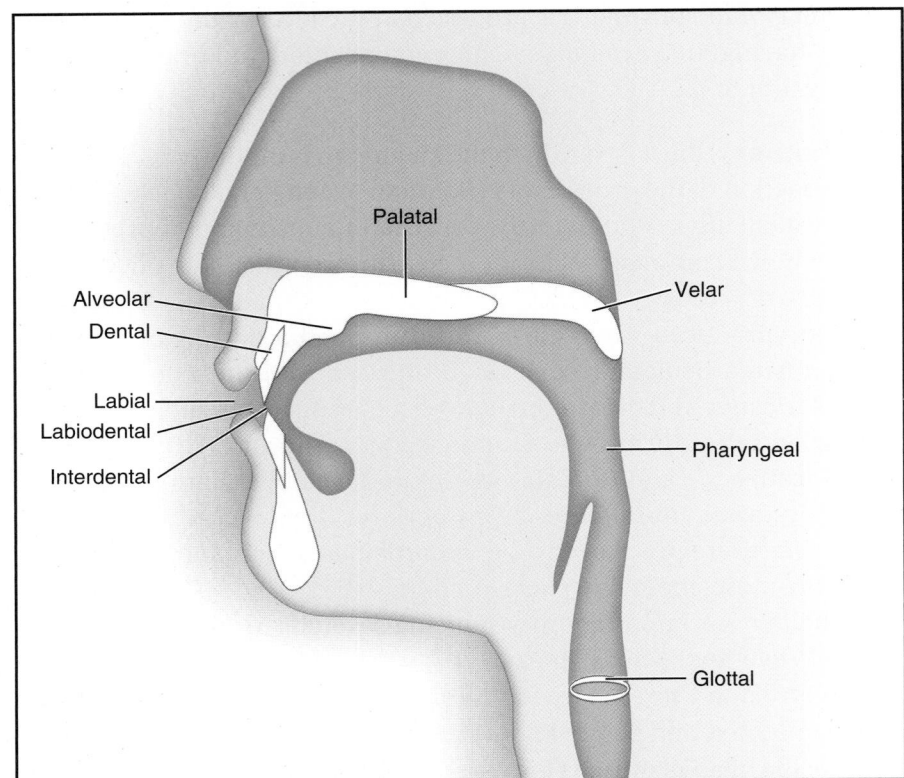

Figure 5-2

The relationship between the articulators and their corresponding places of articulation.

© Cengage Learning 2013.

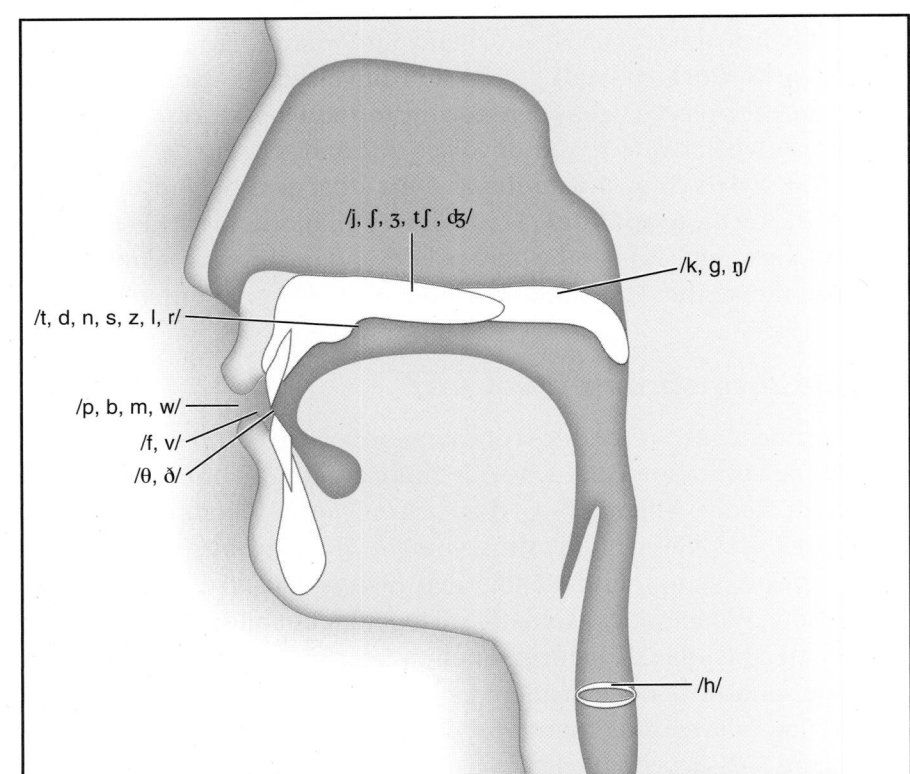

Figure 5-3

General places of articulation for the primary consonants in American English.

© Cengage Learning 2013.

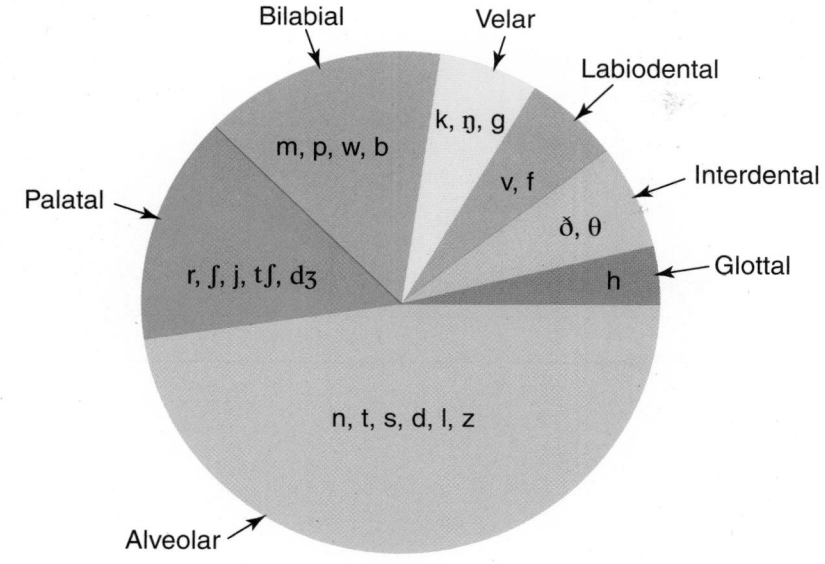

Figure 5-4

Pie chart showing the relative frequency of occurrence of consonants produced at different places of articulation.

Based on data from Dewey, 1923.

Dewey (1923) studied the frequency of occurrence of English consonants by using 100,000 words taken from newspapers, fiction books, speeches, letters, scientific articles, and magazines. A pie chart shows the relative frequency of occurrence of consonants produced at different places of articulation (Figure 5-4). The rank order of frequency of occurrence for place of articulation, from most to least frequent, is alveolar (almost 50% of consonants), palatal, bilabial, velar, labiodental, interdental, and glottal. Also, the individual consonants are listed in rank order of frequency of occurrence. For example, /n/ is the most frequent alveolar consonant (it is the most frequent of *all* consonants). Knowing the frequency of occurrence for place of articulation of consonants is important clinically; for example, by helping children who have difficulty with alveolar sounds, we can help them improve the articulation of almost half of all consonants they speak. Bilabial sounds and labiodental sounds are often relatively easy to remediate; therefore, by helping children improve the articulation of the alveolar, bilabial, and labiodental sounds, approximately 75% of consonants will be correctly articulated.

ETIOLOGIES OF COMMUNICATION DISORDERS

There are three general etiologies, or causes, of communication disorders (articulation, phonology, and language) in children: normal variation, environmental problems, and physical impairments or differences. In many cases, a combination of etiologies affects a child. Often the cause or causes of a communication disorder remain elusive, even with a careful case history, review of all educational and medical records, and extensive testing of the client.

labiodental

The /f/ and /v/ sounds, where the upper front teeth are in contact with the lower lip.

linguadental (interdental)

Voiced and unvoiced /th/ sounds with the tongue tip placed lightly between the top and the bottom front teeth.

linguapalatal

The /ʃ/ [sh] and /ʒ/ [zh] sounds, where the top center of the tongue is near the hard palate.

linguavelar

The /k/ and /g/ consonants, where the back of the tongue moves near the soft palate.

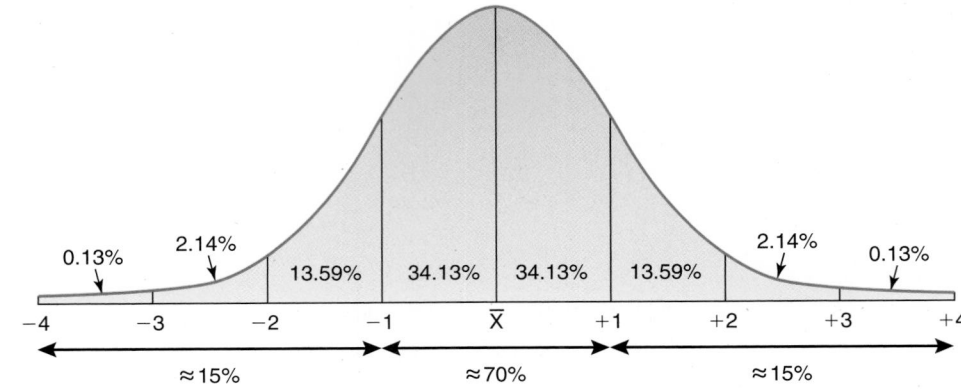

Figure 5-5

Normal distribution.

Adapted from Nicolosi, Harryman,
& Kresheck, 2004.

Normal Variation

If we consider the basic bell-shaped curve that reflects the normal distribution of any trait or ability, it helps us realize that most children (approximately 70%) are within the normal range of speech and language development and that relatively few are outside of the normal range by one, two, or three standard deviations (see Figure 5–5). This is an important concept for SLPs and Auds because it is possible to lose the perspective of normalcy if we are not around normal-speaking children enough to keep our ears and perception finely tuned to what is within the normal range and what is outside of it. As clinicians, we work with individuals who are one, two, or more standard deviations below the mean in hearing, speech, language, and cognitive functioning. If a clinician works with many children who have moderate to severe impairments (two or three standard deviations below the mean) and then evaluates a child who is just one standard deviation below the mean, the clinician may feel and report to the parents that the child is doing "just fine" or even "great." However, when compared to normal children of the same age rather than to children with **significant** communication problems, the child is not doing "just fine" or "great."

All parts of our bodies and their functioning may be considered inside or outside normal variation. A body structure or system outside of normal variation could cause or contribute to communication impairments. However, another structure or system may compensate to prevent communication impairments from manifesting. A classic example is a moderate or even severe dental malocclusion that would appear to significantly affect an individual's speech intelligibility; however,

significant

A term often used to specify the impairment level a child must exhibit before he is considered to have a speech or language disorder; no "gold standard" is available to use to define this term as it applies to speech and language disorders. In statistics, the probability that a given finding (e.g., an individual test score) may have occurred by chance; usually a finding that occurs fewer than 5 times in 100 by chance alone ($p < .05$).

because of the remarkable adaptability of the tongue, an individual may have normal or near-normal speech intelligibility.

"Functional" versus "Organic" Disorders

SLPs and Auds have long debated the distinction between **functional** and **organic** communication disorders. They are considered labels of convenience because communication disorders may be neither all organic nor all functional. That is, "functional" disorders may have some organic elements, and "organic" disorders may have some functional elements.

The terms *speech impediment* or *defect* and *tongue-tie* have long been used by lay people (individuals not educated in speech-language pathology or audiology, including parents, teachers, nurses, and physicians) in reference to individuals of all ages who have some speech impairment. These terms suggest that there is a structural cause of a speech problem even though there is no apparent structural (organic) problem that can be found when an evaluation is conducted. The terms *speech impediment* or *defect* and *tongue-tie* are considered obsolete terms for *speech disorder* or *speech impairment (problem)*.

functional

An incorrect production of standard speech sounds for which there is no known anatomical, physiological, or neurological basis.

organic

The inability to correctly produce standard speech sounds because of anatomical, physiological, or neurological causes.

Tongue-tie (ankyloglossia)

"Tongue-tie" is a term that has been applied to a variety of communication problems, including impaired articulation, stuttering, and shyness. However, tongue-tie (*ankyloglossia*) is caused by a restrictive lingual **frenum** or **frenulum** that is abnormally short or is attached too close to the tip of the tongue (see Figure 5–6). This causes difficulty elevating and protruding the tongue tip, which affects production of some sounds (e.g., /t, d, l, th/).

frenum/frenulum

A fold of mucous tissue connecting the floor of the mouth to the midline underside of the tongue.

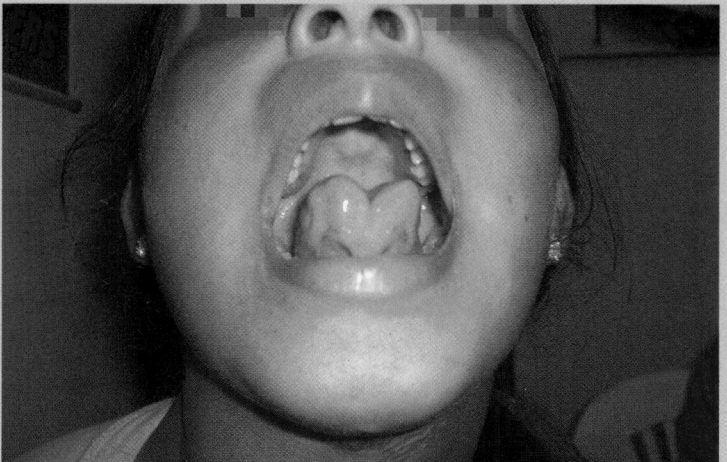

Paul Fogle, Ph.D., Rotaplast International Cleft Palate Mission, Cumaná, Venezuela, 2008

Figure 5–6
Restrictive lingual frenum (tongue-tie).

Environmental Problems

Even though a person may have the best of genetic potential at the moment of conception, the embryo and fetus's prenatal environment may seriously affect the realization of that potential. Furthermore, when genetic potential is good and the embryo or fetus develops in an ideal prenatal environment, the postnatal environment may seriously or even profoundly diminish a person's potential in life.

Prenatal Environment

In a way, the prenatal environment begins at the moment of conception and is affected by the combination of genetic material. It is also influenced by both the mother's and the father's physical health at that moment and thereafter by the mother's self-care and general health throughout the pregnancy. Unfortunately, even women who take excellent care of themselves during their pregnancies may have health problems that predispose a child to developmental delays and disorders; examples include pre-pregnancy obesity, type II diabetes mellitus, insufficient amounts of folic acid in the diet, the need to take seizure medication, and the human immunodeficiency virus (HIV) found in those with AIDS. During the embryo's first trimester of life, it is most susceptible to medical complications.

Apgar Scores

Apgar scores (named after Virginia Apgar, an American obstetric anesthesiology specialist, 1909–1974) evaluate an infant's physical condition at 1 minute and again at 5 minutes after birth. The attending pediatrician rates five factors: skin color, heart rate, respiratory effort, muscle tone, and reflex irritability. The rating procedure now utilizes an acronym based on Virginia Apgar's name: A (appearance), P (pulse), G (grimace), A (activity), and R (respiration). Each factor is scored with a low value of 0 to a normal value of 2, and the scores are totaled for each evaluation; for example, a newborn may have an Apgar of 8 at 1 minute and of 10 at 5 minutes. Most newborns have a score of 7–9 at 1 minute. Scores of 5–6 are borderline, and scores of 4 or less mean the newborn requires immediate assistance with breathing and possible transfer to a *neonatal intensive care unit* (NICU) (Apgar, 1953). Infants with low Apgar scores may be considered high risk for various developmental delays and disorders that may not be noticeable until the child begins to walk, develop speech and language, or has difficulty reading and learning. Most mothers and fathers do not know their children's Apgar scores and, therefore, may not make the connection that the early minutes after birth may set the stage for the child being at risk for developmental problems through the years and challenges throughout adulthood.

Syndromes

Various syndromes can cause or contribute to communication delays and disorders. A few examples of syndromes that may significantly affect communication development include (1) *Down syndrome*, the most common chromosomal disorder, which is characterized by a small head, flat face, upward slanting eyes, and short fingers; (2) *fetal alcohol syndrome* (FAS), characterized by prenatal and postnatal growth retardation, facial abnormalities, heart defects, joint and limb abnormalities, and intellectual impairment; (3) *Asperger's syndrome*, which is a pervasive developmental disorder similar to autistic disorder, characterized by severe impairment of social interactions and by restricted interests and behaviors, although speech, language, and cognitive development may be near normal. Many syndromes, including those mentioned here, also include mild to severe speech, language, and cognitive delays or disorders.

Maternal Substance Abuse

The most likely etiology of prenatal problems of all kinds is the mother's abuse of illegal drugs, alcohol, and nicotine (Center on Addiction and Substance Abuse, 2005). Approximately 35% to 40% of women in the United States abuse illegal drugs, alcohol, or nicotine sometime during pregnancy. In addition, approximately 75% of pregnant women who abuse one substance abuse other substances that could be harmful to the unborn child. Maternal substance abuse resulting in neurological and other damage to newborns is perhaps the only cause of communication and other impairments that is 100% preventable.

When maternal substance abuse is the cause of or a contributor to a child's communication problems, the child's potential for developing normal or merely functional communication abilities and skills for independent living may be significantly reduced, even with the best long-term professional involvement. The long-term consequences for these children are not always clear and ongoing therapy is usually necessary. Figure 5–7 presents risks of prenatal drug exposure for physical and communicative development.

Low Birth Weight and Prematurity

In the United States, approximately 8.5% of infants have **low birth weight** (Rossetti, 2001); this percentage may be significantly higher in less-developed countries. Seventy percent of low birth weight infants (weight less than 5.5 pounds or 2,500 grams) are **premature**. In the United States, 97% of newborns weigh between ≈5.5 pounds (2,500 grams) and ≈10 pounds (4,500 grams), with an average of ≈7.5 pounds (3,500 grams) (Mosby, 2009). Unlike normal birth weight infants, premature and low birth weight infants have fragile and underdeveloped vascular systems, including in their brains. Infants may have strokes in utero (primarily *hemorrhagic* strokes where a blood vessel in the brain ruptures and blood leaks or flows into the brain tissue). Prematurity and low birth weight put an infant at risk for communication problems, including learning disabilities that may not be evident until early elementary school when the child is learning to read (Grunau, Kearney, & Whitfield, 1990).

low birth weight

An infant whose weight at birth is less than 5.5 pounds (2,500 grams), regardless of gestational age.

premature (infant)

Any infant born before the gestational age of 37 weeks; often associated with low birth weight that results in high risk for incomplete organ system development, causing poor temperature regulation, respiratory disorders, and poor sucking and swallowing reflexes.

Physical Risks
- Small head circumference
- Low birth weight from prematurity or intrauterine growth retardation
- Small strokes or heart attacks (intrauterine cerebral and cardiac infarctions) before birth
- Congenital malformations of the heart, genitourinary tracts, and limbs
- AIDS and other infections

Behavioral Risks

Infancy
- Irritability
- Hypertonicity or hypotonicity
- Hyperactivity
- Tremulousness
- Deficiencies in organization of state and interactive abilities
- Seizures

Childhood
- Reduced self-regulation
- Distractibility (ADD or ADHD)
- Reduced pretend play
- Flat affect
- Attachment problems

Figure 5-7

Risks of prenatal drug exposure for physical and communicative development.

Adapted from Sparks, 1993.

perinatal

Pertaining to the time and process of giving birth or being born.

infantile hypoxia

In newborns and infants, inadequate oxygenation of the blood leading to *tachycardia* (rapid heart rate) and rapid, shallow breathing that quickly affects the brain and other organs and systems; severe hypoxia can result in cardiac failure.

anoxia

A complete lack of oxygen to the brain that is relatively rare but causes devastating neurological disorders.

Perinatal Environment

Perinatal (time of birth) problems occur because of complications at birth and often result in multiple severe handicaps. **Infantile hypoxia**, a partial or significantly diminished supply of oxygen to the brain that results in neurological damage, is the most common perinatal complication. **Anoxia**, a complete lack of oxygen reaching the brain, is a relatively rare but devastating cause of neurological disorders. When hypoxia or anoxia occurs, the cerebral cortex is most severely damaged because it is furthest from where the blood enters the brain. In many cases, the brainstem and midbrain may be relatively well preserved, allowing the major body systems and organs to function; however, the cortical damage may cause severely impaired communication, cognition, and swallowing abilities.

Postnatal Environment

Our environment influences or determines the sounds we produce for individual words and the words we use to express ourselves. In most cases, children are about as intelligible as the parents who have helped them learn speech and language. Some home and community environments for children are not conducive to good speech and language development. When a child has limited environmental stimulation (deprivation),

Chanel

Chanel was 2 years old when her parents contacted me to evaluate their daughter who was not yet saying her first intelligible words. The case history revealed that the child had been adopted as a newborn in another state and was a **failure-to-thrive** infant. Chanel had inefficient sucking and swallowing reflexes, and the parents went through extraordinary measures to provide sufficient nutrition for the infant, including **gavage feeding** for 7 months. Metabolically, Chanel was unable to accept food. The parents eventually were able to contact the obstetrician who delivered the infant and learned that the mother "may have" used illegal drugs during the pregnancy, which likely was the etiology of Chanel's failure to thrive and other developmental problems.

I worked with the child three times a week in the family home on a blanket on the living room floor demonstrating to the mother and grandmother, who were always present, how to maximize speech and language development throughout the day and techniques to improve muscle tone of the various speech systems (the child had been diagnosed by a pediatrician as having cerebral palsy). I eventually discontinued working with Chanel when she entered a public preschool program for severely handicapped children where she would receive more extensive therapy throughout the day; however, I maintained intermittent contact with the parents to follow the child's progress.

At 8 years of age, Chanel was the size of a 2-year-old. She underwent a magnetic resonance imaging (MRI) examination, which revealed that during the birthing process she had sustained an *occlusive stroke* (blockage of an artery in the brain) that had cut off all of the blood supply to the pituitary gland (the "master gland" that controls growth and the secondary production of other hormones and functioning of organ systems). The stroke that caused the lack of pituitary functioning also severely complicated the developmental problems she had from the mother's use of illegal drugs during the pregnancy. Over the years, Chanel developed slow but steady communication abilities, including a simple sign language system. As clinicians we sometimes work with children who have extraordinary and complicated medical problems. ■

failure to thrive

The abnormal retardation of growth and development of an infant resulting from conditions that interfere with normal metabolism, appetite, and activity.

gavage feeding

The use of a **nasogastric (NG) tube** to provide sufficient nutrition and hydration for newborns who have a failure-to-thrive condition, with infant milk or specialized formulas (e.g., PediaSure®) inserted into the tube.

nasogastric (NG) tube

A medical device consisting of a long flexible tube that is passed through the nose, down the esophagus, and into the stomach for the delivery of liquids, nutrition, and medications.

especially interaction with adults, then fewer synaptic connections may be made in the brain. This can significantly affect development of speech, language, and cognition. However, in most cases of limited environmental stimulation, there are only gaps in speech and language development compared to children who have normal experiences. Cases of extreme environmental and sensory deprivation are rare.

CASE STUDY

Genie

On November 4, 1970, a 13-year-old girl was taken into custody by officials in Los Angeles, California. The child had been kept in such isolation by her parents that she never learned to talk. Genie was locked in a closet and tied to a potty chair most of her life. Completely restrained, she was forced to sit alone with little to look at and no one to talk to for more than 10 years. When she was discovered by a social worker, she was functioning as an infant and uttering only infantile noises. Genie was placed at a children's hospital for care, training, and education. By May 1971 she was beginning to imitate and repeat single words, although not clearly. By the end of spring, the 13-year-old child could say more than 100 words. When given a new item, she looked at it carefully, often putting it to her mouth (much like an infant), as though she was investigating it because she had little or no experience with common, everyday objects.

Genie was eventually placed with a foster family, the psychologist who had been working with her at the children's hospital and his wife, who was a graduate student in human development. Genie's foster parents became her full-time teachers. Genie eventually developed simple language to help her describe what her life had been like for 10 years in the tiny room. Her foster parents began to feel that Genie was successfully learning a first language even though she had passed the early years of normal language development. Because Genie was more inclined to use gestures to communicate than to use speech, her therapists decided to bring in a teacher who taught sign language. Over the next few years, it became clear that Genie was able to learn vocabulary and to sign or say words but she was not able to use words in sequence to form grammatical language. Genie was eventually placed in an adult foster care home in southern California where she continues to live. (For more information on the language intervention attempts with Genie, see Curtis, 1977.) ■

Application Question

What are five things parents can do to help provide a rich communication environment for their children?

Hearing Impairments

Among the variables that influence speech and language development, perhaps none is as crucial as hearing (Martin & Clark, 2012). One of the most important factors in the development of speech and language is an intact auditory system sensitive to the frequency range within which most speech sounds occur (500 to 4,000 Hz). Hearing impairments almost always result in delays and disorders of speech and language. When infants cannot hear at normal intensity levels (*conductive hearing loss*) or the sounds are distorted or misperceived from a damaged or poorly functioning cochlea or auditory pathway to the brain (*sensorineural* or *central hearing loss*), articulation and language development will likely be impaired. (See Chapter 14, Hearing Disorders in Children and Adults, for a more complete discussion of this topic.)

Physical Impairments or Differences in the Central and Peripheral Nervous Systems

Infants may be born with neurological disorders (e.g., cerebral palsy) and children at any age can acquire a neurological disorder from a traumatic brain injury that results in communication and cognitive impairments (see Chapter 13, Special Populations with Communication Disorders). Communication disorders also can be caused by diseases such as *bacterial* or *viral meningitis*.

Integration of Factors

For most children with communication problems, we cannot determine a single factor as a cause. In most cases, several factors (**multifactorial**) may come into play. For some children genetic and congenital syndromes contribute; for others, they do not. Some children have sensory problems and others have normal acuity and perceptual abilities. Some children come from home environments in which there is a lack of speech and language stimulation and good *modeling* (verbally or physically demonstrating a good example of a behavior, such as production of a sound or correct grammar), but many others come from normal home environments or even language-enriched environments.

Even if the contributing causes of communication disorders can be determined, we cannot alter a child's genetic make-up or eliminate a syndrome. We often can help a child's auditory acuity problems with hearing amplification, but we have to work within a child's auditory perceptual abilities and limitations. We cannot change a child's impoverished home life, and seldom can we do much to change the parents' language stimulation and modeling skills (some parents would benefit from speech and language therapy themselves). Most of the time clinicians are left to work with children's communication disorders no matter the cause or current contributing factors. We do the best we can with what we are presented with and, perhaps surprisingly, often we help children in remarkable ways.

ARTICULATION DISORDERS

Articulation involves very rapid and accurate direction of movement, placement, timing, pressure, and coordination of the mandible, lips, tongue, and soft palate. Therefore, an articulation disorder is the incorrect *production* (pronouncing) of speech sounds because a child is (1) not moving an articulator in the correct direction, (2) not placing it in the correct position in the mouth (e.g., the tongue tip not being placed on the alveolar ridge properly), (3) not having precise timing and speed of movement of the articulators (down to milliseconds), (4) having inadequate pressure or too much pressure of one

multifactorial

Referring to the likelihood of two or more causes contributing to the etiology or development of an impairment or disorder, including genetic influences.

articulator against another, or (5) having difficulty coordinating the movements of the articulators.

The term *articulation disorder* implies that a child has a motor component to the disorder that affects an ability to clearly articulate specific sounds and syllables in words. Articulation disorders are often developmental disorders in which sounds are produced incorrectly or inadequately compared to normative standards for a child's age. Articulation disorders may occur as an isolated problem or as part of other delays or disorders, including language disorders, cognitive impairments, neurological disorders such as cerebral palsy or brain injuries, and orofacial anomalies such as cleft lip and cleft palate.

Four primary types of articulation errors can be made on any one sound: **s**ubstitutions, **o**missions, **d**istortions, and **a**dditions (S.O.D.A.). Articulation errors can occur in the initial, medial, or final position of words. A sound **substitution** is the replacement of one *standard speech sound* by another (a standard speech sound can be represented by a phonetic symbol). When a child has a sound substitution she has produced a wrong sound in place of the correct sound, such as "thoup" for *soup* (a *frontal lisp*), "shoup" for *soup* (a *lateral lisp*), or "wed" for red (/w/ for /r/). Sound substitutions are probably the most common type of articulation errors children have. A sound **omission** is the absence of a speech sound where one should occur in a word; for example, "k-on" for *crayon*, or "ba" for *box*. Some children will have both a substitution and an omission in the same word, for example, "sketty" for spaghetti, where there is an omission of the /p/ and schwa sound /ə/, and substitution of /k/ for /g/. A sound **distortion** is a sound that does not have a phonetic symbol to represent the sound that is produced in place of the intended sound, such as a lateral lisp that is not a clear "sh" sound, or a distorted /r/ sound that cannot be clearly represented by a phonetic symbol. Sound distortions are commonly heard in children who have neurological disorders such as cerebral palsy or traumatic brain injuries when the articulators are weak and cannot make rapid or precise movements. An **addition** is the insertion of a sound or sounds that are not part of the word itself, such as *animamal* for *animal*.

PHONOLOGICAL DISORDERS

As discussed previously, a phonological disorder (also referred to as *developmental phonological disorder* or *phonological impairment*) can be defined as errors of several phonemes that form patterns and are the result of a child simplifying individual sounds and sound combinations. Children with phonological disorders may be able to physically produce all of the speech sounds that are appropriate for their age. Their difficulty relates to the use of particular sounds in particular contexts within words. Phonology is a subsystem of *linguistics*, the scientific study of language, and phonological disorders involve a child's lack of knowledge and development of the phonological (sound) system of a language.

substitution

The replacement of one standard speech sound by another, e.g., /th/ for /s/.

omission

The absence of a speech sound where one should occur in a word, e.g., *k-on* for *crayon*.

distortion

A sound that does not have a phonetic symbol to represent the sound that is produced in place of the intended sound (e.g., a lateral lisp that is not a clear "sh" sound, or a distorted /r/ sound that cannot be clearly represented by a phonetic symbol).

addition

The insertion of a sound or sounds not part of the word itself, such as *animamal* for *animal*.

This difficulty with the acquisition of the sound system is intricately connected to a child's overall growth in language.

A child with a phonological disorder has not learned all of the linguistic rules to properly produce and combine sounds into syllables, even though the motor movements can be executed adequately. Examples of phonological errors are when a child uses a /t/ for /s/ but uses /s/ for /sh/ and /sh/ for /ch/ (Gordon-Brannan & Weiss, 2007). However, it is possible that a child may have a combination of a phonological disorder and an articulation disorder; they are not mutually exclusive. In such cases it is difficult to determine where one disorder leaves off and the other begins. The two problems compound one another, resulting in a child not knowing the sound system and not being able to easily and accurately move the articulators. A child's therapy often focuses on both articulation and phonology.

When a child has not acquired certain phonemes by a particular age that would be expected and there are patterns to her speech errors, the child may be said to be exhibiting *phonological processes*. For example, if a child has the pattern of omitting final consonants in words, she is said to have a *final consonant deletion process*. There are approximately 35 phonological processes that may affect a child's speech intelligibility; however, approximately 10 are considered common phonological processes (see Table 5–3).

EVALUATION OF ARTICULATION AND PHONOLOGY

When a child's articulation and phonology are going to be evaluated, initial interactions with a clinician typically involve rapport building, with the hope that the child will like and trust the clinician enough to be willing to cooperate during the structured evaluation portion. The clinician will visit with the child, ask about home, school, and other involvements of the child, and show genuine interest in the child. The clinician may have some age-appropriate toys and games for the child to play with to help make the time more enjoyable. However, throughout this apparently unstructured time with the child, the clinician is making mental notes of the child's respiratory, phonatory, resonatory, and articulatory systems to develop an impression of whether there may be an anatomical or physiological cause for the child's delayed or disordered speech. Other observations important to make are the child's general speech intelligibility and receptive and expressive language abilities. (Note: Sometimes a child's articulation or phonological problems may be the first sign of language or cognitive problems. Sometimes parents will refer a child for a speech evaluation when there may be significant problems in other areas of the child's development.) The clinician may tape-record the interaction for a later analysis of a **spontaneous (connected, running) speech sample** (usually 50 to 100 utterances)

spontaneous (connected, running) speech sample

A sample of a child's oral discourse in conversation or while describing a picture, usually 50 to 100 consecutive utterances.

TABLE 5-3   Common Phonological Processes in Typical Speech Development

PHONOLOGICAL PROCESS	DESCRIPTION	EXAMPLE
Context sensitive voicing	A voiceless sound is replaced by a voiced sound.	*p*ig → *b*ig, *c*ar → *g*ar
Final consonant devoicing	A final voiced consonant in a word is replaced by a voiceless consonant.	re*d* → re*t*, ba*g* → ba*k*
Final consonant deletion	The final consonant in many words is omitted.	ho*me* → h*oe*, ca*t* → c*a*
Velar fronting	A velar consonant is replaced with a consonant produced at the front of the mouth.	*k*iss → *t*iss, *g*ive → *d*iv
Palatal fronting	The sibilant consonants /ʃ/ and /ʒ/ are replaced by alveolar sibilants made on the alveolar ridge.	*sh*ip → *s*ip, mea*s*ure → me*zz*a
Consonant harmony	The pronunciation of the whole word is influenced by a single sound in the word.	*d*og → *g*og hat → *t*at
Weak syllable deletion	Unstressed or weak syllables are omitted.	te*l*ephone → teffone, *ba*nana → _nana
Cluster reduction	Part of a consonant cluster is omitted.	*s*pider → pider, *f*riend → fend
Gliding of liquids	The liquid consonants /l/ and /r/ are replaced with /w/ or /j/ (y).	*r*eal → *w*eal, *l*eg → *y*eg
Stopping	A fricative or affricate is replaced by a stop consonant.	*f*unny → *p*unny *j*ump → *d*ump

Adapted from Bowen (1998) and Grunwell (1997).

(see Figure 5-8). Several areas of speech may be analyzed from the spontaneous speech sample, including the following:

- Correctly produced sounds
- Errored speech sounds
- Number of sound errors
- Types of errors
- Consistency of errors between the speech sample and the articulation test
- Intelligibility in conversation
- Speech rate
- Prosody

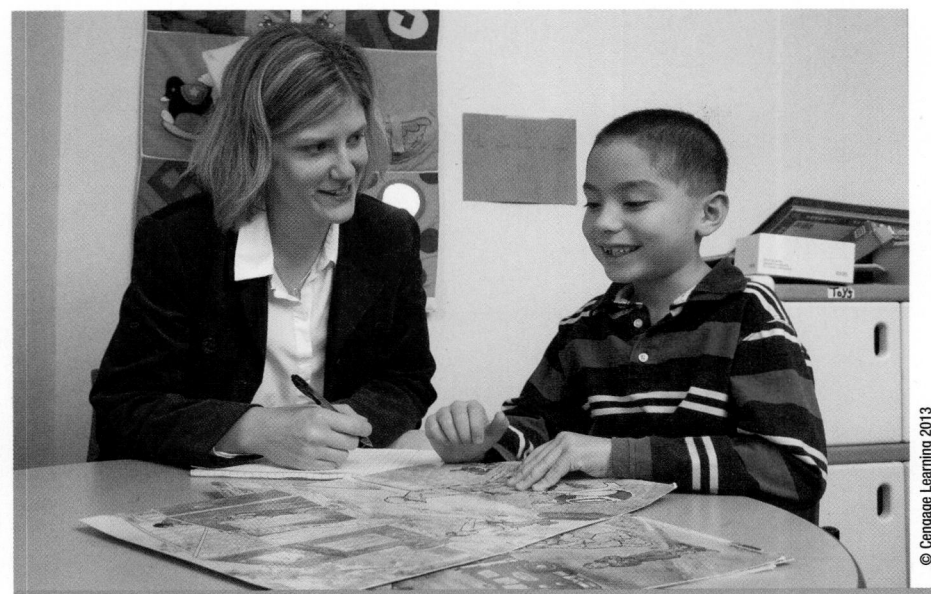

© Cengage Learning 2013

Figure 5-8

Collecting a spontaneous speech and language sample.

During the speech sample the clinician listens for the child's level of speech intelligibility in single words, short phrases, sentences, and conversation and makes note of her intelligibility (e.g., ≈80% accurate [intelligible] with single words, ≈70% with phrases and sentences, and ≈60% in conversation). When a child has inconsistent errors on a particular sound (i.e., sometimes says it correctly and sometimes does not), it may mean that the sound is *emerging* and that with a little therapy the sound may be *established*. Speech-language pathologists and audiologists may be considered "trained listeners"; therefore, a child may be somewhat more intelligible to clinicians than to people who may have only occasional opportunities to hear the child speak.

The clinician will assess the child's articulatory system during an *oral-mechanism* or *oral-peripheral examination*. This somewhat methodical examination notes the anatomy (structure) of the mandible, lips, tongue, and hard and soft palates to determine whether they are within normal limits in size and **symmetry** for the child's chronological age. The physiology (function) of each articulator will be assessed for range of motion (ROM), strength, coordination, and rate of movement to determine whether they are within normal limits for the child's age (see Figure 5-9). A child may have articulators within normal limits in structure and they may function within normal limits during *nonspeech* tasks (e.g., *protruding, retracting, elevating, depressing,* and *lateralizing* the tongue), but the child may not be able to coordinate all of the speech systems together—respiratory, phonatory, resonatory, and articulatory. In many cases, however, it is just the articulators (mandible, lips, and tongue) that children have difficulty coordinating during the rapid, precise movements needed for good articulation.

Clinicians usually have several tasks to formally and informally evaluate a child's speech; that is, structured and unstructured evaluation tasks.

symmetry (symmetrical)

Both sides (e.g., the lips) in balanced proportions for size, shape, and relative position.

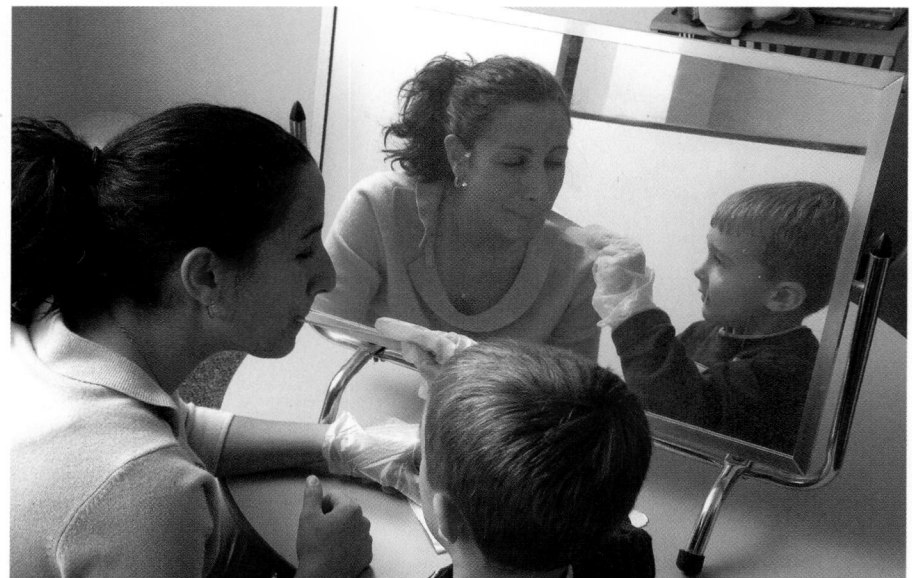

Figure 5–9

A clinician during an oral-mechanism examination (showing the child what she wants him to do).

Clinicians administer *standardized (norm-referenced) assessments* (formal tests) of articulation to collect samples of children's speech productions of individual sounds in the initial, medial, and final positions of words. The clinician asks the child to name or describe a set of test pictures, while carefully listening to the child's production of the individual sounds in the words. When evaluating a child's articulation of sounds in words, clinicians make notations on the test *protocol* (test form) to indicate the correct production of sounds and which sounds are in error in a word, in what way they are in error, and in what positions of a word they are in error. For example:

SOUND	INITIAL	MEDIAL	FINAL
p	p	b	– (omitted)
t	t	t	–
r	w	w	w
s	ʃ/s	ʃ/s	dist. (distorted)
br	b–	b–	

Note: Not all sounds occur in all three positions of words, particularly blends.

stimulability

The evaluation of a child's ability to produce a correct (or an improved) sound in imitation after the clinician models the sound for the child or after the child is given specific instructions on the articulatory placement or manner of production.

When a child has an errored sound, it is often reasonable to check the child's **stimulability** for the sound before beginning therapy. Stimulability refers to the child's ability to produce the correct (or an improved) sound in imitation after the clinician models it for the child or after the child is given specific instructions on the articulatory placement or manner of production. If a child is stimulable for a sound, the prognosis is often good that the child will be trainable for the sound without the need for extensive therapy.

In writing a report about a child's articulation errors, a clinician may make a statement such as "Jennifer demonstrated 6 sound errors in the initial position, including /s/, /z/ /r/, and initial /s/ blends, /sl/ and /st/; sound errors in the medial position, including /s/, /z/, /r/, /f/, /θ/, and /dʒ/; and 8 sound errors in the final position, including /s/, /z/, /r/, and /dʒ/, and omission of the final consonants /s/, /z/, /t/, and /d/."

A clinician who has completed an evaluation of articulation may determine that a child's speech problems go beyond the motor learning and skills for articulation. In such cases the clinician may choose to further assess the child's phonological development. Phonological evaluation may involve either tests specifically designed to assess phonology or special ways of analyzing standard articulation tests. Phonological evaluations measure performance of *sound processes* (i.e., the sound system) of a language. Results gathered from a test of phonology are reported as *phonological process errors* with a statement such as, "Michelle demonstrated errors in cluster reduction (e.g., friend → fɛnd) and final consonant deletion (bed → bɛ)."

Multicultural Considerations

The United States has a large population of immigrants from other countries, and many of the children in public schools have learned English as a second language (ESL) and are bilingual. Bilingual children often speak the parents' native language in the home environment and speak American English in school or other environments. This is frequently seen in the Hispanic culture. Spanish is the second-most-common language in the United States, with approximately 58% of the Spanish-speaking population speaking the Mexican dialect. There are also several large Asian immigrant populations in the United States, including Japanese, Mandarin Chinese, Cantonese, and Vietnamese (U.S. Census Bureau, 2010). When English is acquired after the native language, the sound system of the first language can significantly influence the pronunciation of the second language (Bauman-Waengler, 2009; Shipley & McAfee, 2009; Wyatt, 2002).

Many clinicians attempt to assess ESL children using tests standardized on native American English speakers. Two general problems may arise when clinicians use these norm-referenced tests with children who use English as a second language: (1) overinterpreting the scores obtained on the tests, and (2) using norms from a population other than the child being tested, which can cause incorrect interpretation of the child's abilities (Shipley & McAfee, 2009; Wyatt, 2002). Clinicians are confronted daily with children of all ages whom they cannot assess in their first or native language. Pena-Brooks & Hegde (2007) state that clinicians need to acquire special expertise in assessing and treating children who speak one of the following:

- A language other than English
- English as a second language acquired some time after the acquisition of their primary language
- A dialectical variety of American English (e.g., African American English)
- A different form of English (e.g., Australian English)

THERAPY FOR ARTICULATION AND PHONOLOGICAL DISORDERS

When working with any type of disorder with any age group, clinicians need to be three people rolled into one. First, we need to be *scientists*. We need to have a good understanding of the anatomy and physiology of the speech systems (respiratory, phonatory, resonatory, and articulatory), as well as the nervous system. We also need a thorough understanding of speech and language development to know when a client is within normal limits for each area of development. We need to base our therapy on well-researched data, considering each client as a *single-subject research design*. That is, we need to *develop a hypothesis* (e.g., the child has an articulation disorder), *test the hypothesis* (collect the data—the evaluation results), *analyze the data* (determine what the evaluation results mean), and *develop a treatment plan* based on the best available evidence.

Second, we must be *humanists.* We work with people, and a good understanding of people is essential to be an effective clinician. Beyond an understanding of the psychology of people, we need to be empathic and try to understand clients from their own point of view—that is, try to understand what they are thinking, feeling, and experiencing. We need to be congruent— genuine. We need to be in touch with our thoughts and feelings and to communicate them in the most appropriate (and often sensitive) way that we can. We need to have unconditional positive regard for the people we try to help. We need to convey a sense of acceptance and respect for all people.

Third, we must be *artists.* The artistic aspects of our work include being flexible and creative. Timing is often a crucial factor in our therapy; that is, saying the right thing at the right time and doing the right thing at the right time. Without the art, we may be functioning more as technicians. As clinicians, we need to "think on our feet." No textbook or therapy manual can tell us what to say and do at any given moment; it is our clinical skills, savvy, and intuition that help us from moment to moment go beyond robotic therapy to creative therapy that both the client and the clinician enjoy and benefit from.

All three of these "beings" take years of education, training, and experience to develop. Most clinicians begin their direct clinical experience with children who have articulation and phonological disorders. From there, clinicians usually begin gaining experience with children who have language disorders. Many training institutions help clinicians develop their clinical skills in an orderly sequence. Speech-language therapy is all about communication; we want our clients to develop their skills to be better communicators, and we want to develop our own skills to be better communicators and clinicians.

Therapy Approaches

Articulation therapy (sometimes referred to as *phonetic [motor] treatment*) focuses on the mechanics of producing the speech sounds. There are several treatment approaches, and there is considerable commonality among the approaches. However, some approaches incorporate **auditory discrimination training** or **ear training** (teaching a child to distinguish individual sounds from other sounds) and others do not; some begin production at the *sound isolation level* (teaching a child to produce a phoneme by itself before adding vowels) and others at the syllable level or even the word level; some include practice of the target speech sounds in nonmeaningful combinations (*"nonsense syllables,"* e.g., "bap"), and some practice only meaningful syllables and contexts (Gordon-Brannan & Weiss, 2007).

Articulation and phonology therapy with children require the clinician to listen very closely to a child's every production of a target sound and provide immediate feedback for the child to know when the sound is improving. The clinician may have the child imitate what the clinician says, have the child name pictures, read individual words or sentences, or use other methods to *elicit* (have the child produce) the targeted sound. Clinicians provide *corrective feedback* (letting the child know that a sound was produced correctly or incorrectly) and give generous **positive reinforcement** or **social reinforcers** for correct productions, such as *verbal praise* (e.g., "Good job!", "Great!", "Excellent!", "Perfect!", "Way to go!", "That's it!", "You got it!", "I knew you could do it!", "That was your best one!", "Yes! High five!").

The position of a word where an error is made is important in the analysis of a child's articulation. Most sounds in English can be produced in the initial, medial, or final position of words. For this reason, most articulation tests assess each consonant separately in those three positions (e.g., *pan, puppy, mop; soap, messy, bus*). A child may have an errored production of the sound in the middle and final positions of words but not in the initial position.

Many children with relatively minor articulation problems can have several sounds in error, and these children often benefit from "traditional" articulation therapy approaches (Bernthal, Bankson, & Flipsen, 2009; Gordon-Brannan & Weiss, 2007). In articulation therapy, the focus is on individual sounds in isolation and nonsense syllables, *phonetic drills* (practicing numerous repetitions producing specific sounds), and small increments of change. Articulation approaches tend to emphasize working with articulator movements to produce a sound correctly.

The general goals of traditional treatment approach are as follows:

- To become aware of characteristics of the standard phoneme (auditory discrimination).
- To recognize characteristics of misarticulations and how they differ from the target sound.

auditory discrimination training (ear training)

The ability to distinguish sounds from one another; involves a comparison of heard sounds with other sounds; a technique used in articulation therapy that stresses careful listening to differentiate among speech sounds.

positive reinforcement (positive feedback, reward)

A technique used to encourage a desired behavior by presenting something the person wants soon after the desired behavior is made.

social reinforcer

A word, phrase, or short statement said with warmth and enthusiasm as a reward and encouragement for an accurate response or good attempt at a specific task or target.

- To produce the standard sound at will, and to stabilize or strengthen the use of the target sound in isolation, syllables, words, phrases, and sentences.

- To use the standard sound in spontaneous speech of all kinds and under all conditions; that is, to *achieve carryover*.

The above goals may be condensed into two main components of articulation therapy: *perceptual training* and *production training*. Clinicians tend to follow an often-used sequence for remediating articulation errors (Bernthal, Bankson, & Flipsen, 2009; Gordon-Brannan & Weiss, 2007): (1) establish or improve auditory discrimination of the target sound so that the child can easily recognize the sounds said by others as correct or incorrect, as well as recognize the accuracy of his own productions; (2) produce the sound in isolation by imitating the clinician; (3) produce the sound in various consonant-vowel, vowel-consonant, and consonant-vowel-consonant combinations; (4) establish the sound first in the initial position, then the final position, and then the medial position of single syllable, *bisyllable* (two syllable), and *multisyllable* words; (5) establish the sound in simple phrases and sentences; (6) establish the sound in controlled discourse (e.g., storytelling); and (7) develop **generalization** of the sound to spontaneous conversation. These seven steps may be condensed into three basic steps: (1) listen, (2) experiment, and (3) practice (see Figure 5–10). The challenge, however, has always been the consistent generalization (*carryover*) to spontaneous conversational speech of the newly acquired and correctly articulated sounds.

generalization

The transfer of learning from one environment to other environments; usually considered the therapy or classroom to a natural environment, such as the home.

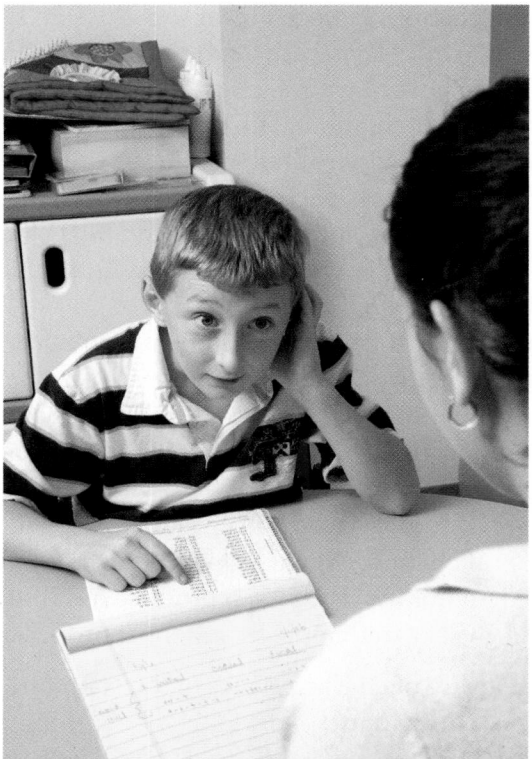

© Cengage Learning 2013

Figure 5–10

"Traditional" speech therapy often involves extensive drill of correct production of a sound in words.

Hunter

Hunter was a 7-year-old boy seen for therapy by a speech-language pathologist in private practice because of his difficulty being understood by friends, family, and even his parents. His parents had resorted to using a simple sign language system to better understand his communications. An evaluation of his speech systems revealed that his respiratory, phonatory, and resonatory systems functioned within normal limits for the development of normal speech. His articulatory system (mandible, lips, and tongue) were within normal limits in structure and symmetry, as well as for function (range of motion, strength, coordination, and rate of movement). Analysis of his speech errors did not reveal a phonological disorder. Neurologically, Hunter appeared intact; he was an excellent student with no apparent attention or behavioral problems, and he was motivated to improve his speech. The cause of his articulation problems could not be determined. However, following a traditional articulation therapy approach over time helped Hunter to become 95%–100% intelligible to his family, friends, and strangers. ■

Phonology therapy applies a different approach compared to articulation therapy. The basic treatment principles for phonological therapy include: (1) intervention begins at the word level; (2) treatment focuses on the phonological system of the child; and (3) groups of sounds or sound classes, rather than individual speech sounds are targeted (Bauman-Waengler, 2007). There are several phonological approaches; however, the *distinctive features approach* is frequently used by clinicians. The general goals of the distinctive features approach are to teach children how to produce specific distinctive features in the context of phonemes and to teach the rules for correct use of a particular distinctive feature (see Table 5–2). Therapy is often begun at the isolation level, that is, the phoneme without a vowel, followed by progressively more advanced levels: syllables, words, phrases, sentences, stories, and finally spontaneous conversation.

Application Question

Why could it be helpful to begin therapy with auditory discrimination training with a child?

MOTOR SPEECH DISORDERS

According to the ASHA, 2010 *Schools Survey Report*, in 2001 (the most recent data available on motor speech disorders in children) approximately 80% of school-based clinicians reported that their caseloads include an average of four children with a motor speech disorder, either childhood apraxia of speech (CAS) or dysarthria. As defined in Chapter 1, a motor speech disorder is impaired speech intelligibility that is caused by a neurological impairment that affects the motor (movement) planning or the strength of the articulators needed for rapid, complex movements in smooth, effortless speech. Motor speech disorders are often considered **sensorimotor** *disorders* because both sensory and motor

sensorimotor

The combination of input of sensations and output of motor activity; motor activity reflects what is happening to the sensory systems.

CASE STUDY

Jonathan: A Multihandicapped Child

Jonathan was a 16-year-old student who was medically diagnosed with Alstrom syndrome, which is a rare disease in which a child progressively loses visual and hearing acuities and has other organ and system disorders, including infantile obesity, baldness, and diabetes type 2. Jonathan's vision was monochromatic—everything he saw was the same color. He eventually learned to read *Braille*. Even with the use of hearing aids, he had a mild hearing loss. His auditory processing skills and memory were both in the average range. Jonathan was unable to identify or produce vowel sounds in isolation. He also had difficulty accurately identifying words in which he had to distinguish between /f/ and /th/ and /m/ and /n/, which correlated with his hearing impairment. Jonathan tended to "fill in the blanks" with what he thought he had heard instead of asking for clarification. This caused him to make numerous mistakes and inappropriate comments to his teachers and peers.

Jonathan had decreased range of motion of his mandible, lips, and tongue, which affected his overall speech intelligibility. He had difficulty placing his tongue in the positions requested by the clinician, so he was allowed to put on a latex glove and feel the clinician's mouth when unable to understand what was wanted for a specific task. He was enrolled in articulation and phonological processing therapy to work on speech intelligibility. His speech clinician began at the single-sound level, and after 3 years, Jonathan was able to segment sounds (recognize individual sounds in words) and spell lengthy words. Vowels remained the most difficult for him to recognize because of his hearing impairment. Extensive modeling and repetitions were needed in therapy to help him achieve the smallest goals. This case study reflects the complexity of working with multihandicapped children. ■

Source: Vic Trierweiler, M.A., CCC-SLP, California School for the Blind, Fremont. Used with permission.

---

childhood apraxia of speech (CAS)

A childhood motor speech disorder in the absence of muscle weakness that affects planning, programming, sequencing, coordinating, and initiating motor movements of the articulators that interferes with articulation and prosody.

perseverate/ perseveration

Automatic and involuntary repetition of a behavior, including repetition of a sound, syllable, word, or phrase when speaking.

neurological systems are involved. These children often have other developmental language and cognitive problems that make evaluation and treatment more challenging.

Childhood Apraxia of Speech

Childhood apraxia of speech (CAS) involves disruptions of planning (programming), sequencing, coordinating, and initiating motor movements of the articulators, which affect articulation and *prosody* (voice inflections such as stress, intonation, and rhythm) (Yorkston, Beukelman, Strand, & Hakel, 2010). CAS causes difficulty moving the articulators into their correct positions to produce sounds; words with more sounds and syllables may create more difficulty for a child. Children with apraxia sometimes **perseverate** (i.e., repeat) sounds, syllables, or words in a somewhat disfluent manner. Childhood apraxia of speech has many similarities to apraxia of speech in adults. ASHA (ASHA, 2007) defines childhood apraxia of speech as:

> A neurological childhood speech-sound disorder in which the precision and consistency of movements underlying speech are impaired in the absence of neuromuscular deficits (e.g., abnormal reflexes, abnormal tone). CAS may occur as a result of known neurological impairment, in association with complex neurobehavioral disorders of known or unknown origin, or as an **idiopathic** neurogenic speech-sound disorder. The core impairment in planning and/or programming spatiotemporal parameters of movement sequences results in errors in speech sound production and prosody.

idiopathic

A disease or disorder of unknown etiology.

Unlike acquired apraxia of speech in adults where damage to Broca's area in the left hemisphere of the brain is the generally accepted site of lesion (see Chapter 11, Neurological Disorders in Adults), the neuropathology for CAS has not been well documented, which creates some controversy among some theorists and clinicians about the legitimacy of the disorder and has been discussed by various authors (Forrest, 2003; Maassen, 2002; Moriarty, Gillon, & Moran, 2005). It is not as easy to diagnose a child as it is to diagnose an adult as having apraxia of speech, although many characteristics of the disorders and the principles of evaluation and treatment are similar for children and adults.

Although there may be tentativeness to the diagnostic term, there is clinical value in differentiating the speech characteristics of CAS from articulation and phonological disorders. However, to complicate these diagnoses and the development of appropriate therapy strategies, children may have a combination of articulation problems, phonological problems, and apraxia of speech (Gordon-Brannan & Weiss, 2007; Velleman, 2003).

Speech Characteristics of Childhood Apraxia of Speech

Characteristics of CAS were first described by Morley in 1957 and have been discussed in the literature since that time. We need to keep in mind that speech involves all speech systems—which includes planning, sequencing, coordinating, and initiating respiratory, phonatory, and resonatory movements, as well as articulatory movements. Some children may perform adequately on isolated articulator movements (e.g., rapid protrusion and retraction of the tongue) but when the complex interactions of the speech systems are added to produce speech, the articulatory system is overtaxed and difficulty becomes apparent. A variety of articulatory errors and speech characteristics have been ascribed to children

Personal Story

Karen: A Child with Developmental Childhood Apraxia of Speech

diadochokinetic (diadochokinesis, diadochols)

In speech, the ability to execute rapid repetitive or alternating movements of the articulators; *diadochokinetic rate* is the speed at which the movements can be performed.

Karen was a very sweet 7-year-old girl who had severe CAS. She received speech therapy at her school; however, her parents felt that she needed more help and called me. I saw Karen twice a week in her home. We typically worked in her bedroom sitting on small chairs in front of the large mirror on her little makeup table. Her mother was often present to watch us work, and the door was always open so she could peek in or come in at any time. Karen was almost unintelligible and had difficulty with even rudimentary oral movements such as placement of her tongue in her mouth and slow **diadochokinetic** movements of her mandible and lips—so that is where we began therapy. I was aware of the conflicting data about the use of oral-motor exercises in therapy; however, for this child I felt it was important to begin at that level. It paid off. The development of oral-motor coordination laid the foundation for the much more complex coordination of respiration, phonation, resonation, and articulation for speech. The combination of school therapy and private therapy helped this child to develop intelligible speech over time. ▪

who may be diagnosed with CAS (Bauman-Waengler, 2000; Campbell, 2003; Downing & Chamberlain, 2006; Gordon-Brannan & Weiss, 2007):

- More errors are made in the sound classes involving more complex oral movements (e.g., consonant clusters, fricatives, and affricates).
- Errors increase with increasing length of word or utterance, and articulation breaks down more in sentences and conversation than in single words.
- A large percentage of omission errors occur (e.g., omission of individual sounds in mono- and bisyllabic words but omission of syllables in multisyllabic words).
- Vowel and diphthong errors occur.
- Well-practiced utterances are produced or imitated more easily than unfamiliar utterances.
- Groping behavior and silent posturing of the articulators occur when the child attempts to articulate some words (e.g., abnormal movements of the articulators in an attempt to find the desired position for a specific sound).
- Prosodic impairments occur (e.g., inappropriate stress on sounds and syllables).

- There is a lack of progress in articulation and phonological therapy over a long period (e.g., many children are highly unintelligible and may be seen for several or many semesters of therapy with one or more clinicians with minimal progress).

Overall, a broad cluster of symptoms represents CAS. ASHA's Ad Hoc Committee on Childhood Apraxia of Speech (2007) narrowed the core symptoms down to (1) inconsistent errors on consonants and vowels when a child is asked to repeatedly produce individual words (i.e., the child makes different errors during different productions of the same word), (2) abnormal transitions between sounds and words (i.e., the child has difficulty with sequencing sounds and syllables, has abnormal breaks between consonants and vowels, and has increasing difficulty as the number of sounds and syllables increase in a word), and (3) inappropriate prosody during production of individual words and phrases (i.e., stress and intonation are abnormal). Bauman-Waengler (2000) says that not all symptoms must be present for a child to have apraxia of speech. Furthermore, no one characteristic or symptom must be present within a child's constellation of symptoms for a child to have CAS.

Childhood Dysarthria

Dysarthria may be caused by damage to either the central nervous system (brain and brainstem) or the peripheral nervous system (cranial nerves that supply the articulators [V, VII, IX, XI, and XII], and branches off of the vagus [X] cranial nerve that supply the larynx and diaphragm). For example, the speech disorder related to **cerebral palsy** is dysarthria caused by damage to the central nervous system (see Chapter 13, Special Populations with Communication Disorders).

Symptoms of dysarthria vary depending on the location and extent of the neurological damage. Dysarthria in children has many similarities to dysarthria in adults, with various combinations of **hypotonicity** and **hypertonicity** in the muscles that control respiration, phonation, resonation, and articulation. Dysarthria may affect each of the speech systems. Interaction of the systems causes a child's speech to be more severely impaired than if just the articulatory system is impaired. Dysarthria usually affects the range of motion, strength, coordination, and rate of movement of the muscles used for speech, often resulting in sound distortions that have no phonetic symbol that clearly represents the error.

Speech Characteristics of Childhood Dysarthria

Dysarthric speech is sometimes referred to as "hot potato speech" because it sounds somewhat like a person trying to talk with hot potatoes in his mouth–speech sounds "mushy." The following are some common characteristics of childhood dysarthria seen in each of the speech

---

dysarthria

A group of motor speech disorders caused by *paresis* (weakness), *paralysis* (complete loss of movement), or incoordination of speech muscles as a result of central and/or peripheral nervous system damage that may affect respiration, phonation, resonation, articulation, and prosody; dysarthric speech sounds "mushy" because of distorted consonants and vowels.

cerebral palsy (CP)

A developmental neuromotor disorder that is caused by damage to the central nervous system *prenatally* (before birth), *natally/perinatally* (during birth), or *postnatally* (during childhood) and results in a nonprogressive, permanent neuromuscular disorder; dysarthria affecting all speech systems is the most common speech problem.

hypotonicity

Weakness or absence of muscle tone or tension in a muscle or muscle group (e.g., laryngeal muscles, velar muscles).

hypertonicity

Excessive tone or tension in a muscle or muscle group (e.g., chest muscles, articulatory muscles).

Application Question

Like all other health care and educational specialists, speech-language pathologists and audiologists sometimes cannot determine the exact cause or make a clear diagnosis of a disorder. How comfortable will you be with some ambiguity in the cause, diagnosis, or specific course of treatment for a child's or an adult's communication disorder?

Personal Story — Mandy

Mandy was a beautiful and perfectly normal girl until she was 8 years old and was hit by a drunk driver as she was crossing a street near her home. She sustained a broken leg, abrasions, and a head trauma that affected her cerebellum. The brain damage affected her balance and her speech, which was moderately dysarthric. Although Mandy received speech therapy at her school, the parents wanted additional therapy for their daughter and contacted me. I worked with Mandy in her home at the kitchen table twice a week for about 12 months. I coordinated my therapy with what the SLP was working on at her school. My goal in therapy was to maximize her speech intelligibility, which required (1) improving her respiratory support for adequate inhalation and controlled exhalation for speech; (2) increasing her loudness and duration of voicing with variations in pitch when speaking; and (3) increasing her range of motion, strength, coordination, and rate of movement of each of the articulators. Prosody was focused on once she made significant gains in the other areas. When therapy was eventually ended, Mandy's speech was 95%–100% intelligible, although not all speech sounds were precise and she had her most difficulty when she was sleepy or fatigued. ∎

systems (Morgan, Mageandran, & Mei, 2010; Yorkston, Beukelman, Strand, & Hakel, 2010):

- *Respiratory*—Low intensity and speech that is limited to short phrases because of decreased respiratory support.
- *Phonatory*—Breathy phonation because of unilateral or bilateral vocal fold paresis or paralysis.
- *Resonatory*—Hypernasality because of weak or absent movement of the soft palate, causing velopharyngeal incompetence.
- *Articulatory*—Distorted, imprecise consonants because of weakness and incoordination of the mandible, lips, and tongue.

EMOTIONAL AND SOCIAL EFFECTS OF ARTICULATION AND PHONOLOGICAL DISORDERS

Children of all ages with mild or moderate articulation or phonological disorders may hear negative comments about their speech and be the target of teasing, ridiculing, mocking imitation, labeling ("He talks like a baby."), and even exclusion and ostracism from conversations, games, parties, and clubs. Children who have such experiences are emotionally hurt, embarrassed, and frustrated with themselves for not being able to speak normally. They often suffer in silence. They may develop negative attitudes about themselves, such as feeling different, inadequate,

Mike's Apraxia

During the first 2 years after earning my master's degree, I worked in what was then called an "aphasia classroom" with adolescents who had "childhood aphasia" (a term no longer used). The class was limited to eight students. One student was Mike, who had been a normal (actually, above normal) boy before a sledding accident when he was on a snow trip with his Boy Scout troop. Mike had been a good student and a good Scout, and he loved playing Little League baseball. During the sledding accident, he hit his head on a tree and received a traumatic brain injury.

Mike's TBI resulted in moderate to severe aphasia and profound apraxia. He was extremely frustrated and angry about his impairments and newly acquired limitations. He tried to play baseball but no longer had the motor skills to play well. He now had learning disabilities, whereas learning used to come easy for him. His greatest frustration, however, was not being able to speak intelligibly. In the classroom my job was to teach academic subjects at the level at which each child could learn and to provide speech, language, and cognitive therapy.

Mike continued being as active in Boy Scouts as he could, but he was sometimes teased by the other boys. His mother asked if I would be willing to come to one of his evening Scout meetings to talk to the Scoutmaster and the other Scouts about Mike's problems. I was happy to do that. On the evening of the meeting, Mike proudly wore his full Scout uniform. He knew I was going to be talking about him. The Scoutmaster and other Scouts listened attentively and asked some very good questions as I tried to explain Mike's complex problems in layperson's terms. I could see that they were beginning to understand Mike's problems and were developing some empathy. Mike's mother and the Scoutmaster felt that the evening was a success. As clinicians, we need to learn how to explain our many professional terms and complex concepts in layperson's terms and be willing to go beyond our therapy rooms or classrooms to meet some of the most important needs of the children we help. ■

disliked, and socially incompetent. Children with more severe articulation and phonological disorders likely experience the most severe emotional and social consequences. Parents report that approximately 55% of their children with speech disorders also exhibit social competence problems, and 70% of the children have behavioral problems 10 years after they were initially diagnosed in preschool as having communication impairments (Aram & Hall, 1989; Rice, Hadley, & Alexander, 1993).

Communication skills are essential for students to be successful in school. Children with speech disorders may limit their willingness to speak up in class and avoid peer interactions for fear of being teased and embarrassed. Also, their articulation and phonological problems may be only part of their overall difficulties communicating. Of preschoolers, 75% to 85% with articulation and phonological disorders also experience disorders of language, and 50% to 70% of school age children with speech disorders also have academic difficulties in all grade levels, particularly with reading, writing, spelling, and mathematics (Bernthal, Bankson, & Flipsen, 2009; Gordon-Brannan, & Weiss, 2007). In order to help children become better communicators and successful in school and life, speech-language pathologists need to be willing and able to help children with their academic, emotional, and social struggles (Flasher & Fogle, 2012).

CHAPTER SUMMARY

General American English ("American English") is spoken by the majority of Americans and is considered not to have a regional dialect. SLPs use phonetics to describe the individual sounds in a language and use the International Phonetic Alphabet (IPA) transcription symbols to identify specific sounds for any language or dialect. Vowels are voiced speech sounds from the unrestricted passage of the air stream through the mouth without audible stoppage or friction. Consonants are speech sounds articulated by either stopping the outgoing air stream or creating a narrow opening of resistance using the articulators. Consonants are commonly described by their distinctive features—voice, manner, and place.

The three general etiologies of communication disorders in children are: normal variation, environmental problems, and physical impairments or differences. In many cases, there may be a combination of etiologies affecting any one child. Often the cause or causes of a communication disorder cannot be determined. Hearing impairments almost always result in delays and disorders of speech and language.

Four primary types of articulation errors can be made on any one sound: substitutions, omissions, distortions, and additions (S.O.D.A.). A phonological disorder involves errors of several phonemes that form patterns and is the result of a child simplifying individual sounds and sound combinations. An evaluation of a child's speech involves assessing all of the speech systems, focusing on the articulatory system, administering a standardized articulation and sometimes a phonological test, and analyzing the test results. Articulation therapy focuses on the mechanics of producing the speech sounds.

Childhood apraxia of speech is a motor speech disorder in the absence of muscle weakness that affects the planning, programming, sequencing, coordinating, and initiating motor movements of the articulators that interferes with articulation and prosody. Childhood dysarthria is a group of motor speech disorders caused by weakness, paralysis, or incoordination of speech muscles as a result of central and/or peripheral nervous system damage that may affect respiration, phonation, resonation, articulation, and prosody; dysarthric speech sounds "mushy" because of distorted consonants and vowels. As clinicians, we need to be aware of and concerned about possible emotional and social effects of articulation and phonological disorders on children.

STUDY QUESTIONS

Knowledge and Comprehension

1. Explain each of the three distinctive features (voice, manner, and place) that determine the production of sounds.

2. What are the three primary etiologies of articulation, phonological, communication, and cognitive problems?

3. How can hearing loss affect development of communication?

4. Explain substitution and distortion, and provide two examples of each.

5. Define and describe childhood apraxia of speech.

Application

1. Why is it important to consider a child's articulation errors in all three positions of words, that is, initial, medial, and final positions of words?

2. Why might you consider the frequency of sounds in our language when trying to determine which sounds to target with children who have developmental articulation delays?

3. How can clinicians maintain a perspective of normal children to help them better recognize and treat children with communication delays and disorders?

4. What could a clinician be informally assessing during the unstructured rapport-building time?

5. Which speech systems would you want to evaluate if you suspected childhood dysarthria? Why?

Analysis/Synthesis

1. When analyzing speech sounds, why might it be helpful to first consider whether a sound is voiced or unvoiced (voicing), then whether it is oral or nasal (manner), and finally, the location (place) in the oral cavity where the articulators make contact?

2. Why is it important for speech-language pathologists and audiologists working in the school systems to have a good background in syndromes and developmental and medical complications of children?

3. How could auditory discrimination problems cause articulation problems?

4. Why is a spontaneous speech sample important in determining a child's level of speech intelligibility?

5. Why would errors increase as the length of a word or utterance increases and articulation break down more in sentences and conversation than in single words for children who have apraxia of speech?

REFERENCES

American Speech-Language-Hearing Association. (2007). *Childhood apraxia of speech* [Position Statement]. Available from www.asha.org/policy.

American Speech-Language-Hearing Association. (2010). *School Survey report: Caseload characteristics.* Rockville, MD: ASHA.

Apgar, V. (1953, July/August). A proposal for a new method of evaluating the newborn infant. *Current Research in Anesthesiology and Analgesia,* 260.

Aram, D. M., & Hall, N. E. (1989). Longitudinal follow-up of children with pre-school communication disorders: Treatment implications. *School of Psychology Review, 19,* 487–501.

Bauman-Waengler, J. (2012). *Articulatory and phonological impairments: A clinical focus* (4th ed.). San Antonio, TX: Pearson/Allyn & Bacon.

Bernthal, J. E., Bankson, N. W., & Flipsen, P. (2009). *Articulation and phonological disorders* (6th ed.). San Antonio, TX: Pearson/Allyn & Bacon.

Bowen, C. (1998). *Developmental phonological disorders: A practical guide for families and teachers.* Melbourne, Australia: ACER Press.

Campbell, T. F. (2003). *Childhood apraxia of speech: Clinical symptoms and speech characteristics: Proceedings of the childhood apraxia of speech research symposium.* Carlsbad, CA: Hendrix Foundation, 37–40.

Center on Addiction and Substance Abuse. (2005). *Substance abuse and the American woman.* New York, NY: Columbia University.

Curtis, S. (1977). *Genie: A psycholinguistic study of a modern-day "wild child."* New York: Academic Press.

Dewey, G. (1923). *Relative frequency of English speech sounds.* Cambridge, MA: Harvard University Press.

Downing, R. S., & Chamberlain, C. E. (2006). *The source for childhood apraxia of speech.* East Moline, IL: LinguiSystems.

Edwards, H. T. (2003). *Applied phonetics: The sounds of American English* (3rd ed.). Clifton Park, NY: Delmar Cengage Learning.

Flasher, L. V., & Fogle, P. T. (2012). *Counseling skills for speech-language pathologists and audiologists* (2nd ed.). Clifton Park, NY: Delmar Cengage Learning.

Forrest, K. (2003). Diagnostic criteria of developmental apraxia of speech used by clinical speech-language pathologists. *American Journal of Speech-Language Pathology, 12*(3), 376–380.

Gelfer, M. P. (1996). *Survey of communication disorders: A social and behavioral perspective.* New York, NY: McGraw-Hill.

Gordon-Brannan, M. E., & Weiss, C. E. (2007). *Clinical management of articulatory and phonological disorders.* Philadelphia, PA: Lippincott, Williams & Wilkins.

Grunau, R., Kearney, S., & Whitfield, M. (1990). Language development at 3 years in pre-term children of birth weight below 1000 grams. *British Journal of Disorders of Communication, 25,* 173–182.

Grunwell, P. (1997). Natural phonology. In M. Ball & R. Kent (Eds.), *The new phonologies: Developments in clinical linguistics.* Clifton Park, NY: Delmar Cengage Learning.

Maassen, C. (2002). Issues contrasting adult acquired versus developmental apraxia of speech. *Seminars in Speech and Language, 23*(4), 257–267.

Martin, F. N., & Clark, J. G. (2012). *Introduction to audiology* (10th ed.). San Antonio, TX: Pearson/Allyn & Bacon.

Morgan, A. T., Mageandran, S. D., & Mei, C. (2010). Incidence and clinical presentation of dysarthria and dysphagia in the acute setting following pediatric traumatic brain injury. *Child: Care, Health, and Development, 36*(1), 44–53.

Moriarty, B., Gillon, G., & Moran, C. (2005). Assessment and treatment of childhood apraxia of speech (CAS): A clinical tutorial. *New Zealand Journal of Speech-Language Therapy, 60*, 18–30.

Morley, M. E. (1957). *The development and disorders of speech in children.* London, England: Livingston.

Mosby. (2009). *Mosby's dictionary of medicine, nursing, & health professions* (8th ed.). St. Louis, MO: Mosby Elsevier.

Pena-Brooks, A., & Hegde, M. N. (2007). *Assessment and treatment of articulation and phonological disorders in children.* Austin, TX: Pro-Ed.

Rice, M. L. , Hadley, P. P., & Alexander, A. L. (1993). Social biases toward children with specific language impairment: A correlative causal model of language limitations. *Applied Pyscholinguistics, 13*, 443–472.

Rossetti, L. (2001). *Communication intervention: Birth to three.* Clifton Park, NY: Delmar Cengage Learning.

Shipley, K. G., & McAfee, J. G. (2009). *Assessment in speech-language pathology: A resource manual* (4th ed.). Clifton Park, NY: Delmar Cengage Learning.

Small, L. H. (2012). *Fundamentals of phonetics: A practical guide for students* (2nd ed.). San Antonio, TX: Pearson/Allyn & Bacon.

U.S. Census Bureau. (2010). *Census summary file 3: 2010 census population and housing technical documentation.* Available at http://www.census.gov/newsroom/minority_links/asian.html.

Velleman, S. (2003). *Childhood apraxia of speech: Resource guide.* Clifton Park, NY: Delmar Cengage Learning.

Wyatt, T. A. (2002). Assessing the communicative abilities of children from diverse cultural and language backgrounds. In D. E. Battle (Ed.), *Communication disorders in multicultural populations* (3rd ed.). Boston, MA: Butterworth-Heinemann.

Yavas, M. (1998). *Phonology development and disorders.* Clifton Park, NY: Delmar Cengage Learning.

Yorkston, K. M., Beukelman, D. R., Strand, E. A., & Hakel, M. (2010). *Management of motor speech disorders in children and adults* (3rd ed.). Austin, TX: Pro-Ed.

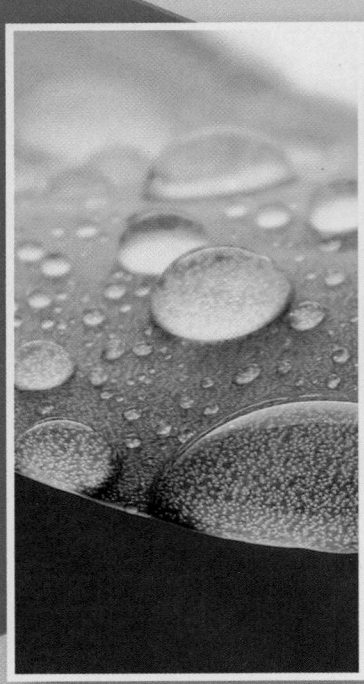

CHAPTER 6
Language Disorders in Children

LEARNING OBJECTIVES

After studying this chapter, you will:

- Be able to define language disorder.
- Be able to discuss language disorder versus language difference.
- Understand the various problems seen in children with specific language impairments.
- Understand the characteristics of language-learning disabilities.
- Be able to discuss the basic process of assessing a child's language.
- Be able to discuss the basic process of therapy for language disorders.
- Be familiar with multicultural considerations of children with language disorders.
- Appreciate the emotional and social effects of language disorders on children.

KEY TERMS

attainable treatment
chronological age
circumlocution
client-specific measurements (clinician devised assessments)
context
developmental coordination disorder
diagnosis

effective treatment
elicit
evidence-based treatment (best practices)
fine motor skills
functional treatment
goal (target behavior)
gross motor skills
heterogeneous
incidence

KEY TERMS continued

language arts
language comprehension
language-learning disability
language sample
learning disabilities (LD)
mean length of utterance (MLU)
measurement
metalinguistics
normative data (norms)
operationally defined goal

prevalence
reliable/reliability
replicate
screening
specific language impairment (SLI)
standardized test (norm-referenced test)
utterance
valid/validity

CHAPTER OUTLINE

heterogeneous

Consisting of dissimilar or diverse individuals or constituents.

INTRODUCTION

Children with language impairments are a **heterogeneous** group who vary in numerous ways. Their language problems may be exacerbated as they progress in age and educational level. For a preschooler, a "mild" language disorder may create greater challenges as he progresses in school and is expected to understand increasingly difficult information presented by teachers and to verbally express himself with more complex language. These problems are again magnified when the child is expected to learn to read and then read to learn, as well as to be able to express himself proficiently in writing.

DEFINITIONS OF LANGUAGE DISORDER

The ASHA's Ad Hoc Committee on Service Delivery in the Schools (1993, p. IV) presented the following definition of language disorder:

> A language disorder is impaired comprehension and/or use of spoken, written (graphic), and/or other symbol systems. The disorder may involve (1) the form of language (phonology, morphology, and syntax), (2) the content of language (semantics), and/or (3) the function of language in communication (pragmatics) in any combination (p. 40).

The ASHA definition identifies the scope of practice for speech-language pathologists in reference to language disorders: we work with both receptive and expressive language disorders that may involve the form, content, and/or function of language in both the spoken and the written modalities. Although researchers and clinicians may discuss components of language separately (i.e., phonology, morphology, syntax, semantics, and pragmatics), in actuality all components interact at one time, with each component affecting the others (Reed, 2012).

Owens (2008) defines a language disorder (impairment) as a heterogeneous group of developmental and/or acquired disorders, delays, or both that are principally characterized by deficits, immaturities, or both in the use of spoken or written language for purposes of comprehension, production, or both that may involve the form, content, and/or function of language in any combination. This definition emphasizes the vast differences in the language problems of children and adolescents and that the impairments may manifest at any time (e.g., acquired language disorders from traumatic brain injuries).

Language disorders may be more apparent in some contexts and learning tasks than in others. The deficits or delays may exist in some or all modes of communication, such as listening, speaking, reading, or writing. Language disorders may be classified according to the areas of language that are impaired: *form* (phonology, morphology, and syntax), *content* (semantics), and *use* (pragmatics); their severity (mild, moderate, severe, profound); and whether they affect comprehension (receptive language), production (expressive language), or both.

Other terms may be used in place of *disorder,* such as impairment or disability. The terms *language disorder* and *language impairment* are often used interchangeably. However, the term *language disability* suggests that a child's language difficulties significantly affect communication and daily activities in both home and school. In addition, various terms may be used by different school districts or states, for example, *specific language disorder, language-learning disability,* or other combinations of these words (the designation used is often determined by children's age, as well as funding available for the provisions of services to children). The term *primary language impairment* suggests a significant impairment of language when there is no other disability, such as cognitive impairment or traumatic brain injury. A *secondary language impairment* accompanies more pervasive disabilities, such as developmental (intellectual) disabilities or developmental delays (see Chapter 13, Special Populations with Communication Disorders).

Language Disorder versus Language Delay

The term *language delay* implies that children may have a slow start at developing language but that they will eventually catch up with their peers (Hegde & Maul, 2006). Parents often refer to these children as "slow talkers" and "late bloomers." Although some children who exhibit early mild language delays eventually develop normal language skills, they are more likely to have residual language impairments and related disabilities throughout childhood (Johnson, Beitchman, Young, Escobar, Atkinson, & Wilson 1999). Children with language disorders do not eventually catch up with their peers; more commonly, the gap in language skills between children developing normally and those with language disorders widens over time (Pence & Justice, 2008).

Language Disorder versus Language Difference

Children's culturally and linguistically diverse backgrounds may significantly affect their expressive communication. However, expressive language affected by cultural and linguistic diversity is not a disorder—it is a *difference.* As discussed in Chapter 4 under Cultural and Linguistic Diversity Perspective, American English includes a variety of social dialects, such as variations of phonology, morphology, syntax, semantics, and pragmatics. No one dialect is better than another within the language.

When determining whether a particular child's language is disordered or different, we must consider two norms: the referenced norms of General American English (GAE) and the cultural norms or expectations of the child. Clinicians who work with children who are bilingual, are learning English as a second language (ESL), or who speak an English dialect that differs from the mainstream dialect need to be careful during their assessments. Many standard language tests are not sensitive enough to differentiate between children who are typically developing and those who have a language impairment (Dollagham & Horner, 2011). For example, the grammatical morphology of children who are learning ESL may look similar to that of children with language impairment, particularly their omission of grammatical morphemes (Hegde & Maul, 2006; Paradis, 2005; Roseberry-McKibbin, 2001).

Prevalence and Incidence of Language Disorders

prevalence

The number of individuals diagnosed with a particular disorder at a given time.

incidence

The rate at which a disorder appears in the normal population over a period, typically 1 year.

Prevalence refers to the number of individuals diagnosed with a particular disorder at a given time. **Incidence** is the rate at which a disorder appears in the normal population over a period of time, typically one year. The prevalence of language disorders is more clinically relevant and, therefore, more commonly reported than is the incidence.

The few large studies available (more than 1,000 children) report that 7% to 8% of children entering kindergarten are recognized as having specific language impairment (SLI) with no other complicating conditions and that approximately 2% more boys than girls have SLI (Erwin, 2001). In terms of actual numbers, more than 1 million children in American schools receive special education services for primary speech or language disorders, and another approximately 700,000 school children receive services for secondary language impairments resulting from cognitive impairments, developmental delays, autism spectrum disorders, and traumatic brain injuries (U.S. Department of Education, 2008).

Severity Levels of Language Disorders

Severity levels for communication disorders (both speech and language) and cognitive disorders range from mild to profound. However, any one child may have different severity levels depending on the communication input or output modality (e.g., auditory or visual input or verbal, gestural, or graphic output). As mentioned earlier, depending on the communication demands, a child may appear to have mild problems when his receptive and expressive language functioning are only minimally challenged. However, when the challenges are more taxing, his true levels of difficulty may become apparent. For example, a child may have only moderate problems with auditory receptive and verbal expressive language but severe problems learning how to read and write. Paul (2011) provides a description of severity ratings that are clinically, educationally, and socially useful (see Figure 6–1).

Mild	Mild language disorders have some effect on a child's ability to perform in social or educational situations but do not preclude participation in normal, age-appropriate activities in school or community.
Moderate	Moderate language disorders involve a significant degree of impairment that necessitates some special accommodations for the child to participate in mainstream community and educational settings.
Severe	Severe language disorders usually make it difficult for a child to function in community and educational activities without extensive support.
Profound	Profound language disorders imply that a child has little or no ability to use language to communicate and is unable to function in community and educational activities.

Figure 6–1

Variations in severity of language disorders.

Adapted from Paul, 2011.

SPECIFIC LANGUAGE IMPAIRMENT (SLI)

As noted previously, **specific language impairment** (sometimes called *primary language disorder*) refers to significant receptive and/or expressive language impairments that cannot be attributed to any general or specific cause or condition (Pence & Justice, 2008; Tomblin, Zhang, Buckwalter, & O'Brian, 2003). These children have hearing within normal limits (although many have histories of middle ear infections), there are no obvious perceptual or neurological disorders, and their nonverbal intelligence is within normal limits. Specific language impairments are characterized more by the absence of other disorders than by some clearly identifiable set of observable traits (Bishop, 2006; Leonard, 2000; Owens, 2008). SLI is the most frequent reason for administering early intervention and special education services to preschool and early primary school children (Pence-Turnbul & Justice, 2012).

Children who are considered "slow talkers" by parents often have some "red flags" that can alert parents and clinicians to a young child's potential specific language impairments (Bishop, 2006; Hegde & Maul, 2006; Leonard, 2000):

- Slow development of speech sounds
- Does not say "Mama" or "Dada" by 12–18 months of age
- Significant late appearance of the first true word (i.e., after approximately 18 months of age)
- Significant late use of two-word combinations (i.e., after approximately 30 months of age)

specific language impairment (SLI)

Significant receptive and/or expressive language impairments that cannot be attributed to any general or specific cause or condition.

- Restricted vocabulary in both comprehension and production
- Reliance on gestures for getting needs met
- Infrequent use of verbs and poor development of verbs
- Lack of yes-or-no responses to questions
- Difficulty initiating interactions with age peers
- Difficulty with turn-taking during conversations
- Difficulty rhyming words
- Difficulty naming letters

Most children under 3 years of age who may have mild to moderate SLI are not recognized as having a significant problem by their parents, although the parents may voice concern to their pediatrician regarding the child's development. Pediatricians often take a "wait and see" approach and encourage parents to be patient, saying that they can expect their "late talker" or "late bloomer" to be a "chatterbox" sometime soon. After another 6 to 12 months pass, the parents' concerns *may* be reinforced by their pediatrician, who then *may* suggest the parents seek an evaluation of the child's speech by a speech therapist. Some pediatricians will again encourage the parents to be patient, particularly if the child is a boy because boys are generally expected to develop language slower than girls. This 6- to 12-month delay (or longer) in seeking services from an SLP can result in important time being lost that could have been used to help the child's speech and language development.

Physicians' Education of Speech-Language Pathology and Audiology

Physicians (e.g., general practitioners, pediatricians, otolaryngologists, and neurologists) in their education and training do not take specific course work on speech and language development or speech and language disorders of children and adults. Some of their textbooks may include cursory discussions of the many disorders that speech-language pathologists and audiologists assess and treat, but physicians do not have specific texts that discuss in detail the theory or SLP or Aud assessment and treatment of any disorders. Because of this lack of education and knowledge about our work, many physicians do not refer patients to us that we could help, leaving patients without the habilitation or rehabilitation we could provide and the gains they could make to improve their quality of life. As professionals, we need to educate physicians about what speech-language pathologists and audiologists can do to benefit patients.

Seldom can we clearly determine the cause of a child's specific language impairment, and it is unlikely that specific language impairment has a single cause. However, genetic makeup may exert a strong influence in determining which children develop SLI. Most researchers agree it is a complex disorder that may have multiple genetic influences that interact with environmental factors (Bishop, 2006). In some children with SLI, there may be subtle impairments of cognitive skills such as auditory perception, memory, and sequencing, although the relationship between cognition and language is not fully established (Choudhury & Benasich, 2003).

Receptive Language

Receptive language (**language comprehension**) is a process by which a listener infers the meaning of a message based on the **context** of the information and long-term stored memory that relates to what is being heard. Children with SLI commonly have difficulty with receptive language. In general, they have impaired ability to understand and integrate information, whether presented verbally or nonverbally. Their slow processing of auditory information can contribute to their difficulty understanding; that is, spoken words may be "coming at them too fast" and they are not able to keep up with a normal rate of conversation (Pence-Turnbull & Justice, 2012). Children with SLI may have difficulty understanding direct questions (e.g., "Do you want to go to McDonald's for lunch?") and even more difficulty understanding indirect questions (e.g., "McDonald's for lunch might be good."). Poor comprehension of individual words and the subtleties of language make it difficult for children to understand connected speech and contribute to their weak expressive vocabularies and impaired expressive language.

Children in primary and junior high school with SLI continue to have weak receptive vocabularies for their ages. They understand direct statements and requests easier than those that are indirect. They are often quite literal in their interpretation of statements and idioms, and misunderstand and misuse metaphors and similes (Pence-Turnbull & Justice, 2012). They have difficulty understanding abstract concepts and expressing their wants, needs, thoughts, and feelings even in rudimentary ways, which may result in frustration and behavioral outbursts.

Expressive Language

Expressive language at all ages is difficult for children with specific language impairments. From their earliest days of communicating, they have difficulty expressing their wants and needs, often leaving parents guessing and frustrated. Not only do they have language problems, they frequently have speech problems that make communicating even more difficult.

Articulation and Phonological Problems

Children 3 and 4 years of age who are difficult to understand often have specific language impairments (Leonard, 2000; Reed, 2012). Their reduced speech intelligibility affects their use of expressive language and their interactions with family and peers. As these children enter primary

language comprehension

An active process in which, from instant to instant, a listener infers the meaning of an auditory message based on the context of the information and long-term stored memory of words and general knowledge.

context

The immediate environment of the speaker and listener, including the topic being discussed and past experiences each person brings to the communication encounter.

In speech, any gross measure used to identify individuals who may require further assessment in a specific area (e.g., articulation, language, hearing, fluency, or voice).

mean length of utterance (MLU)

The average length of oral expressions as measured by representative sampling of oral language (e.g., 50–100 spontaneous utterances [Pence & Justice, 2008]); usually calculated by counting the number of morphemes per **utterance** and dividing by the number of utterances; e.g.,

$$\frac{150 \text{ morphemes}}{50 \text{ utterances}} = 3.0 \text{ MLU}.$$

utterance

A unit of vocal expression that is preceded and followed by silence; may be made up of a word or words, phrases, clauses, or sentences.

school they are recognized through **screening** or teacher referral as having articulation problems and are assessed and enrolled in therapy.

Morphological and Syntactic Problems

Morphological and syntactic problems are common in children with SLI. When morphological elements are missing, children's language is grammatically incomplete or incorrect. Children with SLI are late in developing syntactic structures and using them consistently (Owens, 2008; Paul, 2011). These problems usually are evident by 3 to 4 years of age in their **mean length of utterance (MLU)**, morphological markers, and sentence complexity. MLU is considered a valid and reliable indication of general language development (Rice, Redmond, & Hoffman, 2006). Children with morphological and syntactic problems often speak in short, incomplete sentences (e.g., "Milk!") or with simple, active, declarative sentences (e.g., "Me want milk."). As children grow older and have increasingly more complex information to communicate, their numerous morphological and syntactic problems interfere with conveying their messages and listeners become confused or lost. Such morphologic and syntactic problems result in children having difficulty with discourse and pragmatics. The consequences of such difficulty may be frustration and emotional pain for both the children and their parents.

Vocabulary Development and Semantic Problems

Children who have delays in using their first true words and who are slow to develop additional vocabulary (fewer than approximately 20 words by 24 months of age and fewer than approximately 200 words by 36 months of age) are at risk for specific language impairments. Normal children 24 months of age typically are using noun-verb constructions for sentences. Most children have a dramatic increase of new words between 24 and 36 months of age; however, children with SLI often have negligible increases during this time. Children with SLI may be able to name some objects but not be able to use adjectives to describe the objects (e.g., *big, brown,* and *noisy*) or verbs to indicate their actions (e.g., *"Doggy!"* versus *"Doggy bark!"*).

Vocabulary development and concept development are strongly related. Children who have weak vocabulary development typically have poor concept development, which may result in difficulty "making sense" of their world. Many nouns are also concepts; for example, the word *ball* has several concepts that may be related to it. There are many kinds of balls (baseball, basketball, beach ball, etc.), and each kind of ball has numerous concepts that relate to it. A ball is round (shape); it may be big (size) and red (color); it can be rolled, bounced, thrown, hit, or kicked (actions). The noun *ball,* then, can have various parts of speech related to it, such as adjectives, verbs, and prepositions. Children with SLI may not understand or use words that express concepts of shape, size, color, quantity, and quality, or verbs that may relate to an object.

In addition, verb markers (e.g., *-ed* and *-ing*) are particularly difficult for these children (Conti-Ramsden & Windfuhr, 2002). Children with specific language impairments commonly have significant difficulty with literacy skills, that is, learning to read, reading to learn, and writing (see Chapter 7, Literacy Disorders in Children).

Word-finding problems are a characteristic of many children with specific language impairments, that is, they are not able to think of a specific word they want to say (Bayne & Moran, 2005). A study conducted in England found that 23% of children receiving language support services had word-finding problems (Dockrell, Messer, George, & Wilson, 1998). Word-finding problems are commonly characterized by (1) unnatural pauses or *latency* (delays while trying to think of a word), (2) *fillers* (um-um, uh-uh), (3) *nonspecific words* (thing, stuff), (4) *substitutions* of a less desired word for the desired word, (5) the use of *excessive pronouns* that leave the listener uncertain of who or what is being referred to, (7) *repetitions* of a word or phrase until the desired (or an acceptable) word is recalled, (8) *topic avoidance* (avoiding topics for which the child may have difficulty recalling words), (9) **circumlocutions** ("talking around words"), and (10) difficulties with *confrontation naming* (naming objects shown or described to them). These children often say "You know" hoping that listeners can fill in missing words or can guess the meanings of their messages. Because children with SLI cannot provide correct nouns, verbs, and adjectives in conversation, listeners are often confused by their messages.

Asking questions is also difficult for these children and many have problems understanding when to use the "wh"-question words (*who, what, when, where, why, how*). Therefore, they may not get information they need and have difficulty asking for clarification of information for which they are uncertain. They have particular difficulty understanding how to form questions using inverted auxiliaries (e.g., "He is going."— declarative sentence; "Is he going?"—interrogative sentence).

Relating *narratives* (stories with a sequence of events) is one of the most challenging skills for these children. Narratives require (1) recall of the event or events, including the time, place, people, and other important details involved, (2) recall of specific words that could help relate the experience to a listener, (3) formulation of the language structures to communicate the experience as accurately and completely as possible, and (4) pragmatic skills to recognize whether the listener is understanding or even interested in the story. Children with specific language impairments may have breakdowns in all of these skills (Colozzo, Gillam, Wood, et al., 2011).

Metalinguistics

Metalinguistics refers to the ability to think about and eventually talk about language. Metalinguistics goes beyond the ability to understand word meanings and grammar. It is the conscious awareness and use of language as a tool. Metalinguistics encompasses the ability to (1) recognize and interpret multiple meanings in words and sentences, (2) make

circumlocution

The use of a description or "talking around" a word when the specific word cannot be recalled.

metalinguistics

The ability to think about and talk about language.

multiple inferences, (3) interpret figurative language, and (4) plan and organize sentences, paragraphs, and narratives (Nicolosi, Harryman, & Kresheck, 2004). Students with specific language impairments generally have poor metalinguistics skills and are at considerable disadvantage when they reach the middle school years (Cairns, Waltzman, & Schlisselberg, 2007).

language arts

Academic activities such as listening, speaking, reading, handwriting, spelling, and written composition.

In the classroom environment, metalinguistics is often included in **language arts** (i.e., listening, speaking, reading, handwriting, spelling, and written composition). Metalinguistics is a significant linguistic achievement that emerges during primary school and develops through junior and senior high school. It is a skill involved with both spoken and written language and facilitates children's acquisition of independent problem-solving abilities (Cairns, Waltzman, & Schlisselberg, 2004).

As learners of semantics, children must be able to understand and explain word definitions, understand and use similarities and differences, and distinguish between literal and figurative meanings. They must be able to recognize and use various types of sentences (e.g., declarative, interrogative, imperative, and exclamatory, as well as simple, compound, and complex). For children with specific language impairments, metalinguistics is a daunting, increasingly complex task. They are struggling with language basics (comprehension, phonology, morphology, vocabulary, syntax, semantics, discourse, narratives, and pragmatics), and now they need to start thinking about the nebulous concept of language to learn more about language (Botting & Adams, 2005).

Pragmatic Problems

You will recall that pragmatics are the rules governing the use of language in social situations. Many children with specific language impairments have a variety of difficulties with the pragmatic aspects of language, which can significantly interfere with family interactions and friendships (see Figure 6–2). These children have difficulty knowing how to initiate a conversation and when they do initiate a conversation, it may be at the wrong time and in the wrong way, with inappropriate ways of attracting the listener's attention (e.g., shouting or hitting). They tend to have difficulty knowing how to gain access into conversations, so they appear to be interrupting or rude. They have difficulty sustaining topics over several conversational turns, often abruptly trying to change a topic. They usually do not ask for clarification when they misunderstand someone (Pence-Turnbull & Justice, 2012; Reed, 2012).

Multicultural Considerations

About 55% of 3- and 4-year-old children in the non-Latino white population are enrolled in preschool programs, but only 43% of Latino children attend preschool. In addition, 13% more non-poor children 3–5 years of age are enrolled in preschool programs than poor children. The lower the parental education, the younger the mother, the

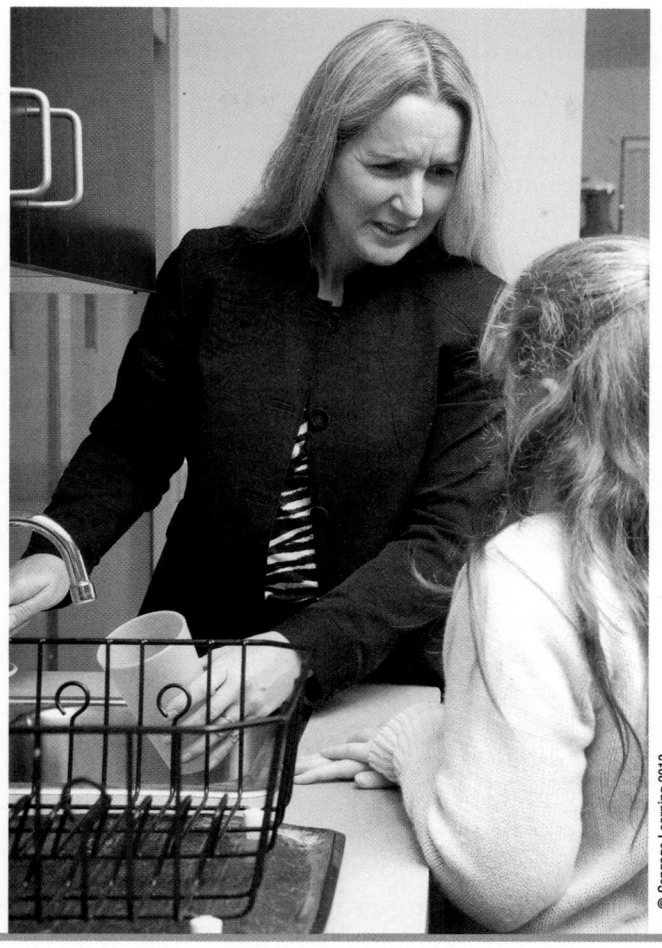

© Cengage Learning 2013

Figure 6-2

Parents sometimes become frustrated with their children who have difficulty communicating.

greater the family's mobility (moving from city to city), the lower the income, and the poorer the English-speaking ability, the less likely children will be enrolled in preschool (U.S. Department of Education, National Center for Education Statistics, 2007).

Bedore & Leonard (2001) found significant grammatical and morphological deficits in Spanish-speaking children with specific language impairments. Without being enrolled in preschool programs, many Latino and poor children do not have the opportunity to be identified and treated for specific language impairments (this is likely true for other non-English-speaking immigrants). Also, because many Latino parents tend to be young and poorly educated, they miss the opportunity to receive information from professionals about things they can do at home to help their children's speech and language development.

LANGUAGE DISORDERS AND LEARNING DISABILITIES

Many children with language disorders also have **learning disabilities (LD)**. Learning disabilities are not diagnosed until a child enters primary school; therefore, preschool children are usually diagnosed as having

learning disability (LD)

A disorder in one or more of the basic psychological processes involved in understanding or using language, spoken or written, that may manifest itself as difficulty listening, speaking, reading, writing, spelling, mathematical calculations, reasoning, and problem solving.

CASE STUDY

Joshua

Joshua was a 4-year-2-month-old boy seen by a speech-language pathologist in a Head Start program. The case history provided by the mother revealed a few of the early "red flags" that indicate a specific language impairment. Joshua did not say his first word until almost 20 months of age and did not combine two words (noun + verb) until 3 years of age. His gestural language was well developed and he often relied on gestures to obtain what he wanted or needed. He had significant difficulty naming objects and using the correct verbs associated with common objects. He did not interact or converse with children his own age.

Joshua's hearing and vision were normal. He had minimal auditory comprehension skills and benefited from gestures that accompanied requests or any communication. The evaluation revealed obvious articulation and phonological problems, some of which interfered with morphological endings (e.g., plurals and past tense). He was inconsistent in his use of various irregular plurals and past-tense forms. His sentences were typically two or three words in length, with occasional four- to six-word sentences; however, the longer his sentences, the more difficult they were to understand.

Joshua had limited receptive and expressive vocabularies, understanding more words than he could use verbally. The *Bracken Basic Concept Scale–Revised* (1998) revealed that he had not yet acquired many of the basic concepts expected for a child his age. His syntax was more like a 2- to 3-year-old child than a 4-year-old child. His sentences were mostly nouns, with some common verbs and occasional adjectives. He tended to avoid discourse and relating stories (narratives), apparently aware that his listener would not likely understand him. He showed some frustration when his parents could not effectively use their "20-question" routine to find out what he wanted or needed. He seemed to avoid frustrating himself by decreasing his verbal interactions. Both mother and father said they were "beside themselves" trying to figure out how to help Joshua communicate.

Therapy was multifaceted, including work on articulation and phonological processes, developing auditory comprehension, vocabulary, concepts, and sentence structure. The parents were encouraged to read simple stories with Joshua and to emphasize the enjoyment of sounds and words and of understanding the sentences and paragraphs in the stories. The parents also were encouraged to require Joshua to use words when he asked for things he wanted or needed rather than allowing him to point or use gestures. Within one year, Joshua was communicating his wants, needs, thoughts, and feelings more completely and accurately, which decreased his frustration significantly. The parents began enjoying their son more and Joshua was interacting more often and appropriately with children his age. ■

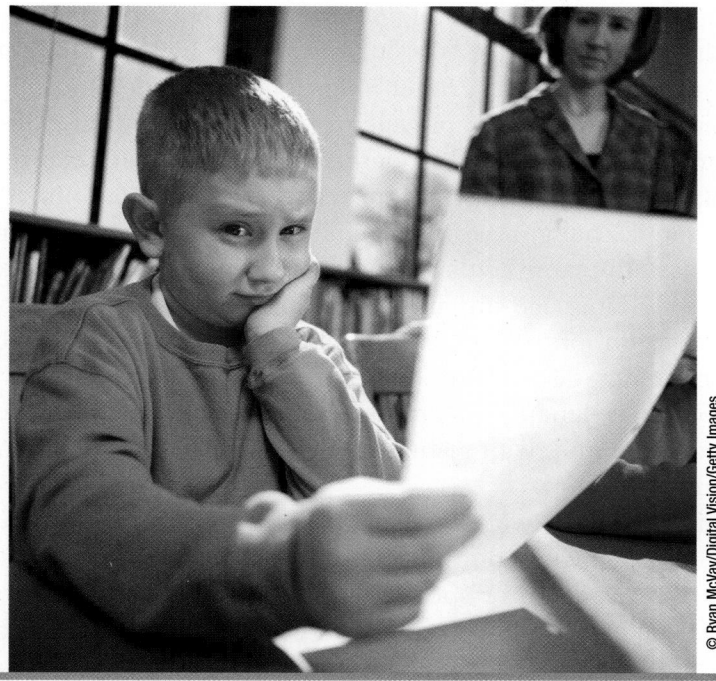

© Ryan McVay/Digital Vision/Getty Images

Figure 6–3
School-age children who have language-learning disorders often show signs of frustration when doing schoolwork.

specific language impairments and this term is often carried over into their school years. After children enter school and struggle academically, an evaluation may reveal that they have a learning disability along with their language impairment. The diagnostic term may be changed to **language-learning disability**, particularly when children are experiencing difficulties with academic achievement in areas associated with language, such as reading, writing, and spelling (Heward, 2008; Pence-Turnbull & Justice, 2012). More than 75% of children with learning disabilities have difficulty understanding and using verbal or graphic language (see Figure 6-3). In many cases a child's learning disability may have as its foundation a language disorder and, therefore, working with an SLP may be essential to helping remediate the child's learning problems (Nelson, 2010; Vinson, 2011).

Children's language problems often manifest themselves differently as they advance through the grades; that is, differences in symptoms and severity levels are reflected in the different communication demands throughout children's education (both auditory–verbal and reading–writing). Because of the increasing demands on children's language abilities as they progress through the grades, various symptoms become apparent that could not be seen in the preschool years. These symptoms often include difficulty (1) understanding increasingly complex verbal information; (2) communicating narrative information in the classroom (e.g., talking during "show and tell time" or making verbal reports on subject matter); (3) learning to read and write (*literacy skills*); and (4) reading to learn (reading for information). When children begin primary school, it becomes clear how their language disorders can impact their academic abilities.

language-learning disability

An impairment of receptive and/or expressive linguistic symbols that affects learning and educational achievement and, consequentially, possible occupational and professional choices and success, in addition to emotional and social development.

Language-learning disabilities tend to run in families. Sixty percent of children with language-learning disabilities have a family member with similar problems, and for 38% it is a parent (Dale, Price, Bishop, & Plomin, 2003). The general prevalence of language-learning disabilities is 12% to 13% for 5-year-old kindergarten children, with approximately 4.5% of children also having speech disorders (Tomblin, Records, Buckwalter, & Zhang, 1996). Most children with language-learning disabilities have the same kinds of problems as younger children diagnosed with specific language impairments; that is, problems with language comprehension, phonology, morphology, syntax, vocabulary development, semantics, discourse or dialogue, narratives, and pragmatics. The severity of these language-learning disabilities may be mild, moderate, severe, or profound, with some areas of language learning being more involved than others.

Many children who receive speech and language therapy also require other special education services, remedial instruction, tutoring, special classroom or special school placement, or a combination of these. The children SLPs work with commonly have more than just speech and language problems, or perhaps their speech and language problems contribute to or exacerbate other academic and social problems. In all cases, however, SLPs are part of a team of professionals doing their best to maximize children's potential.

Motor Skills

Approximately 15% of children with learning disabilities have major difficulty with **gross** and **fine motor skills** and coordination (i.e., **developmental coordination disorder**) (Kurtz, 2007). Fine motor coordination problems also may cause difficulty with articulatory movements, as is seen in *childhood apraxia of speech* (see Chapter 5). Developmental coordination disorders can affect a child's interactions with peers, which complicate the social development of children who already have difficulty with communication.

Adolescents with Language-Learning Disabilities

Some (perhaps many) children who have been diagnosed with specific language impairments or language-learning disabilities have communication problems that persist into secondary school and, probably at some level, throughout life. In addition, their communication problems increasingly affect their educational achievements, choice of vocational and professional careers, potential earning power, and marital and peer relationships. In some cases, language problems may emerge during adolescence because of involvement with drugs. However, many adolescents with language disorders remain unidentified, unserved or underserved, and neglected (Beitchman, Wilson, Douglas, Young, & Adlaf, 2001; Ehren, 2002; Nippold, 2001; Reed, 2012).

---

gross motor skills

Involvement of the large muscles of the body (e.g., trunk, legs, arms) that require tone, strength, and coordination that enable such functions as standing, lifting, walking, and throwing a ball.

fine motor skills

Movements that require a high degree of dexterity, control, and precision of the small muscles of the body that enable such functions as grasping small objects, drawing shapes, cutting with scissors, fastening clothing, and writing.

developmental coordination disorder

Impairment of groups of gross and fine muscles that prevents smooth and integrated movements, which results in clumsiness during walking, jumping, and athletic movements, and during more refined movements such as using eating utensils and writing; often associated with learning disabilities and complicated by low self-esteem, repeated injuries from accidents, and weight gain as a result of avoiding participating in physical activities.

Receptive Language Problems

Adolescents who had receptive language problems at an earlier age often continue to have significant problems throughout their high school years. In general, they (1) have weak single-word receptive vocabularies, (2) experience problems understanding abstract words and words with multiple meanings, (3) often find figurative language expressions puzzling (including slang and jargon), (4) have difficulty following directions, (5) have difficulty understanding questions, (6) experience problems with semantics, (7) face challenges following rapid speech, (8) have poor listening skills, (9) experience difficulty grasping the essential messages of lectures, and (10) misinterpret facial expressions, body postures, and gestures.

Expressive Language Problems

Expressive language may be even more of a challenge than receptive language for adolescents with language disorders. Because there is a reasonably good chance they do not fully understand a question, message, instructions or directions, their responses or behaviors are likely to be incomplete, inaccurate, and sometimes inappropriate. They have weak vocabularies compared to their normal peers, although they may be able to use teenage figurative language easily (not being able to use more adult vocabulary to express themselves may be an indication of inadequate language development). They often use low-content or no-content words such as *thing* or *stuff*. They use pronouns without clear referents so that listeners are uncertain about who or what is being talked about.

Their syntax tends to be simple and they use fewer compound and complex sentences than other adolescents. Verb tense is often a problem for adolescents with language disorders. They frequently use fragmented sentences that do not clearly convey their messages and leave their listeners confused. They may know what questions they want to ask or what answers they want to give, but do not know how to express them or to do so tactfully. They may have abrasive conversational speech. They violate rules for social distance. They do not know or cannot easily use the necessary concepts and vocabulary needed in community businesses, such as banks, grocery stores, and employment agencies.

Many adolescents with language-learning disabilities who graduate from high school are able to go to college. At the university level, learning disability was the fastest growing category among students with disabilities between 1988 and 2000. In 2000 approximately 40% of university freshmen with disabilities cited a learning disability, compared with only 16% in 1988 (Henderson, 2001).

Overall, preschool children who have specific language disorders may become primary schoolchildren with language-learning disabilities; these schoolchildren may become adolescents with language-learning disabilities, who also may become college students

Application Question

There is a reasonably good chance that a fellow student in the class you are in has a learning disability. Although students with disabilities cannot be pointed out by professors, what could you do to be of assistance to a student with a learning disability?

with language-learning disabilities. Whether or not these adolescents go to college or work, they are likely to enter adulthood with some level of language impairment and they must learn to work and live within their limitations. However, some of these adults become surprisingly and extraordinarily successful despite their language and learning problems.

Multicultural Considerations

In 2006, 11% of people aged 18–24 years were high school dropouts. However, in states where there is a high Hispanic or poor population such as Arizona, New Mexico, Nevada, Texas, Louisiana, Mississippi, and Georgia, the dropout rates are at or above 14% (U.S. Census Bureau, 2008: School Enrollment in the United States, 2006). In some communities within these states the dropout rate is much higher. Teens who drop out of high school are three times more likely to live in poverty than those who complete high school, with the added risk of getting in trouble with the law.

The high dropout rate for Hispanic and poor children may have its roots at the preschool level. Recall that significantly fewer Hispanic and poor children attend preschool and do not have the opportunity to be identified as having or being at risk for communication impairments, including hearing loss. Furthermore, 80% of Hispanic children in the public schools are learning English as a second language. If the 12%–13% of children in the general population having language-learning impairments holds true for the Spanish-speaking population, a significant number of Latinos have language impairments that likely contribute to their educational failures.

ASSESSMENT OF LANGUAGE

As mentioned in Chapter 2, Speech-Language Pathologists and Audiologists, the terms *assessment* and *evaluation* are often used interchangeably; however, *assessment* appears to be the general preference for authors of texts on language disorders in children (e.g., Hegde & Maul, 2006; Owens, 2008; Reed, 2012). Typically the term **diagnosis** is distinguished from *assessment*. Assessment is the work or activity that leads to a clinical decision—the diagnosis. A diagnosis is the determination that there is or is not a disorder, and the label or professional term for the disorder is based on the results of valid and reliable measurements of relevant abilities and skills. However, the intervening part is the **measurement** within the assessment process. Clinicians need to obtain **valid** and **reliable** measures during the assessment to have accurate results from which they can have confidence in their decisions for diagnosis and development of an effective treatment plan. Clinicians need to measure observable behaviors that they, as well as others, can see and hear, and if necessary, **replicate** for research purposes.

---

diagnosis

The determination of the type and possible cause of a hearing, speech, language, cognitive, or swallowing disorder based on the signs and symptoms of a client obtained through case history, interviews, observations, and formal and informal evaluations.

measurement

Procedures that quantify observed behaviors and can be calculated as mathematical results, such as percentages and percentiles.

valid/validity

The extent to which a test measures what it is intended to measure.

reliable/reliability

The dependability of a test or treatment procedure as reflected in the consistency of its scores on repeated measurements of the same group.

replicate

Evaluation or treatment procedures that can be repeated by either the same investigator or other investigators to determine reliability of the data.

Assessment serves numerous purposes:

- It determines whether a child has problems of clinical concern and qualifies for services.
- In some cases, the assessment may help identify the cause or causes of a child's problems.
- It allows the clinician to describe patterns that are both present and absent in a child's language (it is important to observe what the child can and cannot do well).
- Factors that may be associated with the language problems may be noted.
- A diagnosis of the child's communication problems can generally be made.
- A treatment plan should be devised from the assessment, including what further assessment is needed.
- A general prognosis may be made as to the child's improvement.

Adequate evaluation of a child's language is one of the most difficult and demanding tasks faced by speech-language pathologists. The goal is to describe the complex language system of a child. Each child has a unique pattern of language rules and behaviors that need to be revealed and described (Owens, 2008). In order to understand a child's language abilities it is essential to describe the child's strengths and weaknesses. Standard deviation units and other statistical measures (see Chapter 5, Figure 5–5) derived from **standardized tests (norm-referenced tests)** do not fully explain a child's receptive and expressive language abilities. In addition, a serious limitation of standardized tests is that they are often inappropriate for children from ethnically and culturally diverse backgrounds because they have not been standardized on these populations (Dollagham & Horner, 2011; Nelson, 2010; Owens, 2008; Reed, 2010). In many cases, SLPs use **client-specific measurements (clinician devised assessments)** to help "fill in the gaps" that standardized tests might leave in the understanding of a child's communication abilities. Overall, it is the information from the case history and parent interview, interpretations of test scores, analysis of client-specific measurements, and descriptions of the child's language behaviors that provide direction for intervention or, in some cases, further assessment. However, assessment is an ongoing process throughout treatment; that is, we are always collecting data on a child's communication behaviors to make appropriate adjustments in therapy.

Referral and Screening

A child may be referred to a speech-language pathologist soon after birth or during early infancy if there is an identifiable syndrome or physical anomaly, such as a cleft lip or palate (see Chapter 10, Cleft Lip and Palate). Parents and preschool teachers may refer children to an SLP when they are as young as 2 or 3 years of age, but more commonly

standardized test (norm-referenced test)

A test that has been administered to a large group of individuals to determine uniform or standard procedures and methods of administration, scoring, and interpretation, and has adequate **normative data** on validity and reliability; tests that are administered to compare one child's performance to others the same age.

normative data (norms)

Data that characterize what is usual in a defined population and that describe rather than explain a particular occurrence; an average of performance of a sample drawn randomly from a population.

client-specific measurements (clinician devised assessments)

Assessments that are not standardized tests that a clinician constructs to make decisions about a specific client's communication abilities.

by 4 or 5 years of age. Parents and teachers also may refer children for a screening at any age while they are in school. Clinicians need to be cautious about the interpretation of screening results when a child uses a dialect such as African American English or is not proficient in English because standardized screening tests do not always contain sufficient numbers of these children for their standardization. We need to remember that there are many individuals from diverse ethnic and linguistic backgrounds who have no problem with language. If an SLP determines there is a problem that needs further investigation, she will recommend the child have a speech, language, and/or hearing evaluation. An interdisciplinary team may become involved in a child's overall evaluation, including an audiologist, a psychologist, special education teacher, physical therapist, occupational therapist, pediatrician, and pediatric neurologist.

Case History and Interview

A complete evaluation of a child includes more than just assessment of language; the process usually includes the following steps:

- Conducting an interview with the parents (the "informants") or other family members (e.g., grandparents) to obtain a detailed case history
- Developing rapport with the child before actual testing begins to help the child "warm up" to the clinician and be willing to participate in the various tasks
- Noting the child's articulation, voice, resonance, and fluency during the rapport-building time
- Evaluating the child's articulation and phonological development
- Examining the orofacial structures and functioning
- Screening hearing
- Evaluating the child's receptive and expressive language, including a language sample
- Meeting with the parents to review the clinician's findings and recommendations

The purposes of a case history and interview are to gather information to help understand the child and his communication problems, to help provide direction of the formal testing, and, ultimately, direction for therapy (Flasher & Fogle, 2012). When possible, one or both parents or other important caregivers of the child are met with in private. The clinician has a list of questions she wants to ask the parents about the child's (1) prenatal and birth history, medical history, speech and language development, (2) hearing ability, (3) the language environment in the home, educational history, (4) possible causes of the communication problem, (5) the child's current communication problems, (6) the child's general behavior, and (7) the parents' feelings about the child's problems.

Developing Rapport and Observing the Child Informally

Before a clinician begins administering tests to a child, she will want to build rapport through relaxed, casual conversation and, when necessary, some play time. Rapport is essential to help a child feel comfortable with the clinician and be willing to participate in the various assessment tasks. The moment the child enters the room, the clinician begins making observations of the child that are important in the overall evaluation. It is during the first several minutes with a child that a clinician often observes many of the strengths and weaknesses of the child's communication abilities. During the initial rapport-building time, the clinician may playfully ask the child to *show me*, *give me*, *hand me*, or *draw me* different objects. This gives the clinician an opportunity to see some of the nouns, verbs, and adjectives the child understands. She may try to "interview" the child, asking about school or play activities, his favorite toys and games, and so on. To the child, what the clinician is doing and asking may appear to make her just a new person in his life who is nice and fun to be with; however, everything the clinician is doing is designed to help understand the child and his communication abilities.

These informal observations can confirm that formal assessment is needed in some additional areas (e.g., a child's voice may be unusually hoarse, his resonance hypernasal, or he may have occasional disfluencies that need to be investigated). Beyond the child's speech and language, the clinician also notes the child's general motor skills and coordination (children with developmental coordination impairments tend to have learning and/or language-learning disabilities [Missiuna, Gaines, Soucie, & McLean, 2006; Webster, Majnemer, Platt, & Shevell, 2005]). During rapport building, screening, and assessment, clinicians must use excellent observational skills. Clinicians become trained listeners and observers—foundational skills for being good speech-language pathologists.

Behavioral Challenges

Not every child is easy to evaluate, usually because of behavioral challenges. As speech-language pathologists we need to learn various methods of behavior modification and techniques to motivate children of all ages to attend to assessment tasks, respond as well as they can, and, ideally, enjoy their time working with the clinician. A positive evaluation session for a child sets him up to be willing to return to the clinician for future therapy.

Evaluating Receptive Language

As discussed earlier, a child with impaired receptive language abilities will often have impaired expressive language abilities. Therefore, a clinician must develop a good impression of a child's receptive language abilities at several levels, including the following:

- Single-word receptive vocabulary and basic concepts
- Morphological structures
- Short sentences
- Longer sentences
- One-, two-, and three-part commands (requests, instructions, and directions)
- Questions
- Conversational speech appropriate for the child's chronological age

A large number of language tests are standardized for different age levels, with some tests targeting specific aspects of receptive language, such as single-word receptive vocabulary. *Comprehensive tests* include evaluations of both receptive and expressive language.

Evaluating Expressive Language

During their education and training SLPs gain experience administering numerous language tests in order to select what they feel are the most appropriate tests to administer to an individual child. SLPs learn to be very flexible and adept in their ability to administer, score, and interpret tests.

Clinicians need to assess many general and specific expressive language abilities, either formally or informally, including the following:

- Spontaneous sounds and words the child uses to communicate
- Morphological units, such as *-ing,* plural *-s,* and past tense *-ed,* used by the child
- Gestures and signs the child often uses to communicate
- Imitation of simple words and phrases
- Vocabulary
- Words, syntax, and semantics the child appears to use easily and others that he appears to have some difficulty using
- Answering of simple questions
- Narrative skills (e.g., describing a picture or telling a story)
- Pragmatic language
- Conversational abilities at an age-appropriate level

Standardized tests are available for assessing each of these areas of expressive language and they are often part of comprehensive language tests. However, as with assessment of receptive language, client-specific measurements are usually needed to fully understand a child's expressive language. A **language sample** is often used as a

language sample

An audio recording of a child's spontaneous conversation or naturalistic verbal interaction with the clinician, family member, or both that is later analyzed.

client-specific measurement. A language sample involves an audio or video recording of a child's spontaneous conversation or verbal interaction with the clinician, family member, or both. However, the interaction is not entirely spontaneous because the clinician designs and guides it to make specific observations. The audio or video recording allows the clinician to later analyze the child's speech and language that was **elicited** during play activities or while having the child describe selected pictures or relate experiences. Open-ended questions (e.g., What did you do last weekend? What is happening in this picture?) allow for more spontaneous elicited language than close-ended questions (e.g., Did you see a movie last weekend? Is the boy throwing the ball?). Clinicians normally attempt to gather 50 to 100 utterances from a child to get an adequate language sample to analyze.

Because context significantly affects the language a child uses, a clinician takes notes on the context of various utterances during the language sample. During the sampling the clinician provides opportunities for the child to demonstrate various pragmatic skills such as greeting, asking questions, *topic initiation* (the skill of introducing new topics for conversation), *topic maintenance* (continuous conversation on the same topic without abrupt interruptions or changing topics), *conversational turn-taking* (talking and listening in an alternating manner), *conversational repair strategies* (verbal behaviors both listeners and speakers use when there are breakdowns in communication), *narrative skills* (telling stories or personal experiences with sufficient details, temporal sequence, characterization, etc.), and *eye contact* (maintenance of mutual eye gaze during conversation) (Hegde & Maul, 2006).

The SLP will transcribe and analyze the language sample in several ways, including phonology, morphology, syntax, semantics, and pragmatics. The clinician will note the frequency of various language skills, including the *comprehension* and *production* (intelligibility) of words, *morphological productions* (e.g., plural -s, past tense -ed, present progressive -ing), *sentence types* (simple, compound, complex, questions), and *conversation skills* (e.g., turn taking, conversational repair). The child's mean length of utterance will be calculated and compared to that of children his **chronological age** (CA). The child's use of vocabulary will be analyzed; for example, naming pictures and objects, objects by category (e.g., foods, clothing), and the use of verbs and adjectives (Hegde & Maul, 2006; Owens, 2008).

Throughout a speech and language evaluation the SLP will attempt to identify possible effective therapy procedures and strategies that will help improve the child's language abilities. Not only is the SLP trying to determine the characteristics of the child's language problems but also what might help remediate them. Any evaluation is a dynamic process where the clinician is always "thinking on her feet," trying to determine from moment to moment what will be the most effective thing to say and do to better understand a child's communication problems and what might be helpful to remediate them.

elicit

Behavior that is drawn out of a person by presenting certain stimuli, e.g., asking a child to name or describe objects to observe his speech and language.

chronological age

The actual age of a person that is derived from date of birth and expressed in days, months, and years.

Diagnosis

It is the responsibility of SLPs to make diagnoses of children's speech and language disorders. This is often not an easy decision and, in reality, a clear diagnosis cannot always be made. All of the information gathered from the case history, parent interviews, and analysis of the assessment results is described, discussed, and included in the clinician's diagnostic report. This information is usually sufficient to provide an understanding of the child's communication strengths and weaknesses, and the clinical decision as to the diagnostic term that best fits the child's communication disorder. Depending on the work setting, certain guidelines may need to be followed when making a diagnosis and qualifying a child for services. For example, public school clinicians may diagnose a language disorder if a child falls below a specified standard deviation below the mean.

SLPs must be able to explain to parents and other family members, as well as to the child himself, what are the child's speech and language strengths and weaknesses. This takes skill in explaining complex speech and language processes in layperson's terms. It also takes considerable tact and good counseling skills when discussing sensitive issues that reveal to parents the type and extent of speech and language problems their child has. Parents can never be objective about their children and parents always have some level of emotional response to hearing the "bad news" (Flasher & Fogle, 2012).

Multicultural Considerations

The challenges of educating children for whom English is their second language are formidable. However, the challenges of learning for these children are formidable as well, including learning to understand, speak, read, and write in English, learning the content of academic subjects, and adjusting to new cultural and linguistic environments. When children have speech and language impairments, in addition to the challenges mentioned here, the tasks are compounded for the teachers, the children, and the speech-language pathologists.

The average percentage of English language learners on school-based speech-language pathologists' caseloads varied from approximately 7% in the Midwest to approximately 20% in the West (Roseberry-McKibbin, Brice, & O'Hanlon, 2005). For example, an estimated 85% of the 1.5 million English language learners enrolled in the California public school system during the 2004–2005 academic year spoke Spanish as their first or home language (California Department of Education, 2006). However, in addition to Spanish, 55 other home languages were reportedly used by families in California schools, including Vietnamese, Hmong, and Cantonese. Nationally, the number of children speaking a language other than English in the United States is increasing rapidly. According to the 2010 U.S. Census, in 2007 62% of people speaking a language other than English in the home reported speaking Spanish. Other languages spoken in American homes include 19% Indo-European (e.g., German, French, Swedish, Italian, Portuguese, Polish, Punjabi); 15% Asian and Pacific Island (e.g., Chinese, Korean, Japanese, Vietnamese, Hmong, Thai, Tagalog), and 4% other languages (e.g., Arabic, Hebrew, languages of Africa).

When bilingual children struggle or fail in their classrooms, SLPs are often involved in assessment teams to determine whether a language disorder or a language difference may be involved. Goldstein (2004) stated that the rapid growth of English language learners has greatly challenged our present system for assessing and treating children who have communication disorders, including such challenges as:

- An inadequate supply of educators and health care providers with knowledge of cultural and linguistic factors that influence communication development

- A paucity of speakers of languages other than English in the provider workforce, along with a lack of trained interpreters and translators

- Health care and early education systems that often are difficult to access for low-income and/or diverse families

- Inadequate assessment tools appropriate for culturally and linguistically diverse children, resulting in over- and underidentification of disabilities

- A mismatch between the cultures of families and those of teachers, with the latter expecting children of these families to fit the dominant culture's expectations

ASHA (1989, p. 93) has provided guidelines for competent clinicians who can provide services in the native language of the child (client):

> Speech-language pathologists who present themselves as bilingual for the purposes of providing clinical services must be able to speak their primary language and to speak (or sign) at least one other language with native or near-native proficiency in lexicon (vocabulary), semantics (meaning), phonology (pronunciation), morphology/syntax (grammar), and pragmatics (uses) during clinical management. To provide bilingual assessment and remediation services in the client's language, the bilingual speech-language pathologist or audiologist should possess: (1) the ability to describe the process of normal speech and language acquisition for bilingual and monolingual individuals and how those processes are manifested in oral (or manually coded) and written language; (2) the ability to administer and interpret formal and informal assessment procedures to distinguish between communication differences and communication disorders in oral (or manually coded) and written language; (3) the ability to apply intervention strategies for treatment of communication disorders in the client's language; and (4) the ability to recognize cultural factors that affect the delivery of speech-language pathology and audiology services to the client's language community.

Whenever a test is standardized (the normative sample) there is always risk of biases in the standardization. Wyatt (2002) discusses biases of standardized tests in America. For example, many of the tests that SLPs use are standardized on middle-class individuals from white backgrounds who speak General American English (GAE). The scores of individuals from other socioeconomic, ethnic, cultural, racial, and dialect backgrounds (e.g., African American English) are often grouped with the white, middle-class GAE speakers, which masks group differences.

Kayser (2002) presents three principles concerning the speech and language evaluation of bilingual children:

1. Both languages should always be evaluated, even when the child understands only the home (native) language.

2. If one of the languages is within normal limits, then a language disorder probably does not exist.

3. A concomitant disorder may exist, such as oral–motor disorders, developmental apraxia of speech, phonological impairment, or developmental delay.

THERAPY FOR LANGUAGE DISORDERS

The terms *therapy*, *treatment*, and *intervention* are often used interchangeably by authors, although most SLPs when talking among themselves use the term *therapy* (e.g., "I have some therapy to do."). Therapy methods should be **evidence-based treatment (best practices)**. Treatment methods also should be **effective** (treatment with a particular method or approach has been shown by research to be better than no treatment), **functional** (the treatment results in improved communication abilities useful to the child in natural environments, such as home and school), and reasonably **attainable** (it is expected the child can achieve the specific targeted goals within a reasonably specified time). In all areas of speech-language pathology, including treatment for language disorders in children, more clinically based research is needed. Such research is conducted by clinicians "in the trenches" daily, conducting language therapy with children in the variety of settings in which SLPs work.

By knowing and understanding a child's particular communication problems a clinician can refine general and specific therapy approaches, therapy techniques, individual stimuli, order of presentation of stimuli, and specific types of reinforcement that a child needs. Although the formal assessment may have been completed, therapy is an ongoing assessment process because a clinician is constantly observing, noting, measuring, collecting data (*daily documentation*), analyzing data, and adjusting therapy to the changing needs of each child. Language therapy should be a well-integrated whole in which various aspects of language combine to enhance communication. The purpose of therapy should be to stimulate overall language development and to teach a repertoire of

evidence-based treatment (best practices)

The integration of (a) clinical expertise, (b) the current best evidence based on controlled and replicated research, and (c) the client's values, needs, and choices to provide high-quality service.

effective treatment

Treatment with a particular method or approach that has been shown by research to be better than no treatment.

functional treatment

Treatment results that improve communication abilities useful in a person's natural environments (e.g., home, school, community, and job).

attainable treatment

The expectation that an individual can achieve a specific target within a reasonably specified time.

linguistic features that can be used to communicate in all contexts and in all environments (Owens, 2008).

Selecting Goals (Target Behaviors)

A **goal (target behavior)** is any verbal or nonverbal skill a clinician tries to teach a child. The target behaviors clinicians try to "hit" are based on axioms, such as the following:

- The language development of normal children can guide the general selection of therapy targets; that is, there is a hierarchical sequence that helps us know what the child has and needs to acquire. However, for any child, the normative sequence may not be what is "normal" for that child.

- Simple language rules are acquired before complex rules. This is the classic idea that a child needs to learn to walk before he learns to run.

- Certain concepts need to be developed before certain vocabulary can be meaningful. For example, a child who does not have the general notion (concept) of *one* and *more than one* will have difficulty learning plurals.

- Although all verbal skills are important, some are more important than others for a child's developmental and language ages. It is important for clinicians to choose language targets that will be most helpful in a child's family, school, and social environments.

Operationally Defined Goals (Targets)

An **operationally defined goal (target)** means that a specific behavior is observable and measurable. That is, a clinician can observe and measure the accuracy and frequency of a particular language behavior (e.g., *-ing* verbing) before therapy begins, as therapy progresses, and when therapy is terminated. Goals that are operationally defined require several specific points:

- A *specific behavior* that is both observable (can be heard or seen) and measurable (e.g., The child will use *-ing verbing* . . .)
- The *setting* or *environment* in which the target behavior is to be observed (e.g., The child will use *-ing* verbing *in the clinic setting* . . .)
- The *number of times* the particular target behavior is to be observed (e.g., The child will use *-ing* verbing in the clinic setting *10 times* . . .)
- The *percent accuracy* criterion chosen (e.g., The child will use *-ing* verbing in the clinic setting 10 times *with 90% accuracy* . . .)
- The *therapy stimuli* to be used (e.g., The child will use *-ing* verbing in the clinic setting 10 times with 90% accuracy *when shown pictures of actions of people and objects and asked, "What is this person [object] doing?"*)

goal (target behavior)

Any verbal or nonverbal skill a clinician tries to teach a child (client).

operationally defined goal (target)

A specific behavior that is observable (can be heard or seen) and measurable.

In this example, the *long-term goal* is for the child to use *-ing* verbing with 100% accuracy in naturalistic environments (home, school, playground, etc.). In reality, it is impossible for a clinician to observe a child in all natural environments and hear whether *-ing* verbing is used accurately 100% of the time. Therefore, we try to obtain feedback from teachers and parents about how the child is doing with a particular goal in the classroom and home environments.

In most cases, to reach a long-term goal, *short-term goals* are needed. Short-term goals may be thought of as "baby steps" to reach the long-term goal. A short-term goal is operationally defined using language similar to that of the long-term goal; however, the short-term goal usually has a lower percent accuracy rate: for example, "The child will use *-ing* verbing in the clinic setting 10 times with 70% accuracy when shown pictures of actions of people and objects and asked, What is this person [object] doing?" Short-term goals may be written without percentages as well, such as, "The child will use *-ing* verbing without modeling or prompting when shown pictures of actions of people and objects."

Most children with whom SLPs work already have some or even a considerable amount of verbal language; however, there are some children for whom our job is to teach both basic and more advanced language skills. A way to think of *basic* is *functional;* for example, we want young children to learn functional vocabulary words that are important in their home environment and preschool children to learn vocabulary words that are important not only for their home environment but also for their school and community environments (see Figure 6–4). The eventual goal of each is natural, spontaneous conversational speech. As children progress in their language learning, increasing time and emphasis are placed on conversations and narratives.

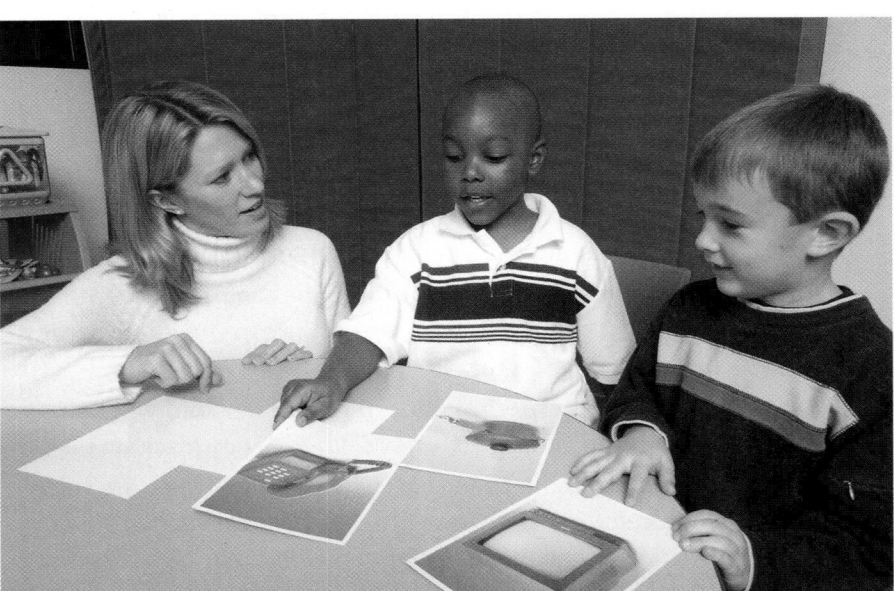

Figure 6–4

A clinician working on functional vocabulary.

© Cengage Learning 2013

There are three primary models that clinicians may choose to follow when working with an individual child who has a communication disorder:

- *Within-discipline model:* The clinician works primarily independently with relatively little interaction with other professionals (classroom teachers, resource teachers, reading specialists, physical therapists, occupational therapists, etc.) who also are working with a child.

- *Interdisciplinary model:* The clinician works with other disciplines and participates in regular (usually weekly) meetings with other professionals to share information about a child's progress in the various intervention programs.

- *Transdisciplinary model:* The various professionals working with a child learn the therapy programs a child is involved in and incorporate information and procedures from all programs into each therapeutic discipline.

Clinicians also may choose combinations of the three. The model or models selected depend on the needs of the individual child. The transdisciplinary model is particularly helpful when working with children who have multiple impairments, such as a child with cerebral palsy who has physical impairments, speech and language problems, and learning disabilities (see Figure 6–5).

Organization and Structure of Therapy Sessions

A few general principles help clinicians determine the organization and structure of individual therapy sessions. In general, young children and children just beginning therapy benefit from well-organized and tightly structured therapy sessions. Tightly structured sessions are more efficient when establishing target behaviors, especially at the morpheme, word, phrase, short-sentence, and simple-question levels. Also, children who have moderate to severe language impairments and behavioral challenges from various neurological causes (e.g., attention deficit disorders, developmental delays, autism spectrum disorders, or traumatic brain injury) benefit from well-organized and highly structured therapy.

A *well-organized therapy session* means that the clinician has carefully preplanned the structure and sequence of therapy tasks and the materials that will be used. She has materials readily available so there are no unnecessary and distracting delays moving from one task to another. She has carefully chosen *tangible reinforcers* (stickers, stamps, bubbles, etc.) that are easily accessible but usually out of sight so that the child is not constantly distracted by them while trying to focus on therapy tasks. The clinician knows how she is going to start the session, what will likely be the middle parts, and how she wants to end the session.

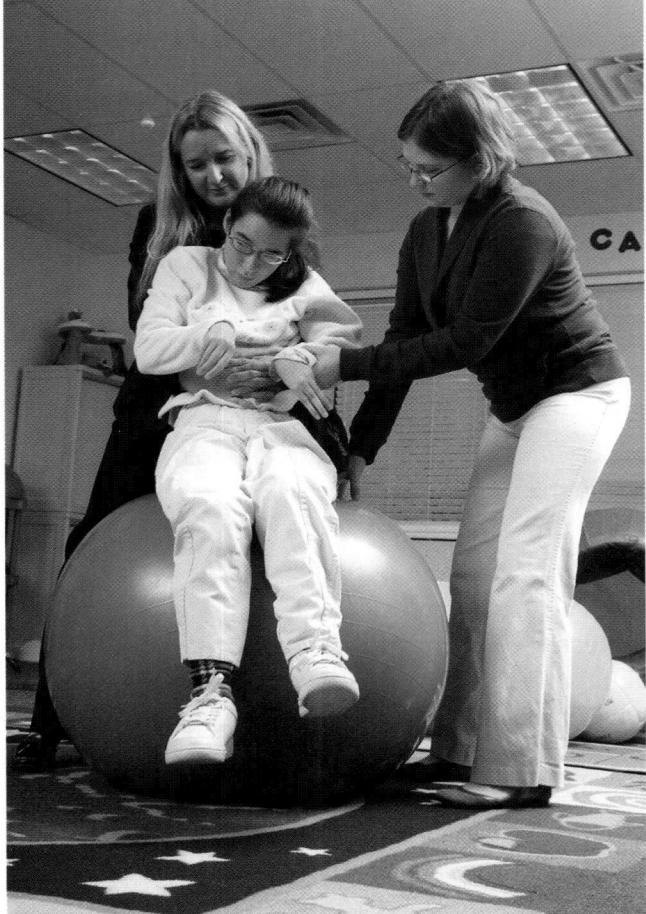

© Cengage Learning 2013

Figure 6–5

A child with cerebral palsy working with a transdisciplinary team.

Nevertheless, the clinician remains flexible throughout the session to accommodate the child's needs, unpredictable behaviors, inability to perform that day as had been expected, internal distractions of the child (e.g., being upset for having gotten in trouble at home or school before coming to therapy), and so on. A clinician's flexibility allows her to make the most of what may otherwise turn out to be a minimally productive session. Clinician flexibility is a hallmark of a good speech-language pathologist at all levels of training and throughout a professional career.

A General Therapy Session Model

It is helpful for clinicians to have in mind a general therapy session model that will likely be functional when working with most children. Within the general therapy session model, there is considerable flexibility that allows clinicians to adapt to the ever-changing and sometimes unpredictable needs of a child. A general therapy session model that works well for many clinicians is the following:

1. *Start the session with a minute or two of general conversation,* asking, for example, how the day is going, how the child did on a recent test, or anything that the clinician can think of that is applicable or

pertinent to the child. This moment or two may provide considerable information that is valuable to the clinician. The clinician will likely receive an answer to the question that was asked; however, she also may hear how the child is producing particular sounds or using certain morphemes, vocabulary, syntactic structures, or pragmatic skills they have been working on. That is, she may be able to see and hear how well the child is generalizing the targeted speech and language skills into connected, spontaneous speech.

Beyond those benefits, the clinician also may get a sense of how the child is feeling about school, classmates and playmates, and other important areas of the child's life. Special bonds are often developed between a child and his "speech teacher," and sometimes a child may share important information with a clinician that is appropriately and necessarily (sometimes mandated) shared with a supervisor, parent, teacher, or other professional (see Flasher & Fogle, 2012, for a discussion of confidentiality as it relates to children).

2. *Review what the child has worked on that he is generally successful with.* This helps reinforce and strengthen what he has been accomplishing, but it also helps him feel that he already has a good start with his speech therapy session for that day. This review time may take just a few minutes, with the child receiving reinforcements for his successes.

3. *Work on new or more difficult therapy targets that need structured teaching and careful monitoring by both the clinician and the child.* This is the hard work of the session that needs intense focus, and the child deserves frequent rewards for his hard work even before he is having correct responses.

4. *Do a quick review of another speech or language skill to give the child a break from the intense focus of the previous task.* The child should be able to respond rapidly and accurately to each stimulus and earn reinforcements for his successes. If time does not allow further work, this is a good way to end the session, with the child feeling he has demonstrated what he has learned, and learned (or started to learn) some new skills.

5. *Work on another challenging task to keep the child working hard and learning new language skills.* At this time, reinforcement is more for hard work than accuracy with such challenging tasks.

6. *End the session on a high note.* A moment of review or going over some skill the child will have high success with helps the child feel that no matter how hard some of the therapy tasks were, he did a great job at the end. This is always appreciated by children.

Eliciting Large Numbers of Responses

For a child to make gains in speech and language abilities, it is important for the clinician to elicit large numbers of responses. As discussed in

Chapter 3, "Anatomy and Physiology of Speech and Language," all therapy involves working with the brain, literally down to the neuron and synapse levels. For a child to learn new vocabulary, morphemes, syntax, semantics, and pragmatics, information (stimuli) must get into the brain and the brain must use or process the information in various locations within the cortex, integrate the information with other language concepts, and be able to retrieve and use the information appropriately when needed. For example, a child may learn some new vocabulary words quickly, such as *male* and *female* for *man* and *woman;* however, the understanding of the appropriate times to use the synonyms may take a considerable amount of additional learning.

Form, content, and use of language a child has not learned automatically through his environment may take a considerable amount of time, effort, and "brain work" in therapy. The concept of making a footpath through grass may clarify this. When you walk across some grass once, the grass quickly springs back up and in a short time there is no trace that you had even walked across it. However, if you walk across the grass many times, you eventually develop a pathway. That is similar to what happens inside the brain; we need to present numerous stimuli and receive numerous responses to develop strong neural pathways.

Multicultural Considerations

In 1998, ASHA adopted the following position statement on the role of speech-language pathologists in providing services to individuals learning English as a second language (ESL):

> It is the position of the American Speech-Language-Hearing Association that speech-language pathologists who possess the required knowledge and skills to provide English as a second language (ESL) instruction in school settings may provide direct ESL instruction. ESL instruction may require specialized academic preparation and competencies in areas such as second-language acquisition (SLA), comparative linguistics, and English as a second language (ESL) methodologies, assessment and practicum. Speech-language pathologists who do not possess the requisite skills should not provide direct instruction in ESL but should collaborate with ESL instructors in providing preassessment, assessment, and/or intervention with English as second-language speakers in school settings.

Battle (2011) offers several points that clinicians need to consider when providing services to individuals with cultural and linguistic differences, some of which are as follows:

- When providing clinical services to all individuals, it is important to consider one's own personal cultural beliefs, attitudes, and values and to be aware that they contribute to and are a major factor in the multicultural, cross-cultural clinical encounter.

- Do not use generic terms as substitutes or synonyms for more descriptive racial or ethnic terms. For example, avoid using *minority* to refer to African Americans, *bilingual* to refer to Hispanics, or *culturally diverse* or *multicultural* to refer to individuals. Note: *African American* does not apply to all black individuals in North America. For example, individuals from Haiti or the Caribbean often want to be referred to based on their home country (Haitian, Bahamian, etc.). Likewise, *Hispanic* does not apply to all individuals from Latin backgrounds. For example, individuals from Puerto Rico or Cuba often want to be referred to based on their home country (Puerto Rican, Cuban, etc.) (Kanzki-Veloso, 2006).

- Be aware that some terms have questionable or negative racial, ethnic, or socioeconomic connotations, such as *culturally deprived* and *culturally disadvantaged.*

EMOTIONAL AND SOCIAL EFFECTS OF LANGUAGE DISORDERS

Language disorders in children can affect them both emotionally and socially throughout their education and possibly into adulthood. The research on psychosocial problems on children dates back to the 1980s. For example:

- Of approximately 300 consecutive intakes of children to a community-based speech and language clinic, 95% of the children with expressive language problems had some form of psychosocial difficulties according to 1980 criteria used by the American Psychiatric Association (Baker & Cantwell, 1982).

- Of 40 consecutive admissions to a child psychiatric unit, 50% of the children had language problems (Gualtieri, Koriath, Van Bourgondien, & Saleeby, 1983).

- Of the children consecutively admitted because of behavioral or emotional problems to an inpatient facility, 67% failed a speech and language screening (Prizant, Audet, Burke, et al., 1990).

As clinicians we need to assess and treat all manner of communication disorders in children, but we also need to recognize that not all children we work with are emotionally stable and may have psychological problems concurrent with their communication disorders. As SLPs, we do not work with the psychological problems of children or other clients, but try to work with individuals in ways that their psychological problems do not interfere with our therapy (Flasher & Fogle, 2012). SLPs need to refer clients to the proper mental health professionals when we feel there are psychological or emotional concerns outside of our scope of practice.

The communication disorders of children often result in parents being in a quandary about what is different about their children, what they might have done to cause or contribute to their children's problems (a considerable amount of soul-searching is done by parents), and what they can do to help their children (parent support groups are often helpful in these areas). Parents naturally want to boast to family and friends about their children's academic achievements; however, parents of children who have communication and learning problems may find it difficult to talk about the school struggles of their children.

The effects of language disorders on the education of children at all ages can be devastating. Good receptive and expressive language skills are essential for learning, and anything less than good skills can affect a child's academic performance and potential success in life. Being undereducated and underemployed are common results of adults having language disorders that were unidentified or undertreated in school. It also has been recognized for years that there is a relationship between juvenile delinquency and adolescent language disorders, and now there is increasing awareness of communication disorders in the adult prison population (Castrogiovanni, 2002; U.S. Department of Education, 2005).

Addendum

As speech-language pathologists, we seldom know the long-term (lifelong) benefits of the work we do with children. After many years of work, we may occasionally come across adults whom we had in therapy as children, and they may remember us. Often we are gratified with how well they are doing. Although we do not try to take credit for their successes in their education, work, and life, we may feel that we were a small part of all of the help they needed to get them where they are.

> For the want of a horseshoe nail the shoe was lost; for want of a shoe the horse was lost; for want of a horse the rider was lost; for want of a rider the battle was lost; for want of the battle, the war was lost—all for the want of a horseshoe nail.
> Sometimes we might be the nail—and that makes all the difference.

CHAPTER SUMMARY

Speech-language pathologists work with children who have both receptive and expressive language delays and disorders that may involve the form, content, and function of language. Specific language impairments (SLI) refer to significant receptive and/or expressive language impairments that cannot be attributed to any general or specific cause or condition.

SLI may include problems with receptive language, morphology, vocabulary, syntax, semantics, discourse, narratives, and pragmatics. When children enter primary school and their SLI begins to interfere with their educational achievement they will likely be diagnosed as having a language-learning disability (language disorder). Clinicians need to obtain valid and reliable measures during their assessments of children to have accurate results from which they can have confidence in their decisions about diagnosis and development of an effective treatment plan. Treatment methods should be effective, functional, and reasonably attainable. Multicultural issues need to be taken into consideration with many of the children identified and treated. As clinicians, we need to be aware of and concerned about possible emotional and social effects of language disorders on children.

STUDY QUESTIONS

Knowledge and Comprehension

1. What is ASHA's definition of a language disorder?
2. Define *specific language impairment*.
3. Define *language-learning disability*.
4. What are three purposes of an assessment of language?
5. What elements need to be included in an operationally defined goal (target)?

Application

1. How does ASHA's definition of language disorder help clinicians understand their professional scope of practice?
2. What are some of the "red flags" parents should note during an infant's first year of life that may indicate the infant is at risk for developing a language disorder?
3. How could understanding a preschool child's specific language impairments help you understand his current language-learning disability?
4. What are some strengths and weaknesses of a child's language that you might observe during the rapport-building time?
5. Outline an organized, structured general therapy session model.

Analysis/Synthesis

1. How can you apply the information about specific language impairments to children with language-learning disabilities?
2. How could language impairments affect children throughout primary and secondary education?

3. How could a high school student's language-learning disability influence decisions about further education and choice of occupations and professions?

4. What are the differences between an assessment and a diagnosis?

5. Discuss the importance of eliciting large numbers of responses during therapy.

REFERENCES

ASHA. (1989). Bilingual speech-language pathologists and audiologists. *ASHA, 31*, 93.

ASHA's Ad Hoc Committee on Service Delivery in the Schools. (1993). Definitions of communication disorders and variations. *ASHA, 35*(Supplement 10), 40–41.

Baker, L., & Cantwell, D. P. (1982). Psychiatric disorders in children with different types of communication disorders. *Journal of Communication Disorders, 15*, 113–126.

Battle, D. (2011). *Communication disorders in multicultural populations* (4th ed.). Boston, MA: Butterworth-Heinemann.

Bayne, G., & Moran, C. (2005). The effect of single word semantic-phonological intervention on developmental word finding difficulties at single word and discourse levels. *New Zealand Journal of Speech-Language Therapy, 60*, 31–44.

Bedore, L. M., & Leonard, L. B. (2001). Grammatical morphological deficits in Spanish-speaking children with specific language impairments. *Journal of Speech, Language, and Hearing Research, 44*, 905–924.

Beitchman, J., Wilson, B., Douglas, L., Young, A., & Adlaf, E. (2001). Substance abuse disorders in young adults with and without LD: Predictive and concurrent relationships. *Journal of Learning Disabilities, 34*, 317–332.

Bishop, D. V. (2006). What causes specific language impairment in children? *Association for Psychological Science, 15*(5), 217–221.

Botting, N., & Adams, C. (2005). Semantics and inferencing abilities in children with communication disorders. *International Journal of Language and Communication Disorders, 40*(1), 49–66.

Cairns, H. S., Waltzman, D., & Schlisselberg, G. (2004). Detecting the ambiguity of sentences: Relationship to early reading skills. *Communication Disorders Quarterly, 25*, 68–78.

Cairns, H. S., Waltzman, D., & Schlisselberg, G. (2007). Development of a metalinguistics skill: Judging the grammaticality of sentences. *Communication Disorders Quarterly, 27*, 213–220.

California Department of Education. (2006). *Dataquest* (online). Available at http://www.cde.ca.gov/ds/sd/cb/dataquest.asp.

Castrogiovanni, A. (2002). *Special populations: Prison populations - 2002 edition*. Rockville, MD: ASHA.

Choudhury, N., & Benasich, A. (2003). A family aggregation study: The influence of family history and other risk factors on language development. *Journal of Speech, Language, and Hearing Research, 46*, 261–272.

Conti-Ramsden, G., & Windfuhr, K. (2002). Productivity with word order and morphology: A comparative look at children with SLI and children with normal language abilities. *International Journal of Language and Communication Disorders, 37*(1), 17–30.

Colozzo, P., Gillam, R. B., Wood, M., Schnell, R. D., Johnston, J. R. (2011). *Journal of Speech, Language, and Hearing Research, 54,* 1609–1627.

Dale, P. S., Price, T. S., Bishop, D., & Plomin, R. (2003). Outcomes of early language delay, I: Predicting persistent and transient language difficulties at 3 and 4 years. *Journal of Speech, Language, and Hearing Research, 46*, 544–560.

Delange, F. (2000). The role of iodine in brain development. *Proceedings of the Nutrition Society, 59*(1), 75–79.

Dockrell, J., Messer, D., George, R., & Wilson, G. (1998). Children with word-finding difficulties: Prevalence, presentation, and naming problems. *International Journal of Language and Communication Disorders, 33*, 445–454.

Dollagham, C. A., & Horner, E. A. (2011). Bilingual language assessment: A meta-analysis of diagnostic accuracy. *Journal of Speech, Language, and Hearing Research, 54*, 1077–1088.

Ehren, B. J. (2002). Speech-language pathologists contributing significantly to the academic success of high school students: A vision for professional growth. *Topics in Language Disorders, 10*, 192–203.

Erwin, M. (2001). Specific language impairments: What we know and why it matters. *ASHA Leader, 6*, 4.

Flasher, L. V., & Fogle, P. T. (2012). *Counseling skills for speech-language pathologists and audiologists* (2nd ed.). Clifton Park, NY: Delmar Cengage Learning.

Gualtieri, L., Koriath, U., Van Bourgondien, M., & Saleeby, N. (1983). Language disorders in children referred for psychiatric service. *Journal of the American Academy of Child Psychiatry, 22*, 165–171.

Goldstein, B. A. (2004). *Bilingual language development and disorders.* Baltimore, MD: Paul H. Brookes.

Hegde, M. N., & Maul, C. A. (2006). *Language disorders in children: An evidence-based approach to assessment and treatment.* Boston, MA: Pearson Allyn and Bacon.

Henderson, C. (2001). *College freshmen with disabilities: A biennial statistical profile.* Washington, DC: American Council of Education.

Heward, W. L. (2008). *Exceptional children: An introduction to special education* (9th ed.). Upper Saddle River, NJ: Merrill Prentice Hall.

Johnson, C., Beitchman, J., Young, A., Escobar, M., Atkinson, L., & Wilson, B. (1999). Fourteen-year follow-up of children with and without speech/language impairments: Speech-language stability and outcomes. *Journal of Speech and Hearing Research, 42*(3), 744–760.

Kanzki-Veloso, E. (2006). *Counseling skills for difficult conversations with supervisees, staff, clients, and families.* ASHA Convention Workshop.

Kayser, H. R. (2002). Bilingual language development and language disorders. In D. E. Battle (Ed.), *Communication disorders in multicultural populations* (3rd ed.). Boston, MA: Butterworth-Heinemann.

Kurtz, L. A. (2007). *Understanding motor skills in children with dyspraxia, ADHD, autism, and other learning disabilities: A guide to improving coordination.* Philadelphia, PA: Jessica Kingsley Publishers.

Leonard, L. B. (2000). *Children with specific language impairment.* Cambridge, MA: MIT Press.

Missiuna, C., Gaines, R., Soucie, H., & McLean, J. (2006). Parental questions about developmental coordination disorder: A synopsis of current evidence. *Pediatric Child Health, 11*(8), 507–512.

Nelson, N. W. (2010). *Language and literacy disorders: Infancy through adolescence.* Boston, MA: Pearson Allyn and Bacon.

Nicolosi, L., Harryman, E., & Kresheck, J. (2004). *Terminology of communication disorders: Speech-language-hearing* (5th ed.). Philadelphia, PA: Lippincott Williams & Wilkins.

Nippold, M. A. (2001). Adolescents with language disorders: An underserved population. *New Zealand Journal of Speech-Language Therapy, 55,* 27–32.

Owens, R. E. (2008). *Language disorders: A functional approach to assessment and intervention* (5th ed.). Boston, MA: Pearson Allyn and Bacon.

Paradis, J. (2005). Grammatical morphology in children learning English as a second language: Implications of similarities with specific language impairment. *Language, Speech, and Hearing Services in the Schools, 36,* 172–187.

Paul, R. (2011). *Language disorders from infancy through adolescence: Assessment and intervention* (4th ed.). St. Louis, MO: Mosby.

Pence-Turnbull, K. L., & Justice, L. M. (2012). *Language development from theory to practice.* Upper Saddle River, NJ: Pearson Prentice Hall.

Prizant, B., Audet, L., Burke, G., Hummel, L., Maher, S., & Theadore, G. (1990). Communication disorders and emotional and behavioral disorders in children and adolescents. *Journal of Speech and Hearing Disorders, 55,* 179–192.

Reed, V. A. (Ed.). (2012). *An introduction to children with language disorders* (4th ed.). Boston, MA: Pearson Allyn and Bacon.

Rice, M. L., Redmond, S. M., & Hoffman, L. (2006). Mean length of utterance in children with specific language impairment and in young control children shows concurrent validity and stable and parallel growth trajectories. *Journal of Speech, Language, and Hearing Research, 49*, 793–808.

Roseberry-McKibbin, C. (2001). *The source for bilingual students with language disorders.* East Moline, IL: LinguiSystems.

Roseberry-McKibbin, C., Brice, A., & O'Hanlon, L. (2005). Serving English language learners in public school settings: A national survey. *Language, Speech, and Hearing Services in the Schools, 36*, 48–61.

Tomblin, J. B., Records, N. L., Buckwalter, P., & Zhang, X. (1996). Prevalence of specific language impairment in kindergarten children. *Journal of Speech, Language, and Hearing Research, 40*, 1245–1260.

Tomblin, J. B., Zhang, X., Buckwalter, O., & O'Brian, M. (2003). The stability of primary language disorder: Four years after kindergarten diagnosis. *Journal of Speech, Language, and Hearing Research, 46*, 1283–1296.

U.S. Census Bureau. (2010). *Language use in the United States: 2007.* Available at http://www.census.gov/prod/2010pubs/acs-12.pdf.

U.S. Census Bureau. (2008). *School enrollment in the United States: 2006.* Washington, DC: U.S. Census Bureau.

U.S. Department of Education. (2008). *Twenty-eighth annual report to Congress on the implementation of the Individuals with Disabilities Education Act (IDEA), 2006, Vol. 1.* Washington, DC: U.S. Department of Education.

U.S. Department of Education, National Center for Education Statistics. (2007). *The condition of education: 2005.* Washington, DC: U.S. Department of Education.

Vinson, B. P. (2011). *Language disorders across the lifespan* (3rd ed.). Clifton Park, NY: Delmar Cengage Learning.

Webster, R. I., Majnemer, A., Platt, R. W., & Shevell, M. I. (2005). Motor function at school age in children with a preschool diagnosis of developmental language impairment. *Journal of Pediatrics, 146*, 80–85.

Wyatt, T. A. (2002). Assessing the communicative abilities of children from diverse cultural and language backgrounds. In D. E. Battle (Ed.), *Communication disorders in multicultural populations* (3rd ed.). Boston, MA: Butterworth-Heinemann.

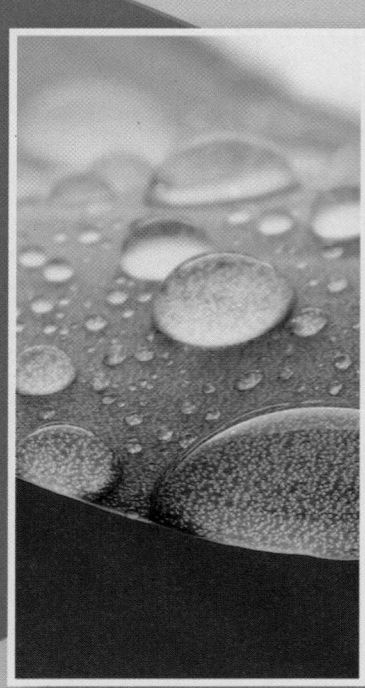

CHAPTER 7
Literacy Disorders in Children

LEARNING OBJECTIVES

After studying this chapter, you will:

- Be familiar with the ASHA guidelines for the roles and responsibilities of speech-language pathologists with respect to literacy for children and adolescents.

- Understand the justification for speech-language pathologists' involvement in literacy.

- Be aware of possible contributions of the English language to reading difficulties.

- Be able to discuss common problems of children with reading and writing disabilities.

- Recognize the multicultural considerations related to literacy problems.

KEY TERMS

alphabetic principle

conventional literacy

dysgraphia

emergent literacy (preliteracy) skills

literacy (reading, writing)

literacy disorder (disability)

orthography

phonics method

phonological awareness

reading disability (dyslexia, developmental dyslexia)

scaffolding

CHAPTER OUTLINE

INTRODUCTION

Students beginning their studies of speech-language pathology and audiology are usually familiar with only the basics of what these professions study and work with clinically—that is, speech, language, and hearing. They are always surprised to find out how much these three areas of study involve. When students learn that speech-language pathologists work with cognition and cognitive disorders, there is an increased realization of the scope and depth of practice of the profession. However, when students learn that speech-language pathology includes learning about **literacy (reading, writing)** and literacy problems (*dyslexia*), they sometimes think these areas are tangential or unrelated to what the profession works with or perhaps *should* work with.

Literacy development is within the scope of practice of speech-language pathologists (ASHA, 2001). When we consider that speech-language pathologists are communication specialists (both normal and impaired communication) and that reading and writing are essential components of communication, it becomes clear that we must learn about and work with literacy and disorders of literacy (Manzo, Manzo, & Thomas, 2009; Nelson, 2010). Kamhi and Catts (2012) and Goldsworthy (2003; Goldsworthy & Lambert, 2010) emphasize that reading and writing are extensions of a child's auditory perception, receptive language, and verbal expressive language skills. In the past, it was assumed that reading disorders were primarily caused by visual perceptual deficits. However, no other factor better justifies speech-language pathologists' involvement in literacy than the research-supported view that reading and writing are *language-based* activities; therefore, language delays, disorders, or both can contribute to or cause literacy problems (Hegde & Maul, 2006).

literacy (reading, writing)

The ability to communicate through written language, both reading and writing.

THE DIFFERENCES BETWEEN LEARNING TO UNDERSTAND SPEECH AND LEARNING TO READ

Kamhi and Catts (2012) discuss three main differences between learning to understand speech and learning to read.

- The human auditory perceptual system is biologically adapted to process spoken words (Lieberman, 1973). In contrast, the human visual system is not biologically adapted to process written words. Learning to read requires specific knowledge of the phonological system of the language; that is, a reader must first know the sounds (phonemes) that correspond with the letters (*graphemes*) in the alphabet (remember, however, that there are many more sounds in the English language than there are letters in the alphabet, which complicates the pronunciation of written words).

- Reading is a comparatively new human ability for which there is no specific biological adaptation. That is, learning to talk is *caught,* but learning to read must be *taught.*

- The nature of the reading system children develop depends on the relative proficiency of all aspects of language, not just phonology.

Geffner (2005), a dual certified speech-language pathologist and audiologist, emphasizes the interrelationship among hearing, phonological processing, reading, and dyslexia. The brain's auditory system and visual system are interconnected by complex pathways of nerve fibers (*sensory–neural integration*). Because of these interconnections, children who have problems in one mode of communication often have problems in another mode. Longitudinal studies have consistently shown that 50% or more of children with language impairments in preschool or kindergarten go on to have reading disabilities in primary or secondary grades and that another 20% of these children are classified as poor readers (Catts, Fey, Tomblin, & Zhang, 2002).

EMERGENT LITERACY/PRELITERACY PERIOD (BIRTH–KINDERGARTEN)

Emergent literacy skills or **preliteracy skills** are terms that have been applied to the skills developed during the preschool years that prepare children for learning to read and write. During the early years, children lack the knowledge of the phoneme–grapheme (sound–letter) correspondence that they later learn. The path to proficient reading and writing skills begins well before children have formal reading and writing instruction in classrooms (Snow, Scarborough, & Burns, 1999).

Before babies can even talk or walk, they may be turning pages of books and spending considerable time looking at pictures in books. Parents often make a big deal about which book they think their child wants to have read, talking animatedly about each book. Children learn that books must be interesting things because there is so much talk about them and parents become excited about reading them. Through *shared book reading,* over time, children begin to learn the names of letters, their shapes, and the sounds they make. For some preschoolers these can lead to the discovery of the underlying **alphabetic principle**—that words consist of discrete sounds represented by letters in print. This principle becomes the foundation of reading.

The National Early Literacy Panel (2004) analyzed several hundred research studies on emergent literacy to identify skills that consistently

emergent literacy (preliteracy) skills

Early skills developed in the preschool years that precede or are presumed prerequisites for later-developing reading and writing skills.

alphabetic principle

Letters and combinations of letters represent speech sounds; speech can be turned into print; and print can be turned into speech.

Application Question

If you are a parent, can you recall when you first started to read to your baby? Can you recall some of the things you did to try to make the experience fun and interesting? If you are not a parent, can you imagine some benefits of reading to a baby at an early age?

and most strongly related to literacy achievement. It found the following to be the strongest skills:

- *Phonological awareness*—Sensitivity to the sound structure of spoken language
- *Oral language*—Grammatical, lexical, and narrative abilities
- *Alphabet knowledge*—Receptive and expressive knowledge of the individual letters of the alphabet
- *Concepts about print*—Knowledge of the rules governing how print is used and organized across various genres, including books and general print in the home and community environments (e.g., labels on boxes, newspapers, and billboards)
- *Name writing*—Representation of one's own name in print

Adult involvement (**scaffolding**) during the emergent literacy and early literacy periods is essential for children to develop these skills in a timely manner (Justice, 2006). Scaffolding involves adults providing whatever supports are needed for children to achieve competence in an activity (such as reading and writing). Gradually, these supports are removed until the child is able to perform independently. Quality emergent literacy assistance involves scaffolding children's achievements in language development, phonological awareness, print knowledge, and writing.

Phonological Awareness

Phonological awareness has an important role in the development of reading skills (Gillon, 2004; Hogan, Catts, & Little, 2005). Phonological awareness is not a simple concept to define. It involves recognizing and understanding (1) sound–letter associations; (2) that individual sounds can be combined to form words; (3) that a single-syllable word (e.g., *dog*) is heard as one word but can be segmented into its beginning, middle, and ending sounds; and (4) that longer words have more "middle" sounds (Foy & Mann, 2003).

The single best predictor of reading success is phonological awareness and the ability to accurately process sounds and words auditorily. Children need to be aware of sounds in speech to acquire sound–letter correspondence knowledge and use this knowledge to *decode* (understand) the printed word. Because phonemes are the fundamental elements of the language system, they are the essential building blocks of all spoken and written words.

Before words can be identified, understood, stored in memory, or retrieved from it, they must be broken into phonemes. When first learning a word, the individual phonemes are processed by the brain's language system. Readers need to convert the letters of words on a page into their corresponding sounds and appreciate that words are composed of smaller segments or phonemes. Children learning to read must rely on hearing sounds to make letter–sound associations to "sound out the word" (the basis of the **phonics method** of reading) and identify the

---

scaffolding

Support that adults provide to children for them to achieve competence in an activity (e.g., reading and writing), with the support gradually removed until the child is able to perform independently.

phonological awareness

Recognition and understanding of sound–letter associations; that individual sounds can be combined to form words; that a single-syllable word is heard as one word but can be segmented into its beginning, middle, and ending sounds; and that longer words have more "middle" sounds.

phonics method

The method of teaching reading and pronunciation by learning the sounds of letters and groups of letters ("sounding out words"); the association of the sounds (phonemes) of a language with the equivalent written forms (graphemes).

first, middle, and last sounds in words. Phonics is heavily influenced by phonological awareness. Children who learn the phonics approach develop *word-attack skills* that allow them to take complex words and sound out each letter and syllable (*letter–sound association*) and to hear themselves say the word. When they can blend the sounds and syllables together, they can often pronounce a word that they have never seen in print or perhaps even heard before. Children who are unable to make such associations are at risk for reading disabilities (Culatta & Hall, 2006; Ehri et al., 2001).

Proficient Word Recognition

When confronted with a new word while reading, we typically try to sound it out in order to say it. However, when it becomes part of our lexicon we visually recognize the word rather than sound out the letters and syllables. For example, we see and read the word *computer;* however, when reading it silently we are not likely to hear ourselves say *c-ah-m-p-ew-t-r,* or even *com-put-er.* Accurate, effortless word recognition requires the ability to use a direct visual route without phonological mediation to access semantic memory and word meaning. It is not surprising that it is unclear how children become automatic, fluent readers.

Emergent Writing: Preschool

Scribbling is likely the beginning of early writing. From about their first birthday, children achieve the fine motor control required to handle a crayon. Most children make horizontal lines before they make vertical lines, and later circular motions are added. Children appear to get considerable pleasure from watching the lines or the colors appear on paper. Then, from about their second birthday, controlled scribbling starts. Children produce patterns of simple shapes: rough circles, crosses, and starbursts. They also begin to arrange shapes and patterns on paper. Learning to hold a crayon and make purposeful lines may be considered the beginnings of **orthography**—learning how to write (print).

LEARNING TO READ AND READING TO LEARN

Although children are expected to understand the spoken language and be able to proficiently verbally express their basic wants, needs, thoughts, knowledge, and feelings well before they enter elementary school, they are not expected to be able to read and write. Not all children attend preschool or are provided the benefit of emergent literacy skills. Schools, therefore, are expected to provide the training and education for children to learn to read and write and later read to learn and write to communicate. To eventually become a proficient reader, a

orthography

The part of language study concerned with letters and spelling; the representation of the sounds of a language by written or printed symbols.

child must be able to visually recognize words accurately and with little effort, which requires knowledge of letter sequences and orthographic patterns (Kamhi and Catts, 2012). Although phonological skills are essential in learning to read and in sounding out new words, mature, fluent readers rely more on their visual systems. That is, during rapid silent reading people do not "sound out" words through the auditory system (*subvocalize*—hear themselves say the words in their heads), but visually process words as units.

Good Raedres Can Raed Tihs

I culod not blveiee taht I cluod aulaclty uesdnatnrd waht I was rdanieg. The pha-onmeanl pweor of the hamun bairn to raed no mttaer in waht oredr the ltteers in a wrod are. Wahts iprmoatnt tohguh is taht the frist and lsat ltteer be in the rghit pclae. The rset can be a taotl mses and you can sitll raed it wouthit a rael porbelm. Tihs is bcuseae the biarn deos not raed ervey lteter by istlef, but the wrod as a wlohe. And I awlyas tghuhot slpelnig was ipmorantt!

Children reach **conventional literacy** when they can read and write according to the rule-governed system using the alpha-betic principle and are able to read to learn. For most children, this occurs around 8 years of age or the third grade. By this age, they have a considerable sight vocabulary, as well as sophisticated word-attack skills. When children are able to automatically read many words they encounter or can easily sound out and figure out a new word through word-attack skills, they are able to shift important cognitive processes from a focus on decoding and word recognition to the act of reading for understanding and acquiring new knowledge (Feifer & De Fina, 2000). When children's cognitive processes are occupied with basic reading tasks and each word must be individually processed, there may not be sufficient cognitive reserve to fully appreciate the meaning of a sentence, paragraph, or story.

LITERACY DISORDERS IN CHILDREN

In the definition of **literacy disorder (disability)** used by speech-language pathologists, both reading and writing disabilities are in-cluded. However, the International Dyslexia Association (IDA) definition of **reading disabilities (dyslexia, developmental dyslexia)** does not include writing disabilities or disorders (**dysgraphia**). Dyslexia is defined by the IDA (Lyon, Shaywitz, & Shaywitz, 2003) in the following manner:

conventional literacy

Reading and writing according to the rule-governed system of the alphabetic principle and being able to read to learn.

literacy disorder (disability)

Reading and writing impairments in a heterogeneous population of children.

reading disability (dyslexia, developmental dyslexia)

An inability or difficulty reading that is of neurological origin.

dysgraphia

A developmental motor and/or literacy disorder that affects a child's or adult's ability to write, characterized by messy or illegible handwriting, misspellings, and difficulty with grammar and organizing sentences; note: *agraphia* is a loss of ability to write resulting from injury to the brain.

Dyslexia is a specific learning disability that is neurological in origin. It is characterized by difficulties with accurate and/or fluent recognition and by poor spelling and decoding abilities. These difficulties typically result from a deficit in the phonological components of language that is often unexpected in relation to other cognitive abilities and the provision of effective classroom instruction. A few of the secondary consequences may include problems in reading comprehension and reduced reading experience that can impede growth of vocabulary and background knowledge.

Dyslexia is the most common learning disability in both children and adults, and 75%–85% of all children with learning disabilities have reading impairments (Nelson, 2010; Reed, 2012). To be diagnosed as having dyslexia, hearing and vision acuity problems must be excluded (this includes with amplification such as hearing aids, corrected vision with eyeglasses or contact lenses, or both). The problem is more prevalent in males, with a ratio of about four boys to every one girl with the disability. The cause or causes of a reading impairment for any one child usually cannot be determined. However, reading disabilities have long been recognized as tending to run in families and are often seen in siblings, parents, and grandparents (Stevenson, Graham, Fredman, & McLoughlin, 1987).

Considerable evidence suggests a strong and reciprocal link between language development and emergent literacy development in preschool children (Goldsworthy, 2003; Justice, Invernizzi, & Meier, 2002). Kamhi & Catts (2012) and Hesketh (2004) maintain that reading disabilities are best characterized as developmental language disorders. That is, reading is a language activity that relies on a person's knowledge of the phonological, morphological, syntactic, semantic, and pragmatic aspects of language. Therefore, impairment in one or more of these aspects of auditory or verbal language, could lead to significant disruptions in the ability to read and communicate effectively in writing (see Figure 7–1).

ASHA (2001) published guidelines for the roles and responsibilities of speech-language pathologists with respect to reading and writing (literacy) for children and adolescents. Our roles and responsibilities include designing and implementing programs to do the following:

1. Prevent reading and writing language problems by fostering language acquisition and emergent literacy.

2. Identify children at risk for reading and writing problems.

3. Assess reading and writing.

4. Provide intervention and document outcomes for reading and writing intervention programs.

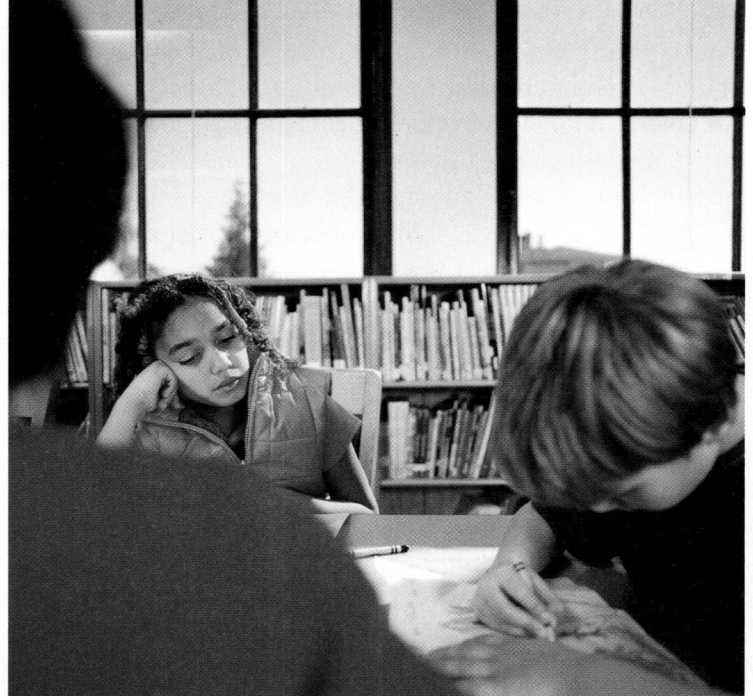

Figure 7–1

Some children find letters, printed words, and reading incomprehensible.

5.   Provide assistance to general education teachers, parents, and students.

6.   Advocate effective literacy practices and advance the knowledge base.

Insufficient opportunities for children during their first 5 years of life to be exposed to the printed word have become an important issue in speech-language pathology (Justice, 2006; Snow, 2006).

POSSIBLE CONTRIBUTIONS OF THE ENGLISH LANGUAGE TO READING DIFFICULTIES

The causes of children's literacy problems may be the same as those that cause speech and language delays and disorders, including heredity (Snowling, Gallagher, & Firth, 2003) (see Chapter 5). However, for children with speech and language delays and disorders, learning to read and write can be even more challenging, especially because of the numerous inconsistencies in pronunciation of words based on the context, inconsistencies in letter–sound correspondence, and even in shapes of letters (consider the number of type fonts a child has to become accustomed to).

Inconsistencies in Pronunciation of Words Based on the Context

Understanding of the intended meaning of a written statement can be affected by pronunciation of words depending on the context. For example, we can use two different pronunciations of the same word in a single sentence: "He couldn't read what she read" (i.e., *read* is pronounced "reed" and "red"). Likewise, the stress on words changes the meaning: "*Maybe* he *may be* willing to do it." and "It is *apparent* he is a *parent*." In the phrases "He is going to *be wilder*" and "He is going to *bewilder*," the change in the pronunciation of the vowel "i" in the last word significantly changes the meaning. Even adult readers sometimes have to reread a sentence to place the proper pronunciation and stress on some words in order to understand the intended meaning.

Inconsistencies in Letter–Sound Correspondence

English is challenging to read due to frequent inconsistencies of the letters in a word and the sounds that correspond to them. This lack of one-to-one letter-to-sound correspondence makes spelling even more difficult for children (and adults). Some classic examples are our use of *ph* to represent the sound *f* (e.g., *phone*) and the many silent consonants and vowels we use in printed words, such as *talk, write,* and *though.* Children's misspellings often reflect the spelling of words as they hear them. Irregularities of English spelling present another obstacle. There are 251 spellings for the 42 phonemes in English (Horn, 1926). There are, for example, 7 spellings for the sound /i/: *e, ie, ei, i, y, ea,* and *ee.* Likewise, the consonant /f/ has 4 spellings: *f, ff, gh,* and *ph.*

Inconsistencies in Shapes and Styles of Letters

Children learning to read usually start with large print that is *sans-serif* (in typography, letters that do not have *serifs*—terminal strokes at the top and bottom of main strokes. The large, plain letters of sans-serif are easier for young children to read. However, usually by second or third grade children are able to read both sans-serif and serif print. Most all casual reading (newspapers, magazines, novels) and formal reading (textbooks) are in serif; however, telephone text messages and computer e-mails are typically in sans-serif. Children must eventually be able to easily shift back and forth from sans-serif to serif while reading different material. Students and other writers have scores of *font* choices on their computers. Publishers of children's books and textbooks for all educational levels make critical choices as to what will be the primary font to use for a book and its *point size* (the size of the letters), as well as which fonts will be selected to highlight or emphasize certain information or illustrations.

COMMON PROBLEMS OF CHILDREN WITH LITERACY DISABILITIES

The International Dyslexia Association's definition of dyslexia provided earlier in this chapter highlights several general and specific areas commonly seen in children with reading disabilities. Any one area may have an interacting and compounding effect on the other areas.

Deficits in Phonological Processing

The IDA definition of dyslexia states that difficulties in word recognition and spelling are typically the result of a deficit in the phonological component of language. As discussed earlier, phonological processing deficits are considered the foundation of dyslexia (Culatta & Hall, 2006; Geffner, 2005; Goldsworthy, 2003). Research has shown that phonological processing deficits are inheritable; however, a common cause of phonological problems (auditory processing disorders) is middle ear infections (Musiek & Chermak, 2007; Olson & Bryne, 2005).

Leitao and Fletcher (2004) stated that phonological processing disorders may be detected before children are challenged to learn to read. This has some important educational and therapeutic implications for early identification of risk factors. That is, if children can be recognized and diagnosed with an auditory processing disorder and can receive appropriate intervention for the disorder, it may help prevent them from developing reading problems. This is a proactive approach rather than a reactive approach; the child receives help to prevent likely problems that would need help anyway (Kamhi & Catts, 2012).

Problems in Word Recognition and Spelling

Historically, the word *dyslexia* has been associated with visual processing deficits that resulted in disturbances such as letter reversals (e.g., *b–d* and *p–q*), letter confusion (e.g., *m–n, s–z,* and *O–Q*), sequencing errors (e.g., *was–saw*), and "misreading" (e.g., *house–horse* and *boy–toy*) that had been seen in children with reading problems. Children with reading problems have significant difficulty decoding printed words, which results in problems recognizing and figuring out new words and building good *sight vocabularies* (words that can be automatically recognized without needing to sound them out). With sufficient help, many children with dyslexia can improve their word-reading accuracy (particularly by developing *word-attack skills*); however, most do not become *fluent readers* (i.e., reading effortlessly).

Children with reading problems typically have difficulty with spelling, which may be a lifelong struggle. Problems with spelling may be the result of several interacting factors, such as phonological problems with sound–letter correspondence, inconsistencies in letter–sound correspondence, and the need to memorize the spelling of words with silent letters.

Underachievement Unrelated to Other Factors

Children with reading disabilities often do not achieve the academic levels that may be expected based on their general intellectual abilities.

However, the use of IQ is controversial when diagnosing or trying to relate intelligence to reading abilities. IQ tests do not directly measure potential for reading achievement; rather, they assess current cognitive abilities, some of which overlap with abilities important for reading. In addition, poor readers generally read fewer books and other materials than good readers and, therefore, acquire less of the knowledge measured by verbal IQ tests, resulting in lower IQs for the poor readers (Siegel, 1989).

Secondary Consequences

Children with reading disabilities face numerous secondary consequences. Secondary consequences include academic difficulties, possible influences on occupation and career choices (with resulting effects on future income), difficulty using reading as a leisure-time activity, and possible effects on interpersonal relationships (Justice, 2006; Stothard, Snowling, Bishop, Chipchase, & Kaplan, 1998).

Reading Comprehension and Academics

Children who have difficulty learning to read also have difficulty reading to learn; that is, reading comprehension and, likely, memory for what they have read may be seriously impaired because the information has not been coded well. As children progress through school, increasing amounts of learning come from independent reading. Thus, children with reading problems learn less, and what they do learn may be partly, largely, or totally in error. These children may argue that what they are saying is what they understood (or misunderstood) from their readings. They wonder why they receive poor grades on tests because they are certain they had written what their textbook said. Their reading and writing problems become more evident in each new grade as learning and grading increasingly depend on these skills.

Reading to learn, among other things, requires the ability to find the main ideas in a passage or story. Finding the main ideas is a complex task involving a child's knowledge of language and text conventions on many levels. A child who cannot determine the main ideas in material he reads has difficulty answering the questions, "What is this story about?" and "What are the important points?"

Reading disabilities affect all areas of academic learning. Consequently, these children have poor academic performance even though they may put out extreme effort to do well. Many of these children become disheartened and eventually develop an "I don't care" attitude as a self-defense for their failures. Their self-esteem and self-confidence deteriorates, and they may create problems in the classroom, interfering with other children's learning. Reading disabilities commonly determine how much children enjoy school and how far they go in school (Institute of Community Integration, 2000).

Application Question

Imagine that you had a reading disability. How would that have affected your education? Your choice of profession? Your life?

Writing Problems

Throughout children's educations, reading and writing are inextricably connected. First and second graders are asked to read aloud the short stories they write. However, by third grade and throughout the rest of their education, students read to find out what to write and write to demonstrate that they understood what they read.

Different types of writing call on different cognitive abilities, use different vocabulary, and employ different sentence forms. For example, writing a narrative story about a personal experience is quite different from writing a cogent argument about a point of view for a controversial topic, and both of these forms of writing are different from writing text material for a book. Children of all ages who have reading and writing problems write shorter compositions than do other children. This is a consistently good predictor of quality of writing; that is, shorter compositions usually do not have well-developed compound or complex sentence structure and often have missing components needed to make a good composition (see Figure 7–2). Overall, writing is a formidable mental process for individuals of all ages (Feifer & De Fina, 2000; Sun & Nippold, 2012). Compared to speaking, writing requires a higher level of abstraction, elaboration, conscious reflection, and self-regulation (we may speak without careful thought, but we seldom write without it).

Common writing problems seen in children (and adults) include inadequate or incorrect reference to the subject (i.e., the reader cannot easily determine who or what is being written about); inconsistent or inaccurate noun–pronoun agreement; inconsistent or inaccurate gender words; shifting inappropriately between first and third person; and inaccurate subject–verb agreement. Punctuation problems are common for individuals with writing disorders, particularly inconsistent or inaccurate use of periods and commas and lack of capitalization.

Figure 7–2

Writing complete sentences seems a nearly impossible task to some children.

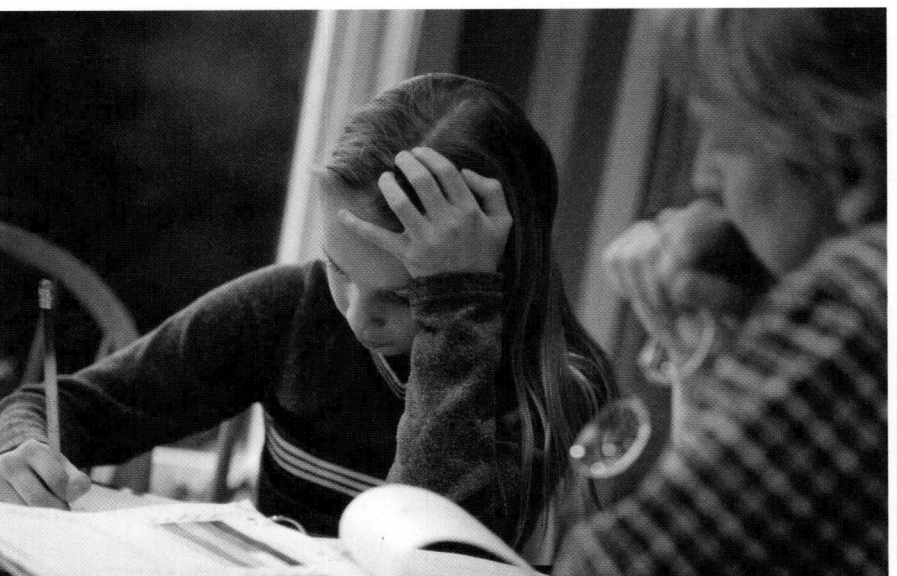

© Keith Brofsky/Photodisc/Getty Images

These problems result in sentences that are fragmented and unclear. In addition, spelling errors are abundant.

ASSESSMENT OF READING AND WRITING SKILLS

We need to keep in mind that not all children come from home environments that foster emergent literacy by having books and other reading material readily available, nor are there drawing and writing utensils easily available, such as crayons, markers, pencils and paper. Although SLPs may gently inquire about such things during parent interviews or even make an occasional home visit, other than encouraging parents to provide a literacy enriched environment, little can be done to change the home milieu.

Assessing Pre-reading and Reading Skills

Preschool children are referred to SLPs for evaluations of speech and language rather than for literacy problems. Therefore, before assessing reading and writing skills, SLPs should assess a child's receptive and expressive language skills. The initial investigation of a child's literacy skills may be more of a screening than an actual assessment, with more in-depth assessment carried out after the child is enrolled in therapy for language problems.

When children enter primary school and are screened for speech, language, and hearing problems, a clinician may detect possible literacy problems as well. These children should be referred to a *reading specialist* (a specially trained teacher who works with students experiencing reading difficulties) for a complete evaluation. However, because there is an important relationship between phonological awareness and reading, phonological awareness needs to be probed by the SLP (Hogan, Catts, & Little, 2005). At the emergent level, children as young as age 3 should be able to detect and produce rhyming words and recognize alliteration, which can be screened in the context of verbal play, nursery rhymes, songs, and books (Schuele, Skibbe, & Rao, 2007). At the kindergarten and early primary levels, children should be able to isolate a phoneme within a word (e.g., the first sound of *dog*); recognize the same sound in different words (e.g., *cat, car, can*); segment phonemes (e.g., *d-, o-, g-* for *dog*); delete sounds (e.g., saying the word *phone* without the /f/ sound); and substitute sounds (e.g., "Say '*can*.' Now say it again but change the /c/ to /m/.") (Hegde & Maul, 2006).

At the kindergarten and early primary levels, children can be assessed for their ability to name letters (*letter identification* or *alphabet knowledge*) (Schatschneider et al., 2002). *Sound–letter (alphabetic principle) association* also can be assessed; for example, asking what sound different letters make and asking children to "sound out" three-letter printed words and then to say the sounds fast and tell what the word is or means (e.g., *man* [*m-a-n*]). Some children become fluent readers although their comprehension of words, sentences, and paragraphs is weak. Comprehension of words, sentences, and short paragraphs can be assessed by having children read both aloud and silently, and then asking them to explain what they have read. Alternatively, clinicians can ask them specific questions about the material they read to see if they understood it.

Assessing Writing Skills

A clinician may ask children to print individual letters or the letters that correspond with certain sounds presented by the clinician. Children may be asked to write (print) short words. If they cannot do this independently, the clinician may ask them to copy letters and words, and if this is too difficult, clinicians can ask them to trace a letter outlined either with dots or dashes. It is important for children to be able to write basic identification information, such as their name, age, telephone number, address, and names of parents or primary caregivers. For more advanced writing skills, the SLP may assess children's legibility of individual letters and words, spelling, word usage, grammar, and punctuation. Content of sentences and paragraphs may be evaluated for cohesiveness, logical sequences, and ability to communicate information. When an SLP obtains information about children's reading and writing abilities, the information should be shared with the children's teachers and reading specialists.

INTERVENTION FOR READING AND WRITING PROBLEMS

Speech-language pathologists' academic training relating to early language and literacy development help prepare them to be an important member of the team that works with children who have reading and writing problems. Other members of the team include the child, classroom teacher, and parents, and, when available, a reading specialist and resource teacher. The ASHA National Outcomes Measurement (NOMS) (2009) data indicate that more than 70% of teachers who responded to a survey believed that students who received speech-language pathology services demonstrated improved pre-reading, reading, or reading comprehension skills. A majority of teachers also cited improvements in the students' listening, written language skills, and ability to communicate in socially appropriate ways (pragmatics). We need to keep in mind that most of our training is in the area of speech and language disorders rather than reading disorders; reading specialists (when available) are specifically trained to work with children who have literacy problems. Some SLPs, however, take additional course work and training in literacy assessment and treatment and provide direct services to children and consultation to other clinicians and teachers.

Teaching Reading Skills in the Context of Speech and Language Therapy

As discussed previously, because reading and writing are language-based activities and auditory processing is an important factor in developing reading skills, speech-language pathologists are appropriate professionals to help children develop their literacy skills. We can be part of the team that involves the child, parents, classroom teacher, and reading specialist. Because literacy is directly linked to speech and language, intervention provided for phonologic, morphologic, syntactic, and semantic aspects of language may improve literacy. Integrating reading and writing skills training can be accomplished within the context of traditional speech and language therapy, although oral communication skills should remain the priority for most speech-language pathologists (ASHA, 2001; Goldsworthy, 2003; Goldsworthy & Lambert, 2010; Hegde & Maul, 2006; Nelson, 2010).

SLPs can pair written material with pictured and modeled verbal stimuli at every level of therapy—from isolated speech sounds paired with printed letters to verbal stimuli of words, phrases, and sentences paired with those words in print. Specifically selected storybooks can be used in conjunction with both speech and language therapy. For older children, *guided reading* (having a child read aloud while providing direct feedback) can simultaneously work on articulation, syntax, semantics, and pragmatics (Hegde & Maul, 2006; National Reading Panel, 2000, 2001; Nelson, 2010). We need to encourage parents to be actively involved with their children's literacy opportunities such as reading to their children (*shared book reading*), patiently listening to their children read aloud, and reading their children's school writing assignments and providing appropriate feedback (Senechal & Cornell, 1993).

Teaching Writing Skills in the Context of Speech and Language Therapy

Young children learning how to write (print) can be asked to write the letter representing a speech sound they are working on. This may initially require helping guide their hands, tracing individual letters, or using "dot-to-dot" outlines. At the word level, children can be asked to write the words they are practicing saying. For older children, writing phrases and sentences can work on spelling, syntax, semantics, and pragmatics. This writing practice can reinforce their work on articulation and language. Consultation with teachers and parents is helpful to devise lists of words and syntactical structures that are important to classroom work and communication at home.

MULTICULTURAL CONSIDERATIONS

Children from culturally and linguistically diverse backgrounds have a greater likelihood than most other groups of children beginning school inadequately prepared to learn to read and to become successful readers (Culatta, Aslet, Fife, & Setzer, 2004; Justice, Chow, Capellini, Flanigan, & Colton, 2003; Thomas-Tate, Washington, & Edwards, 2004). In 2005, the National Assessment for Educational Progress (NAEP) reported that by fourth grade, 59% of African American children and 56% of Latino or Hispanic children read below basic levels, compared with 25% of majority-culture children. The 2005 NAEP report also stated that 54% of children living in poverty demonstrated reading proficiency below basic reading levels.

For preschoolers who are known to be at risk for language and literacy problems, it is essential to provide appropriate interventions so that they may enter kindergarten on par with other children (Rosin, 2006). This should include providing emergent literacy opportunities that respect and build on children's home culture while simultaneously preparing them to succeed in the majority culture.

Ample evidence supports early proactive interventions that focus intensively on promoting emergent literacy and language skills in minority cultures, as well as in children living in poverty. In addition, early intervention for children with language difficulties, rather than focusing exclusively on language acquisition, should include reciprocal and similarly intensive focus on emergent literacy development (Justice et al., 2002; Washington, 2006).

Several differences in narrative writing of children from culturally and linguistically diverse backgrounds are reported by Fiestas and Pena (2004), including story length, level of description, content, sequence and structure of the story, and prominent verb forms used (e.g., past tense versus present progressive). Support may be provided along a continuum for helping these children develop their narrative skills, from labeling pictures with a single word, to telling and retelling stories based on shared book reading, to personal accounts and language–experience activities in which a child's experiences are used as the foundation of the written narrative (e.g., a trip to the zoo), to development of imagined stories.

EMOTIONAL AND SOCIAL EFFECTS OF LITERACY DISORDERS

Although it is a real issue, little is written about the emotional and social effects of literacy disorders on children and adults. Most early elementary school children who are learning to read are aware of the ease or difficulty they are experiencing with this new skill. They fairly easily recognize what reading "group" they are in and take pride in being known as a good reader or feel embarrassment and sometimes rejection in being a poor reader. They soon realize the effects of their reading and writing difficulties when studying various subject matter and writing stories and answering questions on tests. They are confronted with their reading and writing problems on a daily basis at school and often at home. For these children, reading and writing difficulties are a daily frustration that can take a toll on their self-confidence, self-image, and self-esteem throughout their education and determine how much and how good of an education they receive. Their reading and writing impairments can affect the kinds of occupations and professions they pursue and even their social lives. (I am aware of one woman [a speech-language pathologist] who chose to end a relationship because the gentleman was a "nonreader.") The quality of life of people who have literacy problems can be significantly affected because they miss the enjoyment of reading recreational material and struggle with reading daily (Alexander-Passe, 2010).

CHAPTER SUMMARY

Reading disabilities are the most common learning disability in both children and adults. Reading disabilities are best characterized as developmental language disorders. Emergent literacy is the reading and writing behaviors of young children before they become readers and writers in the conventional sense. Adult involvement (scaffolding) during the emergent literacy and early literacy periods is essential for children to develop these skills in a timely manner. Speech-language pathologists need to take a proactive role in preventing reading difficulties among children with whom they work, as well as in the more general population of at-risk children for whom emergent literacy intervention may be the most powerful mechanism for improving the likelihood that they will become lifelong readers.

For many children, English is a challenging language to learn to read, especially because of the numerous inconsistencies in pronunciation of words based on the context, in letter–sound correspondence, and even in shapes of letters. There are numerous secondary consequences for children with reading disabilities, including academic difficulties, possible influences on occupation and career choices (with resulting effects on future income), difficulty using reading as a leisure-time activity, and possible effects on self-esteem and interpersonal relationships. An SLP can be an important member of the team to help children with literacy problems, including providing assessment and remediation.

Children from culturally and linguistically diverse backgrounds have a greater likelihood than most other groups of children of beginning school inadequately prepared to learn to read. For those preschoolers who are known to be at risk for language and literacy problems, it is essential to provide appropriate interventions so that they may enter kindergarten on par with other children.

STUDY QUESTIONS

Knowledge and Comprehension

1. Define *literacy disorder.*

2. What must be excluded for a child to be diagnosed as having a literacy disorder or dyslexia?

3. What is emergent literacy?

4. Explain *scaffolding.*

5. What are some secondary consequences of reading disabilities?

Application

1. What does ASHA say are the roles of speech-language pathologists in regard to working with children who have reading disabilities?

2. How could speech-language pathologists incorporate storybook reading into their work with children who have language disorders?

3. In what areas might scaffolding be used other than reading development?

4. Why is it important to encourage parents to read to their children?

5. What are two methods speech-language pathologists could use to integrate literacy skills while working on speech and language?

Analysis/Synthesis

1. Why are reading disabilities best characterized as developmental language disorders?

2. Discuss ways in which the English language may contribute to reading difficulties.

3. How can children's automatic recognition of many words and development of word-attack skills help them in their learning the content of written material?

4. How could reading problems set up children for academic problems and other problems throughout their lives?

5. Why would children with reading problems be likely to have problems with writing, particularly expository and narrative compositions?

REFERENCES

Alexander-Passe, N, (2010). *Dyslexia and depression: The hidden sorrow.* London South Bank University: London.

ASHA. (2001). *Roles and responsibilities of speech-language pathologists with respect to reading and writing for children and adolescents: Practice guidelines.* Rockville, MD: ASHA.

ASHA. (2009). *National Outcomes Measurement System Fact Sheet: Do SLP services have an impact on students' classroom performance? What teachers think.* Rockville, MD: ASHA.

Catts, H. W., Fey, M. E., Tomblin, J. B., & Zhang, X. (2002). A longitudinal investigation of reading outcomes in children with language impairments. *Journal of Speech, Language, and Hearing Research, 45*, 1142–1157.

Culatta, B., Aslet, R., Fife, M., & Setzer, L. A. (2004). Project SEEL: Part I. Systemic and engaging early literacy instruction. *Communication Disorders Quarterly, 25*, 79–88.

Culatta, B., & Hall, K. A. (2006). Phonological awareness instruction in early childhood settings. In L. M. Justice (Ed.). *Clinical approaches to emergent literacy intervention*. San Diego, CA: Plural Publishing.

Ehri, L., Nunes, S., Willows, D., Schuster, B., Uagoub-Zadeh, K., & Shanahan, T. (2001). Phonic awareness instruction helps children learn to read: Evidence from the National Reading Panel's meta-analysis. *Reading Quarterly, 36*(3), 250–287.

Feifer, S. G., & De Fina, P. A. (2000). *The neuropsychology of reading disorders: Diagnosis and intervention*. Washington, DC: National Association of School Psychologists.

Fiestas, C., & Pena, E. (2004). Narrative discourse in bilingual children: Language and task effects. *Language, Speech, and Hearing Services in Schools, 35*, 155–168.

Foy, J., & Mann, V. (2003). Home literacy environment and phonological awareness in preschool children: Differential effects for rhyme and phoneme awareness. *Applied Psycholinguistics, 24*, 59–88.

Geffner, D. (2005). What is the role of audition in literacy? *The ASHA Leader, 10*(13), 8–9, 33.

Gillon, G. (2004). *Phonological awareness: From research to practice*. New York, NY: Guilford Press.

Goldsworthy, C. (2003). *Developmental reading disabilities: A language-based treatment approach* (2nd ed.). Clifton Park, NY: Delmar Cengage Learning.

Goldsworthy, C., & Lambert, K. (2010). *Linking the strands of language and literacy: A resource manual*. San Diego, CA: Plural Publishing.

Hegde, M. N., & Maul, C. A. (2006). *Language disorders in children: An evidence-based approach to assessment and treatment*. Boston, MA: Allyn and Bacon.

Hesketh, A. (2004). Early literacy achievement of children with a history of speech problems. *International Journal of Language and Communication Disorders, 39*(4), 453–468.

Hogan, T. P., Catts, H. W., & Little, T. D. (2005). The relationship between phonological awareness and reading. *Language, Speech, and Hearing Services in Schools, 36*, 285–293.

Horn, E. (1926). *A basic writing vocabulary*. University of Iowa Monographs in Education, No. 4. Iowa City, IA: University of Iowa Press.

Institute of Community Integration. (2000). *Impact: Feature issue on postsecondary education supports for students with disabilities*. Minneapolis, MN: University of Minnesota Press.

Justice, L. M. (2006). *Clinical approaches to emergent literacy intervention.* San Diego, CA: Plural Publishing.

Justice, L. M., Chow, S., Capellini, C., Flanigan, K., & Colton, S. (2003). Emergent literacy intervention for vulnerable preschoolers: Relative effects of two approaches. *American Journal of Speech-Language Pathology, 12,* 320–332.

Justice, L. M., Invernizzi, M., & Meier, J. (2002). Designing and implementing an early literacy screening protocol: Suggestions for speech-language pathologists. *Language, Speech, and Hearing Services in Schools, 33*(2), 84–101.

Kamhi, A. G., & Catts, H. W. (2012). *Language and reading disabilities* (3rd ed.). San Antonio, TX: Pearson/Allyn & Bacon.

Leitao, S., & Fletcher, J. (2004). Literacy outcomes for students with speech impairments: Long-term follow-up. *International Journal of Language and Communication Disorders, 39*(2), 245–256.

Lieberman, P. (1973). On the evolution of language: A unified view. *Cognition, 2,* 59–94.

Lyon, G., Shaywitz, S., & Shaywitz, B. (2003). A definition of dyslexia. *Annals of Dyslexia, 53,* 1–14.

Manzo, U. C., Manzo, A. V., & Thomas, M. M. (2009). *Content area literacy: Strategic teaching for strategic learning* (5th ed.). New York, NY: Wiley.

Musiek, F. E., & Chermak, G. D. (2007). *Handbook of (central) auditory processing disorders: Vol. 1, Auditory neuroscience and diagnosis.* San Diego, CA: Plural Publishing.

National Assessment for Educational Progress. (2005). *The nations report card* [online]. Available at http://nces.ed.gov.nationsreportcard/reading/.

National Early Literacy Panel. (2004). *The National Early Literacy Panel: A research synthesis on early literacy development.* Paper presented at the National Association of Early Childhood Specialists Conference, Anaheim, CA.

National Reading Panel. (2000). *Teaching children to read: An evidence-based assessment of the scientific research literature on reading and its implications for reading instruction* (NIH Pub. No. 00–4769). Washington, DC: National Institutes of Child Health and Human Development.

National Reading Panel. (2001). *Put reading first: The research building blocks for teaching children to read.* Washington, DC: U.S. Department of Education.

Nelson, N. W. (2010). *Language and literacy disorders: Infancy through adolescence.* Boston, MA: Allyn and Bacon.

Olson, D., & Bryne, B. (2005). Hereditability of word reading and phonological skills. In H. W. Catts, T. P. Hogan, & S. M. Adolf (Eds.). *Connections between language and reading disabilities.* Mahwah, NJ: Erlbaum.

Reed, V. A. (2010). *An introduction to children with language disorders* (4th ed.). Boston, MA: Pearson Allyn and Bacon.

Rosin, P. (2006). Literacy intervention in culturally and linguistically diverse worlds: The Linking Language and Literacy Project. In L. M. Justice (Ed.*), Clinical approaches to emergent literacy intervention.* San Diego, CA: Plural Publishing.

Schatschneider, C., Carlson, C. D., Francis, D. J., Floorman, R., & Fletcher, J. M. (2002). Relationship between rapid automatized naming and phonological awareness in early reading development: Implications for the double-deficit hypothesis. *Journal of Learning Disabilities, 35*(3), 245–257.

Schuele, C. M., Skibbe, L. E., & Rao, P. K. S. (2007). Assessing phonological awareness. In K. L. Pence (Ed.). *Assessment in emergent literacy.* San Diego, CA: Plural Publishing.

Senechal, M., & Cornell, E. H. (1993). Vocabulary acquisition through shared reading experiences. *Reading Research Quarterly, 28,* 360–375.

Siegel, L. S. (1989). IQ is irrelevant to the definition of learning disabilities. *Journal of Learning Disabilities, 22,* 469–478.

Snow, C. E., Scarborough, H. S., & Burns, M. S. (1999). What speech-language pathologists need to know about early reading. *Topics in Language Disorders, 20*(1), 48–58.

Snow, K. L. (2006). Measuring school readiness: Conceptual and practical considerations. *Early Education Development, 17,* 7–14.

Snowling, M. J., Gallagher, A., & Firth, U. (2003). Family risk of dyslexia is continuous: Individual differences in precursors of reading skills. *Child Development, 74,* 358–373.

Stevenson, J., Graham, P., Fredman, G., & McLoughlin, V. (1987). A twin study of genetic influences on reading and spelling ability and disability. *Journal of Child Psychology and Psychiatry, 28,* 229–247.

Stothard, S., Snowling, M., Bishop, D., Chipchase, B., & Kaplan, C. (1998). Language-impaired preschoolers: A follow-up into adolescence. *Journal of Speech, Language, and Hearing Research, 41,* 407–418.

Sun, L., & Nippold, M. A. (2012). *Narrative writing in children and adolescents: Examining the literate lexicon.* Language, Speech, and Hearing Services in Schools, *43,* 2–13.

Thomas-Tate, S., Washington, J., & Edwards, J. (2004). Standardized assessment of phonological awareness skills in low income African American first graders. *American Journal of Speech-Language Pathology, 13,* 182–190.

Washington, J. (2006). *Emergent literacy in high-risk communities: Research considerations.* Presentation at the Department of Communicative Disorders, University of Wisconsin-Madison, Madison, WI.

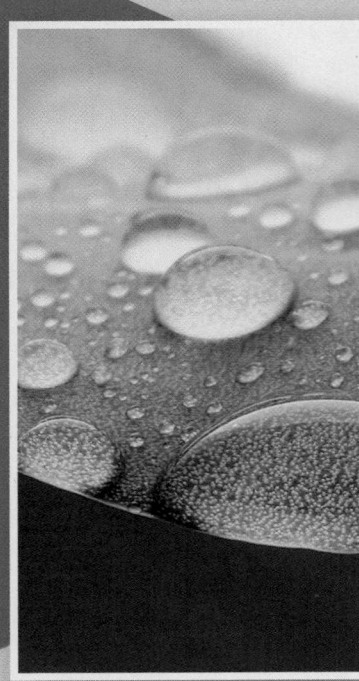

CHAPTER 8
Fluency Disorders

LEARNING OBJECTIVES

After studying this chapter, you will:

- Be able to define stuttering.
- Understand normal disfluency.
- Know some of the audible and visible overt behaviors of stutterers.
- Be familiar with general information about stuttering.
- Be familiar with the general theories of stuttering.
- Understand some multicultural considerations regarding stuttering.
- Be able to discuss the evaluation and treatment of children and adults who stutter.
- Appreciate the emotional and social effects of stuttering.

KEY TERMS

affect/affective

biofeedback

cluttering

cognitive behavioral therapy

congruent/congruence

external motivation

family systems therapy

fluency shaping (modification)

internal motivation

normal disfluency

secondary/overt/concomitant stuttering behaviors

stuttering (disfluency)

stuttering modification

CHAPTER OUTLINE

INTRODUCTION

Stuttering (disfluency) is probably the most common problem people think of when they think of a speech disorder. The problem has been discussed since the earliest days of recorded history with Chinese writings from 4000 B.C.E., Egyptian hieroglyphs from 3500 B.C.E., and early Biblical references (Bobrick, 1995). The earliest work in speech pathology focused on the causes and treatments of stuttering (Travis, 1931). Even then, theorists and therapists "projected their observations with a definiteness that suggests that they believe the problem to be solved" (West, 1942). The same may be said today.

Stuttering is perhaps the most researched of all speech disorders. In addition to SLPs, professionals such as psychologists, psychiatrists, pediatricians, neurologists, and others have investigated and written about this fascinating problem. It is no wonder there are so many views of what stuttering is, what causes it, what maintains it, and what can be done to help children and adults who do it.

stuttering (disfluency)

A disturbance in the normal flow and time patterning of speech characterized by one or more of the following: audible or silent blocks; sound, syllable, or word repetitions; sound prolongations; interjections; broken words; circumlocutions; or sounds and words produced with excessive tension.

Most speech-language pathologists refer to the disorder as either *stuttering* or *disfluency*—a disorder of fluency (note: most authors use the Latin prefix *dis* whereas some use the Greek prefix *dys*). The term *stammering* is now rarely used in the United States but is often used in Europe, Great Britain, and other countries. Even among those who have the disorder, there is disagreement about what to call people who stutter. Many people who stutter say "I am a stutterer," and others are adamant that they only be referred to as a "person who stutters" (i.e., a person-first reference—the person is not the disorder but is a person *with* a disorder). Some people want to say they are *disfluent* rather than say they stutter. For some clinicians and individuals who stutter, perhaps the word *stutter* sounds too harsh and has too many automatic negative connotations or mental images. Although ASHA emphasizes *person-first* when referring to individuals with any disorder, speech-language pathologists who stutter and are considered experts in the area of stuttering and author articles and texts on this disorder commonly use the term *stutterer* (Bloodstein & Berstein Ratner, 2008; Gregory, 2003; Conture, 2001; Guitar, 2006; Van Riper, 1982). This chapter follows the convention of well-known SLPs who are themselves stutterers and author texts on stuttering.

NORMAL DISFLUENCY

All children and adults are disfluent to some degree. Essentially all verbally disfluent behaviors that clinicians attribute to individuals who stutter may be heard in normal-speaking children and adults but not necessarily with the same frequency or degree (Ward, 2006). As children are simultaneously developing speech, language, and fluency, their rates of development can be significantly different (Zebrowski & Kelly, 2002). **Normal disfluencies** include occasional repetitions of syllables or words once or twice, li-li-like this. Disfluencies also may include hesitations and the use of fillers such as "uh," "er," and "um." Such disfluencies occur most often between 1½ and 5 years of age and they tend to come and go. They are usually signs that a child is learning to use language in new ways. Sometimes disfluencies will disappear for several weeks and then return, which means the child may be going through another stage of learning (Gregory, 2003; Guitar, 2006; Manning, 2010). Children do not begin to stutter on their first attempts to speak. Children who go on to stutter do not seem to have difficulty with the earliest speech sounds such as cooing and babbling. Most children develop a considerable vocabulary and grammatical base before exhibiting abnormal disfluency (Ramig & Dodge, 2010; Yairi & Ambrose, 2005).

normal disfluency

The repeating, pausing, incomplete phrasing, revising, interjecting, and prolonging of sounds that are typical in the speech of young children.

Some children and adults are remarkably fluent and articulate, and we may envy their communication abilities. Other children and adults may be particularly disfluent much of the time and have moderate to severe difficulty communicating with ease. However, a person can have significant disfluencies and still may not be considered a stutterer. The question for parents and SLPs is whether a child's disfluencies are normal or abnormal. It is not always easy to say.

DEFINING STUTTERING

One of the historical and ongoing problems of stuttering is how to define the disorder. Van Riper (1982, p. 15) provided a definition that continues to be appreciated by many clinicians: "Stuttering occurs when the forward flow of speech is interrupted by a motorically disrupted sound, syllable, or word, or by the speaker's reactions thereto." Guitar (2006) defines stuttering as an abnormal high frequency or duration of stoppages in the forward flow of speech affecting its continuity, rhythm, rate, and effortfulness. In 1977 the World Health Organization (WHO) provided a definition of stuttering that states stuttering includes "disorders in the rhythm of speech in which the individual knows precisely what he wishes to say, but at the time is unable to say it because of an involuntary repetitive prolongation or cessation of a sound" (p. 202). This definition uses the word "disorders" to imply that the symptoms of stuttering can take many forms and have more than one etiology (Manning, 2010).

Gregory (2003) says that stuttering is a problem related to the fluency of a person's speech or the way in which the sounds, syllables, and words of speech flow together in a forward-moving temporal sequence, and that a definition should consider both *overt behaviors* (audible and visible characteristics) and *covert reactions* (thoughts and feelings). The overt behaviors and covert reactions are essential elements to describing, understanding, and treating stuttering. We cannot change the cause of a child's stuttering, but we can work with the child who stutters and, when appropriate and possible, the parents or other caregivers important in a child's life.

Secondary/Overt/Concomitant Stuttering Behaviors

The **secondary, overt, or concomitant (accompanying) behaviors** of stuttering refer to the quantitative and qualitative audible and visible characteristics of the disorder. They are what most people think of when they think of stuttering. However, the difficulty is deciding what constitutes stuttering based on *which behaviors occur* (qualitative) and *how often these behaviors occur* (quantitative).

Audible Overt Behaviors

Audible refers to what is heard. Stutterers have "core behaviors" (Guitar, 2006; Van Riper, 1982) that are the basic speech behaviors of

secondary/overt/ concomitant stuttering behaviors

Extraneous sounds and facial and body movements a person who stutters uses during moments of stuttering; e.g., repetitions of "uh" or "um," eye blinks, and unusual head, hand, or other body part movements.

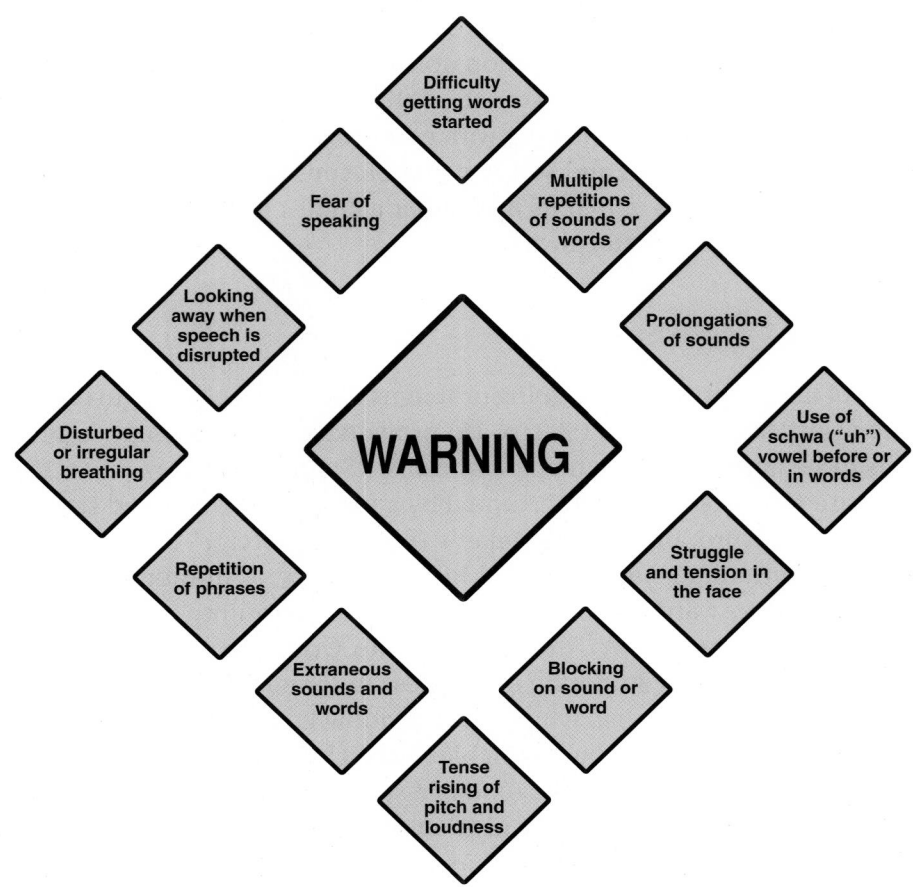

Figure 8–1

Warning signs of stuttering.

© Cengage Learning 2013.

stuttering: repetitions of sounds, prolongations of sounds, and "silent blocks." Repetitions of a sound, syllable, or single-syllable word are the core behaviors observed most frequently among children who are just beginning to stutter. Prolongations of voiced or voiceless sounds for as brief as a half second to a minute or more (with pauses for breaths) usually appear somewhat later in the speech of children who are beginning to stutter. Silent blocks are the inappropriate stopping of the flow of air or voice and often movements of the articulators that may last an instant to several minutes. (I once had a 19-year-old male client have a 10-minute silent block on the word "I.") Blocks may occur at each level of the speech production mechanism—respiratory, phonatory, or articulatory. Blocks are usually the last core behavior to appear in children as they are developing stuttering. As stuttering persists, blocks often become longer and more tense and tremors may be noticed in the lips or mandible (Guitar, 2006). (See Figure 8–1.)

The following audible overt behaviors indicate stuttering and are described by Bloodstein & Berstein Ratner, 2008; Conture, 2001; Gregory, 2003; Guitar, 2006; Manning, 2010; Ramig & Dodge, 2010; Reardon-Reeves & Yaruss, 2004; Ward, 2006; Zebrowski & Kelly, 2002. All of these audible overt behaviors may be repeated once, twice, or numerous times, and accompanied by visible signs of tension.

- *Part-word repetitions*—Sound or syllable repetitions that are involuntary and occur at the beginning of words (e.g., "M-m-m-mommy's home to make d-d-dinner!")
- *Whole-word repetitions*—Repetitions of an entire word (e.g., "Mommy-mommy-mommy's home to make dinner!")
- *Phrase repetitions*—Repetitions of units consisting of two or more words (e.g., "Mommy's home-mommy's home to make dinner.")
- *Interjections of sounds, syllables, words, and phrases*—Sounds or words that occur between words in a sentence that do not have a linguistic purpose in messages, such as "uh" (schwa [ə] vowel), "um," "well," and "you know" (e.g., "Mommy's-uh-uh-home to make-um-um-um-dinner! I'm well you know really hungry.")
- *Revisions of phrases and sentences*—A change in the content or the intended message, grammatical form, or pronunciation of a word (e.g., "Mommy's home to make lunch-dinner," "Mommy's home to have-make dinner," and "Mommy's home to take-make dinner!")
- *Prolongations of sounds and syllables*—Inappropriate lengthening of sounds and syllables, which may be accompanied by pitch change (often a tense rising pitch) (e.g., "Mmmmommy's home to mmmake dinner!")
- *Blocks*—Inappropriate timing in the initiation of a sound that is often accompanied by tension (a tense pause that may be just an instant to many seconds—or longer) (e.g., ". . . . . Mommy's home to make dinner!")
- *Dysrhythmic phonations*—Disturbances in the normal rhythm of speech that may include a variety of behaviors, such as a break between syllables ("Mom—my"), unusual timing (rapid "Mommy's home to" slow "make dinner!"), or any abnormal rhythm in speech that draws attention to how the person is speaking rather than what is being said.

Curlee (2007, p. 3) gives the following advice to parents to help them recognize whether their child is stuttering:

> First, children who stutter often have problems getting words started, and many of these disruptions occur at the beginning of sentences. When they stutter, they tend to repeat parts of words, for example, sounds or syllables, rather than whole words or phrases. In addition, they frequently repeat portions of words two or more times before they are able to say what they want. Sometimes a child may exaggerate or prolong a sound in a word. The child may seem to be stuck with no sound or word coming out, perhaps working hard at speaking, or look away just as his speech is disrupted.

Visible Overt Behaviors

Stuttering is not just about verbal disfluencies; it is also about what the person is doing literally from head to toe that is associated with stuttering behaviors. Some people are verbally fluent by using countless extraneous and often subtle body movements. The overt or secondary stuttering behaviors are often the true handicap of stuttering because listeners (observers) are usually more distracted by what they see a stutterer doing than by what they hear the stutterer saying (Sheehan, 1970). Overt stuttering behaviors may include losing eye contact at the moment of stuttering, blinking the eyes rapidly, furrowing the forehead, tensing facial muscles, jerking the head, tensing or raising the shoulders, swinging an arm, jerking the arm or hand, clenching the fist, pressing the thumb and a finger together, tensing the chest muscles (which affects breathing), moving the upper or lower part of a leg, pulling the foot up toward the shin, tapping a foot, tensing the toes, and countless other almost imperceptible "tricks and crutches to be fluent" (Bloodstein & Berstein Ratner, 2008; Gregory, 2003; Guitar, 2006; Manning, 2010; Ramig & Dodge, 2010; Sheehan, 1970; Ward, 2006). As Williams (1979, 2004) pointed out, trying not to stutter usually involves some form of physical struggle or interference with talking.

Covert Reactions

Covert (i.e., emotional and cognitive) reactions to stuttering include feelings and thoughts such as frustration, anxiety, anger, guilt, hostility, shame, and expectations of difficulty talking, which leads to inhibitory and avoidance behaviors (Conture, 2001; Gregory, 2003; Guitar, 2006; Iverach, Menzies, O'Brian, Packman, & Onslow, 2011; Ramig & Dodge, 2010). Gregory (2003) said that as the overt behaviors of stuttering increase, the covert reactions grow stronger. Furthermore, increased negative emotions associated with speaking lead to more tension and stuttering, and more stuttering results in more negative emotions. However, it is difficult to know which comes first: the stuttering or the emotional effects of stuttering (see Figure 8–2). The covert reactions of individuals who stutter can be some of the most serious challenges they face while in therapy.

Figure 8–2

It is difficult to know which comes first: the stuttering or the emotional effects of stuttering.

© Cengage Learning 2013.

Which Comes First?

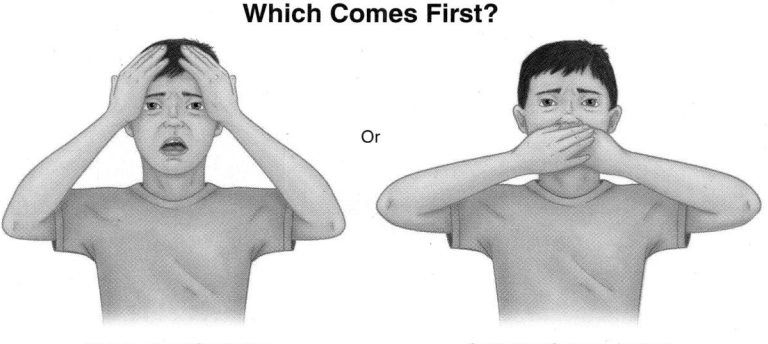

Or

Anxiety about Stuttering

Stuttering Causes Anxiety

GENERAL INFORMATION ABOUT STUTTERING

Much information about stuttering has been obtained over the decades. Areas of general concern include such things as the incidence of stuttering, the male–female ratio, family history of stuttering, physiological characteristics of stutterers, and psychological characteristics of stutterers.

- **Incidence:** The general incidence of stuttering is 1% in the population (Bloodstein & Berstein Ratner, 2008; Yairi & Ambrose, 2006).

- **Age of Onset:** Ninety percent of disfluent children begin to stutter between 2 to 6 years of age, and only 10% begin to stutter after 6 years of age (Ramig & Dodge, 2010).

- **Male–Female Ratio:** In cultures around the world, slightly more boys than girls begin to stutter, but girls are more likely to recover so that by school age and beyond, there are 3 or 4 males to every 1 female who stutter (Goldman, 1967; Yairi & Ambrose, 2005).

- **Family History of Stuttering:** Stuttering tends to run in families and stuttering appears to have a genetic basis in many individuals, although genes must interact with environmental factors for stuttering to appear (Buck, Lees, & Cook, 2002; Guitar, 2006; Yairi & Ambrose, 2005).

- **Stuttering and Other Speech and Language Disorders:** Many children who stutter have concurrent communication disorders, including articulation, phonology, and language disorders (Blood, Ridenour, Qualls, & Hammer, 2004; Ntourou, Conture, & Lipsey, 2011; Paden, 2005).

- **Physiological Characteristics:** Bloodstein & Berstein Ratner (2008) reviewed the literature on physiological characteristics of stutterers (e.g., respiration, cardiovascular, biochemical) and found that, in general, there are no significant differences between stutterers and nonstutterers other than just preceding and during the moment of stuttering (e.g., respiratory and pulse rates increase). That is, on average, stutterers are normal physiologically other than when they stutter. As these authors state, the "necessary and sufficient [physiological] conditions for stuttering" have not yet been found (p. 190).

- **Brain Function and Stuttering:** The general themes of the available research are that (1) the neural systems of individuals when stuttering can be distinguished from those when they are not stuttering; (2) areas known to be associated with motor speech and language production are found to show differences in levels of activity among individuals who stutter compared to individuals who do not stutter; (3) stuttering is not necessarily related to one structure or neural pathway; and (4) stuttering is particularly associated with hemispheric asymmetry, including increased activity in motor centers in the nondominant (typically the right) hemisphere (DeNil, 2004; Manning, 2010; Ward, 2006). However, whether the differences that have been observed represent the underlying problem that leads to stuttering or reflect the speakers' attempts to compensate for the deficit is unclear (Bloodstein & Berstein Ratner, 2008).

- **Cognitive and Personality Characteristics:** The general cognitive abilities of children who stutter are similar to those of their non-stuttering peers (Yairi & Ambrose, 2005). Sufficient research over the decades that has compared stutterers to nonstutterers has shown that people who stutter are generally adequately adjusted and that there are no specific character and personality traits of stutterers; that is, stuttering is not the symptom of a basic personality disorder (Bloodstein & Berstein Ratner, 2008).

Stutterers Are in Good Company

Many successful and famous people have stuttered at some time in their lives (De Keyser, 1973; Silverman, 2004; Tillis & Wager, 1984; see also www.stutteringhelp.org):

- *Actors and TV personalities*—Jane Seymour, Julia Roberts, Marilyn Monroe, Mike Rowe (*Dirty Jobs*), Anthony Quinn, Bruce Willis, Harvey Keitel, James Earl Jones (voice of Darth Vader), Nicholas Brendon, Jimmy Stewart, Peggy Lipton, Samuel L. Jackson, Emily Blunt, John Stossel (broadcast journalist)
- *Authors*—Aesop (*Aesop's Fables*), Andrew Lloyd Weber (playwright—*Phantom of the Opera, Cats*), Lewis Carroll (*Alice in Wonderland*), Jim Davis (cartoonist—*Garfield*), John Updike, Washington Irving, Somerset Maugham
- *Politicians*— President George Washington, President Thomas Jefferson, President Theodore Roosevelt, Joseph Biden (U.S. Vice President), Prince Albert of Monaco, King George VI of England (1895–1952 [film—"The King's Speech"]), Napoleon the 1st, Winston Churchill, Demosthenes (ancient Greek statesman)
- *Scientists*—Charles Darwin, Isaac Newton, Steven Hawking, Alan Rabinowitz
- *Singers*—Marc Anthony, Carly Simon, Mel Tillis, Nat King Cole, B. B. King
- *Sports figures*— Tiger Woods (world-champion golfer), Bill Walton (professional basketball player), Bo Jackson (football and baseball), Bob Love (basketball), Horace Grant (basketball), Johnny Damon (baseball), Ken Venturi (champion golfer), Herschel Walker (football Heisman Trophy winner), Sophie Gustafson (champion golfer), Kenyon Martin (basketball), Lester Hayes (football), Darren Sproles (football), Gordie Lane (hockey), Michael Spinks (heavyweight boxing champion), Ron Harper (basketball), Rubin "Hurricane" Carter (professional boxer), Ty Cobb (baseball)
- *Other prominent figures*—Alan Turning (founder of computer science), Annie Glenn (wife of U.S. Senator and astronaut John Glenn), Aristotle (ancient Greek orator), Arthur Blank (cofounder of Home Depot and owner of the NFL's Atlanta Falcons), Clara Barton (American founder of the Red Cross), Henry Luce (founder of *Time* magazine and *Sports Illustrated*), Jack Welch (former head of General Electric), John Scully (executive at Apple Computers), Moses (biblical Hebrew prophet)

THEORIES OF THE ETIOLOGY OF STUTTERING

Numerous theories of the etiology of stuttering and what occurs at the moment of disfluency have been proposed and there have been strong disagreements among authorities on the factors involved. The number of proposed etiologies by different authorities suggests that there is no certainty about the cause or the moment of stuttering, and no one theory fully explains these for all individuals.

Many factors, including characteristics of the child and characteristics of the environment, come into play when considering the etiology of stuttering. For example, characteristics of the child include genetic, gender, physiological, neurological, psychological, and linguistic. Characteristics of the environment include parental attitudes and behaviors such as expectations of the child's speech and other behaviors. Essentially all major theorists believe that environmental factors are important in the development and maintenance of stuttering (Bloodstein & Berstein Ratner, 2008; Conture, 2001; Gregory, 2003; Guitar, 2006).

Theories of the etiology and moment of stuttering are divided into *breakdown theories, repressed need theories,* and *anticipatory struggle behavior theories* (Bloodstein & Berstein Ratner, 2008; Silverman, 2004). Within each theory, more specific hypotheses help explain the cause of stuttering and, ideally, lead to some direction for its treatment. However, rather than focusing on possible individual etiologies of stuttering, it may be more productive to consider stuttering as having *multifactorial* causes for many children; that is, two or more potential causes may need to come into play for any one child to develop stuttering.

The *breakdown theories* of the onset of stuttering attribute the disorder to the effects of early environmental stress and usually assign an important role to neurological predisposition factors. Increasing evidence supports the theory of a neurological predisposition to stutter (Biermann-Ruben, Salmelin, & Schnitzler, 2005; DeNil, 2004; Ingham, 2001). That is, if a child had a stressful environment but did not have the predisposition to stutter, he would not likely stutter; likewise, if he had a predisposition to stutter but did not have a stressful environment, he would not likely stutter (Ramig & Dodge, 2010). (See Figure 8–3.)

Repressed need theories of the etiology of stuttering tend to merge with theories of the etiology of neurotic behavior. That is, a stutterer has an emotional need that has not been met, and the stuttering behaviors are a symbolic expression or symptom of that repressed need (Bloodstein & Berstein Ratner, 2008).

Anticipatory struggle behavior theories attribute stuttering to parental penalties for normal disfluency or to pressures extending to other speech failures. That is, stuttering is a learned behavior somehow precipitated by the child anticipating and fearing it, and the struggle is to avoid it, with the struggle itself becoming the stuttering (Silverman, 2004).

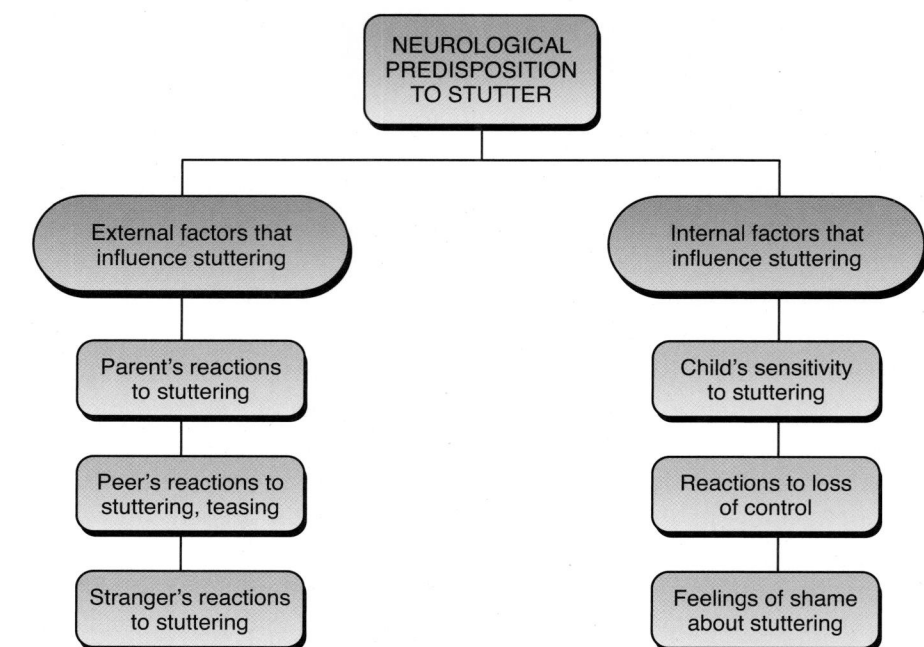

Source: Ramig & Dodge, 2010/
© Cengage Learning 2013.

Figure 8–3

External and internal factors that influence a child's neurological predisposition to stutter.

Guitar (2006) integrates these theories with a two-stage model. The first stage is primary stuttering, which involves repetitions and prolongations that are frequently the first signs of stuttering. These signs are thought to be the result of constitutional factors: a "dyssynchrony" at some level of the speech and language production process. The second stage is secondary stuttering, which involves the tension, struggle, escape, and avoidance behaviors that are often present in persistent stuttering. These behaviors may be the result of a separate constitutional factor: a reactive temperament that triggers a defense response that makes the individual more emotionally conditioned than the average speaker (see Figure 8–4).

Conditions That Increase Stuttering

Two of the most challenging words for stutterers to say are their own name and the word *I*. Many (most) stutterers will avoid saying their name at all costs, including simply not identifying themselves. Having to take a turn reading aloud to a class or having to wait to speak (particularly having to wait to introduce himself when in a group) creates increased anxiety and pressure for stutterers, which increases their likelihood of stuttering. Speaking to authority figures (the disciplinary parent, the bully in the classroom, or a teacher, principal, supervisor, or boss) is particularly difficult for stutterers. Speaking on the telephone can be terrifying to many stutterers, and they will sometimes try to convince other

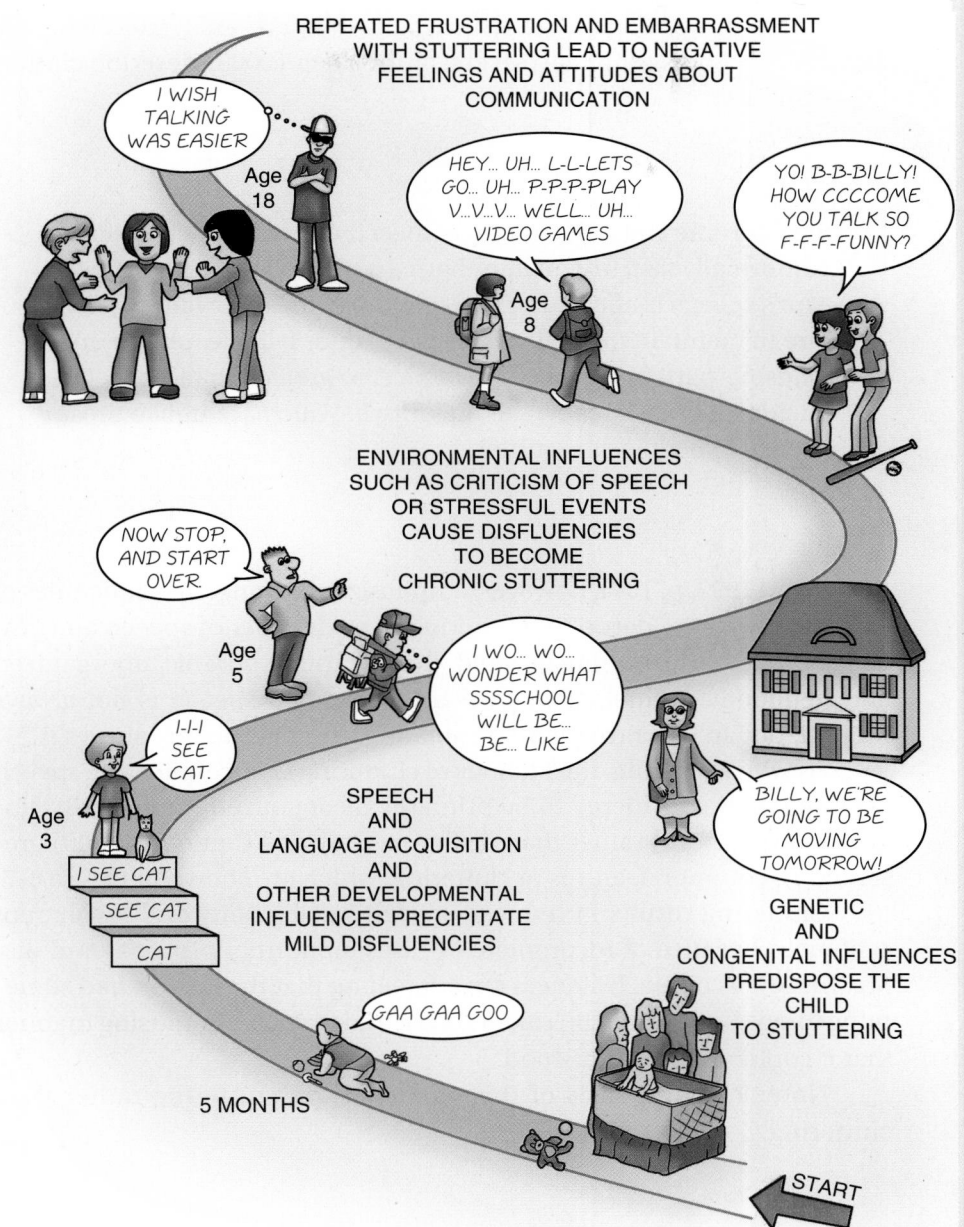

Figure 8–4

A developmental pathway to stuttering.

Source: Figure 1–1, p. 6 In Guitar, B. (2006). *Stuttering: An integrated approach to its nature and treatment.* Baltimore, MD: Lippincott Williams & Wilkins. Copyright © 2006 by Lippincott Williams & Wilkins. Adapted with permission. http://lww.com.

people to make calls for them to avoid confronting one of their worst fears (Gregory, 2003; Ramig & Dodge, 2010).

CLUTTERING

Cluttering is a speech and language disorder that shares some of the characteristics of stuttering but differs in many important ways (Ward, 2006). Although stuttering has been well researched, cluttering has not. Like stuttering, however, cluttering is difficult to define because of

cluttering

A fluency disorder characterized by a speech rate that is abnormally fast or irregular that may be affected by (1) failure to maintain normally expected sound, syllable, phrase and pause patterns, and (2) evidence of greater than expected incidences of disfluency, the majority of which are unlike those typical of people who stutter.

differences in opinions as to which behaviors are associated with the disorder. St. Louis, Raphael, Myers, and Bakker (2003) describe cluttering as follows:

> A syndrome characterized by a speech delivery which is either abnormally fast, irregular, or both. In cluttered speech the person's speech is affected by one or more of the following: (1) failure to maintain normally expected sound, syllable, phrase and pausing patterns, and (2) evidence of greater than expected incidents of disfluency, the majority of which are unlike those typical of people who stutter.

Daly (1992, p. 107), however, emphasizes the language difficulties of clutterers when he describes cluttering as a "disorder of speech and language processing resulting in rapid, dysrhythmic, sporadic, unorganized and frequently unintelligible speech. Accelerated speech is not always present, but an impairment in formulating language almost always is."

As with stuttering, the etiology of cluttering is uncertain. The speech of clutterers is considered to be primarily disorganized (motorically, linguistically, or both) rather than disfluent. Daly and Cantrelle (2006) presented 10 common features of cluttering, which are shown in Figure 8–5.

Cluttering results in reduced speech intelligibility and incoherent sentences because of incomplete phrases, abnormal prosody, and disorganized discourse. Listeners are left feeling that the person had something to say, but the person said it so fast and in such a confusing manner that it could not be understood.

Note: The emphasis of this chapter is on stuttering rather than cluttering.

Figure 8–5

Ten common features of cluttering.

Adapted from Daly & Cantrelle, 2006.

1. Telescoping or condensing of words (e.g., omission of sounds)
2. Lack of effective self-monitoring of speech
3. Lack of pauses
4. Lack of awareness of speech difficulties
5. Imprecise consonants (e.g., distortion of sounds)
6. Irregular rate of speech; speaking in spurts (staccato-like speech)
7. Use of numerous interjections, revisions, and filler words
8. Compulsive talking, verbosity, and circumlocutions (i.e., talking around words rather than using a specific word)
9. Disorganized language with confused wording
10. Apparent verbalization before adequate thought formulation

WORKING WITH CHILDREN WHO STUTTER

Before clinicians can provide intervention (therapy) for a child who stutters, they need to interview the parents and evaluate the child's general speech and language development. In a way, the initial parent interview, which always involves answering their questions about stuttering and their child's speech, is the beginning of therapy. A clinician's first meeting with the parents and child often establishes the future working relationship with the family. Throughout the working relationship with a family, the **family systems therapy, family-centered service delivery**, and **cognitive behavioral therapy** models are helpful (Gregory, 2003; Guitar, 2006; Maul, 2011; Yu & Kashinath, 2011; Zebrowski, 2002). Family systems therapy emphasizes collaboration with all family members who have significant involvement with the child. The child is the person who is brought into therapy but other family members are essential in the overall treatment of the child's fluency problem. Cognitive behavioral therapy emphasizes that there are numerous perspectives or interpretations of any given event or behavior. Furthermore, the way in which people think about events and behaviors (their perceptions) determine how they feel about themselves, others, and the future. The essential purpose of cognitive therapy is to help individuals recognize and examine tightly held but problematic beliefs and replace them with more adaptive and flexible ways of thinking (Flasher & Fogle, 2012).

Evaluation of a Child

Depending on the environment in which a clinician works, the setting for an evaluation may differ significantly. In a university clinic, the evaluation usually takes place in a relatively small, often somewhat "sterile" clinic room with the child and at least one parent present. In the schools, the speech therapy room is used and the clinician and child are likely surrounded by many colorful posters and therapy materials, although a parent is not likely present to give information and be asked questions. In hospital settings, one or both parents usually bring the child and the evaluation may be done in an office environment or therapy room. In private practice, the evaluation may be done in an office setting, a therapy room, or the family home (with all of the variables you can imagine) with one or both parents present. In all settings, excellent interviewing and counseling skills are essential when questioning and talking to parents and children about such sensitive issues as a child's fluency. Some parents and children become emotional and clinicians need to know how to handle such emotions professionally and gracefully (Flasher & Fogle, 2012).

During the evaluation of a child, the clinician will observe the types and frequency of his disfluencies under different conditions, such as interacting with his parents and interacting with the clinician during play, conversation, direct questioning, reading (if he is a reader), and

family systems therapy/ family-centered service delivery

Models of counseling and service delivery that focus on variables regarding the family unit as a whole; i.e., each family member is part of a system (the family), each member affects the others, and the system is interdependent; that is, within the system there are sub-systems: e.g., mother–father, mother–son, father–son, grandparent–grandchild.

cognitive behavioral therapy

A model of counseling designed to help individuals recognize and examine problematic beliefs and replace them with more adaptive and flexible ways of thinking.

Figure 8-6

A clinician evaluating a preschool child who stutters. (Notice that the child is sitting to the side of the clinician rather than across the table so there is not a physical or psychological barrier between them.)

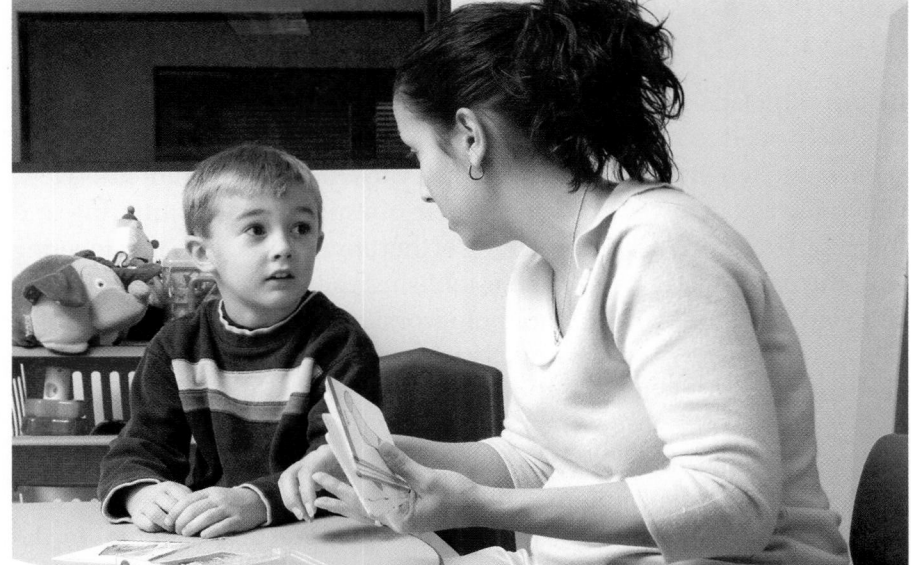

© Cengage Learning 2013

even talking on a telephone. Audio- or video-recording is important for a later analysis. Requesting the parents to bring an audio- or video-recording of the child talking in various situations at home is very helpful in getting a more true-to-life example of the child's speech.

Beyond the interview and fluency evaluation, the clinician will want to evaluate the speech systems (respiratory, phonatory, resonatory, and articulatory) and may choose to administer standardized articulation and language assessments. Upon completion of the evaluation of the child, the clinician should be able to diagnose whether stuttering is occurring and its severity level. Impressions also need to be made about the child's covert reactions to his stuttering, such as frustration, anger, shame, and inhibitory and avoidance behaviors (see Figure 8–6).

Analysis of the child's disfluencies may include the *percent disfluency rate* (e.g., 54 disfluent words divided by 318 words in a speech sample, equals 17% disfluency rate). The actual percent disfluency may not be as clinically significant as what the child is doing at the moment of disfluency; that is, what he tries to do to prevent being disfluent (e.g., avoiding talking or long pauses); what he does during the disfluency (e.g., rapid repetitions or prolongations of a sound, blinking his eyes and looking away); and what he does to end the disfluency (e.g., jerks his head and finishes the word in a high-pitched, tense voice). The clinician should take notes on all of the "core stuttering" and verbal and secondary stuttering behaviors that she observes to include in her analysis and evaluation report.

The first major decision the clinician needs to make is whether the child's speech has normal disfluencies. Guitar (2006) uses the following criteria for determining normal disfluencies: (a) the child has fewer than 10 disfluencies per 100 words; (b) the disfluencies consist mostly of multisyllabic word and phrase repetitions, revisions, and interjections;

(c) when disfluencies are repetitions, they have two or less repeated units per repetition that are slow and regular in tempo; (d) the ratio of stuttering-like disfluencies to total disfluencies is less than 50%; (e) all disfluencies will be relatively relaxed and the child will seem to be hardly aware of them and is not upset when he is aware.

Severity Levels

When a child is diagnosed as having abnormal disfluencies (i.e., stuttering), it is important to determine the severity level to help guide the direction of therapy. Guitar (2006) says children may be considered to have *borderline stuttering* if they have more than 10 disfluencies per 100 words, but the disfluencies are loose and relaxed. The disfluencies may be part-word repetitions, single-syllable word repetitions, prolongations, and/or repetitions with two repeated units (sounds, syllables, words, or phrases) per instance.

Key features of *beginning stuttering* include rapid, abrupt repetitions; pitch rises during repetitions and prolongations; difficulty with airflow or phonation; and tension while talking. Beginning stutterers appear to be aware of their difficulty talking and may be frustrated by it. They may use escape behaviors such as head nods or eye blinks to try to end stuttering blocks. They may begin avoiding words by substituting more easily spoken words for words they have difficulty with (e.g., using "me" for "I").

Children at the *intermediate stuttering* level have most of the characteristics of children who are at the beginning level, but repetitions and prolongations of sounds and syllables are more common. In addition, they may use a variety of starters (e.g., "uh uh uh," "um um," "You know") to begin sentences and look away (lose eye contact) or appear embarrassed about their difficulty talking. They may have "silent blocks." They appear to anticipate stuttering and use *avoidance behaviors*, that is, extraneous behaviors such as eye blinking before saying *feared words* (words they expect to stutter on). Children may use *escape behaviors* to terminate blocks, such as head jerking or forcing the word out using excessive tension, as though the word explodes from the mouth. They anticipate feared people (people with whom they expect to do considerable stuttering), places (e.g., talking in front of the class), and situations (e.g., having to answer questions or large family gatherings).

Advanced stuttering includes longer and more tense blocks, often with tremors of the lips, tongue, or jaw. Numerous repetitions and prolongations of sounds and syllables occur. Complex patterns of avoidance and escape behaviors may be so well habituated that stutterers are unaware they are doing them. Stuttering behaviors may be suppressed in some individuals through extensive avoidance behaviors, making them appear more fluent than they really are. Emotions, fears, embarrassment, and shame are very strong in advanced stuttering. Stutterers usually have negative feelings about themselves as competent speakers and these feelings may be pervasive in their self-concept.

Personal Story

Jonathan

I received a call from a mother who sounded intense and somewhat desperate. She had been referred to me by the mother of another child who stuttered whom I had worked with the previous year. The mother explained that Jonathan was 4 years old, a sweet and bright little boy who was stuttering. The father was a fairly new police officer and the mother was a librarian with a degree in English. I scheduled an appointment to see the family in their home.

When first meeting the parents, I had the impression of meeting Ken and Barbie in person. Both parents looked perfect in every way, with manners that seemed to have come from a manual on etiquette. The house was neat and clean (spotless), and there was a nicely circumscribed area in the family room for Jonathan's play area. Jonathan was polite and well mannered. He shook my hand as though he had been well trained. After visiting with the parents for a few minutes, the parents asked Jonathan to show me his room. A nice room it was; neat and orderly. When Jonathan finished playing with one toy, he put it back in its place and took out another. Jonathan was definitely exhibiting some signs of disfluency.

Over the next 2½ months, I met with the family once or twice a week in the family home. Both parents were always present and if one could not make the scheduled appointment, they rescheduled. I worked with Jonathan for a while in his room during each visit, with the parents just outside the door to listen. The parents and I then sat around the formal dining room table to discuss stuttering in general, their child's stuttering in particular, and specific things the parents could do during the week that could help Jonathan's speech. Never had parental perfectionism been so helpful. They did every assignment perfectly and began to see that the little changes they needed to make in their daily family lives could have big benefits for Jonathan. The parents began to accept Jonathan's occasional disfluencies and not react to them; his imperfect, but normal for his age, articulation of sounds and words; and his normal 4-year-old playfulness and other behaviors of a child his age. The parents eventually became less perfect (i.e., "lightened up"), and Jonathan's speech became more fluent. This story helps illustrate the importance of working with the parents of children who stutter. ■

Treatment of Children Who Stutter

When a child is at risk for stuttering but is not yet stuttering, a speech-language pathologist can focus on prevention strategies, rather than providing direct therapy. ASHA (1988) published a position statement on applying prevention strategies, stating that speech-language pathologists should play a significant role in the development and application of prevention strategies in all areas of communication disorders. Hill (2003) describes primary prevention strategies for children at risk for stuttering.

Primary prevention refers to SLPs being involved in eliminating or inhibiting the onset and development of stuttering by changing the susceptibility of children or modifying exposure conditions that may lead to the development of the disorder (ASHA, 1988; Nelson, 1999). The goal of primary prevention is educating parents so they can support the development of communication skills in their children by understanding normal speech, language, and fluency development; providing appropriate language stimulation; identifying signs of speech, language, and fluency concerns; and seeking advice from knowledgeable resources—such as speech-language pathologists. Of particular help to parents of children at risk for stuttering are publications from the Stuttering Foundation of America (www.stutteringhelp.org [Spanish: www.tartamudez.org]), especially *Stuttering and Your Child: Questions and Answers* (2002a), *Stuttering and the Preschool Child: Help for Families* (2002b), *Stuttering: Straight Talk for Teachers* (2002c), and *Fundación Americana de la Tartanudez* (2002d) (information in Spanish).

Although parents may not be the cause of the stuttering problem, they can be an important part of the solution. Some helpful points for parents include (Stuttering Foundation of America, 2002a–c):

- Speak with your child in an unhurried manner, pausing frequently. Wait a few seconds after your child finishes speaking before you begin to speak so that the child does not feel the conversation is being rushed.

- Refrain from making remarks such as "Slow down," "Take a breath," "Relax," or "Think before you talk." Such advice can feel demeaning to a child and it is not helpful.

- Refrain from finishing his sentences or filling in words when your child is having trouble talking.

- Maintain natural eye contact and try not to look embarrassed when he is disfluent. Just wait patiently and naturally until your child is finished.

- Let your child know by your manner and actions that you are listening to *what* he is saying, not *how* he is saying it.

- Reduce the number of questions you ask your child. Instead of asking questions, simply comment on what your child has said.

- Set aside a few minutes at a regular time each day when you can give your undivided attention to your child.

- Help all members of the family learn to take turns talking and listening.

- Accept your child and find ways to show your child that you love and value him and that you enjoy your time together.

Ramig and Dodge (2010) have several major emphases in their stuttering program for children and adolescents, including (a) counseling and helping parents learn about stuttering; (b) assessment of the

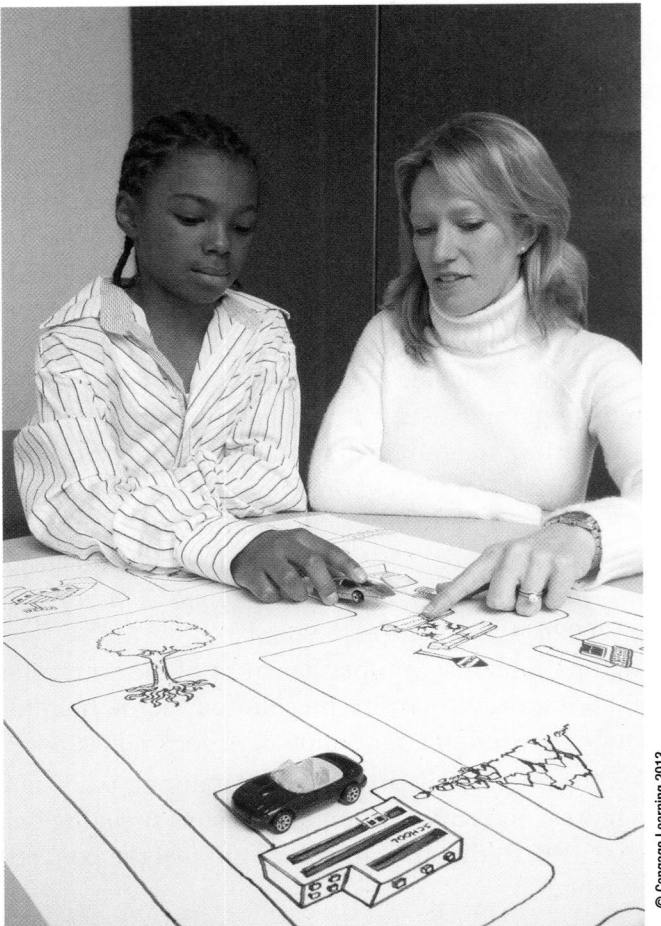

Figure 8-7

A speech-language pathologist playing "On the Road" with a child who stutters.

© Cengage Learning 2013

child's disfluencies; (c) working with teachers so they will understand stuttering and how to be supportive of a child who stutters; (d) direct therapy approaches with children, such as fluency shaping and stuttering modification; and (e) transference and maintenance. Ramig and Dodge emphasize a cooperative model of stuttering treatment that includes the child, the parents or caregivers, and the speech-language pathologist.

Zebrowski and Kelly (2002, pp. 75–76) provide a creative way of helping children identify and then learn to change their stuttering behaviors. The authors call it "On the Road" (illustrated in Figure 8–7). The clinician draws or sets up objects to form a roadway that has smooth stretches and various obstacles, including railroad tracks, a mud slick or oil spill, a drawbridge, and a closed roadway with a detour. For every obstacle, there should be an alternative path or way to move through the obstacle. The child and clinician use their vehicles to go "on the road." Each obstacle represents a type of disfluency; for example, bumpy speech for railroad tracks, mud slick or oil spill for sound prolongations, drawbridge for broken words, and closed roadway for silent "blocks." Using the child's own terms for the various types of disfluencies, the clinician shows the child how to take the smooth detour around or through all obstacles by using easy speech techniques.

Therapy for children who stutter requires a sound base of knowledge and understanding of the problem based on the best available literature, insight into both children and adults (parents), and creativity. To become confident and successful when working with children who stutter, you will need to take a genuine interest in the problem and seek every opportunity to expand your education and training in this complex area. The rewards for the children and families you help, and for you, can be enormous.

Direct Therapy

Stuttering therapy is a dynamic process, meaning that the goals and procedures used are determined by the child's behaviors and needs and the specific goals are likely to change during the process. A clinician typically fine-tunes the overall therapy plan as she becomes familiar with the child's abilities, attitudes, and concerns during the early stages of treatment. The work with the parents is likewise fine-tuned as trust is developed and the parents further understand stuttering in general and their child's in particular (Zebrowski & Kelly, 2002).

The relationship we develop with the child is important in our ability to help him. We work to develop an open child–clinician relationship as an important component for building trust, confidence, and understanding (Ramig & Dodge, 2010; Reardon-Reeves & Yaruss, 2004). Our general approach is to be understanding and accepting so that the child views us as someone who is genuinely interested in him and accepting of whatever he says and however he says it. By having a good child–clinician relationship, our social reinforcement will be more important to the child. It is important for the therapist to model for the parents what will be helpful to the child's speech. Our calm, warm, and accepting manner along with our relaxed, easygoing way of talking with the child may be quite different from how the parents normally interact and communicate with their child.

Building the child's self-confidence is important throughout therapy (Chmela & Reardon, 2005). Providing the child with successful speaking activities and opportunities, such as single-word and phrase-level tasks, can be helpful. Therapy activities may be built around child-level conversations and games. Games are not therapy; rather, therapy lies in the speech and communication that occurs while games are being played. Blocks, memory-matching card games (e.g., Go Fish), toy trains, and action figures can be used in creative ways. The goal of a game is not to see who wins but for the clinician to model easy speech and for the child to have numerous opportunities for successful, easy, and relaxed speech attempts.

Some clinicians choose to use published fluency therapy packages. Some of these programs provide speech modification games, drill activities, role-playing scenarios, and counseling activities that can

Personal Story   Shot in the Heart

Jared was 7 years old when he was referred to me by a public school speech therapist. Jared was a severe stutterer and had been in therapy for more than a year with only minimal progress. The therapist was going to continue, but then something drastic happened. On a Saturday morning, Jared was playing in the front yard of his house when a teenager who lived across the street fired a BB gun through his screen door and hit Jared. The BB went through Jared's T-shirt, passed through his skin and chest muscles between two ribs, and entered his heart. Jared did not fall but quickly grabbed his chest. His mother saw that something was wrong and ran to him. She saw the hole in his T-shirt and some blood. She immediately called 911, and within minutes the fire department ambulance was at the home.

Jared was rushed to the hospital. In the emergency room, the doctor tried to extract the BB from Jared's heart, but he could not find it. From Jared's chest X-rays, the doctor discovered the BB lodged in his right shoulder. Apparently, the BB had entered Jared's heart directly into the left ventricle and was pumped out through the aorta and then traveled to the right subclavian artery that carried it to his right shoulder, where it lodged in a smaller artery. The doctor removed the BB from Jared's shoulder and "patched him up."

After the shooting incident, Jared was seen by a psychologist who was helpful with him "working through" the incident. However, after Jared returned to school, his speech therapist thought he needed a different approach to help his stuttering, as well as someone who could work with the parents. Working with the parents was essential, and I spent many hours in Jared's home talking with them about stuttering in general and Jared's stuttering in particular. Because Jared was aware of his stuttering and motivated to work on it, a direct approach was used. Although Jared made significant improvements in his fluency, he continues even now to have some difficulty with stuttering. It is important for clinicians to appreciate that even when we provide our best therapy, not all outcomes are what we or the clients and their families hope for. ▪

be adapted to or integrated with other approaches. General therapy approaches have been used with preschool and school-age children who stutter to teach a slow, smooth, relaxed pattern of speech through clinician and parent modeling. The usual practice is to progress systematically from one- or two-word utterances to longer and more complex sentences (Conture, 2001; Gregory, 2003; Guitar, 2006; Ramig & Dodge, 2010; Reardon-Reeves & Yaruss, 2004).

Fluency Shaping (Modification)

With both children and adults, **fluency shaping (modification)** therapy attempts to directly train stutterers to speak with relaxed respiration, relaxed vocal folds, and relaxed articulation muscles. The goal is to teach stutterers how to talk fluently. Fluency shaping therapy tends to be highly structured behavior modification that works directly on the physical aspects of speech and fluency, that is, respiratory, phonatory, and articulatory movements. Fluency controlling techniques are used through a series of exercises that are usually implemented within a slow-speech framework, which fundamentally changes the way that respiration, phonation, and articulation are coordinated for speech (Ward, 2006). Essentially, the stutterer is taught to do the opposite of what he does when he stutters. That is, rather than speaking with (a) tense, shallow intake of breaths, he learns to take relaxed full breaths; (b) tense and tight vocal mechanism, he learns to relax the vocal folds and laryngeal muscles; (c) tense articulatory system, he learns to relax the articulators; and (d) rapid and tense rate of speech, he learns to speak with a slower and more relaxed rate.

Fluency shaping uses various direct modifications of the speech act. The speech act starts with an intake of air followed by controlled exhalation, and a smooth continuous airflow is needed to produce fluent speech. The clinician teaches the child to have a *smooth airflow* by using diaphragmatic breathing to help him learn to fill his lungs so that he does not run out of breath while talking. This can be demonstrated by placing the hand on the upper abdomen and feeling the abdomen rise during inhalation and lower during exhalation. The child also learns to exhale a small amount of air a second or two before he starts to speak, which initiates a smooth exhalation that helps produce smooth phonation.

A *soft glottal onset* or *gentle initiation of sound* builds on the smooth airflow technique. The soft glottal onset helps decrease tension of the vocal folds and other muscles of the larynx. The soft glottal onset is used primarily with vowels and glides (semivowels) as an attempt to make the smooth airflow technique carry over into a gentle initiation of vocal fold vibration so that the sound emerges rather than being abruptly produced. Initially this may sound as though an /h/ has been placed before the initial vowel of a word, for example, *am* may sound like *hhaam*; however, with further development of the technique the /h/ is less noticeable and the person acquires a steady yet inaudible airflow while speaking.

Soft consonant contacts are taught to reduce the force of the contact between articulators and reduce tension in the articulatory system. The initial consonants of words are produced by bringing the two articulators lightly together. Clients can practice by attempting a soft contact consonant and contrasting that with the production of a hard contact, for example, on the word *big*. However, the client must simultaneously use a smooth air flow and soft glottal onset so that all three systems are working smoothly and effortlessly. The fluency shaping approach tends

fluency shaping (modification)

A therapy approach for children and adult stutterers that attempts to directly train individuals to speak with relaxed respiration, relaxed vocal folds, and relaxed articulation muscles; the approach attempts to teach stutterers how to talk fluently.

to slow the stutterer's speech rate, although the clinician also may work with the stutterer to intentionally slow his speech rate by prolonging syllables in words. Later, as the stutterer increases and habituates his fluency a more natural speech rate may be used.

Stuttering Modification

stuttering modification

A therapy approach for children and adult stutterers that requires the speaker to recognize and confront his fears, avoidances, and struggles to escape his stuttering, and the speaker reducing and managing those fears, avoidances, and struggles.

The **stuttering modification** therapy approach was first developed by Charles Van Riper in his early writings (Van Riper, 1939; 1971) and has continued to be the foundation of many fluency experts since that time (Gregory, 2003; Ramig, 1997; Sheehan, 1970; Williams, 2004). A primary premise of this approach is the stutterer recognizing and confronting his fears, avoidances, and struggles to escape his stuttering, and, therefore, a primary focus of therapy is the reduction and management of his fears, avoidances, and struggle behaviors. The acronym "MIDVAS" (Van Riper, 1971, 1982) outlines the principle components of stuttering modification therapy:

- *Motivation* of the stutterer is the most important underlying factor throughout the therapy process, and the stutterer must be an active participant in the therapy. The stutterer is changed by what he does, not by what he thinks about.

- *Identification* of the stuttering behaviors, both verbal and secondary, is essential before they can be changed or eliminated. The stutterer needs to identify, analyze, and confront his specific patterns of stuttering (most stutterers have never looked at themselves in a mirror to see what they do when they stutter). Beyond looking at his behaviors he also needs to confront his anxieties and fears associated with his stuttering.

- *Desensitization* is partly achieved by a stutterer's willingness to examine what he has always avoided—his stuttering behaviors. The stutterer is expected to talk openly to family and friends about his stuttering problem. Negative practice (stuttering voluntarily but in a new and easier way) further helps desensitize the feelings of frustration, guilt, and shame.

- *Variation* provides the individual alternative stuttering behaviors to increase speaking control. The stutterer goes from his old, reflexive, and automatic pattern of stuttering to small but important changes that he intentionally uses to vary his stuttering behaviors.

- *Approximation* of increasingly "normal" fluency includes using specific techniques such as "cancellations" (after finishing a stuttered word, saying the word again but in an easier, less tense manner) and "pull-outs" (changing the stuttering behavior as it is occurring).

- *Stabilization* is the transference of the speaker's new perceptions and skills to situations outside of the therapy setting. From the earliest therapy sessions the client is asked to do assignments in his home, community, school, and work place. The goal is for the speaker to become resilient in responding to the variety of communicative pressures encountered in daily speaking situations.

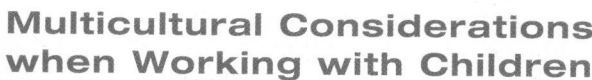

Multicultural Considerations when Working with Children

Stuttering exists in all known cultures, with some having a higher or lower incidence than others (Bloodstein & Berstein Ratner, 2008; Botterill & Fry, 2005; Ezrati-Vinacour & Amir, 2005; Kenjo, 2005; Limongi, 2005; Lundstrom & Garsten, 2005; Robinson & Crowe, 2002; Subramanian & Prabhu, 2005; Yang, 2005). Proctor, Yairi, Duff, & Zhang (2008) in their study on the prevalence of stuttering in African American preschoolers (2,223 African American children compared with 941 European American children) found no statistically significant difference in the incidence of stuttering between the two groups.

Watson and Kayser (1994) discussed several fluency issues in bilingual and bicultural children that should be considered when evaluating and treating children who stutter:

- Bilingual children may exhibit pauses, repetitions, revisions, or a combination of these related to second-language acquisition.
- Distinguish true stuttering from disfluencies associated with second-language acquisition.
- Disfluencies observed only in a second language that are not accompanied by secondary behaviors are most likely not stuttering behaviors.
- Monolingual clinicians should be able to identify tension and secondary characteristics in a bilingual child even if they do not understand the child's language.

WORKING WITH ADOLESCENTS AND ADULTS WHO STUTTER

Adolescents and adults who stutter come to a speech-language pathologist because they want help (**internal motivation**) or because someone else, such as a parent, spouse, or employer, wants the person to receive help (**external motivation**). Internal motivation is essential; however, some external motivation can be helpful to keep the person in therapy. Treatment of adolescents and adults who stutter is sometimes the result of earlier (preschool or school-age) therapy that was not successful. Therapy's success relies on numerous variables, including the readiness of the person to receive help, motivation and maturity, and having the right therapist with the right therapy at the right time.

Adult stutterers come for help at all ages (I have worked with some adults in their 60s who decided that they wanted to "conquer" their stuttering before they die); however, many adults appear to seek therapy when they recognize that their stuttering problem is interfering with or holding them back in their occupations and professions. Sometimes when a stutterer is promoted to a job with more speaking responsibilities (e.g., a managerial position) and increased pressure to communicate fluently, the person recognizes that the stuttering problem is going

internal motivation

Motivation that is self-generated or intrinsic in which a person decides what is important and needed.

external motivation

Motivation that is provided by the encouragement of someone else, often family or an employer.

to become obvious to others and that something needs to be done—even starting therapy.

Evaluation of Adolescents and Adults

The evaluation of adolescents and adults is considerably different from that of preschool and school-age children. (Note: Because of the wide range of maturity levels from early adolescence to late adolescence, evaluation and therapy techniques may overlap from the childhood-adolescence group and the adolescence-adult group.) When evaluating adolescents, the parents may play a role in providing some history of the adolescent's stuttering and some family background information; however, the emphasis is on the stutterer and her problem and her perceptions of the problem. With adults, however, there is typically no parental involvement, with the only information about the parents and family history being provided by the client.

The interview and evaluation of both adolescents and adults are direct. As mentioned previously, interviewing is an essential skill for clinicians to develop, and all interviewing involves counseling skills. Interviewing and therapy require clinicians to be **congruent**; that is, our thoughts, feelings, words, tone of voice, and body language all need to be in agreement. Our clients are probably going to "read" us better than we can read ourselves. They can tell if we are faking knowledge, understanding, and confidence. People most readily trust us when we are congruent (Flasher & Fogle, 2012). In a university clinic setting, clients realize that their student clinicians are "learning on them," and they tacitly accept that students probably do not really know what they are doing, but hope that the supervisor behind the mirror does know and is giving the student good direction.

Knowledge about stuttering is not sufficient to be a good or excellent clinician; it also takes the ability to enter into the person's world and develop a strong therapeutic relationship. The relationship has dynamics that are inevitably affected by what the client and clinician bring to it. Variables contributing to the therapeutic relationship are illustrated in Figure 8–8. The client–clinician relationship emphasizes the **affective**

Application Question

What kind of motivation (internal or external) would you most likely need to seek professional help for a personal problem?

congruent/congruence

The agreement among a person's thoughts, feelings, words, tone of voice, and body language; communication in which a person sends the same message on both verbal and nonverbal levels.

affective/affect

Relating to, arising from, or influencing feelings or emotions; *affect* is revealed by facial expressions, body posture and gestures, tone of voice, and choice of words.

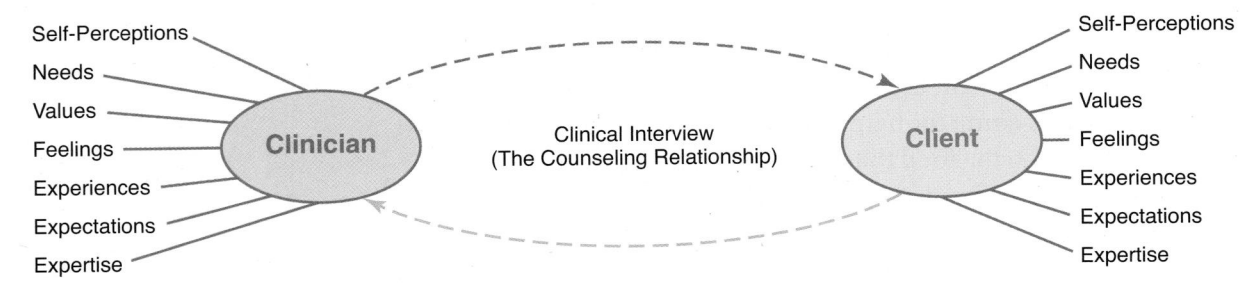

Figure 8–8

Variables contributing to the therapeutic relationship.

Adapted from Brammer & McDonald, 1999.

Too Good at Hiding

Two of my recent adult male clients who stuttered had both "successfully" hidden their stuttering from their wives and employers for years. One stutterer had been a forklift driver for several years (he chose the job because he did not need to talk much), and the other was a police officer who liked working in the toughest areas of a well-known high-crime city. However, both men said that their stuttering was "eating them up inside." Even though to other people they appeared fluent and generally normal speakers, they both knew they were "faking" having fluent speech. One of the early assignments both men were given was to talk to their wives about their stuttering. Although both men found this a very challenging assignment, they were extremely relieved for their wives to learn about their problems and to find out how accepting their wives were and how supportive they were of therapy.

mode because, like any relationship, there is an emotional quality to the interaction. The client and clinician influence each other as their relationship evolves. How clients behave toward us is invariably linked to how we think, feel, and behave toward them. The relationship can change subtly or even significantly from session to session and sometimes from moment to moment. However, mutual respect and trust help the client and clinician through the "rocky" times of their therapeutic relationship.

During the interview, the clinician takes notes about stuttering behaviors she sees and hears. Often, as the interview progresses, the clinician can begin to recognize stuttering patterns. For example: *When she stutters she tends to repeat the first sound of the word three times, then stops, then looks away (usually up and to her right), then clenches her left hand, then clears her throat, then tries to say the word again as she is looking around the room, and then says the word.* Clinicians develop astute behavioral observation skills.

Some stutterers will be remarkably fluent—too fluent—during the evaluation. The clinician may wonder where the stuttering is. The client has found such subtle tricks for concealing her stuttering from others (even family members) that she can be as fluent—or more fluent—than nonstutterers. However, the stutterer knows she stutters, and her hiding and dishonesty with herself can be tormenting. It is unlikely that an adult would come for stuttering therapy if she did not stutter. If there is not a legitimate problem, therapy is too time and emotionally consuming and financially expensive to pursue. Therefore, when a fluent adult enters therapy, believe her when she says she stutters.

When adolescents and adults talk about their stuttering, be aware of the emotions that may be released (having a box of tissues handy is helpful).

> **Application Question**
>
> How important do you think having a strong background in counseling would be to becoming an excellent clinician?

> **Application Question**
>
> What do you like friends to do when you are crying? What would you want someone you did not know well to do if you are crying?

You may be the first person they have ever been open with about their problem, and that may open the floodgates. Most people are not comfortable with the tears of people they do not know well, and even experienced clinicians are not always certain just what to say or do. Flasher and Fogle (2012) provide suggestions on managing such delicate times.

A stuttering evaluation with an adult usually lasts an hour. During that time the clinician should have enough information to decide on the direction of therapy. Most adults are not particularly keen on long, protracted evaluations of every nuance of their stuttering (much less their receptive and expressive language abilities) before starting to work on their problem. Still, in a sense, all therapy involves continual evaluation of the client—and the therapy itself.

Treatment of Adolescents and Adults

Adolescents and adults do not enter therapy with a clean slate. That is, they have some preconceived notions about what will help and what will not. They (especially adults) have beliefs and often strong opinions about therapy based on their past experiences with it or what they have imagined. It is helpful to learn about their beliefs and opinions. Your therapy may reinforce what they think might help, or it may run counter to what they had imagined. The one certainty is that they will be asked to do things that they are uncomfortable doing and may resist doing. It is important for clinicians to appreciate that behind resistance is fear; often the fear of change.

If therapy is to be successful, change is required. People change in essentially three ways (Flasher & Fogle, 2012):

1. *Evolution*—A person slowly, sometimes almost imperceptibly, changes over time (e.g., normal maturation and growth, education, and rehabilitation).

2. *Revolution*—A significant event in a person's life changes the way she thinks, believes, or behaves (e.g., marriage, parenthood, loss of a loved one, or a stroke).

3. *Resolution*—A person decides that it is now time to change (e.g., going back to school, stopping drinking or taking drugs, or starting therapy or taking responsibility for improvements in therapy).

As clinicians, we know that the person's stuttering evolved over time and is, in a way, still evolving as the person develops new tricks and crutches to replace (or add to) the old ones that no longer help her be fluent. We also know that therapy is an *evolutionary* process and that it will take time for the stutterer to change old beliefs and attitudes and behaviors. We are aware that most stutterers are impatient with therapy. They want a *revolutionary* change: "I want to take care of this problem I've had all of my life in the next couple of months." As clinicians, we know that for the stutterer to improve she needs to have *resolve* (a *resolution*); she needs to stay with therapy even when she most wants to quit.

Brian

Brian was a fluent stutterer who had "successfully" hidden his stuttering from everyone, including his wife and employer. Brian was also a veteran police officer who preferred to work the night shift in the roughest, high-crime areas of a large city. He had done plenty of "take downs" and had "taken men out." During one therapy session, he told me about an experience he had just the night before. He was in hot pursuit on foot of an armed robber. He knew the robber could turn at any moment and shoot at him. Brian admitted that his greatest fear was not whether he might be shot by the man he was chasing but whether he would stutter badly at the moment he caught him. ■

Gregory (2003) describes four areas of emphasis in therapy for adolescents and adults who stutter. There is a sequence to therapy, but fairly soon the client will be working on the stuttering in all four areas during each therapy session.

1. *Developing insight into attitudes, thoughts, and feelings about stuttering.* Stutterers have strong feelings about their stuttering, and they have conjured and imagined how other people must think about stuttering and stutterers, although they most likely have never asked people what they think about stuttering. Part of therapy may involve a "reality check" in which the stutterer asks family, friends, and others their opinions about stuttering and stutterers. Most clients find that people do not think nearly as much or as negatively about stuttering and stutterers as what clients have imagined. In therapy, speech changes accompany attitude changes.

2. *Increasing awareness of muscular tension through the use of relaxation exercises.* Stutterers are aware that they have muscular tension, but for many of them the tension is so chronic that it becomes their "norm" and they hardly notice the tension in their face, throat, shoulders, chest, and back. Some stutterers who have been placed on **biofeedback** instruments have been able to see graphically displayed the sometimes extraordinary tension in some muscles. Stutterers often need to become aware of muscle tension in the large muscle groups before they can become aware of and modify the tension in their speech and facial muscles. Many stutterers do not know what normal muscle tension feels like, and it comforts them to begin their first perceptions of normalcy.

3. *Analyzing and modifying speech.* Early in therapy, audio and videotaping may be used to help the client hear and see what she does when she stutters. Stutterers often initially deny that certain

biofeedback

The process of becoming aware of various physiological functions of the body using instruments that provide information on the activity of muscles or systems being monitored, with the goal of being able to control or manipulate those muscles or systems voluntarily.

behaviors (tricks and crutches to help them be fluent) are part of their stuttering: "It's just the way I talk." These tricks and crutches are "avoidance" behaviors. But when they try to talk without using some of these behaviors, they discover that they become more disfluent. What the clinician knows, the stutterer has to learn. As therapy progresses, clients learn to modify their stuttering and overall speech production.

A speech modification technique that has been used by many clinicians is referred to as "voluntary stuttering" or "voluntary disfluency," in which the person is asked to do the very thing she does not want to do—stutter. The difference is that the person learns that she has a choice as to *when* she stutters, *how* she stutters, and *how long* she stutters—voluntarily (Gregory, 2003; Guitar, 2006; Sheehan, 1970; Van Riper, 1982). By using voluntary stuttering, the client is performing an "approach" behavior, which will decrease fear and tension. Stutterers learn that *monitoring* (paying attention to their speech) and *modifying* are continuous processes. Stuttering modifications need to be carried from the clinic room to the real world if they are going to be used in daily conversations.

4. *Building new speech skills.* Therapy does not focus only on stuttering but includes communication in general. We work with stutterers head to toe and even sometimes with their articulation and use of language. The more confidence stutterers can develop that they are good communicators, despite some disfluencies, the better they feel about themselves. Stutterers learn that they can say what they want and not resort to saying whatever is easiest at the moment (stutterers have eaten countless meals in restaurants that they did not want; stutterers often order what they can say easily rather than what they really want).

Clinicians need to have a clear organization in their therapy so that they know where they have come from, where they are, and where they are going with therapy. However, therapy is unscripted; it is not, "If she says that, I'll say this." Therapy requires moment-to-moment decision making about what is the best thing to say, when to say it, and how to say it. The ability to integrate all of your perceptions of the client at the moment and your knowledge and understanding of stuttering and the ability to "think on your feet" are essential in stuttering therapy.

Stuttering therapy is a marathon, not a sprint. To be most successful, stuttering therapy needs to be long-term. After a foundational period of therapy (usually 3 to 6 months), a follow-through program of 12 to 18 months is most beneficial. People who stutter need to realize that they will continue to experience challenging situations that will require time to process. Many concepts not well understood during therapy are clarified with further experience. Stutterers develop new insights into their feelings and behaviors, and therapy techniques they resisted earlier are used more effectively and more willingly.

A $40,000 Phone Call

A private client of mine who was in his late 20s was already success- ful farming orchard crops. John had avoided the telephone all of his life; he even had his wife make the initial phone call to set up the first appointment with me. After several weeks of therapy, John was increasingly working on overcoming his feared situations, especially those involving the telephone. At the beginning of one appointment, he smiled, shook my hand, and thanked me for helping him make $40,000 that week. He told me that for the first time he made a phone call to talk directly to one of his buyers and from that conversation landed an additional $40,000 contract that he had never expected to obtain. Beyond all of the emotional and psychological "costs" of stuttering, for many people their fears and avoidances can be finan- cially costly. ■

Success of Therapy

How successful therapy will be for a stutterer depends on many variables. If the therapy approach is well researched and understood, appropriate, and well presented by the clinician, the variables that determine suc- cess mostly depend on the individual stutterer. Many stutterers do not stay with therapy for the entire time that it takes to fully understand and integrate the principles and techniques they learn from their clinician. Many drift away or in and out of therapy, perhaps because they develop some level of comfort. For those who stay with therapy, are reasonably diligent in following the principles and techniques they learn, and do the exercises, there is a good chance they will have long-lasting benefits. Gregory, in his Adult Stuttering Program at Northwestern University and in his private practice, has found that approximately 8 out of 10 clients are pleased with the results of therapy and consider it successful. Success is defined as gaining sufficient confidence to be comfortable about communication, being able to speak easily in most situations, and having a program for continuing to work on speech goals.

EMOTIONAL AND SOCIAL EFFECTS OF STUTTERING

Clinicians who have considerable experience working with children and adults who stutter recognize that stuttering is a communication disorder that is fraught with emotional and social distress (which are different from emotional and social disorders) (Gregory, 2003; Guitar, 2006; Zebrowski, 2002). As a group, children and adults who stutter have a more sensitive temperament, which may be associated with more physical tension in laryngeal muscles (Guitar, 2006). Children and adults have anxiety about their stuttering, and stuttering causes anxiety (Iverach et al., 2011). They tend to have low self-esteem and excessive needs for social approval. Individuals who stutter often feel punished by their disfluency and avoid certain speaking situations (e.g., speaking up in class or speaking in meetings) and talking to certain people (particularly people they perceive as "authority figures"). One of the indications of strong emotional reactions to stuttering is habitual avoidance of speaking (Bloodstein & Berstein Ratner, 2008). Most stutterers have spent most of their lives trying to hide their stuttering from others and even from themselves—denying that it is a problem. Many people who stutter choose their daily social interactions based on how fluent they feel they will be when they start their day.

People who stutter may choose their occupations or professions based on their fluency, preferring jobs in which speaking is a minimal part of their work. Parents often wonder whether they may have caused or contributed to their child's stuttering problem, and frequently feel some guilt and embarrassment about their child's stuttering (Flasher & Fogle, 2012; Guitar, 2006; Zebrowski, 2002). However, in spite of the emotional toll their stuttering takes, many people who have been and are stutterers have had remarkably happy and successful lives.

CHARLES VAN RIPER (1905–1994)

Perhaps no single person has had a greater effect on the profession of speech-language pathology, and stuttering therapy in particular, than Charles Van Riper. In speech-language pathology, he was a legend in his own time. The first quarter-century of his life was plagued by profoundly severe stuttering (perhaps the most profoundly severe stuttering of any person known to the profession). His stuttering led him to become a pioneering founder of this new profession and widely recognized world authority on stuttering. Dr. Van Riper was a prodigious author, with more than 200 publications spanning seven decades. His *The Nature of Stuttering* (1982) and *The Treatment of Stuttering* (1973) are classics in the specialty.

Beyond his professional writing, he also was a poet. While an undergraduate at Northern Michigan College in an honors class with the resident poet, Robert Frost, the renowned Frost awarded Van Riper first prize for his poetry, which was later published. Van Riper earned his master's degree at the University of Michigan with a specialty in Old English literature and Elizabethan ballads. He earned his doctoral degree in clinical psychology at the University of Iowa. During his years at Iowa, he worked with Lee Edward Travis and others to help his stuttering, and it was there that he developed his theories of and therapy for stuttering. After leaving Iowa, he taught at Western Michigan University in Kalamazoo and remained there most of his professional career. As Van Riper once wrote, "The potential in any living thing is immense, but to release that potential someone has to intervene. . . . After a bum beginning, I've had a very rewarding life—love to see the human flowers bloom, and take no credit except for the weeding and fertilizing."

> **A Sun**
>
> For reasons that I do not know,
> I am a sun, a small, small sun
> Whose warmth helps others grow,
> Bear fruit and seed
> So other human suns
> May glow.
>
> —Charles Van Riper

CHAPTER SUMMARY

Stuttering typically comprises both verbal overt behaviors and visible overt behaviors. The covert, emotional, and social reactions of individuals who stutter can be some of the most serious challenges they face in therapy. The incidence of stuttering is generally considered to be 1% of the childhood population. The gender ratio is three or four males to one female stutterer. Stuttering tends to run in families. Physiologically, the only difference between stutterers and nonstutterers occurs just before and at the moment of stuttering. Stutterers are within the norms for intelligence. There do not appear to be any particular personality traits that are typical of individuals who stutter.

Throughout the working relationship with a family, the family systems model coupled with a cognitive therapy counseling model is helpful. Not all children who are disfluent need direct therapy, particularly those who are at risk for stuttering but are not yet stuttering. The function of the speech-language pathologist with such children is in the area of prevention. In direct therapy with children and adolescents, our general approach is to be understanding and accepting so that the child views us as someone who is genuinely interested in him and accepting of whatever he says and however he says it. Providing children with successful speaking activities and opportunities can be helpful. Fluency shaping and stuttering modification approaches are used with both children and adults.

Four areas of emphasis in therapy for adolescents and adults who stutter may include developing insight into attitudes, thoughts, and feelings about stuttering; increasing awareness of muscular tension through the use of relaxation exercises; analyzing and modifying speech; and building new speech skills. To be most successful, stuttering therapy needs to be long-term. Success is defined as gaining sufficient confidence to be comfortable about communication, being able to speak easily in most situations, and having a program for continuing to work on speech goals.

STUDY QUESTIONS
Knowledge and Comprehension

1. What are normal disfluencies?
2. What is family systems therapy and what does it emphasize?

3. Discuss what a clinician should be able to do after completion of a fluency evaluation.

4. What is primary prevention?

5. What might be a reasonable definition of success in therapy for adults who stutter?

Application

1. How could covert reactions contribute to a person's disfluency?

2. Explain why stuttering therapy is a dynamic process.

3. What are some helpful points for how parents should react when their child is disfluent?

4. Discuss the importance of the relationship a clinician develops with a child who is disfluent.

5. Why is interviewing an essential skill for clinicians to develop?

Analysis/Synthesis

1. Why are visible overt behaviors considered part of stuttering?

2. Why would no one theory fully explain the cause of stuttering in all children?

3. What are the similarities and differences between fluency shaping and stuttering modification approaches?

4. Why is the *affective* mode so important in understanding the variables that contribute to the therapeutic relationship?

5. Discuss the three essential ways people change and how these may be applied to stuttering therapy.

REFERENCES

American Speech-Language-Hearing Association. (1988, March). *Position statement: Prevention of communication disorders.* Washington, DC: ASHA.

Biermann-Ruben, K., Salmelin, R., & Schnitzler, A. (2005). Right rolandic activation during speech perception in stutterers: A MEG study. *NeuroImage, 25,* 793–801.

Blood, G. W., Ridenour, C., Qualls, C. D., & Hammer, C. S. (2004). Co-occurring disorders in children who stutter. *Journal of Communication Disorders, 36,* 427–488.

Bloodstein, O., & Berstein Ratner, N. (2008). *Handbook on stuttering* (6th ed.). Clifton Park, NY: Delmar Cengage Learning.

Bobrick, B. (1995). *Knotted tongues: Stuttering in history and the quest for a cure.* New York, NY: Kodansha International.

Botterill, W., & Fry, J. (2005). Stuttering research and treatment around the world: United Kingdom. *ASHA Leader, 9,* 41.

Buck, S. M., Lees, R., & Cook, F. (2002). The influence of family history of stuttering on the onset of stuttering in young children. *Folia Phoniatrica, 54,* 117–124.

Chmela, K. A., & Reardon, N. (2005). *The school-age child who stutters: Working effectively with attitudes and emotions: A workbook.* Memphis, TN: Stuttering Foundation of America.

Conture, E. G. (2001). *Stuttering: Its nature, diagnosis, and treatment.* Boston, MA: Allyn and Bacon.

Curlee, R. F. (2007). Does my child stutter? In *Stuttering and your child: Questions and answers,* Publication no. 0022. Memphis, TN: Stuttering Foundation of America.

Daly, D. A. (1992). Helping the clutterer: Therapy considerations. In F. L. Meyers & K. O. St. Louis (Eds.), *Cluttering: A clinical perspective.* Kibworth, England: Far Communications.

Daly, D. A., & Cantrelle, R. P. (2006). *Cluttering: Characteristics identified as diagnostically significant by 60 fluency experts.* Paper presented at the 5th International Fluency Association World Congress on Disorders of Fluency, Dublin, Ireland.

De Keyser, J. (1973). The stuttering of Lewis Carroll. In Y. Lebrun & T. Hoops (Eds.), *Neurolinguistic approaches to stuttering.* The Hague: Mouton.

DeNil, L. (2004). Recent developments in brain imaging research in stuttering. In B. Maassen, R. D. Kent, H. F. Petters, P. H. van Lieshout, & W. Hulstijn (Eds.), *Speech motor control in normal and disordered speech.* Oxford: Oxford University Press.

Ezrati-Vinacour, R., & Amir, O. (2005). Stuttering research and treatment around the world: Israel. *ASHA Leader, 9,* 8–9.

Flasher, L. V., & Fogle, P. T. (2012). *Counseling skills for speech-language pathologists and audiologists* (2nd ed.). Clifton Park, NY: Delmar Cengage Learning.

Goldman, R. (1967). Cultural influences on the sex ratio in the incidence of stuttering. *American Anthropologist, 69,* 78–81.

Gregory, H. H. (2003). *Stuttering therapy: Rationale and procedures.* Boston, MA: Allyn and Bacon.

Guitar, B. (2006). *Stuttering: An integrated approach to its nature and treatment* Baltimore, MD: Lippincott Williams & Wilkins.

Hill, D. G. (2003). Differential treatment of stuttering in the early stages of development. In H. H. Gregory, *Stuttering therapy: Rationale and procedures.* Boston, MA: Allyn and Bacon.

Ingham, R. (2001). Brain imaging and studies of developmental stuttering. *Journal of Communication Disorders, 34,* 493–516.

Iverach, L., Menzies, R. G., O'Brian, S., Packman, A., & Onslow, M. (2011). Anxiety and stuttering: Continuing to explore a complex relationship. *American Journal of Speech-Language Pathology, 20,* 221–232.

Kenjo, M. (2005). Stuttering research and treatment around the world: Japan. *ASHA Leader, 9*, 36.

Limongi, F. P. (2005). Stuttering research and treatment around the world: Brazil. *ASHA Leader, 9*, 6.

Lundstrom, C., & Garsten, M. (2005). Stuttering research and treatment around the world: Sweden. *ASHA Leader, 9*, 36–37.

Manning, W. H. (2010). *Clinical decision making in fluency disorders* (3rd ed.). Clifton Park, NY: Delmar Cengage Learning.

Maul, C. A. (2011). *Family-centered service delivery: Is there an evidence base*? CSHA Magazine, 41(1), 8–9.

Nelson, L. A. (1999). How does our home life influence his stuttering? In *Stuttering and your child: Questions and answers*. Memphis, TN: Stuttering Foundation of America.

Ntourou, K., Conture, E. G., & Lipsey, M. W. (2011). Language abilities of children who stutter: A meta-analytical review. *American Journal of Speech-Language Pathology, 20*, 163–179.

Paden, E. (2005). Development of phonological ability. In E. Yairi & N. Ambrose (Eds.). *Early childhood stuttering: For clinicians by clinicians*. Austin, TX: Pro-Ed.

Proctor, A., Yairi, E., Duff, M. C., & Zhang, J. (2008). Prevalence of stuttering in African American preschoolers. *Journal of Speech, Language, and Hearing Research, 51*(6), 1465–1479.

Ramig, P. R. (1997). Various paths to long-term recovery from stuttering. Paper presented at 2nd World Congress on Fluency Disorders, San Francisco, CA.

Ramig, P. R., & Dodge, D. M. (2010). *The child and adolescent stuttering treatment and activity resource guide* (2nd ed.). Clifton Park, NY: Delmar Cengage Learning.

Reardon-Reeves, N. A., & Yaruss, J. S. (2004). *The source for stuttering: Ages 7-18*. East Moline, IL: LinguiSystems.

Robinson, T. L., & Crowe, T. A. (2002). Fluency disorders. In D. E. Battle (Ed.), *Communication disorders in multicultural populations* (3rd ed.). Boston, MA: Butterworth-Heinemann.

Sheehan, J. G. (1970). *Stuttering: Research and therapy*. New York, NY: Harper & Row.

Silverman, F. H. (2004). *Stuttering and other fluency disorders*. Long Grove, IL: Waveland Press.

St. Louis, K. O., Raphael, L. J., Myers, F. L., & Bakker, K. (2003). Cluttering updated. *ASHA Leader, 18,* 4–5, 20–21.

Stuttering Foundation of America. (2002a) *Stuttering and your child: Questions and answers*. Memphis, TN: Stuttering Foundation of America.

Stuttering Foundation of America. (2002b). *Stuttering and the preschool child: Help for families*. Memphis, TX: Stuttering Foundation of America.

Stuttering Foundation of America. (2002c). *Stuttering: Straight talk to teachers*. Memphis, TN: Stuttering Foundation of America.

Stuttering Foundation of America. (2002d). *Foudacion Americana de la tartanudez*. Memphis, TN: Stuttering Foundation of America.

Subramanian, U., & Prabhu, B. (2005). Stuttering research and treatment around the world: India. *ASHA Leader, 9,* 7–8.

Tillis, M., & Wager, W. (1984). *Stutterin' boy*. New York, NY: Rawson Associates.

Travis, L. E. (1931). Diagnosis and treatment of stuttering cases. *Proceedings of the American Speech Correction Association, 1,* 121–127.

Van Riper, C. (1939). *Speech correction, principles and methods*. New York, NY: Prentice-Hall.

Van Riper, C. (1971). *The nature of stuttering*. Englewood Cliffs, NJ: Prentice Hall.

Van Riper, C. (1982). *The nature of stuttering* (2nd ed.). Englewood Cliffs, NJ: Prentice Hall.

Ward, D. (2006). *Stuttering and cluttering: Framework for understanding and treatment*. East Sussex, England: Psychology Press.

Watson, J., & Kayser, H. (1994). Assessment of bilingual/bicultural children and adults who stutter. *Seminars in Speech and Language, 15,* 149–164.

West, R. (1942). The pathology of stuttering. *The Nervous Child, 2*(2), 96–106.

Williams, D. E. (1979). A perspective on approaches to stuttering therapy. In H. Gregory (Ed.), *Controversies about stuttering therapy*. Baltimore, MD: University Park Press.

Williams, D. E. (2004). *The genius of Dean Williams* (compiled by the Stuttering Foundation of America). Memphis, TN: Stuttering Foundation of America.

World Health Organization. (1977). *Manual of the international statistical classification of diseases, injuries, and causes of death* (Vol. 1). Geneva: World Health Organization.

Yairi, E., & Ambrose, N. (2005). *Early Childhood Stuttering*. Austin, TX: Pro-Ed.

Yang, E. (2005). Stuttering research and treatment around the world: Taiwan. *ASHA Leader, 9,* 37–38.

Yu, B., & Kashinath, S. (2011). *Family-centered care and other labors of love: Culturally competent service delivery for young children and their families*. CSHA Magazine, 41(1), 12–13.

Zebrowski, P. M. (2002). Counseling: An approach for speech-language pathologists. *Contemporary Issues in Communication Sciences and Disorders, 29,* 91–100.

Zebrowski, P. M., & Kelly, E. M. (2002). *Manual of stuttering intervention*. Clifton Park, NY: Delmar Cengage Learning.

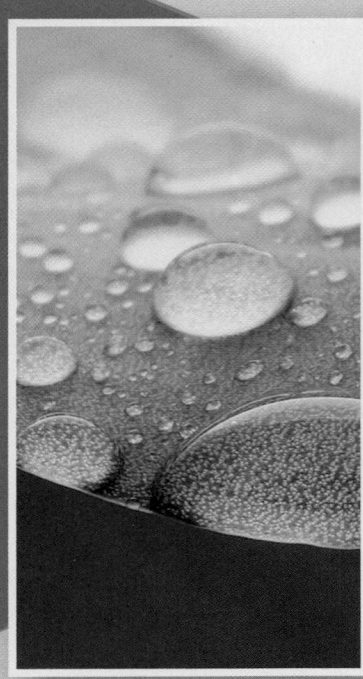

CHAPTER 9
Voice Disorders in Children and Adults

LEARNING OBJECTIVES

After studying this chapter, you will:

- Be able to describe the major voice disorders.
- Be able to discuss the evaluation of voice disorders by the otolaryngologist and speech-language pathologist.
- Be familiar with two of the foundational voice therapy approaches.
- Be able to discuss voice therapy for patients who have had laryngectomy surgery.
- Be aware of the emotional and social effects of voice disorders on clients.

KEY TERMS

acute
acute laryngitis/
    traumatic laryngitis
breathiness
cancer (carcinoma)
chronic
chronic laryngitis
contact ulcer
conversion reaction
    (disorder)
diplophonia
direct laryngoscopy
dystonia
edema
electrolarynx/
    artificial larynx

endoscopy
esophageal speech
facilitating techniques
functional aphonia
functional
    dysphonia
hard glottal attack
harshness
hoarseness
holistic
hyperadduction
hyperfunction
hypoadduction
hypofunction
indirect
    laryngoscopy

intubation
laryngectomy
laryngitis
laryngopharyngeal
    reflux (LPR)
lesion
malignant
muscle tension
    dysphonia (MTD)
mutational falsetto
    (puberphonia)
otolaryngologist/
    otorhino-
    laryngologist
    (ear, nose, and
    throat [ENT]
    doctor)

KEY TERMS continued

papilloma
  (papillomatosis)

phonotrauma

polypoid thickening
  (degeneration)

referred pain

spasmodic
  dysphonia (SD)

stoma

tracheoesophageal
  prosthesis
  (TEP)

vocal abuse

vocal fold paralysis

vocal hygiene

vocal misuse

vocal nodule

vocal polyp

voice disorder
  (dysphonia)

CHAPTER OUTLINE

Introduction
Classification of Voice Disorders
Voice Disorders Related to Functional Etiologies
    and Faulty Usage
    Laryngitis
    Vocal Nodules
    Vocal Polyps
    Contact Ulcer
    Functional Dysphonia
    Functional Aphonia
    Mutational Falsetto/Puberphonia
Voice Disorders Related to Organic Etiologies
    Papillomas
    Blunt, Penetrating, and Inhalation Traumas
    Cancer/Carcinoma
Voice Disorders Related to Neurological Etiologies
    Hypoadduction Vocal Fold Problems
    Hyperadduction Vocal Fold Problems
Multicultural Considerations
Assessment of the Voice
    The Otolaryngologist's Examination
    The Speech-Language Pathologist's Assessment
Voice Therapy
    Voice Therapy Approaches
    Laryngectomy
Emotional and Social Effects of Voice Disorders
    Young Children
    Adolescents
    Adults
Chapter Summary
Study Questions
References

**voice disorder
(dysphonia)**

Any deviation of loudness, pitch, or quality that is outside the normal range of a person's age, gender, or geographic or cultural background that interferes with communication, draws unfavorable attention to itself, or adversely affects the speaker or listener.

INTRODUCTION

Voice disorders (dysphonias) have been recognized for more than 3,500 years. The Edwin Smith Papyrus from an ancient Egyptian burial tomb, dated about 1600 B.C., described in some detail a crushing injury to the neck, which caused the loss of speech. The Egyptian writings contained a hieroglyph portraying the lungs and trachea, although the larynx was not pictured because no organ for voice had yet been identified (Fink, 1975). To treat recognized voice disorders, different cultures used treatments such as gargles derived from fruit juices, cabbage, garlic, the juice of crabs, centipedes, owl's brain, and the urine of sacred cows. Other remedies included wearing beads of various kinds or a black silk cord around the throat (Stevenson & Guthrie, 1949; Wright, 1941). In more modern times, before speech-language pathologists began working with voice disorders, singing teachers, phoneticians (recall Henry Higgins [Rex Harrison] working with Eliza Doolittle [Audrey Hepburn] in the movie *My Fair Lady*), and voice and diction teachers worked with trained and untrained singers and other individuals with voice problems (Curry, 1940). Since that time, speech-language pathologists have become the professionals who work with disorders of the speaking voice.

The voice has long been considered a mirror of the person—the inner self. The voice is a reflection of an individual's personality and is a sensitive indicator of emotions, attitudes, and the roles we play. People can recognize the typical voice of intense, hard-driving people and the nasal, singsong voice of the constant whiner. We detect a depressed or withdrawn person's monotone, deenergized voice and we know the voice of the outgoing, charismatic, happy person. A soft, soothing voice tends to calm an agitated person, and a tense, strident voice tends to be discomforting (Andrews, 2006; Boone, McFarlane, & Von Berg, 2009; Colton, Casper, & Leonard, 2011).

The loudness, pitch, and quality of voice are influenced by multiple factors involving the anatomy and physiology of the respiratory system, the vocal folds, and the *supraglottal vocal tract's* (above the vocal folds) tuning characteristics (Scherer, 2006; Stemple, Glaze, & Klaben, 2009; Titze, 2000). A variety of terms are used to subjectively describe the quality of dysphonia, such as *hoarse, breathy, harsh, husky, raucous, grating, strident, thin, strained, tense, weak, tremulous,* and *monotone.* The subjective term *hoarse* is the most commonly used by professionals who work with voice disorders.

TABLE 9–1	Voice Disorders Speech-Language Pathologists Work With	
FUNCTIONAL	**NEUROLOGICAL**	**ORGANIC**
Diplophonia	Ataxic dysarthria	Cancer
Falsetto	Essential tremor	Congenital abnormalities
Functional aphonia	Guillain-Barré syndrome	Contact ulcers
Functional dysphonia	Hyperkinetic (spasmodic dysphonia, essential tremor)	Endocrine changes
Muscle tension dysphonia	Hypokinetic (Parkinson's disease)	Granuloma
Nodules	Lower motor neuron (LMN)	Hemangioma
Phonation breaks	Mixed (amyotrophic lateral sclerosis, TBI, multiple sclerosis)	Hyperkeratosis
Pitch breaks	Myasthenia gravis	Infectious laryngitis
Polyps	Resonance disturbance	Laryngectomy
Reinke's edema	Spasmodic dysphonia	Leukoplakia
Traumatic laryngitis	Spastic dysarthria	Papilloma
Ventricular dysphonia	Sulcus vocalis	Pubertal changes
Vocal cord thickening	Unilateral dysarthria	Reflux
Vocal fold paralysis	Upper motor neuron (UMN)	Webbing

Adapted from Boone, McFarlane, and Von Berg, 2009.

CLASSIFICATION OF VOICE DISORDERS

Boone, McFarlane, and Von Berg (2009) use a three-way classification of voice disorders: functional, neurological, and organic (see Table 9–1). *Functional voice disorders* usually are considered to be caused by faulty use of a normal vocal mechanism. *Neurological voice disorders* are related to muscle tone and control of the muscles used for respiration and phonation. *Organic voice disorders* are related to some physical abnormality in the larynx. However, many voice disorders also include an emotional or psychological component. Two other important classifications are vocal **hyperfunction** and vocal **hypofunction**. Hyperfunction describes a pervasive pattern of excessive effort and tension that affects many different structures and muscles in the phonatory system, as well in some cases in the respiratory, resonatory, and articulatory systems (Andrews, 2006). Signs of hyperfunction include a tense sounding voice and **hard glottal attacks**. Hypofunction describes inadequate muscle

hyperfunction

A pervasive pattern of excessive effort and tension that affects many different structures and muscles in the phonatory system and, in some cases, the respiratory, resonatory, and articulatory systems; signs of hyperfunction include a tense sounding voice and hard glottal attacks.

hypofunction

Inadequate muscle tone in the laryngeal mechanism and associated structures, including the muscles of respiration; signs of hypofunction include breathiness because of inadequate closure of the vocal folds, weak vocal power that can affect speech intelligibility, and reduced vocal endurance.

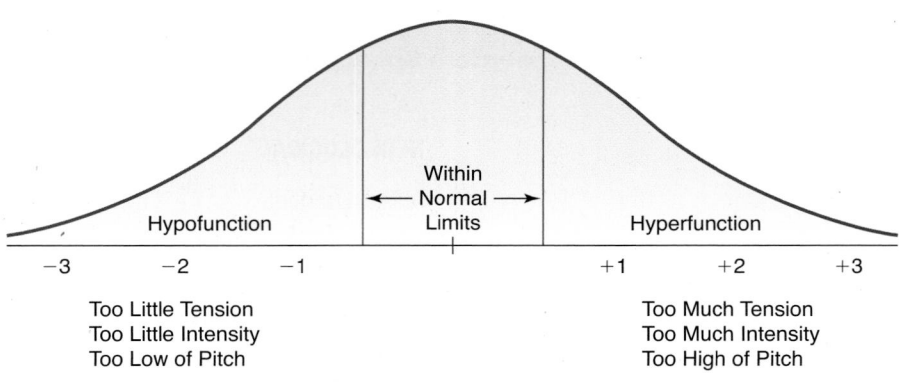

Figure 9-1

Bell-shaped curve with examples of hyperfunctional and hypofunctional voice problems.

© Cengage Learning 2013.

hard glottal attack

Forceful *approximation* (closing) of the vocal folds during the initiation of phonation.

vocal nodule

A *benign* (nonmalignant or not cancerous) vocal fold growth that tends to be *bilateral* (both sides, i.e., both vocal folds) and occurs at the same location as vocal polyps (i.e., juncture of the anterior 1/3 and middle 1/3 of the vocal folds), caused by continuous vocal fold hyperfunction (abuse and misuse).

phonotrauma

Deleterious acute or chronic vocal behaviors, such as excessive yelling, screaming, cheering, coughing, throat clearing, inappropriate pitch or loudness, singing beyond the range of the vocal mechanism, hard glottal attacks, inadequate respiratory support, talking loudly over noise, poor hydration, and smoking that are damaging to the vocal folds and the laryngeal and pharyngeal muscles and tissues.

tone in the laryngeal mechanism and associated structures, including the muscles of respiration. Signs of hypofunction include breathiness because of inadequate closure of the vocal folds, weak vocal power that can affect speech intelligibility, and reduced vocal endurance (Andrews, 2006). Some voice disorders (e.g., **vocal nodules**) may be caused by hyperfunctional vocal activity (e.g., **phonotrauma**) and result in a hypofunctional (e.g., breathy, weak) voice.

It may be helpful to visualize a bell-shaped curve, where hyperfunction refers to excess tension or forcing in the laryngeal region (i.e., +1, +2, or +3) and hypofunction refers to decreased or inadequate tension or reduced vocal capacity (i.e., –1, –2, or –3) (see Figure 9-1). The two concepts can be extended to hyperfunction referring to too much intensity, too high of a pitch, too much talking, too much **vocal abuse** and **misuse**, and so on. Hypofunction can refer to too low of intensity, too low of a pitch, too little vocal fold vibration, and so on. For a person diagnosed with a hyperfunctional voice disorder, the general therapeutic goal is to teach and train the person to use more hypofunctional behaviors to bring the voice closer to normal limits. When someone has a hypofunctional voice disorder, the goal is to teach and train the person to use more hyperfunctional behaviors to bring the voice closer to normal limits.

Many cases of voice disorders have both functional and organic components that may be causing and maintaining the disorder. For example, individuals with vocal nodules may have originally caused the voice problem (e.g., **hoarseness**) from either **acute** or **chronic** phonotrauma (also referred to by some authorities as *vocal abuse* and *misuse* [Boone et al., 2009; Colton et al., 2011]), such as excessive yelling, screaming, cheering, coughing, throat clearing, chronic loudness, use of the wrong pitch, and hard glottal attacks. Smoking is also considered to cause phonotrauma. These could be considered "functional" behaviors that may lead to an "organic" disorder—the vocal nodules (Andrews, 2006; Boone et al., 2009; Colton et al., 2011). Individuals with neurologically based voice disorders also may have organic and functional components to their voice problems.

VOICE DISORDERS RELATED TO FUNCTIONAL ETIOLOGIES AND FAULTY USAGE

The concepts of hyperfunction and hypofunction, as discussed previously, are important to understanding the various voice disorders that are related to functional etiologies and faulty usage. Many of these disorders have a hyperfunctional component (e.g., tension) that can include a hypofunctional component (e.g., breathiness).

Laryngitis

Laryngitis is a general term that refers to an acute or chronic voice disorder that may have a variety of etiologies, such as phonotrauma or bacterial or viral infections of the larynx. The term *laryngitis* is used to describe an inflammation of the vocal fold mucosa that causes mild to severe dysphonia with lowered pitch and *intermittent phonation breaks* (the voice cuts in and out randomly). Laryngitis is one of the most common hyperfunctional laryngeal problems that results in a voice disorder. The vocal quality that is typically heard in laryngitis is hoarseness, that is, a combination of **harshness** and **breathiness** (Stemple et al., 2009; Swigert, 2005).

Acute Laryngitis/Traumatic Laryngitis

Acute laryngitis (traumatic laryngitis) is often caused by yelling, screaming, and cheering (e.g., at sports events). When in large, noisy crowds, people try to talk over the noise and cheer loud enough so others can hear them (drinking alcohol also decreases inhibitions and awareness of irritation and pain). Many people, after they start to lose their voice, will try to yell or cheer harder to make up for their decreased loudness and vocal control, thereby traumatizing their vocal folds even more and causing **edema** (see Figure 9–2; compare to Figures 3–5 and 3–6). Acute laryngitis also may be caused by bacterial or viral infections that result in *membranous laryngitis*.

Chronic Laryngitis

Chronic laryngitis is laryngitis that lasts more than 10 days and may be caused by a variety of behaviors; for example, (1) acute laryngitis where the vocal folds were not allowed to return to their normal healthy condition because of continued vocal abuses and misuse behaviors; (2) allergies and chemical irritants (including **laryngopharyngeal reflux [LPR]**) that may result in irritation and chronic coughing (Boone et al., 2009; Rees & Belafsky, 2008); (3) singing excessively at damaging intensity levels and in vocal registers outside of a singer's normal range (rock singers sometimes have severely dysphonic voices that become part of their singing style); and (4) smoking, which has numerous effects on the larynx and lungs, such as drying and irritating the vocal folds and irritation of the lungs, both of which can cause chronic coughing and

---

vocal misuse

Deleterious chronic vocal behaviors that may have a cumulative effects on the structure and functioning of the laryngeal mechanism, such as chronic inappropriate loudness or pitch, singing beyond the range of the vocal mechanism, frequent hard glottal attacks, and speaking with inadequate respiratory support.

hoarseness

A common dysphonia that is a combination of breathiness and harshness that may affect loudness (usually decreased loudness or a monoloudness), pitch (usually a low pitch with reduced pitch range), and quality (usually decreased "pleasantness" of the sound of the voice).

acute

Intense and of short duration, usually referring to a disease or injury.

chronic

Of long duration with slow progress, usually in reference to a disease or disorder.

laryngitis

An acute or chronic inflammation of the mucous membranes of the larynx that often results in hoarseness or loss of voice.

harshness

A "rough" sounding vocal quality resulting from a combination of hard glottal attacks, low pitch, and high intensity caused by *overadduction* (hyperfunction) of the vocal folds.

breathiness

Incomplete closure of the vocal folds during phonation that results in excessive unvibrated air escaping.

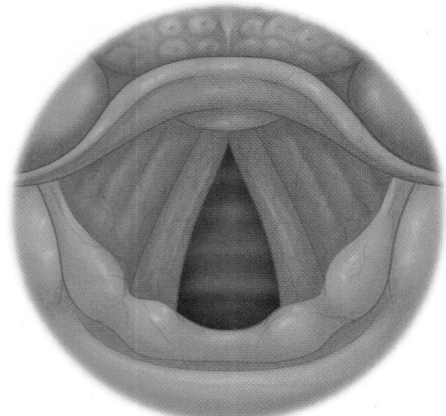

Acute Laryngitis

Figure 9–2

Acute traumatic laryngitis; compare to Figures 3–5 and 3–6.

© Cengage Learning 2013.

acute laryngitis/ traumatic laryngitis

An abrupt, intense, and usually relatively brief inflammation of the mucous membrane lining in the larynx, accompanied by edema of the vocal folds with hoarseness and loss of voice that is often caused by severe vocal abuse.

edema

Accumulation of excessive fluid in tissue that is associated with inflammatory conditions and results in swelling of the tissue.

chronic laryngitis

A persistent laryngitis lasting more than 10 days with inflammation of the mucous membrane lining in the larynx, accompanied by edema of the vocal folds with hoarseness and loss of voice that is often caused by heavy smoking, coughing, allergies and chemical irritants, and ongoing vocal abuse and misuse.

vocal fold trauma (not to mention the potential for laryngeal cancer, lung cancer, or both). It is standard practice that anyone with chronic dysphonia in the absence of a throat infection or *upper respiratory infection* (common cold) needs to undergo a laryngeal examination by an **otolaryngologist** to determine the possible cause or causes of the problem and to rule out serious laryngeal disease (e.g., cancer).

Vocal Nodules

Vocal nodules are the most common benign **lesions** of the vocal folds in both children and adults (Sataloff, 2005). They have been referred to as "cheerleaders' nodes," "screamers' nodes," and "singers' nodes" in reference to the individuals who sometimes develop them. They are a vocal hyperfunction problem caused by continuous abuse and misuse of the voice. Common causes of vocal nodules are yelling and screaming, hard glottal attacks, singing in an abusive manner, frequent speaking in noisy environments, coughing, and excessive throat clearing. Nodules are usually bilateral, but may be *unilateral* (one side).

In the early stage of development, nodular masses are soft and pliable; however, with continuous abuse and misuse of the vocal mechanism, the masses may become larger, harder, and more fibrous. Upon direct visual examination of the vocal folds, nodules generally look like whitish *protuberances* (bumps) on the edges of the vocal folds, typically at the juncture of the anterior one-third and middle one-third of the folds (Boone et al., 2009) (see Figure 9–3). Nodules occur at this location because this is the point on the vocal folds where there is the greatest impact during phonation. As miniscule as the difference may be in terms of pressure on that point compared to any other location on the vocal folds during vibration, if we consider the average number of times the vocal folds vibrate per second (in adult males approximately 120 Hz and in females approximately 225 Hz), we can see that over time the vocal folds may adduct millions of times over months and years.

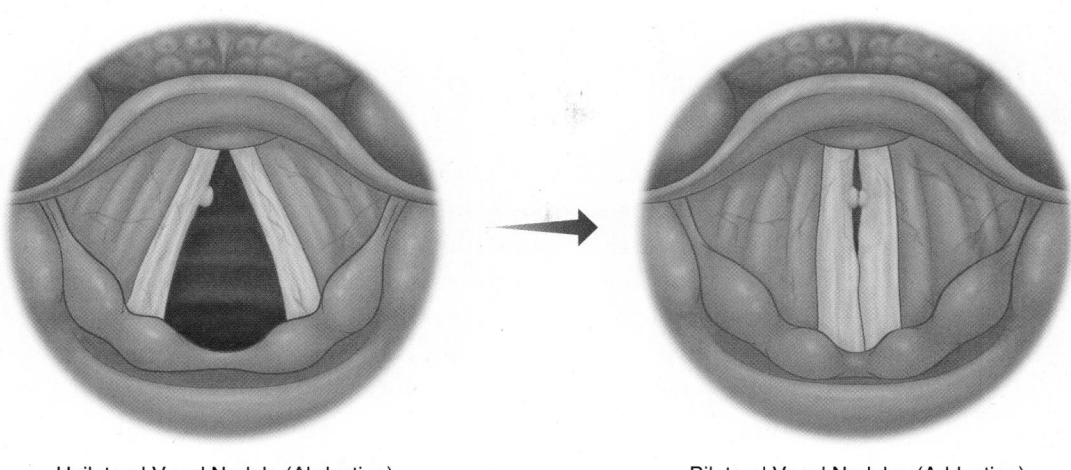

Unilateral Vocal Nodule (Abduction)   Bilateral Vocal Nodules (Adduction)

Figure 9–3

Vocal nodules.

© Cengage Learning 2013.

Individuals with vocal nodules have a hoarse voice quality caused by the nodules preventing the vocal folds from completely adducting. The nodules allow excessive air to escape during phonation, resulting in a breathy quality. The harshness is the result of the extra mass on the vocal folds causing *aperiodicity* (irregular vocal fold vibration). The added mass of tissue (as minute as it is) also can cause the pitch to lower slightly compared to what is optimal for a person (Andrews, 2006; Swigert, 2005).

Evaluation of individuals with vocal nodules involves a detailed case history; perceptual judgments of the loudness, pitch, and quality of the voice; and instrumental evaluations. Voice therapy for vocal nodules is a behavioral, symptomatic approach, often following a four-step program: (1) identifying abuses and misuses of the voice; (2) reducing the occurrence of the abuses and misuses; (3) searching with the patient for various voice therapy facilitating approaches that seem to produce an easy, optimal vocal production; and (4) using the **facilitating techniques** that work best as a practice method (Boone et al., 2009; Stemple et al., 2009). Voice therapy with an SLP is usually needed for at least 6 to 8 weeks. For many children and adults, there is a need for strong psychological and counseling support by the SLP (Andrews, 2006). With appropriate symptomatic behavioral therapy and counseling, surgical removal of vocal nodules is generally not needed.

Vocal Polyps

Vocal polyps are benign vocal fold lesions that tend to be unilateral and typically occur at the same location as vocal nodules; that is, the juncture of the anterior one-third and middle one-third of the vocal folds.

laryngopharyngeal reflux (LPR)

Gastric reflux (stomach acids causing heartburn) that flows through the esophagus, past the upper esophageal valve, and into the larynx or pharynx; reflux may spill over onto the vocal folds and irritate them, causing coughing and inflammation.

otolaryngologist/ otorhinolaryngologist (ear, nose, and throat [ENT] doctor)

A medical doctor who specializes in diseases of the ears, nose, and throat; often referred to as an "ear, nose, and throat" (ENT) doctor.

lesion

A wound, injury, or area of pathological change in tissue.

facilitating techniques

The selected therapy exercises that help to achieve a "target" or a more optimal vocal response by the patient.

Beverly was a 45-year-old woman who was referred to me by an otolaryngologist for voice therapy to help with her vocal nodules. Beverly had been an elementary school teacher for 20 years. She loved teaching and loved the children. She was a single mother struggling financially to support 14- and 17-year-old daughters. She was active in her church and sang in the choir. She was, in many ways, typical of many adults with vocal nodules: she had a job that required excessive use of her voice, sometimes with vocal abuses such as yelling to children on the playground; she had a variety of stresses in her life, from financial pressures to trying to raise teen-age children; and she tried to reach the extremes of her vocal range during choir practice, choir performances, and singing around the house. She had little time to take care of herself and relax and she felt guilty when she tried to do something for herself. She was both intense and tense.

Besides symptomatic voice therapy and **vocal hygiene** education, I used considerable counseling skills to help Beverly learn to take better care of herself. She eventually began to appreciate that if she "used herself up and burned herself out" she would not be able to continue teaching or singing and she may have difficulty using her voice when trying to talk with her family and friends and on the job. As she learned to balance her life better and manage her stresses better, some of her generalized tension—as well as the tension in her larynx—began to diminish. Voice therapy helped prevent Beverly from requiring surgery to remove the vocal nodules. ■

vocal hygiene

Behaviors that are helpful to achieve and maintain a healthy vocal mechanism and prevent or decrease vocal pathologies, such as eliminating phonotrauma, speaking in an appropriate pitch, turning the television or radio down while talking, using amplification when speaking to an audience in a large room, and singing within the optimal pitch range.

vocal polyp

A benign vocal fold growth that may take various forms and is caused by vocal abuse and misuse and results in vocal hoarseness.

polypoid thickening (degeneration)

A condition in which a vocal fold becomes edematous, flabby, and almost jelly-like as the result of vocal hyperfunction, making the voice chronically low pitched and hoarse.

Polyps may take various forms and are caused by vocal hyperfunction (abuse and misuse). For otolaryngologists, the observable distinctions and *histological* (microscopic study of tissue) differences are not always clear between vocal nodules and vocal polyps, and occasionally one may be mistaken for the other (Colton et al., 2011; Sataloff, 2005).

Polyps may be *pedunculated* (attached to the vocal fold only by a slim stalk of tissue), *sessile* (a broad-based mass adhering to the mucosa of the vocal fold) (see Figure 9–4), or *hemorrhagic* (appearance of a blood blister). Vocal polyps are often precipitated by a single hyperfunctional vocal episode, much like what causes acute laryngitis. The hyperfunctional vocal episode may cause a small capillary to hemorrhage (*intracordal hemorrhage*) in the membranous covering of a vocal fold. A polyp may form out of the hemorrhagic irritation by adding mass that is filled with blood. Further vocal abuse or misuse will cause increased irritation that results in the formation of **polypoid thickening (degeneration)**. If the growth is diffuse, it may cover half to two-thirds of the length of a

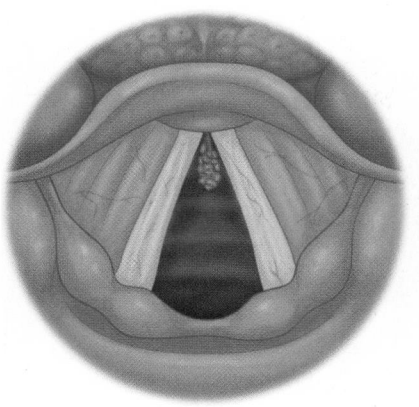

Pedunculated Polyp
at Anterior Commissure

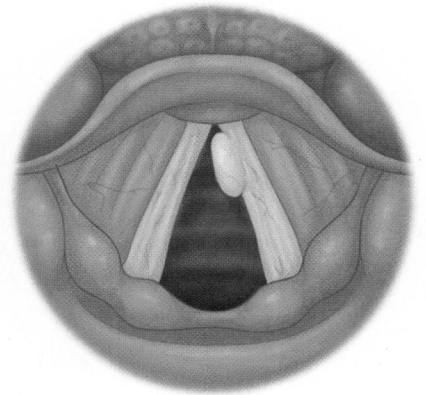

Sessile Polyp

Figure 9–4

Pedunculated and sessile vocal polyps.

© Cengage Learning 2013.

vocal fold (Case, 2002). The polyp, like a vocal nodule, interferes with vocal fold vibration, causing breathiness and harshness and results in a severe hoarse voice quality (Zhang & Jiang, 2004).

The evaluation and therapy for vocal polyps is much the same as it is for vocal nodules. To avoid surgery as the initial management of a vocal polyp, the "sandwich approach" may be used by some otolaryngologists. That is, voice therapy from an SLP to eliminate the kinds of vocal behaviors that cause a vocal polyp, and then surgery only if necessary. If surgery is still needed to remove the vocal polyp, the patient will likely benefit from follow-up voice therapy to reinforce the vocal hygiene techniques that were taught before the surgery (Andrews, 2006; Colton et al., 2011; Stemple et al., 2009).

Contact Ulcer

A **contact ulcer** is a small ulceration that develops in the posterior region on the *medial surface* of a vocal fold (i.e., the edge of one vocal fold that makes contact with the edge of the other vocal fold) (see Figure 9–5). They are usually caused by hyperfunctional use of the voice with persistent and excessive slamming together of the arytenoid cartilages during production of a chronic low-pitched voice in conjunction with hard glottal attacks and other vocal fold abuses and misuses. Contact ulcers tend to occur in hard-driving males who frequently experience gastroesophageal reflux (GERD) that spills over onto the vocal folds causing irritation, coughing, and frequent throat clearing. They may have pain in the laryngeal region that radiates out to one ear (**referred pain**) (Andrews, 2006; Colton et al., 2011; Rubin & Sataloff, 2006).

Surgical removal of contact ulcers is usually not needed; however, medical management of the gastric reflux is essential. These individuals often respond well to voice therapy, where elimination of vocal

contact ulcer

A benign vocal fold ulceration at the juncture of the middle one-third and posterior one-third of a fold that is caused by persistent and excessive vocal hyperfunction that is most commonly seen in adult males.

referred pain

Pain felt at a site different from that of an injured or diseased organ or part of the body, e.g., *angina*, the pain of coronary artery insufficiency, may be felt in the left shoulder, arm, or mandible.

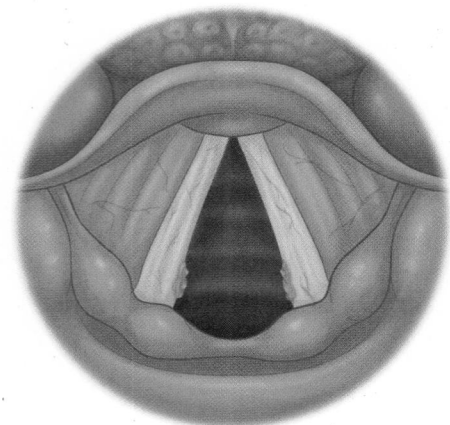

Contact Ulcers

Figure 9–5

Contact ulcers.

© Cengage Learning 2013.

---

functional dysphonia

A voice disorder that may be either hyperfunctional or hypofunctional and has no organic, physical, or neurological cause but is heard in patients with extreme tension in both the laryngeal and the supralaryngeal regions; the voice may have hypofunctional qualities such as low-pitch and breathy or hyperfunctional qualities such as high-pitch, strident, or hoarse.

---

abuses and misuses (including using an abnormally low-pitched voice) and learning how to initiate the voice gently without hard glottal attacks. Teaching voice conservation techniques is also essential (Ferrand, 2012).

Functional Dysphonia

Functional dysphonia may be the diagnosis when an otolaryngologist has determined that there is no organic, physical, or neurological cause for a voice disorder. Patients with functional dysphonia may have severely disturbed voices with a range of vocal symptoms, from hypofunctional vocal folds that produce a low-pitched, breathy voice to hyperfunctional vocal folds that produce a high-pitched, tense, strident, harsh, or hoarse vocal quality. Functional dysphonia is the result of extreme tension in both the laryngeal and the *supralaryngeal* (vocal tract above the larynx) regions. There is no medical or surgical treatment for functional dysphonia. The voice therapist (SLP) works on dimensions that directly help improve the sound of the voice, including appropriate vocal intensity for the speaking environment (e.g., a quiet conversational environment), helping establish the patient's best pitch, and improving the quality of the voice. Considerable counseling, similar to individuals with vocal nodules, is often needed. The person's motivation and commitment to improving the voice are key factors in the success of therapy (Andrews, 2006; Boone et al., 2009; Ferrand, 2012; Rubin & Sataloff, 2006).

Individuals with functional dysphonia often benefit from psychological support from the clinician. Although few individuals need referral for specialized professional counseling from a psychologist or psychiatrist, speech-language pathologists need to take into consideration the psychological correlates of functional dysphonia (Andrews, 2006; Boone et al., 2009; Colton et al., 2011; Mirza, Ruiz, Baum, & Staub, 2003).

Margaret

Margaret was a successful attorney and prominent person in the community. Her husband had held a high political office in the state and together they made a dynamic team. Margaret also had functional dysphonia and was referred to me by an otolaryngologist for voice therapy. After the evaluation and several therapy sessions in the client's home, she asked to have a session in her office so that I could see the environment she worked in.

The office was large and imposing with a massive desk. When she sat behind her desk and I sat where her clients normally would, I noticed that she automatically raised the loudness of her voice. I also noticed a noisy heater and air conditioner vent directly over her desk, which may have contributed to her automatically raising her voice loudness. Margaret agreed to try talking with clients in a small conference room adjacent to her office where it was quieter and she did not have to raise her loudness level to be easily heard. Often when therapists are working with clients with functional dysphonia, clients can make many small changes in their vocal behaviors that, together, make significant improvements in their voices. ■

Muscle Tension Dysphonia

In a type of functional dysphonia called **muscle tension dysphonia (MTD)** the voice is adversely affected by excessive muscle tension that ranges from mild to severe (Boone et al., 2009; Andrews, 2006). MTD is a hyperfunctional voice disorder. Various subtypes of MTD have been discussed in the literature but are beyond the scope of this text. In general, individuals who demonstrate MTD tend to have weak voices with a lack of intensity range and variation. A rough, hoarse, or thin vocal quality that lacks resonance and carrying power, along with a voice that fatigues easily are common. Differential diagnosis depends on clear evidence that the dysphonia does not have an organic etiology. MTD is generally responsive to voice therapy from an SLP who specializes in voice disorders (Andrews, 2006).

Functional Aphonia

Functional aphonia is a hyperfunctional voice disorder, although it first may appear to be hypofunctional because patients speak with a whisper (i.e., the vocal folds are held in an abducted position during phonation). As with all voice disorders, an otolaryngologist needs to evaluate these patients to determine whether there are structural or neurological causes of the voice problem. Functional aphonia may have a variety of causes, most of which have some psychological foundation.

muscle tension dysphonia (MTD)

A hyperfunctional voice disorder in which the voice is adversely affected by excessive muscle tension that ranges from mild to severe; characteristics include a weak voice that lacks intensity, range and variation, a rough, hoarse, or thin vocal quality that lacks resonance, and a voice that fatigues easily.

functional aphonia

A hyperfunctional voice disorder in which a person speaks mostly with a whisper although is able to use a normal voice when laughing, coughing, clearing the throat, and humming; often associated with psychological stressors or conflicts.

CASE STUDY

Irene

Irene had suffered with intermittent functional aphonia for several years, and the aphonia was becoming more persistent. When her lack of voice began to threaten her job security, she sought help from a speech-language pathologist who specialized in voice disorders. The therapist saw Irene for one session, and she was able to achieve some phonation during various nonspeech tasks. However, before proceeding further, the therapist requested that Irene be seen by an otolaryngologist. She scheduled an appointment with an otolaryngologist at a time the voice therapist could be present. The physician, therapist, and client were all able to view her vocal folds clearly with *videostroboscopy* (to be discussed later). There were no apparent organic or neurological causes for her aphonia. Within two more therapy sessions, Irene was able to achieve and sustain good phonation but with intermittent phonation breaks when talking about certain job stresses. The therapist recognized that she needed to work with another professional to help her manage some personal stresses in her life and that by having a functional and generally reliable voice she would be able to better communicate with a professional counselor. Sometimes as voice therapists we can help prepare clients to work with other professionals who can work on areas outside of our scope of practice (Flasher & Fogle, 2012). It is difficult for mental health professionals to provide "talk" therapy when an individual does not have a voice for communicating. Speech-language pathologists can help clients achieve voice so that they can more fully benefit from the help of other professionals. ■

---

conversion reaction (disorder)

An ego defense mechanism in which *intrapsychic conflict* (mental struggle of opposing impulses or wishes within oneself) is expressed symbolically through physical symptoms that may manifest as actual illness or delusions of illness or incapacity (including voice disorders); causal factors may include a conscious or unconscious desire to escape from or avoid some unpleasant situation or responsibility, or to obtain sympathy or some other secondary gain.

The disorder has been referred to as a **conversion reaction (disorder)** because of its association with psychological stressors or emotional conflicts that produce such emotional pain that a physical symptom such as aphonia is more tolerable to the individual than dealing with the emotional pain directly (Rubin & Sataloff, 2006). Individuals with aphonia may receive reinforcing gains from their loss of voice by not having the ability to use their voice to assume personal responsibilities for life problems (Andrews, 2006; Baker, 2003; Case, 2002).

When patients with functional aphonia are able to produce some sound, it is usually high pitched, strident, weak, and breathy. Paradoxically, patients are able to use a normal voice during nonspeech vocalizations such as laughing, coughing, clearing the throat, and even humming, as though they do not associate these voice uses with the same voice needed for talking. That is, individuals with functional aphonia often do not recognize that these sound productions reveal that the vocal folds are physiologically capable of vibrating to produce sound. Therapeutically, these nonspeech sounds can be used to help patients "merge" into vocalization for speech. Most patients with functional aphonia respond well to voice therapy, often achieving a normal functioning voice in either the first therapy session or within the first few sessions (Andrews, 2006; Case, 2002; Stemple et al., 2009).

Mutational Falsetto/Puberphonia

Mutational falsetto (puberphonia) is a high-pitched, breathy voice produced by the vibration of the anterior one-third of the vocal folds, with the posterior two-thirds held tightly in a slightly open position or else so tightly adducted that little or no posterior vibration occurs (Colton et al., 2011; Seikel et al., 2010). Falsetto is the voice quality produced at the upper end of the normal range and represents the highest register of the voice (e.g., some songs sung by James Blunt, Aaron Neville, Robin Thicke, and Greg Pritchard are in falsetto, also the Bee Gees singing group used their falsetto voices for many of their songs in *Saturday Night Fever* with John Travolta).

Falsetto voice occurs in adolescent males where psychological factors may lead to inhibition of the transitional events that produce a lower-pitched, more masculine voice (Andrews, 2006). A falsetto voice in a male projects a female vocal quality. These males may have occasional downward pitch breaks, although they quickly resume their more habituated high-pitched falsetto voice. The social penalties for this kind of voice can be significant.

Voice therapy focuses on helping these patients lower their pitch to produce a more natural male voice. *Digital manipulation* (using the fingertips to lower the larynx while the person is phonating or using light finger pressure on the thyroid cartilage) can often bring the vocal pitch down so the patient can hear and feel the more natural and appropriate pitch. Another therapy approach is to use *masking* (a *white noise* [sound that contains energy at all frequencies in the audible spectrum] that is fed through headphones) while the person is reading aloud. Typically, the person will quickly and automatically begin to use a more normal adult male's voice. Once the more appropriate male pitch is established (often in the first or at least the first few sessions), the patient has little or no difficulty maintaining it.

VOICE DISORDERS RELATED TO ORGANIC ETIOLOGIES

There are a variety of voice disorders related to organic etiologies and in most cases medical management, including surgery, is needed. However, as a member of the team who specializes in helping children and adults with voice disorders, a speech-language pathologist is often involved in the rehabilitation of the voice.

Papillomas

Papillomas (papillomatosis) are wartlike growths on the vocal folds. They have a viral origin and occur mostly in young children 4 to 6 years

mutational falsetto (puberphonia)

A high-pitched, breathy voice produced by the vibration of the anterior one-third of the vocal folds, with the posterior two-thirds held tightly in a slightly open position or else so tightly adducted that little or no posterior vibration occurs.

papilloma (papillomatosis)

Soft, wartlike, benign growths on the vocal folds of children that have a viral origin and may grow to a size that can obstruct the airway.

Personal Story — Jason

Jason was a 17-year-old adolescent referred to me by an otolaryngologist. He had the highest-pitched voice of any adolescent male I had ever heard (almost 290 Hz), plus being tense and strained. He was cooperative and said he wanted to achieve a normal-sounding male voice. After interviewing Jason and evaluating his voice, I decided to ask him to do something that I believed he did not expect. Rather than asking him to try to lower his voice pitch, I asked him to try to raise his pitch "just a little." With some effort, he was able to raise his pitch noticeably. I then had him lower back to his "normal" voice, which he did easily. I had him practice raising his pitch a little higher several times and then back down to his accustomed (*habitual*) pitch level. When he had developed some control of his pitch, I asked him to lower it just a little below his normal pitch, which he was able to. After numerous successful attempts at raising his pitch quite a lot and then lowering it just a little, he was able to start lowering it significantly. By the third session, his voice was at a comfortable (optimal) 120–130 Hz. We discussed his new "voice image" and how he was going to manage when his friends made comments about his new voice.

Often in therapy we use several well-researched techniques to establish which technique evokes the desired response from the client. This information then is helpful in designing approaches for stabilizing the individual client's new voice behaviors. Sometimes we may try a new technique that we have not seen in the literature. If the new technique or approach is beneficial, it may be added to our therapy repertoire, and perhaps eventually be included in our professional literature. ■

of age but may occur up to the age of puberty (much like warts that occur on the hands of children and tend to end by puberty because by that age children have developed a natural immunity to the virus that causes both warts and papillomas). Although papillomas can cause severe voice disorders because the masses produce breathiness and harshness that results in chronic severe hoarseness, the major threat is to the child's airway (see Figure 9–6). The glottis is very small in children, and it takes only small masses to potentially occlude it, which can be life threatening. Because of the potential of papillomas for airway obstruction, children who are hoarse for more than 10 days, independent of a cold or allergy, should have a laryngeal examination by an otolaryngologist to rule out papillomas (Lindman, Gibbons, Morleir, & Wiatrak, 2004).

When papillomas are identified, they need to be removed surgically or through other medical procedures. Beyond the removal of the

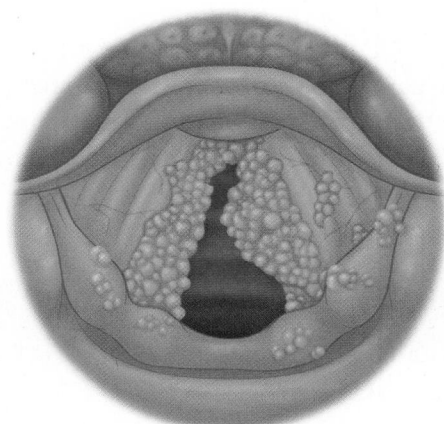

Juvenile Papillomatosis

Figure 9–6

Juvenile papillomas.

© Cengage Learning 2013.

tissue mass, the goal is to prevent damage to the vocal folds that can cause more permanent voice problems. SLPs are often needed to help the children develop their best voices and to teach vocal hygiene techniques. On a more long-term basis, it is helpful to monitor children's voices for early detection of hoarseness caused by recurrence of papilloma growths (Swigert, 2005).

Blunt, Penetrating, and Inhalation Traumas

A variety of traumatic injuries may affect the larynx, including the larynx being compressed or crushed by the steering wheel of a car (this tends to occur when individuals are in accidents while not wearing seat belts), attempted strangulation, and penetrating neck wounds such as from bullets or other projectiles that occur in war (Kleinsasser, Priemer, Schulze, & Kleinsasser, 2000). The trauma can immediately compromise the airway and needs emergency medical or surgical treatment. Later, voice therapy is needed to help patients achieve their most functional voice within the limits of their altered larynges.

Inhalation injuries may occur from inhalation of gases, steam, and smoke (all of which may occur during a house fire). The reflexive closure of the vocal folds is brief and then a person will gasp for air, causing the chemicals and heat to penetrate the larynx, trachea, and lungs. Likewise, *thermal injuries* from hot smoke or steam (sometimes seen in children with severe scald injuries) can damage the larynx and entire respiratory system. Within moments of inhaling hot fumes, the laryngeal and supraglottal structures usually have extensive edema, which can occlude the airway (Belanger, Scott, Scholten, Curtiss, & Vanderploeg, 2005; Casper, Clark, Kelley, & Colton, 2002). Severe edema of the respiratory tract may appear immediately or may develop within hours, and it can quickly lead to bronchial obstruction and death. Emergency *tracheotomy* and **intubation** are needed for survival. Voice therapy can be a concern

intubation

The passage of a breathing tube through the mouth, through the nose, or directly into the trachea through a *tracheotomy* (endotracheal intubation) to ensure a *patent* (open; pronounced "pAtent") airway for delivery of oxygen.

only after treatment of the bodily and organ injuries. However, speech-language pathologists can be helpful to the patient, family, and medical staff during the early stages of medical management by providing a functional and efficient means for the burn victim to communicate through *augmentative* or *alternative systems* (see Chapter 13).

> **Fires**
>
> During my years working as an EMT in ambulances in Southern California and my tour of duty as a combat medic in Vietnam in 1969, I saw many cases of burn (thermal) injuries. In those days, my first concern was pulling people out of the fires and to safety, making certain their airways were open, and treating the burns as best I could before moving them to the hospital or *medevac* (medical evacuation [usually by helicopter]) for further treatment. I remember breathing in the hot, smoky, noxious air and fumes and how drying and irritating they were to my throat, sometimes causing severe coughing spasms afterward. When I began studying voice disorders as a student of speech-language pathology, I began to more fully understand the effects of smoke, heat, and fumes on my larynx and lungs and those of the people I was trying to rescue and help. The study of speech-language pathology provides us information that helps us understand experiences in our own lives well beyond what we do in our professional work.

Cancer/Carcinoma

Cancer or **carcinoma** in the vocal tract is a life-threatening disease that requires medical and surgical management. If a **malignant** lesion affects one or both vocal folds, the vocal symptom will be hoarseness (Colton et al., 2011) (see Figure 9–7). For this reason, all voice cases speech-language pathologists work with must be evaluated by an otolaryngologist to determine whether there is a malignant mass on the vocal folds causing the voice problem. As is well known, cigarette smoking is a major cause of cancers of the lungs, larynx, and oral cavity (Stewart & Semmler, 2002; Zhang, Morgenstern, & Spitz, 2000). However, cancer may be caused by other agents, including environmental irritants, chemicals and other contaminants, metabolic disorders, and unknown causes.

VOICE DISORDERS RELATED TO NEUROLOGICAL ETIOLOGIES

As mentioned earlier, neurological voice disorders are related to muscle control and innervation of nerves into the muscles of respiration and phonation. Many neurological voice disorders are associated with dysarthrias, with either **hypoadduction** or **hyperadduction** of the vocal folds (Colton et al., 2011; Stemple et al., 2009).

---

cancer (carcinoma)

A malignant *neoplasm* (new growth) characterized by uncontrolled growth of cells that tend to invade surrounding tissue and *metastasize* (spread) to distant body sites.

malignant

A neoplasm with uncontrollable growth and dissemination that invades and destroys neighboring tissue.

hypoadduction

Difficulty making the vocal folds close strongly enough or long enough for normal phonation that results in a weak, breathy voice that often deteriorates with increasing amounts of vocal use throughout the day.

hyperadduction

Difficulty with the vocal folds closing too tightly or for too long that results in a voice that sounds tense and strained and tends to fatigue with use as a result of hypertonicity.

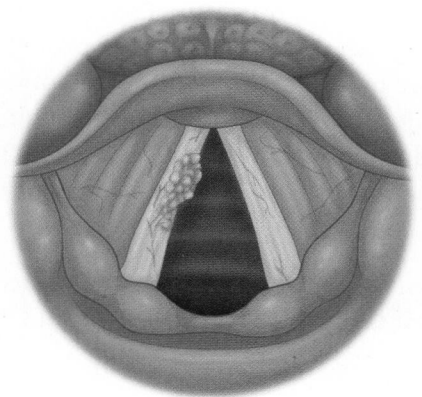 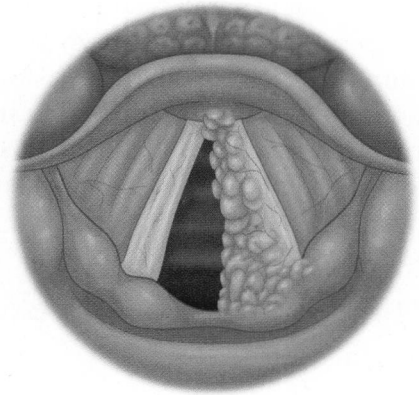

Early Carcinoma of
Right Vocal Fold

Extensive Carcinoma of Left Vocal
Fold Involving Arytenoid Region

Figure 9–7

Laryngeal cancer.
© Cengage Learning 2013.

Hypoadduction Vocal Fold Problems

Individuals with hypoadduction voice problems have difficulty making the vocal folds close strongly enough or long enough (Shrivastav & Sapienza, 2003). Their voices are often weak and breathy and deteriorate with increasing amounts of vocal use throughout the day. Their voices are often stronger in the morning than in the afternoon, making jobs that require extensive voice use (e.g., teaching) more difficult (Rubin & Sataloff, 2006). Various neurological disorders have hypoadduction problems, including muscular dystrophy and Parkinsonism (these disorders are discussed in more detail in Chapter 11).

Vocal Fold Paresis and Paralysis

One or both vocal folds may be paretic or paralyzed. Vocal fold paresis or paralysis may be caused by damage to one or more areas of the central and peripheral nervous systems, such as the motor strip in the cerebral cortex, the pyramidal tract, cerebellum, brainstem, vagus nerves, and recurrent laryngeal nerves (Loughran, Alves, & MacGregor, 2002; Marchant, Supiot, Choufani, & Hassid, 2003; Segas, Stravroulakis, Monolopoulos, Yiotakis, & Adamopoulus, 2001). Patients with unilateral **vocal fold paralysis** present with varied vocal symptoms, ranging from mild to severe dysphonias, depending on the *resting position* (the position of the folds during quiet breathing) of the paralyzed vocal fold. When a unilateral paralyzed vocal fold is positioned in the midline, voice quality is less impaired than when it is further from the midline because the healthy vocal fold comes closer to approximating the paralyzed fold. Typically, the voice is characterized by breathiness, low intensity, and **diplophonia**.

Bilateral vocal fold paralysis is often the result of damage to the brainstem, such as strokes, tumors, carcinoma, or trauma. If both vocal

vocal fold paralysis

Unilateral or bilateral loss of laryngeal movements (including vocal fold opening or closing) that may be caused by damage to the brainstem, vagus (X cranial) nerves, recurrent laryngeal nerves, or the neuromuscular junctions (where the nerve fibers connect with the muscle tissue), resulting in a weak, breathy voice, or possible difficulty breathing if the vocal folds are paralyzed in the closed position.

diplophonia

Two distinct pitches perceived simultaneously during phonation that is caused by the two vocal folds vibrating under different degrees of tension (as in unilateral vocal fold paralysis) or vibration of the ventricular folds concurrently with the true vocal folds.

folds become paralyzed in the midline position, the immediate medical concern is respiratory survival; that is, the closed vocal folds prevent normal respiration. If the vocal folds are paralyzed in the abducted position, there is increased risk of aspiration of food or liquid because the vocal folds are not adequately closed during swallowing (see Chapter 12, Swallowing Disorders/Dysphagia for a discussion of vocal fold closure during swallowing).

Hyperadduction Vocal Fold Problems

Patients with hyperadduction problems have difficulty with the vocal folds closing too tightly or for too long. Their voices are often tense and strained and tend to fatigue with use as a result of hypertonicity. Individuals with spastic dysarthria are good examples of hyperadduction problems (see Chapter 11, Neurological Disorders in Adults). However, the most striking cases with hyperadduction disorders are those with spasmodic dysphonia.

Spasmodic Dysphonia

spasmodic dysphonia (SD)

A relatively rare voice disorder that may have either or both neurological and psychological etiologies; characterized by a strained, strangled, harsh voice quality, or an absence of voice because of tight abduction of the vocal folds; clients typically do not respond well to voice therapy.

Spasmodic dysphonia (SD) is relatively rare. Individuals with this voice disorder exhibit a strained, strangled, harsh voice quality with observable effort to push air through the vocal folds to obtain useable voice. The vocal folds are typically held closed with such extreme tension while trying to phonate that normal vibration is prevented. In many cases, the false vocal folds also are adducted tightly. In some cases, however, the vocal folds may be held rigidly in an open position during efforts to phonate, resulting in an absence of vibration of the vocal folds and a tense, breathy sounding "voice." The voice disorder is usually insidious in onset and progresses over months or years. Schweinfurth, Billante, and Courey (2002), in a study of 168 patients with spasmodic dysphonia, found that 79% of the patients were female and 21% were male, with an average age of 45 years. Thirty percent of patients directly associated the onset of spasmodic dysphonia symptoms with an upper respiratory tract infection, and 21% to a major life stress. However, the general consensus in the medical and voice disorder literature, as well as the National Spasmodic Dysphonia Association (NSDA; www.dysphonia.org) is that spasmodic dysphonia is a central nervous system disorder and a form of **dystonia** (Haslinger, Erhard, Dresel, et al., 2005; Simonyan, & Ludlow, 2010; Sulica, 2004).

dystonia

A general neurological term for a variety of problems characterized by excessive contraction of muscles with associated abnormal movements and postures.

Regretfully, most individuals with spasmodic dysphonia do not respond well to voice therapy approaches alone. Most success for the voices of these individuals occurs when medical-surgical approaches are used, such as injection of *botulinum toxin* (botox) into one vocal fold to create weakness of the fold that temporarily (usually months) decreases vocal fold tension, or the severing of the recurrent laryngeal nerve that innervates one vocal fold to permanently decrease vocal fold tension. Voice therapy from an SLP is needed to maximize the benefits of the medical-surgical techniques (Andrews, 2006; Boone et al., 2009; Stemple et al., 2009).

MULTICULTURAL CONSIDERATIONS

There is little literature investigating multicultural considerations and voice disorders. Haller and Thompson (1975), in their study of 1,000 African American children in Harlem, New York, found that 22% of the children exhibited dysphonia marked by hoarseness (compared to Ramig and Verdolini's 1998 estimated 3%–6% of school-age children with dysphonia). However, Duff, Proctor, and Yairi (2004), in their study of the prevalence of voice disorders in 2,445 African American and European American young children (1,246 males and 1,199 females, 2 to 6 years of age), hoarseness was identified in 3.9% of the total sample, with no statistically significant differences among those children in age, gender, or race. Holland and DeJarnette (2002) did an extensive review of the literature on voice-related pathologies in minority groups in the United States, health issues related to voice dysfunction, ethnographic and racial factors related to voice, and the role of the speech-language pathologist in prevention, assessment, and intervention. Their review of the literature on *epidemiology* (the study of the determinants of disease in different populations) of voice-related pathologies in minority groups revealed the need for increased research on the incidence and prevalence of causal factors and types of disorders among minority populations. However, the available literature suggests that health risk factors include occupational and daily living exposure to *teratogens* (any substance that interferes with normal prenatal development, causing developmental abnormalities in a fetus) in pregnant women, substance abuse, and possible predisposition to certain disease processes that are the combined effect of biological inheritance and environmental conditions. Holland and DeJarnette (2002, p. 329) state, "Developing culturally sensitive, client centered, and relevant approaches to voice service delivery permits speech-language pathologists to fulfill their roles and responsibilities as preventionists, diagnosticians, and interventionists in working with multicultural groups."

ASSESSMENT OF THE VOICE

An otolaryngologist (ENT) is essential in the diagnosis of a person with a voice disorder and often in the treatment. However, the speech-language pathologist (with clients who have voice disorders, we are often referred to as *voice therapists*) frequently needs to be on the team who evaluates and treats voice disorders. The ENT may refer a patient to an SLP after her initial evaluation and diagnosis of a patient. However, in other cases a person with a voice disorder may first contact an SLP for help and the therapist may conduct an evaluation and initiate therapy; however, therapy cannot continue until an ENT has evaluated the patient and referred the patient back to the voice therapist. In the schools an SLP can screen, evaluate, and initiate therapy with a child who has a voice disorder, but therapy cannot continue unless the child also is evaluated by an ENT.

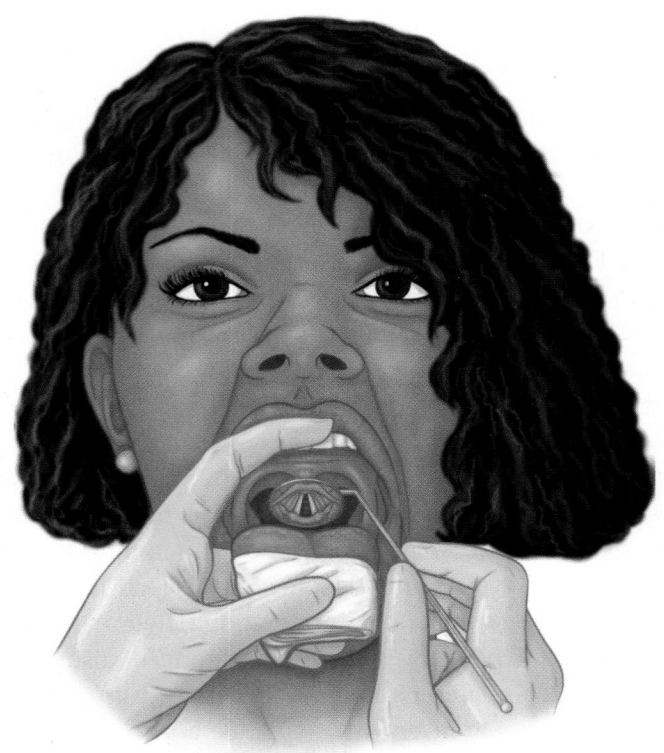

Technique

Figure 9-8

Indirect laryngoscopy with
a laryngeal mirror.
© Cengage Learning 2013.

indirect laryngoscopy

A method of examining the larynx
and vocal folds by placing a
laryngeal mirror (a small round
mirror attached to a long handle)
into the back of the mouth and
directing a reflected light source
onto the mirror to shine on the
vocal folds.

direct laryngoscopy

Examination by an ENT physician
of the interior of the larynx by
direct vision with the aid of a
laryngoscope, usually while the
patient is anesthetized.

laryngoscope

A hollow tube used by an ENT
physician that is inserted into
the larynx through the mouth for
examining or operating on the
interior of the larynx.

The Otolaryngologist's Examination

Otolaryngologists use three primary procedures to view the vocal folds (*laryngoscopy*): **indirect laryngoscopy, endoscopy**, and **direct laryngoscopy**. The indirect laryngoscopy examination is usually the first method the ENT specialist uses to view the vocal folds. During this procedure, the physician attempts to view the larynx and vocal folds using a laryngeal mirror (see Figure 9–8). Indirect laryngoscopy is considered a fairly noninvasive procedure because it does not require anesthesia or cause any pain or trauma to the patient (Colton et al., 2011). The ENT physician also may choose to evaluate the laryngeal mechanism by using endoscopy with a rigid scope that is passed through the oral cavity with the tip of the scope reaching near the posterior pharyngeal wall, and the physician viewing the vocal folds and laryngeal region on a monitor (see Figure 9–9). A video recording (*videoendoscopy*) or video recording with strobe lighting (*videostroboscopy*) may be chosen for later study of the images. The physician also may choose to use a *flexible fiberoptic scope* that is passed *transnasally* (through the nose and down to the level of the epiglottis) to view the vocal folds and laryngeal area (Woo, 2006) (see Figures 9–10 and 9–11). *Direct laryngoscopy* is less commonly used by ENT physicians and is the most invasive of the laryngeal examination procedures. It is usually performed in a hospital with

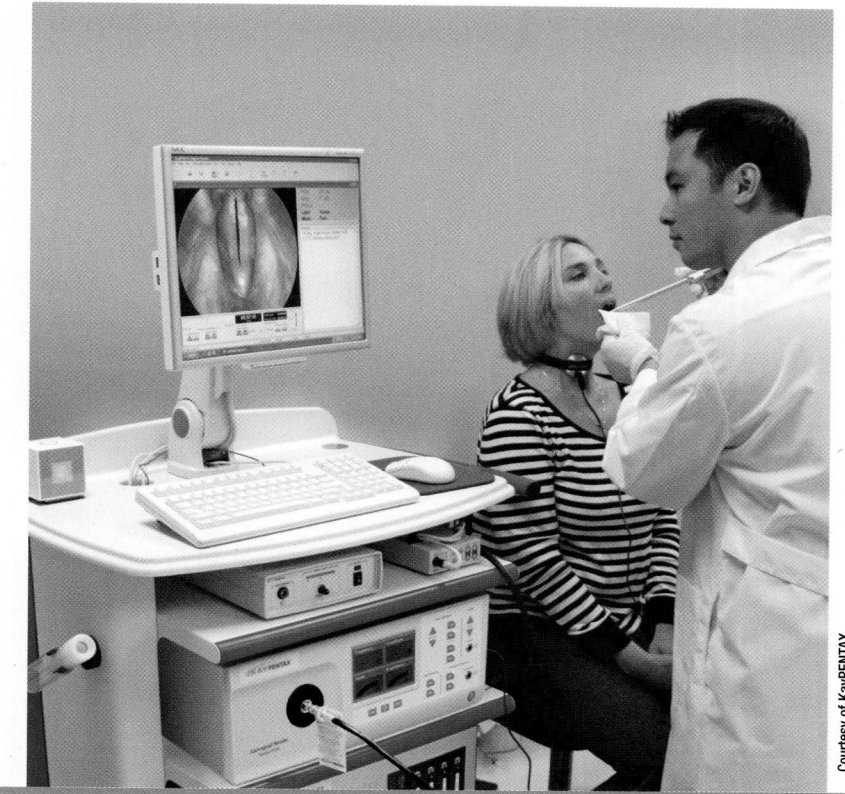

Courtesy of KayPENTAX

Figure 9–9
Videoendoscopy using a rigid scope through the oral cavity (note the microphone pressed against the neck to record the patient's voice simultaneously while the vocal folds are being viewed).

a patient under general anesthesia. Direct laryngoscopy allows an ENT physician to examine the laryngeal structures in more detail and, when necessary, obtain a biopsy of a lesion (Colton et al., 2011).

The Speech-Language Pathologist's Assessment

A complete voice evaluation includes numerous components, and the entire evaluation may not be completed on the first *visit* (appointment) with a client. The SLP must do a thorough evaluation of the person's respiratory and phonatory systems to determine the best course of therapy. However, the voice evaluation and voice therapy cannot be separated. Effective voice therapy is an ongoing, continuous evaluation process (Boone et al., 2009; Shipley & McAfee, 2009). This is necessary to be continually listening to subtle changes in the client's voice, as well as to incorporate increased understanding of the person as the client reveals more information about what may have contributed to the voice problem and what is maintaining it.

Case History

If the client already has been examined by an ENT physician, then the speech-language pathologist should read the medical report before seeing the client the first time. The first meeting between the client and

endoscopy

Methods of viewing the velopharyngeal mechanism, vocal tract, or both that use a rigid endoscope introduced *intraorally* (through the mouth) or flexible fiberoptic endoscope *transnasally* (through the nose) with a camera lens and fiber-optic light source at the tip of the scope that can illuminate the nasopharynx, oropharynx, and larynx; the structures may be videotaped (*videoendoscopy*), and the light source can be put in *strobe mode* (rapid flashing) so that the vibrating vocal folds appear to move in slow motion for more detailed viewing (*videostroboscopy*); (note: SLPs may be trained to perform endoscopic evaluations and in most states are allowed to perform them).

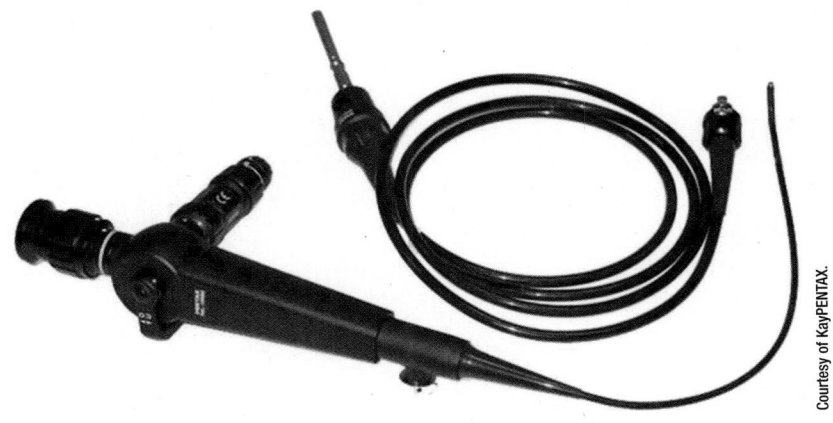

Figure 9-10

Flexible fiberoptic endoscope that can be passed transnasally to view the velopharyngeal mechanism, vocal folds, and laryngeal region.

Courtesy of KayPENTAX.

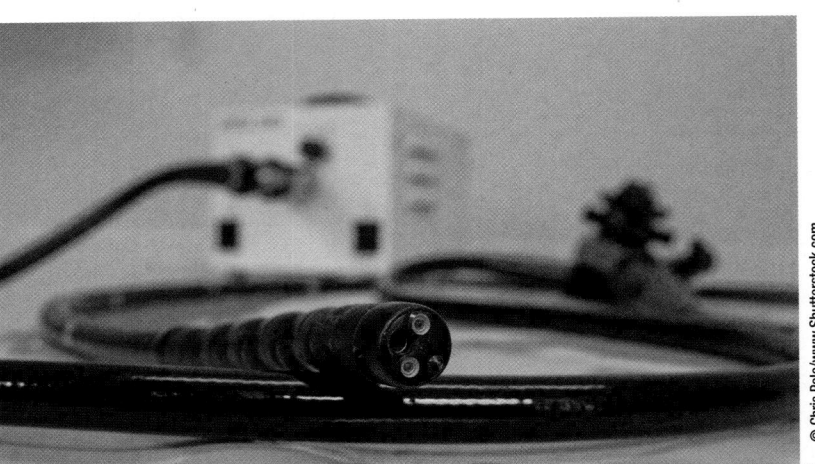

Figure 9-11

Tip of a flexible fiberoptic endoscope showing the very small light source and camera lens.

© Chris Pole/www.Shutterstock.com

Application Question

Have you ever had a voice problem? If you have, what do you recall about it? How was it evaluated? How was it treated?

the clinician is important because rapport must be established for open and honest sharing of information. The interview with a client who has a voice disorder requires some of the most sensitive skills we use during any interaction with clients (Flasher & Fogle, 2012). An individual's voice is a personal expression of the individual, and most people feel that it represents them as individuals. The kinds of questions we ask and the way we ask them can significantly influence the responses we receive.

During the interview, we want the client to describe the problem, what she feels may have caused it, and what is contributing to its continuation. We want to learn when the voice is at its best and worst; for example, during various times of the day, in different environments (home, work, etc.), with different people, and when talking about different topics. We want information about any vocal abuses and misuses. We also need to know about medications the client takes (some may have effects on the voice) and any smoking and drinking habits. As you can imagine, considerable tact is needed to investigate certain areas.

Throughout the interview, we also are listening to and observing the client's vocal behaviors. For example, we are noting the loudness, pitch, and quality of the voice; vocal abuses such as frequent throat clearing or coughing; and tension in the voice, face, and body. During the interview we are using some of our most astute observational and listening skills to understand the person and the voice problem. It is the *observational skills* (auditory, visual, and sometimes even tactile) that help clinicians recognize nuances of attitudes, feelings, and behaviors that indicate relaxation and tension in a person's body and throat. Keen listening skills help the clinician hear the subtleties in the voice that indicate positive or negative changes, or no changes.

Quantification of the Voice

A clinician may choose from several voice rating scales that are commercially available to help quantify the various characteristics of the voice. Most published voice rating scales quantify several key areas of voice based on the evaluator's perceptual judgments. During a voice evaluation, the clinician is trying to investigate the *perceptual*, *acoustic*, and *physiologic* correlates. The perceptual correlates refer to what we hear, such as loudness, pitch, and quality. The *acoustic* correlates refer to the biomechanical characteristics of the vocal folds, such as *habitual pitch* (what the person typically uses), *pitch range* (highest pitch and lowest pitch), *optimal pitch* (the most comfortable and appropriate pitch for the person's vocal mechanism), and *maximum phonation time* in seconds (how long a person can hold a sound). To measure the acoustic correlates, sophisticated computerized instruments such as the Visi-Pitch™ or the Computerized Speech Lab™ (CSL) by KayPentax may be used. The physiologic correlates of the vocal folds refer to *aerodynamic features* and *vibratory behavior*, such as *airflow rates* (volume of air passing between the vibrating vocal folds in a fixed period of time), *airflow pressures* (force of the air passing between the vocal folds), *abnormal movements* of the vocal folds during vibration, and *masses on the vocal folds* (ASHA, 2004a). Sophisticated computerized instruments may be used to measure the physiologic correlates.

Resonance of the voice, from the posterior pharyngeal wall through the nasal passages, influences the quality of the voice. Individuals who use their articulators in a constricted manner (e.g., speaking with their mandible nearly closed or with their teeth clenched) affect their ability to project their voice because they are not using the "megaphone effect" of their mouth, which results in the need for increased laryngeal tension to achieve adequate loudness to be easily heard. A hearing screening should always be a part of a complete assessment.

During the assessment, in addition to the interview and formal voice evaluation, it is important to try various voice therapy stimulability techniques to hear how they may affect the voice. In a way, the voice evaluation and voice therapy merge into one another when we say to a client, "I want you to try . . . to see what happens." When we have tried a few therapy techniques that give a positive change to the client's voice, we have a better idea of the direction of therapy.

Application Question

How would you rate the loudness, pitch, and quality of your voice compared to that of your friends of the same age and gender?

VOICE THERAPY

Voice therapy usually involves a multifaceted approach that integrates several areas of knowledge, training, skills, and understanding. Voice clinicians rely on several strong foundations: (1) a thorough understanding of the anatomy and physiology of all speech systems, but especially the respiratory and phonatory systems; (2) knowledge of the many voice disorders; (3) a thorough evaluation of the client or patient; (4) knowledge and understanding of the various voice therapy approaches and techniques; (5) training in both auditory and visual perceptual discrimination; and (6) good listening skills and a "good ear" to help recognize nuances of voice. Technical expertise is essential in our work with individuals who have voice disorders (or any disorder); however, it is not sufficient for being a good or excellent clinician. A good background in psychology and counseling is essential when working with individuals (Flasher & Fogle, 2012). Almost all skills of a well-trained speech-language pathologist come into play when working with people who have voice disorders. In voice therapy, we are confronted with the job of trying to disentangle the organic, psychological, and social factors that are intertwined in the person with a voice disorder (Andrews, 2006; Boone et al., 2009; Case, 2002; Colton et al., 2011; Rubin & Sataloff, 2006; Stemple et al., 2009) (see Figure 9–12).

Voice Therapy Approaches

A number of factors influence the design of voice therapy programs, including the age of the person, the type and severity of the disorder, the patient's personality and understanding of the problem, and the person's commitment to change. Clinician variables also are important. Some clinician variables include education and training in voice disorders, previous experience working with a variety of individuals and types of voice disorders, interest in voice disorders, and personality. Some voice

Figure 9–12

A speech-language pathologist helping a client with a voice disorder understand how the vocal folds work.

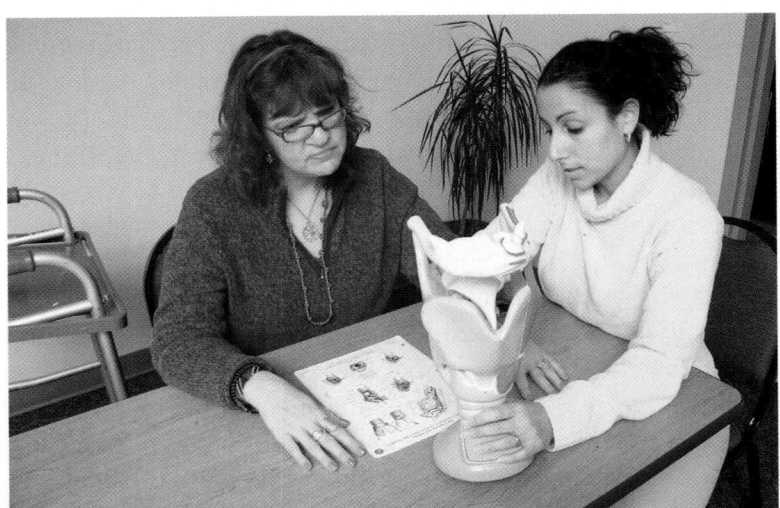

Using Metaphors in Therapy | Personal Story

Beth was a 43-year-old woman who was diagnosed by an ENT physician as having functional dysphonia and was referred to me for an evaluation and therapy. I noticed that Beth tended to talk rapidly and to change subjects often, as well as to be unusually animated, all in a somewhat tense manner. She also liked to describe herself using metaphors, such as "I feel like a turtle in mud" (i.e., she felt she could never talk fast enough or say everything she wanted). I realized that Beth would relate well to metaphors and used them to illustrate various concepts about voice and her voice problem. For example, I told her that the conversation reminded me of a race-horse rider who kept changing horses in the middle of a race; each horse rode a little differently, but she never stayed on one horse long enough to get a real "feel" for it—to finish a topic. Beth liked that metaphor and thought about it often in her conversations outside of therapy. As therapy progressed, she recognized that she was "staying on one horse longer" in a conversation and eventually "rode one horse all the way to the finish" (the end of a topic of conversation). Over time, and with the use of various therapy approaches, she decreased her overall tension and had a more relaxed-sounding voice. This example illustrates how, as clinicians, we always need to be "thinking on our feet" and finding novel ways to help our clients understand subtle (and not so subtle) concepts that help them make attitudinal and behavioral changes to improve their voices. ■

clinicians are more physiological and instrumentation oriented and their therapy tends to have more emphasis in those directions. Other clinicians are more psychosocially oriented and their therapy may have more emphasis on the psychological and emotional aspects of the voice disorder. Most clinicians, however, are probably somewhat balanced in their orientation to therapy and draw on a combination of approaches (Andrews, 2006; Stemple et al., 2009). Although various approaches may be used, voice therapy has been demonstrated to be an effective treatment for dysphonia (MacKenzie, Millar, Wilson, Sellars, & Deary, 2001). Three of the foundational voice therapy approaches are *physiologic voice therapy, hygienic voice therapy,* and *symptomatic voice therapy*.

Physiologic Voice Therapy

Physiologic voice therapy attempts to directly alter or modify the physiology of the vocal mechanism. Normal voice production relies on normal functioning and balance of the respiratory, phonatory, and resonatory systems; that is, their anatomy and physiology. A disturbance in the physiologic balance of these systems may lead to a voice disorder. The causes of the disorders may be mechanical, neurological, or psychological. In physiologic voice therapy, addressing the cause of the voice problem is not the focus of therapy. Modification of the inappropriate physiologic activity through exercises and manipulation of the respiratory, phonatory, and resonatory systems is the focus. This approach uses objective data obtained through physiologic measurements of laryngeal functioning to guide the direction of therapy for altering the function of the laryngeal musculature and the respiratory support of voice production (Andrews, 2006; Stemple, Glaze, & Klaben, 2009).

Hygienic Voice Therapy

Hygienic voice therapy (i.e., vocal hygiene education) is often the first step in many voice programs. For many individuals, poor vocal hygiene may contribute to their voice disorder. Some examples of poor vocal hygiene include shouting, screaming, yelling, coughing, frequent throat clearing, talking loudly over noise, and poor hydration. These behaviors are often considered *vocal abuses*. Other damaging behaviors include frequently speaking too loudly or for prolonged periods, speaking or singing with a pitch outside of the person's best pitch range, poor phonatory habits such as hard glottal attacks, making playful animal sounds or sounds of motors, and speaking with inadequate respiratory support. These behaviors are often referred to as *vocal misuses*.

Vocal hygiene therapy strives to instill healthy vocal behaviors in the person's habitual speech patterns. *Internal hydration* (i.e., drinking plenty of fluids) is often a key component of vocal hygiene therapy. Therapy is usually behaviorally oriented; that is, determining what vocal abuses, misuses, or both a person has; helping the person become aware of the damaging behaviors; and helping the person eliminate the inappropriate or damaging vocal behaviors.

Symptomatic Voice Therapy

Symptomatic voice therapy is based on the premise that most voice disorders are caused by the functional misuse or abuse of the respiratory, phonatory, or resonatory systems, as well as inappropriate loudness, vocal pitch, and rate of speaking. When identified through the evaluation process, the abuses and misuses are reduced or eliminated through various voice therapy facilitating techniques. The focus of symptomatic voice therapy is on the modification of a person's vocal symptoms, finding the person's "best" voice in the presence of the disorder, and facilitating techniques to stabilize the improved voice production. A few of the facilitating techniques used by voice clinicians include the following (Boone et al., 2009):

- Auditory feedback: Used to enhance a client's listening of her voice with *real-time amplification* (client uses an amplifier, microphone, and headset to hear her own voice as she phonates), or

Mathew and Mark

Mathew and Mark were both 8-year-old boys attending a private school who were referred to me by an ENT doctor for voice therapy because of their chronic laryngitis and vocal nodules. They were in the same class, lived near each other, and did most everything together, including, as their mothers said, "yelling their voices away." Initially I saw them individually in their homes for the evaluations and the first several therapy sessions. One of the fathers was on the school board and made arrangements for me to see the boys together twice a week for half-hour sessions at the school. They needed to learn what they were doing that caused them to lose their voices, develop vocal nodules, and then make the slow behavioral changes so that they could regain and maintain their voices and eliminate the nodules. With the support of their teacher and parents, the boys began remembering some voice therapy techniques that helped them have successful outcomes. Voice therapy is a team approach, and for children it is helpful to have both teachers and parents who are supportive and willing to help the children monitor their vocal abuses. ■

loop feedback (client uses a device that provides immediate feedback by replaying a tape or digital recording of her voice).

- Counseling: Explanation of the voice problem is essential for the client to understand her voice disorder, but explanations must be made in ways a client can understand them and in ways that will not make a client defensive (Flasher & Fogle, 2012).

- Elimination of abuses (phonotrauma): Therapy cannot be successful for many clients until contributory vocal abuses and misuses are significantly reduced, which first requires identifying the abuses and misuses and then consciously attempting to decrease and then eliminate them.

Laryngectomy

There are various medical and surgical approaches to treating laryngeal cancer, including radiation, chemotherapy, and partial or total **laryngectomy** (Back & Sood, 2005; Zeitels, Jarboe, & Franco, 2001). (Note: A person who has had a laryngectomy surgery is commonly referred to as a *laryngectomee* and does not always follow the person-first rule.) There are a variety of types of laryngeal cancer and some respond better to one mode of treatment than another, but all have consequences for the voice. The effect of voice production capability will depend on the extent and nature of the surgery performed. For example,

laryngectomy

Surgical removal of the larynx because of cancer and includes the trachea being brought forward and sutured to the skin in the lower midline of the neck to create a permanent stoma; the pharynx is closed as a separate tract for swallowing.

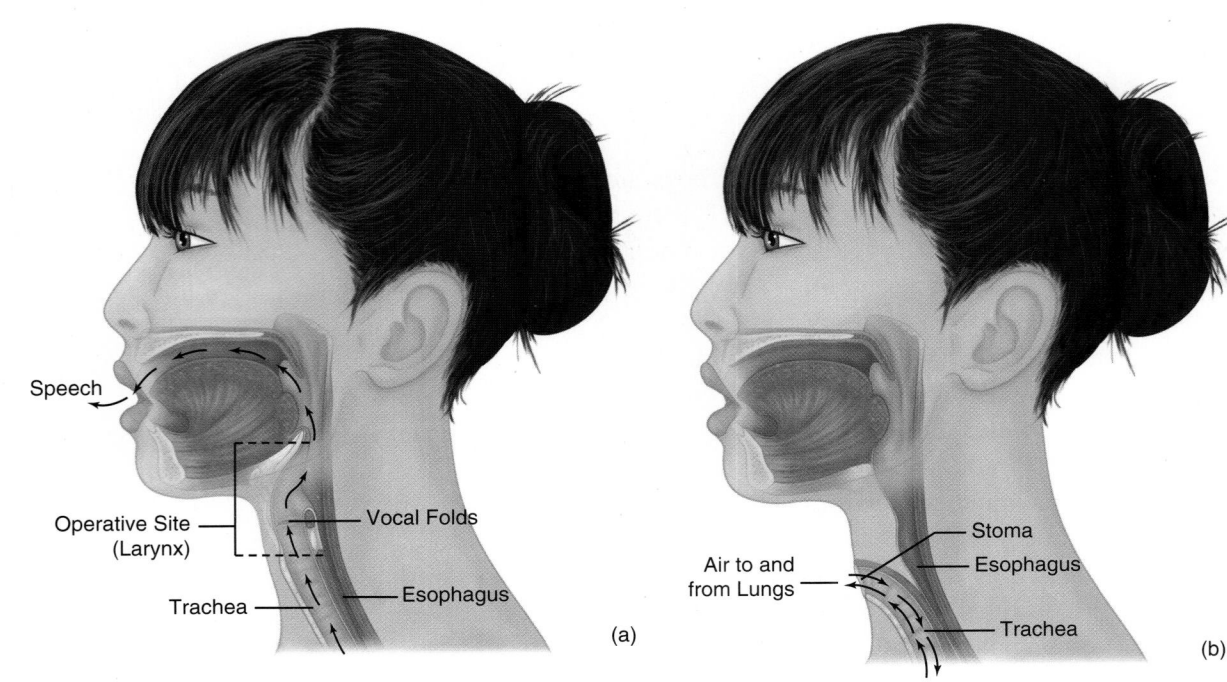

Figure 9-13

(a) Larynx before laryngectomy and (b) after laryngectomy.

© Cengage Learning 2013.

stoma

An opening about the diameter of a finger or thumb made surgically into the neck that allows a person to breathe directly through the trachea.

tracheoesophageal prosthesis (TEP)

A surgical procedure (*tracheoesophageal puncture*) in which an incision through the trachea and esophageal walls is created to fit a one-way plastic valve (*prosthesis*) that directs air from the trachea into the esophagus where it can reach the oral cavity and be articulated for speech.

some patients may be able to have just a small cancerous growth *excised* (cut out), others may have a *partial laryngectomy* with part of the larynx removed or a *hemilaryngectomy* with half of the larynx removed, and still others may need to have the entire larynx removed—a *total* or *complete laryngectomy*. In a total laryngectomy surgery a **stoma** is created in the neck just above the *sternum* (breastbone). A stoma is an opening about the diameter of a finger or thumb that connects to the trachea through which the patient will breathe for the rest of her life (see Figure 9-13).

Speech-language pathologists have important roles both before and after laryngectomy surgery. Before surgery, it is helpful for the SLP to meet with the patient and family to discuss the clinician's role in vocal rehabilitation and the various choices the patient has for eventual voice production. It is also important for both the patient and the family to understand that after the surgery the patient will not be able to make *any* vocal sound, not even crying or whispering (patients do not always realize that). Establishing some form of communication, such as writing or a communication board will assist the patient in communicating important medical and personal needs. Providing the patient and family members with information about the *International Association of Laryngectomees* (IAL) and its website (http://www.theial.com) can help them feel that they are not alone and will have a means to communicate with other laryngectomees both locally and around the world. The three general postlaryngectomy alaryngeal speech options (listed in the order most commonly used) are: **tracheoesophageal prosthesis (TEP)**, esophageal speech, and electrolarynx (Brown, Hilgers, Irish, & Balm, 2003).

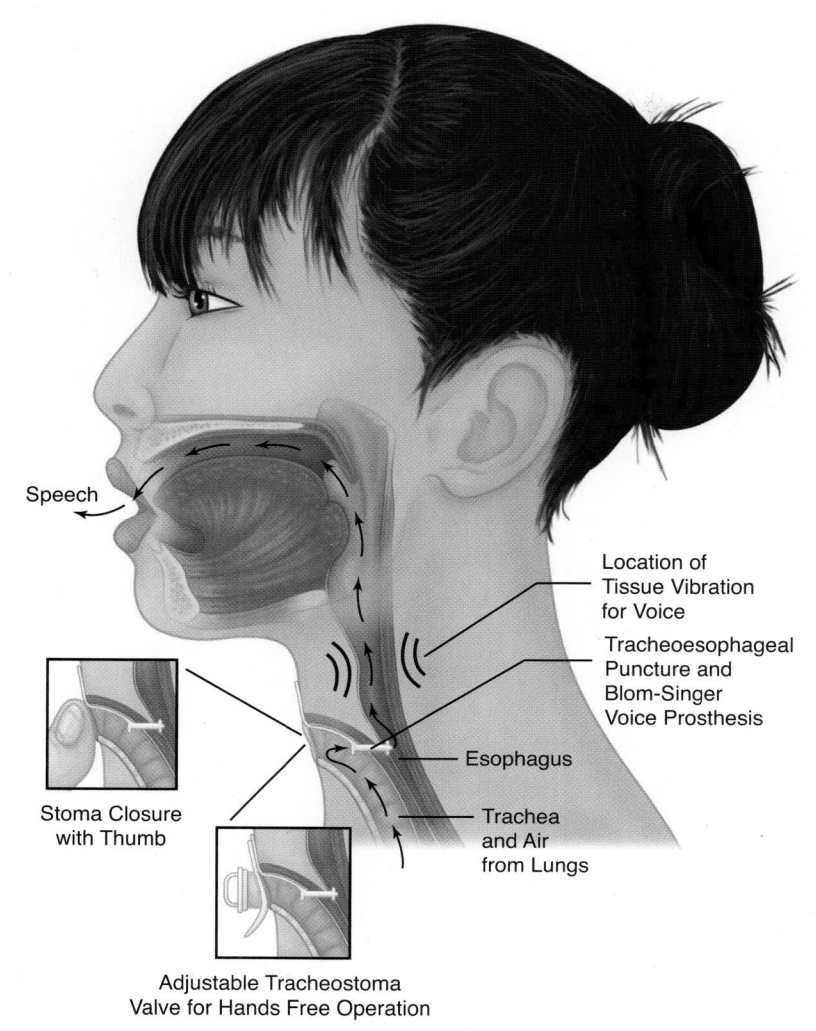

Speech

Location of
Tissue Vibration
for Voice

Tracheoesophageal
Puncture and
Blom-Singer
Voice Prosthesis

Esophagus

Trachea
and Air
from Lungs

Stoma Closure
with Thumb

Adjustable Tracheostoma
Valve for Hands Free Operation

Figure 9-14

Representation of speech
being produced using
a tracheoesophageal
puncture (TEP) shunt,
and examples of various
prostheses.

© Cengage Learning 2013.

Tracheoesophageal Prosthesis (TEP)

Many laryngectomees today are candidates for the tracheoesophageal prosthesis and many have the tracheosphageal (TE) puncture
performed at the time of the laryngectomy surgery (ASHA, 2004b). In
the TE puncture procedure, the surgeon makes an incision (puncture)
through the tracheal and esophageal walls, creating a *fistula* (passageway). A one-way plastic valve (*prosthesis*) is inserted into the fistula that
allows the laryngectomee to cover the stoma with his fingers or thumb.
With the stoma covered, air coming up the trachea is directed into the
prosthesis that sends the air into the esophagus. From there, it travels
up to the pharynx and into the mouth, where it is articulated for speech
(see Figure 9–14).

Esophageal Speech

When a patient uses **esophageal speech**, she must be trained to take
air into the esophagus by compressing the air within the *oropharynx*

esophageal speech

The compression of air within
the oropharynx and injection of it
into the esophagus, followed by
the rapid expelling of the air out
of the esophagus that causes it
to vibrate the upper esophageal
valve, which produces a low-
pitched, monotone "voice" that
is shaped by the articulators to
produce "burp" speech.

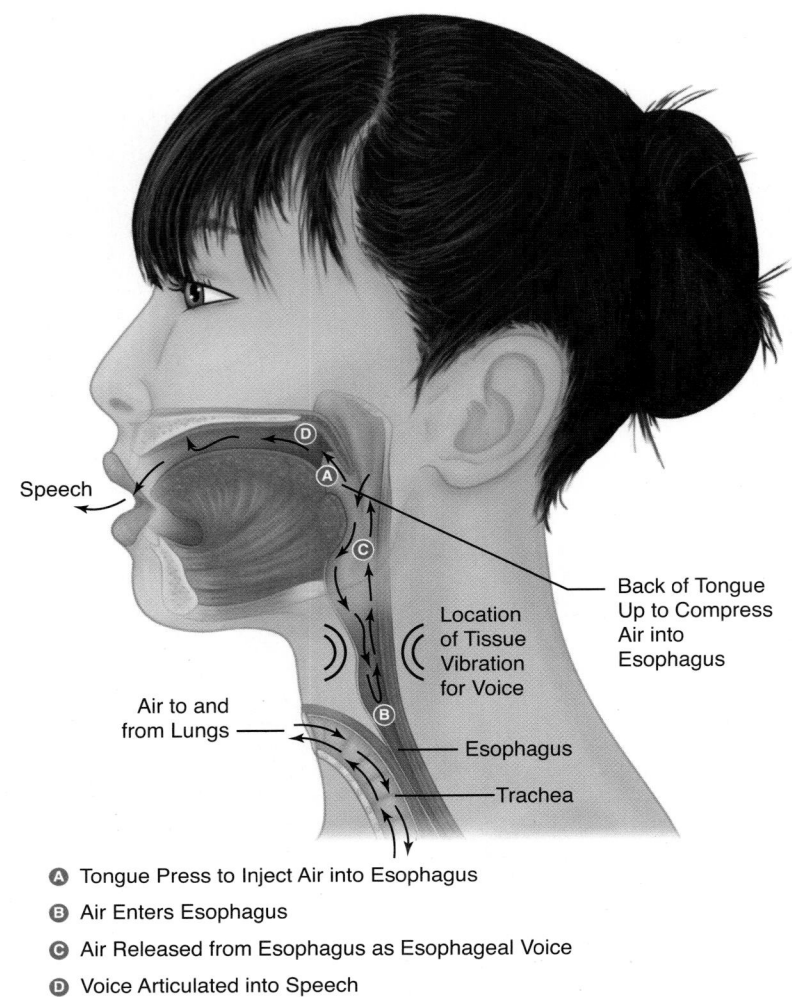

Figure 9-15

Representation of speech being produced using esophageal speech.

© Cengage Learning 2013.

Speech

(D)
(A)

(C)

Location of Tissue Vibration for Voice

Back of Tongue Up to Compress Air into Esophagus

Air to and from Lungs

(B)

Esophagus

Trachea

(A) Tongue Press to Inject Air into Esophagus

(B) Air Enters Esophagus

(C) Air Released from Esophagus as Esophageal Voice

(D) Voice Articulated into Speech

(back of mouth and top of pharynx), injecting it into the esophagus (but not down into the stomach), and then expelling the air out of the esophagus. This causes the air to vibrate the *pharyngoesophageal segment/upper esophageal valve* (top of the esophagus), which produces a low-pitched, monotone "voice." The patient then learns how to shape the sound by using the articulators to produce "burp" speech (see Figure 9–15).

Two methods for teaching esophageal speech are commonly used: the *injection method* and the *inhalation method*. Both methods compress air within the oropharynx and inject the compressed air into the space of the esophagus. Once the compressed air flows into the esophagus, the greater pressure from the elasticity of the esophageal walls forces the air back up the esophagus, through the pharyngoesophageal segment, and into the oral cavity where the air can be articulated. As an analogy, consider blowing up a balloon (compressed air from the lungs flowing into the balloon), holding the neck of the

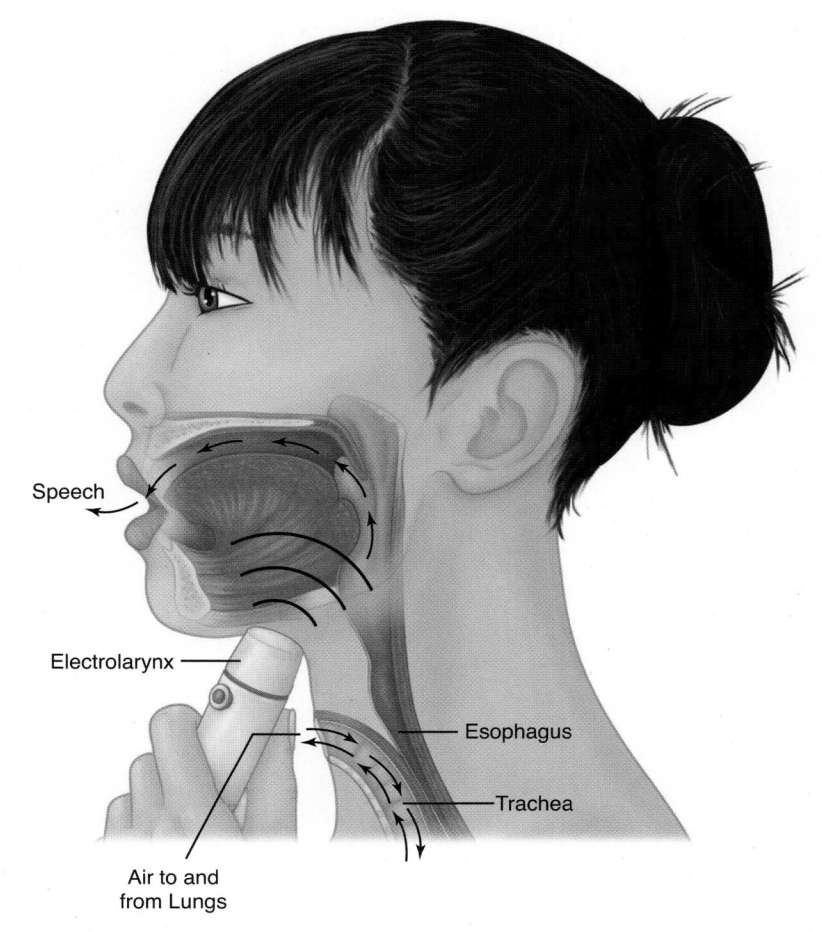

Speech

Electrolarynx

Esophagus

Trachea

Air to and
from Lungs

Figure 9–16

Representation of speech
being produced with a
neck-type electrolarynx.

© Cengage Learning 2013.

balloon closed for a second, and then releasing the hold slightly. The
walls of the balloon (esophagus) force the air out of the balloon and
through the mouth of the balloon (PE segment), producing a rather
raucous sound. The sound that the PE segment produces in the laryngectomee is then modified and resonated by the oropharyngeal and
oral cavities for speech. (A detailed discussion of the specifics of the
injection and inhalation methods of teaching esophageal speech is
beyond the scope of this text.)

Electrolarynx/Artificial Larynx

The use of an **electrolarynx (artificial larynx)** during the first few
days following surgery can provide patients a voice while healing, and
some individuals choose to continue using the device as their main
source of oral communication. There are a variety of brands and types
of artificial larynges and usually one or more will work well for a patient.
Most are neck-type devices with a vibrating source within the electrolarynx that produces the sound. The head of the device is placed against a
spot on the neck (sometimes called the "sweet spot") where the sound
is transferred into the pharyngeal region (see Figure 9–16). The sound in

**electrolarynx/artificial
larynx**

An electronic (battery powered)
device used by laryngectomees
that produces a vibrated
mechanical sound that is held
against the neck, with the sound
entering the pharynx and oral cavity
where it is articulated for speech.

the pharyngeal region moves into the oral cavity where it is articulated in a normal manner. When an electrolarynx is used, all sounds (vowels, voiced and unvoiced consonants) are voiced because of the continuous vibration of the electrolarynx; however, listeners fairly easily become accustomed to this continuous voicing, and most laryngectomees are at least moderately intelligible using an electrolarynx (Liu, Wan, Wang, & Niu, 2004; Watterson, Cox, & McFarlane, 1998).

Regardless of the method of speech a person eventually uses, all individuals with a laryngectomy benefit from counseling support provided by a speech-language pathologist. Patients undergo adjustment difficulties with acceptance of themselves as being cancer survivors, permanently losing their normal way of producing voice, their way of communicating with family and friends, social obstacles, and possible loss of employment they may have had for decades. These individuals benefit from meeting other individuals who have successfully adjusted to their laryngectomy and can encourage the new laryngectomee. Successful voice and speech rehabilitation includes the person's overall life adjustment, coping skills, and general well-being (Schuster et al., 2003).

EMOTIONAL AND SOCIAL EFFECTS OF VOICE DISORDERS

Our normal voices can reflect our emotions from moment to moment and our reactions to our voice disorders can cause us emotional distress. A person's facial expressions and voice are the two most important ways of communicating emotions. Because we know that our voices can reveal our feelings, we learn how to suppress emotionally charged cues. We want to communicate our thoughts but we do not always want to communicate all of the feelings behind our thoughts (Andrews, 2006; Rammage et al., 2001).

Young Children

Most preschool children with hyperfunctional voice disorders appear unaware of or unconcerned about the problems that clinicians hear. Voice therapy for young children is often deferred until they are in kindergarten or first grade; however, the parents may be counseled about how they can encourage their children to be less abusive to their voices when talking and playing. Even when children are in the early elementary grades they typically have little concern about the quality of their voices; to them, a hoarse voice is as acceptable as a clear voice. It is SLPs and perhaps ENT doctors and parents who have to try to instill in children enough emotional concern about their voice problems to motivate them to participate in therapy. As children get older they usually become increasingly aware of their voices and are better candidates for voice therapy (Andrews, 2006; Boone et al., 2009).

To change their behaviors, people of all ages need to be sufficiently emotionally concerned and engaged to carry out the often long-term tasks to accomplish the changes. This takes a level of emotional maturity, the cognitive abilities to understand the need for the changes, the memory to carry out the tasks, and the ability to accept delayed gratification ("If I do what I need to now, then later on I will have the rewards.").

Adolescents

It is usually during adolescence when children begin focusing on their every little imperfection that they begin to be concerned about their voices. Adolescent boys and girls may "yell their voices away" while cheering at football, soccer, or rugby games. In a way, the acute laryngitis they develop is a badge of honor—they had cheered their team on. It is only when adolescents develop chronic voice problems that interfere with verbal communication that they may be sufficiently motivated to follow a voice therapy regimen. However, adolescents are able to do much of their communicating now without their voices, using instant messages (IMs) on their computers and text messages on their mobile phones, which may have a secondary benefit of providing some voice rest.

Adolescent boys with falsetto voices may have serious emotional reactions to their voice disorders (most individuals with falsetto voices have sought help by early adulthood). The social penalties can be significant for adolescent boys and men who sound effeminate or child-like. They typically feel rejected and isolated, and are ridiculed by their peers. Because of the social penalties most individuals with falsetto voices are highly motivated and have good prognoses for change (Andrews, 2006; Boone et al., 2009; Peppard, 2000).

Adults

It is normal for the voice to change in some ways as a person grows older; however, normal voice changes should not be in the direction of a pathology (Stathopoulos, Huber, & Sessman, 2011). According to Boone (1997), approximately 25% of adults in the United States are displeased with the sound of their voices and believe that their social lives and/or careers have been affected. However, the incidence of voice disorders in the United States is estimated to be 3% to 9% of the adult population (Ramig & Verdolini, 1998). It is unknown whether some adults may attribute lack of social and/or career success to their voices, over which they may feel they have little control.

Many adults with hyperfunctional voice disorders have considerable stress in both their home and work place, and stressors in either location can contribute to a voice disorder. The voice is often a mirror of a person's reactions to what is going on in the person's life. As clinicians, our understanding of the voice's reflection of the person and of the human condition in general allows us to help many people regain their voices and then maintain them by better coping with life's vicissitudes.

holistic

A philosophic concept in which an entity (e.g., person) is seen as more than the sum of its parts; a prominent approach to psychology, biology, nursing, medicine, and other scientific, sociologic, and educational fields of study and practice (including speech-language pathology and audiology).

Application Question

If you ever had a voice disorder, what emotional effects do you recall it having on you?

By considering our clients and patients **holistically**, we can better address both the physical and emotional causes of their voice disorders and their reactions to their disorders (Merrill, Anderson, & Sloan, 2011).

CHAPTER SUMMARY

A voice disorder (dysphonia) occurs when the loudness, pitch, or quality is outside the normal range for voice use for a person's age, gender, or both. The quality of voice relies on multiple factors involving the anatomy and physiology of the respiratory system, the vocal folds, and the supra-glottal vocal tract resonating characteristics. Functional voice disorders usually are considered to be caused by faulty use of a normal vocal mechanism. Neurological voice disorders are related to the muscle control and innervation of the muscles of respiration and phonation. Organic voice disorders are related to some physical abnormality. With many cases of voice disorders, both functional and organic factors may be causing and maintaining the disorder. Hyperfunctional voice disorders refer to too much tension, intensity, breathiness, talking, vocal abuse and misuse, and too high of a pitch. Hypofunctional voice disorders refer to too low of intensity or pitch and too little vocal fold vibration. Some individuals have laryngectomy surgery to remove laryngeal cancer and must learn an alternative method of producing a functional voice. Our normal voices can reflect our emotions from moment to moment and our reactions to our voice disorders can cause us emotional distress.

STUDY QUESTIONS
Knowledge and Comprehension

1. Define voice disorder.
2. Explain hoarseness.
3. What is an otolaryngologist?
4. Why might the interview of a client with a voice disorder be sensitive?
5. What is acute (traumatic) laryngitis, and what are some common causes?

Application

1. Discuss why many voice disorders have both functional and organic components or factors that may be causing and maintaining the disorders.
2. What are some of the observations a clinician would want to make during an interview with a client who has a voice disorder?
3. Explain the use of the bell-shaped curve in understanding voice disorders.

4. Why is effective voice therapy an "ongoing, continuous evaluation process"?

5. Why are preschool children and many early elementary school children not good candidates for voice therapy?

Analysis/Synthesis

1. Discuss the similarities and differences between vocal abuse and vocal misuse.

2. Compare and contrast hyperfunction and hypofunction.

3. Discuss the similarities and differences between vocal nodules and contact ulcers.

4. What is meant by *perceptual, acoustic,* and *physiologic correlates* of the vocal folds?

5. Explain mutational falsetto (puberphonia) voice and why adolescents and young adults with falsetto voices may have serious emotional reactions to their voice disorders?

REFERENCES

Andrews, M. L. (2006). Manual of voice treatment: Pediatrics through geriatrics (3rd ed.). Clifton Park, NY: Delmar Cengage Learning.

ASHA. (2004a). Knowledge and skills for speech-language pathologists with respect to vocal tract visualization and imaging. *ASHA (Supplement 24),* 184–192.

ASHA. (2004b). Evaluation and treatment for tracheoesophageal puncture and prosthesis: Technical report. *ASHA (Supplement 24),* 135–139.

Back, G., & Sood, S. (2005). The management of early laryngeal cancer: Options for patients and therapists. *Current Opinions in Otolaryngology and Head and Neck Surgery, 13,* 85–91.

Baker, J. (2003). Psychogenic voice disorders and traumatic stress experience: A discussion paper with two case reports. *Journal of Voice, 17*(3), 308–313.

Belanger, H., Scott, S., Scholten, J., Curtiss, G., & Vanderploeg, R. (2005). Utility of mechanism-of-injury-based assessment and treatment: Blast injury program case illustration. *Journal of Rehabilitation Research and Development, 42*(4), 403–412.

Boone, D. R. (1997). *Is your voice telling on you* (2nd ed.). Clifton Park, NY: Delmar Cengage Learning.

Boone, D. R., McFarlane, S. C., & Von Berg, S. L. (2009). *The voice and voice therapy* (8th ed.). Boston, MA: Pearson Allyn and Bacon.

Brown, D. H., Hilgers, F., Irish, J., & Balm, A. (2003). Postlaryngectomy voice rehabilitation: State of the art at the millennium. *World Journal of Surgery, 27*(7), 824–831.

Case, J. L. (2002). *Clinical management of voice disorders* (4th ed.). Austin, TX: Pro-Ed.

Casper, J., Clark, W., Kelley, R., & Colton, R. (2002). Laryngeal and phonatory status after burn/inhalation injury: A long-term follow-up study. *Journal of Burn Care and Rehabilitation, 23*(4), 235–243.

Colton, R. H., Casper, J. K., & Leonard, R. (2011). *Understanding voice problems: A physiological perspective for diagnosis and treatment* (4th ed.). Philadelphia, PA: Lippincott Williams & Wilkins.

Curry, R. (1940). *The mechanism of the human voice.* New York, NY: Longmans, Green & Co.

Duff, M. C., Proctor, A., & Yairi, E. (2004). Prevalence of voice disorders in African American and European American preschoolers. *Journal of Voice, 18*(3), 348–353.

Ferrand, C. T. (2012). *Voice disorders: Scope of theory and practice.* San Antonio, Tx: Pearson/Allyn & Bacon.

Fink, R. (1975). *The human larynx: A functional study.* New York, NY: Raven Press.

Flasher, L. V., & Fogle, P. T. (2012). *Counseling skills for speech-language pathologists and audiologists* (2nd ed.). Clifton Park, NY: Delmar Cengage Learning.

Haller, R. M., & Thompson, E. A. (1975). Prevalence of speech, language, and hearing disorders among Harlem children. *Journal of the National Medical Association, 4*, 299–306.

Haslinger, B., Erhard, P., Dresel, C., Castrop, F., Roettinger, M., & Ceballos-Baumann, A. (2005). Silent event-related fMRI reveals reduced sensorimotor activation in laryngeal dystonia. *Otolaryngology—Head and Neck Surgery, 133*(5), 654–656.

Holland, R. W., & DeJarnette, G. (2002). Voice and voice disorders. In D. Battle (Ed.). *Communication Disorders in Multicultural Populations* (3rd ed.). Boston, MA: Butterworth-Heinemann.

Kleinsasser, N., Priemer, F., Schulze, W., & Kleinsasser, O. (2000). External trauma to the larynx: Classification, diagnosis, therapy. *European Archives of Oto-Rhino-Laryngology, 257*(8), 439–444.

Lindman, J., Gibbons, M., Morleir, R., & Wiatrak, B. (2004). Voice quality of prepubescent children with quiescent recurrent respiratory papillomatosis. *International Journal of Pediatric Otorhinolaryngology, 68*(5), 529–536.

Liu, H., Wan, M., Wang, S., & Niu, H. (2004). Aerodynamic characteristics of laryngectomee breathing quality and speaking with the electrolarynx. *Journal of Voice, 18*(4), 567–577.

Loughran, S., Alves, C., & MacGregor, F. B. (2002). Current etiology of unilateral vocal fold paralysis in a teaching hospital in the West of Scotland. *Journal of Laryngology and Otology, 116*(11), 907–910.

MacKenzie, K., Millar, A., Wilson, J., Sellars, C., & Deary, I. (2001). Is voice therapy an effective treatment for dysphonia? A randomized controlled trial. *British Medical Journal, 323*, 658–663.

Marchant, H., Supiot, F., Choufani, G., & Hassid, S. (2003). Bilateral vocal fold palsy caused by chronic axonal neuropathy. *Journal of Laryngology and Otology, 117*(5), 414–416.

Merrill, R. M., Anderson, A. E., & Sloan, A. (2011). Quality of life indicators according to voice disorders and voice-related conditions. *Laryngoscope, 121*(9), 2004–2010.

Mirza, N., Ruiz, C., Baum, E. D., & Staub, J. P. (2003). The prevalence of major psychiatric pathologies in patients with voice disorders. *Ear, Nose, and Throat Journal, 82*(10), 808–814.

Peppard, R. C. (2000). Functional falsetto. In J. C. Stemple (Ed.), *Voice Therapy: Clinical Studies*. Clifton Park, NY: Delmar Cengage Learning.

Ramig, L. O., & Verdolini, K. (1998). Treatment efficacy: Voice disorders. *Journal of Speech-Language-Hearing Research, 41*, 101–116.

Rammage, L., Morrison, M., & Nichol, H. (2001). *Management of the voice and its disorders* (2nd ed.). Clifton Park, NY: Delmar Cengage Learning.

Rees, C. J., & Belafsky, P. C. (2008). Laryngopharyngeal reflux. In R. Leonard & K. Kendall (Eds.), *Dysphagia assessment and treatment: A team approach*. San Diego, CA: Plural Publishing.

Rubin, J. S., & Sataloff, R. T. (2006). *Diagnosis and treatment of voice disorders* (3rd ed.). San Diego, CA: Plural Publishing.

Sataloff, R. T. (Ed.). (2005). *Professional voice: The science and art of clinical care* (3rd ed.). Clifton Park, NY: Delmar Cengage Learning.

Scherer, R. C. (2006). Laryngeal function during phonation. In J. S. Rubin & R. T. Sataloff (Eds.), *Diagnosis and treatment of voice disorders* (3rd ed.). San Diego, CA: Plural Publishing.

Schuster, M., Lohscheller, J., Kummer, P., Hoppe, U., Eysholdt, U., & Rosanowski, F. (2003). Quality of life in laryngectomees after prosthetic voice restoration. *Folia Phoniatrica, 55*(5), 211–219.

Schweinfurth, J. M., Billante, M., & Courey, M. S. (2002). Risk factors and demographics in patients with spasmodic dysphonia. *Laryngoscope, 112*(2), 220–223.

Segas, J., Stravroulakis, P., Monolopoulos, L., Yiotakis, J., & Adamopoulus, G. (2001). Management of bilateral vocal fold paralysis: Experience at the University of Athens. *Otolaryngology—Head and Neck Surgery, 124*, 68–71.

Seikel, J. A., King, D. W., & Drumright, D. G. (2010). *Anatomy & physiology for speech, language, and hearing* (4th ed.). Clifton Park, NY: Delmar Cengage Learning.

Shipley, K. G., & McAfee, J. G. (2009). *Assessment in speech-language pathology: A resource manual* (4th ed.). Clifton Park, NY: Delmar Cengage Learning.

Shrivastav, R., & Sapienza, C. (2003). Objective measures of breathy voice quality obtained during an auditory model. *Journal of Acoustical Society of America, 114*(4), 2217–2224.

Simonyan, K., & Ludlow, C. L. (2010). Abnormal activation of the primary somatosensory cortex in spasmodic dysphonia: An fMRI study. *Cerebral Cortex 20*(11), 2749–2759.

Stathopoulos, E. T., Huber, J. E., & Sessman, J. E. (2011). Changes in acoustic characteristics of the voice across the life span: Measures from individuals 4–92 years of age. *Journal of Speech, Language, and Hearing Research, 54,* 1011–1021.

Stemple, J., Glaze, L., & Klaben, B. (2009). *Clinical voice pathology* (4th ed.). San Diego, CA: Plural Publishing.

Stevenson, S., & Guthrie, G. (1949). *A history of otolaryngology.* Edinburgh, Scotland: E. & S. Livingston.

Stewart, B. W., & Semmler, P. C. (2002). Establishing causation of laryngeal cancer by environmental tobacco smoke. *Medical Journal of Australia, 176,* 113–116.

Sulica, L. (2004). Contemporary management of spasmodic dysphonia. *Current Opinion in Otolaryngology & Head and Neck Surgery, 12*(6), 543–548.

Swigert, N. B. (2005). *The source for children's voice disorders.* East Moline, IL: Lingui Systems.

Titze, I. R. (2000). *Principles of voice production* (2nd ed.). Iowa City, IA: National Center for Voice and Speech.

Watterson, T. L., Cox, T., & McFarlane, S. C. (1998). Speech intelligibility using four different electric-neck larynges. *Phonoscope, 1,* 21–26.

Woo, P. (2006). *Stroboscopy.* San Diego, CA: Plural Publishing.

Wright, J. (1941). *A history of laryngology and rhinology* (2nd ed.). Philadelphia, PA: Lea and Febiger.

Zeitels, S. M., Jarboe, J., & Franco, R. A. (2001). Phonosurgical reconstruction of early glottic cancer. *The Laryngoscope, 111*(10), 1862–1865.

Zhang, Z. F., & Jiang, J. J. (2004). Chaotic vibration of a vocal fold model with a unilateral polyp. *The Journal of the Acoustical Society of America, 115*(3), 1266–1269.

Zhang, Z. F., Morgenstern, H., & Spitz, M. R. (2000). Environmental tobacco smoke, mutant sensitivity and head and neck squamous cell carcinoma. *Cancer Epidemiology Biomarkers Prevention, 9,* 1043–1049.

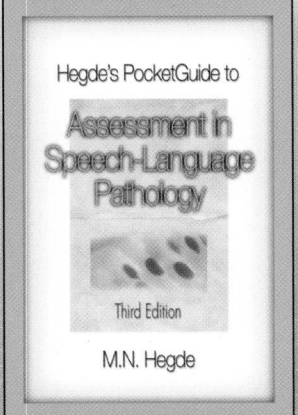
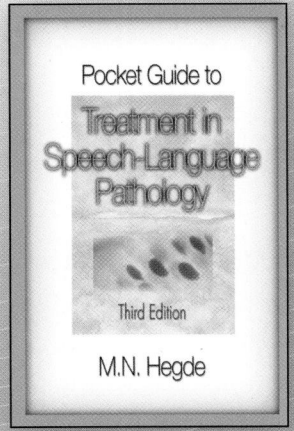
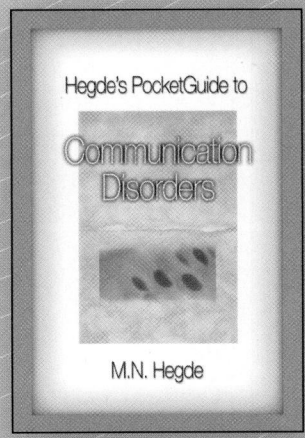
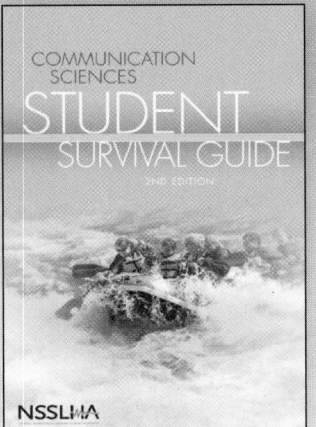

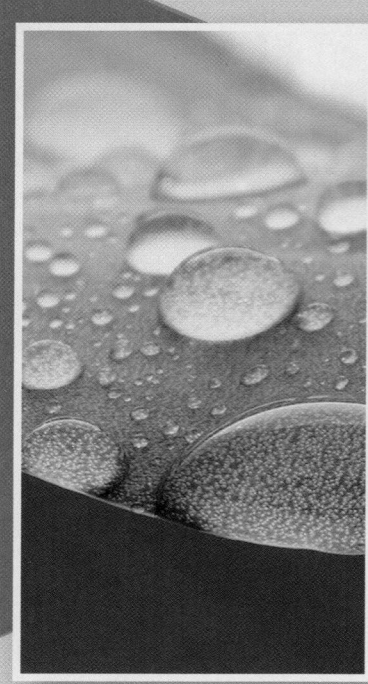

CHAPTER 10
Cleft Lip and Palate

LEARNING OBJECTIVES

After studying this chapter, you will:

- Know how to describe the various types of clefts of the lip and palates.

- Be able to discuss the anomalies and disorders associated with clefts.

- Understand the need for a team approach to help the child and family.

- Be aware of the complexity of cleft lip and palate repair.

- Understand the involvement of the speech-language pathologist from the formation of the team into, in some cases, the patient's adulthood.

- Describe common speech-language pathology evaluation techniques.

- Be familiar with general therapy techniques for children with structurally competent velopharyngeal mechanisms to help them use more normal oral resonance.

- Understand some of the emotional and social effects of a child's cleft lip or palate on the parents and the child.

KEY TERMS

anesthesia
atrophy
cul-de-sac resonance
denasal/denasality
Eustachian (auditory) tube
glottal stops
hypernasal/hypernasality

hyponasal/hyponasality
interdisciplinary team
intraoral breath pressure
nasal air emission/nasal escape
nasometer
nasopharyngoscopy
palatal fistula

KEY TERMS continued

palatal lift

palatal obturator

palatoplasty

pharyngeal fricatives

pharyngoplasty

pressure-airflow technique

prosthetic device (prosthesis)

rule of 10s

social worker

speech bulb obturator

submucous cleft

teratogen

velopharyngeal incompetence
(inadequacy, insufficiency,
dysfunction)

CHAPTER OUTLINE

Introduction

Etiologies of Cleft Lip and Palate

Clefts of the Lip and Alveolar Ridge

Clefts of the Hard and Soft Palates

   Submucous Clefts

Multicultural Considerations

Associated Problems with Cleft Lip and Palate

   Feeding

   Hearing

   Dental Anomalies

   Resonance Disorders

   Articulation and Phonological Disorders

   Language Delays and Differences

Surgical Management of Cleft Lip and Palate

   Cleft Lip and Nose Repair

   Primary Surgery for Cleft Palate Repair

Speech and Resonance Evaluation

   Noninstrumental Tests

   Instrumental Procedures

Speech Therapy

   The First Years

   Preschool Through School Age

Speech Appliances (Prosthetic Devices, Prostheses)

Multicultural Considerations

Emotional and Social Effects of Cleft Lip and Palate

   Parents' Initial Shock and Adjustment

   Children's Preschool and Early Elementary School Years

   School-Age Years

   Adolescents

   Adults

Chapter Summary

Study Questions

References

INTRODUCTION

Hippocrates (400 B.C.) mentioned cleft lip but not cleft palate in his writings. For centuries clefts were considered to be caused by syphilis, and it was not until 1556 that Pierre Franco recognized that clefts of the lip and palate were congenital disorders. Cleft lip is sometimes referred to as "harelip," a term now considered inaccurate and insensitive. The term originated in the 16th century when a French doctor referred to a patient with a cleft as having the "lip of a hare [rabbit]," which was later shortened in English to "harelip." During the dark ages of history and into the 17th century, there was superstition that children born with cleft lips were born to women who, when pregnant, were frightened by the devil, who had assumed the shape of a hare. A woman who gave birth to an infant with a cleft lip was assumed to have had relations with the devil, and both she and the infant were put to death.

A variety of clefts can occur. Some clefts affect just the lip, either unilaterally or bilaterally; others affect the hard palate; and still others affect just the soft palate. The most severe clefts occur when all three structures are involved. One other form of cleft may occur when the mucosal tissue covering the hard palate is intact but there is a small hole (*fistula*) in the hard palate. A cleft of any type is not painful to the infant because the cleft is not a wound but a malformation; therefore, the tissue around the cleft is not tender or sore to touch.

The latest worldwide data (30 countries) from the WHO reveals that the overall prevalence of cleft lip and/or cleft palate is approximately 1 in 1,000 births (9.92 per 10,000) (International Perinatal Database of Typical Oral Clefts, 2011).

Hippocrates

Hippocrates (460–377 B.C.) was a Greek physician. He is called the "father of medicine" because he introduced a scientific approach to healing by seeking physical causes of disease rather than magic, superstition, possession of evil spirits, or disfavor of the gods. He also compiled case records of illnesses, including results of treatments administered, and developed the art of ethical bedside care. He believed that the body must be treated as a whole and not just a series of parts (the beginning of *holistic* [wholistic] medicine, a philosophic approach that considers a person is more than the sum of his parts). He believed in the natural healing process of rest, good diet, fresh air, and cleanliness. He was also the first physician to hold the belief that thoughts, ideas, and feelings come from the brain and not the heart (Asimov, 1982).

The "Hippocratic oath" is attributed to Hippocrates and serves as an ethical guide for all medical professions, including speech-language pathology and audiology. The oath reads, in part, as follows (Collier, 1910):

To consider dear to me as my parents him who taught me this art . . . I will prescribe regimen for the good of my patients according to my ability and my judgment and never do harm to anyone. . . . In every house where I come I will enter only for the good of my patients, keeping myself far from all intentional ill-doing. . . . All that may come to my knowledge in the exercise of my profession or outside of my profession or in daily commerce with men, which ought not to be spread abroad, I will keep secret and will never reveal. If I keep this oath faithfully, may I enjoy my life and practice my art, respected by all men and in all times, but if I depart from it or violate it, may the contrary be my lot.

Note: The basis of the ASHA Code of Ethics is the Hippocratic Oath.

ETIOLOGIES OF CLEFT LIP AND PALATE

No single cause or etiological model can explain the occurrence of cleft lip, cleft palate, or both. Clefts may be caused by single genes, chromosomal disorders, or intrauterine environmental factors. A cleft is a feature in more than 300 genetic syndromes (e.g., Apert syndrome, Crouzon syndrome, Pfeiffer syndrome, Pierre Robin sequence, Rett syndrome, Stickler syndrome, Treacher Collins syndrome, and velocardiofacial syndrome). When a child has a cleft lip, cleft palate, or both, it is reasonable to consider the possibility that a syndrome is involved. Likewise, when a child has a syndrome, it is wise to look closely for any type of clefting. People without syndromes may have clefts and their clefts may be the result of a single *mutant* (abnormal) gene (Sekhon, Ethunandan, Markus, Krishnan, & Rao, 2011; Mitchell & Risch, 1992).

Most human traits, however, are *multifactorial;* that is, there are probably several genes, possibly combined with environmental factors (e.g., maternal nutrition), that determine the expression of traits such as height, hair color, and eye color, as well as intelligence and other cognitive traits. The multifactorial model suggests that there is a "threshold" at which sufficient predisposing factors (genetic and environmental) cause an abnormality to occur, whether it is a cleft or some other abnormality. The multifactorial model is widely accepted as an explanation of clefts without accompanying syndromes (Peterson-Falzone, Hardin-Jones, & Karnell, 2010; Rahimov, Jugessur, & Murray, 2012).

During the first trimester of pregnancy, the embryo is particularly vulnerable to the influences of harmful agents or **teratogens**, including cigarettes, alcohol, drugs, and some medications (e.g., antiseizure medications) (Diehl & Erickson, 1997; Ericson, Kallen, & Westeholm, 1979; Khoury, Gomez-Farias, & Mulinare, 1989; Koren, Pastuszak, & Ito, 1998; Sampson, 2000). Peterson-Falzone et al. (2010) state that the influence of various illegal drugs on the incidence of birth defects has been under investigation for years. Many babies with structural (e.g., clefts) and neurological deficits have parents who abuse multiple substances

teratogen

Any substance, agent, or process that interferes with prenatal development, causing the formation of one or more developmental abnormalities in a fetus.

(tobacco, alcohol, marijuana, cocaine, heroin, etc.). For this reason, it is nearly impossible to segregate the effects of these various substances. Maternal nutritional deficiencies have been implicated in causing clefts and other malformations. In particular, inadequate folic acid in the maternal diet may affect embryonic and fetal development (Rosenblatt, 1995).

CLEFTS OF THE LIP AND ALVEOLAR RIDGE

Recall that the central (*median*) and side (*lateral*) portions of the upper lip have fused by eight weeks gestation and have formed the three segments of the lip: left side, middle (philtrum), and right side (the small philtril ridges are the fusion lines). There are various types of cleft lip and different degrees of severity. An *incomplete cleft lip* can be as minor as a small notch in the lip tissue with no involvement of the alveolar ridge (see Figure 10–1a). In more severe cases, the cleft may extend on one side through what would have been the philtral ridge up to the floor of the nostril (*unilateral complete cleft lip*) (Figure 10–1b and 10–1c). More severe yet is when there are clefts through both sides of the lip that extend to the floor of the nostrils (*bilateral complete cleft lip*) (Figure 10–1d). The more severe the cleft of the lip, the more likely the alveolar ridge will be involved as well as the hard and soft palates. When a bilateral cleft lip extends through the alveolar ridge, the tissue that would have formed the philtrum and alveolus is often a mass that protrudes and may cover the nostrils. In these cases, the nose is often involved and is wide, flat, and malformed.

In a cleft lip, the orbicularis oris muscle that forms the upper lip is divided and misaligned as it curves upward with the cleft. A cleft lip that extends through the alveolar ridge results in disunity of the orbicularis oris muscle in unilateral, and more severely in bilateral, clefts. Clefting can affect an infant's ability to suck and nurse. If a cleft lip is not repaired in infancy (as is the case in many countries around the world), articulation can be affected where the child is not able to develop normal **intraoral breath pressure** to produce pressure consonant sounds such as plosives (e.g., /p/, /b/), fricatives (e.g., /f/, /th/, /z/, /sh/), and affricates (e.g., /ch/). Numerous complicated dental anomalies, including missing teeth, rotated teeth, and misaligned teeth, require the services of dentists and orthodontists (see Figure 10–1e).

intraoral breath pressure

A buildup of air pressure in the oral cavity that provides the force for the production of oral consonants, particularly plosives, fricatives, and affricates.

CLEFTS OF THE HARD AND SOFT PALATES

Between the 8 and 12 weeks of gestation, the roof of the mouth is formed and fused together with the fusion occurring in an anterior to posterior direction (see Chapter 3, Figure 3–8). This direction of fusion allows for normal development of the anterior portions of the hard and soft palates

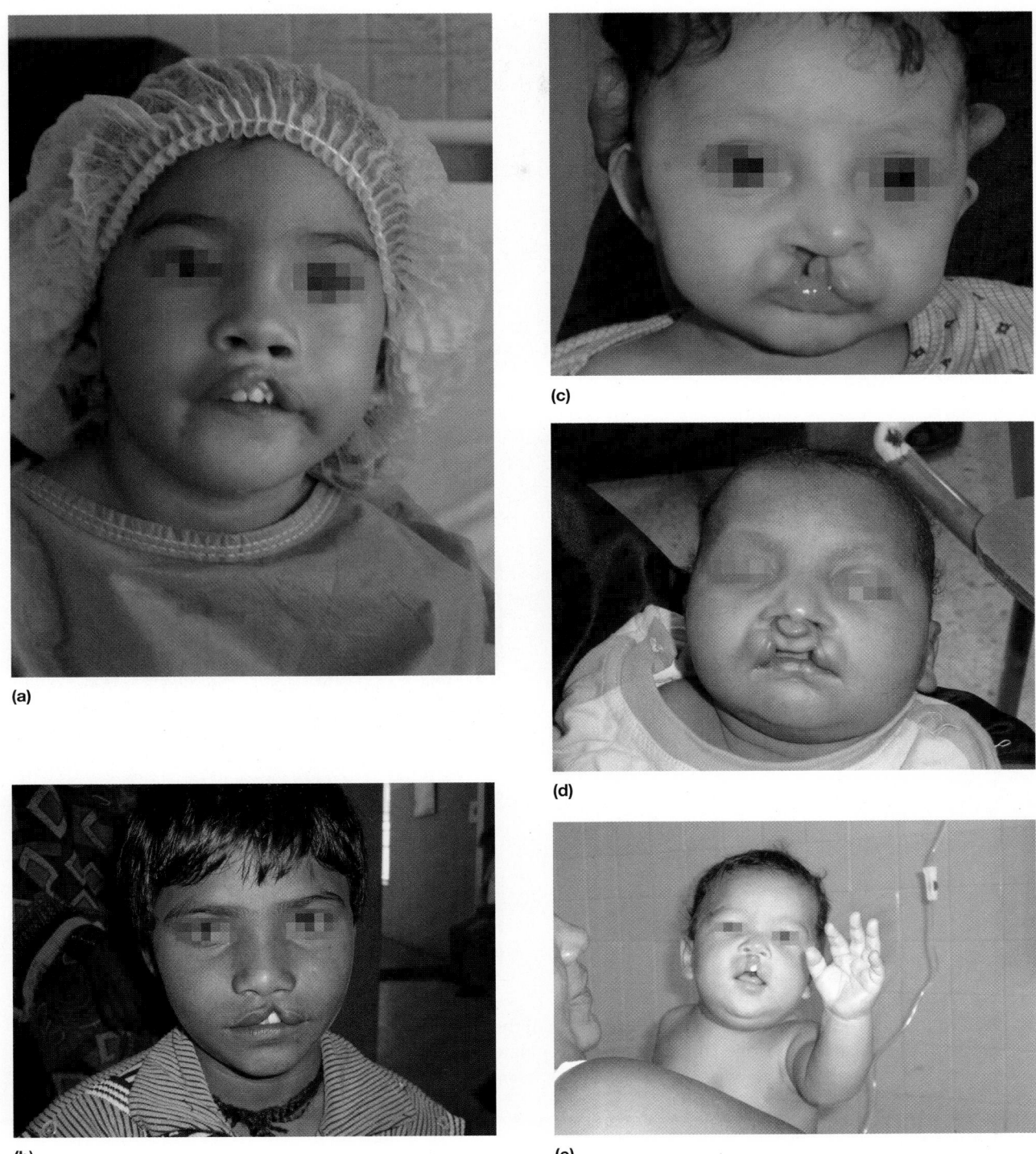

(a)

(b)

(c)

(d)

(e)

Figure 10–1

(a) Mild incomplete unilateral cleft left. (b) Unilateral complete cleft lip. (c) Unilateral complete cleft of the lip and alveolar ridge. (d) Bilateral complete cleft lip. (e) Dental anomalies are common with cleft lips and palates.

Source: All images courtesy of Paul Fogle, Ph.D., Rotaplast (Rotary) International Cleft Palate Missions, Cumaná, Venezuela, 2008, Sohag, Egypt, 2010, Nagamangala, India, 2011.

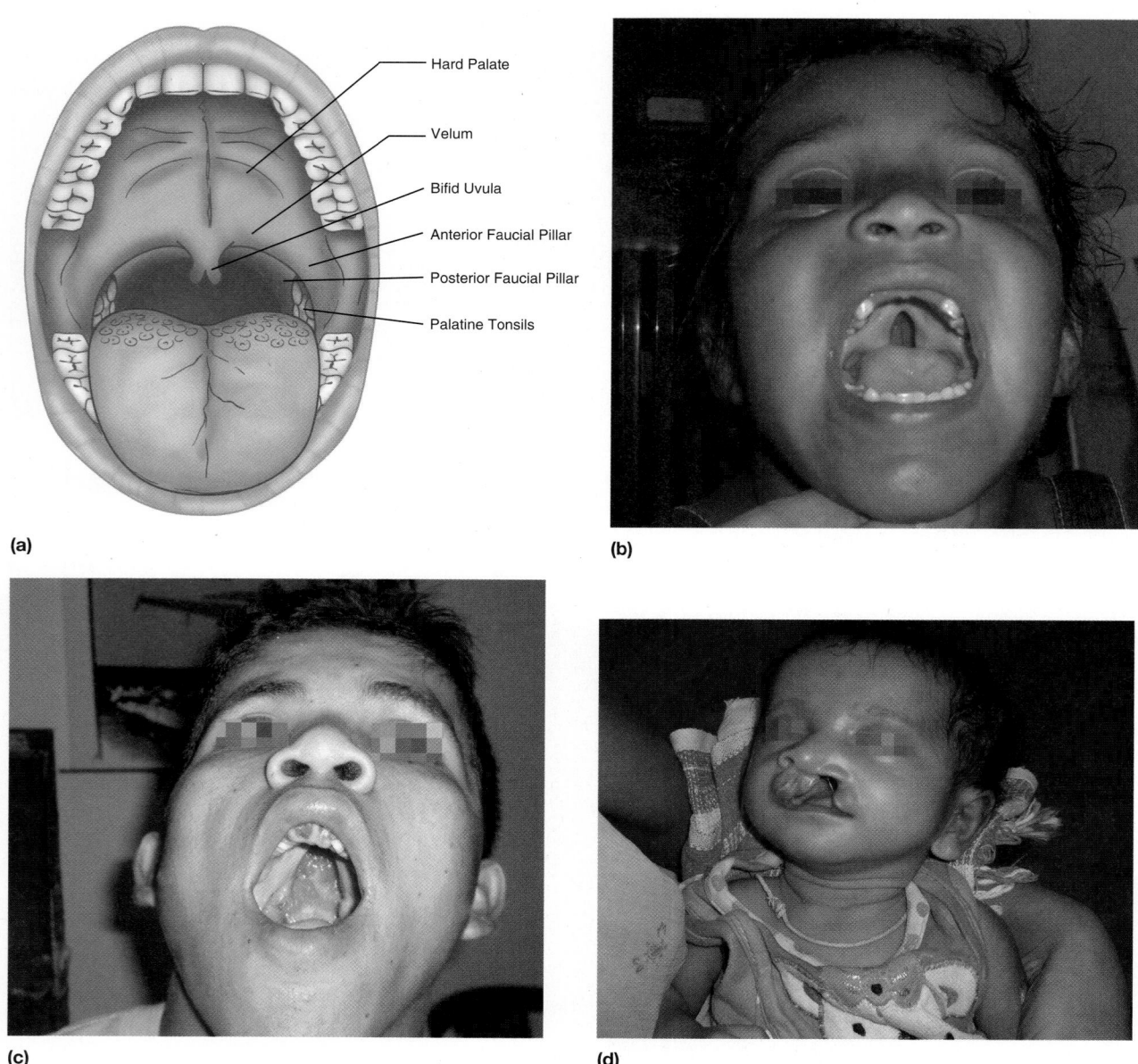

Figure 10-2

(a) A bifid uvula. (b) Cleft of the soft palate. (c) Clefts of the hard and soft palates—*complete cleft palate*.
(d) Clefts of the lip, alveolar ridge, and hard and soft palates.

Source: Image (a) © Cengage Learning 2013; Images (b) through (d) courtesy of Paul Fogle, Ph.D., Rotaplast (Rotary) International Cleft Palate Missions, Cumaná, Venezuela, 2008, Sohag, Egypt, 2010, Nagamangala, India, 2011.

and only a minor defect of the uvula, resulting in a *bifid uvula* (divided uvula) (see Figure 10–2a). Clefts of the soft palate may occur (Figure 10–2b), of the hard and soft palates (referred to as a *complete cleft palate*) (Figure 10–2c), of the alveolar ridge and hard and soft palates, or of the lip, alveolar ridge and hard and soft palates (Figure 10–2d).

A cleft of the soft palate results in *velopharyngeal inadequacy/ insufficiency* (i.e., the palate does not have adequate or sufficient tissue to make contact with the posterior pharyngeal wall), which results in **velopharyngeal incompetence (VPI)** and is heard as hypernasal speech. In the literature on cleft palate and velopharyngeal closure, the terms velopharyngeal "incompetence," "inadequacy," "insufficiency," and "dysfunction" are often used interchangeably (Peterson-Falzone et al., 2010).

Submucous Clefts

A **submucous cleft** (sometimes referred to as *occult submucous cleft*) is a defect in the hard palate in the absence of an actual opening into the nasal cavity; that is, the mucosal tissue of the palate covers the defect. A defect in the muscles of the soft palate that cannot be seen through the mucosal tissue also may be considered a submucous cleft (Peterson-Falzone et al., 2010). Indications that a submucous cleft may be present are a bifid uvula and a bluish tint in the midline of the soft palate. Although the hard and soft palates may appear intact, there may be some disunity of the muscles of the soft palate that results in velopharyngeal incompetence and hypernasality. However, some individuals do not have any noticeable speech problems and the submucous cleft may go undetected throughout life.

Famous People with Repaired Clefts

There are several contemporary famous people with repaired cleft lips, cleft palates, or both, including Blaise Winter (football player); Jesse Jackson (reverend and politician); Cheech Marin (actor and comedian, in comic duo Cheech and Chong); Gale Gordon (actor); Nikki Payne (comedian from Canada); Jason Robards (actor); Lee Raymond (CEO of Exxon); Mary Crosby (actress, daughter of Bing Crosby); Nick Palmer (British Member of Parliament); Rita McNeil (country-western singer); Joaquin Phoenix (actor); Stacy Keach (actor who always wore a heavy mustache); Tom Brokaw (TV news anchor); and Tom Burke (British actor).

MULTICULTURAL CONSIDERATIONS

Vanderas (1987) examined the literature on *epidemiological* (study of the determinants of diseases or disorders in populations) studies of cleft lip, cleft palate, and cleft lip and cleft palate in African Americans, American Indians, Chinese, and Japanese using both U.S. and international studies. Clefts vary in different racial groups, but in general there are twice as many clefts in Asians than in Caucasians and twice as many clefts in Caucasians than in blacks (Chung & Kau, 1985; Vanderas, 1987; Peterson-Falzone et al., 2010). The causes of the variations of incidence of cleft lip and palate among various racial groups have not been clearly determined.

Application Question

If you were a new mother or father and your newborn infant with a bilateral cleft lip was presented to you for the first time, what do you think your reaction would be?

velopharyngeal incompetence (inadequacy, insufficiency, dysfunction)

A term generally used to describe abnormal velopharyngeal function, regardless of the cause (i.e., an anatomical or structural defect [e.g., a cleft] or a neuromotor or physiological disorder [e.g., weakness of the soft palate caused by a CVA or TBI]) that typically results in hypernasality and/or nasal emission; various authors use different terms, such as *incompetence*, *inadequacy*, *insufficiency*, and *dysfunction*.

submucous cleft

A defect in the hard palate in the absence of an actual opening into the nasal cavity or a defect in the muscles of the soft palate that cannot be seen through the mucosal tissue but may cause disunity of the velar muscles, resulting in velopharyngeal incompetence and hypernasality.

Personal Story

Working with Philanthropic Organizations

I have been involved with philanthropic organizations that provide cleft lip and palate care to infants, children, adolescents, and adults in countries around the world. These organizations send complete teams to hospitals, including plastic surgeons, anesthesiologists, surgical and recovery room nurses (my wife Carol, a recovery nurse, was on a mission to Sohag, Egypt in 2010), pediatricians, dentists, a speech-language pathologist, and nonmedical volunteers such as instrument sterilizers, logisticians, team directors, and others. The working conditions are always less than ideal, including no air conditioning (except for surgical suites), unsterile work areas, ventilation provided by open windows that allow dust, dirt, and insects into work areas, and long hours—usually 12- to 14-hour days for a typical two-week "mission" (see Figure 10–3). In this setting, team members from different countries quickly build a sense of camaraderie and pride for providing assistance to those who would never have surgical and speech management of their clefts without their help.

If the SLP does not speak the language of the country, a translator works with the SLP during all interactions with patients and family members. Most countries have speech-language pathologists who also act as translators. The SLP's roles typically include evaluating and helping determine the best candidates (*triage*) for surgery, working with family members prior to and after the patient's surgery, instructing families about feeding techniques post-surgery to help prevent damaging the sutured areas, providing parents information about speech and language development, and helping the surgeons evaluate the success of the surgical repairs of the palates.

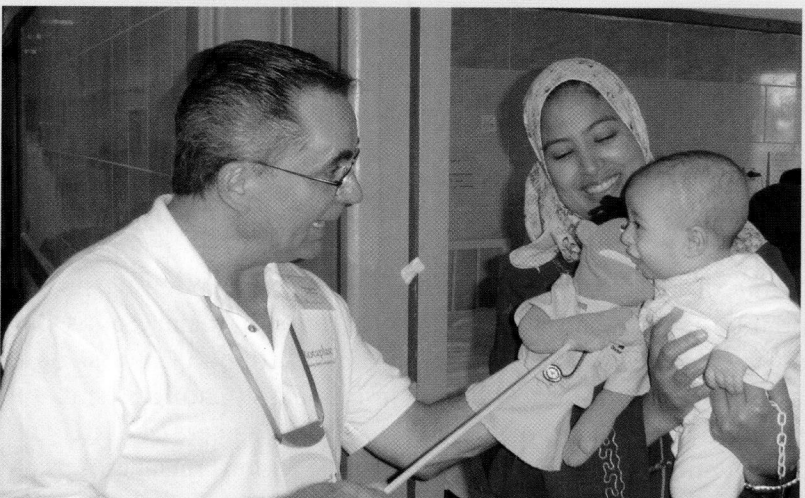

Figure 10–3

Dr. Fogle with mother, child, and "Mohammed" in Sohag, Egypt, 2010.

Paul Fogle, Ph.D., Rotaplast (Rotary) International Cleft Palate Mission, Sohag, Egypt, 2010.

Teaching and training resident SLPs and providing inservices and workshops for SLPs and medical staff is often a part of missions. SLPs who want to be members of international teams need considerable expertise and experience working with individuals who have cleft lips and palates. Several philanthropic organizations provide cleft lip and palate and oral–facial anomaly surgery in many parts of the world. Examples include Operation Smile (www.operationsmile.org); Rotaplast International Cleft Palate Team (www.rotaplast.org); and Smile Train (www.smiletrain.org). ■

Culture and country of origin must be considered when developing a complete profile of people with clefts. In many cases, these factors influence families' attitudes toward treatment and even the availability of treatment (Middleton & Pannbacker, 1997). In some developing countries, treatment for cleft lip and palate may be a relatively low priority because of economics, availability of treatment, and other factors. In addition, social, cultural, and religious attitudes about birth defects affect both societal willingness to provide medical treatment to individuals with all types of disabilities and individual willingness to seek treatment (Strauss, 1985).

Because of individual, family, cultural, and socioeconomic differences, it is important for the cleft palate team to be sensitive to the family's culture and values and to listen carefully to the parents' perceptions about the cause of the cleft, preferred treatments, and expectations for improvement (Mollar & Glaze, 2009; Strauss, 1991). However, it is important to avoid stereotyping individuals' attitudes based on their cultural identity. Not all individuals adhere to traditional values and beliefs, and these values and beliefs may be influenced by, among other things, a person's or a family's level of education and acculturation into a society. It is, therefore, important not only to understand the beliefs of a cultural group but also to understand how closely the family identifies with and subscribes to these beliefs (Salas-Provance, 2012).

ASSOCIATED PROBLEMS WITH CLEFT LIP AND PALATE

Feeding difficulties, middle ear infections, and dental anomalies are some of the myriad problems associated with cleft lip and palate. Resonance disorders caused by velopharyngeal incompetence are the hallmarks of cleft palate. Speech and language problems are common for children with clefts, particularly when associated with syndromes (e.g., Treacher Collins syndrome and Pierre-Robin sequence). Even after surgical management of a cleft palate, many children are left with some velopharyngeal dysfunction that can significantly affect speech intelligibility.

Feeding

Difficulty or inability to feed efficiently is an immediate problem for infants born with cleft lip, cleft palate, or both. Severe clefts present significant oral feeding problems, resulting in low volumes of oral intake, decreased nutrition, and poor weight gain (Kummer, 2008; Redford-Badwal, Mabry, & Frassinelli, 2003). Adequate nutrition and weight gain are necessary before lip and palatal surgery can be performed. Infants born with clefts resulting in feeding problems may have other pediatric feeding and swallowing problems that can complicate the already-challenging task of acquiring adequate nutrition for growth and weight gain. Such problems include gastroesophageal and gastrointestinal tract disorders, respiratory disorders, central and peripheral nervous system damage, and cardiac defects, particularly when syndromes are involved (see Chapter 12, "Normal Swallow Function and Dysphagia," for more information).

Feeding problems for these infants typically include poor oral suction, poor intake that causes inadequate nutrition, lengthy feeding times, excessive energy expenditure, *nasal regurgitation* (reflux of milk or other material into the nasopharynx and nasal cavity during feeding), gagging, choking, excessive air intake, discomfort with feeding, and stressful feeding interactions between the infant and the caregivers (Carlisle, 1998; Kummer, 2008).

New mothers have to learn specialized feeding techniques for the infant to receive sufficient nutrition for growth and health. No single feeding method is successful for infants with clefts. A variety of special bottles and nipples are commercially available to help with feeding problems. Feeding specialists (including speech-language pathologists trained and specialized in this area) can help mothers find the best method of providing nutrition to their infants.

Hearing

Children with various craniofacial anomalies may have ear deformities, particularly when syndromes are involved. The *auricle* (outer ear) as well as the middle ear and *ossicles* (3 small bones in the middle ear) may be abnormally formed. Conductive hearing losses are common. The maxilla and mandible also may be severely deformed, typically on one side. The facial nerve may be damaged unilaterally, resulting in weak or flaccid muscles on one side of the face.

Middle Ear Infections

Infants and children with cleft palates are considered to be at high risk for *otitis media* (*middle ear infections*) and associated conductive hearing loss (Kwan, Abdullah, Liu, van Hasselt, & Tong, 2011; Antonelli, Jorge, Feniman, et al., 2011). (Hearing loss is discussed in detail in Chapter 14.)

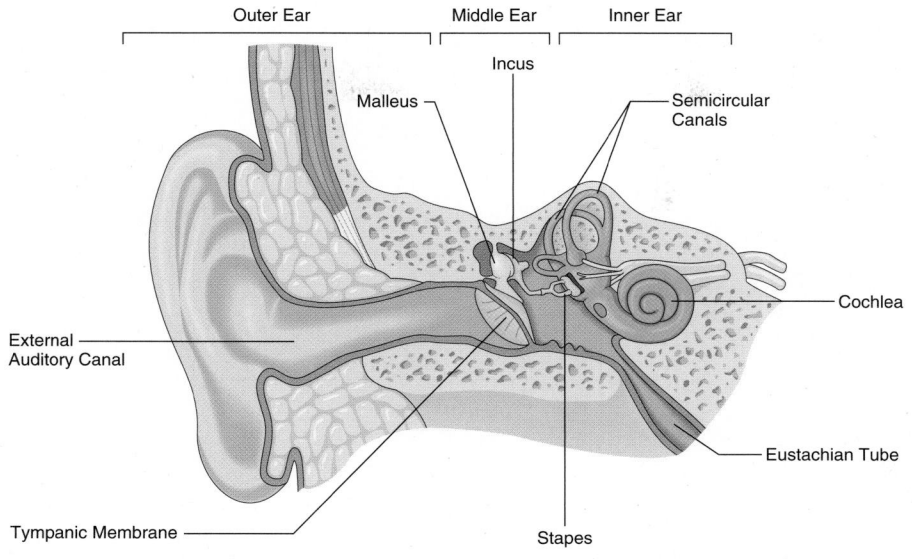

| Outer Ear | Middle Ear | Inner Ear |

Incus

Malleus — — Semicircular Canals

— Cochlea

External Auditory Canal

— Eustachian Tube

Tympanic Membrane — — Stapes

Figure 10-4

Eustachian (auditory) tube and the ear.

© Cengage Learning 2013.

The otitis media is the result of malfunction of the **Eustachian (auditory) tubes** that connect the nasopharynx to the middle ear (see Figure 10–4).

Dental Anomalies

Cleft lip and palate can contribute to dental anomalies (Kummer, 2008; Al Jamal, Hazza, & Rawashdeh, 2010). One of the most common problems is missing teeth. One or more teeth are often absent from clefts in the alveolar ridge; however, when teeth are present, they may be smaller than normal, misshapen, or malformed. Children with clefts have various problems with their bite as a result of maxillary and mandibular misalignment. *Pedodontists* (dentists who specialize in children) and *orthodontists* are essential professionals on the cleft palate team (see Figure 10–5).

Resonance Disorders

Resonance is the quality of the voice that results from the vibration of sound in the pharynx, oral cavity, and nasal cavity. Resonance disorders are commonly seen in children with clefts of the hard and soft palates. Functional hard and soft palates are necessary for normal oral–nasal resonance balance. Velopharyngeal incompetence can affect speech and resonance in a variety of ways, but in particular it can cause hypernasality and nasal air emission. The speech intelligibility of many individuals with cleft palate is severely affected by velopharyngeal incompetence. The term "*cleft palate speech*" is often used to describe the typical consonant productions, abnormal nasal resonance, abnormal nasal airflow, altered laryngeal voice quality, and nasal or facial grimaces of children with clefts of the hard and/or soft palates.

Eustachian (auditory) tube

A tube lined with mucous membrane that joins the nasopharynx and the middle ear cavity; normally closed but opens during yawning, chewing, and swallowing to allow equalization of air pressure in the middle ear with atmospheric pressure (named after Bartolomeo Eustachio, an Italian anatomist, 1524–1574).

DENTAL CLASSIFICATION	EXAMPLE	SKELETAL CLASSIFICATION	EXAMPLE
Class I Occlusion The mesiobuccal cusp of the upper molar occludes in the buccal groove of the lower molar. The remaining teeth are arranged upon a smoothly curving line.	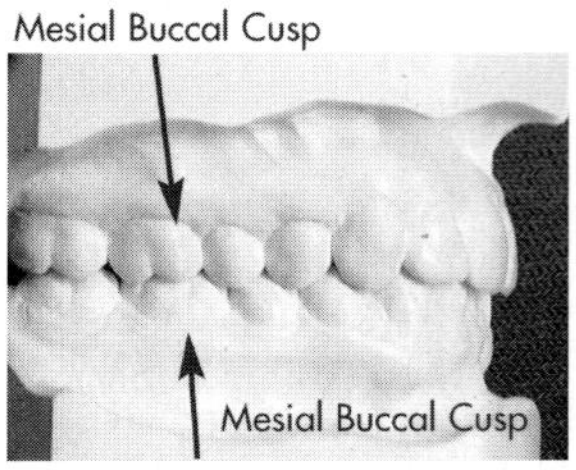 Mesial Buccal Cusp / Mesial Buccal Cusp	Class I–Normal	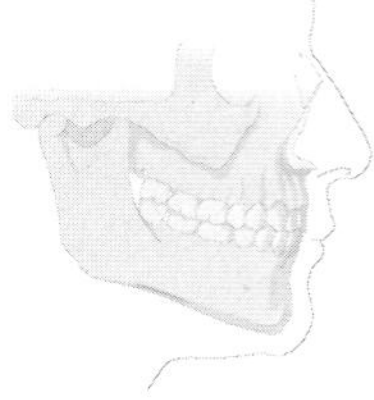
Class I Malocclusion Normal relationship of the molars, but line of occlusion is incorrect because of malpositioned teeth, rotations, or other causes.	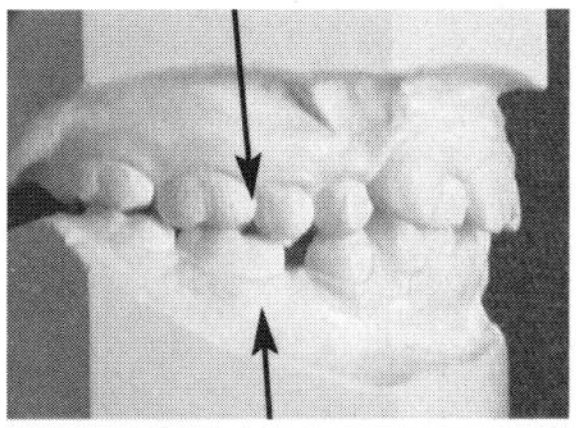	Class I–Normal	
Class II Malocclusion Lower molar distally positioned relative to upper molar; line of occlusion is not specified.	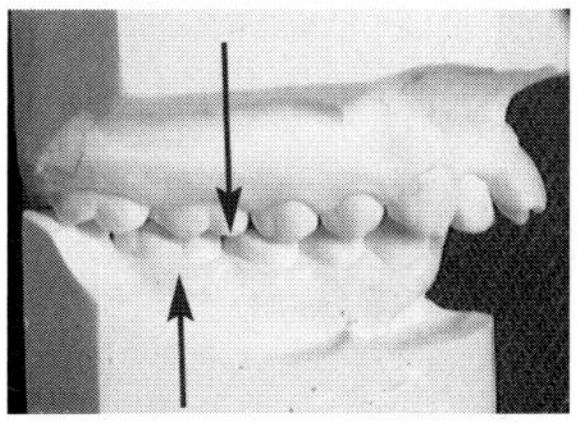	Class II– Mandibular Retrusion and/or Maxillary Protrusion	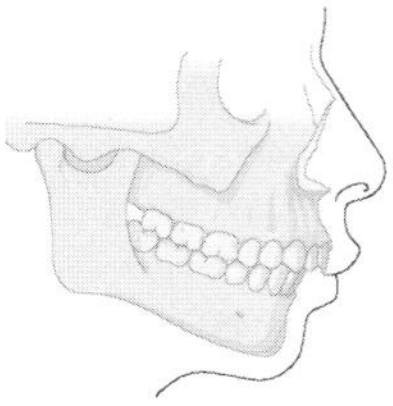
Class III Malocclusion Lower molar mesially positioned relative to upper molar; line of occlusion is not specified.	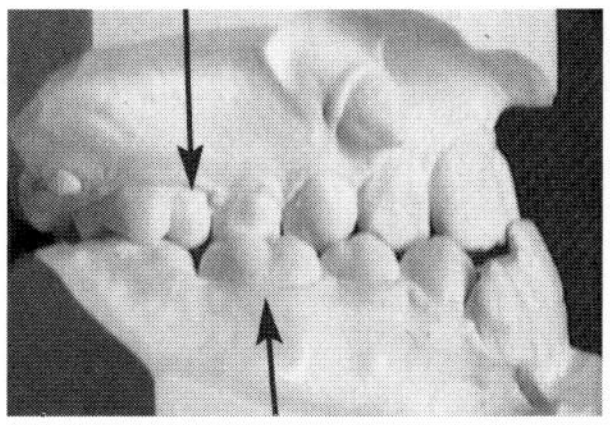	Class III– Mandibular Protrusion and/or Maxillary Retrusion	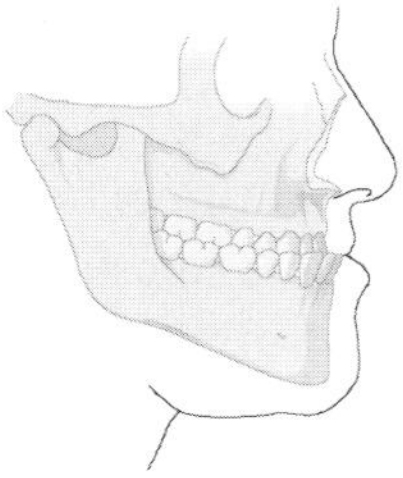

Figure 10–5

Angle's classification of occlusion and skeletal relationships.

Adapted from Kummer, 2008. © Cengage Learning 2013.

Hypernasality

Hypernasality refers to an excessive and undesirable amount of perceived nasal cavity resonance during speech. Hypernasality occurs when there is abnormal coupling of the oral and nasal cavities, resulting in distorted or nasal-sounding vowels and oral consonants. In general, consonants that require more intraoral breath pressure will force more air into the nasal cavity and increase the perception of hypernasality (e.g., voiced plosives /b/, /d/, /g/; fricatives /z/, /v/; and affricates /ʧ/ [ch]). The voiced plosives often sound as if they are substituted with their nasal cognates (/m/ for /b/, /n/ for /d/, and /n/ for /g/). Hypernasality is easiest to perceive in connected speech; it often increases during faster rates of speech (Ha & Kuehn, 2011).

Nasal Air Emission/Nasal Escape

Nasal air emission refers to the inappropriate release of air pressure through the nose during speech, causing distortion of speech. Nasal air emission occurs primarily on voiceless consonants (e.g., plosives /p/, /t/, /k/ and fricatives /s/, /f/) because voiceless consonants require more intraoral breath pressure than voiced consonants. (This can be tested by placing your hand in front of your mouth and producing the /p/ sound and then the /b/ sound. On which sound do you feel more air pressure on your hand?) Velopharyngeal incompetence affects consonants by causing decreased intra oral air pressure, nasal emission, or both. The combination of hypernasality, decreased intraoral air pressure, and nasal air emission on the phonemes of any single word can seriously affect a word's intelligibility Baylis, Munson, & Moller (2011).

Hyponasality/Denasality

Hyponasality (**denasality**) refers to a reduction in nasal resonance during speech that is caused by partial blockage (*occlusion*) in the nasopharynx or the posterior entrance to the nasal passages, as might occur when the *adenoids* (masses of lymphoid tissue on the posterior pharyngeal wall of the nasopharynx) are enlarged. Hyponasality particularly affects the nasal consonants (/m/, /n/, and /ŋ/ [ng]), often distorting them.

Cul-de-sac Resonance

Cul-de-sac resonance is a variation of hyponasality. It differs in the place of obstruction and in the way the speech sounds. The nasal sounds are trapped in a blocked passage with only one outlet: back the direction it came and then out through the mouth. The speech has a muffled characteristic, which you can hear in your own speech if you repeat the consonant–vowel (CV) combination "me, me, me" and then, continuing to produce the sounds, pinch your nostrils together tightly. You will hear and feel the air stream necessary for the nasal sounds as it enters the open posterior nasal passage, but you will trap it by the tight anterior constriction. The resonating cavity, which is normally an open tube, becomes a cul-de-sac with the consequent changes in nasal resonance.

Articulation and Phonological Disorders

The various associated problems with cleft lip and palate can have cascading effects on speech. For example, the middle ear problems and infections can negatively affect the development of speech sounds and the phonetic repertoire that are the building blocks for words, sentences, and language. Clefts can severely affect the development of many sounds. Studies have revealed that during speech development young children with clefts have a smaller phonetic repertoire and use restricted syllables and structures in the formation of their early words, although there is considerable variation among children (Chapman & Hardin, 1992; Salas-Provance, Kuehn, & Marsh, 2003). Severe dental anomalies can negatively affect sound productions (Peterson-Falzone et al., 2010).

Compensatory Articulation Errors

In individuals with cleft palate, some articulation errors appear to develop to compensate for velopharyngeal incompetence. **Glottal stops** are the most common compensatory articulations produced by individuals with cleft palate (Peterson-Falzone, 1989; Sulprizio, 2010). Glottal stops are compensatory articulation productions primarily for plosive sounds (e.g., /p/, /b/, /t/, /d/). Individuals with velopharyngeal incompetence are unable to build the necessary intraoral air pressure to produce stop sounds because the air escapes into the nasal passages, resulting in hypernasality and nasal emission. Glottal stops are characterized by the forceful adduction of the vocal folds and the buildup and release of air pressure under the glottis, resulting in a grunt-type sound (Kummer, 2008). **Pharyngeal fricatives** also are used as compensatory articulation patterns. Pharyngeal fricatives are produced when the tongue is retracted so that the base of the tongue approximates, but does not touch, the pharyngeal wall, which causes a friction sound as air pressure passes through the narrow opening during production of fricatives and affricates (e.g., /f/, /v/, /s/, /z/, /ʃ/ [sh], and /tʃ/ [ch]).

glottal stops

Compensatory articulation productions primarily for plosive sounds (e.g., /p/, /b/, /t/, /d/) used by individuals with velopharyngeal incompetence; characterized by the forceful adduction of the vocal folds and the buildup and release of air pressure under the glottis, resulting in a grunt-type sound.

pharyngeal fricatives

Compensatory articulation productions primarily for fricatives and affricates (e.g., /f/, /v/, /s/, /z/, /ʃ/ [sh], and /tʃ/ [ch]) used by individuals with velopharyngeal incompetence; characterized by tongue retraction so that the base of the tongue approximates, but does not touch, the pharyngeal wall, which causes a friction sound as air pressure passes through the narrow opening.

CASE STUDY

Daddy Wanted to Hear "Daddy"

I was conducting a research study on the speech-sound development of 11-month-old babies with cleft palate. One of the babies produced many glottal stops. The parents were proud of their daughter because she produced this sound to communicate in an expressive manner. It sounded like "uh uh uh." She was a "daddy's girl," and Daddy was happy with the glottal stops but was hurt because the baby had only one recognizable word, "mamma." No matter how hard the father worked with her, she would never say "daddy." When I explained to him that it was physically impossible at this time for her to make a /d/ sound, he was so relieved he just squeezed his little girl and said, "You do love daddy, I knew you did!" In addition, I took the opportunity to tell the parents not to reinforce the glottal stop sounds and taught them how to help their daughter make other speech sounds with her lips and tongue. ■

Source: Marlene Salas-Provance, Ph.D.

Language Delays and Differences

Children with cleft palates are at risk for various language delays and disorders compared with children without clefts, particularly when clefts are associated with syndromes or other disorders. Children with clefts tend to have poor receptive and expressive language skills, shorter mean length of utterance, reduced structural complexity, smaller vocabularies, and poor reading skills (Broen, Devers, Doyle, Prouty, & Moller, 1998; Chapman, 2011; Scherer & D'Antonio, 1997). In general, the poorer the speech intelligibility, the poorer the expressive language (Pannbacker, 1975).

SURGICAL MANAGEMENT OF CLEFT LIP AND PALATE

Management of children with cleft lip and palate, as well as other craniofacial anomalies, requires an **interdisciplinary team** approach in which the team members collaborate and coordinate the care of the patient and family (Hodgkinson et al., 2005; Moller & Glaze, 2009; Taub & Lampert, 2011). The parents are always essential members of the team. Various other team members are involved at different stages of the care of the infant and child. Team members who may be involved at various times include an audiologist, geneticist, neurosurgeon, nurse, nutritionist, ophthalmologist, oral surgeon, orthodontist, otolaryngologist, pediatrician, pedodontist, plastic or craniofacial surgeon (Gk. *plastikos,* to mold or form), prosthodontist, psychologist, radiologist, social worker, and a speech-language pathologist (see Figure 10–6). The American Cleft

interdisciplinary team

A group of professionals from various disciplines who work together to coordinate the care of a patient through collaboration, interaction, communication, and cooperation.

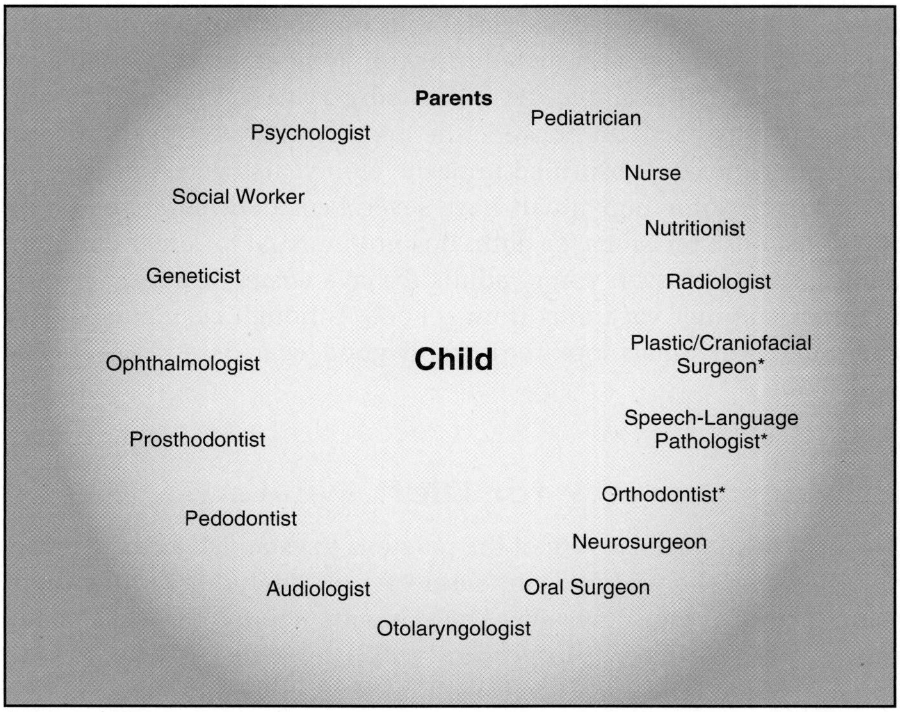

Figure 10–6

Potential members of a cleft palate–craniofacial anomalies team (* indicates essential team members).
© Cengage Learning 2013.

rule of 10s

A guideline for the appropriate time for a cleft lip repair, which says that the infant must be at least 10 weeks of age, weigh 10 pounds, and have a hemoglobin count of 10 grams before the lip repair.

anesthesia

The administration of a topical, local, regional, or general drug or agent capable of producing a partial or complete loss of sensation or consciousness.

palatoplasty

The surgical repair of a cleft palate.

pharyngoplasty

A surgical procedure of the pharynx that is designed to correct velopharyngeal dysfunction.

Palate–Craniofacial Association has established basic standards for what constitutes a professional cleft palate or craniofacial team. The minimum core professionals must include a surgeon, speech-language pathologist, and orthodontist who are qualified by virtue of their education, experience, and credentials to provide craniofacial and cleft care (American Cleft Palate-Craniofacial Association, 1996).

Cleft Lip and Nose Repair

Many plastic surgeons follow the **rule of 10s** guidelines to determine an infant's readiness for lip repair. This rule says that the infant should be at least 10 weeks of age, weigh 10 pounds, and have a hemoglobin count of 10 grams. By doing the initial cleft lip surgery sometime between the 2nd and 3rd month of life, physicians have more time to investigate other potential problems the infant may have, such as syndromes or medical complications. The infant also will have established a feeding technique that allows weight gain. However, the most important reason is for the surgery team to be assured that the infant will survive the long period (usually 1 to 2 hours) under general **anesthesia**. The goals of cleft lip surgery are to achieve unity of the orbicularis oris muscle and normal lip configuration with a cupid's bow. The size of the cleft (incomplete vs. complete) and whether the cleft is unilateral or bilateral determine the complexity of the surgery (Lazarus et al., 1998; Kuehn & Henne, 2003) (see Figure 10–7).

Most children with cleft lips undergo some *secondary surgery* (revisions) in early childhood to reduce scar tissue on the lip, improve the symmetry of the lip, and improve the symmetry and appearance of the nose. Other secondary surgeries may not be performed until there is more complete facial growth during the elementary school and adolescent years. For example, secondary surgery to straighten the *nasal septum* (fleshy partition between the nostrils) and improve the nasal airway may not be performed until the teen years (Peterson-Falzone et al., 2010). Some individuals have several cosmetic surgeries for lip revisions, nose revisions, or both. It is not unusual for older children, adolescents, and even young adults to have cosmetic surgeries during their summer vacations from school. Although cosmetic surgery can make individuals look remarkably good, scar tissue may still be noticeable.

Primary Surgery for Cleft Palate Repair

The goal of surgical closure of the palate is to establish an intact division between the oral and the nasal cavities, including a fully functional velopharyngeal system. The patient's age for the cleft palate repair (**palatoplasty**, **pharyngoplasty**) depends on whether the surgeon follows the early (between 6 months and 15 months) or late (between 15 months and 24 months) surgery philosophy (Kuehn &

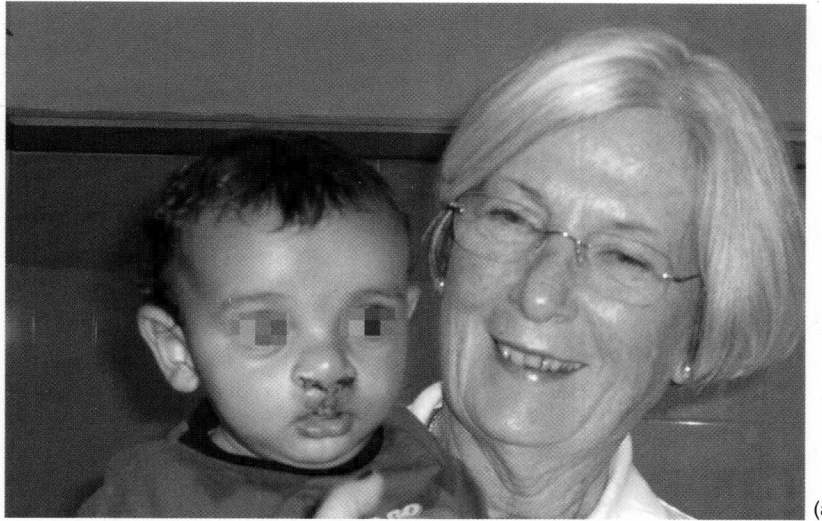

(a)

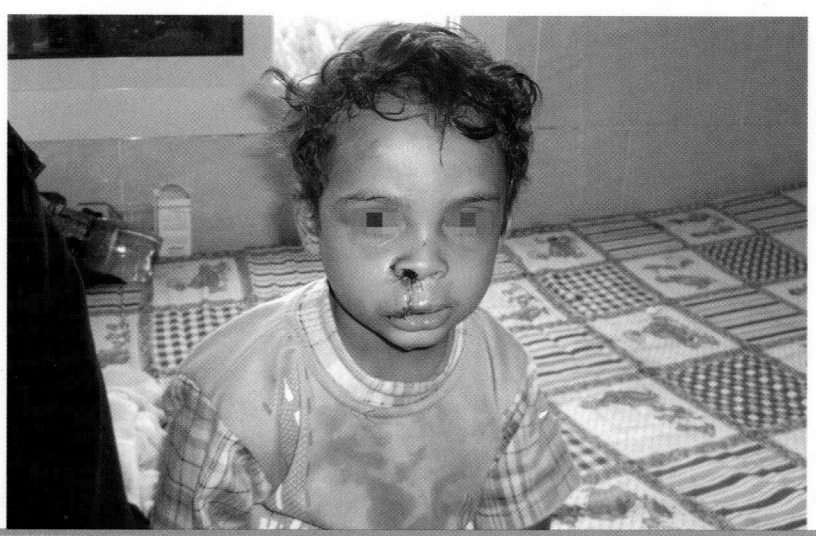

(b)

Figure 10-7

(a) Post-cleft-lip-repair patient with operating room nurse. (b) Post cleft lip repair.

Source: Paul Fogle, Ph.D., Rotaplast (Rotary) International Cleft Palate Missions, Cumaná, Venezuela, 2008, Sohag, Egypt, 2010.

Henne, 2003). Primary palatal surgery performed before 12 months of age is more likely to prevent compensatory articulation behavior, such as the production of glottal stops (Murthy, Sendhilnathan, & Hussain, 2010). Achieving a good result with palatal surgery is often more difficult than achieving a good result with lip surgery. Palatal surgery is technically more challenging with potentially more complications. In addition to closing the hard and soft palates so that they form a barrier between the mouth and the nasal passages, the surgeon needs to repair the soft palate so that it functions dynamically (i.e., is able to move) for normal speech. Surgeons may choose from various types of repairs, such as a *Von Langenbeck* repair or a *Wardill-Kilner* repair (see Figure 10-8 and Figure 10-9).

When the primary palatal repair does not provide adequate velopharyngeal closure, or when closure appears adequate for speech in

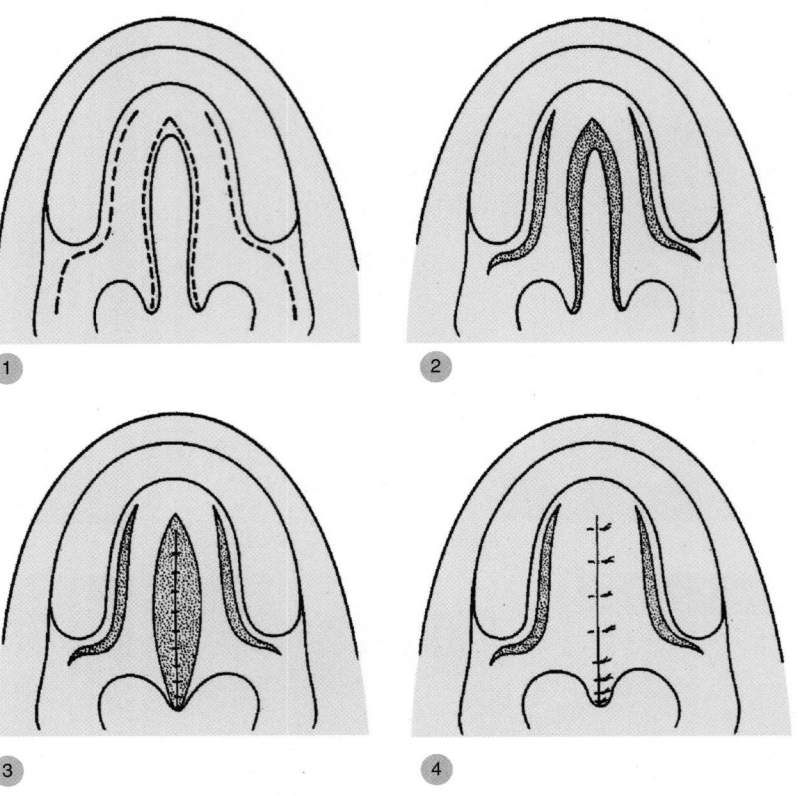

Figure 10-8

The Von Langenbeck surgical technique of palatal repair. Note the markings on the palate where incisions will be made and the illustrations of how the tissue will be moved to close the cleft.

From *Plastic Surgery*, by Joseph McCarthy, 1990, Vol. 4, Fig. 54–12. Orlando, FL: W.B. Saunders Company. Reprinted with permission.

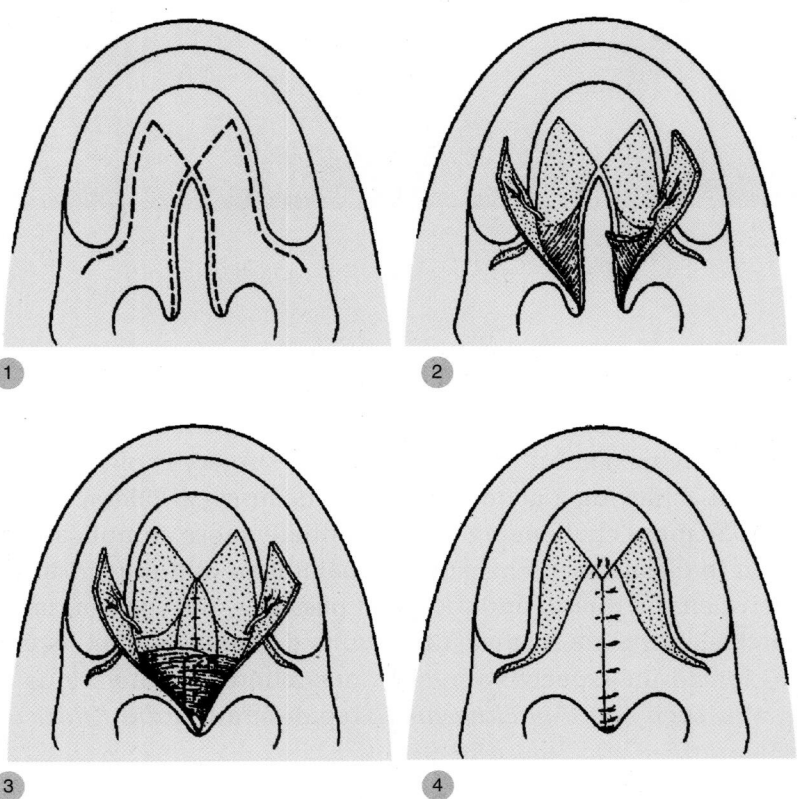

Figure 10-9

The Wardill-Kilner surgical type of palatal repair. Note the markings on the palate where incisions will be made and the illustrations of how the tissue will be moved to close the cleft.

From *Plastic Surgery*, by Joseph McCarthy, 1990, Vol. 4, Fig. 54–11. Orlando, FL: W.B. Saunders Company. Reprinted with permission.

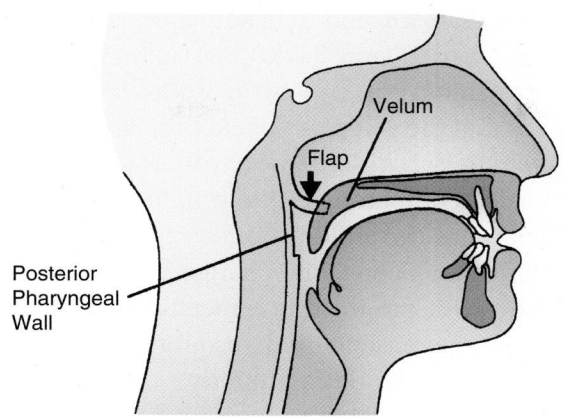

Figure 10–10

A lateral view of a pharyngeal flap.

© Cengage Learning 2013.

early childhood but then changes to inadequate closure as a result of natural growth of the craniofacial bones or **atrophy** of the adenoids, the craniofacial team needs to consider how to best reestablish good velo-pharyngeal function (Peterson-Falzone et al., 2010). Surgical approaches include creation of a *pharyngeal flap;* that is, sewing a flap of tissue from the back of the throat (posterior pharyngeal wall) into the soft palate, leaving an opening (*port*) on either side for breathing and nasal drain-age (see Figure 10–10). A few surgical options are available to alter the position and function of the pharyngeal muscles (Liedman-Boshki, Lohmander, Persson, Lith, & Elander, 2005).

SPEECH AND RESONANCE EVALUATION

The speech-language pathologist is always in an evaluation process of an infant, child, adolescent, and even adult who has had a cleft palate. The emphasis changes as the child matures. The first concern is feed-ing for nutrition and growth, followed by language development, and then speech development and intelligibility. Ongoing counseling with the parents and later with the child is part of the evaluation process (Flasher & Fogle, 2012).

Noninstrumental Tests

Speech-language pathologists have several simple noninstrumental, low-tech techniques to evaluate children for velopharyngeal incom-petence and nasal emission (Kuehn & Henne, 2003; Kummer, 2008; Peterson-Falzone et al., 2010). These techniques include the mirror test, nostril pinching, and air paddle. During the *mirror test,* the clinician places a small mirror, such as a dental mirror, under the child's nostrils and asks the child to produce nonnasal voiceless and voiced consonants (e.g., /p/, /t/, /k/, /b/, /d/, /g/, /s/, /z/) and several words loaded with these consonants (e.g., *badges, boat, cookie, cupcake, dishes, foot, juices,*

atrophy

A shrinking in size or wasting away that is usually caused by injury, disease, lack of use (e.g., muscles), or natural reduction in size over time (e.g., adenoids and tonsils).

kitty, pipe, safety, shoes, tooth, and *top*). Sentences also may be used, such as "Take the dog to the park" and "I like Coca Cola." The clinician watches for fogging (condensation) of the mirror from either nostril. If fogging occurs, it indicates that the velopharyngeal port is not closing properly.

Nostril pinching (occluding) is another technique to evaluate for velopharyngeal incompetence. While lightly pinching the nostrils closed, the clinician has the child produce nonnasal words (see earlier examples). The clinician listens for a change in perceived nasality compared to the sound with the nostrils unoccluded. If there is increased oral resonance and decreased nasal resonance, it indicates that the velopharyngeal port is not working properly.

Nasal emission can be detected by using an *air paddle.* An air paddle can be cut from a piece of paper and placed underneath each nostril individually while the child is rapidly producing pressure-sensitive voiceless consonants (e.g., "pa pa pa, ta ta ta, ka ka ka"). If the paddle moves during the production of these sounds, it indicates that there is nasal air emission.

Instrumental Procedures

If hypernasality or nasal emission is detected, further assessment of velopharyngeal function is indicated. **Nasopharyngoscopy** is a minimally invasive procedure that is commonly used by SLPs that allows visual observation and analysis of the velopharyngeal mechanism (Garrett & Deal, 2002; Kummer, 2008). See Figure 10–11. Nasopharyngoscopy uses the same flexible fiberoptic endoscopic equipment as is used for laryngoscopy (see Figure 9–10 and Figure 9–11). However, the purpose of nasopharyngoscopy is to view the nasal surface of the velum and all of the structures of the velopharyngeal valve during speech.

nasopharyngoscopy

A minimally invasive procedure commonly used by SLPs for evaluation of velopharyngeal dysfunction that allows visual observation and analysis of the velopharyngeal mechanism during speech; equipment includes a flexible fiberoptic endoscope, the same that is used in laryngoscopy.

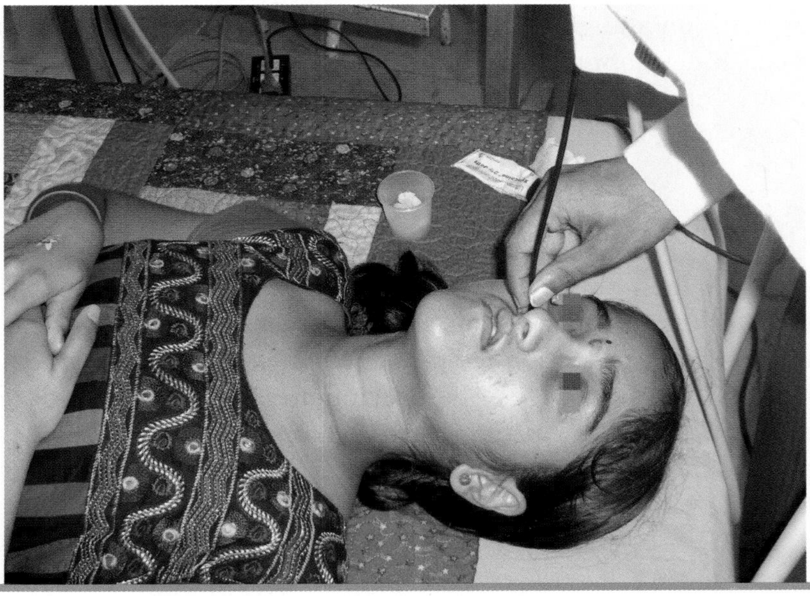

Paul Fogle, Ph.D., Rotaplast (Rotary) International Cleft Palate Team Mission, Nagamangala, India, 2011

Figure 10–11

Nasopharyngoscopy being performed by an ENT on a 13-year-old girl to determine feasibility of pharyngeal flap surgery.

Other instrumental evaluations (e.g., *nasometry*) may be conducted before recommendations for further surgery designed to improve speech (Peterson-Falzone et al., 2010). A **nasometer** is a computer-based instrument that measures the relative amount of nasal acoustic energy in an individual's speech, resulting in a *nasalance* score. **Pressure-airflow techniques** may detect various pressures in the oral and nasal cavities.

SPEECH THERAPY

Most children with cleft palates will need the services of a speech-language pathologist at some time in their lives. Speech therapy can improve their articulation or phonological development, general expressive language abilities, or a combination of these. For many of these children, the course of speech and language therapy will be complex. Clinicians must determine when it is appropriate to initiate therapy, when it is appropriate to refer for physical management, and when it is prudent to defer management of all kinds. The initial assessment will not always provide the information needed to develop a long-term course of management. The therapy process itself often must provide the information needed to arrive at a diagnosis and ongoing modifications in clinical management (Peterson-Falzone et al., 2010).

The First Years

During the first year, the primary speech pathology concerns are feeding and the development of the prerequisites for verbal communication (Kummer, 2008; Moller & Glaze, 2009; Sulprozio, 2010). Nursing staff and speech-language pathologists help train the parents on feeding techniques of the baby; however, if feeding continues to be a problem, the speech-language pathologist needs to evaluate the infant's swallowing abilities so that the problem can be resolved quickly (see Chapter 12, Dysphagia/Swallowing Disorders).

The speech-language pathologist does considerable teaching, explaining, and training with the parents on methods of speech and language stimulation. During the first 3 years, language development is the primary focus, rather than good intelligible speech; that is, during the early years, the quantity of speech is more important than the quality of speech. During these years, the clinician will likely meet with the parents periodically (at least annually) to assess the child's language development, provide further information to the parents, and answer their questions. Most clinicians are able to spend only 1 to 2 hours per week working directly with a patient and family (there are 168 hours in a week, leaving 166 without direct clinician involvement); therefore, extensive parent participation is essential to successful speech and language development—not only for children with clefts, but other communication disorders (Pamplona & Ysunza, 1999; Pamplona, Ysunza, & Uriostegui, 1996; Scherer & D'Antonio, 1997).

Infants and young children with cleft palates should be given normal language stimulation. Parents should talk to their children frequently

---

nasometer

A computer-based instrument that measures the relative amount of nasal acoustic energy in a person's speech.

pressure-airflow technique

A procedure using *aerodynamic instrumentation* to evaluate the dynamics of the velopharyngeal mechanism during speech; also used to evaluate nasal respiration and to quantify upper airway obstruction through measurements of nasal airway resistance.

and listen to them. Parents should avoid using nonsense words and should speak clearly, using correctly formed words and short phrases. Infants with cleft palates should be allowed to babble freely and naturally. Children should be encouraged to communicate using speech. Even though the speech sounds of children born with cleft palates will be nasally produced before primary palatal surgery, these sounds are preferred over glottal stops. Orally produced sounds, or attempts at orally produced sounds, should be reinforced even though they are produced nasally. Glottal stops should be ignored and not reinforced. Once glottal stops become habitual, they may be difficult to change with therapy as the child grows older (Golding-Kushner, 2001; Kuehn & Henne, 2003; Kuehn & Moller, 2000).

About age 3, the child should receive a comprehensive evaluation of speech and language. Parents' reports of their child's speech and language progress are good indications of the child's communication development. Resonance and velopharyngeal function can be assessed in the child's connected speech through perceptual (i.e., listening) evaluations described above.

Preschool Through School Age

Most children with clefts require intervention to improve their articulation, phonological development, or expressive language development (Blakely & Brockman, 1995; Chapman, 1993; Peterson-Falzone et al., 2010; Sulprizio, 2010). The speech therapy techniques used with articulation disorders related to resonance disorders (compensatory productions) are similar to those used in basic articulation and phonology therapy (see Chapter 5, Articulation and Phonological Disorders). Kummer (2008) provides several general therapy techniques that may be helpful to encourage children with structurally competent velopharyngeal mechanisms to use more normal oral resonance:

- Auditory discrimination training to hear the difference between normal oral speech and hypernasal speech
- Visual feedback using instruments (e.g., nasometer or pressure-flow instrumentation) that allow a child to see increases in oral resonance
- Tactile-kinesthetic training to allow the child to increase awareness and sensation of soft palate movement
- Tactile feedback using the child's fingers on the side of her nose to feel for vibration during the production of oral and nasal phonemes
- Increasing oral activity and using an open-mouth approach when talking to reduce intraoral resistance and increase oral resonance

Chapman, Hardin-Jones, and Halter (2003) made the following additional recommendations for speech and language therapy for children with clefts:

- When evaluating, be sure to include whether or not the sound inventories contain stops and other true consonants.

- These sounds should be targeted in early treatment because the ability to produce them early can affect later speech development.
- Therapy goals should focus not only on acquisition of new words but also on acquisition of new sounds.

Overall, the goal for children who have had successful cleft palate repairs and have achieved functional velopharyngeal mechanisms is normal speech. The team approach is essential in the successful management of children with clefts. Speech and language therapy should continue as long as a child is making progress (Blakely & Brockman, 1995; Hardin-Jones, Chapman, & Scherer, 2006; Sulprizio, 2010).

SPEECH APPLIANCES (PROSTHETIC DEVICES, PROSTHESES)

When surgical correction of velopharyngeal dysfunction is not an option or when surgical management and speech therapy have not been able to sufficiently improve oral-nasal resonance balance, prosthetic management may be used (Kummer, 2008; Peterson-Falzone et al., 2010). **Prosthetic devices (prostheses)** can be fabricated out of acrylic (plastic) and metal to close the palate or the velopharyngeal port for speech. Various types of speech appliances may be used to lift the soft palate to hold it in place close to or against the posterior pharyngeal wall (**palatal lift**), to cover an open defect in the hard palate (**palatal obturator**), or occlude the velopharyngeal port during speech (**speech bulb obturator**) (see Figure 10–12).

prosthetic device (prosthesis)

An artificial device to replace or augment a missing or impaired part of the body.

palatal lift

A prosthetic appliance that can be used to raise the velum for speech if the velum is long enough to achieve velopharyngeal closure but does not move well, often because of central or peripheral neurological impairment.

palatal obturator

A prosthetic appliance that can be used to cover an open palatal defect, such as an unrepaired cleft palate or a **palatal fistula**; it can be used to improve an infant's ability to achieve compression of the nipple for suction or can be used to close a palatal defect for speech.

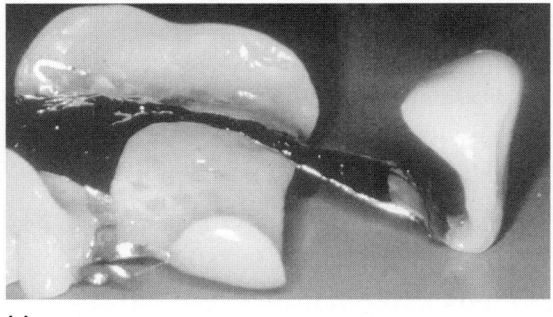

(a)

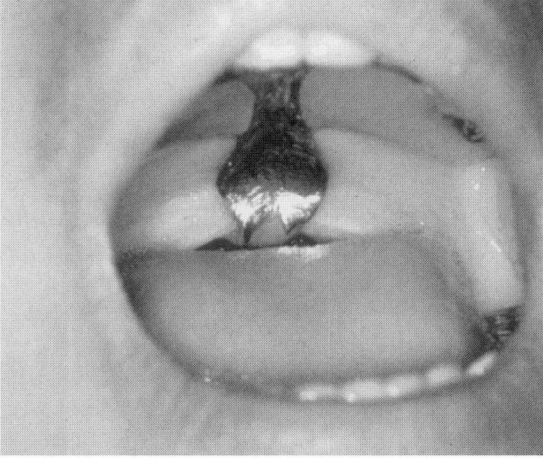

(b)

Figure 10–12

(a) A speech bulb obturator, and (b) the speech bulb obturator in place. The bulb sits in the nasopharynx to occlude the velopharyngeal port during speech. This improves speech and can improve swallowing because it eliminates nasal regurgitation.

Source: Kummer, 2008.

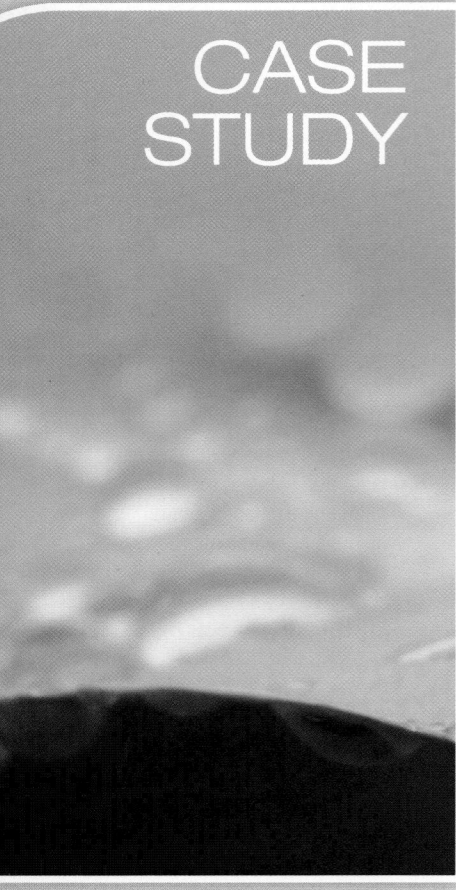

CASE STUDY

Marty

Marty was a 4-year-old boy referred to a speech-language pathologist in private practice. He was born with a bilateral cleft lip and complete cleft of the hard and soft palates. He had undergone repair of the lip and palates but likely would need more than one lip revision. He met the guideline for being a candidate for speech therapy. He was seen twice weekly for 1-hour sessions in his home, primarily to help him use the velopharyngeal structures that were functioning adequately and to learn appropriate articulatory placement and oral airflow. The parents were concerned about Marty developing good speech before entering kindergarten. The parents were obviously proud of Marty and had a series of framed portraits of him on the wall, both before his initial lip surgery and about every 6 months after to show his growth.

Marty had become accustomed to getting his way in his home and tried to avoid working in therapy, even when play therapy and a variety of motivators and reinforcers were incorporated. The therapist had to make numerous adjustments in the therapy approach, always keeping in mind the goals and targets of therapy. Marty made significant gains over time in use of his velopharyngeal mechanism and articulatory placement and airflow despite himself. Although "drill" is an essential component of much of therapy, the clinician's creativity in making the drill "palatable" is an important skill that needs to be developed. ■

speech bulb obturator

A prosthetic device that may be considered when the velum is too short to close completely against the posterior pharyngeal wall; it consists of a retaining appliance and a bulb (usually made of acrylic) that fills in the pharyngeal space for speech.

palatal fistula

Usually a small opening or passage between the oral cavity and the nasal cavity that allows air or sound to escape from the oral cavity into the nasal cavity, causing some hypernasality.

EMOTIONAL AND SOCIAL EFFECTS OF CLEFT LIP AND PALATE

A baby born with a serious facial disfigurement sets in motion an array of emotions in everyone related to or involved with the newborn. The delivery team's first concern is the physical well-being of both the infant and the mother, but the team also knows there will be emotionally trying times for the family who will be taking home a less than perfect baby (Fallowfield & Jenkins, 2004). This section is about the parents who must adjust to their disappointments and fears and about the children who develop increasing awareness that they look and sound different from everyone in their family and, likely, all of their playmates.

Parents' Initial Shock and Adjustment

Probably all soon-to-be-parents have said, "I don't care if it's a boy or girl; I just want my baby to be healthy." In some cases, because of increasingly refined ultrasound techniques, a cleft lip or other craniofacial anomaly may be detected in utero. Learning about their baby's cleft at this stage of development is emotionally shocking for the parents, and from that point on they need to receive information and counseling from the obstetrician and pediatrician (Despars, Peters, Borghini, et al., 2011). The early knowledge that the unborn child is not perfect—that it has a cleft—allows the parents time to learn about the problem and perhaps develop some adjustment to the reality of the birth.

Most parents, however, have no advanced warning and opportunity to prepare for the birth of a child with a cleft; the baby is born, and the parents' first awareness of the facial anomaly is when they are shown their new baby (Strauss et al., 1995). Many parents of babies with clefts have never heard of or seen pictures of clefts ("harelip" is usually the term adults have heard) before their child's birth.

Parental reactions to first seeing their baby's birth defect include disbelief, shock, anger, guilt, depression, feelings of inadequacy, resentment, grief, frustration, anxiety, fear, and protectiveness—all common reactions to any serious physical defect of a newborn (Bradbury & Hewison, 1994; Dolger-Hafner, Bartsch, Trimbach, Zobel, & Witt, 1997; Van Staden & Gerhardt, 1995). These emotions are not just fleeting feelings. Because a cleft is a "chronic" problem, the parental reactions may become chronic too, sometimes being externalized (e.g., frustration and anger) to the spouse or team of professionals involved in trying to help the child and family. Realizing that this might occur, it is wise not to take the parents' frustration and anger personally but to appreciate that it is the entire situation and all of the stressors around it that are frustrating and anger-producing for the parents. While the SLP plays an important role in assisting a child with a cleft to develop speech and language properly, another team member, such as a **social worker** or psychologist, would be better equipped to deal with the parents' feelings about having a child with a disability.

We do not want to forget that the newborn may have older brothers and sisters who also will be reacting to the baby's appearance. The grieving behavior of a child will often be similar to that of the same-gender parent. For example, a son may try to be stoic and "strong," much as he sees his father trying to be (Flasher & Fogle, 2012; Sanders, 1998). Likewise, grandparents have their own reactions but do the best they can to be supportive of the new parents and the other grandchildren. A *family systems counseling model* is usually the most helpful in these cases (see Chapter 8).

A major cause of stress for many parents is the cost of a cleft palate team, surgery, and the care needed for these children. A family's health insurance, Health Maintenance Organization (HMO), or various other third-party payers may cover the cost of certain aspects of an infant's and child's care. However, parents need to be advocates for their child and themselves when insurance companies and HMOs deny claims because they are considered "cosmetic" surgeries, dental problems rather than medical problems, "preexisting" conditions, or because the claims agent feels that an entire cleft palate team is not necessary. In addition, beyond what might be covered by third-party payers, there are always numerous expenses that come out of the pockets of the family.

Many parents have had little experience with hospitals before the birth of their baby, and now they must learn to navigate the complexities

social worker

A professional who helps families coordinate appointments, deal with insurance and other funding sources, and manage their stress and emotional reactions to the many problems associated with a patient's treatment.

Application Question

How do you think you might react if your baby was born with a serious physical defect? What can you do to try to develop some empathy for the new parents of a baby born with a cleft or other serious physical defect?

of the medical system, as well as insurance companies. A knowledgeable and compassionate social worker can be most helpful to the parents at this time. As the first surgery time (usually closing the lip) approaches, the stress and anxiety of the parents and family increase.

Parent–infant attachment and bonding have been a concern for years (Koepp-Baker & Harkins, 1936). The more severe the cleft, the more likely the following behaviors will occur: parents perceive their infants as irritable and having less pleasing personality characteristics; mothers delay in touching their babies; and mothers are less interactive (less playful, less responsive, and less facially expressive) with their babies (Coy, Speltz, & Jones, 2002; Slade, Emerson, & Freedlander, 1999).

Children's Preschool and Early Elementary School Years

During the preschool years, children's self-images and feelings about themselves are influenced primarily by the attitudes and behaviors of their parents. The relationship between parents' attitudes and a child's self-concept is crucial during the preschool years. As children's interactions with the community expand in the school years, the effects on self-image, socialization, school adjustment, and academic achievement become more complex (Collett & Speltz, 2006; Endriga, Jordan, & Speltz, 2003). How children look and sound when entering elementary school affects how they perceive themselves and their social interactions. A child's facial appearance is strongly correlated with attractiveness and social acceptance (Krueckeberg, Kapp-Simon, & Ribordy, 1993; Turner, Rumsey, & Sandy, 1998).

A number of studies have looked at how early elementary school children with craniofacial anomalies perceive themselves. In general, the children felt more alienated, sadder, and more scared, angry, and upset than the normal-appearing control groups (Elder, 1995; Slifer et al., 2006). Parents and teachers often need help to realize that many children with clefts feel rejected and are rejected by their peers and that children with clefts may need special training and experiences in ways to positively handle teasing and ridiculing and to develop good social skills. Parents may want to discuss with their children how to handle negative social situations related to their clefts. A child who is entering school should learn the proper (and age-appropriate) terms related to the cleft. The ability to confidently explain the condition to others may limit feelings of awkwardness and embarrassment and reduce negative social experiences.

School-Age Years

Self-perceptions and self-concepts of children during the elementary school years become increasingly complex, with many factors influencing how they feel about themselves almost moment to moment. Children with clefts generally have a significantly lower self-concept than their noncleft peers. They generally perceive themselves as less socially adept and more often sad and angry than children without clefts. They report significantly greater dissatisfaction with their appearance, less success in school, and greater general unhappiness and anxiety than do other children (Millard & Richman, 2001; Warschausky, Kay, Buchman, Halberg, & Berger, 2002). Richman and Millard (1997) found that girls with clefts tend to be more socially inhibited than boys. Pillemer and Cook (1989) found that for school-age children with a history of cleft, better physical attractiveness correlated with better overall adjustment.

Overall, clinicians need to be aware of the potential for children and adolescents with repaired or unrepaired clefts to have self-concept and self-esteem issues and need to be willing to listen when they want to talk about how they feel about themselves. Being empathic is more helpful to these children than being sympathetic, and working on social skills (particularly on handling teasing) as part of pragmatic language development can be helpful.

Adolescents

The adolescent years are a tremendous challenge—even for individuals with no apparent physical or other abnormality. Adolescents view appearance as the most important characteristic, above intelligence and humor (Prokhorov, Perry, Kelder, & Klepp, 1993). Physical appearance concerns are consistently higher in adolescents with a history of clefts, particularly in girls (Berger, Hons, & Dalton, 2011).

Adolescents with repaired clefts have the same challenges as other adolescents, plus the likely addition of some that are related to residual surgical scars, facial features, and speech patterns associated with cleft lips and palates. Adolescents are susceptible to comments and ridicule because they cannot hide their facial differences from their peers. Males often deal with their concerns about their facial appearance by internalizing and developing anxiety and depression. They often externalize by withdrawing from others, becoming aggressive, or both. Females also often develop problems relating to self-image with anxiety and depression, and withdrawing from others, but they are less likely to become aggressive. Both males and females typically rate their *quality of life* as lower than that of their peers (Pope & Snyder, 2004; Slifer et al., 2004). Psychosocial functioning of individuals with clefts often improves after further surgery, but the positive outlook may be short-lived due to unrealistic expectations of the surgery (Topolski, Edwards, & Patrick, 2005). Not all adolescents with clefts have significant psychosocial problems; still, it is important for parents to be aware of psychosocial challenges their adolescents may face and to know where to turn if problems arise (Persson, Aniansson, Becker, & Svensson, 2002).

Adults

Among adults, an indication of self-satisfaction and feelings of success in social interactions is their dating and marrying patterns. Several studies have reported that adults with repaired clefts marry later and less often than other adults. There also are more childless couples and fewer children per marriage (Yttri, Christensen, Knudsen, Bille, 2011). Individuals with repaired clefts tend to rely on extended family for support and social activities, often having just a few close friends. They tend to have a high rate of persistent dissatisfaction with their appearance, teeth, hearing, speech, and social life (Havstam, Laakso, Lohmander, & Ringsberg, 2011; Marcusson, 2002; Marcusson, Akerlind, & Paulin, 2001). However, Clifford (1987) and Hunt, Burden, Hepper, and Johnston (2005) reviewed the psychosocial literature on this area and concluded that individuals with repaired clefts generally assume a reasonable position in society and typically fall within the norms in their educational levels, employment, psychosocial adjustment, and social integration.

Although adults with repaired clefts generally are in the norms and mainstreams of society, there is strong agreement among cleft palate and craniofacial team members that the parents of children born with clefts would benefit from access to a psychologist and that children and adolescents, every 2 to 3 years, should receive a psychological consultation, particularly before and after each major surgery (Krueckeberg, Kapp-Simon, & Ribordy, 1993; Pope & Ward, 1997; Strauss, 1991).

CHAPTER SUMMARY

There are a variety of clefts that can occur, with some affecting just the lip, others affecting the hard palate, and still others affecting just the soft palate. The severest kind of cleft occurs when all three structures are involved. A submucous cleft occurs when there is a defect in the hard palate in the absence of an actual opening into the nasal cavity. Velopharyngeal incompetence is the inability to achieve adequate separation of the nasal cavity from the oral cavity by velar and pharyngeal action, resulting in hypernasal resonance.

Many infants have difficulty feeding and children have middle ear infections and dental anomalies. Resonance disorders caused by velopharyngeal incompetence are the hallmark of a cleft palate. Speech and language problems are common for children with clefts.

Management of children with cleft lip and palate requires an interdisciplinary team approach. The goal of surgical closure of the palate is to establish an intact division between the oral and the nasal cavities, including a fully functional velopharyngeal system. Most children with cleft palates need therapy to improve their articulation or phonological development, as well as general expressive language abilities. During the first year, the primary speech pathology concerns are feeding and the development of the prerequisites for verbal communication. For the next couple of years, language development is the primary focus. The preschool and school-age years usually require the SLP to focus on articulation and phonological development and expressive language development.

A baby born with a serious facial disfigurement sets in motion an array of emotions in everyone related to or involved with the newborn. Elementary school children have significantly greater dissatisfaction with their appearance, less success in school, and greater general unhappiness and anxiety than other children. Adolescent males and females with repaired clefts typically rate their quality of life as lower than that of their peers. Adults with repaired clefts tend to have a high rate of persistent dissatisfaction with their appearance, teeth, hearing, speech, and social life. However, individuals with repaired clefts generally assume a reasonable position in society and typically fall within the norms in their educational levels, employment, psychosocial adjustment, and social integration.

STUDY QUESTIONS

Knowledge and Comprehension

1. What is velopharyngeal incompetence (VPI)?
2. What is hypernasality?
3. Define *interdisciplinary team* and list the essential (core) members of a cleft palate team.
4. What are the primary concerns of the speech-language pathologist during the child's first year?
5. What are some of the parental reactions that may be expected when first seeing their baby's cleft?

Application

1. How can a cleft lip cause articulation problems?
2. Why is it important to evaluate the receptive and expressive language of a child who has a cleft lip, cleft palate, or both?
3. Explain three of the noninstrumental tests a speech pathologist might use during an evaluation of a child for velopharyngeal incompetence.
4. Why is a speech-language pathologist always in an evaluation process when working with individuals who have cleft palates?
5. As a clinician, how can being aware that parents may "externalize" their reactions to various professionals help you better work with their frustrations and anger?

Analysis/Synthesis

1. Explain the similarities and differences between hypernasality and nasal emission.
2. Discuss the similarities and differences between hypernasality and hyponasality.
3. Discuss the differences in emphasis of the speech-language pathologist's work during the first years and those of preschool through school age.

4. How does the focus of counseling change from the initial work with the parents to later work with the child and adolescent?

5. Explain why the cleft palate team members may need to continue their involvement into a person's adulthood.

REFERENCES

Al Jamal, G., Hazza, A., Rawashdeh, M. (2010). Prevalence of dental anomalies in a population of cleft lip and palate patients. *The Cleft Palate-Craniofacial Journal, 47*(4), 413–420.

American Cleft Palate–Craniofacial Association (1996). The cleft and craniofacial team. Available at http://www.acpa-cpf.org.

Antonelli, P., Jorge, J., & Feniman, M. (2011). Otologic and audiologic outcomes with the Furlow and von Langenbeck with intravelar veloplasty palatoplasties in unilateral cleft lip and palate. *The Cleft Palate-Craniofacial Journal, 48*(4), 412–418.

Asimov, L. (1982). *Asimov's biographical encyclopedia of science and technology* (2nd ed.). Garden City, NY: Doubleday.

Baylis, A. L., Munson, B., & Moller, K. (2011). Perceptions of audible nasal emission in speakers with cleft palate: A comparative study of listener judgement. *The Cleft Palate-Craniofacial Journal, 48*(4), 399–411.

Berger, Z. E., Hons, D., & Dalton, L. J. (2011). *Coping with a cleft: Factors associated with psychological adjustment of adolescents with a cleft lip and palate and their parents.* The Celft Palate-Craniofacial Journal, *48*(1), 82–90.

Blakely, R. W., & Brockman, J. H. (1995). Normal speech and hearing by age 5 as a goal for children with cleft palate: A demonstration project. *American Journal of Speech-Language Pathology, 4*, 25–32.

Bradbury, E., & Hewison, J. (1994). Early parental adjustment to visible congenital disfigurement. *Child Care Health and Development, 20*(4), 251–266.

Broder, H. L., Smith, F., & Strauss, R. (1994). Effects of visible and invisible orofacial defects on self-perception and adjustment across developmental eras and gender. *Cleft Palate–Craniofacial Journal, 31*, 429–436.

Broen, P., Devers, M., Doyle, S., Prouty, J. M., & Moller, K. (1998). Acquisition of linguistic and cognitive skills by children with cleft palate. *Journal of Speech, Language, and Hearing Research, 41*, 676–687.

Carlisle, D. (1998). Feeding babies with cleft lip and palate. *Nursing Times, 94*(4), 59–60.

Chapman, K. L. (2011). The relationship between early reading skills and speech and language performance in young children with cleft lip and palate. *The Cleft-Palate Craniofacial Journal, 48*(3), 301–311.

Chapman, K. L. (1993). Phonologic processes in children with cleft palate. *Cleft Palate–Craniofacial Journal, 30*, 64–71.

Chapman, K. L., & Hardin, M. A. (1992). Phonetic and phonological skills of two-year-olds with cleft palate. *Cleft Palate-Craniofacial Journal, 29*, 435–441.

Chapman, K. L., Hardin-Jones, M. A., & Halter, K. A. (2003). The relationship between early speech and later speech and language performance for children with cleft lip and palate. *Clinical Linguistics and Phonetics, 17*(3), 173–197.

Chung, C. S., & Kau, M. C. (1985). Racial differences in cephalometric measurements and incidence of cleft lip with or without cleft palate. *Journal of Craniofacial Genetics and Developmental Biology, 5*, 341–349.

Clifford, E. (1987). *The cleft palate experience: New perspectives on management.* Springfield, IL: Charles C Thomas.

Collett, B. R., & Speltz, M. L. (2006). Social–emotional development of infants and young children with orofacial clefts. *Infants and Young Children, 19*(4), 262–291.

Collier, P. F. (1910). *Oath and law of Hippocrates.* Available at http://www.medword.com/hippocrates.html.

Coy, K., Speltz, M. L., & Jones, K. (2002). Facial appearance and attachment in infants with orofacial clefts: A replication. *Cleft Palate-Craniofacial Journal, 39*, 66–72.

Depars, J., Peters, C., Borghini, A., Pierrehumbert, B., Habersaat, S., et al. (2011). Impact of a cleft lip and/or palate on maternal stress and attachment representations. *The Cleft Palate-Craniofacial Journal, 48*(4), 419–424.

Diehl, S. R., & Erickson, R. P. (1997). Genome scan for teratogen-induced clefting susceptibility in the mouse: Evidence of both allelic and locus heterogeneity distinguishing cleft lip and cleft palate. *Proceedings of the National Academy of Science, 94*, 5231–5236.

Dolger-Hafner, M., Bartsch, A., Trimbach, G., Zobel, I., & Witt, E. (1997). Parental reactions following the birth of a cleft child. *Journal of Orofacial Orthopedics, 58*(2), 124–133.

Doyle, W. J., Cantekin, E. I., & Bluestone, C. D. (1980). Eustachian tube function in cleft palate children. *Annals of Otology, Rhinology, and Laryngology Supplement, 89*(3, Pt. 2), 34–40.

Elder, R. A. (1995). Individual differences in young children's self-concepts: Implications for children with cleft lip and palate. In R. A. Elder (Ed.), *Developmental perspectives on craniofacial problems.* New York, NY: Springer-Verlag.

Endriga, M. C., Jordan, J., & Speltz, M. L. (2003). Emotion self-regulation in preschool children with and without orofacial clefts. *Journal of Developmental and Behavioral Pediatrics, 24*(5), 336–344.

Ericson, A., Kallen, B., & Westeholm, P. (1979). Cigarette smoking as an etiologic factor in cleft lip and palate. *American Journal of Obstetrics and Gynecology, 135*, 348–351.

Fallowfield, L., & Jenkins, V. (2004). Communicating sad, bad, and difficult news in medicine. *Lancet, 363*(9405), 312–319.

Farrall, M., & Holder, S. (1992). Familial recurrence pattern analysis of cleft lip with or without cleft palate. *American Journal of Human Genetics, 50*, 270–277.

Flasher, L. V., & Fogle, P. T. (2012). *Counseling skills for speech-language pathologists and audiologists* (2nd ed.). Clifton Park, NY: Delmar Cengage Learning.

Garrett, J. D., & Deal, R. E. (2002). Endoscopic and perceptual evaluation of velopharyngeal insufficiency and hypernasality. *Journal of Medical Speech-Language Pathology, 19*, 194–200.

Golding-Kushner, K. J. (2001). *Therapy techniques for cleft palate speech and related disorders.* Clifton Park, NY: Delmar Cengage Learning.

Ha, S., & Kuehn, D. P. (2011). Temporal characteristics of nasalization in speakers with and without cleft palate. *The Cleft Palate-Craniofacial Journal, 48*(2), 134–144.

Hardin-Jones, M., Chapman, K., & Scherer, N. J. (2006). Early intervention in children with cleft palate. *ASHA Leader, 11*(8), 8–9, 32.

Havstam, C., Laakso, K., Lohmander, A., & Ringsberg, K. C. (2011). *Taking charge of communication: Adults' descriptions of growing up with a cleft-related speech impairment.* The Cleft Palate-Craniofacial Journal, *48*(6), 717–726.

Hodgkinson, P., Brown, S., Duncan, D., Grant, C., McNaughton, A., Thomas, P., & Mattick, C. (2005). Management of children with cleft lip and palate: A review describing the application of a multidisciplinary team working in this condition based upon the experiences of a regional cleft lip and palate centre in the United Kingdom. *Fetal and Maternal Medicine Review, 16*, 1–27.

Hunt, O., Burden, D., Hepper, P., & Johnston, C. (2005). The psychological effects of cleft lip and palate. *European Journal of Orthodontics, 27*(3), 274–285.

International Perinatal Database of Typical Oral Clefts Working Group (IPDTOC). (2011). Prevalence at birth of cleft lip with or without cleft palate: Data from the IPDTOC. *The Cleft Palate-Craniofacial Journal, 48*(1), 66–81.

Khoury, M., Gomez-Farias, J., & Mulinare, J. (1989). Does maternal cigarette smoking during pregnancy cause cleft lip and palate in offspring? *American Journal of Diseases in Children, 143*, 333–337.

Koepp-Baker, H., & Harkins, C. (1936). *The [cleft palate] child we have forgotten.* Philipsburg, PA: The Women's Club of Philipsburg.

Koren, G., Pastuszak, A., & Ito, S. (1998). Drugs in pregnancy. *New England Journal of Medicine, 338*, 1128–1137.

Krueckeberg, S., Kapp-Simon, K., & Ribordy, S. (1993). Social skills of preschool children with and without craniofacial anomalies. *Cleft Palate–Craniofacial Journal, 30*, 475–481.

Kuehn, D. P., & Henne, L. J. (2003). Speech evaluation and treatment for patients with cleft palate. *American Journal of Speech-Language Pathology, 12*, 103–109.

Kuehn, D. P., & Moller, K. T. (2000). Speech and language issues in the cleft palate population: The state of the art. *Cleft Palate-Craniofacial Journal, 37*, 348–383.

Kummer, A. W. (2008). Cleft palate and craniofacial anomalies: Effects on speech and resonance (2nd ed.). Clifton Park, NY: Delmar Cengage Learning.

Kwan, W. M., Abdullah, V. J., Liu, K., van Hasselt, C. A., & Tong, C. F. (2011). Otitis media with effusion and hearing loss in Chinese children with cleft lip and palate. *The Cleft Palate-Craniofacial Journal, 48*(6), 684–689.

Lazarus, D., Hudson, D., van Zyl, J., Fleming, A., & Fernandes, D. (1998). Repair of unilateral cleft lip: A comparison of five techniques. *Annals of Plastic Surgery, 41*(6), 587–594.

Liedman-Boshki, J., Lohmander, A., Persson, C., Lith, A., & Elander, A. (2005). Perceptual analysis of speech and the activity in the lateral pharyngeal walls before and after velopharyngeal flap surgery. *Scandinavian Journal of Plastic and Reconstructive Surgery and Hand Surgery, 39*, 22–32.

Marcusson, A. (2002). Facial appearance in adults who had cleft lip and palate treated in childhood. *Scandinavian Journal of Plastic and Reconstructive Surgery and Hand Surgery, 35*(1), 16–23.

Marcusson, A., Akerlind, I., & Paulin, G. (2001). Quality of life in adults with repaired complete cleft lip and palate. *Cleft Palate-Craniofacial Journal, 38*(4), 379–385.

Middleton, G., & Pannbacker, M. (1997). *Cleft palate and related disorders*. Bisbee, AZ: Imaginart International.

Millard, T., & Richman, L. C. (2001). Different cleft conditions, facial appearance, and speech: Relationship to psychological variables. *Cleft Palate-Craniofacial Journal, 38*, 68–75.

Mitchell, L. E., & Risch, H. (1992). Mode of inheritance of nonsyndromic cleft lip with or without cleft palate: A reanalysis. *American Journal of Human Genetics, 51*, 323–332.

Moller, K., & Glaze, L. (2009). Cleft lip and palate: interdisciplinary issues and treatment (2nd ed.). Austin, TX: Pro-Ed.

Murthy, J., Sendhilnathan, S., Hussain, A. (2010). *Speech outcomes following late primary palate repair.* The Cleft Palate-Craniofacial Journal, *47*(2), 156–161.

Pamplona, M., & Ysunza, A. (1999). Active participation of mothers during speech therapy: Improved language development of children with cleft palate. *Scandinavian Journal of Plastic and Reconstructive Surgery, 33*, 1–6.

Pamplona, M., Ysunza, A., & Uriostegui, C. (1996). Linguistic interaction: The role of parents in therapy for cleft palate patients. *International Journal of Pediatric Otorhinolaryngology, 37*, 17–27.

Pannbacker, M. (1975). Oral language skills of adult cleft palate speakers. *Cleft Palate Journal, 12*, 95–106.

Persson, M., Aniansson, G., Becker, M., & Svensson, H. (2002). Self-concept and introversion with cleft lip and palate. *Scandinavian Journal of Plastic and Reconstructive Surgery and Hand Surgery, 36*(1), 24–27.

Peterson-Falzone, S. J. (1989). Compensatory articulations in cleft palate speakers: Relative incidence by type. Proceedings of the International Congress on Cleft Palate and Related Craniofacial Anomalies, Jerusalem, Israel.

Peterson-Falzone, S. J., Hardin-Jones, A., & Karnell, M. P. (2010). *Cleft palate speech* (4th ed.). St. Louis, MO: Mosby.

Pillemer, F. G., & Cook, K. V. (1989). The psychosocial adjustment of pediatric craniofacial patients after surgery. *Cleft Palate Journal, 26*(3), 201–207.

Pope, A. W., & Snyder, H. T. (2004). Psychosocial adjustment in children and adolescents with a craniofacial anomaly: Age and sex patterns. *Cleft Palate-Craniofacial Journal, 42*, 4–12.

Pope, A. W., & Ward, J. (1997b). Self-perceived facial appearance and psychosocial adjustment in preadolescents with craniofacial anomalies. *Cleft Palate–Craniofacial Journal, 34*, 396–401.

Prokhorov, A. V., Perry, C., Kelder, S., & Klepp, K. (1993). Lifestyle values of adolescents: Results from the Minnesota Heart Health Youth Program. *Adolescence, 28*, 119–127.

Rahimov, F., Jugessur, A., & Murray, J. C. (2012). Genetics of nonsyndromic orofacial clefts. *The Cleft Palate-Craniofacial Journal, 49*(1), 73–91.

Ramstad, T., Ottem, E., & Shaw, W. (1995). Psychosocial adjustment in Norwegian adults who had undergone standardized treatment of complete cleft lip and palate. *Scandinavian Journal of Plastic and Reconstructive Surgery, 29*, 251–257.

Redford-Badwal, D. A., Mabry, K., & Frassinelli, J. D. (2003). Impact of cleft lip and/or palate on nutritional health and oral-motor development. *Dental Clinics of North America, 47*(2), 305–317.

Richman, L. C., & Millard, T. (1997). Cleft lip and palate: Longitudinal behavior and relationships of cleft conditions to behavior and achievement. *Journal of Pediatric Psychology, 22*, 487–494.

Rosenblatt, C. B. (1995). Effects of folate deficiency on embryonic development. *Braillieres Clinical Hematology, 8*(3), 617–637.

Salas-Provance, M. (2012). Counseling in a multicultural society. In L. V. Flasher & P. T. Fogle, *Counseling skills for speech-language pathologists and audiologists* (2nd ed.). Clifton Park, NY: Delmar Cengage Learning.

Salas-Provance, M. B., Kuehn, D., & Marsh, J. (2003). Phonetic repertoire and syllables characteristics of 15-month-old babies with cleft palate. *Journal of Phonetics, 31*, 23–38.

Sampson, P. D. (2000). On categorization in analyses of alcohol teratogenesis. *Environmental Health Perspectives, 108*, 421–428.

Sanders, C. (1998). Gender difference in bereavement expression across the life span. In K. Doka & J. Davidson (Eds.), *Living with grief: Who we are, how we grieve*. Washington, DC: Hospice Foundations of America.

Scherer, N. J., & D'Antonio, L. L. (1997). Language and play development in toddlers with cleft lip and/or palate. *American Journal of Speech-Language Pathology, 6*(4), 48–54.

Sekhon, P., Ethunandan, M., Mrkus, A., Krishnan, G., & Rao, C. (2011). Congenital anomalies associated with cleft lip and palate: An analysis of 1623 consecutive patients. *The Cleft Palate-Craniofacial Journal, 48*(4), 371–378.

Slade, P., Emerson, D. J., & Freedlander, E. (1999). A longitudinal comparison of the psychological impact on mothers or neonatal and 3-month repair of cleft lip. *British Journal of Plastic Surgery, 52*, 1–5.

Slifer, K., Amari, B., Diver, T., Hilley, L., Beck, M., Kane, A., & McDonnel, S. (2004). Social interaction patterns of children and adolescents with and without oral clefts during a videotaped analogue encounter. *Cleft Palate–Craniofacial Journal, 41*, 175–184.

Slifer, K., Pulbrook, M., Amari, B., Vona-Messersmith, M., Cohen, J., Ambadar, Z., Beck, M., & Piszczor, R. (2006). Social acceptance and facial behavior in children with oral clefts. *Cleft Palate–Craniofacial Journal, 43*(2), 226–236.

Snyder, H. T., Bilboul, M. J., & Pope, A. W. (2005). Psychosocial adjustment in adolescents with craniofacial anomalies: A comparison of parent and self-reports. *Cleft Palate–Craniofacial Journal, 42*, 5–16.

Strauss, R. P. (1985). Culture, rehabilitation, and facial birth defects: International case studies. *Cleft Palate Journal, 22*(1), 56–62.

Strauss, R. P. (1991). Culture, health care, and birth defects in the United States: An introduction. *Cleft Palate Journal, 27*(3), 275–278.

Strauss, R. P., Sharp, M., Lorch, S., & Kachalia, B. (1995). Physicians' communication of "bad news"—Parent experiences of being informed of their child's cleft lip/palate. *Pediatrics, 96*(1), 82–89.

Sulprizio, S. L. (2010). *The source for cleft palate and craniofacial speech disorders*. East Moline, IL: LinguiSystems.

Taub, P. J., & Lampert, J. A. (2011). Pediatric craniofacial surgery: A review for the multidisciplinay team. *The Cleft Palate-Craniofacial Journal, 48*(6), 670–683.

Topolski, T. D., Edwards, T. C., & Patrick, D. L. (2005). Quality of life: How do adolescents with facial differences compare with other adolescents? *Cleft Palate–Craniofacial Journal, 42*, 1, 19–24.

Turner, S. R., Rumsey, N., & Sandy, J. R. (1998). Psychological aspects of cleft lip and palate. *European Journal of Orthodontics, 20*(4), 407–415.

Vanderas, A. P. (1987). Incidence of cleft lip, cleft palate, and cleft lip and palate among the races: A review. *Cleft Palate Journal, 24*(21), 216–225.

Van Staden, F., & Gerhardt, C. (1995). Mothers of children with facial cleft deformities: Reactions and effects. *South American Journal of Psychology, 25*(1), 39–46.

Warschausky, S., Kay, J., Buchman, S., Halberg, A., & Berger, M. (2002). Health-related quality of life in children with craniofacial anomalies. *Plastic and Reconstructive Surgery, 110*(2), 409–41.

Yttri, J. E., Christensen, K., Knudsen, L. B., & Bille, C. (2011). Reproductive patterns among Danish women with oral clefts. *The Cleft Palate-Craniofacial Journal, 48*(5), 601–607.

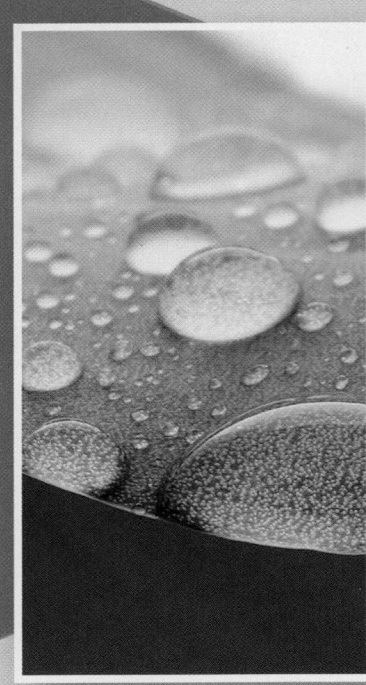

CHAPTER 11
Neurological Disorders in Adults

LEARNING OBJECTIVES

After studying this chapter, you will:

- Know the etiologies of neurogenic communication disorders and the various types of strokes.
- Be able to discuss the common characteristics of the aphasias.
- Be familiar with cognitive disorders caused by closed and open head injuries.
- Know the common characteristics of right-hemisphere syndrome.
- Understand basic information about dementia and Alzheimer's disease.
- Be familiar with principles of assessment of aphasia and cognitive disorders.
- Be able to discuss general principles of therapy for aphasia and cognitive disorders.
- Be familiar with the emotional and social effects of neurological disorders on patients and their families.

KEY TERMS

activities of daily living (ADLs)
agrammatic (agrammatism)
agraphia
alexia (acquired dyslexia)
Alzheimer's disease (AD)
aneurysm
anomia
anomic aphasia
anosognosia
aphasia (dysphasia)
arteriosclerosis

atherosclerosis
attention impairments
autopsy (postmortem)
board and care home
Broca's aphasia
cerebral embolism (embolus)
cerebral hemorrhage (hemorrhagic stroke)
cerebral thrombosis (thrombus)
chronic traumatic encephalopathy (CTE)

circumlocution
closed head injury (CHI) (nonpenetrating brain injury)
cognitive disorder
coma
computerized tomography (CT) scan
concussion
contrecoup injury
cortical atrophy
custodial care
degenerative disease

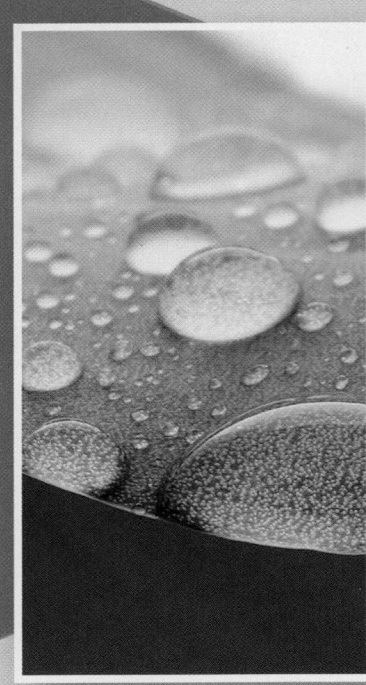

KEY TERMS continued

dementia
edema
expressive aphasia
family therapy
fluent aphasia
functional outcomes
global aphasia
high blood pressure
  (hypertension)
incontinence
infarction (necrosis)
integrate (integration)
jargon aphasia
literal or phonemic
  paraphasia
loss of consciousness
  (LOC)
magnetic resonance
  imaging (MRI)
mental status
  examination
metastasis
neologism

neuritic (senile) plaques
neurofibrillary tangles
neuropsychologist
nonfluent aphasia
occlusive (ischemic)
  stroke
open head injury (OHI)
perseverate/
  perseveration
persistent vegetative
  state (PVS)
positive emission
  tomography (PET)
postconcussion
  syndrome (PCS)
post-traumatic stress
  disorder (PTSD)
premorbid
prognosis
prosody (prosodic)/
  melody (melodic)
prosopagnosia
quality of life

receptive aphasia
residential care facility
right-hemisphere
  syndrome
senility
spontaneous recovery
stroke (cerebrovascular
  accident, CVA)
toxin
transient ischemic attack
  (TIA)
traumatic brain injury
  (TBI) (head trauma,
  acquired brain injury
  [ABI])
tumor (neoplasm)
vegetative state
verbal or semantic
  paraphasia
visual–spatial
  impairments
Wernicke's aphasia
working memory

CHAPTER OUTLINE

INTRODUCTION

Neurological disorders may occur at any age, but most commonly occur in people over 65 years of age. With improved medical care and the increasing "graying of America," there is an increase in individuals with neurological disorders. Speech-language pathologists work with individuals who have neurological impairments in settings such as hospitals (acute care, subacute care, and convalescent [sometimes called a *nursing home, skilled nursing facility—SNF,* or *long-term care facility—LTC*]), inpatient and outpatient clinics, rehabilitation centers, home health care, private practices, and university clinics.

ETIOLOGIES OF NEUROGENIC SPEECH, LANGUAGE, COGNITIVE, AND SWALLOWING DISORDERS

Neurogenic communication and swallowing problems have many possible etiologies. The causes vary somewhat by age group; for example, young adults are more likely to have traumatic brain injuries from motor vehicle accidents (MVAs) or altercations, and older individuals are more likely to have strokes, brain tumors, or degenerative disorders. Understanding the causes of patients' speech, language, cognitive, and swallowing problems can be helpful in both assessment and treatment. However, we base therapy not on just the neurological cause of the communication or swallowing impairments but on the signs and symptoms we see during our assessment and ongoing work with patients. In some cases our assessment and therapy may be initiated before we are able to obtain a clear medical or radiological cause of a patient's disorders. Also, our prognosis for an individual patient's rehabilitation and recovery is based more on what we see during our assessment and treatment than what may be predicted based on a neurologist's or radiologist's findings (Cherney, 2004; Davis, 2007; Huckabee & Pelletier, 2003; LaPointe, 2005; Murray & Clark, 2006; Papathanasiou, Coppens, & Potagas, 2012). Many patients make progress far beyond what might be predicted based on the cause and extent of neurological damage, and some make less progress.

Strokes (Cerebrovascular Accidents)

Strokes or **cerebrovascular accidents (CVAs)** are the third-leading cause of death in the United States and the world for people over 45 years of age, with the first- and second-leading causes of death being heart attacks and cancer. The average age to have a first stroke is approximately

stroke (cerebrovascular accident, CVA)

A disruption of blood supply to the brain caused by an occluded (blocked) artery or an artery that has.

67 years. Men have a higher risk for stroke, with an incidence of 1.25 times higher than that of women; however, women are more likely to die from stroke (of every five deaths caused by stroke, two are men and three are women) (American Heart Association, 2012 [Note: the American Stroke Association is a division of the American Heart Association].

Nearly 150,000 people in the United States die from strokes each year, with about 600,000 survivors experiencing various forms and degrees of speech, language, cognitive, swallowing, and physical impairments affecting all parts of their bodies (strokes are the leading cause of disability in the United States). Approximately 85% of stroke survivors are able to return to their prestroke living environment with various levels of permanent impairments, and about 15% of survivors must be admitted to long-term care facilities (Goldstein, 2009; American Heart Association 2012).

The number of strokes in the United States has been increasing from approximately 550,000 per year in the 1970s to about 730,000 per year in the 1990s. The reasons for this increase are uncertain, although they may be related to dietary and stress factors (American Heart Association, 2012). A physiological manifestation of stress is **high blood pressure (hypertension)**, which causes increased susceptibility to strokes.

Strokes result in brain damage because of the disruption of blood flow that prevents oxygenated blood and nutrients from reaching areas of the brain. This can result in a range of problems, from *localized lesions* (relatively small damaged areas) to widespread, diffuse damage. Strokes can occur in any area of the central nervous system: the brain, cerebellum, brainstem, and even spinal cord. The *site* (location) and size of the lesion are what generally determine the characteristics and extent of neurological damage. Beyond the stroke itself, edema of brain tissue can develop that increases pressure inside the brain, causing further damage.

Since the 1990s, the National Stroke Association and the American Heart Association have attempted to increase public awareness about the eminent dangers of strokes by calling them "*brain attacks.*" This term was adopted because of the public's awareness of the need for immediate medical attention for heart attacks. People who have heart attacks are susceptible to strokes because the same vascular problems that occur in heart attacks can cause brain attacks.

Numerous risk factors predispose a person for a stroke; for example, being male, smoking, being overweight, a fatty diet, lack of exercise, heavy alcohol consumption, diabetes mellitus, high blood pressure, getting older, family history of stroke or heart attack, and lack of regular health checkups. Risk factors for strokes are also risk factors for heart attacks (American Heart Association, 2012) (see Figure 11–1).

Occlusive (Ischemic) Strokes

An **occlusive (ischemic) stroke** means that an area of the brain is deprived of blood because of a blocked (*occluded*) artery. Occlusive strokes make up about 80% of the strokes in people. If the occlusion

high blood pressure (hypertension)

A common disorder in middle age and later (although now often being seen in obese children and young adults) in which blood pressure is chronically above 140 over 90 mm Hg (120/80 is considered normal).

occlusive (ischemic) stroke

A partial or complete blockage (occlusion) of a cerebral artery, causing decreased blood supply to brain tissue.

Application Question

Considering your age and gender, what risk factors might you have for a stroke or heart attack? What do you do regularly to decrease your risk factors?

It is important for everyone to know warning signs of stroke. If you become aware of any of the following symptoms in yourself or another person, emergency medical care is essential:

 Sudden numbness or weakness of the face, arm, or leg, especially on one side of the body

 Sudden confusion or difficulty speaking or understanding

 Sudden difficulty seeing in one or both eyes

 Sudden difficulty walking, dizziness, and loss of balance or coordination

Sudden, severe headache with no known cause

A quick test to recognize if a person is having a stroke uses the acronym **F.A.S.T.:**

 Face: Ask the person to smile. A stroke can cause one side of the face to droop. Abrupt dimming of vision and a sudden, severe headache with no known cause are also warning signs.

 Arms: Ask the person to raise both arms. If one arm drifts downward or it cannot be raised, a stroke may be causing weakness, numbness, or paralysis. Individuals may also have a loss of balance or a sudden fall.

 Speech: Ask the person to repeat a simple sentence. Listen for slurred words and trouble speaking or understanding speech.

 Time: If the person has any symptoms, call 911 immediately. Time is of the essence!

Figure 11-1

General warning signs of stroke and F.A.S.T.

Adapted from the American Stroke Association, 2012; and Kothari, Pancioli, Liu, Brott, & Broderick, 1999.

---

infarction (necrosis)

A localized area of necrotic (dead) tissue resulting from lack of blood supply and oxygen to the tissue.

transient ischemic attack (TIA)

An episode of cerebral vascular insufficiency with partial occlusion of a cerebral artery by atherosclerotic plaque or an embolus; disturbances of vision in one or both eyes, dizziness, weakness, numbness, dysphasia, or unconsciousness may occur; TIA (sometimes called "ministroke") usually lasts a few minutes, and in rare cases symptoms may continue for several hours.

lasts for more than 3 minutes, death (**infarction**, **necrosis**) of brain tissue is likely. In addition, swelling (edema) of brain tissue develops around the area damaged from the stroke, compressing and causing temporary or permanent damage to more brain tissue. **Transient ischemic attacks (TIAs)** (sometimes called "*ministrokes*") are episodes of cerebral vascular insufficiency with partial occlusion of a cerebral artery by atherosclerotic plaque or an embolus. The symptoms vary with the site and degree of occlusion (Mosby, 2009).

Even the Strong Have Strokes

On February 6, 2005, Tedy Bruschi led the New England Patriots to a 24–21 victory in Super Bowl XXXIX, with six solo tackles and a timely fourth-quarter interception against the Philadelphia Eagles. But 10 days later, at 4 a.m. on February 16, Bruschi awoke with a severe headache, his left arm and leg numb, and loss of vision in his left visual field. After an emergency trip to Massachusetts General Hospital, a CT scan revealed that Bruschi had sustained a stroke caused by a blood clot. However, on October 30, 2005, following months of rehabilitation, Bruschi was back on the football field as a Patriot. That day he made 10 tackles in a win over Buffalo and was named the National Football League's Comeback Player of the Year for the 2005 season.

Cerebral Thrombosis (Thrombus)

A **cerebral thrombosis (thrombus)** occurs when an artery in the brain gradually becomes blocked by debris in the blood. Fatty substances accumulate over decades on the lining of arterial walls. This causes a buildup of atherosclerotic plaque, which may lead to **atherosclerosis**, a type of **arteriosclerosis** (hardening of the arteries). Eventually, 50%–100% of an artery may be blocked. With increased blockage, blood flow decreases to the areas of the brain the artery supplies (see Figure 11–2). The person's functioning may slowly deteriorate over many years, but the person may not have any acute symptoms that alert the need for medical attention until there is a complete blockage. By that time, the person has a dramatic change in functioning and there may be considerable deterioration of tissue in some areas of the brain.

Cerebral Embolism (Embolus)

A **cerebral embolism (embolus)** occurs when a fragment of material travels through the circulatory system and reaches a small artery in the brain, where it occludes a blood vessel. At the location of the occlusion, the embolus begins to function as a thrombus. A variety of material may form as an embolus from most locations in the body (e.g., fragment of atherosclerotic plaque, piece of a blood clot, or tumor material). Many cerebral emboli are associated with coronary artery disease (Mosby, 2009).

Cerebral Hemorrhage

Cerebral hemorrhages (hemorrhagic strokes) account for approximately 20% of strokes. Hemorrhages are the result of a rupture of a blood vessel. People with chronic high blood pressure are most susceptible to hemorrhagic strokes (see Figure 11–3). During a cerebral hemorrhage, blood is forced into the brain tissue and destroys it (blood is toxic to brain tissue). Besides the death of neurons, the blood forms a

cerebral thrombosis (thrombus)

An abnormal condition in which a clot (thrombus) develops within a blood vessel.

atherosclerosis

A common disorder characterized by yellowish plaques of cholesterol and other lipids (fats) in the inner layers of the walls of arteries; often associated with tobacco use, obesity, hypertension, diabetes mellitus, and aging.

arteriosclerosis

A common disorder characterized by thickening, hardening, and loss of elasticity of arterial walls as a result of build-up of atherosclerotic plaque, leading to decreased blood supply.

cerebral embolism (embolus)

An abnormal condition in which a blood clot, piece of tumor, or other material (embolus) circulates in the bloodstream until it becomes lodged in a cerebral blood vessel, causing an occlusion; at the location of the occlusion, the embolus begins to function as a thrombus.

cerebral hemorrhage (hemorrhagic stroke)

The result of a blood vessel under pressure rupturing and sending blood into the brain tissue; hemorrhages may be arterial, venous, or capillary.

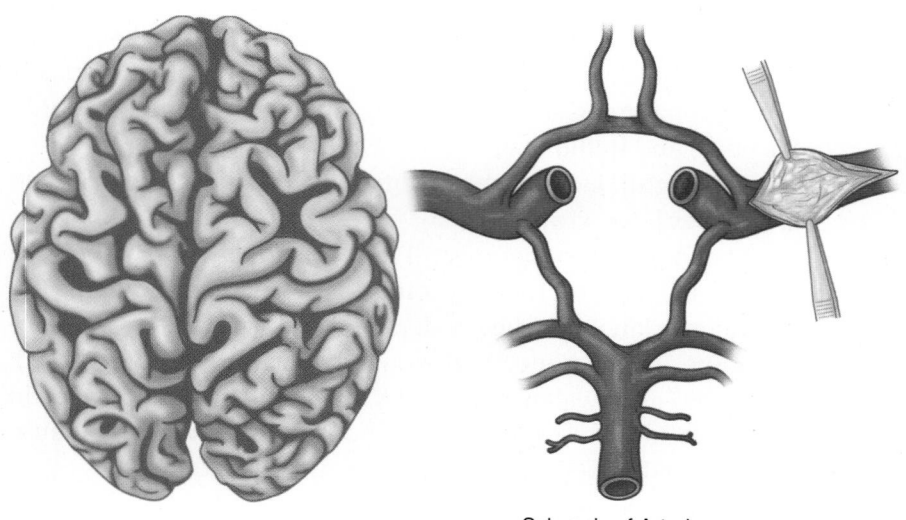

Atrophy of the Brain in Arteriosclerosis

Sclerosis of Arteries in the Base of the Brain

Figure 11–2

Atherosclerotic plaque and arteriosclerosis.

© Cengage Learning 2013.

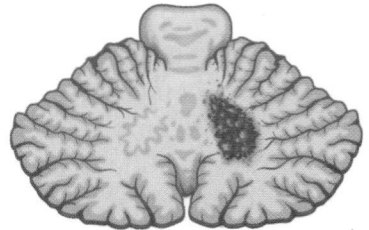

(b)   Cerebellar Hemorrhage

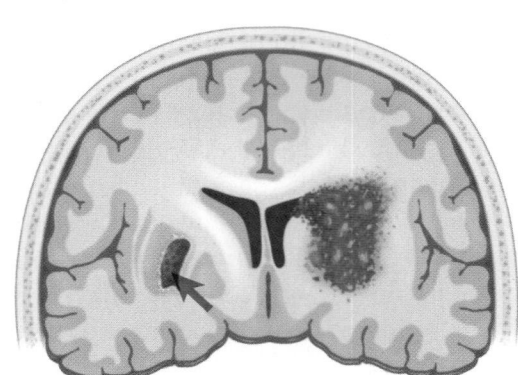

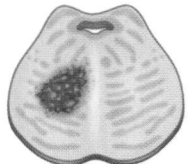

Figure 11-3

Cerebral hemorrhages may occur in different locations in the (a) brain, (b) cerebellum, or (c) brainstem.

© Cengage Learning 2013.

Massive Hemorrhage with Rupture into Ventricle. Scar of Old "Healed" Hemorrhage on Opposite Side.

(a)

(c)   Pontine Hemorrhage

mass (like a clot) that can create pressure on surrounding brain tissue, causing further neurological symptoms that are remote from the area of the hemorrhage. Cerebral hemorrhages are a medical emergency of the highest degree (Broderick, Adams, & Barsan, 1999).

CASE STUDY

Kirk Douglas's Stroke of Luck

A stroke can occur in anyone, regardless of who we are or what we do. In 1994, Kirk Douglas, the famous actor (whose son is another famous actor, Michael Douglas), sustained an occlusive stroke in his left hemisphere. After discharge from the hospital, he received rehabilitation treatment, including speech therapy in his home. Before Douglas's stroke, the Academy of Motion Picture Arts and Sciences had voted to award him an Oscar for Lifetime Achievement. He worked with his speech-language pathologist to be ready to appear on stage in front of 2,000 of his peers and millions of television viewers.

On Oscar night, Douglas was introduced by director Steven Spielberg. Douglas later wrote:

I thought of my speech therapist: "Pause . . . breathe . . . swallow . . . articulate." I started slowly: "I see my four sons. They're proud of the old man." The audience laughed. They understood me! I spotted my wife sobbing. I held up the Oscar. "Anne, this belongs to you. I love you." I paused, took a deep breath and swallowed. "Thank you for 50 wonderful years in the wonderful world of moviemaking." I bowed, thunderous applause engulfing me. I couldn't believe it. They really understood me! ■

Adapted from Douglas, 2002.

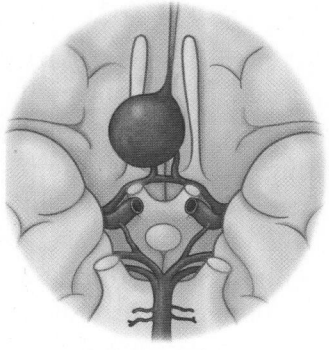

(b)

Aneurysm of Anterior
Cerebral Artery

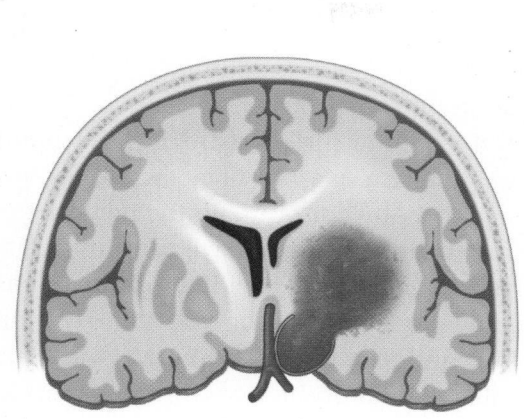

(a)   Aneurysm Ruptured Intracerebrally

Figure 11–4

A cerebral aneurysm:
(a) aneurysm ruptured
intracerebrally and
(b) aneurysm in anterior
cerebral artery.
© Cengage Learning 2013.

An **aneurysm** is a bulging of an artery at its weakest point (much like a chain is only as strong as its weakest link; an artery is only as strong as its weakest point). The walls of the aneurysm are stretched and thinned, increasing the likelihood of hemorrhaging when a person's blood pressure is unusually high (see Figure 11–4).

Multicultural Considerations

Ethnicity and culture appear to have roles in the prevalence of strokes and aphasia. Behind these two factors may lay differences in socioeconomic status and health. However, data on ethnicity and cultural differences for health problems of all kinds, including strokes, are both limited and inconsistent.

Some data are seen as generally reliable. For example, African Americans have a higher incidence of high blood pressure than other populations in the United States and are, therefore, more susceptible to strokes (Singh, Cohen, & Krupp, 1996). In fact, African American men and women are nearly twice as likely to have strokes as the Caucasian population. Mexican Americans have a higher incidence of strokes compared to the non-Hispanic white population. African Americans and Hispanic Americans tend to have strokes younger than the Caucasian population. African American males have the highest death rates from strokes, and Hispanics and American Indians and Alaskan Natives have the lowest. The risk factors for strokes are generally the same for all ethnic and cultural populations—that is, high blood pressure, smoking, high cholesterol, obesity, poor diet, high-sodium diet, lack of exercise, alcohol consumption, and diabetes (American Heart Association, 2012).

aneurysm

A localized dilation of a blood vessel wall, resulting in the thinning of the wall at that site (much like a balloon being blown up) and increasing the likelihood of hemorrhaging, especially with high blood pressure.

Recovery from Strokes

Most people make their greatest gains in **spontaneous recovery** (physiological healing of the brain) during the first few weeks or months after a stroke. The majority of speech and language recovery occurs during the first six months post onset; however, additional but slower recovery may continue for years after (Code, 2001).

Each patient has a limited capacity for reorganizing the brain circuitry, and the limitations are based on a variety of factors; for example, a patient's chronological age (usually, the younger the person, the better the **prognosis**); physical health (a person who is physically healthy without serious organ damage from an accident or illness has a better prognosis than a person who is not well or has serious organ damage); and the site (location) and size of the lesion. Most people who have had strokes have some residual problems with their speech, language, cognitive functioning, or a combination of these. Many individuals have difficulty returning to their previous employment, others become somewhat housebound, and some must be admitted to long-term care facilities.

Traumas

Traumatic brain injury (TBI) (also called *acquired brain injury* or ABI) has its highest incidence in the 15- to 24-year-old age group. It is the leading cause of death of people under 35 years of age and the leading cause of neurological disability of people under the age of 50. About one in three people are left with permanent disabilities; consequently, many individuals who sustain a TBI must cope with communicative and cognitive difficulties for the greater part of their adult lives (Guerrero, Thurman, & Sniezek, 2000).

Approximately one-half to two-thirds of all head traumas are caused by motor vehicle accidents, and many of these are alcohol related, particularly with younger drivers. Assaults that are often related to alcohol or drugs (particularly in the young male adult population) and falls (in the older population) account for most other TBIs. The frontal lobes are the most commonly damaged area of the brain in TBIs (see Figure 11–5). Males are nearly twice as likely to receive TBIs as females (Guerrero, Thurman, & Sniezek, 2000; Tate, McDonald, & Lulham, 1998).

Closed Head Injury (CHI) (Nonpenetrating Brain Injury)

Closed head injuries (nonpenetrating brain injuries) are the most common type of head injury in the civilian population. In CHIs, the skull receives a severe impact and may be fractured, but it is not penetrated. The most common causes of CHIs in adults are motor vehicle accidents and assaults. In CHIs, damage is usually caused either by a blunt object (e.g., the head hitting the windshield of a vehicle) or by a sudden stopping of the head's movement in a particular direction (e.g., the head

---

spontaneous recovery

The physiological healing of the brain's damaged tissue, including reduction of cerebral edema, development of collateral blood vessels, and rerouting of neural pathways.

prognosis

A prediction of the probable course, duration, recovery, or termination of a disease or disorder; a prediction of the outcome of a proposed course of treatment, its effectiveness and duration, and the individual's progress.

traumatic brain injury (TBI) (head trauma, acquired brain injury [ABI])

An acquired injury to the brain caused by an external force and resulting in partial or total functional disability, including psychosocial impairment; applies to both closed and open head injuries, affecting speech, language, cognition, psychosocial behavior, and physical functioning.

closed head injury (CHI) (nonpenetrating brain injury)

Severe impact to the skull, often with a blunt object such as the windshield of a vehicle or a bat, or the head striking the ground after a fall; the skull may be fractured but is not penetrated (e.g., by a bullet).

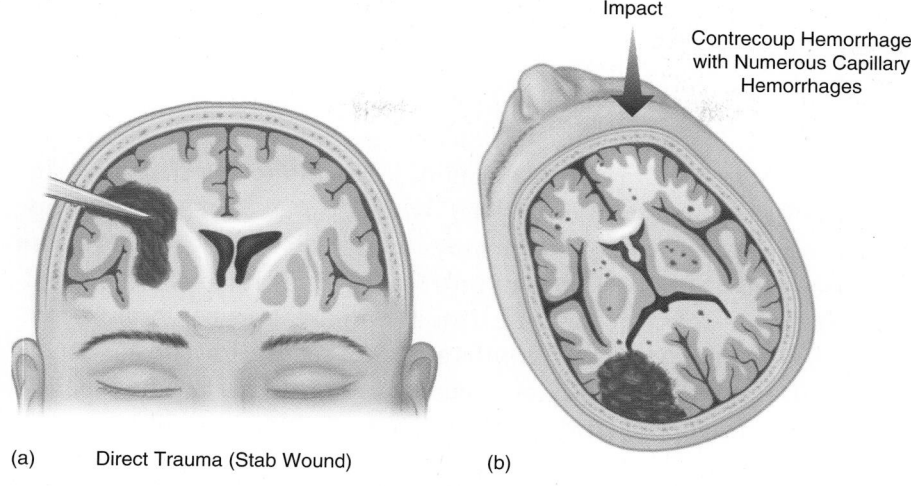

Impact

Contrecoup Hemorrhage
with Numerous Capillary
Hemorrhages

(a)   Direct Trauma (Stab Wound)   (b)

Figure 11–5

Traumatic brain injuries
can occur in countless
ways, including (a) direct
trauma such as a stab
wound causing an open
head injury or (b) closed
head injury from a motor
vehicle accident that
may result in contrecoup
hemorrhage.

© Cengage Learning 2013.

hitting the ground during a fall). The sudden stopping of the head's momentum sets off a cascade of physiological events. Closed head injuries sometimes result in **contrecoup damage** (pronounced "contra-coo") in which there is damage to the brain at both the site of impact and the opposite side because the brain "flows" and causes intense compression (see Figure 11–5). After a CHI, the brain tissue swells, causing sustained compression of the neurons and damaging them further. The edema may not subside for several days to weeks, during which time the person will present as more severely impaired than after the edema has diminished (Kochanek, Clark, & Jenkins, 2007; Tate, McDonald, & Lulham, 1998).

In motor vehicle accidents, *whiplash injury* often occurs at the same instant as the brain damage because of the rapid forward and backward or rotational movement of the head. Whiplash injuries damage the cervical vertebrae or their supporting ligaments and muscles. Whiplash injuries also can damage the brainstem, resulting in weakness or paralysis of the muscles of the speech systems causing in dysarthria and/or dysphagia (see Chapter 12), as well as bodily impairments.

Mild Traumatic Brain Injury (mTBI)

More than two-thirds of all head injuries are classified as mild, where there is **concussion** but no **loss of consciousness (LOC)** (lack of awareness and wakefulness), or no more than 30 minutes of LOC (other medical criteria are used as well). There is an increased awareness of concussions that occur in sports, causing **chronic traumatic encephalopathy (CTE)**. At the high school level, 15% of injuries among athletes are concussions, with some athletes sustaining more than one concussion in the same year. High school football is the most likely sport for males to receive concussions, followed by soccer and ice hockey. For females, high school soccer and lacrosse are the most likely sports to receive concussions (Meechan, d'Hemecourt, Collins, & Comstock, 2011).

contrecoup injury

In closed head injuries damage to the brain occurring on the opposite side of the trauma site; for example, when an impact to the right frontal side of the skull results in brain damage on the left posterior side.

concussion

Mild traumatic brain injury caused by a violent jarring or shaking that often occurs during a closed head injury and results in at least a brief loss of consciousness.

loss of consciousness (LOC)

Impaired responsiveness, usually caused by diffuse brain dysfunction or damage to the brainstem and the reticular activating system; duration is often used as a measure of traumatic brain injury severity.

chronic traumatic encephalopathy (CTE)

A degenerative brain disease caused by repeated brain traumas (particularly concussions) that results in behaviors similar to Alzheimer's disease.

CASE STUDY

Haitham

Haitham was a 26-year-old man referred by a physician to a speech-language pathologist in private practice. He was a civil engineer who had been born and raised in Amman, Jordan, and his first language was Arabic. Haitham sustained a TBI when he was 23 years old during a motor vehicle accident. **Computerized tomography (CT) scan** and **magnetic resonance imaging (MRI)** of his head revealed multiple brain traumas with diffuse axonal damage and cerebral edema. Haitham was in a coma for 8 months and after recovering consciousness was transferred to a rehabilitation center in Amman where he received physical, occupational, and speech therapy. Eighteen months after the motor vehicle accident he was flown to London, England, where he was seen at a neurological rehabilitation center as an outpatient. A **mental status examination** by a **neuropsychologist** revealed that Haitham remained at considerable risk for emotional difficulties, particularly when the somewhat unrealistic goals he had set for himself could not be realized (i.e., returning to his work as a civil engineer).

Haitham eventually came to California with his mother to live with a relative and to continue receiving speech, language, and cognitive therapy. Evaluation of Haitham by the speech-language pathologist revealed severe dysarthria, mild-to-moderate receptive and expressive aphasia, and severe cognitive impairments that interfered with independent functioning in a consistently safe manner in the home and community. He worked with the therapist twice weekly for several months, making significant gains in most areas, and then returned to his home in Amman, Jordan. Haitham remained unrealistic about his potential to return to his previous work as a civil engineer. ■

Because most concussions do not result in loss of consciousness, they are typically more difficult to detect and can be under-diagnosed in athletes (Moser, Iverson, Echemendia, et al., 2007).

Postconcussion syndrome (PCS) is a constellation of symptoms seen in some patients with mild traumatic brain injury, including headache, poor concentration, short-term memory deficits, and affective disturbances (e.g., anxiety, depression, and irritability). However, when loss of consciousness occurs and is prolonged (hours to years) the person is comatose and the length and depth of the **coma** has some prognostic implications for long-term recovery. Patients who have longer and deeper comas generally have a poorer recovery than patients who have shorter and lighter comas (Guthrie, Mast, McQuaid, & Pavlakis, 1999; Johnson & Jacobson, 2007). The term **vegetative state** differs from coma; whereas there is neither awareness nor wakefulness in coma, in a vegetative state a patient may have some minimal level of wakefulness but has not regained awareness (i.e., there is no observable cognitive function).

Persistent vegetative state (PVS) is applied to individuals who survive extensive and irrevocable brain damage but are highly unlikely ever to achieve higher functioning above a vegetative state (Giacino & Whyte, 2005; Hirsch, 2005; Golper, 2010).

Even when head injuries are mild, there are often long-lasting subtle impairments, including difficulty concentrating under distracting conditions (e.g., reading with a television on) or multitasking (trying to do more than one task at a time, such as preparing a meal while talking with someone, or driving—the ultimate challenge in multitasking). Individuals who have had mild traumatic brain injuries often have ongoing difficulty with attention, memory, and higher-level cognitive functioning, particularly when there is frontal lobe damage. Motivation is frequently impaired, and these individuals often have increased anxiety, depression, and irritability (Iverson, Lange, Gatz, & Zasler, 2007; McDonald, 2007; Ponsford, 2004; Sohlberg & Mateer, 2001).

People with mild TBIs are usually discharged from the acute-care hospital after only a short stay, and they may receive some outpatient rehabilitation. However, their real impairments often do not become apparent until they try to return to work and find that they cannot easily perform at the same level as they did before their TBI. Problems also start developing at home. Because people with brain injuries cannot perform at their **premorbid** level on the job, they may be demoted or lose their jobs, causing financial strain on the family. Marital relationships often deteriorate. The individuals may feel guilty that they cannot be the same husband or wife or father or mother they were before the accident. If they are able to maintain a job, they come home exhausted with little or no reserve energy for family life. Resentment may build up within the family because injured people prefer to rest rather than do family activities on weekends. Old friends may begin to stay away because injured people often lose interest or are unable to continue activities they had enjoyed all of their lives. As rehabilitation specialists, we need to always keep in mind that the effects of neurological damage on individuals affect everyone with whom they are associated (Flasher & Fogle, 2012; McDonald, 2007; Tanner, 2007).

Open Head Injury (OHI)

Open head injuries (OHI) are the result of the skull and brain being penetrated either by severe impact or by projectiles (e.g., bullets, fragments of glass, or shrapnel from explosions). In many cases, there is a single trajectory (path) of the projectile (e.g., bullet), and it is mainly the tissue damaged along the path that causes the *cognitive-linguistic impairments* we see. Patients with OHIs often continue to have significant impairments the rest of their lives. In civilian life, OHIs occur less often than CHIs.

War Wounds

Traumatic brain injuries may cause CHIs or OHIs, and the injuries are often different from typical TBIs in civilian life (Lew, Poole, Alvarez, &

neuropsychologist

A Ph.D. psychologist specialized in the area of practice in clinical psychology and neurogenic disorders who assesses cognitive functioning, discriminates between psychiatric and neurological conditions, distinguishes among different neurological conditions, and predicts the course of a patient's recovery; however, most of the cognitive-linguistic therapy is provided by SLPs.

postconcussion syndrome (PCS)

A constellation of symptoms seen in some patients with mild traumatic brain injury, including headache, poor concentration, short-term memory deficits, and affective disturbances (e.g., anxiety, depression, and irritability).

coma

A prolonged period of unconsciousness in which a patient has minimal, if any, purposeful responses to stimuli.

vegetative state

A condition in which a person may have some minimal level of wakefulness but has not regained awareness (i.e., they lack observable cognitive function).

persistent vegetative state (PVS)

A medical diagnosis made only after numerous neurological and other tests that, due to extensive and irrevocable brain damage, a patient is highly unlikely ever to achieve higher functioning above a vegetative state.

premorbid

In medicine, the wellness or functioning of a patient before a significant illness or injury.

Personal Story — Vietnam

As a combat medic in Vietnam in 1969, I knew how uncomfortable and heavy steel helmets were after wearing them for many hours every day and night. I encouraged men to wear their helmets at all times while on the lines or on patrols, but some men chose not to. I saw many men receive head wounds from rifle fire and shrapnel from mortars and rockets that could have been prevented or at least lessened if they had been wearing their helmets. Fortunately, in later wars (e.g., Iraq and Afghanistan) the new helmet material is lighter yet stronger and helmets are worn more consistently because of comfort—and because the soldiers are following strict orders to wear them. This information is particularly important for clinicians who will work in VA hospitals and will see many men and women with war wounds. ■

Application Question

Do you know anyone who had a mild traumatic brain injury or concussion? Were there any differences in how they were as people before and after the head injury?

open head injury (OHI)

Head injury in which the skull and brain are penetrated by a severe impact or by a projectile (bullet, fragment of glass, or shrapnel from an explosion).

post-traumatic stress disorder (PTSD)

A set of symptoms after exposure to a psychologically extreme traumatic stressor that involves intense fear, horror, or helplessness; symptoms include persistent reexperiencing of the traumatic event or events, avoidance of stimuli associated with the trauma, and symptoms of increased arousal (*hypervigilance*).

Moore, 2005). In war wounds, the open head injuries are usually more extensive (partly because the high-velocity bullets from military weapons result in powerful shock waves in the brain, causing more diffuse damage) and the individuals often have multiple severe injuries throughout their bodies, including their face and neck. In civilian life, war wounds are seen in explosions, including terrorist attacks. In all cases, the medical goal is to keep the person alive. Once the person is *stabilized* (physiological and metabolic processes of equilibrium in the body), rehabilitation can begin. Some SLPs and Auds work in Veterans Administration (VA) hospitals where they see terrible wounds in men and women. In some cases, soldiers may be discharged from a VA hospital and moved to a community hospital closer to the soldier's home where rehabilitation can continue. Clinicians need to be aware that these patients may be a "different" type of patient compared to those injured in civilian life (Flasher & Fogle, 2012).

Post-traumatic stress disorder (PTSD) is a problem that can affect combat veterans (whether or not they were physically wounded) in both subtle and obvious ways the rest of their lives. However, providing therapy for veterans is often a pleasure because they are disciplined and motivated, they have a joy of life (perhaps because they have seen so much loss of life), and they appreciate all that is done for them (Fogle, 2009b).

Tumors

Tumors (neoplasms) may grow in the brain and cause various communication, cognitive, and swallowing problems. The sites and sizes of tumors determine the impairments that develop in individuals. Tumors are abnormal masses of tissue that cause compression and displacement of

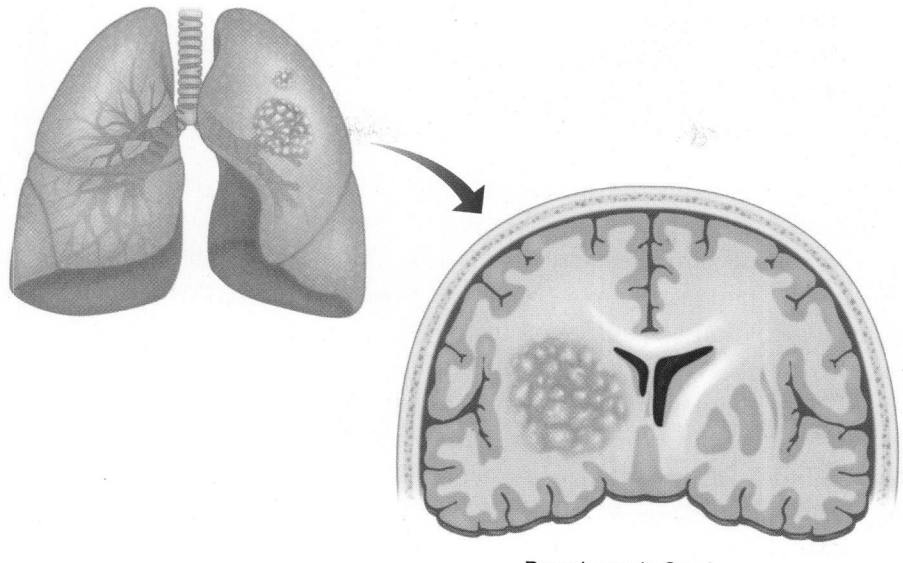

Bronchogenic Carcinoma
Metastasizing to Brain

Figure 11–6

Tumors may metastasize to
the brain from other areas
of the body.

© Cengage Learning 2013.

brain tissue unassociated with the specific site of the tumor. Tumors may be either *primary* (originating in the brain) or *secondary* (originating elsewhere in the body and then traveling to the brain). For example, a tumor may originate in the lungs (the primary tumor), and then cells from that tumor can **metastasize** (travel or spread) by way of the bloodstream to other areas of the body, such as the CNS (see Figure 11–6). Tumors may be either *benign* (not cancerous) or *malignant* (cancerous).

Toxins

SLPs sometimes work with patients who have neurological disorders caused by various toxins, some of which are preventable. **Toxins** are substances that poison or cause inflammation of the CNS. Probably the most commonly used toxic substance is alcohol. Years of excessive alcohol consumption can have severe effects on the CNS. Besides alcohol, many other toxins are self-administered as "recreational" drugs that can have lifelong effects on the nervous system and the person's quality of life. Many patients with neurological damage from various toxins have poor prognoses for significant improvement because much of their brain can be affected, leaving little "healthy" brain tissue available to be used for rehabilitation.

Degenerative Diseases and Disorders

Neurogenic communication disorders may be caused by **degenerative diseases** that affect structures and functions and cause progressive deterioration over time. Degenerative diseases can affect speech, language, cognition, swallowing, hearing, and balance. Examples of degenerative diseases that SLPs see clinically that result in cognitive-linguistic

tumor (neoplasm)

Any abnormal growth of new tissue, either benign or malignant, caused by aberrant increases in the rate of cell reproduction.

metastasis/metastasize

The process by which tumor cells travel or spread to distant parts of the body.

toxin

A substance that poisons or causes inflammation of tissue, including in the central nervous system.

degenerative disease

Any condition that causes gradual deterioration of normal body functions.

"I Wanted To See What Would Happen."

During a graduate internship at Rancho Los Amigos Hospital in Southern California, I was asked by my supervisor to accompany him to a local convalescent hospital to assess a 19-year-old man. The patient had taken an overdose of a drug and was left with severe neurological damage sufficient to cause him to remain hospitalized for the rest of his life. I asked him (probably inappropriately) why he did it, and he answered, "I wanted to see what would happen." As clinicians, we sometimes see individuals who, in a moment of reckless abandon, alter their lives forever. ■

impairments are the dementias (including Alzheimer's disease) (see Cognitive Disorders) and motor speech disorders such as amyotrophic lateral sclerosis (ALS, or Lou Gehrig's disease), Parkinson's disease, and myasthenia gravis (see Chapter 12).

THE APHASIAS

Numerous definitions of **aphasia (dysphasia)** have been used by various authors. Brookshire, in his earlier writings (1992, p. 1), provided a relatively simple but useful definition by saying that "Aphasia is a deficit in language processing that may affect all input modalities (auditory, visual, and tactile) and all output modalities (speaking, writing, and gesturing)." Code (2012) defines aphasia as an acquired language impairment resulting from neurological damage in the absence of **cognitive disorders** or motor and sensory impairments. Most SLPs use the term *aphasia* even though patients typically have impaired or disordered language (*dysphasia*) rather than a complete loss of language.

Classifications and Terminology Associated with the Aphasias

Classifications and terminology influence the way speech-language pathologists communicate with other SLPs, PTs, OTs, physicians, nurses, third-party payers (e.g., Medicare and insurance companies), and with patients and their families (Threats & Worrall, 2004). Although each patient is different, there are sufficient similarities so that we can use classification systems and diagnostic terms that communicate to other professionals of the basic impairments of the person. A diagnostic term implies that a certain set of characteristics apply to a patient.

The two classifications used specifically for aphasia are: **receptive aphasia** and **expressive aphasia**. That is, a person's language

aphasia (dysphasia)

An acquired language impairment resulting from neurological damage in the absence of cognitive, motor, or sensory impairments.

cognitive disorder

Impaired ability to process and use incoming information for memory, organization of information, reasoning, judgment, and problem solving for adequate functioning in activities of daily living, including a person's work. A diagnostic term implies that a certain set of characteristics apply to a patient.

receptive aphasia

Difficulty comprehending verbal, written, and/or gestural language.

expressive aphasia

Difficulty formulating verbal, written, and/or gestural language.

impairments may be narrowed down to difficulty understanding what is being communicated (auditory, reading, or gestural comprehension), difficulty expressing what the person wants to communicate (verbal, written, or gestural expression), or both. The receptive and expressive aphasia classification is roughly equivalent to the *fluent* (receptive) and *nonfluent* (expressive) classification system.

Fluent and Nonfluent Aphasia Classification System

Speech fluency is an important concept for understanding aphasia syndromes; therefore, the **fluent** and **nonfluent aphasia** classification system was devised. The **prosodic** or **melodic** characteristics of speech are the primary distinguishing factors for fluent and nonfluent aphasia. Fluency, when referring to the aphasias, does not connote stuttering (disfluency), although the concept of speech that flows easily (fluent) versus speech that has hesitations and repetitions (nonfluent) is the origin of the concept as it relates to aphasia (LaPointe, 2005).

Fluent aphasias are often associated with lesions posterior to the fissure of Rolando (central sulcus), primarily in and around the language areas in the temporal lobe of the left hemisphere *(perisylvian region)*. Patients with fluent aphasia typically have **auditory comprehension** impairments, difficulty comprehending written information, omission of important nouns, verbs, and adjectives in sentences, and syntactic errors; however, their speaking rate is relatively normal (100–200 words per minute), with normal phrasing (5–8 words per phrase or sentence), and they have relatively normal articulation, inflections, and intonation. Nonfluent aphasias are associated with lesions anterior to the fissure of Rolando, primarily in or around Broca's area in the premotor strip of the left frontal lobe. Nonfluent aphasia is characterized by relatively good auditory and reading comprehension, but difficulty initiating speech and saying the first sound or syllable of a word, reduced rate of speech (less than 50 words per minute), unusual effort when speaking, and omission of *functor* words (e.g., *a, an, the*).

Fluent aphasias include *Wernicke's aphasia, anomic aphasia, conduction aphasia*, and *transcortical sensory aphasia*. Nonfluent aphasias include *Broca's aphasia, transcortical motor aphasia*, and *global aphasia*. The *Boston Classification System* (Goodglass, Kaplan, & Barresi, 2001) has been particularly influential in our understanding of the different types of aphasia and the likely areas of neurological damage (see Figure 11–7).

Major Types of Aphasia

Each type of aphasia has its own characteristics. However, depending on the site and size of the lesion, many patients have two or more types of aphasia, making a simple or clear diagnosis difficult.

fluent aphasia

Aphasia that results from damage to posterior regions of the cortex (i.e., temporal or temporal-parietal lesions) characterized by language with normal pauses and articulation but with frequent syntactic errors, paraphasias, and circumlocutions.

nonfluent aphasia

Aphasia that results from damage to anterior cortical regions (i.e., frontal lobe lesions) characterized by sparse, perseverative language with disturbed prosody, misarticulations, errors in syntax, and a reduction in phrase length.

prosody (prosodic)/ melody (melodic)

The qualities of stress and intonation in the voice that are influenced by the pitch, loudness, and duration of individual speech sounds.

auditory comprehension

The ability to understand spoken language at the single word, phrase, simple sentence, complex sentence, paragraph, and conversational speech levels.

Application Question

A single word can conjure up numerous memories (auditory, visual, tactile, and even taste and smell), associations, thoughts, and feelings. For just a moment, think about the word *mother*. What images, memories, experiences, associations, thoughts, and feelings start coming to mind? Which modalities and lobes of your brain are you using?

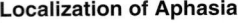

Localization of Aphasia

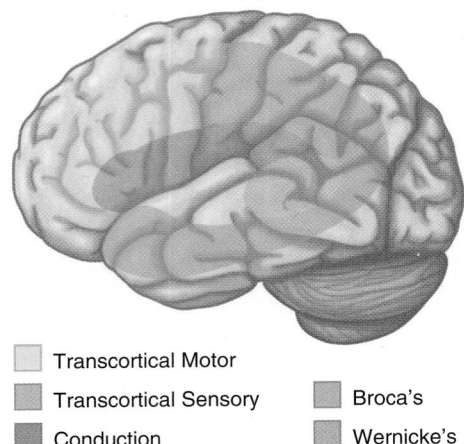

☐ Transcortical Motor
☐ Transcortical Sensory   ■ Broca's
■ Conduction   ■ Wernicke's

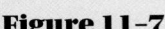

Figure 11–7

General areas of damage for fluent and nonfluent aphasia.

© Cengage Learning 2013.

Wernicke's aphasia

A fluent aphasia characterized by impaired comprehension, integration of information, and formulation of language caused by damage to the perisylvian regions in or around Wernicke's area in the posterior superior left temporal lobe (auditory association cortex).

---

alexia (acquired dyslexia)

Impaired ability to read as the result of neurological damage.

Wernicke's Aphasia

A German neurologist, Karl Wernicke (1848–1905), in 1874 was the first to describe the location of damage and the symptoms of what was later to be called **Wernicke's aphasia** (Geshwind, 1965). Wernicke's aphasia is a fluent aphasia caused by damage to the perisylvian regions in or around Wernicke's area in the posterior superior left temporal lobe (i.e., the *auditory association cortex*). Wernicke's aphasia is characterized by impaired auditory comprehension, integration, and formulation of language (LaPointe, 2005).

Impaired Auditory Comprehension

Impaired auditory comprehension (minimal to profound) is a hallmark characteristic of Wernicke's aphasia (Caspari, 2005; LaPointe, 2005; Morris & Franklin, 2012). Patients often have significant difficulty understanding single words, following simple directions, and understanding conversation. They have increasing difficulty at all levels when there is background noise, conversation, or visual distractions. To comprehend information or a conversation, a variety of areas in the brain may be actively involved to understand individual words, unique combinations of words in a sentence to convey a message, tone of voice, facial expressions, and body language of the speaker. In essence, *integration* (cognition) is the core of both comprehension and formulation of language. A person's expressive language may be the result of a combination of impaired comprehension and integration of information.

Patients with aphasia often have comprehension problems in more than the auditory modality; typically, they have equal or more severe impairments with reading comprehension (**alexia** or **acquired dyslexia**) (Webb, 2005). Patients may have difficulty associating sounds with letters, recognizing and naming letters, and reading and comprehending individual words, sentences, and paragraph-length information. It is important for SLPs to diagnose and document reading problems of patients. In addition to reading, patients also may have difficulty comprehending other people's gestural and body language. Overall, for many patients there is no intact input modality.

> ### Communication Techniques That May Help a Person Better Understand You
>
> - Have the person watch your face as you speak.
> - Speak clearly, but do not exaggerate your articulation or facial expressions—use a natural tone of voice and inflection as you would talk to any normal adult.
> - Have short pauses between sentences to give the person a little more time to process the information.
> - If the person asks you to repeat something or looks quizzically at you, repeat what you said verbatim and in the same tone of voice so that he does not have to try to compare and comprehend different words or different voice inflections.
> - If the person still does not understand, change just a few words that may help him comprehend.
> - Writing a word or sentence may help the person understand.
> - Avoid becoming frustrated when a person does not understand—he is doing the best he can, and his lack of understanding is always harder on him than it is on anyone else.

Impaired Integration of Information

To **integrate** information (process it at various levels of depth and relate it to information stored in other modalities), numerous areas of the brain need to become actively involved (remember that all processing is occurring at the neuronal and synaptic levels of the brain). Other terms for *integration* are *cognitive processing, cognition,* or *thinking;* that is, the brain's manipulation of stimuli in various lobes and areas to use it. Comprehension and integration cannot be separated—they are occurring in the brain simultaneously and in multiple areas.

Impaired Formulation of Language

Patients with aphasia often have a variety of language-formulation problems, the most common of which is **anomia** (Martin, 2012; Raymer, 2005). Anomia goes by several terms that are more descriptive than the technical diagnostic term; for example, *naming impairments, word-finding problems, word-recall deficits,* and *word-retrieval difficulties* (note that *impairments, deficits, difficulties,* and *problems* are interchangeable). Anomia is often one of several expressive language impairments seen in patients who have aphasia.

Anomia can range from mild to profound, including difficulty remembering a person's own name. When patients cannot name an object, they may try to talk about it or describe it (**circumlocution**), perhaps hoping that listeners will name it for them. People with aphasia experience

---

integrate (integration)

The process of combining into a complete and functional whole; combining and processing information from the various input modalities to store, attach meaning, and respond.

anomia

Impaired ability to retrieve (remember) names of people, places, or things, as well as to retrieve other parts of speech (e.g., verbs and adjectives) while speaking.

circumlocution

Description or "talking around" something when the specific word cannot be recalled.

Personal Story · A Medical–Legal Case

Because of my work in *forensic* speech-language pathology (work with attorneys and courts on legal cases that involve speech, language, cognition, and swallowing) (Fogle, 2000; Fogle, 2003; Fogle, 2006), I receive requests from attorneys around the country to evaluate legal documents of individuals who have had speech-language and swallowing therapy to make various determinations about communicative, cognitive, and swallowing competence.

An attorney from another state contacted me asking if I would review all available medical and rehabilitation documentation on a 72-year-old man who had sustained a left-hemisphere CVA. The patient was diagnosed by an SLP as having receptive and expressive aphasia (including reading impairments), cognitive impairments, and dysphagia (swallowing problems). One hour before undergoing a modified barium swallow study (see Chapter 12, Swallowing Disorders/Dysphagia), the patient was asked by his adult son to sign a significant change in his will. A few days after the modified barium swallow study, the patient died and there was a legal dispute about the change in the will. The legal questions being asked were, "Was the patient able to read and comprehend the changes in his will?," and "Was he cognitively competent to make an informed decision?" After careful review of the patient's entire medical chart, reports, and documentation (including the SLP's reports and daily therapy notes), I determined that the patient was not able to read and comprehend such a complex legal document or cognitively competent to make an informed decision. I wrote an extensive report that supported my conclusions, which was used in the final determination of the case. The case was eventually settled out of court, and I was later contacted by the attorney who informed me about the legal decisions. The patient's wife won the case and the changed will was "thrown out," allowing her to remain the beneficiary of her husband's estate. ■

---

literal (phonemic paraphasia)

Sounds and syllables that are correctly articulated but may be extraneous, transposed, or substituted, usually with the preservation of the vowels and intended number of syllables in a word (e.g., tar for car); often occurring in both speech and writing.

difficulty remembering words whenever they try to communicate, and some people begin to avoid communicating because of embarrassment and frustration.

The language (both spoken and written) of patients with aphasia is often filled with various paraphasias. **Literal** or **phonemic paraphasias** are substitutions of unintended sounds for intended sounds in words; for example, *mat* for *cat* and *hairblane* for *airplane*. (LaPointe, 2005, provided the following literal paraphasia of a former mortician who had aphasia. The mortician attempted to explain a proverb by saying, "Don't put all your eggs in one *casket*.") **Verbal** or **semantic paraphasias** are word errors in which the erred word is often semantically related to the intended word; for example, *salt* for *pepper* and *mother* for *wife*. (LaPointe also provided the following verbal paraphasia of one of his patients who was trying to give his clinician a compliment, "You are very *begoing* today, Nancy.") **Neologisms** are another form of paraphasia in which a person combines consonants and vowels that sound like they could be words and even uses inflection to give them emotional meaning; for example, *bingtema* and *hitican*. A patient using neologisms or other paraphasias may be unaware of the errors and continue talking as though he is making complete sense, which is referred to as **jargon aphasia**. Patients with aphasia may use a variety of paraphasias and actual meaningful words in a sentence, along with appropriate prosody and inflection, so that listeners may get the gist of what is being communicated.

In addition to impaired verbal expression, most patients with aphasia have even more difficulty communicating in writing—**agraphia**. The combination of alexia and agraphia is common (McNeil & Tseng, 2005; Mortensen, 2004; Papathanasiou & Csefalvay, 2012). As with their speech, writing may be copious but meaningless. Such patients write using paraphasias (phonemic, semantic, neologistic, and jargon) and circumlocutions and have syntactic errors.

Anomic Aphasia

Some patients may have primarily a persistent and severe naming (word retrieval) problem when other areas of their language are relatively intact (e.g., auditory comprehension). These patients may be said to have **anomic aphasia**. Anomia is the most common residual symptom of people who have had any type of aphasia (Boyle, 2004; Martin, 2012). Individuals with anomic aphasia have frequent and often severe difficulty remembering most classes of words, not just nouns (names); for example, verbs and adjectives often elude them (Freed, Celery, & Marshal, 2004). Reading comprehension is usually fairly good, but they have significant difficulty describing what they read because of the word-finding impairment.

Broca's Aphasia

Broca's aphasia was first described in 1863 by Paul Broca (1824–1880), a French neurosurgeon (he called the impairment *aphemia*) after studying the impaired speech and language of several patients, followed by autopsies of their brains after death (one patient became known as "Tan" because that was the only word he could say) (Berker, Berker, & Smith, 1986). The site of lesion that impaired the speech and language of these patients was in the lower posterior region of the left frontal lobe in the premotor cortex (premotor strip), the area that later became known as *Broca's area*. However, since that time it has been discovered that damaged cortex around Broca's area also may cause signs and symptoms of Broca's aphasia (Kearns, 2005).

verbal (semantic paraphasia)

Unintended substitution of one word for another word that is often semantically related to the intended word (e.g., *sister* for *brother* and *horse* for *dog*); often occur in both speech and writing.

neologism

A form of paraphasia in which a person combines consonants and vowels that sound like they could be words and uses inflection to give them emotional meaning; for example, *bingtema* and *hitican*.

jargon aphasia

Continuous but unintelligible speech with various combinations of literal and verbal paraphasias and neologisms, with little or no conveying of information; often with the speaker having little awareness of the problem and occurring in both speech and writing.

agraphia

An acquired disorder of writing resulting in difficulty writing letters, words, and sentences.

anomic aphasia

A disorder whose primary feature is persistent and severe difficulty retrieving names of people, places, and objects, as well as all classes of words (e.g., verbs and adjectives).

Application Question

What strategies do you use when you cannot remember a word, for example, on an exam?

CASE STUDY

A Nurse's Aphasia

A male nurse in his early 40s had a CVA that resulted in receptive and expressive aphasia, cognitive impairments, and right-side hemiparesis (weakness on one side). He received physical therapy, occupational therapy, and speech therapy at the acute-care hospital and in the rehabilitation unit. After being discharged from rehabilitation, he learned that because of his impairments he had lost his job at the convalescent hospital where he had worked for several years. He was unmarried and had difficulty taking care of himself in his small apartment, but he was determined to be as independent as possible.

He began therapy at a university speech-language clinic and worked diligently and consistently for several semesters. His goal and motivation were always to return to nursing. He even brought in nursing textbooks to use as part of his therapy. The client made significant improvement during his semesters in the clinic, although he continued having difficulty with auditory comprehension, verbal expression, and cognition, as well as right-side hemiparesis and balance problems. He eventually became more realistic about returning to nursing work. He stopped attending therapy when he had accepted and adjusted to his communication problems and his new self. As SLPs, we need to keep in mind that clients and patients will sometimes remain in therapy only until they reach their personal goals or have accepted their limitations, even though they may have potential for further improvement. ■

Broca's aphasia

A nonfluent expressive aphasia characterized by agrammatic language with omissions of articles, conjunctions, prepositions, plurals, possessives, and verb morphemes and auxiliary verbs; speech is often limited to high-frequency content words, making it sound telegraphic; apraxia of speech, dysarthria, or both often coexist.

agrammatic (agrammatism)

Impairment of the ability to produce words in their correct sequence and with all necessary morphemes.

Patients with Broca's aphasia often have right-side weakness (*paresis, hemiplegia*) or complete loss of movement (*paralysis, hemiplegia*) of the face (including the articulators) because the damage around Broca's area also can affect the *precentral gyrus* (motor strip controlling the face and articulators). These patients also may have paresis or paralysis of the right arm and hand and of the leg and foot.

Many patients with Broca's aphasia have problems with auditory comprehension, although not as severe as that of patients with fluent aphasias. They have particular difficulty understanding syntactical morphemes and structures (e.g., *-ing, -ed, have been*) and relational words (e.g., *heavier–lighter*), much like their difficulty using grammatical structures.

Patients with Broca's aphasia often use **agrammatic** expressive language because they tend to omit the grammatical function (*functor*) words such as articles (*the, a, an*), conjunctions (e.g., *and, but*), prepositions (e.g., *in, out, on, off*), plurals and possessives (*-s, -'s*), verb morphemes (e.g., *-ing, -ed*), and auxiliary verbs (e.g., *have, has, is, are, was, were*). The expressive language of these patients often sounds *telegraphic* (i.e., language that is condensed so that only the most essential words and morphemes are used—much like the language used in a telegram) (Kearns, 2005; Marshall, 2012).

Patients who have Broca's aphasia without other complications tend to have a relatively good prognosis. However, Broca's aphasia often occurs with the motor speech disorders of apraxia of speech, dysarthria, or both. Patients with multiple diagnoses often have *"guarded" prognoses*, that is, there is considerable uncertainty in the potential for significant recovery.

The speech of patients with Broca's aphasia is often slow and effortful because of trial-and-error groping for the intended articulatory movements. Such patients frequently use substitutions, omissions, and repetitions of sounds with little consistency in their errors. Patients have increasing difficulty as the length of a word becomes longer (e.g., *live— lively—liveliest*).

Patients with Broca's aphasia commonly have difficulty with both reading and writing. Their oral reading is effortful and nonfluent. They may understand the content words (e.g., nouns, verbs, and adjectives) easier than the syntactical morphemes and structures (much like their auditory comprehension abilities). Their writing, like their speech, is slow, laborious, and halting. Their written language is similar to their spoken language—that is, agrammatic (Kearns, 2005).

Global Aphasia

Global aphasia is a combination of fluent and nonfluent aphasia and is generally considered the most severe form of aphasia. Global aphasia is usually caused by occlusion of the left middle cerebral artery, causing diffuse damage to the temporal, frontal, and parietal lobes. The occlusion can severely impair all language processing and speech production. Patients have severe impairments of comprehension, integration, and formulation of language in all modalities, as well as significant cognitive impairments. They may have apraxia of speech, resulting in severe difficulty with planning articulatory movements. They also may have severe weakness in the speech systems (respiratory, phonatory, resonatory, and articulatory), causing profound distortions of speech (dysarthria). The prognosis for these patients is often poor because of the extent of the neurological damage and the severity of the combination of disorders (Collins, 2005; Portagas, Kasselimis, & Evdokimidis, 2012).

Cognitive Impairments Associated with Aphasia

Patients with receptive, expressive, or both types of aphasia also may have cognitive impairments. People use more than just their left hemisphere when comprehending, integrating, and formulating language. People use language when consciously thinking (cognition); therefore, when individuals have aphasia, they will likely have some level of difficulty with the various components of cognition (Portagas, Kasselimis, & Evdokimidis, 2012).

global aphasia

A severe-to-profound aphasia resulting from a diffuse lesion involving portions of the left temporal, frontal, and parietal lobes that is characterized by severely impaired receptive and expressive language in all input and all output modalities, with motor speech disorders of apraxia of speech, dysarthria, or both.

Principles of Assessment of Aphasia

When working in hospitals or other medical settings, assessment of patients with neurological damage usually follows a general format. After the SLP receives the referral (*consult*) from the patient's physician, she reads the patient's medical chart that is usually located at the nurses' station. Reviewing all parts of the chart is essential to understand as much as possible about the patient.

After reviewing the medical chart, the clinician interviews the patient and obtains a case history. Speaking with family members can be helpful to add to or corroborate information the patient has provided. The interview is the initiation of the evaluation and the clinician should note the patient's hearing acuity (a formal hearing evaluation may be needed later), assess the speech systems (respiratory, phonatory, resonatory, articulatory), and evaluate receptive and expressive language abilities. In many cases, some cognitive assessment may be appropriate. The purpose of an assessment is always to identify and document general and specific strengths and impairments using relevant functional items so that a diagnosis can be made and a treatment program can be developed and implemented (Helm-Estabrooks & Albert, 2004; Larkins, Worrall, & Hickson, 2004; Murray & Clark, 2006). The following are the most commonly assessed areas of patients with neurological disorders (note that these areas apply to most individuals with communication impairments, regardless of etiology):

Receptive language abilities

- Hearing acuity (with and without hearing aid devices)
- Visual acuity (with and without glasses or contacts)
- Pointing to objects or pictures named by the clinician
- Answering simple to complex questions
- Following simple to complex spoken directions
- Answering questions about spoken discourse
- Following conversational speech

Expressive language abilities

- Evaluation of the speech systems (respiratory, phonatory, resonatory, articulatory)
- Naming common objects (*confrontation naming*)
- Providing the verb (action) associated with common objects
- Providing the word that commonly completes a phrase spoken by the clinician (*responsive naming*; e.g., salt and _____)
- Word fluency (e.g., naming all the animals the patient can think of in 1 minute)
- Repeating words, phrases, and sentences of different lengths spoken by the clinician
- Producing automatic speech (e.g., days of the week or months of the year)

- Producing a sentence using a word provided by the clinician
- Describing what is happening in a picture
- Engaging in conversation (*discourse*)

Ability to communicate nonverbally (through body language)

- Imitation of common facial expressions and gestures
- Following simple commands for facial expressions and gestures

Reading abilities

- Matching pictures, letters, and geometric forms
- Matching printed words to pictures
- Reading aloud printed numbers, letters, words, phrases, and sentences
- Verbally answering printed questions
- Silently reading a paragraph or story and verbally answering questions about it

Writing abilities

- Copying geometric forms, letters, and words
- Writing letters, words, and sentences spoken by the clinician
- Writing biographical information (e.g., name, age, phone number, address, and names of close relatives)
- Writing names of common objects and their functions
- Formulating and producing written narratives

Multicultural Considerations

Assessment and treatment of patients from diverse ethnic, cultural, and linguistic backgrounds present significant challenges for clinicians because most tests have not included a representative number of people from diverse backgrounds in their standardization (Edwards & Bastiannse, 2007; Penn, 2007). Moreover, standardized aphasia tests have not been systematically translated into other languages. Some SLPs are bilingual (usually English and Spanish); however, most clinicians struggle to assess patients in any language other than English (Tonkovich, 2002).

Interpreters and translators can help by removing many of the language barriers between clinicians and patients; however, something is often "lost" in the interpretation or translation from the clinician to the patient and from the patient back to the clinician (Kayser, 2006; Wallace 1997). Centeno (2005) and Hegde and Davis (2010) present several suggestions for clinicians working with individuals from varied ethnic, cultural, and linguistic backgrounds:

- If the use of a standardized instrument is necessary even though it may not be totally appropriate for a given patient, interpret the test results cautiously, considering the patient's ethnic, cultural, and linguistic background.

- While working with certain ethnocultural groups, beliefs about health, illness, disability, and disorders, as well as medical care and rehabilitation, may need to be explored because beliefs affect motivation to seek and continue services.
- If possible, consult with another SLP who belongs to the same or a similar ethnocultural background as the patient.
- Avoid multicultural stereotyping and consider whether your own ethnic, cultural, and linguistic background is influencing your interactions with and assessment of the patient.

General Principles of Therapy

Successful treatment of individuals with neurological disorders is based on numerous and complex interacting factors, including the following:

- *Age of the patient*—Usually the younger, the better.
- *Premorbid language and literacy skills*—The higher the level of premorbid language and literacy, the better.
- *Nature of neuropathology (size and site of lesion)*—The smaller the lesion in a less crucial area, the better.
- *Severity of the impairments*—The less severe, the better.
- *General physical health*—The healthier the patient, the better.
- *Timing of therapy*—The sooner therapy is initiated, the better.
- *Length of therapy*—Generally, the lengthier and more extensive the therapy, the better.
- *Intensity of therapy*—Within reasonable limits, the more intensive (the number of hours per week) of therapy, the better.
- *Appropriateness and effectiveness of therapy goals and procedures*—The more appropriate and effective, the better.
- *Family involvement*—The more supportive and willing to take direction from the clinician, the better.

Clinicians mainly use the *restorative* or the *compensatory* approach when treating individuals with neurological impairments (Ben-Yishay & Diller, 1993; Code, 1991). The restorative approach focuses on improving the underlying processes that are impaired. For example, when patients have word-finding problems, improving their word-finding abilities (e.g., teaching strategies to recall words, not just teaching single words) will likely help them develop functional communication more than trying to recall individual words. Clinicians can enlist conversational partners (e.g., family and friends) to help support patients' attempts to interact and communicate (Fogle, 2009a; Kagan, Black, Duchan, Simmons-Mackie, & Square, 2001). *Aphasia Couples Therapy* (ACT) (Boles, 2009) empowers spouses and other caregivers to become involved in a practical way in the care and therapy of their loved one in ADLs outside of the clinic.

A compensatory approach may be used to provide strategies for persistent language deficits. For example, patients with severe word-finding problems who have not benefited significantly from a restorative approach may need to be taught to use gestures or a communication board to communicate their basic wants, needs, thoughts, and feelings (see Chapter 13, Augmentative and Alternative Communication).

Therapy Goals and Rationales

Therapy goals are determined by the assessment results, the clinician's observations of the patient during the interview and evaluation, and the goals the patient identifies for herself. The bottom line is always to improve the person's **quality of life** (Fogle & Reece, 2006; Hilari & Byng, 2001; Murray & Clark, 2006). The clinician's goals for the person and the person's goals for himself need to be in agreement, and therapy should be designed to meet those goals. This encourages shared decision making with a client-focused treatment approach (Cruice, Worrall, & Hickson, 2000).

We need to have good rationales for our therapy goals, and it is essential to consider the **functional outcomes** that will most benefit the patient (Code & Muller, 1995; Fogle, 2009a; Helm-Estabrooks & Albert, 2004). The rationales for functional outcomes answer the question, What are we going to do in therapy that will have direct effects on the patient's ability to communicate? That is:

- In the hospital setting with medical and rehabilitation staff
- In the home, performing **activities of daily living (ADLs)**
- In the community
- On the job (if he returns to work)

Clinicians also need to ask, Will an insurance company or Medicare reviewer recognize that we are working on goals that will actually improve the person's daily functioning and quality of life and merit reimbursement?

COGNITIVE DISORDERS

Cognitive disorders are seen in many individuals with neurological disorders from various etiologies. Three of the most common etiologies are traumatic brain injuries (TBIs), right-hemisphere damage, and the dementias. Cognitive impairments create some interesting and challenging behaviors that need to be understood and managed by individuals who are working and living with these individuals.

Traumatic Brain Injury

The nature or type of head injury an individual has can significantly affect the symptoms seen during assessment and therapy. It is important to carefully read the hospital medical chart for information on the type of head injury the patient sustained and any bodily injuries he may have. Head injuries are divided into two main classifications: closed head injuries (CHIs) and open head injuries (OHIs).

quality of life

A global concept that is difficult to measure but often is considered to involve a person's standard of living, personal freedom, and the opportunity to pursue happiness; a measure of a person's ability to cope successfully with the full range of challenges encountered in daily living; the characterization of health concerns or disease effects on a person's lifestyle and daily functioning.

functional outcomes

The results of treatment intended to clearly show a person's improved ability to communicate in the hospital setting with medical and rehabilitation staff; at home, performing activities of daily living (ADLs); in the community; and on the job (if the person returns to work).

activities of daily living (ADLs)

The normal activities and tasks people perform in the course of a day, such as ablutions (washing, bathing, brushing the teeth, toileting), dressing, and eating.

Cognitive Impairments Resulting from Traumatic Brain Injury

Traumatic brain injuries can result in numerous cognitive impairments. As with CVAs, the site and size of the lesion determine the symptoms seen (Constantinidou & Kennedy, 2012; Eslinger, Zappala, Chakara, & Barrett, 2007). Many patients with severe TBIs are initially in a comatose state.

Coma

Coma (prolonged period of unconsciousness) may occur with severe brain damage. The patient has minimal, if any, purposeful responses to environmental stimuli. When a patient is in a deep coma, he has no observable response to touch, pain, sound, or movement. In lighter stages of coma, the patient may respond with generalized body movements to strong stimuli. The length and depth of a coma is a fairly reliable indicator of eventual recovery. Patients with longer and deeper comas generally have a poorer recovery than patients with shorter and lighter comas (Mysiw, Fugate, & Clinchot, 2007).

Be Careful of What You Say

Clinicians (really, all people) need to be careful of what they say around patients who are comatose or semicomatose because some patients, when able to eventually communicate, have described both appropriate and inappropriate comments they had heard, understood, and remembered while in their comatose states.

Attention

Patients with damage to various areas of the brain may have impaired *attention* as seen in decreased readiness to respond to stimuli and difficulty with *selective attention* (attending to specific stimuli and ignoring others); *alternating attention* (shifting focus of attention between tasks); *divided attention* (responding simultaneously to more than one task); and *sustained attention* to a task for a reasonable length of time.

Memory

Memory is a complex and controversial area. Many models of memory have been developed within different disciplines (e.g., cognitive psychologists, neuropsychologists, and speech-language pathologists), each with its own preferred terminology (Loring, 1999). In general, patients with neurological disorders have impairments in the acquisition and retention of information (Constantinidou & Kennedy, 2012; McDonald, 2007; Moran & Gillon, 2004; Turkstra, 2001).

Orientation

Orientation is typically divided into four areas: person, place, time, and purpose (i.e., *oriented* $\times 4$). This sequence roughly represents increasingly complex cognitive processing. Patients with TBIs often are disoriented to person (who and what the person is and what the person is doing); place (where the person is and the surrounding environment, including the room, building, city, state, and country); time (month, season, and year, and approximate time, day, and date); and purpose (understanding and being able to reason why something has occurred or is occurring) (Johnson & Jacobson, 2007).

Reasoning and Problem Solving

In all aspects of daily living and working, *abstract reasoning* and *problem solving* are important. Reasoning and problem solving are considered high-level thought processes that rely on all previously discussed cognitive functions; that is, a person has to have functional attention, memory, and be oriented $\times 4$.

Reasoning involves drawing conclusions based on general knowledge or principles or forming solutions from information that supports a conclusion. Problem solving involves (1) recognition of a problem, (2) the ability to select a strategy to solve the problem, (3) the use of the strategy to solve it, and (4) evaluation of the outcome. Patients with neurological disorders, particularly those with right-hemisphere damage and TBIs, often have impaired abstract reasoning and problem solving (Constantinidou & Kennedy, 2012; Fogle, Reece, & White, 2008; Sohlberg & Mateer, 2001).

Executive Functions

Executive functions are controlled by the executive system, a nonspecific region of the prefrontal cortex. This area is thought to coordinate input from all other regions of the brain and, therefore, is important for coordinating and *actualizing* (making things happen) activities involved in cognitive processes (Ponsford, 2004). Executive functions refer to abstract thinking and our ability to (1) anticipate needs, (2) set goals to meet those needs, (3) plan strategies to achieve those goals, (4) implement those strategies, and (5) use feedback to determine the success of the plan and strategies. Executive functions are important in regulating our behaviors (including abstract reasoning and problem solving) and emotions (Chapey, 2008; Sohlberg & Mateer, 2001).

Individuals with executive function impairments have difficulty with ADLs in the home and community, including maintaining personal safety (Fogle, Reece, & White, 2008). They have difficulty in the work environment because they cannot anticipate what needs to be done, figure out ways to do it, and clearly determine that they accomplished what they wanted. Many people are in work environments where safety risks are always a concern and good executive functioning is essential. Executive functions, more than any other cognitive dimension, determine the extent of social and vocational recovery and the ability to live independently (McDonald, 2007; Ponsford, 2004).

Speech and Language Disorders

Along with cognitive impairments, patients with both CHIs and OHIs can have localized lesions that affect speech and language. This combination of impairments may occur for a couple of reasons. In both CHI and OHI, the left hemisphere's Broca's area, precentral gyrus, and Wernicke's area may be damaged, resulting in apraxia of speech, dysarthria, or classic aphasia symptoms. Language impairments, however, may be confused with problems caused by impaired attention, memory, and other cognitive processes. For example, comprehension disorders may be the result of attention and memory problems. In addition, it is difficult to clearly separate language and cognition during comprehension, integration, and formulation of language because many areas of the brain may need to be involved at any instant during communication.

Auditory comprehension abilities, anomia, pragmatics, and reading and writing problems are the most common language impairments seen in individuals with TBIs (McDonald, 2007; Murdoch & Theodoros, 2001). SLPs do not typically administer aphasia tests to patients with TBIs but recognize the possibilities of receptive and expressive language impairments during the interview and through the responses of patients during assessment of cognition.

General Principles of Assessment of Traumatic Brain Injury

Initially, some patients may be comatose or semicomatose and unable to respond to verbal or visual stimuli. However, for most patients during our assessments we often see that they are inconsistent, disorganized, disoriented, confused, restless, and irritable. Both formal and informal assessments of a patient with a TBI are needed to evaluate his cognitive, linguistic, and speech abilities (Murdoch & Whelan, 2007).

General Principles of Therapy for Traumatic Brain Injury

Therapy for patients with TBIs requires maximum teamwork with other medical and rehabilitation specialists. Patients often have unique medical complications, including external and internal injuries, cognitive-linguistic impairments, and behavioral disorders because of disinhibition. SLPs typically use the following approaches with patients who have TBIs: *environmental control, behavioral management, orientation therapy, cognitive retraining,* and *compensatory training.* The cognitive-linguistic approaches used by clinicians are usually determined by the stage of recovery or cognitive level of functioning of the patient.

SLPs may combine two or more approaches in any one therapy session to maximize the benefits of the therapy (Chapey, 2008; Murdoch & Whelan, 2007; Togher, 2007).

Environmental Control

Patients who are confused and agitated after TBIs are not responsible for their own behaviors; therefore, the professionals involved with these patients must try to make their environments stable, secure, and predictable. This helps minimize confusion and agitation and allows patients to use their cognitive energy to better manage themselves. This can be accomplished, in part, by having a consistent, organized daily routine. For example, meals can be served in the same location daily, and rehabilitation appointments can be scheduled at the same time, in the same place, and with the same therapists each day.

Behavioral Management

Behavioral management is used with environmental controls. Therapists attempt to increase adaptive behaviors and decrease maladaptive behaviors. Controlling the environment and reinforcing appropriate behaviors allow patients to begin to function more appropriately in structured environments. *Tangible reinforcements* are needed for these patients, for example, allowing patients to briefly listen to some favorite music or providing food reinforcement, such as a small bowl of ice cream for accomplishing a specific task.

Orientation Therapy

Most patients with TBIs are at least moderately disoriented to person, place, time, and purpose. Therapy is devised to help patients increase their orientation $\times$ 4, which also helps them increase their ability to manage themselves. For example, much repetition is needed to help patients realize and remember that they have weakness on one side of their body or that they must lock the brakes on their wheelchair before attempting to stand up.

Cognitive Retraining

In a sense, all rehabilitation involves cognitive retraining. However, more specifically, therapy is directed at increasing each of the components of cognition. Attention is often the first cognitive function targeted in therapy because that is the foundation of the rest of therapy; if the patient is not attending, he cannot receive maximum benefit from any therapy task. Increasing memory is needed for the patient to recall specific tasks, sequences, and behaviors, as well as important biographical information. Therapy to help patients redevelop their ability to organize information prepares them for problem-solving tasks for ADLs and to act in a reasonable and safe manner in their homes and communities. A collaborative approach is essential to help patients return to some level of functioning in the home, school, and/or work environments. Collaboration with family and friends who can help the patient carry over the rehabilitation program into the home and community environments is important for the patient to maximize his independence (Fogle, 2009a).

Compensatory Training

Few patients with moderate-to-severe TBIs return to their previous levels of functioning in their home, community, and work environments; therefore, they need to learn compensatory strategies to manage tasks that they could have managed independently premorbidly. For example, patients may be taught to keep daily notebooks with them to remind them of appointments or find a quiet room to be alone for a while if they begin to feel agitated.

Right-Hemisphere Syndrome

Recall from the discussion in Chapter 3, Anatomy and Physiology of Speech and Language, that the right hemisphere is particularly important in attention, orientation (e.g., self-awareness, where the person is, time of day, etc.), emotions, and cognition. Approximately half of all strokes and other neurological damage occur in the right hemisphere of the brain. **Right-hemisphere syndrome** is the result of a person having damage to the right hemisphere with impairments of its normal functions.

Cognitive Impairments

Right-hemisphere damage typically results in a variety of characteristics that comprise right-hemisphere syndrome, including several cognitive impairments (Blake, 2005; Myers, 2008). Right-hemisphere impairments are often subtle but may have profound effects on a person's daily life. Patients may be unaware of or do not appreciate the severity of their disorders (**anosognosia**). When a patient does not appreciate the severity of the impairments, the person may not be sufficiently motivated to work hard in therapy to make significant gains.

Visual–Spatial Impairments

Patients with right-hemisphere damage often have **visual–spatial impairments** and become disoriented and easily confused or lost, particularly in unfamiliar places such as the maze of hospital corridors or in grocery stores or shopping centers. When these patients are discharged from the hospital and are eager to begin driving, their visual–spatial impairments could prove to be life-threatening (Mackenzie & Paton, 2003; Tanner, 2007). These patients also may have difficulty recognizing familiar faces (**prosopagnosia**), including those of family members, medical personnel, and rehabilitation staff (e.g., they may not recognize you and may say they have never seen you before even though you have worked with them many times), however, they may recognize your voice.

---

right-hemisphere syndrome

Damage to the right hemisphere of the brain that can result in impairments of attention, visual–spatial abilities, orientation to person, place, time, and purpose, emotions, cognition, subtle to overt communication problems, and left-side neglect.

anosognosia

Decreased awareness of deficits or disabilities often seen in right-hemisphere damage; impairment of an individual's ability to relate to parts of his body.

visual–spatial impairments

Difficulty associating seen objects with their spatial relationships, that is, what is around the objects and the environment; often results in disorientation.

prosopagnosia

Difficulty recognizing familiar faces (including those of family members) and famous people.

Attention Impairments

Attention impairments occur with both right-hemisphere and left-hemisphere damage, but they are particularly noticeable in patients with right-hemisphere damage. Patients with attention impairments have difficulty staying focused on tasks and difficulty appropriately shifting attention from one task to another. Patients also may **perseverate**, that is, continue a thought or behavior after it is no longer appropriate.

Left-Side Neglect (Visual Hemi-inattention)

Neglect (i.e., lack of awareness and attention) of the left side of the body or space around the body is common in individuals who have right-hemisphere damage, particularly with damage to the parietal-temporal region (Davis, 2007). Individuals with *left neglect* tend to bump into things on their left, not notice food on the left side of the plate or tray, apply make-up on only the right side of the face, and draw only the right side of an object. Individuals also may have reading difficulties related to not attending to the left side of words or the left side of a page (*neglect dyslexia*), and, likewise, may have writing problems (*neglect dysgraphia*) where they have large margins on the left side of a page and use a right upward slant when writing words and sentences (Murray & Clark, 2006).

Communication Impairments

Subtle and sometimes overt receptive and expressive communication impairments are commonly seen in patients with right-hemisphere damage (Myers, 2008; Sohlberg & Mateer, 2001). These patients tend to be literal in their interpretation of messages, without realizing subtleties of meaning conveyed by choice of words, voice inflection, facial expressions, and body language. Metaphors (e.g., "The stars look like little diamonds in the sky."), idioms (e.g., "He kicked the bucket."), and proverbs (e.g., "Every cloud has a silver lining.") are often taken literally. People with right-hemisphere damage frequently violate the social and interactional aspects of communication (pragmatics), such as *turn-taking* (rambling on without regard to the listener), *topic maintenance* (frequent changes in the direction of conversation without regard to the topic of conversation), and *social conventions* (interrupting another person who is talking, not showing interest and respect for another's point of view, etc.). Patients typically interject irrelevant, tangential, and inappropriate comments into conversations. Their communication also may be devoid of emotion, have decreased prosody, and have an overall flat affect (Myers, 2008; Sohlberg & Mateer, 2001).

Individuals with right-hemisphere damage may have naming problems. They may be able to name several objects in a category (e.g., car, truck, and motorcycle), but have difficulty naming the category itself (e.g., transportation). When describing pictures, they may be able describe what they see but have difficulty giving a holistic view of what is occurring in the scene.

attention impairments

Difficulty staying focused on a task, difficulty appropriately shifting attention from one task to another, and dividing attention between auditory and visual stimuli.

perseverate/ perseveration

An automatic and often involuntary continuation of a thought or behavior after it is no longer appropriate.

General Principles of Assessment and Therapy for Right-Hemisphere Syndrome

Assessment for patients with right-hemisphere damage is similar to that of aphasia and cognitive disorders; however, assessments for attention and visual-perceptual disturbances are frequently included. Both formal and informal assessment procedures may be used. In general, we can apply the principles of therapy for aphasia and cognitive disorder to patients with right-hemisphere damage, with additional focus on the characteristics of this syndrome. Also, just as with patients with aphasia and cognitive disorders, we need to consider the functional outcomes and benefits for each patient's ADLs.

Dementia

dementia

A medical term for a syndrome caused by a progressive neurological disease that involves intellectual, cognitive, communicative, behavioral, and personality deterioration that is more severe than what would occur through normal aging.

senility

A medical term that refers to the normal loss of cognitive functioning with advanced age.

Alzheimer's disease (AD)

A disease that causes progressive dementia that usually begins after age 65 and in many cases is related to genetic factors that cause neuronal degeneration, cerebral atrophy, neurofibrillary tangles, neuritic plaques, white matter changes, and diminished neurotransmitters; characterized by decline in memory, intellect, disorientation, delusions, personality changes, and communication impairments.

cortical atrophy

Shrinkage and wasting away of cortical (brain) tissue that is common in dementia.

Dementia is a medical term for a syndrome caused by a progressive neurological disease that involves intellectual, cognitive, communicative, behavioral, and personality deterioration that is *more severe* than would occur through normal aging (Mahendra & Hopper, 2012). Dementia is perhaps the most devastating cognitive problem associated with aging. **Senility**, however, refers to *normal loss* of cognitive functioning with advanced age. It is dementia, not senility that we are concerned about (American Psychological Association, 2000; Bourgeois, 2005; Pachalska, 2007).

Dementia has numerous causes and types, with Alzheimer's type being the most common cause. Two other causes and types of dementia include *vascular dementias* (the second most common cause) in which atherosclerosis in the brain develops from deposits of fats and other debris that form on the inside of arteries and partially or completely block the flow of blood. Blockages cause multiple occlusive strokes (*multi-infarct dementia*) and interruptions of blood flow to the brain. Dementia also may be a late-onset symptom of Parkinson's disease, with memory, judgment, reasoning, and speech most affected.

Alzheimer's Disease

Alzheimer's disease (AD) (dementia of the Alzheimer type, or DAT) is the most common and probably the best-known progressive dementia. Approximately one-half of individuals with dementia have Alzheimer's disease. Alois Alzheimer (1864–1915), a German professor of neuropsychiatry, described the behaviors of a 55-year-old woman who had been institutionalized for several years in an asylum for the insane in Frankfurt, Germany. She was disoriented, confused, severely demented, and used "perplexing language." Alzheimer performed the autopsy of her brain and discovered that she had extensive cortical tissue loss (**cortical atrophy**), as well as other neuronal cell changes that have become the hallmarks of the disorder. Alzheimer published his findings in 1906 and described the cognitive and behavioral characteristics, as well as the neuroanatomical changes of the patient (the term *Alzheimer's disease* was first used by another German psychiatrist in 1910 in honor of Alzheimer). Ironically, Alzheimer died of Alzheimer's disease at the young age of 51.

Alzheimer's disease tends be seen in women more than men because of their greater longevity, which puts them in older age groups with greater risks. Alzheimer's disease causes degenerative dementia characterized by slow onset with a progressive and deteriorating course. It is characterized by a decline in intellect, memory, communication, and personality. The DSM-IV-TR (APA, 2000) says the cognitive and intellectual impairments should be severe enough to interfere with social or occupational functioning.

Cortical atrophy may be observed through MRIs in people with Alzheimer's disease, as well as other forms of dementia. **Autopsy (postmortem)** examination of brain tissue is needed to reveal **neuro-fibrillary tangles** and **neuritic (senile) plaques** for a clear diagnosis of Alzheimer's disease. Various medical diagnostic tests (e.g., blood and urine) and brain imaging techniques on patients cannot definitively determine the existence of Alzheimer's disease. However, there are currently attempts to develop diagnostic criteria for Alzheimer's disease in individuals who are living by investigating *biomarkers* (indicators of disease) using various brain scans (e.g., MRI, **positive emission tomography [PET]**), as well as spinal taps that may reveal signs of neurological changes (De Meyer, Shapiro, & Vanderstichele, 2010).

Stages of Alzheimer's Disease

Alzheimer's disease is usually categorized into three stages: mild, moderate, and severe (also called early, middle, and late stages). Each stage has general characteristics that may not apply to all individuals. The signs and symptoms may overlap from one stage to the next, and some signs and symptoms may never occur in some individuals (Bayles & Tomoeda, 2007; Pachalska, 2007; Toner & Shadden, 2011).

Stage I: Mild Alzheimer's, Early-Stage Alzheimer's, Forgetfulness Stage

During the early stage, the warning signs of Alzheimer's disease are often subtle, which makes it difficult for the individual and family members to recognize that something is wrong. Some of the earliest signs and symptoms include: impaired **working memory**; difficulty completing familiar tasks; difficulty remembering common names; misplacing items in inappropriate places (e.g., putting a wallet in the refrigerator); sudden changes in mood or behavior for no apparent reason; showing an indifference to personal appearance; disorientation to place, time, and purpose; and becoming lost while driving on familiar streets.

During the mild stage, people may try to maintain regular routines at work, at home, and in the community. Their difficulties may be thought of as stress related, and they may become frustrated and angry with the increasing difficulties. They may begin to take out their frustration and anger on family, friends, and coworkers.

autopsy (postmortem)

A medical examination performed to determine or confirm the cause of death.

neurofibrillary tangles

Neuronal abnormalities seen in Alzheimer's disease where there are filamentous bodies (fine, threadlike fibers) in nerve cells, axons, and dendrites.

neuritic (senile) plaques

Neuronal abnormalities and degeneration seen in cortical and subcortical brain regions of people with Alzheimer's disease.

positive emission tomography (PET)

A computerized radiographic scanning technique that examines metabolic activity, blood flow, and biochemical activity of the brain and other body parts.

working memory

Temporary information storage that is limited in capacity and requires rehearsal; often thought of as "what is on your mind" at any given moment.

Personal Story | "That's—That's My Wife!"

I had been working in a convalescent hospital during the summer. One of my residents was Mr. McAdams, an 84-year-old man with cognitive-linguistic impairments. I had worked with him for several sessions when I learned from another staff member that his wife was in the residential care facility across the parking lot from the convalescent hospital we were in. I also learned that Mr. McAdams had probably not seen his wife in at least 2 months because no staff member had taken the time or effort to bring her to the convalescent hospital.

After working through the normal nursing and administrative channels to no avail to try to arrange a visit of Mrs. McAdams to see her husband, I took it upon myself to make all of the arrangements. The following day at 2 p.m., I rolled Mr. McAdams in his wheelchair into the empty dining room that was light and cheery and had little vases of flowers on the tables. I placed Mr. McAdams beside a table with two glasses of water on it and turned his chair to face the open door. I told him I would be back in a few minutes. I walked across the parking lot and found Mrs. McAdams in her room, where she had put on her best dress and had her hair and make-up done. She was beaming as I rolled her across the parking lot to the convalescent hospital where she would see her husband for the first time in more than 2 months.

When we got to the door of the dining room, Mrs. McAdams sat up straight and had a big smile on her face. I wheeled her directly to her husband and she had tears in her eyes. When Mr. McAdams could clearly see her, he said, "That's—that's my wife!" I placed Mr. and Mrs. McAdams beside one another in their wheelchairs. They started to hug and cry. I left the room and closed the door.

After that day, I brought Mrs. McAdams over to see her husband twice a week, sometimes during craft time so that they could work on crafts together. When it was time for me to leave the hospital at the end of the summer to return to teaching, I wrote in the patient care plan in Mr. McAdams's medical chart that his wife was to be brought over twice a week for visits. By having this officially written in his medical chart, it was then nursing's professional obligation to carry out the visits, along with all that was written in the patient's Care Plan. As speech-language pathologists, we can sometimes "go beyond the call of duty" and help people by simply being extra caring. ■

Depression is common in the forgetfulness stage, although it is often under-diagnosed and undertreated (Reynolds, Alexopoulos, & Katz, 2002). Although individuals in stage I could benefit from therapy that targeted their deteriorating cognitive functioning, few people receive help.

Stage II: Moderate Alzheimer's, Middle-Stage Alzheimer's, Confusion Stage

The warning signs of Alzheimer's disease are more apparent at the middle stage. Beyond obvious memory loss, the person is not thinking clearly or using good judgment. This is when family members are likely to take the person to see the doctor and the diagnosis of Alzheimer's disease is made. Some signs and symptoms of the moderate stage include: increased loss of working memory; significantly diminished vocabulary; conversation is increasingly empty, meaningless; loss of reading and writing ability; difficulty with tasks that require skilled movements, such as tying shoelaces or using utensils (see Figure 11–8); aggressiveness, outbursts of anger, or withdrawal; inappropriate public behavior; and hallucination or delusions.

At this stage, the person is not responsible for his personal safety and others need to monitor and manage any safety concerns (Fogle, Reece, & White, 2008). For example, the person should no longer be allowed to drive or have access to vehicle keys. Any firearms that may have been available to the person should be removed or locked up. The person

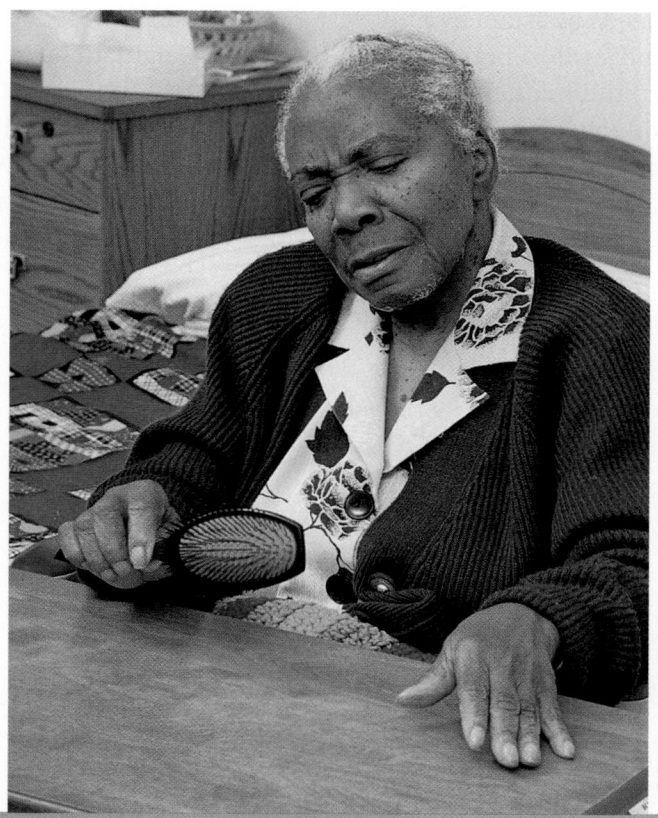

© Cengage Learning 2013

Figure 11–8

A patient with moderate Alzheimer's disease may forget how common objects are used and have problems with normal activities of daily living.

should be carefully watched when trying to cook or using any appliance that becomes hot, including irons and hairdryers. This is an emotionally trying time for the family, which needs to develop a new perspective of the relationship with the person with Alzheimer's disease. A "24-7" monitoring and caregiving approach needs to be established. An individual's independence is partly determined by the confidence caregivers have in the person's ability to act in a safe and reasonable manner. When the caregivers can no longer provide a safe environment and maintain a person's health and hygiene, placement in a convalescent or nursing home may need to be considered. Speech-language pathologists are often the professionals who educate and train family members and caregivers about strategies that are helpful for maximizing individuals' cognitive-linguistic abilities, as well as providing the safest environments for these individuals.

Stage III: Severe Alzheimer's, Late-Stage Alzheimer's, Terminal Stage

The progress of Alzheimer's disease to the severe stage may take a few years to many years. By this time, the person is no longer able to think and reason or consistently communicate wants and needs. The person likely needs maximum assistance for all ADLs, including dressing, eating, and toileting. Some signs and symptoms of the severe, late stage include: little or no memory; difficulty speaking and understanding simple sentences and individual words; expresses little or no emotion; minimal verbal discourse; difficulty recognizing others and sometimes himself in a mirror; needs assistance for all ADLs and personal care; and difficulty chewing and swallowing that results in loss of weight, dehydration, and risks for aspiration pneumonia (see Figure 11–9).

Individuals in stage III Alzheimer's disease are not candidates for speech and language therapy. Because of their frequent swallowing problems, many people with Alzheimer's disease develop aspiration pneumonia, which causes death more often than the Alzheimer's itself.

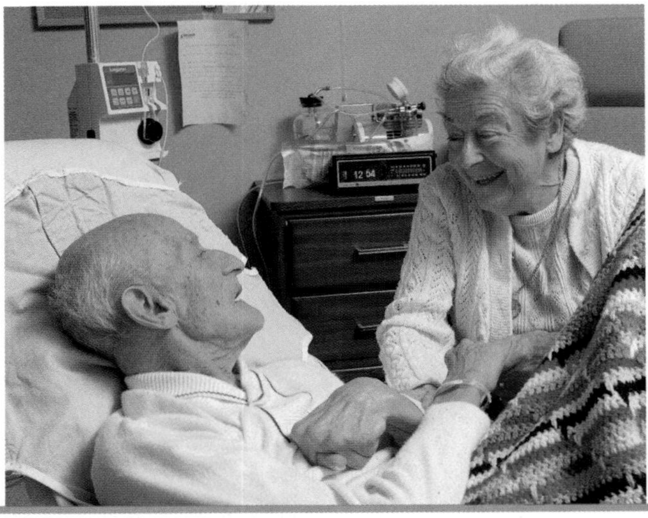

Figure 11–9

A convalescent hospital or nursing home may be the only option when the caregiver of an individual with dementia can no longer provide a safe environment or sufficient care.

© Cengage Learning 2013

Daisy

Some residents I work with in convalescent hospitals particularly touch my heart. Because few residents have anything to cuddle, hug, and "care for," many times I have given them little stuffed animals. Daisy was a resident I worked with who had both dementia and swallowing problems. She told me she liked little dogs. I found a cute little stuffed dog at a toy store, and just before I had to discharge Daisy from therapy I gave her the stuffed animal. She loved it. She began keeping it with her all of the time. Her dog "slept" with her at night and was on her lap or beside her when she was in her wheelchair. One day I had a nurse take a picture of us together, with her "pet" beside her (see Figure 11–10).

A couple of months after I returned to my fall teaching, I received a note from one of Daisy's daughters saying that Daisy had died. The family buried the little stuffed dog with her. Over the years, I occasionally thought about Daisy. Then in the fall of 2004, a new graduate student in my department (Vanessa) said that she recognized me as soon as she first saw me. Daisy was her great-grandmother and the student had seen the picture of Daisy and me together (it was also the last picture taken of Daisy alive). Vanessa told me about her visits with Daisy at the convalescent hospital when she was young and that "Daisy loved her speech therapist!" ■

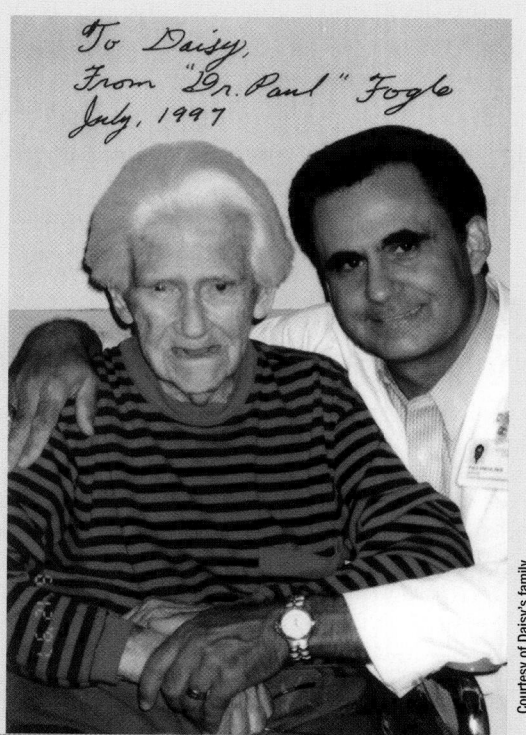

Courtesy of Daisy's family

Figure 11–10

The author with Daisy.

Death occurs, on average, about 8 to 10 years after the initial diagnosis of Alzheimer's disease by a physician.

General Principles of Assessment and Treatment of Cognitive-Linguistic Functioning of People with Dementia

The purpose of the speech-language pathologist's evaluation of individuals with dementia is not to diagnose dementia or Alzheimer's disease (although our evaluations may help confirm a diagnosis), but to assess their cognitive, linguistic, and swallowing abilities and from the assessment determine what, if any, therapy is appropriate. The actual diagnosis of dementia and Alzheimer's disease is made by physicians and psychologists.

People who are in the mild-to-moderate stages of Alzheimer's disease, and even some in the severe stage, may still be living at home, in a **board and care home**, or in a **residential care facility**. Family members and caregivers need to learn specific strategies for maximizing the abilities of individuals with dementia to communicate and function in their environments.

The speech-language pathology therapy goals for individuals with dementia (primarily those in stages I and II) are to help maximize their current cognitive-linguistic abilities and slow the inevitable deterioration of those abilities. Clinicians also need to help patients with awareness and problem solving for safety issues in the hospital and home environments (Fogle, Reece, & White, 2008). Much of what we do involves counseling and educating the caregivers (including family) on ways to manage and cope with the progressive cognitive and behavioral deterioration of the patient. The therapy goals, as with all individuals with neurological impairments, need to be functional—for both the patient and the caregivers. Ultimately we are trying to improve the quality of life of the patient and, by doing so, improve the quality of life of the people involved with the patient (Worrall & Hickson, 2003).

board and care home

A homelike environment where there may be a few to several elderly or physically impaired individuals residing and meals, laundry, and other services are provided.

residential care facility

Often a fairly large complex of small "apartments" where individuals or couples live; there is communal dining, and various services (e.g., security, trips to the mall, and outings) are provided to residents.

custodial care

Services and care of a nonmedical nature (e.g., bathing and feeding) provided long term, usually for convalescent and chronically ill patients.

incontinence

The inability to control or retain urination or defecation.

Alzheimer's Units

The question may be asked, What happens to people with advanced stage Alzheimer's disease or dementia? In the United States and most industrialized countries where health care is available from birth to end of life, these individuals may be placed in "Alzheimer's units" of specialized convalescent hospitals or care facilities. At this time in the progression of Alzheimer's disease or dementia, patients often need **custodial care** because of **incontinence** of bowel and bladder. They need protection from wandering away from the facility; therefore, the unit can only be entered or exited through a locked door. Psychosis also can occur as a secondary syndrome in Alzheimer's disease; therefore, patients often need protection from harming themselves and others (Palmer, Folsom, Bartels, & Jeste, 2002).

End-of-Life Care

End-of-life care is something many people think about as they get older: How do I want to be cared for in my final months, weeks, and days of life? Patients may choose either palliative care or hospice care. *Palliative care* is designed to relieve or reduce discomfort and pain, and patients may choose to pursue aggressive medical therapy aimed at curing a disease. Palliative care may continue for years to decades. *Hospice care* is normally intended for those who have a *life-limiting illness* (i.e., a *terminal condition*) where the prognosis is 6 months or less, should the disease follow a normal progression. Hospice care is family-focused care, and "family" is whomever the patient considers is family—not just blood relatives. Hospice care is interdisciplinary and may include physicians, nurses, social workers, chaplains, aides, and trained volunteers. Much of the care of the patient is pain management and attempts to maintain the patient's comfort and dignity (Jenko & Moffit, 2006; Roffi, 2007).

EMOTIONAL AND SOCIAL EFFECTS OF NEUROLOGICAL DISORDERS

Beyond the communication and cognitive impairments of individuals with neurological impairments, there are always emotional effects for both the patient and the family. As clinicians, we always need to keep in mind the entire person (and the family) with whom we are working, not just the disorder or disorders the person has. We need to place considerable importance on developing good, caring, working relationships with clients and families, without which our therapy could not be carried out optimally. The clinician's understanding of the emotional and social effects on the patient and family can help during the evaluation of the patient and the sensitive time of discussing the results of the evaluation. Understanding and appreciating the emotional and social effects can help clinicians maintain empathy during the process of treatment. It also helps patients and families feel that the clinician understands the realities of the challenges the patient and family face (Flasher & Fogle, 2012; Sander, 2007).

When an individual has a neurological injury, it often sets into motion a chain of events for the patient and family. Initially, after a neurological insult, a person may be comatose or semicomatose and, therefore, not aware of significant changes in his communication and cognitive functioning. However, when awareness emerges, the person begins to realize that he is not only having difficulty communicating, remembering, and recognizing other people but also may have obvious bandages and scars on his body, face, and head from a motor vehicle accident or neurosurgery after a stroke. His self-image (self-concept) takes a blow, and mental confusion may add to his lack of understanding of why he is in the hospital with tubes entering and exiting his body (e.g., a nasogastric tube for feeding and a catheter for urinary excretion).

The person with the neurological impairment has an immediate alteration of his self-image; the family does also. Family members likely will see themselves in a passive role during the medical treatment to keep their loved one alive and to minimize the brain damage. Like the impaired person, family members will feel fear and confusion. The experience is likely nothing they can relate to: a family member being rushed to the hospital; anxious time in an emergency room; admission to the hospital, possibly to a critical care unit; possible neurosurgery and wondering if it will be successful; weeks to months of rehabilitation; and having a loved one's levels of functioning altered forever.

Family systems theory and family-centered service delivery models are particularly applicable to individuals and families when a neurological disorder has occurred. When an individual in a family has a neurological impairment, the family system as a whole is affected. Elisabeth Kübler-Ross's five *stages of grief* (denial, anger, bargaining, depression, and acceptance) apply to their experiences. In addition to the emotional effects of the neurological impairment on the patient and family, social and financial effects add to the distress of each person (Flasher & Fogle, 2012; Roberts, 2011).

CHAPTER SUMMARY

This chapter on neurological (neurogenic) disorders in adults has covered an extensive amount of information on a challenging population of individuals that many speech-language pathologists work with full-time in acute-care hospitals, outpatient clinics, subacute hospitals, convalescent hospitals, rehabilitation centers, home health care, and private practices.

Strokes are the most common cause of neurological disorders in adults and they can occur at any age, not just in older adults. The two main types of strokes are occlusive and hemorrhagic. The site and size of the stroke usually determine the symptoms seen. Other common causes of neurogenic disorders are traumatic brain injuries, tumors, toxins, and degenerative diseases and disorders. Aphasia is a common disorder after a stroke in the left hemisphere's temporal lobe in or around the perisylvian area. Aphasia is a deficit in language processing that affects all input modalities (auditory, visual, and tactile) and all output modalities (speaking, writing, and gesturing). Aphasia is generally classified as receptive aphasia (difficulty with auditory comprehension) and expressive aphasia (difficulty formulating and verbally expressing language). Wernicke's aphasia is a fluent aphasia characterized by impaired comprehension, integration, and formulation of language; Broca's aphasia is a nonfluent aphasia with symptoms of impaired initiation of sound sequences, restricted grammar, and vocabulary that limits verbal expression to high-frequency content words (nouns, verbs, and adjectives). Patients with global aphasia have severely impaired receptive and expressive language in all input and output modalities. Assessment of aphasia involves evaluating a patient's auditory reception and verbal expression language abilities, as well as reading and writing abilities.

Therapy focuses on strengthening the impaired modalities with an emphasis on functional communication in activities of daily living.

Cognitive disorders are typically the result of traumatic brain injuries, right-hemisphere syndrome, and dementia. Patients with TBIs often have a variety of cognitive impairments affecting their attention, memory, orientation, reasoning, and problem-solving abilities. Patients with TBIs can be some of the most challenging people speech-language pathologists work with. Therapy often includes environmental control; behavioral management techniques; orientation to person, place, time, and purpose; cognitive retraining; and compensatory retraining.

Right-hemisphere syndrome is characterized by decreased awareness of deficits, visual–spatial impairments, attentional impairments, decreased awareness of emotions of other people, and cognitive impairments. Patients with right-hemisphere damage also may have communication impairments, including both receptive and expressive language disorders.

Dementia involves declining cognitive and social abilities that are more severe than what would occur through normal aging. Alzheimer's disease is the most common and best-known form of dementia. Alzheimer's disease has three commonly recognized stages, each with increasingly severe symptoms. The SLP's goals are to maximize the patient's current cognitive-linguistic abilities and slow the inevitable deterioration of those abilities, and help with their swallowing problems.

Regardless of the cause or severity of the neurological disorder, we are always working with a person and the person's family. Individual who have neurological injuries often awaken to discover that they are not the person they were a moment before the injury. They may not have the physical, communication, or cognitive abilities that they had relied on every minute of their lives. Both patients and their families typically go through the stages of grief—denial, anger, bargaining, depression, and, hopefully, acceptance of their new circumstances. Neurological damage takes a major toll on the person and all the people the individual associates with.

STUDY QUESTIONS

Knowledge and Comprehension

1. What are five warning signs of stroke?

2. Define receptive aphasia and expressive aphasia.

3. Discuss any three cognitive impairments that may be seen with a traumatic brain injury.

4. What are some of the interacting factors that may affect successful treatment of patients with neurological disorders?

5. What is the difference between dementia and senility?

Application

1. Why is it important to know the warning signs of stroke when working with patients of any age, but particularly those at risk for stroke?

2. What are the general areas that are normally evaluated when assessing a patient with a neurological impairment?

3. Why do important areas for therapy include a patient's awareness and problem-solving abilities for safety issues in the hospital and home?

4. What are any five general principles of therapy for aphasia?

5. Why is it important to understand the emotional and social effects of a neurological disorder on a patient and the family?

Analysis/Synthesis

1. Why is a speech-language pathologist's therapy based on her own evaluation more than on the neurological cause of the communication impairment?

2. In Wernicke's aphasia, how could impaired auditory comprehension contribute to problems with integration and formulation of language?

3. Discuss the similarities and differences between closed and open head injuries.

4. Discuss the stages of Alzheimer's disease that would most benefit from therapy.

5. Why is it important to always keep in mind functional outcomes when working with patients?

REFERENCES

American Heart Association. (2005). *Heart disease and stroke statistics: 2005 update.* Dallas, TX: American Heart Association. Available at http://www.strokeassociation.org.

American Psychological Association. (2000). *Diagnostic and statistical manual of mental disorders* (DSM-IV-TR) (4th ed., text rev. ed.). Washington, DC: APA.

Bayles, K. A., & Tomoeda, C. K. (2007). *Cognitive-communicative disorders of dementia: Definition, diagnosis, and treatment.* San Diego, CA: Plural Publishing.

Ben-Yishay, Y., & Diller, L. (1993). Cognitive remediation in traumatic brain injury: Update and issues. *Archives of Physical Medicine and Rehabilitation, 74,* 204–213.

Berker, E. A., Berker, A. H., & Smith, A. (1986). Translation of Broca's 1865 report: Localization of speech in the third frontal convolution. *Archives on Neurology (Chicago), 43,* 1065–1072.

Blake, M. L. (2005). Right hemisphere syndrome. In L. LaPointe (Ed.), *Aphasia and related neurogenic language disorders* (3rd ed.). New York, NY: Thieme.

Boles, L. (2009). *Aphasia couples therapy (ACT) workbook.* San Diego: Plural Publishing.

Bourgeois, M. S. (2005). Dementia. In L. LaPointe (Ed.), *Aphasia and related neurogenic language disorders* (3rd ed.). New York, NY: Thieme.

Boyle, M. (2004). Semantic feature analysis treatment for anomia in two fluent aphasia syndromes. *American Journal of Speech-Language Pathology, 13*(3), 236–249.

Broderick, J. P., Adams, H., & Barsan, W. (1999). Guidelines for the management of spontaneous intracerebral hemorrhage. *Stroke, 30,* 905–915.

Brookshire, R. (1992). *Introduction to neurogenic communication disorders* (4th ed.). Minneapolis, MN: Brookshire.

Caspari, I. (2005). Wernicke's aphasia. In L. LaPointe (Ed.), *Aphasia and related neurogenic language disorders* (3rd ed.). New York, NY: Thieme.

Centeno, J. (2005). Working with bilingual individuals with aphasia: The case of a Spanish–English bilingual client. *Perspectives on Communication Disorders and Sciences in Culturally and Linguistically Diverse Populations. ASHA, Division 14, 12*(1), 2–5.

Chapey, R. (Ed.). (2008). *Language intervention strategies in adult aphasia and related neurogenic disorders* (5th ed.). Baltimore, MD: Lippincott Williams & Wilkins.

Cherney, L. R. (Ed.). (2004). *Clinical management of dysphagia in adults and children.* Gaithersburg, MD: Aspen.

Code, C. (1991). *Aphasia therapy: Studies in disorders of communication.* Clifton Park, NY: Delmar Cengage Learning.

Code, C. (2001). Multifactorial processes in recovery from aphasia: Developing the foundations for a multilevel framework. *Brain and Language, 77,* 25–44.

Code, C. (2012). Significant landmarks in the history of aphasia and its therapy. In I. Papathanasiou, P. Coppens, & C. Potagas (Eds.). *Aphasia and related neurogenic communication disorders.* Burlington, MA: Jones & Bartlett Learning.

Code, C., & Muller, D. (Eds.). (1995). *The treatment of aphasia: From theory to practice.* Clifton Park, NY: Delmar Cengage Learning.

Collins, M. (2005). Global aphasia. In L. LaPointe (Ed.). *Aphasia and related neurogenic language disorders* (3rd ed.). New York, NY: Thieme.

Constantinidou, F., & Kennedy, M. (2012). Traumatic brain injury in adults. In I. Papathanasiou, P. Coppens, & C. Potagas (Eds.). *Aphasia and related neurogenic communication disorders.* Burlington, MA: Jones & Bartlett Learning.

Cruice, M., Worrall, L., & Hickson, L. (2000). Quality of life measurement in speech pathology and audiology. *Asia Pacific Journal of Speech, Language and Hearing, 5,* 1–20.

Davis, G. (2007). Aphasiology: *Disorders and clinical practice.* Boston, MA: Allyn and Bacon.

De Meyer, G., Shapiro, F., & Vanderstichele, H. (2010). Diagnosis-independent Alzheimer disease biomarker signature in cognitively normal elderly people. *Archives of Neurology, 67,* 949–956.

Douglas, K. (2002). *My stroke of luck.* New York, NY: William Morrow.

Edwards, S., & Bastiannse, R. (2007). Assessment of aphasia in a multi-cultural world. In M. Ball & J. S. Damico (Eds.). *Clinical aphasiology: Future directions: A festschrift for Chris Code.* London: Psychology Press, Taylor & Francis Group.

Eslinger, P., Zappala, G., Chakara, F., & Barrett, A. (2007). Cognitive impairments after TBI. In N. Zasler, D. Katz, & R. Zafonte (Eds.). *Brain injury medicine: Principles and practice.* New York, NY: Demos Medical Publishing.

Flasher, L. V., & Fogle, P. T. (2012). *Counseling skills for speech-language pathologists and audiologists* (2nd ed.). Clifton Park, NY: Delmar Cengage Learning.

Fogle, P. T. (2000, February). Forensic speech-language pathology: A practical guide for the expert witness. In *ADVANCE for speech-language pathologists and audiologists.* King of Prussia, PA: Merion Publications.

Fogle, P. (2003). A practical guide for the expert witness. *Vital Resources for Medical-Legal Solutions, 4*(6), 2.

Fogle, P. (2006). Forensic speech-language pathology: Court testifying as an expert witness. Paper presented at New Zealand Speech Therapy Association Convention, Canterbury, New Zealand.

Fogle, P. T. (2009a). Cognitive Rehabilitation: Collaborative Brain Injury Intervention. Paper presented at the Asia Pacific Society for the Study of Speech, Language, Hearing Conference, Honolulu, HI, July 2009.

Fogle, P. T. (2009b, March). Being a veteran and speech-language pathologist. *Advance for Speech-Language Pathologists and Audiologists.* King of Prussia, PA. Merion Publications.

Fogle, P. T., & Reece, L. (2006). *Classic aphasia therapy stimuli.* San Diego, CA: Plural Publishing.

Fogle, P. T., Reece, L., & White, J. (2008). *The source for safety: Cognitive retraining for independent living.* East Moline, IL: LinguiSystems.

Freed, D., Celery, K., & Marshall, R. C. (2004). Effectiveness of personalized and phonological cueing on long-term naming performance by aphasic subjects: A clinical investigation. *Aphasiology, 18*(8), 743–757.

Geshwind, N. (1965). Wernicke's contribution to the study of aphasia. *Cortex, 3*, 449–463.

Giacino, J., & Whyte, J. (2005). The vegetative and minimally conscious states: Current knowledge and remaining questions. *Journal of Head Trauma Rehabilitation, 20*, 30–50.

Goldstein, L. B. (Ed.). (2009). *A primer on stroke prevention and treatment: An overview based on the American Heart Association/ American Stroke Association Guidelines.* New York, NY: Wiley-Blackwell.

Golper, L. A. (2010). *Medical speech-language pathology: A desk reference* (3rd ed.). Clifton Park, NY: Delmar Cengage Learning.

Goodglass, H., Kaplan, E., & Barresi, B. (2001). *The Boston diagnostic aphasia examination* (3rd ed.). Philadelphia, PA: Lea & Febiger.

Guerrero, J., Thurman, D., & Sniezek, J. (2000). Emergency department visits associated with traumatic brain injury: United States, 1995–1996. *Brain Injury, 14*, 181–186.

Guthrie, E., Mast, J., McQuaid, M., & Pavlakis, S. (1999). Traumatic brain injury in children and adolescents. *Child and Adolescent Psychiatric Clinics of North America, 8*, 807–826.

Hegde, M. N., & Davis, D. (2010). *Clinical methods and practicum in speech-language pathology* (5th ed.). Clifton Park, NY: Delmar Cengage Learning.

Helm-Estabrooks, N., & Albert, M. L. (2004). *Manual of aphasia and aphasia therapy* (2nd ed.). Austin, TX: Pro-Ed.

Hilari, K., & Byng, S. (2001). Measuring quality of life in people with aphasia: The stroke specific quality of life scale. *International Journal of Language & Communication Disorders, 36*, 86–91.

Hirsch, J. (2005). Raising consciousness. *Journal of Clinical Investigation, 115*(5), 1102–1112.

Huckabee, M. L., & Pelletier, C. A. (2003). *Management of adult neurogenic dysphagia.* Clifton Park, NY: Delmar Cengage Learning.

Iverson, G., Lange, R., Gatz, M., & Zasler, N. (2007). Mild traumatic brain injury. In M. Zasler, O. Kats, & R. Zafonte (Eds.). *Brain injury medicine: Principles and practice.* New York, NY: Demos Medical Publishing.

Jenko, M., & Moffit, S. (2006). Transcultural nursing principles: An application to hospice care. *Journal of Hospice and Palliative Nursing, 8*(3), 172–180.

Johnson, A. F., & Jacobson, B. H. (2007). *Medical speech-language pathology: A practitioner's guide* (2nd ed.). New York, NY: Thieme.

Kagan, A., Black, S. E., Duchan, J. F., Simmons-Mackie, N., & Square, N. (2001). Training volunteers as conversation partners using "supportive conversation for adults with aphasia" (SCA): A controlled trial. *Journal of Speech, Language, and Hearing Research, 44,* 623–638.

Kayser, H. (2006). Service delivery issues for culturally and linguistically diverse populations. In R. Lubinski, L. E. Golper, & C. Frattali (Eds.), *Professional issues in speech-language pathology and audiology* (3rd ed.). Clifton Park, NY: Delmar Cengage Learning.

Kearns, K. P. (2005). Broca's aphasia. In L. LaPointe (Ed.), *Aphasia and related neurogenic language disorders* (3rd ed.). New York, NY: Thieme.

Kochanek, P., Clark, R., & Jenkins, L. (2007). Traumatic brain injury: Pathobiology. In M. Zasler, O. Kats, & R. Zafonte (Eds.). *Brain injury medicine: Principles and practice.* New York, NY: Demos Medical Publishing.

LaPointe, L. L. (2005). Mixed metaphors. *Journal of Medical Speech-Language Pathology, 13*(3), vii–viii.

Larkins, B., Worrall, L., & Hickson, L. (2004). Use of multiple methods to determine items relevant for a functional communication assessment. *New Zealand Journal of Speech-Language Therapy, 59,* 13–18.

Lew, H. L., Poole, J. H., Alvarez, S., & Moore, W. (2005). Soldiers with occult traumatic brain injury. *American Journal of Physical Medicine and Rehabilitation, 84*(6), 393–398.

Loring, D. (Ed.). (1999). *International neuropsychological society dictionary of neuropsychology.* Oxford: Oxford University Press.

Mackenzie, C., & Paton, G. (2003). Resumption of driving following stroke. *Aphasiology, 17*(2), 107–122.

Mahendra, N., & Hopper, T. (2012). Dementia and related cognitive disorders. In I. Papathanasiou, P. Coppens, & C. Potagas (Eds.). *Aphasia and related neurogenic communication disorders.* Burlington, MA: Jones & Bartlett Learning.

Marshall, J. (2012). Disorders of sentence processing in aphasia. In I. Papathanasiou, P. Coppens, & C. Potagas (Eds.). *Aphasia and related neurogenic communication disorders.* Burlington, MA: Jones & Bartlett Learning.

Martin, N. (2012). Disorders of word production. In I. Papathanasiou, P. Coppens, & C. Potagas (Eds.). *Aphasia and related neurogenic communication disorders.* Burlington, MA: Jones & Bartlett Learning.

McDonald, S. (2007). The social and neuropsychological underpinnings of communication disorders after severe traumatic brain injury. In M. Ball & J. S. Damico (Eds.). *Clinical aphasiology: Future directions: A festschrift for Chris Code.* London, England: Psychological Press, Taylor & Francis Group.

McNeil, M. R., & Tseng, C. H. (2005). Acquired neurogenic agraphias: Writing problems. In L. LaPointe (Ed.), *Aphasia and related neurogenic language disorders* (3rd ed.). New York, NY: Thieme.

Meechan, W. P., d'Hemecourt, P., Collins, C., & Comstock, R. (2011). Assessment and management of sport-related concussions in United States high schools. *American Journal of Medicine, 20*(10), 2311–2318.

Moran, C., & Gillon, G. (2004). Working memory influences on traumatic brain injury: A tutorial. *New Zealand Journal of Speech-Language Therapy, 59,* 4–12.

Morris, J., & Franklin, S. (2012). Disorders of auditory comprehension. In I. Papathanasiou, P. Coppens, & C. Potagas (Eds.). *Aphasia and related neurogenic communication disorders.* Burlington, MA: Jones & Bartlett Learning.

Mortensen, L. (2004). Perspectives on functional writing following acquired brain impairment. *Advances in Speech-Language Pathology, 6*(1), 15–22.

Mosby. (2009). *Mosby's dictionary of medicine, nursing, & health professions* (8th ed.). St. Louis, MO: Mosby Elsevier.

Moser, R., Iverson, G., Echemendia, R., Lovell, M., Schatz, P., et al. (2007). Neuropsychological evaluations in the diagnosis and management of sports-related concussions. *Archives of Clinical Neuropsychology, 22,* 909–916.

Murdoch, B. E., & Theodoros, D. G. (2001). *Traumatic brain injury: Associated speech, language and swallowing disorders.* Clifton Park, NY: Delmar Cengage Learning.

Murdoch, B. E., & Whelan, B. (2007). Assessment and treatment of speech and language disorders in TBI. In N. Zasler, D. Katz, & R. Zafontel (Eds.). *Brain injury medicine: Principles and Practice.* New York, NY: Demos Medical Publishing.

Murray, L. L., & Clark, H. M. (2006). *Neurogenic disorders of language: Theory driven clinical practice.* Clifton Park, NY: Delmar Cengage Learning.

Myers, P. S. (2008). Communication disorders associated with right hemisphere brain damage. In R. Chapey (Ed.). *Language intervention strategies in adult aphasia and related neurogenic disorders* (5th ed.). Baltimore, MD: Lippincott Williams & Wilkins.

Mysiw, W., Fugate, L., & Clinchot, D. (2007). Assessment, early rehabilitation intervention, and tertiary prevention. In N. Zasler, D. Katz, & R. Zafontel (Eds.). *Brain injury medicine: Principles and Practice.* New York, NY: Demos Medical Publishing.

Pachalska, M. (2007). Progressive language and speech disorders in dementia. In M. Ball & J. S. Damico (Eds.). *Clinical aphasiology: Future directions: A festschrift for Chris Code.* London, England: Psychology Press, Taylor & Francis Group.

Palmer, B., Folsom, D., Bartels, S., & Jeste, D. (2002). Psychotic disorders in late life: Implications for treatment and future directions for clinical services. *Generations: Journal of the American Society of Aging, 26*(1), 39–43.

Papathanasiou, I., Coppens, P. & Potagas, C. (Eds.). (2012). *Aphasia and related neurogenic communication disorders.* Burlington, MA: Jones & Bartlett Learning.

Papathanasiou, I., & Csefalvay, Z. (2012). Written language and its impairments. In I. Papathanasiou, P. Coppens, & C. Potagas (Eds.). *Aphasia and related neurogenic communication disorders.* Burlington, MA: Jones & Bartlett Learning.

Penn, C. (2007). Cultural dimensions of aphasia: Adding diversity and flexibility to the question. In M. Ball & J. S. Damico (Eds.). *Clinical aphasiology: Future directions: A festschrift for Chris Code.* London: Psychology Press, Taylor & Francis Group.

Ponsford, J. (2004). *Cognitive and behavioral rehabilitation: From neurobiology to clinical practice.* New York, NY: Guilford Press.

Portagas, C., Kasselimis, D. S., & Evdokimidis, I. (2012). Elements of neurology essential for understanding the aphasias. In I. Papathanasiou, P. Coppens, & C. Potagas (Eds.). *Aphasia and related neurogenic communication disorders.* Burlington, MA: Jones & Bartlett Learning.

Raymer, A. M. (2005). Naming and word-retrieval problems. In L. LaPointe (Ed.), *Aphasia and related neurogenic language disorders* (3rd ed.). New York, NY: Thieme.

Reynolds, C., Alexopoulos, G., & Katz, I. (2002). Geriatric depression: Diagnosis and treatment. *Generations, Journal of the American Society of Aging, 26*(1), 28–31.

Roberts, S. D. (2011). Patient- and family-centered care: Today's standard of care delivery. *CSHA Magazine, 41*(1), 6–7.

Roffi, B. (2007, February). End-of-life care. *Advance for Nurses.* King of Prussia, PA: Merion Publications.

Sander, A. (2007). A cognitive-behavioral intervention for family members of persons with TBI. In N. Zasler, D. Katz, & R. Zafonte (Eds.). *Brain injury medicine: Principles and practice.* New York, NY: Demos Medical Publishing.

Singh, R., Cohen, S. N., & Krupp, R. (1996). Racial differences in cerebrovascular disease. *Neurology, 46*(Supplement 21), A440–A441.

Sohlberg, M. M., & Mateer, C. A. (2001). *Introduction to cognitive rehabilitation theory and practice* (2nd ed.). New York, NY: Guilford Press.

Tanner, D. C. (2007). *Surviving traumatic brain injury and communication disorders: A professional and family guide.* San Diego, CA: Plural Publishing.

Tate, R. L., McDonald, S., & Lulham, J. L. (1998). Traumatic brain injury: Severity of injury and outcome in an Australian population. *Journal of Australia and New Zealand Public Health, 22,* 11–15.

Threats, T., & Worrall, L. (2004). Classifying communication disability using the ICF. *Advances in Speech-Language Pathology, 6*(1), 53–62.

Togher, L. (2007). Traumatic brain injury rehabilitation: Advanced communication perspectives. In M. Ball & J. S. Damico (Eds.). *Clinical aphasiology: Future directions: A festschrift for Chris Code.* London, England: Psychology Press, Taylor & Francis Group.

Toner, M. A., & Shadden, B. B. (2011). *Aging and communication: For clinicians by clinicians* (2nd ed.). Austin, TX: Pro-Ed.

Tonkovich, J. D. (2002). Multicultural issues in the management of neurogenic communication and swallowing disorders. In D. E. Battle (Ed.), *Communication disorders in multicultural populations* (3rd ed., pp. 233–265). Boston, MA: Butterworth-Heinemann.

Turkstra, L. S. (2001). Treating memory problems in adults with neurogenic communication disorders. *Seminars in Speech and Language, 22*(2), 147–155.

Wallace, G. L. (1997). Working with interpreters and translators. In G. L. Wallace (Ed.), *Multicultural neurogenics: A resource for speech-language pathologists providing services to neurologically impaired adults from culturally and linguistically diverse backgrounds.* San Antonio, TX: Communication Skill Builders.

Webb, W. G. (2005). Acquired dyslexia: Reading disorders associated with aphasia. In L. LaPointe (Ed.). *Aphasia and related neurogenic language disorders* (3rd ed.). New York, NY: Thieme.

Worrall, L. E., & Hickson, L. M. (2003). *Communication disability in aging: From prevention to intervention.* Clifton Park, NY: Delmar Cengage Learning.

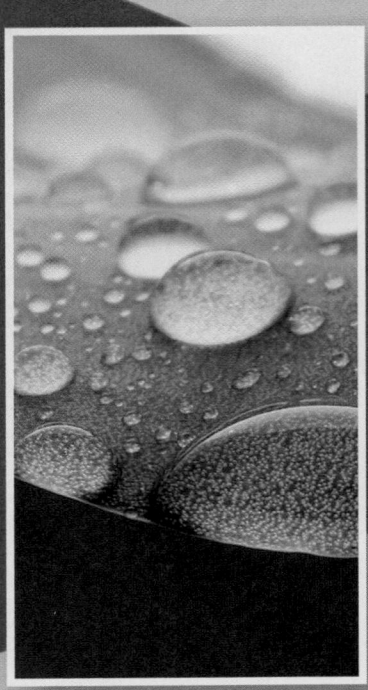

CHAPTER 12
Motor Speech Disorders and Dysphagia/ Swallowing Disorders

LEARNING OBJECTIVES

After studying this chapter, you will:

- Know the essentials of motor speech disorders—dysarthria and apraxia.

- Be familiar with principles of assessment of dysarthria and apraxia of speech.

- Be able to discuss general principles of therapy for dysarthria and apraxia of speech.

- Understand the essentials of dysphagia.

- Recognize the need for a team approach to dysphagia.

- Be able to explain each of the four phases of swallowing.

- Be able to discuss disordered swallowing in each of the four phases.

- Understand essential procedures for evaluating adults with swallowing disorders.

- Be able to describe treatment of adults with swallowing disorders.

- Be familiar with the emotional and social effects of motor speech disorders and swallowing disorders on patients and their families.

KEY TERMS

amyotrophic lateral sclerosis (ALS, Lou Gehrig's disease)
anarthria
apraxia of speech (speech apraxia, verbal apraxia, acquired apraxia)
aspiration
aspiration pneumonia

automatic speech
autonomy
bioethics
differential diagnosis
dysarthria
dysphagia (swallowing disorder)
enteral feeding

KEY TERMS continued

evidence-based practice
fiberoptic endoscopic evaluation
   of swallowing (FEES)
gastroenterologist
modified barium swallow study
   (MBSS)
motor speech disorders
myasthenia gravis
NPO (nothing by mouth)

oral apraxia (nonverbal apraxia,
   facial apraxia, buccofacial
   apraxia)
plateau
range of motion (ROM)
silent aspiration
treatment effectiveness
treatment efficacy
tremors at rest

INTRODUCTION

Dysarthria, speech apraxia, and dysphagia are frequently seen as problems in the same patient (Duffy, 2005; Duffy, 2006; Logemann, 1998). Dysarthria is a neurological speech disorder that is a result of weakness, paralysis, or inability to coordinate the articulatory, resonatory, phonatory, and/or respiratory systems. All of these systems also are important in swallowing. Speech apraxia is the result of an impaired ability to plan, sequence, coordinate, and initiate motor movements of the articulators, which also can affect voluntary initiation of swallowing. The same neurological insults (e.g., CVAs, TBIs, degenerative diseases) that cause dysarthria and apraxia can cause dysphagia. This is not only true for adults, but also true for children (Morgan & Skeat, 2010; Morgan, Mageandran, & Mei, 2010).

MOTOR SPEECH DISORDERS

Disordered speech is sometimes the first sign of neurological disease. Because speech is normally such an automatic process, a sudden disturbance requires immediate attention. Darley, Aronson, and Brown (1975) estimated that for every second a person is talking, approximately 140,000 neuromuscular contractions and relaxations occur in the speech production muscles (i.e., muscles of the respiratory, phonatory, resonatory, and articulatory systems).

Motor speech disorders result from neurological impairments affecting the motor planning, programming, neuromuscular control, execution of speech, or a combination of these. They include the dysarthrias and apraxia of speech. Motor speech disorders have a sensory component and should be thought of as *sensorimotor*, not just motor, in character (Duffy, 2005; Weismer, 2006). Motor speech disorders often accompany aphasia, cognitive impairments, or both when the lesion is extensive; however, motor speech disorders can occur alone.

Dysarthria

Dysarthria is a general term for a collection of speech disorders characterized by weakness in the muscles that control respiration, phonation, resonation, and articulation (see Figure 12–1). The weakness may have a minimal-to-profound effect on all speech systems, depending on the site and size of the lesion or lesions. In general, the **range of motion (ROM)**, strength, coordination, and rate of muscle movement may be affected in each of the speech systems, which have an overall affect on the prosody of speech (Duffy, 2005; Weismer, 2006; Yorkston, Beukelman, Strand, & Hakel, 2010). Individuals with severe dysarthria may have no

motor speech disorders

Neurological impairments that affect the motor planning, programming, neuromuscular control, and/or execution of speech and include the dysarthrias and apraxia of speech; they typically have a sensory component and should be thought of as sensorimotor disorders.

dysarthria

A group of motor speech disorders caused by *paresis* (weakness), *paralysis* (complete loss of movement), or incoordination of speech muscles as a result of central and/or peripheral nervous system damage that may affect respiration, phonation, resonation, articulation, and prosody; dysarthric speech sounds "mushy" because of distorted consonants and vowels.

range of motion (ROM)

For speech, the limits the mandible can open and close, the lips can protrude and retract, and the tongue can protrude and retract, elevate and lower, and move side to side (*lateralize*).

- *Respiration*—Low intensity and speech that is limited to short phrases caused by decreased respiratory support
- *Phonation*—Breathy phonation caused by unilateral or bilateral vocal fold paresis or paralysis (weakness)
- *Resonation*—Hypernasality caused by weak movement of the soft palate leading to velopharyngeal incompetence
- *Articulation*—Distorted, imprecise consonants caused by weakness and incoordination of the mandible, lips, and tongue

Figure 12-1
Speech dimensions of dysarthria.
Adapted from Duffy, 2005.

functional intelligible speech, and many of these individuals would benefit from augmentative and alternative communication (AAC) systems.

Dysarthria may have the same etiologies as aphasia and cognitive disorders (e.g., CVAs, TBIs, tumors, toxins, degenerative diseases, and others). Sometimes, however, dysarthria has no clearly identifiable cause. Of the two motor speech disorders (apraxia and dysarthria), dysarthria is the more prevalent, primarily because a variety of areas in the CNS and PNS may be damaged and result in dysarthria (Duffy, 2005; Weismer, 2006).

Application Question

Have you ever listened to a person who was drinking alcohol and becoming progressively drunk? The slurred speech of some people who have been drinking is similar to that of some individuals with dysarthria.

Neuromuscular Disorders Commonly Associated with Dysarthria

Certain neuromuscular conditions or disorders are commonly associated with dysarthria. Some of these conditions may be seen in relatively young adults; however, in general, the older a person becomes, the more susceptible the person is to neurological diseases and disorders that may result in dysarthria (Golper, 2010).

Parkinson's Disease

Parkinson's disease (PD) is caused by a gradual deterioration of certain nerve centers in the brain that are important in the delicate balance of chemicals needed for transmission of nerve impulses for control of movement of the body, including the articulators. Arms and legs become stiff and do not swing or move in a smooth manner because opposing muscles (e.g., biceps and triceps in the arms) are contracting simultaneously. The face may become masklike with little expression, although the person has all of the same emotions as before the Parkinson's disease. A common symptom of Parkinson's disease is **tremors at rest**, for example tremors of the hands or head when the person does not consciously move them. Speech-language pathologists become involved with these individuals when their Parkinson's disease begins to affect their speech, swallowing, or both. Dysarthria is the speech disorder associated with the disease (McAuliffe, Ward, & Murdoch, 2007).

tremors at rest

Tremors that occur when the head, limbs, hands, or fingers are not intentionally being moved; when movement is initiated, the tremors subside until the body part is again no longer moving.

Michael J. Fox

The actor Michael J. Fox (recall the *Back to the Future* movies) has suffered from Parkinson's disease for many years, including when he was the star of the television series *Spin City.* He was able to hide his Parkinson's disease from the viewing audience by constantly being in motion, which he incorporated into the character he played. When his Parkinson's disease became so severe that he could not make his movements appear to be part of a normal functioning person, he made his problem known publicly. Since then, he has been an important advocate and spokesperson for research into Parkinson's disease. (Note: Mr. Fox has not yet developed any noticeable dysarthria.)

Myasthenia Gravis

myasthenia gravis

A neuromuscular disorder more commonly seen in women than men; characterized by chronic fatigue and muscle weakness, especially in the facial and articulatory muscles, resulting in dysarthria.

Myasthenia gravis is a disease that affects women twice as often as it affects men, with an incidence of approximately 1 in 10,000. The disease often begins in women in their 30s, and in men the onset is usually in their 60s. Symptoms of myasthenia gravis appear first and most noticeably in the face. The eyelids begin to droop, double vision occurs, and weakness in the articulators causes slurred speech (dysarthria), dysphonia, and difficulty swallowing (Chang, Lee, & Kuo, 2004). The arms and legs may be affected, making it difficult to comb the hair or stand without being wobbly. A key diagnostic feature is decreasing muscle function with use and easy fatigability. With medication, some transmission of nerve impulses can be restored, but myasthenia gravis cannot be cured.

Amyotrophic Lateral Sclerosis

amyotrophic lateral sclerosis (ALS, Lou Gehrig's disease)

A rare, rapidly progressive degenerative disease of motor neurons that control movement of all muscle systems, including the speech systems.

Amyotrophic lateral sclerosis (ALS) is commonly called *Lou Gehrig's disease* (named after the famous New York Yankee's baseball player who retired in 1939 because of ALS after playing 2,130 consecutive games). ALS is a rare, rapidly progressive degenerative disease of the motor neurons that control movement of all muscle systems, including the speech systems. ALS usually begins in middle age, with the age of initial symptoms occurring as early as the 40s and as late as the 70s. Males are affected more often than females. Death usually occurs within 5 years from wasting of the body, with pneumonia typically being the final illness. There is no known medical treatment.

anarthria (anarthric)

The complete inability to articulate or speak that is usually caused by brain lesions or damage to peripheral nerves that innervate the articulatory muscles.

Every physical function of the body can be affected, including breathing, swallowing, speaking, and walking (Hillel et al., 1989). Speech-language pathologists are likely to see patients with ALS for swallowing disorders, speech disorders, or both. As the disease progresses, the speaking rate of most patients diminishes. During the last years or months of life, they experience a severe communication disorder, with some individuals being **anarthric**.

TABLE 12-1	Characteristics of the Six Types of Dysarthrias		
TYPE	**DISEASE/DISORDER CHARACTERISTICS**	**SITE OF LESION**	**SPEECH CHARACTERISTICS**
Spastic	Pseudobulbar palsy	Upper motor neuron	Imprecise articulation, slow rate, harsh voice quality
Ataxic	Cerebellar or Friedrich's ataxia	Cerebellum	Phoneme and syllable prolongation, slow rate, abnormal prosody
Flaccid	Bulbar palsy, myasthenia gravis	Lower motor neuron	Audible inspiration, hypernasality, nasal emission, breathiness
Hyperkinetic	Huntington's chorea, dystonia	Extrapyramidal system	Imprecise articulation, prolonged pauses, variable rate, impaired prosody
Hypokinetic	Parkinson's disease	Extrapyramidal system	Monoloudness, monopitch, reduced intensity, short rushes of speech
Mixed	Multiple sclerosis, amyotrophic lateral sclerosis	Multiple motor systems	Dependent on motor systems affected

Adapted from Gillam, Marquardt, & Martin, 2000.

Multiple Sclerosis (MS)

Multiple sclerosis (MS) is a debilitating disease in which the body's immune system slowly destroys the protective sheath (*myelin*) that covers the nerves. This interferes with the communication between the brain and the muscles and organs of the body. MS is most often seen in females between 20 and 40 years of age whose families originated in northern Europe, but it can occur at any age. Signs and symptoms of MS vary depending on the nerve fibers affected and may include numbness or weakness in one or more limbs, tingling or pain in parts of the body, tremors and lack of coordination or unsteady gait, fatigue, dizziness, and partial or complete loss of vision. Over time, speech, language, cognition, and swallowing may be affected. In the early stages of the disease individuals typically experience exasperation of symptoms that are followed by partial or complete remission. There is no known cure for MS, although medical management can modify the course of the disease and treat its symptoms.

Types of Dysarthrias

Six types of dysarthria have been described in the literature (Darley et al., 1975; Duffy, 2005; Weismer, 2006): spastic dysarthria, ataxic dysarthria, flaccid dysarthria, hyperkinetic dysarthria, hypokinetic dysarthria, and mixed dysarthria (see Table 12–1).

General Principles of Assessment of Dysarthria

A diagnosis of a motor speech disorder is made after a thorough evaluation of a patient's motor speech abilities. Sometimes evaluation results are unambiguous and a clear diagnosis can be made. More commonly, there are several possible interpretations and the clinician has to rank the possibilities. The process of narrowing possibilities and reaching conclusions about the nature of a deficit is known as **differential diagnosis**. A thorough evaluation of the speech systems (respiratory, phonatory, resonatory, and articulatory) is completed, with emphasis on the oral mechanism. Careful visual, auditory, and even tactile perceptual evaluations are essential, with emphasis on the auditory. Perceptual evaluations are the "gold standard" for clinical differential diagnosis, judgments of severity, many decisions about management, and assessment of functional change (Duffy, 2005; Weismer, 2006; Yorkston et al., 2010).

General Principles of Therapy for Dysarthria

The primary goal of speech therapy for dysarthria is to maximize the effectiveness, efficiency, and naturalness of communication (Swigert, 2010; Yorkston et al., 2010). Depending on the severity of the dysarthria, patients and clinicians together may choose different approaches. For example, patients with mild dysarthria may focus on efficient and natural-sounding speech; patients with moderate dysarthria may choose to work on speech intelligibility and efficiency (i.e., manageable physical effort); and for those with severe dysarthria, the emphasis may be on effective and efficient alternative means of communication (Duffy, 2005).

Speech pathologists treat dysarthria by using *behavioral management*, with its primary goal to maximize communication (McAuliffe, 2006; Weismer, 2006). When improving speech intelligibility is the focus of therapy, clinicians attempt to reduce the patient's impairments by increasing physiological support for speech; for example, modifying or improving posture and increasing range of motion, muscle tone, strength, and rate of movement. *Drill* (the systematic practice of specially selected and ordered exercises) is a foundation of therapy. Patients with motor speech disorders must speak to improve their speech. When speech muscles are not exercised sufficiently, muscle strength may further decline (this is similar to general body deconditioning when patients are confined to bed) (Covertino, Bloomfield, & Greenleaf, 1997). When speaking, patients need to make speech highly conscious so that their focus is on being heard and understood rather than on how quickly they can communicate their messages.

Apraxia of Speech

Apraxia of speech (speech apraxia, verbal apraxia, acquired apraxia) is caused by damage in the region of the posterior inferior left frontal lobe in or around Broca's area (Duffy, 2005; Yorkston et al., 2010).

---

differential diagnosis

The process of narrowing possibilities and reaching conclusions about the nature of a deficit.

---

apraxia of speech (speech apraxia, verbal apraxia, acquired apraxia)

A deficit in the neural motor planning and programming of the articulatory muscles for voluntary movements for speech in the absence of muscular weakness; primarily interferes with articulation and prosody.

The most common cause of apraxia of speech is stroke. The important motor functions of Broca's area are planning and programming for voluntary movements of the articulators. Speech apraxia is the result of an impaired ability to plan, sequence, coordinate, and initiate motor movements of the articulators. When only Broca's area is damaged, the speech errors are not the result of weakness; however, when the adjacent precentral gyrus or the pyramidal tract also is damaged, weakness can contribute to impaired speech intelligibility. A patient may have both speech apraxia and dysarthria (to be discussed in more detail later).

Characteristics of Apraxia of Speech

The characteristics of apraxia of speech were first described by Darley et al. (1975), and further described by Wertz, LaPointe, and Rosenbek (1991):

- Articulation errors are not the result of muscle weakness or paralysis.
- Articulation errors are highly variable.
- Sound errors are more often substitutions than distortions, omissions, or additions.
- Consonant errors are more common than vowel errors.
- Errors occur most often on the initial consonant of words.
- Consonant clusters (e.g., /bl, sp, st, tr/) are more likely to be in error than single consonants.
- Errors increase with increasing word length (i.e., number of sounds and syllables).
- There are trial-and-error "gropings" for the correct placement of the articulators to produce sounds, causing the person to look like he is working hard or struggling to talk.
- Front-of-the-mouth sounds (e.g., /b, d, z/) are more likely to be correct than back-of-the-mouth sounds (e.g., /k, g, ch, sh/).
- There are "islands" of fluent, error-free words, phrases, and sentences amid effortful, struggling speech.

Individuals with severe apraxia of speech may be able to say a few "stock" (*stereotypic*) phrases, such as "I'm fine. How are you?," or even "I know what I want to say, but I can't say it," or "I know I want to say 'I work in construction,' but I can't say it." In the last instance, the person actually says automatically and effortlessly the very word, phrase, or sentence that could not be said when intentionally trying to say it. Once the patient is able to volitionally say the word or phrase correctly, he usually thinks that he will be able to say it again without difficulty, but his next attempt may be as difficult and off target as his first attempt (Duffy, 2005; Weismer, 2006; Yorkston et al., 2010).

One of the hallmark characteristics of apraxia of speech is its inconsistency. Patients may be able to say complex, multisyllabic words and

Personal Story Profanity

One of my patients at a university medical center was the wife of a professor. She always had been known by her family and friends as a rather demure and proper lady who never used profanity. However, after having a stroke and developing moderate-to-severe speech apraxia, many of her attempts to communicate were punctuated with a variety of scatological words and other profanities. Her family and friends were surprised and she was embarrassed, saying that she sounded like a "drunken sailor." Fortunately, as her speech apraxia diminished, so did her profanity. ■

automatic speech

Over-learned sequences of words that can be recited without much conscious thought, such as counting to 10; saying the days of the week, months of the year, and the alphabet; and singing some songs (e.g., the birthday song).

oral apraxia (nonverbal apraxia, facial apraxia, buccofacial apraxia)

Difficulty with volitional nonspeech movements of the articulators (e.g., puffing the cheeks, clicking the tongue, protruding the tongue, whistling, or smiling).

then may have difficulty with simple, single-syllable words. They often can say sequences of **automatic speech**, such as counting to 10 and saying the days of the week or the months of the year. However, when a patient is trying to say *Thursday,* for example, he may not be able to say it alone, so he gets a "running start" by starting with *Sunday* and when he reaches *Thursday* he stops and says, "That's it." Many people also can sing very familiar songs (e.g., the birthday song) even though they may have difficulty saying "happy birthday." Another fairly common characteristic of speech apraxia is the ability to fluently use profanity and strings of profane words (even individuals who claim to never use profanity may spontaneously and almost uncontrollably use profane words). This automatic and difficult-to-control behavior is embarrassing to some individuals.

Patients with a pure speech apraxia (i.e., no aphasia or cognitive disorders) typically recognize their errors and try to repair them, but to their chagrin the harder they try the more difficult it is for them to say their intended words. Patients often become frustrated and angry with themselves. Individuals with severe apraxia may begin to avoid talking and feel that the effort and embarrassment are not worth trying to communicate.

Patients with speech apraxia also may have **oral apraxia (nonverbal apraxia, facial apraxia, buccofacial apraxia)**. They have difficulty with nonspeech movements of their articulators; for example, intentionally blowing through the lips, clicking the tongue, protruding the tongue, whistling, and smiling. They have effortful groping of the articulators or inconsistent trial-and-error attempts. They usually are confused, frustrated, embarrassed, and sometimes even amused by their difficulty with seemingly easy tasks. However, these same individuals may automatically and spontaneously do any of these movements and be unaware they just performed them (Duffy, 2005; Yorkston et al., 2010).

Limb Apraxia

The articulators are not the only muscles in the body that may be apraxic. *Limb apraxia* (considered the result of damage to the posterior region of the frontal lobe, particularly the left frontal lobe near Broca's area) is seen when a patient cannot perform volitional movements of an arm, hand, or fingers. Limb apraxia is typically more severe with the hand and fingers than with the arm. For example, a patient is likely to have more difficulty showing you how to snap his fingers, flip a coin, or wind a watch than showing you how to salute or drink from a glass. This symptom is important to speech-language pathologists because when a patient has a moderate-to-severe speech apraxia, we cannot rely on the patient having sufficient control of finger movements to write what he cannot say. In addition to writing being nonfunctional, teaching a patient to use finger spelling or a complex sign system such as *American Sign Language* (ASL) may not be practical. However, a sign system such as *American Indian Hand Talk (Amerind)* (Skelly, 1979), which relies on somewhat universal "natural gestures" (e.g., raising the fingers to the mouth as if eating to represent *hunger, food,* or *eat*) may be functional for the person to learn for basic communication.

General Principles of Assessment of Apraxia of Speech

As with dysarthria, a thorough evaluation of the speech systems is completed. When an apraxia of speech is suspected, the patient's speech and oral mechanism are the target of the evaluation. The previously described signs and symptoms are noted and, when appropriate, a diagnosis of apraxia of speech is made. Many patients have combinations of other impairments, such as dysarthria, aphasia, cognitive disorders, and dysphagia.

General Principles of Therapy for Apraxia of Speech

The primary goal of therapy for apraxia of speech is to maximize the effectiveness, efficiency, and naturalness of communication. Therapy focuses on restoring or compensating for impaired functions, as well as helping the person emotionally adjust to the loss of abilities that cannot be restored. *Behavioral intervention* is at the heart of therapy for apraxia of speech (Duffy, 2005; Weismer, 2006; Yorkston et al., 2010).

Therapy for individuals with apraxia of speech should start as early as possible. The various approaches to therapy emphasize carefully selecting the stimuli (functional words) the clinician wants the patient to work on during any one session, an orderly progression of therapy tasks (generally from easiest to hardest), and the use of intensive and systematic drill (practicing repeatedly).

Many individuals with apraxia of speech benefit from watching their face and articulators in a mirror while they are talking. The visual feedback helps compensate for their lack of awareness of where their articulators are and where they want to move them. Apraxia therapy often uses a multimodality approach.

CASE STUDY

John: A Speech-Language Pathologist with Aphasia and Apraxia of Speech

John, a prominent retired speech-language pathologist, had surgery on his lower esophageal valve to help manage his severe gastric reflux. The surgery was successful; however, while in his hospital room resting, he had an occlusive stroke that resulted in severe receptive and expressive aphasia and speech apraxia (global aphasia). He received the amount of speech, physical, and occupational therapy his insurance authorized and was then discharged home. John's wife, Ginger, contacted a speech-language pathologist who taught the courses in neurological disorders in adults and motor speech disorders at a university about an hour away. Ginger wanted to discuss John's problems and try to "make sense" of them.

As a speech-language pathologist, John certainly knew what aphasia and apraxia were, but because of the severity of his aphasia, he could understand little of what was said to him and could communicate only minimally his wants, needs, thoughts, and feelings. The speech-language pathologist decided to show John and Ginger a professionally produced videotape that was made to help laypeople understand strokes, aphasia, and motor speech disorders. The video showed a variety of stroke survivors talking about their problems. While John and Ginger watched the video with the speech-language pathologist, one or the other would occasionally and excitedly point to the television and say, "That's it! That's it!" The video was able to help them see and understand from other survivors' perspectives the problems John was experiencing.

Because of the distance the couple lived from the university, the speech-language pathologist referred them to a university speech-language clinic that was closer to them and had a stroke support group that met weekly. John became a regular member of that group for several years and, although his recovery **plateaued** (still at a severe "global" level), he continued with the group because he enjoyed being around other people that he could relate to. ■

plateau

A patient's general leveling off of improvement in rehabilitation, after which gains are slower and less easily documented; often the reason for discharging from rehabilitation.

DYSPHAGIA/SWALLOWING DISORDERS

dysphagia (swallowing disorders)

Difficulty swallowing that occurs when impairments affect any of the four phases of swallowing (oral preparatory, oral, pharyngeal, or esophageal); puts a person at risk for aspiration of food and/or liquid and potential aspiration pneumonia.

Dysphagia refers to difficulty swallowing (*deglutition* [L. *deglutire,* to swallow]) that occurs when impairments affect any of the four phases of swallowing (oral preparatory, oral, pharyngeal, or esophageal) and put a person at risk for **aspiration**—food, liquid, or both entering the larynx, trachea, and lungs—and potential **aspiration pneumonia**. It is the area of rehabilitation that speech-language pathologists have most recently encompassed. Dysphagia is not part of communication, but it is intimately connected to the speech systems (respiratory, phonatory, resonatory, and articulatory) that serve verbal communication. Speech-language pathologists are recognized by the medical community as the professionals most knowledgeable and directly responsible for the evaluation and treatment of dysphagia (Corbin-Lewis, Liss, & Sciortino, 2005; Miller & Groher, 2005). Dysphagia assessment and treatment are within our scope of practice (see ASHA's "Scope of Practice for Speech-Language Pathologists" on their website, www.asha.org).

Dysphagia requires a team approach, with the speech-language pathologist typically the coordinator or head of the team (Davies, Taylor, MacDonald, & Barer, 2001; Homer, 2003; Leonard & Kendall, 2008; Swigert, 2007). Team members may include (in alphabetical order): a *dentist* for making dental appliances and dentures; a *dietician* or *nutritionist* who checks the patient's daily intake of liquids and food and tries to make the various food textures as palatable (edible) as possible and makes certain the patient is receiving adequate nutrition for maintaining and improving health; various *family* members who may be involved with feeding the patient and making decisions about the level of care a patient may be able to return to; a *gastroenterologist* for evaluating esophageal problems and inserting nasogastric and stomach feeding tubes; a *neurologist* for assessing and treating some aspects of the patient's neurological impairments; *nurses* who can manage the patient's day-to-day medical needs and inform the team members about a patient's medical changes; an *occupational therapist* for helping with positioning the patient for meals and assessing and managing the patient's ability to retrieve food from a plate and bring it to the mouth; an *otolaryngologist* to examine laryngeal function; a *pharmacist* for providing information about side effects of the patient's medications that may influence swallowing adversely; a *physical therapist* who assesses and manages postural problems and finds the best wheelchair for the patient; one or more *physicians* who are managing the patients medical problems; a *pulmonologist* who can assess respiratory functions and treat respiratory problems such as aspiration pneumonia; a *radiologist* for performing and helping read modified barium swallowing studies; a *respiratory therapist* who can carry out various respiratory treatments, sometimes several times a day; and a *social worker* who is involved in patient advocacy and works with insurance companies, Medicare, and other third-party payers (see Figure 12–2).

The work of SLPs with patients who have dysphagia is in some ways the most challenging and high-risk work we do because a patient's physical health (indeed, life) may be determined by our evaluation, correct diagnosis, and appropriate management of the swallowing disorder (Logemann, 1998; Murry & Carrau, 2006). Beyond basic academic course work on dysphagia during graduate training, there must be considerable hands-on training during hospital internships and additional training through professional workshops and seminars to become competent to work independently with patients who have swallowing disorders. It is essential that clinicians develop the skills outlined by ASHA (2000a; 2000b;

aspiration

A term in reference to material (food, liquid, saliva, etc.) penetrating the larynx and entering the airway below the true vocal folds; food or liquid entering the lungs rather than the stomach after the swallow.

aspiration pneumonia

An acute inflammation of the lungs caused by foreign material (e.g., food or liquid) entering the lung tissue and resulting in infection; alveolar and bronchiole congestion with substances discharged from the alveolar walls as a protection against foreign material.

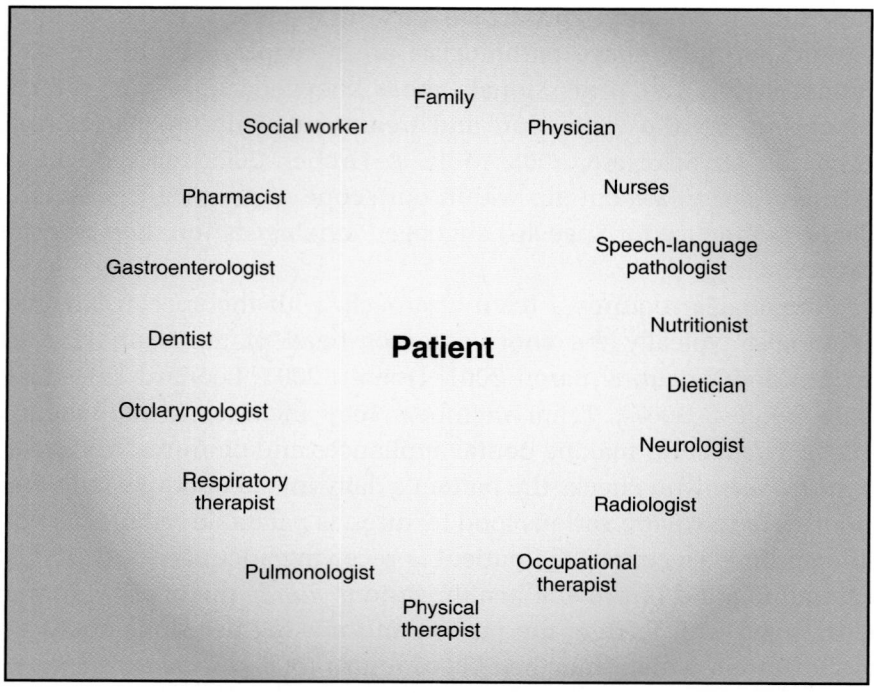

Figure 12-2

Potential members of a
dysphagia team.

© Cengage Learning 2013.

2002; 2004a; 2004b) for providing services to patients and clients with
dysphagia:

- Identify people at risk for dysphagia.
- Conduct and interpret clinical assessments of oral–pharyngeal
  and respiratory functions related to feeding.
- Conduct and interpret instrumental-based evaluations of swallowing.
- Develop intervention strategies (i.e., safe feeding recommenda-
  tions, swallowing precautions, and therapeutic interventions).
- Document care and discharge planning.
- Provide education, counseling, and training to patients and all
  other relevant individuals (e.g., family and health professionals).

Causes of Dysphagia

Swallowing disorders may occur at any age—from newborns to the end
of life. Essentially, the same neurological causes of motor speech disorders and cognitive disorders in children and adults may cause dysphagia.
However, in addition to neurological etiologies, cancer (lingual, oral,
pharyngeal, and laryngeal) may cause swallowing problems. The treatment of these cancers (surgical removal, radiation, chemotherapy) also
may cause or contribute to swallowing impairments. Side effects of some
medications may cause swallowing problems. Muscle relaxants may
affect muscle tone of the swallowing muscles (Carl & Johnson, 2006).
HIV and AIDS in children and adults are associated with dysphagia

(Crary & Groher, 2003; Finley, Clifton, Stewart, Graham, & Worsley, 2001; Huckabee & Pelletier, 2003).

Speech-language pathologists work with dysphagia in all clinical settings, plus home health care. In a U.S. study of acute care hospital patients, it was found that approximately one-third of patients with new strokes have dysphagia (Teasell, Foley, Fisher, & Finestone, 2002). Dysphagia has become the primary focus of the acute care hospital work for speech-language pathologists in Australia and England (Armstrong, 2003; Code & Heron, 2003). In some hospitals, speech-language pathologists become known as *swallowing therapists* more than speech pathologists. School-based SLPs are increasingly finding that their caseloads include children with medical complications and even swallowing problems, particularly those with orthopedic handicaps (e.g., cerebral palsy) (Ratner, 2006; Kurjan, 2000; Rempel & Moussavi, 2005).

THE NORMAL SWALLOW

To understand when a patient has a swallowing problem, we must first understand the anatomy and physiology of a normal swallow. What we take for granted every time we unconsciously swallow is the complex interaction of several muscle groups with split-second timing to allow us to effortlessly, automatically, and safely carry out one of the most mundane functions of our bodies. People generally swallow approximately 600 times a day (we even automatically swallow our saliva during sleep), which is almost 220,000 times a year. If we multiply that by, say, 50 years, it means that the average 50-year-old person has swallowed automatically and mostly unconsciously more than 10 million times. Each swallow has four phases (stages): (1) oral preparatory phase, (2) oral phase, (3) pharyngeal phase, and (4) esophageal phase. Patients may have difficulty with any or all of the phases and even specific problems within each portion of a phase (Corbin-Lewis et al., 2005; Kendall, 2008; Logemann, 1998).

Oral Preparatory Phase

All of our senses come into play during the oral preparatory phase—that is, vision, hearing (e.g., the sound of food cooking or popcorn popping), touch, smell, and taste (Fogle, 1998). The oral preparatory phase may be considered to begin with a person's cognitive level of awareness that food or drink is available to be consumed. The next cognitive process is to decide how to bring the food or liquid to the mouth. Once food enters the mouth, it must be chewed sufficiently to prepare it to be swallowed (it is referred to as a *bolus* [Gk. *bolos,* lump] when it is in the mouth). How we chew and how long we chew depends on the temperature of the food and the size, texture, and consistency of the bite. As we prepare the food inside our mouth, we tighten our cheeks slightly to prevent food

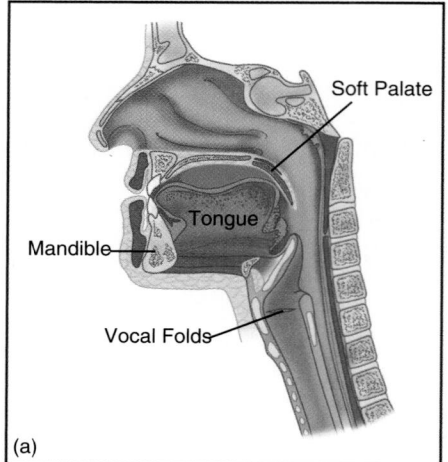

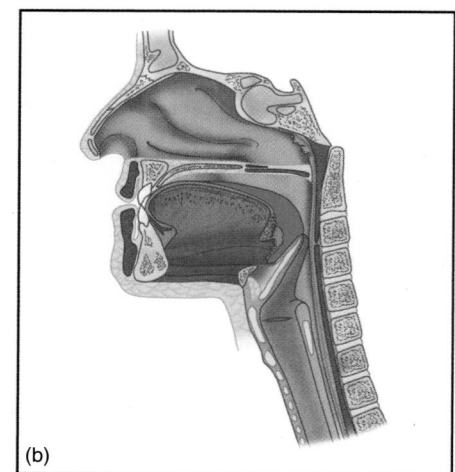

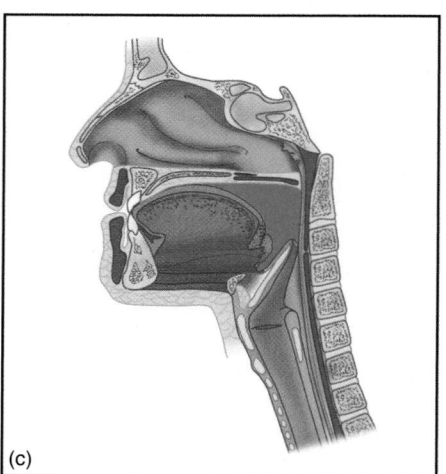

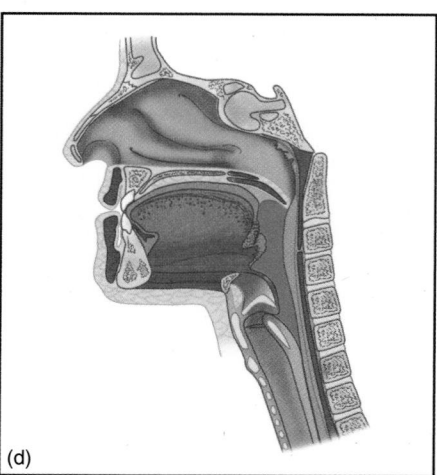

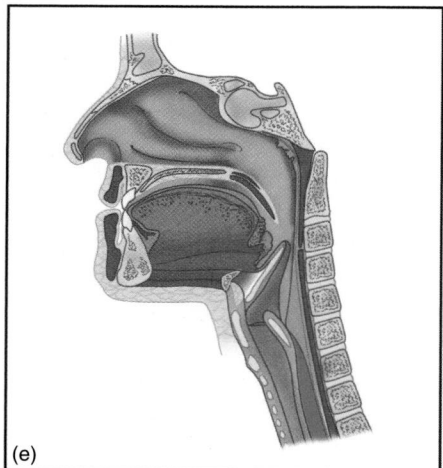

Figure 12-3

The normal swallow involves four separate phases that are interdependent and highly coordinated: the oral preparatory phase, the oral phase, the pharyngeal phase, and the esophageal phase. This series demonstrates a lateral view of bolus propulsion during the swallow: (a) The tongue begins the voluntary initiation of the swallow; (b) this triggers the pharyngeal swallow; (c) the bolus moves to the vallecula; (d) the tongue base then moves anteriorly and the pharyngeal walls begin peristalsis; and (e) the bolus moves to the cervical esophagus and the cricopharyngeal region.

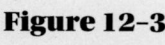

© Cengage Learning 2013.

from lodging between our gums (*gingiva*) and our cheeks. We also pull the soft palate down firmly against the base of the tongue to prevent food from falling past the tongue into the open airway. We use our tongue to move the food around inside our mouth and between our teeth to chew the food (see Figure 12-3).

Oral Phase

The oral phase begins when we stop chewing and the tongue tip elevates to touch the alveolar ridge. The food is on top of the tongue and the tongue quickly sweeps back, pulling the food to the back of the mouth and toward the pharynx. The soft palate moves up to make contact with the posterior pharyngeal wall to prevent food from accidentally entering the nasal passage (*nasal regurgitation*). The oral phase normally takes 1 second.

Pharyngeal Phase

Passage of food through the pharynx and into the esophagus occurs during the pharyngeal phase of swallowing. Four physiological responses occur during the pharyngeal phase. First, as the bolus flows over the base of the tongue, there is a squeezing action (*peristalsis*) caused by contraction of the muscles in the pharynx that helps move the bolus downward. Second, the thyroid cartilage of the larynx rises, which causes the epiglottis to drop down over the opening into the larynx to shield it and prevent food or liquid falling into the open airway (*aspiration*), and initiates the opening of the *upper esophageal valve* (UEV) so the bolus can enter the esophagus. Third, the true and false vocal folds adduct tightly, which provides two more levels of protection (defense) from food or liquid entering the trachea. And fourth, the upper esophageal sphincter at the top of the esophagus relaxes and opens, allowing the bolus that has flowed around the epiglottis to enter into the esophagus. All of the pharyngeal phase normally takes 1 second.

Esophageal Phase

When the bolus passes the upper esophageal sphincter, the sphincter closes and the peristaltic squeezing action of the esophageal muscles carries the bolus to the *lower esophageal sphincter* at the bottom of the esophagus, which then briefly opens to allow the bolus to enter the stomach. When the bolus has passed, the sphincter again closes to prevent gastric contents from reentering the esophagus. The esophageal phase may take 8 to 20 seconds.

DYSPHAGIA—DISORDERED SWALLOWING

Individuals may have problems in any or all four of the phases of swallowing, and a problem at an earlier phase may cause a problem during a later phase (Corbin-Lewis et al., 2005; McCulloch & Jaffe, 2006). When thinking about swallowing disorders, it is helpful to organize your thinking by considering each phase in sequence.

Application Question

Try swallowing one or two sips of water. What do you notice? When you are going to eat some food, think about each of the four phases of swallowing. What do you notice?

Oral Preparatory Phase Problems

Many patients have decreased cognition because of neurological damage from a stroke or head trauma. Some patients have impaired awareness and do not realize that there is food in front of them or what to do with it if they are aware. Some patients, particularly those with TBIs, are impulsive and will take dangerously large bites of food and keep putting more spoonfuls into their mouths before adequately chewing (*masticating*) and swallowing the previous bites. Patients also may have weak mandible, lip, and tongue muscles that make it difficult to hold food in their mouths and to chew and control it adequately.

Oral Phase Problems

This phase involves the final movement of the bolus to the posterior oral cavity on its way to the pharynx. If the lips do not have a good seal, *anterior spillage* (drooling) may occur. When there is a poor posterior seal between the soft palate and the base of the tongue, food or liquid may spill over the base of the tongue before the swallow is initiated (*premature spillage*). A weak tongue, particularly the tip, will cause discoordinated and impaired posterior movement of the bolus to the back of the mouth. *Pocketed food* between the cheek and the gums (*sulcus*) may leave *residue* or *stasis* (food that is not cleared and swallowed). In some patients, the force used to propel the bolus is insufficient and the bolus will not move efficiently through to the next phase.

Pharyngeal Phase Problems

Numerous problems may occur in this phase. There may be a *delayed swallow response* from a few seconds to many seconds after the patient attempts to swallow. Timing and coordination of the oral–pharyngeal structures may be impaired. The soft palate may be too weak to close the velopharyngeal port to prevent material from entering the nasal passages. Muscles that raise the larynx may be weak causing the epiglottis not to drop down to cover the open airway, causing *penetration*, and the upper esophageal valve may not open, preventing food or liquid entering the esophagus. The true and false vocal folds may not have strong closure, allowing material that may enter the larynx to pass below the vocal folds (aspiration).

Patients with swallowing disorders may not have normal sensation in the laryngeal region, and material may penetrate the larynx without a protective cough or choking occurring, resulting in **silent aspiration**. That is, material enters the larynx, passes below the vocal folds, and moves down the trachea into the lungs without the patient having any sensation of something in the airway. Without sensation, there are no protective maneuvers such as coughing and choking (Ramsey, Smithard, & Kalra, 2003; Murry & Carrau, 2006). Other individuals may attempt to cough, but the cough is too weak to be protective and effective; therefore, the material is able to pass below the vocal folds into the trachea and down into the lungs.

silent aspiration

Penetration of food or liquid (including saliva) into the larynx and passing below the vocal folds without a protective cough or choking occurring.

Esophageal Phase Problems

Esophageal problems may be the result of the upper esophageal sphincter not opening at the precise time or not remaining open for the entire bolus to flow through. Slow or absent *esophageal peristalsis* may not carry the bolus through the esophagus in an efficient and complete manner, causing discomfort or pain in the chest and leaving residue on the esophageal walls that can cause infection. In some patients, the lower esophageal valve (LEV) does not sufficiently relax to allow the food in the esophagus to flow into the stomach causing *achalasia* (abnormal constriction of the lower portion of the esophagus). **Gastroenterologists** are the medical professionals who treat esophageal disorders.

gastroenterologist

A physician who specializes in diseases of the gastrointestinal tract.

DIAGNOSIS OF DYSPHAGIA

When an SLP begins her day at a hospital, she may be given a physician's order to "evaluate and treat" a particular new admission for swallowing problems. These medical orders should be taken care of as soon as possible because in some instances a patient's meals may be held up until the SLP can make a decision about swallowing safety. Also, legally the clinician has a certain window of time to complete an assessment and written report. The SLP is a hospital's main resource on swallowing function and disorders, and nurses and other medical staff members follow the SLP's recommendations. Referrals to a speech-language pathologist to evaluate a patient's swallowing typically are based on three general areas of concern:

- The patient appears to be at risk for aspirating food or liquid based on the medical diagnosis.
- Difficulties have been observed related to feeding and the intake of food or liquid.
- The patient appears not to be taking in adequate nourishment (Cherney, 2004; Logemann, 1998; Swigert, 2007).

Bedside (Clinical) Swallow Evaluation

The evaluation of a patient who may have dysphagia begins with a careful review of the patient's medical chart. The next step is screening the patient, which includes interviewing the patient to understand her perceptions of the problem and to determine whether the patient has a sufficiently strong protective cough to clear food or liquid from the airway. A multistep clinical or "bedside" evaluation is performed, including an oral-mechanism examination with careful observation of the anatomy and physiology of the articulatory structures, the *symmetry* of the structures (i.e., are both left and right sides equal in dimension and function), volitional movements, range of motion, strength, and coordination of each articulator. The clinician needs to observe the patient drinking different consistencies or thicknesses of liquids (i.e., *regular* [thin], *nectar, honey,* and *pudding*) and foods of different textures (i.e., *regular* [normal diet with all textures], *mechanical soft* [food easily chewed into a cohesive bolus], and *puree* [blended food or baby-food texture] (Rodriquez & Borelli, 2003). Some signs and symptoms that a patient is at risk for aspiration and needs an *instrumental evaluation* are: coughing or choking during the evaluation, difficulty managing oral secretions, multiple attempts to swallow a bolus of food, and others. When there is risk for aspiration an instrumental evaluation is needed to clarify the kind of swallowing disorder the patient has (e.g., oropharyngeal) and the underlying physiological deficits. It is essential to document in the patient's medical chart all assessment procedures and results (ASHA, 2005a; Swigert, 2007).

Modified Barium Swallow Study

modified barium swallow study (MBSS)

A dynamic (moving) imaging radiographic (x-ray) procedure focusing on the mouth, pharynx, larynx, and cervical esophagus used to examine the process of swallowing; a video recording of real-time movement of a bolus from entering the mouth to entering the stomach.

The **modified barium swallow study** (MBS study or MBSS; also known as a *videofluoroscopy swallow study,* or VFSS) is considered the "gold standard" instrumental evaluation for viewing the physiology of the swallow and determining the presence or absence of aspiration (see Figure 12–4). It is a *dynamic* (moving) imaging *radiographic* (x-ray) procedure to examine the process of swallowing; that is, a video recording of real-time movement of the bolus from entering the mouth to entering the stomach. The MBSS provides the most thorough information on the physiology of the swallowing process (ASHA, 2004a; Becker, McLeroy, & Carpenter, 2005; DeMatteo, Matovich, & Hjartarson, 2005). It is performed in the radiology (x-ray) suite with the speech-language pathologist and radiologist working as a team. The clinician presents to the patient various liquid consistencies that have been mixed with *barium* (a *radiopaque* substance that stops the passage of x-rays and is used to outline the interior of hollow organs, e.g., the esophagus) and food textures that have been

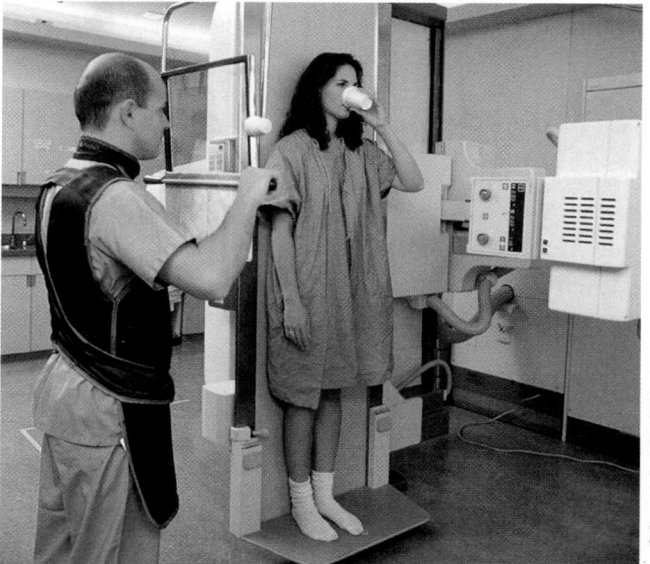

© Cengage Learning 2013

Figure 12–4

A radiologist conducting a modified barium swallow study with a patient.

coated with barium. The clinician carefully observes on the video screen the patient's oral preparatory, oral, pharyngeal, and esophageal phases of swallowing. Beyond diagnosing oropharyngeal dysphagia, the clinician also has the patient try various compensatory swallowing techniques to see which techniques allow for a safe and efficient swallow; for example, modified liquid consistencies and food textures, postural adjustments of the patient, and swallowing maneuvers. These techniques can later be trained during the dysphagia therapy (Swigert, 2007).

Fiberoptic Endoscopic Evaluation of Swallowing

Fiberoptic endoscopic evaluation of swallowing (FEES) is a procedure used to provide information about the pharyngeal phase of swallowing (ASHA, 2002a; Langmore, 2003). During the FEES procedure, the patient sits in a chair and a flexible endoscope with a light source (see Figures 9–10 and 9–11) is passed through the nasal passageway into the nasopharynx and down to just below the epiglottis. FEES studies are video-recorded for detailed analysis. A selected texture of food is dyed green (e.g., applesauce) to provide a clear color contrast from the laryngeal tissue and is given to the patient to chew and swallow. The laryngopharynx is viewed through the endoscope to determine whether food material remains in the pharynx, penetrates into the larynx, or is aspirated into the airway with or without attempts to clear the throat through coughing or choking (see Figure 12–5). The FEES procedure allows the clinician to view the movement of the vocal folds and the pharyngeal and laryngeal structures only before and after the swallow.

fiberoptic endoscopic evaluation of swallowing (FEES)

A procedure used to provide visual information about the pharyngeal phase of swallowing; a flexible endoscope is passed through the nasal passageway into the nasopharynx to view the laryngopharynx and the patient is asked to swallow food or liquid that has been dyed green for contrast.

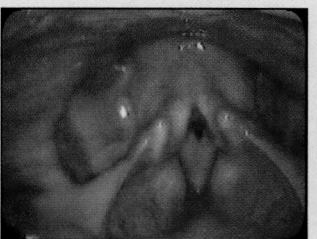

Courtesy of KayPENTAX

Figure 12–5

Fiberoptic Endoscopic Evaluation of Swallowing (FEES). Note the green colored applesauce on the right side of the larynx but not in the glottal region, i.e., there is no penetration into the airway.

TREATMENT OF DYSPHAGIA

A complete evaluation of dysphagia does not end at diagnosing a swallowing disorder in the oral or pharyngeal phases; in a sense, the clinician is reevaluating the patient during every therapy session. Treatment planning requires numerous careful decisions. The first decision is to choose a long-term functional goal based on the prognosis of the patient. *Long-term functional goal* refers to treatment results that improve a patient's swallowing ability in *natural environments* (home, community) or in a patient's future *lowest level of care* (e.g., skilled nursing facility). For most patients with dysphagia the long-term goals are "Patient will achieve safe and efficient swallowing to sustain adequate nutrition and hydration orally" or "Patient will be able to eat a regular diet safely" (Swigert, 2007). The emphasis in safety is important in many areas of our work with patients who have neurological disorders, but it is particularly important for patients who have swallowing problems (Fogle, Reece, & White, 2008).

As discussed previously, the SLP's decision to provide dysphagia therapy must be based on firm anatomical and physiological findings that indicate skilled intervention is necessary for a patient to eat safely and adequately to provide sufficient nutrition to maintain body weight.

Treating adults and children with dysphagia is interesting and challenging work. *Best practices* have been established and are continually refined for our treatment of dysphagia (ASHA, 2004b). In all therapy, clinicians need to consider **treatment efficacy**, which involves the extent to which an intervention can be shown to be beneficial under optimal (or ideal) conditions, and **treatment effectiveness**, which involves the extent to which services are shown to be beneficial under typical (or real-world) conditions (ASHA, 2004a, 2005; El Dib & Atallah, 2006; Frymark, Schooling, Mullen, et al., 2009; Logemann, 2004).

treatment efficacy

The extent to which an intervention can be shown to be beneficial under optimal (or ideal) conditions.

treatment effectiveness

The extent to which services are shown to be beneficial under typical (or real-world) conditions.

evidence-based practice

The quality of treatment that is measurable in terms of some form of functional outcomes and maintained in the face of cost-containment efforts.

Evidence-Based Practice

Evidence-based practice refers to quality of treatment that is measurable in terms of some form of functional outcomes and maintained in the face of cost-containment efforts. Evidence-based practice is an approach that deemphasizes both clinician intuition and unsystematic approaches to clinical care. It requires decisions to be made through a scientific process rooted in the examination of clinical research. Clinicians must be effective literature researchers and return to their academic roots. In this manner, clinical work may be supported with clinical evidence and literature (Lubinski, Golper, & Frattali, 2007).

Third-party payers (Medicare, health maintenance organizations [HMOs], etc.) do not want to know a test score; they want to know if a patient can be discharged, go home, recover, and return to work. Payers want those outcomes for the least amount of money and in the least amount of time. In other words, providers need to keep costs down, keep quality high, achieve maximum patient satisfaction, and be able to measure it and prove it. Health care delivery has become a process that balances costs and risks yet affords an acceptable outcome and level of quality (Lubinski, Golper, & Frattali, 2007).

For patients who have swallowing problems, therapy can include *compensatory treatment techniques, facilitation treatment techniques, compensatory and facilitation techniques, and diet modification techniques* (Swigert, 2007).

Compensatory Treatment Techniques

Compensatory treatment techniques help optimize a patient's ability to use his current swallowing abilities. The hospital staff and family may be taught to use these techniques when they are preparing or helping the patient to eat or drink.

Postural Techniques

Postural techniques are used to control the flow of the food or liquid bolus and reduce the risk of the patient's symptoms; for example, while attempting to swallow, tucking the chin downward or rotating the head to one side. Patients with communication and cognitive problems usually find postural techniques the easiest to learn (Leonard & Kendall, 2008; Murry & Carrau, 2006).

Food Placement

Food is normally placed in the midline of the tongue; however, some patients benefit from having food placed on the stronger side of the mouth, especially if it is food that needs to be chewed. Controlling bolus size is also important, usually limiting it to a small amount such as 5cc ($\approx$ 1 tsp.).

Facilitation Treatment Techniques

Facilitation treatment techniques are designed to improve the function of the swallowing mechanism and include techniques that help increase vocal fold adduction and teaching the patient to intentionally hold his breath just prior to and during the swallow, among other techniques. Oral-motor exercises for strengthening the muscles of the articulators have not been clearly effective for individuals with muscle weakness from dysarthria; however, there is indication they may be helpful for increasing muscle tone and strength to help improve swallowing (Clark, 2003; Hind, Nicosia, Roecker, Carnes, & Robbins, 2001; Murry & Carrau, 2006). Shaker (pronounced "shakeer") exercises help to increase laryngeal elevation and opening of the upper esophageal sphincter.

Compensatory and Facilitation Techniques

Compensatory and facilitation techniques are intended to help a patient's swallow become more functional. *Swallow maneuvers* try to bring aspects of the pharyngeal phase of the swallow into conscious awareness and voluntary control. A few swallowing maneuvers have been developed, a couple of which are the *supraglottic swallow* that is designed to close the airway at the level of the true vocal folds before and during the swallow, and the *effortful swallow* that is designed to increase posterior motion of the tongue base during the pharyngeal swallow phase (Cherney, 2004; Huckabee & Pelletier, 2003; Logemann, 1998). (Note: It is beyond the scope of this text to include descriptions of the various swallow maneuvers.)

Diet Modification Techniques

Diet modification techniques are often needed for patients with oral and/or pharyngeal phase swallowing problems (Logemann, 1998; Swigert, 2007). The National Dysphagia Diet Task Force (2002) standardized dietary modifications for patients based on a graded series of four levels of food textures and four levels of liquid consistencies (see Table 12–2). SLPs can choose which of the food textures and liquid consistencies they feel are best and safest for a particular patient who has dysphagia.

Although our treatment for dysphagia can be challenging, many patients benefit from the treatment and many can return to relatively

TABLE 12-2	Textures of Foods and Consistencies of Liquids

FOODS	LIQUIDS
Regular: No restrictions in foods but meats and some vegetables may be chopped; includes baked potatoes, rice, cooked or uncooked vegetables, fruits, fruit pies, cookies, cooked or dry cereals.	**Thin:** No restrictions.
Dysphagia advanced: Ground or chopped tender meat, potatoes (no skin), pasta, cooked vegetables, beans, canned fruits, apple slices (no peel), cookies, fruit pies, fried eggs, hot cereal.	**Nectar-like:** All liquids (including water) must be thickened to a nectar consistency; fruit nectars, V8 juice, eggnog.
Dysphagia mechanical soft: Ground or finely chopped tender meat with gravy, mashed potatoes with gravy, pasta, soft cooked vegetables, canned fruits, soft cookies, scrambled eggs, cooked cereals.	**Honey-like:** All liquids (including water) must be thickened to a honey consistency, usually with a commercial thickener.
Dysphagia pureed: Pureed meat, mashed potatoes with gravy, pureed vegetables, strained soups thickened to pudding consistency, pureed fruits, pudding, cooked cereals.	**Spoon-thick:** All liquids (including water) must be thickened to a pudding consistency, usually with a commercial thickener.

© Cengage Learning 2012.

normal eating and drinking. Early identification of and intervention for swallowing disorders reduce the risk of aspiration, shorten the hospitalization time, and improve quality of life. Overall, treatment for dysphagia has been reported to be cost effective compared to the cost of hospitalization and treatment of aspiration pneumonia (Evidence Reports/Technology Assessments, 1999; Johns Hopkins, 2000).

NPO (Nothing by Mouth)

Some patients have such severe swallowing disorders that they must be placed on **NPO (nothing by mouth)**, at least temporarily. NPO is a patient care instruction advising that the patient is prohibited from orally ingesting food, beverage, or medicine. Usually, after having swallowing therapy, patients are able to eat orally again. Patients who are on NPO may receive their nutrition through **enteral feeding**, which is the delivery of nutrition and hydration into the gastrointestinal (GI) tract by way of tube feedings through the nose (*nasogastric tube* [NG-tube]) or the stomach (*gastrostomytube* [G-tube]) (Johnson & Jacobson, 2007) (see Figure 12–6). Enteral feeding may be a temporary or permanent source of nutritional support. A common source of nutrition and hydration for patients on enteral feeding is the lactose-free nutrition supplement Ensure™ (Pediasure™ for children) that contains protein, carbohydrates, fat, vitamins, and minerals. Ensure™ and Pediasure™ can be purchased in local supermarkets and pharmacies.

NPO (nothing by mouth)

A patient care instruction advising that a patient is prohibited from orally ingesting food, beverage, or medicine; patients must receive nutrition through enteral feeding.

enteral feeding

The delivery of hydration and nutrition into the gastrointestinal (GI) tract by way of tube feedings through the nose or stomach.

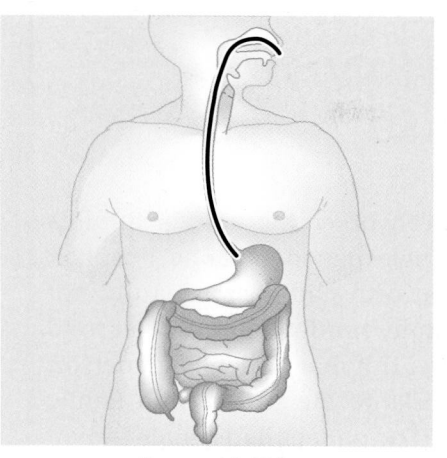

Nasogastric Tube

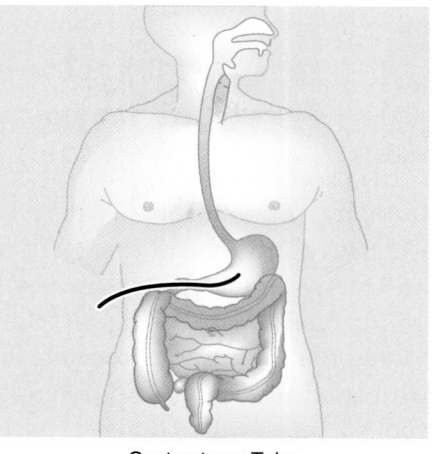

Gastrostomy Tube

Figure 12–6

Nasogastric tube (NG tube) and gastrostomy tube (G tube) feeding for patients who are NPO.

© Cengage Learning 2013.

Rachelle

CASE STUDY

Rachelle was a 29-year-old female and a single mother of three children. Rachelle had been in a motor vehicle accident while driving alone. She sustained a moderately severe head injury with contrecoup damage. The patient was impulsive, as well as confused and agitated. The speech-language pathologist's bedside evaluation revealed moderate receptive and expressive language impairments, severe cognitive impairments (which likely were contributing to her language problems), and significant impulsivity. She had bilateral weakness, worse on the left side of her body. There was moderate dysarthria affecting each of the speech systems. She had an adequate but not a strong protective cough. The bedside swallowing evaluation using a mechanical soft diet revealed an impaired oral preparatory phase as a result of impulsivity (trying to eat too fast) and discoordinated lingual movements with pocketing of food in the left lateral sulcus. She was not able to tolerate (manage) thin liquids but did well with nectar consistency. The oral phase was slow with poor posterior lingual movement. During the pharyngeal phase of swallowing, there was slow laryngeal elevation because of apparent weakened suprahyoid muscles. An MBSS confirmed the preceding findings and revealed residue on the left side pharyngeal wall likely caused by decreased pharyngeal peristalsis. She received a diagnosis of moderate oropharyngeal dysphagia and was considered a good candidate for swallowing therapy. With appropriate dysphagia and speech, language, and cognitive therapy, as well as physical and occupational therapy, Rachelle eventually was able to return home and to her job and support her family. ■

Personal Story

Multicultural Work Environments

In many of the hospitals where I have worked, numerous cultures were involved with the care of a single patient. In one hospital, an elderly female Vietnamese patient who had dysphagia did not understand or speak English. Her family routinely brought in food for her that was not appropriate for her dysphagia diet. Each person who tried to explain the potential risks to the patient and family spoke English with a different accent. The patient had a male Indian physician, several female and male Filipino nurses, female and male African American and Hispanic certified nursing assistants, and me, a Caucasian male speech-language pathologist from California. The patient and family may not have understood the message (i.e., no foods or liquids from home that are not of the right texture or consistency), or they made the choice to disregard the recommendations. As clinicians, we need to keep in mind that patients may receive medical care and treatment from a variety of cultures with different first languages, dialects, accents, and worldviews. Also, we need to remember that as speech-language pathologists we not only evaluate and treat patients from many cultures but work with professionals from many cultures. ■

Multicultural Considerations

All cultures have their own food preferences and unique ways of preparing foods. In addition, cultures have rituals around food and meals. There may be religious and dietary preference and taboos related to the use of special spices and food preparation practices, when and where meals are served, and even who is present during meals (some cultures have rigid rules as to whether both males and females can be present) (Shoemaker, 1997). Patients in hospitals are presented "institutional food" that the kitchen staff tries to make as nutritious and enjoyable as possible. However, many patients would agree that the food is often rather bland and not always appetizing or appealing.

For patients who are accustomed to "ethnic" foods because of their ethnic and cultural backgrounds, the hospital food presented may be totally foreign to them. A patient with dysphagia may be a visitor to this country or a long-time resident, but has not adopted the food choices and preparation methods of this country. The hospital kitchen staff cannot provide the desired ethnic foods for every person in the hospital who wants it; therefore, many patients are presented foods that are foreign and even distasteful to them.

Family members sometimes try to bring in food and drinks to a patient that they know their loved one will enjoy. This is a very caring and loving gesture; however, the food and drinks may be the wrong texture and consistency and cause the patient to cough, choke, or aspirate. Patients who have not eaten "real" food for a while may try to eat too fast and cause themselves swallowing problems. As clinicians, it is our job to educate both the patient and family about the hazards of feeding a patient foods and liquids that are unsafe (Provencio-Arambula, Provencio, & Hegde, 2006; Tonkovich, 2002).

EMOTIONAL AND SOCIAL EFFECTS OF MOTOR SPEECH DISORDERS AND DYSPHAGIA

Patients who have motor speech disorders are often very aware of the difficulty they have being understood and attempts to communicate can be fraught with frustration. Individuals may have only motor speech problems and little or no impairment of language or cognition. Some individuals, because of severe difficulty communicating verbally, will avoid verbal communication as much as possible—not wanting to place the burden of understanding on their listener and not wanting to embarrass themselves.

Adults who were very effective verbal communicators and may have even made their living based on their verbal skill, may find that without those skills they can no longer compete in the marketplace or enjoy socializing with colleagues, friends, and family. What they may have taken pride in for decades—their verbal skill—now eludes them and they feel isolated.

Food and eating have strong emotional significance for most people. Our thoughts about food and drink are typically based on acquiring and enjoying it, not on what damage it might do to our health (e.g., aspiration pneumonia or asphyxiation). Eating is a social function that people enjoy as a natural part of their lives. We "break bread together" as a way of establishing, building, and maintaining friendships and relationships. We raise a "toast" at weddings and other celebrations. We have our "comfort foods" and there is chocolate "to die for." People spend considerable time thinking about food: breakfast, midmorning snack, lunch, afternoon snack, dinner, evening snack, and maybe even a midnight snack. We have our favorite foods, meals, restaurants, coffee houses, bars, and pubs.

Eating alone or being fed by hospital staff takes away much of the enjoyment of eating, which can result in patients eating just enough to satisfy their hunger but not enough to get all of the nutrition and hydration they need (Fogle, 1998). What happens to people emotionally and socially when every bite of food and sip of liquid may bring on a "fit of coughing" or choking? How do they manage knowing that they may never again be able to swallow food without needing to consciously think about what they had spent their lives *not* thinking about? Does thinking about the mechanics of chewing and swallowing take away from the pure enjoyment of the taste and texture of food?

I have interviewed and discussed these concerns with numerous patients of mine in acute, subacute, and convalescent hospitals who had swallowing problems. Some of the following information is based on literature, and some of it comes from anecdotal reports from patients from their late teens into their 100s who have had dysphagia. So often when clinicians are working with patients with swallowing disorders, they focus on the anatomy and physiology of the swallowing problem and forget that there are genuine emotional and social concerns that may be helpful to discuss with their patients. The individuals we try to help are always *first* people and only *secondarily* patients or clients.

Quality of Life

A patient's quality of life is always the most important concern in patient care (Chen et al., 2001; Watt & Whyte, 2003). As clinicians and researchers, we are increasingly questioning what constitutes good quality of life from the patient's point of view. What we as professionals may think is good for patients may not be what they think is good for themselves, and ultimately they need to decide. We can inform, advise, and recommend, but they can demand. As clinicians we can provide information to patients about their swallowing problems and give our professional opinion about what we think is safest for their consumption of foods and liquids, but **bioethics** emphasizes that we must respect a patient's **autonomy** (Aiken, 2008; Beauchamp & Childress, 2008).

Food texture is important in the enjoyment of food. (Who would want pureed roast beef?) Decreasing the texture of food or increasing the *viscosity* (thickness) of liquids changes their flavor (Dahl, 2008; Matta, Chambers, Garcia, & McGowan-Helverson, 2006). Patients' complaints that foods do not taste the same when they are pureed are legitimate. Food has five inherent properties: appearance, aroma, flavor, texture, and nutrition. Only nutrition cannot be detected by the senses. It is the inherent qualities of food that we enjoy, and when these are lost (e.g., when finely chopped or pureed) many patients will decrease their consumption even though they understand the need for nutrition (Fogle, 1998).

Anxieties and Fears

Patients with dysphagia may experience anxieties and fears around eating. Examples include fear of: embarrassment in front of family and friends who visit during meal time; an acute or chronic illness (aspiration pneumonia), or even death because of aspiration; discomfort from suctioning of food or liquid out of the oral cavity, trachea, and lungs; never being able to eat their favorite foods (at least with a normal texture) and have normal thin liquids again (Ekberg et al., 2002; Flasher & Fogle, 2012).

bioethics

The attempt to understand and resolve ethical issues and problems in health care setting.

autonomy

Respect for the patient's right to determine his or her own choices in making health care decisions.

Mr. M and His Mittens

Personal Story

After beginning summer work in a skilled nursing facility, I was asked to evaluate an elderly gentleman for potential oral feeding. The patient had had a nasogastric tube (NG-tube) for several months and was wearing thick padded "mittens" on both hands as a restraint to prevent him from pulling out the NG-tube, which he had done many times before being required to wear the mittens. My evaluation revealed that he was not a safe oral feeder and that NPO was the safest method of feeding. He also had severe dysarthria and receptive and expressive aphasia. The patient's wife was present during my evaluation and shared her frustration and sadness about not being able to hold her husband's hand to comfort him because of the interference of the mittens. I suggested that a stomach feeding tube might be a consideration.

I wrote my evaluation results in the patient's medical chart with the recommendation to the physician for the placement of a gastric tube (G-tube). The physician denied my request, so I followed up and spoke with the physician. He told me that the patient was going to die soon and there was no need to change from an NG-tube to a G-tube. The patient's wife also spoke to the physician about wanting the change, but he would not be assuaged. As a speech-language pathologist, I was looking at the patient holistically rather than just physically. Had the patient received a G-tube months before, he could have had the comfort of his wife's hand on his, meeting both of their emotional needs. Sometimes we can only watch in sadness as medical decisions are made that we may feel do not take into consideration the patient as a whole person. ■

Stages of Grief

The stages of grief apply to dysphagia as well as other neurological disorders. Patients may begin with *denial* of their swallowing problem, possibly realizing that if they admit to it the SLP will take away their regular food and give them "baby food." When they realize they are having swallowing problems, they may become *angry* and displace the anger onto us and other people who are trying to help them. When their anger does not get them what they want (back on regular foods and liquids), they may try to *bargain* with the SLP, agreeing to do anything the clinician wants if she will just let them eat "real food" again. *Depression* may be partly the result of moving through the stages of grief, but it also may be compounded by the depression discussed previously. *Acceptance* is more a resignation of how things are and the realization that there are fewer episodes of coughing, choking, and pneumonia while on the new diet and when using the safe swallow techniques taught by the SLP.

When people lose lifelong natural abilities, they lose a sense of self. They have to readjust their self-images and self-concepts, and that takes time. Few patients receive counseling from any professional (including speech-language pathologists) about the emotional struggles they are dealing with around their swallowing problems (Ekberg et al., 2002). Most patients likely struggle in silence, complaining and grumbling sometimes but never "talking through" their sense of loss of who they were as a person.

CHAPTER SUMMARY

Motor speech disorders result from neurologic impairments affecting the motor planning, programming, neuromuscular control, execution of speech, or all of these. They include the dysarthrias and apraxia of speech. Motor speech disorders frequently accompany aphasia, cognitive impairments, and dysphagia; however, motor speech disorders can occur alone. *Dysarthria* is a general term for a collection of speech disorders characterized by weakness in the muscles that control respiration, phonation, resonation, and articulation. Apraxia of speech is the result of impaired ability to plan, sequence, coordinate, and initiate motor movements of the articulators in the absence of muscular weakness. Patients with speech apraxia also may have nonverbal oral apraxia.

Dysphagia refers to difficulty swallowing that occurs when impairments affect any of the four phases of swallowing (oral preparatory, oral, pharyngeal, or esophageal) that puts an individual at risk for aspiration of food and liquid and potential aspiration pneumonia. Dysphagia requires a team approach with numerous medical specialists; typically, the speech-language pathologist is the head of the team. Dysphagia is a major area of our work in hospitals, and children with swallowing disorders may be on the caseloads of school speech therapists. The same neurological causes of motor speech disorders and cognitive disorders can cause dysphagia, plus dysphagia may be caused by oral and laryngeal cancer.

Evaluation of patients with dysphagia includes a careful review of the medical chart, interview of the patient, a cursory assessment of the patient's speech, language, and cognitive functioning, an evaluation of the speech systems (respiratory, phonatory, resonatory, and articulatory), a bedside (clinical) evaluation of a patient's ability to tolerate various food textures and liquid consistencies, and possibly an instrumental evaluation such as modified barium swallow study (MBSS).

During treatment for dysphagia, the clinician works with the feeding environment, postural techniques, modifications of foods and liquids, oral motor exercises, and swallow maneuvers. Some patients are not able to tolerate any oral presentation of food and must be placed on NPO (nothing by mouth). These patients receive their nutrition and hydration through enteral (tube) feeding, either through the nose (nasogastric tube [NG-tube]) or through the stomach (gastric tube [G-tube]).

The quality of life of the patient is always the most important question in all aspects of patient care. Patients with swallowing problems have anxiety and fear about the possibility of choking or developing pneumonia. People with swallowing problems may become depressed, and they likely will go through the stages of grief.

STUDY QUESTIONS

Knowledge and Comprehension

1. Define dysarthria.
2. What are five characteristics of apraxia of speech?
3. Define dysphagia.
4. What is a modified barium swallow study (MBSS)?
5. Based on the National Dysphagia Diet, what are the four textures of food and four consistencies of liquids?

Application

1. Why is it important to evaluate each of the speech systems (respiratory, phonatory, resonatory, and articulatory) when differentially diagnosing dysarthria?
2. Why is it important to assess nonspeech movements of the articulators in patients who may have apraxia of speech?
3. Why would oral–pharyngeal (oropharyngeal) dysphagia be the most common diagnosis for a swallowing disorder?
4. Why is it essential to determine whether a patient has a protective cough during the evaluation?
5. Why is silent aspiration particularly dangerous for patients?

Analysis/Synthesis

1. Why might the severity of the dysarthria help determine the therapeutic approach?
2. Why is it important to consider the possibility of a limb apraxia in a patient who has apraxia of speech?
3. Why is it essential to have a thorough understanding of the process of normal swallowing in order to help patients with swallowing disorders?
4. What is evidence-based practice and why is it important to our profession?
5. What are the stages of grief and how do they relate to patients with dysphagia?

REFERENCES

Aiken, T. D. (2008). *Legal and ethical issues in health occupations* (2nd ed.). Philadelphia, PA: Saunders.

American Speech-Language-Hearing Association. (2000a). Clinical indicators for instrumental assessment of dysphagia. *ASHA Desk Reference, 3*, 225–233.

American Speech-Language-Hearing Association. (2000b). Skills needed by speech-language pathologists providing services to dysphagic patients/clients. *ASHA, 32*(Supplement 2), 7–12.

American Speech-Language-Hearing Association. (2002). Knowledge and skills for speech-language pathologists performing endoscopic assessment of swallowing functions. *ASHA* (Supplement 22), 107–112.

American Speech-Language-Hearing Association. (2004a). Preferred practice patterns for the profession of speech-language pathology. Available at ASHA website: preferred practice patterns for the profession of speech-language pathology.

American Speech-Language-Hearing Association. (2004b). Guidelines for speech-language pathologists performing videofluoroscopy swallowing studies. *ASHA* (Supplement 24), 77–92.

American Speech-Language-Hearing Association. (2005). Clinical guidelines for speech-language pathology services. *ASHA Leader,* May (6–7), 22–23.

Armstrong, E. (2003). Communication culture in acute speech pathology settings: Current issues. *Advances in Speech-Language Pathology, 5*(2), 137–143.

Beauchamp, T. L., & Childress, J. F. (2008). *Principles of bioethics* (6th ed.). Oxford, UK: Oxford University Press.

Becker, S., McLeroy, K., & Carpenter, M. A. (2005). Reliability of observations from modified barium swallow studies. *Journal of Medical Speech-Language Pathology,* June, 28–37.

Carl, L. L., & Johnson, P. R. (2006). *Drugs and dysphagia: How medications can affect eating and swallowing.* Austin, TX: Pro-Ed.

Chang, C., Lee, K., & Kuo, W. (2004). Dysphonia as the initial symptom of myasthenia gravis, *Journal of Otolaryngology, 33*, 57–59.

Chen, A., Frankowski, R., Bishop-Leone, J., Hebert, T., Leyk, S., Lewin, J., & Goepfert, H. (2001). The development and validation of a dysphagia-specific quality-of-life questionnaire for patients with head and neck cancer. *Archives of Otolaryngology Head and Neck Surgery, 127*, 870–876.

Cherney, L. R. (Ed.). (2004). *Clinical management of dysphagia in adults and children.* Gaithersburg, MD: Aspen.

Clark, H. M. (2003). Neuromuscular treatments for speech and swallowing. *American Journal of Speech-Language Pathology, 12*, 400–415.

Code, C., & Heron, C. (2003). Services for aphasia, other acquired adult neurogenic communication and swallowing disorders in the United Kingdom, 2000. *Disability and Rehabilitation, 25*(21), 1231–1237.

Corbin-Lewis, K. M., Liss, J. M., & Sciortino, K. L. (2005). *Clinical anatomy and physiology of the swallowing mechanism.* Clifton Park, NY: Delmar Cengage Learning.

Covertino, V., Bloomfield, S., & Greenleaf, J. (1997). An overview of the issues: Physiological effect of bed rest and restricted physical activity. *Medical Science and Sports Exercise, 29,* 187–194.

Crary, M. A., & Groher, M. E. (2003). *Introduction to adult swallowing disorders.* St. Louis, MO: Butterworth-Heinemann.

Dahl, W. J. (2008). *Modified texture food production: A manual for patient care facilities* (2nd ed.). Toronto, Ontario: Dietitians of Canada.

Darley, F. L., Aronson, A. E., & Brown, J. R. (1975). *Motor speech disorders.* Philadelphia, PA: W. B. Saunders.

Davies, S., Taylor, H., MacDonald, A., & Barer, D. (2001). An interdisciplinary approach to swallowing problems in acute stroke. *International Journal of Language & Communication Disorders, 36,* 357–368.

DeMatteo, C., Matovich, D., & Hjartarson, A. (2005). Comparison of clinical and videofluoroscopic evaluation of children with feeding and swallowing difficulties. *Developmental Medicine and Child Neurology, 47,* 149–157.

Duffy, J. R. (2005). *Motor speech disorders: Substrates, differential diagnosis, and management* (2nd ed.). St. Louis, MO: Elsevier Mosby.

Duffy, J. R. (2006). Apraxia of speech in degenerative neurological disease. *Aphasiology, 20*(6), 511–527.

Ekberg, O., Hamdy, S., Woisard, V., Wuttge-Hannig, A., & Ortega, P. (2002). Social and psychological burden of dysphagia: Its impact on diagnosis and treatment. *Dysphagia, 17*(2), 139–146.

El Dib, R. P., & Atallah, A. N. (2006). Evidence-based speech, language, and hearing therapy and the Cochrane Library's systematic reviews. *Sao Paulo [Brazil] Medical Journal, 124*(2), 51–54.

Evidence Reports/Technology Assessments. (1999). *Diagnosis and treatment of swallowing disorders (dysphagia) in acute-care stroke patients.* Rockville, MD: ECRI Health Technology Assessment Group.

Finley, R., Clifton, J., Stewart, K., Graham, A., & Worsley, D. (2001). Prediction of aspiration in patients with newly diagnosed untreated advanced head and neck cancer. *Archives of Otolaryngology Head and Neck Surgery, 127,* 975–979.

Flasher, L. V., & Fogle, P. T. (2012). *Counseling skills for speech-language pathologists and audiologists* (2nd ed.). Clifton Park, NY: Delmar Cengage Learning.

Fogle, P. T. (1998). Preparing a feast for the senses. *Advance for Speech-Language Pathologists and Audiologists, 8,* 14–16.

Fogle, P. T., Reece, L., & White, J. (2008). *The source for safety: Cognitive retraining for independent living.* East Moline, IL: LinguiSystems.

Frymark, T., Schooling, T., Mullen, R., Wheeler-Hegland, K., Ashford, J., McCabe, D., Musson, N., & Hammond, C. (2009). Evidence-based systematic review: Oropharyngeal dysphagia behavioral treatments: Part I – Background and methodology. *Journal of Rehabilitation Research & Development, 46*(2), 175–184.

Golper, L. A. (2010). *Medical speech-language pathology: A desk reference* (3rd ed.). Clifton Park, NY: Delmar Cengage Learning.

Hillel, A., Miller, R., Yorkston, K., McDonald, E., Norris, R., & Konikow, N. (1989). Amyotrophic lateral sclerosis severity scale. *Neuroepidemiology, 8,* 142–150.

Hind, J., Nicosia, M., Roecker, E., Carnes, M., & Robbins, J. (2001). Comparison of effortful and non-effortful swallows in healthy middle aged and older adults. *Archives of Physical Medicine and Rehabilitation, 82,* 1661–1665.

Homer, E. M. (2003). An interdisciplinary team approach to providing dysphagia treatment in the schools. *Seminars in Speech and Language, 24,* 215–234.

Huckabee, M. L., & Pelletier, C. A. (2003). *Management of adult neurogenic dysphagia.* Clifton Park, NY: Thomson Delmar Learning.

Johns Hopkins. (2000). Help when it's hard to swallow. *Johns Hopkins Medical Letter, Health After 50, 11*(12), 6–7.

Johnson, A. F., & Jacobson, B. H. (2007). *Medical speech-language pathology: A practitioner's guide* (2nd ed.). New York, NY: Thieme.

Kendall, K. (2008). Anatomy and physiology of deglutition. In R. Leonard & K. Kendall (Eds.). *Dysphagia assessment and treatment: A team approach.* San Diego, CA: Plural Publishing.

Kurjan, R. M. (2000). The role of the school-based speech-language pathologist serving preschool children with dysphagia. *Language, Speech, and Hearing Services in Schools, 31,* 42–49.

Langmore, S. E. (2003). Evaluation of oropharyngeal dysphagia: Which diagnostic tool is superior? *Current Opinions in Otolaryngology Head and Neck Surgery, 11,* 485–489.

Leonard, R., & Kendall, K. (2008). *Dysphagia assessment and treatment: A team approach.* San Diego, CA: Plural Publishing.

Logemann, J. A. (1998). *Evaluation and treatment of swallowing disorders* (2nd ed.). Austin, TX: Pro-Ed.

Logemann, J. A. (2004). Evidence-based practice. *Advances in Speech-Language Pathology, 6*(2), 134–135.

Lubinski, R., Golper, L. A., & Frattali, C. (2007). *Professional issues in speech-language pathology and audiology* (3rd ed.). Clifton Park, NY: Delmar Cengage Learning.

Matta, Z., Chambers, E., Garcia, J., & McGowan-Helverson, J. (2006). Sensory characteristics of beverages prepared with commercial thickeners used for dysphagia diets. *Journal of the American Dietetic Association, 106*(7), 1049–1054.

McAuliffe, M. J. (2006). Current approaches to the assessment and treatment of acquired dysarthria. New Zealand Speech-Language Therapists' Association Biennial Conference, Christchurch, New Zealand.

McAuliffe, M. J., Ward, E. C., & Murdoch, B. E. (2007). Intra-participant variability in Parkinson's disease: An electropalatographic examination of articulation. *Advances in Speech-Language Pathology, 9*(1), 13–19.

McCulloch, T. M., & Jaffe, D. (2006). Head and neck disorders affecting swallowing. *GI Motility,* May, 1–12.

Miller, R. M., & Groher, M. E. (2005). Speech-language pathology and dysphagia: A brief historical perspective. *Dysphagia, 8*(3), 180–184.

Morgan, A. T., Mageandran, S. D., & Mei, C. (2010). Incidence and clinical presentation of dysarthria and dysphagia in the acute setting following pediatric traumatic brain injury. *Child: Care, Health and Development (Special Edition on Traumatic Brain Injury), 36*(1), 44–53.

Morgan, A. T., & Skeat, J. (2010). Evaluating service delivery for speech and swallowing problems following pediatric brain injury: An international survey. *Journal of Evaluation in Clinical Practice, 17*(2), 275–281.

Murry, T., & Carrau, R. L. (2006). *Clinical management of swallowing disorders* (2nd ed.). San Diego, CA: Plural Publishing.

National Dysphagia Diet Task Force. (2002). *National dysphagia diet: Standardization for optimal care.* Washington, DC: American Dietetic Association.

Provencio-Arambula, M., Provencio, D., & Hegde, M. N. (2006). *Treatment of dysphagia in adults: Resources and protocols—a bilingual manual.* San Diego, CA: Plural Publishing.

Ramsey, D. J., Smithard, D. G., & Kalra, L. (2003). Early assessment of dysphagia and aspiration risk in acute stroke patients. *Stroke, 34,* 1252–1257.

Ratner, N. B. (2006). Evidence-based practice: An examination of its ramifications for the practice of speech-language pathology. *Language, Speech, and Hearing Services in Schools, 37,* 257–267.

Rempel, G., & Moussavi, Z. (2005). The effect of viscosity on the breath–swallow pattern of young children with cerebral palsy. *Dysphagia, 20*(2), 108–112.

Rodriquez, L., & Borelli, M. (2003). *Dysphagia screening: A training resource pack.* New York, NY: John Wiley & Sons.

Shoemaker, A. (1997). Religious and cultural issues in dysphagia treatment. *Advance for Speech-Language Pathologists & Audiologists, 10,* 19.

Skelly, M. (1979). *American gestural code based on universal American Indian hand talk.* New York, NY: Elsevier.

Swigert, N. B. (2007). *The source for dysphagia* (3rd ed.). East Moline, IL: LinguiSystems.

Swigert, N. B. (2010). *The source for dysarthria* (2nd ed.). East Moline, IL: LinguiSystems.

Teasell, R., Foley, N., Fisher, J., & Finestone, H. (2002). The incidence management and complications with medullary strokes to a rehabilitation unit. *Dysphagia, 17,* 115–120.

Tonkovich, J. D. (2002). Multicultural issues in the management of neurogenic communication and swallowing disorders. In D. E. Battle (Ed.). *Communication disorders in multicultural populations* (3rd ed.). Boston, MA: Butterworth-Heinemann.

Watt, F., & Whyte, M. N. (2003). The experience of dysphagia and its effect on the quality of life of patients with esophageal cancer. *European Journal of Cancer Care, 12*(2), 183–193.

Weismer, G. (2006). *Motor speech disorders.* San Diego: Plural Publishing.

Wertz, R. T., LaPointe, L. L., & Rosenbek, J. C. (1991). *Apraxia of speech in adults: The disorder and its management.* Clifton Park, NY: Delmar Cengage Learning.

Yorkston, K. M., Beukelman, D. R., Strand, E. A., & Hakel, M. (2010). *Management of motor speech disorders in children and adults* (3rd ed.). Austin, TX: Pro-Ed.

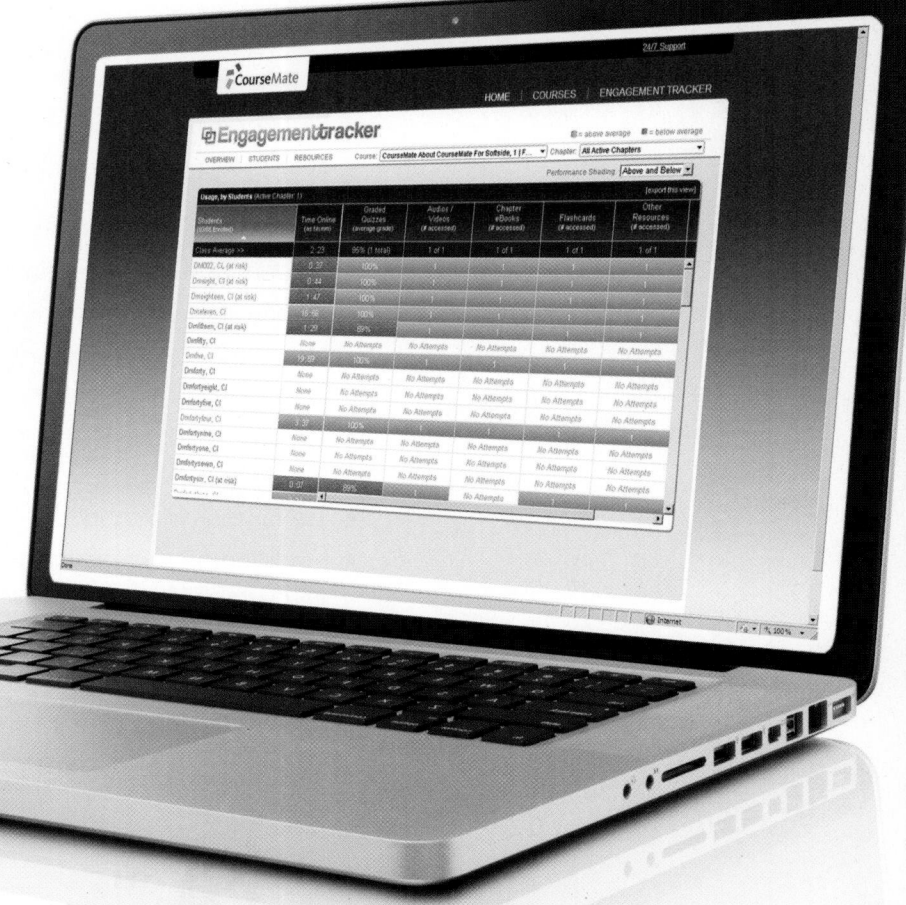
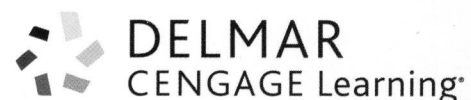

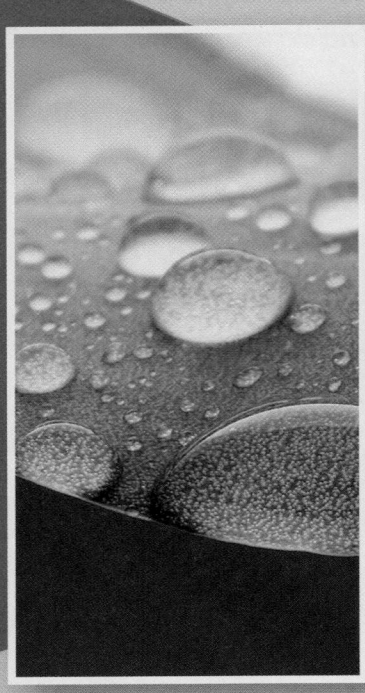

CHAPTER 13
Special Populations with Communication Disorders

LEARNING OBJECTIVES

After studying this chapter, you will:

- Understand the essentials of intellectual disabilities.
- Be familiar with Down syndrome.
- Know the common characteristics of autism and pervasive developmental disorders.
- Be able to discuss attention deficit/hyperactivity disorders (AD/HD, ADD).
- Be familiar with auditory processing disorders (APD).
- Understand the essential information about traumatic brain injury in children.
- Be able to discuss cerebral palsy and its various types.
- Be familiar with augmentative and alternative communication (AAC).

KEY TERMS

adaptive behavior
attention deficit/hyperactivity disorder (AD/HD, ADD)
auditory processing disorder (APD)/central auditory processing disorder (CAPD)
augmentative and alternative communication (AAC) or assistive technology (AT)
autism
autism spectrum disorder (ASD)

bruxing
cerebral palsy (CP)
communication (conversation) board
contracture
developmental disability (DD)
Down syndrome
echolalia
generalization
hypertonicity (hypertonic)

INTRODUCTION

Speech-language pathologists and audiologists may find certain clinical populations particularly interesting and challenging to work with and choose to specialize in assessment and treatment of these populations. To develop expertise in these areas, clinicians need considerable continuing education and training that is offered through ASHA, state, and other organizations. This education and training may include cross-training with other professionals, such as physical and occupational therapists.

Increasingly, SLPs and Auds are working with children who have complex medical problems (sometimes referred to as *medically fragile children*). Clinicians who work in public schools now need knowledge of numerous syndromes and other developmental and medical complications that can contribute to or cause a variety of communication disorders. This chapter provides essential information on special populations of children and adults who have communication and cognitive disorders associated with other disabilities. For some of these individuals, verbal communication is not realistic and augmentative and alternative communication methods are needed.

INTELLECTUAL DISABILITIES

An **intellectual disability (ID)** is a disability characterized by significant limitations in *intellectual functioning* (learning, reasoning, problem solving) and **adaptive behavior** that are apparent before the age of 18. An intellectual disability is under the umbrella term, **developmental disability (DD)** (American Association on Intellectual and Developmental Disabilities, 2010). The term "mental retardation" is generally avoided nowadays when referring to individuals with developmental or intellectual disabilities. For example, what was formerly titled the American Association on Mental Retardation (AAMR) is now the American Association on Intellectual and Developmental Disabilities (AAIDD).

An individual's intellectual functioning is measured by tests of **intelligence** to obtain an **intelligence quotient (IQ)**. Intellectual disability is diagnosed when IQs are below 70 (with 100 being considered the mathematical average). *Mild* intellectual disability is considered as 50 to 70 (≈90% of DD); *moderate* disability falls in the range of 35 to 49 (≈6% of DD); *severe* disability from 20 to 34 (≈3% of DD); and *profound* disability below 20 (≈1% of DD). Children with developmental disabilities are sometimes referred to as *special needs* or *exceptional* children

---

intellectual disability (ID)

A disability characterized by significant limitations in intellectual functioning (learning, reasoning, problem solving) and adaptive behavior that are apparent before the age of 18.

adaptive behavior

The ability to act as independently and responsibly as other people of the same age and cultural background in everyday social and practical skills; includes conceptual skills (e.g., language and money concepts), social skills (e.g., following rules and pragmatics), and practical skills (e.g., dressing appropriately and work skills).

developmental disability (DD)

An umbrella term that relates to some childhood disabilities and includes intellectual disability, physical disabilities (e.g., cerebral palsy or epilepsy), and disabilities that may be both intellectual and physical (e.g., Down syndrome).

(e.g., Special Olympics). According to the World Health Organization (2001), the prevalence of intellectual disability is believed to be between 1%–3% worldwide, with higher rates in developing countries because of the higher incidence of injuries and anoxia around birth and early childhood neurological damage, in part because of poor nutrition. Intellectual disabilities occur about twice as often in males than in females. Numerous syndromes have developmental disabilities as a prominent characteristic, including Down syndrome.

A syndrome is a complex of signs and symptoms resulting from a common etiology. A few examples of syndromes that may significantly affect communication and cognitive development include (1) *Down syndrome* (discussed later); (2) *fetal alcohol syndrome* (FAS) (characterized by prenatal and postnatal growth retardation, facial abnormalities, heart defects, joint and limb abnormalities, and intellectual impairment); and (3) *Asperger's syndrome* (a pervasive developmental disorder with similarities to autistic disorder, characterized by severe impairment of social interactions and by restricted interests and behaviors, although speech, language, and cognitive development may be near normal). Many syndromes, including those mentioned here, also include mild to severe speech, language, and cognitive delays or disorders.

American Association on Intellectual and Developmental Disabilities

The American Association on Intellectual and Developmental Disabilities (AAIDD (formerly known as the American Association on Mental Retardation [AAMR]), was founded in 1876 and is an international multidisciplinary association of professionals. Since 1921, the association has had the responsibility of defining intellectual disability and providing information and support to individuals with developmental disabilities and their families, as well as professionals.

Language Delays and Disorders

Children with intellectual disabilities typically have both receptive and expressive language delays and disorders. They generally understand single words better than sentences because the syntax may be confusing for them. They understand concrete information better than abstract information. They understand speech better when the rate is slightly slower than normal and pauses between sentences are slightly longer than normal. In general, the "rule of fives" is helpful when communicating in sentences with individuals with intellectual delays; that is, use five-letter words (i.e., one- or two-syllable words) in five-word sentences (i.e., simple declarative or interrogative sentences).

Expressive language is usually one of the most impaired areas for children with intellectual disabilities. Individuals with intellectual disabilities commonly have limited vocabularies and some difficulty

intelligence

A global construct involved in the collective capacity to act purposely, think rationally, and deal effectively with the environment.

intelligence quotient (IQ)

An estimate of intellectual status based on an index determined by dividing the *mental age* (MA) in months by the *chronological age* (CA) in months and reducing the result to a percentage; 100 is considered the mathematical average.

recalling words they have used frequently. Their vocabularies tend to be filled with concrete words (things they can see, hear, or touch) and basic verbs to describe the most common actions of nouns. They have limited synonyms for words and difficulty describing characteristics of objects (e.g., size, color, shape, texture, composition), so they tend to repeat a specific word (until they are emphatic) because they cannot provide another word with the same meaning or describe what they are talking about. Depending on their level of intellectual disability, they may communicate in single words, simple sentences, or even complex sentences.

Pragmatics for most individuals with intellectual disabilities are a problem. They often do not initiate conversation, so they have fewer peer interactions than would be normal. When they do initiate conversation, they tend to use *imperative sentences* (sentences that give demands or make requests). They often have difficulty appreciating a listener's "personal space" and may move an uncomfortable distance toward the listener (Adams, Lloyd, Aldred, & Baxendale, 2006; Farmer & Oliver, 2005).

These individuals (both children and adults) may be aware when listeners do not understand them and may attempt conversational repairs by repeating what they have said. However, because of their limited vocabulary, they seldom can go beyond repetition. **Generalization** of language skills taught in therapy is often limited. Children with intellectual disabilities may be able to demonstrate their improved use of language in the clinical setting but may not be able (perhaps not remember) to use these skills in other settings.

Speech

Speech intelligibility problems are common among children and adults with intellectual disabilities because of articulation and phonological disorders. There also may be a motor component such as apraxia or dysarthria. In general, the severity of speech intelligibility depends on the degree of intellectual disability; that is, the more severe the intellectual disability, the more severe the articulation problems. Many children with intellectual disabilities also have hearing losses, which contribute significantly to their speech impairments (Martin & Clark, 2009).

Down Syndrome

Down syndrome is the most common chromosomal cause of developmental (both intellectual and physical) disabilities, with an estimated 1 in every 800 to 1,000 infants born with this condition. A woman's chances of giving birth to a child with Down syndrome increases with age. For a woman 25 years old, the chance is 1 in 1,250; for a 35-year-old woman, it is 1 in 400; and for a 40-year-old woman, it is 1 in 100. Intellectual disability levels are typically in the mild to moderate range. Their speech and language delays may range from mild to severe, with many at the moderate level.

Application Question

If you have had interactions with individuals who have intellectual disabilities, what pragmatic problems have you noticed during the interactions?

generalization

The transfer of learning from one environment (e.g., therapy room or classroom) to a natural environment (e.g., home or community).

Down syndrome

A common chromosome disorder due to an extra chromosome number 21 (trisomy 21) that results in intellectual disability, small head, small ears, flat face with upward slant of the eyes, and abnormal physical development.

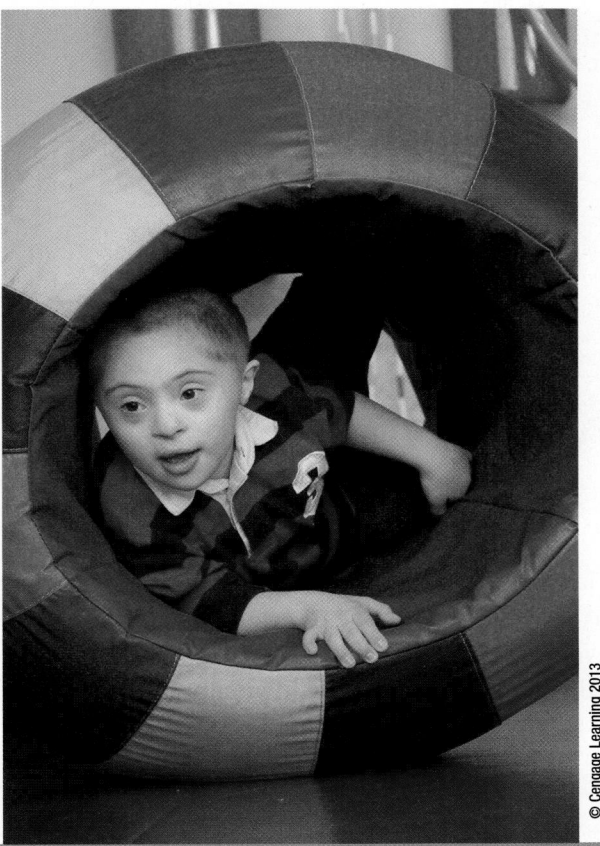

© Cengage Learning 2013

Figure 13-1
Facial features of someone with Down syndrome.

Hearing loss is common, both conductive and sensorineural. Down syndrome has distinctive physical characteristics, including a small head, small ears, flat face, and upward slanting eyes. Many children with Down syndrome are happy, affectionate, and easygoing (see Figure 13–1). Many go to school, learn to read and write, find jobs, and live relatively independent or semi-independent lives (Mayo Clinic, 2009).

Speech and Language

Children with Down syndrome have inconsistent and distorted speech that may be attributed to *hypotonicity* (weakness) and delayed motor development. They usually develop most sounds of other children but at a slower rate. Children with Down syndrome often have *macroglossia* (an abnormally large tongue) that can interfere with articulation because the tongue fills the oral cavity, not allowing normal range of movement and precise articulation points.

Children and adults with Down syndrome have language comprehension roughly equivalent to their mental age. Their vocabulary comprehension is usually better developed than their comprehension of syntax. In general, their comprehension abilities exceed their expressive language and speech abilities. These children often show relatively good language development during infancy and toddlerhood, particularly when involved in early-intervention programs. However, after this age,

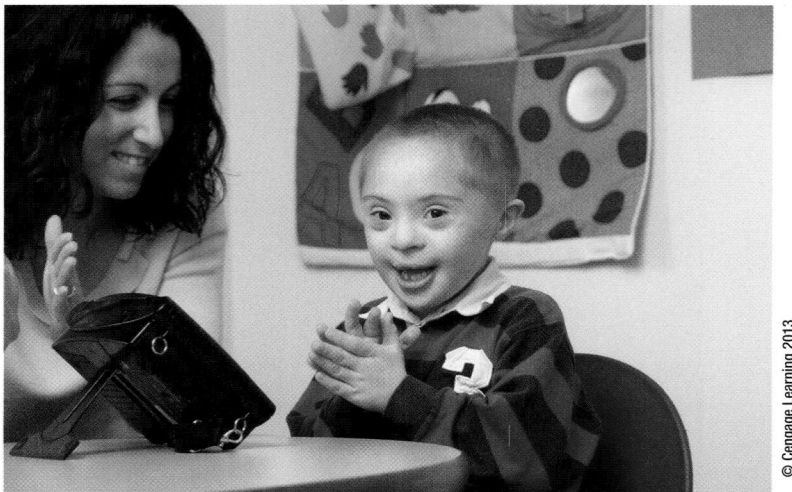

© Cengage Learning 2013

Figure 13-2
Children with Down syndrome are often a joy to work with.

autism (autistic disorder)

A highly variable neurodevelopmental disorder in the broad *autism spectrum disorders (ASD)*, which is in the still broader group of *pervasive developmental disorders*. Autism is a lifelong complex behavioral syndrome that appears by 3 years of age, with children having a markedly absent interest in social interactions and relationships; severely impaired communication skills; and repetitive, stereotyped movements; and restricted interests that are often obsessive or fixated.

autism spectrum disorder (ASD)

A range of developmental disorders from mild to severe, with autism being the most severe form.

pervasive developmental disorder (PDD)

Serious multiple developmental impairments typically diagnosed in children before the age of 3 and occurs in males approximately four times as often as in females; autism spectrum disorders are the more severe extreme.

their rate of language learning continues at a slower pace into the early school years (see Figure 13-2). Many children appear to plateau in their language development around 8 years of age or as late as adolescence, with further development primarily in vocabulary.

AUTISM AND PERVASIVE DEVELOPMENTAL DISORDERS

Autism (autistic disorder) falls within the broader diagnostic category of **autism spectrum disorder (ASD)**, which in turn is within the still broader diagnostic category of **pervasive developmental disorder (PDD)** (see Figure 13-3). Autism was first described in the literature in 1943 (Kanner, 1943). Until the 1970s, Kanner and other mental health experts believed that autism was an emotional or psychiatric disorder generally attributed to environmental influences in the child's home, with the parents—unfairly—being held responsible for their child's disorder. Since the 1970s, autism has been viewed as a developmental disorder rather than an emotional disorder (American Psychiatric Association, 2000). It is now considered a developmental disability that has a genetic or unknown origin and is present from birth. The prevalence of autism is about 1–2 per 1,000 people worldwide; however, the Center for Disease Control and Prevention (CDC) reports approximately 9 per 1,000 children (≈1 in 110) in the United States are diagnosed within the autism spectrum disorder. The number of children diagnosed with autism has increased dramatically since the 1980s, partly due to changes in diagnostic practice; however, it is not certain whether the actual prevalence has significantly increased (Newschaffer, Croen, Daniels, et al., 2007; Tonge, 2002).

Autism is described as a complex behavioral syndrome that appears by 3 years of age with children having (1) a markedly absent interest in social interactions and relationships; (2) severely impaired communication skills; and (3) repetitive, **stereotyped movements**, combined with

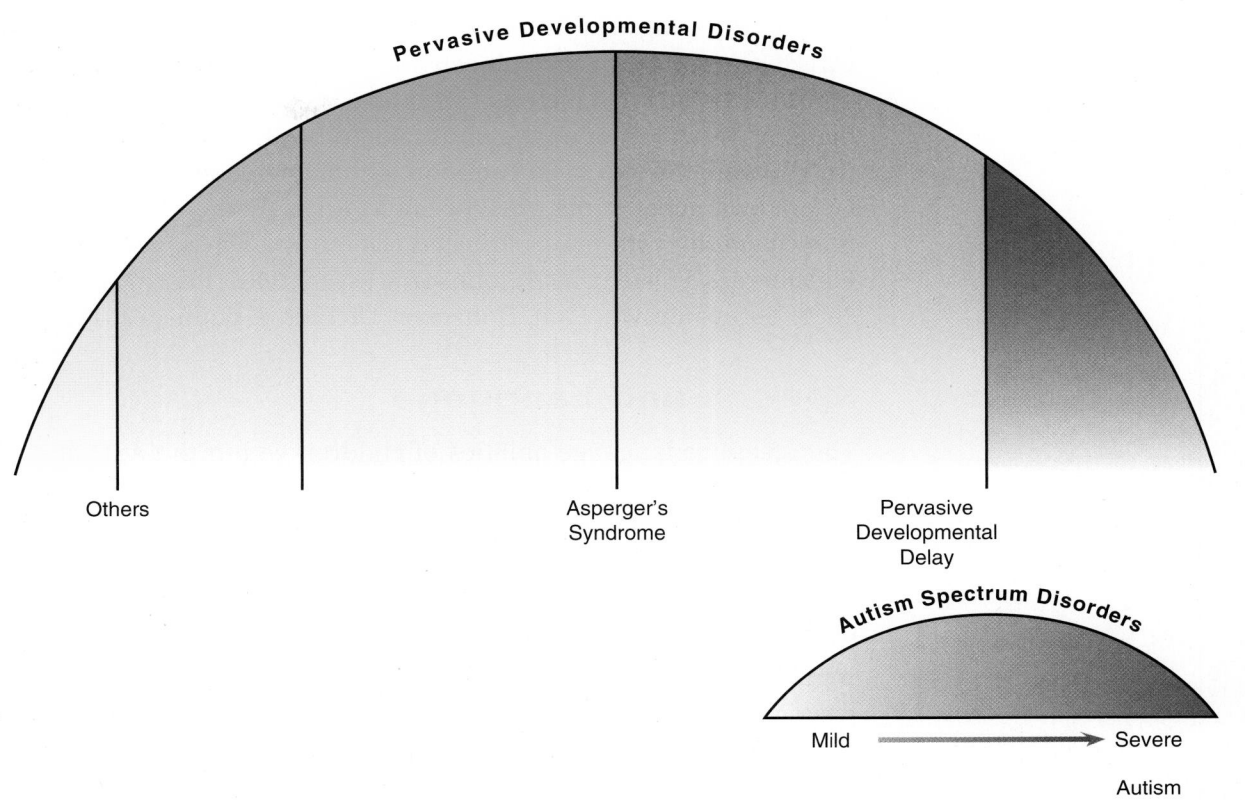

Figure 13-3

Pervasive developmental disorders.
© Cengage Learning 2013.

restricted interests that are often obsessive or fixated. Some individuals demonstrate extraordinary skills, such as memory for numbers or being able to mentally calculate dates (**savant syndrome**) (Heaton & Wallace, 2004). Early symptoms often appear by 18 months of age, such as lethargy, preferring solitude, or being highly irritable (Kupperman, 2006).

Numerous problems associated with autism have been reported, including intellectual deficiencies in approximately three-quarters of all children, with most cases at the moderate level (IQ 35–49). Most individuals have poor physical coordination and seizures occur in approximately one-third of individuals (seizures can deteriorate motor coordination). Individuals who are autistic often have *hyposensitivity* or *hypersensitivity* to certain stimuli; for example, they may be oblivious to heat, cold, or pain but show extreme distress when they are touched unexpectedly. Some show *hyperacusis* (abnormal intolerance for normal environmental sounds), for example, having a catastrophic reaction to a person's whispering but not reacting to very loud noises. They tend to prefer sounds they produce themselves, such as unusual vocalizations or teeth grinding (**bruxing**).

Many individuals have self-stimulating behaviors, for example twisting or twirling objects in front of their face (particularly shiny objects), spinning, rocking, hand flapping, toe walking, sniffing objects,

stereotyped movements

Persistent and inappropriate mechanical repetition of actions, body postures, or speech patterns, often seen in autism.

savant syndrome

The co-occurrence with autism of unexpected or unusual high-level skills with generally limited intelligence (e.g., mathematical calculations, days and dates in history or the future, or remarkable memory for unrelated information).

bruxing

A compulsive, unconscious clenching and grinding of the teeth, especially during sleep or as a mechanism for releasing tension during periods of extreme stress in waking hours.

repetitive feeling of the texture of materials, and attachment to and carrying around unusual objects. Some children have frequent self-injurious behaviors, such as self-biting, scratching, hitting, and head banging. However, of all the unusual and bizarre behaviors of children with autism, the two most common identifying behaviors are a marked lack of awareness of the existence of feelings of others and a persistent preoccupation with parts of objects (Dominick, Davis, Lainhart, Tager-Flushberg, & Folstein, 2007; Johnson & Myers, 2007; Reece & Challenner, 2006; Turner-Brown, Lam, Holtzclaw, Dichter, & Bodfish, 2011).

Speech and Language

The receptive language abilities of children within the ASD and PDD categories are generally similar to their mental age; for example, a 5-year-old child may have a mental age of 2 years. However, the comprehension abilities of any one child in the spectrum at any specific moment are particularly difficult to determine because of inconsistent or absent responses to both test and normal stimuli. That is, a child may understand what was said but not respond accurately or appropriately.

Approximately 50% of children with autism are considered non-verbal, with *selective* or *elective* **mutism** occurring in some cases; however, children who are nonverbal do not necessarily try to compensate with gestures or mime. Children with autism who are verbal are well known for their abnormal verbal behavior (Reed, 2010; Richard, 2008; Tager-Flusberg & Caronna, 2007). Children with PDDs tend to be more verbal than children within the autism spectrum, depending on their severity levels. One of the most striking verbal traits of children who are autistic is **echolalia**—the automatic repeating of words, phrases, or sentences said to them or to someone else. Although these children may repeat what is said, they often do it without normal accompanying facial expressions and gestures.

Although children with autism do not appear to have significant difficulty understanding pronouns, they have particular difficulty using pronouns correctly. They often make errors in gender (*he* for *she, him* for *her*) and singular and plural (*it* for *they* and *them*). They often use *you* to refer to themselves and *I* or *me* to refer to others.

The expressive language of some children with autism may be grammatically adequate but have unusual or bizarre semantics and pragmatics. They often use **idiosyncratic language**; that is, their choice of words and use of words in sentences have unique meanings, which may or may not be interpretable to a listener (e.g., "They're having a meal and then they're finishing and *siding the table,*"—interpreted as "clearing the table," and "He's seriously wounded like *cutes and bloosters,*"—interpreted as "cuts and bruises"). Sometimes they use *neologisms* (e.g., "She's *bawcet,*"—interpreted as "She's bossy") (Volden & Lord, 1991, p. 118).

Impaired pragmatics, social deficits, and inappropriate behaviors are hallmark characteristics of children with autism. The following behavioral characteristics are adapted from the American Psychiatric

mutism

The inability or unwillingness to speak; usually used in reference to voice disorders where an individual may use selective or elective mutism, that is, unconsciously or consciously not be able to use voice or speak.

echolalia

The automatic and involuntary repetition of another person's utterance that is normal for 18–24-month-old children, but which also can occur at later ages (including adulthood) in individuals who are autistic or have neurological damage.

idiosyncratic language

An individual's choice of words and use of words in sentences that have their own unique meaning, which may or may not be interpretable to a listener.

Association's *Diagnostic and Statistical Manual of Mental Disorders, 4th edition, Text Revision* (DSM-IV TR) (2000): nonverbal and verbal behaviors that include inadequate or inappropriate eye gaze, facial expressions, and general body language; general lack of initiating verbal interaction; frequent inappropriate whispering; unusual fluctuations of loudness; limited pitch range resulting in monotonous speech; excessive nasal resonance; voice inflections not in agreement with their meaning; repetition of television commercials verbatim; difficulty pointing to or showing objects to their parents; difficulty or inability to "read" the mood, needs, or intentions of others; and mechanical imitation of other people's actions or voices.

The speech of children in the autism spectrum or who have PDDs is generally intelligible but sounds much like the mental age of the child. There are frequent distortions of consonants in their speech throughout their lives. Overall, it is not their speech intelligibility that makes them difficult to understand but their idiosyncratic language and inappropriate speech inflections and pragmatics that leave listeners confused and bewildered.

ATTENTION DEFICIT DISORDERS

Attention deficit/hyperactivity disorder (AD/HD) was first described in 1845 by Heinrich Hoffman, a German physician who wrote texts in medicine and psychiatry. Hoffman also wrote children's books, with one titled *The Story of Fidgety Philip* that was translated into English and which accurately described a boy with characteristics of AD/HD. However, it was not until Sir George F. Still published a series of lectures that he presented to the Royal College of Physicians in England in 1902 that described a group of impulsive children with significant behavioral problems that AD/HD began to be accepted as a true disorder (Still, 1902). Attention deficit disorders are not new problems.

The DSM-IV TR (2000) is the standard and authoritative source for U.S. practitioners, researchers, and others in the field of mental disorders. The DSM-IV TR provides definitions, criteria, descriptions, and prevalence information for *attention deficit/hyperactivity disorder*. "ADD," as it is often written, is a broad syndrome relating to individuals who demonstrate three primary problems: inattention, impulsivity, and hyperactivity. *Inattention* refers to difficulty either in selecting what to attend to or in keeping attention focused as long as necessary to perform an age-appropriate task. *Impulsivity* means that the individual has difficulty properly controlling or regulating behavior. *Hyperactivity* relates to excesses in physical movement, especially excesses that have a purposeless, poorly directed, or driven quality. Approximately 3%–5% of school-age children in the United States have ADD, and boys are approximately four times more likely to have the problem than girls. Risk factors for ADD include being male, a possible hereditary component, and pregnancy and birth complications. ADD occurs in a heterogeneous population

attention deficit/ hyperactivity disorder (AD/HD, ADD)

A broad syndrome relating to children who demonstrate three primary problems: inattention, impulsivity, and hyperactivity.

of children and adults and from all family economic and educational backgrounds.

The DSM-IV TR states that the following four conditions must be met for a child to be diagnosed with attention deficit/hyperactivity disorder:

- Presence of a minimum number of symptoms (six or more) of inattention, hyperactivity–impulsivity, or both (see the complete symptom list in the DSM-IV TR, 2000)
- Presence of symptoms for 6 months or longer
- Presence of symptoms before 7 years of age
- Impaired functioning in two or more settings caused by ADD symptoms (usually home and school)

Barkley (2006), a professor of psychiatry and neurology, says attention is a global construct that is difficult to define; however, the construct includes:

- Arousal (becoming alert)
- Selective attention (choosing what to attend to)
- Sustained attention (staying focused)
- Short-term (working) memory (seconds to minutes)
- How much information can be attended to or processed at one time

Barkley says that children with ADD are distractible because they become bored with a task much sooner than normal children. Once they become bored, which may take only seconds, they shift their attention to something else.

Frequent Coexisting Disorders with Attention Deficit Disorders

Language disorders and ADD often coexist. The DSM-IV TR criteria for diagnosis of ADD include several behaviors that SLPs would assess as receptive language impairments and pragmatic problems. Children diagnosed by psychologists, psychiatrists, or pediatricians as having ADD would benefit from evaluations by SLPs to determine whether these children also have receptive and/or expressive language disorders and then to receive appropriate therapy (Schonwald & Lechner, 2006; Tetnowski, 2004).

ADD and **auditory processing disorders (APD)** coexist, making it difficult for these children when they are attending to clearly understand what is being said (Bellis, 2002, 2003; Stach, 2010). Learning disabilities also are a common problem for children with ADD and they are often referred to as "academic underachievers." ADD is estimated to co-occur in 20%–50% of children with learning disabilities, depending on how the disorders or disabilities are defined or assessed. Children's learning disabilities extend to reading and writing problems (Byrnes, 2008).

auditory processing disorder (APD)/central auditory processing disorder (CAPD)

A disorder in children and adults who have difficulty using auditory information to communicate and learn; may affect their abilities to listen, understand speech, develop language, and have academic success.

An ADD Support Group — *Personal Story*

My wife, a registered nurse (RN), and I ran a support group for three years for parents of children with ADD, APD, and learning disabilities. We met every other Wednesday evening in a high school classroom. (When I do seminars around the United States on ADD and APD, I tell the speech-language pathologists, audiologists, psychologists, teachers, and parents who attend that I speak from three perspectives: an academic who studies the problems, a therapist who works with children who have these problems, and a parent with a child [now adult] with these problems.) We had many parents who came to the support group almost in panic, saying, "My child was just diagnosed with ADD! What is ADD?" Other parents who had known about their children's problems for years would share (sometimes commiserate) stories about the trials of family life with a child (or two) who has ADD, APD, a learning disability, or a combination of these. We talked about strategies to help our children and ways for parents to cope with the sometimes unusual challenges they present. With enough of the right kinds of support (family, educational, psychological, and if needed, pharmacological), many of these children become productive and often unusually creative adults. ■

Some children with ADD have co-existing anxiety, depression, or both. If the anxiety and depression are treated, the child will be better able to manage the daily challenges that accompany ADD. Additionally, effective treatment of ADD can have a positive effect on anxiety and depression because these children are better able to succeed academically and in their family and social lives (Wilens, Biederman, & Spencer, 2002). Effective treatment often includes a multimodality approach: (1) behavioral intervention, (2) educational intervention, (3) psychological (counseling) intervention, and (4) medical (pharmacological) intervention. Children who have ADD grow up to be adults who have ADD, and the effects on their personal and occupational or professional lives can be incalculable (Wender, 2000).

AUDITORY PROCESSING DISORDERS

The term *auditory processing disorder (APD)* refers to children and adults who have difficulty using auditory information to communicate and learn (Jerger & Musiek, 2000). The auditory processing problems occur during different listening tasks and are made worse in noisy environments. APDs are associated with difficulty listening, understanding speech, developing language, and learning. APDs have been recognized by audiologists and speech-language pathologists for more than 50 years; however, it has only been since the 1990s that APDs have taken a prominent role in the work of many speech-language pathologists (ASHA, 1995; Bellis, 2003; Musiek & Chermak, 2007; Richard, 2004).

Factors Commonly Associated with Auditory Processing Disorders

Several factors are commonly associated with people who are diagnosed with an auditory processing disorder (Bellis, 2003; Geffner & Ross-Swain, 2007; Kelly, 2001; Musiek & Chermak, 2007; Richard, 2001):

- APD occurs in a heterogeneous population of children and adults and from all family economic and educational backgrounds.
- There is a complex of symptoms with no two children having precisely the same problems to the same degree.
- Most children have normal hearing, but there is typically a history of middle ear infections and *upper respiratory infections* (colds, flu, and sinus allergies).
- Children and adults with APD typically have difficulty understanding what is being said when there is background noise, for example, in noisy classrooms and work environments.
- They have difficulty following multipart directions.
- Children are often considered underachievers by teachers and parents.

A history of middle ear infections is the problem most consistently associated with APDs in children (middle ear infections will be discussed in some detail in Chapter 14, Hearing Disorders in Children and Adults). Middle ear infections also are associated with phonological disorders, language disorders, learning disabilities, and reading problems. These problems often require the services of speech-language pathologists and audiologists (Geffner & Ross-Swain, 2007; Hay & Flynn, 2004; Musiek & Chermak, 2007; Richard, 2001).

As mentioned previously, to complicate matters APD and ADD can coexist (Bellis, 2002, 2003; Stach, 2010). Determining which is the primary problem and which is the secondary problem is not easy. Ideally, when a child has problems with auditory processing and attention, both problems are diagnosed and treated. However, because it is often difficult to obtain a clear diagnosis of either APD or ADD, children who have both of these problems are fortunate if they receive a diagnosis of one or the other disorder and get appropriate follow-up treatment (Geffner & Ross-Swain, 2007). Stach (2010) states that it is necessary to have the combined efforts of an audiologist and speech-language pathologist during the diagnosis and treatment of APD.

Auditory Processing and Attention Deficit Disorders Beyond the United States

Personal Story

In 2004, I was invited by two separate organizations to Singapore to speak about auditory processing disorders and attention deficit disorders. The May conference was organized for parents of children who had been diagnosed with either APD or ADD (about 90% of the population in Singapore is Asian, but almost 100% of the people speak English as well as their primary language—Chinese, Malaysian, and others). I was surprised to be speaking to more than 200 Asian parents about problems that I had thought were primarily American.

In August, I returned to present an all-day seminar to the Speech-Language-Hearing Association of Singapore, titled "Evaluation and Treatment of APD/ADD/ADHD: A Cognitive-Linguistic Approach." I learned from the speech-language pathologists and audiologists present that they had received their professional training in various countries, including Australia, England, India, New Zealand, and Poland. The audiologist from India said that she had an entire academic course on auditory processing disorders and that APD is a recognized disorder in that country. The SLPs all stated that in whatever country they were from or wherever they received their training, ADD/ADHD and APD were increasingly being recognized, diagnosed, and treated. ■

Children with APD, ADD, or both may have cascading problems that result in various other difficulties. Either APD or ADD may contribute to language disorders and learning disabilities. Some children with learning disabilities develop emotional reactions, such as anxiety, depression, or both, as a result of their difficulties in school. Some children also may develop **psychophysiological (psychosomatic) disorders**, such as headaches, gastrointestinal problems, or both (Egger, Costello, Erkanli, & Angold, 1999; Santalahti, Aromaa, Sourander, Helenius, & Piha, 2005). As speech-language pathologists and audiologists, we must recognize the often pervasive effects of APD and ADD on the lives of children and their families. When we are helping children increase their auditory processing and attentional abilities, we may also be helping with other areas of their lives. Figure 13–4 is a model of how APD, ADD/ADHD, language disorders, learning disabilities, some psychological disorders, and some psychophysiological disorders may interact.

psychophysiological (psychosomatic) disorder

A disorder with physical signs and symptoms that have a psychological origin, often with common ailments such as tension headaches, gastrointestinal disorders, or both that are attributed to psychological stress.

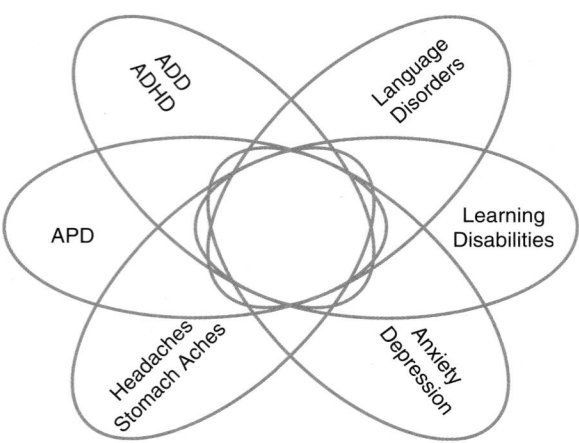

Figure 13–4

APD, ADD/ADHD, language disorders, learning disabilities, psychological disorders, and psychophysiological disorders may interact.

© Cengage Learning 2013.

TRAUMATIC BRAIN INJURY IN CHILDREN

Pediatric traumatic brain injury (TBI) (head trauma) can occur at any age, from newborns through adolescents. Infants may be dropped, may fall, or be abused; children have bicycle accidents, sports injuries, and unbelievable other ways of being injured; adolescents get into altercations and are beaten or shot; and any age may be in motor vehicle accidents (MVAs) (most TBIs in all ages are from MVAs) (Krause, 1995).

Shaken Baby Syndrome

One of the most tragic causes of pediatric TBI is shaken baby syndrome. Shaken baby syndrome is a condition of whiplash-type injury (which often damages the brainstem) caused by violent shaking. Damage ranges from bruises on the arms and trunk where the infant was firmly grasped to retinal hemorrhages in the eyes, seizures, intracranial bleeding from tearing of cerebral blood vessels, coma, and death (Mosby, 2009).

TBIs are particularly tragic because children may be normal one instant and the next instant severely impaired in all ways for the rest of their lives. Children and adolescents are especially susceptible to TBIs because of normal childhood impulsiveness and lack of awareness or concern about *cause and effect* (i.e., "If I do this, this is what could happen").

Speech, Language, Cognitive, and Swallowing Disorders

Depending on the location and severity of brain damage, a variety of speech, language, cognitive, and swallowing problems may be present (Blosser & DePompei, 2003; Lebby & Asbell, 2007; Savage & Callahan, 2003; Ylvisaker, 1998). A child may have apraxia, dysarthria, or both affecting speech intelligibility (see Chapter 5, Articulation and Phonological Disorders in Children). Receptive and expressive language problems

Being an Emergency Medical Technician in Ambulances

Personal Story

During my years of work as an emergency medical technician (EMT) in ambulances in Southern California, I saw countless infants, children, and adolescents who were injured in sometimes unbelievable ways. Many had multiple injuries to their bodies, in addition to their heads (especially in MVAs). In emergency work the goals are to keep the person alive by maintaining an open airway, stop profuse bleeding, splint broken bones, and prevent further injury during transportation to a hospital emergency room. That is not always easy with injured children who are crying and hysterical.

Because of remarkable advances in emergency care, more children are surviving serious traumas, which also means that the work of the rehabilitation team is that much more complex and challenging. The rehab team sees the children who have survived and been "cleaned up." We need to appreciate, however, that somebody had to extricate the children out of crushed automobiles, stop the bleeding, bandage the injuries, splint the broken bones, and transport the children to the next level of care.

(see Chapter 6, Language Disorders in Children) are commonly seen in children with traumatic brain damage. Both language and cognitive disorders that result from TBI can result in learning problems and behavioral problems (see Chapter 11, Neurological Disorders in Adults). Dysphagia may be present that causes a child to have difficulty swallowing foods and liquids and may require a feeding tube (see Chapter 12, Motor Speech Disorders and Dysphagia/Swallowing Disorders).

Generally, children with mild TBIs have good recovery, with the brain's **neural plasticity** likely being a significant factor. However, children with moderate to severe brain damage tend to experience long-term speech and language deficits, particularly in word-finding abilities. Children with moderate to severe brain injuries have more diffuse neuronal and axonal damage, which may affect the amount of neural plasticity potential (Chapman, Gamino, Cook, et al., 2009; DePompei, 2010).

The most devastating problems, however, are the cognitive impairments, including attention, memory (immediate or working memory, recent memory, and long-term memory), orientation (to person, place, time, and purpose), reasoning, judgment, and problem solving. The cognitive impairments affect intellectual abilities and academic performance. Children with such impairments are often placed in special education classes or one grade lower than before the head injury (Babikian & Asarnow, 2009; Chapman, 2006; Gamino & Chapman, 2009).

neural plasticity

The brain's ability to reorganize itself throughout life by forming new neural connections. Neural plasticity allows neurons to compensate for injury and disease and to adjust their activities in response to new situations or to changes in their environment.

Behavioral Effects of Traumatic Brain Injury

Beyond the speech, language, and cognitive impairments seen in children with TBIs, various behavioral effects can interfere with rehabilitation, resocialization, and success upon reentry into school. Clinicians need to be aware that there is a natural progression of behavioral changes throughout the recovery period, which may take months to years (Feeney & Ylvisaker, 2008; Lebby & Asbell, 2005; Turkstra, Williams, Tonks, & Frampton, 2008; Yeates & Taylor, 2006; Yen & Wong, 2007).

Children with TBIs often are not aware of the seriousness of their impairments and may try to do things they are not physically or cognitively capable of, which puts them at risk for additional injuries (e.g., riding a bicycle or driving a vehicle). They are often more impulsive and lack awareness of cause and effect than they were before the trauma, again putting themselves at risk for more injuries. (The person most likely to have a head injury is the person who already has had a head injury.) Their pragmatic skills are frequently severely impaired, and they may become verbally abusive to their family, caregivers, and rehabilitation staff. They often have difficulty getting along with even their best friends, which can cause the end of friendships. They eventually may feel isolated and despondent. However, over time, many of the more normal behaviors of these children begin to reemerge. They typically have to develop new friendships, often with children one or two years younger than themselves because they now relate better to those ages (Hawley, Ward, Magnay, & Mychalkwiw, 2004; Turkstra, et al., 2008).

CEREBRAL PALSY

Cerebral palsy (CP) is the neuromotor impairment that is the most frequent cause of dysarthria in children. Cerebral palsy is one of the more common disorders caused by central nervous system damage in newborns, with an incidence of about 1 in 500 children in developed (industrialized) countries. However, because of increased survival rates of low-birth-weight infants, there has been an increase in the prevalence of cerebral palsy in these countries since the mid-1970s (Pharoah, Platt, & Cooke, 1996). The incidence of cerebral palsy may be even higher in developing countries than in developed countries because of poor prenatal care and inadequate medical care following cerebral infection (e.g., meningitis) and *febrile convulsions* often caused by malaria in infants, and TBIs in children of all ages (Stanley, Blair, & Alberman, 2000; Winter, Autry, Boyle, & Yeargin-Allsopp, 2002).

Causes of Cerebral Palsy

Cerebral palsy may be caused by damage to the central nervous system at different times in the *prenatal* (before birth), *natal/perinatal* (during birth), or *postnatal* (during childhood) history of the child. Some children

---

cerebral palsy (CP)

A developmental neuromotor disorder that can occur prenatally, natally, or perinatally and result in a *nonprogressive* (does not worsen over time), permanent motor function disorder; dysarthria affecting all speech systems is the most common speech problems.

"Something Changed"

Personal Story

A local physician called me to ask if I would work with his 2-year-old son who recently had been diagnosed with severe spastic quadriplegic cerebral palsy. During my first meeting with the mother and father in their home, I interviewed them and asked questions about Samuel's (Sammy's) prenatal, natal, and postnatal history. The mother told me that the pregnancy was going well with no complications and then at 6 months she felt "something changed." She did not know what had changed, and her obstetrician could not detect anything that had gone wrong, but still the mother felt there was something "different" about the baby.

The labor and delivery were normal, and the newborn's birth weight was within normal limits, but his muscle tone was somewhat below normal. He had an Apgar score of 6 (moderate distress) at 1 minute and a score of 7 (borderline distress) at 5 minutes. Sammy's initial growth was normal, but muscle tone was abnormal. Sammy was not officially diagnosed with cerebral palsy until he was almost 2 years old (pediatricians and pediatric neurologists are often "conservative" when making a diagnosis of cerebral palsy). I worked with Sammy for almost 3 years twice a week in his home, typically on the living room floor or with him on his *incline board*, in his *corner chair*, or in his special wheelchair. A team approach was used and I consulted and interacted regularly with both a physical therapist and an occupational therapist. Sammy eventually entered a school for children with **orthopedic** disabilities, where he could receive further physical, occupational, and speech therapy. ■

orthopedic

A branch of health care concerned with the prevention and correction of disorders of the musculoskeletal systems of the body; an *orthopedist* is a physician who specializes in orthopedics.

may have damage that occurs at more than one time in their developmental history. Individuals who sustain damage to the brain (e.g., TBI) in later childhood, before anatomical and physiological maturation of the brain is complete, can have *acquired cerebral palsy.*

Some of the prenatal causes of cerebral palsy include mothers who take illegal drugs before pregnancy, during pregnancy, or both. *Fetal intracranial hemorrhages* (rupture of a blood vessel in the brain, cerebellum, or brainstem during gestation) are fairly common in preterm infants weighing less than 1,500 grams (≈3½ pounds). Infants born with various respiratory problems are also more likely to have intracranial hemorrhages (Wood, Marlow, Costeloe, et al., 2001).

A natal/perinatal cause of cerebral palsy is *fetal distress* (i.e., a compromised condition of the fetus during labor). When the heart is not beating normally, insufficient blood and oxygen reach the brain. Fetal distress may occur during a *breach delivery* (buttocks first) or *precipitous* (very rapid) *delivery. Traumatic forceps deliveries* are now rare because *cesarean sections* are performed more often to prevent the need for forceps (Mosby, 2009).

Traumatic brain injuries (falls, MVAs, assaults [e.g., shaken baby syndrome]) are the most common postnatal causes of cerebral palsy. Hypoxic and anoxic conditions such as *near drowning* are also common causes. Another postnatal cause is neurological diseases such as *encephalitis,* which is an inflammatory condition of the brain that can be caused by *lead poisoning* (most often caused by eating flakes of lead paint, as occurs in some children who live in dwellings painted with lead-based paints).

Classifications (Types) of Cerebral Palsy

Cerebral palsy may be classified by the muscle tone of the limbs. Some children with cerebral palsy have too much muscle tone (**hypertonicity**), making voluntary movements difficult, whereas other children have too little muscle tone (**hypotonicity**), making it difficult to maintain posture, balance, and grasp. Children may have a combination of hypertonicity in their limbs and hypotonicity in their trunks, with weak back, chest, and abdominal muscles (weak trunk muscles are associated with impaired respiratory support).

Another classification method relates to the limbs *involved* (affected or impaired). When one side of the body is affected, it is referred to as *hemiplegia;* when only the legs are involved, it is called *paraplegia;* when only one limb is involved, it is *monoplegia* (rare); when three limbs are involved, it is *triplegia* (rare); and when all four limbs are involved, it is *quadriplegia.* The most common classification system includes spastic type, athetoid type, ataxic type, and mixed type.

Spastic Type

Spastic (Gk. *spastikos,* drawing in) *cerebral palsy* (*spasticity*) is the most common form of the disorder (60%–70% of the cerebral palsy population). The most common symptom is increased muscle tone (hypertonicity) of flexor muscles (e.g., biceps), resulting in stiff, inflexible muscles and joints. Individuals have jerky, abrupt, rigid, and slow, labored movements. **Infantile (primitive) reflexes** (brainstem and midbrain level reflexes) are often present long after they should have been "overridden" by higher cortical areas of the brain. Some individuals develop **contractures** as a result of an *agonist* muscle (e.g., bicep of the arm) being in a constant, strong state of contraction that stretches and weakens an *antagonist* muscle (e.g., tricep of the arm).

Usually both sides of the body are involved, but often one side is more involved than the other. The person's arms, legs, and feet are rotated inward. The heels of the feet are pulled up, causing the person to be a "toe walker." One or both arms are raised with the wrists flexed (pulled down). The head may be drawn back and rotated to one side with the neck and back arched posteriorly (*extensor thrust pattern*). The mouth

hypertonicity/hypertonic

Excessive tone or tension in a muscle or muscle group (e.g., bicep or back muscles).

hypotonicity/hypotonic

Weak or absent tone or tension in a muscle or muscle group (e.g., tricep or abdominal and chest muscles).

infantile (primitive) reflex

Inborn behavioral patterns that develop during intrauterine life, are present at birth and are automatic, uncontrolled movements that normally disappear (become "integrated"—inhibited by higher centers in the brain) by about 6 months of age.

contracture

An abnormal, usually permanent condition of a muscle group (e.g., bicep and muscles of the forearm) characterized by flexion and fixation of the limb that may be caused by shortening of muscle fibers; in severe cases, the bone (e.g., humerus [upper arm]) may develop an abnormal curvature.

is usually open because the head is pulled back and the mandibular muscles are weak, resulting in *anterior spillage* of saliva (drooling). The facial muscles look tense and strained.

Athetoid Type

Athetoid (Gk. *athetos,* not fixed) *cerebral palsy* (*athetosis*) occurs in 20%–30% of the cerebral palsy population. It is a neuromuscular condition characterized by slow, writhing, "wormlike," continuous, and involuntary movements of the extremities. The feet and knees are often rotated inward, causing the person to walk on the outer edges of the feet and making balance difficult. The arms are flexed and the fingers are extended back at an awkward angle. The head is drawn back and rotated to one side. The person has to look down and to one side to see forward. An open mouth with drooling and the tongue protruding are common. Athetoid movements are often exaggerated when the person is excited or emotionally upset.

Ataxic Type

Ataxic (Gk. *ataxia,* without order) *cerebral palsy* (*ataxia*) occurs in 5%–10% of the cerebral palsy population. Ataxia is seen as an impaired ability to coordinate movements and maintain balance. The person keeps his legs spread wide in an attempt to maintain balance, resulting in an awkward, abnormal gait. He may push his head forward while his arms are drawn backward in a further effort to maintain balance. His arm and hand movements are clumsy, awkward, and uncoordinated. He often moves his arms and hands in the wrong direction and is continually correcting or overcorrecting his movements. His muscles are generally hypotonic and weak.

Mixed Type

Some children have symptoms of more than one of the common types of cerebral palsy, particularly if there is extensive neurological damage. The most common combination is spasticity and athetosis, with varying degrees of each type. Other combinations are also possible.

Speech, Language, Cognitive and Swallowing Problems

Most children and adults with cerebral palsy have speech impairments, primarily dysarthria. Because all speech systems may be involved simultaneously, the speech of many of these individuals is moderately to severely unintelligible. Sounds that require tongue-tip movements are usually most affected because of the rapid and fine coordinated movements required for speech. In addition, many children with cerebral palsy also have swallowing difficulties because of the weak and poorly coordinated swallowing mechanism.

The Tokyo Taxi

In 1969 I had a military leave to Tokyo, Japan. Among my memories is an incident that occurred on a rainy spring day on a busy city street. I happened to watch a man who had obvious cerebral palsy and was drenched from the rain (he could not hold an umbrella over his head) try to get a taxi. A taxi eventually pulled up to let him in, but when the taxi driver saw the man's abnormal, and to him perhaps bizarre movements, he harshly closed the door on the man and sped away, leaving him standing in the rain experiencing one more indignity and rejection that was probably a part of his daily life. ▪

Children with cerebral palsy typically have receptive and expressive language delays or disorders, or both. Cognitive impairments are also common and they affect all areas of children's lives, including their ability to learn. Parents of children who have cerebral palsy commonly have difficulty getting them dressed and ready to take on outings, which means the children have fewer life experiences to learn language and develop cognition (Pennington & McConachie, 2001). In addition, children and adults may not interact and play normally with children who have cerebral palsy, causing countless missed normal language and social interactions, not just during childhood but throughout life. Most people in communities have had little experience with adults who have cerebral palsy. When people encounter an individual who has awkward or strange movements of the body, unusual facial contortions when trying to talk, and speech that is difficult to understand, a common reaction is confusion and sometimes even fear. The individual with moderate to severe cerebral palsy does not lead a normal life, or at least a life that most other people would want to lead.

Associated Problems

Most children and adults with cerebral palsy have various other problems or impairments, including intellectual disabilities, hearing impairments, visual impairments, and seizure disorders (Reed, 2010; Workinger, 2005). Children with cerebral palsy, therefore, require management of a variety of problems beyond speech. A team approach with a number of different professionals is essential in helping these children maximize their potential. (Historically, children and adults with cerebral palsy often were treated cruelly and even horrendously, being imprisoned and chained because it was felt that their abnormal movements and speech indicated they were possessed by demons.)

Intellectual Disabilities

Intellectual disabilities occur in approximately 75% of individuals with cerebral palsy. However, about 25% of individuals with cerebral palsy have normal or even superior intellectual abilities (Surveillance of Cerebral Palsy in Europe, 2002). It is difficult to measure the intellectual functioning of most children with cerebral palsy because their impaired speech intelligibility interferes with examiners' (usually psychologists) accurate understanding of responses. Likewise, their arm and hand coordination impairments affect their ability to demonstrate intellectual capacities on the performance portions of IQ tests.

Seizure Disorders

Seizure (epilepsy, convulsion) disorders occur in almost 45% of individuals with cerebral palsy (Workinger, 2005). A seizure may be *tonic* (a temporary state of constant involuntary muscle contraction) or *clonic* (rapid, alternating involuntary contraction and relaxation of muscles); *unilateral* (one side) or *bilateral* (both sides); and *focal* (localized or limited to one area or region of the body), or *generalized* (all or most of the body involved). Antiseizure medications are used to prevent seizures. It is important for clinicians to be aware of a client's history of seizures because a seizure may occur during an evaluation or therapy. Clinicians need to learn (usually in a first aid course) how to recognize and assist an individual having a seizure.

Evaluation and Treatment of Cerebral Palsy

Cerebral palsy is a complex neuromuscular disorder that requires a team of professionals specialized in the evaluation and treatment. Evaluations by **physical therapists (PTs), occupational therapists (OTs)**, and speech-language pathologists are extensive and ongoing. Evaluations by PTs and OTs include the central nervous system's primitive reflexes that are normal in infants up to approximately six months of age, and beyond that are considered abnormal. SLPs assess the **oral reflexes** such as the *rooting reflex* (triggered when an infant's cheek is touched or stroked, causing the infant to turn his head and open his mouth for nursing) and *sucking* and *swallowing reflexes*. Because abnormal primitive reflexes throughout the body may affect speech development, the information gained by the physical and occupational therapists' evaluations is crucial to the SLP; likewise, the SLP's information is important to the physical and occupational therapists.

The physical therapist is usually the lead member of the treatment team. The PT can provide important information about the best postures and positions for the child to be in during various therapy tasks. *Neurodevelopmental therapy* (NDT) is a commonly used approach for treatment of cerebral palsy (originally known as the Bobath method, named after Karl and Berta Bobath, a physician and a physical therapist in England who pioneered the method [Bobath & Bobath, 1952, 1967]). Neurodevelopmental therapy emphasizes the inhibition or integration of primitive postural patterns and promotes the development of normal

---

seizure (epilepsy, convulsion)

A hyperexcitation of neurons in the brain that causes a sudden, sometimes violent, involuntary series of contractions of groups of muscles.

physical therapist (PT)

A rehabilitation specialist who is licensed to evaluate and treat developmental and physical impairments through the use of special exercises or other modalities to assist individuals to maximize independence and mobility, self-care, and functional skills necessary for daily living.

occupational therapist (OT)

A rehabilitation specialist who is licensed to evaluate and treat developmental, physical, and cognitive impairments that interfere with functional independence for daily living and work skills by facilitating the development of **sensory–motor (sensorimotor) integration**, perceptual functioning, and neuromuscular functioning.

oral reflex

Infantile primitive reflexes that are present at birth or soon after that are specifically designed to assist the infant in finding and obtaining oral nutrition; for example, the *rooting reflex*, *sucking reflex*, and *swallowing reflex*.

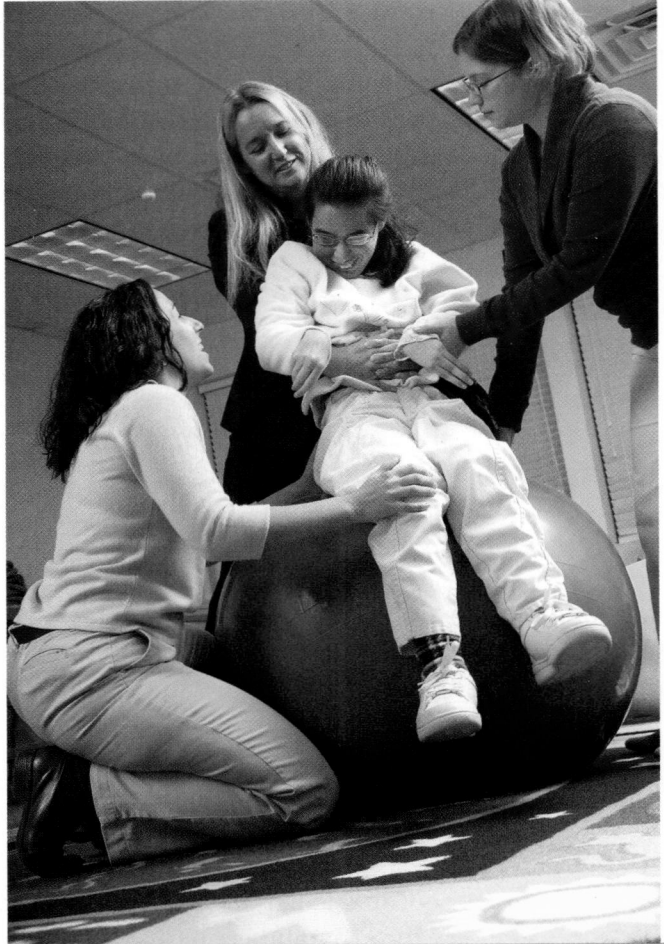

© Cengage Learning 2013

Figure 13-5

Children with cerebral palsy need to be correctly positioned during therapy.

sensory–motor (sensorimotor) integration

The ability to take information (*stimuli*) in through the senses of vision, hearing, touch, taste, and smell, and to combine the information with previously stored memories to develop a coherent concept or appropriate motor response.

postural reactions and achievement of normal muscle tone. Speech therapy initially focuses on *prespeech* abilities—that is, helping the child develop the ability to control and "override" primitive oral reflexes that are interfering with functional articulator movements for speech development (see Figure 13-5).

Many children and adults who cannot develop functional oral communication are able to use various augmentative and assistive devices to communicate. Despite their sometimes severe difficulty with communication and their substantial movement disorders, most children and adults with cerebral palsy appear to be generally happy individuals who are perhaps surprisingly accepting of their physical limitations (although, no doubt, they have many times of frustration and aggravation). My experience with every child and adult with cerebral palsy whom I have worked with clinically or gotten to know personally has consistently shown me that people with even severe challenging physical and communication handicaps can have joyful personalities and be magnanimous in the face of adversity. They are an inspiration to those of us who sometimes complain about the challenges in our own lives.

AUGMENTATIVE AND ALTERNATIVE COMMUNICATION (AAC)

Augmentative and alternative communication (AAC), also known as **assistive technology (AT)**, is any approach designed to support, enhance, or supplement the communication of individuals who are not independent verbal communicators in all situations. AAC is described in a document produced by the Augmentative and Alternative Communication (AAC) Special Interest Division 12 of ASHA (2005, p. 1) as follows:

> AAC refers to an area of research, clinical, and educational practice. AAC involves attempts to study and when necessary compensate for temporary or permanent impairments, activity limitations, and participation restrictions of persons with severe disorders of speech-language production and/ or comprehension, including spoken and written modes of communication.

AAC is a multidisciplinary field in which individuals who use devices and their families, along with computer programmers, educators, engineers, linguists, occupational therapists, physical therapists, speech-language pathologists, and many other professionals, contribute to the knowledge and practice base (Beukelman & Mirenda, 2005; Schlosser, Wendt, Angermeier, & Shetty, 2005). AAC technology is developed and used internationally and there are members of the International Society for Augmentative and Alternative Communication (ISAAC) from more than 50 countries (Forbat, 2003).

AAC systems involve nonelectronic and electronic systems, and there are many advances in technology and new products every year. Children and adults who use AAC systems are sometimes referred to as individuals with *complex communication needs.* The AAC website hosted and updated regularly by the Barkley AAC Center at the University of Nebraska-Lincoln (http://aac.unl.edu) provides links to the websites of manufacturers and publishers in the AAC field.

The field of AAC incorporates three general areas of information: (1) *people* with disabilities who may benefit from AAC; (2) *processes,* such as messages, symbols, alternative access, assessment, and intervention; and (3) *procedures* developed to serve individuals with developmental disabilities who require AAC systems (Beukelman & Mirenda, 2005; Cook, 2011). We begin our discussion of the people, both young and old, who may use and benefit from augmentative and alternative communication.

augmentative and alternative communication (AAC) or assistive technology (AT)

Any approach designed to support, enhance, or supplement the communication of individuals who are not independent verbal communicators in all situations.

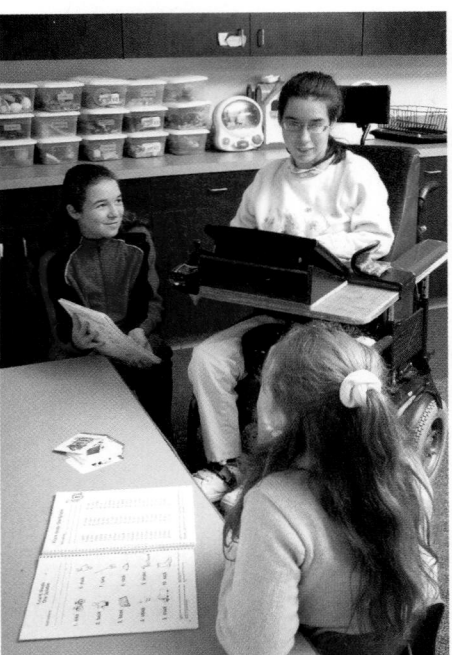
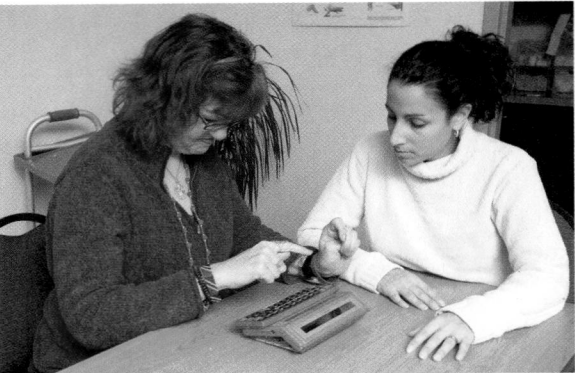
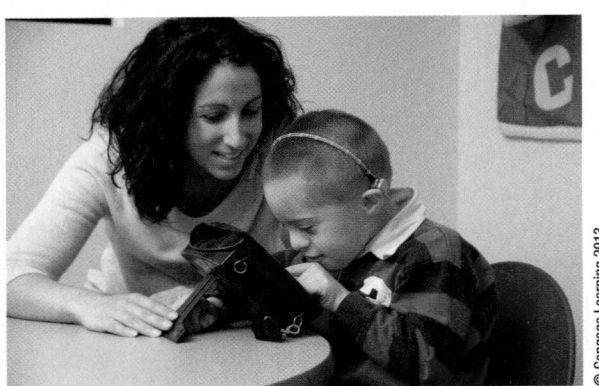

© Cengage Learning 2013

Figure 13–6
Individuals with a variety of developmental disabilities may benefit from AAC.

Children and Adults with Developmental and Motor Disabilities

Children and adults with a variety of severe physical and communication impairments may benefit from AAC, and some begin using assistive devices fairly early in life (see Figure 13–6). Children and adults with cerebral palsy are often the people who come to mind when thinking about who might benefit from AAC; however, individuals with severe apraxia of speech, intellectual disabilities, autism, and pervasive developmental disorders also may benefit (Harris, 2004; Johnston, Reichle, & Evans, 2004; Light & Drager, 2007; Sadao & Robinson, 2010; Wishart, 2010).

For children and adults to receive maximum benefits from sophisticated AAC systems, some level of literacy is essential. At a communication level, literacy skills improve the ability to participate in face-to-face interactions and allow individuals a means of self-expression and a way to develop personal independence. In addition, literacy skills provide access to educational and vocational opportunities, which can be limited due to the physical and communication impairments of these children and adults (Kent-Walsh & Rosa-Lugo, 2006; Sturm & Clendon, 2004). AAC can be mutually beneficial and mutually supportive for both communication and literacy development. That is, when individuals are able to use AAC to communicate, it can facilitate interactions with

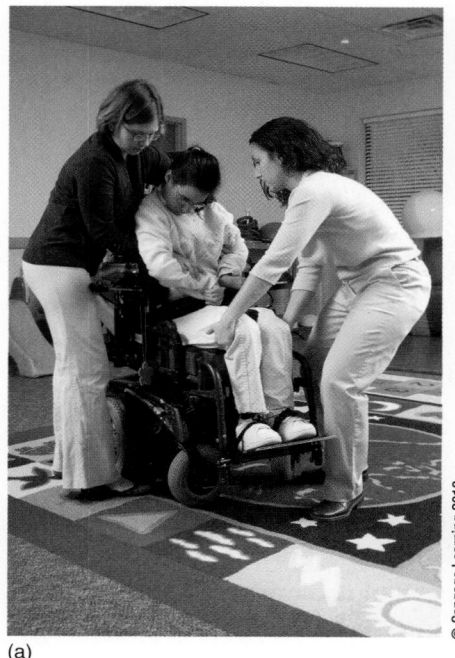

(a)

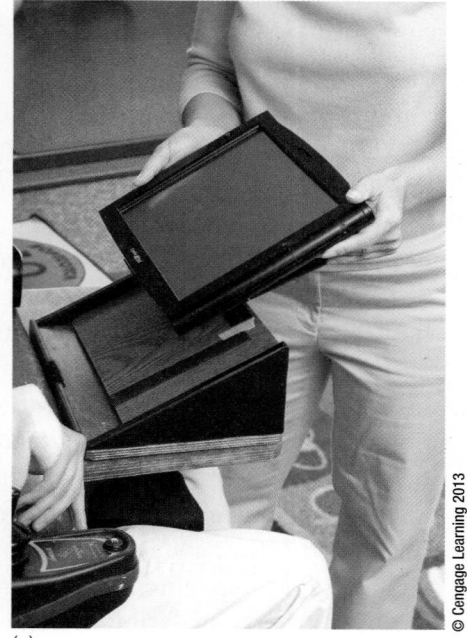

(c)

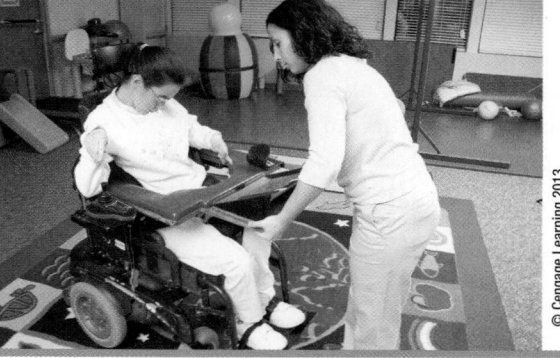

(b)

Figure 13–7

A team approach is necessary when fitting individuals with cerebral palsy with an AAC device: (a) A physical therapist and speech-language pathologist may work together to position a client in her wheelchair; (b) the speech-language pathologist places the tray that holds an AAC device; and (c) the speech-language pathologist then places the AAC device for the client to use.

parents and other caregivers, teachers, and others who are trying to help develop literacy skills. Likewise, developing literacy skills may allow children and adults to use more sophisticated AAC systems for better communication and may open the world of the Internet to them for educational growth, interpersonal communication, and entertainment (Poulson & Nicolle, 2004).

Children and adults with cerebral palsy have difficulty exploring the world on their own because of their motor dysfunctions. Because of their limited physical independence and speech impairments, they often are isolated from social environments. To become competent communicators, individuals with severe cerebral palsy need to acquire expressive symbolic and linguistic skills in communication modes within their own physical and cognitive limitations (Millar, Light, & Schlosser, 2006; Sutherland, Gillon, & Yoder, 2005) (see Figure 13–7).

Beukelman and Mirenda (2005) emphasize the need for a "balanced approach" to communication programs for people with severe expressive communication disorders. This means that emphasis on AAC

CASE STUDY

James

Samuel was a 37-year-old man who was living alone in the family home after his mother had died. An SLP in private practice was called by his aunt to help him obtain an assistive device. Samuel had already been assessed by a specialist in AAC, so the device had already been chosen for him; however, the specialist lived some distance from Samuel and could not continue working with him. Samuel had completed high school and had some community college education (cognitive functioning was not a problem). His communication impairment was severe dysarthria, plus he had ambulatory and moderate-to-severe general motor incoordination. He had an expensive powered wheelchair that he used when he left his home and went into the community.

The major challenge to acquiring the appropriate assistive communication device was the expense and the approval through various agencies for the payment of the device. It took months of reports, paperwork, and red tape to obtain the assistive device and the apparatus that allowed a connection to the client's wheelchair so that he could communicate with people when he was out in the community. Samuel was genuinely excited when the device and wheelchair attachments were all in place and working, and he was in his wheelchair ready to make his first excursion into the community on his own. It was a proud day, indeed. (Although the SLP had spent many hours involved with this client, he felt that it was appropriate to do the work pro bono [time and expertise donated]). ■

needs should be balanced with motor development training, speech therapy, and academic instruction to maximize each person's overall potential. AAC systems may provide individuals an immediate ability to communicate their basic wants, needs, thoughts, and feelings; however, a systematic speech therapy program to train more complex skills may lay a firm foundation for developing more complex and balanced communication (Reichert Hoge & Newsome, 2002; Millar et al., 2006; Sadao & Robinson, 2010; Treviranus & Roberts, 2003).

Adults with Acquired Communication Disorders

Adults with acquired communication impairments (e.g., severe aphasia, apraxia, or dysarthria) from CVAs, TBIs, and other neurological disorders who are not able to develop functional speech and language can benefit from AAC. Other adults can benefit who have progressively deteriorating central and peripheral nervous system diseases, such as Parkinson's disease, amyotrophic lateral sclerosis (ALS),

Application Question

Have you ever tried to communicate with an adult who could not understand or speak effectively and did not have an AAC device? What did you do to try to make the person's communication easier?

Dorothy

Dorothy was a woman in her late 60s who had developed Parkinson's disease and had increasingly severe dysarthria. I was called by a daughter-in-law, Sharon, and asked to be her speech-language pathologist. I saw Dorothy twice a week in her home for many months. Initially, her speech was moderately dysarthric and I was able to help her maximize her intelligibility. However, the Parkinson's disease was stronger than her determination and therapy combined, and she began to deteriorate further. Emphasis in speech intelligibility changed from short phrases to two words and finally to single-word intelligible speech. Before she could no longer utter single words intelligibly, I helped her acquire an assistive device that allowed her to type, albeit slowly, messages that others could read; synthesized speech could also be heard. Eventually there was nothing more that I could do for Dorothy and I had to end therapy with her.

I did not hear from the daughter-in-law for several months. Then one day I received a telephone call from Sharon, letting me know that Dorothy had died. Sharon then asked if I would do the eulogy at Dorothy's funeral. I was humbled and honored to be asked to perform this important task at the funeral of such a prominent woman in the community. I agreed, and a few days later I was doing the eulogy at a funeral home chapel filled to standing room only, with people outside seated and listening to the service through a loudspeaker. However, not only was I to do the eulogy, I was told just before the service began that I would be "officiating" the service (i.e., introducing the singers and speakers, and leading all parts of the service). After the service was finished and all had gone well, I thought my job was over. Then the funeral home director told me that I would be conducting the graveside service as well—and that is what I did. Although I could have refused all that was asked of me, I felt it was important to accept the unusual requests and to step out of the role of a speech-language pathologist and into the role of a friend who the family felt they could rely on to perform a difficult task with dignity and equanimity. Sometimes a client comes back into our lives in unexpected ways and we have the choice to be of additional service. ■

multiple sclerosis, Guillain-Barré syndrome, or dementia (Armstrong, Jans, & MacDonald, 2000; Ball, 2003; Ho, Weiss, Garrett, & Lloyd, 2005; Purdy & Dietz, 2010). The AAC systems can be designed to accommodate each person's physical limitations. For these individuals, AAC can help them participate more fully in important life activities.

AAC SYSTEMS

Numerous areas need to be considered in an AAC assessment, including the person's positioning and seating, neuromotor impairments, motor capabilities, sensory and perceptual abilities (vision and hearing), communication abilities, cognitive abilities, functional symbols that can be used, and literacy skills. From the evaluation and understanding of the person— and some trial-and-error—the best AAC system can be developed (Reichert Hoge & Newsome, 2002).

Communication Boards

Communication (conversation) boards are the most widely used type of AAC system that are functional for many users in a variety of settings. They may be an apparatus, electronic device, or simple board upon which common communication symbols and messages are represented. They may be no-tech, low-tech, or sophisticated (and expensive) high-tech electronic devices. Basic communication boards typically have the alphabet, numbers 1–10, and a few key words and phrases a person can point to in order to communicate basic messages (see Figure 13–8). Some individuals use communication boards to "supplement" their speech. When a listener has not understood a verbal message, the individual can point to letters, numbers, words, or phrases to help the listener.

Because all communication involves symbols (spoken words are just arbitrary symbols [sounds] that represent whatever we say they represent), individuals employing AAC simply use a system of symbols different from that used by other people to communicate their messages. Representational symbols are some of the most common forms of communication used with AAC.

Photographs and Simple Illustrations

Simple black and white or color photographs or illustrations are excellent for representations of people, objects, and actions. Photographs for

---

communication (conversation) board

An apparatus or simple board upon which common communication symbols and messages (e.g., alphabet, numbers, pictures, symbols, and common words and expressions) are represented, allowing expressive communication by pointing or gazing; communication boards may be no-tech, low-tech, or sophisticated high-tech electronic devices.

Figure 13–8

A simple, "no-tech" communication board.

© Cengage Learning 2013.

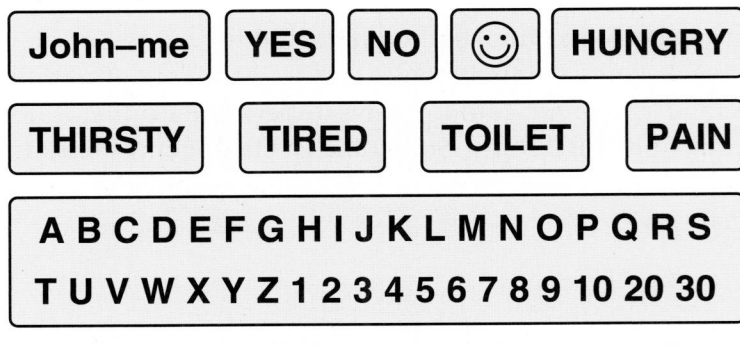

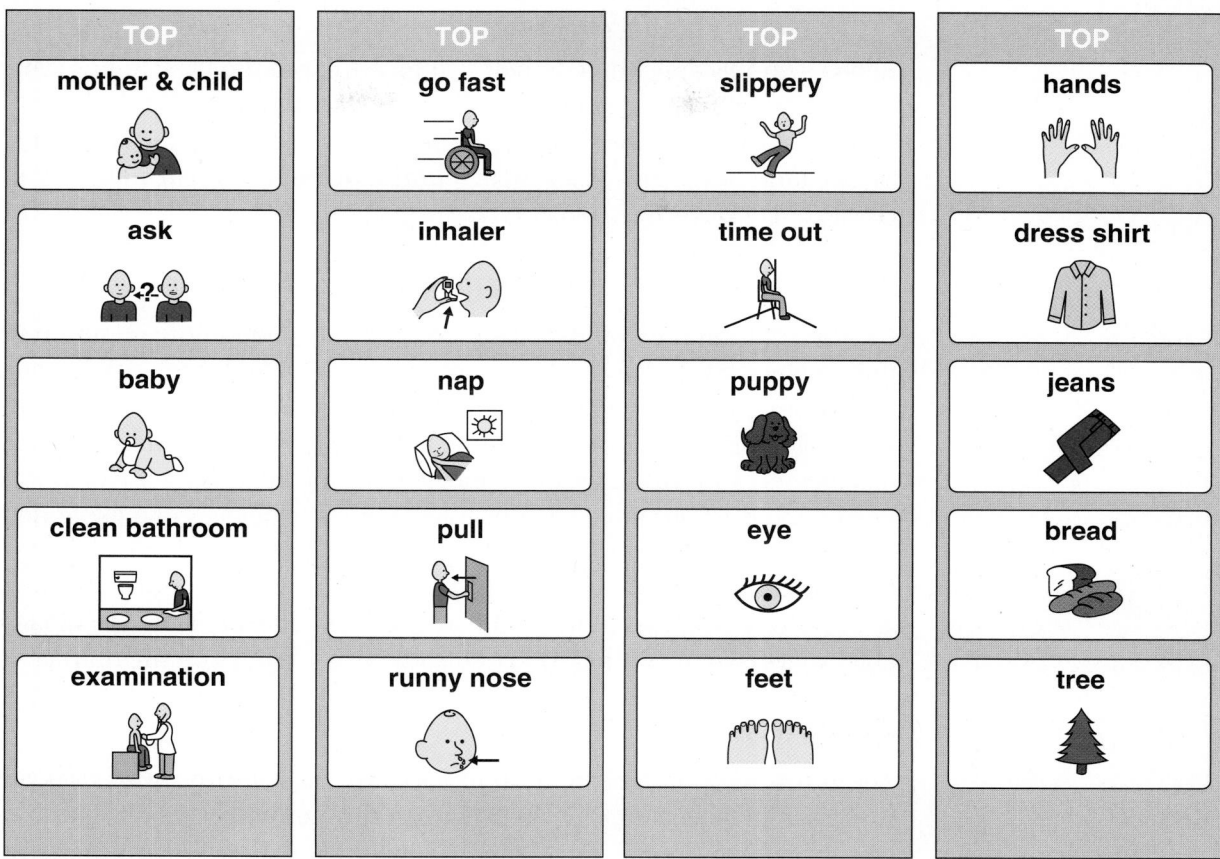

Figure 13–9

Examples of Picture Communication Symbols © (PCS) using Boardmaker™ software.

communication boards may be taken of people, objects, or locations in the client's environment or cut out of magazines, catalogs, advertisements, and so on. Users of AAC need to have sufficient visual acuity and visual perceptual abilities to recognize who or what is being shown in the photographs. No-tech communication boards can easily be made by clinicians by simply cutting out pictures, pasting or taping them to a piece of heavy stock paper or cardboard, and covering the board with a plastic protector.

Picture Communication Symbols

The Picture Communication Symbols© (PCS) developed by Johnson (1994) has more than 7,000 clear, simple black-and-white or color line drawings (including more than 500 verbs) that are available as Boardmaker™ software through Mayer-Johnson for both Windows and Macintosh (see Figure 13–9). The words displayed above the drawings are available in 24 languages and several that use non-Roman alphabets (e.g., Hebrew, Japanese, and Hmong).

Application Question

If you needed to use a simple communication board for a while, what would you like included on it?

Rebus Symbols

Rebus symbols are simple line drawings similar to the PCS. Rebus symbols were originally designed by Woodcock, Clark, and Davies (1968) to help nonhandicapped children read, but they were later developed in England for individuals with communication impairments (Van Oosterum & Devereux, 1985).

Applications for Smartphones and Pads

As smartphones and tablet computers (pads) become more common in the wireless market, so do applications for individuals with AAC needs (e.g., *Communicating Basic Needs App* for the iPod Touch, iPhone, and iPad). The proliferation of downloadable applications for smartphones has created opportunities for people with physical and cognitive limitations, including enhanced accessibility of mobile devices and expanded ability to engage in daily activities through the use of smartphones (Hallett, 2011; Steele & Woronoff, 2011). There is strong appeal for such applications because they would be relatively inexpensive downloadable "apps" when compared to dedicated AAC devices on the market.

Selection Techniques

The term *selection techniques* refers to the way a person who uses an AAC system selects or identifies items from the pictures, symbols, and words on a communication board. There are two basic selection methods, direct and scanning. Depending on the physical abilities of an individual, one or both methods may be used. For example, Figure 13–10 shows the Talara-32 system that is manufactured by Zygo Industries. This digital recording AAC device is designed for easy use and can be customized for both children and adults with wide ranging abilities and needs. The user can scan the numerous figures in the various overlays using the scanning mode that is best suited to the individual.

Most people using AAC systems use finger pointing or touch to indicate messages. More sophisticated and somewhat more challenging methods are headsticks and light pointers, including safe laser head pointers. Some people who do not have the motor control to point to

Figure 13–10

The Talara-32 AAC device.

Source: Courtesy of ZYGO-USA.

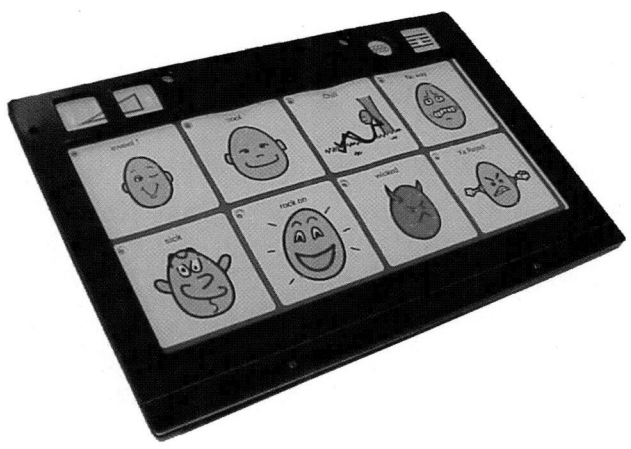

Steven

Steven is a typical 16-year-old adolescent who likes football, watching television, and talking to girls. He attends regular high school in Houston, Texas. Other than having severe spastic quadriplegic cerebral palsy, being in a powered wheelchair, and using an AAC device to communicate, Steven is normal. The AAC device doubles as his mode of vocal and written communication and a computer on which he can do his homework. He powers both the device and the head pointer system from his wheelchair battery. Steven makes maximum use of his AAC device and powered wheelchair to enjoy school and numerous activities. He socializes and feels most students in his school are his friends. He is planning to attend college and earn a degree in computer programming, hoping to help develop even more sophisticated AAC devices for other people. ■

individual symbols may use scanning devices. With a scanner, the person activates the electronic board and then when the desired symbol is highlighted indicates in some way that the symbol has been selected. This can be a slow, laborious process but still the most efficient method of communicating for some people (Bedrosian, Hoag, & McCoy, 2003).

CHAPTER SUMMARY

A intellectual disability is a disability that originates before 18 years of age and is characterized by significant limitations in intellectual functioning and adaptive behavior, and is under the umbrella term of developmental disability. Most children with intellectual disabilities have significant problems with speech and language, and essentially all have impairments of cognition. Down syndrome and autism are two of the best-known developmental disabilities. ADD/ADHD is a broad syndrome relating to children who demonstrate three primary problems: inattention, impulsivity, and hyperactivity. APD is a disorder in some children and adults who have difficulty using auditory information to communicate and learn that affects their abilities to listen, understand speech, develop language, and have academic success. Pediatric TBI can occur at any age, from newborns through adolescents. Depending on the location and severity of brain damage, a variety of speech, language, and cognitive problems may be present. Cerebral palsy is a developmental neuromotor disorder that can occur prenatally, natally, or perinatally and results in a nonprogressive, permanent motor function disorder. Cerebral palsy is the neuromotor impairment that is the most common cause of dysarthria in children.

Augmentative and alternative communication (AAC) systems involve nonelectronic and electronic systems that may be no-tech, low-tech, or high-tech devices. The field of AAC incorporates three general areas of information: (1) people, (2) processes, and (3) procedures. Children with a variety of severe physical and communication impairments may benefit from AAC, and some children begin using assistive devices fairly early in life. Adults who have congenital or acquired communication disabilities also benefit from AAC.

STUDY QUESTIONS

Knowledge and Comprehension

1. Define autism.

2. Describe the three primary problems that children with ADD demonstrate?

3. What are four factors that are often associated with auditory processing disorders?

4. Describe the behavioral effects of traumatic brain injury in children.

5. Discuss two problems that are associated with cerebral palsy.

Application

1. Why might it be valuable for speech-language pathologists working in various settings (e.g., schools, clinics, hospitals) to have a copy of the American Psychiatric Association's *Diagnostic and Statistical Manual of Mental Disorders, 4th edition, Text Revision* (DSM-IV TR)?

2. What are some of the behaviors you would look for that could indicate a child might be in the autism spectrum?

3. Discuss three examples of syndromes that may significantly affect communication and cognitive development.

4. How could speech, language, and/or cognitive problems caused by a TBI affect a child's learning?

5. Discuss the concept that people who use augmentative and alternative communication (AAC) systems need a "balanced approach" to communication.

Analysis/Synthesis

1. How can you apply information from the chapter on Language Disorders in Children to children with Down syndrome?

2. What could be the effects of an auditory processing disorder and an attention deficit disorder occurring in the same child?

3. How could you apply your knowledge about neurological disorders in adults (aphasia, traumatic brain injury, and cognitive disorders) to help you diagnose and treat children with traumatic brain injuries?

4. How can you apply information from the chapter on Motor Speech Disorders and Dysphagia/Swallowing Disorders to children who have cerebral palsy?

5. Why is some level of literacy essential for children to receive maximum benefits from sophisticated augmentative or alternative communication (AAC) systems?

REFERENCES

Adams, C., Lloyd, J., Aldred, C., & Baxendale, J. (2006). Exploring the effects of communication intervention for developmental pragmatic language impairments: A signal-generation study. *International Journal of Language and Communication Disorders, 41*(1), 41–65.

American Association on Intellectual and Developmental Disabilities. (2010). *Intellectual disability: Definition, classification, and systems of support* (11th ed.) Washington, DC: AAIDD.

American Psychiatric Association. (2000). *Diagnostic and statistical manual of mental disorders* (DSM-IV-TR) (4th ed., text rev. ed.). Washington, DC: APA.

American Speech-Language-Hearing Association. (1995). *Central auditory processing: Current status of research and implications for clinical practice. A report from the ASHA task force on central auditory processing.* Rockville, MD: ASHA.

American Speech-Language-Hearing Association. (2005). Roles and responsibilities of speech-language pathologists with respect to augmentative and alternative communication: Position statement. *ASHA* (Supplement 25).

Armstrong, L., Jans, D., & MacDonald, A. (2000). Parkinson's disease and aided AAC: Some evidence from practice. *International Journal of Language and Communication Disorders, 35*(3), 377–389.

Babikian, T., & Asarnow, R. (2009). Neurocogitive outcomes and recovery after pediatric TBI: Meta analysis of the literature. *Neuropsychology, 23*(3), 283–296.

Ball, H. (2003). AAC transitions for persons with ALS: A "classic" example. *ASHA Leader, 13,* 207.

Barkley, R. A. (2006). *ADHD: What do we know?* New York, NY: SR Publications.

Bellis, T. J. (2002). *When the brain can't hear: Unraveling the mystery of auditory processing disorder.* New York, NY: Atrira Books.

Bellis, T. J. (2003). *Assessment and management of central auditory processing disorders in the educational setting: From science to practice* (2nd ed.). Clifton Park, NY: Delmar Cengage Learning.

Beukelman, D. R., & Mirenda, P. (2005). *Augmentative and alternative communication: Supporting children and adults with complex communication needs* (3rd ed.). London, England: Paul H. Brookes.

Blosser, J. L., & DePompei, R. (2003). *Pediatric traumatic brain injury* (2nd ed.). Clifton Park, NY: Delmar Cengage Learning.

Bobath, K., & Bobath, B. (1952). The neuro-developmental treatment of spastic children. *British Journal of Physical Medicine, 5,* 87–94.

Bobath, K., & Bobath, B. (1967). The neuro-developmental treatment of cerebral palsy. *Journal of the American Physical Therapy Association, 47,* 1039–1041.

Byrnes, J. P. (2008). *Cognitive development and learning in instructional contexts* (3rd ed.). Boston, MA: Allyn and Bacon.

Chapman, S. B. (2006). Neurocognitive stall: A paradox in long term recovery from pediatric brain injury. *Brain Injury Professional, 3*(4), 10–13.

Chapman, S. B., Gamino, J. F., Cook, L. G., Hanten, G., Li, X., & Levin, H. S. (2009). Impaired discourse gist and working memory in children after brain injury. *Brain and Language, 97,* 178–188.

Cook, A. M. (2011). It's not about the technology, or is it? Realizing AAC through hard and soft technologies. *Perspectives on Augmentative and Alternative* Communication, *20*(2), 64–68.

DePompei, R. (2010, November). Pediatric traumatic brain injury: Where do we go from here? *The ASHA Leader.*

Dominick, K. C., Davis, N., Lainhart, J., Tager-Flushberg, H., & Folstein, S. (2007). Atypical behaviors in children with autism and children with a history of language impairment. *Journal of Developmental Disabilities, 28*(2), 145–162.

Egger, H., Costello, E., Erkanli, A., & Angold, A. (1999). Somatic complaints and psychopathology in children and adolescents: Stomach aches, musculoskeletal pains, and headaches. *Journal of the Academy of Child and Adolescent Psychiatry, 38*(7), 852–860.

Farmer, M., & Oliver, A. (2005). Assessment of pragmatic difficulties and socioemotional adjustment in practice. *International Journal of Language and Communication Disorders, 40*(4), 403–429.

Feeney, T. J., & Ylvisaker, M. (2008). Context sensitive cognitive-behavioral supports for young children with TBI: A second replication study. *Journal of Positive Behavioral Interventions, 10*(2), 115–128.

Forbat, L. (2003). Communicating without speech: Practical augmentative and alternative communication. *British Journal of Learning Disabilities, 31*(3), 140–144.

Gamino, J. F., & Chapman, S. B. (2009). Strategic learning in youth with traumatic brain injuy: Evidence for stall in higher-order cognition. *Topics in Language Disorders, 24*(3), 1–12.

Geffner, D., & Ross-Swain, D. (2007). *Auditory processing disorders: Assessment, management and treatment.* San Diego, CA: Plural Publishing.

Hallett, T. (2011, November). *IPods, IPads, & IPhones: Applications for teachers, supervisors, & researchers.* Paper presented at the American Speech-Language-Hearing Association convention, San Diego, CA.

Harris, M. D. (2004). Impact of aided language stimulation of symbol comprehension and production in children with cognitive disabilities. *American Journal of Speech-Language Pathology, 13,* 155–167.

Hawley, C., Ward, A. B., Magnay, A., & Mychalkwiw, W. (2004). Return to school after brain injury. *Archives of Disease in Childhood, 89,* 136–142.

Hay, E., & Flynn, M. (2004). Pediatric auditory processing disorder and its implications for speech-language therapists. *New Zealand Journal of Speech-Language Therapy, 59,* 35–39.

Heaton, P., & Wallace, G. L. (2004). The savant syndrome. *The Journal of Child Psychology and Psychiatry, 45,* 899–911.

Ho, K., Weiss, S., Garrett, K., & Lloyd, L. (2005). Effect of remnant and pictographic books on the communicative interaction of individuals with global aphasia. *Augmentative and Alternative Communication, 21*(3), 218–232.

Jerger, S., & Musiek, F. (2000). Report on the consensus conference on the diagnosis of auditory processing disorders in school-aged children. *Journal of the Academy of Audiology, 11*(9), 467–474.

Johnson, C. P., & Myers, S. M. (2007). Identification and evaluation of children with autism spectrum disorders. *Pediatrics, 12*0(5), 1183–1215.

Johnson, R. (1994). *The Picture Communication Symbols combination book.* Solana Beach, CA: Mayer-Johnson.

Johnston, S. S., Reichle, J., & Evans, J. (2004). Supporting augmentative and alternative communication use by beginning communicators with severe disabilities. *American Journal of Speech-Language Pathology, 13*(20), 1044–1058.

Kanner, L. (1943). Autistic disturbances of affective contact. *Nervous Child, 2,* 217–250.

Kelly, D. (2001). *Central auditory processing disorders: Identification and intervention.* Gaylord, MI: Northern Speech Services/National Rehabilitation Services.

Kent-Walsh, J., & Rosa-Lugo, L. (2006). Communication partner interventions for children who use AAC: Storybook reading across culture and language. *ASHA Leader, 11*(3), 6–7, 28–29.

Krause, J. F. (1995). Epidemiological features of brain injury in children: Occurrence, children at risk, causes and manner of injury, severity and outcomes. In S. Broman & M. Michel (Eds.), *Traumatic head injury in children.* New York, NY: Oxford University Press.

Kupperman, P. (2008). *The source for intervention in autism spectrum disorders.* East Moline, IL: LinguiSystems.

Lebby, P. C., & Asbell, S. J. (2005). *The source for traumatic brain injury: Children and adolescents.* East Moline, IL: LinguiSystems.

Light, J., & Drager, K. (2007). AAC technologies for young children with complex communication needs: State of the science and future research directions. *Augmentative and Alternative Communication, 23*(3), 204–216.

Martin, F. N., & Clark, J. G. (2009). *Introduction to audiology* (10th ed.). Boston, MA: Pearson.

Mayo Clinic. (2009). *Mayo Clinic family health book.* Rochester, MN: Mayo Clinic.

Millar, D., Light, J., & Schlosser, R. (2006). The impact of augmentative and alternative communication intervention on the speech production of individuals with developmental disabilities: A research review. *Journal of Speech-Language-Hearing Research, 49,* 248–264.

Mosby. (2009). *Mosby's medical, nursing, and allied health dictionary* (8th ed.). St. Louis, MO: Mosby.

Musiek, F. E., & Chermak, G. D. (2007). *Handbook of (central) auditory processing disorder: Vol 1. Auditory neuroscience and diagnosis.* San Diego, CA: Plural Publishing.

Newschaffer, C., Croen, L., Daniels, J., Giarelli, E., Grether, J., et al. (2007). The epidemiology of autism spectrum disorders. *Annual Review of Public Health, 28,* 235–258.

Pennington, L., & McConachie, H. (2001). Interaction between children with cerebral palsy and their mothers: The effects of speech intelligibility. *International Journal of Language and Communication Disorders, 36*(3), 371–393.

Pharoah, P., Platt, M., & Cooke, T. (1996). The changing epidemiology of cerebral palsy. *Archives of Disease in Childhood (fetal and neonatal ed.), 75,* 169–173.

Poulson, D., & Nicolle, C. (2004). Making the Internet accessible for people with cognitive and communication impairments. *Universal Access in the Information Society, 3*(1), 48–56.

Purdy, M., & Dietz, A. (2010). Factors influencing AAC usage by individuals with aphasia. *Perspectives on Augmentative and Alternative Communication, 19*(3), 70–78.

Reece, P. B., & Challenner, N. C. (2006). *The source for behavior management in autism.* East Moline, IL: LinguiSystems.

Reed, V. A. (2010). *An introduction to children with language disorders* (4th ed.) Boston, MA: Pearson Allyn and Bacon.

Reichert Hoge, D., & Newsome, C. A. (2002). *The source for augmentative alternative communication.* East Moline, IL: LinguiSystems.

Richard, G. J. (2001). *The source for processing disorders.* East Moline, IL: LinguiSystems.

Richard, G. J. (2004). Redefining auditory processing disorder: A speech-language pathologist's perspective. *ASHA Leader, 7*(March), 21.

Richard, G. (2008). Autism spectrum disorders in the schools. *The ASHA Leader, 13*(13), 26–28.

Sadao, K. C., & Robinson, N. B. (2010). *Assistive technology for young children: Creating inclusive learning environments.* Baltimore, MD: Brookes Publishing.

Santalahti, P., Aromaa, M., Sourander, A., Helenius, H., & Piha, J. (2005). Have there been changes in children's psychosomatic symptoms? A 10-year comparison from Finland. *Pediatrics, 115*(4), 434–442.

Savage, R. C., & Callahan, C. D. (2003). Review: Pediatric traumatic brain injury proactive intervention. *Journal of Head Trauma Rehabilitation, 18*(3), 303–304.

Schlosser, R. W., Wendt, O., Angermeier, K. L., & Shetty, M. (2005). Searching for evidence in augmentative and alternative communication: Navigating a scattered literature. *Augmentative and Alternative Communication, 21*(4), 233–255.

Schonwald, A., & Lechner, E. (2006). Attention deficit/hyperactivity disorder: Complexities and controversies. *Current Opinions in Pediatrics, 18*(2), 189–195.

Stach, B. A. (2010). *Clinical audiology: An introduction* (2nd ed.). Clifton Park, NY: Delmar Cengage Learning.

Stanley, F., Blair, E. & Alberman, E. (2000). *Cerebral palsies: Epidemiology and causal pathways.* London, England: Mac Keith Press.

Steele, R., & Woronoff, P. (2011). Design challenges of AAC apps on wireless portable devices for person's with aphasia. *Perspectives on Augmentative and Alternative Communication, 20*(2), 41–51.

Still, G. F. (1902). Some abnormal physical conditions in children: The Goulstonian lectures. *Lancet, 1,* 1008–1012.

Sturm, J., & Clendon, S. A. (2004). Augmentative and alternative communication, language, and literacy: Fostering the relationship. *Topics in Language Disorders, 24*(1), 76–91.

Surveillance of Cerebral Palsy in Europe. (2002). Prevalence and characteristics of children with cerebral palsy in Europe. *Developmental Medicine and Child Neurology, 44,* 633–640.

Sutherland, D., Gillon, G., & Yoder, D. (2005). AAC use and service provision: A survey of New Zealand speech language therapists. *Augmentative and Alternative Communication, 21*(4), 295–307.

Tager-Flusberg, H., & Caronna, E. (2007). Language disorders: Autism and other pervasive developmental disorders. *Pediatric Clinics of North America, 54*(3), 469–481.

Tetnowski, J. A. (2004). Attention deficit hyperactivity disorder and concomitant communicative disorders. *Seminars in Speech and Language, 25*(3), 215–223.

Tonge, B. J. (2002). Autism, autism spectrum and the need for better definition. *Medical Journal of Australia, 176*(9), 412–413.

Treviranus, J., & Roberts, V. (2003). Supporting competent motor control of AAC systems. In J. Light & D. Beukelman, *Communication competence for individuals who use AAC.* Baltimore, MD: Brookes.

Turkstra, L. S., Williams, W. H., Tonks, J., & Frampton, I. (2008). Measuring social cognition in adolescents: Implications for students with TBI returning to school. *NeuroRehabilitation, 23*(6), 501–509.

Turner-Brown, L. M., Lam, K., Holtzclaw, T. N., Dichter, G. S., & Bodfish, J. W. (2011). Phenomenology and measurement of circumscribed interests in autism spectrum disorders. *Autism, 15,* 437–456.

Van Oosterum, J., & Devereux, K. (1985). *Learning with Rebuses.* Black Hill, Ely, Cambridgeshire, England: WAEO, The Resource Centre.

Volden, J., & Lord, C. (1991). Neologisms and idiosyncratic language in autistic speakers. *Journal of Autism and Developmental Disorders, 21,* 109–130.

Wender, P. H. (2000). ADHD: *Attention-deficit hyperactive disorder in children, adolescents, and adults.* Oxford: Oxford University Press.

Wilens, T. E., Biederman, J., & Spencer, T. J. (2002). Attention deficit/hyperactivity disorder across the lifespan. *Annual Review of Medicine, 52,* 113–131.

Winter, S., Autry, A., Boyle, C., & Yeargin-Allsopp, M. (2002). Trends in the prevalence of cerebral palsy in a population-based study. *Pediatrics, 110,* 1220–1225.

Wishart, K. (2010). Clinical impressions of how young children use AAC at home and in child care settings: A Canadian perspective. *Perspectives on Augmentative and Alternative Communication, 19*(1), 21–28.

Wood, N. S., Marlow, N., Costeloe, K., Gibson, A., & Wilkinson, A. (2001). Neurologic and developmental disability after extremely preterm birth. *Obstetrics & Gynecology, 56*(1), 13–15.

Woodcock, R., Clark, C., & Davies, C. (1968). *Peabody Rebus reading program.* Circle Pines, MN: AGS Publishing.

Workinger, M. S. (2005). *Cerebral palsy resource guide for speech-language pathologists.* Clifton Park, NY: Delmar Cengage Learning.

World Health Organization. (2001). *International classification of functioning, disability, and health.* Geneva, Switzerland: WHO.

Yeates, K. O., & Taylor, G. H. (2006). Behavior problems in school and their educational correlates among children with traumatic brain injury. *Exceptionality, 14*(3), 141–154.

Yen, H. L., & Wong, J. T. (2007). Rehabilitation for traumatic brain injury in children and adolescents. *Annals, Academy of Medicine, Singapore, 36,* 62–6.

Ylvisaker, M. (1998). *Traumatic brain injury rehabilitation: Children and adolescents* (2nd ed.). Boston, MA: Butterworth-Heinemann.

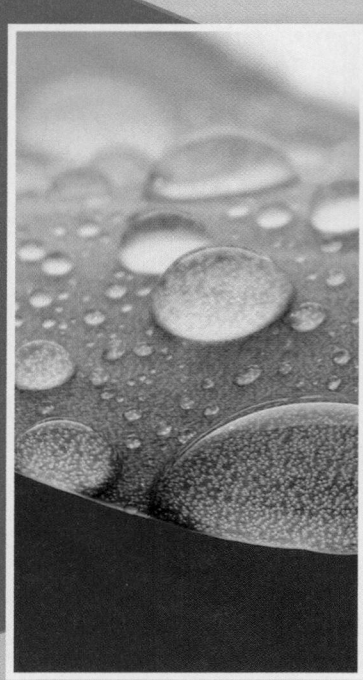

CHAPTER 14
Hearing Disorders in Children and Adults

LEARNING OBJECTIVES

After studying this chapter, you will:

- Be able to discuss the anatomy and physiology of the hearing mechanism.
- Understand hearing sensitivity and auditory nervous system impairments.
- Be familiar with newborn hearing screening.
- Understand the essentials of pure-tone and speech audiometry.
- Be able to discuss the essentials of amplification and assistive devices for individuals who are hearing impaired.
- Be familiar with aural rehabilitation.
- Appreciate that the Deaf culture has long been established in countries around the world.
- Understand the essentials of the emotional and social effects of hearing loss in children, adults, and their families.

KEY TERMS

acoustic trauma (noise-induced hearing loss)
adenoids (pharyngeal tonsils)
admittance
air conduction
American Sign Language (ASL)
assistive listening device
audiogram
audiometer
auditory brainstem response (ABR)
auditory nervous system impairment

auditory training
aural habilitation
aural rehabilitation
bone conduction
cerumen
cochlea
cochlear implant
compliance
conductive hearing loss
Deaf community
Deaf culture
differential threshold
Eustachian (auditory) tubes
finger spelling

hearing aid
hearing sensitivity impairment
hearing threshold
immittance audiometry
impedance
lipreading
manualism
manually coded English
masking
mastoiditis
Meniere's disease
middle ear
mixed hearing loss
oralism

KEY TERMS continued

ossicular chain
otitis media with effusion
otosclerosis
ototoxic
outer (external) ear
palatine tonsils
presbycusis
pressure-equalizing
 (PE) tube

proprioception/
 proprioceptive
pure-tone audiometry
retrocochlear hearing
 loss
sensorineural hearing
 loss
sign language
speech audiometry

speechreading
tinnitus
total communication
tympanic membrane
 (eardrum)
tympanometry
Valsalva maneuver
vestibular system

CHAPTER OUTLINE

INTRODUCTION

The hearing mechanism is a system that takes physical energy and transforms it into chemical and electrical activity for us to hear the sounds in our environment. The auditory system includes the outer, middle, and inner ear structures and the auditory nervous system. Hearing loss is the most common of all physical impairments. The two major types of hearing impairments in children and adults are hearing sensitivity impairments and auditory nervous system impairments. Hearing screening of newborn infants is increasingly being performed in many hospitals. Hearing evaluations of children and adults attempt to determine the nature and extent of hearing loss. The evaluation information can provide important direction for rehabilitation. The goal of hearing rehabilitation is to limit the extent of any communication disorder that results from a hearing loss. Hearing aids and now cochlear implants may be used by individuals of most any age. Sign language (*manualism*) is a natural form of communication for many deaf children and adults when communicating among themselves. There are always emotional and social effects on children and adults who have a hearing loss.

ANATOMY AND PHYSIOLOGY OF THE HEARING MECHANISM

The hearing mechanism and auditory (L. *auditorius,* hearing) system are remarkable in both their simplicity and complexity. They take physical energy (i.e., acoustic air pressure waves) and transform it into chemical and electrical activity to allow us to hear the world around us. They continually monitor the environment for potential danger (e.g., the sound of footsteps behind you) while processing acoustic signals as complex as speech or music. (Note: Although the hearing mechanism is bilateral, descriptions usually refer to the singular, with most illustrations and models being of the right ear.)

Hearing is a distance sense unaffected by many barriers that interfere with sight, touch, smell, and taste. Sound can bend around corners with little distortion, and in many conditions it is possible to tell the direction of the source of the sound (*localization*). It is the millisecond difference between when a sound coming from the side reaches one ear and when it reaches the other ear that allows us to know from which direction it is coming. However, when a sound *reverberates* (reflects off of other surfaces), it is more difficult to distinguish the location of the source.

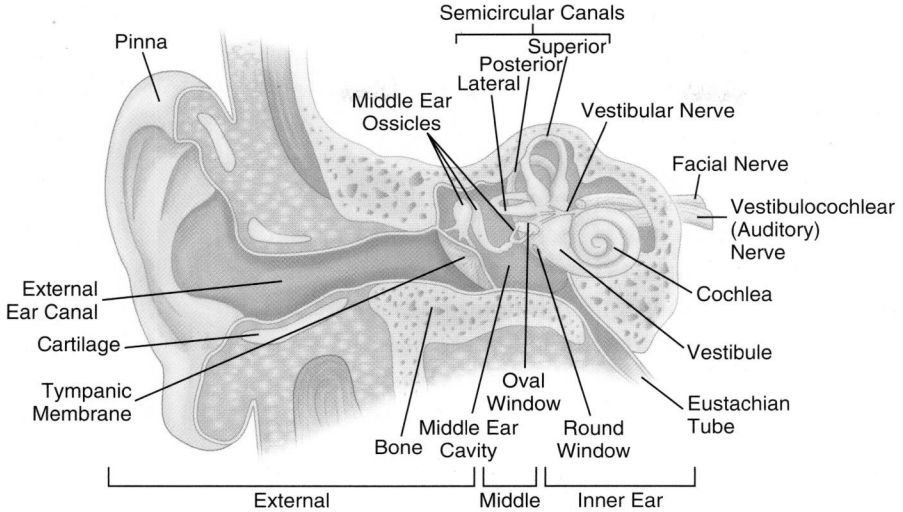

Figure 14–1

The human peripheral auditory system has three divisions: external, middle, and inner ear. The external ear consists of the pinna (auricle) and the external ear canal (external auditory meatus). The tympanic membrane (eardrum) closes off the medial end of the external ear canal. The middle ear is an air-filled cavity that contains the three middle ear ossicles. The middle ear cavity is connected to the nasopharynx by the **Eustachian tube**. The inner ear includes the cochlea, vestibule, and three semicircular canals. The cochlea contains the end organ for hearing. The vestibule and three semicircular canals contain the end organs for balance and motion detection.

© Cengage Learning 2013.

The physical processing of acoustic (Gk. *akoustikos,* hearing) information occurs in three groups of structures, commonly known as the outer, middle, and inner ear (see Figure 14–1). Physiological processing begins in the inner ear and continues along the *auditory nerve* (VIII cranial nerve) to the central auditory nervous system.

Outer Ear

The **outer (external) ear** collects and resonates sound, assists in localizing the direction from which sound is coming, and helps protect the middle ear. The three main parts of the outer ear are the *auricle* (L. *auricula,* little ear) or pinna (L. *pinna,* feather; the cartilaginous portion you see), the *ear canal (external auditory canal)*, and the outer surface of the **tympanic membrane (eardrum)**. The upper rim of the ear is the *helix* (Gk. coil), and the lower flabby portion is the *lobule* (Gk. *lobos,* lobe).

The external ear canal is a narrow channel or tube with a slight upward angle. It leads from an opening in the side of the temporal bone in the skull to the tympanic membrane, a distance of approximately 1 inch (2.5 cm) in adults. Rather than round, the canal is oval, with its height greater than its width. The canal contains sebaceous glands that secrete

Eustachian (auditory) tube

A tube lined with mucous membrane that joins the nasopharynx and the middle ear cavity that is normally closed but opens during yawning, chewing, and swallowing to allow equalization of air pressure in the middle ear with atmospheric pressure.

outer (external) ear

The concave, somewhat funnel-like structure that collects, resonates, and directs sound waves to the tympanic membrane, assists in localizing the direction from which sound is coming, and helps protect the middle ear; composed of the auricle (pinna), ear canal, and outer layer of the tympanic membrane.

tympanic membrane (eardrum)

A thin, semitransparent membrane that separates the ear canal from the middle ear and transmits sound vibrations into the middle ear.

cerumen

A yellowish or brownish waxy secretion produced by ceruminous glands in the ear canal that protects the ear canal from intrusion by insects.

hearing threshold

In audiometry, the level at which a stimulus sound, such as a pure tone, is barely perceptible; usual clinical criteria demand that the level be just high enough for the subject to be aware of the sound at least 50% of the time it is presented.

middle ear

An air-filled chamber located within the temporal bone of the skull; beginning at the inner side of the tympanic membrane and attaching the ossicular chain to the oval window of the cochlea.

ossicular chain

The three small bones (ossicles) of the middle ear named after their basic shapes: *malleus*, for the mallet or hammer; *incus*, for the anvil; and *stapes*, for the stirrup.

cerumen (*sebum* or *earwax*), which helps discourage insects from entering the canal. Men tend to have hair near the opening of the canal, which also helps keep insects out. The length of the canal helps protect the tympanic membrane from trauma and keep it at a constant temperature and humidity. The ear canal directs sound to the tympanic membrane.

The tympanic membrane is a thin, nearly oval, semitransparent membrane with a vertical diameter of about 10 mm (a little less than 1/2 inch) that separates the ear canal from the middle ear and transmits sound waves (vibrations) into the middle ear. The tympanic membrane is fairly taut, like a drum, and it vibrates at the same rate (*frequency*) and magnitude (*intensity*) as the sound waves that reach it. It is an extremely efficient vibrating surface. Movement of one-billionth of a centimeter is sufficient to produce a **hearing threshold** response in normal-hearing individuals in the 800- to 6000-Hz range (i.e., the level at which a sound is just sufficient to produce a sensation—the person can barely detect the sound) (Harris, 1986).

Middle Ear

The **middle ear** is an air-filled chamber located within the temporal bone of the skull for protection (see Figure 14–2). It begins at the inner surface of the tympanic membrane and extends to the *oval window*. The entire middle ear, including the tympanic membrane, is lined with mucous membrane.

The middle ear contains the **ossicular chain**, which consists of three joined bones named after their basic shapes: the *malleus*, for the mallet or hammer; the *incus*, for the anvil; and the *stapes*, for the stirrup. The ossicles are suspended in the middle ear cavity and connect the tympanic membrane to the oval window of the *cochlea*. The ossicles provide a bridge between the tympanic membrane and the cochlea,

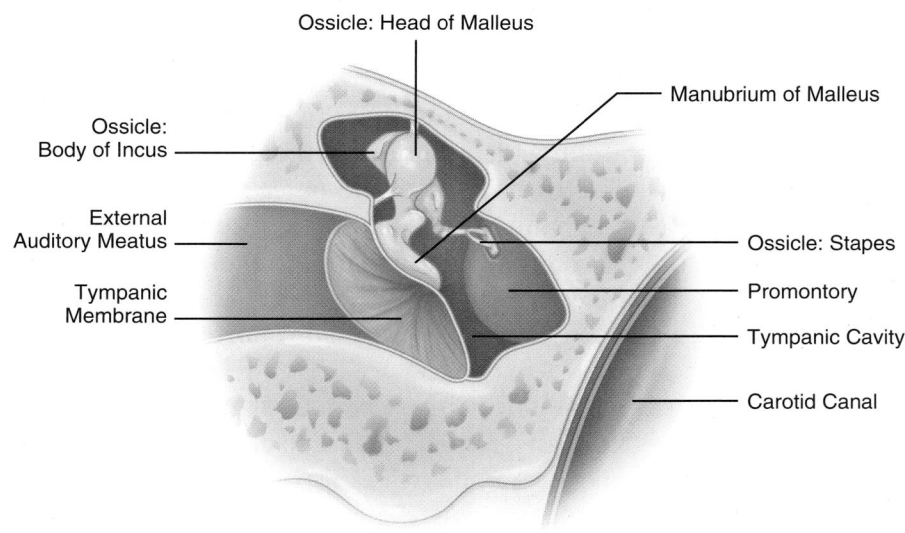

Figure 14–2

Tympanic membrane, middle ear, and ossicles.
© Cengage Learning 2013.

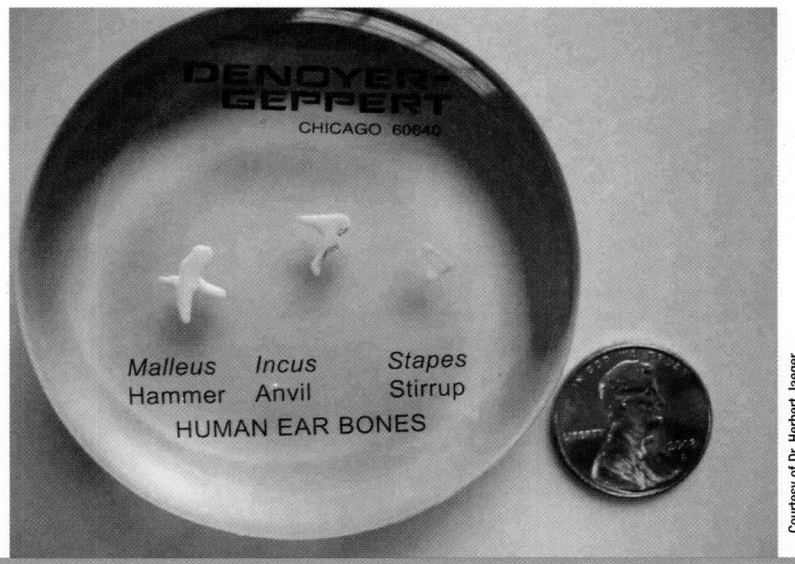

Figure 14–3

The size of the ossicles in relation to a penny (a penny is 20 mm [≈¾ inch] in diameter).

and they are set into vibration by the eardrum. Each of the ossicles is so delicately poised by its ligament connections within the middle ear that their collective function is unaltered by gravity when the head changes in position (Martin & Clark, 2012). The photograph in Figure 14–3 illustrates the size of the ossicles in relation to a penny. Vibrations of the tympanic membrane are conducted along the ossicular chain to the oval window of the cochlea. It is the action of the ossicles that provides the energy transformation for which the middle ear is designed.

The Eustachian Tubes

Air in the left and right middle ear cavities is kept at atmospheric air pressure by way of the Eustachian tubes. The Eustachian tubes lead from the middle ear to the nasopharynx at a downward angle of approximately 30 degrees in adults for a distance of about 35 mm (≈1¼ inches) (see Figure 14–1). In infants, the Eustachian tubes are shorter and in a more horizontal plane than they are in adults. The tubes are bone in the superior one-third and cartilage in the inferior two-thirds. The *orifices* (openings) of the Eustachian tubes are normally closed at the nasopharyngeal ends; however, they tend to remain open in infants until the age of about 6 months. They normally open with the oral and pharyngeal movements used during chewing, swallowing, yawning, and sneezing to allow air to enter the tubes and flow into the middle ear cavities, equalizing the atmospheric and middle ear pressure (*pressure equalization*) to maximize mobility of the tympanic membrane (recall from Chapter 12, Motor Speech Disorders and Dysphagia/Swallowing Disorders, that we swallow approximately 600 times a day, giving many opportunities for equalization of middle ear pressure, plus all of those provided by chewing). However, when atmospheric air pressure changes suddenly (e.g., going up or down in an elevator or ascending or descending in an airplane), the middle ear cavities will have relatively more or less pressure and

Valsalva maneuver

The procedure of closing the mouth and pinching the nostrils closed with the fingers and forcefully exhaling air, usually causing the Eustachian tubes to open and air to flow into the middle ear to equalize middle ear cavity air pressure with atmospheric air pressure, for example, when going up or down in an elevator or ascending or descending in an airplane, causing the ears to "pop"; any exhaling of air against tightly closed vocal folds, as when lifting heavy objects.

cochlea

The part of the inner ear containing the sensory mechanism of hearing; a spiral tunnel with 2¾ turns about 30 mm (about 1¼ inches) long, resembling a tiny snail shell.

vestibular system

The inner ear structures associated with balance and position sense, including the vestibule and semicircular canals of the vestibular mechanism, with interactions of the visual and **proprioceptive** systems and connection to the cerebellum.

proprioception/ proprioceptive

The sensation of body position and movement using sensory signals from muscles, joints, and skin.

Figure 14-4

The cochlea and semicircular canals are surrounded by the temporal bone for protection (view is looking from above down onto the cochlea and semicircular canals).

© Cengage Learning 2013.

a feeling of "fullness" in the middle ear can occur. The tympanic membrane is pressed outward as atmospheric air pressure decreases (ascending altitude) and pressed inward as atmospheric air pressure increases (descending altitude). A method of intentionally opening the Eustachian tubes is the **Valsalva maneuver**, where the mouth and nose are held closed while forcing air into the Eustachian tubes, causing the ears to "pop."

Flying and the Eustachian Tubes

Some people have had their eardrums rupture on airplane flights when their Eustachian tubes were not functioning normally because they were ill with an *upper respiratory infection* (URI) (common cold). They may have attempted to use the Valsalva maneuver to equalize the changing air pressure when they were ascending or descending, although without success, resulting in one or both tympanic membranes rupturing. Although this is relatively rare, anyone with an upper respiratory infection should give flying a second thought when their ears are "plugged up."

Babies unintentionally use the Valsalva maneuver when they start to cry when in an airplane that is ascending or descending. The loud crying causes the Eustachian tubes to open and equalize the middle ear cavity pressure with the changing air pressure inside the cabin of the plane. Once the plane has leveled out, the air pressure is stabilized and the baby is comfortable again.

Inner Ear

The inner ear consists of two important structures; the **cochlea** and the **vestibular system** (see Figure 14-4). The delicate cochlea is protected by being housed inside the temporal bone of the skull. The cochlea is the

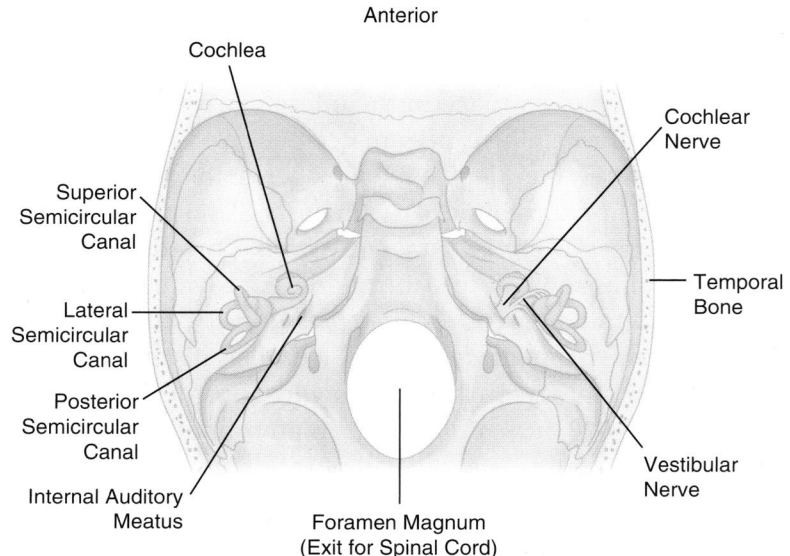

part of the inner ear that contains the sensory mechanism of hearing. It resembles a tiny snail shell with its 2¾-turn spiral tunnel and, uncoiled, is about 30 mm (about 1¼ inches) long. The cochlea is actually full size at the time of birth, which is important for the anatomical feasibility of **cochlear implants** in infants and young children. The cochlea has two fluid-filled tubes that are separated by the *basilar membrane*. The cochlea has over 15,000 tiny hair cells that are stimulated by movement of the cochlear fluid in response to sound.

The vibration of the stapes in the middle ear against the oval window of the cochlea creates motion of the fluid in the cochlea, resulting in stimulation of the hair cells that send neural impulses to the *auditory nerve* (*VIII cranial nerve*). Hair cells in different portions of the cochlea are stimulated by different frequencies of sound (higher frequencies are nearer the oval window and lower frequencies are farther from the oval window).

The Vestibular Mechanism

The vestibular mechanism of the inner ear acts as a motion detector and is affected by forces of gravity and inertia. The immediate entryway into the inner ear is the vestibule, which is filled with fluid. It is within the vestibular portion of the inner ear that the organs of equilibrium are housed. The vestibular system maintains a person's balance and interacts with the visual and proprioceptive systems that send their inputs to the cerebellum.

The vestibular mechanism's three *semicircular canals* contain fluid. Each semicircular canal lies at a different angle (plane), and as a person moves the head or body the fluid stimulates different portions of the semicircular canals, sending the sensation to the vestibulocochlear nerve (see Figure 14–5). When a person is tumbled around (e.g., in the ocean by heavy waves), the vestibular system becomes "confused" and

Application Question

Have you ever pinched your nose tightly to stifle a sneeze? What do you think could happen to some mucus that would normally be blown out of your nose?

cochlear implant

A device that enables individuals with profound hearing loss to perceive sound through an array of electrodes that are surgically implanted in the cochlea and deliver electrical signals to the vestibularcochlear (VIII cranial) nerve, and an external amplifier that activates the electrode array.

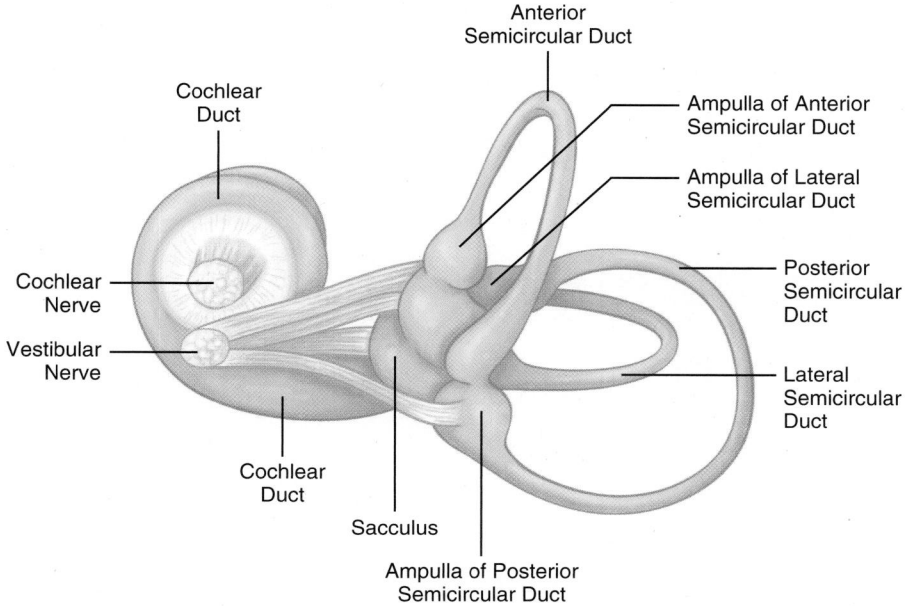

Figure 14–5

The semicircular canals of the vestibular mechanism.

© Cengage Learning 2013.

does not know which way is up (people have drowned because of that). Motion sickness (*kinesia*) is caused by erratic or rhythmic motions (such as in a boat or car) that stimulate the semicircular canals and can result in nausea, headache, and *vertigo* (a sensation of instability, loss of equilibrium, or spinning). Note: Some audiologists include in their practices *vestibular (balance) disorders*, although these disorders are beyond the scope of this text.

AUDITORY NERVOUS SYSTEM

The auditory nervous system is primarily an afferent system that sends neural (electrical) impulses from the cochlea to the auditory cortex in the temporal lobes of the brain. The hair cells have axons that leave the cochlea and form the cochlear branch of the vestibulocochlear nerve and synapse in the medulla of the brainstem. Approximately 75% of the impulses from the right ear are transmitted to the left hemisphere, and 75% of the impulses from the left ear are transmitted to the right hemisphere. The other 25% of impulses from each ear ascend to the *ipsilateral* (same side) hemisphere of the brain, allowing for *redundant pathways* (i.e., most information is sent to one hemisphere of the brain but some information also is sent to the other hemisphere). However, what is received in the right hemisphere must be sent by way of the corpus callosum to the temporal lobe in the left hemisphere for further auditory processing because in most people the left hemisphere is dominant for processing speech and language (Hixon, Weismer, & Holt, 2008; Seikel, King, & Drumright, 2010).

Central Auditory Nervous System

The central auditory nervous system has several synaptic junctions before reaching the primary auditory cortex (*Heschl's gyrus*) (see Figure 14–6)

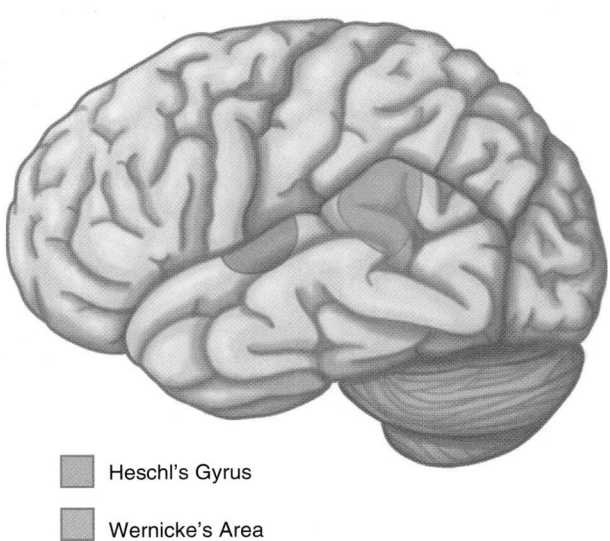

Figure 14–6

The primary auditory cortex (Heschl's gyrus) and Wernicke's area.

© Cengage Learning 2013.

    Heschl's Gyrus

    Wernicke's Area

in the temporal lobe of each hemisphere (Katz, Medwetsky, Burkard, & Hood, 2009). What begins as a pressure wave striking the tympanic membrane sets into motion a complex series of neural responses that spread throughout the auditory system. Processing of speech information occurs throughout the central auditory system, although its primary language processing occurs in the left temporal lobe. Recall from the section on language processing in Chapter 3, Anatomy and Physiology of Speech and Language, that auditory processing, auditory comprehension, and language processing involve numerous levels of skills that overlap and are essentially inseparable (Bellis, 2003; Geffner & Ross-Swain, 2007). Briefly, these skills include sensation, auditory attention, auditory discrimination, auditory association, auditory memory, and auditory cohesion.

HOW WE HEAR

The auditory system is able to both detect the smallest of pressure waves causing the faintest of sounds (*hearing sensitivity*) and discriminate minute changes in the nature of sound, such as pitch and intensity (*hearing acuity*). Hearing sensitivity involves hearing threshold and **differential threshold** (the smallest difference that can be detected between two auditory signals).

Stach (2010, p. 75) describes hearing in the following way:

differential threshold

The smallest difference that can be detected between two auditory signals.

> Our ability to hear relies on this very sophisticated series of structures that process sound. The pressure waves of sound are collected by the pinna and funneled to the tympanic membrane by the external auditory canal. The tympanic membrane vibrates in response to the sound, which sets the ossicular chain into motion. The mechanical movement of the ossicular chain then sets the fluids of the cochlea in motion, causing the hair cells on the basilar membrane to be stimulated. These hair cells send neural impulses from the VIII cranial nerve to the auditory brainstem. From the brainstem, networks of neurons act on the neuronal stimulation, sending the signals to the auditory cortex.

TYPES AND CAUSES OF HEARING IMPAIRMENTS

Hearing loss often has been called an "invisible condition" or "invisible handicap," yet its effect may be anything but invisible. The consequences of hearing loss may be seen in almost all aspects of a person's life.

Normal, everyday communication may be difficult or impossible as a consequence of hearing loss. A *communication handicap* involves the psychosocial disadvantages that result from hearing loss (Tye-Murray, 2009). The age of onset, type, and severity of the hearing impairment are the first considerations when working with an individual with a hearing loss. Because of hearing loss, a young child may have delays in development of speech, language, social skills, and educational achievement.

The term *impairment* is used to describe an abnormality in the structure or function of the ear. There are two primary types of hearing impairments in children and adults: hearing sensitivity impairments and auditory nervous system impairments. **Hearing sensitivity impairments** and *peripheral hearing loss* are the most common type of hearing loss (Bess & Humes, 2008; Martin & Clark, 2012). They are a reduction in the sensitivity of the auditory mechanism that results in sounds needing to be a higher intensity than normal before they can be heard by the listener. Auditory nervous system impairments are the result of reduced ability to hear sounds above the *hearing threshold* (the level at which a sound is barely detectable). **Auditory nervous system impairments** or *(central) auditory processing disorders* occur less often and individuals with them may have hearing sensitivity impairments concurrently, causing a dual auditory problem.

Incidence

Hearing loss is the most common of all physical impairments. Among infants and children, approximately 1 in every 22 newborns in the United States has some kind of hearing problem, and 1 in every 1,000 infants has a severe to profound hearing loss (ASHA, 2008a). Of school-age children, 83 out of 1,000 have an "educationally significant hearing loss" (National Information Center for Children and Youth with Disabilities, 2004). In a 2003–2004 study of 5,742 Americans ages 20 to 69 years, 16% (29 million) had hearing loss in one ear (9%) or both ears (7%). Men were 5.5 times more likely than women to have a hearing loss. Hearing loss prevalence occurred earlier among research participants who smoked, had noise exposure, or cardiovascular disease (Agrawal, Platz, & Niparko, 2008). The National Institute of Deafness and Communication Disorders (2002) reported that 54% of individuals over 65 years of age have some degree of hearing loss. In the Scandinavian countries of Denmark, Finland, Norway, and Sweden and in the United Kingdom, hearing loss also has a high incidence, with 20% in the general population having some degree of loss (Barton et al., 2001).

Hearing Sensitivity Impairments

When sound is not conducted normally through the outer ear, middle ear, or both, the result is a **conductive hearing loss**. When the sensory

---

hearing sensitivity impairment

The most common type of hearing loss; a reduction in the sensitivity of the auditory mechanism that results in sounds needing to be a higher intensity than normal before they can be heard by the listener.

auditory nervous system impairment

The result of reduced ability to clearly hear sounds above the hearing threshold; occurs less often than hearing sensitivity impairments, which may occur concurrently, causing a dual hearing problem.

conductive hearing loss

A reduction in hearing sensitivity because of a disorder of the outer or middle ear.

or neural cells or their connections within the cochlea are absent or are not functioning normally, a **sensorineural hearing loss** occurs. When both the conductive mechanism (outer ear, middle ear, or both) and the cochlea are not functioning normally, there is a **mixed hearing loss**. **Retrocochlear hearing loss** is a hearing disorder resulting from a *neoplasm* (tumor) or other lesion located on cranial nerve VIII or beyond in the auditory brainstem or cortex.

Conductive Hearing Loss

A decrease in the strength of a sound is referred to as *attenuation*. When a soft sound is attenuated because of poor conduction through the outer or middle ear, it may not have sufficient magnitude to reach the cochlea. A conductive hearing loss is easily experienced when you cover your ears tightly with your hands and try to listen to a conversation. Some words you hear clearly because they are spoken louder or there is more acoustic energy in the sounds of the words, other words may be misunderstood, and still other words are not heard at all.

Hearing Loss and the Outer Ear and the External Auditory Canal

Some disorders or malformations of the outer ear may occur that result in hearing loss, for example malformations of the *auricle (pinna)*. *Otic atresia* (Gk. *ous,* ear, *a-,* without, + *tresis,* opening) of the external auditory canal may occur where some or all of the canal is congenitally malformed or absent. Some otic atresias may occur because of traumas or severe burns. Otic atresia, unless surgically repaired, causes conductive hearing loss. Surgical procedures for correction of otic atresia are often successful, particularly when the cartilaginous portion of the canal and the tympanic membrane are normal.

External otitis (L. *externus,* outward, Gk. *ous,* ear, + *itis,* inflammation) is an infection that occurs in the skin of the external auditory canal. The condition is often seen in people who have had water trapped in their ear canals and is referred to as *swimmer's ear.* External otitis is usually caused by bacterial infection, but it can be caused by fungus (*otomycosis*). Itching is a common complaint with mild infections, and extreme pain often accompanies advanced infections. Edema of the ear canal may be present, but the canal usually is not completely occluded. There typically is not a noticeable loss of hearing during the infection. Medical treatment includes irrigating the ear canal with warm salt water, drying it carefully, and applying a topical antibiotic (Mosby, 2009).

Some people have copious amounts of cerumen that occludes the ear canal, creating a conductive hearing loss. However, when people try to remove the earwax themselves, they may end up pushing it further into the ear canal (*impacted cerumen*), even against the tympanic membrane. The cerumen needs to be properly removed. It is now within the

sensorineural hearing loss

A reduction in hearing sensitivity because of a disorder of the cochlea.

mixed hearing loss

A reduction in hearing because of a combination of a disordered outer or middle ear and inner ear.

retrocochlear hearing loss

A hearing disorder resulting from a *neoplasm* (tumor) or other lesion located on cranial nerve VIII or beyond in the auditory brainstem or cortex.

Application Question

Have you ever experienced a temporary conductive hearing loss? What was it like? What were some of your thoughts and feelings about it that you can recall?

scope of practice of audiologists who are specifically trained to perform this procedure (Wilson & Roeser, 1997).

Foreign bodies in the external ear canal are common, particularly in children. If something can fit into the ear canal, some child has probably gotten it stuck in there. In some cases, when an object has been in the canal for too long, swelling and infection may occur. Surgical removal of the foreign object under a microscope is sometimes required. When the external ear canal is occluded by a foreign object, there is a conductive hearing loss on that side.

Perforation (rupture) of the tympanic membrane can occur in many ways. Direct trauma from pointed objects such as hairpins during attempts to remove earwax has occurred. The tympanic membrane may be perforated by concussion from explosions or a hand clapped hard over the ear. The tympanic membrane also may be perforated when there is excessive buildup of fluid in the middle ear during a middle ear infection. Conductive hearing loss occurs with perforation of the tympanic membrane.

Hearing Loss and the Middle Ear

Several causes of middle ear problems result in hearing loss. The age of the person tends to determine the likely causes, with young children commonly having *otitis media* and *otosclerosis* being an adult problem. We discuss only the most common problems of the various ages.

otitis media with effusion

Any inflammation or infection of the middle ear; particularly common in childhood and often associated with a common cold, allergies, sinus infections, and sore throats; Eustachian tube malfunction typically is the physiological cause; effusion— the escape of fluid from tissue as a result of seepage.

Otitis Media (Middle Ear Infection)   Otitis media with effusion (middle ear infection) is one of the most common disorders of the middle ear. Otitis media is any inflammation, infection, or both of the mucous membrane lining the interior of the middle ear, commonly with *purulent* (pus-producing) organisms resulting in *effusion* (fluid in the middle ear) (see Figure 14–7). Middle ear infections occur in almost 70% of children born in the United States before they are two years old, with many of these children experiencing more than one episode (Siegel & Bien, 2004). In a Chinese study of more than 3,000 children 3 to 6 years old, otitis media was present in almost 10% of the children (Chen, Lin, Hwang, & Ku, 2003).

Children who are exposed to tobacco smoke are more likely to have middle ear infections than other children (Kraemer et al., 1983). *Upper respiratory infections* (common colds), allergies, sinus infections (*sinusitis*), and sore throats caused by infections are also common contributors to otitis media. Often the infection is literally blown through the orifice of the Eustachian tube and into the middle ear by a stifled sneeze or by blowing the nose too hard (keeping the mouth open during sneezing and blowing the nose with just moderate force can help prevent forcing bacterial or viral infections into the Eustachian tube and middle ear).

Although otitis media is primarily a disease of childhood, it can occur at any age. When a Eustachian tube is infected, it becomes swollen, interfering with its middle ear pressure-equalization function. With a swollen Eustachian tube, the air inside the middle ear is trapped

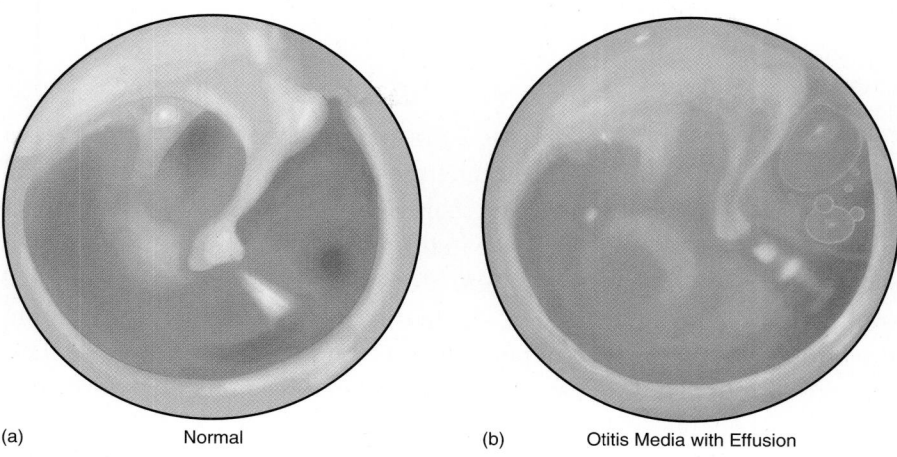

(a)   Normal   (b)   Otitis Media with Effusion

Figure 14–7

Illustrations of a normal tympanic membrane (a), and during an episode of otitis media with effusion (b). The normal membrane is sufficiently translucent that some underlying structures can be seen. The ear with otitis may show considerable redness, distention of the membrane, and the presence of fluid, ranging from clear to amber. Underlying structures are not typically visible as they are in the normal state.

© Cengage Learning 2013.

and begins to be absorbed by the mucosa (walls) of the middle ear cavity. This creates a slight vacuum effect (negative pressure) in the middle ear. The lining of the middle ear then becomes inflamed. If allowed to persist, fluid from the inflamed tissue begins to seep through the mucosal walls into the middle ear cavity (effusion). A conductive hearing loss results once this fluid is sufficient to impede normal movement of the tympanic membrane and ossicles. Harmful bacteria in the fluid can cause a middle ear infection.

Some behaviors of children with middle ear infections include irritability, difficulty hearing normal conversational levels, and turning up the television volume. As the infection worsens, children usually have elevated temperatures and are visibly ill. It is important for parents to take their child to a physician *as soon as possible* because by the time symptoms are apparent the infection may already have been present for a few days and a course of antibiotics may take a week to 10 days to be completed (recall from the discussion on "Auditory Processing Disorders" in Chapter 13 that middle ear infections are often associated with auditory processing disorders).

Medical treatment of otitis media is imperative, and without it there can be permanent damage to the middle ear structures. If the condition continues even further, the tympanic membrane may rupture (Klein, 2000). Pus that cannot find its way out of the middle ear may invade the *mastoid bone* (a protrusion of the temporal bone behind the outer ear), causing **mastoiditis**. Untreated mastoiditis can result in *meningitis* and sometimes death (Bess & Humes, 2008; Martin & Clark, 2012).

mastoiditis

An infection of one of the mastoid bones (just behind the ear) that is usually an extension of a middle ear infection, characterized by earache, fever, headache, and malaise; medical treatment may require intravenous antibiotics for several days, and residual hearing loss may follow the infection.

CASE STUDY

Jennifer

Jennifer was a 4-year-old girl when she experienced her first middle ear infection. She also suffered from allergies and began having occasional sinus infections, which may have contributed to the middle ear infections. The child's pediatrician treated her several bouts of otitis media with effusion with antibiotics and decongestants—common medical treatments. However, on one occasion the child had a severe reaction to the antibiotic, a derivative of penicillin, and had to be hospitalized for a few days. From that point, she could no longer have penicillin-derivative antibiotics because of a future life-threatening allergic reaction to them. The parents, both professionals in the medical field, took Jennifer to a local *otologist* (a physician who specializes in ear diseases and disorders) for placement of PE tubes. Over the next few years, Jennifer had six sets of PE tubes but continued to have allergies, sinus infections, and middle ear infections.

The parents began to feel that the adenoids might be the "culprits" in contributing to the middle ear infections, and they took Jennifer (now age 7) to an otolaryngologist who took x-rays of the nasopharyngeal region to determine the size of the adenoids. They were significantly enlarged and were occluding the opening of the Eustachian tubes and preventing normal aeration of the middle ear. The enlarged adenoids also prevented the child from being a normal nasal breather, forcing her to breathe through her mouth (an indication of enlarged adenoids is if a child cannot chew food with the mouth closed, even with repeated encouragement). The child was scheduled for an adenoidectomy and tonsillectomy in outpatient, short-stay surgery at a local hospital. The otolaryngologist did a postoperative visit with the parents and told them that Jennifer's adenoids were "the size of oysters." The removal of the adenoids took care of most of the middle ear infections, although the child later needed sinus surgery for more complete removal of sinus drainage to help end the sinus infections. A 3-year course of allergy shots helped take care of the chronic allergy problems that contributed to her sinus infections. As many parents learn, much of the ongoing expense of raising children is centered on the eyes (glasses and contacts), ears (middle ear infections), nose (allergies and sinus infection), and mouth (dental care and orthodontia). ■

Surgical Management for Otitis Media   When a child has had *recurrent otitis media* (usually a series of three to five middle ear infections in a 1-year period), many otolaryngologists or *otologists* (physicians who specialize in diseases and disorders of the ear) will consider surgical management. The primary purpose of surgery for patients with middle ear infections is to eliminate disease, and in some cases reconstruction of a damaged hearing mechanism is needed. The procedures are typically performed in an outpatient surgical setting and the patient is allowed to go home that same day.

Dormant Otitis Media

When the proper type and sufficient dosage of antibiotics are not used, the infection may move into a dormant state rather than being eliminated (*resolved*). Because the overt symptoms may disappear, the patient and family may assume that the otitis media has been cured. However, a few to several weeks later the patient may experience what seems like a new bout of otitis media, which is in reality an exacerbation of the same condition experienced earlier but allowed to lie dormant. Many patients discontinue their own antibiotic treatment when their symptoms abate, leaving some of the hardier bacteria alive. Then, when the condition flares up again, it is the result of a stronger strain, one less susceptible to medication (Martin & Clark, 2012). There is increasing concern among physicians and medical scientists about both children and adults having decreased benefits from antibiotics because of improper use of them and overreliance on them for a variety of illnesses, allowing some forms of bacteria to develop immunity to antibiotics (Lutter, Currie, Mitz, & Greenbaum, 2005; Samore et al., 2001).

A *myringotomy* (L. *myringa,* eardrum, + Gk. *temnein,* to cut) is performed in which a small surgical incision is made into the tympanic membrane to relieve pressure and release fluid or pus from the middle ear (see Figure 14–8a). A small suction device may be inserted through the incision to delicately suction out the fluid and pus. Antibiotics are given before and continued afterward to manage the infection (Mosby, 2009).

Following the myringotomy and cleaning of the middle ear, the otolaryngologist may insert a **pressure-equalizing (PE) tube** through the incision in the tympanic membrane (see Figure 14–8b and Figure 14–9). The tube is plastic, tiny, and hollow with a flange on each

pressure-equalizing (PE) tube

A small silicone tube inserted into the tympanic membrane following a myringotomy to equalize air pressure between the middle ear cavity and the atmosphere as a substitute for a nonfunctional Eustachian tube.

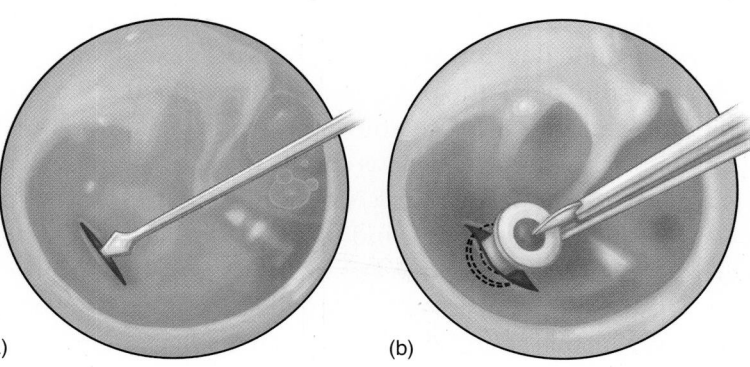

(a)   (b)

Figure 14–8

(a) A myringotomy incision. (b) A pressure-equalizing tube positioned through the tympanic membrane to allow middle ear ventilation.

© Cengage Learning 2013.

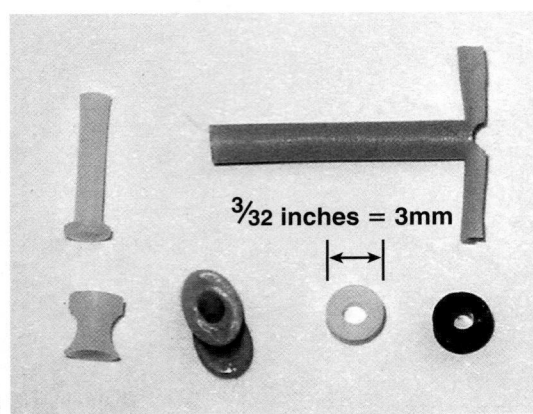

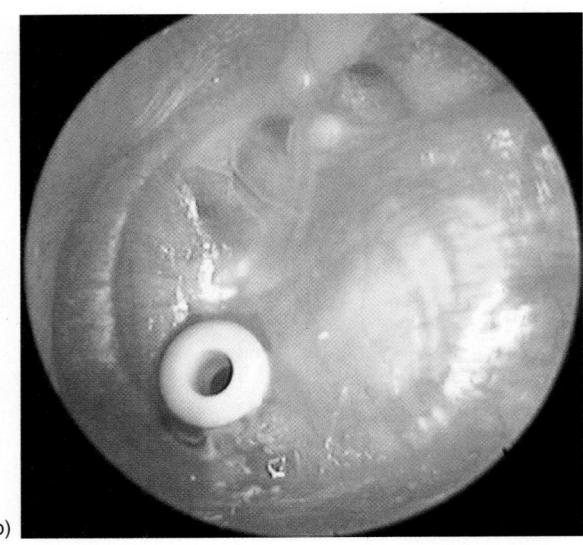

3/32 inches = 3mm

(a)

(b)

Figure 14–9

(a) Types of pressure-equalizing tubes. (b) Photo of a pressure-equalizing tube inserted in the tympanic membrane.

Copyright http://www.entusa.com. Used with permission.

end that prevents the tube from falling into the middle ear or falling out of the tympanic membrane prematurely. The tube allows direct ventilation of the middle ear and functions as an artificial Eustachian tube to maintain normal middle ear air pressure. The tube may remain in place from several weeks to several months, after which time it *extrudes* (pushes out) naturally into the external auditory canal, usually without the child noticing. Newer-designed tubes may remain in place indefinitely.

Some children with middle ear infections have enlarged **adenoids (pharyngeal tonsils)** that may be occluding the openings to the Eustachian tubes and preventing aeration of the middle ear, leading to middle ear infections. Adenoids are made of *lymphoid tissue* (tissue that produces lymphocytes that are helpful in fighting infection) and are found in the *nasal–pharyngeal region* (on the pharyngeal wall above the soft palate, which does not allow them to be seen during an oral examination). They begin to develop about 6 months of age and may continue to grow and possibly block the passage of air from the nasal cavity into the pharynx, preventing nasal breathing and requiring mouth breathing (during an oral examination, clinicians should always determine whether a child is a nasal or mouth breather). Mouth breathing is a good indicator of enlarged adenoids. Another indicator of a child having enlarged adenoids is whether he has enlarged **palatine tonsils** (see Figure 3–10 for normal tonsils). Both the adenoids and the palatine tonsils normally have *atrophied* (decreased in size) and essentially disappeared by early adolescence.

Adenoidectomy and Tonsillectomy

Adenoidectomy and *tonsillectomy* are surgical procedures that may be performed because the adenoid tissue, tonsillar tissue, or both are enlarged, chronically infected, or causing obstruction. Normal adenoids may be *excised* (cut out) as a *prophylactic* (preventive) measure during a tonsillectomy. The surgery is performed under general anesthesia in children, but a local anesthesia may be used with adults. When the patient has recovered from the anesthesia, ice chips or clear liquids without a drinking straw may be offered (Mosby, 2009). Most of these procedures are now done in the outpatient surgical setting.

Otosclerosis

Otosclerosis is a common problem in adults and is typically hereditary (Chen et al., 2002). Otosclerosis occurs when there is growth of bony tissue around the footplate of the stapes that presses against the oval window, resulting in a conductive hearing loss. The otosclerosis prevents normal vibration and causes attenuation in the cochlea. Otosclerosis usually occurs bilaterally, although the two ears may not begin to be affected at the same time. It is a progressive disorder with onset ranging from mid-childhood to late–middle adulthood. Some individuals in early adolescence begin to notice some hearing loss. Women are more likely to be diagnosed with otosclerosis than men, and its onset is often related to pregnancy (Martin & Clark, 2012).

Auditory Nervous System Impairments

Auditory nervous system impairments may occur in the cochlea, auditory nerve and various synaptic junctions (*retrocochlear*), as well as in the primary auditory cortex (*Heschl's gyrus*) in the temporal lobe of each hemisphere. A problem at a lower level (e.g., cochlea) will send the distorted or errored neural impulses through the rest of the auditory system. Sensorineural hearing loss from cochlear disorders may arise from many causes. Newborns may have inherited disorders that affect the nervous system, as well as congenital malformations of the cochlea. Many disorders may occur at any age, such as infections, acoustic trauma, and *ototoxicity* (harmful effects of certain substances on the VIII cranial nerve or the organs of hearing and balance). *Presbycusis* is a common problem with aging.

Hearing Loss and Disorders of the Inner Ear

Abnormalities and diseases of the cochlea are probably the largest cause of sensorineural hearing impairments, with the delicate hair cells usually being involved. Although the hair cells are damaged, the auditory nerve

---

adenoids (pharyngeal tonsils)

Lymphoid tissue (tissue that produces lymphocytes, which are helpful in fighting infection) found on the pharyngeal wall in the nasal–pharyngeal region; begin to develop about 6 months of age and may continue to grow and possibly interfere with or occlude the openings of the Eustachian tubes; when enlarged, they may block the passage of air from the nasal cavity into the pharynx, preventing normal nasal breathing and requiring mouth breathing; sometimes removed to allow nasal breathing and help prevent middle ear infections.

palatine tonsils

Two almond-shaped masses of lymphoid tissue between the anterior and the posterior faucial pillars.

otosclerosis

Typically a hereditary condition that occurs when there is growth of bony tissue around the footplate of the stapes that presses against the oval window, resulting in a conductive hearing loss, and causing attenuation in the cochlea.

fibers connected to the hair cells often remain intact (this is an important fact with cochlear implants). When there is damage or abnormality in the cochlea, decreased hearing sensitivity is not the only symptom. Individuals often complain of difficulty understanding speech—more specifically, auditory discrimination problems. Drawing primarily from Martin and Clark (2012), and Stach (2010), the following discussions are based on ages of onset.

Prenatal Causes

Prenatal causes refer to adverse effects on the cochlea during embryological and fetal development, resulting in congenital hearing loss. Development of the external, middle, and inner ear takes place between the 4th and 8th weeks of gestation. Some infants have hereditary factors that predispose them to hearing loss. In some cases, there are associated genetic abnormalities that accompany the hearing loss, including skull, facial, and external ear deformities; cleft palate; visual disorders; abnormal skin pigmentation; thyroid disorders; disorders of the heart; musculoskeletal anomalies; cognitive disabilities; difficulty with balance and coordination; and a variety of sensorimotor impairments. In many cases, there may be a combination of genetic and in-utero environmental factors that come into play—that is, *multifactorial genetic considerations.*

Teratogens   As discussed in Chapter 10, Cleft Lip and Palate, teratogens are environmental substances or agents that result in malformations and anomalies of specific organs and systems that are undergoing rapid development in the embryo or fetus. Exposure to teratogens during these periods may result in major congenital anomalies. For example, exposure to teratogens between 21 and 27 days gestation is associated with anomalies of the external ear (Hayes & Northern, 1997). Exposure before the 3rd week of gestation may result in death and spontaneous abortion. There are numerous teratogens, such as drugs and alcohol, congenital HIV and AIDS, *rubella, cytomegalovirus* (CMV), *herpes simplex-type virus, toxoplasmosis,* and *congenital syphilis.*

Perinatal Causes

Perinatal causes of hearing loss are those that occur during the process of birth. Handicapping sensorineural hearing loss occurs in 2% to 4% of neonatal intensive care units (NICU) survivors (Amatuzzi, Northrop, Bento, & Eavey, 2005). Hearing loss in infants who were in NICUs is often associated with the identifiable disorders that caused the need for the NICU or treatment for the disorders, such as low birth weight and hypoxia. *Respiratory distress syndrome* (RDS; also called *hyaline membrane disease*) is the most common respiratory disease in premature infants. Infants who have RDS and become *septic* (generalized infection) are typically treated with antibiotics with potential **ototoxic** properties that place them at risk for hearing loss. *Congenital heart disease* (CHD) is among the most common birth defects; infants with congestive heart

ototoxic

Drugs that have harmful effects on the central auditory nervous system, including aspirin, aminoglycoside antibiotics, furosemide, and quinine.

disease often experience failure-to-thrive and feeding problems. Although CHD in newborns does not cause hearing problems, infants with CHD often have syndromes associated with hearing loss. Numerous central nervous system disorders may have hearing loss as one component of the disorder, including cerebral hemorrhage, hydrocephalus, and *neonatal seizures*. Any disorder that results in hypoxia may affect an infant's neurological status and hearing. Neurological dysfunction by itself does not affect hearing, but it can cause significant auditory processing, speech, and language development problems (Stach, 2010; Tye-Murray, 2009).

Postnatal and Childhood Causes

Postnatal causes of cochlear hearing loss are any factors occurring after birth. *Bacterial meningitis* may cause total deafness. Numerous childhood infections may affect hearing, such as *measles, mumps, chicken pox, influenza,* and *viral pneumonia.* Most virus-producing hearing losses are bilateral, except mumps. The body's natural reaction to infection is elevation of temperature; however, when fever becomes excessive, cellular damage can occur, including cells of the cochlea. Treatment of bacterial infections may necessitate use of ototoxic antibiotics. *Diabetes mellitus* and *kidney disease* have been implicated in sensorineural hearing loss. *Head traumas* may occur at any age and may result in both neurological disorders and hearing loss.

Older Children and Adults

Hearing loss in older children and adults has numerous causes, one of which is mostly preventable (i.e., noise-induced hearing loss). Most people are likely to have reduced hearing as they grow older (particularly after age 60); however, people can do many things to try to preserve their hearing. Hearing is usually one of the things in our lives that we do not think much about until we lose it.

Noise-Induced Hearing Loss and Acoustic Trauma

Noise-induced hearing loss and **acoustic trauma** dates back hundreds (thousands) of years. When World War II soldiers returned from battlefields with hearing impairments, this type of noise-induced hearing loss began attracting attention. Airports to construction sites, street repairs to lawn mowers, and even some large restaurants where you have to talk over the noise, create sustained loud noise, particularly for the workers (see Table 14–1). Noise-induced hearing loss can be temporary or permanent. Exposure to excessive sound results in a change in the threshold of hearing sensitivity. However, the length of time of exposure is also important; the longer the exposure level, the greater the possibility of damage to the hearing mechanism.

Acoustic trauma from a single exposure may cause permanent hearing loss. Gradual hearing loss from repeated exposure to excessive

noise-induced hearing loss

A permanent sensorineural hearing loss caused by exposure to excessive loud noise, often over long periods of time.

acoustic trauma

Damage to hearing from a transient, high-intensity sound.

TABLE 14-1	Decibel Levels of Common Sounds
DECIBELS	**SOUND**
130+	Jet takeoff, gunfire (pain threshold)
120+	Rock concert speaker sound, sandblasting, thunderclap, fireworks, pneumatic drill
110+	Dance club, snowmobile, powerboats, hammering metal
100+	Chain saw, bulldozer
90+	Subway trains, motorcycle, workshop tools (e.g., belt sander), lawn mower
80+	Heavy city traffic, factory noise, vacuum cleaner, garbage disposal, Niagara Falls
70+	Dog barking, noisy restaurant, busy traffic
60+	Ringing telephone, baby crying, alarm clock 2 feet away
50+	Quiet automobile 10 feet away
40+	Everyday conversation
30+	Quiet street at night with no traffic
20+	Whispered conversation
10+	Soft rustle of leaves, birds singing, dripping water faucet
0	Just audible sound

Based on data from: Northern & Downs, 2012; Van Bereijk, Pierce, & David, 1960; and the American Industrial Hygiene Association, 2007.

sound can damage or destroy the delicate hair cells in the cochlea. There is evidence that children and adolescents are suffering increased amounts of hearing loss from toys, phones, stereo systems, musical instruments, and a variety of other noise makers, some of which produce sound up to 155 dB, resulting in self-induced hearing loss (Nadler, 1997). Shargorodsky, Curhan, Curhan, and Eavy (2010) in an article on "Change in Prevalence of Hearing Loss in U.S Adolescents" in the *Journal of the American Medical Association* reported that 12- to 19-year-old U.S. adolescents had a 31% increase in hearing loss from 1988–1994 to 2005–2006, and that one in five adolescents had a hearing loss (6.5 million teens). The most likely cause of such an alarming increase in hearing loss among teens, as well as college students, is the use of MP3 players and earbuds that can present loud music to the ears without disturbing other people around the users (Hoover & Krishnamurti, 2010; Moore, 2010; Shafer, 2006).

The Author's Experience — Personal Story

During my military service in the U.S. Army, the many hours of training on the firing range with a variety of weapons (M16 rifles, 45-caliber pistols, M60 machine guns, M70 grenade launchers, and hand grenades) exposed me to countless sharp, very loud noises and explosions. Further training as a tank driver, with a 90-mm cannon firing directly over my head, exposed me to more painfully loud noise. During my time of service as a combat medic in Vietnam in 1969, not only did I need to fire many rounds with my M16 and an M60, but there were countless mortars and rockets that came in on us—sometimes like rain—with explosions all around. Our personnel would return fire with their "quad-4s" (four 50-caliber machine guns mounted on a turret) and various artillery (it is hard to describe the deafening sounds). Flying in noisy medevac (medical evacuation) helicopters (HU1s ["Hueys"]) with the side door off and insufficient ear protection added to the noise exposure. Realistically, protecting our hearing is not an important concern in combat—survival and doing our "job" are important. I now have some trouble hearing in my right ear—the side only inches from my weapons. I am a normal war veteran. Men and women who survive combat in all wars (currently and in the future) will likely suffer from some hearing loss. ■

What You Can Do to Protect Your Hearing

1. *Know which noises can cause damage.* Noises above 85 dB are most damaging. Whenever possible, avoid loud noises.

2. *Turn down the volume.* Today, many people play their TV sets, home and car stereos, and MP3 players unnecessarily loud (high school and college age are particularly inclined). Consider lowering the volume. When purchasing headphones, look for sets with volume limiters that keep the sound at safe levels. This is especially important when buying them for children and teenagers.

3. *Protect yourself.* Earplugs are inexpensive and come in a variety of types, sizes, and colors.

4. *Reduce your exposure.* Some situations are inherently noisy, but you can decrease the risk of noise-induced hearing loss by avoiding or limiting your time in loud restaurants and clubs. When riding motorcycles, personal watercraft, or other loud vehicles, limit the time you spend on them and wear ear protection.

5. *Remember your neighbors.* Noise from your personal recreation affects not only you but also everyone around you.

Based on information from the American Industrial Hygiene Association, 2007.

Hearing conservation programs can help protect workers from ongoing loud noises. The first line of defense against occupational noise is to diminish loud sounds at the source. Blocking noise with hearing protection devices such as earplugs or earmuffs can help the wearer—but only if they are worn correctly and when necessary. Noise-induced hearing loss is generally painless, progressive, permanent—and preventable. As speech-language pathologists and audiologists, part of our "mission" as professionals is to protect our hearing and to encourage others to protect theirs. Most people are going to lose some of their hearing sooner or later; there is no need for them to lose it sooner than they have to.

Tinnitus

tinnitus

A subjective noise sensation, often described as a ringing, roaring, or swishing in the ear that may be heard in one or both ears; associated with a variety of hearing disorders in both adults and children; can affect concentration, sleep, education, employment, personal relationships, and social functioning, and sometimes is debilitating; treatment success varies.

Tinnitus is a subjective noise sensation that is often described as a ringing, roaring, or swishing in the ear that may be heard in one or both ears. Although tinnitus is more commonly associated with cochlear diseases, it can occur with some middle ear problems, including otosclerosis. The actual source of tinnitus within the auditory system is uncertain; it can likely rise from various sites, from the external ear to the auditory cortex (Sandlin & Olsson, 2000). It may be a sign of otosclerosis, acoustic trauma, Meniere's disease, presbycusis, or an accumulation of cerumen impinging on the eardrum or occluding the external auditory canal. It sometimes occurs for no reason. Many children with hearing loss requiring amplification experience some tinnitus (Gold, 2003). Tinnitus is common enough that tinnitus support groups have been formed in countries around the world (e.g., American Tinnitus Association, Australian Tinnitus Association, British Tinnitus Association, and Tinnitus Association of Canada—see the list of websites provided at the end of this chapter). Although tinnitus may not have a significant deleterious effect on hearing, it can affect concentration, sleep, education, employment, personal relationships, and social functioning. For some people, it may be socially debilitating (Davis & Refaie, 2000). Many treatments have been developed, but all have varying success.

Meniere's Disease

Meniere's disease

A chronic disease of the inner ear characterized by recurrent episodes of vertigo, tinnitus, and sensorineural hearing loss may that be bilateral.

Meniere's disease is a common disorder with an unknown etiology that may involve both the cochlea and the vestibular system. Meniere's disease has a constellation of symptoms, including episodic *vertigo* (sensation of instability or rotation caused by disturbance in the semicircular canals of the inner ear), vomiting, tinnitus, pressure in the involved ear with a feeling of "fullness," and progressive, fluctuating, sensorineural hearing loss that is normally unilateral. The initial recommended medical treatment may be a change in diet, adherence to a low-sodium diet, diuretics, steroids, and/or other medications (Campbell, 2007).

Presbycusis

presbycusis

Hearing loss associated with old age, usually involving both a loss of hearing sensitivity and a reduction in clarity of speech.

Presbycusis (also spelled *presbyacusis*) is a progressive hearing loss as a result of the aging process. Age takes its toll on the entire auditory system (actually, all bodily systems), including the tympanic membrane, ossicular chain, cochlea, and central auditory nervous system. Symptoms of presbycusis are usually seen by age 60. A common characteristic of presbycusis is difficulty understanding speech, although speech is usually more easily understood when it is slower rather than louder. Speech is also more difficult to understand when there is background noise. Some comments made by people with presbycusis (Pichora-Fuller, 1997) are:

- "I hear but I have trouble understanding."
- "I understand when it's quiet but have trouble in a group."
- "People seem to talk too fast; I need more time to make sense of what they're saying."
- "I don't know for sure when I hear correctly and when I don't."

Neural Disorders

Neural disorders can affect the auditory system. *Neuritis,* or inflammation of the auditory nerve, can cause temporary or permanent hearing loss. Multiple sclerosis and brainstem tumors can affect hearing function. *Neoplastic* growths, including carcinoma and various other types of tumors can affect the auditory system.

COMMUNICATIVE DISORDERS OF INDIVIDUALS WITH HEARING IMPAIRMENTS

Several variables affect the type and degree of communication disorders seen in hearing impaired individuals (Hull, 2009; Lee, 2012; Stach, 2010; Tye-Murray, 2009):

1. *Age*—Infants born with hearing impairments (congenital impairments) have more problems with communication than children who have already acquired speech and language.

2. *Severity*—Individuals of any age have more communication problems when the hearing loss is severe rather than mild.

3. *Configuration of the hearing loss*—*Low frequency* hearing loss will affect hearing some consonants and vowels (e.g., /z, v, b, d, m, n, l, i, u, e, o, ɔ/), *middle frequency hearing loss* will affect hearing other sounds (e.g., /a, æ, ʃ, ʧ, p, g, k/), and *high frequency loss* will affect still others (e.g., /f, θ, ð, s/) (see Figure 14–10).

4. *Type of hearing loss*—Individuals with conductive hearing losses may benefit from hearing aids in ways that individuals with sensorineural hearing losses may not.

5. *Beginning of professional care*—When a newborn is identified as having a hearing loss and professional care is initiated, the infant has a better opportunity for speech and language development than an infant who is not identified until 1 year of age or older. The younger and sooner children are identified and begin to receive

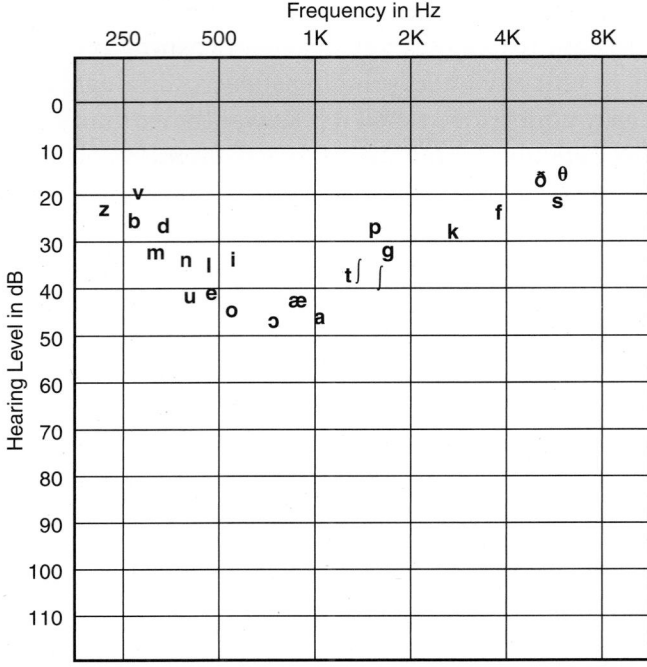

Figure 14–10

Generalized phonetic representations of speech sounds occurring at normal conversational levels plotted on an audiogram.

© Cengage Learning 2013.

comprehensive services, the better their opportunities to develop speech and language. Also, the more involved the parents are with their child's habilitation, the better the child's communication development will likely be.

6. *Presence of other handicaps*—Some children with hearing impairments also have other handicapping conditions, such as developmental delays and auditory processing disorders that compound the difficulty developing speech, language, and cognitive skills.

Speech

The sounds that cannot be heard well are the sounds most difficult to develop. Normal-hearing and normal-speaking individuals sometimes speak with a low intensity, making hearing conversation that much more difficult for individuals with hearing impairments. Final consonants are often spoken with such low intensity that there is barely a "hint" of the sound (e.g., the word *sound* may be spoken by many people so that it is heard more like *soun*). The person with a hearing impairment is unlikely to hear final consonants when there is little stress placed on them and, therefore, to produce them in conversation. Other sounds the person with a hearing impairment does not hear easily are also likely to be omitted, particularly unstressed sounds in blends; for example, *stream* may be heard as *stea*.

Individuals with severe hearing impairments often are confused about voiced and voiceless sounds (*cognates*) and substitute one for the other. For example, /p/ and /b/ may be inconsistently substituted for one another (e.g., *pat* becomes *bat* and *bat* becomes *pat*), as well as

/d/ and /t/ (e.g., *time* becomes *dime* and *dime* becomes *time*). Oral and nasal cognates are sometimes substituted, such as /m/ and /b/ (e.g., *meat* becomes *beat* and *beat* becomes *meat*). Children who develop some lipreading skills tend to recognize "visible" sounds more easily than "invisible" sounds (e.g., /p/ is easier to recognize than /k/).

Stress, speaking rate, breath control, pitch, and intensity (*supra-segmentals*) are common problems for children with significant hearing losses. They tend to have a distinct speech quality. Their speech often sounds breathy, labored, staccato, and arrhythmic. They may place equal stress on all syllables or stress syllables inappropriately (e.g., *baby* may have the stress on the second syllable, sounding like "bah-BEE") (Tye-Murray & Folkins, 1990). Children with severe-to-profound hearing losses typically speak slowly (approximately half the rate of normal-hearing children) and pause often, both within words and between words. Most children who are hard-of-hearing or deaf produce relatively few syllables per breath and use their breath inefficiently. They often let out more breath during connected speech than do children with normal hearing (Forner & Hixon, 1977). The voice quality of severely hearing impaired individuals is often unpleasant. Their pitch may sound excessively high or variable, or they may use a monotone. They often have pitch breaks, with the pitch abruptly changing from high to low. They often speak too softly or too loudly for the situation or environment, and their intensity may fluctuate inappropriately (Tye-Murray, 2009). (See Table 14–2 for more on hearing impairment levels.)

TABLE 14-2	Degree of Hearing Loss and Its Effects on Communication as Indicated by Pure-Tone Audiograms
HEARING LEVEL	**HEARING ABILITY**
Normal (-10 to 10 dB)	Can hear speech normally
Minimal (10 to 25 dB)	Has difficulty hearing faint speech in a noisy place
Mild (25 to 40 dB)	Has difficulty hearing faint or distance speech, even in a quiet environment
Moderate (40 to 55 dB)	Hears conversational speech only at a close distance
Moderately severe (55 to 70 dB)	Hears loud conversational speech
Severe (70 to 90 dB)	Cannot hear conversational speech
Profound (>90 dB)	May hear loud sounds; hearing is not the primary communication channel

Adapted from Stach, 2010.

Language

Regardless of which communication mode children with severe hearing impairments use (aural and oral or signing), most children who are profoundly deaf and who use hearing aids do not learn their native language well (Mahshie, Moseley, Scott, & Lee, 2006; Stiles, McGregor, & Butler, 2012; Vinson, 2011). Ninety percent of children with significant hearing loss are born to parents who have normal hearing. As a result, many children are not exposed to language early because they do not have access to the auditory signal and their parents have not learned sign language to communicate with these children (Tye-Murray, 2009). The grammar of adults with significant hearing loss is usually about the level of 8-year-old normal-hearing children, and their vocabulary development is normally at the fourth-grade level (Bamford & Saunders, 1985). We briefly look at form (syntax and morphology), content (semantics and vocabulary), and pragmatics (use).

Form

Children with hearing impairments tend to use primarily content words (nouns and verbs) and rarely use adverbs, prepositions, or pronouns. They often omit function words (*a, an, the,* etc.). They usually use short subject–verb–object sentences and rarely use compound or complex sentences. Their sentences often sound "telegraphic." Likewise, children with hearing impairments have difficulty understanding the compound and complex sentences used by normal-hearing people (Lee, 2012; Tye-Murray, 2009).

Content

Children with significant hearing losses consistently have weak vocabularies. Weak vocabularies typically mean poor understanding of basic concepts. They may, for example, understand and be able to use a word as a verb (e.g., *stand,* as in *stand up*) but not be able to use the same word as a noun (e.g., *stand,* as in *music stand* or *band stand*). They typically know and use few synonyms and antonyms. Understanding common idioms is a major problem for the hearing impaired. They understand and use concrete words more easily than abstract words (Lee, 2012; Tye-Murray, 2009).

Pragmatics

Children with hearing impairments often do not know how to initiate or maintain a conversation or how to repair breakdowns in communication. They have difficulty with turn-taking and changing topics. They often try to pretend that they are understanding when they are not and, therefore, have inappropriate responses (Tye-Murray, 2009).

Literacy

Children with significant hearing impairments have difficulty not only understanding and using oral language but also reading and writing.

This contributes significantly to their communication problems because they do not have a modality that they can use to clearly understand or communicate their wants, needs, thoughts, and feelings. As discussed in Chapter 7, Literacy Disorders in Children, learning to read and write is more challenging for children than learning to understand and use oral language. This is particularly true for children with hearing impairments.

Reading

Children who are hard of hearing or deaf and use hearing aids often have delays or differences with reading. The average reading and writing skills of high school students who are deaf are at a third- or fourth-grade level, which is barely adequate for reading a newspaper (Allen, 1986). Several interacting factors likely cause reading problems for children who are hearing impaired:

1. They have inadequate aural–oral language systems with deficits in vocabulary and compound and complex sentence structures that interfere with their ability to understand printed text.

2. Children with significant hearing losses do not develop an auditory basis for mapping sound to print (Golding-Meadow & Mayberry, 2001). When hearing impaired children do not have a normal phonological code, they have difficulty "sounding out words" in print that they are unfamiliar with.

3. Many children with hearing impairments do not have normal experiences with world knowledge (e.g., hearing and seeing TV news reports) with which to relate printed stories (e.g., newspaper articles). Many other factors, no doubt, are involved that affect children with hearing impairments abilities to read (Tye-Murray, 2009).

Writing

In general, poor syntax, vocabulary, and word spelling reflect the expressive language abilities of children and adults with hearing impairments. Their writing samples often contain syntactic errors such as omission of articles, inappropriate use of pronouns, and omission of bound morphemes (e.g., -'s and -ed). Most written sentences are simple subject–verb–object forms; rarely are there compound and complex syntactic structures. Synonyms, antonyms, and metaphors are seldom used. Topics are often introduced but not developed or elaborated. Writing narratives where there is a clear beginning, middle, and end to the story are difficult for children with hearing impairments. They are better at writing some factual details about a topic than explaining the theme or the main points of a topic (Shirin & Reed, 2005; Tye-Murray, 2009). Adults with hearing impairments commonly do not feel confident to write sentences to communicate with people who have normal hearing and literacy skills.

AUDITORY PROCESSING DISORDERS

Auditory processing disorders (APD) are mentioned briefly here because they are rather controversial among some audiologists, as they are among some speech-language pathologists; that is, not all of these professionals believe these disorders exist. The term *central auditory processing disorders* (CAPD) has been replaced by *auditory processing disorders* by most speech-language pathologists to emphasize the interactions of disorders at both the peripheral and the central sites without necessarily attributing difficulties to a single anatomical location (Bellis, 2003; Geffner & Ross-Swain, 2007; Jerger, & Musiek, 2000, Musiek & Chermak, 2007). Accurate diagnosis of auditory processing disorders requires a team approach and should include an audiologist, speech-language pathologist, psychologist, and educators. Auditory processing disorders were discussed in some detail in Chapter 13, Special Populations with Communication Disorders.

HEARING ASSESSMENT

The main purpose of a hearing evaluation is to define the nature and extent of the hearing impairment. From this information, decisions can be made about appropriate steps in the rehabilitation of the hearing disorder and handicaps that may result from the impairment. Several questions that need to be answered as part of a hearing evaluation include (Stach, 2010):

- Why is the person being evaluated?
- Should the person be referred for medical consultation?
- What is the person's hearing sensitivity?
- How well does the person understand speech?
- How well does the person process auditory information?
- Does the hearing impairment cause a hearing handicap?

People seek hearing evaluations by audiologists for various reasons. Parents want to find out if their child has a hearing problem. Older people seek evaluations to confirm their suspicion that they have developed a hearing problem. Adults may be referred to audiologists because of long-term noise exposure in the workplace or an accident with a view toward compensation for any hearing loss. Patients may be referred for audiological evaluations by otolaryngologists to determine the nature and extent of hearing impairments that result from active disease processes. Otolaryngologists will likely want audiological evaluations both before and after treating the disease process with drugs or surgery.

The fundamental purpose of an audiological evaluation is similar for most children and adults, although the specific focus of the evaluation can vary considerably depending on the nature of the individual and problem. We begin our discussion of hearing assessment at the beginning—with newborns.

Newborn Hearing Screening

Each year there are approximately 4 million babies born in the United States and an unknown number born around the world. Many children are born with significant hearing impairments but are not identified and provided with appropriate intervention. These children lose their ability to acquire fundamental speech, language, cognitive, and social skills required for later schooling and success in society. Early intervention for youngsters with hearing impairments is needed for them to develop communication skills on par with their normal-hearing peers (Vaughn, 2005; Yoshinaga-Itano & Gravel, 2001). Mohr, Feldman, Dunbar, et al. (2000), estimated that lifetime costs to society for individuals with prelingual (before speech development) onset of hearing loss exceeds $1 million, including costs of educational resources, reduced work productivity and earning capacity, social services (e.g., unemployment compensation), and other expenses and loss of income generating potential. The high cost associated with prelingual onset of severe to profound hearing impairment shows that interventions aimed at infants and children, such as early identification and aggressive medical and audiological intervention, can have a substantial payback.

Hearing screening is likely a low priority in many countries where the very survival of infants is the primary concern. Hearing screening may be a luxury in many nations, but it is becoming increasingly important in nations with the resources to provide the procedures. The challenge for the United States and many other countries is having qualified personnel who can perform the screening procedures accurately and reliably. Increasingly, hospitals are relying on supportive technicians and volunteers to carry out this important task. The use of supportive personnel for newborn screenings frees valuable time for audiologists whose efforts may be more meaningfully used for provision of follow-up, diagnostic, and intervention services (Katz, Medwetsky, Burkard, & Hood, 2009; Mahshie, Moseley, Scott, & Lee, 2006; Martin & Clark, 2009).

Newborn hearing screening did not become fairly common until the 1970s and 1980s for infants who were determined to be at risk for potential hearing impairment. Screening the hearing of newborn infants is now a routine procedure and compulsory in most states, and is both beneficial and justifiable. Hayes and Northern (1997) stated that the prevalence of significant hearing disorders in newborns may be as high as 6 in every 1,000 live births. Infants with low Apgar scores are considered at risk for hearing impairments. Some newborns may pass a hearing screening and still be at high risk for hearing loss; therefore, based on hereditary history, it is important to perform regular follow-up hearing screenings for at least several months (Mann, Cuttler, & Campbell, 2001). Detection of hearing loss in newborns may help alert medical professionals to the possibility of other complications. There appears to be a biological relationship between newborn hearing loss and other conditions, including *sudden infant death syndrome* (SIDS). Both may be caused by congenital deficiencies of certain important enzymes,

Application Question

If you are a parent, did your baby have a hearing screening before going home? If you are a possible future parent, would you request that your newborn have a hearing screening?

which can lead to a variety of disorders of other systems, such as vision, cardiopulmonary, and musculoskeletal, and a predisposition to infection (Walker, 2003).

Sudden Infant Death Syndrome (SIDS)

Sudden infant death syndrome (SIDS, formerly called *crib death*) is the unexpected and sudden death of an apparently normal and healthy infant that occurs during sleep and with no physical evidence of disease. It is the most common cause of death in children between 2 weeks and 1 year of age, with an incidence rate of 1 in every 300 to 350 live births in the U.S. The origin of SIDS is unknown, but multiple causes have been proposed. SIDS occurs most often in infants 2 to 4 months old, and in 95% of cases it occurs before 6 months of age. It is more common in infants born prematurely and most often occurs in the fall and winter months. SIDS is more prevalent in boys than girls and tends to occur more often among infants who have recently had a minor illness such as an upper respiratory infection. SIDS occurs more often among babies born to women who are in lower socioeconomic status groups, who are less than 20 years of age, who have at least one previous child, who begin prenatal care in the 3rd trimester, and/or who smoke, use drugs, or are anemic. SIDS is more common in infants who sleep in the prone (face down) or side-lying position; who have soft bedding, loose articles, or both in the sleeping environment; who are overheated (thermal stress); and who sleep with adults, especially on a sofa. There is a lower incidence of SIDS among breast-fed babies (Mosby, 2009).

Application Question

If you had an infant, what are some things you could do that could help prevent SIDS?

Newborn hearing screening requires the use of techniques that can be performed without active participation of the patient. One procedure that is frequently used is **auditory brainstem response (ABR)**, which is an electrophysiologic technique that involves attaching electrodes to an infant's scalp and recording electrical responses of the brain to sound. For screening purposes, the technique is often automated to limit testing interpretation errors (Stach, 2010).

auditory brainstem response (ABR)

An *electrophysiological response* (the relationship between electrical activity and biologic function, in this case, brain activity) to sound that consists of five to seven identifiable peaks that represent neural function of auditory pathways.

Pediatricians and Family Medicine (Practice) Physicians

Pediatricians and family medicine physicians are usually the first professionals to see a child with ear or hearing problems (Isaacson & Vora, 2003). The physician will take a thorough history and conduct a careful physical examination to diagnose and treat ear problems. The physical examination begins with visualization and palpation of the auricle and *periauricular* (around the auricle) tissue. A handheld *otoscope* (a device with a light source that permits visualization of the ear canal and eardrum) is used to examine the external auditory canal for *cerumen* (earwax), foreign bodies, and abnormalities of the canal skin (see Figure 14–11). The mobility, color, and surface anatomy of the tympanic

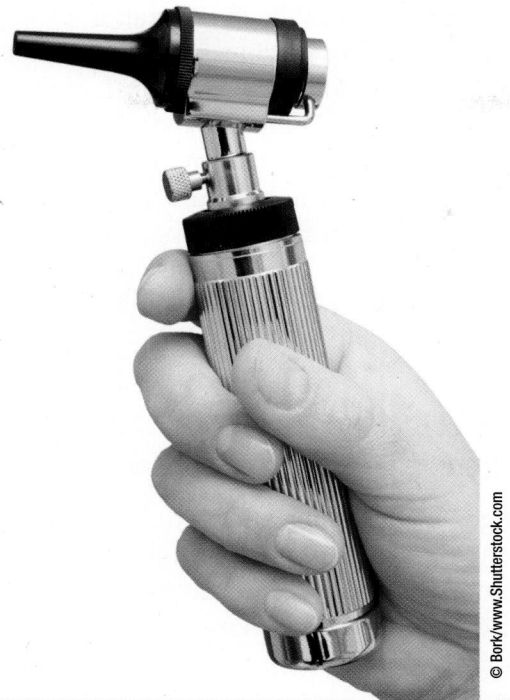

© Bork/www.Shutterstock.com

Figure 14-11
A handheld otoscope.

membrane are examined. A pneumatic bulb is used to test the movement of the tympanic membrane.

If the pediatrician or family medicine physician cannot treat or chooses not to treat the ear problem, she will likely refer the patient to an otolaryngologist for further evaluation and treatment. The otolaryngologist will likely perform many of the same examination techniques as the referring physician, plus others that he is more specialized in administering. Otolaryngologists often make referrals to audiologists for hearing evaluations.

Audiologists' Case History and Interview

Before evaluating pediatric or adult clients, audiologists typically gather a complete case history. A good case history guides an audiologist in several ways. It provides important information about the following:

- The patient's complaints about her hearing
- The family's complaints about the patient's hearing
- Whether the hearing problem is unilateral or bilateral
- Whether the problem is acute or chronic
- The duration of the problem
- What may be contributing to the hearing problem

Many audiologists use case history and questionnaire forms that can be completed by the patient or parents of a patient. Audiologists are sometimes the entry point into the health care system for individuals and it is important that they be knowledgeable about warning signs that indicate the need for a medical referral. For example, a patient's responses to questions about dizziness, numbness, weakness, tinnitus, and other signs indicate potential otological, neurological, or other medical problems. Experienced audiologists take advantage of the interview not only to obtain information from the client or patient but also to make important observations. For example, does the person have articulation or language problems, and is the person relying on lipreading to understand the audiologist? Getting a sense about how the person feels about a possible hearing loss helps the audiologist direct his counseling efforts (Mahshie et al., 2006).

Evaluating the Structures of the Outer and Middle Ear

Structural changes in the outer and middle ear can cause functional changes that result in hearing impairments. The auricle is inspected for shape, size, location on the head, and any visible abnormalities that may indicate possible syndrome involvement. Careful visual inspection of the external auditory canal can be done with an otoscope. The external ear canal is inspected for any obvious inflammation, obstruction from foreign objects, and excessive cerumen. The tympanic membrane is inspected for inflammation, perforation, or any other obvious structural abnormalities in structure. If disease processes are suspected, the patient should be referred for a medical assessment following the audiological evaluation.

Pure-Tone Audiometry

Pure-tone audiometry is built on the concept of tuning forks. Tuning forks are made of metal and are sometimes used by singers to match certain pitches or musicians to tune musical instruments (see Figure 14–12). A tuning fork produces a precise pitch and has a clear musical quality,

pure-tone audiometry

Audiometry using tones of various frequencies and intensities as auditory stimuli to measure hearing using both air conduction and bone conduction.

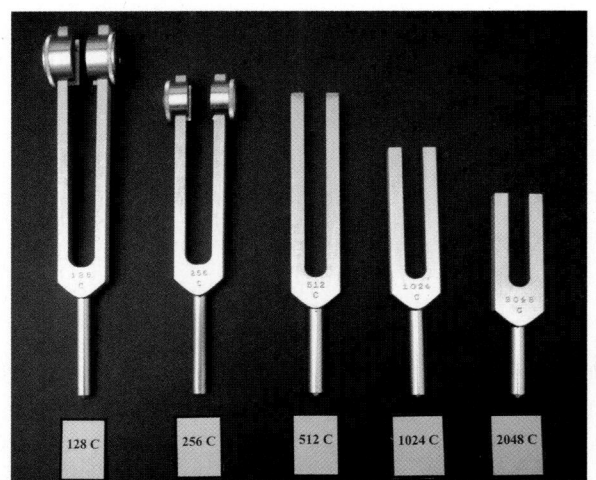

Figure 14–12

Tuning forks. The larger the tuning fork, the lower the frequency produced.

Courtesy of Elizabeth Jardine, Au.D.

usually corresponding to the musical scale of C. The tuning fork was used to test hearing more than a century ago, long before the development of audiometers.

Pure-tone audiometry uses tones of various frequencies and intensities as auditory stimuli to measure hearing and is performed with an **audiometer**, ideally in a sound-proof audiology booth (see Figure 14–13 and Figure 14–14). The purposes of pure-tone audiometry are to establish

audiometer

An electronic device designed to measure the sensitivity of hearing of pure-tone frequencies (*hertz*) and *intensities* (decibels); sounds are delivered to the ears either through earphones or *free field* (i.e., through loudspeakers in a testing environment with no reverberating surfaces) in an audiometry booth.

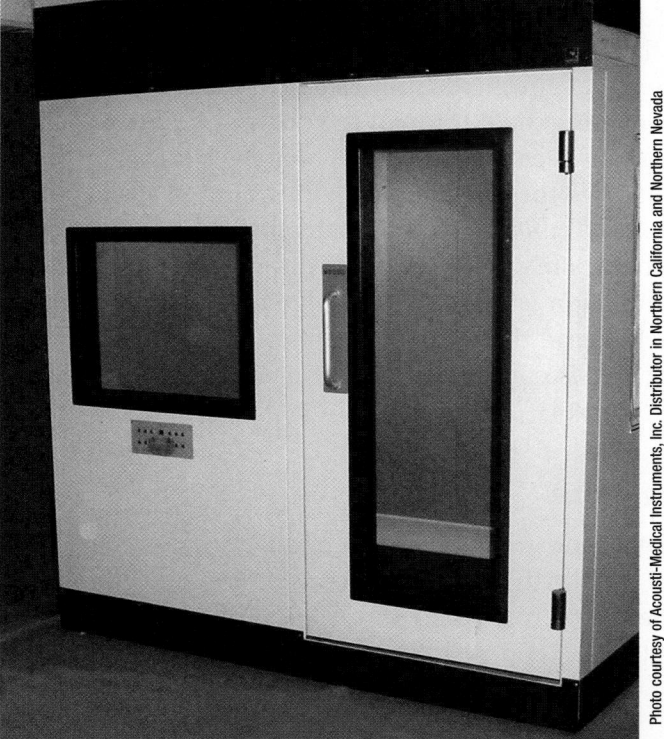

Photo courtesy of Acousti-Medical Instruments, Inc. Distributor in Northern California and Northern Nevada

Figure 14–13

A commercial, double-room, sound-treated audiometric test booth.

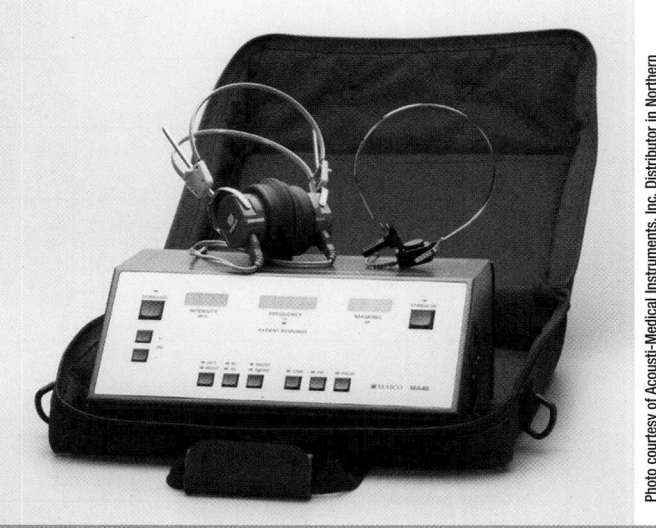

Photo courtesy of Acousti-Medical Instruments, Inc. Distributor in Northern California and Northern Nevada

Figure 14–14

Portable audiometers allow children and adults to be screened or tested away from sound-treated audiometric test booths.

hearing threshold sensitivity across the range of audible frequencies important for human communication, and to determine the lowest intensity that a person can "just barely hear"; that is, the *hearing threshold*. All newer audiometers are computerized with sophisticated microprocessors. To be accurate and reliable, audiometers need to be calibrated regularly by the manufacturer. Assessment reliability is based on the interrelationships among calibration of the equipment, test environment, patient performance, and experience of the examiner.

All audiometers can measure air conduction and bone conduction. **Air conduction** is the transmission of sound to the inner ear through the external auditory canal and the structures of the middle ear. Air-conduction thresholds are tested by transmission of sounds using earphones or free field through the outer and middle ear to determine auditory acuity (see Figure 14–14). **Bone conduction** is the transmission of sound to the inner ear through vibration applied to the bones of the skull. Bone conduction allows determination of the cochlea's hearing sensitivity while bypassing any outer or middle ear abnormalities. Bone conduction is tested by stimulation of the inner ear by placing a bone oscillator on the mastoid bone or forehead to determine whether a hearing loss is conductive, sensorineural, or mixed (i.e., both types) (see Figure 14–14).

Audiograms

Audiograms are graphs with a frequency-versus-intensity plot to show threshold sensitivity changes across the frequency range. *Audiometric frequencies* for conventional pure-tone audiometry are usually 250, 500, 1000, 2000, 4000, and 8000 Hz (see Figure 14–15).

---

air conduction

The transmission of sound to the inner ear through the external auditory canal and the structures of the middle ear.

bone conduction

Transmission of sound to the inner ear through vibration applied to the bones of the skull; allows determination of the cochlea's hearing sensitivity while bypassing any outer or middle ear abnormalities.

audiogram

A standard graph used to record pure-tone hearing thresholds with air- and bone-conduction thresholds graphed by frequency in hertz (Hz) and hearing level (HL) in decibels (dB).

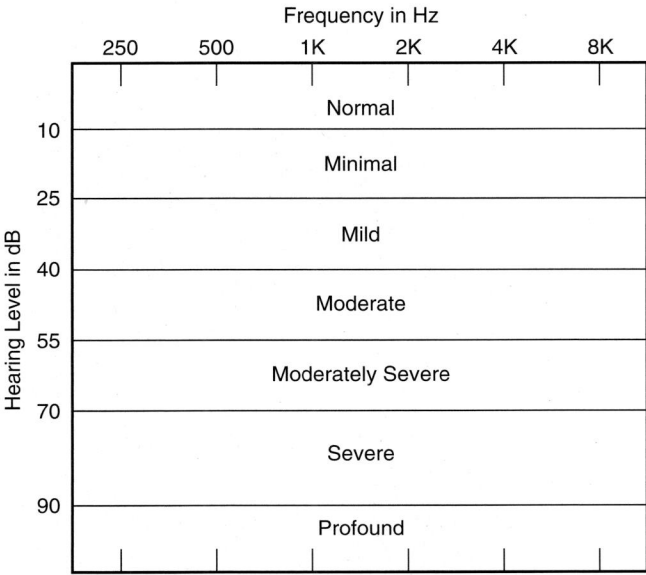

Figure 14–15

Degrees of hearing loss plotted on an audiogram.

© Cengage Learning 2013.

In clinical audiometry, intensity is expressed on a decibel scale relative to *average normal hearing*. The zero line running horizontally across the top of an audiogram is the sound intensity corresponding to average normal hearing at each of the test frequencies. Some people hear better than normal; therefore, –10 represents hearing at frequencies that a normal-hearing individual may not be able to hear. Pure-tone audiograms provide important information in several ways:

1. Audiograms indicate the degree of loss and its effects on communication. The effects on communication of a hearing loss may be considered the *functional results of the hearing loss*; that is, how the loss may affect a person's daily interactions with other people and the environment.

2. There are three basic shapes of loss on audiometric configurations. For example, a hearing loss may be the same at all frequencies and have a *flat configuration;* the degree of loss may decrease as the curve moves from the low-frequency region to the high-frequency region and have a *rising configuration;* or the loss may increase as the curve moves from the low-frequency region to the high-frequency region and have a *downward sloping configuration* (see Figure 14–16).

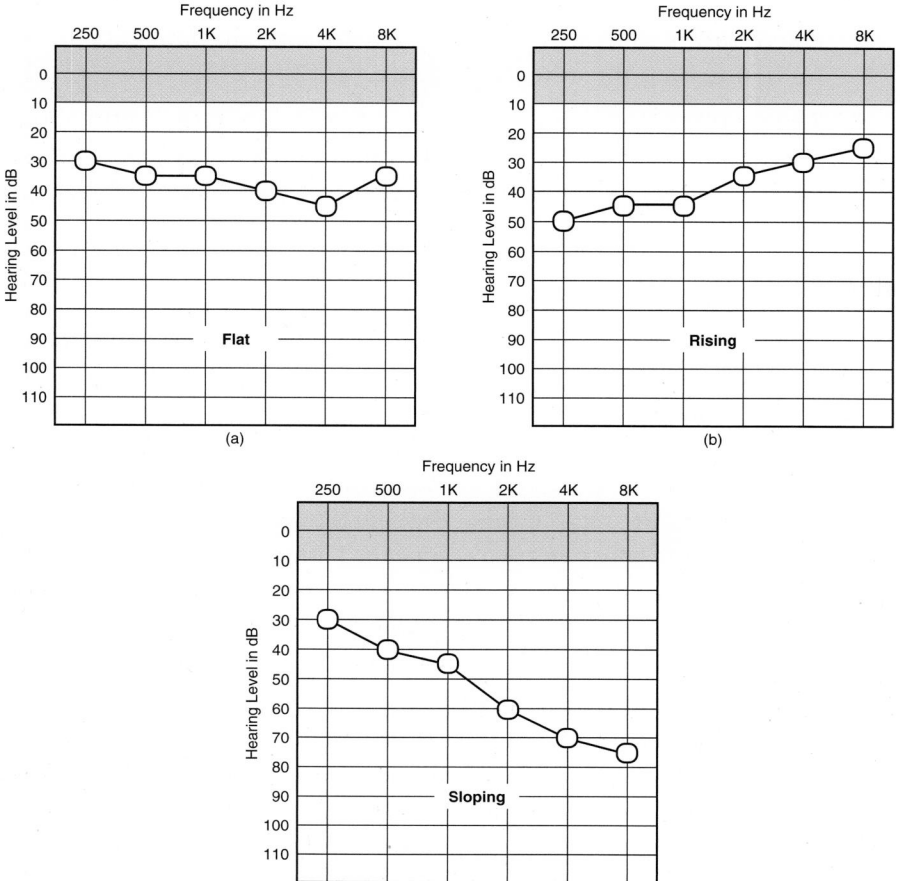

Figure 14–16

Three audiometric configurations: (a) flat, (b) rising, and (c) sloping.

© Cengage Learning 2013.

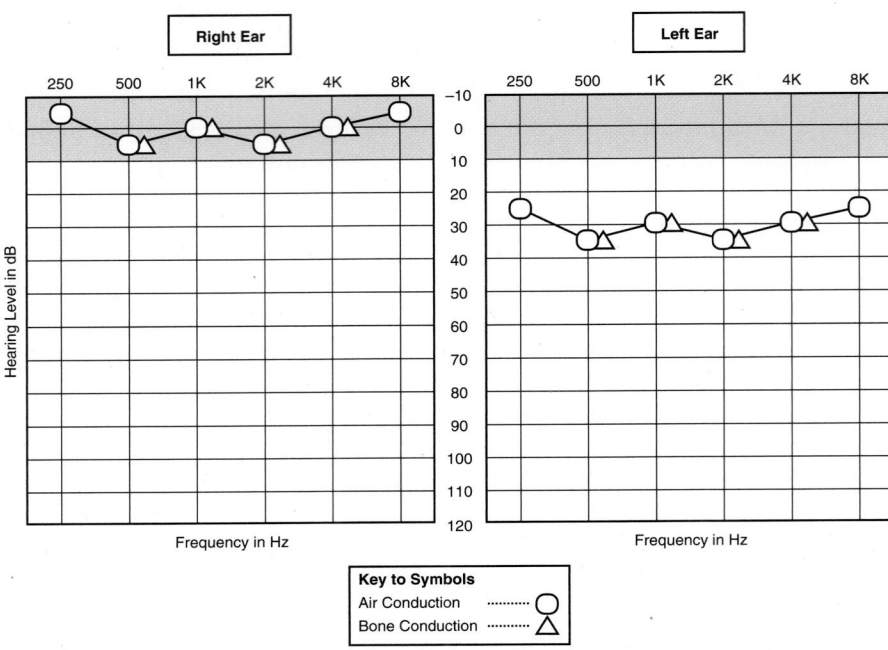

Figure 14–17

An audiogram representing asymmetrical hearing loss.

© Cengage Learning 2013.

---

3. The audiogram provides a measure of *interaural symmetry,* or the extent to which hearing sensitivity is the same in both ears or better in one than the other (see Figure 14–17).

4. The combination of air- and bone-conduction audiometry allows the differentiation of peripheral hearing loss into one of three types: conductive, sensorineural, or mixed (see Figure 14–18).

Masking

When two sounds are heard simultaneously, the intensity of one sound may be sufficient to cause the other to be inaudible. This change in the threshold of a sound caused by a second sound with which it occurs simultaneously is called **masking**. We all know what it is like not to hear someone speaking (or at least not clearly) because of background (*ambient*) noise. At such times, the background noise is *masking* (drowning out) the other person's speech. Light that has equal energy at all frequencies in the light spectrum is referred to as *white light.* This concept has been adapted to sound; that is, sound that has equal energy at all frequencies in the audible spectrum is referred to as *white noise.* Audiologists have various ways of using white noise as masking noise while performing pure-tone audiometry.

When an audiometric tone is presented to the test ear through an earphone at an intensity level that may cause the sound to "cross over" to the nontest ear, the nontest ear may allow the person to hear the sound. Whenever cross-hearing is suspected, it is necessary to remove the nontest ear from the test procedure to determine whether the original

masking

In audiology, the process that occurs when two sounds occur simultaneously and one sound is sufficiently loud to cause the other to be inaudible.

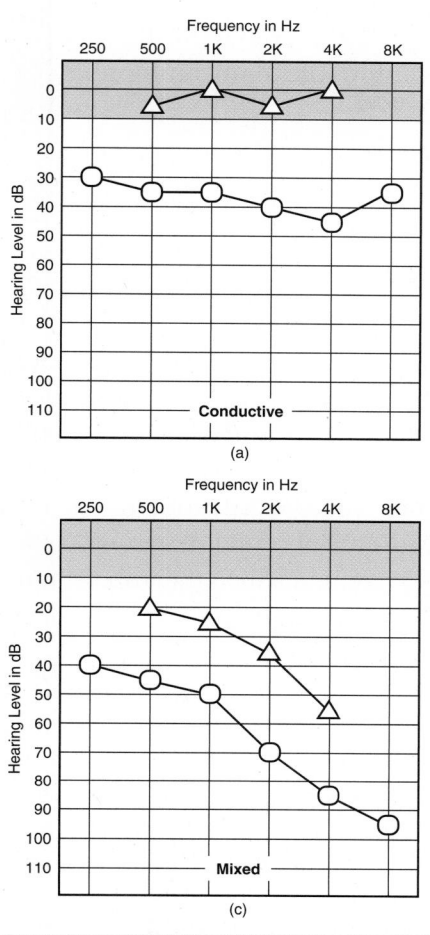

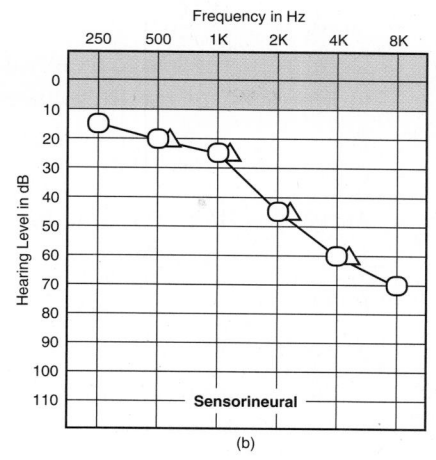

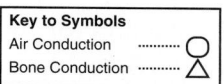

Figure 14–18

Audiograms representing three types of hearing loss: (a) conductive, (b) sensorineural, and (c) mixed.

© Cengage Learning 2013.

responses were obtained through the nontest ear and, if they were, what the true threshold of the test ear really is. This is accomplished by masking (Bess & Humes, 2008; Stach, 2010).

Speech Audiometry

Pure-tone audiometry provides valuable information about an individual's hearing; however, it does not yield clear insights into the degree of disability the individual has understanding speech. **Speech audiometry** uses the kinds of auditory signals present in everyday communication and, therefore, provides a more realistic assessment of how a hearing disorder might affect normal communication. Speech-language pathologists find that information obtained from speech audiometry is particularly helpful in planning therapy and client and family counseling (Bess & Humes, 2008; Mahshie et al., 2006; Martin & Clark, 2012). The influence of speech processing can be detected at all levels of the auditory system: middle ear, cochlea, auditory nerve, brainstem pathways, and auditory centers in the cortex. Speech audiometry is used to:

- Measure thresholds for speech
- Cross-check pure-tone sensitivity

speech audiometry

A key component of audiological assessment that uses auditory signals present in everyday communication; assessment involves, in part, the presentation of single-syllable words at a fixed intensity level above the threshold with the client aurally discriminating the sounds in the words to correctly say words aloud for the examiner to score.

tympanometry

A measurement of middle ear pressure that is determined by the mobility of the tympanic membrane as a function of various amounts of positive and negative air pressure in the external ear canal (the more positive or negative the air pressure in the external ear canal, the more the normal middle ear system becomes immobilized).

compliance

The ease with which the tympanic membrane and middle ear mechanism function.

impedance

The opposition of sound-wave transmission, which includes frictional resistance, mass, and stiffness, and is influenced by frequency.

immittance audiometry

A routinely used objective assessment of the functioning of the middle ear; a general term to describe measurements made of tympanic membrane impedance, compliance, or **admittance**.

admittance

The ease and flow of energy transmission through a system; the reciprocal of impedance.

- Quantify *suprathreshold* (above threshold) speech recognition
- Determine the range from most comfortable to uncomfortable loudness levels for an individual
- Determine the ability to recognize and discriminate speech sounds
- Assist in differential diagnosis
- Assess central auditory processing ability
- Estimate communicative function

A *speech threshold* is the lowest level at which speech can be detected or recognized; that is, the *speech awareness threshold* (SAT). A basic form of speech recognition testing involves the presentation of single-syllable words at a fixed intensity level above the threshold. The client has to hear and aurally discriminate the sounds in the words to correctly say the words aloud for the examiner to score. Differential diagnosis as to the location or locations in the auditory system in which the impairment is occurring can be determined from speech audiometry.

Tympanometry

Tympanometry is a measurement of middle ear **compliance** and **impedance** that is determined by the mobility of the tympanic membrane as a function of various amounts of positive and negative air pressure in the external ear canal. The tympanic membrane vibrates most efficiently when the pressure on both sides is equal (i.e., atmospheric air pressure). Tympanometry is performed using a *tympanometer*, which generally is part of **immittance audiometry** that performs immittance assessments (see Figure 14–19).

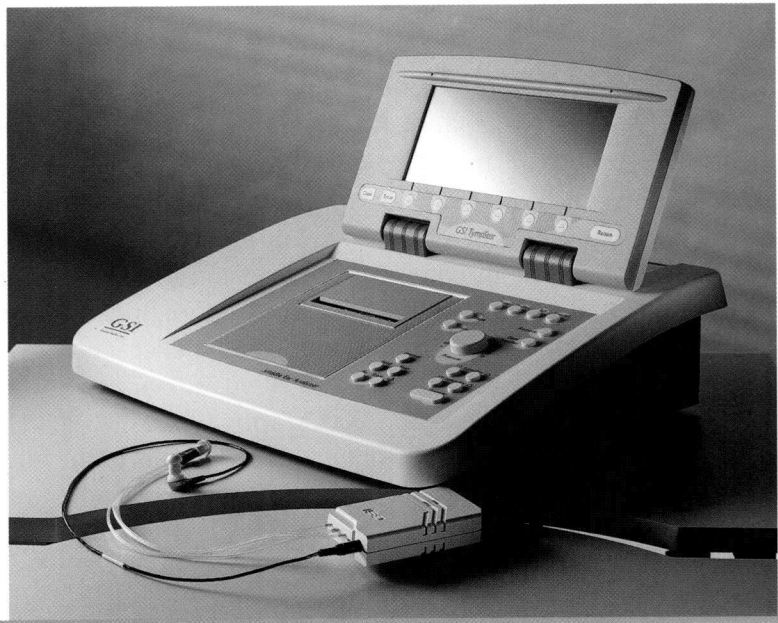

Figure 14–19

An immittance meter with insert earplugs (tips) for tympanometry.

Photo courtesy of Acousti-Medical Instruments, Inc. Distributor in Northern California and Northern Nevada

During tympanometry assessment, an insert earplug is placed in one ear with a good seal obtained to prevent leakage of air pressure, creating a "closed system" with the earplug on one end of the canal and the tympanic membrane on the other. The tympanometer pumps air into the external ear canal to a particular level, creating a positive pressure against the tympanic membrane while measurements are taken by the tympanometer that reflect the compliance of the tympanic membrane (i.e., the ease of movement of the tympanic membrane under pressure). After the peak pressure and movement of the tympanic membrane are reached, the air pressure is decreased by the tympanometer and successive measurements are again taken. After the pressure in the external ear canal is again at atmospheric air pressure, the tympanometer creates negative pressure and additional compliance measurements are made. The purpose of tympanometry is to determine the point and magnitude of the greatest compliance of the tympanic membrane. These measurements are valuable in understanding the condition of the tympanic membrane and middle ear structures.

Evaluating the Functioning of the Cochlea and Auditory Nervous System

From the time acoustic stimuli reach the inner ear, what is transmitted to the brain is not "sound" but rather a series of *neuroelectrical* impulses. Measurement of the electrical responses generated within the cochlea establishes an objective measure of hearing sensitivity. *Electrocochleography* (ECoG) was developed to measure the electrical responses generated within the cochlea. In addition, whenever a sound is heard (perceived) by a person, there is some change in the ongoing electrical activity of the brain. Because electrical signals are transmitted extremely rapidly, they are measured in terms of milliseconds (one-thousandth of a second). *Auditory evoked potential audiometry* has been developed to extract the tiny voltages (*electrical potentials*) produced in the brain by acoustic stimulation. Discussion of electrocochleography or auditory evoked potential and electrophysiological testing methods is beyond the scope of this text. Refer to Bess and Humes (2008), Martin and Clark (2012), Stach (2010), or any other audiology introductory text for a discussion of these assessment procedures.

AMPLIFICATION FOR INDIVIDUALS WITH HEARING IMPAIRMENTS

Audiological habilitation (for children who did not have hearing pre-linguistically) or *rehabilitation* (for children and adults who developed speech and language before losing their hearing) usually encompasses the diagnosis of hearing loss and the provision of listening devices, often with the emphasis on follow-up of **hearing aids** and less on communication strategies and speech perception training (Tye-Murray, 2009).

hearing aid

Any electronic device (usually battery operated) designed to amplify and deliver sound to the ear and consists of a microphone, amplifier, and receiver.

CASE STUDY

A Stroke and a Hearing Loss

A 23-year-old man sustained two hemorrhagic cerebrovascular accidents (CVAs) in an 18-month period. His first stroke involved the right temporal and parietal lobes and resulted in left arm and leg paresis. During his second stroke, he became confused and disoriented and began having seizures. His speech, language, and cognition were impaired, and for several days the patient had no hearing in either ear. During the 2nd week after the CVA, he began to hear loud sounds. Although he began to regain his hearing sensitivity, he could not understand conversational speech. About 6 months after the CVA, he could discern some speech in everyday situations, partly because of developing speechreading skills. Background noises were disturbing to him.

Computerized tomography (CT) scans and magnetic resonance imaging (MRI) revealed that both the right and the left hemispheres' Heschl's gyri and the temporal lobes were severely damaged by the two strokes. Audiological testing revealed profound central nervous system hearing losses bilaterally, likely caused by the severely damaged right and left Heschl's gyri. However, later pure-tone testing revealed fluctuating hearing losses bilaterally, and speech detection thresholds began to approach normal after several months. The patient did not begin to consistently understand single words until 14 months after the CVAs.

Long-term follow-up (over an 8-year period) indicated that this was a case of complete central deafness in that, initially, the patient could not perceive any environmental or speech sounds and had no response to standard pure-tone audiometric testing at the maximum output of the audiometer. The patient was young (23 years), which allowed him to benefit from plasticity of his brain for some recovery of auditory functions. Recovery of perception of environmental sounds (e.g., music) significantly preceded his ability to perceive speech sounds. The speech of familiar voices of people was more easily recognized than speech of unfamiliar speakers. As with many people who have impaired central auditory nervous systems, background noise, competing speech, and generally poor acoustics had a significant effect on his comprehension abilities. The partial recovery of this patient's central auditory nervous system was significantly enhanced by working with a speech-language pathologist on auditory identification and discrimination of speech sounds and adjusting the environment to decrease distracting background noises. Because of the long-term auditory rehabilitation, the efforts put forth by the patient, the speech-language pathologist, and the benefit of his young age and plasticity of his brain, the patient made significant progress in his communication abilities. (Adapted from Musiek, Baran, & Pinheiro, 1994.) ■

The fundamental goal of hearing rehabilitation is to limit the extent of any communication disorder that results from a hearing loss. The first step in reaching that goal is to maximize the use of *residual hearing*. That is, every effort is made to put the remaining hearing that a person has to its most effective use. Once this has been accomplished, treatment often proceeds with some form of aural rehabilitation (Mahshie, Moseley, Scott, & Lee, 2006; Stach, 2010; Tye-Murray, 2009). We begin our discussion where we began hearing assessment—with newborns.

Amplification for Infants

When an infant with a hearing impairment is identified before 3 months of age, the intervention process should begin before 6 months of age (Diefendorf, 2005; Yoshinaga-Itano & Gravel, 2001; Yoshinaga-Itano, Sedey, Coulter, & Mehl, 1998). This requires a comprehensive hearing evaluation as well as a team of professionals working closely with both the infant and the family (Munos, Nelson, Goldgewicht, & Odell, 2011). Over the course of a child's development, the professional team will likely include various pediatricians, otolaryngologists, audiologists, speech-language pathologists, early childhood specialists, social workers, counselors, educational psychologists, and special and regular educators. The head of the team is always the parents or primary caregivers—they are the ultimate determiners of what will or will not be done.

Federal law requires that when hearing loss is suspected in a newborn or young child, evaluation and early intervention services must be provided in accordance with the *Individuals with Disabilities Education Act (IDEA),* Part H (birth to 3 years of age) of Public Law 102-1119. The law provides for statewide, comprehensive, coordinated multidisciplinary, interagency programs of early intervention services for all children with disabilities and their families. In many cases, the professionals involved with the infant who has a hearing problem are more in tune to the reality of the problem than the parents.

The Role of the Parents and Family

Parent and family involvement with a newborn with a hearing impairment is crucial. The basic components related to early intervention include (1) counseling to support the parents' adaptation to the diagnosis and provide a forum in which they can express and work through their feelings; (2) fitting hearing aids to supplement the infant's impaired auditory reception; and (3) giving encouragement to early development of a rich symbolic communication system between the infant and the family (ASHA, 2008b; Bess & Humes, 2008; Tye-Murray, 2009).

Parental feelings must be considered and worked with before there can be successful intervention of the infant. Parents may not readily accept the diagnosis of a hearing loss or deafness of their baby. There may be few real signs of a hearing impairment and the parents must rely on the results of the audiologist's evaluation of the infant over several sessions. Most people have had no association with an audiologist and may not even know what an audiologist does. The parents now are expected to accept the diagnosis and take the recommendations from an unknown professional (and an unknown profession) that have turned their world upside down.

A family-centered treatment philosophy assumes that social support affects family functioning; the child's needs are best met by meeting the family's needs; and families have the right to retain as much control as they desire over the intervention process (Clark & English, 2004; Tye-Murray, 2009). We are, as always, working with the entire family constellation, and the person with the hearing loss is the center of the constellation.

Hearing Aids and Cochlear Implants for Infants and Young Children

Hearing aids or a cochlear implant should be considered and possibly provided as soon as the audiologist is firmly convinced that a hearing loss is present (Hayes & Northern, 1997; Katz, 2001; Mahshie et al., 2006). The evaluation and fitting of hearing aids is an ongoing process, and several changes may need to be made before the "final" fitting. In addition, if the infant or child has a progressive sensorineural loss, periodic monitoring and adjustments in aids will likely be required.

Binaural ear-level hearing aids are available in small sizes to fit behind the ears. The older, bulky body-type hearing aids with cord and external receiver are now seldom used. The newer aids are custom fitted and electronically tuned for the specific pattern of hearing loss identified for each ear. The audiologist may need to adjust the limit of the *gain* (the difference between the input signal and the output signal) of the hearing aids because aids that provide too much intensity (sound pressure level) may potentially cause further hearing loss. *Ear molds* can be made for an infant, but because of growth of the infant they need to be remade every few months.

Although it is the infant or young child who wears the hearing aids, it is the parents who are responsible for their care and daily use. The parents need to be willing and able to take on this critical responsibility (regretfully, not all parents are). Hearing aids and the batteries that power them are serious potential swallow hazards and careful monitoring of the infant and child is needed to be certain they are not ingested. In addition, parents or other caregivers need to be certain that the hearing aids are positioned correctly in the child's ear or ears, kept clean and dry, are in good working order, and have good batteries.

In addition to hearing aids, cochlear implants are the latest technology that has been developed to help young children with profound bilateral sensorineural hearing loss. Cochlear implants have been successfully used with children as young as 10 months of age (Hayes & Northern, 1997; Tomblin, Barker, Spencer, Zhang, & Gantz, 2005). For young children to be candidates for cochlear implants, they need to have normal intelligence, not have other handicaps that would contraindicate their use, and have dedicated family support (Cohen & Waltzman, 1996).

Application Question

What might be your reaction and feelings if you were a new parent and your infant was diagnosed as deaf or hard of hearing?

Application Question

If your infant or young child had to wear hearing aids, how might you prevent the child from accidentally swallowing an aid or battery?

Hearing Aids for Children and Adults

Attempts to amplify sound have existed as long as people have cupped their hands behind their ears to momentarily improve their hearing. What we consider primitive attempts at mechanical devices to improve hearing were "high tech" in their early days of development. Likewise, what we consider state-of-the-art now will someday be considered crude attempts at sophisticated technology. The advent of miniature batteries allowed behind-the-ear hearing aids and in-the-temple eye-glass hearing aids. The development of microbatteries and microprocessors allows in-the-ear aids and now aids completely in the ear canal. The following provides a basic understanding of hearing aids.

Components of Hearing Aids

A hearing aid is a miniature electronic amplifier that has three main components: a microphone, an amplifier, and a speaker (receiver). A battery is the power source and a volume adjuster (*gain control* or *attenuator*) allows the wearer to increase or decrease the hearing aid gain. The microphone is a vibrator that moves in response to the pressure waves of sounds in the environment (much like a person's tympanic membrane). The electrical signal is boosted by the amplifier and then delivered to the speaker. The speaker then converts the electrical signal back into an acoustic signal to be delivered to the person's eardrum.

Conventional Hearing Aids

Figure 14–20 shows the four most common styles of hearing aids used today:

- Behind the ear (BTE)
- In the ear (ITE)
- In the canal (ITC)
- Completely in the canal (CIC)

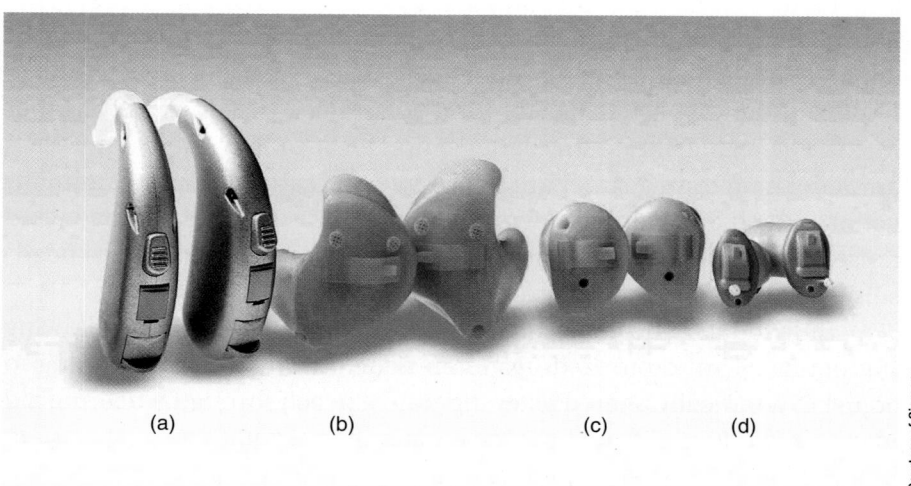

(a)   (b)   (c)   (d)

Courtesy of Siemens

Figure 14–20

Four common types of hearing aids: (a) behind the ear (BTE), (b) in the ear (ITE), (c) in the canal (ITC), and (d) completely in the canal (CIC).

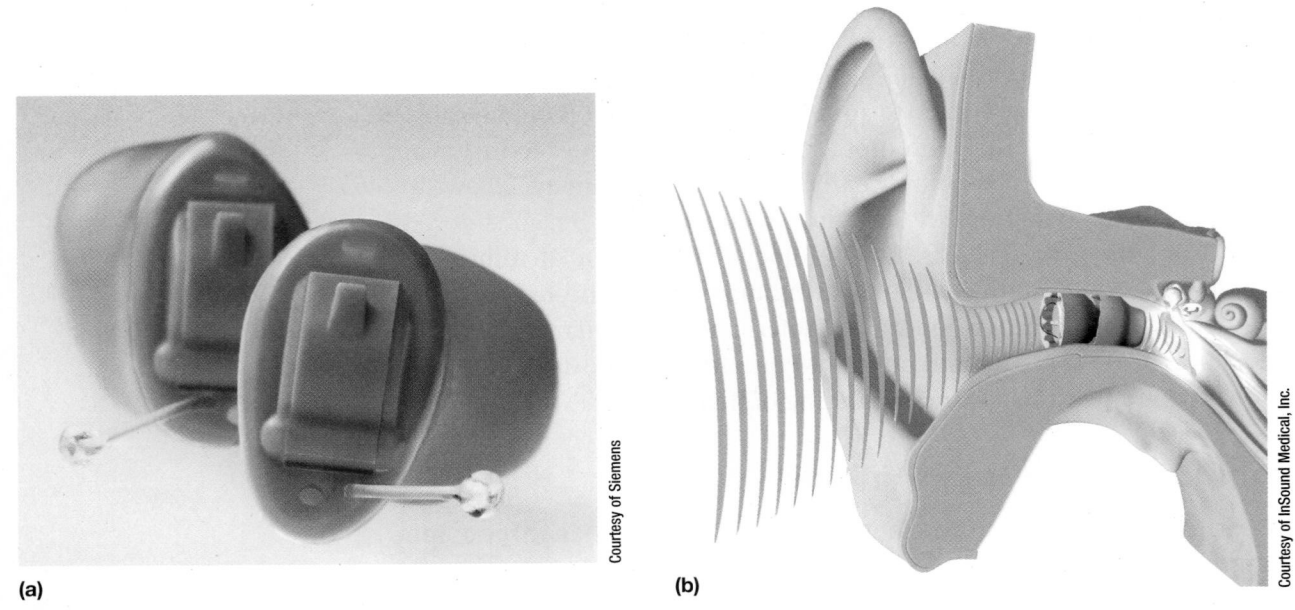

Figure 14-21

(a) A completely-in-the-canal (CIC) hearing aid. (b) The Lyric is the first hearing aid designed to fit deep in the ear canal and be invisible from the outside. It can be worn for up to three months without removal or replacement.

A BTE hearing aid is worn over the ear and is held in place by a plastic "hook" that fits over the top of the ear. The amplified sound is delivered to the ear canal through a tube that leads to a custom-fitted ear mold. An ITE hearing aid is in a custom-fitted case that fits into the outer ear. An ITC hearing aid is a smaller version of an ITE, which fits mostly into the ear canal. A CIC hearing aid is an even smaller version of an ITE and is custom-fitted to sit 1 to 2 mm (approximately ¼ inch) inside the opening of the ear canal so that it is almost invisible.

The CIC type is the smallest and most inconspicuous hearing aid available at this time (see Figure 14-21). It is designed for mild-to-moderate hearing losses. The CIC aids have some advantages over larger aids. Because they sit completely in the ear canal, they receive the natural benefit of the auricle's collection and resonance properties that enhance sound in the higher frequencies, which is particularly helpful in understanding speech in background noise. Because CIC aids sit further into the ear canal, they allow better sound localization. They require less amplifier gain than a larger aid to produce the same amount of amplification, which also permits increased battery life. CIC aids reduce wind noise, improve ease of telephone use, and enhance listening with headsets (Martin & Clark, 2012; Strom, 2004).

Individuals who have incurred a sudden hearing loss following trauma or use of ototoxic drugs often benefit from auditory training to adjust to a radically altered listening state. Speech through a hearing aid may sound different from how they remember it, and they must learn to interpret what they hear. After successful fitting of a hearing aid, individuals benefit from support and training to maximize the benefits of the aid.

Application Question

If you had to wear a hearing aid, which type do you think you might prefer? Why?

Assistive Listening Devices

Amplification systems other than conventional hearing aids have been designed for more specific listening situations. These devices are known as **assistive listening devices** (ALDs). Among the devices considered ALDs are personal amplifiers, telephone listeners, and frequency modulation (FM) systems. All of these systems are designed to enhance speech signals over background noise by use of a remote microphone. That is, rather than the microphone being built into the same case as the amplifier and receivers as it is in hearing aids, it is separated in some way to close the physical distance between the speaker and the listener.

Some individuals choose ALDs to supplement their hearing aids in certain situations, for example, in the workplace. Some people need ALDs just when talking on the telephone, watching television, or attending church. Others may benefit from these devices because of auditory processing disorders when they have difficulty understanding speech in background noise, for example, in a classroom.

A *personal amplifier (pocket talker)* consists of a microphone connected by a cord to a case about the size of a deck of cards that houses the battery, amplifier electronics, and volume control. The microphone is held by the person who is talking. Typically a set of lightweight headphones or earbud transducers are worn by the listener (see Figure 14–22). By separating the microphone from the amplifier, it can be moved close to the speaker's mouth, which enhances the signal-to-noise ratio (i.e., there is more speech signal and less background noise). Many speech-language pathologists working in hospital settings carry their own personal amplifiers when going to see a patient with a known hearing loss. Many patients with hearing losses do not have their hearing aids with them, or their hearing aids have been lost.

Telephone amplifiers are popular ALDs and are available in several forms (see Figure 14–23). Some telephone handsets have built-in amplifiers with a volume control. Many portable telephone amplifiers can be attached to any phone. Telephone receivers also can be adapted

assistive listening device

Amplification systems, other than conventional hearing aids, that are designed for specific listening situations (e.g., personal amplifiers, telephone amplifiers, personal text telephones, and personal FM systems).

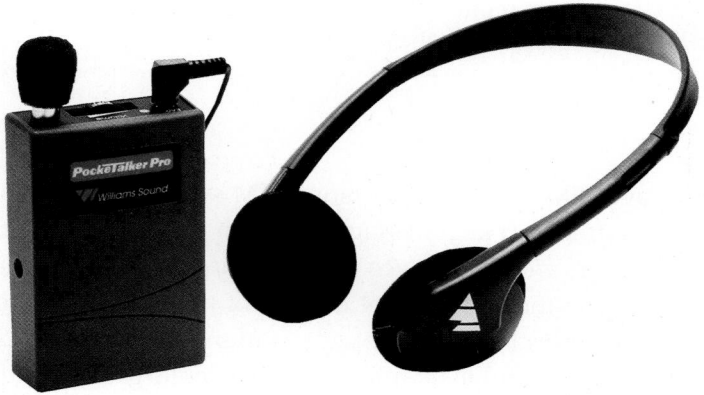

Courtesy of Williams Sound Corp.

Figure 14–22

A personal amplifier (pocket talker).

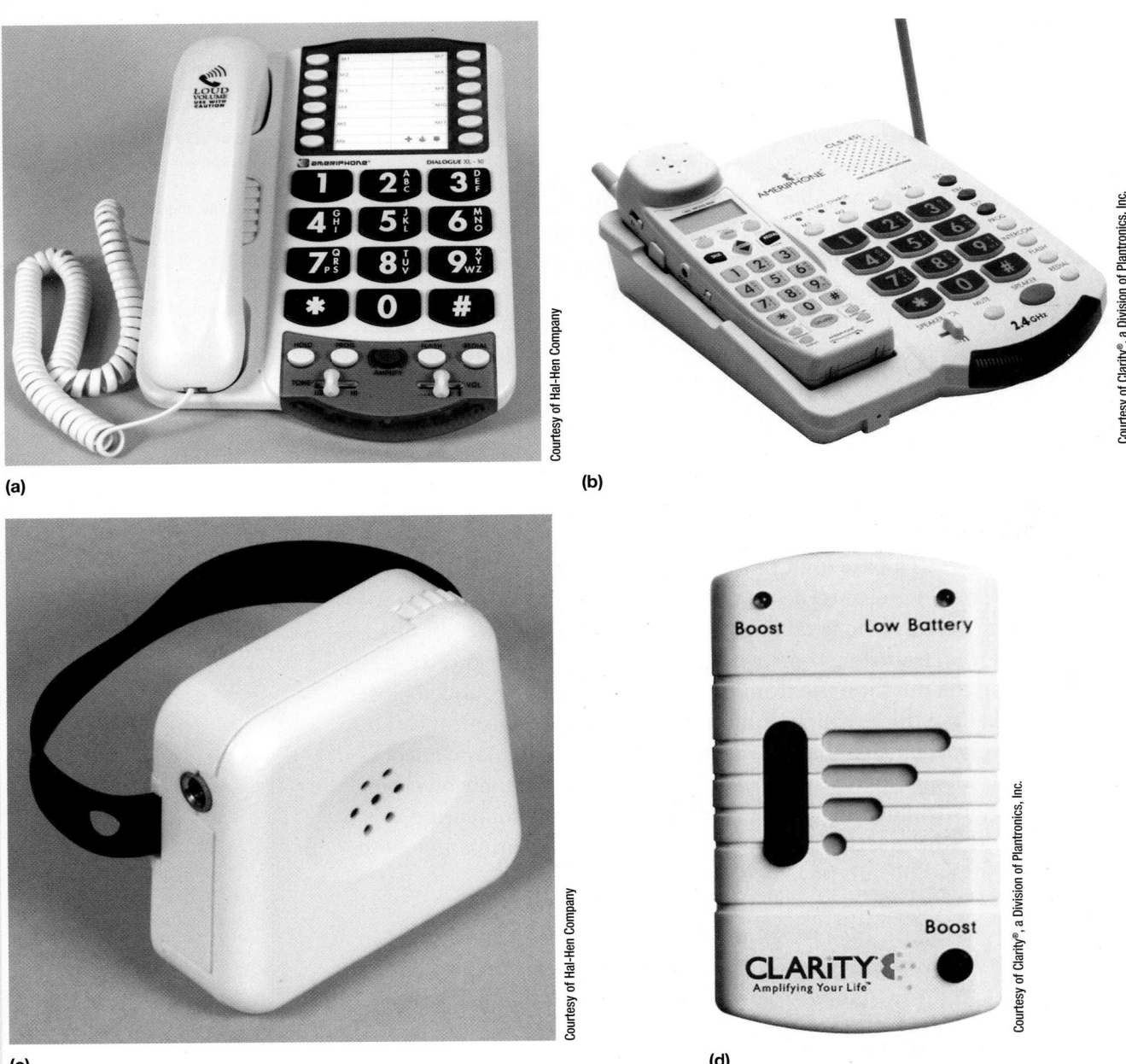

(a)

Courtesy of Hal-Hen Company

(b)

Courtesy of Clarity®, a Division of Plantronics, Inc.

(c)

Courtesy of Hal-Hen Company

(d)

Courtesy of Clarity®, a Division of Plantronics, Inc.

Figure 14–23

Examples of telephone amplifiers: (a) amplified telephone model XL-30, (b) built-in amplified telephone from Clarity®, (c) mini portable telephone amplifier, and (d) portable high-frequency amplifier.

to transmit over FM waves to a personal FM system. Telephones lines may be used to transmit text messages through a *personal text telephone* (TT) or *telecommunication device for the deaf* (TDD, also abbreviated TTY for teletypewriter) for a visual display of typed messages over the telephone, which are also available with printers (see Figure 14–24). *Text messaging* through cellular telephones is particularly easy and convenient for many hearing impaired individuals.

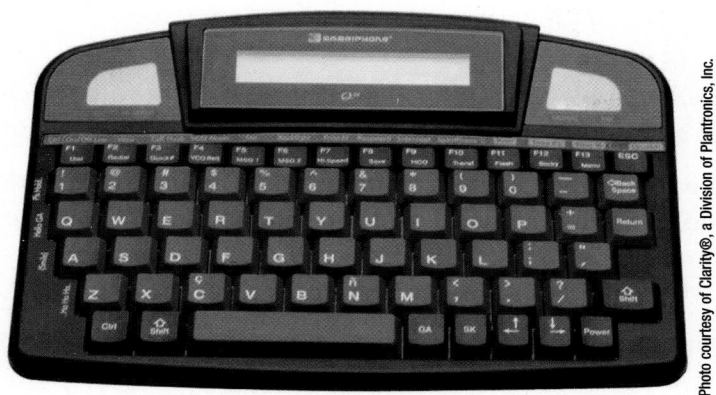

Photo courtesy of Clarity®, a Division of Plantronics, Inc.

Figure 14-24

The Ameriphone TTD is an example of a text telephone.

Personal FM systems consist of two parts, a microphone-transmitter and amplifier-receiver. The microphone is connected to, or is a part of, the case that contains the FM transmitter. The person who is talking (e.g., a teacher) wears the microphone and transmitter. Signals from the transmitter are sent to a receiver using FM radio waves. The listener wears the amplifier receiver, which acts like an FM radio and "picks up" the transmitted signal. The receiver is usually attached to the listener's ear by means of earphones or to hearing aid transmitter coils by means of a neck loop that transmits the signal. FM systems are particularly helpful for children with auditory processing disorders who find that normal classroom noises are distracting to them (Chermak & Musiek, 2007; Geffner & Ross-Swain, 2007; Tye-Murray, 2009). With the teacher wearing the microphone, the teacher's voice is no further away than her mouth from the child's ears. For individuals who also have hearing acuity problems, entire FM receiver systems can be integrated into conventional BTE or ITE hearing aids.

Application Question

Have you ever spoken on the telephone with a person who is hard of hearing? What do you recall of the experience?

Other Assistive Devices for Hearing Impaired Individuals

Other assistive devices are available for hearing impaired people that do not amplify sound but add another modality to the stimulus; these include the following:

- *Closed captioning* provides written text to match the spoken words on a TV program.
- *Vibratory pagers* vibrate against the user to alert the person to an incoming telephone call that can be read as a text message.
- *Vibrating alarm clocks* have a vibrator that can be placed under the user's pillow.
- *Flashing alarm clocks* use a flashing lamp or strobe light to signal the alarm.
- A *doorbell signal* can be coupled to a lamp that flashes when the doorbell is rung.

- A *smoke detector* can have a light that flashes a signal to alert for the presence of smoke.
- A *baby cry alert system* can have a flashing light with which a parent can be signaled if a baby begins to cry in another room.

These devices provide personal convenience for the hearing impaired, as well as some safety features for alerting of possible danger.

Cochlear Implants

Cochlear implants are the latest and most sophisticated devices to help children and adults with severe or profound bilateral hearing losses. Some individuals, however, benefit from having a cochlear implant in one ear while using a hearing aid in the other. Severe-to-profound deafness results from a loss of hair cell functioning in the cochlea. As a result, neural impulses are not generated and electrical activity in the auditory nerve is not initiated. Cochlear implants are designed to stimulate the auditory nerve directly.

The internal components of cochlear implants are the receiver and the electrode array. The surgery to insert a unilateral cochlear implant usually requires 2 to 3 hours and an overnight stay in the hospital. Under general anesthesia, a skin flap behind the auricle is elevated and a *partial mastoidectomy* performed (removing part of the mastoid bone directly behind the ear). The bone tissue removed makes room for the receiver component of the implant. The middle ear is entered, and the cochlea is opened. A tiny, flexible tube with an electrode array (up to 40 electrodes) is surgically implanted 22 to 24 mm (almost 1 inch) into the spiral tunnel of the cochlea (see Figure 14–25).

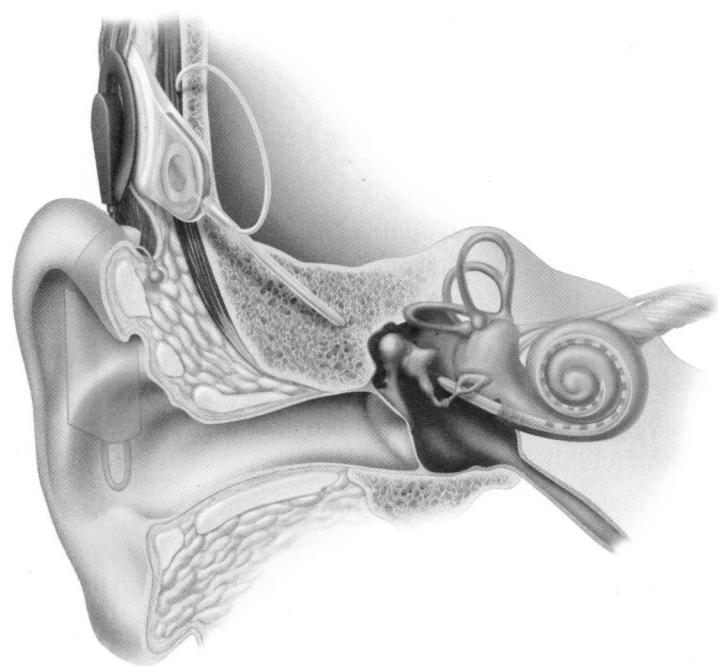

Figure 14–25

A view of the outer, middle, and inner ear, with an internal receiver and stimulator (electrode array) coiled in the cochlea.

Image courtesy of Cochlear Limited.

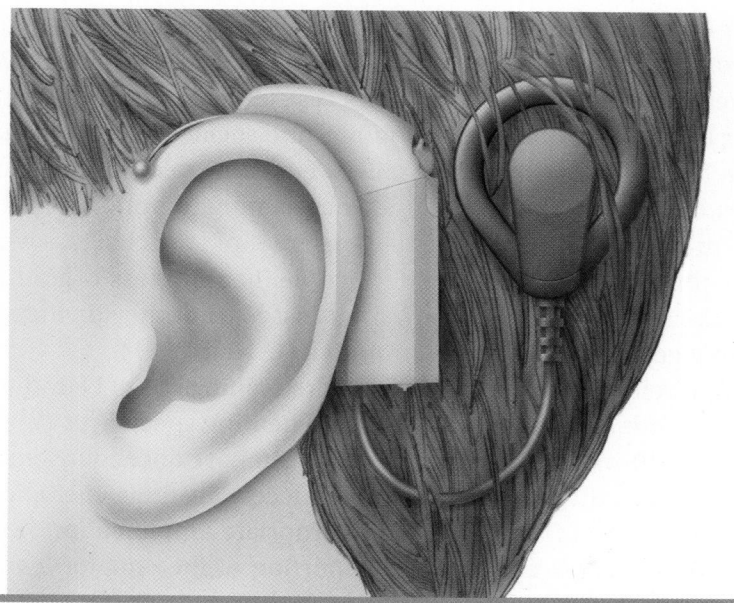

Figure 14–26

The external components with an ear-level speech processor and the transmitter, which is held in place by a magnet against the internal receiver. The transmitter is about the size of a nickel (20mm).

Image courtesy of Cochlear Limited.

The external components of a cochlear implant are similar to those of a conventional hearing aid (see Figure 14–26). The microphone is located in an ear-level device. Output from the microphone is routed to an amplifier that uses digital signal processing. The amplified signal is delivered to a receiver that sends signals to a transmitter coil. The transmitter coil has a magnet that holds it against the skin opposite the internal receiver. The signal is then transmitted electromagnetically across the skin. The receiver then transmits these signals to the proper electrodes in the array, where they can stimulate the intact auditory nerve fibers.

In sensorineural hearing impairments, although the hair cells are damaged, the auditory nerve fibers connected to the hair cells often remain intact. It is because of the intact auditory nerve fibers that cochlear implants can be successful. The nerve fibers can be stimulated to fire by applying the appropriate electrical currents using the cochlear implant. The actively propagated nerve impulses are sent through the auditory nerve and auditory pathway to the auditory cortex in the temporal lobe of the brain, where the impulses are interpreted as sound. Hearing success for the person improves with time and experience using a cochlear implant (Ertmer, 2005; Nicholas & Greers, 2003; Stach, 2010; Tye-Murray, 2009).

AURAL REHABILITATION

Aural rehabilitation is a broad term that involves intervention aimed at minimizing and alleviating the communication difficulties associated with hearing loss. It may include identification and diagnosis of hearing loss and communication handicaps, patient and family counseling and education, selecting and fitting amplification devices, communication

> **Application Question**
>
> If you were considering a cochlear implant for a hearing impairment, what questions might you ask the audiologist and the physician?

aural rehabilitation

A broad term that involves intervention aimed at minimizing and alleviating the communication difficulties associated with hearing loss; includes identification and diagnosis, patient and family counseling and education, selection and fitting amplification devices, communication training strategies, speech perception training, speech-language therapy, promotion of literacy, and educational management.

training strategies, speech perception training, speech-language therapy, promotion of literacy, and educational management (ASHA, 2008b). Aural rehabilitation not only includes assistance to improve or manage hearing loss but also includes emotional and social support for individuals with hearing loss and their families. For some people, a minor hearing loss can have significant, if not devastating, emotional and social effects on their lives, particularly if there is a rapid onset of loss with little time to adjust to it. For most older people, hearing loss is gradual and they make subtle adjustments to their losses until they or their family can no longer overlook or work around it (O'Neil, 2007).

Aural rehabilitation emphasizes three main areas: (1) understanding the individuals served by speech and hearing specialists; (2) providing them with appropriate professional support and counseling; and (3) maximizing their communication success in their everyday environments once they have received appropriate amplification (Mahshie et al., 2006; Tye-Murray, 2009). This portion of the chapter focuses on the third area.

Auditory Training

aural habilitation

Sometimes used synonymously with *aural rehabilitation*; intervention for people who have not developed listening, speech, and language skills; may include diagnosis of communication and hearing-related difficulties, speech perception training, speech and language therapy, manual communication, and educational management.

auditory training

Aural rehabilitation methods designed to optimize use of residual hearing by structured practice in listening, altering the environment, and use of hearing aids to increase sound awareness, sound discrimination, identification of words, and comprehension of spoken messages.

The goal of **aural habilitation** and **auditory training** for children with hearing loss is to develop their ability to recognize speech using auditory signals and to interpret auditory information (Tye-Murray, 2009). Auditory training helps children use their residual hearing to their maximum capability. Children should be fitted with appropriate amplification before starting an auditory training program. Hearing aids can enhance hearing, but the act of listening is a behavior that must be learned. In addition, auditory training will not change hearing sensitivity but will enhance a child's ability to use whatever sound is available. Children who are deaf since birth (*prelingual*) have no memory or concept of sound, but young children who acquire a hearing loss after developing some speech and language often have the concept and memory of sound, as well as some speech and language. The key elements to auditory training include detection, discrimination, identification, and comprehension (Hull, 2009).

Detection or Awareness of Sounds

Detection involves children becoming aware of sound and learning to attend to sounds. At the detection level, the child simply responds to the presence or absence of sound. For most hearing impaired children, this only occurs when there is adequate amplification. In addition, the parents play a crucial role in helping draw their child's attention to the linguistic and nonlinguistic sounds in the environment—for example, the mother pointing out to the child that he is hearing (as well as seeing) his daddy laugh or that the child is hearing the noisy blue jay bird in the backyard.

Discrimination of Sounds

Discrimination develops as children learn to perceive the differences in sounds. Suprasegmental discrimination of intensity, duration, pitch, and timing appear first. Discrimination allows children to tell whether auditory patterns are the same or different from others. How sounds differ and what sounds mean comes later in the child's development.

Identification of Sounds

Identification is the stage at which children can repeat or point to what sounds and words represent. Identification requires memory but not necessarily understanding of the sounds. It is when understanding accompanies memory that comprehension begins to develop.

Comprehension

Comprehension of speech and language is the most complicated stage of auditory development. Comprehension is a higher auditory skill level in which the child understands the meaning of spoken messages. Comprehension requires various areas of the brain to integrate the individual words in a message that express concepts that may require auditory, visual, tactile, smell, or taste sensory systems. For example, the word *popcorn* can conjure auditory sensations of the popping sounds; the visual sensations of the kernels before and after they pop; the olfactory sensation of freshly popped corn; the tactile sensations of warm popcorn in the hand and the feeling of crunching it between the teeth; and the taste sensations of delicious salted or buttered popcorn in the mouth.

Lipreading and Speechreading

During **lipreading**, a person relies only on the visual cues provided by the speaker's mouth and face for recognizing speech. For most people, this is a difficult task. Researchers have studied eye movement patterns during lipreading using instruments that track the center of the pupil. During **speechreading**, a person uses residual hearing and attends carefully to the speaker's visual messages (nonverbal communication, such as facial expressions and body language), clues from the setting of the conversation, and the likely conversational topics in the setting. Good lip-readers are likely good speech-readers. Normal-hearing people rely on speechreading in probably most conversations each day. Because people often are not tuned into every word that is said in a conversation, they use speechreading to fill in the "blanks" that they do not fill from an auditory message (Hull, 2009; Tye-Murray, 2009). The **oralism** philosophical approach in the education of the deaf maintains that language should be oral, that is, from the mouth, and sign language and teachers who are deaf should be excluded from the classroom.

lipreading

The process of recognizing speech using only the visual cues from the speaker's mouth and face.

speechreading

The process of recognizing speech by attending to the speaker's auditory and visual messages (nonverbal communication, such as facial expressions and body language), clues from the setting of the conversation, and the likely conversational topics in those settings.

oralism

A philosophy in the education of the deaf that maintains language should be oral, that is, from the mouth, and sign language and teachers who are deaf should be excluded from the classroom.

Application Question

Have you ever tried to read someone's lips while the person was talking? How difficult was it? How do you use speechreading in conversation?

Speech Skills

The speech skills of children with hearing impairments need to be determined. In Chapter 5, the section on Assessment of Articulation and Phonology provides general information for assessing speech intelligibility of children with hearing impairments. Standardized articulation and phonology tests are appropriate; however, it is particularly important to assess spontaneous, continuous speech to determine conversational intelligibility.

Goals for a comprehensive speech development program may include the following (Carney & Moeller, 1998; Hull, 2009; Tye-Murray, 2009):

- Increase vocalizations that have appropriate timing characteristics and that require numerous vocal tract movements
- Expand phonetic and phonemic repertoires
- Establish links between audition and speech production
- Improve suprasegmental aspects of speech
- Increase speech intelligibility

Phonetic and phonological process errors are targeted in therapy. Therapy goals, for example, may focus on increasing a child's phonetic repertoire and reducing phonological process errors. Auditory modeling, often combined with visual and tactile input, is used extensively.

Ling (1976) developed a program based on the premise that there is a hierarchy of speech skills. The most effective and efficient way to learn these is to build new skills on existing skills. For example, a child should be able to rapidly say a sequence such as *bee-bee-bee-bee* before being expected to say a sequence such as *bee-boo-bee-boo.* Following a natural sequence of progression in therapy allows hearing impaired children to develop speech skills in a similar sequence as normal-hearing children.

Language Skills

The language skills of children with hearing impairments need to be determined. Analyzing a child's receptive and expressive language using language samples can be informative. Therapy goals in language development may include the following (Carney & Moeller, 1998; Hull, 2009; Tye-Murray, 2009):

- Increase communication between parents and child
- Promote an understanding of complex concepts and discourse units
- Enhance vocabulary growth
- Increase world knowledge
- Enhance self-expression
- Enhance growth in use of language syntax and pragmatics
- Develop narrative skills

Therapy goals are often based on information about the language development of normal-hearing children. For preschool children, the emphasis may initially be on vocabulary development and simple sentences. For school-age children, the focus is on development of syntax and semantics. Throughout therapy, form, content, and pragmatics are developed. *Naturalistic methods* are typically used in which language instruction optimizes everyday events and structuring the environment so that certain events occur to promote the growth of form, content, and pragmatics.

Sign Language and Manual Communication

The use of gestures and hands, as well as facial expressions and body language, are as much a part of natural communication as is speaking. Facial expressions (*microgestures*) and gestures of the hands, arms, and body posture (*macrogestures*) are used almost unconsciously in everyday conversation for illustration, emphasis, and emotional content. *Nonverbal communication* or *body language* has been recognized as a form of communication since the beginning of human communication. In a way, it is our first language. Infants communicate with parents through facial expressions and body language long before they can communicate with spoken words. Likewise, infants recognize their parents' nonverbal communications before they clearly recognize the meanings of words and sentences.

Sign language is a natural form of communication for many deaf children and adults when communicating among themselves. Sign language has two main forms of communicating with the fingers and hands: finger spelling and signing. **Finger spelling** is the use of certain finger and hand shapes to represent letters of the alphabet and spell individual words. Sign language is a visual means of communication using hand and arm shapes and gestures to represent words and concepts, along with some finger spelling. Sign language users typically use the force or speed of a sign along with facial expressions to help communicate the emotional content of their messages (e.g., No! or Stop!). Sign language does not depend on spoken language and is used within Deaf communities and learned naturally by interaction with other signers. **Manualism** is a philosophy in the education of the deaf that emphasizes the learning and use of sign language and finger spelling as a natural form of communication among the deaf.

Many countries have their own sign language systems (e.g., **American Sign Language** or **ASL**; British Sign Language, or BSL; Chinese Sign Language, or CSL; French Sign Language, or FSL; German Sign Language, or GSL; Swedish Sign Language, or SSL, etc.), and within countries there are often various systems of sign language used (e.g., in America there is ASL, Signing Exact English, Seeing Exact English, and others). Many normal-hearing people take courses in sign language out

sign language

A visual means of communication using finger, hand, and arm shapes and gestures to represent words and concepts, along with some finger spelling; communication that does not depend on spoken language and is used within Deaf communities and learned naturally by interaction with other signers.

finger spelling

The use of certain finger and hand shapes to represent letters of the alphabet and spell individual words.

manualism

A philosophy in the education of the deaf that emphasizes the learning and use of sign language and finger spelling as a natural form of communication among the deaf.

American Sign Language (ASL)

A manual system of communication commonly used by members of the Deaf culture in the United States; sometimes referred to as *Ameslan*.

of interest or, in some cases, with the intention of becoming sign language interpreters in various settings where deaf individuals may be a part of a larger hearing community, such as in a church service.

ASL is unique to the Deaf community and is its own language that closely follows the French Sign Language system. A person does not use ASL and speak at the same time because ASL has a different grammar than spoken English. One ASL sign might represent a concept that would require several English words to express. Facial expressions and body language can impart a variety of shades of meanings to the signs. In both ASL and manually coded English, finger spelling may be used if there is no sign for a particular word or concept (Tye-Murray, 2009).

Manually coded English (*signed English*) is composed of manual signs corresponding to the words of English, and it has the same syntactic structures. Typically, a person using manually coded English speaks simultaneously while signing, signing each word that she says, including articles such as *the, a,* and *an.* The combined use of sign and speech as an educational philosophy is referred to as *simultaneous communication.*

The Deaf Community Today

(Note: In keeping with Woodward, 1972, *Deaf* with a capital "D" refers to a linguistic and cultural minority of people and *deaf* with a lowercase "d" is related to an audiometric hearing level.)

Normal-hearing people in countries around the world have long tried to determine how deaf individuals should communicate, and there are strong opinions from manualists and oralists. Some teachers of the deaf advocate that all deaf people need to learn and become proficient in speechreading to integrate within the normal-hearing community. On the other hand, manualists recognize that the **Deaf community** is a genuine culture (i.e., **Deaf culture**, and a culture in which they should take pride) and that they should be allowed to communicate in the language of their choosing and not be forced into being marginalized into the hearing world. Whether born into Deaf culture or enculturated later in life, the Deaf have chosen sign language as their primary method of communication and associate primarily with those who have made the same choice (Clark & English, 2004). Another opinion is that deaf individuals should learn sign language to communicate with one another but also learn speechreading and develop speech the best they can to communicate with hearing individuals to some degree (**total communication**).

Most children who are deaf have normal-hearing parents, and most deaf parents have children with normal hearing. Only about 10% of children born deaf have parents who are also deaf (Miles, 2005). Deaf children who have deaf parents are brought up learning the sign language of their parents as their first language. They become a part of the Deaf community from babyhood. Some deaf individuals can trace their deaf ancestors back generations.

In many communities around the world there are Deaf social clubs where sign language is the natural form of communication.

manually coded English

A form of communication in which manual signs correspond to English words and syntax.

Deaf community

Those deaf and hard of hearing individuals who share a common language (usually manual communication), common experiences and values, and a common way of interacting with each other and with hearing people.

Deaf culture

Ideology, beliefs, and customs shared by many individuals with prelinguistic deafness that may include communication, social protocol, entertainment, art, recreation, worship, and other aspects of culture.

total communication

A philosophy calling for every possible means of communication to be used by deaf individuals, including hearing aids and assistive devices, speechreading, signing, and spoken English.

Notable scenes in Deaf culture include the standing joke of the club committee trying to push people out at closing time and crowds standing around in the street signing for a good hour afterward, or of people of all ages staying up half the night together telling jokes and stories (a major part of Deaf culture), signing songs or poems or playing sign language games, or of a regional rally, where a town center is taken over by sign language for a weekend and people from all over the country greet old school friends across the street without a word spoken. Overall, although educators of the deaf may try to be multiculturally sensitive to various cultures and ethnic groups, they may still have difficulty accepting the natural communication system of the Deaf culture (Miles, 2005).

EMOTIONAL AND SOCIAL EFFECTS OF HEARING IMPAIRMENTS

The parents and family of newborns with hearing impairments have emotional reactions (challenges) to the news of their baby's loss and must work through the stages of grief (denial, anger, bargaining, depression, and acceptance). The emotional and social effects of hearing loss can be influenced by the different stages of life. Each stage (infancy, preschool, school age, adolescence, young adulthood, late adulthood, old age) has unique problems for both the hearing impaired person and the family (Tye-Murray, 2012).

Infants with hearing impairment do not respond normally to parent-initiated verbal play or attempts to be soothed when crying or distraught, leaving the parents feeling rejected, inadequate, and like failures. Infant–parent bonding can be significantly affected. Children with hearing loss are more likely than other children to have poor self-concepts, feel unlikeable, overly shy, and socially isolated. Hearing impaired adolescents feel covert or overt rejection from peers, and these feelings can continue throughout the rest of their lives (DeLuzio & Girolametto, 2011; Hull, 2009; Tye-Murray, 2009; Tye-Murray, 2012).

Young adults who have acquired hearing losses from listening to very loud music (Shafer, 2006) or being exposed to loud noises (e.g., from being in the military [Chandler, 2006]), or from traumatic brain injuries from motor vehicle accidents typically feel angry and frustrated. Acquired hearing loss during the early years of adulthood causes many people to reevaluate their life expectations and goals. Adults with severe-to-profound hearing losses often feel that they do not fit into any social group: they are not part of the Deaf community because they have a newly acquired hearing loss, and they are no longer comfortably a part of their normal social group because they are out of touch with normal conversation. Compared to normal hearing elderly people, elderly people with hearing losses who choose not to wear hearing aids or are unable to get them report feeling more sad or depressed, anxious, insecure, irritable, fearful, tense, and isolated (National Council on Aging, 1999) (see Figure 14–27).

- DO be facially expressive when communicating.
- DO NOT break eye contact when communicating with Deaf people. Lack of eye contact is considered rude when communicating with a visually oriented person.
- DO get a Deaf person's attention by tapping the shoulder, waving your hand in the person's line of sight, blinking the lights, and so on.
- DO NOT take offense at direct questions regarding qualifications or personal life. Direct questions between one Deaf person and another Deaf person are culturally quite common and can spill over into interactions with hearing people with no attempt to be rude.
- DO be conscious of hearing-loss terminology. Within Deaf culture, the norm is *profound deafness* and a *mild hearing loss* may mean "hard of hearing" to the Deaf person.
- DO NOT touch the Deaf person's hands while that person is signing.
- DO define Deaf individuals by their abilities rather than their disabilities—for example, not by their inability to perform well on a standard speech-reception test, but rather by their abilities in auditory pattern perceptions or environmental sound identification.
- DO NOT talk with another hearing person in the presence of a Deaf person without signing or ensuring a clear line of sight for speechreading. Just as those with acquired hearing loss may be suspicious when they do not understand what others are saying, so may Deaf individuals. Use sign language, use written communication, or ensure the Deaf person can speech-read what is said.
- DO attempt to use sign language with the Deaf. Any attempt is appreciated, but if you are not fluent, the services of an interpreter should be obtained.
- DO NOT use the term *oral* as it implies oral ideologies (*oralists*). Rather, use the term *spoken English* or *spoken communication*. Similarly, *communication training* may be preferred to *aural rehabilitation* because the former implies improvements in aspects of communication, such as written communication, that are not aurally based.

Figure 14-27

Some dos and don'ts when communicating with deaf and hard of hearing people and individuals in the Deaf community.

Adapted from Kaplan, 1996.

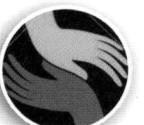

Multicultural Considerations

Clark and English (2004) state that audiologists often feel insecure in their counseling interactions with the hearing impaired and even more so when working with multicultural patients. In addition, the Deaf culture is nearly as foreign to audiologists as might be any other cultural group, and few audiologists are fluent in sign language. Clark and English (2004, p. 173) further state:

> Our own [audiology] professional culture and its very trappings are diametrically opposed to the Deaf culture. Audiologists are heavily steeped within a pathology model of health care. We perform diagnostic measures to characterize hearing loss, assess the impact of hearing loss on the individual and family, help those with hearing loss find effective means to overcome the negative impact of the loss with which they suffer, and refer to those we see as "patients."

In contrast, the Deaf culture views deafness as a difference and not as a pathology, disorder, or defect that needs treatment. A person is considered a member of the Deaf culture not on the basis of an audiometric profile but rather on the basis of a chosen identity through adoption of its values, practices, and natural language—signing (Kaplan, 1996). To be a part of the Deaf community does not require deafness. Many normal-hearing individuals are fluent signers and are actively involved in the Deaf culture, including being proponents of its goals and causes.

Just as there are minority groups within the hearing community, there are minority groups in the Deaf community, and these groups can have as much diversity in cultural values and beliefs as any multicultural group. The common denominator among these heterogeneous and international communities is that they all use sign language (Schirmer, 2001; Clark & English, 2004). Just as racial and cultural status among people with normal hearing can affect a person's socioeconomic status, being a minority within a minority in the Deaf community tends to have a far greater effect (MacLeod-Gallinger, 1993; Schirmer, 2001).

Application Question

What are some things you could do to become involved in the Deaf culture?

CHAPTER SUMMARY

The hearing mechanism and auditory system are remarkable in their simplicity and complexity. They take physical energy (i.e., acoustic air pressure waves) and transform it into chemical and electrical activity to allow us to hear the world around us. The physical processing of acoustic information occurs in the outer, middle, and inner ear. Physiological processing begins primarily in the inner ear and continues along the auditory nerve (VIII cranial nerve) to the central auditory nervous system.

Hearing loss is the most common of all physical impairments. A hearing loss can involve a communication handicap with psychosocial disadvantages, including delays in development of speech, language, social skills, and educational achievement. There are two primary types of hearing impairments in children and adults: hearing sensitivity impairments and auditory nervous system impairments. Hearing sensitivity impairments and peripheral hearing loss are the most common type of hearing loss. When the sensory or neural cells or their connections within the cochlea are absent or not functioning normally, a sensorineural hearing loss occurs. When both the conductive mechanism (outer ear, middle ear, or both) and the cochlea are not functioning normally, there is a mixed hearing loss.

The main purpose of a hearing evaluation is to define the nature and extent of the hearing impairment. From this information, decisions can be made about appropriate steps in the rehabilitation of the hearing disorder and handicaps that may result from the impairment. The fundamental purpose of an audiological evaluation is similar for most children and adults, although the specific focus of the evaluation can vary considerably depending on the nature of the individual and the problem. Screening the hearing of newborn infants is now a routine procedure in many hospitals and is both beneficial and justifiable. Detection of hearing loss in newborns may help alert medical professionals to the possibility of other complications.

The fundamental goal of hearing rehabilitation is to limit the extent of any communication disorder that results from a hearing loss. The first step in reaching that goal is to maximize the use of residual hearing.

A hearing aid is a miniature electronic amplifier that has three main components: a microphone, an amplifier, and a speaker. Cochlear implants are the latest and most sophisticated devices to help children and adults with severe or profound bilateral hearing losses. Sign language has two main forms of communicating with the fingers and hands: finger spelling and signing. The Deaf community is a genuine culture and the community has chosen sign language as its primary method of communication.

STUDY QUESTIONS

Knowledge and Comprehension

1. Describe the tympanic membrane and its functions.

2. Explain pure-tone audiometry.

3. Explain the three major types of hearing impairments seen in children and adults.

4. What are the adenoids and how might they contribute to middle ear infections and mouth breathing?

5. Briefly explain aural rehabilitation.

Application

1. How might you explain the hearing mechanism to a client?

2. What are the signs and symptoms of middle ear infections that you might alert a parent to watch for in her child?

3. What can you do to protect your hearing?

4. What are some emotional challenges (reactions) parents may have when an infant is diagnosed with a hearing impairment, and what treatment philosophy may be most helpful when working with parents?

5. What are five dos and don'ts when relating to culturally Deaf people?

Analysis/Synthesis

1. Explain the similarities and differences between air conduction and bone conduction.

2. Compare and contrast a conductive hearing loss and a sensorineural hearing loss.

3. What are the similarities and differences between otitis media with effusion and dormant otitis media?

4. What are the differences between audiologists' professional culture and the Deaf culture?

5. How might hearing impairments affect young adults and older adults emotionally and socially?

REFERENCES

Agrawal, Y., Platz, E. A., & Niparko, J. K. (2008). Prevalence of hearing loss and differences by demographic characteristics among US adults. *Archives of Internal Medicine, 168*(14), 1522–1530.

Allen, T. E. (1986). Patterns of academic achievement among hearing impaired students: 1973–1974. In A. N. Schildroth & M. A. Karchmer (Eds.), *Deaf children in America.* San Diego, CA: College-Hill Press.

Amatuzzi, M. G., Northrop, C., Bento, R. F., & Eavey, R. (2005). Histopathological patterns of hearing loss. *International Archives of Otorhinolaryngology, 9*(3), 213–219.

American Industrial Hygiene Association. (2007). Available at http://www.aiha.org/Content/AccessInfo/consumer/.

American Speech-Language-Hearing Association. (2008a). *Incidence and prevalence of hearing loss and hearing aid use in the United States—2008 edition.* Rockville, MD: ASHA.

American Speech-Language-Hearing Association. (2008b). *Guidelines for audiologists providing adjustment counseling to families of infants and young children with hearing loss birth to 5 years of age.* Available from www.asha.org/policy.

Bamford, J., & Saunders, E. (1985). *Hearing impairment, auditory perception, and language disability.* London: Edward Arnold.

Barton, G., Davis, A., Mair, I., Parving, A., Rosenhall, U., & Sorri, M. (2001). Provision of hearing aid service: A comparison between the Nordic countries and the United Kingdom. *Scandinavian Audiology, 30*(3), 16–20.

Bellis, T. (2003). *Assessment and management of central auditory processing disorders in the educational setting: From science to practice* (2nd ed.). Clifton Park, NY: Delmar Cengage Learning.

Bess, F. H., & Humes, L. E. (2008). *Audiology: The fundamentals* (3rd ed.). Philadelphia, PA: Lippincott Williams & Wilkins.

Campbell, K. C. M. (2007). *Pharmacology and ototoxicity for audiologists.* Clifton Park, NY: Delmar Cengage Learning.

Carney, A., & Moeller, M. P. (1998). Treatment efficacy: Hearing loss in children. *Journal of Speech, Language, and Hearing Research, 41*(Supplement), S61–S84.

Chandler, C. W. (2006, July 11). Blast-related ear injury in current U.S. military operations: Role of audiology on the interdisciplinary team. *The ASHA Leader.*

Chen, W., Campbell, C., Green, G., Van Den Bogaert, K., Komodikis, L., Manolidis, et al. (2002). Linkage of otosclerosis to a third locus (OTSC3) on human chromosome 6p21.3-22.3. *Journal of Medical Genetics, 39,* 473–477.

Chen, W., Lin, C., Hwang, Y., & Ku, C. (2003). Epidemiology of otitis media in Chinese children. *Clinical Otolaryngology and Allied Sciences, 28*(5), 442–445.

Chermak, G. D., & Musiek, F. E. (2007). *Handbook of (central) auditory processing disorders: Comprehensive intervention* (Vol. II). San Diego, CA: Plural Publishing.

Clark, J. G., & English, K. M. (2004). *Counseling in audiologic practice: Helping patients and families adjust to hearing loss.* Boston, MA: Pearson Allyn and Bacon.

Cohen, N., & Waltzman, S. (1996). Cochlear implants in infants and young children. *Seminars in Hearing, 17*(2), 215–222.

Davis, A., & Refaie, A. E. (2000). Epidemiology of tinnitus. In R. Tyler (Ed.), *Tinnitus handbook.* Clifton Park, NY: Delmar Cengage Learning.

DeLuzio, J., & Girolametto, L. (2011). Peer interactions of preschool children with and without hearing loss. *Journal of Speech, Language, and Hearing Research, 54*, 1197–1210.

Diefendorf, A. O. (2005). Early hearing detection and intervention: New ASHA guidelines available on children, ages birth to 5. *The ASHA Leader, 7*, 13.

Ertmer, D. J. (2005). *The source for children with cochlear implants.* East Moline, IL: LinguiSystems.

Forner, L., & Hixon, T. (1977). Respiratory kinematics in profoundly hearing-impaired speakers. *Journal of Speech and Hearing Research, 66*, 383–408.

Geffner, D., & Ross-Swain, D. (2007). *Auditory processing disorders: Assessment, management and treatment.* San Diego, CA: Plural Publishing.

Gold, S. L. (2003). Clinical management of tinnitus and hyperacusis. *ASHA Leader,* Nov. 4–5, 23–25.

Golding-Meadow, S., & Mayberry, R. I. (2001). How do profoundly deaf children learn to read? *Learning Disability Research and Practice, 16*, 222, 229.

Harris, J. D. (1986). Anatomy and physiology of the peripheral auditory system. In *The Pro-Ed studies in communication disorders.* Austin, TX: Pro-Ed.

Hayes, D., & Northern, J. L. (1997). *Infants and hearing.* Clifton Park, NY: Delmar Cengage Learning.

Hixon, T. J., Weismer, G., & Holt, J. D. (2008). *Preclinical speech science: Anatomy, physiology, acoustics, perception.* San Diego, CA: Plural Publishing.

Hoover, A., & Krishnamurti, S. (2010). Survey of college students' MP3 listening: Habits, safety issues, attitudes, and education. *American Journal of Audiology, 19*, 73–83.

Hull, R. H. (2009). *Introduction to aural rehabilitation.* San Diego, CA: Plural Publishing.

Isaacson, J. E., & Vora, N. M. (2003). Diagnosis and treatment of hearing loss. *American Family Physician, 68*(6), 1125–1134.

Jerger, J., & Musiek, F. (2000). Report of the consensus conference on the diagnosis of auditory processing disorders in children. *Journal of the American Academy of Audiology, ii*, 467–474.

Kaplan, H. (1996). The nature of Deaf culture: Implications for speech and hearing professionals. *Journal of the Academy of Rehabilitative Audiology, 25,* 71–84.

Katz, J. (2001). *Handbook of clinical audiology.* Philadelphia, PA: Lippincott Williams & Wilkins.

Katz, J., Medwetsky, L., Burkard, R., & Hood, L. (2009). *Handbook of clinical audiology.* Philadelphia, PA: Lippincott Williams & Wilkins.

Klein, J. O. (2000). The burden of otitis media. *Vaccine, 8*(19), 2–8.

Kraemer, M., Richardson, M., Weiss, N., Furukawa, C., Shapiro, G., Pierson, W., & Bierman, C. (1983). Risk factors for persistent middle ear effusions. *Journal of the American Medical Association, 249,* 1022–1025.

Lee, K. (2012). Language and children with auditory impairment. In V. A. Reed, *An introduction to children with language disorders* (4th ed.). Boston: Pearson Allyn & Bacon.

Ling, D. (1976). *Speech and hearing-impaired child: Theory and practice.* Washington, DC: Alexander Graham Bell Association for the Deaf.

Lutter, S., Currie, M., Mitz, L., & Greenbaum, L. (2005). Antibiotic resistance patterns in children hospitalized for urinary tract infections. *Archives of Pediatric and Adolescent Medicine, 159*(10), 924–928.

MacLeod-Gallinger, J. (1993). *Deaf ethnic minorities: Have they a double liability?* Paper presented at the annual meeting of the American Educational Research Association, Rochester, NY: Office of Postsecondary Career Studies in Deafness, National Technical Institute of the Deaf.

Mahshie, J., Moseley, M. J., Scott, S. M., & Lee, J. (2006). *Enhancing communication skills of deaf and hard of hearing children in the mainstream.* Clifton Park, NY: Delmar Cengage Learning.

Mann, T., Cuttler, K., & Campbell, C. (2001). Newborn hearing screens may give a false sense of security. *Journal of the American Academy of Audiology, 12,* 215–219.

Martin, F. N., & Clark, J. G. (2009). *Introduction to Audiology* (10th ed.). Boston, MA: Pearson Allyn and Bacon.

Miles, D. (2005). *British Sign Language: A beginner's Guide.* London: BBC Books.

Mohr, P. E., Feldman, J. J., Dunbar, J., McConkey-Robbins, A., Niparko, J., Rittenhouse, R., & Skinner, M. (2000). The societal costs of severe to profound hearing loss in the United States. *International Journal of Technology Assessment in Health Care, 16*(4), 1120–1135.

Moore, M. (2010, September 21). Teens at risk: We're on the edge of an epidemic: Research on hearing loss has long-term implications for audiologists. *The ASHA Leader.*

Mosby. (2009). *Mosby's dictionary of medicine, nursing, & health professions* (8th ed.). St. Louis, MO: Mosby Elsevier.

Munos, K., Nelson, L., Goldgewicht, N., & Odell, D. (2011). Early hearing detection and intervention: Diagnostic hearing assessment practices. *American Journal of Audiology, 20,* 123–131.

Musiek, F. E., Baran, J. A., & Pinheiro, M. L. (1994). *Neuroaudiology case studies.* Clifton Park, NY: Delmar Cengage Learning.

Musiek, F. E., & Chermak, G. D. (2007). *Handbook of (central) auditory processing disorders: Auditory neuroscience and diagnosis* (Vol. I). San Diego, CA: Plural Publishing.

Nadler, N. (1997). Noisy toys: Hidden hazards. *Hearing Health,* November/December, 18–21.

National Council on Aging. (1999). *The consequences of untreated hearing loss in older persons.* Washington, DC: National Council on Aging.

National Information Center for Children and Youth with Disabilities. (2004, January). *Deafness and hearing loss* (Pub. No. FS3). Washington, DC: Author.

National Institute of Deafness and Communication Disorders. (2002). Report of the ad hoc committee on epidemiology and statistics in communication. Bethesda, MD: National Institutes of Health.

Nicholas, J. G., & Greers, A. E. (2003). Personal, social, and family adjustment in school-aged children with cochlear implants. *Ear and Hearing, 24,* 69–81.

Northern, J. L., & Downs, M. P. (2012). *Hearing in children* (6th ed.). Baltimore, MD: Lippincott Williams & Wilkins.

O'Neil, J. (2007). Audiologic/Aural rehabilitation is valued and necessary. *The ASHA Leader,* June 19, 5–6.

Pichora-Fuller, M. K. (1997). Language comprehension in older listeners. *Journal of Speech-Language Pathology and Audiology, 21,* 125–142.

Samore, M., Magill, M., Adler, S., Severina, E., Morrison, L., De Boer, L., Lyon, L., & Carroll, K. (2001). High rates of multiple antibiotic resistance in streptococcus pneumonia from healthy children living in isolated rural communities. *Pediatrics, 108*(4), 856–865.

Sandlin, R. E., & Olsson, R. T. (2000). Subjective tinnitus: Its mechanism and treatment. In M. Valente, H. Hossford-Dunn, & R. Roeser (Eds.), *Audiology treatment.* New York, NY: Thieme.

Schirmer, B. (2001). *Psychological, social, and educational dimensions of deafness.* Boston, MA: Allyn and Bacon.

Seikel, J. A., King, D. W., & Drumright, D. G. (2010). *Anatomy and physiology for speech, language, and hearing* (4th ed.). Clifton Park, NY: Delmar Cengage Learning.

Shafer, D. N. (2006, April 11). Noise-induced hearing loss hits teens: ASHA holds national press club event to highlight dangers of MP3 players, media coverage goes worldwide. *The ASHA Leader.*

Shargorodsky, J., Curhan, S. G., Curhan, G. C., & Eavy, R. (2010). Change in prevalence of hearing loss in U.S. adolescents. *Journal of the American Medical Association, 304*(7), 772–778.

Shirin, D. A., & Reed Susanne. (2005). Written language of deaf and hard-of-hearing students in public schools. *Journal of Deaf Studies and Deaf Education, 10*(3), 244–255.

Siegel, R. M., & Bien, J. P. (2004). Acute otitis media in children. *Pediatrics in Review, 25,* 187–193.

Stach, B. A. (2010). *Clinical audiology: An introduction* (2nd ed.). Clifton Park, NY: Delmar Cengage Learning.

Stiles, D. J., McGregor, K. K., & Bentler, R. A. (2012). Vocabulary and working memory in children fit with hearing aids. *Journal of Speech, Language, and Hearing Research, 55,* 154–167.

Strom, K. E. (2004, March). A brightening Future? A review of today's hearing instrument market. *Hearing Review.*

Tomblin, J. B., Barker, B. A., Spencer, L. J., Zhang, X., & Gantz, B. J. (2005). The effect of age at cochlear implant initial stimulation on expressive language growth in infants and toddlers. *Journal of Speech, Language, and Hearing Research, 48,* 853–867.

Tye-Murray, N. (2009). *Foundations of aural rehabilitation: Children, adults, and their family members* (3rd ed.). Clifton Park, NY: Delmar Cengage Learning.

Tye-Murray, N. (2012). Counseling for adults and children who have hearing loss. In L. V. Flasher & P. T. Fogle, *Counseling Skills for Speech-Language Pathologists and Audiologists.* Clifton Park, NY: Delmar Cengage Learning.

Tye-Murray, N., & Folkins, J. (1990). Jaw and lip movements of deaf talkers producing utterances with known stress patterns. *Journal of the Acoustical Society of America, 87,* 2675–2683.

Van Bereijk, W., Pierce, J., & David, E. (1960). Waves and the ear. *Science, 131* (339), 219–220.

Vaughn, L. (2005, February 8). Diagnosis and follow-up of hearing loss in infants. *ASHA Leader, 1,* 4.

Vinson, B. P. (2011). *Preschool and school-aged language disorders.* Clifton Park, NY: Delmar Cengage Learning.

Walker, J. D. (2003). *Universal newborn screening: Saving money, saving lives.* Annual meeting of the Texas Chapter of the American Academy of Pediatrics, Galveston, TX.

Wilson, P. L., & Roeser, R. J. (1997). Cerumen management: Professional issues and techniques. *Journal of the American Academy of Audiology, 8,* 421–430.

Woodward, J. (1972). Implications of sociolinguistic research among the deaf. *Sign Language Studies, 1,* 1–7.

Yoshinaga-Itano, C., & Gravel, J. S. (2001). The evidence for universal newborn hearing screening. *American Journal of Audiology, 10,* 62–64.

Yoshinaga-Itano, C., Sedey, A., Coulter, D., & Mehl, A. (1998). Language of early- and later-identified children with hearing loss. *Pediatrics, 102*(5), 1161–1171.

Epilogue

Congratulations! You have completed your introductory course on speech-language pathology and audiology and have read this textbook on the essentials of these professions—not an easy task. There likely were some surprises in what you learned about the professions. For one, there is much more to these professions than what anyone can imagine who has not studied them. The scope, breadth and depth of information that you will use as your daily base of knowledge includes understanding what is normal and what is abnormal about human communication. Within this understanding, you have knowledge of the anatomy and physiology of each of the speech systems: respiratory, phonatory, resonatory, articulatory, and auditory. You also have a foundational understanding of the neurology that makes the speech systems function independently and together.

Appreciating the complex interactions of these systems adds to the amazement of what it takes to understand the simplest messages we hear and to provide the simplest responses. Fortunately, in our everyday communication we are able to take all of these for granted and hardly give them a second thought. If we had to consciously think of all that takes place every second while we are communicating, we would be continually stumbling over our thoughts, words, and muscle movements that are required to talk.

Another surprise for many students is how much of the study of speech-language pathology and audiology can be applied to their everyday lives. To truly appreciate the knowledge you acquire, it helps to relate it to your personal life. From my perspective, studying speech-language pathology and audiology are the best majors for preparation for adult life and parenthood. You learn about normal and abnormal development of infants and children. You learn how to work with children one-on-one and in small groups of two or three. You learn how to motivate children to work hard to improve their communication and academic skills. You learn how to manage the sometimes delicate task of talking with parents about their concerns regarding their children. You learn how to work with adults and elderly people with a variety of neurological problems and the sensitive issues that accompany impairment or loss of communication abilities. You learn about the problems of hearing impairments at all ages and the effects on not only the person with a loss but the family. And you learn how to be a patient, active listener—a trained listener—which is perhaps the most important interpersonal skill you can develop. On a personal level, it is inevitable that sometime in your life you will be confronted with a few of the disorders discussed within this text. What problems you escape, someone you care about may not.

If you choose not to take further course work in speech-language pathology, consider that you can always draw on the information you have learned and apply it to yourself and people you care about when needed. There is also a possibility that you may be a resource to your family and friends by having some basic education in this area, as well as having a textbook that you can keep for reference. This textbook was written and designed to be "a keeper." The book can be a valuable reference when someone asks you a question that relates to anything you studied in the course. You cannot present yourself as an "armchair" speech-language pathologist or audiologist, but you can speak with some knowledge that could help another person recognize the importance of seeking help from a professional speech-language pathologist or audiologist who is state licensed and nationally certified. For example, over the years, you may refer to this text to refresh your memory on middle ear infections in your own children or problems in speech and language development. Some years down the line, you may be amid the "sandwich generation"—trying to raise your own family at the same time you are taking care of elderly parents or grandparents. Having an understanding of neurological disorders and dementia can help you communicate with medical and rehabilitation staff.

This text also was written to be "a keeper" for SLP and Aud majors. The extensive glossary was carefully developed to provide a resource for terms and definitions for students to have many of the important words used in our professional vocabularies. Another reason for holding on to this text is that it can be helpful when taking graduate courses. For example, when beginning a graduate course on neurological disorders, a quick rereading of Chapter 11, Neurological Disorders in Adults, will be an excellent memory refresher for many of the concepts you will learn in graduate-level textbooks. Likewise, rereading that chapter can get you off to a good start in the clinic with your first client who has had a CVA or TBI if you have not yet completed your coursework in that area. Clinical supervisors are impressed when they hear a student say, "I reread the chapter on neurological disorders in adults in the text we used in the intro course and I think I have a basic understanding of aphasia, but there is still a lot more for me to learn."

Beyond the academic preparation for your profession, so often it seems that when there is a fully qualified SLP or Aud in a family, that person becomes an important resource to other family members. SLPs and Auds know a considerable amount about the human body and various medical problems that can result in disorders and handicaps of various kinds. SLPs and Auds also learn how to negotiate many of the complexities of the medical system, including how to talk with doctors and nurses at a professional level. SLPs and Auds learn about the educational system and how to talk to and interact with teachers and administrators at a professional level—a valuable skill for parents.

Not to sound overly dramatic, but your education and training in speech-language pathology and audiology will change you for the better. Your best character traits will be enhanced. If you consider yourself a patient, understanding, caring, and insightful person, those traits will become stronger. Your character weaknesses may become apparent as well. For example, if you have difficulty tolerating ambiguity—not being able to handle knowing there are few absolutes when working with people who have complex problems—that trait will be magnified and will likely result in considerable frustration. Having disorders neatly contained in boxes with specific therapy approaches and techniques to help empty the boxes is an ideal that is not based on reality.

If communication disorders were mechanical problems where parts could be repaired or replaced, our work would be "cleaner." However, it is the human elements such as emotions, motivation, amount of physical energy, and even the will to want to improve that can make the difference in the success of therapy. The final section of each chapter in this text was always about the emotional and social effects of the disorder. No matter how much we know about a disorder, the variables that determine success in therapy often depend on the emotional makeup and social support of the people who need our help.

Finally, you the student and future clinician are an essential variable in a child's or an adult's success in therapy. If, while taking this course, you continually found it difficult to devote time to studying the material because it did not grab your interest, there is a reasonably good chance that this is not the kind of information you want to spend the next few years delving deeper into, much less spending decades working with. If, on the other hand, you found most chapters of study interesting and even fascinating and could hardly wait to reach the next chapter to see what lies in store, this could be the kind of information you could find endlessly intriguing and captivating. There is an added joy to life when your chosen profession never becomes boring or "old," where you are always interested in the new discoveries, want to learn new ways of viewing familiar problems, and can hardly wait to try new therapy procedures and materials on your clients and patients.

SLPs or Auds whom you happen to meet while on vacation or holiday any place in the country or the world are never strangers; you always have common bonds and things to talk about. It seems that SLPs and Auds never tire of talking about their favorite subject. I have seen people marvel at watching SLPs and Auds who have just met talk animatedly and with a sense of camaraderie about the subject that binds them together. The bottom line for SLPs and Auds is always the children and adults we are trying to help. The treatment approaches, techniques, and materials we use are merely tools for helping people communicate and improve their quality of life. It is hoped that your study of speech-language pathology and audiology further enhances *your* quality of life.

Best wishes to you all,
Paul T. Fogle, Ph.D., CCC-SLP

A

abduct/abduction—The opening of the vocal folds away from the midline; (L. *abducto,* to take away).

accent—Usually considered the speech pronunciation and inflections used by nonnative American English speakers (foreign accent); (L. *ac-* [variation of *ad-*], to, + *cantus,* song; i.e., to sing).

acoustic trauma—Damage to hearing from a transient, high-intensity sound; (Gk. *akoustikos,* hearing, + *trauma,* wound).

acquired disorder—A disorder that begins after an individual has developed normal communication abilities, such as a hearing loss from loud noise exposure or a speech, language, or cognitive disorder caused by a traumatic brain injury; (L. *acquirere,* to seek in addition to; *dis,* apart or impaired, + *ordo,* rank).

activities of daily living (ADLs)—The normal activities and tasks people perform in the course of a day, such as ablutions (washing, bathing, brushing the teeth, toileting), dressing, and eating.

acute—Intense and of short duration, usually referring to a disease or injury; (L. *acutus,* sharp).

acute care hospital—A hospital where patients are treated for brief but severe episodes of illness, injury, trauma, or during recovery from surgery; (L. *acutus,* sharp; Old Ger. *chara,* lament; L. *hospitium,* guesthouse).

acute laryngitis/traumatic laryngitis—An abrupt, intense, and usually relatively brief inflammation of the mucous membrane lining in the larynx, accompanied by edema of the vocal folds with hoarseness and loss of voice that is often caused by severe vocal abuse.

adaptive behavior—The ability to act as independently and responsibly as other people of the same age and cultural background in everyday social and practical skills; includes conceptual skills (e.g., language and money concepts), social skills (e.g., following rules and pragmatics), and practical skills (e.g., dressing appropriately and work skills); (L. *adaptare,* to fit).

addition—The insertion of a sound or sounds not part of a word itself, such as *animamal* for *animal;* (L. *ad-,* before, + *dere,* to put).

adduct/adduction—The closing of the vocal folds toward the midline; (L. *adducto,* to bring to).

adenoids (pharyngeal tonsils)—Lymphoid tissue (tissue that produces lymphocytes, which are helpful in fighting infection) found on the pharyngeal wall in the nasal–pharyngeal region; begin to develop about 6 months of age and may continue to grow and possibly interfere with or occlude the openings of the Eustachian tubes; when enlarged, they may block the passage of air from the nasal cavity into the pharynx, preventing normal nasal breathing and requiring mouth breathing; sometimes removed to allow nasal breathing and help prevent middle ear infections; (Gk. *aden,* gland, + *eidos,* form; Gk. *pharynx,* throat, L. *tonsillae,* tonsil).

admittance—The ease and flow of energy transmission through a system; the reciprocal of impedance; (L. *admittere,* to allow in).

affect/affective—Relating to, arising from, or influencing feelings or emotions; *affect* is revealed by facial expressions, body posture and gestures, tone of voice, and choice of words; (L. *afficio,* to have influence on).

agrammatic/agrammatism—Impairment of the ability to produce words in their correct sequence and with all necessary morphemes; (Gk. *agrammatos,* unlearned; from *a-,* without, + *grammatikos,* letters).

agraphia—A disorder of writing resulting in difficulty writing letters, words, and sentences; (Gk. *a-,* without or loss of, + *graphos,* write).

air conduction—The transmission of sound to the inner ear through the external auditory canal and the structures of the middle ear; (L. *con* [variation of *com*], together, + *ducere,* to lead).

alexia (acquired dyslexia)—Impaired ability to read as the result of neurological damage; (Gk. *a-,* without or loss of, *dys,* impairment or disorder, + *lexis,* word; L. *acquirere,* to seek or obtain).

allophone—Slight variation in the way different people produce individual phonemes that can be affected by the initial, middle, or final position of a word, or what sounds precede or follow an individual phoneme; (Gk. *allos,* other or different, + *phonema,* sound).

alphabetic principle—Letters and combinations of letters represent speech sounds; speech can be turned into print; and print can be turned into speech; (L. *alpha,* letter *a,* + *beta,* letter *b*; L. *princep,* first or chief).

alveolar ridge—The upper portion of the mandible and the lower portion of the maxilla that contain sockets for the roots of the teeth; (L. *alveolus,* little hollow—in reference to the sockets for the teeth).

Alzheimer's disease (AD)—A disease that causes progressive dementia that usually begins after age 65 and in many cases is related to genetic factors that cause neuronal degeneration, cerebral atrophy, neurofibrillary tangles, neuritic plaques, white matter changes, and diminished neurotransmitters; characterized by decline in memory, intellect, disorientation, delusions, personality changes, and communication impairments (named after Alois Alzheimer, German neuropsychiatrist, 1864–1915).

American Sign Language (ASL)—A manual system of communication commonly used by members of the

Deaf culture in the United States; sometimes referred to as *Ameslan*.

American Speech-Language-Hearing Association (ASHA)—The professional organization that represents speech-language pathologists and audiologists and sets standards for their education, training, and certification. The organization was formerly called the American Speech and Hearing Association, and retained the ASHA abbreviation.

amyotrophic lateral sclerosis (ALS, Lou Gehrig's disease)—A rare, rapidly progressive degenerative disease of motor neurons that control movement of all muscle systems, including the speech systems; (Gk. *a-*, without, + *myo*, muscle, + *trophe*, nourishment; *latus*, side; *sklerosis*, hardening).

anarthria/anarthric—The complete inability to articulate or speak that is usually caused by brain lesions or damage to peripheral nerves that innervate the articulatory muscles; (L. *an-*, without, + Gk. *arthron*, joined; i.e., [speech] that is not joined).

anesthesia—The administration of a topical, local, regional, or general drug or agent capable of producing a partial or complete loss of sensation or consciousness; (Gk. *an-*, without or loss of, + *aisthesis*, feeling, sensation, or perception).

aneurysm—A localized dilation of a blood vessel wall, resulting in the thinning of the wall at that site (much like a balloon being blown up) and increasing the likelihood of hemorrhaging, especially with high blood pressure; (Gk. *aneurysma*, to dilate).

anomia—Impaired ability to retrieve (remember) names of people, places, or things, as well as to retrieve other parts of speech (e.g., verbs and adjectives) while speaking; (Gk., *a-*, without, + *noma*, name).

anomic aphasia—A syndrome whose primary feature is persistent and severe difficulty retrieving names of people, places, and objects, as well as all classes of words (e.g., verbs and adjectives); (Gk. *a-*, without or loss of, + L. *nomen*, name; *a-*, without or loss of, + *phasos*, to speak).

anosognosia—Decreased awareness of deficits or disabilities often seen in right-hemisphere damage; impairment of an individual's ability to relate to parts of the body; (Gk., *a*, without, + *nosos*, disease, + *gnosis*, knowledge).

anoxia—A complete lack of oxygen to the brain that is relatively rare and is usually caused by asphyxiation (e.g., near-drowning or loss of airway from choking) or inadequate blood circulation (e.g., heart attack) that results in unconsciousness and death of brain tissue; (Gk. *a*, without, + *oxys*, sharp).

aphasia (dysphasia)—A deficit in language processing that may affect all input modalities (auditory, visual, and tactile) and all output modalities (speaking, writing, and gesturing); (Gk. *a-*, without or loss of, + *phasos*, to speak; *dys*, impairment or disorder, + *phasos*).

aphonia—A complete loss of voice followed by whispering for oral communication that typically has psychological causes such as emotional stress; (Gk. *a-* without or loss of, + *phone*, voice).

apraxia of speech (speech apraxia, verbal apraxia, acquired apraxia)—A deficit in the neural motor planning and programming of the articulatory muscles for voluntary movements for speech in the absence of muscular weakness; primarily interferes with articulation and prosody; (Gk. *a-* loss, + L. *praxis*, movement or action).

arteriosclerosis—A common disorder characterized by thickening, hardening, and loss of elasticity of arterial walls as a result of build-up of atherosclerotic plaque, leading to decreased blood supply; (Gk. *arteria*, artery, + *sklerosis*, hardening).

articulation/articulator—In speech, the mandible, lips, tongue, and soft palate are the articulators; *articulation* refers to the movements of the articulators for speech sound production that involves accuracy in placement, timing, direction of movement, and pressure of the articulators on one another; the totality of motor processes involved in the planning and execution of speech; (L. *articulatus*, joined).

articulation disorder—The incorrect production of speech sounds due to faulty placement, timing, direction, pressure, speed, or integration of the movements of the mandible, lips, tongue, or velum; (L. *articulatus*, joined; L. *dis-* apart or impaired, + *ordo*, arrangement or group; i.e., arrangement apart from what is [normally] joined—misarticulated).

arytenoid cartilages—A pair of pyramid-shaped cartilages that sit on top of the posterior edge of the cricoid cartilage and rotate to open and close the vocal folds and pivot back and forth to help change the pitch of the voice; (Gk. *arytaina*, ladle, + *eidos*, form; L. *cartilago*, cartilage).

aspiration—A term in reference to material (food, liquid, saliva, etc.) penetrating the larynx and entering the airway below the true vocal folds; food or liquid entering the lungs rather than the stomach after the swallow; (L. *aspirare*, to breathe upon).

aspiration pneumonia—An acute inflammation of the lungs caused by foreign material (e.g., food or liquid) entering the lung tissue and resulting in infection; alveolar and bronchiole congestion with substances discharged from the alveolar walls as a protection against foreign material; (L. *aspirare*, to breathe upon; (Gk. *pneumon*, lung, + *-ia*, suffix meaning disease).

assessment—See *evaluation*.

assistive listening device—Amplification systems, other than conventional hearing aids, that are designed for specific listening situations (e.g., personal amplifiers, telephone amplifiers, personal text telephones, and personal FM systems); (L. *ad-*, to or toward, + *sistere*, take a stand or cause to stand).

atherosclerosis—A common disorder characterized by yellowish plaques of cholesterol and other lipids (fats) in the inner layers of the walls of arteries; often associated with tobacco use, obesity, hypertension, diabetes mellitus, and aging; (Gk. *athere*, meal, + *sklerosis*, hardening).

atrophy—A shrinking in size or wasting away that is usually caused by injury, disease, lack of use (e.g., muscles), or natural reduction in size over time (e.g., adenoids and tonsils); (Gk. *atrophia*, wasting away [*a-*, not, + *trophe*, nourishment]).

attainable treatment—The expectation that an individual can achieve a specific target within a reasonably specified time; (L. *at-*, before, + *tangere*, to touch, + *abilis*, capable; L. *tractare*, to handle or deal with, + *mentum*, result).

attention deficit/hyperactive disorder (AD/HD, ADD)—A broad syndrome relating to children who demonstrate three primary problems: inattention, impulsivity, and hyperactivity; (L. *addendere*, to stretch; *deficere*, to want; Gk. *hyper-*, excess, + L. *activus*, active).

attention impairments—Difficulty staying focused on a task, difficulty appropriately shifting attention from one task to another, and dividing attention between auditory and visual stimuli; (L. *prejorare*, make worse).

audiogram—A standard graph used to record pure-tone hearing thresholds with air- and bone-conduction thresholds graphed by frequency in hertz (Hz) and hearing level (HL) in decibels (dB); (L. *audire*, to hear, + Gk. *gramma*, record).

audiologist—A professional who is specifically educated and trained to identify, evaluate, treat, and prevent hearing disorders, plus select and evaluate hearing aids, and habilitate or rehabilitate individuals with hearing impairments; (L. *audire*, to hear, + *logia*, study of).

audiometer—An electronic device designed to measure the sensitivity of hearing of pure-tone frequencies (*hertz*) and *intensities* (decibels); sounds are delivered to the ears either through earphones or *free field* (i.e., through loudspeakers in a testing environment with no reverberating surfaces) in an audiometry booth; (L. *audio-*, to hear, + Gk. *metron*, measure).

auditory brainstem response (ABR)—An *electrophysiological response* (the relationship between electrical activity and biologic function, in this case, brain activity) to sound that consists of five to seven identifiable peaks that represent neural function of auditory pathways.

auditory comprehension—The ability to understand spoken language at the single word, phrase, simple sentence, complex sentence, paragraph, and conversational speech levels; (L. *com*, with, + *prehendere*, to grasp).

auditory discrimination training (ear training)—The ability to distinguish sounds from one another; involves a comparison of heard sounds with other sounds; a technique used in articulation therapy that stresses careful listening to differentiate among speech sounds; (L. *dis-*, apart, + *crimin*, distinction).

auditory nervous system impairment—The result of reduced ability to clearly hear sounds above the hearing threshold; occurs less often than hearing sensitivity impairments, which may occur concurrently, causing a dual hearing problem.

auditory processing disorder (APD)/central auditory processing disorder (CAPD)—A disorder in children and adults who have difficulty using auditory information to communicate and learn; may affect their abilities to listen, understand speech, develop language, and have academic success; (L. *auditorius*, hearing; *pro-*, forward, + *cedere*, to go; *centrum*, center).

auditory training—Aural rehabilitation methods designed to optimize use of residual hearing by structured practice in listening, altering the environment, use of hearing aids, etc.

augmentative and alternative communication (AAC) or assistive technology (AT)—Any approach designed to support, enhance, or supplement the communication of individuals who are not independent verbal communicators in all situations; (L. *augmentum*, increase, + *ativus*, tending to; *alter*, other or another; *assistere*, cause to stand; Gk. *techne*, art or skill, + *logos*, study of).

aural habilitation—Sometimes used synonymously with *aural rehabilitation*; intervention for people who have not developed listening, speech, and language skills; may include diagnosis of communication and hearing-related difficulties, speech perception training, speech and language therapy, manual communication, and educational management.

aural rehabilitation—A broad term that involves intervention aimed at minimizing and alleviating the communication difficulties associated with hearing loss; includes identification and diagnosis, patient and family counseling and education, selection and fitting amplification devices, communication training strategies, speech perception training, speech-language therapy, promotion of literacy, and educational management; (L. *auris*, ear, *-alis*, related to; L. *re-* again, + *habitare*, make fit).

autism—A highly variable neurodevelopmental disorder in the broad *autism spectrum disorders (ASD)*, which is in the still broader group of *pervasive developmental disorders*. Autism is a lifelong complex behavioral syndrome that appears by 3 years of age, with children having a markedly absent interest in social interactions and relationships; severely impaired communication skills; and repetitive, stereotyped movements; and restricted interests that are often obsessive or fixated; (Gk. *autos*, self).

autism spectrum disorder (ASD)—A range of developmental disorders from mild to severe, with autism being the most severe form; (Gk. *autos*, self; L. *specere*, to look at or appearance).

automatic speech—Over-learned sequences of words that can be recited without much conscious thought, such as counting to 10; saying the days of the week, months of the year, and the alphabet; and singing some songs (e.g., the birthday song); (Gk. *auto-*, self, + *matos*, thinking).

autonomy—Respect for the patient's right to determine his or her own choices in making health care decisions; (Gk. *auto-*, self, + *nomos*, custom or law).

autopsy (postmortem)—A medical examination performed to determine or confirm the cause of death; (Gk. *auto*, self, + *opsis*, view; L. *post*, after, + *mors*, death).

axon—The cellular extension of a neuron that carries impulses away from the cell body; (Gk. *axon*, axis or axle).

B

babbling—The production of a consonant and vowel in the same syllable, either reduplicated (*ba-ba, gaa-gaa*) or nonreduplicated (*baa-da-gi*), that tends to appear about 6 or 7 months of age; (L. *babulus*, prattle).

behavioral theory (behaviorism)—In reference to speech and language, a perspective of development that asserts that speech and language are behaviors learned through operant conditioning.

Bernoulli's law—A law in physics that states when air flowing through a tube (e.g., trachea) reaches a constriction (e.g., vocal folds) there is an increase in speed of the flow of air that causes decreased pressure on the walls of the constriction that results in a slight negative pressure (i.e., slight vacuum) at the constriction; in voice, this slight negative pressure contributes to the vocal folds closing during vibration; (Daniel Bernoulli, Swiss scientist, 1700–1782).

bilabial—Referring to the two lips; (L. *bi-* two, + *labia*, lips).

bilingual—Children who often speak the parents' native language in the home environment and speak American English in school or other environments; (L. *bi-*, two, + *lingua*, tongue).

bioethics—The attempt to understand and resolve ethical issues and problems in the health care setting; (*bio-*, life, + Gk. *ethos*, moral character).

biofeedback—The process of becoming aware of various physiological functions of the body using instruments that provide information on the activity of muscles or systems being monitored, with the goal of being able to control or manipulate those muscles or systems voluntarily.

blend (consonant cluster)—A blend or consonant cluster occurs when two or more sounds appear together with no vowel separation (e.g., /tr, sp, bl, str, spl, str, skw/).

board and care home—A homelike environment where there may be a few to several elderly or physically impaired individuals residing and meals, laundry, and other services are provided.

bone conduction—Transmission of sound to the inner ear through vibration applied to the bones of the skull; allows determination of the cochlea's hearing sensitivity while bypassing any outer or middle ear abnormalities.

brainstem—The structure (pons and medulla oblongata) that connects the brain to the spinal cord; it is important in sensory and motor functions and contains neurons for the cranial nerves that exit the pons and medulla.

breathiness—Incomplete closure of the vocal folds during phonation that results in excessive unvibrated air escaping.

Broca's aphasia—A nonfluent expressive aphasia characterized by agrammatic language with omissions of articles, conjunctions, prepositions, plurals, possessives, and verb morphemes and auxiliary verbs; speech is often limited to high-frequency content words, making it sound telegraphic; apraxia of speech, dysarthria, or both often coexist; (named after Paul Broca, French neurosurgeon, 1824–1880).

Broca's area—The center for motor speech control (planning, sequencing, coordinating, and initiating) of the articulators located in the lower posterior portion of the left hemisphere's frontal lobe.

bruxing—A compulsive, unconscious clenching and grinding of the teeth, especially during sleep or as a mechanism for releasing tension during periods of extreme stress in waking hours; (Gk. *brychein*, to gnash the teeth)

C

cancer (carcinoma)—A malignant *neoplasm* (new growth) characterized by uncontrolled growth of cells that tend to invade surrounding tissue and *metastasize* (spread) to distant body sites; (L. *cancer*, crab; Gk. *karkinos*, crab, + *oma*, tumor).

cartilage—Firm, fibrous, and strong connective tissue that does not contain blood vessels; (L. *cartilage*, gristle).

central nervous system (CNS)—The brain, cerebellum, brainstem, and spinal cord; (Gk. *kentron*, center; *neuron*, nerve; *systema*, system).

cerebellum—The CNS structure largely concerned with the coordination of muscles and the maintenance of balance and body equilibrium; (L. *cerebellum*, little cerebrum; i.e., little brain).

cerebral embolism (embolus)—An abnormal condition in which a blood clot, piece of tumor, or other material (embolus) circulates in the bloodstream until it becomes lodged in a cerebral blood vessel, causing an occlusion; at the location of the occlusion, the embolus begins to function as a thrombus; (Gk. *embolus*, wedge-shaped object used as a stopper).

cerebral hemisphere—Either of the two halves of the brain that contains a frontal lobe, parietal lobe, occipital lobe, and temporal lobe; (L. *cerebrum*, brain; Gk. *hemi*, half, + *sphaira*, ball).

cerebral hemorrhage (hemorrhagic stroke)—The result of a blood vessel under pressure rupturing and sending blood into the brain tissue; hemorrhages may be arterial, venous, or capillary; (Gk. *haimo*, blood, + *rrhagia*, to break or burst).

cerebral palsy (CP)—A developmental neuromotor disorder that is caused by damage to the central nervous system *prenatally* (before birth), *natally/perinatally* (during birth), or *postnatally* (during childhood) and results in a nonprogressive, permanent neuromuscular disorder; dysarthria affecting all speech systems is the most common speech problem; (L. *cerebrum*, brain; Gk. *para*, beyond, + *lysis*, loosening; *palsy* is a modification of the word *paralysis*).

cerebral thrombosis (thrombus)—An abnormal condition in which a clot (thrombus) develops within a blood vessel; (Gk. *thrombos*, clot).

cerumen—A yellowish or brownish waxy secretion produced by ceruminous glands in the ear canal that protects the ear canal from intrusion by insects; (L. *cera*, wax).

childhood apraxia of speech (CAS)—A childhood motor speech disorder in the absence of muscle weakness that affects the planning, programming, sequencing, coordinating, and initiating motor movements of the articulators that interferes with articulation and prosody; (Gk. *a-*, loss, + *praxis*, movement or action).

chronic—Of long duration with slow progress, usually in reference to a disease or disorder; (Gk. *chronos*, time).

chronic laryngitis—A persistent laryngitis lasting more than 10 days with inflammation of the mucous membrane lining in the larynx, accompanied by edema of the vocal folds with hoarseness and loss of voice that is often caused by heavy smoking, coughing, allergies and chemical irritants, and ongoing vocal abuse and misuse; (Gk. *chronos*, time, *larynx*, larynx, + *itis*, inflammation).

chronic traumatic encephalopathy (CTE)—A degenerative brain disease caused by repeated brain traumas (particularly concussions) that results in behaviors similar to Alzheimer's disease; (Gk. *chromos*, time; *trauma*, wound; *enkephalos*, brain, + *pathos*, disease).

chronological age—The actual age of a person that is derived from date of birth and expressed in days, months, and years; (Gk. *khronos*, time, + *logia*, study of).

circumlocution—The use of a description or "talking around" a word when the specific word cannot be recalled; (L. *circum*, around, + *locutio*, speech).

client-specific measurements (clinician devised assessments)—Assessments that are not standardized tests that a clinician constructs to make decisions about a specific client's communication abilities; (L. *clientem*, follower; *species*, sort; *mensurare*, to measure).

Clinical Fellowship—A 36-week full-time (35 hours per week) or the equivalent part-time mentored clinical experience totaling a minimum of 1,260 hours begun after all academic coursework and university clinic training are completed; required by ASHA to be eligible for the Certificate of Clinical Competence (CCC).

clinical intuition—A decision-making process that is used unconsciously by experienced clinicians that is rapid, subtle, and based on the entire context of the situation, but does not follow simple, cause-and-effect logic; (L. *intuititus*, look at or consider).

clinicians—Health care professionals, such as physicians, nurses, physical therapists, occupational therapists, speech-language pathologists, audiologists, psychiatrists, or psychologists involved in clinical practice who base their practice on direct observation and treatment of a patient or client; (Gk. *kline*, bed).

closed head injury (CHI) (nonpenetrating brain injury)—Severe impact to the skull that damages the brain, often with a blunt object such as the windshield of a vehicle or a bat, or the head striking the ground after a fall; the skull may be fractured but is not penetrated (e.g., by a bullet).

cluttering—A fluency disorder with speech that is abnormally fast with omission of sounds and syllables of words, abnormal patterns of pausing and phrasing, and often spoken in bursts that may be unintelligible; frequently includes abnormalities in syntax, semantics, and pragmatics; (ME, *clotteren*, to clot).

cochlea—The part of the inner ear containing the sensory mechanism of hearing; a spiral tunnel with 2¾ turns about 30 mm (about 1¼ inches) long, resembling a tiny snail shell; (L. *cochlea*, snail shell).

code switching—An occurrence for bilingual individuals in which sounds, words, semantics, syntactic, or pragmatic elements from one language are included when speaking another language, either automatically or intentionally; also can be expanded to include nonstandard and standard dialects; (L. *caudex*, book).

cognate—Two sounds that differ only in voicing (e.g., /p/ - /b/); (L. *cognatus*, of common descent; from *co-*, with, + *gnatus* [*natus*], to be born).

cognition—The act or process of thinking or learning that involves perceiving, memory, abstraction, generalization, reasoning, judgment, and problem solving; closely related to intelligence; (L. *cognitio*, knowledge; *co-*, with or together, + *gnoscere*, to know).

cognitive behavioral therapy—A model of counseling designed to help individuals recognize and examine problematic beliefs and replace them with more adaptive and flexible ways of thinking.

cognitive development—The progressive and continuous growth of perception, memory, imagination, conception, judgment, and reasoning; it is the intellectual counterpart of a person's biological adaptation to the environment; (L. *cognitio*, knowledge; Fr. *desvoluper*, to unwrap or expose).

cognitive disorder—An impairment of attention, perception, memory, reasoning, judgment, and/or problem solving (i.e., thinking) to allow adequate functioning in activities of daily living (L. *cognitio*, knowledge; *dis*, apart or impaired, + *ordo*, rank).

coma—A prolonged period of unconsciousness in which a patient has minimal, if any, purposeful responses to stimuli; (Gk. *koma*, deep sleep).

communicate/communication—Any means by which individuals relate their wants, needs, thoughts, knowledge, and feelings to another person; (L. *communicare*, to share).

communication (communicative) disorder—Speech, language, voice, resonance, cognitive, or hearing that noticeably deviates from that of other people, calls attention to itself, interferes with communication, or causes distress in both the speaker and the listener; any speech, language, voice, resonance, cognitive, or hearing impairment, disability, or handicap that interferes with a person conveying his wants, needs, thoughts, knowledge, and feelings to another person; (L. *communicare*, to share; *dis-*, apart or impaired, + *ordinare*, to order; i.e., communication that is not in order).

communication (conversation) board—An apparatus or simple board upon which common communication symbols and messages (e.g., alphabet, numbers, pictures, symbols, and common words and expressions) are represented, allowing expressive communication by pointing or gazing; communication boards may be no-tech, low-tech, or sophisticated high-tech electronic devices.

communicative competence—A child's grammatical knowledge of phonology, morphology, syntax, semantics, and pragmatics; (L. *com* [variation of *cum*] with or together, + *petitio*, request or seek).

compliance—The ease with which the tympanic membrane and middle ear mechanism function; (L. *complere*, to complete).

computerized tomography (CT) scan—A radiographic technique to visualize body tissue not able to be seen on standard X-ray images; formerly called computerized axial tomography (CAT) scan; (L. *com-*, with or together, + *putare*, to consider; Gk. *tomos*, section, + L. *graphos*, write).

concussion—Mild traumatic brain injury caused by a violent jarring or shaking that often occurs during a closed head injury and results in at least a brief loss of consciousness; (L. *concutere*, to shake violently).

conductive hearing loss—A reduction in hearing sensitivity because of a disorder of the outer or middle ear; (L. *conducere*, to conduct).

congenital disorder—A disorder that is present at birth; (L. *congenitus*, born with; *dis*, apart or impaired, + *ordo*, rank).

congruent/congruence—The agreement among a person's thoughts, feelings, words, tone of voice, and body language; communication in which a person sends the same message on both verbal and nonverbal levels; (L. *con*, with, + *gruere*, to suit; i.e., to suit with—to be in agreement).

consonant—Speech sounds articulated by either stopping of the outgoing air stream or creating a narrow opening of resistance using the articulators; (L. *con* [variation of *cum*], with or together, + *sonare*, to sound; literally, sound together).

contact ulcer—A benign vocal fold ulceration at the juncture of the middle one-third and posterior one-third of a fold that is caused by persistent and excessive vocal hyperfunction that is most commonly seen in adults males; (L. *contactus*, contact; *ulcus*, sore).

context—The circumstances or events that form the environment within which something exists or takes place; also, the words, phrases, or narrative that come before and after a particular word or phrase in speech or a piece of writing that helps to explain its full meaning; (L. *contextus*, join together).

continuing education units (CEUs)—Additional education or training required by ASHA and most states throughout a professional's career to help the professional remain current in the field.

contracture—An abnormal, usually permanent condition of a muscle group (e.g., bicep and muscle of the forearm) characterized by flexion and fixation of the limb that may be caused by shortening of muscle fibers; in severe cases, the bone (e.g., humerus [upper arm]) may develop an abnormal curvature; (L. *contractura*, pulling together).

contrecoup injury—In closed head injuries damage to the brain occurring on the opposite side of the trauma site; for example, when an impact to the left frontal side of the skull results in brain damage on the right posterior side; (L. *contra*, in opposition, + F. *coup*, impact or blow).

convalescent hospital—A medical facility, such as a skilled nursing facility, extended care facility, or nursing home, that provides extended medical, nursing, or custodial care for individuals over a prolonged period, e.g., during the course of a chronic illness or the rehabilitation phase after an acute illness or injury; (L. *convalescere*, to grow strong; *hospitium*, guesthouse).

conventional literacy—Reading and writing according to the rule-governed system of the alphabetic principle and being able to read to learn; (L. *con-*, with or together, + *venire*, to come; *litterae*, letters).

conversion reaction (disorder)—An ego defense mechanism in which *intrapsychic conflict* (mental struggle of opposing impulses or wishes within oneself) is expressed symbolically through physical symptoms that may manifest as actual illness or delusions of illness or incapacity (including voice disorders); causal factors may include a conscious or unconscious desire to escape from or avoid some unpleasant situation or responsibility, or to obtain sympathy or some other secondary gain; (L. *convertere*, to turn around; *re*, again, + *agrere*, to act).

cooing—The production of vowel-like sounds (usually /u/ and /oo/ with occasional brief consonant-like sounds similar to /k/ and /g/; usually produced by infants when feeling comfort or pleasure and interacting with a caregiver; (the term is in reference to the low, soft sounds of doves).

cortex (gray matter)—The outer layer (approximately one-fourth to one-half inch) of brain tissue containing nerve cell bodies (neurons); (L. *cortex*, bark).

cortical atrophy—Shrinkage and wasting away of cortical (brain) tissue that is common in dementia; (Gk. *a*, without, + *trophe*, nourishment).

cricoid cartilage—A solid circle of *cartilage* (nonvascular dense supporting connective tissue) shaped like a signet (class) ring located below and behind the thyroid cartilage and on top of the first tracheal ring; (Gr. *krikos*, ring, + *edios*, form).

cul-de-sac resonance—A variation of hyponasality that differs in the place of obstruction (anterior, compared to posterior in hyponasality or denasality), resulting in distortion (a muffled quality) of the nasal consonants /m/, /n/, and /ng/; (Fr. *cul-de-sac*, bottom of the sack).

cultural—linguistic diverse (CLD) theory—A perspective of language development that emphasizes the similarities and differences of the people and the languages spoken around the world, and that stresses how one language or dialect is no better than another.

culture—The philosophies, values, attitudes, perceptions, religious and spiritual beliefs, educational values, language, customs, child-rearing practices, lifestyles, and arts shared by a group of people and passed from one generation to the next; (L. *cultura*, culture).

custodial care—Services and care of a nonmedical nature (e.g., bathing and feeding) provided long term, usually for convalescent and chronically ill patients; (L. *custodia*, guarding).

D

Deaf community—Those deaf and hard of hearing individuals who share a common language (usually manual communication), common experiences and values, and a common way of interacting with each other and with hearing people.

Deaf culture—Ideology, beliefs, and customs shared by many individuals with prelinguistic deafness that may include communication, social protocol, entertainment, art, recreation, worship, and other aspects of culture.

decibel (dB)—A basic unit of measure of the intensity of sound; it is one-tenth of 1 bel (B); an increase in 1 bel is perceived as a 10-fold increase in loudness; (L. *decimus*, one-tenth, + *bel*, named after Alexander Graham Bell, American inventor, 1847–1922).

deciduous teeth—The set of 20 teeth that appear during infancy and early childhood (10 uppers, 10 lowers), with the front teeth appearing (erupting) through the gums about 6 months of age; all 20 teeth normally have erupted by 18–24 months. Shedding (losing) the deciduous teeth occurs between 6 and 13 years of age; (L. *decidere*, to fall off).

degenerative disease—Any condition that causes gradual deterioration of normal body functions; (L. *de-*, down from, + *generare*, to produce [i.e., decreased production]; *dis-*, opposite of; Fr. aise, ease).

deglutition—The act of swallowing; (L. *de-*, down, + *gluttire*, swallow).

dementia—A medical term for a syndrome caused by a progressive neurological disease that involves intellectual, cognitive, communicative, behavioral, and personality deterioration that is more severe than what would occur through normal aging; (L. *de-*, loss of, + *mens*, mind).

dendrite—A branching extension of a neuron that carries impulses to the cell body; (Gk. *dentron*, tree).

dentition—The type, number, and arrangement of teeth in the maxilla and mandible, including the incisors, cuspids (canines), bicuspids (premolars), and molars; (L. *dens*, tooth).

developmental coordination disorder—Impairment of groups of gross and fine muscles that prevents smooth and integrated movements, which results in clumsiness during walking, jumping, and athletic movements, and during more refined movements such as using eating utensils and writing; often associated with learning disabilities and complicated by low self-esteem, repeated injuries from accidents, and weight gain as a result of avoiding participating in physical activities.

developmental (intellectual) disability (DD or ID)—A disability that originates before 18 years of age and is characterized by significant limitations in intellectual functioning (intelligence) and adaptive behavior as expressed in conceptual, social, and practical skills.

diadochokinetic (diadochokinesis, diadochols)—In speech, the ability to execute rapid repetitive or alternating movements of the articulators; *diadochokinetic rate* is the speed at which the movements can be performed; (Gk. *diadochos*, successive, + *kinesis*, motion or movement).

diagnosis—The determination of the type and cause of a speech, language, cognitive, swallowing, or hearing disorder based on the signs and symptoms of the client or patient obtained through case history, observations, interviews, formal and informal evaluations, and other methods; (Gk. *dia*, through, + *gnosis*, knowledge).

dialect—A specific form of speech and language used in a geographical region or among a large group of people (social or ethnic dialects) that differs significantly from the standard of the larger language community in pronunciation, vocabulary, grammar, and idiomatic use of words; (Gk. *di-*, two, + *logos*, word or speech, becoming *dialecktos*, conversation).

diaphragm—A large, dome-shaped muscle that separates the thoracic and abdominal cavities and is the main muscle of respiration; during inspiration it moves down to increase the volume in the thoracic cavity, and during expiration it moves up to decrease the volume; (Gk. *diaphragma*, partition).

differential diagnosis—The process of narrowing possibilities and reaching conclusions about the nature of a deficit.

differential threshold—The smallest difference that can be detected between two auditory signals.

diphthong—A combination of two vowels in which one vowel glides continuously into the second vowel;

in American English: /eɪ/, /aɪ/ /oʊ/, /ɔɪ/ and /aʊ/; (Gk. *di-*, two, + *phthongos*, voice or sound).

diplophonia—Two distinct pitches perceived simultaneously during phonation that is caused by the two vocal folds vibrating under different degrees of tension (as in unilateral vocal fold paralysis) or vibration of the ventricular folds concurrently with the true vocal folds; (Gk. *diplos*, double, + *phone*, voice).

direct laryngoscopy—Examination by an ENT physician of the interior of the larynx by direct vision with the aid of a laryngoscope, usually while the patient is anesthetized; (L. *directus*, straight, + Gk. *larynx*, larynx, + *skopein*, to look).

disability—Any restriction or lack (resulting from an impairment) of ability to perform an activity in the manner or within the range considered normal for a human being (World Health Organization [WHO]); the impairment, loss, or absence of a physical or intellectual function; *physical disability* is any impairment that limits the physical functions of limbs or gross or fine motor abilities; *sensory disability* is impairment of one of the senses (e.g., hearing or vision); *intellectual disability* encompasses intellectual deficits that may appear at any age; (L. *dis*, apart, + *ablen*, to make fit, + *-itas*, suffix for condition or state).

discourse—An extended verbal exchange on a topic (i.e., a conversation or long narrative); (L. *dis-*, apart, + *currere*, to run).

disorder—A disruption of or interference with normal functions; (L. *dis*, apart, + *ordo*, rank).

distinctive feature—The smallest individual differences required to differentiate one phoneme from another in a language; (L. *distinctus*, separate [*dis-*, apart, + *tinct*, colored or tinged]; L. *facere*, to make).

distortion—A sound that does not have a phonetic symbol to represent the sound that is produced in place of the intended sound (e.g., a lateral lisp that is not a clear "sh" sound, or a distorted /r/ sound that cannot be clearly represented by a phonetic symbol); (*dis-*, apart, + *torquere*, to twist).

Down syndrome—A common chromosome disorder due to an extra chromosome number 21 (trisomy 21) that results in intellectual disability, small head, small ears, flat face with upward slant of the eyes, and abnormal physical development; (named after the English physician John Down, 1828–1896).

dysarthria—A group of motor speech disorders caused by *paresis* (weakness), *paralysis* (complete loss of movement), or incoordination of speech muscles as a result of central and/or peripheral nervous system damage that may affect respiration, phonation, resonation, articulation, and prosody; dysarthric speech sounds "mushy" because of distorted consonants and vowels; (Gk. *dys-*, difficult, impaired, + *arthroo*, articulate).

dysgraphia—A developmental motor disorder that affects a child's or adult's ability to write, characterized by messy or illegible handwriting, misspellings, and difficulty with grammar and organizing sentences; note: *agraphia* is a loss of ability to write resulting from injury to the brain; (Gk. *dys*, impaired or difficult, + *graphein*, write).

dysphagia (swallowing disorders)—Difficulty swallowing that occurs when impairments affect any of the four phases of swallowing (oral preparatory, oral, pharyngeal, or esophageal); puts a person at risk for aspiration of food and/or liquid and potential aspiration pneumonia; (Gk. *dys*, difficult or impaired, + *phagein*, to eat).

dysphonia—A general term that means a voice disorder, with the person's voice typically sounding rough, raspy, or hoarse; (Gk. *dys-*, impaired, + *phonia*, voice).

dystonia—A general neurological term for a variety of problems characterized by excessive contraction of muscles with associated abnormal movements and postures; (Gk. *dys-*, impaired, + L. *tonus*, sound).

E

echolalia—The automatic and involuntary repetition of another person's utterance that is normal for 18–24-month-old children, but which also can occur at later ages (including adulthood) in individuals who are autistic or have neurological damage; (Gk. *ekhe*, sound + *lalia*, talk).

edema—Accumulation of excessive fluid in tissue that is associated with inflammatory conditions and results in swelling of the tissue; (Gk. *oidema*, swelling).

effective treatment—Treatment with a particular method or approach that has been shown by research to be better than no treatment; (L. *effectus*, to bring about; L. *tractare*, to handle or deal with, + *mentum*, result).

electrolarynx/artificial larynx—An electronic (battery powered) device used by laryngectomees that produces a vibrated mechanical sound that is held against the neck, with the sound entering the pharynx and oral cavity where it is articulated for speech.

elicit—Behavior that is drawn out of a person by presenting certain stimuli, e.g., asking a child to name or describe objects to observe his speech and language; (L. *elicitus*, draw forth).

emergent literacy (preliteracy) skills—Early skills developed in the preschool years that precede or are presumed prerequisites for later-developing reading and writing skills; (L. *e-* out, + *mergere*, to plunge).

endoscopy (videoendoscopy, videostroboscopy)—Methods of viewing the velopharyngeal mechanism, vocal tract, or both that use a rigid endoscope introduced *intraorally* (through the mouth) or flexible fiberoptic endoscope *transnasally* (through the nose) with a camera lens and fiberoptic light source at the tip of the scope that can illuminate the nasopharynx, oropharynx, and larynx; the structures may be videotaped (*videoendoscopy*), and the light source can be put in *strobe mode* (rapid flashing) so that the vibrating vocal folds appear to move in slow motion for more detailed viewing (*videostroboscopy*); (note: SLPs may be trained to perform endoscopic evaluations and in most states are allowed to perform them); (Gk. *endon*, within, + *skopein*, to look).

English as a second language (ESL)—Learning English after a child's native (home) language has been established.

enteral feeding—The delivery of hydration and nutrition into the gastrointestinal (GI) tract by way of tube feedings through the nose or stomach; (Gk. *enteron*, bowel).

epiglottis—A large cartilage that is wide at the top and narrow at the bottom that is attached to the anterior edge of the cricoid cartilage and drops over the vocal folds like a lid to prevent food and liquid from entering the trachea and lungs when swallowing; (Gk. *epi*, on or upon, + *glossa*, tongue).

esophageal speech—The compression of air within the oropharynx and injection of it into the esophagus, followed by the rapid expelling of the air out of the esophagus that causes it to vibrate the upper esophageal valve, which produces a low-pitched, monotone "voice" that is shaped by the articulators to produce "burp" speech; (Gk. *oisophagos*, gullet).

etiology—The cause of an occurrence (e.g., a medical problem that results in a disorder or disability); (Gk. *aitia*, cause, + *logos*, science; i.e., the science of causes).

Eustachian (auditory) tube—A tube lined with mucous membrane that joins the nasopharynx and the middle ear cavity; normally closed but opens during yawning, chewing, and swallowing to allow equalization of air pressure in the middle ear with atmospheric pressure (named after Bartolomeo Eustachio, an Italian anatomist, 1524–1574).

evaluation/assessment—The overall clinical activities designed to understand an individual's communication abilities and disabilities before a treatment program is determined and established; (L. *e-* [variation of *ex-*], missing or absent, + *valuer*, value, i.e., missing value; *assidere*, to sit beside).

evidence-based practice—The quality of treatment that is measurable in terms of some form of functional outcomes and maintained in the face of cost-containment efforts (L. *evidentia*, proof; *practicare*, to do or perform).

evidence-based treatment (best practices)—The integration of (a) clinical expertise, (b) the current best evidence based on controlled and replicated research, and (c) the client's values, needs, and choices to provide high-quality service; (L. *evidentia*, proof; *tractare*, manage or handle).

executive functions—A composite of the following activities related to goal completion: anticipation, goal selection, planning, initiation of activity, self-regulation or self-monitoring, and use of feedback to adjust for future responses; (L. *executio*, accomplish; *functio*, performance).

expiration (exhalation)—The process of breathing air out of the lungs; (L. *ex*, out, + *spirare*, to breathe).

expressive aphasia—Difficulty formulating verbal, written, and/or gestural language; (L. *expressus*, clearly presented; Gk. *a-*, without or loss of, + *phasos*, to speak).

expressive language—The words, grammatical structures, and meanings that a person uses verbally; (L. *ex-*, out of or from, + *pressare*, to press; *pro-*, before, + *-ducere*, leading to; *in-*, in, + *codex*, trunk of a tree [originally, document carved from wooden tablets]).

external motivation—Motivation that is provided by the encouragement of someone else, often family or an employer; (L. *externus*, beyond or outside; *motus*, move).

F

facilitating techniques—The selected therapy exercises that help to achieve a "target" or a more optimal vocal response by the patient; (L. *facilis*, easy to do; Gk. *tekhne*, art, skill, or method).

failure to thrive—The abnormal retardation of growth and development of an infant resulting from conditions that interfere with normal metabolism, appetite, and activity.

false vocal folds (ventricular folds)—Paired, thick folds of mucous membranes with few muscle fibers that lie just above the true vocal folds in the larynx at the level of the Adam's apple; they do not vibrate during speech but close tightly during swallowing to prevent material from entering the trachea; (L. *ventriculus*, little belly).

family systems therapy—A model of counseling in which each family member is part of a system (the family), each member affects the others, and the system is interdependent; within the system there are sub-systems: e.g., mother–father, mother–son, father–son, grandparent–grandchild; (L. *familia*, household; Gk. *syn-* with or together, + *histanai*, to stand; L. *consilium*, consult; *modulus*, small measure).

family therapy—The counseling theory that emphasizes that a person's emotional reactions and problems must be viewed in the context of the family's roles and communication and interaction patterns; the focus is on family relationships and interdependent family systems (e.g., husband-wife, parent-child) rather than individuals within the family.

fiberoptic endoscopic evaluation of swallowing (FEES)—A procedure used to provide visual information about the pharyngeal phase of swallowing; a flexible endoscope is passed through the nasal passageway into the nasopharynx to view the laryngopharynx and the patient is asked to swallow food or liquid that has been dyed green for contrast; (L. *fibra*, fiber, + Gk. *optikos*, sight, Gk. *endon*, inward, within, + *skopia*, to look).

fine motor skills—Movements that require a high degree of dexterity, control, and precision of the small muscles of the body that enable such functions as grasping small objects, drawing shapes, cutting with scissors, fastening clothing, and writing.

finger spelling—The use of certain finger and hand shapes to represent letters of the alphabet and spell individual words.

fluency shaping (modification)—A therapy approach for children and adult stutterers that attempts to directly train individuals to speak with relaxed respiration, relaxed vocal folds, and relaxed articulation muscles; the approach attempts to teach stutterers how to talk fluently; (L. *fluens*, relaxed; *modificare*, to limit or restrain).

fluent aphasia—Aphasia that results from damage to posterior regions of the cortex (i.e., temporal or temporal-parietal lesions) characterized by language with normal pauses and articulation but with frequent syntactic errors, paraphasias, and circumlocutions (L. *fluens*, relaxed; Gk. *a-*, without or loss of, + *phasos*, to speak).

formulate—In language, the choice of words and grammatical structures in the construction of a meaningful verbal expression; (L. *formula*, form or rule).

frenum/frenulum—A fold of mucous tissue connecting the floor of the mouth to the midline underside of the tongue; (L. *frenum*, bridle, reins, and bit used to control a horse; *frenulum* is the diminutive for *frenum*).

frequency—In speech, the number of complete cycles (opening, closing) per second that the vocal folds vibrate; *pitch* is the psychological perception of frequency; (L. *frequens*, repeated).

fricative—A sound formed by forcing the air stream through a narrow opening between articulators (tongue-teeth - /θ/, /ð/ [th]; lips - /f/, /v/; tongue-alveolar ridge /s/, /z/, and tongue-hard palate /ʃ/).

functional—An incorrect production of standard speech sounds for which there is no known anatomical, physiological, or neurological basis; (L. *functico*, to perform).

functional aphonia—A hyperfunctional voice disorder in which a person speaks mostly with a whisper although is able to use a normal voice when laughing, coughing, clearing the throat, and humming; often associated with psychological stressors or conflicts; (Gk. *a-*, without or loss of, + *phone*, sound or voice).

functional disorder—A problem or impairment with no known anatomical, physiological, or neurological basis that may have behavioral or emotional causes or components; (L. *functico*, to perform; *dis*, apart or impaired, + *ordo*, rank).

functional dysphonia—A voice disorder that may be either hyperfunctional or hypofunctional and has no organic, physical, or neurological cause but is heard in patients with extreme tension in both the laryngeal and the supralaryngeal regions; the voice may have hypofunctional qualities such as low-pitch and breathy or hyperfunctional qualities such as high-pitch, strident, or hoarse; (L. *functio*, performance; Gk. *dys-*, disturbance or impaired, + *phonia*, voice).

functional outcomes—The results of treatment intended to clearly show a person's improved ability to communicate in the hospital setting with medical and rehabilitation staff; at home, performing activities of daily living (ADLs); in the community; and on the job (if the person returns to work).

functional treatment—Treatment results that improve communication abilities useful in a person's natural environments (e.g., home, school, and community); (L. *functio*, performance; L. *tractare*, to handle or deal with, + *mentum*, result).

functor (function) words—Words whose grammatical functions are more obvious than their semantic content and that serve primarily to give order to a sentence, such as articles, conjunctions, determiners, prepositions, and modal and auxiliary verbs.

G

gastroenterologist—A physician who specializes in diseases of the gastrointestinal tract; (Gk. *gaster*, stomach, + *enteron*, intestine, + *logos*, science).

gavage feeding—The use of a *nasogastric (NG) tube* (see definition) to provide sufficient nutrition and hydration for newborns who have a failure-to-thrive condition, with infant milk or specialized formulas (e.g., PediaSure®) inserted into the tube; (Fr. *gaver*, to gorge).

General American English (GAE)—The speech of native speakers of American English that is typical of the United States and that excludes phonological forms easily recognized as regional dialects (e.g., Northeastern or Southeastern) or limited to particular ethnic or social groups, and that is not identified as a nonnative American accent; the norm of pronunciation by national radio and television broadcasters.

generalization—The transfer of learning from one environment to other environments; usually considered the therapy or classroom to a natural environment, such as the home and community); (L. *generalis*, relating to all).

glide/semivowel—A type of consonant that has a gradual (gliding) change in an articulator (lips or tongue) position and a relative long production of sound; /w/, /j/.

global aphasia—A severe-to-profound aphasia resulting from a diffuse lesion involving portions of the left temporal, frontal, and parietal lobes that is characterized by severely impaired receptive and expressive language in all input and all output modalities, with motor speech disorders of apraxia of speech, dysarthria, or both; (L. *globus*, globe; Gk. *a-*, without or loss of, + *phasos*, to speak).

glottal stops—Compensatory articulation productions primarily for plosive sounds (e.g., /p/, /b/, /t/, /d/) used by individuals with velopharyngeal inadequacy; characterized by the forceful adduction of the vocal folds and the buildup and release of air pressure under the glottis, resulting in a grunt-type sound.

goal (target behavior)—Any verbal or nonverbal skill a clinician tries to teach a child; (OF *targe'*, shield, i.e., a warrior would try to hit what a shield was trying to protect).

grammar—The rules of the use of morphology and syntax in a language; (Gk. *grammatikos,* letter, + L. *ars,* art; literally, the art of letters).

gross motor skills—Involvement of the large muscles of the body (e.g., trunk, legs, arms) that require tone, strength, and coordination that enable such functions as standing, lifting, walking, and throwing a ball; (L. *grossus,* thick or course).

H

habilitation/habilitate—The process of developing a skill in order to function within the environment; the initial learning and development of a new skill; (L. *habilitatus,* ability, to make able).

handicap—Loss or limitation of opportunities to take part in the life of the community on an equal level with others (World Health Organization [WHO]); a congenital or acquired physical or intellectual limitation that hinders a person from performing specific tasks; (*hand in cap,* 17th-century game of betting).

hard glottal attack—Forceful approximation (closing) of the vocal folds during the initiation of phonation.

hard palate—The bony anterior two-thirds of the roof of the mouth that separate the oral cavity from the nasal cavity; (L. *palatum,* palate).

harshness—A "rough" sounding vocal quality resulting from a combination of hard glottal attacks, low pitch, and high intensity caused by *overadduction* (hyperfunction) of the vocal folds.

hearing aid—Any electronic device (usually battery operated) designed to amplify and deliver sound to the ear and consists of a microphone, amplifier, and receiver.

hearing impairment—Abnormal or reduced function in hearing resulting from an auditory disorder; (L. *im-* [variation of *in-*], in or into, + *pejorare,* make worse).

hearing sensitivity impairment—The most common type of hearing loss; a reduction in the sensitivity of the auditory mechanism that results in sounds needing to be a higher intensity than normal before they can be heard by the listener; (L. *sentire,* feel or perceive).

hearing threshold—In audiometry, the level at which a stimulus sound, such as a pure tone, is barely perceptible; usual clinical criteria demand that the level be just high enough for the subject to be aware of the sound at least 50% of the time it is presented.

hertz (Hz)—The unit of vibration adopted internationally to replace *cycles per second* (CPS); 1 hertz = 1 cycle per second = fundamental frequency (1 Hz = 1 CPS = f_0); (Heinrich R. Hertz, German physicist, 1857–1894; first person to broadcast and receive radio waves).

heterogeneous—Consisting of dissimilar or diverse individuals or constituents; (Gk. *heteros,* other or different, + *genos,* kind).

high blood pressure (hypertension)—A common disorder in middle age and later (although now often being seen in obese children and young adults) in which blood pressure is persistently above 140 over 90 mm Hg (120/80 is considered normal).

hoarseness—A common dysphonia that is a combination of breathiness and harshness that may affect loudness (usually decreased loudness or a monoloudness), pitch (usually a low pitch with reduced pitch range), and quality (usually decreased "pleasantness" of the sound of the voice).

holistic—A philosophic concept in which an entity (e.g., person) is seen as more than the sum of its parts; a prominent approach to psychology, biology, nursing, medicine, and other scientific, sociologic, and educational fields of study and practice; (Gk. *holos,* whole).

holophrastic language—The use of a single word to express a complete thought; (Gk. *holos,* whole, + *phrazein,* to declare; i.e., to declare the whole [meaning]).

hyperadduction—Difficulty with the vocal folds closing too tightly or for too long that results in a voice that sounds tense and strained and tends to fatigue with use as a result of hypertonicity; (Gk. *hyper-,* excess, + *adducere,* to bring to).

hyperfunction—A pervasive pattern of excessive effort and tension that affects many different structures and muscles in the phonatory system and, in some cases, the respiratory, resonatory, and articulatory systems; signs of hyperfunction include a tense sounding voice and hard glottal attacks; (Gk. *hyper,* over or beyond; + L. *functio,* performance or execution).

hypernasal/hypernasality—A resonance disorder that occurs when oral consonants and vowels enter the nasal cavity because of clefts of the hard and soft palates or weakness of the soft palate, causing a person to sound like he is "talking through his nose"; (Gk. *hyper-,* excess, + L. *nasus,* nose).

hypertonicity—Excessive tone or tension in a muscle or muscle group (e.g., chest muscles, articulatory muscles); (Gk. *hyper,* over or above [normal], + *tonos,* tone).

hypoadduction—Difficulty making the vocal folds close strongly enough or long enough for normal phonation that results in a weak, breathy voice that often deteriorates with increasing amounts of vocal use throughout the day; (Gk. *hypo-,* under, + L. *adducere,* to bring to).

hypofunction—Inadequate muscle tone in the laryngeal mechanism and associated structures, including the muscles of respiration; signs of hypofunction include breathiness because of inadequate closure of the vocal folds, weak vocal power that can affect speech intelligibility, and reduced vocal endurance; (*hypo,* under; + L. *functio,* performance).

hyponasal/hyponasality (denasal/denasality)—Lack of normal resonance caused by partial or complete obstruction in the nasal tract resulting in the three English phonemes /m/, /n/, and /(ŋg)/ being perceived as /b/, /d/, or /g/ respectively; (Gk. *hypo-* under, [L. *de-,* down], + L. *nasus,* nose).

hypotonicity—Weak or absent tone or tension in a muscle or muscle group (e.g., laryngeal muscles or abdominal muscles); (Gk. *hypo,* under or below [normal], + *tonos,* tone).

I

idiom—An expression in the usage of a language that is peculiar to itself either grammatically (e.g., "Zip your lip.") or in having a meaning that cannot be derived from the normal combination of words (e.g., "Keep your eyes on the ball, your shoulder to the wheel, and your nose to the grindstone."); (Gk. *idioma,* to appropriate or acquire).

idiopathic—A disease or disorder of unknown etiology; (Gk. *idio,* own or personal, + *pathos,* suffering).

idiosyncratic language—An individual's choice of words and use of words in sentences that have their own unique meaning, which may or may not be interpretable to a listener; (Gk. *idios,* one's own, + *syn,* together, + *krasis,* to blend or mix; i.e., blending together one's own [language]).

immittance audiometry—A routinely used objective assessment of the functioning of the middle ear; a general term to describe measurements made of tympanic membrane impedance, compliance, or admittance; (a combination of *impedance* and *admittance*; L. *audio-,* to hear, + Gk. *metron,* measure).

impairment—Any loss or abnormality of psychological, physiological, or anatomical structure or function that interferes with normal activities (World Health Organization [WHO]); (L. *impejorare,* to make worse).

impedance—The opposition of sound-wave transmission, which includes frictional resistance, mass, and stiffness and is influenced by frequency; (L. *impedire,* to entangle).

incidence—The rate at which a disorder appears in the normal population over a period, typically 1 year; (L. *incidere,* to fall into).

incisors—The four front upper and lower teeth (central and lateral incisors); (L. *incidere,* to cut into, as in *incision*).

incontinence—The inability to control or retain urination or defecation; (L. *incontinentia,* inability to retain).

indirect laryngoscopy—A method of examining the larynx and vocal folds by placing a *laryngeal mirror* (a small round mirror attached to a long handle) into the back of the mouth and directing a reflected light source onto the mirror to shine on the vocal folds; (L. *in-,* not, + *directus,* straight; Gk. *laryngos,* upper windpipe, + *skopein,* to look).

infantile hypoxia—In newborns and infants, inadequate oxygenation of the blood leading to *tachycardia* (rapid heart rate) and rapid, shallow breathing that quickly affects the brain and other organs and systems; severe hypoxia can result in cardiac failure; (L. *infans,* unable to speak; Gk. *hypo,* below or deficient, + *oxys,* sharp or quick).

infantile (primitive) reflex—Any reflex normal in infants that is an automatic, uncontrolled movement; normally disappears (becomes "integrated") by about 6 months of age; (L. *infans,* unable to speak; *primivus,* primitive; *reflectere,* to bend back).

infarction (necrosis)—A localized area of necrotic (dead) tissue resulting from lack of blood supply and oxygen to the tissue; (L. *in* + *farctus,* to fill; Gk. *nekros,* dead).

inner speech (internal discourse, stream of consciousness)—The nearly constant internal monologue a person has with himself at a conscious or semi-conscious level that involves thinking in words; a conversation with oneself.

inpatient—A patient who has been admitted to a hospital or other health care facility for at least an overnight stay.

inspiration (inhalation)—The process of drawing air into the lungs; (L. *in,* in, + *spirare,* to breathe).

integrate—In neurology, the process of combining information from various input modalities, attaching meaning and interpreting the information, storing (remembering), and making decisions about responding; (L. *integrare,* to make whole).

intelligence—A global construct involved in the collective capacity to act purposely, think rationally, and deal effectively with the environment; (L. *intelligentia,* intelligent).

intelligence quotient (IQ)—An estimate of intellectual status based on an index determined by dividing the *mental age* (MA) in months by the *chronological age* (CA) in months and reducing the result to a percentage; 100 is considered the mathematical average; (L. *intellentia,* intelligent; *quot,* how many).

intelligible—The degree to which a person's utterances are understood by the average listener; influenced by articulation, rate of speech, fluency, vocal quality, and intensity of voice.

intensity—In reference to voice, the force with which the vocal folds open and close and the amount of air that escapes between the open vocal folds; *loudness* is the psychological perception of intensity; (L. *intensus,* strained or tight).

interdisciplinary team—A group of professionals from various disciplines who work together to coordinate the care of a patient through collaboration, interaction, communication, and cooperation; (L. *inter,* between, + *disciplina,* teaching).

internal motivation—Motivation that is self-generated or intrinsic in which a person decides what is important and needed; (L. *internus,* between; *motus,* move).

International Phonetic Alphabet (IPA)—Specially devised signs and symbols designed to represent the individual speech sounds of all languages.

intonation—Variations in pitch on syllables, words, and phrases that produce *stress* to give emphasis and meaning to utterances; (L. *in-,* in or into, + Gk. *tonus,* tone).

intraoral breath pressure—A buildup of air pressure in the oral cavity that provides the force for the production of oral consonants, particularly plosives, fricatives, and affricates; (L. *intra,* within, + *os,* mouth).

intubation—The passage of a breathing tube through the mouth, through the nose, or directly into the trachea through a *tracheotomy* (endotracheal intubation) to ensure a *patent* (open; pronounced "pAtent") airway for delivery of oxygen; (L. *in,* in or within, + *tubus,* tube, + *atio,* process).

J

jargon aphasia—Continuous but unintelligible speech with various combinations of literal and verbal paraphasias and neologisms, with little or no conveying of information; often with the speaker having little awareness of the problem and occurring in both speech and writing; (O.Fr. *gargon,* gibberish).

L

labia—Pertaining to the lips; (L. *labia,* lips).

labiodental—The /f/ and /v/ sounds, where the upper front teeth are in contact with the lower lip; (L. *labia,* lips, + *dentes,* teeth).

language—A socially shared code or conventional system for representing concepts through the use of arbitrary symbols [sounds and letters] and rule-governed combinations of those symbols [grammar]; (L. *lingua,* tongue or language).

language arts—Academic activities such as listening, speaking, reading, handwriting, spelling, and written composition.

language comprehension—An active process in which, from instant to instant, a listener infers the meaning of an auditory message based on the context of the information and long-term stored memory of words and general knowledge; (L. *com-,* with, + *prehendere,* to grasp or seize).

language delay—An abnormal slowness in developing language skills that may result in incomplete language development; (L. *de-,* down or from, + Fr. *laier,* leave).

language development—The progressive growth of a receptive and expressive communication system for representing concepts using arbitrary symbols (sounds and words) and rule-governed combinations of those symbols (grammar); (L. *lingua,* tongue or language; Fr. *desvoluper,* to unwrap or expose).

language differences—Variations in speech and language production that are the result of a person's cultural, linguistic, and social environments; (L, *differentia,* diversity).

language disorder—An impairment of receptive and/ or expressive linguistic symbols (morphemes, words, semantics, syntax, or pragmatics) that affects comprehending what is said or verbally expressing wants, needs, thoughts, information, and feelings; (L. *dis,* apart or impaired, + *ordo,* rank).

language-learning disability—An impairment of receptive and/or expressive linguistic symbols that affects learning and educational achievement and, consequentially, possible occupational and professional choices, in addition to emotional and social development.

language sample—An audio recording of a child's spontaneous conversation or naturalistic verbal interaction with the clinician, family member, or both.

laryngectomy—Surgical removal of the larynx because of cancer and includes the trachea being brought forward and sutured to the skin in the lower midline of the neck to create a permanent stoma; the pharynx is closed as a separate tract for swallowing; (Gk. *larynx,* larynx, + *ektome,* excision).

laryngitis—An acute or chronic inflammation of the mucous membranes of the larynx that often results in hoarseness or loss of voice; (Gk. *larynx,* larynx, + *-itis,* disease or inflammation).

laryngopharyngeal reflux (LPR)—Gastric reflux (stomach acids causing "heart burn") that flows through the esophagus, past the upper esophageal valve, and into the larynx or pharynx; reflux may spill over onto the vocal folds and irritate them, causing coughing and inflammation; (L. *refluere,* to flow back).

larynx (pl. larynges)—Located just above the trachea, the structure that contains cartilages, muscles, and membranes that produce voice by air passing between the vocal folds; (Gk. *larynx,* larynx).

learning disability (LD)—A disorder in one or more of the basic psychological processes involved in understanding or using language, spoken or written, that may manifest itself as difficulty listening, speaking, reading, writing, spelling, mathematical calculations, reasoning, and problem solving; (L. *dis-,* apart or impaired, + *habilitas,* aptitude or easy to manage).

lesion—A wound, injury, or area of pathological change in tissue; (L. *laesus,* injury).

letter—An arbitrary written or printed symbol or character representing a speech sound (L. *littera,* letter of the alphabet).

lexicon—Refers to all morphemes, including words and parts of words, that a person knows; (Gk. *lexikos,* of words).

linguadental (interdental)—Voiced and unvoiced /th/ sounds with the tongue tip placed lightly between the top and the bottom front teeth; (L. *lingua,* tongue, + *dens,* tooth).

linguapalatal—The /ʃ/ [sh] and /ʒ/ [zh] sounds, where the top center of the tongue is near the hard palate; (L. *lingua,* tongue, + *palatum,* palate).

linguavelar—The /k/ and /g/ consonants, where the back of the tongue moves near the soft palate; (L. *lingua,* tongue, + *velum,* curtain or veil).

linguistics—The scientific study of the structure and function of language and the rules that govern language; includes the study of phonemes, morphemes, syntax, semantics, and pragmatics; (L. *lingua,* tongue).

lipreading—The process of recognizing speech using only the visual cues from the speaker's mouth and face.

literacy (reading, writing)—The ability to communicate through written language, both reading and writing; (L. *litterae,* letters; Old English [OE] *raedan,* to advise; OE *writan,* to scratch).

literacy disorder (disability)—Reading and writing impairments in a heterogeneous population of children; (L. *litterae,* letters).

literal or phonemic paraphasia—Sounds and syllables that are correctly articulated but may be extraneous, transposed, or substituted, usually with the preservation of the vowels and intended number of syllables in a word (e.g., *tar* for *car*); often occurring in both speech and writing; (L. *littera,* of a letter;

Gk. *phonema,* sound or voice; *para,* near or alongside, + *phasos,* speech).

loss of consciousness (LOC)—Impaired responsiveness, usually caused by diffuse brain dysfunction or damage to the brainstem and the reticular activating system; duration is often used as a measure of traumatic brain injury severity; (L. *conscius,* to know).

low birth weight—An infant whose weight at birth is less than 5.5 pounds (2,500 grams), regardless of gestational age.

M

magnetic resonance imaging (MRI)—An imaging study that does not expose the patient to radiation and often provides images with sharper detail than those from computerized tomography (CT) scans; medical imaging based on the resonance of atomic nuclei in a strong magnetic field; (Gk. *magnesia,* lodestone [a type of iron that attracts other iron]; *resonare,* to sound again; *imago,* image).

malignant—A neoplasm with uncontrollable growth and dissemination that invades and destroys neighboring tissue; (L. *mal-,* bad, poor, or abnormal + *ignari,* disposition).

malocclusion—Misalignment of the maxillary teeth with the mandibular teeth; (L. *malus,* bad, poor, or abnormal, + *occludere,* to shut).

mandible—The lower jaw that is hinged to the temporal bone for opening and closing and contains sockets for the lower teeth; (L. *mandibula,* jaw).

manner—The way in which the air stream is modified as a result of the interaction of the articulators; direction of airflow (e.g., oral or nasal sounds), or the degree of narrowing of the vocal tract by the articulators in the various places; (L. *manus,* hand, in reference to how a sound is made; [*manufactured,* made by hand]).

manualism—A philosophy in the education of the deaf that emphasizes the learning and use of sign language and finger spelling as a natural form of communication among the deaf; (L. *manus,* hand, + *-isma,* feature).

manually coded English—A form of communication in which manual signs correspond to English words and syntax.

masking—In audiology, the process that occurs when two sounds occur simultaneously and one sound is sufficiently loud to cause the other to be inaudible; (L. *maschera,* mask).

mastication—The act of chewing food in preparation for swallowing and digestion; (L. *masticare,* to chew).

mastoiditis—An infection of one of the mastoid bones (just behind the ear) that is usually an extension of a middle ear infection, characterized by earache, fever, headache, and malaise; medical treatment may require intravenous antibiotics for several days, and residual hearing loss may follow the infection; (Gk. *mastos,* breast [e.g., mastectomy], + *edios,* form, + *itis,* inflammation).

maxilla—The upper jaw that includes the hard palate and contains sockets for the upper teeth; forms much of the midfacial structure; (L. *maxilla,* upper jaw).

mean length of utterance (MLU)—The average length of oral expressions as measured by representative sampling of oral language (e.g., 50–100 spontaneous utterances); usually calculated by counting the number of morphemes per utterance and dividing by the number of utterances; e.g.,

$$\frac{150\ \text{morphemes}}{50\ \text{utterances}} = 3.0\ \text{MLU}.$$

measurement—Procedures that quantify observed behaviors and can be calculated as mathematical results, such as percentages and percentiles; (L. *mensurare,* to measure).

Meniere's disease—A chronic disease of the inner ear characterized by recurrent episodes of vertigo, tinnitus, and sensorineural hearing loss, which may be bilateral; (named after Prosper Meniere, French physician, 1799–1862).

mental status examination—A structured interview and observations conducted by a psychologist or neuropsychologist of a patient's orientation, attention, concentration, memory, language comprehension and expression, visual–spatial skills, abstraction abilities, general cognitive functioning, and insight into problems, with impairments typically treated by an SLP.

metalinguistics—The ability to think about and talk about language; (Gk. *meta-,* changed or beyond, + L. *lingua,* tongue).

metastasis—The process by which tumor cells travel or spread to distant parts of the body; (Gk. *methistanai,* to change; from *meta,* beyond, + *stasis,* standing).

middle ear—An air-filled chamber located within the temporal bone of the skull; beginning at the inner side of the tympanic membrane and attaching the ossicular chain to the oval window of the cochlea.

mixed hearing loss—A reduction in hearing because of a combination of a disordered outer or middle ear and inner ear.

modality—Any sensory avenue through which information may be received, i.e., auditory, visual, tactile, taste, and olfactory (smell); (L. *modus,* measure or quantity).

modified barium swallow study (MBSS)—A dynamic (moving) imaging radiographic (x-ray) procedure focusing on the mouth, pharynx, larynx, and cervical esophagus used to examine the process of swallowing; a video recording of real-time movement of a bolus from entering the mouth to entering the stomach.

morpheme—The smallest unit of language having a distinct meaning, for example, a prefix, root word, or suffix; (Gk. *morphe,* form, + *pheme,* sound).

morphology—The study of the structure (form) of words; (Gk. *morphe,* form, + *logia,* study of).

motor—Pertaining to motion or movement; nerve cells that initiate and regulate contracting and relaxing of muscle fibers; (L. *movere,* to move).

motor speech disorders—Neurological impairments that affect the motor planning, programming, neuromuscular control, and/or execution of speech and include the dysarthrias and apraxia of speech; they typically have a sensory component and should be thought of as sensorimotor disorders.

multicultural—A society characterized by a diversity of cultures, languages, traditions, religions, and values, as well as socioeconomic classes, sexual orientations, and ability levels; ideally, where individuals are respected and valued for their contributions to the whole of that society; (L. *multus,* many, + *cultura,* culture).

multifactorial—Referring to the likelihood of two or more causes contributing to the etiology or development of an impairment or disorder; (L. *multi,* many, + *factus,* made by hand; i.e., many hands [causes] make the disorder).

muscle tension dysphonia (MTD)—A hyperfunctional voice disorder in which the voice is adversely affected by excessive muscle tension that ranges from mild to severe; characteristics include a weak voice that lacks intensity, range and variation, a rough, hoarse, or thin vocal quality that lacks resonance, and a voice that fatigues easily; (L. *musculus,* little mouse; *tension,* stretch; *dys,* impaired or difficult, + Gk. *phone,* sound or voice).

mutational falsetto (puberphonia)—A high-pitched, breathy voice produced by the vibration of the anterior one-third of the vocal folds, with the posterior two-thirds being held tightly in a slightly open position or else so tightly adducted that little or no posterior vibration occurs; (L. *falsus,* false, + *ete,* small; L. *puberatus,* age of maturity, + Gk. *phonia,* voice).

mutism—The inability or unwillingness to speak; usually used in reference to voice disorders where an individual may use selective or elective mutism, that is, unconsciously or consciously not be able to use voice or speak; (L. *mutus,* mute).

myasthenia gravis—A neuromuscular disorder more commonly seen in women than men; characterized by chronic fatigue and muscle weakness, especially in the facial and articulatory muscles, resulting in dysarthria.

myofunctional therapy—Treatment designed to correct a tongue thrust or habitual forward-resting position of the tongue against the front teeth; (Gk. *myos,* muscle, + L. *functio,* performance).

N

narrative—The orderly, sequenced relating of accounts or events; (L. *narratus,* to know).

nasal—Sound resulting from the closing of the oral cavity, preventing air from escaping through the mouth, with a lowered position of the soft palate and a free passage of air through the nose (/m/, /n/, and /ŋ/ [ng]); (L. *nasus,* nose).

nasal air emission/nasal escape—The inappropriate release of air pressure through the nose during speech, causing distortion of the speech; (L. *e-,* out, + *mittere,* to send).

nasogastric (NG) tube—A medical device consisting of a long flexible tube that is passed through the nose, down the esophagus, and into the stomach for the delivery of liquids, nutrition, and medications; (L. *nasus,* nose, + Gk. *gastros,* stomach).

nasometer—A computer-based instrument that measures the relative amount of nasal acoustic energy in a person's speech; (L. *nasus,* nose, + Gk. *metron,* measure).

nasopharyngoscopy—A minimally invasive procedure commonly used by SLPs for evaluation of velopharyngeal dysfunction that allows visual observation and analysis of the velopharyngeal mechanism during speech; equipment includes a flexible fiberoptic endoscope, the same that is used in laryngoscopy; (L. *nasus,* nose, + Gk. *pharynx,* throat, + *skopein,* to look).

National Student Speech-Language-Hearing Association (NSSLHA)—The preprofessional association for students interested in the study of communication sciences and disorders.

nativistic theory—A perspective of language development that emphasizes the acquisition of language as an innate, physiologically determined, and genetically transmitted phenomenon; (L. *nativus,* innate, produced by birth).

natural processes—The processes that are common in the speech development of children across languages.

neologism—A form of paraphasia in which a person combines consonants and vowels that sound like they could be words and uses inflection to give them emotional meaning; for example, *bingtema* and *hitican;* (Gk. *neos,* new, + L. *logos,* word).

neonate—A child within the first 28 days after birth; (Gk. *neos,* new, + L. *natus,* born).

neural plasticity—The brain's ability to reorganize itself throughout life by forming new neural connections. Neural plasticity allows neurons to compensate for injury and disease and to adjust their activities in response to new situations or to changes in their environment; (Gk. *neuro,* nerve; *plastikos,* to mold).

neuritic (senile) plaques— Neuronal abnormalities and degeneration seen in cortical and subcortical brain regions of people with Alzheimer's disease.

neurofibrillary tangles—Neuronal abnormalities seen in Alzheimer's disease where there are filamentous bodies (fine, threadlike fibers) in nerve cells, axons, and dendrites.

neuron—The basic nerve cell of the nervous system, containing a nucleus within a cell body and extending an axon and multiple dendrites (Gk. *neuron,* nerve).

neuropsychologist—A Ph.D. psychologist specialized in the area of practice in clinical psychology and neurogenic disorders who assesses cognitive functioning, discriminates between psychiatric and neurological conditions, distinguishes among different neurological conditions, and predicts the course of a patient's recovery; however, most of the cognitive-linguistic therapy is provided by SLPs (Gk. *neuron,* nerve, + *psyche,* breath, life, or soul).

noise-induced hearing loss—A permanent sensorineural hearing loss caused by exposure to excessive loud noise, often over long periods of time.

nonfluent aphasia—Aphasia that results from damage to anterior cortical regions (i.e., frontal lobe lesions) characterized by sparse, perseverative language with disturbed prosody, misarticulations, errors in syntax, and a reduction in phrase length (L. *non*, not, + *fluens*, relaxed; Gk. *a-*, without or loss of, + *phasos*, to speak).

normal disfluency—The repeating, pausing, incomplete phrasing, revising, interjecting, and prolonging of sounds that are typical in the speech of young children; (L. *normalis*, according to pattern).

normative data (norms)—Data that characterize what is usual in a defined population and that describe rather than explain a particular occurrence; an average of performance of a sample drawn randomly from a population; (L. *norma*, rule or pattern; *datum*, thing given).

NPO (nothing by mouth)—A patient care instruction advising that a patient is prohibited from orally ingesting food, beverage, or medicine; patients must receive nutrition through enteral feeding; (L. *nil per os*, nothing by mouth).

O

occlusion—The process of bringing the upper and lower teeth into contact; (L. *occludere*, to shut).

occlusive (ischemic) stroke—A partial or complete blockage (occlusion) of a cerebral artery, causing decreased blood supply to brain tissue; (L. *occludere*, to close up; Gk. *ischein*, to hold back, + *haima*, blood).

occupational therapist (OT)—A rehabilitation specialist who is licensed to evaluate and treat developmental, physical, and cognitive impairments that interfere with functional independence for daily living and work skills by facilitating the development of sensory-motor (sensorimotor) integration, perceptual functioning, and neuromuscular functioning; (L. *occupare*, work; Gk. *therapia*, treatment).

omission—The absence of a speech sound where one should occur in a word, e.g., *k-on* for *crayon*; (L. *omittere*, to let go).

open bite—An abnormal vertical space between the anterior maxillary and mandibular teeth that often allows the tongue tip to be seen when a person smiles.

open head injury (OHI)—Head injury in which the skull and brain are penetrated by a severe impact or a projectile (bullet, fragment of glass, or shrapnel from an explosion).

operant (instrumental) conditioning—A learning model for changing behavior in which a desired behavior is reinforced immediately after it spontaneously occurs; (L. *opera*, work; *instruere*, to arrange; *condicio*, agreement or stipulation).

operationally defined goal—A specific behavior that is observable (can be heard or seen) and measurable; (L. *opera*, work, + *-atio*, action or process).

oral apraxia (nonverbal apraxia, facial apraxia, buccofacial apraxia)—Difficulty with volitional nonspeech movements of the articulators (e.g., puffing the cheeks, clicking the tongue, protruding the tongue, whistling, or smiling; (L. *buccus*, cheeks, + *facies*, make or form).

oralism—A philosophy in the education of the deaf that maintains language should be oral, that is, from the mouth, and sign language and teachers who are deaf should be excluded from the classroom; (L. *os*, mouth, + *isma*, feature).

oral reflex—Infantile primitive reflexes that are present at birth or soon after that are specifically designed to assist the infant in finding and obtaining oral nutrition; for example, the *rooting reflex*, *sucking reflex*, and *swallowing reflex*; (L. *os*, mouth; *reflexus*, bending back).

orbicularis oris—The muscle surrounding the opening of the mouth; the muscular structure of the lips; (L. *orbis*, circle, + *biculus*, little; *or*, mouth; i.e., the little circle of the mouth).

organic—Inability to correctly produce standard speech sounds because of anatomical, physiological, or neurological causes; (L. *organum*, to work).

organic disorder—A problem or impairment with a known anatomical, physiological, or neurological basis; (L. *organum*, to work; *dis*, apart or impaired, + *ordo*, rank).

orthography—The part of language study concerned with letters and spelling; the representation of the sounds of a language by written or printed symbols; (Gk. *orthos*, correct or straight, + *graphe*, to write).

orthopedic—A branch of health care concerned with the prevention and correction of disorders of the musculoskeletal systems of the body; an *orthopedist* is a physician who specializes in orthopedics; (Gk. *orthos*, straight, + *pais*, child).

ossicular chain—The three small bones (ossicles) of the middle ear named after their basic shapes: *malleus*, for the mallet or hammer; *incus*, for the anvil; and *stapes*, for the stirrup; (L. *os*, bone; *ossiculum*, small bone).

otitis media with effusion—Any inflammation or infection of the middle ear; particularly common in childhood and often associated with a common cold, allergies, sinus infections, and sore throats; Eustachian tube malfunction typically is the physiological cause; effusion—the escape of fluid from tissue as a result of seepage (Gk. *ous*, ear, + *itis*, inflammation, L. *medius*, middle; *effundere*, to pour out).

otolaryngologist/otorhinolaryngologist—A medical doctor who specializes in diseases of the ears, nose, and throat; often referred to as an "ear, nose, and throat" (ENT) doctor; (Gk. *ot-*, ear, + *rhin-*, nose, + *larynx*, larynx, + *logos*, study of).

otosclerosis—A hereditary condition of unknown cause in which irregular ossification occurs in the ossicles of the middle ear, especially of the stapes, causing hearing loss; typically first observed between 11 and 30 years of age; women are affected twice as often as men and may begin during pregnancy; (Gk. *ous*, ear, + *skelos*, hard, + *osis*, condition).

ototoxic—Drugs that have harmful effects on the central auditory nervous system, including aspirin, aminoglycoside antibiotics, furosemide, and quinine; (Gk. *ous*, ear, + *toxikon*, poison).

outer (external) ear—The concave, somewhat funnel-like structure that collects, resonates, and directs sound waves to the tympanic membrane, assists in localizing the direction from which sound is coming, and helps protect the middle ear; composed of the auricle (pinna), ear canal, and outer layer of the tympanic membrane.

outpatient—A patient who is not hospitalized but is being treated in an office, clinic, or medical facility.

P

palatal fistula—Usually a small opening or passage between the oral cavity and the nasal cavity that allows air or sound to escape from the oral cavity into the nasal cavity, causing some hypernasality; (L. *palatum*, palate; *fistula*, pipe).

palatal lift—A prosthetic appliance that can be used to raise the velum for speech if the velum is long enough to achieve velopharyngeal closure but does not move well, often because of central or peripheral neurological impairment.

palatal obturator—A prosthetic appliance that can be used to cover an open palatal defect, such as an unrepaired cleft palate or a palatal fistula; it can be used to improve an infant's ability to achieve compression of the nipple for suction or can be used to close a cleft palate for speech; (L. *palatum*, palate; obturare, to close).

palatine tonsils—Two almond-shaped masses of lymphoid tissue between the anterior and the posterior faucial pillars; (L. *palatum*, plate, *tonsillae*, tonsil).

palatoplasty—The surgical repair of a cleft palate; (L. *palatum*, palate, + Gk. *plastikos*, to mold or form).

papilloma—Soft, wart-like, benign growths on the vocal folds of children that have a viral origin and may grow to a size that can obstruct the airway; (L. *papilla*, nipple, + Gk. *oma*, tumor).

parallel speech—Naming, describing, and explaining what the child is experiencing and probably feeling, almost as if the caregiver is the child; a technique used by some parents, as well as clinicians, to help children develop receptive and expressive language; (Gk. *para*, beside, + *allos*, one another).

parentese (motherese, baby talk, child-directed speech)—The often automatic speech pattern of parents and caregivers with infants in which the person uses a high pitched voice with an unusual amount of inflection, one- and two-syllable words in short, simple sentences, and a slower than normal rate of speech with clear articulation that sometimes emphasizes every syllable.

perception—The process of detecting, discriminating, and recognition of a stimulus; (L. *per*, through, + *capere*, to grasp or take).

perinatal—Pertaining to the time and process of giving birth or being born; (Gk. *peri*, around, + L. *natus*, birth).

peripheral nervous system (PNS)—The cranial nerves that exit the brainstem and the spinal nerves that exit the spinal cord that allow the body to communicate sensory information to the brain and the brain to communicate motor information to the body; (Gk. *peripheria*, circumference).

perseverate/perseveration—An automatic and involuntary repetition or continuation of a thought or behavior after it is no longer appropriate, including repetition of a sound, syllable, word, or phrase when speaking; (L. *perseverare*, to persist; *per*, through, + *severus*, severe).

persistent vegetative state (PVS)—A medical diagnosis made only after numerous neurological and other tests that, due to extensive and irrevocable brain damage, a patient is highly unlikely ever to achieve higher functioning above a vegetative state; (L. *persistere*, continue steadfastly; *vegere*, to be alive; *status*, condition).

pervasive developmental disorder (PDD)—Serious multiple developmental impairments typically diagnosed in children before the age of 3 and in males approximately four times as often as in females; autism spectrum disorders are the more severe extreme; (L. *per-*, through, + *vadere*, to go).

pharyngeal fricatives—Compensatory articulation productions primarily for fricatives and affricates (e.g., /f/, /v/, /s/, /z/, /ʃ/ [sh], and /ʧ/ [ch]) used by individuals with velopharyngeal inadequacy; characterized by tongue retraction so that the base of the tongue approximates, but does not touch, the pharyngeal wall, which causes a friction sound as air pressure passes through the narrow opening.

pharyngoplasty—A surgical procedure of the pharynx that is designed to correct velopharyngeal dysfunction; (Gk. *pharynx*, throat, + *plastikos*, to mold or form).

phonation—The vibration of air passing between the two vocal folds that produces sound that is used for speech; (Gk. *phone*, voice; L. *vox*, voice).

phoneme—The shortest arbitrary unit of sound in a language that can be recognized as being distinct from other sounds in the language; (Gk. *phone/phonema*, voice or sound).

phonetics—The study of speech-sound production and the special symbols that represent speech sounds.

phonics method—The method of teaching reading and pronunciation by learning the sounds of letters and groups of letters ("sounding out words"); the association of the sounds (phonemes) of a language with the equivalent written forms (graphemes).

phonological awareness—Recognition and understanding of sound–letter associations; that individual sounds can be combined to form words; that a single-syllable word is heard as one word but can be segmented into its beginning, middle, and ending sounds; and that longer words have more "middle" sounds.

phonological disorder—Errors of phonemes that form patterns in which a child simplifies individual sounds or sound combinations; (Gk. *phonos*, sound + *logia*, study of).

phonological processes—The simplification of sounds that are difficult for children to produce in an adult manner; phonological processes help explain errors of substitution, omission, and addition that children may use to simplify the production of difficult sounds.

phonology—The study of speech sounds and the system of rules underlying sound production and sound combinations in the formation of words; (Gk. *phone/phonema*, voice or sound, + *logia*, study of).

phonotrauma—Deleterious acute or chronic vocal behaviors, such as excessive yelling, screaming, cheering, coughing, throat clearing, inappropriate pitch or loudness, singing beyond the range of the vocal mechanism, hard glottal attacks, inadequate respiratory support, talking loudly over noise, poor hydration, and smoking that are damaging to the vocal folds and the laryngeal and pharyngeal muscles and tissues; (Gk. *phone*, sound or voice, + *trauma*, wound).

physical therapist (PT)—A rehabilitation specialist who is licensed to evaluate and treat developmental and physical impairments through the use of special exercises or other modalities to assist individuals to maximize independence and mobility, self-care, and functional skills necessary for daily living; (Gk. *physikos*, body; *therapia*, treatment).

place—The location in the mouth where two articulators come together (constrict) to produce specific sounds; places may include the lips, teeth, alveolar ridge, tongue, and hard and soft palates.

plateau—A patient's general leveling off of improvement in rehabilitation, after which gains are slower and less easily documented; often the reason for discharging from rehabilitation; (Fr. *plateau*, platter).

polypoid thickening (degeneration)—A condition in which a vocal fold becomes edematous, flabby, and almost jelly-like as the result of vocal hyperfunction, making the voice chronically low pitched and hoarse; (L. *poly*, many, + Gk. *oeides*, form).

positive emission tomography (PET)—A computerized radiographic scanning technique that examines metabolic activity, blood flow, and biochemical activity of the brain and other body parts; (L. *positivus*, positive; *emissio*, send out; Gk. *tomos*, slice or section, + *graphia*, describe).

positive reinforcement (positive feedback, reward)—A technique used to encourage a desired behavior by presenting something the person wants soon after the desired behavior is made; (L. *positivus*, positive; L. *re-*, again, *en*, in, + *fortis*, strong).

postconcussion syndrome (PCS)—A constellation of symptoms seen in some patients with mild traumatic brain injury, including headache, poor concentration, short-term memory deficits, and affective disturbances (e.g., anxiety, depression, and irritability); (L. *post*, after, + *concussio*, shaking; Gk. *syn-* with, + *dromos*, running or course).

post-traumatic stress disorder (PTSD)—A set of symptoms after exposure to a psychologically extreme traumatic stressor that involves intense fear, horror, or helplessness; symptoms include persistent reexperiencing of the traumatic event or events, avoidance of stimuli associated with the trauma, and symptoms of increased arousal (*hypervigilance*); (L. *post*, after; *trauma*, wound).

pragmatics—The rules governing the use of language in social situations; includes the speaker–listener relationship and intentions and all elements in the environment surrounding the interaction—the context; (L. *pragmaticus*, skilled in law or business).

prelinguistic (preverbal) vocalizations—The sounds produced by an infant before the production of true words (e.g., crying, cooing, babbling, and echolalia); vocal behaviors that precede the acquisition of true language; (L. *prae*, before, + *lingua*, tongue; L. *vocalis*, sound).

premature (infant)—Any infant born before the gestational age of 37 weeks; often associated with low birth weight that results in high risk for incomplete organ system development, causing poor temperature regulation, respiratory disorders, and poor sucking and swallowing reflexes; (L. *prae*, before, + *maturare*, to ripen; i.e., before ripe).

premorbid—In medicine, the wellness or functioning of a patient before a significant illness or injury; (L. *prae-*, before, + *morbus*, disease).

presbycusis—Hearing loss associated with old age, usually involving both a loss of hearing sensitivity and a reduction in clarity of speech; (Gk. *presbys*, old man, + *akousis*, hearing).

pressure-airflow technique—A procedure using *aerodynamic instrumentation* to evaluate the dynamics of the velopharyngeal mechanism during speech; also used to evaluate nasal respiration and to quantify upper airway obstruction through measurements of nasal airway resistance; (L. *pressus*, to press).

pressure-equalizing (PE) tube—A small silicone tube inserted into the tympanic membrane following a myringotomy to equalize air pressure between the middle ear cavity and the atmosphere as a substitute for a nonfunctional Eustachian tube; (L. *pressus*, to press; *aequalis*, uniform or equal).

prevalence—The estimated total number of individuals diagnosed with a particular disorder at a given time in a population, or the percent of people in a population with the disorder; (L. *praevalere*, to be powerful).

process—In reference to neurological functioning, the activation of neurons (hundreds to millions at any instant) with their impulses sent through axons and dendrites to other neurons to bring about general and specific cognitive, linguistic, and motor activity; (L. *processus*, process).

produce—In speech, to create an utterance (sound, syllable, word, sentence, or longer) that is spontaneous or imitated; (L. *productus,* lead forth).

prognosis—A prediction of the probable course, duration, recovery, or termination of a disease or disorder; a prediction of the outcome of a proposed course of treatment, its effectiveness and duration, and the individual's progress; (Gk. *pro,* first or before, + *gnosis,* knowledge).

prosody (prosodic)/melody (melodic)—The qualities of stress and intonation in the voice that are influenced by the pitch, loudness, and duration of individual speech sounds; (Gk. *prosoidia,* song sung to music).

prosopagnosia—Difficulty recognizing familiar faces (including those of family members) and famous people; (Gk. *prosopon,* mask; + *gnosis,* knowledge).

prosthetic device (prosthesis)—An artificial device to replace or augment a missing or impaired part of the body; (Gk. *pros-,* in addition to, + *tithenai,* to put).

protrude—In speech, the puckering of the lips forward or the movement of the tongue forward past the lips; (L. *pro-,* in front of or forward, + *trudere,* to thrust).

psychophysiological (psychosomatic) disorder—A disorder with physical signs and symptoms that have a psychological origin, often with common ailments such as tension headaches, gastrointestinal disorders, or both that are attributed to psychological stress; (Gk. *psyche,* breath, life, or soul, + *physikos,* of nature; *somatikos* [soma], body).

pure-tone audiometry—Audiometry using tones of various frequencies and intensities as auditory stimuli to measure hearing using both air conduction and bone conduction.

Q

quality of life—A global concept that is difficult to measure but often is considered to involve a person's standard of living, personal freedom, and the opportunity to pursue happiness; a measure of a person's ability to cope successfully with the full range of challenges encountered in daily living; the characterization of health concerns or disease effects on a person's lifestyle and daily functioning; (L. *qualis,* of what sort).

R

range of motion (ROM)—For speech, the limits the mandible can open and close, the lips can protrude and retract, and the tongue can protrude and retract, elevate and lower, and move side to side (lateralize).

reading disability (dyslexia, developmental dyslexia)—An inability or difficulty reading that is of neurological origin; (OE *raedan,* to advise or interpret; Gk. *dys,* impaired or difficult, + *lexis,* word).

receptive aphasia—Difficulty comprehending verbal, written, and/or gestural language; (L. *recipere,* to receive; Gk. *a-,* without or loss of, + *phasos,* to speak).

receptive language—What a person understands of what is said; (L. *recipere,* to receive; *lingua,* tongue or language).

referred pain—Pain felt at a site different from that of an injured or diseased organ or part of the body, e.g., *angina,* the pain of coronary artery insufficiency, may be felt in the left shoulder, arm, or mandible; (L. *referre,* to bring back; *poena,* punishment).

reflex—An involuntary response to a sensory input, such as the corneal reflex in which both eyes blink in response to something irritating an eye; the gag reflex, caused by something touching the posterior wall of the pharynx; and the knee jerk (deep tendon) reflex, caused by a sharp tap just below the knee; (L. *reflectere,* to bend back).

rehabilitation—Restoration of impaired functions and abilities to normal or to as satisfactory a status as possible; (L. *re-,* back or return, + *habilitatus,* ability, to make able).

reliable/reliability—The dependability of a test or treatment procedure as reflected in the consistency of its scores on repeated measurements of the same group; (L. *re-,* again, + *ligare,* to bind).

replicate—Evaluation or treatment procedures that can be repeated by either the same investigator or other investigators to determine reliability of the data; (L. *re-,* again, + *plicare,* to make parallel).

residential care facility—Often a fairly large complex of small "apartments" where individuals or couples live; there is communal dining, and various services (e.g., security, trips to the mall, and outings) are provided to residents; (L. *residere,* to rest).

resonance—The quality of the voice that results from the vibration of sound in the vocal tract (i.e., spaces and tissues of the pharynx, oral cavity, and nasal cavity); (L. *resonantia,* echo; *re-,* again, + *sonare,* to sound).

resonance disorder—Abnormal modification of the voice by passing through the nasal cavities during production of oral sounds (*hypernasality*) or not passing through the nasal cavities during production of nasal sounds (*hyponasality*).

respiration (ventilation, pulmonary ventilation, breathing)—The movement of air into and out of the lungs that allows for the exchange of oxygen and carbon dioxide; (L. *respirare,* to breathe).

retract—In speech, the pulling back of the lips past their neutral or resting position, or the movement of the tongue back into the oral cavity after protrusion or past the neutral, resting position; (L. *re-,* back or again + *trudere,* to thrust).

retrocochlear hearing loss—A hearing disorder resulting from a *neoplasm* (tumor) or other lesion located on cranial nerve VIII or beyond in the auditory brainstem or cortex; (L. *retro-,* back or behind, + *cochlea,* snail shell).

right-hemisphere syndrome—Damage to the right hemisphere of the brain that can result in impairments of attention, visual–spatial abilities, orientation to person, place, time, and purpose, emotions, cognition, subtle to overt communication problems, and left-side neglect.

rule of 10s—A guideline for the appropriate time for a cleft lip repair, which says that the infant must be at least 10 weeks of age, weigh 10 pounds, and have a hemoglobin count of 10 grams before the lip repair; the purpose of the rule is to help insure the infant will survive the anesthesia during surgery.

S

savant syndrome—The co-occurrence with autism of unexpected or unusual high-level skills with generally limited intelligence (e.g., mathematical calculations, days and dates in history or the future, or remarkable memory for unrelated information); (Fr. *savoir,* to know).

scaffolding—Support that adults provide to children for them to achieve competence in an activity (e.g., reading and writing), with the support gradually removed until the child is able to perform independently.

scope of practice—ASHA's delineation of the general and specific areas in which speech-language pathologists and audiologists may engage with the appropriate and necessary education, training, and experience.

screening—In speech, any gross measure used to identify individuals who may require further assessment in a specific area (e.g., articulation, language, hearing, fluency, or voice).

secondary/overt/concomitant stuttering behaviors—Extraneous sounds and facial and body movements a person who stutters uses during moments of stuttering; e.g., repetitions of "uh" or "um," eye blinks, and unusual head, hand, or other body part movements.

seizure (epilepsy, convulsion)—A hyperexcitation of neurons in the brain that causes a sudden, sometimes violent, involuntary series of contractions of groups of muscles; (Fr. *saisir,* to seize; Gk. *epilepsia,* seizure; L. *convulsion,* to cramp).

semantic-cognitive theory—A perspective of language development that emphasizes the interrelationship between language learning and cognition, that is, the meanings conveyed by a child's productions; (Gk. *semantikos,* meaning; L. *co-,* with, + *gnosticus,* knowledge).

semantics—The study of meaning in language conveyed by words, phrases, and sentences; (Gk. *semantikos,* to mean or signify).

senility—A medical term that refers to the normal loss of cognitive functioning with advanced age; (L. *senilis,* old or aged).

sensorimotor—The combination of input of sensations and output of motor activity; motor activity reflects what is happening to the sensory systems; (L. *sentire,* to perceive or feel, + *movere,* to move).

sensorineural hearing loss—A reduction of hearing sensitivity produced by disorders of the cochlea and/or the auditory nerve fibers of the vestibulocochlear (VIII cranial) nerve; (L. *sentire,* to perceive or feel, + Gk. *neuron,* nerve).

sensory—Pertaining to sensation or awareness of stimuli that are received in the central nervous system; (L. *sentire,* to feel).

sensory–motor (sensorimotor) integration—The ability to take information (*stimuli*) in through the senses of vision, hearing, touch, taste, and smell, and to combine the information with previously stored memories to develop a coherent concept or appropriate motor response; (L. *sentire,* to perceive or feel; *movere,* to move; *integrare,* make whole).

sibilant—A fricative sound whose production is accompanied by a "hissing" sound (/s/, /z/, /ʃ/ [sh], and /ʒ/ [dj]); (L. *sibilare,* to hiss).

sign—An objective finding of a disease or change in condition as perceived by an examiner, such as a physician; (L. *signum,* mark).

significant—A term often used to specify the impairment level a child must exhibit before he is considered to have a speech or language disorder; no "gold standard" is available to use to define this term as it applies to speech and language disorders. In statistics, the probability that a given finding (e.g., an individual test score) may have occurred by chance; usually a finding that occurs fewer than 5 times in 100 by chance alone (*p.* < .05).

sign language—A visual means of communication using hand and arm shapes and gestures to represent words and concepts, along with some finger spelling; communication that does not depend on spoken language and is used within Deaf communities and learned naturally by interaction with other signers.

silent aspiration—Penetration of food or liquid (including saliva) into the larynx and passing below the vocal folds without a protective cough or choking occurring; (L. *aspirare,* to breathe upon).

social-pragmatic theory—A perspective of language development that considers communication as the basic function of language.

social reinforcer—A word, phrase, or short statement said with warmth and enthusiasm as a reward and encouragement for an accurate response or good attempt at a specific task or target; (L. *socius,* companion, associate; *re-,* again, + *en-,* in, + *fortis,* strong).

social worker—A professional who helps families coordinate appointments, deal with insurance and other funding sources, and manage their stress and emotional reactions to the many problems associated with the child's treatment.

soft palate (velum)—The muscular tissue in the posterior one-third of the roof of the mouth that separates the oral cavity from the nasal cavity when raised and in contact with the posterior pharyngeal wall; (L. *palatum,* palate; *velum,* curtain or veil).

spasmodic dysphonia (SD)—A relatively rare voice disorder that may have either or both neurological and psychological etiologies; characterized by a strained, strangled, harsh voice quality, or an absence of voice because of tight abduction of the vocal folds; clients typically do not respond well to voice therapy; (Gk. *spasmodes,* spasm or convulsion; *dys-,* disturbance or impaired, + *phonia,* voice).

specific language impairment (SLI)—Significant receptive and/or expressive language impairments that cannot be attributed to any general or specific cause or condition.

speech—The production of oral language using phonemes for communication through the process of respiration, phonation, resonation, and articulation.

speech audiometry—A key component of audiological assessment that uses auditory signals present in everyday communication; assessment involves, in part, the presentation of single-syllable words at a fixed intensity level above the threshold with the client aurally discriminating the sounds in the words to correctly say words aloud for the examiner to score.

speech bulb obturator—A prosthetic device that may be considered when the velum is too short to close completely against the posterior pharyngeal wall; it consists of a retaining appliance and a bulb (usually made of acrylic) that fills in the pharyngeal space for speech; (L. *obturare,* to close).

speech development—The progressive evolving and shaping of individual sounds and syllables that are used as arbitrary symbols and applied in rule-governed combinations to produce words to communicate a person's wants, needs, thoughts, knowledge, and feelings; (Fr. *desvoluper,* to unwrap or expose).

speech disorder—Any deviation of speech outside the range of acceptable variation in a given environment; (L. *dis,* apart or impaired, + *ordo,* rank).

speech-language pathologist/speech pathologist/ speech therapist—A professional who is specifically educated and trained to identify, evaluate, treat, and prevent speech, language, cognitive, and swallowing disorders; (Anglo Saxon *speche,* to speak; [Gk. *spharageisthai,* to crackle]; Anglo Saxon *langue,* tongue; [Gk. *lingua,* tongue]; Gk. *pathos,* suffering or disease; Gk. *logia,* study of).

speech-language pathology assistant (SLPA)—A support person who performs tasks as prescribed, directed, and supervised by ASHA certified SLPs.

speechreading—The process of recognizing speech by attending to the speaker's auditory and visual messages (nonverbal communication, such as facial expressions and body language), clues from the setting of the conversation, and the likely conversational topics in those settings.

spinal cord—A thick "cord" of nerve fibers that passes through the vertebral column that conducts sensory and motor impulses to and from the brain and controls many body reflexes; (L. *spina,* backbone).

spontaneous (connected, running) speech sample—A sample of a child's oral discourse in conversation or while describing a picture, usually 50 to 100 consecutive utterances; (L. *sponte,* voluntary).

spontaneous recovery—The physiological healing of the brain's damaged tissue, including reduction of cerebral edema, development of collateral blood vessels, and rerouting of neural pathways.

Standard American English (SAE)—See *General American English* (GAE).

standard dialect—The dialect of a language that is commonly spoken or established by individuals with considerable formal education; (Gk. *dia-,* two or apart, + *lektos,* discourse, way of speaking).

standardized test (norm-referenced test)—A test that has been administered to a large group of individuals to determine uniform or standard procedures and methods of administration, scoring, and interpretation, and has adequate normative data on validity and reliability; tests that are administered to compare one child's performance to others the same age.

stereotyped movements—Persistent and inappropriate mechanical repetition of actions, body postures, or speech patterns, often seen in autism (Gk. *stereos,* solid, + *typos,* mark).

stimulability—The evaluation of a child's ability to produce a correct (or an improved) sound in imitation after the clinician models the sound for the child or after the child is given specific instructions on the articulatory placement or manner of production; (L. *stimulare,* to goad).

stoma—An opening about the diameter of a finger or thumb made surgically into the neck that allows a person to breathe directly through the trachea; (Gk. *stoma,* mouth).

stop—Sound made by building up air pressure in the mouth and then suddenly releasing it; the airflow can be blocked momentarily by pressing the lips together (bilabial—/p, b/) or by pressing the tongue against either the gums (lingua [tongue]-alveolar—/t, d/) or the soft palate (linguavelar—/k, g/).

stress—Variations in intensity, frequency, and duration on one syllable more than another in a word, which usually results in the syllable sounding both louder and longer than other syllables in the same word.

stroke (cerebrovascular accident, CVA)—A disruption of blood supply to the brain caused by an occluded (blocked) artery or an artery that has hemorrhaged; (from the concept that a person has been *stricken*).

stuttering (disfluency)—A disturbance in the normal flow and time patterning of speech characterized by one of more of the following: repetitions of sounds, syllables, or words; prolongations of sounds; abnormal stoppages or "silent blocks" within or between words; interjections of unnecessary sounds or words; circumlocutions (talking around an intended word); or sounds and words produced with excessive tension; (Teutonic, *steut,* stop; L. *dis-,* apart or impaired + *fluere,* to flow [i.e., impaired flow]).

stuttering modification—A therapy approach for children and adult stutterers that requires the speaker to recognize and confront his fears, avoidances, and struggles to escape his stuttering, and the speaker reducing and managing those fears, avoidances, and struggles.

subacute hospital—A level of care needed by patients who do not require acute care but who are medically fragile and require special services, e.g., respiratory therapy, intravenous tube feeding, and complex wound management care; (L. *sub*, under or beneath; *hospitium*, guesthouse).

submucous cleft—A defect in the hard palate in the absence of an actual opening into the nasal cavity or a defect in the muscles of the soft palate that cannot be seen through the mucosal tissue but may cause disunity of the velar muscles, resulting in velopharyngeal inadequacy and hypernasality; (L. *sub*, under or beneath, + *mucus*, slime).

substitution—The replacement of one standard speech sound by another, e.g., /th/ for /s/; (L. *substituere*, to put in place of).

suprasegmentals/paralinguistics/prosody (prosodic) features—Voice inflections used in a language such as stress, intensity, changes in pitch, duration of a sound, and rhythm that help listeners understand the true intent of a message and that convey the emotional aspects of a message, such as happiness, sadness, fear, or surprise; (L. *supra*, above or beyond, + *segmentum*, cut or divide).

swallow/swallowing—The process of moving food from the mouth to the stomach via the esophagus that involves smooth coordination of muscles in the mouth, pharynx, and esophagus.

syllable—Either a single vowel (V) or a vowel and one or more consonants (C); e.g., V+ consonant (VC), VCC, CV, CCV, CVC, etc.; (Gk. *syn-* together, + *lambanein*, to take).

symmetry (symmetrical)—Both sides (e.g., the lips) in balanced proportions for size, shape, and relative position; (Gk. *syn*, with or together, + *metron*, measure).

symptom—A subjective indication of a disease or change in condition as perceived by the patient or other nonmedical or rehabilitation specialist, such as a family member; (Gk. *symptoma*, that which happened).

synapse—The junction at which two neurons communicate with each other; (Gk. *syn*, with or together, + *haptein*, to fasten).

syndrome—A complex of signs and symptoms resulting from a common etiology or appearing together that presents a clinical picture of a disease or inherited anomaly; (Gk. *syn*, together, + *dromos*, course).

syntax—Rules that dictate the acceptable sequence and combination of words in a sentence to convey meaning; the study of sentence structure; (Gk. *syntaktos*, order or arrange together).

T

telecommunication devices for the deaf (TDD)—Telephone systems used by those with significant hearing impairments in which a typewritten message is transmitted over telephone lines and is received as a printed message; (Gk. *tele-*, afar, + L. *commicare*, to share).

telegraphic speech (language)—Condensed language in which only the essential words are used, such as nouns, verbs, and adjectives; often used by 3-year-old children and college students taking lecture notes (Gk. *tele*, afar, + *graphos*, written).

teratogen—Any substance, agent, or process that interferes with prenatal development, causing the formation of one or more developmental abnormalities in a fetus; (Gk. *teras*, monster, + *genein*, to produce).

therapy/treatment—The care of any significant condition to prevent, alleviate, or cure it; (Gk. *therapeia*, medical treatment; L. *tractare*, manage, handle, or deal with, + *mentum*, result.

thoracic cavity—The upper part of the trunk that contains the organs of respiration (lungs) and circulation (heart); (Gk. *thorax*, chest; *cavus*, hollow).

thyroid cartilage—The largest of the *laryngeal cartilages* that is the main structure of the larynx and encloses and protects the vocal folds; its *anterior* (front) point is popularly referred to as the "Adam's apple"; (Gk. *thyreos*, shield; L. *cartilago*, cartilage).

tinnitus—A subjective noise sensation, often described as a ringing, roaring, or swishing in the ear that may be heard in one or both ears; associated with a variety of hearing disorders in both adults and children; can affect concentration, sleep, education, employment, personal relationships, and social functioning and sometimes is debilitating; treatment success varies; (L. *tinnire*, to tinkle).

tongue (lingua, glossus)—The primary articulator, whose movement creates consonants and vowels as well as performs biological functions; (L. *lingua*, tongue; Gk. *glossa*, tongue).

tongue thrust—The habitual pushing of the tongue against the inner surface of the front teeth (incisors), or the protrusion of the tongue between the upper and the lower teeth.

total communication—A philosophy calling for every possible means of communication to be used by deaf individuals, including hearing aids and assistive devices, speechreading, signing, and spoken English.

toxin—A substance that poisons or causes inflammation of tissue, including in the central nervous system; (Gk. *toxikon*, poison).

trachea (windpipe)—The tube that begins just below the larynx and continues down to where it divides into the lungs; (Gk. *tracheia*, rough [from the appearance of the numerous tracheal rings]).

tracheoesophageal prosthesis (TEP)—A surgical procedure (*tracheoesophageal puncture*) in which an incision through the trachea and esophageal walls is created to fit a one-way plastic valve (*prosthesis*) that directs air from the trachea into the esophagus where it can reach the oral cavity and be articulated for speech; (Gk. *tracheia,* rough, + *oisophagos,* gullet; Gk. *prostithenai,* add to).

transient ischemic attack (TIA)—An episode of cerebral vascular insufficiency with partial occlusion of a cerebral artery by atherosclerotic plaque or an embolus; disturbances of vision in one or both eyes, dizziness, weakness, numbness, dysphasia, or unconsciousness may occur; TIA (sometimes called "ministroke") usually lasts a few minutes, and in rare cases symptoms may continue for several hours; (L. *transire,* to go through; Gk. *ischein,* to hold back; L. *attacco,* attack).

traumatic brain injury (TBI) (head trauma, acquired brain injury [ABI])—An acquired injury to the brain caused by an external force and resulting in partial or total functional disability; applies to both closed and open head injuries, affecting speech, language, cognition, psychosocial behavior, and physical functioning; (Gk. *trauma,* wound; L. *injurus,* injury).

treatment effectiveness—The extent to which services are shown to be beneficial under typical (or real-world) conditions.

treatment efficacy—The extent to which an intervention can be shown to be beneficial under optimal (or ideal) conditions; (L. *tractare,* manage, handle, or deal with; *efficacere,* accomplish or efficiency).

tremors at rest—Tremors that occur when the head, limbs, hands, or fingers are not intentionally being moved; when movement is initiated, the tremors subside until the body part is again no longer moving; (L. *tremere,* to shake).

true vocal folds—Paired muscles (thyroarytenoid and vocalis) covered with mucous membranes with a pearly white appearance inside the thyroid cartilage at the level of the Adam's apple that open and close extremely rapidly to produce voice; closure during swallowing protects the trachea and lungs from penetration of food and liquid.

tumor (neoplasm)—Any abnormal growth of new tissue, either benign or malignant, caused by aberrant increases in the rate of cell reproduction; (L. *tumor,* swelling; Gk. *neos,* new, + *plasma,* something formed).

tympanic membrane (eardrum)—A thin, semitransparent membrane that separates the ear canal from the middle ear and transmits sound vibrations into the middle ear; (Gk. *tympanon,* drum; L. *membrana,* thin skin or covering).

tympanometry—A measurement of middle ear pressure that is determined by the mobility of the tympanic membrane as a function of various amounts of positive and negative air pressure in the external ear canal (the more positive or negative the air pressure in the external ear canal, the more the normal middle ear system becomes immobilized); (Gk. *tympanon,* drum, + *metron,* measure).

U

utterance—A unit of vocal expression preceded and followed by a pause or silence; may be a single sound, word or words, phrase, clauses, or sentence; (ME. *utter,* outward, + L. *ans,* relating to).

uvula—The cone- or teardrop-shaped structure that hangs from the back of the soft palate but does not have any known function; (L. diminutive or *uva,* cluster of grapes; i.e., one grape).

V

valid/validity—The extent to which a test measures what it is intended to measure; (L. *validus,* strong).

Valsalva maneuver—The procedure of closing the mouth and pinching the nostrils closed with the fingers and forcefully exhaling air, usually causing the Eustachian tubes to open and air to flow into the middle ear to equalize middle ear cavity air pressure with atmospheric air pressure, for example, when going up or down in an elevator or ascending or descending in an airplane, causing the ears to "pop"; any exhaling of air against tightly closed vocal folds, as when lifting heavy objects; (named after Antonio Valsalva, Italian surgeon, 1666–1723).

vegetative state—A condition in which a person may have some minimal level of wakefulness but has not regained awareness (i.e., they lack cognitive function).

velopharyngeal closure—The upward and backward movement of the soft palate to make contact with the posterior pharyngeal wall to close off the coupling of the oral and nasal cavities; (L. *velum,* curtain or veil, + Gk. *pharyngos,* throat; L. *clausura,* closing).

velopharyngeal incompetence—A term generally used to describe abnormal velopharyngeal function, regardless of the cause (i.e., an anatomical or structural defect [e.g., a cleft] or a neuromotor or physiological disorder [e.g., weakness of the soft palate caused by a CVA or TBI]) that typically results in hypernasality and/or nasal emission; various authors use different terms, such as *incompetence, inadequacy, insufficiency,* and *dysfunction*; (L. *velum,* curtain, + Gk. *pharyngos,* throat; L. *in,* variation of *im,* not, + *competere,* able).

ventricular folds—See *false vocal folds.*

verbal or semantic paraphasia—Unintended substitution of one word for another word that is often semantically related to the intended word (e.g., *sister* for *brother* and *horse* for *dog*); often occur in both speech and writing; (Gk. *semantikos,* significant; *para,* near or alongside, + *phasos,* speech).

vestibular system—The inner ear structures associated with balance and position sense, including the vestibule and semicircular canals of the vestibular mechanism, with interactions of the visual and proprioceptive systems and connection to the cerebellum; (L. *vestibulum,* courtyard).

visual–spatial impairments—Difficulty associating seen objects with their spatial relationships, that is, what is around the objects and the environment; often results in disorientation.

vocal abuse—Deleterious acute or chronic vocal behaviors that are damaging to the vocal folds and laryngeal and pharyngeal muscles and tissue, such as yelling, screaming, cheering, coughing, frequently clearing the throat, and talking loudly over loud noise; (L. *vocalis*, sound; *abusus*, to use or consume).

vocal fold paralysis—Unilateral (one side) or bilateral (two sides) loss of laryngeal movements (including vocal fold opening or closing) that may be caused by damage to the brainstem, vagus (X cranial) nerves, recurrent laryngeal nerves, or the neuromuscular junctions (where the nerve fibers connect with the muscle tissue), resulting in a weak, breathy voice, or possible difficulty breathing if the vocal folds are paralyzed in the closed position; (L. *vocalis*, sound; Gk. *paralyein*, disable or feeble).

vocal hygiene—Behaviors that are helpful to achieve and maintain a healthy vocal mechanism and prevent or decrease vocal pathologies, such as eliminating phonotrauma, speaking in an appropriate pitch, turning the television or radio down while talking, using amplification when speaking to an audience in a large room, and singing within the optimal pitch range; (L. *vocalis*, sound; Gk. *hygieinos*, healthful).

vocal misuse—Deleterious chronic vocal behaviors that may have a cumulative effects on the structure and functioning of the laryngeal mechanism, such as chronic inappropriate loudness or pitch, singing beyond the range of the vocal mechanism, frequent hard glottal attacks, and speaking with inadequate respiratory support (L. *vocalis*, sound).

vocal nodule—A *benign* (nonmalignant or not cancerous) vocal fold growth that tends to be *bilateral* (both sides, i.e., both vocal folds) and occur at the same location as vocal polyps (i.e., juncture of the anterior 1/3 and middle 1/3 of the vocal folds), caused by continuous vocal fold hyperfunction (abuse and misuse); (L. *nodus*, knot).

vocal play—The longer strings of syllables that extend babbling (e.g., *baa-da-gi-daa-um-ma*).

vocal polyp—A benign vocal fold growth that may take various forms and is caused by vocal abuse and misuse and results in vocal hoarseness; (Gk. *polys*, many, + *pous*, foot).

voice—The distinctive feature that refers to a sound produced either with the vocal folds vibrating (*voiced*) or not vibrating (*unvoiced*); (L. *vox* and *vocalis*, voice).

voice box—See *larynx*.

voice disorder (dysphonia)—Any deviation of loudness, pitch, or quality of voice that is outside the normal range of a person's age, gender, or geographic cultural background that interferes with communication, draws unfavorable attention to itself, or adversely affects the speaker or listener; (L. *vox*, voice or sound; *dis-* apart or impaired, + *ordinare*, to order).

voice quality—The auditory aspects of the function of the vocal folds that is affected by adequate closure, efficient timing of closure, and the amount of muscle tone of the vocal folds; normal voice quality is a described as nontense, no extraneous noise, nonbreathy, and easily produced and sustained throughout phonation.

vowel—Voiced speech sounds from the unrestricted passage of the air stream through the mouth without audible stoppage or friction; (L. *vocalis*, voice).

W

Wernicke's aphasia—A fluent aphasia characterized by impaired comprehension, integration, and formulation of language caused by damage to the perisylvian regions in or around Wernicke's area in the posterior superior left temporal lobe (auditory association cortex); characteristics include impaired auditory comprehension, integration of information, and formulation of language; (named after Karl Wernicke, German neurologist, 1848–1905).

working memory—Temporary information storage that is limited in capacity and requires rehearsal; often thought of as "what is on your mind" at any given moment.

World Health Organization (WHO)—An agency of the United Nations established in 1948 to further international cooperation in improving health conditions throughout the world.

Index

Page numbers in italics indicate figures, tables, and boxes.

Energy: Management, Supply and Conservation

Clive Beggs

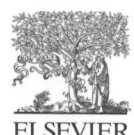

Amsterdam • Boston • Heidelberg • London • New York • Oxford
Paris • San Diego • San Francisco • Singapore • Sydney • Tokyo
Butterworth-Heinemann is an imprint of Elsevier

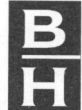

Butterworth-Heinemann is an imprint of Elsevier
Linacre House, Jordan Hill, Oxford OX2 8DP, UK
30 Corporate Drive, Suite 400, Burlington, MA 01803, USA

First published 2002
Reprinted 2003, 2005
Second edition 2009

British Library Cataloguing in Publication Data
Beggs, Clive.
 Energy: management, supply and conservation. — 2nd ed. 1. Buildings—Energy Conservation. 2. Buildings—Power supply.
I. Title
696—dc22

Library of Congress Control Number: 2009925900

ISBN: 978-0-7506-8670-9

For information on all Butterworth-Heinemann publications
visit our website at elsevierdirect.com

Typeset by Macmillan Publishing Solutions
(www.macmillansolutions.com)

Printed and bound in Great Britain

09 10 11   10 9 8 7 6 5 4 3 2 1

Working together to grow
libraries in developing countries

www.elsevier.com | www.bookaid.org | www.sabre.org

ELSEVIER   BOOK AID International   Sabre Foundation

Contents

CHAPTER 1

Energy and the Environment

Society in the developed world is built on the assumption that energy is both freely available and relatively cheap. However, there are environmental costs associated with the continued use of fossil fuels and these are causing a reappraisal of the way in which energy is used. This chapter investigates the global use of energy and its impact on economies and the environment.

1.1 Two Worlds

Those of us who live in developed countries take energy very much for granted. Although we may not understand exactly what it is, we certainly know how to use it. Indeed, never before has there been a society, which is as reliant on energy as our own. Consider for a moment the number of everyday items of equipment, tools and appliances that run on electricity – lamps, washing machines, televisions, radios, computers and many other 'essential' items of equipment – which all need a ready supply of electricity in order to function. Imagine what life would be like without electricity. Both our home and our working lives would be very different. Indeed, our high-tech, computer-reliant society would cease to function; productivity would fall drastically and gross domestic product (GDP) would also be greatly reduced, a fact highlighted by the power cuts that brought California to its knees in 2001 [1]. Similarly, if oil supplies ceased, then the fabric of our society would very quickly fall apart. Those living in the UK may remember the events of September 2000, when a relatively small number of 'fuel protesters' managed to almost stop petroleum supplies to the UK's petrol stations, resulting in the economy grinding to a halt within days; people could not get to work and the supermarkets ran out of food. Those in the UK with longer memories might also recall how a combination of striking coal miners, power workers and crude oil price rises in the 1970s brought the UK to a standstill; electricity power cuts were commonplace, vehicle speed restrictions were introduced, and ultimately the government was forced to introduce a three-day working week in order to save energy. Clearly, although all too often taken for granted, cheap and available energy is essential to the running of any advanced industrialized society. Understanding the nature of energy, its supply and its utilization is therefore a subject of great importance. For without energy we in the developed world face an uncertain future.

To some reading this book, the society that has just been described may seem alien. Those living in developing countries will be all too aware that energy is a very finite resource. In many poorer countries, electricity is supplied only to major towns, and even then, power cuts are commonplace. This not only reduces the quality of life of those living in such countries, but also hampers productivity and ultimately ensures that those countries have a low GDP. If you live in one of these poorer nations, then you are in the majority – a majority of the world's population that consumes the minority of its energy. This is indeed a great paradox. One-third of the world's population lives in a consumer society which squanders energy all too easily, while the other two-thirds live in countries which are often unable to secure enough energy to grow economically – a fact highlighted by the USA which consumes approximately 21% of the all world's primary energy [2], while having only about 4% of the world's population.

The inequalities between developed and developing countries are real and should be cause for great concern to the whole world. Unfortunately, political self-interest is often much stronger than altruism, and the gap between the rich and the poor nations has widened in recent years. However, when confronted with unpalatable facts about gross inequalities between rich and poor nations, our usual response is to assume that the problem is altogether too large to solve and to forget about it. After all, most of us have many other pressing needs and problems to worry about. This, of course, is a very understandable response. However, forgetting about the problem does not mean that it will go away. In fact, the reality is that as the economies of the developing world grow, so their demand for energy will also grow. This will increase pressure on the Earth's dwindling supply of fossil fuel and will also increase greenhouse gas emissions and atmospheric pollution in general. It is worth remembering that the Earth is a relatively small place and that atmospheric pollution is no respecter of national boundaries. Indeed, issues such as climate change and third-world debt are now impinging on the comfort and security of the developed world. Indeed, it is the perceived threat of global climate change that has been the driving force behind all the intergovernmental environmental summits of the late twentieth century. In historical terms, the summits at Montreal, Rio and Kyoto were unique – never before had so many nations sat down together to discuss the impact of humans on the environment. In fact, it could truthfully be said that never before in the history of the world have so many sat down together to discuss the weather! Collectively these summits produced protocols which set targets for reducing ozone depletion and greenhouse gas emissions, and have forced governments around the world to reappraise policies on energy supply and consumption. The collective agreements signed at these summits have impacted, to varying degrees, on the signatory nations and manifest themselves in a variety of ways. For example, in the UK, a large proportion of the electricity supply sector has switched from coal, a high carbon intensity fuel, to natural gas, which has a much lower carbon content. In the construction industry, so-called 'green buildings' are being erected which are passively ventilated and cooled with the express intention of minimizing energy consumption and eliminating the use of harmful refrigerants. In addition, the high-profile nature of the various intergovernmental summits has meant that concern about energy and its utilization is now at the forefront of public consciousness.

Because most lay people focus on the consumption of energy it is often forgotten that the supply of energy is itself a large and important sector of the world's economy. For example, the energy industry in the UK is worth 5% of GDP and employs 4% of the industrial workforce (1999 data) [3], making it one of the largest industries in the UK. The energy supply sector is also very multinational in nature. For example, crude oil is transported all around the globe, with a total of 52,561 barrels being transported daily in 2006 alone [2]. Similarly, large quantities of natural gas are piped daily over long distances and across many international borders, and electricity is traded between nations on a daily basis. Given the size of the energy supply industry, its multinational nature and its importance to the world economy, it should come as no surprise that many parties have a vested interest in promoting energy consumption and that this often leads to conflict with those driven by environmental considerations.

1.2 Politics and Self-Interest

Any serious investigation of the subject of energy supply and conservation soon reveals that it is impossible to separate the 'technical' aspects of the subject from the 'politics' that surround it. This is because the two are intertwined; an available energy supply is the cornerstone of any economy and politicians are extremely interested in how economies perform. Politicians like short-term solutions and are reluctant to introduce measures that will make them unpopular. Also, many political parties rely on funding from commercial organizations. Consequently, political self-interest often runs counter to collective reason. For example, in many countries (although not all), politicians who put forward policies which promote congestion charging, or petrol price increases, become unpopular, and are soon voted out of office. As a result, measures which might at first sight appear to be extremely sensible are discarded or watered down due to political self-interest. It is of course far too easy to blame politicians for hypocrisy, while ignoring the fact that we as individuals are also often culpable. Consider the case of a rapidly growing large city which has traffic congestion problems; journey times are long and air quality is poor. Clearly the quality of life of all those in the city is suffering due to the road congestion. The solution is obvious. People need to stop using their cars and switch to public transport. If questioned on the subject, car drivers will probably agree that the city is too congested and that something should be done to reduce the number of cars on the roads. However, when it is suggested that they, as individuals, should stop using their own cars, then self-interest tends to win over reason; objections are raised, sometimes violently, that such a measure is too extreme and that the freedom of the individual is being compromised. From this we can only conclude that it is impossible for politicians alone to bring about changes in 'energy politics' without changes in public opinion. In many ways it is true to say that we all get the leaders we deserve!

The road congestion example discussed above is a good illustration of the contradiction between reason and self-interest, which is often manifest within individuals. However, exactly the same contradiction is often all too evident at a governmental and international level. When it comes to environmental issues, governments often refuse to implement sound policies because in so doing they might inhibit economic growth. To those concerned with environmental issues, the idea of putting national 'self-interest' before the environmental health of the planet might seem absurd. However, the issue is not as clear-cut as it would appear at first sight. There is a strong link between energy consumption and GDP. Without a cheap and available energy supply, the economic growth of many nations will be restricted. Consequently, any enforced reduction in GDP due to environmental control measures is going to be much more painful to the inhabitants of poorer countries than an equivalent cut in a developed country. Indeed, to many poorer nations, the notion of rich, developed countries telling them to reduce greenhouse gas emissions is hypocritical; after all, the advanced nations of North America and Europe only became rich through intensive manufacturing. Since the eighteenth century, the developed countries have consumed large amounts of primary energy and produced high levels of pollution. So in the twenty-first century when – having created many environmental problems – these same nations turn to their poorer neighbours and expect them to restrict economic growth in the name of environmentalism, it is not surprising that to many in the developing world this approach appears high-handed. Therefore, perhaps it is up to those of us in the developed world to lead by example and alter our approach towards energy consumption.

1.2.1 Human Nature

From the discussion above it is clear that the management and conservation of energy is strongly influenced by the collective mindset of society. With respect to this, we cannot ignore the role played by human nature, as it influences both politicians and consumers alike, and does not necessarily lead to outcomes that benefit either society or the environment. Consider, for example, the case of Easter Island, a small and remote rocky outcrop in the Pacific Ocean. As one commentator has aptly pointed out:

> The Easter Islanders, aware that they were almost completely isolated from the rest of the world, must surely have realized that their very existence depended on the limited resources of a small island. After all, it was small enough for them to walk round the entire island in a day or so and see for themselves what was happening to the forests. Yet they were unable to devise a system that allowed them to find the right balance with their environment. [4]

Faced with dwindling timber resources, the ancient tribal groups on Easter Island fought each other for control of supply and ultimately consumed all the timber on the island, with disastrous consequences for their society. Unfortunately, rather than acting cooperatively, societies, groups and individuals tend to act out of self-interest and consume as much as they can. This has led some to postulate that all societies evolve to degrade as much energy as possible. Consequently, governments, societies and individuals tend to use their power (be it political, military or financial) to maximize their consumption of energy and other finite resources. One only has to look at the global conflicts of the twentieth and early twenty-first centuries to see that many have considered scarce commodities well worth fighting over. Indeed, in 1999 US Secretary of Energy, Bill Richardson, stated:

> Oil has literally made foreign and security policy for decades. Just since the turn of this century, it has provoked the division of the Middle East after World War I; aroused Germany and Japan to extend their tentacles beyond their borders; the Arab Oil Embargo; Iran versus Iraq; the Gulf War. This is all clear. [5]

Oil is an extremely high-quality fuel, which has a higher energy content per unit weight than coal and which can be burnt at a higher temperature. It is easier to transport than coal and can be used to power internal combustion engines. No other primary energy source has oil's intrinsic qualities of extractability, transportability and versatility, at relatively low cost. Given this, and the fact that people and commodities throughout the world are transported by oil-powered vehicles, it is not surprising that individuals and governments will go to extreme lengths to secure its supply. In short, the unhappy truth appears to be that human nature will seek to maximize consumption while stocks last – only when oil runs out will things change! Perhaps we are not too different from the Easter Islanders after all?

1.3 What is Energy?

Before discussing global energy production and consumption, it is perhaps wise to first look at the physics associated with energy. Although most are familiar with the term *energy*, surprisingly few people fully appreciate its true nature. In everyday language, the word *energy* is used very loosely; words like *work*, *power*, *fuel* and *energy* are often used interchangeably and, frequently, incorrectly. To the physicist or an engineer, energy is a very specific term which is perhaps best explained by means of an illustration.

Consider a mass of 1 kg which is raised 1 m above a surface on which it was originally resting. It is easy to appreciate that in order to raise the weight through the distance of 1 m, someone, or some machine, must have performed work. In other words, work has been put into the system to raise the mass from a low level to a higher level. This work is the amount of energy that has been put into the system. So, when the weight is in the raised position, it is at a higher energy level than when on the surface. Indeed, this illustration forms the basis for the International System (SI) unit of energy, the 'joule', which can be defined as follows:

> One joule (J) is the work done when a force of 1 newton (N) acts on an object so that it moves 1 metre (m) in the direction of the force.

and

> One newton (N) is the force required to increase or decrease the velocity of a 1 kg object by 1 m per second every second.

The number of newtons needed to accelerate an object can be calculated by:

$$F = m \times a \qquad (1.1)$$

where m is the mass of the object (kg) and a is the acceleration (m/s^2). Given that the acceleration due to gravity is 9.81 m/s^2, a mass of 1 kg will exert a force of 9.81 N (i.e. 1 kg $\times$ 9.81 m/s^2). Therefore the energy required to raise it through 1 m will be 9.81 J.

If the 1 kg mass is released it will fall through a distance of 1 m back to its original position. In doing so the *potential energy* stored in the 1 kg mass when it is at the higher level will be released. Notice that the energy released is equal to the work put into raising the weight. For this reason the term *work* is sometimes used instead of *energy*. Perhaps a good way of viewing energy is to consider it as stored work. Therefore, *potential energy* represents work that has already been done and stored for future use.

Potential energy can be calculated by:

$$\text{Potential energy} = m \times g \times h \qquad (1.2)$$

where m is the mass of the object (kg), g is the acceleration due to gravity (i.e. 9.81 m/s^2) and h is the height through which the object has been raised (m).

As the weight falls it will possess energy because of its motion and this is termed *kinetic energy*. The kinetic energy of a body is proportional to its mass and to the square of its speed. Kinetic energy can be calculated by:

$$\text{Kinetic energy} = 0.5 \times m \times v^2 \qquad (1.3)$$

where v is the velocity of the object (m/s).

We can see that during the time the mass takes to fall, its potential energy decreases whilst its kinetic energy increases. However, the sum of both forms of energy must remain constant during the fall. Physicists and engineers express this constancy in the 'law of conservation of energy', which states that the total amount of energy in the system must always be the same.

It should be noted that the amount of energy expended in raising the weight is completely independent of the time taken to raise the weight. Whether the weight is raised in 1 second or 1 day makes no difference to the energy put into the system. It does, however, have an effect on the 'power' of the person or machine performing the work. Clearly, the shorter the duration of the lift, the more powerful the lifter has to be. Consequently, power is defined as the rate at which work is done, or alternatively, the rate of producing or using energy. The SI unit of power is the watt (W). Therefore, a machine requires a power of 1 W if it uses 1 J of energy in 1 second (i.e. 1 W is 1 J per second). In electrical terms, 1 W is the energy released in 1 second by a current of 1 ampere passing through a resistance of 1 ohm.

It is well known that if two rough surfaces are rubbed together, the work required in overcoming the friction produces heat. Also, it is known that electricity can be used to perform mechanical work by utilizing an electric motor. Therefore, it is clear that energy can take a number of forms (e.g. electrical energy, mechanical work and heat) and that it can be easily converted between these various forms. For example, fossil fuel can be burnt to produce heat energy in a power station. The heat energy produced is then converted to mechanical energy by a turbine, which in turn produces electrical energy through a generator. Finally, the electricity is distributed to homes and factories where it can be converted to mechanical work using electric motors, heat using resistance elements and light using electric lamps.

1.3.1 Units of Energy

For myriad reasons (too numerous to mention here), a bizarre array of units for energy has evolved. Books, articles and papers on energy quote terms such as 'kWh', 'therms', 'joules', 'calories', 'toe' and many more. This makes things very complicated and confusing for the reader. This section is, therefore, included to introduce some of the units more commonly in use.

Kilowatt-hour (kWh)

The kilowatt-hour (kWh) is a particularly useful unit of energy which is commonly used in the electricity supply industry and, to a lesser extent, in the gas supply industry. It refers to the amount of energy consumed in 1 hour by the operation of an appliance having a power rating of 1 kW. Therefore:

$$1\,kWh = 3.6 \times 10^6\,J$$

British thermal unit (Btu)

The British thermal unit (Btu) is the old imperial unit of energy. It is still very much in use and is particularly popular in the USA:

$$1\,Btu = 1.055 \times 10^3\,J$$

Therm

The therm is a unit that originated in the gas supply industry. It is equivalent to 100,000 Btu:

$$1\,therm = 1.055 \times 10^8\,J$$

Tonne of oil equivalent (toe)

The 'tonne of oil equivalent' (toe) is a unit of energy used in the oil industry:

$$1\,toe = 4.5 \times 10^{10}\,J$$

Barrel

The barrel is another unit of energy used in the oil industry. There are 7.5 barrels in 1 toe:

$$1\,barrel = 6 \times 10^9\,J$$

Calorie

In the food industry the calorie is the most commonly used unit of energy. It is in fact the amount of heat energy required to raise 1 g of water through 1°C:

$$1 \text{ calorie} = 4.2 \times 10^3 \text{ J}$$

1.3.2 The Laws of Thermodynamics

Thermodynamics is the study of heat and work, and the conversion of energy from one form into another. There are actually three laws of thermodynamics, although the majority of thermodynamics is based on the first two laws.

The first law of thermodynamics

The first law of thermodynamics is also known as the law of conservation of energy. It states that the energy in a system can neither be created nor destroyed. Instead, energy is either converted from one form to another, or transferred from one system to another. The term 'system' can refer to anything from a simple object to a complex machine. If the first law is applied to a heat engine, such as a gas turbine, where heat energy is converted into mechanical energy, then it tells us that no matter what the various stages in the process are, the total amount of energy in the system must always remain constant.

The second law of thermodynamics

While the first law of thermodynamics refers to the quantity of energy that is in a system, it says nothing about the direction in which it flows. It is the second law that deals with the natural direction of energy processes. For example, according to the second law of thermodynamics, heat will always flow only from a hot object to a colder object. In another context, it explains why many natural processes occur in the way they do. For example, iron always turns to rust; rust never becomes pure iron. This is because all processes proceed in a direction which increases the amount of disorder, or chaos, in the universe. Iron is produced by smelting ore in a foundry, a process which involves the input of a large amount of heat energy. So, when iron rusts it is reverting back to a 'low-energy' state. Although it is a difficult concept to grasp, disorder has been quantified and given the name 'entropy'. Entropy can be used to quantify the amount of useful work that can be performed in a system. In simple terms, the more chaotic a system, the more difficult it is to perform useful work.

In an engineering context it is the second law of thermodynamics that accounts for the fact that a heat engine can never be 100% efficient. Some of the heat energy from its fuel will be transferred to colder objects in the surroundings, with the result that it will not be converted into mechanical energy.

The third law of thermodynamics

The third law of thermodynamics is concerned with absolute zero (i.e. −273°C). It simply states that it is impossible to reduce the temperature of any system to absolute zero.

The first and second laws of thermodynamics are well illustrated by the ideal heat engine shown in Figure 1.1. Heat engines are devices, such as internal combustion

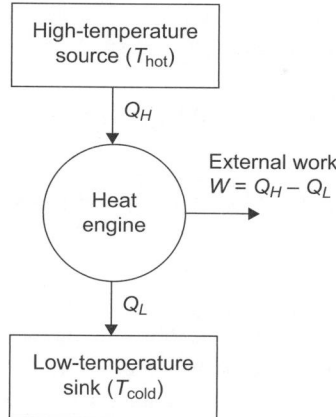

FIG 1.1 Schematic diagram of an ideal heat engine.

engines and gas turbines, which convert thermal energy into mechanical work. They do this by exploiting the temperature gradient between a hot 'source' and a cold 'sink'. As heat flows from the hot 'source' to the cold 'sink' it passes through the 'working' part of the engine where it is converted into mechanical energy.

If it is assumed that no energy is stored, then by applying the first law of thermodynamics it is possible to write down an energy balance for the system:

$$W = Q_H - Q_L \qquad (1.4)$$

where W is the mechanical work produced by the engine (J), Q_H is the heat absorbed from the high-temperature 'source' (J), and Q_L is the heat rejected to the low-temperature 'sink' (J).

Similarly, the efficiency, η, of the heat engine can be expressed thus:

$$\eta = \frac{\text{work output}}{\text{work input}} = \frac{W}{Q_H} = 1 - \frac{Q_L}{Q_H} \qquad (1.5)$$

Because the respective heat flows are proportional to the absolute temperature of the hot 'source' and the cold 'sink', it is possible to express the efficiency of an ideal heat engine as:

$$\eta = 1 - \frac{T_L}{T_H} \qquad (1.6)$$

where T_H is the absolute temperature of the hot 'source' (K), and T_L is the absolute temperature of the cold 'sink' (K).

Given that the second law of thermodynamics dictates that heat must flow from hot to cold, it can be seen from Eqn 1.6 that if no temperature difference exists between the hot 'source' and the cold 'sink', then heat cannot flow and the efficiency of the engine must therefore be zero. Conversely, if a large temperature difference exists between the hot 'source' and the cold 'sink', then the heat flow will be much greater, with the result that the efficiency of the cycle will be high.

1.3.3 Ecology, Society and the Second Law of Thermodynamics

Although often forgotten by policy makers and those involved in the management and conservation of energy, the second law of thermodynamics is of profound importance. Indeed, Albert Einstein stated:

> A theory is the more impressive the greater the simplicity of its premises, the more varied the kinds of things that it relates and the more extended the area of its applicability. Therefore classical thermodynamics has made a deep impression on me. It is the only physical theory of universal content which I am convinced, within the areas of the applicability of its basic concepts, will never be overthrown. [6]

So all-embracing is the second law of thermodynamics that it can be used to explain how the communities and ecosystems on Earth behave when they consume energy [7]. Consider for example, a large, sealed, clear container placed in sunlight, which contains air, water, soil, plants, microorganisms and animals all in carefully controlled proportions. As long as the sun shines, the ecosystem in the vessel will survive with no external maintenance. The biomass inside the container will increase until a steady state is reached in which the ecosystem is stable. If, however, the vessel is removed from the sunlight then the second law of thermodynamics will take over and the biomass will very quickly decompose into a foul-smelling high-entropy mess. Similarly, if pollution and toxins are allowed to build up in the vessel when it is placed in sunlight, the second law of thermodynamics tells us that the entropy (i.e. chaos) in the ecosystem will also increase.

The Earth behaves in much the same way as the sealed vessel described above. It is a sealed ecosystem, with negligible exchange of matter between its surface and space. It is also a balanced system, receiving all its energy from the sun in the form of short-wavelength radiation, which it then re-radiates to space as long-wavelength heat. Over millions of years the Earth has developed a stable ecosystem with a highly ordered low-entropy biomass, sustained wholly by the sun's energy. Solar energy not only heats the Earth, but also drives its atmosphere. Wind, rain, ocean currents and Earth's biomass all arise directly from the action of solar energy striking the Earth's surface.

If environmental pollution is low and only renewable energy sources are used, then the Earth should remain relatively stable, allowing a low-entropy ecosystem to survive and prosper. If, however, fossil fuels, such as petroleum, coal and natural gas, are consumed, then 'concentrated energy' from the sun, laid down in biomass hundreds of thousands of years ago, is suddenly released into the atmosphere. In thermodynamic terms, the energy trapped in fossil fuels is in a highly ordered low-entropy form. When burnt, this highly ordered energy is dispersed into the environment raising its entropy, which is exactly what the second law of thermodynamics predicts. So as more and more non-renewable fossil fuels are consumed the *Second Law* tells us that entropy-related problems, such as pollution and global warming, will inevitably increase.

It is impossible to 'buck' the second law of thermodynamics – entropy will always increase in the end! Even nuclear power, which some think might solve the Earth's energy crisis, conforms to the second law of thermodynamics. While nuclear power offers almost unimaginable amounts of energy from very small masses of uranium, the *Second Law* tells us that once this highly ordered energy is consumed it will inevitably be dispersed into the environment raising its overall entropy. This increase in entropy may, in part, explain why the safe disposal of nuclear waste has proven to be a considerable problem. Perhaps after all there is no such thing as a free lunch!

As well as explaining global behaviour, the second law of thermodynamics can be used to explain the behaviour of the various societies found on Earth. Those of us who live in the developed countries of Europe and North America are used to institutions, utilities and infrastructures that are reliable and function efficiently. By comparison, those in the developing world may be used to infrastructures and institutions that are less robust and more chaotic. In such countries, the infrastructure may be at best patchy and in many places non-existent. This suggests that these countries have higher-entropy societies compared to their more ordered low-entropy counterparts in the developed world. This is self-evident when one considers that the developed economies are amongst the highest consumers of energy on the planet. However, what is perhaps not so clear is the huge amount of energy consumed by these nations in maintaining robust institutions and infrastructures. One only has to observe the level of street lighting in Western Europe to realize that the governments of these countries consider an efficient infrastructure to be something of importance. What is less obvious, but nonetheless true, is the vast amount of energy consumed in schools, hospitals, universities and government organizations, ensuring that the institutions in these countries are run and maintained by healthy, highly educated individuals who are equipped to function in an efficient manner. By comparison, in the developing world much less energy is focused on health, education and the infrastructure, with the result that the economies of these countries are less efficient. In short, it takes huge amounts of focused energy to create a 'low-entropy' first-world society. The implications of this are far reaching. According to the second law of thermodynamics, while it is possible to have 'regions' of low entropy within a system, order can only increase in these zones if it decreases elsewhere within the system. When this is applied to the Earth as a whole, it implies that the low-entropy societies of Europe and North America have become so at the expense of less-developed societies in Africa and Asia – as the developed countries have become more ordered, so the developing nations have become more chaotic! It also implies that it is impossible for all the societies on Earth to acquire very low-entropy characteristics. Indeed, common sense tells us that this is true – as oil reserves dwindle, it will not be possible for every family in Africa and Asia to have two cars, like many in Europe and North America. The uncomfortable truth, according to the *Second Law*, is that entropy in the developing world can only be reduced if it increases in the developed world.

1.4 Energy Consumption and GDP

In the introduction to this chapter it was stated that it is almost impossible to remove politics from any discussion or study of energy. This is because the GDP of any nation is

TABLE 1.1   Historical overview of per capita energy consumption [8]

Period and location	Type of society	Characteristics	Daily per capita energy consumption, kCal (MJ)
Very early	Gatherers	Gathered wild fruit, nuts and vegetables	2000 (8.2)
1,000,000 BC	Hunter-gatherers	Gathered wild fruit, etc., hunted and cooked food	4000 (16.4)
4000 BC (Middle East)	Settled farmers	Sowed crops and kept animals	12,000 (49.2)
1500 AD (Europe)	Agricultural with small-scale industry	Agricultural society with specialized industries producing metal, glass, etc.	21,000 (88.2)
1900 AD (Europe)	Industrialized society	Large-scale industry, mass production and large cities	90,000 (378)
1990 AD (USA, Western Europe)	Advanced industrialized society	Consumer society, mass transport, many labour-saving devices	250,000 (1000)

related to its energy consumption. Perhaps the best way to illustrate this link is to look at energy consumption from a historical viewpoint. Table 1.1 shows the estimated average daily consumption of people in various historical societies.

From Table 1.1 it can be seen that per capita energy consumption has increased (almost exponentially) as societies have become more advanced and industrialized. The first humans were simple gatherers who lived off wild fruit, nuts and vegetables. However, as people began to hunt and live in less-hospitable regions, they learnt to use fire for cooking and heating. As time progressed, societies developed – first came agriculture and then industrial practices, such as the smelting and working of metals and increased trading of goods and materials. With these technological and social advances came increased energy consumption; buildings needed heating, food needed cooking and manufacturing processes required fuel. It is estimated that per capita energy consumption rose from approximately 4000 kilocalories per day, in the age of the hunter-gatherer, to approximately 21,000 kilocalories per day, in Europe prior to the Industrial Revolution [8]. The Industrial Revolution, first in Europe and later in North America, resulted in a rapid increase in per capita energy consumption during the nineteenth century. Populations grew rapidly and became concentrated in large towns and cities. Mass production became commonplace and with it more transportation of goods, raw materials and people. This dramatic increase in energy consumption continued throughout the twentieth century as more and more societies became industrialized, to such an extent that in technologically advanced countries such as the USA, per capita energy consumption has reached approximately 250,000 kilocalories per day [8].

From the above historical review, it is clear that there is a strong link between per capita energy consumption and economic growth. In simple terms, less-developed agrarian societies consume much less energy than their advanced industrial counterparts. Figure 1.2 shows data derived from the IEA Key World Energy Statistics 2006 [9]. These data

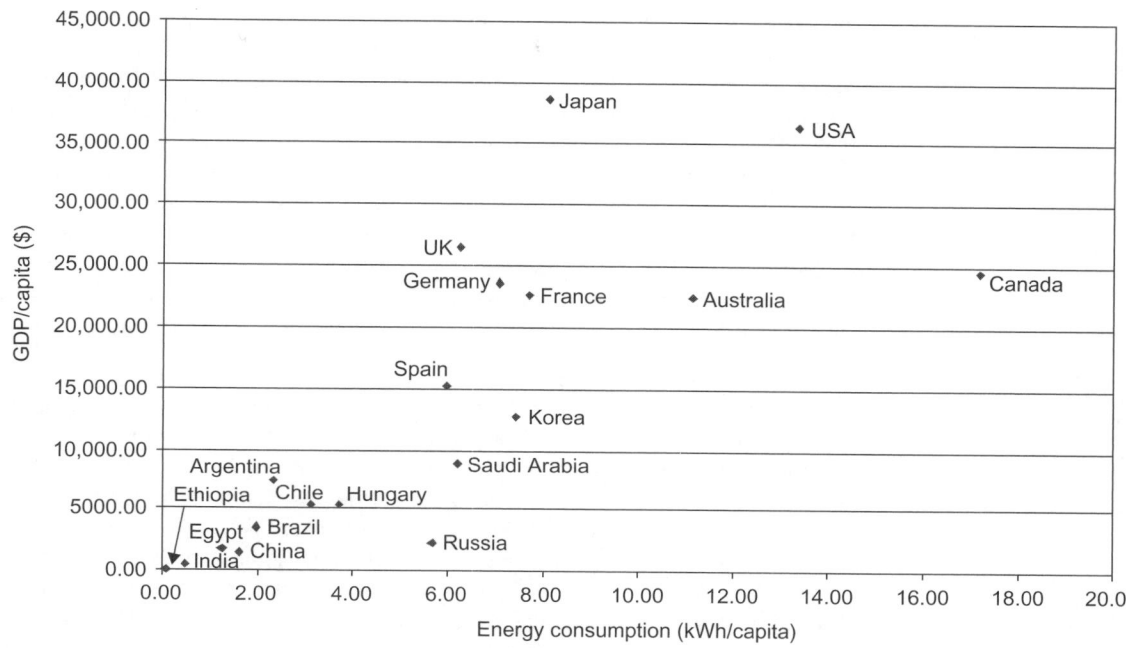

FIG 1.2 Per capita GDP versus energy consumption of various sample nations [9].

illustrate the relationship between per capita GDP and energy consumption for some of the world's nations. Although energy consumption is influenced by factors such as population density, weather and location, it can be seen from Figure 1.2 that for most nations, particularly developing countries, there is still a strong correlation between GDP and energy consumption. Broadly speaking in most societies, energy consumption and economic growth tend to move in parallel. However, comparison between countries can be complicated by geographical factors. For example, larger countries tend to expend higher levels of energy on freight transportation in order to ensure nationwide distribution of goods. Countries with cold climates may consume as much as 20% more energy per capita compared with countries which have moderate climates. Likewise, hot countries may expend 5% more energy per capita due to demand for air conditioning. In addition, due to the high energy intensity associated with processing raw materials, countries which produce large amounts of raw material expend considerably more energy per unit of manufacturing output than those which mainly import processed materials. For example, Canada has a high ratio of energy consumption to GDP, due to the fact that it is a large, cold country with a substantial raw materials processing sector. By comparison, Japan, which has a milder climate, a small land mass, and processes much fewer raw materials, has a lower ratio of energy use to GDP.

Although there has been a strong historical link between GDP and energy consumption, in recent years there has been a decoupling of this relationship in many of the more advanced countries. It has been observed that since the 1970s in these countries, increased GDP has not been accompanied by a pro-rata increase in energy consumption.

Indeed, in the UK and a number of other European countries, energy consumption has plateaued and remained relatively constant in recent years [8]. The reasons for the plateau effect are, in part, due to the adoption of energy-efficient technologies and partly because many older energy-intensive manufacturing industries have been replaced by high-tech and service sector industries, which consume much less energy. However, from a global perspective, it is simplistic to argue that this move towards the service sector is conserving energy, since in reality these countries are effectively exporting their manufacturing and heavy industry requirements to other parts of the world where wage costs are lower. Indeed, there is evidence that many advanced 'consumer' nations are simply exporting their 'dirty' energy-intensive industries to countries in which environmental legislation is much weaker, with the result that in gross terms environmental pollution is increasing.

The ratio of energy used to GDP is known as the *energy intensity* of an economy. It is a measure of the output of an economy compared with its energy inputs, in effect a measure of the efficiency with which energy is used. Manufacturing nations, with old or relatively poor infrastructures, like many of the East European and former Soviet Union (FSU) countries, often exhibit very high *energy intensities*, while the more energy-efficient 'post-industrialized' nations have much lower intensities. The link between infrastructure and *energy intensity* is very strong indeed. In developing countries, development of an infrastructure leads to growth in energy-intensive manufacturing industries. In industrialized economies, *energy intensity* is strongly influenced by the efficiency of the infrastructure and capital stock such as power stations, motor vehicles, manufacturing facilities and end-user appliances. The energy efficiency of capital stock is, in turn, influenced by the price of energy relative to the cost of labour and the cost of borrowing capital. If energy costs are high in relation to these other costs, then it is much more likely that investments will be made in energy-efficient technologies. Conversely, if energy prices are low, then little incentive exists for investment, or indeed research, in more energy-efficient technologies.

While energy intensity is strongly influenced by the price of energy, it is also affected by factors which are not directly attributable to price effects. For example, changes in technology and changes in the composition of world trade can influence energy intensity. Geographical location has a strong influence; cold northerly countries tend to exhibit high energy intensities. Other factors include changes in fashion and preferences. For example, if the practice of cycling to work becomes popular with enough people, then it is possible that this will influence the energy intensity of an economy. In short, there are many factors which influence energy intensity.

1.5 Environmental Issues

A full investigation of the environmental problems facing the Earth, although very interesting, is well beyond the scope of this book. However, because environmental considerations, in particular the perceived threat of global warming, are influential in shaping the energy policy of many countries, it is essential that the issue be discussed in some detail. Indeed, it is the threat of climate change, above any other issue, which is changing the attitudes towards energy consumption. Although there is much scientific debate on the precise nature and extent of the twin threats of global warming and ozone depletion, the fact remains that these threats are generally perceived to be real, with the result that both national and international energy policies are now being driven by an environmental agenda. It is therefore important to have an understanding of pertinent environmental issues. Ignorance of the facts relating to environmental issues is surprisingly widespread amongst politicians, professionals and the public at large. Concepts such as global warming and ozone depletion are often confused and interchanged. Indeed, some individuals committed to environmentally green lifestyles exhibit very woolly thinking when it comes to the science of the environment. This section is, therefore, written with the sole intent of presenting the relevant facts and explaining the pertinent issues relating to global warming and ozone depletion.

1.5.1 Global Warming

There is growing scientific evidence that greenhouse gas emissions caused by human activity are having an effect on the Earth's climate. The evidence suggests that the Earth's climate has warmed by 0.8°C since 1882 [10], and that the pace of this warming is increasing. Globally, the 1990s were the warmest years on record, with seven of the ten warmest years being recorded in that decade [10]. Indeed, in 1998 the global temperature was the highest since 1860 and this was the twentieth consecutive year with an above normal global surface temperature. Figure 1.3 illustrates the steady rise in global temperature that has occurred over the past 125 years.

The effects of the rise in global temperature have been wide ranging and profound. Perhaps the most visible effect of global warming has been the rapid decrease in glaciation experienced over the past 50 years. This phenomenon is well illustrated in Figure 1.4, which shows the change in the Alaskan Muir and Riggs glaciers between 1941 and 2004. The Muir glacier, parts of which were more than 65 m thick in 1941,

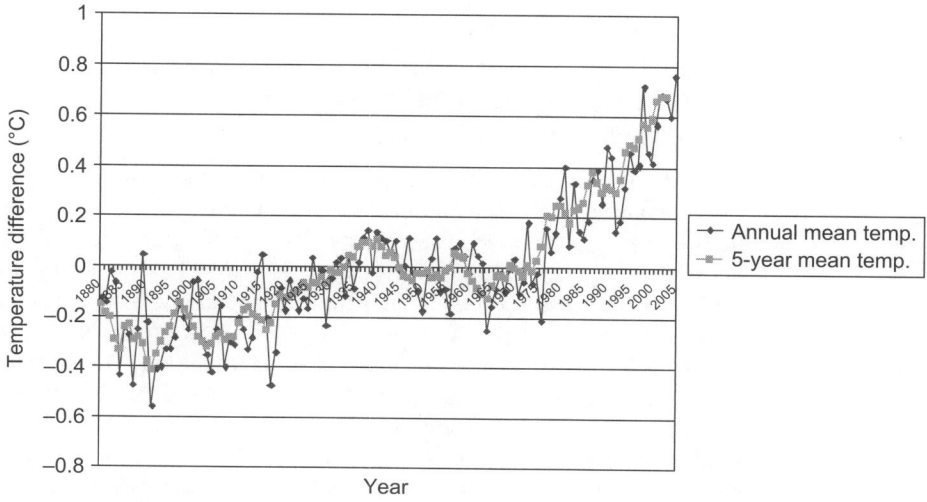

FIG 1.3 Global mean surface air temperature anomaly [10].

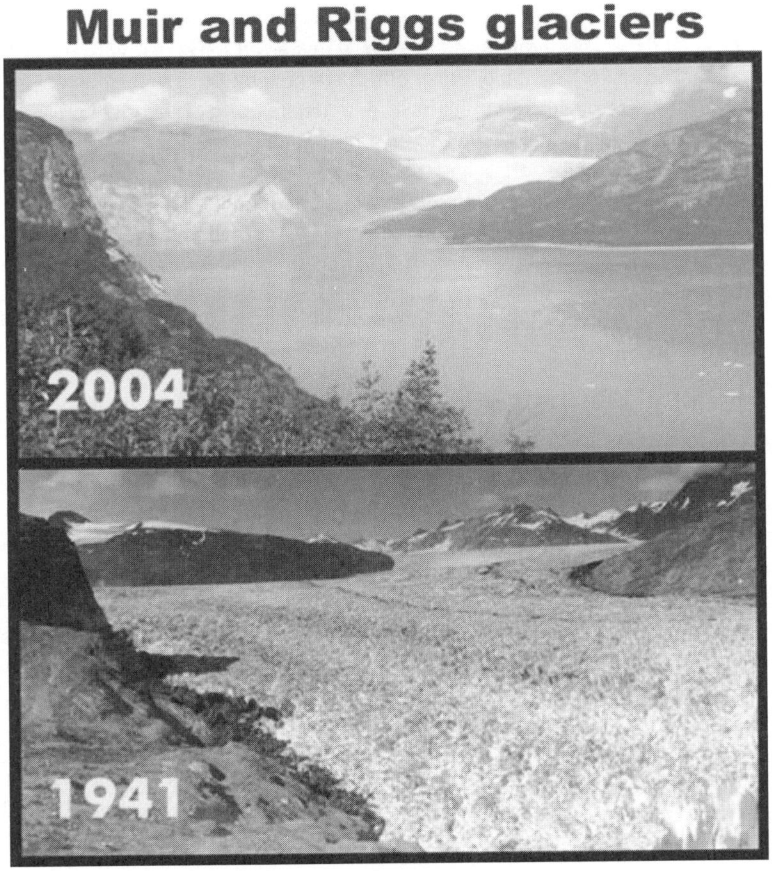

Muir and Riggs glaciers

FIG 1.4 Comparison of Muir and Riggs glaciers (1941 and 2004).

retreated more than 20 km during this period – in the 2004 picture this glacier is out of sight (towards the upper left). Likewise the Riggs glacier, which is still visible (upper right) in the 2004 image, has greatly receded.

It is generally accepted that the rapid rise in global temperature experienced during the latter part of the twentieth century is due, in part, to atmospheric pollution arising from human activity, which is accelerating the Earth's greenhouse effect. The greenhouse effect is a natural phenomenon which is essential for preserving the 'warmth' of the planet. It is caused by trace gases in the upper atmosphere trapping long-wave infrared radiation emitted from the Earth's surface. The Earth's atmosphere allows short-wave solar radiation to pass relatively unimpeded. However, the long-wave radiation produced by the warm surface of the Earth is partially absorbed and then re-emitted downwards by greenhouse gases in the atmosphere. In this way an energy balance is set up, which ensures that the Earth is warmer than it would otherwise be. Without the greenhouse effect it is estimated that the Earth's surface would be approximately 33°C cooler [11], and almost uninhabitable. Although the greenhouse effect is essential to the well-being

TABLE 1.2 Contribution to global warming of various gases

Greenhouse gas	CO_2 equivalent per molecule	Pre-1800 concentration	1990 concentration	Growth rate (%/year)	Atmospheric life (years)
CO_2	1	280 ppmv	353 ppmv	0.50	50–200
Methane	21	0.8 ppmv	1.72 ppmv	0.90	10
CFC-12	7300	0.0 ppmv	484 pptv	4.00	130
CFC-11	3500	0.0 ppmv	280 pptv	4.00	65
Nitrous oxide	290	288 ppbv	310 ppbv	0.25	150

of human populations, if greenhouse gas levels rise above their natural norm, the consequent additional warming could threaten the sustainability of the planet as a whole.

The main naturally occurring greenhouse gases in the Earth's atmosphere are water vapour and CO_2. Of these, it is water vapour which has the greatest greenhouse action. While CO_2 concentrations are strongly influenced by human activity, atmospheric water vapour is almost entirely determined by climatic conditions and not human action. Human activity is responsible for production of a number of other potent greenhouse gases, including methane, nitrous oxide, chlorofluorocarbons (CFCs) and hydrochlorofluorocarbons (HCFCs). From the late eighteenth century onwards, concentrations of 'man-made' greenhouse gases (with the exception of CFCs and HCFCs, which were first introduced in the 1930s) have steadily increased. Table 1.2 shows the pre-industrial and 1990 levels of various greenhouse gases. For each gas it can be seen that there has been a substantial rise in the atmospheric concentration. For example, CO_2 concentrations have grown from 280 ppm in the middle of the eighteenth century to approximately 353 ppm in 1990: a rise of about 26%, leading to a current rate of increase of about 0.5% a year [11]. Indeed, the Intergovernmental Panel on Climate Change (IPCC) forecast that a likely doubling of atmospheric CO_2 will occur by 2050, leading to an average global temperature increase of between 1.5°C and 4.5°C [11,12].

Although CO_2 is the single 'man-made' gas which contributes most towards overall global warming (i.e. in excess of 50%), it is by no means the most potent of the greenhouse gases. Methane, for example, is approximately 21 times as potent as CO_2. In other words, methane has a relative global warming potential (GWP) of 21 compared with that of CO_2, which is 1. Incredibly, CFC-11 has a GWP of approximately 3500 and CFC-12 has a GWP of approximately 7300 [11], making CFCs the most potent of greenhouse gases. CFCs were first introduced in the 1930s and were widely used as refrigerants, solvents and aerosol propellants, until they were withdrawn in the mid-1990s. They are very stable and remain in the upper atmosphere for considerable periods of time, as much as 130 years in the case of CFC-12 [11]. Given that they are also potent ozone depletors, it is not surprising that the control and elimination of CFCs became one of the major environmental targets in the 1990s.

The extent to which global warming is likely to occur as a result of the build-up of greenhouse gases is a matter of much scientific debate. The Hadley Centre of the UK

Meteorological Office predicts that, under the 'business as usual' scenario, the world's climate will warm by about 3°C over the next 100 years [13], which is in keeping with the IPCC's forecast of a 1.5°C–4.5°C rise by 2050 [11]. Although there is general agreement that climate change is the most serious environmental threat facing the world today, the precise nature of this 'climate change' is open to debate. It is predicted that as global warming progresses, sea levels will rise by over 400 mm by 2080 [13] due to the combined effects of thermal expansion of the oceans and melting of polar ice. This will put the lives of millions of people at risk, with an additional 80 million people particularly threatened with flooding in the low lying parts of southern and South-East Asia [13]. It is probable that droughts will occur due to increased temperatures and that Africa, the Middle East and India will all experience significant reductions in cereal crop yields [13]. Increased drought will mean that by 2080 an additional 3 billion people could suffer increased water stress, with Northern Africa, the Middle East and the Indian subcontinent expected to be the worst affected [13]. It is ironic that it will be the poorest countries, often ones which have contributed the least to global warming, which are most likely to be vulnerable to the effects of climate change.

1.5.2 Carbon Intensity of Energy Supply

Carbon intensity is a measure of the amount of CO_2 that is released into the atmosphere for every unit of energy produced. As such it is wholly dependent on the type of fuel used. For example, electricity produced from nuclear power plants produces no CO_2 emissions, whereas that produced from coal-fired power station has a high carbon intensity. Table 1.3 shows the relative carbon intensities for electricity produced from a variety of fuels.

While renewable energy sources such as wind, solar and hydropower emit no CO_2, the carbon content of fossil fuels varies greatly. It can be seen from Table 1.3 that electricity produced in a typical coal-fired power station produces approximately 2.4 times as much CO_2 as that produced by a combined cycle gas turbine (CCGT) plant [14]. Indeed, it has been demonstrated that the carbon intensity of delivered mains electricity is not constant, but varies considerably with time and with the generation plant mix [15]. For example, in England carbon intensity is at its lowest during the night-time in summer, when the bulk of the power is produced from nuclear energy.

TABLE 1.3 CO_2 emissions per kWh of delivered electrical energy [14]

Primary fuel	Kilogram of CO_2 per GJ of primary energy	Average gross efficiency of power plant (%)	Kilogram of CO_2 per GJ of delivered electrical energy	Kilogram of CO_2 per kWh of delivered electrical energy
Coal	90.7	35	259.1	0.93
Oil	69.3	32	216.6	0.78
Gas (CCGT)	49.5	46	107.6	0.39

It is possible to achieve significant reductions in carbon intensity simply by switching from a fuel such as coal, which has a high carbon intensity, to one with a much lower intensity, such as natural gas. This is in fact what happened in the UK during the 1990s when there was a massive switch from coal to natural gas as the fuel of choice for electricity generation.

Because carbon intensity is wholly dependent on the type of fuel used, it differs across regions and also over time. During the 1990s coal became less important as a source of energy in western Europe, with the shutting down of lignite production in Germany and of hard coal production in the UK [16]. For example, in England and Wales the switch from coal to natural gas which accompanied deregulation of the electricity supply industry meant that coal consumption dropped from 65 million tonnes of oil equivalent (mtoe) in 1989 to only 35.6 mtoe in 1999 [2]. This has resulted in a 45% decrease in the UK's carbon intensity from 1980 to 1998. By contrast in the USA during the 1990s the electricity generators continued to use coal extensively and as a result the carbon intensity for western Europe has dropped below that of North America in recent years [16].

1.5.3 Carbon Dioxide Emissions

It has been estimated that global CO_2 emissions will reach approximately 42.9 billion tonnes per annum by 2030 – an increase of 103% on 1990 levels [17]. Amongst the OECD countries of Europe, the increase in CO_2 emissions is predicted to be small (see Figure 1.5) at about 0.3% per year [17]. Similarly, the rate of increase for Japan is predicted to be only 0.1% per year. This reflects the overall maturity of the energy infrastructure in these economies and their willingness to adopt low-energy technologies. By comparison,

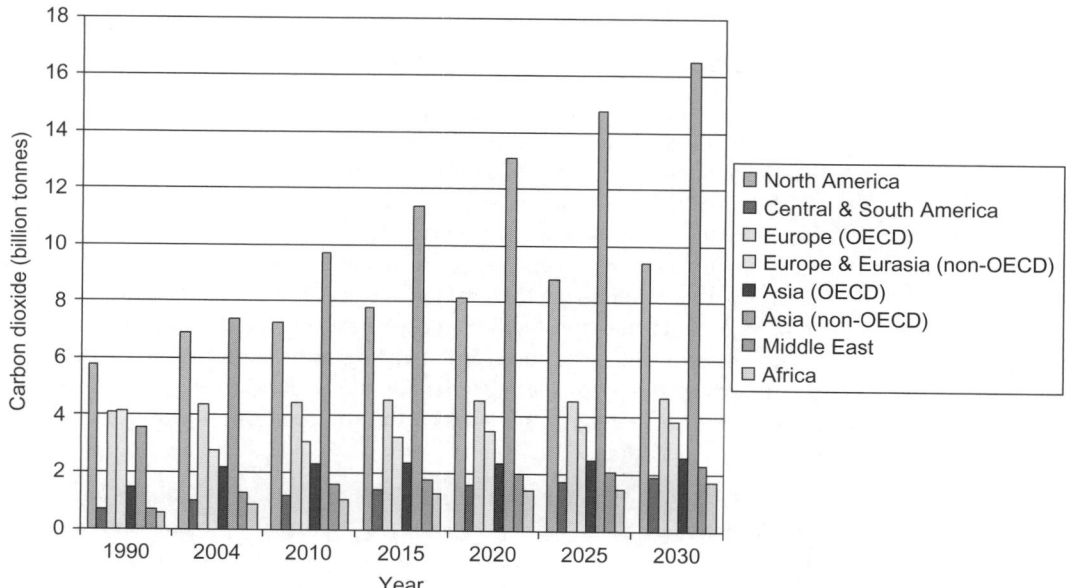

FIG 1.5 Historical and predicted CO_2 emissions by region [17].

growth amongst the OECD nations of North America is likely to be somewhat greater, at 1.2% per annum, due in part to predicted growth in the Mexican economy and a general reluctance to switch to low-carbon technologies. The USA, for example, is expected to remain the largest source of petroleum-related CO_2 emissions, with projected emissions of 3.3 billion tonnes in 2030, 66% above the corresponding projection for China [17]. In comparison to the OECD countries, growth in CO_2 emissions for the non-OECD nations is predicted to be much larger (see Figure 1.5), with the predicted annual rate of increase for the period 2004–2030 being 2.6% [17]. This rapid growth is predicted because of the high growth rate of the non-OECD Asian economies and their heavy dependence on coal. CO_2 emissions for India are predicted to rise at 2.6% per annum, while the growth rate for China is anticipated to be a staggering 3.4% [17].

The implications of the data presented in Figure 1.5 are both profound and far reaching, because they suggest that the greatest room for reducing CO_2 emissions lies not in the OECD countries, but rather in the emerging non-OECD economies. This is an important point, because to date most attention (both in technological and policy terms) has been firmly focused on reducing CO_2 emissions in the developed OECD countries. While there is plenty of room for improvement in North America, the scope for cutting CO_2 emissions in Europe appears to be much more limited and it is debatable whether increased 'green' effort in this region will have much effect on global warming. By comparison, the non-OECD countries have largely been ignored, despite the fact that many of the rapidly industrializing Asian economies pose a much greater threat. Indeed, the situation is compounded by the fact that much of the manufacturing output of countries like China is consumed in the OECD countries. Clearly, therefore, if global CO_2 emissions are to be controlled in any meaningful way, it will be necessary to tackle the rise in emissions in the non-OECD countries.

1.5.4 Depletion of the Ozone Layer

Ozone (O_3) in the Earth's stratosphere performs the vital function of protecting the surface of the planet from ultraviolet (UV) radiation which would otherwise be extremely harmful to human and animal life. The stratosphere is a layer approximately 35 km thick which has its lower limit at an altitude of 8–16 km. Ozone is produced in the stratosphere by the absorption of solar UV radiation by oxygen molecules (O_2) to produce ozone through a series of complex photochemical reactions [18]. The ozone produced absorbs both incoming solar UV radiation and also outgoing terrestrial long-wave radiation. In doing so, the ozone in the stratosphere is converted back to oxygen. The process is, therefore, both continuous and transient, with ozone continually being created and destroyed. The process is dependent on the amount of solar radiation incident on the Earth; consequently, ozone levels in the stratosphere are strongly influenced by factors such as altitude, latitude and season.

In the late 1970s a 'hole' was first discovered in the ozone layer above Antarctica [19]. Observations over a number of decades reveal that each September and October up to 60% of the total ozone above Antarctica is depleted [19]. In addition, progressive thinning of stratospheric ozone in both the northern and the southern hemispheres has been observed, with record low global ozone levels being recorded in 1992 and 1993

[19]. The average ozone loss across the globe has totalled about 5% since the mid-1960s, with the greatest losses occurring each year in the winter and spring [19]. This degradation of the ozone layer has resulted in higher levels of UV radiation reaching the Earth's surface. Increased UV radiation in turn leads to a greater incidence of skin cancer, cataracts and impaired immune systems.

Blame for the recent and rapid deterioration of the ozone layer has been placed on escaping gases such as CFCs and nitrous oxide. Until recently CFCs were widely used in many applications including aerosol propellants, refrigerants, solvents and insulation foam. CFCs, especially CFC-11 and CFC-12, as well as being strong greenhouse gases, are also potent ozone depletors. The lifetime of CFC-11 in the stratosphere is about 65 years, while that for CFC-12 is estimated to be 130 years [11]. In recent years, intergovernmental agreements, particularly the Montreal Protocol (1987), have phased out the production and use of CFCs. However, CFCs are very long lived in the stratosphere and hence any reduction in CFC release will have little effect in the near future. The phasing out of CFCs has caused a greater reliance on HCFCs, in particular HCFC-22, which although much more ozone friendly is still a potent greenhouse gas. Under the Montreal Protocol, HCFC-22 is being phased out and as a result the chemical companies are developing new generations of ozone 'friendly' refrigerants. Ozone depletion has caused many designers of buildings in Europe to question the need for vapour compression refrigeration machines to air condition buildings, with the result that alternative passive ventilation strategies are now being adopted in many new buildings.

1.5.5 Intergovernmental Action

In the 1980s governments around the world became aware of some of the environmental problems associated with atmospheric pollution, and the first, in a series of, intergovernmental summits was held in a concerted effort to combat the perceived problems. In many ways the Montreal Protocol, signed in September 1987, marks a turning point in global environmental policy. The leading industrialized nations signed the Montreal Protocol with the aim of limiting emissions of certain ozone-depleting gases, such as CFCs and halons. The original intention of the Protocol was to reduce consumption of these ozone-degrading gases by 50% below the 1986 level by 1999 [18]. Since its original signing, the Protocol has been reviewed regularly and such has been the concern about ozone depletion that the Protocol was expanded to cover HCFCs (i.e. HCFC-141b, HCFC-142b and HCFC-22) and the phase-out schedule was also accelerated. In 1992, the parties to the Protocol agreed to accelerate the 100% phase out of CFCs, carbon tetrachloride and methyl chloroform to the end of 1995 and halons to the end of 1993 [20]. The parties to the Protocol also agreed to phase out HCFCs so that a 90% reduction in production would be achieved by 2010 and a complete phase out by 2030 [21].

Having made a concerted effort to tackle the problem of ozone depletion, the world's leading industrialized nations then turned their attention to the problem of global warming. Through a series of summits, notably Rio in 1992 and Kyoto in 1997, the nations formulated an international framework for reducing global CO_2 and other greenhouse gas emissions. At the Kyoto conference in December 1997, attended by 160 countries, the so-called 'Annex I' countries (which included the USA, Canada, the

European Union [EU] countries, Japan, Australia and New Zealand) agreed to reduce their emissions of six greenhouse gases (i.e. CO_2, nitrous oxide, methane, hydrofluoro-carbon gases [HFCs], perfluorocarbons [PFCs] and sulphur hexafluoride) by at least 5% compared with 1990 levels between 2008 and 2012 [22]. However, the EU aims to reduce its emissions of the main six greenhouse gases (from 1990 levels) by 8% by 2012 [23,24]. In order to meet this target, the EU member states have taken various steps, including tightening building regulations and the introduction of carbon taxes.

1.5.6 Carbon Credits and Taxes

In order to meet their obligations under the Kyoto agreement a number of countries, notably The Netherlands, Sweden, Finland, Norway, Denmark and the UK have intro-duced 'carbon taxes'. These taxes are designed to penalize high carbon intensity energy consumption and promote the use of renewable energy sources. For example, the UK introduced its Climate Change Levy in 2001 with the express intention of increas-ing the share of its electricity generated by renewables from 2% to 10% by 2010. Nevertheless, many economists are sceptical about the use of carbon taxes, preferring instead a system of tradable emission permits. Under the Kyoto Protocol, flexibility was introduced into the agreement through 'Kyoto mechanisms' which allow countries to partake in emissions trading. It is argued that tradable permits are superior to carbon taxes, because unlike carbon taxes, they are a form of rationing which should ensure that targets are achieved. Permits are also more applicable to the international nature of the problem, since a regime of international carbon taxes would be extremely difficult to enforce.

The concept of trading in greenhouse gas emissions may seem very strange to many, so perhaps an analogy would be helpful at this point. Consider the case of a home-owner who wakes up one morning to find that a pipe has burst and that a flood has occurred. Imagine also that this particular homeowner runs a profitable law firm and is also very good at mending burst pipes. The homeowner is, therefore, faced with a dilemma. He can take a day off work to mend the pipe, or alternatively, he can employ a professional plumber to repair the damaged pipe. If the homeowner repairs the pipe, then a day's fees will be lost; it is a much cheaper option to employ a plumber. Realizing this, the homeowner opts for the financially expedient solution and employs the plumber. As a result both parties benefit from the transaction; the plumber gets paid a fee and the lawyer is able to earn more money in court. This analogy is very similar to trading greenhouse gas emission permits, insomuch as those parties buying emission *permits* or *credits* are actually paying someone else to reduce greenhouse gas emissions who can do it more cheaply than they can themselves. However, in order for a trading scheme to work there must be something forcing the participants to make emission reductions, in much the same way that the homeowner was forced to act because the burst pipe would have created a considerable amount of damage if left unattended. Therefore, at the heart of any trading scheme there must be an obliga-tion on the part of the participants to achieve greenhouse gas emission reductions; the obligations under the Kyoto Protocol are forcing countries to reduce greenhouse gas emissions. However, it does not matter geographically where these reductions are made. It is, therefore, possible for participating companies to trade all or part of their obligation without any detrimental environmental effects. This can be achieved by issuing permits which allow the holder to emit a given quantity of greenhouse gas.

One possible advantage of tradable emission permits is that they can be rationed. Permits could be issued which would give the parties involved in the scheme the right to emit at their 1990 emissions levels for free. If every year a proportion of permits were to be withdrawn and then sold either by direct sale or by auction, incentives would be created for the participants in the scheme to reduce emissions. Also, if permits were tradable and banking was to be permitted then a market would be created. However, it is essential that a single, central authority be created which could control the system and fine parties who exceeded their quotas.

1.6 Energy Consumption

Global energy consumption has steadily increased over the past 40 years from 3826.6 mtoe in 1965 to 10,878.5 mtoe in 2006 [2]. This is graphically illustrated in Figure 1.6, which shows the breakdown of global energy consumption, by fuel type. From these data it can be seen that although growth was relatively steady over the period 1965–2000, there was a significant increase (i.e. 1315.3 mtoe) in consumption from 2000 to 2005. In addition, it can be seen that over the period 1965–2005, growth occurred for all fuel types, with none declining in popularity.

While global energy consumption has steadily increased in recent years, in regional terms this growth has been somewhat uneven. From Figure 1.7 it can be seen that energy consumption in North America has increased by only a modest amount in recent years, while that in Europe has actually fallen. By comparison, energy consumption in Asia has rocketed with the industrialization of China and India, so that now that region consumes more energy than either Europe or North America [2].

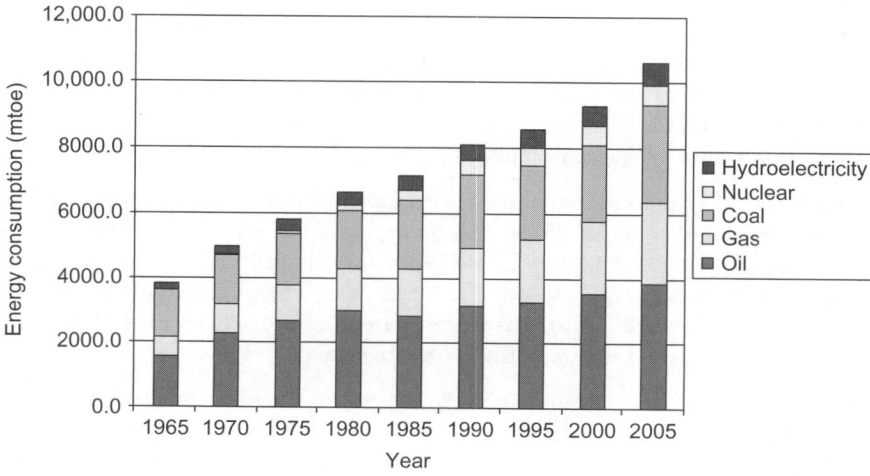

FIG 1.6 Global energy consumption by fuel type (1965–2005) [2].

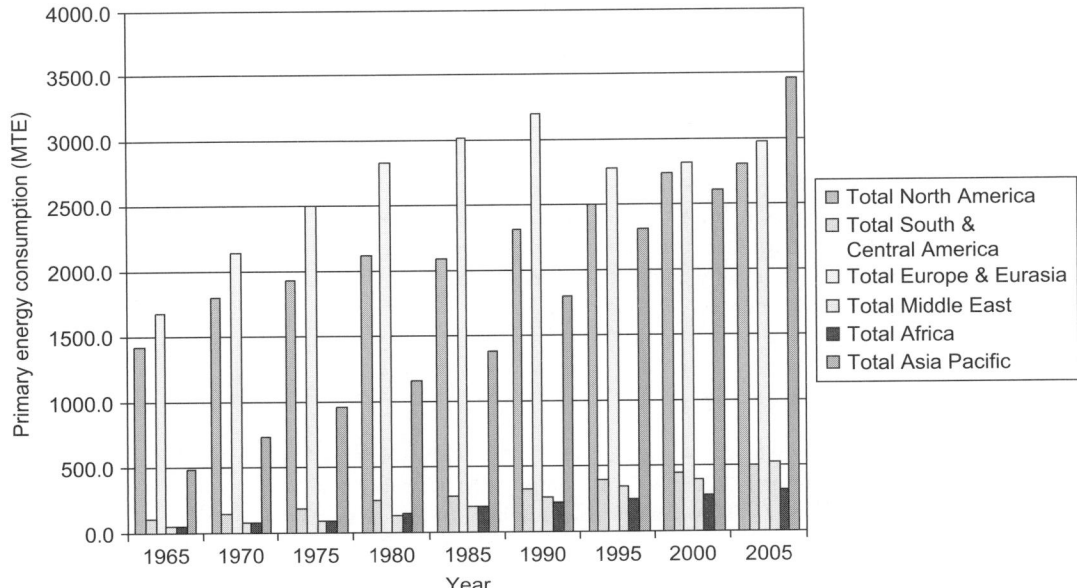

FIG 1.7 Primary energy consumption by region (1965–2005) [2].

Global energy consumption data for 2006 is presented in Table 1.4. These data give a detailed breakdown of energy consumption on a country-by-country and fuel-by-fuel basis. It can be seen from Table 1.4 that in 2006 global energy consumption was approximately 10,879 mtoe. Of this total, only 51.1% is consumed in the OECD countries, with 21.4% consumed in the USA and 15.8% in the EU. While this means that over half the world's energy is still consumed in the OECD countries, it represents a significant shift from the position in 1999, where 59.1% was consumed by the OECD economies [2]. This reduction reflects the rapid industrialization that has occurred in China and India in recent years – a process that has been driven, in part, by the outsourcing of manufacturing capacity to these countries by many corporate organizations in Europe, Japan and North America. In 2006 China and India accounted for 15.6% and 3.9% respectively of global consumption.

From Table 1.4 it can be seen that the fuel mix and hence the carbon intensity varies greatly from region to region. In the USA, for example, the ratio of coal to natural gas consumption is 1.00:1.00, whereas in the UK the ratio is 1.00:1.87, while in China the ratio is only 1.00:0.04 and in India it is 1.00:0.15. These figures reflect, firstly, the shift away from coal towards natural gas that occurred in the UK during the 1990s and, secondly, the heavy reliance on coal in China and India.

The Energy Information Administration (EIA) in the USA predicts that in the twenty-first century there will be substantial increases in energy demand, based mostly on fossil fuels [16]. This is expected to occur mainly because of economic growth in the developing economies of Asia and South America. In developing countries, energy and

TABLE 1.4 Global primary energy consumption by fuel type for 2006 (compiled from BP energy data) [2]

Country	Oil (mtoe)	Natural gas (mtoe)	Coal (mtoe)	Nuclear energy (mtoe)	Hydroelectric (mtoe)	Total consumption (mtoe)	Percentage of total (%)
USA	938.8	566.9	567.3	187.5	65.9	2326.4	21.39
Canada	98.8	87.0	35.0	22.3	79.3	322.3	2.96
Mexico	86.9	48.7	9.3	2.5	6.8	154.2	1.42
Total North America	1124.6	702.5	611.6	212.3	152.0	2803.0	25.77
Argentina	21.1	37.6	0.9	1.7	9.7	71.0	0.65
Brazil	92.1	19.0	13.1	3.1	79.2	206.5	1.90
Chile	11.4	6.8	3.0	–	6.7	27.9	0.26
Colombia	10.3	6.6	2.4	–	9.6	28.9	0.27
Ecuador	8.1	0.2	–	–	1.9	10.3	0.09
Peru	7.5	1.6	0.9	–	4.1	14.1	0.13
Venezuela	26.1	25.8	*	–	18.4	70.4	0.65
Other South & Central America	59.8	19.9	1.5	–	18.3	99.5	0.91
Total South & Central America	236.5	117.5	21.8	4.9	147.9	528.6	4.86
Austria	14.2	8.5	3.0	–	8.1	33.7	0.31
Azerbaijan	4.7	8.6	*	–	0.6	13.9	0.13
Belarus	8.0	17.6	0.1	–	*	25.7	0.24
Belgium & Luxembourg	41.0	15.3	6.1	11.0	0.6	73.9	0.68
Bulgaria	5.0	2.7	7.4	4.4	0.8	20.3	0.19
Czech Republic	9.8	7.6	19.4	5.9	0.7	43.5	0.40
Denmark	9.5	4.6	5.5	–	*	19.6	0.18
Finland	10.6	3.8	5.2	5.4	2.6	27.6	0.25
France	92.8	40.6	13.1	102.1	13.9	262.6	2.41
Germany	123.5	78.5	82.4	37.9	6.3	328.5	3.02
Greece	22.1	2.9	8.8	–	1.4	35.2	0.32
Hungary	7.4	11.3	2.9	3.0	*	24.7	0.23
Iceland	1.0	–	0.1	–	1.6	2.7	0.02
Republic of Ireland	9.3	4.0	1.8	–	0.2	15.4	0.14
Italy	85.7	69.4	17.4	–	9.7	182.2	1.67

Continued

TABLE 1.4 (Continued)

Country	Oil (mtoe)	Natural gas (mtoe)	Coal (mtoe)	Nuclear energy (mtoe)	Hydroelectric (mtoe)	Total consumption (mtoe)	Percentage of total (%)
Kazakhstan	10.6	18.2	29.7	–	1.8	60.3	0.55
Lithuania	2.8	2.9	0.2	2.0	0.2	8.0	0.07
Netherlands	49.6	34.5	7.5	0.8	*	92.3	0.85
Norway	10.0	4.0	0.4	–	27.1	41.5	0.38
Poland	23.1	12.3	58.4	–	0.7	94.5	0.87
Portugal	16.8	3.7	3.7	–	2.7	26.7	0.25
Romania	10.5	15.3	7.6	1.3	4.2	38.8	0.36
Russian Federation	128.5	388.9	112.5	35.4	39.6	704.9	6.48
Slovakia	3.9	5.0	3.8	4.1	1.0	17.8	0.16
Spain	78.1	30.0	18.3	13.6	5.7	145.8	1.34
Sweden	14.9	0.8	2.2	15.4	14.0	47.3	0.43
Switzerland	12.6	2.7	0.1	6.3	7.4	29.0	0.27
Turkey	28.5	27.4	28.8	–	9.9	94.7	0.87
Turkmenistan	5.2	17.0	–	–	–	22.3	0.20
Ukraine	15.0	59.8	39.6	20.4	2.9	137.8	1.27
United Kingdom	82.2	81.7	43.8	17.0	1.9	226.6	2.08
Uzbekistan	6.9	38.9	1.1	–	1.6	48.5	0.45
Other Europe & Eurasia	26.5	13.2	22.0	1.9	17.2	80.8	0.74
Total Europe & Eurasia	970.1	1031.7	552.9	287.8	184.6	3027.2	27.83
Iran	79.3	94.6	1.1	–	3.8	178.8	1.64
Kuwait	14.0	11.6	–	–	–	25.6	0.24
Qatar	4.4	17.6	–	–	–	21.9	0.20
Saudi Arabia	92.6	66.3	–	–	–	158.9	1.46
United Arab Emirates	19.7	37.5	–	–	–	57.2	0.53
Other Middle East	70.2	32.7	7.8	–	1.1	111.8	1.03
Total Middle East	280.1	260.3	8.9	–	4.9	554.2	5.09
Algeria	11.5	21.4	0.6	–	*	33.5	0.31

Continued

TABLE 1.4   (Continued)

Country	Oil (mtoe)	Natural gas (mtoe)	Coal (mtoe)	Nuclear energy (mtoe)	Hydroelectric (mtoe)	Total consumption (mtoe)	Percentage of total (%)
Egypt	29.1	25.8	1.0	–	2.9	58.8	0.54
South Africa	23.2	–	93.8	2.4	0.8	120.2	1.11
Other Africa	66.7	21.0	7.5	–	16.4	111.5	1.03
Total Africa	130.5	68.2	102.8	2.4	20.2	324.1	2.98
Australia	40.3	25.8	51.1	–	3.6	120.8	1.11
Bangladesh	4.1	13.7	0.4	–	0.3	18.5	0.17
China	349.8	50.0	1191.3	12.3	94.3	1697.8	15.61
China Hong Kong SAR	13.2	2.2	7.5	–	–	22.9	0.21
India	120.3	35.8	237.7	4.0	25.4	423.2	3.89
Indonesia	48.7	35.6	27.7	–	2.3	114.3	1.05
Japan	235.0	76.1	119.1	68.6	21.5	520.3	4.78
Malaysia	23.0	36.2	6.3	–	1.6	67.0	0.62
New Zealand	7.2	3.3	2.2	–	5.2	18.0	0.17
Pakistan	18.4	27.6	4.0	0.6	7.4	58.0	0.53
Philippines	14.4	2.3	6.5	–	1.9	25.2	0.23
Singapore	44.0	5.9	–	–	–	50.0	0.46
South Korea	105.3	30.8	54.8	33.7	1.2	225.8	2.08
Taiwan	52.5	10.7	39.5	9.0	1.8	113.6	1.04
Thailand	44.3	27.5	12.4	–	1.8	86.1	0.79
Other Asia Pacific	27.3	10.9	31.6	–	10.2	80.0	0.74
Total Asia Pacific	1148.0	394.7	1792.1	128.2	178.6	3641.5	33.47
Total world	3889.8	2574.9	3090.1	635.5	688.1	10,878.5	100.00

In this table, primary energy comprises commercially traded fuels only.
*Less than 0.05.

economic growth tend to move in parallel. Economic development is an energy-intensive process which ultimately raises living standards and facilitates broad access to electricity and motorized transportation. Economic development of the infrastructure also causes growth in energy-intensive manufacturing industries. In contrast to the developing countries, in advanced industrialized countries the link between economic growth and energy consumption is relatively weak, with energy demand growth lagging behind economic growth. In advanced economies per capita energy use tends to be relatively stable, with old energy-intensive appliances and equipment often being replaced by newer more energy-efficient equipment. Consequently it is predicted that the percentage growth in energy demand will be considerably lower in the developed countries compared with the developing countries.

It is predicted by the EIA that the trend towards the increased use of natural gas in the 1990s will continue in the twenty-first century [16]. This is because natural gas is increasingly perceived as the fuel of choice for electricity generation: it has a much lower carbon intensity than coal; the electricity generation process is more efficient; it is free from the industrial disputes which are often associated with coal production; and it is much cheaper and quicker to construct gas-fired power plants. Oil demand is predicted to grow with the increased use of motorized transport in developing countries.

1.7 Energy Reserves

One of the major concerns of environmentalists and economists alike is the rate at which 'precious' fossil fuel reserves are being expended. It has been estimated that crude oil could remain plentiful and cheap for at least 40 years [25]. However, this prediction assumes that production volumes remain constant, and that production rates can be maintained as reserves decline – an assumption that appears optimistic given that demand for oil is increasing with economic growth in the developing world. It has been predicted that world demand for petroleum will grow from 83 million barrels oil equivalent per day in 2004 to 118 million in 2030 [17], with much of the overall increase projected for the nations of non-OECD Asia. Indeed, the unprecedented rise in the price of oil that occurred in 2008 [26] suggests that increased demand is already making the era of cheap oil a thing of the past.

Even if oil remains plentiful until the middle of the twenty-first century, geophysical surveys indicate that massive new oil deposits are unlikely to be found [25]. In future new oil finds are likely to be much smaller than those already discovered and the cost of extracting the oil much higher. In other words, the law of diminishing returns is likely

TABLE 1.5   Proven energy reserves by fuel type for 2006 (compiled from BP energy data) [2]

Proved reserves at the end of 2006	Oil		Natural Gas		Coal	
	Thousand million barrels	Share of total (%)	Trillion cubic metres	Share of total (%)	Million tonnes	Share of total (%)
Total North America	59.9	5.0	7.98	4.4	254,432	28.0
Total South & Central America	103.5	8.6	6.88	3.8	19,893	2.2
Total Europe & Eurasia	144.4	12.0	64.13	35.3	287,095	31.6
Total Middle East	742.7	61.5	73.47	40.5	419	>0.05
Total Africa	117.2	9.7	14.18	7.8	50,336	5.6
Total Asia Pacific	40.5	3.4	14.82	8.2	296,889	32.7
Total world	1208.2	100.0	181.46	100.0	909,064	100.0

to apply. Although this should mean that oil will continue to be extracted from the earth for many years to come [27], its market price is likely to be much greater than that experienced throughout much of the twentieth century. Consequently, there should be a trend towards the use of more energy-efficient technologies and alternative sources of fuel for motorized transportation.

Although there is considerable debate about the global oil reserves, it is generally agreed that conventional oil production outside the Middle East will start to decline before that in the Middle East, implying a greater reliance on Middle Eastern oil [2]. Table 1.5 shows global proven energy reserves at the end of 2006. From these data it can be seen that approximately 62% of proven oil reserves are located in the Middle East. It is, therefore, not surprising that as existing supplies become depleted the rest of the world will become reliant on Middle Eastern oil suppliers.

It is likely that as global oil stocks become depleted, natural gas will replace oil, since gas can be converted into liquid fuels which can be used for automotive purposes at relatively low cost. Indeed, the EIA predict that natural gas would be the fastest-growing primary energy source between 1996 and 2020 [16].

References

[1] Clark WW, Lund H. Civic markets: the case of the California energy crisis. Int J Global Energy Issues 2001;16(4):328–44.
[2] BP: BP Statistical Review of World Energy, June; 2007.
[3] DTI: Digest of United Kingdom Energy Statistics; 2000.
[4] Ponting C. A green history of the world: the environment and the collapse of great civilizations: Penguin; 1993. New York.
[5] Heinberg R. The party's over: oil, war and the fate of industrial societies. Clairview Books; Forest Row, East Sussex; 2005.
[6] Einstein A; 1949. Autobiographical Notes. In: P. A. Schlipp (Ed). Albert Einstein: Philosopher and Scientist; New York: The Library of Living Philosophers.
[7] Schneider ED, Kay JJ. Life as a manifestation of the Second Law of Thermodynamics. Math Comput Model 1994;19:25–48.
[8] Hill R, O'Keefe P, Snape C. The future of energy use: Earthscan; 1995. London.
[9] IEA. Key world energy statistics 2006. Paris: International Energy Agency; 2006.
[10] GISS. Global annual mean surface air temperature change. New York: Goddard Institute for Space Studies; 2008.
[11] WMO/UNP. Climate change: The IPCC scientific assessment. In: WMO/UNP Intergovernmental panel on climate change; 1990.
[12] May R. Global warming needs action. Energ Explor Exploit 1998;16(1):93–102.
[13] Climate Change. Action to tackle global warming: Department of the Environment; 2000. London. HMSO.
[14] Shorrock LD, Henderson G. Energy use in buildings and carbon dioxide emissions: Building Research Establishment; 1990. Watford, UK.
[15] Beggs CB. A method for estimating the time-of-day carbon dioxide emissions per kWh of delivered electrical energy in England and Wales. Building Serv Eng Res Technol 1996;17(3):127–34.
[16] DOE/EIA. International Energy Outlook 1999: environmental issues and world energy use; 1999.
[17] DOE/EIA. International Energy Outlook 2007.
[18] Harrison RM. Pollution: causes, effects and control: Royal Society of Chemistry; 1990. Cambridge, UK.

[19] Environmental indicators: ozone depletion. USEP; 1996.

[20] The accelerated phase out of class I ozone-depleting substances. USEP; 1999.

[21] HCFC phase out schedule. USEP; 1998.

[22] OECD. Energy in the 21st-century: the return of geopolitics?; 1999.

[23] Greenhouse gases and climate change – Environment in EU at the turn of the century; 2001.

[24] Svendsen GT. Towards a CO_2 market in the EU: the case of electric utilities. Eur Environ 1998;8(4):121–28.

[25] Campbell CJ, Laherrère JH, George RL, Anderson RN, Fouda SA. Preventing the next oil crunch. Sci Am 1998;278(3):59–77.

[26] BBC. Oil price soars as US woes mount; 2008.

[27] Allwright A. Simplistic predictions of looming oil drought are wide of the mark. Irish Times 31st May 2008.

CHAPTER 2

Utility Companies and Energy Supply

Energy costs are strongly influenced by the policies of utility companies and fuel suppliers. It is therefore important to have a good understanding of the supply side of the energy industry. This chapter explains the fundamental issues associated with the supply of fuel and energy, and explains how utility companies recover their costs.

2.1 Introduction

This chapter is not intended to be a text on the chemical properties of various fuels, or indeed a work on the geographical aspects of energy supply, rather it is written from the point of view of the end-user, who may also be the energy purchaser. The aim of this chapter is to explain the ways in which utility companies operate and also to highlight key issues which influence the supply of fuel and energy.

When investigating the subject of energy supply it is necessary to understand the process by which energy is delivered to the consumer. In general terms, most facilities consume one or more of the following 'fuels':

- Coal
- Oil

- Natural gas
- Electricity

Natural gas and electricity are delivered to consumers by utility companies via extensive pipe and cable infrastructures. By contrast, coal and oil are purchased on the open market and require vehicular delivery and storage facilities. Each 'fuel' therefore has its own set of peculiarities and limitations, and these strongly influence both usage and energy costs. Some fuels, such as natural gas, are unavailable in many locations because nearby pipelines do not exist. Other fuels, such as coal and oil, are perceived as dirty and difficult to handle, and also require considerable storage space. Since all these factors influence energy costs, it is important to be familiar with the costs associated with each type of fuel. Fuel and energy costs can be categorized as:

- Direct costs associated with the purchase of the 'fuel';
- Indirect costs associated with the use of the 'fuel'; and
- Indirect environmental costs.

Direct fuel costs are those costs specifically associated with the purchase of the fuel, such as unit energy charges and standing charges, and indirect costs are those costs associated with the storage and handling of fuels such as coal and oil. Indirect environmental costs also exist, but the end-user does not always perceive their existence. Environmental costs can take an obvious form, such as an environmental tax on fossil fuel consumption (see Chapter 1). However, it is more often the case that environmental costs are absorbed and disguised within other costs. For example, if an electricity company is required to invest in expensive desulphurization equipment to clean up its generating plant, it will probably pass this environmental related cost on to its customers in the form of higher energy prices.

2.2 Primary Energy

Three fuels – oil, coal and natural gas – dominate the world's primary energy market. In 1999, 40.6% of the world's primary energy came from oil, 25.0% from coal, 24.2% from natural gas, 2.7% from hydroelectricity and 7.6% from nuclear power [1]. Although oil is currently the principal source of the world's energy, consumption is outstripping supply and known oil reserves are dwindling. It has been estimated that at current rates of consumption, cheap available oil supplies will be exhausted in approximately 40 years' time [2]. However, unlike oil, the Earth's coal reserves are in a much healthier state, with worldwide reserves of anthracite and bituminous coal alone exceeding 200 times annual coal consumption [1]. One might therefore assume that coal could fill the 'vacuum' which will be created as oil reserves diminish. This, however, is a simplistic assumption, since oil is primarily used in the transport sector and coal, unless synthesized, is unsuitable for this purpose. Also, coal is perceived as being environmentally unfriendly, producing large quantities of carbon dioxide (CO_2) and sulphur dioxide (SO_2) when burnt. By contrast, natural gas is clean when burnt and is relatively easy to handle. Consequently, worldwide natural gas consumption is increasing. For example, in the UK, natural gas consumption rose from 52.4 billion cubic metres in 1990 to 92.0 billion cubic metres in 1999 [1]. The expansion in the natural gas sector in the UK was mainly due to the construction of a large number of new combined cycle gas turbine power stations in the 1990s. The rise in the UK's gas consumption was matched by a steep decline in its coal consumption, which was only 35.6 mtoe in 1999, compared with 64.9 mtoe in 1990 [1]. This scenario has been matched elsewhere in Europe. In France, for example, coal production fell by 59.0% from 1990 to 1999 [1] and in Germany the corresponding fall was 51.3% [1].

In terms of global energy consumption, natural gas is the fastest growing primary fuel. This is primarily because natural gas reserves are large and the cost of production is relatively low. In the former Soviet Union (FSU) countries alone, proven gas reserves are 56.7 trillion cubic metres (1999 data), enough to supply their own, together with the whole of Europe's, requirements for at least 50 years [1]. One important attribute of natural gas is that it is very clean compared with more carbon-intensive fuels such as oil and coal. Following the 1997 Kyoto agreement many nations have sought to reduce the CO_2 emissions by increased utilization of natural gas. It is also a more manageable fuel than coal, which has to be mined and involves expensive handling. Consequently, in many parts of the world, electricity companies are turning away from coal and switching to natural gas. One added bonus to the generating companies is that gas-fired power stations are not prone to industrial action by miners, as coal-fired stations are.

2.3 Delivered Energy

It is important to appreciate the difference between primary energy and delivered energy. For example, natural gas is a primary fuel which can be burnt in a power station to produce electricity (i.e. a 'secondary' fuel) or instead piped straight to the consumer as a primary fuel. By contrast, electricity is always a 'secondary' fuel, which is produced from a primary source, often by a very inefficient conversion process. Therefore for every unit (i.e. kWh) of electricity which is delivered to a property, several units of primary energy must be consumed.

The price paid by the consumer for energy usually reflects closely the cost of its production and its general availability. Consider the case of electricity produced from natural gas in a combined cycle power station, with thermal efficiency of 47%. It is not difficult to see that the cost to the utility company of producing the electricity must be over twice the cost of the natural gas. Indeed, when all the other maintenance, transportation and management costs are factored in, then the cost of the delivered electricity will be much higher. In fact, in the UK the unit price of electricity is generally three to five times the price of natural gas, depending on the type of consumer.

2.4 Electricity Supply

Consider the generic model of an electricity supply network shown in Figure 2.1. The saleable commodity, electricity, is generated in power stations, from a variety of primary energy sources. These power stations are all connected to a high voltage transmission grid, which is used to transmit the electricity over long distances. At various points in the system, electricity is drawn from the transmission grid and distributed to

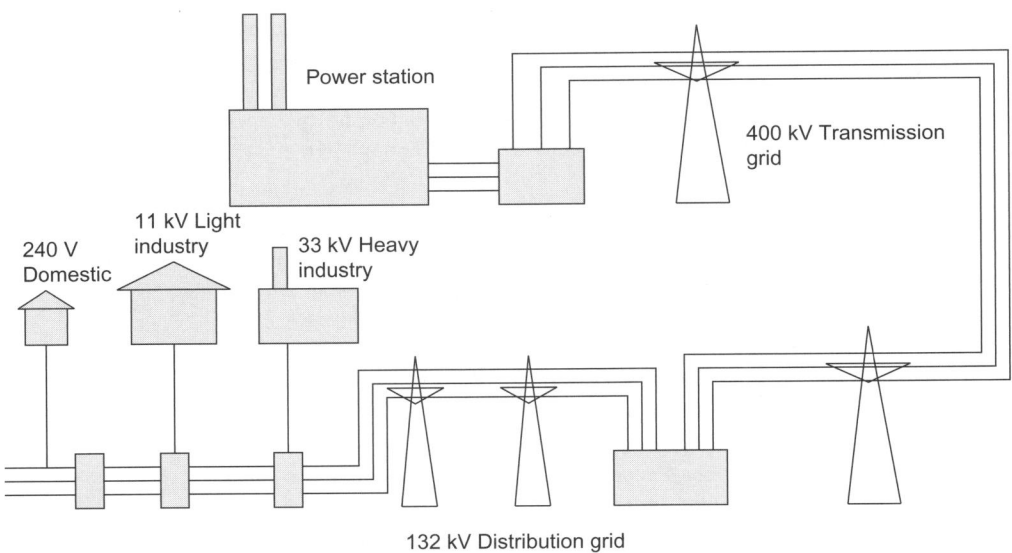

FIG 2.1 A generic electricity supply network.

consumers. This involves the use of a local distribution network which distributes the electricity at a reduced voltage, say 33 kV or 11 kV, to local substations, where the voltage is further reduced, say 415 V, before being supplied to the consumer. Finally, the electricity is sold to consumers and the amount consumed recorded using meters.

In broad terms, the various component parts of an electric supply industry can be categorized as follows:

(i) *The generation process*: This takes place in the power stations and involves the conversion of primary energy from fossil fuels into electricity. It is at the generating stage that all the pollution associated with electricity production is created. Electricity generation is a complex and costly business, which involves the construction, operation and maintenance of large power stations and the purchase, transportation and storage of primary fuels. Because electricity cannot be stored easily, it is necessary for the generating companies to have enough spare capacity to cope with the high peaks in demand which occur at certain times of the year. Therefore, many smaller and less-efficient power stations are rarely used and only operate when demand on the transmission grid is high. This situation is very uneconomic because even though these power stations are infrequently used, they still need to be maintained. Consequently, the generating companies have to recover the cost of maintaining inactive power stations from the electricity produced by the active ones.

(ii) *The transmission process*: This is the process whereby electricity is transported through a transmission grid over long distances around a region or country. The transmission grid is operated at a very high voltage, for example, 400 kV, in order to minimize the energy wastage. Operating a transmission grid involves the

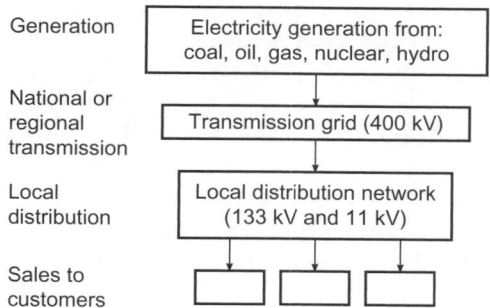

FIG 2.2 Typical structure of an electricity supply network.

construction and maintenance of a very large piece of infrastructure, which may extend for thousands of miles, sometimes over very inhospitable terrain. Naturally large costs are involved in operating such a network and these must be recovered from the sale of any electricity which is transmitted through the grid.

(iii) *The distribution process*: Once electricity has been transmitted over a long distance at high voltage, it must then be distributed to the various end-users. At various points along the transmission grid electricity will be 'siphoned' off into local distribution networks. These distribution networks are regional grids, operating at a lower voltage (e.g. 132 kV and 33 kV), which distribute the electricity around a city or a particular locality. During the distribution process the voltage of the electricity is stepped down (through the use of substations) to the voltage required by the consumers (e.g. 240V, 415V or 11 kV). As with the transmission grid, the costs involved in maintaining and operating a distribution network must be recouped from the revenue received from the electricity sold.

(iv) *The sales process*: The sales process is not as easy to identify as the other processes because it does not involve any obvious hardware, but it is no less important. All utility companies have to market their product in order to attract customers, and once customers have been found, a utility company must monitor and record all the energy that is consumed, so that customers can be billed and the revenue collected. There are therefore considerable administration costs associated in managing each customer's account. These costs are usually recovered by levying a periodic standing charge on each customer.

The relationship between the various processes in a typical electricity supply industry is shown in Figure 2.2.

Although the processes described above are common to all electricity supply industries, the way in which they are achieved in practice varies considerably around the globe. In some countries all the four processes are performed by a single vertically integrated utility company, which generates, transmits and distributes electricity, and bills its own customers. Examples of vertically integrated utility companies exist in many parts of the USA. In other countries such as in England and Wales a horizontal structure exists in which the various processes are fragmented, with a number of utility companies performing different roles within the whole supply industry. For example, in

England and Wales, electricity generation is performed by a number of competing generating companies such as National Power and PowerGen. Another independent company, the National Grid Company, which levies rental charges for using its power lines, performs the transmission process. Finally, regional utility companies such as Yorkshire Electricity and London Electricity purchase electricity from the national grid and distribute it to their customers. They also read their customers' meters and invoice them for the electricity consumed. This horizontal approach can result in extremely complex trading mechanisms (see Chapter 3). No matter how complex the structure, it is important to understand that the component processes described above and their related costs are the same the world over. Consequently the tariffs levied by all electricity utility companies tend to follow a similar format.

2.4.1 Electricity Charges

From the discussion in Section 2.4 it can be seen that many costs are incurred in generating and supplying electricity, and these must be recovered from the end-user. They can be summarized as:

- The cost of purchasing the primary energy and converting it to electricity;
- The cost of transporting electricity around a region or country;
- The cost of distributing electricity to the customer; and
- The cost involved in meter reading, billing and managing customers' accounts.

Because electricity cannot be stored, the size, and hence the cost, of the supporting infrastructure is governed by the maximum instantaneous load on the system and not the amount of energy which is consumed. Consider the electricity demand profiles for 1993 for the national grid in England and Wales presented in Figure 2.3. It can be seen from these profiles that the greatest demand for electricity in 1993 occurred in winter, reaching a peak of 48 GW at approximately 18.00 hours on 29 November [3]. However, for most of the year the demand was considerably less. In fact at 06.00 hours on 1 August 1993 demand on the grid dropped to a low of approximately 16 GW. The only conclusion which can be drawn from this is that for most of the year the transmission and distribution grids are working at a level well below their maximum capacity. Although a considerable amount of generating capacity is idle for much of the year, it still has to be maintained on standby, ready to be used should demand on the grid rise to a high level. In fact, if excess capacity is not built into the system, when demand for electricity rises to a higher level, one of two things will happen:

1. There may not be enough generating capacity to meet demand; or
2. The cables in the transmission grid may become overloaded.

If either of these happen, then power cuts will occur, which is highly undesirable. Given this, the utility companies are faced with a decision, either to:

- Build more power stations and reinforce their transmission and distribution networks, which is a very costly solution; or
- Discourage their customers from consuming large amounts of electricity at times when electricity demand is high.

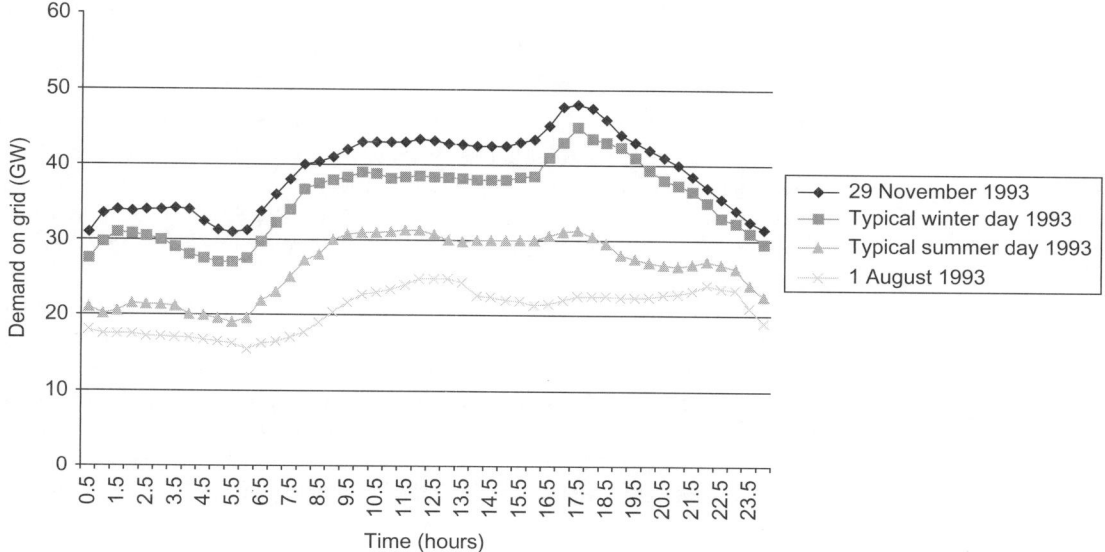

FIG 2.3 Electricity demand profiles for England and Wales for 1993 [3].

Given this choice it is not surprising that most electricity utility companies opt for the latter solution. In practice they discourage high electricity usage by levying large demand charges on customers who use electricity during periods of peak demand. In northern Europe the period of peak demand is in the winter months, but in the southern states of the USA the peak occurs in summer due to the increased use of air-conditioning equipment [4]. From this it can be seen that utility companies can influence demand on their network by altering the charges levied on customers under tariffs.

Although tariffs can be used to discourage customers, they can also be used to encourage them. Figure 2.3 demonstrates that electrical demand is much higher in the day time than at night-time. Consequently, generating plant is underutilized at night. In an attempt to remedy this situation, utility companies often offer night-time (i.e. off-peak) electricity at a discounted rate as an incentive to customers to use off-peak electricity. This is a common practice worldwide. Some utility companies even divide the day into 3 or 4 bands and charge various unit energy rates for each band, depending on the demand experienced on their network. Utility companies also use tariffs to discourage building designers from over-designing their electrical installations by levying availability charges. When a building is constructed the local electrical utility company is generally obliged to supply it with electricity. This usually involves laying a new power cable to the building and may involve the construction of a new transformer and sub-station. In some cases, if the facility is large, it might even involve reinforcing the whole local electrical distribution network. The capital cost involved in all this work is borne by the utility company. Not surprisingly the utility company does not look kindly on end-users who overestimate their power requirements as this results in them incurring large capital costs. One solution is therefore to levy a supply availability charge on the power demand (i.e. system-rated capacity) requested by the end-user. This charge is levied each month on every 1 kW (or 1 kVA) of the system-rated capacity. Clearly a deterrent to overcautious building designers!

Some utility companies meter their customers in kW and kWh rather than kVA and kVAh. At school we are taught that electrical power (measured in watts) is the product of voltage (measured in volts) and current (measured in amps). So at first sight there appears to be no difference between kW and kVA. There is, however, a subtle and very important difference between the two. If an electric current is passed through a reactive load, such as a fluorescent lamp fitting or an induction motor, the current will become out of phase with the voltage and lag behind it. This subject is discussed at length in Chapter 14, so here it suffices to say that reactive loads consume more power than is usefully used. Therefore, a reactive load such as an induction motor will draw a larger current than would be anticipated by its useful power rating. Consequently, if a utility company meters its customers in kW, then it must levy an additional reactive power charge in kVAh. This ensures that the utility is paid for all the power it supplies to the site, and not penalized for the customer's poor power factor.

2.4.2 Electricity Tariffs

Electricity utility companies offer tariffs to their customers which reflect the various costs incurred. These tariffs are published in advance and are standard for all customers. Although tariffs differ from one utility company to another, they are all structured to recover the various costs incurred in generating, transmitting, distributing and selling electricity.

Domestic tariffs are probably the simplest form of electricity tariff that exists. They are offered to domestic and other small consumers, and are usually billed quarterly. In their simplest form they consist of a fixed standing charge levied every quarter and on a standard unit charge, as shown in Table 2.1. A more sophisticated version of the simple domestic tariff is the introduction of peak and off-peak unit charges, designed to encourage off-peak consumption of electricity. In the UK this tariff is known as an 'Economy 7 tariff', a typical example of which is shown in Table 2.1.

For larger non-domestic customers with demands below 50 kW, 'block tariffs' are usually offered. Block tariffs are similar in structure to domestic tariffs with the exception

TABLE 2.1 Domestic electricity tariffs

General domestic tariff	
Quarterly standing charge	£8.25
Unit charge	6.53p/kWh
Economy 7 domestic tariff	
Quarterly standing charge	£10.78
Off-peak unit charge (00.30–07.30 hours)	2.28p/kWh
Peak unit charge (all other times)	6.89p/kWh

that the first tranche of energy consumed, usually a 'block' of approximately 1000 kWh, is charged at a higher unit rate. Some utility companies may even offer tariffs with more than one block. As with the domestic tariff, peak/off-peak variants are usually offered. Table 2.2 shows the structure of a typical block tariff.

For larger commercial and industrial consumers the most commonly offered type of tariff is probably the 'maximum demand tariff', which is offered in various guises by many utility companies around the world. Table 2.3 shows a typical 'maximum demand' tariff used by a UK electricity utility company.

Under a maximum demand tariff shown in Table 2.3 the billing and administrative costs are recovered through a monthly standing charge which is constant and independent of the amount of electricity consumed. The unit charge covers the cost of providing electrical energy and therefore is levied on every kVAh of electricity consumed. The unit charge is generally made up of two components: a larger component, which covers the cost of producing the electricity, and a smaller component, which covers the operating costs associated with its transmission and distribution. In order to encourage off-peak electricity consumption, a reduced off-peak unit charge is offered nightly from 00.30 to

TABLE 2.2   Block electricity tariff

General block tariff	
Quarterly standing charge	£8.69
Unit charge for the first 1000 kWh consumed	8.94p/kWh
Unit charge for additional kWh consumed	6.70p/kWh
Economy 7 block tariff	
Quarterly standing charge	£11.22
Off-peak unit charge (00.30–07.30 hours)	2.28p/kWh
Peak unit charge for the first 1000 kWh consumed	8.94p/kWh
Peak unit charge for additional kWh consumed	7.05p/kWh

TABLE 2.3   Typical maximum demand tariff

	Tariff
1. Monthly charge	£32.00
2. Supply availability charge per month for each kVA of chargeable supply capacity	£1.40
3. Maximum demand charge per month for each kVA of monthly maximum demand in the months of: December and January November and February	£5.40 £2.70
4. Unit charges for maximum demand tariffs (p/kVAh) For each unit supplied For each unit supplied between the hours of 00.30 and 07.30 each night	2.65p

07.30 hours. This encourages customers to load shift and thus reduce the demand on the network during periods of peak demand.

The capital costs associated with the distribution network are recovered through the maximum demand charge, which is levied to penalize consumers who have a high power demand (in kW or kVA) during periods in which demand for electricity is high. In the case of the tariff shown in Table 2.3, the 'peak power demand' period lasts from 1 November to 28 February. During this period a demand charge is levied on every kVA of the peak instantaneous demand recorded in any particular month. During the colder months of December and January the charge is £5.40 per kVA. However, this drops to £2.70 per kVA during November and February. For the rest of the year, no demand charges are levied.

The supply availability charge is designed to deter customers and building designers from requesting oversized supply cables to their facilities. If a customer overestimates their required supply capacity, then the utility company will incur additional expense. If the customer's high demand estimates do not materialize, then the utility company will have spent money which it cannot recoup through either maximum demand or unit charges. Consequently, an availability charge is levied monthly on each kVA or kW of the requested supply capacity, in order to penalize overambitious customers.

A variation on the maximum demand tariff described above is the seasonal time of day (STOD) tariff which is illustrated in Table 2.4.

Under a STOD tariff, monthly standing and availability charges are levied as in the maximum demand tariff. However, there are no demand charges, and instead the unit charges reflect the demand on the utility company's network, penalizing very heavily those customers who consume electricity during periods of peak demand.

Variations on the tariffs described above can be found throughout the world. One novel variation occurs in Finland, where IVO, the country's largest supplier, has a triple band tariff. This reflects the nature of, and the production costs associated with, the various types of generating plant required to meet demand [5]. The base tariff is linked to hydro and nuclear power, the middle tariff is related to coal-based power production and the peak tariff is based on oil-fired and gas turbine power production. In many hotter regions, such as in the southern states of the USA, peak demand occurs during the summer months due to the intensive use of air-conditioning plant. Therefore utility companies in these regions levy maximum demand charges in the summer months and not during the winter.

It should be noted that in many countries some form of 'value added tax' (VAT) is levied on energy consumption. If this applies in a particular region or country, it is important that this is considered when estimating and analysing electrical energy bills.

The discussion above demonstrates that the overall price per kWh or kVAh paid by the consumer depends greatly on the end-user's consumption profile. Indeed, in some circumstances it can be considerably greater than the unit energy charge quoted by a utility company. Example 2.1 illustrates the technique which should be used in order to accurately calculate electrical energy costs.

TABLE 2.4 Typical seasonal time of day tariff

	Tariff
1. Monthly charge	£32.00
2. Supply availability charge per month for each kVA of chargeable supply capacity	£1.40
3. Winter unit charges (p/kVAh) (November to March inclusive)	
(i) For each unit supplied between 16.00 and 19.00 hours each day on Mondays to Fridays inclusive during	
(a) December and January	30.50p
(b) November and February	17.60p
(ii) For each unit supplied between 08.30 and 20.00 hours each day on Mondays to Fridays inclusive during the months of December to February inclusive, other than charged at rates (i) (a) or (b) above	7.45p
(iii) For other winter day units supplied between 07.30 and 00.30 hours	5.30p
(iv) For winter night units supplied between 00.30 and 07.30 hours	2.65p
4. Summer unit charges (p/kVAh) (April to October inclusive)	
(i) For each summer day units supplied between 07.30 and 00.30 hours	4.50p
(ii) For summer night units supplied between 00.30 and 07.30 hours	1.90p

Example 2.1

The monthly electricity consumption data for a hotel building for a calendar year is as follows:

Month	Electricity peak units (kVAh)	Electricity off-peak units (kVAh)	Monthly maximum demand (kVA)
January	223,475	63,031	592
February	214,718	57,076	552
March	186,845	46,711	476
April	185,513	40,722	471
May	174,103	33,162	427
June	165,988	27,021	381
July	163,181	24,383	365
August	150,089	26,486	372
September	164,746	31,380	410
October	174,983	41,045	452
November	189,752	47,438	486
December	222,952	55,738	623
Total	2,216,345	494,193	n.a.

Given that the declared maximum supply capacity of the hotel building is 650 kW and that the maximum demand tariff shown in Table 2.3 applies, determine the annual electricity bill, and hence an average price for each unit (kVAh) of electricity consumed (exclusive of VAT).

Solution

Elemental charge	Calculation	Cost (£)
Monthly standing charge	£32.00 × 12	384.00
Supply availability charge	650 kVA @ £1.40 per kVA × 12	10,920.00
Maximum demand charges		
December	623 kVA @£5.40	3364.20
January	592 kVA @ £5.40	3196.80
November	486 kVA @ £2.70	1312.20
February	552 kVA @ £2.70	1490.40
Energy charges		
Peak rate	2,216,345 kVAh @ 6.15p/kVAh	136,305.22
Off-peak	494,193 kVAh @ 2.65p/kVAh	13,096.11
	Annual electricity cost	**170,068.93**

$$\text{Average unit price of electricity} = \frac{170,068.93 \times 100}{(2,216,345 + 494,193)} = 6.274\text{p/kVAh}$$

2.5 Natural Gas

Gas utility companies are similar to electricity utility companies insomuch as they both supply energy directly to buildings via pipes or cables. Both types of utility companies have therefore to construct, operate and maintain large transmission and distribution networks. In addition, both types of utility companies have to invoice customers and maintain customer accounts. However, there are some distinct and influential differences between the two 'fuels':

- Unlike electricity, natural gas is a primary fuel which must be removed from the ground by some means.
- Natural gas can be stored in large quantities, while electricity cannot.
- Unlike electricity, which is required all year round, the market for natural gas is very seasonal and is weather dependent.

Natural gas consists almost entirely of methane (see Table 2.5) and has a net calorific value of approximately 38.6 MJ/m³; its density is about 0.73 kg/m³. As such it has a low energy density compared with oil. In fact, 1 m³ of natural gas contains approximately one-thousandth of the energy of the same volume of crude oil. Consequently, transportation of natural gas is an expensive and difficult operation, involving substantial networks of large-diameter pipelines. Gas transportation is therefore usually by high-pressure pipeline, although gas can be liquefied and then transported by ship. Both methods usually require large-scale storage near to consumers to balance out fluctuations in demand.

Figure 2.4 shows an example of a supply chain for gas produced from an offshore platform [7]. From the platform the gas is sent through an offshore pipeline to a landing terminal. From there, it is either sent through transmission pipelines to serve the domestic market, or transferred to another country via an international transmission pipeline. At some stage the gas will end up in a regional distribution pipeline before eventually being supplied to domestic users, large industrial users or electricity generators.

Gas supply chains vary depending on their location and often involve a large number of parties. The gas producers may not necessarily be the companies who own the offshore pipeline; similarly the transmission company may not be involved in regional and final distribution. Therefore as gas flows along a chain, its ownership may be transferred several times.

TABLE 2.5   Composition of natural gas

Constituent part	Percentage by volume (%)
Methane, CH_4	92.6
Ethane, C_2H_6	3.6
Propane, C_3H_8	0.8
Butane, C_4H_{10}	0.3
Nitrogen, N_2	2.6
Carbon dioxide, CO_2	0.1

From Eastop and Croft (1990) *Energy Efficiency for Engineers and Technologists*, © Longman Group Ltd 1990, reprinted by permission of Pearson Education Ltd [6].

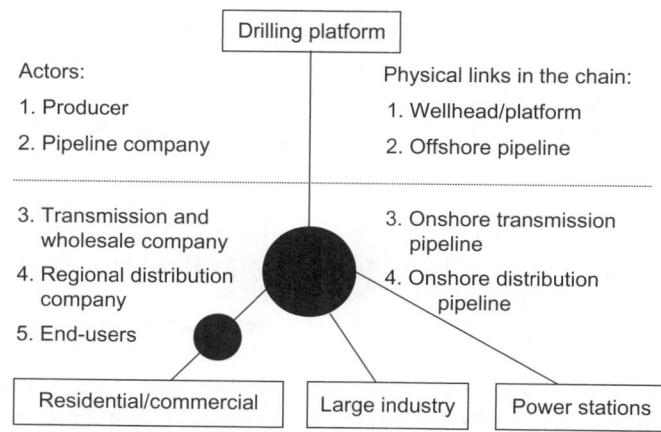

FIG 2.4 Gas chain [7].

2.5.1 Natural Gas Production, Transmission and Distribution

The gas chain in Figure 2.4 shows that a number of distinct processes are involved in bringing the finished product to the customer:

(i) *Gas gathering pipelines*: These link the production fields to the transmission lines and may run undersea or over land. They transport untreated gas which is not usually of marketable quality. Untreated gas may be 'dry' or 'wet'. The gathering pipelines for 'dry gas', which is relatively free of liquids, will be much like any other transmission line. 'Wet gas' contains substantial quantities of liquid; if this is to be transported then it must be treated to prevent line clogging.

(ii) *Gas treatment*: When it is extracted, natural gas is nearly always mixed with impurities such as water, acid gases, nitrogen and helium [7]. In order to prevent corrosion of transmission lines, these impurities must be removed. This process usually takes place in an onshore gas treatment facility.

(iii) *Gas transmission*: Gas transmission pipelines ensure an uninterrupted supply of gas at a set pressure from the gas gathering pipeline to various delivery points. These delivery points are typically the inlets to local utility distribution systems. At their simplest, transmission pipelines can simply be a connection between two points. However, it is more common that transmission pipelines supply several points along their routes, as is the case with the Russian pipelines, which serve several European countries. In transmission pipelines it is necessary to boost the gas pressure at regular intervals by using compressors.

(iv) *Blending*: Depending on their hydrocarbon and nitrogen content, the calorific content of natural gases from different sources may vary. Many gas appliances are designed to run on one type of gas and cannot burn a gas with a different calorific value. Consequently, blending stations are required to mix the various different gases into a blend whose calorific value is within the tolerance of end-users' appliances.

2.5.2 Peak Demand Problems

In Europe and North America, where natural gas is predominantly used for space heating, demand is strongly dependent on outside air temperature. Gas transmission and distribution systems must therefore cope with large swings in seasonal demand, while still maintaining a continuous supply to customers. It is particularly important to ensure that all gas pipelines are maintained well above atmospheric pressure, so that air is not entrained into the system; otherwise a potentially explosive mixture may be created. In order to overcome the problem of fluctuating demand, gas utility companies can employ a number of alternative strategies:

- They can construct a transmission infrastructure which is large enough to cope with the maximum likely demand.
- They can store large reserves of gas near to consumers when gas demand is low, ready for withdrawal when demand is high.
- They can offer interruptible supply tariffs with discounted unit charges. However, under this type of tariff, the utility company does not guarantee to supply gas to customers when demand rises to a high level.

The first solution involves large capital expenditure on infrastructure; an infrastructure which is inevitably underutilized for most of its life, with the result that production and transmission costs are increased. The second solution attempts to balance production and transmission loads and also provides a measure of security against supply disruption. However, it does involve capital expenditure on storage facilities. The third solution involves no capital expenditure and is very popular with utility companies. By offering an interruptible supply to large customers, the utility company is not guaranteeing a gas supply during periods of peak demand. Interruptible supplies are popular with organizations that are able to switch at short notice to another fuel, such as oil, and so are able to reduce the peak demand on the gas utilities network. In return, consumers who opt for an interruptible supply are offered an advantageous tariff. In practice, a combination of all three solutions is often employed to balance a utility company's supply load.

2.5.3　Gas Tariffs

The supply of natural gas to customers involves costs which must be met by the various companies involved. These can be categorized as:

- The cost of collecting, processing and delivering the gas 'onshore';
- The cost of transporting the gas through the transmission pipelines; and
- The costs involved in marketing, billing and managing customers' accounts.

One of the most influential factors in determining the price that customers pay for gas is the transportation levy that gas suppliers have to pay for the use of transmission pipelines. This transportation levy reflects the costs incurred in constructing and operating the transmission network, and is generally determined by the length of the pipeline and the maximum gas-flow rate during periods of peak demand.

Gas tariffs are much simpler than those used for electricity. They tend to follow a fixed pattern of charges, namely: a fixed quarterly standing charge and a charge for every unit (kWh) of gas supplied. Unit charges usually incorporate a transportation charge. For smaller consumers unit charges are generally constant. For larger customers, the unit charge usually decreases as gas consumption increases. Table 2.6 shows a typical gas tariff for a small customer.

It should be noted that in many countries VAT is levied on gas consumption. A variation on this gas tariff shown in Table 2.6 is the introduction of a higher unit charge for the first 'block' of gas consumed, in a similar manner to an electrical block tariff.

Larger customers tend to be offered monthly tariffs in which the unit charge decreases as gas consumption increases. They also have the option of negotiating either firm or

TABLE 2.6　Typical gas tariff for small customer

Standing charge per quarter	£9.57
Unit charge per kWh supplied	1.52p/kWh

interruptible supply contracts. The unit charges associated with an interruptible supply are lower than those for a firm supply and therefore they are an attractive proposition for some customers. Interruptible supply contracts can be negotiated in a variety of forms, with a variable interruption period. Not surprisingly, the longer the permitted period of interruption the lower the unit price of the gas. With an interruptible supply tariff or contract, the customer is given short notice that the gas supply is going to be cut and must therefore be prepared to switch over to another fuel.

2.6 Fuel Oil

Unlike gas and electricity, oil is not supplied under a tariff, but must be purchased on the open market. This means that the price of oil can be extremely volatile. Where possible it is worth using dual burners on boilers, so that if the price of oil gets too high, natural gas can be used as an alternative.

There are a variety of fuel oils on the market, ranging from free-flowing domestic heating oil to thick heavy grade oils. Classification of fuel oils is usually made according to their viscosity (as shown in Table 2.7).

Unlike gas and electricity, which are relatively easy to handle, the use of fuel oil imposes restrictions. It is therefore important to consider the storage and handling facilities required, since these can affect purchasing arrangements and also impact on energy consumption. The storage volume in relation to average and peak consumption rates should be considered. Heavier grades of oil need to be heated in order to facilitate pouring, it is therefore worth considering reducing the volume that is kept heated, in order to reduce standing losses. Whilst it is normal to provide enough storage for approximately 3 weeks' operation [9], in facilities which have an interruptible gas supply it may be necessary to install additional storage capacity.

Storage tanks in which heavier fuel oils are kept heated should be well insulated in order to minimize standing losses. In addition, the lower price of heavier grade oils should be

TABLE 2.7   Fuel oils and their properties

	Domestic heating oil	Gas oil	Light fuel oil	Medium fuel oil	Heavy fuel oil
Class	C	D	E	F	G
Viscosity (Redwood No.1 @ 100 seconds)	–	35	220	950	3500
Density at 16°C (kg/l)	0.79	0.85	0.94	0.97	0.98
Pour point (°C)	–	–6.7	17.0	21.0	21.0
Gross calorific value (MJ/l)	35.5	38.7	40.8	41.6	41.7

From Eastop and Croft (1990) *Energy Efficiency for Engineers and Technologists,* © Longman Group Ltd 1990, reprinted by permission of Pearson Education Ltd, and Porges and Porges (1976) *Handbook of Heating, Ventilating and Air Conditioning,* Newnes-Butterworths [8].

set against the additional costs associated with handling the oil and maintaining it at a pouring temperature. For example, for Class G fuel oil a pumping temperature of 55°C is required.

References

[1] BP energy statistics 2001, BP website www.bp.com/downloads/702/BPwebglobal.pdf; March 2002.
[2] Campbell CJ, Laherrère JH, George RL, Anderson RN, Fouda SA. Preventing the next oil crunch. Sci Am1998; 27(8): 359–77.
[3] The National Grid Company. Seven Year Statement; 1994.
[4] Wendland RD. Storage to become rule, not exception. ASHRAE Journal1987; May.
[5] International Energy Agency/OECD. Electricity supply in the OECD; 1992.
[6] Eastop TD, Croft DR. Energy efficiency for engineers and technologists. Longman Scientific & Technical; 1990. Harlow, Essex.
[7] International Energy Agency/OECD. Natural gas transportation: organisation and regulation; 1994.
[8] Porges J, Porges F. Handbook of heating, ventilating and air conditioning. Newnes-Butterworths; 1976. London.
[9] Energy audits and surveys. CIBSE Applications Manual AM5; 1991.

Bibliography

Department of the Environment. Economic use of electricity in buildings. Fuel Efficiency Booklet 9; 1995
Eastop TD, Croft DR. Energy efficiency for engineers and technologists. (Chapter 9). Longman Scientific & Technical, 1990. Harlow, Essex.
Energy audits and surveys. CIBSE Applications Manual AM5; 1991.
Yuill D. Understanding electricity costs. Energy Manager's Workbook, 2 (Chapter 2). Energy Publications, 1985. Cambridge.

CHAPTER 3

Competition in Energy Supply

In this chapter the concept of competition in the energy sector is examined for both electricity and gas supply industries, and the experience of electricity deregulation in the UK and USA is discussed in detail. The potential role of demand-side management (DSM) is also investigated and comparisons are drawn between experiences in the UK and USA.

3.1 Introduction

It has traditionally been the case that gas and electricity utility companies, irrespective of ownership (i.e. state or privately owned), are natural monopolies, which are regulated by legislative measures. These monopolies evolved partly because of the high infrastructure costs associated with the transmission and distribution of gas and electricity, and partly because it was easier to manage and regulate utility companies which generated/supplied, transmitted and distributed electricity or gas. Indeed, it is difficult to imagine anything other than a monopoly, given that most buildings have only one physical connection to a gas pipe and another to an electricity cable. However, while monopolistic utility companies are relatively easy to control and regulate, they prevent competition in the energy market. Consequently, it is not possible to buy and sell 'bulk' energy in the same way other commodities are traded.

In recent years many governments around the world have begun to investigate alternative solutions which introduce competition into their respective electricity and gas supply industries. This has become possible because of various technical and financial advances made in the late 1980s and 1990s. The UK has been at the forefront in pioneering utility deregulation, and has completely restructured its utility sector. During the 1990s the UK deregulated first its electricity supply industry and then its gas industry, in a long and complex process, which at time of writing is still ongoing. Such has been the radical nature of these changes that in many ways the UK has become the 'pilot study' for the rest of the world. Following the UK's lead a number of countries, including the USA, have deregulated (at least in part) their electricity supply industries and are developing new energy-trading markets. In addition to the UK electricity spot market (i.e. the electricity 'pool'), four other 'pools' have so far been created in Europe; the Amsterdam Power Exchange (covering The Netherlands, Belgium and Germany), the Spanish Pool, the Swiss Pool and the Nordpool in Scandinavia (covering Norway, Sweden and Finland) [1].

3.2 The Concept of Competition

Consider the case of an organization which uses oil to heat its buildings. Under normal circumstances the organization will have a choice of competing fuel suppliers from whom to purchase oil. The organization can negotiate a bilateral supply contract with any one of these suppliers. If one supplier becomes too expensive, then the organization can simply switch to purchase oil from another supplier. If the general demand for fuel oil is high, then the suppliers will be able to raise their prices. Conversely, if demand is low then the price of oil will also be low. Thus a competitive market in fuel oil exists which reflects the demand for oil at any moment in time. As with any other commodity, the oil price will vary because customers have the ability to switch between suppliers. In addition, there is no cross-subsidy of one group of customers by another group of customers. Each fuel supply contract is negotiated on an individual basis between the parties concerned.

Now consider the same organization purchasing electricity under a tariff from a utility company. Since the electricity is supplied through cables owned by the utility company, the customer has no choice of alternative supplier and so the organization is compelled to purchase electricity at a price fixed by the utility company. As a consequence:

- *No competition exists*: The customer is in a weak position since electricity prices are fixed by the utility company.
- *No market exists*: Under a tariff, electricity prices are fixed, with the result that prices do not accurately reflect the fluctuations in demand for electricity. Although many tariffs do have reduced 'off-peak' elements, these are at best only a crude indicator of market demand.
- *The potential for cross-subsidy exists*: The utility company may decide to offer lower electricity prices to its large industrial customers, and recoup some of its

lost income by increasing the prices of its smaller domestic and commercial tariff customers. This is termed 'cross-subsidy', and effectively means that one group of customers is subsidizing another group.

While this monopolistic scenario may suit the utility companies, it does not benefit the customer. The utility companies are in a strong position and the potential exists for artificially high electricity prices. Lack of competition ultimately leads to:

- Manufacturing industry paying a high price for energy, with the result that the unit cost of production increases and the industry becomes less competitive.
- Utility companies becoming overmanned and inefficient.

It is therefore easy to see why many governments are reviewing the monopolistic position of their respective utility companies with a view to introducing a competitive energy market.

3.3 Competition in the Electricity Supply Industry

While it is easy to state that competition in the energy market is a desirable thing, in practice it is difficult to achieve a truly competitive market amongst utility companies. Utility networks, be they gas or electricity, lend themselves to monopolies and are not naturally suited to competition. This is because it is impractical and prohibitively expensive to construct two or more sets of competing transmission/distribution networks. Given this, the simplest and easiest way to organize affairs is to have a 'vertically integrated' structure in which a single utility company is responsible for provision of supply. Figure 3.1 shows the structure of a typical vertically integrated electricity supply industry.

In a vertically integrated electricity supply industry the various utility companies have monopolies over their 'franchise' regions. Within its franchise region a utility company will be responsible for generating, transmitting, distributing and supplying electricity to all its customers. Customers in the utility company's franchise region are forced to

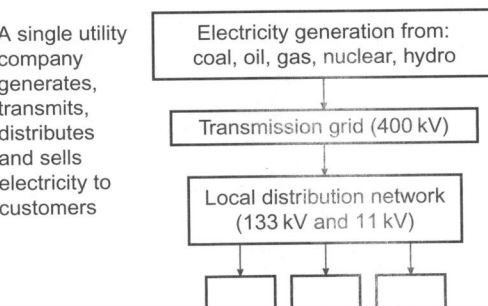

A single utility company generates, transmits, distributes and sells electricity to customers

Electricity generation from: coal, oil, gas, nuclear, hydro

Transmission grid (400 kV)

Local distribution network (133 kV and 11 kV)

FIG 3.1 A vertically integrated electricity supply industry.

purchase their electricity from the regional utility company. Vertically integrated utility companies can exist in both the private and the public sectors. Their monopolistic position is derived solely from their physical location, which excludes competition and means that the utility company has a protected market. Under this scenario energy prices can easily become overinflated if the utility company is not tightly regulated.

In order to promote competition in the electricity supply industry it is necessary to create a market for the commodity which is flexible and yet still robust enough to cope with wide fluctuations in demand. The market should:

- Allow various electricity supply companies and generators to compete with each other to sell electricity direct to customers.
- Allow customers to negotiate electricity supply contracts with various suppliers.
- Be transparent, so that generators, suppliers and customers can see that the market is fair and equitable.
- Create a 'spot market' which accurately reflects both demand for energy and cost of production. This spot market then becomes the market indicator of the real cost of production at any given point in time.
- Facilitate a future's market in electricity trading.

While the above points are relatively easy to achieve in a normal commodity market, they are not easily achieved in a market in which electricity is bought and sold. This is because electricity cannot be stored and must be generated only when it can be consumed. Any potential trading market in electricity must fully accommodate the physical constraints of an electricity supply system. As a result a truly competitive market in electricity is likely to be much more complex than a normal commodities market.

It is impossible to achieve a competitive market with a vertically integrated electricity supply industry. Instead a horizontally integrated structure is required. The introduction of a horizontally integrated electricity supply industry, in which the generation, transmission and distribution roles are all split up from each other, is the key to facilitating competition. By splitting up the roles it is possible to create competition between generators, who then have to bid in a 'spot market' for the right to supply electricity to the transmission grid. If the transmission company acts in a fair and independent manner, purchasing power at 'least cost', then any possible cartel should be eliminated. It then becomes possible for new 'independent power producers' to enter the market to compete with existing generators. This should result in a reduced cost to the customer for each unit of electrical energy produced. Figure 3.2 shows the structure of a typical horizontally integrated electricity supply industry.

Whilst the spot market described above facilitates competition between generators, it does not of itself offer the customer a choice of competing suppliers. In order to achieve this, the customer must be allowed to negotiate supply contracts with individual energy suppliers. This is achieved by allowing 'second tier' electricity 'wholesale' suppliers to purchase 'bulk' electricity from the transmission grid and sell it directly to customers. Under this arrangement the customer purchases electricity from competing supply companies, who pay a fee to the relevant distribution companies for the use of their 'wires'. This 'line rental' fee is then passed on to the customer and included in the

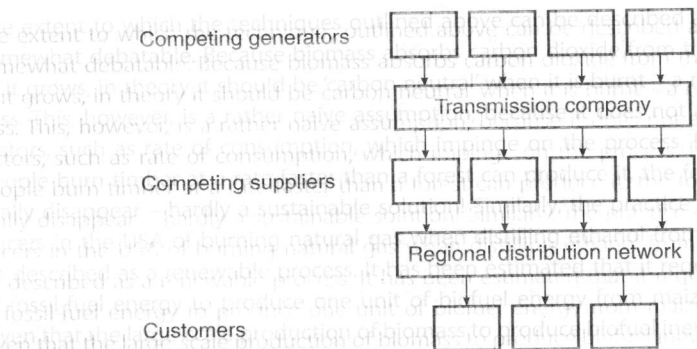

FIG 3.2 A horizontally integrated electricity supply industry.

unit price paid for the electricity. In order to ensure that true competition takes place, the 'line rental' fees should be transparent and equal for all potential electricity suppliers. These fees are usually fixed by some form of statutory regulatory mechanism.

This discussion indicates that facilitating competition in an electricity supply industry involves the setting-up of a complex structure, with many demarcation boundaries. Indeed, there is an inherent conflict of interests between the engineering and financial requirements of a horizontally integrated structure. The transmission company is primarily interested in procuring enough electrical energy from generators in order to meet the instantaneous demand on its grid. It seeks to procure this energy from the cheapest power producers and is not particularly interested in individual supply contracts. Conversely, customers, suppliers and generators are primarily interested in negotiating contracts which ensure secure supply and therefore are not interested in the transmission company's need to meet instantaneous demand. Satisfying these conflicting needs requires the setting-up of complex bidding, pricing and settlement mechanisms. It is the specific nature of these mechanisms and the efficiency with which they are applied which will ultimately determine the success or failure of any electricity market.

In addition to the complex financial and settlement mechanisms required to operate the market, suppliers need to know the 'real-time' electricity consumption of their contract (i.e. non-domestic) customers. This involves the installation of 'smart' meters which measure electricity usage every half hour, and can be read remotely and automatically. The data from these meters are transmitted to remote disseminated centres, from which relevant data are sent to all the parties involved in the supply contract. Contract customers may purchase or lease their metering equipment, but the installation and maintenance of these meters should be carried out by approved operators.

3.4 The UK Electricity Experience

Competition in electricity supply is still in its infancy and many protocols are not yet firmly in place. Most of the electricity power markets which exist around the world are only a few years old and even the UK market, established in 1990, is still undergoing major revisions. This makes it difficult to describe general rules which apply to all electricity markets. In the absence of any firm 'ground rules' it is worthwhile looking in detail at the evolution of the competitive electricity market in England and Wales (the largest part of the UK), since this has been the 'template' for subsequent deregulation schemes in various parts of the world.

In 1990 in England and Wales a daily spot market known as the electricity 'pool' was created. The pool was administered by the National Grid Company (NGC), which owned and operated the transmission grid in England and Wales. Each morning the competing generating companies would submit 'bids' for their various generating sets to NGC for the following day's operation. Each bid included an offer price at which the generating company would be prepared to operate its various generating units for the following day. It also included a declaration of availability of generating plant for the following day. Once the generators had submitted their bids to the pool, the NGC examined its own demand forecast for the following day and ranked each generating unit in order of price (lowest price first), so that finally a merit schedule was produced. This schedule was then published at approximately 15.00 hours, so that the generating companies were notified of the generating units required for the following day. As there was often considerable overcapacity in the system, any generating units for which the offer price was too high were either placed on standby or excluded from the pool and forced to shut down.

As electricity cannot be stored, it is essential that the controllers of the national transmission grid be able to bring online (or download) additional generating capacity at very short notice to cope with fluctuating demand. Figure 3.3 shows the national grid demand profile for a peak 'winter time' weekday, 29 November 1993 [2]. This graph

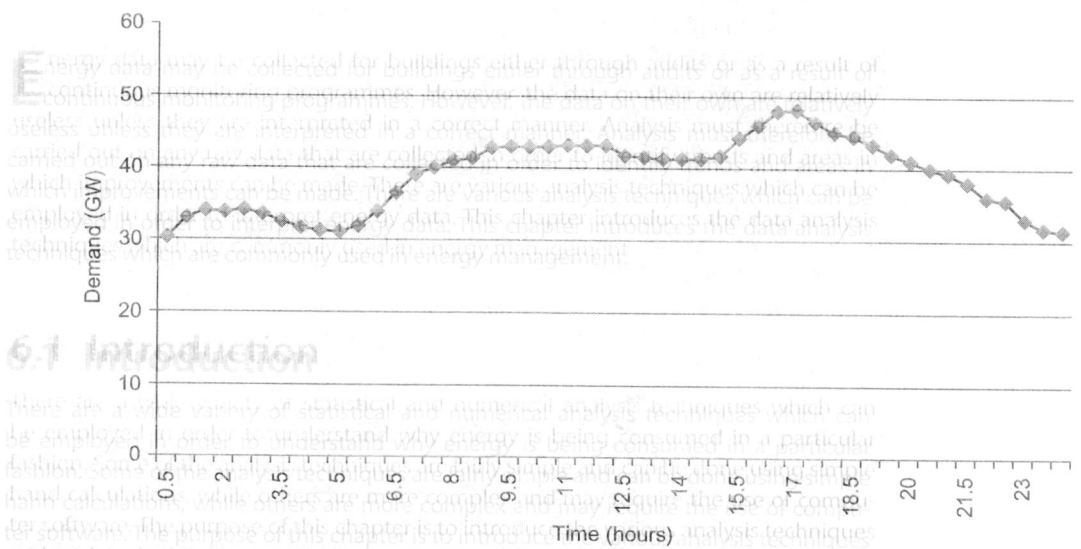

FIG 3.3 Demand experienced by National Grid, 29 November 1993 [2].

shows that demand on that day varied considerably over the 24-hour period. To cope with increases in demand, generating units had to be brought online as and when they were required, but in strict accordance with their ranking in the daily pool merit schedule. In other words, generating sets which bid a low price were brought online first, while the more expensive units had to wait until demand increases before they were allowed to generate. Consequently the pool price varied for each half hour period throughout the day. When demand was high, it generally followed that pool price would also be high. In this way the pool price reflected the demand on the transmission grid.

The bid price submitted for the most expensive generating unit brought online to meet the demand in any given half hour period was known as the 'system marginal price' (SMP). For example, if the highest bid price accepted into the pool for the half hour period 11.00–11.30 hours was 2.5p/kWh, then the SMP would be 2.5p/kWh. It is important to note that it is the SMP, not the bid prices submitted by the individual generators, which became the basis for the eventual pool price for any given half hour, and that all the generators online in that particular half hour were paid the 'pool purchase price' (PPP). Electricity supply companies and large consumers purchasing from the pool had to pay the 'pool selling price' (PSP). Not surprisingly PSP is always greater than PPP, the difference being an uplift to cover the pool operating costs. The electricity pool in England and Wales enabled a competitive market to exist amongst the generators, and gave the market as a whole an indication of the true costs of electricity production at any given time.

While an electricity pool facilitates competition between the various generators, it does not on its own provide the mechanism for promoting a competitive market amongst customers. In order to achieve this, 'second tier' electricity 'wholesale' supply companies must be allowed to purchase electricity from the transmission grid and sell it on directly to customers. These wholesale suppliers negotiate bilateral contracts with the generating companies to purchase 'bulk' electricity at fixed rates, under a series of *contracts for differences* (defined later in this paragraph), and then sell it on to the customer at a marked-up price. These supply companies make their money by purchasing 'bulk' electricity from the generators at a low price and selling it on to their customers at a higher price. This involves considerable financial risk and the supply companies must negotiate contracts which ensure that they make a profit. However, pool price can be extremely volatile, especially in the winter. This volatility increases the element of risk for the supply companies if they purchase from the pool, with the result that they may lose money if they purchase at a high price and have to sell at a low one. The inherent volatility of the pool also makes planning ahead difficult. In an attempt to hedge against the risk of high pool prices, the supply companies take out *contracts for differences* with the individual generating companies. The contracts between the supply companies and the generators operate outside the pool and operate in a similar way to 'futures contracts' traded in the world's commodity markets. Under a typical contract for differences a supply company would contract with a specific generator to buy electricity at a fixed price for a specific time period (usually on a daily five time block basis) [3]. This 'hedges' against the volatility of the pool, and enables both generators and suppliers to predict the future financial risk involved in generating and selling electricity with some degree of confidence. These *contracts for differences* underpin the electricity market. They are called *contracts for differences* because payments are made by the parties involved to make good the difference between the pool price and the agreed contract price. Under this system, if the pool price falls below the contract price, the supply company remunerates the generator for the difference between the two prices, and vice versa if the pool price is above the contract price. The price of most of the electricity bought and sold is fixed in advance by *contracts for differences*. Hence the vast majority of electricity that is traded in England and Wales is purchased outside of the electricity pool.

3.4.1 The Evolution of the UK Electricity Market

The electricity pool described in Section 3.4 has become the basis for a number of other trading pools set up during the 1990s in Europe. However, in the UK, during the late 1990s, concerns were expressed that the pool system:

- Favoured the large generating companies; indeed there was suspicion that these companies were able in some way to control the pool price.
- Inhibited the introduction of new independent energy traders into the market.
- Inhibited the negotiation of bilateral electricity supply contracts between various parties.

The last point is an important one. In most trading deals the customer can state the price at which they wish to purchase a commodity and this has an influence on the overall market price. However, under the pool system the 'market price' (i.e. the pool price) was wholly determined by the sellers (i.e. the generating companies). The pool could therefore be viewed as being in some way only 'half a market' [4].

As a result of the concerns stated above, the UK completely restructured its electricity trading arrangements in 2000 and introduced the 'New Electricity Trading Arrangement' (NETA) [5]. This new arrangement abolished the old centrally regulated pool in favour of a 'free-market' approach which allowed a series of 'power exchanges' (i.e. electricity commodity markets) to be established; the hope being that the exchanges and brokers would create forwards, futures, and short-term bilateral markets. The intention was that the true price of electricity would become established through the power exchanges in much the same way that the commodity markets fix the price of other traded commodities. However, while the power exchanges can facilitate trade in 'bulk' energy, there is no way in which they can satisfy the physical engineering requirements of NGC (the operators of the transmission grid), who need to predict accurately at any point in time the demand on their network. Because electricity cannot be stored, the NGC must bring online more generating capacity as demand rises, otherwise power cuts will occur. Clearly, no commodity market can solve this problem alone! So the NETA arrangements were designed to operate in parallel with the new power exchanges, so that every time a bilateral contract is signed between a generator and a supplier they are required to inform NGC (or its settlements agent) of the quantity of electricity traded and the duration of the contract. It should be noted that parties are not required to notify NGC of the price paid for the electricity. All the supply companies and the generating companies are also required to notify NGC in advance of their expected operating levels for the following day. So by 11.00 hours on the day before trading, both the generators and the suppliers must submit to NGC their forecasts of demand, on a minute-by-minute basis, for the day ahead. They can do this because all parties know the quantity of electricity they have contracted to supply or purchase for the following day. By 'gate closure' (i.e. 3.5 hours before real time) the suppliers and generators must submit finalized demand forecasts to NGC. In this way NGC can effectively manage the transmission grid and inform the individual generators of the generating plant that will be required for the following day.

In theory the demand profiles predicted by the supply companies should exactly match the generation profiles predicted by the generating companies. In reality this never happens because it is difficult to accurately predict demand for electricity on a daily basis. A large number of factors influence electricity consumption, including weather and television scheduling. Since many variables influence electricity consumption, it is inevitable that the true demand for electricity will vary from the demand predicted by the supply companies. This means that NGC will have to bring online (or take offline) at short notice, additional generating plant in order to cope with variations from the predicted values. This of course incurs additional expense on behalf of the generating companies who have either to bring online extra plant or lay off generating plant which it had planned to operate. These 'imbalance costs' (i.e. costs incurred due to deviations from bilateral supply contracts) are calculated by NGC through a complex series of counter 'bids' and 'offers' made by both the generators and the suppliers. In this way NETA determines only the unit price of electricity which is 'traded' at the margins (i.e. outside of the power exchanges). It is intended that the 'imbalance' electricity costs will be higher than the 'bulk' electricity price, thus encouraging both the generators and the suppliers accurately to forecast predicted demand.

From the discussion above it is evident that in order to accommodate the engineering constraints of a transmission grid and facilitate a commodity market in electricity, extremely complex trading arrangements must be set up. Given this, it is understandable that competition in the electricity supply sector has been slow to evolve. Indeed, it would have been impossible without recent rapid advances in information technology (IT) in general and the Internet in particular. Without these IT advances, it would be impossible to rapidly transfer the large amounts of data associated with the bidding process to the many parties involved in a power exchange.

3.4.2 The Californian Experience

From the discussion in Section 3.4.1, it is clear that facilitating a true competitive market in electricity is an extremely complex process. Indeed, the electricity supply industry is of such strategic importance that if the deregulation process goes wrong, it can have a catastrophic effect on the whole economy. With this in mind, the experience of the Californian electricity supply industry should be a salutary lesson to all legislators who might be considering deregulating their utility sector. In January 2001, large parts of the state of California suffered major power cuts, not because of any technical failures, but as a direct result of poorly thought out legislation [6].

In 1996, the California Assembly voted to deregulate the state's electricity indus-try and to dismantle what was considered to be a government-regulated monopoly [7]. Prior to deregulation, the state had a vertically integrated electricity supply industry, with a number of investor-owned utility companies owning and operating their own power stations, transmission grids and distribution networks. With deregulation, a non-profit making organization, the California Power Exchange, was established and the fol-lowing changes were made:

- Operational control of the transmission grids was transferred to a single Independent System Operator who became responsible for the management of the system.
- The investor-owned utility companies, such as Southern California Edison and Pacific Gas and Electric, were forced to sell most of their power stations to other unregulated private companies. This forced the major utility companies to purchase wholesale electricity through the California Power Exchange.
- The California Power Exchange acted as a wholesale commodities market, through which all the state's electricity was bought and sold. An auction process therefore set the price of wholesale electric power.

The investor-owned utility companies did, however, retain ownership and control of their distribution networks.

By making these changes the California legislature created a classic model for a com-petitive, deregulated electricity supply industry. However, there were two critical fac-tors which were to have a significant influence on the events that were to follow:

1. While deregulation forced the utility companies to purchase their power on the open market and pay market prices, it prevented them from passing on any increases in the cost of wholesale electricity to their customers until at least 31 March 2002 [7].
2. Because of environmental concerns the state authorities prevented the building of new power stations. For 20 years or more, there had been no significant increase in California's generating capacity, despite the fact that demand for electricity in the state had been growing at approximately 2% each year [7].

These two critical factors were to have disastrous consequences for California in general and its electricity supply industry in particular. What the state legislature had done was to force the utility companies to buy wholesale electricity on the open market, which can be extremely volatile, while at the same time effectively fixing the price at which the utilities could sell electricity to their customers. The failings of this strategy were compounded by the fact that there was little excess generating capacity in the system. Without excess capacity there was little competitive pressure to keep whole-sale prices low. As a result during the summer of 2000, when demand for power peaked, the utility companies urgently needed power from the electricity wholesal-ers and generating companies, who promptly raised their prices. Bulk electricity prices rose steeply, with the average price of electricity bought through the Power Exchange rising from approximately $30 per MWh in January 2000 to $330 in January 2001 [8]. In fact, in December 2000 the price reached a peak of $1400 per MWh [7]. Unable to recoup these inflated costs from their customers, the utility companies, not surprisingly, started to lose money. They rapidly ran out of money, with the two largest utilities, Southern California Edison and Pacific Gas and Electric, claiming that by January 2001 their combined losses exceeded $9 billion [7]. Indeed, Pacific Gas and Electric filed for bankruptcy in April 2001 [9]. The financial difficulties of the utility companies had two direct consequences:

1. The banks became very reluctant to lend more money to the cash-starved utility companies, who were rapidly becoming insolvent.
2. The wholesale and generating companies became reluctant to sell electricity to utility companies which were obviously in financial difficulties.

Faced with such high financial losses and not wanting to lose any more money, the utility companies took the only course of action available to them: they stopped purchasing electricity and the state of California suffered major power cuts. The state authorities then had to step in and try to pick up the pieces and sort the mess out.

The sorry state of affairs that occurred in California graphically highlights the major problems which can occur if all the issues involved in deregulation are not thought out in advance. Clearly, the combination of a shortage in generating capacity and an unregulated wholesale market, facilitating what is in effect an energy cartel, is a recipe for disaster.

3.5 Competition in the Gas Market

In many ways facilitating competition in the gas market is similar to the electricity market. As with electricity supply, horizontal integration is the key to a competitive gas market. However, there are a number of fundamental differences which make trading in natural gas much simpler than trading electricity:

- Natural gas is not generated; it is pumped out of oil and gas fields at sea or on land and sold to licensed shippers (i.e. wholesale supply companies) who sell it on to customers.
- Unlike electricity, natural gas can be stored to a limited extent.
- Demand for natural gas is very seasonal.

Given the differences between the nature of gas and electricity, a relatively simple horizontally integrated model is required to facilitate a competitive market in gas (as shown in Figure 3.4).

Because there are only three parties involved in the process and also because gas can be stored, the whole structure is much simpler to control and operate than that of an electricity supply industry. However, in order to ensure that the system functions in a fair and equitable manner it is important that the gas transmission company charges equal transportation fees to all suppliers and that all fees should be transparent.

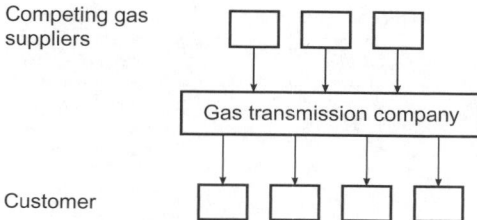

FIG 3.4 Horizontally integrated gas supply industry.

Under a horizontally integrated gas supply structure, individual customers are free to negotiate bilateral supply contracts with various competing suppliers. The price paid by the customer is the price the supplier pays for the gas at the 'beachhead' plus the cost of transportation plus the supplier's profit. However, the price paid by the customer is mainly affected by the cost of gas at the beachhead.

It is the responsibility of the gas transmission company to balance supply and demand on its network on a continual basis. If too much gas enters the network then it must be stored in underground caverns or gasometers. Conversely, if too little enters the network, then gas from the storage vessels will have to be utilized. Suppliers therefore have to ensure that the gas they put into the network is roughly equal to the gas that their customers use. If they miscalculate either way by too great a margin, then the transmission company will levy a penalty charge on them.

3.6 Load Management of Electricity

From the discussions in Section 3.4 it can be seen that the 'true' cost of electricity production varies with demand on the network, and that through the use of pricing mechanisms such as the 'pool' it is possible to introduce real-time electricity pricing. Under this scenario *when electricity is consumed* becomes as important as *how much electricity is consumed*. Those customers who have the ability to manage their electrical load should thus be in a good position to reduce energy costs.

An ability to manage electrical load not only reduces customers' electrical costs, it also enables them to negotiate more competitive electricity supply contracts. If a potential customer wishes to negotiate a supply contract, they will need to furnish potential suppliers with the following information:

- The annual consumption of electricity in kWh.
- The maximum demand in kW.
- The load factor.

The load factor for any given period represents the percentage of time for which plant and equipment operates during that period. It can be calculated as follows:

$$\text{Load factor} = \frac{\text{Energy consumed (kWh)}}{\text{Max. demand (kW)} \times \text{Time period (h)}} \times 100$$

TABLE 3.1 Typical load factors for a variety of applications [10]

Type of organization	Load factor
24-hour operation	0.7–0.85
Two shift system	0.45–0.6
Single shift system	0.25–0.4
Modern hotel complex	0.5–0.6
Hospital	0.6–0.75
Retailing	0.3–0.4
Catering business	0.3–0.5

Table 3.1 shows some typical load factors which might be expected for a various types of organizations [10]. Buildings such as air-conditioned commercial offices, with a high daytime peak and a low night-time demand, will exhibit a low (i.e. poor) load factor. At the other extreme, factories which operate a 24-hour shift system will exhibit a high (i.e. good) load factor.

From the utility companies' point of view, organizations which possess a high load factor are potentially more desirable customers, since they will be buying more electrical energy for a given amount of investment in generation and distribution equipment. Customers who possess high load factors should therefore expect to negotiate better supply contracts than those with low load factors. This provides great potential benefit to contract customers who possess the ability to load shift from day to night by using technologies such as ice thermal storage (see Chapter 13). This should be particularly true for office buildings which would otherwise exhibit a very poor load factor.

3.7 Supply Side and Demand Side

The collective term for the operations performed by utility companies is the 'supply side', whereas energy consumption by customers is referred to as the 'demand side'; so named because customers create a demand for energy which is then supplied by utility companies. These concepts are illustrated in Figure 3.5.

Consider the case of an electricity utility company which experiences an overload of its system during the daytime in the winter months. The company cannot meet the increase in demand with its existing generating plant and is therefore faced with the choice of either building more power stations or encouraging its customers to consume less electricity and thus reduce electrical demand during the daytime. The former solution is a 'supply-side measure' since the solution lies wholly with the utility company (i.e. on the supply side) and the latter is termed a 'demand-side measure' since the solution to the problem lies with the customer. The demand-side solution could be achieved by introducing an electricity tariff offering lower unit charges to customers who are prepared to switch their electricity consumption from the daytime to the night-time. Through management of the 'demand side' in this way it is possible for utility

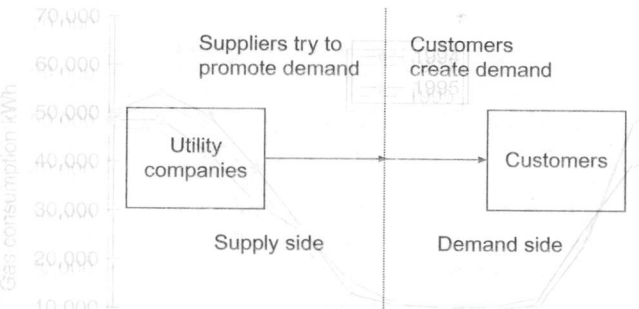

FIG 3.5 Concept of supply side and demand side.

companies to utilize their resources efficiently and thus achieve substantial cost savings. Demand-side measures are therefore concerned with direct intervention in the customer's end use of electricity by the utility company, in a way which affects the planning of the utility company's infrastructure.

Traditionally electricity utility companies have tended to rely on supply-side measures to shape their businesses; that is, the utility companies have tried to influence the way in which their customers use electricity from the supply side of the meter, and have provided the infrastructure to meet the predicted demand. However, in recent years, both in the UK and the USA, there has been increasing interest in the use of demand-side measures.

3.8 Demand-Side Management

The concept of DSM (sometimes referred to as 'least cost planning') was pioneered in the USA during the 1980s, where it has since become an influential force. In some parts of the USA the electrical demand can increase by as much as 40% during the summer months, due to the use of air-conditioning equipment [11]. There is also stiff legislative opposition from the Public Utility Commissioners to the construction of new power stations. Faced with this situation many utility companies in the USA have introduced DSM programmes to encourage customers to conserve energy, and persuade as many as possible to shift their daytime load to the night-time. In the USA, DSM programmes include such measures as financial support for feasibility studies, free advice on techniques, capital grants towards the cost of new equipment and even the free issue to customers of low energy light bulbs. Many utility companies in the USA have found it more economical to persuade their customers to conserve energy, rather than be forced to build new generating plant. A typical example of this is that of Pacific Gas and Electricity, which in 1985 announced that it intended to 'build' a new power plant; a 1000 MW conservation power plant. In other words they intended to buy extra efficiency improvements which would reduce their peak demand by 1000 MW [12].

Simple analysis of energy consumption demonstrates the great benefit of encouraging energy conservation over the construction of new generating plant. If it assumed that a typical thermal power station has an efficiency of 35%, then the overall primary energy saved through the conservation of 1 kWh of delivered electrical energy is:

$$\text{Primary energy saved} = \frac{1}{0.35} = 2.86 \text{ kWh}$$

From this it is obvious that in energy conservation terms, encouraging customers to conserve electrical energy makes much sense. Nevertheless, in order to persuade the utility companies to adopt an energy conservation strategy, it must also make commercial sense. In the late 1980s, Ontario Hydro of Canada estimated that meeting its peak demand obligations through supply-side measures (i.e. constructing new generating plant and reinforcing transmission and distribution networks) would cost the utility four times as much as using demand-side measures [13]. The findings of Ontario Hydro are backed up by Rosenfeld and de la Moriniere [14] who demonstrated in 1985 the cost of constructing new generating capacity to be in the region of $1200–$1500/kW, which compared very poorly with the maximum of $400/kW of electricity saved which could be achieved by using an ice storage system. It is therefore clearly in the interests of vertically integrated utility companies, such as those that exist in many parts of the USA and Europe, to encourage the installation of DSM technologies. To this end, many of the utility companies in the USA offer substantial capital incentives to building users to install technologies such as low energy light fittings and ice thermal storage [12].

Although DSM has become an influential force in the USA, its country of origin, the UK has been slow to adopt it. The UK does not suffer from a shortage of generating capacity, as is the case in some parts of the USA. It also experiences a winter peak, unlike many states in the USA. In addition, in England and Wales the electricity supply industry is not vertically integrated as much of the USA still is, thus making comparisons between the two countries very difficult. However, despite the obvious differences between the electricity supply industries in the USA and England and Wales, the regional distribution companies in the UK have recently become interested in DSM, since it is one method by which they can significantly reduce the demand on their cables and transformers, and thus reduce their operating and capital investment costs.

Because of the complex nature of the UK's horizontally integrated electricity supply industry, the role of DSM in the UK is somewhat ambiguous. In theory the widespread introduction of DSM should:

- Produce a reduction in the fuel burnt at power stations.
- Cause the deferral of the capital and financing costs of new power station construction.
- Cause a reduction in distribution losses.
- Result in the possible deferral of distribution reinforcement.
- Cause a reduction in transmission losses.
- Result in the possible deferral of transmission reinforcement associated with both new power plants and increased loads.
- Lead to a reduction in the emissions of CO_2, SO_2 and NO_2 from power stations.

While at first sight all the above points seem to indicate that there is a strong case for implementing DSM policies in the UK, further analysis casts doubt on the validity of the statement above. In theory all parties in the UK electricity supply industry benefit from the introduction of DSM. Yet, because of the fragmentation of the industry due to horizontal integration it is difficult to initiate and coordinate an effective DSM policy. For example, who will pay for a DSM policy? Are the regional distribution companies going to pay for a policy which arguably gives greatest benefits to the generators and the NGC? It is also difficult for the competing generators to initiate DSM, since they have no 'captive' market and they have little direct influence over the end-users. Also, the structure of the electricity market is such that individual generators are always seeking to generate as much electricity as possible. The benefit to the generators through the implication of a DSM policy is dubious to say the least, since there is overcapacity in the system, and every generator benefits from higher electricity prices when demand is high. Therefore, for DSM to succeed in the UK it must benefit both the regional distribution companies and their customers.

3.8.1 The USA Experience

The US-based energy research body the Electrical Power Research Institute (EPRI) defines DSM as:

The planning, implementation and monitoring of utility activities designed to influence customer use of electricity in ways that will produce desired changes in load shape [15]

In the USA, DSM programmes are often initiated by the Public Utility Commissioners who are intent on minimizing the construction of new generating plant. Utility companies are required to demonstrate to the Commissioners that their proposed course of action is the least expensive option for supplying customers with electricity. The onus is therefore on the utility companies to reduce demand rather than build more power stations. In some states in the USA, utilities are even being awarded bonuses for implementing DSM programmes.

Although DSM programmes in the USA have been initiated as a result of social concern and regulatory pressure, it is the potential for profit to the utility companies that has driven such programmes. In the USA the utilities are permitted to over-recover the costs of DSM programmes through increases in electricity prices. Consequently, the utilities receive a greater marginal return from demand-side measures than they would from supply measures. This has resulted in DSM programmes in North America being used on a large scale. Many North American utility companies spend more than 5% of their total turnover on investment in DSM. Table 3.2 shows the investment levels and targeted energy savings for some DSM programmes, operated by a variety of North American utility companies [16].

Although some of the DSM programmes included in Table 3.2 have not proved to be cost effective, many of the utility companies have reported that their DSM programmes have proved less expensive in total cost terms, when compared with the costs avoided

TABLE 3.2   Examples of North American utilities' expenditure on DSM [16]

Utility company	Current expenditure ($ millions)	Target GWh savings	Target MW savings	MW savings as % of projected peak	Target year for savings
BC Hydro	66	4491	1266	9.4	2000
Hydro Quebec	251	9289	5065	13.2	2000
Manitoba Hydro	8	931	255	4.7	2000
Ontario Hydro	377	14,911	5200	16.0	2000
Consolid. Edison	76	7120	2500	22.5	2008
Florida P & L	66	2800	1884	8.7	1999
Long Island	33	2840	589	11.4	2008
Nevada Power	5	190	147	5.2	2007
New York State	25	2790	846	18.9	2004
Niagara Mohawk	37	2680	849	12	2008
Orange & Rock.	8	191	122	7.6	2008
Pacific G & E	120	5760	2270	11.1	2001
Rochester G & E	7	876	186	10.7	2009
Southern Calif.	107	5170	2780	11.2	2009
Wisconsin Elec.	40	1260	290	5.6	2000

on the supply side. These findings even applied in circumstances where the utility company had an excess of generating capacity.

When a DSM policy is introduced a utility company avoids generating costs, network losses, some administration charges, and may avoid capital expenditure on network reinforcement and expanding generating capacity. However, it also sells less electricity and is therefore liable to a loss of revenue through implementing a DSM programme.

To avoid this situation some form of 'balancing' mechanism must be provided to ensure that the utility company does not lose revenue. In the USA, this balancing mechanism is provided by a regulator, who approves an increase in tariffs for all customers, subject to the utility company demonstrating that the 'average' customer receives an overall reduction in energy costs [17].

In recent years the electricity supply industry in the USA has undergone major restructuring in order to facilitate wholesale trading in electricity in a similar way to the industry in the UK [18]. Despite the uncertainty that surrounds this change, the industry in the USA reported that in 1999, a total of 848 electricity utilities had DSM programmes and of this number, 459 'large' DSM programmes resulted in a 50.6 billion kWh energy saving [19].

3.8.2 The UK Experience

Unlike North America, where DSM programmes have become commonplace, DSM in the UK is still in its infancy. Under the old state-owned electricity supply industry, one of the few examples of a DSM policy in the UK was the introduction of the 'Economy 7' tariffs which were used in conjunction with night storage heaters. Over many years under the nationalized regime, night storage heaters were heavily marketed, the main objective being:

- To achieve better utilization of the nation's generating plant.
- To utilize the electricity distribution network more efficiently.
- To raise useful revenue for the regional electricity boards by selling the night storage heaters to the public.

The marketing of night storage heaters was an extremely successful policy – perhaps too successful. Analysis of the pool price profile for an average weekday in December 1992 (see Figure 3.6) shows that the PSP for some of the night-time is actually greater than the daytime (office hours) price. This was because of the generating capacity required at night-time to satisfy night storage heaters. However, this high night-time PSP was not reflected in the price paid by tariff customers, typically between a third to a half of the daytime price, for both domestic 'Economy 7' customers and a commercial maximum demand tariff customers. In the case of 'Economy 7', the off-peak price was set to compete with gas central heating in the domestic market. As a result the users of night storage heaters were in fact being subsidized by other customers who have to pay higher daytime prices.

The intensive marketing of night storage heaters meant that in some areas of the UK, the regional distribution networks experienced high night-time peaks. This caused problems and resulted in a number of regional distribution companies (who were also electricity suppliers) marketing flexible off-peak domestic tariffs. These flexible off-peak tariffs were designed to replace the old monolithic 'Economy 7' tariff, and offered customers 10 hours of off-peak electricity compared with the old 7-hour period [20]. A sample of one of these flexible tariffs is shown in Table 3.3 from which can be seen that the utility company is trying to utilize more effectively the troughs

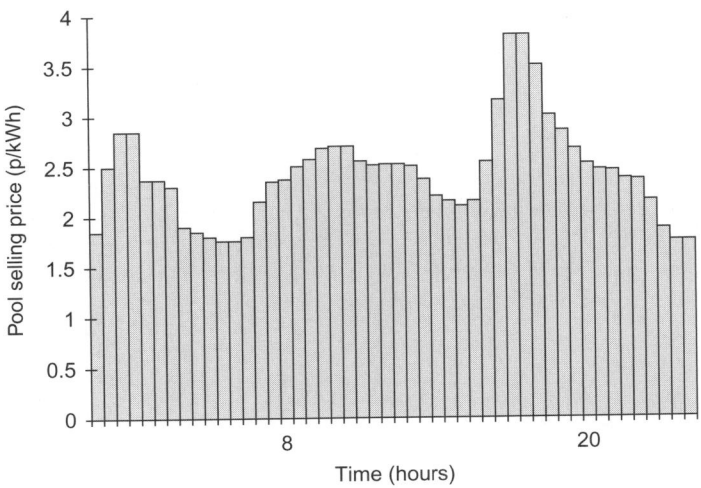

FIG 3.6 Average weekday pool selling price, December 1992.

TABLE 3.3 East Midlands electricity 'heatwise' tariff 1 May 1992 [20]

Off-peak supply is available for 10 hours	Monday to Friday	Saturday and Sunday
Five hours continuously during night	00.00–7.00	00.00–8.00
Three hours continuously during afternoon	13.00–16.30	13.00–17.30
Two hours continuously during evening	17.30–22.00	17.30–22.00
Standing quarterly charge	£3.90	
Unit charges:		
Off-peak	2.90p/kWh	
Peak	7.64p/kWh	

in the UK's daily demand profile, which generally correspond to periods when electricity prices are low.

To the regional distribution companies these flexible tariffs have a number of advantages. They shift much of the off-peak period from its 'traditional' night-time slot to the daytime and evening periods, so that troughs in the daytime demand can be exploited. They also have inherent flexibility which allows the utility company to control the precise start and stop times of the 'off-peak' periods and allows these to be varied from day to day.

The regional distribution companies receive two major benefits from these flexible tariffs:

1. They achieve better utilization of their distribution networks and avoid capital expenditure on network reinforcement.
2. If they are also a supply company, the regional distribution company can purchase electricity from the generators at periods when prices are low and sell it on to their customers for heating purposes at the standard tariff price. Consequently, they have more scope for increasing profit margins in their supply business.

To implement flexible tariffs such as the one outlined above involves the installation of complex metering equipment, which is capable of both recording the electricity consumption at the various periods of the day and also of receiving switching signals from the utility company concerned, to activate the 'off-peak' period on the meter. To achieve this in the domestic market the utility companies offering these tariffs have to use a radio tele-switching system.

If the subject of night storage heaters is set aside, DSM in the UK is being driven primarily by those regional distribution companies which are experiencing network problems [21,22]. The position of the generators towards DSM is ambivalent, since it is unclear how they would benefit commercially. Therefore, the potential benefits of DSM in the UK are perceived to lie in enabling the distribution companies to optimize their existing networks.

Electricity companies always seek to maximize their returns on their investment in generation, transmission and distribution equipment. In the past, increasing electricity demand has ensured that whenever a system needed reinforcement in order to maintain security of supply, the capital investment could be recouped from increased electricity sales. Before deregulation, the electricity supply industry used vigorously to promote the use of electricity in the hope of maximizing sales. This situation has, however, changed. The electricity market in the UK is a mature one. Sales of electricity have steadied and predicted growth is low. In some areas electricity sales are static or even declining. Distribution companies cannot look to increased sales to finance system reinforcement. Under this scenario DSM becomes an important option which the distribution companies must consider.

From the position of the competing generators in the UK, it is unlikely that DSM is going to gain much support. Electricity prices tend to be high when demand is high. Therefore all the generators benefit from high demand. From a generator's point of view, DSM can be viewed as a competitor since it reduces electricity sales.

DSM programmes cost money to implement, especially if they involve capital grants to customers to purchase energy efficient or load shifting equipment. Therefore the utility companies need some mechanism to recoup investment costs. In the USA, utility companies are allowed to increase tariff prices to all their customers to pay for DSM programmes. In effect the ordinary customers of the utility companies are subsidizing those customers benefiting from the DSM measure. In the UK the regulatory authorities will not allow this approach to paying for DSM, since it both distorts the market and is 'unfair' on franchise customers. Indeed, the regulatory authorities in the UK appear to be opposed to the widespread adoption of such schemes on the grounds that they represent a cross-subsidy between customers. The distribution companies must therefore recoup their DSM programme costs from those customers who benefit directly from it.

References

[1] European electricity deregulation progress. www.commodities-now.com.
[2] National Grid Company. Seven Year Statement; 1994.
[3] Business focus. National Power Plc. Issue 3, July; 1992.
[4] Littlechild S. Demand side bidding in the pool. OFFER 1993; 5 May.
[5] Haigh R. An overview of the New Electricity Trading Arrangements V1.0. OFGEM and DTI 2000; 31 May.
[6] Campbell D. Blackouts bring gloom to California. The Guardian 2001; 19 January.
[7] Feldman C. The California power quagmire. CNN.com, January 4. http://www.cnn.com/SPECIALS/views/y/2001/01/feldman.power.jan3, 29 March; 2001.
[8] Feldman C. California power crisis sends shock waves nationwide. CNN.com In-depth specials – power crisis. http://www.cnn.com/SPECIALS/2001/power.crisis, 29 March; 2001.
[9] National Energy Information Center Subsequent Events – California's energy crisis. http://www.eia.doe.gov/cneaf/electricity/california/subsequentevents.html, 12 July; 2001.
[10] Forrester R. Hard bargaining. Electr Rev 1993; 9–29 July: 32–34.
[11] Wendland RD. Storage to become rule, not exception. ASHRAE Journal 1987; May.
[12] Oliver D. The energy efficient way of life. CIBSE Journal 1986; June: 40.
[13] Redford SJ. Demand side management – intervention across the meter. CIBSE Journal 1995; June: 25.
[14] Rosenfeld A, de la Moriniere. The high cost-effectiveness of cold storage in new commercial buildings. ASHRAE Trans 1988: 818.
[15] Duguid T, Mee CA. The drivers behind the UK experience of DSM. Power Eng J 1994; October: 225–28.
[16] Demand side measures – a report to the office of electricity regulation. LE Energy Ltd. SRC International ApS, 12 October; 1992.
[17] Redford SJ. The rational for demand-side management. Power Eng J 1994; October: 211–17.
[18] DOE. U.S. electricity utility demand-side management: trends and analysis, DOE (USA).
[19] DOE. Electricity utility demand-side management. DOE (USA); 1999.
[20] Heatwise. East Midlands Electricity Plc. 1 May; 1992.
[21] Savings on demand. CIBSE Journal 1995; June: 29.
[22] Stanway J. The holyhead experience. Power Eng J 1994; October: 221.

CHAPTER 4

Energy and Transport

Efficient transport is vital to the performance of modern economies. However, oil reserves appear to be dwindling, raising questions about the sustainability of many forms of transport. In this chapter the issue of transport energy is discussed and the environmental impact of various modes of transport is assessed.

4.1 Transport and the Economy

Transport is important. Imagine what life would be like without the internal combustion or jet engine. Getting to work might be a problem, especially if your home is some distance from your place of work. Likewise, visiting family and friends would be much more difficult. This, however, would only be the tip of the iceberg. How would the countless food producers get their products onto the shelves of your local supermarket? Indeed, having managed to walk to the supermarket, how would you get your weekly 'shop' home? Furthermore, overseas travel would be much more difficult and imported goods would be scarce. In short, life would be considerably more difficult and parochial, as it was in Europe before the twentieth century and still is many parts of the developing world. It should therefore come as no surprise that transport is a subject of great importance to governments around the world – for without efficient transport systems, it is difficult for economies to grow, because labour and goods cannot be moved around easily. Efficient transport is therefore of vital importance to all societies as it impacts both

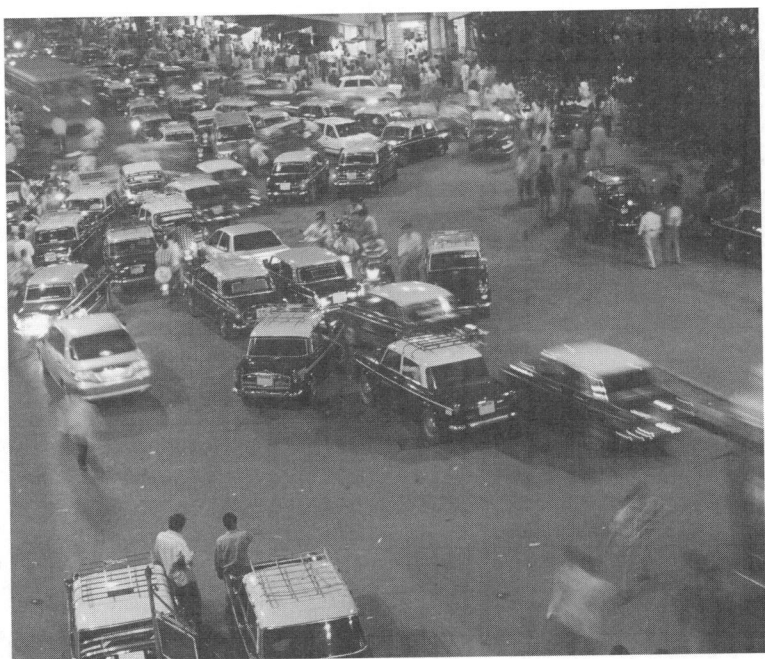

FIG 4.1 Typical urban scene in India illustrating the extent to which the citizens of such cities rely on motorized transport.

on their economic development and the welfare of populations as a whole. Efficient transport systems provide wide-ranging economic and social benefits whereas deficient systems impose economic costs in the form of missed or reduced opportunities.

Improved transport systems can benefit economies in two ways. Firstly, they enable people to gain access to places where they can engage in wealth-generating activities and can consume goods and services, including education and health care facilities. This ultimately leads to a healthier, better-educated society and enables larger markets to develop, thus saving time and reducing costs. Secondly, transport enables companies to access raw materials and parts with greater ease, thus reducing production costs. It also enables them to deliver their products to customers more easily. In so doing it acts as an intermediate input to production. In addition, transport plays an important social role enabling people to network and socialize, ultimately promoting the growth of leisure services and facilities.

Transport promotes mobility, and it is this that is considered by many economists to be a reliable indicator of economic development. Mobility satisfies one of the most basic characteristics of economic activity, the need to transport people, freight and information from one location to another. Economies that exhibit greater mobility therefore tend to have better opportunities to develop than those in which mobility is restricted. Reduced mobility impedes economic development, while greater mobility acts as a

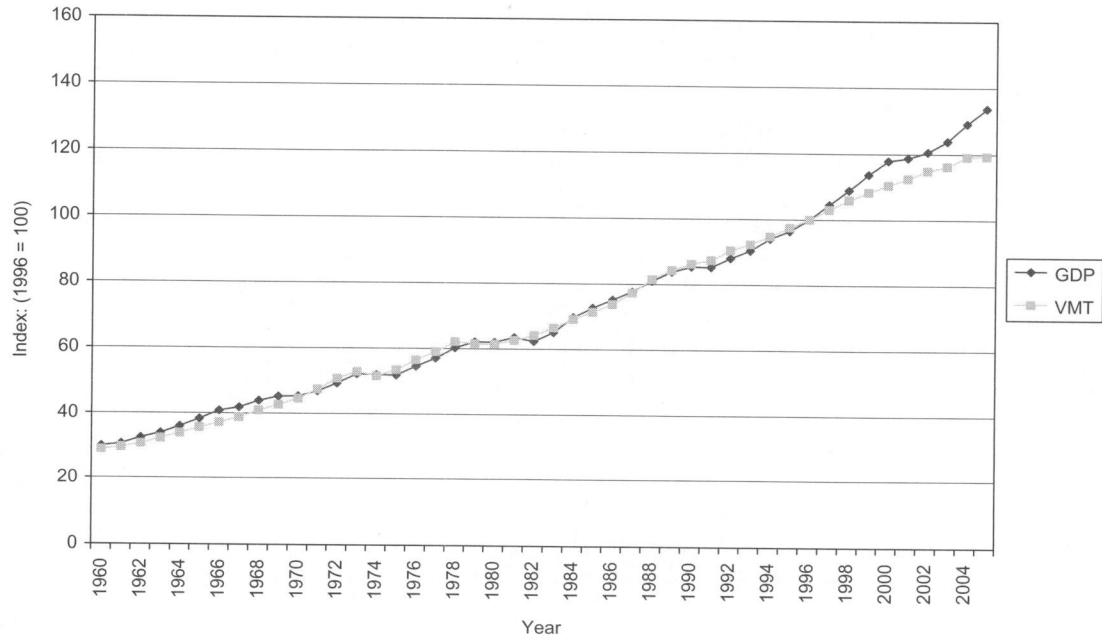

FIG 4.2 US gross domestic product and vehicle miles of travel indexes [1].

catalyst promoting growth. The importance of transport to a nation's economy is well illustrated in Figure 4.2 which shows highway vehicle miles travelled (VMT) in the USA and the US gross domestic product (GDP) [1]. From this it can be seen that there is a striking similarity between the VMT and GDP curves, indicating that a very strong relationship exists between the two. This reflects the fact that the efficient movement of people, raw materials and goods is a vital component of any economy. Without an adequate transport infrastructure and the fuel to power vehicles most economies very soon grind to a halt.

4.2 The History of Transport

For much of human history, travelling overland has been a difficult and dangerous business. Mountains, forests, ravines and other geographical features made land transport a slow and arduous experience. By comparison it was much easier to travel by boat along rivers and across seas. Consequently, early human settlements sprang up along rivers and coastlines. In time this led to the development of large seaports, which enabled nations to trade with each other. These seaports allowed sailors to navigate the globe in large vessels and enabled the maritime nations of Europe to grow wealthy on international trade through their colonial empires. Water transport also played an important role in the early stages of the industrial revolution. In the eighteenth and early nineteenth centuries the development of canal systems in Western Europe enabled companies to transport heavy goods over long distances with relative ease. In so doing they allowed manufacturing centres to flourish, for the first time, in inland locations.

In the mid-nineteenth century the railways emerged. These were much more flexible than the canals which preceded them and were the first truly integrated inland transportation system – enabling, for first time, the mass transport of both people and goods. With the expansion of the railways, the industrial centres of North America and Europe flourished and grew large. The twentieth century saw the development of road transport and automobile manufacturing. While this facilitated individual transportation for the masses, it was not until after the Second World War that automobile ownership became widespread. With this rise in car ownership also came improvements in highway infrastructure, with the result that travelling times were greatly reduced.

The later part of the twentieth century saw the development of global air transport. This enabled the masses, for the first time, to travel abroad and in so doing facilitated growth in international trade. The effect of this was to break down international boundaries and make the world a smaller place, an effect reinforced by the explosion in telecommunications that occurred in the later part of the twentieth century.

From the above, it can be seen that the history of transport mirrors that of the world's economic development. In a few hundred years the world has changed from what was essentially a collection of parochial societies, into an interconnected network dominated by global corporations. International trade is at the heart of this global economy, with countries like China becoming manufacturing powerhouses for the whole planet. Without an efficient international transport system it would be difficult for this global economy to function. Indeed, the economies of the world are now so dependent on international trade that it should come as no surprise that there is strong vested interest in ensuring that international transport continues to thrive.

4.3 Passenger Transport

At a national level the amount of energy consumed on transport depends very much on the distances travelled by passengers and goods, and the type of transport preferred by the population. Table 4.1 presents a breakdown of the modes of passenger transport used in various OECD countries [2]. These data reveal much about the behaviour of people in the various nations. For example, it can be seen that in North America people generally do not travel by bus or train, much preferring to travel by car – in Canada 95.2% of passenger travel is by car, while in the USA this figure is 96.4%. This reflects the petroleum prices in the USA and Canada, which are less than half of those in many OECD countries, making the cost of motoring in North America very cheap. At the other end of the scale, the Japanese appear much happier to travel by public transport, particularly by train, with only 61.6% of passengers travelling by automobile. In western and northern Europe car use is relatively high, whereas in Eastern Europe, where per capita incomes are lower, automobile use is somewhat less. It is also noticeable that in the larger OECD countries more people tend to travel further by automobile.

TABLE 4.1 Passenger transport data for various OECD countries for 2003 (including the average price of petroleum in each country) [2]

	Rail		Buses and coaches		Private cars		Petroleum price
	Billion passenger-kilometres	Percentage of total (%)	Billion passenger-kilometres	Percentage of total (%)	Billion passenger-kilometres	Percentage of total (%)	US dollars per litre
Belgium	8.3	6.3	13.7	10.4	109.9	83.3	1.50
Canada	1.4	0.3	22.0	4.5	462.6	95.2	0.68
Czech Republic	6.5	7.8	9.4	11.3	67.3	80.8	1.08
Denmark	5.6	7.4	9.0	11.9	61.5	80.8	1.51
Finland	3.3	4.7	7.7	10.9	59.6	84.4	1.54
France	72.3	8.5	42.6	5.0	738.6	86.5	1.42
Germany	70.8	7.8	75.8	8.3	764.4	83.9	1.46
Greece	1.6	3.6	6.2	14.2	35.9	82.2	1.14
Hungary	10.3	13.7	18.6	24.7	46.4	61.6	1.30
Italy	45.3	4.8	98.0	10.5	791.4	84.7	1.53
Japan	385.0	31.4	86.0	7.0	757.0	61.6	1.26
Netherlands	14.5	8.2	16.0	9.1	146.1	82.7	1.62
Norway	2.9	4.9	5.9	9.9	50.6	85.2	1.61
Poland	19.6	8.9	30.0	13.6	170.7	77.5	1.20
Portugal	3.6	3.6	10.5	10.5	85.9	85.9	1.38
Slovak Republic	2.3	6.6	7.8	22.0	25.2	71.5	1.17
Spain	21.1	5.1	49.3	11.8	346.5	83.1	1.21
Sweden	9.4	8.3	10.5	9.2	94.0	82.5	1.51
Switzerland	14.2	13.4	6.4	6.0	85.3	80.6	1.29
United Kingdom	40.9	5.6	47.0	6.4	647.3	88.0	1.56
United States	8.9	0.1	238.4	3.5	6543.7	96.4	0.54

This is partly because these nations have larger populations and also because they generally cover a greater geographical area. The longer travelling distances experienced in North America is evidenced by the very high passenger-kilometre values in the USA and Canada.

Although transport systems adhere in many ways to the same laws of supply and demand as those of other industries, they are complicated by network effects and differences in the various modes of transport. In particular, comfort and convenience are influential. For example, in the UK 88% of all passenger trips are made by car [2]. This high figure reflects the importance that individuals in the UK place on personal transport, as opposed to public transport. Cars are used to travel to work, school and the shops, as well as for commercial and leisure purposes. Given that cars can convey travellers and their luggage from door to door in privacy, and also facilitate entertainment on the journey, it is not surprising that so many opt for the comfort afforded by this mode of transport. The inherent dangers and expenses associated with automobiles are either not appreciated or are considered acceptable. Furthermore, for many travellers, particularly those in rural locations, the car is the only option – there is simply no other alternative form of transport.

Given the large number of passenger-kilometres travelled in the OECD countries it is not surprising that the energy consumed on transport in these countries is substantial. Table 4.2 presents a breakdown of the energy consumed by the transport sector in various OECD countries [2]. From this it can be seen that most OECD countries consume in the region of 25%–40% of total energy on transport.

4.4 Energy Consumption and Transport

Most vehicles that travel overland and many ships utilize internal combustion engines. Such engines use oil as fuel and tend to be very inefficient. For example, the thermal efficiency of a typical petrol engine is only about 26%, before mechanical inefficiencies are taken into account. This means that most standard engines have an overall efficiency of only about 20%. In other words, 80% of the fuel energy is lost to atmosphere as heat. By comparison, diesel engines which have a higher compression ratio than petrol engines have efficiencies around 45%, making them a much more energy-efficient option. Given that internal combustion engines are inefficient, automobile manufacturers have made strenuous efforts in recent years to improve the efficiency of petrol engines. However, despite significant improvements in engine efficiency, the average fuel efficiency of petrol-engine cars has remained relatively static [3], simply because more people now own large luxury cars. Indeed, in the USA, due to the growth in popularity of large sports utility vehicles (SUVs), average fuel efficiency has fallen to 20.4 mpg (US) in 2001, a substantial reduction from the 1987–1988 peak of 22.1 mpg [3].

Rail vehicles have become more efficient in recent years. In a recent study comparing a 30-year-old passenger train with a double-deck TGV train of the same capacity, it was found that the newer train exhibited half the aerodynamic drag per seat, when travelling at 150 km/h [4]. However, energy consumption rises dramatically when trains travel at speeds over 200 km/h [3], with the result that fuel savings arising from aerodynamic efficiency are often sacrificed in favour of improved performance.

While manufacturers of cars and trains tend to focus on mechanical efficiency, it can be seen from the above discussion that overall efficiency is strongly influenced by the way in which vehicles are used, something that is wholly dictated by the user. This fact alone makes it very difficult to make energy comparisons between vehicle types, because many user-related variables affect energy performance. While mechanical efficiency is of some relevance, what really matters is the energy consumed per passenger-kilometre – something that depends wholly on the extent to which cars, buses and

TABLE 4.2 Energy consumed by the transport sector in various OECD countries for 2003 [2]

	Industry (mtoe^3)	Industry (%)	Transport (mtoe^3)	Transport (%)	Other (mtoe^3)	Other (%)	Total (mtoe^3)
Australia	25.77	35.66	29.18	40.38	17.32	23.97	72.27
Austria	9.28	33.05	7.81	27.81	10.99	39.14	28.08
Belgium	16.95	39.72	10.42	24.42	15.29	35.83	42.67
Canada	74.42	37.68	54.34	27.52	68.73	34.80	197.49
Czech Republic	10.44	39.35	6.11	23.03	9.98	37.62	26.53
Denmark	3.12	20.37	5.05	32.96	7.15	46.67	15.32
Finland	12.64	48.17	4.76	18.14	8.85	33.73	26.24
France	49.54	28.63	52.82	30.52	70.70	40.85	173.06
Germany	77.36	31.49	64.03	26.06	104.28	42.45	245.67
Greece	5.10	23.62	8.03	37.19	8.46	39.18	21.59
Hungary	4.80	25.26	3.87	20.37	10.33	54.37	19.00
Iceland	0.91	38.56	0.33	13.98	1.12	47.46	2.36
Ireland	2.36	20.22	4.55	38.99	4.76	40.79	11.67
Italy	48.09	34.55	44.36	31.87	46.73	33.58	139.18
Japan	146.89	41.55	93.41	26.42	113.23	32.03	353.53
Korea	66.20	47.09	34.58	24.60	39.79	28.31	140.57
Luxembourg	0.90	22.33	2.39	59.31	0.74	18.36	4.03
Mexico	31.44	32.49	41.63	43.02	23.70	24.49	96.78
Netherlands	24.31	39.13	15.11	24.32	22.71	36.56	62.12
New Zealand	4.94	37.17	5.54	41.69	2.81	21.14	13.29
Norway	9.25	44.19	4.78	22.84	6.90	32.97	20.93
Poland	19.81	33.17	11.49	19.24	28.43	47.61	59.72
Portugal	8.06	38.64	7.31	35.04	5.50	26.37	20.86
Slovak Republic	4.90	43.56	2.21	19.64	4.14	36.80	11.25
Spain	38.07	37.99	37.89	37.81	24.25	24.20	100.21
Sweden	14.16	39.55	8.45	23.60	13.20	36.87	35.80
Switzerland	4.56	21.14	7.03	32.59	9.98	46.27	21.57
Turkey	23.59	39.31	13.20	22.00	23.22	38.69	60.01
United Kingdom	44.10	27.46	53.79	33.49	62.73	39.05	160.62
United States	459.21	29.23	634.60	40.39	477.28	30.38	1571.09

trains are filled with passengers. If a large intercity train carries only a handful of passengers, then the fuel consumption per passenger-kilometre will be much greater than if it was full. Consequently, it is often difficult to make direct energy efficiency comparisons between different forms of transport, and assumptions about passenger loading and engine size must be made, which may, or may not, be realistic.

In an attempt to make a direct comparison between different modes of transport, Kemp [5] undertook a study of the relative energy consumption per seat for a journey from London to Edinburgh. The study was designed to evaluate the energy efficiency of trains travelling at speeds in excess of 200 km/h. In the study, comparison was made between an aeroplane (Airbus A321), a modern diesel-powered car (VW Passat TDI) and two hypothetical trains, running at 225 km/h and 350 km/h, respectively. The results of this study are presented in Figure 4.3, from which it can be seen that the primary fuel consumed per seat by a 225 km/h train is much the same as that used by a modern diesel car (i.e. about 23 litres per seat when both vehicles are 50% full). Surprisingly, the diesel car consumed considerably less energy than the high-speed train travelling at 350 km/h. Even more surprisingly, the aeroplane consumed slightly less fuel than the high-speed train. Indeed, when travelling at the higher speed the train consumed almost twice as much fuel as it did when travelling at 225 km/h [3].

The implications of Kemp's work are far reaching because they challenge the rather simplistic notion, often pervaded, that cars and aircraft are bad and trains are good. Clearly, the amount of primary energy consumed per seat depends on vehicle passenger loading and, in the case of trains, the speed at which they are operated.

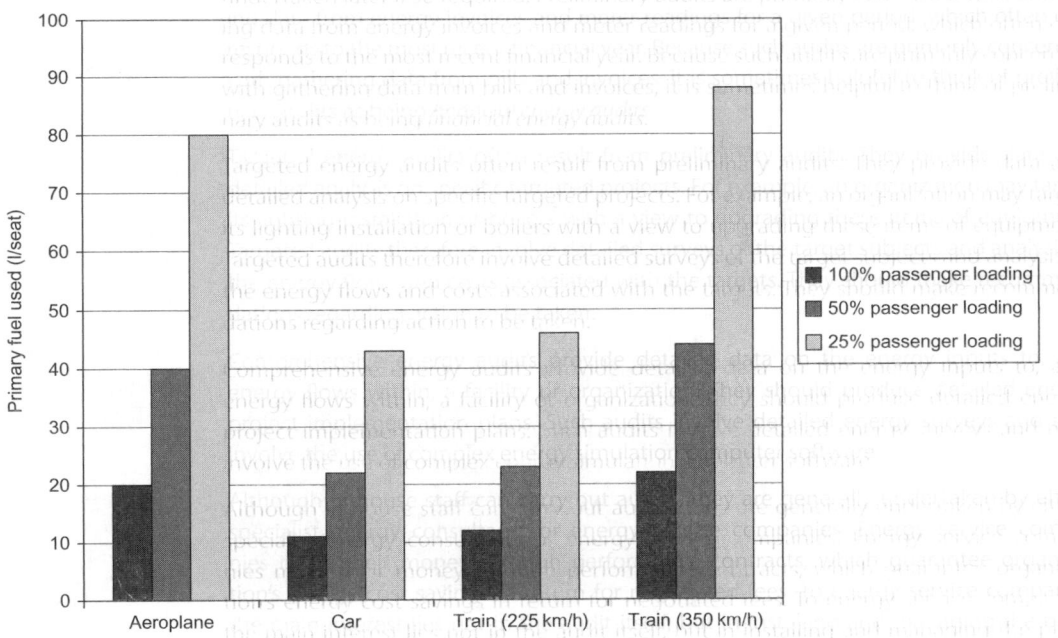

FIG 4.3 Comparison of the energy consumed by various forms of transport from London to Edinburgh [3,5].

4.4.1 Carbon Dioxide Emissions

In 2007 the UK government published 'real-life' carbon dioxide (CO_2) emission data for various types of passenger vehicles [6]. These data were designed to give an accurate indicator of the CO_2 emissions produced by various vehicles under realistic scenarios and allowed for things such as air conditioning and typical driving practice. Table 4.3 presents the real-life CO_2 emissions for various types of motor vehicle. From these data it can be seen that petrol-engine cars produce considerably more CO_2 than diesel cars, with petrol–electric hybrids producing less than both – about the same as a large motorbike.

Table 4.4 shows similar data for aviation transport [6]. These data are presented in terms of CO_2 emissions per passenger-kilometre for domestic, short-haul and long-haul flights, respectively. From these data it can be seen that longer flights tend to produce fewer CO_2 emissions. The reason for this is that large amounts of fuel are consumed

TABLE 4.3   Comparison of the 'real-life' carbon dioxide produced per kilometre travelled for various vehicle types [6]

Vehicle type	Engine size (litres)	Miles per gallon	Grams of CO_2 produced per km
Petrol car	<1.4	35.5	183.1
	1.4–2.0	30.1	216.2
	>2.0	21.9	296.4
Diesel car	<1.7	49.3	150.7
	1.7–2.0	39.5	188.1
	>2.0	28.2	263.5
Hybrid petrol–electric car	Medium	51.5	126.2
Motorbike	<0.125	89.2	72.9
	0.125–0.5	69.2	93.9
	>0.5	50.6	128.6

TABLE 4.4   Comparison of the 'real-life' carbon dioxide produced per passenger-kilometre travelled for various aviation flights [6]

Flight type	Example flight	Load factor (%)	Grams of CO_2 produced per passenger km
Domestic	London to Edinburgh	65	158.0
Short-haul international	London to central Europe	65	130.4
Long-haul international	London to New York	79.7	105.6

during take-off and landing, which makes up a greater component of a domestic flight compared with a long-haul international flight.

Comparison between the data presented in Tables 4.3 and 4.4 reveals the rather surprising finding that air travel is not as environmentally unfriendly as some might think. The data suggest that taking a short-haul international flight (provided that the aircraft is relatively full) is almost as 'environmentally friendly' as travelling to the same destination on a large motorbike. Indeed, the data suggest that a single person travelling in a hybrid petrol–electric car would produce about the same amount of CO_2 as a person travelling on a short-haul international flight. Of course if four persons were to travel in the car, then that would be a much more environmentally friendly option.

If nothing else, the above discussion highlights the difficulties associated with promoting environmentally friendly transport. Small changes in the assumptions made during the calculation process can radically alter the conclusions reached, and it is all too easy to make assumptions which neatly fit current political thinking so that the 'correct' answer is reached. However, history is littered with 'politically correct' answers, which turned out to be failures. It is therefore important to make decisions that are based on sound knowledge and accurate assumptions.

4.5 Oil

As the world's economy grows, so its transport sector continues to expand and with it the demand for oil. Oil is, however, a finite resource, which is being consumed at an increasing rate and which will eventually run out. Consequently, the future is somewhat uncertain and it is difficult to make accurate predictions about how the crude-oil markets will behave. This uncertainty is well illustrated by the '2007 International Energy Outlook' [7] which predicted, under a worst-case scenario, that the price of oil might reach $100 per barrel by 2030, when in fact the price reached $139 per barrel in June 2008 [8]. Clearly gazing into the future is never easy! However, while it might be difficult to predict the future price of crude oil with any degree of accuracy, it is probably safe to assume in the medium/long term that as demand rises and stocks decrease, so the price of oil will increase.

It has been predicted that demand for petroleum will rise from its 2004 level of 83 million barrels oil equivalent per day to 118 million barrels by 2030 [7], with most of this increase being consumed by the transport sector. Two regions in particular, North America and non-OECD Asia, are predicted to experience large increases in demand for oil. Indeed, it is thought that in non-OECD Asia the growth in oil consumption will average 2.7% per year from 2004 to 2030 [7]. Whether or not this prediction will prove to be correct, only time can tell. However, as the economies of China and India rapidly industrialize, it seems reasonable to presume that in these 'thirsty' nations the demand for petroleum will continue to increase.

Given that oil reserves are finite and that demand for oil is increasing, it might seem reasonable to assume that oil will run out in the near future. Indeed, many commentators have spent much time pondering on this doomsday scenario. However, because of market forces, things are not quite as simple as that. While the era of cheap oil may be nearing its end, it would be wrong to assume that oil reserves are going to run out soon. Paradoxically, the very fact that oil prices are likely to rise should ensure that the world will be supplied with oil for many years to come [9]. This is because as the price of crude oil rises, two things happen:

- Firstly, the cost of motoring greatly increases, with the result that motorists will try to reduce petroleum consumption. They may take up cycling, switch to public transport or opt for smaller more energy-efficient cars. Ultimately this will lead to the development of technologies and transport systems that are more energy efficient, resulting in a reduced demand for oil.
- Secondly, as the price of oil increases, so it becomes financially more worthwhile to exploit those reserves that hitherto might have been considered uneconomic. It is important to remember that at any point in time oil reserves are simply a best estimate of how much oil can be economically produced at today's prices using today's technology [9]. Currently (2008), the economic recovery factor for most oil fields is typically about 40% [9], which means that 60% of the oil does not appear on the reserves estimate because its extraction is deemed to be uneconomic. If the price of oil increases, then it becomes worthwhile for the oil companies to exploit these uneconomic oil deposits. Furthermore, it becomes a financially viable proposition to develop new improved technologies for extracting oil deposits that previously might have been too difficult to reach. Consequently, as the price of oil increases, so the reserves of oil also effectively increase [9].

From the above discussion it can be seen that although petroleum is likely to be with us for many years to come, it is unlikely to be the cheap fuel that we have known in the past. However, the very fact that oil is likely to become more expensive should change the behaviour of consumers and result in the development of transport vehicles and systems that are likely to be more fuel efficient.

4.6 Biofuels

With increased concern about global warming there has been a trend in recent years towards the production of so-called biofuels (petroleum and diesel substitutes) from crops such as maize (corn), soybean and sugar cane. Some have hailed these new biofuels as 'green' carbon-neutral fuels, because the crops absorb CO_2 from the atmosphere as they grow. Indeed, such are the green credentials of biofuels that the US government has encouraged farmers to produce crops for biofuel rather than for food – in 2007 around a fifth of the US maize harvest was brewed into ethanol [10]. However, the green credentials of such fuels are somewhat dubious. The problem is that when the crop is fermented it is necessary to distil off the neat ethanol and this process requires considerable heat energy. In the USA it is common practice for ethanol plants to burn natural gas to facilitate distillation – hardly a carbon-neutral practice! Indeed, it has been estimated that it requires 0.77 units of fossil-fuel energy to produce one unit of biofuel energy from maize [10]. By comparison the production of biodiesel from soybeans appears to be a much more environmentally friendly process, with only 0.4 units of fossil-fuel energy required to produce one unit of biodiesel energy [10].

They say that there is no such thing as a free lunch, and this certainly appears to be the case with biofuels. In 2007 global food prices rose steeply, causing much concern around the world. Analysis of the markets revealed that one of the major contributing factors to this situation was the increased use of agricultural land to produce biofuel rather than food [11]. Such was the switch to the production of biofuels that it caused global shortages in food crops, with the result that food prices rose sharply.

References

[1] Energy UDo. Gross domestic product and vehicle travel: how do they relate? Vehicle Technologies Program; 2006.

[2] OECD. Passenger transport data; 2003.

[3] Kemp RJ. Transport energy consumption: a discussion paper; 2004.

[4] Kemp RJ. Rail transport in the next millennium: visions of tomorrow. In: IMechE 150 year symposium, London; July 1997.

[5] Kemp RJ. Environmental impact of high-speed rail. In: IMechE seminar on high speed rail developments; April 2004.

[6] DEFRA. Passenger transport emissions factors; 2007.

[7] DOE/EIA. International Energy Outlook 2007; 2007.

[8] BBC. Oil price soars as US woes mount; 2008.

[9] Allwright A. Simplistic predictions of looming oil drought are wide of the mark. Irish Times 31 May 2008.

[10] Bourne JKJ. Green dreams. National Geographic 2007; 212: 38–59.

[11] Blythe N. Biofuel demand makes food expensive: BBC; 2007.

CHAPTER 5

Renewable Energy

While fossil fuels are still the dominant source of primary energy in the world, concerns about climate change, coupled with high energy prices, have strengthened interest in the exploitation of renewable energy. This chapter presents an overview of renewable energy and discusses the concepts associated with this subject.

5.1 Renewable Energy

Climate change, coupled with concerns about high oil and energy prices, is driving a global trend towards the increased use of renewable energy. Unlike fossil fuels which are rapidly being depleted, renewable energy sources such as sunlight and wind are naturally replenished and therefore sustainable. Indeed, it is the perceived notion of sustainability that is driving governments around the world to introduce legislation promoting the use of renewable energy [1].

Most sources of renewable energy originate either directly or indirectly from the sun. For example, both wind and wave power derive their energy indirectly from the sun. When solar radiation is absorbed by the Earth it is dissipated around the globe in the form of winds and ocean currents. The wind interacts with the oceans and transfers mechanical energy to water thus creating waves. In addition, solar energy promotes evaporation of water from the oceans. This airborne water ultimately falls as rain, creating rivers which may be dammed to produce hydroelectric power. Furthermore, solar energy drives the photosynthesis necessary for the plants that are used to create biofuels.

Currently, only about 18% of the world's energy demand is supplied from renewable energy sources [1]. However, there is great potential to increase this contribution. Indeed, it has been estimated that the technical potential of renewable energy is more than 18 times that of current global primary energy demand [2]. This estimate, however, does not allow for economic and environmental constraints and is therefore somewhat misleading. Owing to constraints, such as economic competitiveness, the potential that is likely to be realized in practice will be only a fraction of this value.

In order to exploit renewable sources of energy it is often necessary to make a considerable capital investment. This is particularly the case with large infrastructure projects such as hydroelectric or tidal barrage schemes. To be economically viable, such projects must absorb large capital costs and still be able to compete on price with traditional sources of energy – something which in most cases it is difficult to do. Furthermore, large infrastructure projects such as hydroelectric dams and tidal barrages may create environmental problems. Consequently, there are major barriers to the widespread exploitation of renewable energy. Indeed, the extent to which renewables may be exploited is not purely a technical issue; rather it depends on a complex raft of economic, political and environmental factors, all of which impinge on the subject.

5.2 Solar Energy

The Earth continuously receives 1.74×10^{17} W of incoming solar radiation at the outer surface of its atmosphere [3]. Of this figure, 31% is reflected back to space, while the rest is absorbed by the atmosphere, oceans and land [4]. The absorbed solar energy promotes convection currents and evaporation of the oceans, which drive the wind and water cycles, respectively. In addition, solar energy is converted into chemical energy via photosynthesis and this produces the biomass from which all fossil fuels are derived.

While the Earth is bathed in sunlight, the solar intensity (W/m^2) experienced around the globe is far from equal. Locations near the equator, being approximately perpendicular to the sun's rays, experience much higher solar intensities than locations nearer the poles, which are only 'glanced' by the sun's rays. In addition, because the Earth's axis is tilted at an angle of 23.5°, it means that higher-latitude regions move towards the sun in summer and away from it in winter, and as a result these locations experience large seasonal variations in solar intensity. By comparison, equatorial regions tend to be hot all year round.

The variations that exist in solar intensity are illustrated in Table 5.1, which shows the direct solar radiation (W/m^2) falling on a horizontal surface and a south-facing vertical surface for various latitudes at different times of the year. From this data, it can be seen that the seasonal variations are much more pronounced at the higher latitudes than those nearer the equator.

TABLE 5.1 Direct solar irradiances (W/m²) on horizontal and south-facing vertical surfaces for various times of the year at various latitudes [5]

Latitude (N)	21 June (12 noon) Horizontal (W/m²)	21 June (12 noon) South (W/m²)	22 September & 21 March (12 noon) Horizontal (W/m²)	22 September & 21 March (12 noon) South (W/m²)	21 December (12 noon) Horizontal (W/m²)	21 December (12 noon) South (W/m²)
0°	830	0	900	0	830	360
5°	870	0	915	80	785	425
10°	900	0	910	160	735	485
15°	915	0	890	240	675	535
20°	915	0	860	315	615	580
25°	910	25	820	380	545	615
30°	915	105	770	445	475	640
35°	905	185	715	500	400	645
40°	880	260	655	550	315	635
45°	845	335	595	595	235	595
50°	805	400	525	625	155	530
55°	755	465	450	645	85	420
60°	700	520	375	645	30	270

TABLE 5.2 Daily solar energy (direct and diffuse) (kWh/m²) falling on a horizontal surface in various locations under bright and dull conditions [6]

Location	Latitude	Bright day (kWh/m²)	Dull day (kWh/m²)
Equator	0.0°	7.5	6.8
Tropics	23.5°	8.3	4.2
Mid-latitudes	45.0°	8.5	1.7
Central UK	52.0°	8.4	0.8
Polar circle	66.5°	7.9	0

Table 5.2 shows the daily solar energy (direct and diffuse) (kWh/m²) falling on a horizontal surface in various locations under bright and dull conditions. While the data presented in this table show the solar energy that is available under bright and dull conditions, they do not give any indication of the annual solar energy that is available. To calculate this it is necessary to take into account the weather conditions – something which is beyond the scope of this book. However, in the northern hemisphere the annual solar energy at ground level is generally thought to be about 900 kWh/m² [6].

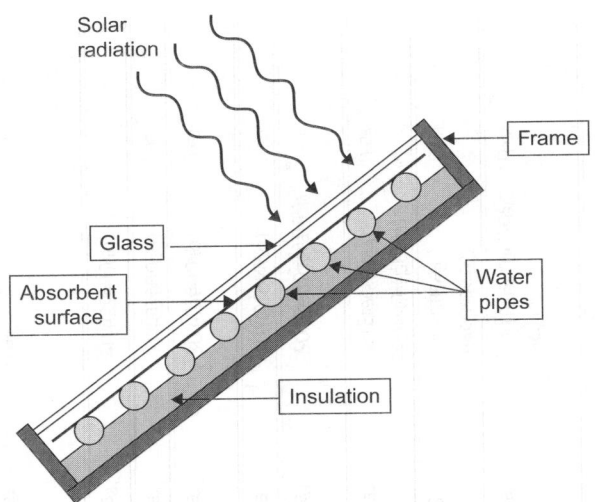

FIG 5.1 Section through a flat-plate solar collector.

5.2.1 Solar Collectors

In many parts of the world, solar energy can be used effectively both for space heating and to heat water. Solar heating systems can be cost effective provided that they are controlled properly and that pump- or fan-operating costs are kept to a minimum. Such systems tend to utilize solar collectors to heat water, which is then circulated around a system. Probably the simplest form of solar collector is the flat-plate collector (see Figure 5.1), which comprises a 'coiled' metal pipe bonded to a metal plate and placed in a glass-fronted box. In order to maximize the solar absorption, the plate and pipe are usually painted matt black – conduction losses are minimized by placing insulation material underneath the plate. The water in such a collector heats up until an equilibrium temperature is reached, where the losses by conduction, convection and radiation are equal to the solar radiation gains.

The heat output from solar flat-plate collectors can be determined using the Hottel–Whillier equation [7]:

$$Q = F[(\tau\alpha)I - U(t_w - t_a)] \tag{5.1}$$

where Q is the rate of delivery of useful energy (W/m^2), I is the intensity of solar radiation (W/m^2), τ is the transmission coefficient, α is the absorption coefficient, U is the overall heat transfer coefficient (W/m^2 K), F is the solar-collector efficiency factor, t_w is the mean water temperature (°C) and t_a is the ambient air temperature (°C).

The efficiency of a solar collector is the ratio of the useful heat output over the solar heat input:

$$\text{Efficiency, } \eta = \frac{Q}{I} \tag{5.2}$$

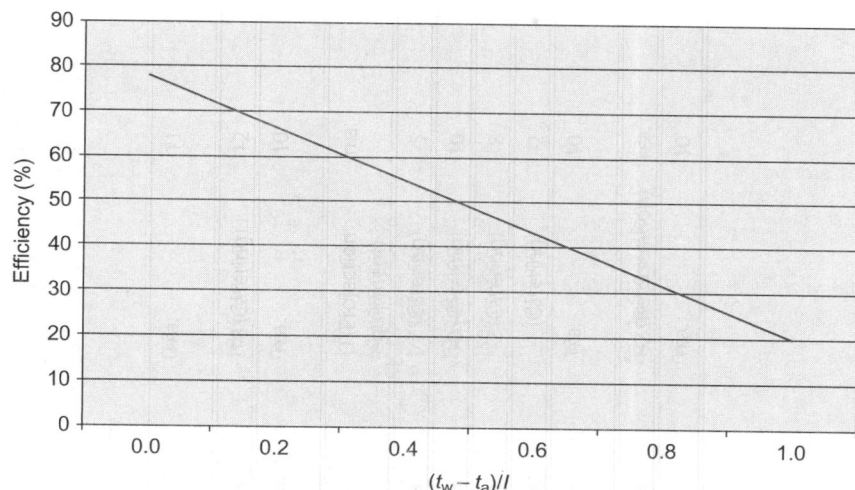

FIG 5.2 Efficiency of a solar water collector.

$$\eta = F(\tau\alpha) - \frac{FU(t_w - t_a)}{I} \tag{5.3}$$

The efficiency of a solar collector is usually represented by plotting efficiency (η) against $[(t_w - t_a)/I]$ on a graph (as shown in Figure 5.2).

For flat-plate collectors typical values of τ are in the region 0.77–0.79, while those for α are 0.95–0.97 [6]. The value of F depends on the design of the collector but is typically in the region 0.85–0.96 [6].

Example 5.1

Experiments on a flat-plate solar collector reveal that:

$$F(\tau\alpha) = 0.8188$$

and

$$FU = 7.0041$$

Given this information and assuming that the collector is located in air at 12°C and that it receives 400 W/m^2 of solar radiation, determine the efficiency and output of the collector when:

(i) Delivering water at a mean temperature of 40°C.
(ii) Delivering water at a mean temperature of 50°C.

Solution

(i) At a mean water temperature of 40°C

$$\eta = F(\tau\alpha) - \frac{FU(t_w - t_a)}{I}$$

$$\eta = 0.8188 - \frac{7.0041 \times (40 - 12)}{400} = 0.3285$$

$$\eta = 32.85\%$$

Therefore,

$$\text{Output, } Q = 400 \times 0.3285 = 131.4 \text{ W/m}^2$$

(ii) At a mean water temperature of 50°C

$$\eta = 0.8188 - \frac{7.0041 \times (50 - 12)}{400} = 0.1534$$

$$\eta = 15.34\%$$

Therefore,

$$\text{Output, } Q = 400 \times 0.1534 = 61.4 \text{ W/m}^2$$

Example 5.1 shows that the efficiency of the solar collector reduces dramatically as the mean water temperature increases. This implies that the value of U is not constant and that it is dependent on the water temperature. At higher water temperatures the value of U increases due to increased radiant heat loss from the collector.

Higher water temperatures can be obtained by using solar collectors with silvered semi-circular or parabolic reflectors, which focus the solar radiation of the collector surface. They also reduce radiant heat losses from the collector. With this type of collector it is important that the reflecting surfaces are clean, otherwise efficiency drops off. This can be a particular problem in dry, dusty environments such as deserts.

5.2.2 Evacuated-Tube Collectors

It is possible to greatly improve solar collection efficiency by using evacuated-tube collectors in which the collector surface is suspended in a glass vacuum tube (see Figure 5.3). In this type of collector the inside surface of the bottom half of a tube is silvered so that the solar radiation is focused on the collector surface. Because a vacuum is maintained within the collector, convection heat losses due to air movement inside the glass tube are significantly reduced. With this type of collector, typical values of $\tau\alpha$ and U are 0.84–0.86 and 0.8 W/m²°C, respectively [6].

Although evacuated-tube collectors can employ liquid as a transfer medium, it is more common for them to utilize a temperature-sensitive fluid, such as methanol, which boils at a relatively low temperature. When solar radiation falls on the surface of the collector, the liquid within the tube vaporizes and rises to the top of the pipe, where it condenses in a heat exchanger. The liquid then flows back down the tube and the whole process is repeated. In the exchanger at the top of the tube the heat from the vapour is transferred to a water–glycol mixture. In order to operate correctly, evacuated-tube collectors must be mounted at a minimum angle of tilt of about 25° – this allows

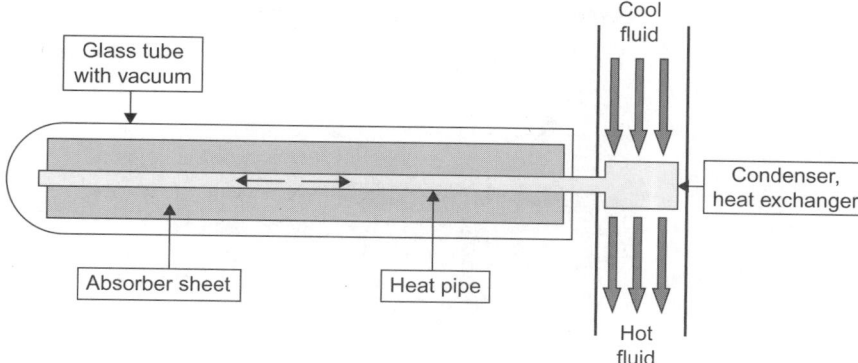

FIG 5.3 Evacuated-tube solar collector.

the heat transfer vapour to rise to the top of the tube and the condensate to fall to the bottom. If evacuated tubes are mounted horizontally, then this cannot happen and heat transfer will not occur.

5.2.3 Photovoltaic Cells

It is possible to produce electricity from light by utilizing a photoelectric process. The term photoelectric is used to describe any effect which produces electricity from light. There are three main photoelectric processes: photoemissivity, photoconductivity and the photovoltaic effect. Photoemissivity occurs when materials emit electrons in the presence of light. The photoconductive effect refers to the phenomenon whereby an electric current flowing through a substance is increased as a result of light falling on it. While both these photoelectric processes are used in specialist applications, it is the photovoltaic effect which is most widely used to produce electricity from sunlight. The photovoltaic effect occurs when light falls on the boundary between two substances and causes electrons to be transferred from one side of the boundary to the other. As a result of this transfer of electrons, one material acquires an excess of electrons and becomes negatively charged, while the other loses electrons and becomes positively charged. In this way a positive–negative (P–N) junction is formed. The resulting imbalance in electrons across the P–N junction produces an electromotive force, which when connected to a circuit causes a current to flow (see Figure 5.4).

Photovoltaic cells comprise solid-state electronic cells, which are fabricated using crystalline silicon wafers as a substrate onto which metal is deposited using a screen-printing process [8]. A photovoltaic cell with an area of $100 \, cm^2$ should produce approximately 3.5 amps in strong sunlight. Manufacturers encapsulate groups of photovoltaic cells under glass covers to form modules. Within these modules, individual cells are interconnected in series and parallel to produce desired voltages and currents. Similarly, photovoltaic modules can be grouped together to form arrays to increase the power output.

Manufacturers subject their photovoltaic modules to a standard test condition of a solar irradiance of $1000 \, W/m^2$ at an operating temperature of 25°C, which is approximately equivalent to the solar radiation which would be experienced by a horizontal surface, at

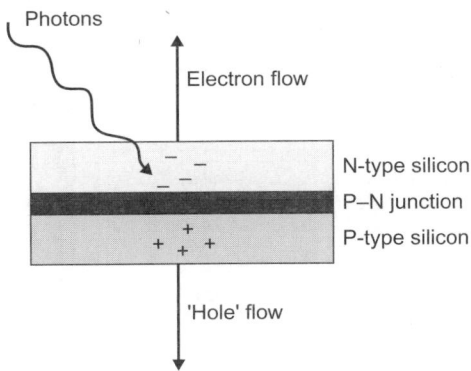

FIG 5.4 Photovoltaic cell.

noon, in June in Saudi Arabia. It should be noted that the performance of photovoltaic modules drops off as the ambient air temperature increases above 25°C. This is of particular importance as photovoltaic modules are often used in environments which are much warmer than 25°C. It has been calculated that operating power reduces by about 0.5% for every 1°C increase [9], thus a 100W module (rated at 25°C) when operating at 41°C would actually produce only 92W.

Photovoltaic cells were first developed in the 1950s in the space industry for use on satellites, but interest in their terrestrial use emerged with the fuel crisis of the early 1970s. Since then, there has been a steady growth in their terrestrial use, mainly limited to remote applications where the provision of mains electricity is prohibitively expensive. However, in recent years reductions in the cost of manufacture of solar cells has meant that the urban use of photovoltaics has become more popular. Currently, photovoltaic cells cost about US $2–3 per peak watt (i.e. power generated when the solar insolation is 1000W/m²) of electricity generated [6]. However, in order to compete with conventionally generated electricity it has been estimated that the installed cost of solar cells would have to be in the region US $0.15–0.3 per peak watt [6]. Clearly, for photovoltaic cells to be truly competitive as a mainstream alternative, the cost of solar cells will have to fall further.

5.3 Wind Power

Although not immediately obvious, wind is a solar-driven process. Solar radiation falling on the equator heats up the air, causing it to rise, while in the polar regions lack of solar energy causes cold air to sink. This sets up a basic pattern of air circulation on the planet, which we experience as wind. The potential of wind power is enormous – it has been estimated that an average of 300,000 nuclear power stations would be required to generate power equal to that produced by winds around the world [9]. Wind therefore represents a substantial source of renewable energy, which can be utilized by populations all over the globe. Indeed, wind power has been utilized by mankind for thousands of years to propel boats and mill grain. For example, in 1750 it was estimated that there were 8000 windmills in operation in the Netherlands, with a further 10,000 in Germany [6].

While the potential of wind power may be enormous, the ability of mankind to harvest energy from this source is limited by a number of constraints. Foremost among these is the fact that the distribution of wind around the planet is not even. The higher latitudes are considerably windier than their equatorial counterparts. Similarly, inland continental areas experience less wind than coastal regions. Consequently, large-scale harvesting of power from the wind is generally only feasible near maritime locations at the higher latitudes, such as those found in North West Europe. However, such locations are often far from population centres, with the result that the potential energy of the wind cannot be fully harnessed. Furthermore, in most regions of the world, even at the higher latitudes, the winds are far from consistent. They may be here today and gone tomorrow. Therefore, wind can only be relied upon to supply part of a population's energy demand, with the rest supplied from another source. Consequently, wind power when utilized tends to be used as a 'top-up' energy resource in an otherwise conventional energy infrastructure. In some circumstances this can make the harnessing of wind energy uneconomic, as it requires the construction of expensive turbines in addition to the provision of a conventional electricity infrastructure.

5.3.1 Power Available in Wind

If one considers the wind, it is not difficult to appreciate that it involves the transport of a large mass of air. So if m is the mass (kg) of the air transported and v is the average velocity of the air (m/s), then the kinetic energy, E_k, of the wind is:

$$E_k = 0.5mv^2 \tag{5.4}$$

If we then consider a window of area, A, through which the air is passing, it can be shown that the power in the wind, P_w, is:

$$P_w = 0.5\rho Av^3 \tag{5.5}$$

where ρ is the density of air (i.e. 1.201 kg/m^3 at 20°C).

So, using eqn (5.5) we can calculate that with 1 m^2 of area, a 4 m/s wind will develop 38.4 W of power, whereas in an 8 m/s wind the power developed will be 307.5 W. It is, however, not possible to extract all this power from the wind. Consider, for example, the air flowing through a wind turbine – the air cannot give up all its energy to the rotors, otherwise it would pile up in front of the turbine and no longer flow through the rotors. Therefore, only a fraction of the wind power can be transferred to the rotor blades. Indeed, it can be shown that the maximum power, $P_{w\,max}$, that the air can deliver to the rotors is:

$$P_{w\,max} = 0.593 \times 0.5\rho A_t v^3 \tag{5.6}$$

where A_t is the face area of the wind turbine.

The figure of 59.3% is known as the *Betz Limit* and this represents the ideal maximum kinetic energy that can be transferred to turbine rotors from the wind. However, in reality, because of aerodynamic and mechanical inefficiencies all wind turbines are less efficient than this. These inefficiencies are generally incorporated into a parameter known as the *power coefficient*, C_p, which is applied to eqn (5.6) as follows:

$$P_{w\,max} = C_p \times 0.5 \rho A_t v^3 \tag{5.7}$$

With commercial wind turbines, C_p is typically in the region 0.3–0.45, which equates to 50%–76% of the ideal theoretical value [10]. The value of C_p, and by inference the efficiency of the wind turbine, varies with the wind speed. If the rotor turns too slowly, then most of the air will pass undisturbed through the gaps in between the rotor blades. Conversely, at very high rotational speeds, due to aerodynamic factors, turbines tend to become inefficient. Therefore, wind turbines are designed to run at an optimum tip speed ratio ($TSR_{p\,max}$) in order to extract as much power out of the wind as possible. The TSR is the ratio between the rotational speed of the tip of the rotor blades and the wind velocity:

$$TSR = \frac{v_{tip}}{v} \tag{5.8}$$

where v_{tip} is the rotor blade tip velocity (m/s), which can be calculated as follows:

$$v_{tip} = 2\pi v_r r \tag{5.9}$$

where v_r is the speed of the rotor blades (rev/s), and r is length of the rotor blades.

Figure 5.5 shows the relationship between C_p and TSR for various types of wind turbine and it can be seen that in each case there is an optimum TSR at which the turbines should run. It is possible to approximately calculate this optimum TSR (i.e. $TSR_{p\,max}$) for each turbine type using the following simple empirical equation:

$$TSR_{p\,max} = \frac{4\pi}{n} \tag{5.10}$$

where n is the number of rotor blades.

From eqn (5.10) it is apparent that the greater the number of rotor blades, the lower the optimum TSR – something that is illustrated in Figure 5.5.

In addition to the inefficiencies associated with the rotors, when wind turbines are used to generate electricity the efficiencies of the gearbox, η_g, and generator, η_e, must be taken into account. For larger turbines η_g is generally in the region 80%–95%, whereas for smaller machines this value drops to 70%–80% [6]. Likewise, the value of η_e is in the region 80%–95% for larger turbines and 60%–80% for smaller machines [6].

Example 5.2

A wind turbine with three rotor blades, each of length 5 m, exhibits a C_p of 0.37 when the TSR is 3. Assuming that η_g is 0.9 and η_e is 0.85, and that the density of air is 1.201 kg/m³, calculate:

(i) The electrical power produced by a turbine operating in a 10 m/s wind.
(ii) The speed of the rotor blades at this wind velocity.

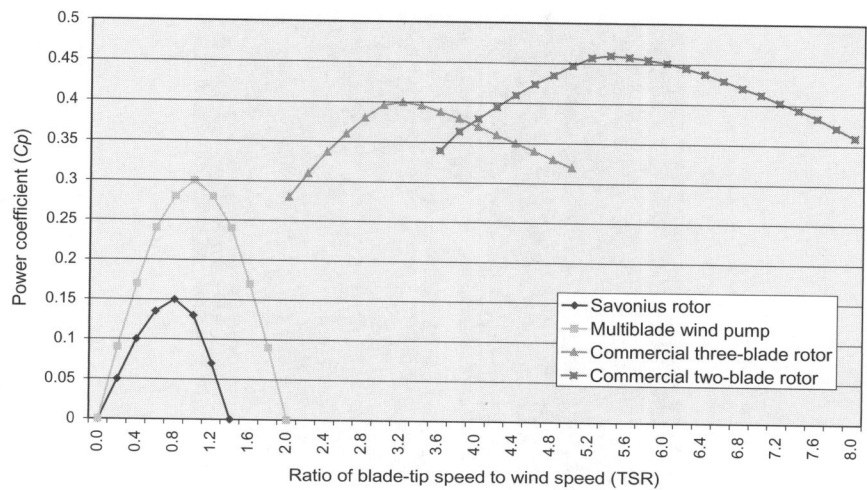

FIG 5.5 Variation in efficiency with tip speed ratio (TSR).

Solution

(i) Area of turbine, $A_t = \pi \times 5^2 = 78.540\,\text{m}^3$

$$\text{Electrical power}, P_e = 0.37 \times 0.9 \times 0.85 \times 0.5\rho A v^3$$

$$P_e = 0.37 \times 0.9 \times 0.85 \times 0.5 \times 1.201 \times 78.54 \times 10^3$$

$$P_e = 13,349.6\,\text{W}$$

(ii) Rotor tip speed, $v_{tip} = \text{TSR} \times v = 3 \times 10 = 30\,\text{m/s}$
and

$$v_{tip} = 2\pi v_r r$$

Therefore,

$$v_r = \frac{30}{2\pi \times 5} = 0.955\,\text{rev/s}$$

5.3.2 Wind Turbines

While they may exhibit many variations, wind turbines can be categorized into two broad groups; those that utilize a horizontal axis, the more common variant, and those whose axis is vertical.

Horizontal-Axis Turbines

Traditionally, wind turbines have been designed along a horizontal axis with the rotor blades facing the wind. With this type of turbine the main rotor shaft is coupled to a gearbox and an electrical generator at the top of a tower (see Figure 5.6). A gearbox is employed to convert the slow rotation of the blades into high-speed rotation suitable for driving a generator.

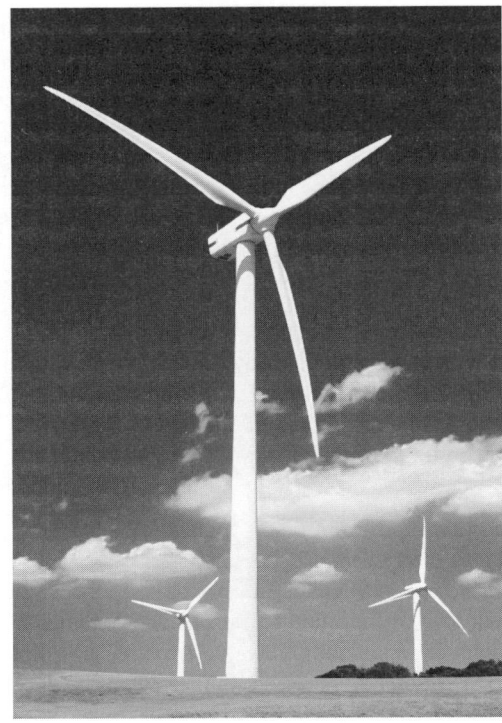

FIG 5.6 Typical commercial horizontal-axis wind turbine.

Larger commercial turbines almost always employ propeller-type rotors on a horizontal axis. Such turbines tend to have low number of blades (i.e. three or less), which are pointed upwind of a support tower. The rotor blades resemble the wings of an aircraft and produce lift perpendicular to the direction of the wind. On commercial turbines, rotor blades can be very long, 20–40 m in length, and it is important that they be both lightweight and strong. Therefore glass fibre–reinforced plastic is generally used to construct rotor blades, with carbon fibre sometimes used as reinforcement.

Although in the nineteenth and early part of the twentieth century multi-blade windmills were widely used, modern commercial horizontal-axis wind turbines tend to have far fewer blades. Two- or three-bladed rotors are the types most commonly used for generating electricity, whereas multi-bladed rotors are generally reserved for tasks such as pumping water. The rotors on modern wind turbines exhibit much higher tip speeds (i.e. up to six times the wind speed) compared with older multi-blade machines. Furthermore, many modern machines utilize variable-speed turbines which enable the TSR to be optimized, thus ensuring maximum efficiency.

Vertical-Axis Turbines
In vertical-axis wind turbines the main rotor shaft is arranged vertically. Compared with their horizontal counterparts, this has the major advantage that the turbine does not need to point into the wind to be effective. This can be an advantage in locations

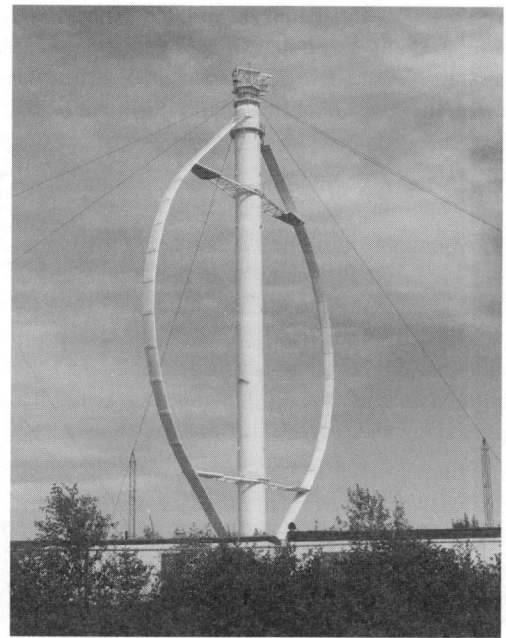

FIG 5.7 Typical vertical-axis wind turbine.

where the wind direction is highly variable. Another advantage is that the generator and gearbox can be located near the ground, negating the need for a support tower. However, because they are frequently mounted on the ground, where wind speeds tend to be lower, there is less wind energy available. In addition, because air flow near the ground is often turbulent, this can cause vibrational issues, with the result that maintenance costs may be increased. Some of these problems can, however, be overcome by installing vertical-axis turbines on the roofs of buildings, where wind speeds tend to be higher than at ground level.

Figure 5.7 shows a typical vertical-axis wind turbine. Such turbines are much less robust than horizontal-axis machines, often requiring guy-wires for support. This lack of structural rigidity can make vertical-axis machines unreliable. Given this it is perhaps not surprising that commercial generators have tended to opt for horizontal turbines instead.

5.4 Power from Water

Mankind's use of water to produce power is not a new phenomenon. The kinetic energy in flowing water has been used for hundreds of years to power water-wheels to produce flour and, in more recent times, to produce hydroelectricity. As such hydroelectric power generation is an established technology, which in 2006 accounted for 6.3% of all the primary energy consumed on Earth [11]. However, while hydropower is well established, other sources of water power, such as waves and tides, remain largely unexploited, with the huge reserves of kinetic energy in the Earth's oceans completely untapped.

Although water power appears to have great potential, it has one major Achilles' heel, namely the environmental impact associated with the infrastructure required to harness the power. Hydroelectric schemes, for example, often require the construction of huge dams, with the result that existing water flows are altered, large areas of land are drowned and populations are displaced. This can have environmental, social and political consequences. For example, the dam at Ilisu in south-east Turkey, construction of which commenced in 2006 [12], has become a source of international tension between Turkey, Syria and Iraq. This was because the dam, located on the Tigris River upstream of the Syrian-Iraq border, will control the flow of water into both Syria and Iraq, and it is feared that the reservoirs associated with the dam may cause a loss of flow to these countries during drier months [13].

In addition to environmental considerations, the infrastructure needed to harness power from water usually requires an expensive civil engineering project. Because of their grand scale, such projects can be inordinately expensive. For example, the Ilisu dam is expected to cost $1.5 billion [13]. It requires considerable political will and determination to commission large projects of this nature. Naturally given the high stakes, politicians tend to be rather hesitant when it comes to committing funds for such projects. Indeed, in the case of tidal barrages it is the exceedingly high infrastructure costs associated with such projects, more than anything else, which has meant that this renewable source of energy has remained largely untapped.

5.4.1 Hydroelectric Power

Most hydroelectric schemes utilize the potential energy in the column of water amassed when a river is dammed. The resulting head of water is used to drive a turbine coupled to a generator (see Figure 5.8). In order to maximize the head of water the turbine chamber is usually located some distance below the level of the dam. Water is then run from the dam to the turbine chamber via a large pipe known as a penstock.

FIG 5.8 Section through a hydroelectric dam and power plant.

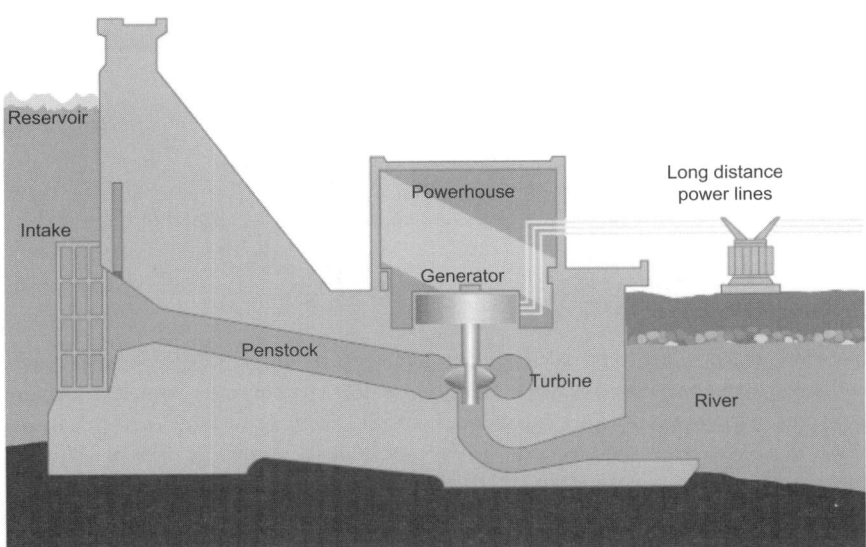

The potential energy in the water contained within the dam depends on its height above the turbine (i.e. the head of water):

$$E_p = \rho g h \qquad (5.11)$$

where ρ is the density of water (i.e. $1000\,\text{kg/m}^3$), g is the acceleration due to gravity (i.e. $9.81\,\text{m/s}^2$) and h is the height of the head of water (m).

Ultimately the potential energy in the head of water (minus any energy losses incurred in the system) is transferred to the turbine. Therefore, the electrical power, P_e, produced can be expressed as follows:

$$P_e = \eta Q \rho g h \qquad (5.12)$$

where η is the overall efficiency of the penstock, turbine and generator, and Q is the volume flow rate of the water (m^3/s).

Example 5.3

The surface of a reservoir is 300 m above a turbine, which is required to produce 200 MW of electricity. If the overall efficiency of the penstock, turbine and generator is 79%, what is the volume flow rate of water required by the turbines?

Solution
The required water flow rate is:

$$Q = \frac{P_e}{\eta \rho g h} = \frac{200,000,000}{0.79 \times 1000 \times 9.81 \times 300} = 86\ \text{m}^3/\text{s}$$

The turbines used in any hydroelectric facility influence its whole design. This is because the type of turbine used determines the overall layout of the facility, the water flow rate and head required. Turbine designs can be grouped into three categories; impulse, reaction and axial flow turbines. Impulse turbines are one of the more common forms of water turbine. They rely on a jet of pressurized water striking open vanes or cups around the perimeter of a wheel (see Figure 5.9). This produces a resultant force on the rotor which is intermittent in nature. Probably the most successful example of an impulse turbine is the Pelton wheel in which water jets are directed against double-hemispherical cups cast on the turbine rotor. Pelton wheel turbines require a large head of water and are suitable for applications which have a head in excess of 360 m [6]. The efficiency of larger commercial wheels can be as high as 90%, whereas with smaller installations it may be as low as 50% [6].

Unlike impulse turbines, which are open, reaction turbines are fully immersed in water and the power comes from the pressure drop across the rotor. With this type of turbine the water acts in a continuous manner, entering radially and leaving axially (see Figure 5.10). The advantage of this type of turbine is that, because high-pressure jets are not required, they do not need a huge head of water to operate.

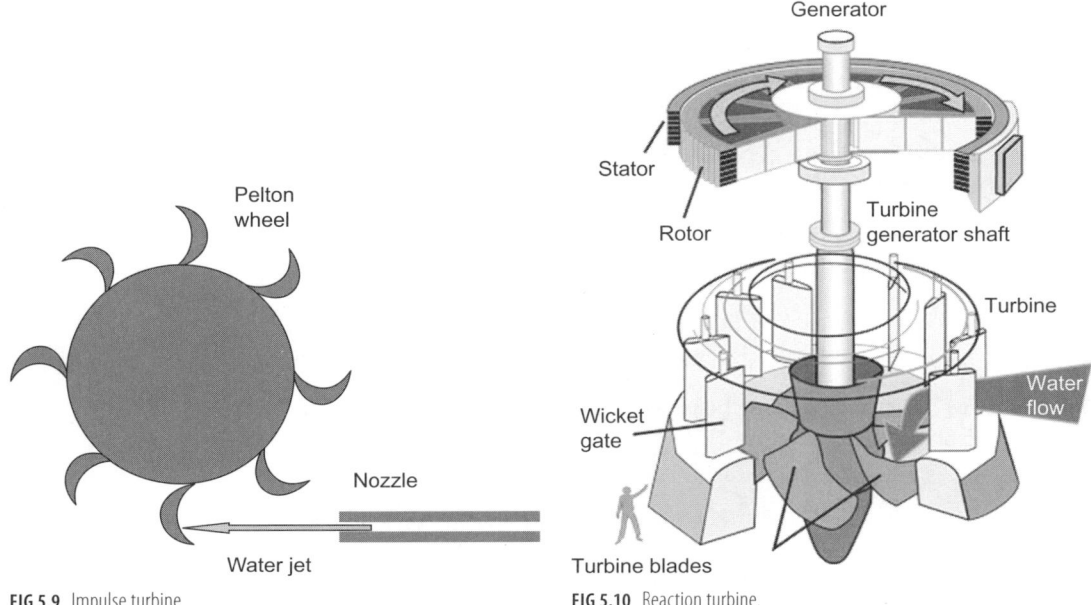

FIG 5.9 Impulse turbine.

FIG 5.10 Reaction turbine.

When only a relatively small head of water (i.e. <30 m) is available, a large volumetric flow of water is required in order to develop significant levels of power [6]. In such circumstances an axial flow turbine is required, in which the water is funnelled through propeller blades to produce mechanical energy.

5.4.2 Tidal Power

Tidal power is the only form of energy that is derived directly from the relative motions of the Earth, the moon and the sun. It is the relative position of the moon and sun, in combination with Earth's rotation, that is responsible for generating the tides. Indeed, it is the gravitational forces produced by the moon and the sun that drag the oceans about on the surface of the Earth on a daily basis. As such, tidal power is probably the most predictable of all the renewable energy sources. Not only can the timing of each tidal event be accurately predicted, but also the potential energy produced. Given this, one might wonder why tidal power has not been widely exploited as an energy source. The simple answer to this is that the infrastructure costs associated with tidal projects are very large, a serious disincentive to would-be investors and something that is well illustrated by the fact that to date there are only three operational tidal barrage plants in existence – at the Rance river in France, the Bay of Fundy in Canada and Kislaya Guba in Russia. Notwithstanding this, tidal barrages are technically feasible. The 240 MW tidal barrage across the Rance river is testament to this. It has been in operation since 1966 [6] and produces on average 600 GWh per year.

Typically tidal power schemes utilize a barrage to dam a tidal river or estuary. This enables the tidal waters to be funnelled using sluice gates through axial hydroelectric

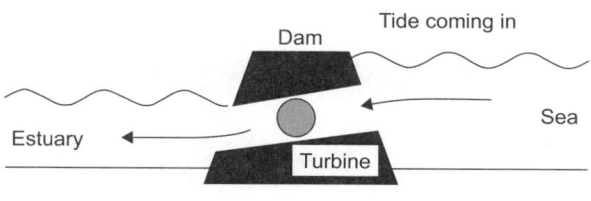

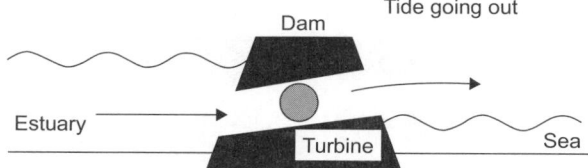

FIG 5.11 Tidal power generation.

turbines (see Figure 5.11). Using this strategy it is possible to generate electricity from both the incoming and outgoing tides.

5.4.3 Wave Power

Waves are produced by the wind passing over the sea. The energy in waves has a kinetic component arising from the mass of water in motion and a potential component associated with the peaks and the troughs that are a feature of waves. The total energy content, E_i, of an ideal deep-water wave must therefore include both potential energy and kinetic energy components. It can be shown that the total energy per metre width of wavefront for an ideal wave is:

$$E_i = \frac{\rho g \lambda H^2}{8} \tag{5.13}$$

where H is the distance between the peak and the trough of the wave (m) and λ is the wavelength of the wave (m).

From eqn (5.13) it can be shown [6] that for an ideal wave the power, P_i, per metre width of wavefront (kW/m) is:

$$P_i = 1.915 \times TH^2 \tag{5.14}$$

where T is the periodic time between wavecrests (s) and

$$T = \left(\frac{2\pi\lambda}{g}\right)^{0.5} \tag{5.15}$$

Sea waves are, however, far from ideal. In reality they come in complicated combinations having different wavelengths and directions. The extractable power in the direction of overall average wave motion in the deep ocean is therefore likely to be only about 10% of the ideal value [6].

Example 5.4

What is the power associated with an ideal deep-sea wave of height 2 m and wavelength 200 m? (Assume $g = 9.81$ m/s^2)

Solution

$$T = \left(\frac{2\pi\lambda}{g}\right)^{0.5} = \left(\frac{2\pi \times 200}{9.81}\right)^{0.5} = 11.32 \text{ s}$$

And the trough–crest height, $H = 2 \times 2 = 4$ m

$$P_i = 1.915 \times TH^2 = 1.915 \times 11.32 \times 4^2 = 346.84 \text{ kW/m}$$

However, given that only 10% of this power is extractable, it is likely that only 35 kW/m will be recoverable.

Because of the prevailing westerly winds, North West Europe is one of the most favourable locations in the world for exploiting wave power. In the North Atlantic, waves have a typical periodic of 10 seconds, which equates to a wavelength of 156 m [6]. This means that they have considerable power. Indeed, it has been estimated that the average power in the waves off the west coast of Scotland is about 70 kW per metre length of wavefront [6].

5.4.4 Wave Power Converters

By their very nature, wave power converters have to be robust and able to cope with extreme weather events. They also have to be able to deal with waves of irregular frequency and amplitude. Furthermore, they have to be economically viable and compete with conventional electricity generators. As a result, the exploitation of wave power is still very much in its infancy, with most technologies being prototypes rather than commercial products. For example, such a prototype has been in operation since 1991 on the island of Islay off the west coast of Scotland (see Figure 5.12) [14]. The 75 kW converter has an energy collector which comprises a sloping reinforced concrete chamber built into the rock face on the shoreline. This has a large inlet, which allows waves to freely enter and leave the central chamber. As waves enter the space, so the level of water rises, compressing the air in the top of the chamber, forcing it through a turbine. In the installation, the turbine is such that it continues to turn in the same way irrespective of the direction of the airflow. Consequently, when the waves draw back and the water level inside the chamber drops, the air is sucked back under pressure into the chamber, keeping the turbine moving. Thus a constant stream of air in both directions is produced by the oscillating column of water, and this is converted into electricity by the turbine which drives a generator.

While most technologies associated with wave power remain prototypes, a few have been utilized on a commercial basis. One example of such a technology is the Pelamis Wave Energy Converter [14] which is an attenuating wave device consisting of a series

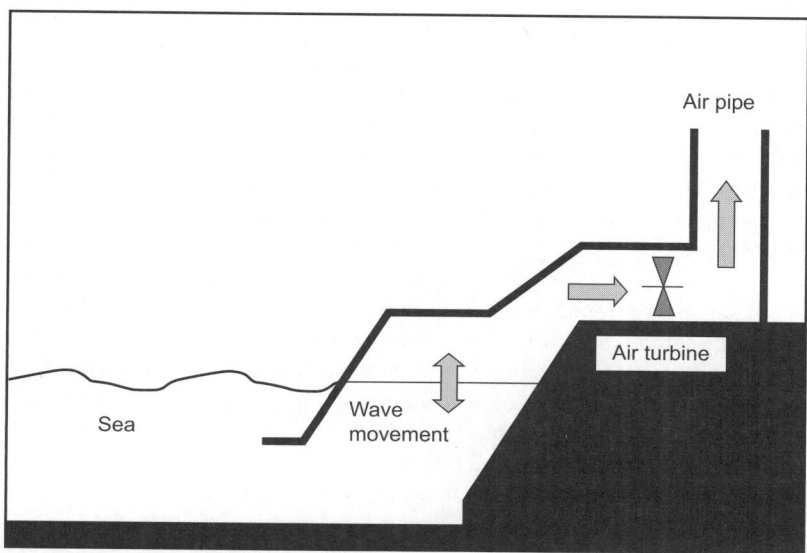

FIG 5.12 Islay shoreline wave converter.

of long, thin cylindrical sections linked by hinged joints. It floats on the surface of the sea and the wave-induced relative motion of the individual sections is resisted by hydraulic rams which pump high-pressure oil through hydraulic motors. The hydraulic motors in turn drive electrical generators which produce electricity. The Pelamis Wave Energy Converter has been used in the world's first commercial wave farm at Aguçadora in Portugal [15].

5.5 Energy from Biomass

The term biomass refers to all living and recently dead biological matter that can be used as fuel. Although this generally refers to plant material grown for use as biofuel, it also includes any biodegradable waste material that can be burnt or used to produce fuel. However, it excludes organic material transformed by geological processes into coal or petroleum.

The simplest use of biomass is to burn it to produce heat energy. Although substances such as cow dung may be burnt, by far the most common fuel used in this way is wood. Indeed, many indigenous societies around the world rely heavily on timber both to cook and to keep warm. A more advanced use of biomass is to process it to produce liquid biofuels, such as ethanol, for use in internal combustion engines. This can be done by fermenting crops, usually maize or sugar cane, to produce alcohol, which is then distilled. An alternative fuel for the internal combustion engine, biodiesel, can be made chemically altering vegetable oils, such as rape seed oil, so that they can be used in an unmodified diesel engine. Finally, it is possible to gasify solid biomass by heating it in the absence of oxygen, to produce a gaseous fuel.

The extent to which the techniques outlined above can be described as *renewable* is somewhat debatable. Because biomass absorbs carbon dioxide from the atmosphere as it grows, in theory it should be 'carbon neutral' when it is burnt – a renewable process. This, however, is a rather naive assumption, because it does not allow for other factors, such as rate of consumption, which impinge on the process. For example, if people burn timber at a rate faster than a forest can produce it, the forest will eventually disappear – hardly a sustainable solution! Similarly, the practice of biofuel producers in the USA of burning natural gas when distilling ethanol from maize cannot be described as a renewable process. It has been estimated that it requires 0.77 units of fossil-fuel energy to produce one unit of biofuel energy from maize [16]. Indeed, given that the large-scale production of biomass to produce biofuel inevitably involves depletion of resources and the consumption of additional energy, it is difficult to see how biomass can be classified as a truly renewable resource. Having said this, if the biomass used is easily replenishable, or is a waste product of another essential process, then the production of energy from biomass may be a sustainable solution, provided that the additional energy consumed in the process is relatively low.

References

[1] Martinot E. Renewable 2007: global status report. Paris: REN21; 2008.
[2] Rogner H. World energy assessment 2001. Part II; 2001.
[3] OU. Discovering science: a temperate earth open university; 1998.
[4] IPCC. Climate change 2001: natural forcing of the climate system. In: Intergovernmental panel on climate change; 2001.
[5] CIBSE. Guide A2, weather and solar data; 1982.
[6] Shepherd W, Shepherd DW. Energy studies. Imperial College Press; 2005. London.
[7] Francis W, Peters MC. Fuels and fuel technology. Pergamon Press; 1980.
[8] Green MA. Photovoltaic solar energy conversion: an update. Australian Academy of Technological Sciences and Engineering, ATSE Focus 1998; 102.
[9] Hill R, O'Keefe P, Snape C. The future of energy use. Earthscan; 1995. London.
[10] Twidell JW, Weir AD. Renewable energy. London: E and F Spon; 1986.
[11] BP. BP statistical review of world energy June 2007. In: BP Plc; 2007.
[12] Smith-Spark L. Turkey dam project back to haunt Kurds. In: BBC News; 2006.
[13] Rohr C. War over water – the case of the Ilisu dam project in Turkey. Pugwash conference: September 7–13 1999; Rustenburg, South Africa; 1999.
[14] Clement A, McCullen P, Falcao A. Wave energy in Europe: current status and perspectives. Renew Sustain Energ Rev 2002;6:405–31.
[15] Wavefarm shipped to Portugal from Scotland. Refocus 7: 12; 2006.
[16] Bourne JKJ. Green dreams. National Geographic 2007;212:38–59.

Bibliography

Hill R, O'Keefe P, Snape C. The future of energy use. Earthscan; 1995. London.
Shepherd W, Shepherd DW. Energy studies: Imperial College Press; 2005. London.

CHAPTER 6

Energy Analysis Techniques

Energy data may be collected for buildings either through audits or as a result of continuous monitoring programmes. However, the data on their own are relatively useless unless they are interpreted in a correct manner. Analysis must therefore be carried out on any raw data that are collected in order to identify trends and areas in which improvements can be made. There are various analysis techniques which can be employed in order to interpret energy data. This chapter introduces the data analysis techniques which are commonly used in energy management.

6.1 Introduction

There are a wide variety of statistical and numerical analysis techniques which can be employed in order to understand why energy is being consumed in a particular fashion. Some of the analysis techniques are fairly simple and can be done using simple hand calculations, while others are more complex and may require the use of computer software. The purpose of this chapter is to introduce the various analysis techniques and explain the practice and theory involved in each.

TABLE 6.1 Energy conversion factors

From	Multiply by factor	To
Therms	29.306	kWh
MJ	0.2778	kWh
GJ	277.778	kWh

TABLE 6.2 Typical gross calorific value of fuels [1]

Fuel type	Typical gross calorific value
Electricity	1 kWh
Natural gas	1.01 therms/100 ft^3
Gas oil (Class D)	38 MJ/l
Heavy fuel oil (Class G)	42 MJ/l
Coal	27–30 GJ/tonne
Propane	92.6 GJ/m^3
Butane	49.3 GJ/m^3

TABLE 6.3 Table of annual energy input for 1998–99

Energy type	Purchased units	Consumption			Cost	
		kWh	%	£	%	p/kWh
Electricity	61,500 kWh	61,500.0	26.0	3075.00	52.58	5.00
Gas	146,800 kWh	146,800.0	62.0	2231.36	38.16	1.52
Oil (Class D)	27,00 l	28,500.0	12.0	541.52	9.26	1.90
Totals	–	236,800.0	100.0	5847.88	100.00	2.47 (av.)

6.2 Annual Energy Consumption

Probably the simplest analysis that can be undertaken is to produce a percentage breakdown of annual energy consumption and cost data. This is a useful technique which enables the overall energy performance of a building quickly and easily to be assessed. The analysis of annual energy consumption should be performed as follows:

(i) Convert all the energy consumption data into standard units (usually the kWh) using the standard conversion factors shown in Table 6.1 and the gross calorific values shown in Table 6.2.

(ii) Produce percentage breakdowns of the total consumption and cost of each energy type, and determine the average unit cost per kWh for each.

(iii) Compile a table similar to the example shown in Table 6.3 showing the total annual energy consumption, cost and percentage breakdown of each fuel type.

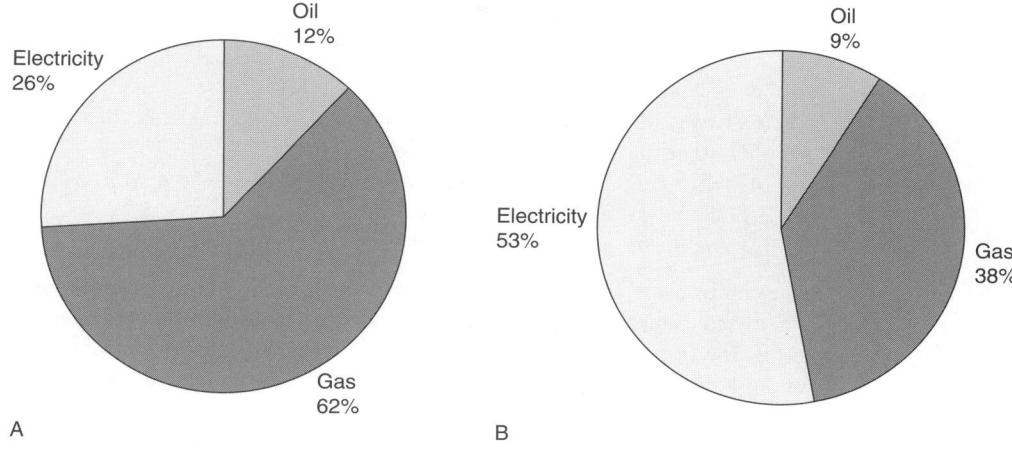

FIG 6.1 Energy consumption (A) and costs (B).

TABLE 6.4   Changes in annual energy use

Year	Consumption (kWh)	Change (%)
1994–95 (base)	201,456.4	n.a.
1995–96	197,562.2	−1.9
1996–97	203,216.2	+0.9
1997–98	220,403.5	+9.4
1998–99	236,800.0	+17.5

(iv) Produce pie charts similar to those shown in Figure 6.1 to show graphically the energy and cost contributions of each energy type.

(v) Where historical energy data are available, comparisons should be made in order to identify any trends, as illustrated in Table 6.4.

It is important to note that although the simple analysis described above may produce energy cost breakdowns and identify possible trends, no allowances have been made for variable factors such as the weather, which may influence the energy performance of the facility. It should therefore be viewed as a rather crude analysis technique, and should not be used when comparing the energy performance of one building against another. If comparison between buildings is required then a more sophisticated analysis approach such as that described in Section 6.3 is required.

6.3 Normalized Performance Indicators

A good indication of the energy performance of a particular building can often be gained simply by comparing actual annual energy consumption and costs with those achieved by buildings of a similar type and function. However, there are a number of inherent problems which must be overcome when comparing the energy performance of one building with another of a similar type in a different location:

- The buildings may be of different sizes.
- The two locations may have different climates. This will influence the amount of energy consumed by the two buildings.
- The two buildings may experience different levels of exposure, which will influence building heat loss.
- The two buildings may experience different operating hours.

In order to overcome these inherent problems it is necessary to correct the building energy consumption data to allow for variables such as weather and occupancy patterns. The concept of the 'normalized performance indicator' (NPI) was developed to address these problems. NPIs enable the energy performance of particular buildings to be compared with others of a similar type and function. They also enable the overall energy performance of a building to be compared with standard energy 'yardsticks' for various building types (see Table 6.6).

Many countries around the world have national energy yardsticks for various building types. These yardsticks are determined by statistical analysis of the results of surveys of measured energy consumption. Energy yardsticks are usually quoted in kWh/m^2 of floor area per annum, although some prefer to use kWh/m^3 of building volume per annum. Yardsticks provide a useful guide against which buildings can be measured. It should be noted that yardsticks are designed to provide useful guidance when establishing priorities; they should not be taken as absolute values to be achieved. In order to determine the actual potential for improving energy performance in a particular facility, it is necessary to undertake further detailed energy surveys. It is also important to remember that performance indicators are only intended to allow comparisons to be made between similar types of building. For example, there is little point in comparing the energy performance of a school with that of a hospital.

The precise energy yardsticks which should be used in various countries will obviously vary widely with the climate experienced and the nature of the construction used. Nevertheless, the principles, which underlie the production of NPIs, are generic and can be applied worldwide. For ease of reference, in this text the energy yardsticks and data applicable to the UK are used to illustrate the process. In the UK, building energy performance is classified as follows:

- *Good:* Generally good controls and energy management procedures although further energy savings are often possible.
- *Fair:* Reasonable controls and energy management procedures, but significant energy savings should be achievable.
- *Poor:* Energy consumption is unnecessarily high and urgent action should be taken to remedy the situation. Substantial energy savings should result from the introduction of energy efficiency measures [1].

Buildings which exhibit a 'poor' performance are most likely to offer the best energy management opportunities, but energy improvements should also be possible for those buildings classified as 'good'.

These broad categories can be assigned to most buildings for energy performance purposes. The process whereby NPI can be determined and building energy performance categorized is based on the CIBSE method [1] and is as follows:

(i) Establish the total building energy use in standard units as described in Section 6.2.
(ii) Ascertain the annual energy use for space heating. This can be determined either by separate sub-metering (see Chapter 7), or by using the analytical techniques described in Section 6.5. If this is not possible, the percentage breakdown data shown in Table 6.5 can be used as an approximate estimation.
(iii) Once the raw annual space heating energy consumption has been established, it must then be corrected to compensate for variations in climate and exposure by applying the following coefficients:

$$\text{Weather coefficient} = \frac{\text{Standard annual heating degree days}}{\text{Annual heating degree days experienced by building}}$$

TABLE 6.5   Proportion of fuel used for space heating and hot water production which is assumed to be attributable to space heating [1]

Building type	Proportion of fuel used for space heating and hot water attributable to space heating (%)
School	75
Hospital, nursing home	50
Other health care	75
Further/higher education	75
Office	75
Sports centre, no pool	75
Sports centre, with pool	65
Swimming pool	55
Library, museum, gallery	70
Church	90
Hotel	60
Bank, agency	75
Entertainment	75
Prison	60
Court, depot, emergency services building	75
Factory	80

In the UK the standard annual number heating degree days is considered to be 2462 (see Appendix 1 for an explanation of degree days). This value will vary with the particular country or region under consideration. Exposure coefficients are as follows:

Exposure	Exposure coefficient
Sheltered (city centre)	1.1
Normal (urban/rural)	1.0
Exposed (coastal/hilly site)	0.9

(iv) The next step is to add the non-heating energy consumption to the corrected space heating energy use to give the raw 'non-time corrected' energy consumption.

(v) The raw annual 'non-time corrected' energy consumption figure should then be multiplied by a coefficient to correct for the 'hours of use' of the building to give the normalized annual energy consumption. This can be done as follows:

$$\text{Hours of use coefficient} = \frac{\text{Standard annual hours of use}}{\text{Actual annual hours of use}}$$

Typical standard annual hours of use values for the UK are shown in Table 6.6.

TABLE 6.6   Yardsticks (kWh/m^2 per year) for annual energy consumption of various building types [1]

Building type	Standard hours of use per year	Fair performance range (kWh/m^2)
Nursery	2290	370–430
Primary school, no pool	1400	180–240
Primary school, with pool	1480	230–310
Secondary school, no pool	1660	190–240
Secondary school, with pool	2000	250–310
Secondary school, with sports centre	3690	250–280
Special school, non-residential	1570	250–340
Special school, residential	8760	380–500
Restaurants	–	410–430
Public houses	–	340–470
Fast-food outlets	–	1450–1750
Motorway service area	–	880–1200
Department/chain store (mechanically ventilated)	–	520–620
Other non-food shops[*]	–	280–320
Superstore/hypermarket (mechanically ventilated)[*]	–	720–830

Continued

TABLE 6.6   (Continued)

Building type	Standard hours of use per year	Fair performance range (kWh/m²)
Supermarket, no bakery (mechanically ventilated)*	–	1070–1270
Supermarket, with bakery (mechanically ventilated)*	–	1130–1350
Small food shop – general*	–	510–580
Small food shop – fruit & veg	–	400–450
University	4250	325–355
Colleges of further education	3200	230–280
Air-conditioned offices, over 2000 m²	2600	250–410
Air-conditioned offices, under 2000 m²	2400	220–310
Naturally ventilated offices, over 2000 m²	2600	230–290
Naturally ventilated offices, under 2000 m²	2400	200–250
Computer centres	8760	340–480
Swimming pool	4000	1050–1390
Sports centre, with pool	5130	570–840
Sports centre, no pool	4910	200–340
Library	2540	200–280
Small hotel	–	240–330
Medium-sized hotel	–	310–420
Large hotel	–	290–420
Banks	2200	180–240
Museum, art gallery	2540	220–310
Cinema	3080	650–780
Theatre	1150	600–900

*Based on sales area.

(vi) The normalized annual energy consumption should be divided by the building floor area to give the NPI. The floor area used in this calculation should exclude completely untreated areas.

(vii) Finally, compare the NPI against the yardsticks given in Table 6.6 and classify the building's energy performance.

Example 6.1 demonstrates the technique involved in calculating an NPI for a library building.

Example 6.1

A library building is situated in an urban location, which experiences 2115 heating degree days per year. It is in use for 2400 hours per year, and consumes 940,000 kWh of natural gas and 28,000 kWh of electricity. If the floor area of the school is 4800 m^2, calculate its NPI and assess its energy performance.

Solution

$$\text{Electrical energy used} = 28,000 \text{ kWh}$$

$$\text{Gas used} = 940,000 \text{ kWh}$$

$$\text{Total energy consumed} = 28,000 + 940,000 = 968,000 \text{ kWh}$$

Table 6.5 shows that 70% of the gas used can be attributed directly to space heating.

Therefore:

$$\text{Space heating energy consumption} = 940,000 \times 0.70 = 658,000 \text{ kWh}$$

By applying weather and exposure coefficients:

$$\text{Corrected space heating energy consumption} = 658,000 \times \frac{2462}{2115} \times 1.0$$
$$= 765,955.6 \text{ kWh}$$
$$\text{Non-heating energy consumption} = 968,000 - 658,000 = 310,000 \text{ kWh}$$

Therefore:

$$\text{Corrected total energy consumption} = 310,000 + 765,955.6 = 1075,955.6 \text{ kWh}$$

and correcting for occupancy (using data from Table 6.6):

$$\text{Normalized annual energy consumption} = 1,075,955.6 \times \frac{2540}{2400} = 1,138,719.7 \text{ kWh}$$

Therefore:

$$\text{NPI} = \frac{1,138,719.7}{4800} = 237.2 \text{ kWh/m}^2$$

According to Table 6.6 the assessed energy performance of the library building is 'fair'. In other words, the building is performing reasonably well, but significant energy saving could still be made.

6.4 Time-Dependent Energy Analysis

If enough energy data are collected it is possible to produce a simple graph in which energy consumption is plotted against time (see Figure 6.2). Through this type of simple time-dependent analysis it is possible to identify general trends and seasonal patterns in energy consumption. This can prove invaluable, since it enables exceptions to the norm to be identified quickly. Although a useful tool, it is important to understand

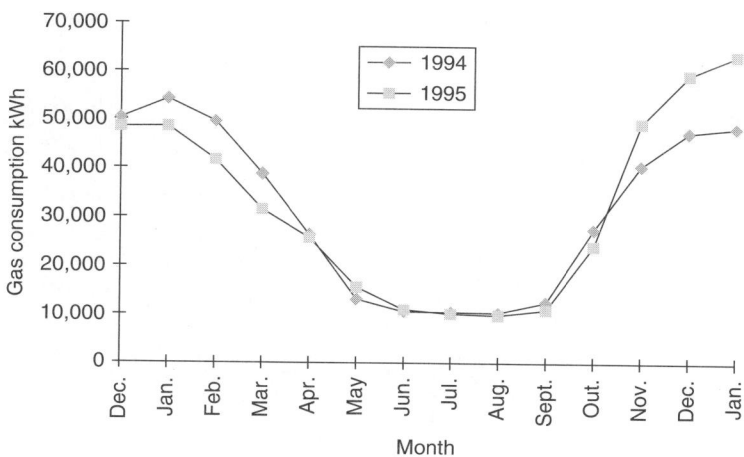

FIG 6.2 Office building gas consumption.

the limitations of this technique, which is best used as a comparative tool and not an absolute one.

Consider the case of the office building represented in Figure 6.2. The time-dependent graph shows monthly gas consumption for the years 1994 and 1995. It can be seen from the graph that:

- Energy consumption during the months of January, February and March of 1995 is consistently less than in the corresponding period in 1994.
- The base load consumption is approximately 10,500 kWh/month. This presumably is the gas consumed in producing domestic hot water and in catering.
- Energy consumption during the months of November and December 1995, and January 1996 appears to have increased significantly compared with the corresponding 1994 figures. This tends to indicate a loss of control in the heating system, which might have arisen as a result of an operative altering the control settings at the end of October.

Although energy consumption in January, February and March of 1995 is consistently lower than that in the corresponding period in 1994, it should be noted that this could be for a variety of reasons, some of which are as follows:

- Improved operating practices.
- Warmer weather in 1995, compared with 1994.
- Fewer hours worked by staff in the office. Perhaps during this period in 1994 the office was open during the weekend, because of a high workload!

It is impossible to identify precisely from Figure 6.2 why the energy consumption for January, February and March 1995 is lower than for the same period in 1994. In order to do this, more sophisticated analytical techniques are required (see Section 6.5). Notwithstanding this, it is possible using a time-related graph to plot more than one variable against time, as in Figure 6.3 where the gas energy consumption figures for 1994 are plotted alongside the relevant degree day data.

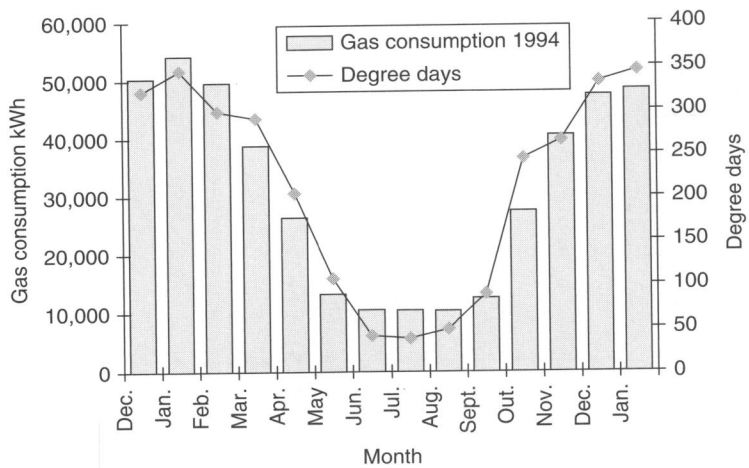

FIG 6.3 Comparison of gas consumption and degree days for 1994.

By generating time-related graphs such as Figure 6.3 it is possible to:

- Identify cyclical patterns which indicate seasonal loads. As the monthly degree day total rises, so gas consumption should also rise.
- Identify general trends which reflect changes in energy consumption. These may arise because of changes in load or efficiency, or alternatively they may be due to changes in operating practice.
- Identify a steady base load, which is the energy consumed when plant is operating at minimum load. For example, in Figure 6.3 a base load of approximately 10,500 kWh per month occurs in June, July and August when no space heating is required. This base load probably represents domestic hot water production and catering gas consumption.
- Identify a lack of any clear pattern. This usually represents a system which is suffering from lack of good control.
- Identify periods of very high or very low energy consumption, which may occur because of unusual changes in plant operation in a particular month. It should always be remembered that anomalies might appear because of errors in logging energy input data.

Most building energy management applications use monthly data. It is therefore recommended that data be based on calendar months, since analysis of data derived from 4- or 5-week periods might cause errors. When using calendar months, the one or two day differences, which occur between successive months, can usually be ignored.

6.5 Linear Regression Analysis

Linear regression analysis is a statistical technique which determines and quantifies the relationship between variables. It is a widely used energy management tool which

TABLE 6.7 Factors which influence energy consumption [2]

Commodity	Duty performed	Possible factors
Electricity	Outside security lighting	Hours of darkness
Water	Swimming pool make-up	Number of bathers (because of evaporation and water removed in swimming costumes)
Gas	Space heating	Heating degree days
Electricity	Air conditioning	Cooling degree days
Oil	Steam-raising in boiler plant	Amount of steam generated
Electricity	Air compressor	Air volume delivered
Diesel	Goods vehicles	Tonne-miles hauled
Steam	Production process	Production volume

enables standard equations to be established for energy consumption, often from data which would otherwise be meaningless.

From Section 6.4 it is clear that although time-dependent analysis is a useful comparative tool, it has its limitations; it is difficult to identify why certain trends occur or, indeed, if perceived trends actually exist at all. Regression analysis overcomes this problem by removing the 'time' element from the analysis and focusing instead on the variables which influence energy consumption. It is a versatile technique which can be used to analyse a wide variety of applications. When used as an energy management tool, the variables commonly compared are [2]:

- Gas consumption versus the number of heating degree days experienced.
- Gas consumption versus the number of units of production.
- Electricity consumption versus the number of units of production.
- Water consumption versus the number of units of production.
- Electricity consumed by lighting versus hours of occupancy.

Regression analysis is very much dependent on the quality of the data used. It should therefore be treated with care. If an analysis indicates the absence of a significant relationship (i.e. $P < 0.05$) between two variables, it does not necessarily mean that no relationship exists. The significance of results depends on the quantity and quality of the data used and, indeed, on the variables used in the analysis. Table 6.7 shows a selection of variables which can influence energy and water consumption.

6.5.1 Single Independent Variable

Consider a case where the monthly gas consumption of an office building (i.e. a dependent variable) and the number of heating degree days experienced (i.e. an independent variable) are plotted against each other on a graph. Since it is well known that building heat losses increase as the outside air temperature gets colder, it is reasonable to expect some sort of relationship between the two. This relationship is in fact linear and it is possible to derive an equation for the *best-fit* straight-line curve through the points plotted on the graph. The *best-fit* straight-line curve is determined by summing the squares of the distances from the straight line of the various data points. Once established, this linear equation can be used to predict future energy consumption. In addition, it can be used as a *standard performance* equation for energy *monitoring and targeting* purposes (see Chapter 9).

The generic equation for a straight-line graph can be represented as:

$$y = c + mx \tag{6.1}$$

where y is the dependent variable (e.g. energy consumption), x is the independent variable (e.g. number of degree days), c is the value at which the straight-line curve intersects the 'y' axis, and m is the gradient of the straight-line curve.

If the straight line $y = c + mx$ is best fitted to a set of data sample points

$$(x_1, y_1)(x_2, y_2)...(x_n, y_n)$$

it can be shown that

$$cn + m\sum x = \sum y \tag{6.2}$$

and

$$c\sum x + m\sum x^2 = \sum xy \tag{6.3}$$

where n is the number of data points.

These equations are known as the normal equations of the problem and they can be used to establish the values of c and m, as illustrated in Example 6.2.

Example 6.2

Consider a hospital building which during a monitoring programme produces the following sample data:

Degree days experienced per month (x)	72	88	95	106	169	204	244	265	290	298	332	345
Gas consumption per month (y) (GJ)	482	520	634	570	671	860	903	940	1007	1210	1020	1131

Therefore:

	x	Y	x^2	xy
	72	482	5184	34,704
	88	520	7744	45,760
	95	634	9025	60,230
	106	570	11,236	60,420
	169	671	28,561	113,399
	204	860	41,616	175,440
	244	903	59,536	220,332
	265	940	70,225	249,100
	290	1007	84,100	292,030
	298	1210	88,804	360,580
	332	1020	110,224	338,640
	345	1131	119,025	390,195
Σ	2508	9948	635,280	2,340,830

Therefore, the normal equations become:

$$12c + 2508m = 9948$$

and

$$2508c + 635,280m = 2,340,830$$

therefore

$$c = \frac{9948 - 2508m}{12}$$

therefore

$$2508\frac{(9948 - 2508m)}{12} + 635,280m = 2,340,830$$

therefore

$$m = 2.355$$

and

$$c = 336.73$$

The *best-fit* straight-line curve equation is therefore:

$$y = 336.73 + 2.355x$$

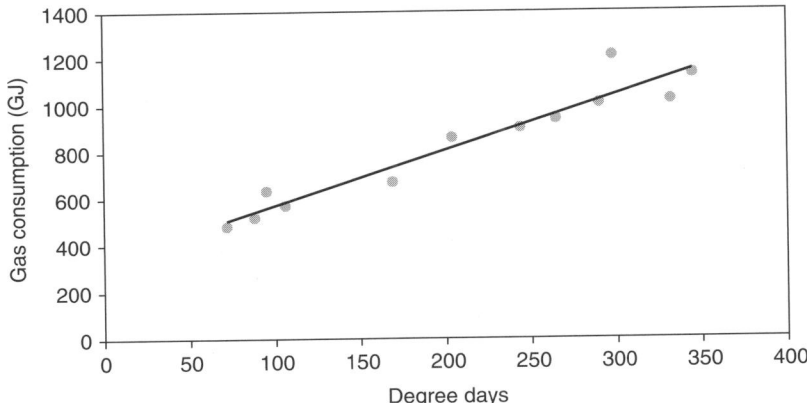

FIG 6.4 Regression analysis for hospital building.

From this equation, it can be seen that the theoretical base load for the building is 336.73 GJ. The graph resulting from the regression analysis is shown in Figure 6.4.

The linear regression curve in Figure 6.4 shows that even when zero degree days are experienced in a particular month, the building still consumes 336.7 GJ of gas. This implies that the theoretical monthly base load gas consumption for catering and hot water production is 336.7 GJ, and that the annual base load consumption is about 4040.4 GJ (i.e. 12 × 336.7 GJ).

6.5.2 Correlation Coefficients

The regression analysis method described in Section 6.5.1 enables a *best-fit* straight line to be determined for a sample data set. However, in some circumstances the sample data points may be very scattered with the result that the derived equation may be meaningless. It is therefore important to determine how well the *best-fit* line correlates to the sample data. This can be done by calculating the Pearson correlation coefficient [3], which gives an indication of the reliability of the line drawn. The Pearson correlation coefficient is a value between 1 and 0, with a value of 1 representing 100% correlation. The Pearson correlation coefficient (r) can be determined using eqn (6.4):

$$r = \frac{\Sigma(x - \bar{x})(y - \bar{y})}{\sqrt{[\Sigma(x - \bar{x})^2 \Sigma(y - \bar{y})^2]}} \tag{6.4}$$

where x, y are the x and y values, and $\bar{x}$, $\bar{y}$ are the average x and y values. Example 6.3 illustrates how the correlation coefficient may be calculated.

Example 6.3

For the data presented in Example 6.2 determine the correlation coefficient.

Therefore:

x	y	$(x - \bar{x})$	$(y - \bar{y})$	$(x - \bar{x})(y - \bar{y})$	$(x - \bar{x})^2$	$(y - \bar{y})^2$
72	482	−137	−347	47,539	18,769	120,409
88	520	−121	−309	37,389	14,641	95,481
95	634	−114	−195	22,230	12,996	38,025
106	570	−103	−259	26,677	10,609	67,081
169	671	−40	−158	6320	1600	24,964
204	860	−5	31	−155	25	961
244	903	35	74	2590	1225	5476
265	940	56	111	6216	3136	12,321
290	1007	81	178	14,418	6561	31,684
298	1210	89	381	33,909	7921	145,161
332	1020	123	191	23,493	15,129	36,481
345	1131	136	302	41,072	18,496	91,204
Σ 2508	9948	0	0	261,698	111,108	669,248

Therefore:

$$r = \frac{261,698}{\sqrt{(111,108 \times 669,248)}} = 0.96$$

Table 6.8 shows minimum acceptable correlation coefficients for the given numbers of data samples.

It can be seen from Table 6.8 that the correlation coefficient in Example 6.3 is very good.

6.5.3 Multivariable Analysis

Often energy consumption can be influenced by several different variables. When this is the case the relationship can be described by the equation:

$$y = c + m_1 x_1 + m_2 x_2 + \cdots + m_n x_n \tag{6.5}$$

where $x_1, x_2, \ldots, x_n$ are the variables that influence y.

Examples of where multiple variables influence energy consumption could be:

- a factory building where electricity consumption is influenced by both the volume of production and the hours of darkness experienced or
- an air-conditioning office building where electricity consumption is influenced by both the cooling degree days and the hours of darkness experienced.

TABLE 6.8   Minimum correlation coefficients [4]

Number of data samples	Minimum correlation coefficient
10	0.767
15	0.641
20	0.561
25	0.506
30	0.464
35	0.425
40	0.402
45	0.380
50	0.362

It is difficult to solve multivariable analysis by hand calculation. It is therefore advisable to use specialist computer software which can be employed to determine the statistical relationship between the variables.

6.6 CUSUM

Regression analysis enables the relationship between energy use and variables such as heating degree days to be established for a given period. It can be used to establish a base line *standard performance* equation, against which subsequent energy consumption can be measured. One technique that can be employed to assess subsequent energy consumption is known as CUSUM, which is an acronym for *cumulative sum deviation method* [2,5]. It is a measure of the progressive deviation from a standard consumption pattern. It is simple to calculate and involves the cumulative summation of the differences between actual energy consumption and target, or baseline, energy consumption. Baseline values should be calculated from a *standard performance* equation which should be derived through analysis of data collected during a monitoring period before any interventions are made.

In order to produce a CUSUM plot the following steps should be taken:

(i) Plot a scatter graph of the two variables under consideration (similar to that shown in Figure 6.4) for the 'baseline' period and derive a *standard performance* equation as described in Section 6.5.1.

(ii) Use the *standard performance* equation to calculate the predicted energy consumption for each month (including the period covered by the baseline and any subsequent study months).

(iii) For each data point (i.e. for each month) subtract the predicted consumption from the actual consumption.

(iv) For each data point obtain the cumulative total deviation from predicted consumption; this gives the CUSUM value for each data point.

(v) Plot the CUSUM values against time.

The CUSUM process is illustrated by Example 6.4, which shows the gas consumption for an office building over a 44-month period.

Example 6.4

An energy audit of an office building for the period August 1989 to December 1990 produced the following gas consumption data:

Year	Month	Gas consumed (kWh)	Heating degree days
1989	August	15,490	18
	September	23,700	36
	October	55,673	109
	November	94,382	199
	December	106,683	239
1990	January	110,745	247
	February	96,458	210
	March	95,903	207
	April	93,265	195
	May	60,045	117
	June	32,267	58
	July	18,849	24
	August	12,435	12
	September	32,775	60
	October	43,924	95
	November	95,012	201
	December	129,505	280

A subsequent monitoring programme found gas consumption for the period January 1991 to March 1993 to be as follows:

Year	Month	Gas consumed (kWh)	Heating degree days
1991	January	140,022	308
	February	180,034	338
	March	118,524	214
	April	112,045	201

Continued

Year	Month	Gas consumed (kWh)	Heating degree days
	May	64,045	108
	June	37,724	67
	July	18,490	24
	August	17,045	21
	September	22,483	35
	October	66,275	140
	November	101,040	219
	December	120,500	262
1992	January	144,240	323
	February	123,140	271
	March	91,500	232
	April	78,041	195
	May	41,004	96
	June	20,549	39
	July	13,461	18
	August	16,062	26
	September	28,740	61
	October	44,467	103
	November	77,206	197
	December	112,442	290
1993	January	98,950	260
	February	98,399	253
	March	97,760	250

Given the information above, produce a CUSUM plot for the building.

Solution

Using the linear regression technique described in Section 6.5.1, the *standard perform-ance* equation for the baseline period is:

$$\text{Monthly gas consumption} = 7744.7 + (427.16 \times \text{degree days})$$

Once this is established it is possible to produce the CUSUM results, as shown in Table 6.9. From the results in Table 6.9 it is possible to produce the CUSUM plot, as shown in Figure 6.5.

TABLE 6.9 CUSUM calculation

Year	Month	Gas consumed (kWh) (1)	Heating degree days (2)	Target gas used (kWh) (3)	Difference (1 − 3) (kWh) (4)	CUSUM (kWh) (5)
1989	August	15,490	18	15,434	56	56
	September	23,700	36	23,122	578	634
	October	55,673	109	54,305	1368	2002
	November	94,382	199	92,749	1633	3635
	December	106,683	239	109,835	−3152	483
1990	January	110,745	247	113,252	−2507	−2024
	February	96,458	210	97,448	−990	−3014
	March	95,903	207	96,166	−263	−3277
	April	93,265	195	91,040	225	−1052
	May	60,045	117	57,722	2323	1270
	June	32,267	58	32,520	−253	1018
	July	18,849	24	17,996	853	1870
	August	12,435	12	12,871	−436	1435
	September	32,775	60	33,374	−599	836
	October	43,924	95	48,325	−4401	−3565
	November	95,012	201	93,603	1409	−2156
	December	129,505	280	127,349	2156	0
1991	January	140,022	308	139,309	713	713
	February	180,034	338	152,124	27,910	28,623
	March	118,524	214	99,156	19,368	47,991
	April	112,045	201	93,603	18,442	66,433
	May	64,045	108	53,878	10,167	76,600
	June	37,724	67	36,364	1360	77,960
	July	18,490	24	17,996	494	78,453
	August	17,045	21	16,715	330	78,783
	September	22,483	35	22,695	−212	78,571
	October	66,275	140	67,547	−1272	77,299
	November	101,040	219	101,292	−252	77,047
	December	120,500	262	119,660	840	77,888

Continued

TABLE 6.9 (Continued)

Year	Month	Gas consumed (kWh) (1)	Heating degree days (2)	Target gas used (kWh) (3)	Difference (1 − 3) (kWh) (4)	CUSUM (kWh) (5)
1992	January	144,240	323	145,716	−1476	76,411
	February	123,140	271	123,504	−364	76,047
	March	91,500	232	106,845	−15,345	60,702
	April	78,041	195	91,040	−12,999	47,703
	May	41,004	96	48,752	−7748	39,955
	June	20,549	39	24,404	−3855	36,100
	July	13,461	18	15,434	−1973	34,127
	August	16,062	26	18,851	−2789	31,339
	September	28,740	61	33,801	−5061	26,277
	October	44,467	103	51,742	−7275	19,002
	November	77,206	197	91,895	−14,689	4314
	December	112,442	290	131,620	−19,178	−14,864
1993	January	98,950	260	118,806	−19,856	−34,720
	February	98,399	253	115,815	−17,416	−52,136
	March	97,760	250	114,534	−16,774	−68,910

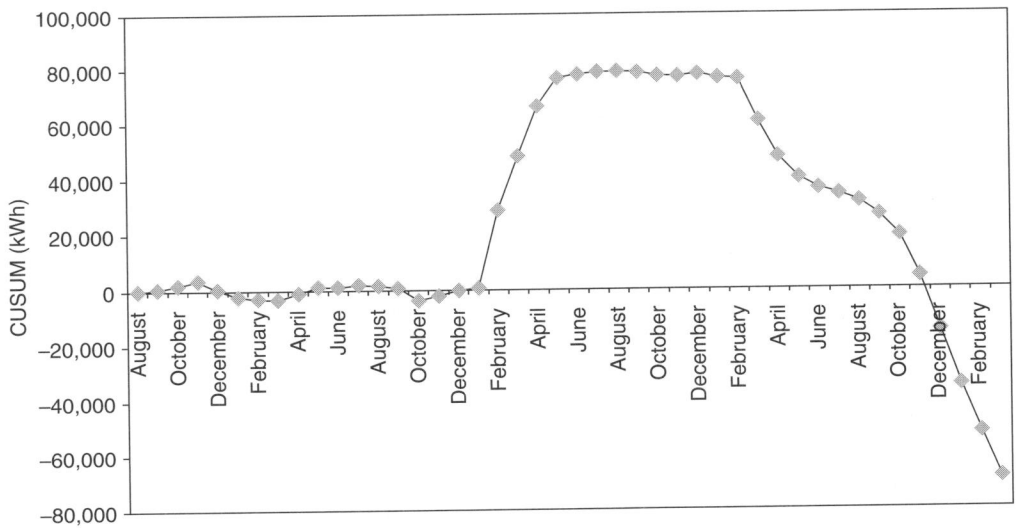

FIG 6.5 CUSUM graph.

A cursory inspection of the CUSUM graph in Figure 6.5 reveals that two major events occurred during the monitoring period – one in February 1991 when the energy consumption dramatically increased and the other in February 1992 when it started to decrease. In fact further investigation revealed that:

- In February 1991 the time clock on the heating system was incorrectly set, so that the heating remained on until 22.00 hours, leading to a dramatic increase in gas consumption. This problem was spotted and rectified in May 1991, at which point the CUSUM plot returns to a similar gradient as that experienced during the baseline period.
- In February 1992 the old single glazing in the office building was replaced by double-glazed windows, thus leading to a fall in energy consumption.

It should also be noted that:

- During the summer months the slope of the CUSUM line became less steep due to the reduced demand for heating.
- The baseline should always be a horizontal line through zero. This is because by definition it is a *best-fit* straight line for the data samples occurring during the baseline period. The actual samples during this period may deviate from the predicted baseline figures, but the CUSUM plot will always fluctuate about zero.
- The greater the slope downwards of the CUSUM line, the more energy efficient the process.

References

[1] Energy audits and surveys. CIBSE Applications Manual AM5; 1991.
[2] Waste avoidance methods. Fuel efficiency booklet 13, Department of the Environment; 1995.
[3] Campbell MJ, Machin D. Medical statistics: a commonsense approach: John Wiley and Sons; 1999. Chichester, West Sussex.
[4] CIBSE. Measurement of energy consumption: CIBSE building energy code part 4; 1982.
[5] Harris P. Monitoring consumption and setting targets (chapter 2). In: Energy manager's workbook, 2: Energy Publications; 1985.

Bibliography

Contract energy management. CIBSE applications manual AM6; 1991.
Eastop TD, Croft DR. Energy efficiency for engineers and technologists (chapters 7 and 9): Longman Scientific & Technical; 1990. Harlow, Essex.
Energy audits and surveys. CIBSE applications manual AM5; 1991.
Harris P. Monitoring consumption and setting targets (chapter 2). In: Energy manager's workbook, 2: Energy Publications; 1985.
Moss KJ. Energy management and operating costs in buildings (chapter 10): E&FN Spon; 1997. London.

CHAPTER 7

Energy Audits and Surveys

Before any energy-saving measures can be undertaken within an organization, it is first necessary to collect comprehensive energy data through an auditing process. This chapter focuses on the mechanics of energy auditing and describes the procedures involved. The differences between preliminary, targeted and comprehensive audits are discussed and the procedures associated with each type highlighted. The subject of energy surveys is also discussed.

7.1 Introduction

There is a strong analogy between the medical profession and the field of energy management. If a patient with a medical complaint presents himself or herself before a doctor, the doctor must first accurately diagnose the condition before taking further steps. The doctor should obtain information from the patient by asking informed questions, possibly carrying out tests, use knowledge and expertise in order to diagnose the complaint and ultimately prescribe treatment. In a similar manner, before any energy 'problems' can be treated it is first necessary to determine the current state of a facility's or organization's energy consumption and thus diagnose any problems that exist. In order to do this, an energy audit must be undertaken and analysis performed on the data collected.

An energy audit is a feasibility study to establish and quantify the cost of the various energy inputs to, and flows within, a facility or organization over a given period. The overall aim of an energy audit is to identify viable and cost-effective energy measures which will reduce operating costs. Energy audits can take a variety of forms, but the process usually involves collecting data from energy invoices and meters, and undertaking surveys of plant, equipment and buildings, as well as collecting information from managers and other staff. The auditing process should identify ways to enhance an organization's operating efficiency and decrease its maintenance costs. In addition, the process should help to resolve any occupant-comfort problem which may exist.

An energy audit should be viewed as the 'foundation' on which any future energy-management programme is built. Energy-management programmes (discussed in detail in Chapter 9) involve the continual monitoring and targeting of energy consumption. Before targets can be set, or effective monitoring undertaken, it is important to establish:

- baseline energy consumption;
- patterns of operation and the work practices used;
- the condition of the organization's buildings, plant and equipment; and
- *energy-management opportunities*, which will result in energy cost reductions.

This information can only be obtained by carrying out a full energy audit of an organization's facilities.

An energy audit should identify those issues which need immediate direct action, as well as those which require further detailed investigation. It should also produce data which can be used to justify future capital investment, and raise, within the organization, general awareness of energy conservation matters. The financial benefits afforded to an organization by an energy audit are both direct and indirect. The direct benefits are fairly obvious; energy cost savings can be achieved by reducing consumption, or simply by changing tariff or fuel type. The indirect benefits are much less obvious; reduced maintenance costs will arise from improved plant utilization and reduced operating hours. Also, improved plant utilization may result in the elimination of excess plant capacity and ultimately reduce capital expenditure.

The auditing process should identify *energy-management opportunities*, which when implemented will result in financial benefit to an organization. The magnitude of these financial benefits is not necessarily dependent on the level of capital investment. In many situations, major cost savings can be achieved through the implementation of 'no cost' or low cost measures, such as:

- changing an energy tariff;
- rescheduling production activities to take advantage of preferential tariffs;
- adjusting existing controls so that plant operation matches the actual requirements of the building or manufacturing process;
- implementing good housekeeping policies, in which staff are encouraged to avoid energy-wasteful practices and
- investing in small capital items such as thermostats and time switches.

Although much can be achieved through low cost measures, it is sometimes necessary to undertake more capital-intensive measures, such as replacing worn-out plant or installing a building management system (BMS). Because of the capital involved in such measures, decisions to invest in them are usually made by senior management (see Chapter 8). In this situation the results of an energy audit can be used to justify capital investment.

7.2 Types of Energy Audit

Although there are many variations, energy audits can broadly be classified as *preliminary, targeted and comprehensive* audits. Each type is distinguished by the level of detail involved and the depth of the analysis undertaken. It is important to select the appropriate audit type for the facility concerned. Comprehensive audits involve detailed energy surveys of plant, equipment and the fabric of buildings, which is a time-consuming and expensive process. They therefore should not be undertaken lightly. It is often better to focus detailed surveys on problem areas highlighted by a preliminary energy audit, otherwise much time and money can be wasted. By carrying out a preliminary audit and methodically applying a range of simple analysis techniques it is often possible to identify major energy problems without the need for expensive and detailed energy surveys.

Preliminary energy audits seek to establish the quantity and cost of each form of energy used in a facility or in an organization. They are relatively quick and are designed to determine a project's potential; more detailed energy audits and surveys can always be undertaken later if so required. Preliminary audits are primarily concerned with obtaining data from energy invoices and meter readings for a given period, which often corresponds to the most recent financial year. Because such audits are primarily concerned with gathering data from bills and invoices, it is sometimes helpful to think of preliminary audits as being *financial energy audits*.

Targeted energy audits often result from preliminary audits. They provide data and detailed analysis on specific targeted projects. For example, an organization may target its lighting installation or boilers with a view to upgrading these items of equipment. Targeted audits therefore involve detailed surveys of the target subjects and analysis of the energy flows and costs associated with the targets. They should make recommendations regarding action to be taken.

Comprehensive energy audits provide detailed data on the energy inputs to, and energy flows within, a facility or organization. They should produce detailed energy project implementation plans. Such audits involve detailed energy surveys and may involve the use of complex energy simulation computer software.

Although in-house staff can carry out audits, they are generally undertaken by either specialist energy consultants or energy service companies. Energy service companies make their money through performance contracts, which guarantee organization's energy cost savings in return for negotiated fees. To energy service companies the main interest lies not in the audit itself, but in installing and managing the plant in accordance with their recommendations. Some companies may even arrange the

TABLE 7.1 Energy audit costs in the USA (1997 rates) [1]

Type of energy audit	Typical cost ($/sq. ft.) (1997 dollar rate)
Preliminary audit	$0.144–0.333 per m^2
Targeted audit	$0.333–0.778 per m^2 (lighting projects)
	$0.556–1.00 per m^2 (HVAC and controls projects)
Comprehensive audit	$2.00–5.556 per m^2 (less than 4500 m^2)
	Less than $1.333 per m^2 (more than 22,500 m^2)

finance for such projects. When using an energy service company it is thus important to remember that they have a vested interest in the outcome of any energy audit and that they may not be totally impartial. By contrast, energy consultants are independent and therefore should provide objective advice.

7.2.1 Audit Costs

Energy audits can be expensive undertakings. Table 7.1 shows data produced by the California Energy Commission for the cost of performing an energy audit in the USA [1].

It can be seen from Table 7.1 that the more complex the audit, the higher the costs involved. It is therefore important to select the appropriate level of audit for any particular application.

Audit costs are affected by the complexity of the facility under consideration. For example, complex facilities such as hospitals or universities are more costly to audit than, say, schools. The age of the facility may also affect the cost. For example, if a mechanical system is complex and the 'as built' drawings are out of date or not available, then the energy auditors may have to produce schematic drawings. This can be very time consuming and obviously greatly increases the audit costs. Given the cost involved, it is important that organizations assist their auditors by preparing in advance for the audit and providing the auditing team with as much relevant information as possible. Energy bills, fuel invoices, meter readings and operational notes should all be collected, together with any relevant system or building drawings. Organizations should also inform their management team that an energy audit is being undertaken and arrange for the auditors to meet with key managers and other relevant staff.

7.3 Why is Energy Wasted?

Before looking in detail at the processes involved in energy auditing, it is perhaps worth looking briefly at the reasons why energy is wasted in so many organizations. Energy is often wasted because of:

- Poorly designed buildings and installations. Buildings may be poorly insulated resulting in high space-heating costs, or mechanical ventilation ducts may be undersized so that fan power consumption is high.

- Inadequate control systems. Heating systems may be installed without any optimum start control.
- Poor control settings. Time clock controllers may be incorrectly set so that buildings are heated when not in use.
- Inefficient plant operation, often arising from the use of old or out-of-date technology, a situation often made worse by poor maintenance practices.
- Poor operating and working practices. Lights are often left on in buildings when they should be switched off.

Although the reasons for energy waste are multifactorial, some of the main reasons are as follows:

- Building designers do not pay energy bills. The design process is closely allied to the construction process, and designers usually select low capital cost solutions, which often result in higher operating costs. This situation is made worse by the fact that the budgets for constructing a facility and running it are usually completely separate.
- Energy consumption is taken for granted. Most building occupants and users do not pay energy bills. They are concerned with their own personal comfort and are not particularly interested in how much energy is consumed in achieving a comfortable environment.
- Most organizations do not have a culture of energy efficiency.
- In many countries the cost of energy is low in comparison with labour costs.

The above list demonstrates that much energy wastage arises from poor strategic and operational management, and also a lack of an energy-saving culture amongst staff. Energy can often be saved at no capital expense simply by improving maintenance procedures and instigating good work practices. This is often referred to as 'good housekeeping' and involves simple measures such as encouraging personnel to switch off lights when they are not required. Initiating good maintenance procedures is also important. For example, if filters in ducted air-handling systems are not replaced regularly, then they become dirty with the result that fan energy consumption increases. It has been estimated that energy bills for organizations can be reduced by approximately 20% through the use of good energy-management practices [2]. It is therefore important that the human and management aspects of energy consumption are investigated in any energy audit. Without a supportive management culture it is difficult to make lasting energy savings in any organization.

7.4 Preliminary Energy Audits

Preliminary audits seek to quantify and cost each form of energy input to a facility or organization over a period of time. They should also identify where the energy is being used within the organization. The main processes involved in such an audit are:

- Collecting data
- Analysing data
- Presenting data
- Establishing priorities and making recommendations.

At the start of any audit process it is important to gather preliminary data about the geographic location of the particular facility concerned, together with any relevant distinguishing features such as its altitude and orientation. Local weather data and degree day data covering the audit period should also be collected. These data will act as a benchmark reference against which the facility's energy consumption can be measured. With manufacturing facilities it will also be necessary to collect data concerning the production output during the audit period, since this will have a considerable impact on energy consumption.

Probably the single most important source of energy data is the energy invoice. It is therefore very important that the audit team has all the relevant energy invoices for the selected audit period. By compiling data from invoices it is possible to build up a clear picture of the pattern of energy consumption and the associated costs to a facility of the various energy inputs. In addition, the total amount spent on energy can be determined from the invoices, thus indicating the upper limit which can ultimately be saved through energy-management measures.

When collecting data from fuel and energy invoices it is important to ensure that copies of all utility invoices for the audit period are collected rather than simply those for which payments were made during the audit period. It is also important to collect all the invoices or delivery notes relating to oil, solid fuel or liquid petroleum gas for the audit period. Due to the time lag between delivery and consumption, it may also be necessary to include deliveries which occurred before the start of the audit period. In addition, it is essential that all the metering and supply points are identified from the invoices, to account for all the energy inputs.

Any estimated meter readings should be identified, since these can result in misleading data. In order to overcome the problems associated with estimated readings, additional invoices should be collected which cover the same months as the estimated invoice, but for years prior to the audit period. These 'real' data can then be compared with the estimated data, to establish realistic data for the audit period. Where possible, data from invoices should be corroborated by independent meter reading data collected over the audit period.

If invoice data are inadequate or unavailable, then it will be necessary to approach the utility companies or fuel suppliers for assistance.

Although for most facilities it will be relatively simple to identify the utility metering points, on large complex sites it may be difficult to account for all the meters. Utility services may come from a variety of sources and this will be reflected in the invoices. Consider a large supermarket site which has an 11 kV electricity supply to the main shopping complex and a separate incoming 415 V supply to a remote petrol station owned by the retailer on the same site. Both supplies will be billed separately and may be on different tariffs. The two supplies might even come from different utility companies!

Preliminary analysis of energy invoices can often be very useful in identifying any anomalies which require further investigation. If a relatively small building on a site consumes as much gas as one of its much larger neighbours, then it would appear that something is wrong.

Further investigation can then be undertaken, which might reveal that the high gas consumption is due to the heating plant in the small building operating at night-time when the building is empty.

Given that the gathering of information from invoices is crucial to the auditing process, it is important that energy invoices be understood. It is also important to understand the peculiarities of the various fuel types and utility services, since these can have a bearing on energy consumption and on the auditing process itself.

7.4.1 Electricity Invoices

The precise nature of electricity tariffs and supply contracts is discussed in detail in Chapter 2. For the purpose of this chapter we will consider only monthly maximum demand tariffs, since many medium-sized and large organizations use tariffs of a similar nature. Figure 7.1 shows a simplified electricity invoice, which illustrates many of the features commonly found in monthly electricity bills.

The monthly electricity invoice shown in Figure 7.1 contains the following information:

- The date of the meter reading.
- The monthly standing charge, which is £30.00 in Figure 7.1.
- The present and previous meter readings with the number of units supplied. These are usually divided into two sets of meter readings, daytime units (i.e. peak rate) and night-time units (i.e. off-peak rate). The difference between the present and previous readings is the units of electricity consumed in the period since the previous meter reading. With some meters a constant may be included on the invoice; multiplication of the meter advances by this constant gives the actual number of units supplied in kVAh or kWh.

Meter readings			Meter reading date: 23/01/2000	
Present	Previous	Units Consumed		
247451	224520	22931		
184530 (Night)	174702 (Night)	9828 (Night)		
Maximum demand this month	270 kVA	**Annual maximum demand**	300 kVA	

Description of charge	No.of units or kVA	Rate	Amount exclusive of tax	Tax (VAT)	% Rate
Monthly charge		£30.00	30.00	5.25	17.50
Availability charge	300.0	£1.41	423.00	74.03	17.50
Max.demand charge	270.0	£5.35	1444.50	252.79	17.50
Unit charge	22931	6.05p	1387.32	242.78	17.50
Night units	9828	2.60p	255.53	44.72	17.50
		Total	3540.35	619.57	
	Total due	£4159.92			

FIG 7.1 Monthly electricity bill.

- The charges for each unit of electrical energy consumed. These are usually different for the daytime and night-time. In Figure 7.1 the peak rate is 6.05p per kVAh and the off-peak rate is 2.60p per kVAh. Sometimes blocks of units are charged at different rates. Some tariffs levy a higher unit charge on the first 1000 kVAh or kWh consumed.
- A monthly maximum demand charge for every kW or kVA of the peak power demand occurring during the billing month. Maximum demand charges are designed to penalize users who make heavy demands on the supply grid during peak periods. They vary throughout the year; in northern countries such as the UK, they are at their highest in December and January and very low, or non-existent, during the summer. In hot countries where air conditioning is extensively used, the situation is reversed with the highest demand charges being levied in summer. Demand charges are often stepped and levied at different rates for various parts of the year. Figure 7.1 shows a maximum demand of 270 kVA, all of which is charged at £5.35 per kVA.
- The supply capacity, for which a monthly availability charge is levied. In Figure 7.1 chargeable supply capacity is 300 kVA, all of which is charged at £1.41 per kVA each month.
- The VAT charged on the bill, together with the total cost due.

7.4.2 Natural Gas

Natural gas invoices are generally much less complicated than their electricity counterparts. Figure 7.2 shows a typical example of a monthly gas invoice.

The gas invoice in Figure 7.2 includes the following:

- The date of meter reading or estimate.
- The calorific value of gas (i.e. 39.6 MJ/m^3 in Figure 7.2);
- The present and previous readings with the amount of gas used, often presented in cubic feet, cubic metres or kWh (and sometimes in therms);
- The unit price per kWh of natural gas (i.e. 1.520p/kWh in Figure 7.2);
- A fixed monthly or quarterly standing charge (i.e. £9.45 per kWh in Figure 7.2).
- The VAT charged on the bill, together with the total cost due.

Date of bill	03/04/2000	Date of meter reading	16/03/2000	Calorific value (MJ/m^3)	39.6

Meter reading		Gas used			Costs
Present	Previous	Cubic feet	Cubic metres	kWh	
3171	2825	346	979.1	10770	163.70

Standing charge
£173.15 at 17.5% VAT

					9.45
					30.30
Unit charge		1.520p/kWh			
				Total	**£203.45**

FIG 7.2 Typical gas bill.

The unit price of natural gas may be fixed as in Figure 7.2, or it may vary depending on the volume of gas consumed. In addition, some large sites may have a combination of firm and interruptible supplies, which may be invoiced separately.

7.4.3 Fuel Oil

Fuel oil is measured by volume, which varies with temperature. Delivery invoices for fuel oils should therefore state the volume corrected to a standard condition of 15.5°C [3]. They should also state the date of delivery, the delivery note reference number, the unit cost per standard litre and the VAT charged on the bill. The calorific value of the oil may be included, but if not, this should be obtained from the supplier. This last point is important because the calorific value varies with the type of fuel oil used.

7.4.4 Solid Fuel

Solid fuel invoices generally state the weight delivered and the cost, but do not always include data on the calorific value. These data can usually be obtained from the supplier. Solid fuels can present particular problems to energy auditors because they are often stock-piled, making accurate short-term assessment of solid fuel consumption a difficult task.

7.4.5 Heat

In many parts of northern Europe buildings and whole towns rely on heat produced in cogeneration plants. The heat is usually supplied in the form of medium- or high-pressure water from a district heating main and transferred to individual buildings via heat exchangers. The heat energy consumption is recorded by heat meters, which record the water flow rate, and the temperatures of the water entering and leaving the facility, thus determining the energy consumed in kWh. It is important to note that the accuracy of heat meters can be affected by variations in temperature and flow rate. At low flow rates or where small temperature differences occur, metering errors can be significant.

7.4.6 Site Records

In larger more complex facilities, especially those which employ an energy manager, it is often the case that site energy records are kept. These can be an important source of information to an audit team and can be used to corroborate data collected from energy invoices. In particular, records of sub-meter readings can be particularly useful, since they give detailed information about energy flows. However, when using data collected from sub-meters, it is important to know where the meters are located and to understand what they are measuring. It should be realized that sub-meters are always 'subordinate' to main meters. In other words, the energy consumption recorded by a sub-meter is always a sub-set of that recorded by the main meter and not additional energy consumption. Failure to recognize this will result in major errors. One good way of avoiding these errors is to construct schematic diagrams showing the respective positions of all the main meters and sub-meters. In addition, it should be remembered that meter records often contain mistakes (see Chapter 9). Care should therefore be taken to validate meter readings.

7.4.7 Data Analysis

The data analysis techniques used in energy audits are described in detail in Chapter 6. For a preliminary energy audit, analysis should be limited to those techniques which enable the auditor to determine:

- How much energy is being consumed;
- What type of energy is being consumed;
- The performance of the facility compared with other similar facilities; and
- The characteristic performance of the building.

These outcomes can be achieved by using the percentage breakdown technique (described in Section 6.2), the normalized performance indicator (NPI) technique (described in Section 6.3) and the linear regression technique (described in Section 6.5).

When all the energy data have been gathered and analysed, they need to be compared against various 'yardsticks' for similar facilities. Table 7.2 gives the NPIs for various building types in the UK, together with percentage breakdowns for typical energy consumption [3]. Example 5.1 illustrates how the analysis for a preliminary energy audit might be performed.

Example 7.1

A preliminary energy audit of a 5000 m² air-conditioned office building has yielded the following energy data:

Month	Heating degree days	Gas consumption (kWh)	Gas cost (£)	Electricity consumption (kWh)	Electricity cost (£)
January	267	90,010	1080.12	68,214	3956.41
February	298	97,160	1165.92	60,312	3437.78
March	250	87,058	1044.70	59,645	3280.48
April	176	71,320	855.84	65,045	3382.34
May	69	47,200	566.40	89,234	4550.93
June	30	38,645	463.74	105,932	5296.60
July	12	33,840	406.08	119,237	5961.85
August	20	34,400	412.80	103,247	5265.60
September	50	44,050	528.60	88,235	4588.22
October	208	75,920	911.04	65,023	3446.22
November	215	78,580	942.96	61,567	3447.75
December	337	106,640	1279.68	70,124	4137.32
Totals	1932	804,823	9657.88	955,815	50,751.50

Given that the office building is located in a city centre and is occupied for 2560 hours per year, perform an analysis which characterizes the building's energy consumption.

TABLE 7.2   Energy breakdown figures and normalized performance indicators for various building types in the UK [3]

Building type	Fair NPI (kWh/m²)	Space heating (%)	Domestic hot water (%)	Lighting (%)	Ventilation (%)	Air conditioning (%)	Other (specified) (%)	Other (unspecified) (%)
School with indoor swimming pool	190–240	43	20	9	n.a.	n.a.	22 (Pool)	6
School without indoor swimming pool	250–310	56	25	12	n.a.	n.a.	n.a.	7
Restaurant	410–430	25	15	15	5	n.a.	40 (Catering)	
Public house	340–470	38	18	12	n.a.	n.a.	11 (Catering)	16
Motorway service area	880–1200	22	32	9	7	n.a.	30 (Catering)	n.a.
Fast-food outlet	1450–1750	4	24	1	n.a.	n.a.	70 (Cooking)	1
Supermarket with bakery	1130–1350	23 (includes ventilation)	2	11	n.a.	n.a.	50 (Refrigeration)	3
Office building (naturally ventilated)	230–290	60	8	20	n.a.	n.a.	12 (Electrical consumption)	n.a.
Office building (air conditioned)	250–410	48	6	16	n.a.	29	1 (Office machines)	n.a.
Sports centre (without swimming pool)	200–340	75	3	11	n.a.	n.a.	11 (Fans, pumps, etc.)	n.a.
Swimming pool	1050–1390	10	3	11	45	n.a.	33 (Pool water heating)	n.a.
Church building	88–169	88	n.a.	6	n.a.	n.a.	n.a.	6

Libraries, museums and art galleries	200–280	60	n.a.	18	n.a.	11	n.a.	11
Large hotel	290–420	50	11	9	n.a.	n.a.	18 (Catering)	12
Bank (non-air conditioned)	180–240	67	4	19	n.a.	n.a.	n.a.	10
Cinema	650–780	77	3	2	15	n.a.	3 (Projection equipment)	n.a.
Bingo hall	631–770	65	5	13	5	n.a.	7 (Catering)	5
Prison	550–689	45	25	10	n.a.	n.a.	10 (Catering)	10
Transport depots	311–381	80	4	6	n.a.	n.a.	2 (Catering)	8
Law court	219–300	84	5	8	n.a.	n.a.	1 (Catering)	2
Factory (excluding process energy)	261–369	72	3	15	n.a.	n.a.	n.a.	10
Cold store	500–675	8	n.a.	10	n.a.	n.a.	82 (Refrigeration)	n.a.
Warehouse	150–269	80	2	8	n.a.	n.a.	n.a.	10

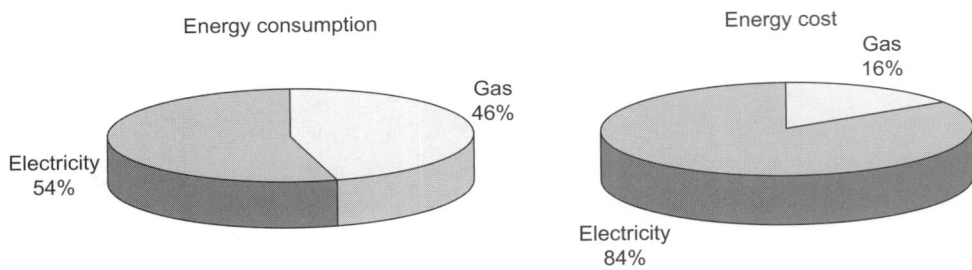

Energy consumption

Gas
46%

Electricity
54%

Energy cost

Gas
16%

Electricity
84%

FIG 7.3 Energy consumption and cost breakdowns.

Solution

The annual energy consumption and energy cost breakdowns are shown in Figure 7.3. It can be seen from the pie charts that although approximately 46% of the energy consumed is natural gas, it only accounts for 16% of the energy costs.

The raw energy consumption and cost figures per m^2 are as follows:

Fuel	Annual energy consumption per m^2	Annual energy cost per m^2
Natural gas	160.965 kWh	£1.93
Electricity	191.163 kWh	£10.15

Using the methodology explained in Section 6.3, the NPI can be established as follows:

$$\text{Electrical energy used} = 955,815 \text{ kWh}$$
$$\text{Gas used} = 804,823 \text{ kWh}$$
$$\text{Total energy consumed} = 955,815 + 804,823$$
$$= 1,760,638 \text{ kWh}$$

From Table 6.5 (see page 105) it can be seen that 75% of the gas consumed can be attributed directly to space heating. Therefore:

$$\text{Space heating energy consumption} = 1760,638 \times 0.75$$
$$= 1,320,478.5 \text{ kWh}$$

By applying weather and exposure coefficients:

$$\text{Corrected space heating energy consumption} = \frac{1,320,478.5 \times 2462 \times 1.0}{1932}$$
$$= 1,682,721.6 \text{ kWh}$$
$$\text{Non-heating energy consumption (kWh)} = 1,760,638 - 1,320,478.5$$
$$= 440,159.5 \text{ kWh}$$

Therefore,

$$\text{Corrected total energy consumption} = 440,159.5 + 1,682,721.6$$
$$= 2,122,881.1 \text{ kWh}$$

and correcting for occupancy (using data from Table 6.6):

$$\text{Normalized annual energy consumption} = 2{,}122{,}881.1 \times \frac{2600}{2560} = 2{,}156{,}051.1\,\text{kWh}$$

Therefore

$$\text{NPI} = \frac{2{,}156{,}051.1}{5000} = 431.21\,\text{kWh/m}^2$$

Because the calculated NPI of 431.21 kWh/m² is above the upper limit of the 'fair' range (i.e. 410 kWh/m² in Table 7.2), for an air-conditioned office building, it can be assumed that the energy performance of the office building is poor.

Using the methodology described in Section 6.5, it is possible to perform a linear regression analysis of the gas data. When such an analysis is performed it yields the following performance equation, which may then be used as the *standard performance* equation for a future monitoring and targeting programme (see Chapter 9).

Monthly gas consumption (kWh) = 31,521.75 + (220.788 × degree days)

This equation shows that the monthly gas base-load consumption is 31,521.75 kWh.

7.5   Comprehensive Energy Audits

It is clear from the analysis presented in Example 7.1 that a considerable amount of useful information can be obtained from a preliminary energy audit. However, without further investigation it is not possible to determine where in the office building the energy is being consumed. In order to do this a more comprehensive audit is required. The analysis techniques used for comprehensive energy audits are essentially much the same as those used for preliminary audits, but the level of detail is much greater. Comprehensive audits require detailed energy surveys to be undertaken, and they often require the installation of additional sub-metering in order to determine accurately component energy flows. Example 7.2 illustrates the auditing benefits which can be gained from installing comprehensive sub-metering.

Example 7.2

Through the installation of sub-meters in the office building in Example 7.1, it has been possible to establish the following data:

Month	Space heating (kWh)	Domestic hot water (kWh)	Catering (kWh)	Lifts (kWh)	Lighting (kWh)	Air conditioning (kWh)	Other (kWh)
January	54,075	13,239	22,696	620	44,016	21,231	2348
February	61,856	12,924	22,380	610	41,082	16,566	2054
March	52,888	11,978	22,191	627	33,746	23,659	1614

Continued

Month	Space heating (kWh)	Domestic hot water (kWh)	Catering (kWh)	Lifts (kWh)	Lighting (kWh)	Air conditioning (kWh)	Other (kWh)
April	38,537	11,348	21,435	631	24,942	27,734	11,738
May	12,841	11,663	22,696	636	19,074	68,013	1511
June	2395	12,293	23,957	640	14,672	88,713	1907
July	427	11,663	21,750	625	15,112	1011,681	1819
August	672	10,717	23,011	621	19,074	81,909	1643
September	14,420	9457	20,174	615	26,410	59,655	1555
October	42,507	11,348	22,065	630	32,719	30,134	1541
November	43,591	11,978	23,011	632	42,549	16,611	1775
December	67,868	13,554	25,217	628	45,483	21,929	2083
Totals	392,077	142,163	270,583	7515	358,877	557,835	31,589

From these data it is possible to produce a comprehensive breakdown of annual energy consumption in each of the component areas (see Figure 7.4).

Example 7.2 makes the bold assumption that extensive sub-metering has been installed in the office building for auditing purposes. While this is possible it would be an expensive option. It is therefore often better to employ other techniques to estimate individual energy flows. In some situations it is possible to deduce energy flows by deducting sub-meter readings from main meter readings. However, other situations may require the members of the auditing team to use their skill and judgement to estimate energy flows.

7.5.1 Portable and Temporary Sub-metering

It may be evident from the outset of an auditing project that the installation of additional sub-metering will yield much useful information about the energy flows within a facility. For example, by placing sub-meters on the energy input side and heat meters on the output side, it is possible to determine the efficiency of individual plant items. Sub-metering should also highlight any imbalances between the consumption

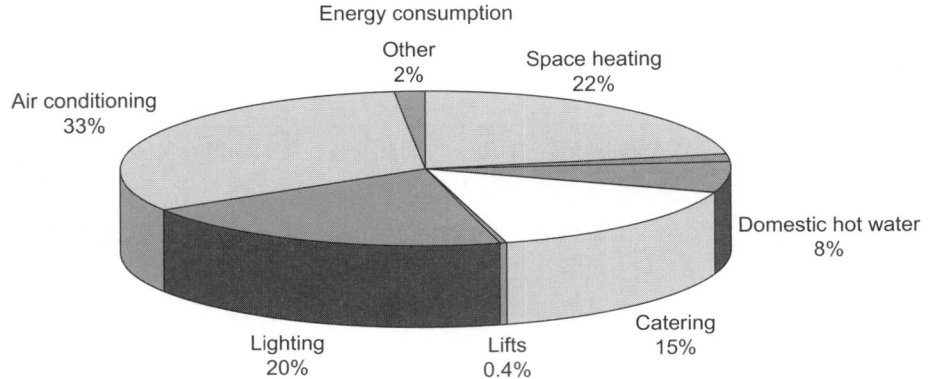

FIG 7.4 Energy consumption breakdown for the office building.

recorded by main meters and the total recorded by the sub-meters. If additional sub-meters are deemed necessary, then the additional cost can usually be justified for items of plant or areas with high loads, particularly in situations where little information exists on current energy consumption.

The process of assessing a facility for additional sub-metering can also highlight short-comings in the facility's existing metering provision. For example, several buildings may be served off a single electricity meter. In such a situation, it may be worth consid-ering the installation of permanent sub-meters, since these would support any future energy-management programme. Permanent metering should also be considered when it is less expensive than the cost of hiring, installing and removing temporary metering equipment. The installation of permanent or temporary meters is invasive and involves the shutting off of energy supplies, which in many circumstances is unsat-isfactory. Instead, it is worth considering the use of portable non-invasive metering. Electricity demand profiles can be monitored using portable clamp-on meters, and heat flows in water pipes can be determined by using clamp-on electronic ther-mometers and portable ultrasonic flow meters.

7.5.2   Estimating Energy Use

In many situations it is either impractical or prohibitively expensive to install comprehen-sive sub-metering and so it is necessary to estimate the energy consumption of various items of plant and equipment. Accurate estimation of equipment energy consumption can be a difficult process and one which relies on skill and judgement. Nevertheless, it is relatively easy to establish an upper limit for energy consumption by using eqn (7.1):

$$\text{Annual energy consumption (kWh)} = \frac{Q_{out}}{\eta} \times T_h \qquad (7.1)$$

where Q_{out} is the plant power output (kW), η is the efficiency of plant and T_h is the number of operating hours per year.

While eqn (7.1) may give an upper limit on plant energy consumption it does not pro-vide the actual operating energy consumption. This problem can be overcome by mon-itoring the actual plant energy consumption for a short period of time, using meters, and then multiplying the average measured load by the annual operating time. In the case of electrical equipment this can be a relatively simple process since the current can be measured using a portable clamp-on meter.

Space heating energy consumption can be estimated using the heat loss and degree day methods described in Chapter 10. The energy consumed in producing domestic hot water can be determined, if the cold feed water is metered, by using eqn (7.2):

$$\text{Annual energy consumption (kWh)} = \frac{m_{cf} \times c_p \times (t_s - t_{cf})}{\eta_s \times 3600} \qquad (7.2)$$

where m_{cf} is the mass of cold feed water used annually (kg), c_p is the specific heat capac-ity of water (i.e. 4.19 kJ/kg K), t_s is the hot water storage temperature (e.g. 60°C), t_{cf} is the cold feed water temperature (e.g. 10°C) and η_s is the seasonal efficiency of system.

The seasonal efficiencies for various domestic hot water–producing systems are given in Table 7.3.

If the cold feed water consumption is not known then it is possible to estimate the energy consumed in producing hot water by using eqn (7.3) [4]:

$$\text{Annual energy consumption (kWh)} = 0.024 \times q_{hws} \times A_f \times N_w \qquad (7.3)$$

where q_{hws} is the mean power requirement (W/m^2), A_f is the floor area (m^2) and N_w is the number of working days.

The power requirement (q_{hws}) can be determined using Table 7.4. The energy consumed by lighting can be estimated simply by counting the number of luminaire fittings and noting their respective power ratings. With all but tungsten filament lamps,

TABLE 7.3 Seasonal efficiencies for water heating systems [3]

System type	Seasonal efficiency
Gas heater with storage cylinder	52
Gas- or oil-fired boiler with storage cylinder	56
Hot water cylinder with immersion heater using off-peak electricity	80
Instantaneous gas multi-point heater	62
District heating with local calorifiers	60
District heating with central calorifiers and distribution	56

TABLE 7.4 Mean power requirements for domestic hot water [3]

Building type	Mean power requirement (q_{hws}) (W/m^2)
Office (5-day occupancy)	2.0
Office (6-day occupancy)	2.0
Shop (5-day occupancy)	0.5
Shop (6-day occupancy)	1.0
Factory (5-day occupancy: single shift)	9.0
Factory (6-day occupancy: single shift)	11.0
Factory (7-day occupancy: multiple shifts)	12.0
Warehouse	1.0
Residential buildings	17.5
Hotels	8.0
Hospitals	29.0
Education	2.0

allowances should be made for control gear losses (see Chapter 14). In most buildings lighting energy consumption lies in the region 10–20 W/m^2 [3].

7.6   Energy Surveys

Energy surveys are an integral part of the auditing process. They enable the auditors to understand the energy flows within facilities and to identify energy wastage. Surveys can be comprehensive, looking in depth at all aspects of a facility's energy consumption, or targeted, in which case they only cover certain specific issues. The main objectives of any energy survey should be to:

- Determine the energy performance of a facility, or in the case of a targeted survey, targeted items of plant and equipment.
- Identify and quantify the principal energy flows.
- Identify and quantify achievable energy cost savings.
- Produce costed recommendations to achieve energy cost savings.
- Make recommendations on the future energy management of the facility.

Energy surveys, with the exception of specifically targeted surveys, should cover all aspects relating to a facility's or organization's energy consumption. This will involve detailed surveys of:

- The management and operation characteristics of a facility or organization.
- The energy supply to an organization's various facilities.
- The energy use within a facility.
- The plant and equipment within a facility.
- The fabric of the organization's buildings.

7.6.1   Management and Operating Characteristics

The management culture within an organization can have a great influence on energy consumption. It is therefore important to determine the management structure and practices relating to energy procurement and consumption. In particular, it is important to identify cost centres clearly, where the managers accountable for operating costs can be made individually responsible for energy consumption. Maintenance practices can also have a direct influence on energy consumption, so it is important to establish the frequency and quality of the maintenance procedures, and to identify new maintenance measures which could improve the energy performance of plant and equipment.

At the auditing stage it is important to survey the operating practices within an organization or facility. Detailed data should be gathered on such factors as:

- The use of a particular space or building.
- The mechanical and electrical services within the building.
- The number and type of occupants. Particular attention should be paid to any special characteristics of occupants. For example, in rooms containing smokers, windows are often opened with the result that space-heating costs are increased.
- The occupancy patterns of building or space.

- The environmental conditions within a space or building. This will include air temperature, dry resultant temperature, relative humidity and illuminance levels.
- The operating practices of major items of plant and equipment.

Knowledge of the above issues will give the auditor a good understanding of how and why energy is consumed within a facility. Particular attention should be paid to situations where actual practice deviates from that stated by the management of an organization. For example, if rooms which are supposed to be heated to 21°C are in fact heated to 23°C, then energy is being wasted on over-heating spaces.

7.6.2 Energy Supply

It is important to identify the tariffs and supply contracts under which any organization purchases its energy. This will enable the energy auditing team to establish whether or not a particular organization is purchasing energy at a low price. If an organization is paying a higher than necessary price for its energy, then the auditor should recommend a change of tariff or fuel supplier.

Because electricity tariffs usually include some form of demand charge, it is important that an organization selects the correct electricity tariff to suite its load profile. Therefore, the audit process should include a survey of the electrical load profile of a facility. For relatively minor loads it may be sufficient to take meter readings at the beginning and end of a selected period, with intermediate readings taken during the daytime, night-time and at the weekend. This will give a good indication of when electrical energy is being consumed and should assist the auditor in recommending an appropriate tariff. For larger electrical loads, it is important to survey the load profile accurately. This can be achieved by using a portable meter to determine demand and consumption at 30-minute intervals over a selected period. Any large peaks in load should be identified and further investigations made in order to establish their cause.

With electricity supply, it is important to determine the power factor of a facility. Many items of equipment, such as fluorescent lamps and electric motors, produce a poor power factor (i.e. a decoupling of the current and the voltage so that they become out of phase with each other). This results in higher than expected electricity bills. If poor power factors are found in a facility then it may be worth considering the installation of power factor correction equipment (see Chapter 14).

7.6.3 Plant and Equipment

Major items of plant, such as boilers and refrigeration chillers, convert energy from one form to another. In doing so energy is wasted. For example, in boilers much of the heat produced by the combustion process can be wasted by allowing it to escape with the flue gases. The more efficient an item of plant, the less energy is wasted. Major items of plant and equipment should therefore be surveyed in order to determine their operating efficiency. It is also important to survey their respective pipe distribution networks since these too can be a major source of energy wastage.

The subjects of energy-efficient heating and refrigeration are dealt with in some detail in Chapters 10 and 13, so the issues involved in a plant survey are only briefly summarized here. With boilers it is essential that they be 'tuned' so that flue gas heat losses are minimized. This involves sampling the CO_2 or O_2 content of the flue gases and adjusting the burner settings so that excess O_2 is minimized, whilst still ensuring that complete combustion takes place. In addition, it is important to identify whether or not flue gas heat recovery is feasible.

The efficiency of refrigeration plant is measured by its coefficient of performance (COP). The higher the COP, the greater the efficiency of the machine. COP varies with the cooling load and the external air conditions. It is therefore necessary to meter the energy input and output over a period of time, if the average COP is to be identified. Note should be taken of the operating pattern of refrigeration plant and also of how it is controlled, since this will tell the auditor much about the operation of the facility. If both boilers and refrigeration chillers are operating at the same time, it could be that the two systems are fighting each other. If this is the case, then the control logic and settings of the system will need adjustment. The feasibility of recovering heat from the hot condenser gases should also be investigated.

In many facilities much energy is wasted from hot water, chilled water and steam distribution pipework because of inadequate or poor quality insulation. Pipework systems should therefore be inspected to establish the quality of the insulation and also to identify any leaks.

Plant surveys should allow for the fact that mechanical equipment has a finite working life and that efficiency often deteriorates badly when plant is old. Therefore one of the important outcomes of such a survey should be a recommendation for the planned replacement of older plant. In many situations it is much more cost-effective to replace old plant, rather than renovate it.

7.6.4 Building Fabric

Although the subject of heat loss through building fabric is covered in detail in Chapter 10, a few words on the subject are timely here. It is important to note the age, size, shape and orientation of the buildings within a facility, since these are all factors which affect energy consumption. In particular, areas of greatest heat loss should be identified. Greatest heat loss will always occur where the building fabric has a high U value (see Chapter 10). If 'as built' drawings exist, these can be used to determine elemental U values. The use of portable infrared thermography can also be very useful, since this enables areas of high heat loss to be instantly identified.

When surveying buildings, it should be appreciated that large amounts of heat can be lost by excess ventilation (see Chapter 10). This is particularly the case in older properties with old fenestration systems. Particular attention should therefore be paid to any poorly fitting window and door frames, or to any space where windows and outside doors remain open for any length of time.

7.7 Recommendations

The energy auditing process should enable recommendations to be made, which will result in cost savings. Although the precise nature of these recommendations will depend on the particular application in question, they can broadly be classified as follows:

(i) *Reducing energy costs by tariff negotiation:* Electricity and gas are supplied either through published tariffs or through negotiated supply contracts. Not all tariffs and supply contracts are suited to every organization and some are better than others. It may therefore be possible to reduce energy costs simply by changing tariff or negotiating a more beneficial supply contract.

(ii) *Good maintenance and work practices:* Energy can often be saved at no capital expense simply by 'good housekeeping' (i.e. improving maintenance procedures and implementing good work practices).

(iii) *Retrofitting and tuning systems:* Energy is often wasted as systems age, because components wear out or become damaged. Also, the controls associated with these systems are often inappropriate or poorly set up with the result that systems perform inefficiently. Significant energy savings can be achieved through modest capital investment to retrofit and re-tune inefficient installations.

(iv) *Capital investment:* In many situations the poor condition of plant and infrastructure makes refurbishment a futile exercise. Under these circumstances major capital investment is required to replace existing plant. In this case, it is often worthwhile reappraising the situation to determine whether or not an alternative installation might be more appropriate. An existing boiler installation could be replaced by a combined heat and power (CHP) plant, thus reducing the need to buy in electrical power. Such measures usually involve large capital investment and careful financial appraisal is therefore required.

7.8 The Audit Report

The audit process should identify potential energy-management opportunities. Since exploitation of these opportunities often involves capital expenditure, maximum effort should be put into investigating those measures which will yield the greatest cost savings. Those energy-management opportunities which result in lesser savings should be given a low priority. However, all energy-management opportunities, identified through the auditing process, should be clearly stated in the final audit report, together with cost/benefit calculations to justify them. The final audit report should include:

- A description of the facility, including layout drawings, construction details, hours of operation, equipment lists and any relevant materials and product flows.
- A description of the various utility tariffs or contracts used.
- A presentation of all the energy data gathered, together with any relevant analysis.
- A detailed statement of potential energy-management opportunities, together with supporting cost/benefit analysis calculations.
- An energy management action plan for the future operation of the facility. This may include an implementation schedule for the recommended energy-management opportunities and a programme for the ongoing energy monitoring and targeting of the facility.

Although the audit report should contain detailed technical information, it is important to remember that its primary purpose is to communicate the principal findings of the audit to an organization's senior management, many of whom may have little understanding of energy matters. It is therefore advisable to include a short executive summary, giving a brief synopsis of the report and highlighting its major findings and recommendations.

References

[1] How to hire an energy auditor to identify energy efficiency projects. California Energy Commission. January; 2000.
[2] Aspects of energy management. General Information Report 12, Department of the Environment. May; 1995.
[3] Energy audits and surveys. CIBSE Applications Manual AM5; 1991.
[4] Measurement of energy consumption: CIBSE Building Energy Code Part 4. CIBSE; 1982.

Bibliography

Capehurst BL, Turner WC, Kennedy WJ. Guide to energy management (Chapter 2). Prentice Hall: The Fairmont Press; 1997.
Eastop TD, Croft DR. Energy efficiency for engineers and technologists (Chapter 9). Harlow: Longman Scientific & Technical; 1990. Harlow, Essex.
Energy audits and surveys. CIBSE Applications Manual AM5; 1991.
Energy audits for buildings, Fuel Efficiency Booklet 1. Department of the Environment; 1993.
How to hire an energy auditor to identify energy efficiency projects. California Energy Commission. January; 2000.
Moss KJ. Energy management and operating costs in buildings (Chapter 9). London: E & FN Spon; 1997.
Thumann A, Mehta PD. Handbook of energy engineering (Chapter 3). Prentice Hall: The Fairmont Press; 1997.

CHAPTER 8

Project Investment Appraisal

It is important to justify any capital investment project by carrying out a financial appraisal. The financial issues associated with capital investment in energy-saving projects are investigated in this chapter. In particular, the discounted cash flow techniques of net present value and internal rate of return are presented and discussed.

8.1 Introduction

When planning an energy-efficiency or energy-management project, the costs involved should always be considered. Therefore, as with any other type of investment, energy-management proposals should show the likely return on any capital that is invested. Consider the case of an energy consultant who advises the senior management of an organization that capital should be invested in new boiler plant. Inevitably, the management of the organization would enquire:

- How much will the proposal cost?
- How much money will be saved by the proposal?

These are, of course, not unreasonable questions, since within any organization there are many 'worthy causes', each of which requires funding and it is the job of senior management to invest capital where it is going to obtain the greatest return. In order to make a decision about any course of action, management needs to be able to appraise all the costs involved in a project and determine the potential returns. However, this is not quite as straightforward as it might first appear. The capital value of plant or equipment usually decreases with time and it often requires more maintenance as it gets older. If money is borrowed from a bank to finance a project, then interest will have to be paid on the loan. Inflation too will influence the value of any future energy savings that might be achieved. It is therefore important that the cost-appraisal process allows for all these factors, with the aim of determining which investments should be undertaken and of optimizing the benefits achieved. To this end a number of accounting and financial appraisal techniques have been developed which help managers make correct and objective decisions. It is these financial appraisal techniques which are introduced and discussed in this chapter.

8.2 Fixed and Variable Costs

When appraising the potential costs involved in a project it is important to understand the difference between fixed and variable costs. Variable costs are those which vary directly with the output of a particular plant or production process, such as fuel costs. Fixed costs are those costs, which are not dependent on plant or process output, such as site-rent and insurance. The total cost of any project is therefore the sum of the fixed and variable costs. Example 8.1 illustrates how both fixed and variable costs combine to make the total operating cost.

Example 8.1

Determine the total cost of a diesel generator operating over a 5-year period. Assume that the capital cost of the generator is £15,000, the annual output is 219 MWh and the maintenance costs are £500 per annum. The cost of producing each unit of electricity is 3.5p/kWh.

Solution

Item	Type of cost	Calculation	Cost (£)
Capital cost of generator	Fixed	n.a.	15,000.00
Annual maintenance	Fixed	£500 × 5	2500.00
Fuel cost	Variable	219,000 × 0.035	7665.00
		Total cost =	25,165.00

From Example 8.1 it can be seen that the fixed costs represent 69.5% of the total cost. In fact, the annual electricity output of 219 MWh assumes that the plant is operating with an average output of 50 kW. If this output were increased to an average of 70 kW, then the fuel cost would become £10,731, with the result that the fixed costs would drop to 62% of the total. Clearly, the average unit cost of production decreases as output increases.

The concept of fixed and variable costs can be used to determine the break-even point for a proposed project. The break-even point can be determined by using eqn (8.1):

$$UC_{util} \times W_{av} \times n = FC + \left(UC_{prod} \times W_{av} \times n\right) \qquad (8.1)$$

where UC_{util} is the unit cost per kWh of bought-in energy (£/kWh), UC_{prod} is the unit cost per kWh of produced energy (£/kWh), FC is the fixed costs (£), W_{av} is the average power output (or consumption) (kW) and n is the number of hours of operation (h).

Example 8.2
Assuming that electricity bought from a local utility company costs an average of 8.1p/kWh, determine the break-even point for the generator described in Example 8.1, when:

(i) the average output is 50 kW and
(ii) the average output is 70 kW.

Solution
(i) Assuming that the average output of the generator is 50 kW:

$$0.061 \times 50 \times n = \left(15,000 + 2500\right) + \left(0.035 \times 50 \times n\right)$$
$$\therefore n = 13,461.5 \text{ hours}$$

(ii) Assuming that the average output of the generator is 70 kW:

$$0.061 \times 70 \times n = \left(15,000 + 2500\right) + \left(0.035 \times 70 \times n\right)$$
$$\therefore n = 9615.4 \text{ hours}$$

Clearly, increasing the average output of the generator significantly reduces the break-even time for the project. This is because the capital investment (i.e. the generator) is being better utilized.

8.3 Interest Charges

In order to finance projects, organizations often borrow money from banks or other lending organizations. Projects financed in this way cost more than similar projects financed from an organization's own funds, because interest charges must be paid on the loan. It is therefore important to understand how interest charges are calculated. Interest charges can be calculated by lending organizations in two different ways: simple interest and compound interest:

(i) *Simple interest*: If simple interest is applied, then charges are calculated as a fixed percentage of the capital that is borrowed. A fixed interest percentage is applied to each year of the loan and repayments are calculated using eqn (8.2).

$$TRV = LV + \left(\frac{IR}{100} \times LV \times P\right) \qquad (8.2)$$

where TRV is the total repayment value (£), LV is the value of initial loan (£), IR is the interest rate (%) and P is the repayment period (years).

(ii) *Compound interest*: Compound interest is usually calculated annually (although this is not necessarily the case). The interest charged is calculated as a percentage of the outstanding loan at the end of each time period. It is termed 'compound' because the outstanding loan is the sum of the unpaid capital and the interest charges up to that point. The value of the total repayment can be calculated using eqn (8.3):

$$\text{TRV} = \text{LV} \times \left(1 + \frac{\text{IR}}{100}\right)^{\text{P}} \tag{8.3}$$

The techniques involved in calculating simple and compound interests are illustrated in Example 8.3.

Example 8.3

A company borrows £50,000 to finance a new boiler installation. If the interest rate is 9.5% per annum and the repayment period is 5 years, determine the value of the total repayment and the monthly repayment value, assuming that:

(i) simple interest is applied and
(ii) compound interest is applied.

Solution

(i) *Assuming simple interest*:

$$\text{Total repayment} = 50,000 + \left(\frac{9.5}{100} \times 50,000 \times 5\right) = \text{£73,750.00}$$

$$\text{Monthly repayment} = \frac{73,750.00}{(5 \times 12)} = \text{£1229.17}$$

(ii) *Assuming compound interest*:

$$\text{Repayment at end of year 1} = 50,000 + \left(\frac{9.5}{100} \times 50,000\right) = \text{£54,750.00}$$

and

$$\text{Repayment at end of year 2} = 54,750 + \left(\frac{9.5}{100} \times 54,750\right) = \text{£59,951.25}$$

Similarly, the repayments at the end of years 3, 4 and 5 can be calculated:

Repayment at end of year 3 is £65,646.62
Repayment at end of year 4 is £71,883.05
Repayment at end of year 5 is £78,711.94.

Alternatively, eqn (8.3) can be used to determine the compound interest repayment value:

$$\text{Total repayment value} = 50,000 \times \left(1 + \frac{9.5}{100}\right)^5 = £78,711.94$$

$$\text{Monthly repayment} = \frac{78,711.94}{(5 \times 12)} = £1311.87$$

It can be seen that by using compound interest, the lender recoups an additional £4962. Not surprisingly lenders usually charge compound interest on loans.

8.4 Payback Period

Probably the simplest technique which can be used to appraise a proposal is payback analysis. The payback period can be defined as 'the length of time required for the running total of net savings before depreciation to equal the capital cost of the project' [1]. In theory, once the payback period has ended, all the project capital costs will have been recouped and any additional cost savings achieved can be seen as clear 'profit'. Obviously, the shorter the payback period, the more attractive the project becomes. The length of the maximum permissible payback period generally varies with the business culture concerned. In some countries, payback periods in excess of 5 years are considered acceptable, whereas in other countries, such as in the UK, organizations generally impose payback periods of less than 3 years. The payback period can be calculated using eqn (8.4):

$$PB = \frac{CC}{AS} \tag{8.4}$$

where PB is the payback period (years), CC is the capital cost of the project (£) and AS is the annual net cost saving achieved (£).

The annual net cost saving (AS) is the cost saving achieved after all the operational costs have been met.

Example 8.4

A new combined heat and power (CHP) installation is expected to reduce a company's annual energy bill by £8100. If the capital cost of the new boiler installation is £37,000, and the annual maintenance and operating costs are £700, what will be the expected payback period for the project?

Solution

$$PB = \frac{37,000}{8100 - 700} = 5.0 \text{ years}$$

8.5 Discounted Cash Flow Methods

The payback method is a simple technique which can easily be used to provide a quick evaluation of a proposal. However, it has a number of major weaknesses:

- The payback method does not consider savings that are accrued after the payback period has finished.
- The payback method does not consider the fact that money, which is invested, should accrue interest as time passes. In simple terms there is a 'time value' component to cash flows. Thus a £100 today is more valuable than £100 in 10 years' time.

In order to overcome these weaknesses a number of discounted cash flow techniques have been developed, which are based on the fact that money invested in a bank will accrue annual interest. The two most commonly used techniques are the 'net present value' and the 'internal rate of return' methods.

8.5.1 Net Present Value Method

The net present value (NPV) method considers the fact that a cash saving (often referred to as a 'cash flow') of £1000 in year 10 of a project will be worth less than a cash flow of £1000 in year 2. The NPV method achieves this by quantifying the impact of time on any particular future cash flow. This is done by equating each future cash flow to its current value today, in other words determining the present value of any future cash flow. The present value (PV) is determined by using an assumed interest rate, usually referred to as a discount rate. Discounting is the opposite process to compounding. Compounding determines the future value of present cash flows, whereas discounting determines the present value of future cash flows.

In order to understand the concept of present value, consider the case described in Example 8.4. If instead of installing a new CHP system, the company invested £37,000 in a bank at an annual interest rate of 8%, then:

$$\text{The value of the end of year } 1 = 37,000 + (0.08 \times 37,000) = £39,960.00$$

and

$$\text{The value of the end of year } 2 = 39,960 + (0.08 \times 39,960) = £43,156.80$$

The value of the investment would grow as compound interest is added, until after n years the value of the sum would be:

$$FV = D \times \left(1 + \frac{IR}{100}\right)^n \tag{8.5}$$

where FV is the future value of investment (£) and D is the value of initial deposit (or investment) (£).

So after 5 years the future value of the investment would be:

$$FV = 37,000 \times \left(1 + \frac{8}{100}\right)^n = £54,365.14$$

So in 5 years the initial investment of £37,000 will accrue £17,365.14 in interest and will be worth £54,365.14. Alternatively, it could equally be said that £54,365.14 in 5 years' time is worth £37,000 now (assuming an annual interest rate of 8%). In other words the present value of £54,365.14 in 5 years' time is £37,000 now. The present value of an amount of money at any specified time in the future can be determined by eqn (8.6):

$$PV = S \times \left(1 + \frac{IR}{100}\right)^{-n} \tag{8.6}$$

where PV is the present value of S in n years time (£), and S is the value of cash flow in n years time (£).

The NPV method calculates the *present value* of all the yearly cash flows (i.e. capital costs and net savings) incurred or accrued throughout the life of a project and summates them. Costs are represented as a negative value and savings as a positive value. The sum of all the present values is known as the NPV. The higher the NPV, the more attractive the proposed project.

The *present value* of a future cash flow can be determined using eqn (8.6). However, it is common practice to use a *discount factor* (DF) when calculating present value. The DF is based on an assumed discount rate (i.e. interest rate) and can be determined by using eqn (8.7):

$$DF = \left(1 + \frac{IR}{100}\right)^{-n} \tag{8.7}$$

The product of a particular cash flow and the *DF is the present value*:

$$PV = S \times DF \tag{8.8}$$

The value of various DFs computed for a range of discount rates (i.e. interest rates) is shown in Table 8.1. Example 8.5 illustrates the process involved in an NPV analysis.

Example 8.5

Using the NPV analysis technique, evaluate the financial merits of the two proposed projects shown in the following table. Assume an annual discount rate of 8% for each project.

Capital cost (£) Year	Project 1 30,000.00 Net annual saving (£)	Project 2 30,000.00 Net annual saving (£)
1	+6000.00	+6600.00
2	+6000.00	+6600.00
3	+6000.00	+6300.00

Continued

Capital cost (£) Year	Project 1 30,000.00 Net annual saving (£)	Project 2 30,000.00 Net annual saving (£)
4	+6000.00	+6300.00
5	+6000.00	+6000.00
6	+6000.00	+6000.00
7	+6000.00	+5700.00
8	+6000.00	+5700.00
9	+6000.00	+5400.00
10	+6000.00	+5400.00
Total net savings at end of year 10	+60,000.00	+60,000.00

TABLE 8.1   Computed discount factors

Year	Discount rate % (or interest rate %)							
	2	4	6	8	10	12	14	16
0	1.000	1.000	1.000	1.000	1.000	1.000	1.000	1.000
1	0.980	0.962	0.943	0.926	0.909	0.893	0.877	0.862
2	0.961	0.925	0.890	0.857	0.826	0.797	0.769	0.743
3	0.942	0.889	0.840	0.794	0.751	0.712	0.675	0.641
4	0.924	0.855	0.792	0.735	0.683	0.636	0.592	0.552
5	0.906	0.822	0.747	0.681	0.621	0.567	0.519	0.476
6	0.888	0.790	0.705	0.630	0.564	0.507	0.456	0.410
7	0.871	0.760	0.665	0.583	0.513	0.452	0.400	0.354
8	0.853	0.731	0.627	0.540	0.467	0.404	0.351	0.305
9	0.837	0.703	0.592	0.500	0.424	0.361	0.308	0.263
10	0.820	0.676	0.558	0.463	0.386	0.322	0.270	0.227
11	0.804	0.650	0.527	0.429	0.350	0.287	0.237	0.195
12	0.788	0.625	0.497	0.397	0.319	0.257	0.208	0.168
13	0.773	0.601	0.469	0.368	0.290	0.229	0.182	0.145
14	0.758	0.577	0.442	0.340	0.263	0.205	0.160	0.125
15	0.743	0.555	0.417	0.315	0.239	0.183	0.140	0.108
16	0.728	0.534	0.394	0.292	0.218	0.163	0.123	0.093
17	0.714	0.513	0.371	0.270	0.198	0.146	0.108	0.080
18	0.700	0.494	0.350	0.250	0.180	0.130	0.095	0.069
19	0.686	0.475	0.331	0.232	0.164	0.116	0.083	0.060
20	0.673	0.456	0.312	0.215	0.149	0.104	0.073	0.051

Solution

The annual cash flows should be multiplied by the annual DFs for a rate of 8% to determine the annual present values, as shown in the following table.

Year	Discount factor for 8%	Project 1		Project 2	
		Net savings (£)	Present value (£)	Net savings (£)	Present value (£)
	(a)	(b)	(a × b)	(c)	(a × c)
0	1.000	−30000.00	−30,000.00	−30000.00	−30,000.00
1	0.926	+6000.00	+5556.00	+6600.00	+6111.60
2	0.857	+6000.00	+5142.00	+6600.00	+5656.20
3	0.794	+6000.00	+4764.00	+6300.00	+5002.20
4	0.735	+6000.00	+4410.00	+6300.00	+4630.50
5	0.681	+6000.00	+4086.00	+6000.00	+4086.00
6	0.630	+6000.00	+3780.00	+6000.00	+3780.00
7	0.583	+6000.00	+3498.00	+5700.00	+3323.10
8	0.540	+6000.00	+3240.00	+5700.00	+3078.00
9	0.500	+6000.00	+3000.00	+5400.00	+2700.00
10	0.463	+6000.00	+2778.00	+5400.00	+2500.20
			NPV = +10,254.00		NPV = +10,867.80

It can be seen that over a 10-year lifespan the NPV for Project 1 is £10,254.00, while for Project 2 it is £10,867.80. Therefore Project 2 is the preferential proposal.

The whole credibility of the NPV method depends on a realistic prediction of future interest rates, which can often be unpredictable. It is prudent therefore to set the discount rate slightly above the interest rate at which the capital for the project is borrowed. This will ensure that the overall analysis is slightly pessimistic, thus acting against the inherent uncertainties in predicting future savings.

8.5.2 Internal Rate of Return Method

It can be seen from Example 8.5 that both projects returned a positive NPV over 10 years, at a discount rate of 8%. However, if the discount rate were reduced there would come a point when the NPV would become zero. It is clear that the discount rate which must be applied, in order to achieve a NPV of zero, will be higher for Project 2 than for Project 1. This means that the average rate of return for Project 2 is higher than for Project 1, with the result that Project 2 is the better proposition. The discount rate which achieves an NPV of zero is known as the internal rate of return (IRR). The higher the IRR, the more attractive the project.

Example 8.6 illustrates how an IRR analysis is performed.

Example 8.6

A proposed project requires an initial capital investment of £20,000. The cash flows generated by the project are shown in the following table.

Year	Cash flow (£)
0	−20,000.00
1	+6000.00
2	+5500.00
3	+5000.00
4	+4500.00
5	+4000.00
6	+4000.00

Given the above cash flow data determine the IRR for the project.

Solution

The NPV should be calculated for a range of discount rates, as shown below.

Year	Cash flow (£)	8% discount rate		12% discount rate		16% discount rate	
		Discount factor	Present value (£)	Discount factor	Present value (£)	Discount factor	Present value (£)
0	−20,000	1.000	−20,000	1.000	−20,000	1.000	−20,000
1	6000	0.926	5556	0.893	5358	0.862	5172
2	5500	0.857	4713.5	0.797	4383.5	0.743	4086.5
3	5000	0.794	3970	0.712	3560	0.641	3205
4	4500	0.735	3307.5	0.636	2862	0.552	2484
5	4000	0.681	2724	0.567	2268	0.476	1904
6	4000	0.630	2520	0.507	2028	0.410	1640
			NPV = 2791		**NPV = 459.5**		**NPV = −1508.5**

It can be clearly seen that the discount rate which results in the NPV being zero lies somewhere between 12% and 16%. The exact IRR can be found by plotting the NPVs on a graph, as shown in Figure 8.1.

Figure 8.1 shows that the IRR for the project is 12.93%. At first sight, both the NPV and the IRR methods look very similar, and in some respects they are. Yet there is an important difference between the two. The NPV method is essentially a comparison tool, which enables a number of projects to be compared, while the IRR method is designed to assess whether or not a single project will achieve a target rate of return.

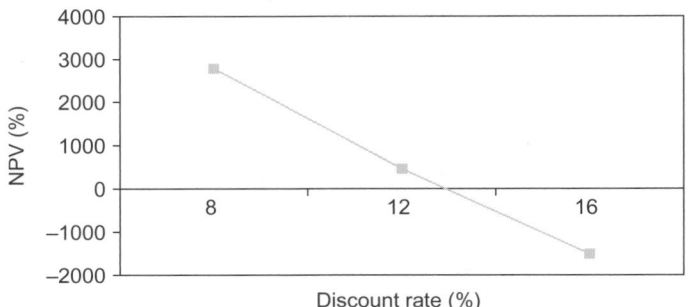

FIG 8.1 NPV versus discount rate.

8.5.3 Profitability Index

Another technique which can be used to evaluate the financial viability of projects is the profitability index. The profitability index can be defined as:

$$\text{Profitability index} = \frac{\text{Sum of the discounted net savings}}{\text{Capital costs}} \qquad (8.9)$$

The higher the *profitability index*, the more attractive the project. The application of the *profitability index* is illustrated in Example 8.7.

Example 8.7

Determine the *profitability index* for the projects outlined in Example 8.5.

Solution

$$\text{Project 1: Profitability index} = \frac{40,254.00}{30,000.00} = 1.342$$

$$\text{Project 2: Profitability index} = \frac{40,867.80}{30,000.00} = 1.362$$

Project 2 is therefore a better proposal than Project 1.

8.6 Factors Affecting Analysis

Although Examples 8.5 and 8.6 illustrate the basic principles associated with the financial analysis of projects, they do not allow for the following important considerations:

- The capital value of plant and equipment generally depreciates over time.
- General inflation reduces the value of savings as time progresses. For example, £100 saved in 1 year's time will be worth more than £100 saved in 10 years' time.

The capital depreciation of an item of equipment can be considered in terms of its salvage value at the end of the analysis period. Example 8.8 illustrates this point.

Example 8.8

It is proposed to install a heat recovery device in a factory building. The capital cost of installing the device is £20,000 and after 5 years its salvage value is £1500. If the savings accrued by the heat recovery device are as shown below, determine the NPV after 5 years. Assume a discount rate of 8%.

Data:

Year	1	2	3	4	5
Savings (£)	7000	6000	6000	5000	5000

Solution

Year	Discount factor for 8% (a)	Capital investment (£) (b)	Net savings (£) (c)	Present value (£) (a) × (b + c)
0	1.000	−20,000.00		−20,000.00
1	0.926		+7000.00	+6482.00
2	0.857		+6000.00	+5142.00
3	0.794		+6000.00	+4764.00
4	0.735		+5000.00	+3675.00
5	0.681	+1500.00	+5000.00	+4426.50
				NPV = +4489.50

It is evident that over a 5-year lifespan the NPV of the project is £4489.50. Had the salvage value of the equipment not been considered, the NPV of the project would have been only £3468.00.

8.6.1   Real Value

Inflation can be defined as the 'rate of increase in the average price of goods and services' [1]. In the UK, inflation is expressed in terms of the retail price index (RPI), which is determined centrally and reflects average inflation over a range of commodities. Because of inflation, the real value of cash flows decreases with time. The real value of a sum of money (S) realized in n years time can be determined by using eqn (8.10):

$$RV = S \times \left(1 + \frac{R}{100}\right)^{-n} \tag{8.10}$$

where RV is the real value of S realized in n years time (£), S is the value of cash flow in n years time (£), and R is the inflation rate (%). As with the 'discount factor' it is common practice to use an 'inflation factor' when assessing the impact of inflation on a project. The inflation factor can be determined by using eqn (8.11):

$$IF = \left(1 + \frac{R}{100}\right)^{-n} \tag{8.11}$$

The product of a particular cash flow and the inflation factor is the real value of the cash flow:

$$RV = S \times IF \tag{8.12}$$

The application of inflation factors is considered in Example 8.9.

Example 8.9

Recalculate the NPV of the energy recovery scheme in Example 8.8, assuming that the discount rate remains at 8% and that the rate of inflation is 5%.

Solution
Because of inflation:

Real interest rate = Discount rate − Rate of inflation

∴ Real interest rate = 8 − 5 = 3%

Example 8.9 shows that when inflation is assumed to be 5%, the NPV of the project reduces from £4489.50 to £4397.88. This is to be expected, because general inflation will always erode the value of future 'profits' accrued by a project.

Year	Capital investment (£)	Net real savings (£)	Inflation factor for 5%	Net real savings (£)	Real discount factor for 3%	Present value (£)
0	−20,000.00		1.000	−20,000.00	1.000	−20,000.00
1		+7000.00	0.952	+6664.00	0.971	+6470.74
2		+6000.00	0.907	+5442.00	0.943	+5131.81
3		+6000.00	0.864	+5184.00	0.915	+4743.36
4		+5000.00	0.823	+4115.00	0.888	+3654.12
5	+1500.00	+5000.00	0.784	+5096.00	0.863	+4397.85
						NPV = +4397.88

References

[1]   Eastop TD, Croft DR. Energy efficiency for engineers and technologists (Chapter 2). Harlow: Longman Scientific & Technical; 1990.

Bibliography

Capehurst BL, Turner WC, Kennedy WJ. Guide to energy management (Chapter 4). Prentice Hall: The Fairmont Press; 1997.

Eastop TD, Croft DR. Energy efficiency for engineers and technologists (Chapter 2). Harlow: Longman Scientific & Technical; 1990.

Investment appraisal for industrial energy efficiency. Good Practice Guide 69. DOE; 1993.

Moss KJ. Energy management and operating costs in buildings (Chapter 8). London: E & FN Spon; 1997.

Sizer J. An insight into management accounting (Chapter 8): Pelican; 1979.

Thumann A, Mehta PD. Handbook of energy engineering (Chapter 2). Prentice Hall: The Fairmont Press; 1997.

CHAPTER 9

Energy Monitoring, Targeting and Waste Avoidance

The concept of monitoring and targeting is discussed in this chapter and techniques for collecting and analysing energy data are explained. A variety of reporting techniques are also presented. The subject of waste avoidance is discussed and practical examples given on how to diagnose and eliminate wasteful energy practices.

9.1 The Concept of Monitoring and Targeting

It is possible to establish the existing energy consumption of a facility or organization through an energy audit (see Chapter 7). However, this only produces a 'picture' of past energy consumption. In order to keep control of subsequent energy consumption, it is necessary to initiate a monitoring programme, although by itself it is only of limited value, as it simply records energy consumption. To achieve improvements in energy performance a targeting programme, in which targets are set, must accompany the monitoring process and planned improvements made. The key elements of a *monitoring and targeting* (M&T) programme are as follows [1]:

- The establishment of Energy Account Centres (EACs) within an organization. These may be departments, processes or cost centres. Operational managers should be accountable for the energy consumption of the EACs for which they are responsible.

- The establishment of *standard energy performance* benchmarks for each EAC. Standard energy performance relates energy consumption to a variable, such as degree days or production output. Standard performance is established through regression analysis of past energy data (see Chapter 6) and it provides a baseline for the assessment of future energy performance.
- Monitoring the energy consumption of each EAC within an organization. This involves setting up procedures to ensure the regular collection of reliable energy data.
- The establishment of energy targets for each EAC. Energy cost savings can only be achieved if improvements are made on standard performance. Achievable targets should therefore be set which improve on standard performance.
- Energy management reports should be produced for each EAC on a regular basis. These reports provide the stimulus for improved energy performance, and should also quantify any improvements that are achieved.

It is important that any proposed M&T programme be designed to suit the needs of its host organization. From an energy point of view, organizations can be characterized in a variety of ways. One useful classification method is, by the number of sites covered and the level of metering adopted, as follows [1]:

- Single site with central utility metering
- Single site with sub-metering
- Multisite with central utility metering
- Multisite with sub-metering.

Single sites with central utility metering are probably best treated as a single EAC, while the introduction of sub-metering enables such sites to be broken-up into a number of separate EACs. Where organizations have a number of separate properties, each with central utility meters, the sites should be treated as separate EACs. If organizations have multiple properties, each containing sub-metering, then it should be possible to divide each site into a number of separate EACs.

9.2 Computer-Based M&T

The use of specially designed computer software is advisable when operating an M&T programme. Computers should not be seen as a replacement for the energy manager, but simply as tools which enable large amounts of data to be stored and analysed in a short period of time. A number of energy management software packages are commercially available, with varying degrees of complexity (discussion of which is beyond the scope of this book). They all tend to share the following generic features:

- A database facility, which is capable of storing and organizing large quantities of data collected over a long period of time.
- The ability to record energy data for all utility types, including data taken from both meters and invoices.

- The ability to handle complex utility tariffs. Tariffs vary from country to country, and are becoming increasingly complex as competition is introduced into the utilities sector.
- The ability to handle other variables such as degree days and production data.
- A data analysis facility. This is achieved by incorporating statistical analysis software into the energy management software.
- A reporting facility, which is capable of quickly producing energy management reports.

With the more sophisticated energy management packages it is possible to interface the software with building management systems (BMS), so that energy data can be automatically recorded on a regular basis (e.g. hourly).

One of the great advantages of computer-based systems is their database facility, which enables historical data and data from many sources to be instantly compared. This facility is particularly useful when comparing site energy costs on a utility basis and enables energy managers quickly to assess the relative performance of various EACs. In this way EACs which are underperforming can be quickly identified and remedial action taken.

9.3 Monitoring and Data Collection

An integral element of any M&T programme is data collection. Ultimately, the accuracy of an energy audit or any M&T programme depends on the collection and input of good quality data. In order to ensure accuracy, robust data collection procedures must be established, but problems can arise for a variety of reasons. If too few data are used, any analysis will be meaningless. Most systems therefore require at least 12 sets of data before any meaningful analysis can be carried out. By contrast, if excessive data are collected it slows down collection and analysis processes, and leads to an over-complex M&T system. In some situations data from various sources may be incompatible, making comparisons very difficult. For example, utility invoices may be collected which cover different time periods. In addition, errors may occur when meters are read incorrectly and also when readings are incorrectly logged.

9.3.1 Data from Invoices

In most applications, energy invoices are the primary source of energy data. Data collection from invoices involves collating various utility and fuel bills, extracting relevant information and inputting data into a computer. Problems arise when invoices are misplaced. It is therefore important to establish good collection procedures which ensure that good quality data are entered into the computer system.

Although an extremely important source of data, in many larger process industries the use of monthly utility invoices is considered inadequate. This is because the data provided by the invoices are of insufficient detail and also because the data collection process is too slow, with the potential for excessive energy wastage. Therefore, in situations where invoice data alone are considered insufficient, it is necessary to establish more detailed data collection systems.

9.3.2 Data from Meters

Meter reading provides another useful source of energy data. Reading of meters should in theory be a relatively simple task, but unfortunately in practice a number of problems can arise. Some of the common faults which may arise are as follows [1]:

- Digits may be recorded in the wrong order.
- Too many digits may be inserted in the recorded reading.
- The recorded reading may be wrong by a factor of 10 or even 100.
- Readings may be lost after being recorded.
- The wrong meter may be read.
- Meters may not be read at all.
- Poor writing may be used when recording readings.

Not surprisingly, poorly recorded meter readings can result in much wasted time and effort. Therefore meter readings should always be validated. Validation checks should include [1]:

- Checking that the correct number of digits is recorded.
- Checking that current readings are higher than previous readings.
- Checking that readings are within predicted energy consumption bands.
- Checking the date of meter readings.

Should a meter reading fail one of the above tests, the most likely source of the discrepancy will be operator error, although the fault cannot always be attributed to the operator. For example, a meter may have been changed, or, for some unknown reason, there may have been a period of abnormally high energy consumption. It is therefore important to establish a robust data validation system, one that alerts the system user as soon as a potential error is detected. Validation can take place either when readings are input or at the initial stages of the data analysis.

The manual reading of meters and the writing down of digits by hand is a time-consuming process which is prone to mistakes. With the advent of smart metering systems, there are a variety of alternatives to the manual approach. For example, data capture units can be employed. These are small portable computer units, into which meter readings can be directly entered. The data collected in this way can later be downloaded to a larger personal computer for analysis. Data capture units can also be programmed to validate data as it is input. Data capture units thus improve the quality of manual meter reading, but they still require an operator to visit all the relevant meters, which is a labour-intensive process. By using pulsed output meters it is possible to carry out remote meter reading automatically. Pulsed output meters send out an electronic signal which can be automatically monitored by an M&T computer. Many BMS also have the capability to monitor energy consumption and data can be downloaded to an M&T computer either as 'ASCII' or spreadsheet files.

In situations where existing metering is unable to provide enough detailed information on energy consumption, it may be necessary to install additional sub-metering (see Chapter 7). This should improve the overall quality of any M&T programme and result in increased energy savings. However, additional metering can be expensive and can also lead to a substantial increase in the quantity of data which must be collected and processed. Therefore any additional metering must be justified, to ensure that potential energy cost savings are not outweighed by the installation costs.

9.4 Energy Targets

At the outset of any M&T programme it is important to set energy targets. Initially, these should be the *standard energy performances* which have been established for the respective EACs [2]. *Standard performance* can be determined through analysis of past energy consumption data (see Chapter 6). If these data do not exist, then it will be necessary to undertake an auditing process to establish credible *standard energy performances* for the respective EACs.

Although the standard energy performance is generally used as an initial target, subsequent energy targets should represent improvements on standard performance. One way of establishing an improved target is to plot a *best-fit* straight line through the lower edge of the points on a scatter diagram (see Figure 9.1). At first sight this might appear as a strange thing to do, but the points on the lower edge of the scatter diagram represent the historical achievement of least energy consumption and therefore should be an achievable target. In other words a straight line through the lower points represents what can actually be achieved in practice and makes an ideal energy target.

Energy targets should be reappraised on a regular basis. This can be done by defining the best historical performance as the target in a similar way to that described above,

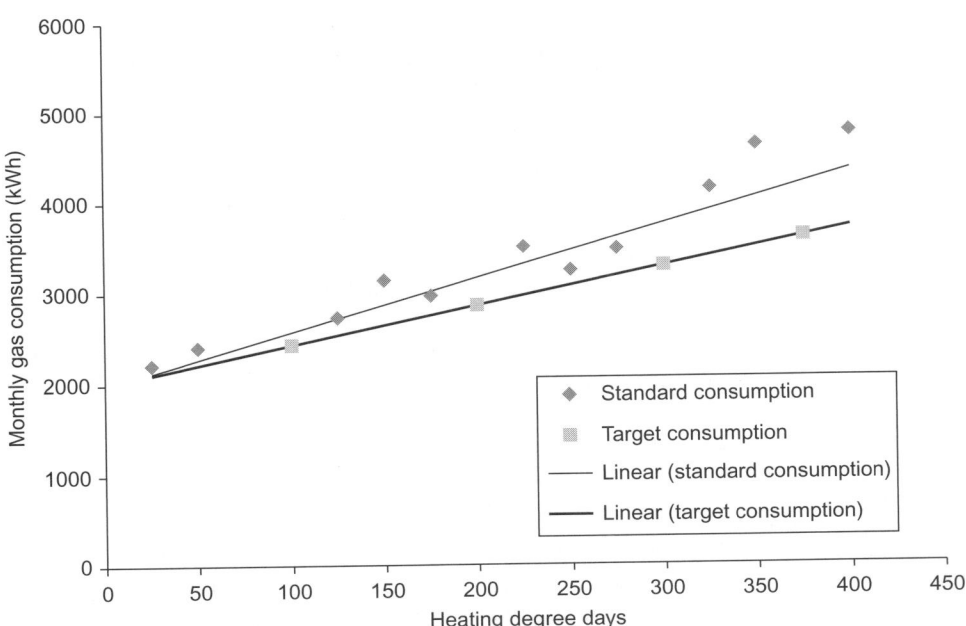

FIG 9.1 Target curve based on best historical performance.

or by basing the target on an agreed action plan that is designed to achieve energy savings. Both these methods have the advantage of being based on real data and so should be achievable. A more arbitrary, and possibly inferior, approach is to set targets based on a percentage improvement on the current energy performance. No matter the approach chosen, all targets should be realistic and achievable otherwise they will lose credibility. They should also be reviewed regularly, in order to maintain pressure to reduce energy consumption.

9.5 Reporting

One of the major outputs of any M&T programme is the production of energy management reports. These reports perform the vital role of communicating key information to senior and operational managers, and are therefore the means by which action is initiated within an organization. In order to ensure that prompt action is taken to minimize wasteful practices, reports should be as simple as possible and should highlight those areas in which energy wastage is occurring. Reports should be published regularly so that energy wasteful practices are identified quickly and not allowed to persist for too long. Reports should be succinct and conform to a standard format which should be generated automatically by a computer. This minimizes preparation time and also familiarizes managers with the information being communicated. Figure 9.2 shows an example of a weekly electricity consumption report produced by an M&T computer program.

Most M&T programmes require reports to be published weekly or monthly. Monthly reports are usually applicable to large organizations with many sites, with weekly

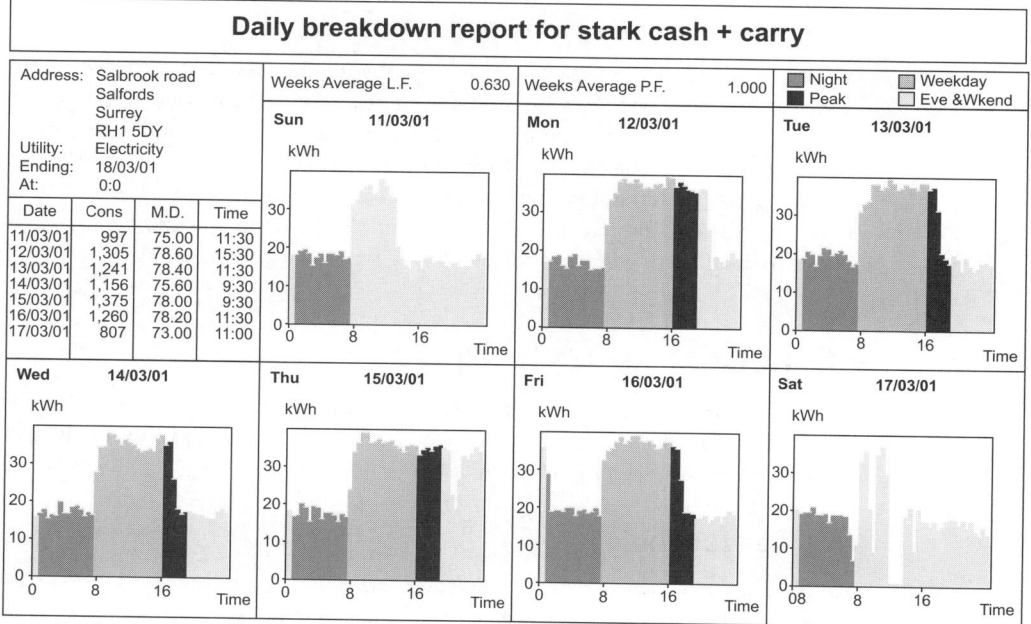

FIG 9.2 Weekly electricity consumption report [3].

Level	Report frequency			
Senior management	Annual	Quarterly		
Department head	Annual		Monthly	
EAC manager	Annual			Weekly
Energy manager	Annual	Quarterly	Monthly	Weekly

FIG 9.3 Relationship between managerial status and report frequency. Crown copyright is reproduced with the permission of the Controller of Her Majesty's Stationery Office and the Queen's Printer for Scotland.

reports being more suitable to complex high energy consuming facilities. In applications where energy consumption is particularly high, reports may be produced daily. If the reporting period is too long, energy may well be needlessly wasted before managers are notified of the problem and remedial action is taken. Yet, if the reporting period is too short this will lead to an over-complex M&T system in which too much irrelevant information requires consideration.

The primary purpose of energy management reports is to communicate effectively with senior and operational managers. They should therefore be tailored to suit the needs of their readers, with different managers within organizations requiring different levels of report. Operational managers may need weekly reports, whereas senior management may only require a quarterly review. Figure 9.3 illustrates the relationship between reporting frequency and managerial status.

One big disadvantage of producing a large number of regular reports is that they can swamp operational managers with what may appear to be irrelevant information. One good way to get around this problem is to adopt a *reporting by exception* system, in which reports are only generated when energy performance falls outside certain predetermined limits. This system has the great advantage that managers only receive reports when energy performance is either poor or very good. In addition, everyone involved in the reporting process benefits from a reduced workload.

9.6 Reporting Techniques

There are a number of reporting techniques which can help energy managers communicate effectively with operational managers. These include the production of league tables and a variety of graphical techniques.

9.6.1 League Tables

League tables can be a particularly effective way of conveying energy performance information. They are most useful when comparing a number of similar EACs. Example 9.1 illustrates this process.

Example 9.1

A retail chain has 12 shops. Table 9.1 shows a league table of the monthly electrical energy consumption and cost of all 12 shops. From the league table, two issues become obvious:

- The shop at Crewe appears to have an abnormally high electricity consumption compared with similar sized shops at Bingley, Burnley and Macclesfield. Further investigation is therefore required to identify the reason for the high electricity consumption.
- The shop at Bingley is paying too much for its electricity, which implies that the tariff needs to be changed.

If an organization has a number of dissimilar EACs then direct comparison by league table is meaningless. However, league tables can still be usefully employed if the EACs are ranked on the basis of variation from target performance, as shown in Table 9.2.

From Table 9.2 it is clear that in energy consumption terms, the Geography department is performing poorly, while the Mechanical Engineering department is performing relatively well.

9.6.2   Graphical Techniques

Graphical techniques, if used correctly, can be an excellent tool for communicating information to managers. However, not all graphical techniques are easy to follow and some can be very misleading. For example, although the *scatter diagram* is an excellent analysis tool (see Chapter 6), it is a poor communication tool because it gives no historical record of energy consumption. Since it is unlikely that senior and operational

TABLE 9.1   League table of shop electrical consumption

Shop	Floor area (m²)	Electrical units consumed (kWh)	Electricity cost (£)	Electrical units per m² (kWh/m²)	Average cost per unit (p/kWh)
Crewe	6560	91,906	4374.72	14.01	4.76
Chester	12,000	149,845	6967.79	12.49	4.65
Leeds	13,600	169,400	6860.70	12.46	4.05
Bingley	6070	73,677	5046.87	12.14	6.85
Macclesfield	6460	74,823	3165.01	11.58	4.23
Huddersfield	9470	108,640	5442.86	11.47	5.01
Stockport	10,800	123,892	4943.29	11.47	3.99
Doncaster	12,500	132,345	5426.15	10.59	4.10
Ashbourne	5780	59,534	2393.27	10.30	4.02
Burnley	7540	74,943	3050.18	9.94	4.07
Halifax	7800	72,513	2806.25	9.30	3.87
Stoke	8670	75,342	3337.65	8.69	4.43

TABLE 9.2 League table of electrical consumption for various university departments

Energy account centre (EAC)	Electrical units consumed (kWh)	Target use (kWh)	Electricity cost (£)	Excess above target (kWh)	Variation from target (%)
Geography dept	11,780	10,484	565.44	+1296	+12.36
Electrical eng. dept	40,056	37,653	1922.69	+2403	+6.38
Civil eng. dept	50,834	48,801	2440.03	+2033	+4.17
Law dept	8893	8982	426.86	−89	−0.99
Chemistry dept	180,567	183,817	8667.22	−3250	−1.77
Mechanical eng. dept	72,004	75,604	3456.19	−3600	−4.76

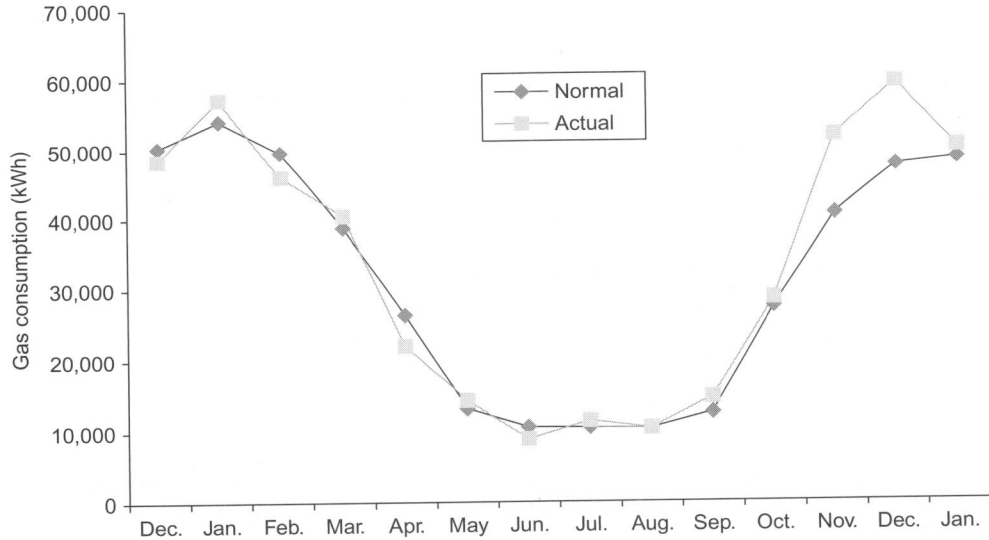

FIG 9.4 Norm chart for gas consumption.

managers will be familiar with energy analysis techniques, it is important that energy performance graphs be of a type that is easily understood by non-energy specialists.

There are a number of graphical techniques which can be used to represent historical energy consumption. Of particular importance are the *norm chart*, the *deviance chart* and the *CUSUM chart*. The *norm chart* is a sequential plot of actual energy consumption overlaid on a plot of target consumption (see Figure 9.4). It is of little value as an analytical tool, but can be very useful for highlighting exceptions and communicating these to managers. Because *norm charts* represent a historical record of energy consumption, senior and operational managers find them relatively easy to understand.

Deviance charts plot the difference between target and actual energy consumption (see Figure 9.5). If, in any one month, energy consumption is above the target value,

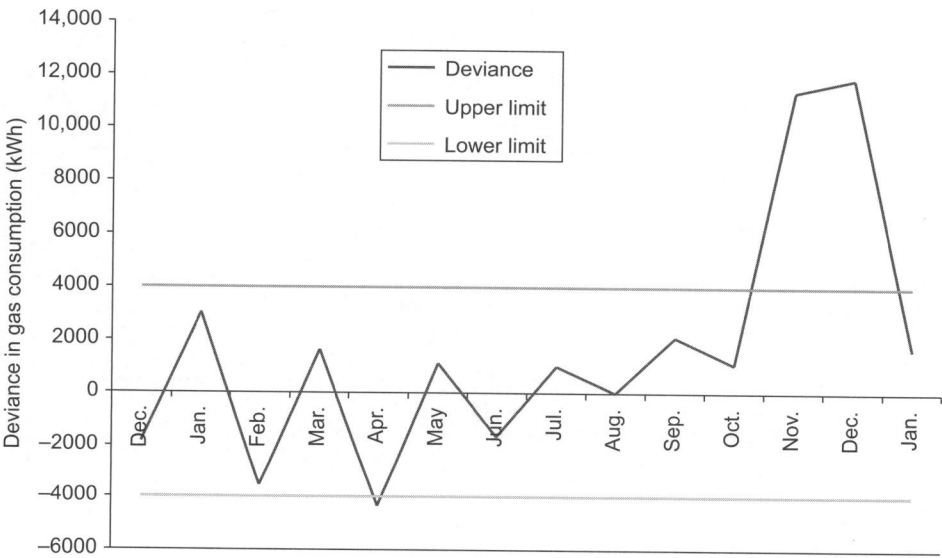

FIG 9.5 Deviance chart for gas consumption.

then the consumption is plotted as a positive value; by contrast a negative value is returned if actual consumption is lower than predicted. When producing a deviance chart it is useful to show on the graph limits of normal operation, since this helps to distinguish between normal background 'noise' and serious deviations from the norm. Deviance charts are particularly good at highlighting problems, so that remedial action can be taken. They can also be used to initiate detailed *exception reports*.

The concept of the CUSUM is discussed in detail in Chapter 6. *CUSUM charts* plot the cumulative sum of the deviation of actual energy consumption from predicted or target consumption. As such they are a useful tool when identifying trends and diagnosing problems. They are also useful when assessing the impact of any remedial action which is taken. While *CUSUM charts* are a useful diagnostic tool, they can be difficult to understand if not fully explained. Care is necessary to ensure that managers understand what is being communicated in a *CUSUM chart*. Figure 9.6 shows a typical *CUSUM chart*.

9.7 Diagnosing Changes in Energy Performance

CUSUM charts can be particularly useful when diagnosing why energy wastage is occurring. This is principally because they identify the date of any change in energy performance. It can be particularly helpful to know when a problem first occurred, as this helps to pinpoint the problem; further analysis can then be undertaken to determine its cause. The diagnostic use of CUSUM is illustrated in Example 9.2.

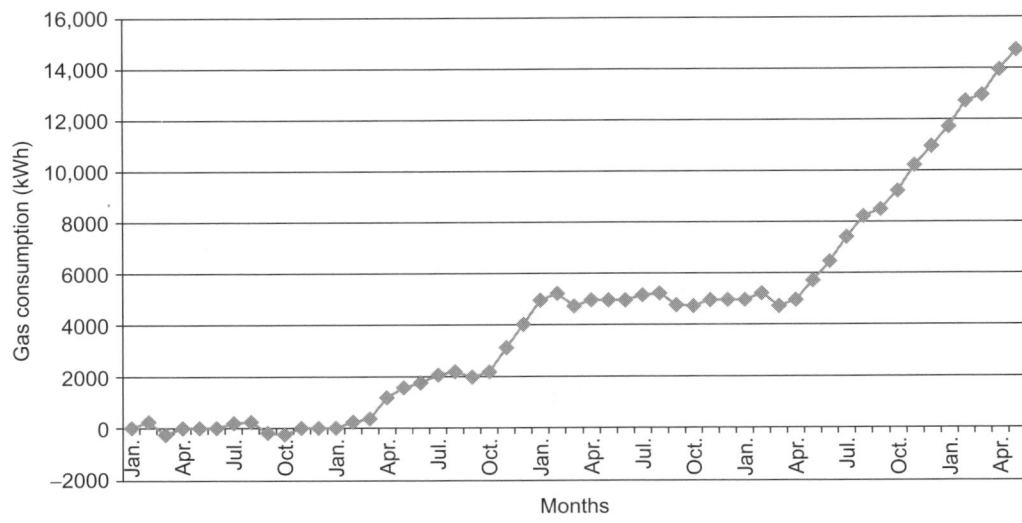

FIG 9.6 CUSUM chart for gas consumption.

Example 9.2

Figure 9.6 shows a CUSUM plot of gas consumption for a residential building for the period January 1997 to May 2001. The CUSUM plot shows that for the period January 1997 to February 1998 the actual energy consumption conformed to *standard energy performance*. However, around March 1998 something happened to change the energy performance of the building dramatically for the worse and the poor performance continued until February 1999 when the problem was rectified. In May 2000 the energy consumption again took a dramatic turn for the worse and this continued unresolved until the end of the analysis period.

In order to determine why the change in performance occurred in March 1998, regression analysis needs to be carried out for periods 'pre and post' the event. Figure 9.7 shows the results of the regression analysis.

From Figure 9.7 it is clear that there is a change in the slope of the *best-fit* straight-line curve which indicates that the increase in energy consumption is weather related. The point at which both lines intersect the *y*-axis is the same, indicating that base-load consumption has not increased. Possible explanations for the increase in weather-related performance could be:

- An increase in the space temperature control setting.
- An increase in the ventilation rate. If the building had a central ducted warm air system, this situation could occur if the fresh air mixing dampers on the main air handling units were incorrectly set.

Now consider the increase in energy consumption which occurred in May 2000. Figure 9.8 shows the regression analysis plot for the periods before and after this date. It can be seen that the slope of the two 'best-fit' straight lines is the same. This indicates that

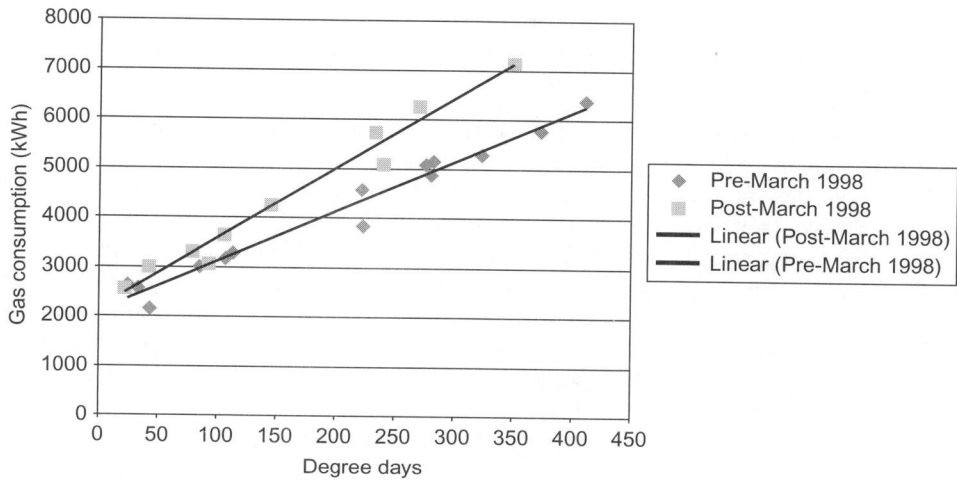

FIG 9.7 Performance lines pre- and post-March 1998, indicating that reduced performance is due to a weather-related matter.

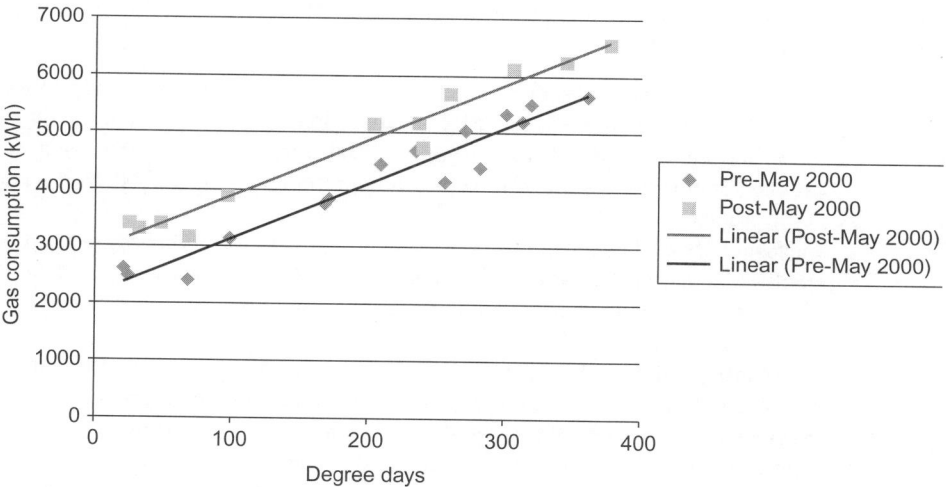

FIG 9.8 Performance lines pre- and post-May 2000, indicating that reduced performance is due to an increased base load.

the increase in energy consumption was not a weather-related issue, but rather caused by a significant increase in the base load. This could have been caused by incorrect setting of the thermostat on the hot water storage cylinders in the building.

9.8 Waste Avoidance

Waste avoidance is a simple concept, which can enable large energy cost savings to be achieved without significant capital investment. As the name implies, *waste avoidance* seeks to minimize avoidable wasted energy. *Waste avoidance* programmes should be quick and inexpensive to implement, since their specific objective is cut out waste that can be easily avoided.

Unlike materials wastage, which is usually relatively easy to detect, energy wastage is not at all easy to spot and identifying it usually requires considerable detective work. It is often the case that large quantities of energy can be wasted over long periods of time, without anybody being aware that wastage is occurring. Consider the case of electric frost protection heaters. These are switched on in winter to protect control panels and other items of equipment from frost damage. Although they may be switched on in winter, it is often the case that they are not switched off when the cold weather has finished. As a result, they remain switched on all year round without anyone noticing. It is not difficult to see that if something like this is detected early enough, large energy savings can be made. Early diagnosis is essential, and a waste avoidance programme utilizing many of the techniques already described in this chapter will facilitate this.

9.9 Causes of Avoidable Waste

Although facilities and organizations may vary widely, many of the causes of avoidable waste are generic and common to most applications. These generic causes include the following [2]:

- Frost protection devices frequently remain in operation for long periods when there is no risk of frost damage. Under-surface heaters often remain on throughout the spring and summer without any perceptible effect. Similarly, pre-heating coils in air handling units often operate all the time, without the system operators being aware of the problem.
- The failure of switches can often cause major energy wastage. Switches are often employed to automatically turn equipment on and off. If for any reason a switch fails in the 'on' position, then the equipment will run continuously, often unnoticed, for a considerable time.
- Time controls can often lead to excessive energy consumption. Time switches are designed to turn off equipment after a pre-set period of operation. If they fail or are overridden, or indeed, if they are simply incorrectly set, it can result in extended plant operation and much excess energy being needlessly consumed.
- Lack of suitable control often results in unnecessarily high energy consumption. Items of equipment such as luminaires and ventilation fans often have no controls other than a manual switch. Such items tend to be left on continuously. Remember, staff and operatives, although quick to switch on items of equipment, often forget to switch them off when they are not needed.
- Leaks of water or steam from pipes often go unnoticed for long periods, since they usually occur out of sight.
- Control valves and dampers, if not correctly monitored and controlled, can result in excessive energy wastage. Air handling systems often employ modulating dampers to vary the quantities of fresh and recirculated air. However, if a damper remains in the 'full fresh air' position for long periods during cold weather, much energy will be wasted in heating up excessive quantities of cold air.

- With air-conditioning systems, much energy can be wasted due to poorly set controls. If the cooling 'set-point' is set below the heating 'set-point', then both the cooling and heating coils will operate at the same time and 'fight' each other. This can occur without the building occupants being aware and always leads to excessive energy consumption.

It should be noted that most of the causes of the energy wastage listed above are due to either incorrect control setting, control failure or the use of insufficient controls. These are failures which can be rectified at relatively little cost.

A good way to detect and solve energy wastage problems is to create checklists which identify common problem areas. Checklists can also assist in the prioritization of energy conservation measures. They should commence with the more obvious and simple energy-saving measures and progress towards those which are more obscure and which may demand capital expenditure.

9.10 Prioritizing

Potential energy-efficiency measures should be prioritized. This involves identifying and quantifying energy costs, and highlighting those measures which offer the greatest potential savings. History is littered with schemes which were embarked upon because they were fashionable or perceived as 'sexy' and which in the long run proved to be ineffective, ultimately becoming 'follies'. Such schemes usually come about because someone at the planning stage did not correctly quantify the potential gains. Very often it is the mundane measures which yield the best returns.

One way to prioritize action areas is to produce league tables as discussed in Section 9.5.1. This enables those EACs requiring most urgent investigation to be identified. When prioritizing measures it is important to assess both the energy consumption and the energy cost. Consider the case of a factory building with a gas-fired heating system, the annual energy and cost breakdowns of which are shown in Figure 9.9.

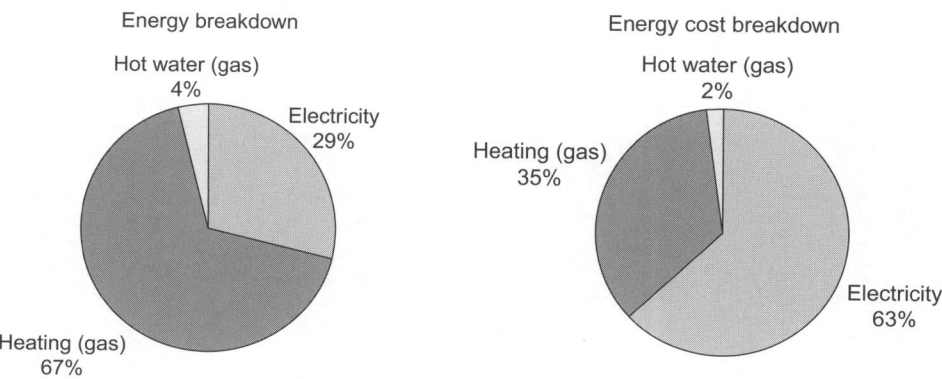

FIGURE 9.9 Factory unit: annual energy and cost breakdown.

It can be seen from Figure 9.9 that although electrical energy use is 29% of total energy use, the cost of the electrical energy represents 63% of the total energy bill, 1.7 times the expenditure on gas. Consequently, priority should be given to reducing electrical consumption rather than gas consumption.

References

1. Computer-aided monitoring and targeting for industry, Good Practice Guide 31. Department of the Environment; 1995.
2. Waste avoidance methods. Fuel Efficiency Booklet 13. Department of the Environment; 1995.
3. Stark energy information systems. http://www.stark.co.uk/, 16 July; 2001.

Bibliography

Computer-aided monitoring and targeting for industry, Good Practice Guide 31. Department of the Environment; 1995.

Eastop TD, Croft DR. Energy efficiency for engineers and technologists (Chapter 9). Harlow: Longman Scientific & Technical; 1990.

Energy audits and surveys. CIBSE Applications Manual AM5; 1991.

Moss KJ. Energy management and operating costs in buildings (Chapter 10). London: E & FN Spon; 1997.

Monitoring and targeting in large manufacturing companies, Good Practice Guide 91. Department of the Environment; 1994.

Waste avoidance methods. Fuel Efficiency Booklet 13. Department of the Environment; 1995.

CHAPTER 10

Energy Efficient Heating

This chapter outlines good practice in the design and operation of building heating systems. It includes a discussion of the types of heating system that should be selected for particular applications. In addition, the concept of building heat loss is discussed, and methodologies presented for predicting heating energy costs and optimizing plant utilization.

10.1 Introduction

For those who live in temperate, cool or cold climates, the provision of adequate heating is essential for large parts of the year in order to maintain comfort and good health. While some may consider good 'central heating' to be a luxury, a recent epidemiological study undertaken in several European countries revealed that death rates amongst those over 50 years of age are proportional to the degree of coldness experienced [1]. In fact, in England and Wales there is a 2% increase in mortality for every 1°C below an outside temperature of 19°C [2]. As a result, weather-related mortality rates in the UK are amongst the highest in Europe, with an estimated 40,000 additional deaths occurring during the winter months each year [1]. One major contributory factor to this sad state of affairs is the poor state of much of the housing stock in the UK [1,3].

In addition to preserving the good health of building occupants, adequate heating of public, commercial and industrial buildings is essential to promote efficient and productive work practices. If people are cold and uncomfortable, they will not perform well and so output will fall. Clearly it is false economy to save a little on fuel costs and lose much in productivity.

Although a building may be heated to a comfortable level, it does not always mean that it is efficiently heated. In many buildings large quantities of heat energy are wasted daily due to a combination of poor design and poor operating and maintenance practices. Broadly speaking, heat can be wasted by any combination of the following:

- Poorly designed heating systems, which are often wrongly selected for particular applications.
- Poorly designed and insulated building envelopes.
- Poorly insulated heating systems.
- Poorly commissioned and maintained boiler plant.
- Poor controls.
- Poor operating practices.

To understand the reasons why heat is so easily wasted in buildings, it is worth considering the case of an old, poorly maintained church hall with a high roof, which is heated by an old low temperature hot water (LTHW) radiator system, served by an oil-fired boiler. Let us assume that the building is used for meetings and social events, mainly in the evenings and at weekends. Without going into too much detail, there are a number of possible ways in which the heating system might be considered to be inefficient:

- The building envelope is probably poorly insulated so heat will be easily lost to the outside by conduction, especially on cold winter nights.
- The building envelope is probably not very well sealed and so large amounts of the warm heated air will be lost through cracks around doors and window frames.
- In the church hall the warm air heated by the radiators will rise up into the high roof space where it will stratify. Consequently, any pigeons that might be in the roof space will be warm, while the occupants at floor level will probably feel cold and uncomfortable.
- The pipework from the boiler to the radiators may not be very well insulated. This will result in major heat losses if the pipes run through unheated spaces, such as floor voids or in the boiler room.
- The boiler will probably be poorly maintained, with the result that some of the heat meant to warm up the water will be lost up the flue with the combustion gases.
- Since the system is old, it is probable that its controls will be inadequate. For example, the system might have a time clock which turns the boiler and pump on at the same time each day, whether or not the hall is occupied. Alternatively, the thermostat in the room space may be set at too high a temperature, so that the hall overheats and the occupants become uncomfortable. It is not uncommon for the occupants of buildings to open windows rather than turn down thermostats. After all, it is often the case that the occupants of a building are not the ones paying the fuel bills.

The illustration of the poorly heated church hall demonstrates four important points:

1. It is essential to take a holistic view when designing a heating system. The building fabric and the mechanical heating system are equally important.
2. It is important to select the correct heating system for the particular application.
3. It is important to have an adequate control system.
4. It is no use designing and installing an excellent heating system, if the building operatives and occupants do not understand how to use it correctly.

10.2 Thermal Comfort

When an individual is in a room, his/her vital organs are maintained at a temperature of 37.2°C through a complex set of heat-transfer mechanisms. The person will lose heat to the surrounding air by convection and to any cold surfaces within the room space by radiation. However, hot surfaces within the room will cause the person to gain heat by radiation. Consider a room in which the air is maintained at 21°C by wall-mounted radiators which have a surface temperature of 70°C. The occupants of the room will lose heat by convection to the air, because the surface of their clothes will be at approximately 30°C. They will also lose heat by radiation to many of the cool surfaces in the room, many of which will be at a temperature of less than 21°C. At the same time they will gain heat by radiation from the hot radiators. The occupants will also lose heat by evaporation through exhalation and perspiration. A small amount of heat will also be lost through their feet by conduction. Consequently, a complex heat balance is set up, which maintains the core temperature of the occupant's bodies at 37.2°C. If for any reason a person becomes hot or cold, in other words uncomfortable, then their body will take involuntary action in order to maintain the core temperature. One such mechanism is perspiration, which increases under warm conditions, so that increased evaporative cooling occurs. If a person is uncomfortable, he/she can also take voluntary steps to rectify the situation. For example, extra/excess clothing can be worn or removed. Equation (10.1) expresses the heat balance between the human body and the surrounding environment [4]. It should be noted that the term for conduction has been omitted from eqn (10.1) because in most normal situations it is negligible:

$$M - W = Q_e \pm Q_c \pm Q_r + S \qquad (10.1)$$

where M is the metabolic rate (W), W is the rate at which energy is expended in mechanical work (W), Q_c is the rate of heat transfer by convection (W), Q_r is the rate of heat transfer by radiation (W), Q_e is the rate of heat loss by evaporation (W), and S is the rate at which heat is stored in the body (W).

Food that is digested by the body is converted into energy. Some of this energy is used to perform mechanical work, but most of it produces heat. In fact, under normal conditions, more heat is produced by the body than it actually requires to maintain its core temperature. Therefore heat is lost from the body by convection, radiation and evaporation. The human body can also gain heat by convection and radiation under hot conditions. It is, however, impossible to gain heat by evaporation, since this is always a cooling mechanism. If a person performs exercises or mechanical work, then the metabolic

TABLE 10.1   Sensible heat outputs and recommended dry resultant temperatures [5]

Type of work	Typical application	Required room dry resultant temperature (°C)	Sensible heat output per person (W)
Light work	Office	20.0	100
Walking slowly	Bank	20.0	110
Light bench work	Factory	16.0	150*
Heavy work	Factory	13.0	200*

*Assumes a dry-bulb temperature of 15°C.

rate increases and the body is required to reject more heat, otherwise it will overheat. Consequently, in rooms such as gymnasia, where vigorous exercise is performed, it is necessary to have a lower room air temperature to compensate for the increased heat production rate of the human body. Table 10.1 shows heat outputs for a range of work rates, together with recommended room temperatures.

The thermal comfort of building occupants can be affected by personal and environmental factors. Personal factors can be defined as those variables which are directly connected with the individual. These include:

- Activity: The higher the level of personal activity, the greater the heat output.
- Clothing: The greater the amount of clothing worn, the lower the heat loss.
- Age: The metabolic rate decreases with age.
- Gender: The resting metabolic rate of women is approximately 10% lower than that of men.
- Health: Illness affects the ability of the body to maintain its core temperature at 37.2°C.

These personal comfort factors should always be considered when designing heating systems for particular applications. For example, because the metabolic rate of the elderly is lower than that of younger people, it is important to maintain air temperatures at a higher than normal level in sheltered accommodation for the elderly. Similarly, when designing the foyer of a railway station, where passengers in transit may be wearing outdoor winter clothes, it is advisable to maintain the air temperature at a lower temperature than, say, an office, where indoor clothing would normally be worn.

The environmental parameters which influence thermal comfort are: air temperature, mean radiant temperature, relative humidity and air velocity. These parameters, in different ways, influence heat transfer by convection, radiation and evaporation. Convective heat transfer is influenced by air temperature and air velocity. It takes place continually, although in most buildings it is imperceptible because air speeds are low (i.e. below 0.1 m/s). To be perceptible, air speeds must exceed approximately 0.2 m/s. Radiant heat transfer occurs between the skin/clothes and those surfaces 'seen' by the human body. It is therefore heavily influenced by the *mean radiant temperature* (t_r) of the surfaces within rooms. For cuboid shaped rooms, the approximate mean radiant temperature at the centre of the room can be determined by:

$$t_r = \frac{a_1 \cdot t_1 + a_2 \cdot t_2 + a_3 \cdot t_3 + \cdots + a_n \cdot t_n}{a_1 + a_2 + a_3 + \cdots + a_n} \tag{10.2}$$

where t_r is the mean radiant temperature (°C), $a_1, a_2, \ldots,$ are the room component surface areas (m^2), and $t_1, t_2, \ldots,$ are the room component surface temperatures (m^2).

Evaporative heat loss is governed by the relative humidity of air and air velocity. If conditions are very humid, as in tropical countries, then evaporative heat losses will be low, since any perspiration produced is unable to evaporate. However, if the air is dry then evaporation readily takes place and the body is cooled. Evaporative cooling becomes an important heat-transfer mechanism at air temperatures above 25°C. At air temperatures above 29°C almost all heat is lost from the body by evaporation [6].

Thermal comfort is determined by a number of environmental factors, particularly mean radiant temperature, air temperature and air velocity. It is thus important that these factors are considered when designing buildings. The concept of *dry resultant temperature* (t_{res}) was developed to make allowances for these considerations. The dry resultant temperature is defined as:

$$t_{res} = \frac{t_r + t_a \cdot \sqrt{10 v_a}}{1 + \sqrt{10 v_a}} \tag{10.3}$$

where v_a is the air velocity (m/s), and t_a is the air temperature (°C).

However, in most buildings, because the air velocity is below 0.1 m/s, eqn (10.3) can be simplified to:

$$t_{res} = 0.5 t_r + 0.5 t_a \tag{10.4}$$

Equation (10.4) tells us that mean radiant temperature is as important as air temperature when maintaining a comfortable environment within buildings. This explains why on returning to an unheated house after some days of absence, the rooms will feel cold and uncomfortable, even though the heating is on and the air up to temperature. The air temperature may be acceptable, but the dry resultant temperature will still be low because the fabric of the building is still cold.

10.3   Building Heat Loss

When a building is heated to a steady internal temperature, an equilibrium is established in which the heat power into the building equals the rate at which heat is lost from the building. Thus to maintain a comfortable internal environment, the output from any heating system must be equal to or greater than the combined effect of the heat loss through the building fabric and the ventilation heat losses. Fabric heat losses are those which occur primarily by conduction through walls, windows, floors and roofs. Ventilation losses are the convective heat losses which occur when warm air is lost from a building and replaced by cold air. A good approximation of the fabric heat losses can be determined using the generic equation:

$$Q_f = U \times A \times (t_{ai} - t_{ao}) \tag{10.5}$$

where Q_f is the fabric heat loss rate (W), U is the thermal transmittance (U value) (W/m^{2}K), A is the area (m^2), t_{ai} is the internal air temperature (°C), and t_{ao} is the external air temperature (°C).

Similarly, the ventilation heat loss can be determined using:

$$Q_v = 0.333 \times n \times V \times (t_{ai} - t_{ao}) \tag{10.6}$$

where Q_v is the ventilation heat loss rate (W), n is the ventilation rate (air changes per hour), and V is the volume (m^3).

From eqns (10.5) and (10.6) it can be seen that both the fabric and the ventilation heat loss rates are directly proportional to the difference between the internal and the external air temperatures. Since the internal air temperature should be maintained at a constant level during the winter, the heat loss therefore varies with the outside air temperature. Boilers and heat emitters should be sized for the 'worst-case' scenario (i.e. a very cold day) and be capable of maintaining the internal design temperature under this extreme weather condition. When operating under less extreme conditions (i.e. under part-load conditions), the output of the heating system can be reduced by using controls. Table 10.2 gives some sample winter external design conditions for various parts of the world.

The simplest way to reduce the energy consumed by a heating system is to create a building envelope which is well insulated and in which ventilation rates are controlled to the minimum required for healthy living. Achieving this usually involves care and attention during both the design and the construction stages, together with increased capital outlay. Not surprisingly, many speculative builders have little incentive to construct energy efficient building envelopes, since they usually do not pay the fuel bills. Therefore most countries have building regulations, of varying degrees of rigour, to force developers to conform to certain minimum thermal insulation standards. Usually these standards are expressed in terms of maximum permissible U values for glazing, walls, floors and roofs.

10.3.1 *U* Values

Thermal insulation standards are usually expressed in terms of U values. The U value, or thermal transmittance, is a measure of the overall rate of heat transfer, under standard conditions, through a particular section of construction. It has units W/m^{2}K and, as can be seen from eqn (10.7), is the inverse of thermal resistance. The lower the U value of an item of construction, the better its thermal insulation performance:

$$U = \frac{1}{\Sigma R} \tag{10.7}$$

where ΣR is the total thermal resistance of the construction (m^{2}K/W).

TABLE 10.2 External winter design temperatures for sample cities around the world [7]

Country	City	Winter external design temperature (°C)
Australia	Perth	6
	Sydney	6
Belgium	Brussels	−7
China	Shanghai	−3
France	Lyon	−10
	Paris	−4
Germany	Berlin	−11
	Hamburg	−9
	Munich	−13
Italy	Milan	−6
	Naples	2
	Rome	1
India	New Delhi	4
Japan	Tokyo	−2
New Zealand	Christchurch	−1
	Wellington	3
Norway	Oslo	−16
Spain	Barcelona	2
	Madrid	−2
Sweden	Stockholm	−13
United Kingdom	Birmingham	−3
	Glasgow	−2
	London	−2
	Manchester	−2.5
USA	Chicago	−20
	Dallas	−6
	Kansas City	−14
	Los Angeles	4
	Miami	8
	New Orleans	1
	New York	−9
	San Francisco	3
	Seattle	−9
	Washington DC	−8

TABLE 10.3 Thermal conductivity of various materials [8]

Material	Density (kg/m³)	Thermal conductivity (W/m K)
Brickwork (outer leaf)	1700	0.84
Brickwork (inner leaf)	1700	0.62
Cast concrete (dense)	2100	1.40
Cast concrete (lightweight)	1200	0.38
Concrete block (heavyweight)	2300	1.63
Concrete block (medium weight)	1400	0.51
Concrete block (lightweight)	600	0.19
Fibreboard	300	0.06
Plasterboard	950	0.16
Plaster (dense)	1300	0.50
Plaster (lightweight)	600	0.16
External rendering	1300	0.50
Screed	1200	0.41
Asphalt	1700	0.50
Tile	1900	0.84
Wood–wool slab	650	0.14
Expanded polystyrene	25	0.035
Glass fibre slab	25	0.035
Phenolic foam	30	0.040

The thermal resistance of each component layer of any construction can be determined by using eqn (10.8):

$$R = \frac{l}{\lambda} \tag{10.8}$$

where R is the thermal resistance of layer (m² K/W), l is the thickness of layer (m), and λ is the thermal conductivity (W/m K).

The total thermal resistance of a construction is the summation of the resistances of all the individual layers, plus the resistances to heat transfer of any surfaces. Table 10.3 gives typical thermal conductivity values for a variety of building materials.

Figure 10.1 illustrates the heat-transfer mechanisms that take place in a typical external wall with an air cavity. While the heat transfer through the solid parts of any construction is by conduction, it is radiation and convection that control the heat transfer at the

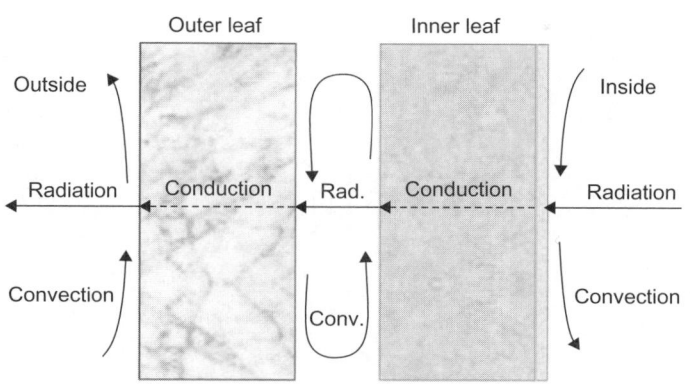

FIG 10.1 Heat transfer through a cavity wall.

surfaces. The resistance to heat transfer of a surface can be calculated using eqn (10.9), which takes into consideration the convective and radiative heat-transfer coefficients, and the emissivity of the surface:

$$R_s = \frac{1}{h_c + (E \times h_r)}$$ (10.9)

where R_s is the surface resistance (m² K/W), h_c is the convective heat-transfer coefficient (W/m² K), h_r is the radiative heat-transfer coefficient (W/m² K), and E is the emissivity factor.

The convective heat-transfer coefficient is the rate at which heat is transferred to or from a 1 m² surface by convection, per 1°C temperature difference between the surface and the neighbouring fluid (i.e. air). The radiative heat-transfer coefficient is the rate of radiant heat transfer to or from a 1 m² surface of a *black body* divided by the difference between the mean temperatures of the radiating surface and that of the surrounding surfaces. The term *black body* refers to a body which absorbs all energy incident on it at every wavelength and conversely emits energy at every wavelength. The emissive power of a black body can be calculated using eqn (10.10):

$$E_b = \sigma \times T^4$$ (10.10)

where E_b is the emissive power (W/m²), σ is the Stefan–Boltzmann constant (i.e. 5.67×10^{-8} W/m² K⁴), and T is the absolute temperature of the black body (K).

Of course, black bodies are theoretical and building materials do not emit and absorb energy at all wavelengths and are therefore non-black bodies. The term *emissivity* is used to describe the ratio of the emissive power of a non-black body to that exhibited by a black body. The emissivity of a black body is 1, while that of all other bodies will be less than 1. Dull surfaces, of the type exhibited by most building materials, have a high emissivity, while shiny metallic surfaces have a low emissivity. High-emissivity surfaces are good emitters and receivers of radiation, while low-emissivity surfaces are not. Table 10.4 gives examples of the emissivity values for typical building materials.

TABLE 10.4 Typical values of emissivity [9]

Surface	Emissivity
Black body	1
Black (non-metallic)	0.90–0.98
Concrete	0.85–0.95
White paint	0.85–0.95
Aluminium (dull)	0.20–0.30
Aluminium (polished)	0.02–0.05

From Smith, Phillips and Sweeney (1987) Environmental Science, © Longman Group UK Ltd (1987), reprinted by permission of Pearson Education Ltd.

TABLE 10.5 Typical internal surface resistances [8]

Building element	Direction of heat flow	Surface resistance (m² K/W)	
		High emissivity factor ($E = 0.97$)	Low emissivity factor ($E = 0.05$)
Walls	Horizontal	0.12	0.30
Ceiling or roofs	Upward	0.10	0.22
Ceiling or floors	Downward	0.14	0.55

The emissivity factor (E) referred to in eqn (10.9) allows for the emissivity and geometrical relationship of both the emitting and the receiving surfaces. The emissivity factor varies with the specific geometrical arrangement of the surfaces involved, but for most building applications it can be taken as being approximately 0.9.

The thermal resistance of any surface is strongly influenced by air velocity. However, for most building applications, room air velocities are not greater than 0.1 m/s and so it is possible to determine typical values for a variety of surfaces (as shown in Table 10.5). Table 10.5 presents typical internal surface resistances for both high- and low-emissivity surfaces.

The resistance of external building surfaces is heavily influenced by wind speed. Table 10.6 gives typical external surface resistances under sheltered, normal and severe conditions.

Unventilated air cavities in walls and roofs offer resistance to heat transfer. For cavities in walls the thermal resistance increases with thickness up to approximately 25 mm. Thereafter the thermal resistance of the air cavity is virtually constant despite any further increase in thickness. Heat transfer across an air cavity is by convection and radiation. Thus the emissivity of the cavity surfaces significantly influences the heat transfer. Table 10.7 gives typical thermal resistances for a variety of air cavities.

Example 10.1 illustrates how the above equation and data can be used to determine the U value of an external wall.

TABLE 10.6   Typical external surface resistances [8]

Building element	Emissivity of surface	Surface resistance (m² K/W)		
		Sheltered	Normal	Severe
Wall	High	0.08	0.06	0.03
	Low	0.11	0.07	0.03
Roof	High	0.07	0.04	0.02
	Low	0.09	0.05	0.02

Sheltered: Applies up to the third floor in city centres.
Normal: Applies to most suburban and rural areas, and from the fourth to the eighth floors on tall buildings in city centres.
Severe: Applies to coastal and hill sites, above the fifth floor in suburban and rural districts and above the ninth in city centres.

TABLE 10.7   Typical resistances of unventilated air cavities [8]

Cavity thickness	Emissivity of surface	Thermal resistance (m² K/W) for stated heat flow direction		
		Horizontal	Upward	Downward
5 mm	High	0.10	0.10	0.10
	Low	0.18	0.18	0.18
25 mm or greater	High	0.18	0.17	0.22
	Low	0.35	0.35	1.06

Example 10.1

An external wall has the following construction:

Element	Thickness (mm)	Thermal conductivity (W/m K)
Plaster	13	0.500
Concrete block (inner leaf)	100	0.200
Air cavity	50	n.a.
Brick (outer leaf)	102	0.840

Assuming that the air cavity has a thermal resistance of 0.18 m² K/W, the internal surface resistance is 0.123 m² K/W and the external surface resistance is 0.055 m² K/W, determine:

(i) The U value of the wall.
(ii) The U value of the wall if the cavity is filled with insulating foam having a thermal conductivity of 0.036 W/m K.

Solution

Using the above data and eqn (10.8), it is possible to determine the total thermal resistance of the cavity wall as follows:

Element	Thickness (m)	Thermal conductivity (W/m K)	Thermal resistance (m² K/W)
Internal surface resistance	n.a.	n.a.	0.123
Plaster	0.013	0.500	0.026
Concrete block (inner leaf)	0.100	0.200	0.500
Air cavity	0.050	n.a.	0.180
Brick (outer leaf)	0.102	0.840	0.121
External surface resistance	n.a.	n.a.	0.055
			Total resistance = 1.005

(i) Therefore:

$$U \text{ value (existing wall)} = \frac{1}{1.005} = 0.995 \text{ W/m}^2 \text{ K}$$

(ii) If the cavity of the wall is filled with foam, then:

$$\text{Thermal resistance of foam} = \frac{0.05}{0.036} = 1.389 \text{ m}^2 \text{ K/W}$$

However, the thermal resistance of 0.18 m² K/W for the air cavity no longer applies, therefore:

$$\text{New thermal resistance of wall} = 1.005 + 1.389 - 0.18 = 2.214 \text{ m}^2 \text{ K/W}$$

Therefore:

$$\text{New } U \text{ value} = \frac{1}{2.214} = 0.452 \text{ W/m}^2 \text{ K}$$

It can be seen from Example 10.1 that by filling the cavity with insulating foam, it has been possible to reduce the U value of the wall by 54.6%.

10.3.2 Heat Loss Calculations

If the U values for the various component parts of a building's fabric are known, then it is possible using eqns (10.5) and (10.6) to determine, with relative accuracy, the wintertime design day heat loss rate and thus ultimately size boiler plant and heat emitters. Example 10.2 illustrates how this calculation should be performed.

Example 10.2

The surface areas and U values of the elements of a building are as follows:

Element	Area (m²)	U value (W/m²K)
Floor	200	0.45
Roof	200	0.28
Single glazing	16	5.60
External doors	8	2.00
External walls	216	0.60

If the internal design temperature is 21°C and the external design temperature is −1°C, determine the design day heat loss rate. (Assume that the building experiences three air changes per hour and that its volume is 800 m³.)

Solution

Under the wintertime design condition, the temperature difference between the inside and outside is 22. Given this, and by applying eqn (10.5) (i.e. $Q_f = UA(t_{ai} - t_{ao})$), it is possible to calculate the heat loss rate through each component element of the building fabric:

Element	Area (m²)	U value (W/m²K)	Temperature difference (°C)	Heat loss (W)
Floor	200	0.45	22	1980.0
Roof	200	0.28	22	1232.0
Single glazing	16	5.60	22	1971.2
External doors	8	2.00	22	352.0
External walls	216	0.60	22	2851.2
			Fabric heat loss =	8386.4

By applying eqn (10.6) it is possible to determine the ventilation heat loss:

$$\text{Ventilation heat loss} = 0.3333 \times 3 \times 800 \times (21 - (-1)) = 17,600 \text{ W}$$

Now:

$$\text{Total heat loss} = \text{Fabric loss} + \text{Ventilation loss}$$

Therefore:

$$\text{Total heat loss} = 8386.4 + 17,600 = 25,986.4 \text{ W}$$

From an energy conservation point of view, one of the advantages of performing a design day heat loss calculation is that it gives an elemental breakdown of the relative heat losses from the building, enabling them to be quickly and easily evaluated. From Example 10.2 it can be seen that 1971.2 W is lost through the single glazing (i.e. 7.6% of the total heat loss). However, the ventilation loss of 17,600 W represents 67.7% of the total heat loss. Given this, it would be folly to install double glazing without first reducing the ventilation heat loss.

While the use of eqns (10.5) and (10.6) gives a relatively accurate value of the winter design day heat loss, it can be inaccurate, especially in applications where radiant heating is used. A superior model, which fully takes into account the radiant heat transfer which occurs within a room space, is described by eqns (10.11) and (10.12):

$$Q_f = F_1 \times \sum (AU) \times (t_c - t_{ao}) \tag{10.11}$$

and

$$Q_v = F_2 \times 0.333 \times N \times V \times (t_c - t_{ao}) \tag{10.12}$$

and

$$Q_p = Q_f + Q_v \tag{10.13}$$

where Q_p is the heating plant output (W), t_c is the dry resultant temperature in the centre of the room (°C), and F_1, F_2 are the characteristic temperature ratios.

The temperature ratios, F_1 and F_2, are defined as:

$$F_1 = \frac{(t_{ei} - t_{ao})}{(t_c - t_{ao})} \tag{10.14}$$

and

$$F_2 = \frac{(t_{ai} - t_{ao})}{(t_c - t_{ao})} \tag{10.15}$$

where t_{ei} is the internal environmental temperature (°C).

The internal environmental temperature is a theoretical construct which is used to calculate the radiative and convective heat transfer to the inside surface of an external wall from the other surfaces in a room. In temperate and hot climates, it can be defined as:

$$t_{ei} = \frac{1}{3} \cdot t_{ai} + \frac{2}{3} \cdot t_m \tag{10.16}$$

where t_m is the mean surface temperature of the room (°C).

The CIBSE publish tables of values for F_1 and F_2 for various heating systems [10]. Tables 10.8, 10.9 and 10.10 show values of F_1 and F_2 for a forced warm air system, a panel radiator system and a high temperature radiant strip system. In each table values of F_1 and F_2 are presented against two variables, $\Sigma(AU)/\Sigma(A)$ and $NV/3\Sigma(A)$.

Once the values of F_1 and F_2 have been established for any system, it is possible to calculate the internal environmental temperature and the mean surface temperature of a room by using eqns (10.17) and (10.18):

$$t_{ei} = (F_1 \times (t_c - t_{ao})) + t_{ao} \tag{10.17}$$

TABLE 10.8 F_1 and F_2 values for 100% convective, 0% radiant heating (i.e. forced warm air heating) [10]

$NV/3\Sigma(A)$	$\Sigma(AU)/\Sigma(A)$							
	0.2		0.4		0.6		0.8	
	F_1	F_2	F_1	F_2	F_1	F_2	F_1	F_2
0.1	0.99	1.03	0.98	1.07	0.97	1.10	0.96	1.13
0.2	0.99	1.03	0.98	1.07	0.97	1.10	0.96	1.13
0.4	0.99	1.03	0.98	1.07	0.97	1.10	0.96	1.13
0.6	0.99	1.03	0.98	1.07	0.97	1.10	0.96	1.13
0.8	0.99	1.03	0.98	1.07	0.97	1.10	0.96	1.13
1.0	0.99	1.03	0.98	1.07	0.97	1.10	0.96	1.13
1.5	0.99	1.03	0.98	1.07	0.97	1.10	0.96	1.13
2.0	0.99	1.03	0.98	1.07	0.97	1.10	0.96	1.13
3.0	0.99	1.03	0.98	1.07	0.97	1.10	0.96	1.13
4.0	0.99	1.03	0.98	1.07	0.97	1.10	0.96	1.13

TABLE 10.9 F_1 and F_2 values for 70% convective, 30% radiant heating (i.e. panel radiators) [10]

$NV/3\Sigma(A)$	$\Sigma(AU)/\Sigma(A)$							
	0.2		0.4		0.6		0.8	
	F_1	F_2	F_1	F_2	F_1	F_2	F_1	F_2
0.1	1.00	1.01	0.99	1.03	0.98	1.05	0.98	1.06
0.2	1.00	1.00	0.99	1.02	0.99	1.04	0.98	1.06
0.4	1.00	0.99	1.00	1.01	0.99	1.02	0.99	1.04
0.6	1.01	0.97	1.00	0.99	1.00	1.01	0.99	1.03
0.8	1.01	0.96	1.01	0.98	1.00	1.00	1.00	1.01
1.0	1.02	0.95	1.01	0.96	1.01	0.98	1.00	1.00
1.5	1.03	0.92	1.02	0.93	1.02	0.95	1.01	0.97
2.0	1.04	0.89	1.03	0.90	1.03	0.92	1.02	0.93
3.0	1.06	0.83	1.05	0.85	1.05	0.86	1.04	0.88
4.0	1.07	0.78	1.07	0.80	1.06	0.81	1.06	0.83

$$t_{ai} = (F_2 \times (t_c - t_{ao})) + t_{ao} \tag{10.18}$$

Rearranging eqn (10.16) gives:

$$t_m = \frac{3}{2} \cdot t_{ei} - \frac{1}{2} \cdot t_{ai} \tag{10.19}$$

Example 10.3 illustrates how eqns (10.11)–(10.13) can be applied to determine the plant output for the building illustrated in Example 10.2.

TABLE 10.10 F_1 and F_2 values for 10% convective, 90% radiant heating (i.e. high temperature radiant systems) [10]

$NV/3\Sigma(A)$	$\Sigma(AU)/\Sigma(A)$							
	0.2		0.4		0.6		0.8	
	F_1	F_2	F_1	F_2	F_1	F_2	F_1	F_2
0.1	1.01	0.97	1.02	0.95	1.02	0.94	1.02	0.93
0.2	1.02	0.95	1.02	0.93	1.03	0.92	1.03	0.91
0.4	1.03	0.91	1.03	0.90	1.04	0.88	1.04	0.87
0.6	1.04	0.87	1.05	0.86	1.05	0.85	1.05	0.84
0.8	1.05	0.84	1.06	0.83	1.06	0.82	1.06	0.81
1.0	1.06	0.81	1.07	0.80	1.07	0.79	1.07	0.78
1.5	1.09	0.74	1.09	0.73	1.09	0.72	1.10	0.71
2.0	1.11	0.68	1.11	0.67	1.11	0.66	1.12	0.65
3.0	1.14	0.59	1.14	0.58	1.14	0.57	1.14	0.57
4.0	1.16	0.52	1.16	0.51	1.17	0.50	1.17	0.50

Example 10.3

For the building described in Example 10.2, determine the heating plant output if the building is heated by:

 (i) A forced warm air heating system.
 (ii) A LTHW panel radiator system.
 (iii) A high temperature radiant strip system.

Assume that the internal design dry resultant temperature is 21°C and that in all other respects the data are unchanged from that shown in Example 10.2.

Solution
In order to quantify F_1 and F_2 the values of the following parameters are determined:

$$\sum(A) = 640 \text{ m}^2$$

$$\sum(AU) = 381.2 \text{ W/K}$$

$$NV/3 = 800 \text{ W/K}$$

Therefore

$$\frac{\sum(AU)}{\sum(A)} = 0.60 \text{ W/m}^2 \text{ K}$$

and

$$\frac{NV}{3\sum(A)} = 1.25 \text{ W/m}^2 \text{ K}$$

By looking up Tables 10.8, 10.9 and 10.10 the values of F_1 and F_2 are found to be:

Option	Heating type	F_1	F_2
(i)	Forced warm air heating	0.970	1.010
(ii)	LTHW panel radiator system	1.015	0.965
(iii)	High temperature radiant strip system	1.080	0.755

Therefore, using eqns (10.11) and (10.13):
(i) Forced warm air heating:

$$Q_f = 0.97 \times 381.2 \times (21-(-1)) = 8134.8 \text{ W}$$

and

$$Q_v = 1.10 \times 0.333 \times 3 \times 800 \times (21-(-1)) = 19,360.0 \text{ W}$$

Therefore

$$Q_p = 8134.8 + 19,360 = 27,494.8 \text{ W}$$

Using eqns (10.17)–(10.19) it is possible to determine the internal air and environmental temperatures, and the mean internal surface temperature of the building:

$$t_{ei} = [0.97 \times (21-(-1))] + (-1) = 20.3°C$$

$$t_{ai} = [1.01 \times (21-(-1))] + (-1) = 23.2°C$$

$$t_m = \frac{3}{2} \times 20.3 - \frac{1}{2} \times 23.2 = 18.9°C$$

Similarly the plant output for options (ii) and (iii) can be established using the above methodology. A summary of the results of the winter design calculation for options (i), (ii) and (iii), together with the results from Example 10.2, is presented in the following table.

Option	Heating type	Q_f (W)	Q_v (W)	Q_p (W)	t_{ai} (°C)	t_m (°C)	t_{ei} (°C)	t_c (°C)
Example 10.2	Non-specific	8386.4	17,600.0	25,986.4	21.0	n.a.	n.a.	n.a.
(i)	Warm air	8134.8	19,360.0	27,494.8	23.2	18.9	20.3	21.1
(ii)	Panel radiators	8512.2	16,983.8	25,496.0	20.2	21.9	21.3	21.1
(iii)	High temp. radiant strip	9057.3	13,287.9	22,345.2	15.6	26.3	22.8	21.0

Comparison of the results from Examples 10.2 and 10.3 indicates that the use of the dry resultant temperature and the F_1 and F_2 coefficients has some effect on the calculated overall plant output. It can be seen that the required output of the high temperature radiant strip system is approximately −5 kW lower than that of the forced warm air system, with the radiator system in the middle. It should also be noticed that the simple method, based on the indoor air temperature, produces a plant output which was similar in magnitude to that required for the LTHW panel radiator system. The margin of error for the less accurate 'air temperature' method was -5.8% when compared with the warm air system, and $+14.0\%$ when compared with the radiant strip system. It can therefore be concluded that while the simple 'air temperature' method is acceptable for sizing standard wall radiator heating systems, the 'F_1 and F_2' method should be used when designing systems which are either 100% convective or almost 100% radiative.

10.4 Heating Energy Calculations

Equations (10.5), (10.6), (10.11) and (10.12) demonstrate that building heat loss is directly proportional to the difference in temperature between the internal and external environments. It follows therefore that buildings which experience harsher winters will, not surprisingly, consume more heating energy during the winter months. It is therefore possible to use the degree day method (see Appendix 1 for a detailed explanation of degree days) to predict annual heating costs.

For a building which is continuously heated and which experiences no substantial continuous heat gains, the annual heating energy consumption can be determined by using eqn (10.20) or (10.21):

$$E = \frac{Q_p}{(t_c - t_{ao})} \times D_{15.5} \times 24 \times \frac{1}{\eta} \tag{10.20}$$

where E is the energy consumed (kWh), Q_p is the heating plant output (kW), $D_{15.5}$ is the number of standard degree days (i.e. to the base temperature 15.5°C), and η is the seasonal efficiency of heating system.

Typical values of η for various types of boiler plant are shown in Table 10.11. As an alternative to eqn (10.20), it is possible to use eqn (10.21) to predict heating energy consumption. However, because eqn (10.21) uses internal air temperature and represents a non-specific heating system, the results calculated are likely to be less accurate than those determined using eqn (10.20). Notwithstanding this, eqn (10.21) is reasonably accurate if buildings are well insulated and a predominantly convective heating system is being used.

$$E = \frac{Q_p}{(t_{ai} - t_{ao})} \times D_{15.5} \times 24 \times \frac{1}{\eta} \tag{10.21}$$

When designing building heating systems it is standard practice to ignore any internal heat gains in the winter design day calculation. In this way the heating system is sized to meet the 'worst-case' scenario (i.e. when the internal heat gain is not present). In reality, if the heating plant is oversized, the heating controls should modulate down the flow water temperature and prevent the building from overheating. However, when performing energy prediction calculations, it may be important to allow for continuous internal heat gains (e.g. from lighting and equipment) in the degree day calculation. This can be achieved by altering the degree day base temperature from 15.5°C to an

TABLE 10.11   Seasonal heating plant efficiencies [11]

Type of system	Seasonal efficiency (%)
Continuous space heating	
Condenser and conventional boilers with weather compensated system	85
Fully controlled gas- or oil-fired boiler with radiator system	70
Fully controlled gas- or oil-fired boiler with radiator system (multiple modular boilers used with sequence controller)	75
Intermittent space heating	
Condenser and conventional boilers with weather compensated system	80
Fully controlled gas- or oil-fired boiler with radiator system	65
Fully controlled gas- or oil-fired boiler with radiator system (multiple modular boilers used with sequence controller)	70

TABLE 10.12 $D_d/D_{15.5}$ ratios for various base temperatures [12]

Base temperature (°C)	$D_d/D_{15.5}$
10	0.33
12	0.57
14	0.82
15	0.94
15.5	1.00
16	1.06
17	1.18
18	1.30

appropriate level. Table 10.12 shows various $D_d/D_{15.5}$ correction factors for various base temperatures.

Internal heat gains can be allowed for in the degree day calculation by determining the temperature rise due to internal gains using eqn (10.22):

$$d = \frac{Q_g}{Q_p} \times (t_c - t_{ao})$$ (10.22)

where d is the average temperature rise which can be maintained by internal heat gains alone (K), and Q_g is the internal heat gain (W).

TABLE 10.13 CIBSE classification of structures by thermal inertia [12]

Weight	Building description
Very heavy	Multi-storey buildings with masonry or concrete curtain walling and sub-divided within by solid partitions.
Heavy	Buildings with large window areas but appreciable areas of solid partitions and floors.
Medium	Single-storey buildings of masonry or concrete, sub-divided within by solid partitions.
Light	Single-storey buildings of a factory type, with little or no solid partitions.

The new base temperature, t_b, can then be determined using eqn (10.23):

$$t_b = t_c - d \qquad (10.23)$$

Equations (10.20) and (10.21) only apply to continuously heated buildings. Most buildings are, however, intermittently occupied and are not heated continuously. When buildings are intermittently occupied it is necessary to allow for the additional heat energy to bring the building structure up to temperature. The amount of preheating required depends on the thermal capacity of the building.

Heavy structures require long preheat periods and, once heated, retain heat well, while lightweight structures tend to heat up and cool quickly. It is therefore impossible to fully consider the impact of intermittent occupation on energy consumption without considering the thermal capacity of the building. The CIBSE classification of structures by thermal inertia is presented in Table 10.13. To allow for intermittent heating when using the degree day method it is necessary to introduce correction factors for:

- The length of the working week.
- The length of the working day.
- The response of the building and plant.

Tables 10.14, 10.15 and 10.16 set out values for these correction factors. Example 10.4 illustrates how the annual heating costs for a building can be calculated.

Example 10.4

A three-storey office building, with a total floor area of 2400 m³, is occupied for 5 days per week and for 8 hours per day. The design day plant output (i.e. heat loss) is calculated to be 190.0 kW when the external temperature is −3.0°C and the dry resultant temperature is 21°C. The building is heated by a series of gas-fired modular boilers connected to a responsive warm air heating system with a seasonal efficiency of 70%.

Given that the building is located in a region which experiences 2354 degree days per year and that the cost of natural gas is 1.5p/kWh, determine the annual heating fuel cost:

(i) Ignoring any internal heat gains (i.e. assuming a base temperature of 15.5°C).
(ii) Allowing for an internal heat gain (from lights and equipment) of 20 W/m².

TABLE 10.14 Correction factor for length of working week [13]

Occupied days per week	Lightweight building	Heavyweight building
7 days	1.0	1.0
5 days	0.75	0.85

TABLE 10.15 Correction factor for length of working day, applies to intermittent use only [13]

Occupied period	Lightweight building	Heavyweight building
4 hours	0.68	0.96
8 hours	1.00	1.00
12 hours	1.25	1.02
16 hours	1.40	1.03

TABLE 10.16 Correction factor for the response of building and plant [13]

Type of heating	Lightweight	Medium weight	Heavyweight
Continuous	1.0	1.0	1.0
Intermittent – responsive plant	0.55	0.70	0.85
Intermittent – plant with a long time lag	0.70	0.85	0.95

Solution

(i) *Ignoring any internal heat gains*: From Table 10.14, the correction factor for length of working week is 0.85. From Table 10.15, the correction factor for length of working day is 1.00. From Table 10.16, the correction factor for response of building and plant is 0.85.

Therefore:

$$\text{Annual heating energy consumption} = \frac{190}{(21-(-3))} \times 2354 \times 24 \times \frac{(0.85 \times 1.00 \times 0.85)}{0.7}$$
$$= 461,636.21 \text{ kWh}$$

and

$$\text{Annual energy cost} = \frac{461,636.21 \times 1.5}{100} = £6924.54$$

(ii) *Allowing for an internal heat gain of* 20 W/m²:

$$\text{Total heat gain} = \frac{2400 \times 20}{1000} = 48.0 \text{ kW}$$

Using eqn (10.22), the temperature rise due to heat gains is:

$$d = \frac{48}{190} \times (21 - (-3)) = 6.06°C$$

Therefore, the new base temperature is:

$$t_b = 21 - 6.06 = 14.94°C$$

From Table 10.12 this corresponds to a $D_d/D_{15.5}$ value of 0.932. Therefore,

Annual heating energy consumption (allowing for heat gains) = $461,636.21 \times 0.932$

$$= 430,244.95 \text{ kWh}$$

Therefore,

$$\text{Annual energy cost} = \frac{430,244.95 \times 1.5}{100} = £6453.67$$

As well as predicting heating energy costs, it is also possible to use the degree day method to evaluate proposed energy-saving measures. Example 10.5 illustrates how this can be achieved.

Example 10.5

An office building has a roof which has a U value of 1.1 W/m² K. It is proposed that additional insulation be installed in the roof to bring its U value down to 0.25 W/m² K.

The office building is located in a region which experiences an annual total of 2350 degree days. Assuming that the efficiency of the building heating system is 70%, the cost of fuel is 1.5p/kWh and the capital cost of installing the roof insulation is £2.00 per m², determine the payback on the investment.

Solution

$$\text{Annual energy saving} = (1.1 - 0.25) \times \frac{2350}{100} \times \frac{24}{0.7}$$
$$= 68.486 \text{ kWh/m}^2$$

Therefore,

$$\text{Annual energy cost saving} = \frac{68.486 \times 1.5}{100} = £1.03 \text{ per m}^2$$

$$\text{Payback period} = \frac{2.00}{1.03} = 1.94 \text{ years}$$

10.5 Intermittent Heating

The degree day calculations in Section 10.4 indicate that the intermittent use of heating plant results in higher energy consumption compared with continuous heating. This is primarily because intermittently occupied buildings, such as office buildings, require the structure to be warmed up after it has been allowed to cool overnight and at weekends. Additional heat energy is therefore required to 'preheat' the building in the mornings, so that its fabric is brought up to a temperature which will be comfortable for the occupants. Buildings with a high thermal mass require greater preheating than buildings with a low thermal mass. However, once heated to the required temperature, heavyweight structures retain their heat for much longer than lightweight ones.

The preheating of a building structure is achieved by running the heating system at full capacity for a preheat period prior to the building's occupation. The heavier the building structure, the longer the preheat period. The preheat period can be reduced in length by oversizing the boiler plant and, to some extent, the heat emitters. It is generally considered more energy efficient to increase the plant margin (i.e. oversize the boiler plant) in order to reduce the preheat period [10]. Table 10.17 gives recommended plant ratios for intermittent heating [10], which should be used in conjunction with eqn (10.24) to determine the intermittent peak heating load. It should be noted that the preheat times in the table assume the use of plant with a short response time, such as a warm air heating system. For slow response heating systems such as underfloor heating the preheating period will be longer:

$$Q_{pb} = F_3 \times Q_p \qquad (10.24)$$

where Q_{pb} is the intermittent peak heating output (W or kW), and F_3 is the plant ratio (i.e. maximum heat output/design day heat output).

When oversizing plant, it is important to consider both boilers and heat emitters. While increased boiler capacity may reduce the preheat time, it can result in poor part-load performance and low seasonal boiler efficiency. It should be remembered that for most of the heating season, the external air temperature will be well above the winter design condition, so for much of the year the boilers will have plenty of excess capacity. It is therefore wise to consider the use of modular boilers.

While increased boiler capacity may be advisable, it is not always necessary to increase individual heat emitters. This is because the following alternative strategies can be employed:

- In buildings which are unoccupied, natural and mechanical ventilation rates can be reduced during the night-time. Reduced ventilation rates will occur naturally during the night-time because doors and windows usually remain closed. With

TABLE 10.17 Recommended plant ratios for intermittent heating [10]

Plant ratio (F_3)	Lightweight building preheat time (hours)	Heavyweight building preheat time (hours)
1.0	Continuous	Continuous
1.2	6	Very long
1.5	3	7
2.0	1	4
2.5	0	2
3.0	0	1

mechanical ventilation systems it is also possible to reduce the ventilation load by fully recirculating the air (i.e. reducing the outside air component of the supply air to 0%) during the preheat period.

- It is possible to elevate the water supply temperature to the heat emitters during the preheat period.

Although a modest oversizing of heat emitters is recommended by the CIBSE, there is no strong economic case for considerable oversizing (i.e. in excess of 25%) of emitter surfaces [10].

10.6 Radiant Heat

The importance of radiant heat transfer in buildings is often misunderstood with the result that potential 'radiant' energy-saving measures are often ignored. It is therefore worth investigating some of the 'radiant' energy-saving techniques that exist.

10.6.1 Radiant Heating

Equation (10.4) shows that the comfort of building occupants is as dependent on the mean radiant temperature as it is on air temperature. This fact can be used to great advantage in applications where a building is poorly insulated and in which ventilation rates are high, such as in old factories or workshops. In such applications, it is often prohibitively expensive to heat up large volumes of air, which are then quickly lost to the outside. It is much better to use some form of radiant heating to warm up the occupants. By using a high temperature radiant heat source it is possible to create a heat balance which enables the occupants to feel comfortable whilst still maintaining the air and fabric at a low temperature.

Radiant heating is particularly well suited to applications in which occupancy is very intermittent and in which the occupants are located in relatively fixed positions. A church building is a classic example of such an application. Such a building is occupied for a relatively short period in every week. Because radiant heating systems react very quickly and warm the occupants rather than the air, they can achieve a good comfort level without any preheating of the building. For this and the other reasons mentioned, radiant heating systems are generally considered to incur lower capital costs and lower operating costs than other comparable systems [13].

In order to achieve high levels of radiant heat transfer it is necessary to have emitters which are at a high temperature, well above 100°C. For safety and comfort reasons, these heat-emitting panels must be placed at high level, well out of the reach of any of the occupants.

10.6.2 Low-Emissivity Glazing

Glazing is often viewed as a thermal 'weak link', because heat is easily conducted through glass from the inside to the outside. This perception is broadly, but not wholly, true. It is often forgotten that much of the heat which is lost through windows occurs because they are, in effect, large flat high-emissivity surfaces which are cold in relation to the other surfaces in a room. All the other surfaces in the room, especially heated surfaces such as radiators and warm bodies, emit long-wave radiation which is readily absorbed by the cool glass. In this way much heat is lost from buildings. It is possible to minimize this problem by installing low-emissivity glazing which reduces the absorption of long-wave radiation. The low-emissivity effect is achieved during the manufacturing process by applying a microscopically thin (i.e. 0.3–0.4 m thick) coating of tin oxide doped with fluorine atoms [14] to the cavity-facing surface of the inner pane of a double-glazed unit. This significantly reduces the radiative heat loss to the cavity and thus reduces the U value of a typical double-glazed unit from approximately $3\,W/m^2\,K$ to $1.8\,W/m^2\,K$.

10.7   Underfloor and Wall Heating

It is possible to heat buildings efficiently by using systems which utilize very low water temperatures. Two effective low temperature systems which can be used are:

*   Underfloor heating, which utilizes flow water temperatures in the range 35–50°C.
*   Wall heating, which utilizes flow water temperatures in the range 30–40°C.

The low water temperatures involved in these systems enable alternative heat sources to be utilized, such as ground source heat pumps or even solar energy. Because both wall and underfloor heating systems involve large heated surfaces, the room mean radiant temperature is increased. This makes it possible to reduce the air temperature within the room space without altering the dry resultant temperature, enabling energy to be saved whilst still maintaining a comfortable environment.

The maximum permissible surface temperature governs the maximum water flow temperature which can be used in both wall and underfloor heating installations. In the case of underfloor heating, occupants feel uncomfortable if the floor surface temperature is above 29°C. For walls the maximum safe surface temperature is about 43°C, since the disassociation temperature for plaster is approximately 45°C.

Underfloor heating systems are best suited to tall spaces, where the use of a conventional warm air or radiator system may lead to stratification of the air (i.e. the warm air becoming trapped at the top of the room space). The use of underfloor heating overcomes this problem and ensures that the air is warmest at ground level, where the occupants are likely to be located.

Underfloor heating systems often consist of a continuous cross-linked polyethylene or polypropylene flexible pipe loop embedded in a floor screed on top of a structural floor [15]. The screed is usually isolated from the structural floor by rigid insulation slabs, which reduce the heat transfer through the slab and help to maintain the screed temperature. The nature of the screed used in underfloor heating systems is of particular importance, since the screed acts as a thermal resistance to the heat transfer from the pipe to the room space and also provides the system with thermal inertia. Screeds can be either cementitious in nature and approximately 75 mm thick or an anhydrite flowing screed which enables the thickness to be reduced to approximately 50 mm. The thermal storage capacity and inertia of a floor screed depend on a number of parameters such as the specific heat capacity, screed thickness, screed density, thermal conductivity, pipe spacing and the water flow and return temperatures. It is therefore difficult to predict exactly how any given floor will perform in practice. However, for a standard 65 mm thick concrete screed floor, with a flow water temperature of 60°C, it has been estimated that the floor screed will take approximately 3 hours to charge and 3 hours to discharge. At lower water temperatures the charging process is considerably extended. The long hysteresis effect of underfloor heating has the disadvantage of being slow to respond and makes it difficult to adjust to sudden changes in the internal environment. Underfloor heating systems are therefore best suited to applications in which occupancy is continuous or well defined and predictable.

Wall heating operates in a similar manner to underfloor heating, with the exception that the pipe coils are generally not located in a material which has a high thermal mass, such as a floor screed. In a typical wall heating system, cross-linked polyethylene pipes are located on the air cavity side of a dry lined plastered wall. The system can be used either with a wet plastered board, or alternatively the pipes can be mechanically bonded to plasterboard using notched battens to make a rigid unit which can then be fixed to the wall. A flexible insulation quilt, such as rock wool, should be placed between the pipes and the structural wall, so that conduction to the building structure is minimized. It is advisable where possible to install the wall heating on internal walls, so that heat losses are minimized.

10.8 Pipework Insulation

Considerable amounts of heat energy can be lost through uninsulated or poorly insulated pipework. It is therefore important to ensure that hot water and steam pipework is properly insulated. A range of insulating materials is available and these can be either inorganic, based on crystalline or amorphous silicon, aluminium or calcium, or organic, based on hydrocarbon polymers in the form of thermosetting/thermoplastic resins or rubbers [16]. They can be either flexible or rigid, both types being available in preformed pipe sections. Table 10.18 lists some of the common types of insulation along with some of their thermal properties.

10.8.1 Pipework Heat Loss

In Section 10.3.1 heat loss through flat surfaces such as walls and roofs is discussed. The geometry of pipework is different from that of flat surfaces, requiring an alternative approach when calculating the heat loss from sections of pipework. The heat transfer through the wall of a pipe can be calculated using eqn (10.25):

$$Q = \frac{2\pi\lambda(t_1 - t_2)}{\ln(r_2/r_1)} \text{ (W per metre length)} \tag{10.25}$$

where λ is the thermal conductivity of pipe wall (W/m K), r_1 is the internal radius of pipe (m), and r_2 is the external radius of pipe (m).

TABLE 10.18   Thermal conductivities of insulating materials [16]

Material	Density (kg/m³)	Thermal conductivity (W/m K)		
		50°C	100°C	300°C
Calcium silicate	210	0.055	0.058	0.083
Expanded nitrile rubber	65–90	0.039	–	–
Mineral wool (glass)	16	0.047	0.065	–
Mineral wool (rock)	100	0.037	0.043	0.088
Magnesia	190	0.055	0.058	0.082
Polyisocyanurate foam	50	0.023	0.026	–

The thermal resistance of the pipe wall (per unit length of pipe) can be determined by:

$$R = \frac{\ln(r_2/r_1)}{2\pi\lambda} \text{ (m K/W)} \tag{10.26}$$

As hot fluid flows along a pipe, heat is transferred to the pipe wall. The rate at which this heat is transferred depends on the thermal resistance of a thin stationary layer of fluid on the pipe wall surface. The heat-transfer rate across this internal surface boundary layer can be expressed as:

$$Q = h \times A \times \Delta t \tag{10.27}$$

where h is the surface heat-transfer coefficient (W/m² K), A is the surface area (m²), and Δt is the temperature difference between the surface and the bulk fluid (°C).

Equation (10.27) can also be applied to the heat transfer across the external surface of a pipe. Consequently, the internal and external surface resistance per unit length of a pipe can be expressed as:

$$R_{\text{so or si}} = \frac{1}{h \times A} \text{ (m K/W)} \tag{10.28}$$

The overall resistance per unit length of a typical insulated pipe can therefore be represented by:

$$R_t = R_{\text{si}} + R_w + R_{\text{ins}} + R_{\text{so}} \tag{10.29}$$

where R_t is the total thermal resistance of pipework per unit length (m K/W), R_w is the thermal resistance of pipe wall per unit length (m K/W), R_{ins} is the thermal resistance of insulation per unit length (m K/W), and R_{si} and R_{so} are the internal and external surface thermal resistances of insulation per unit length (m K/W).

Once the overall resistance of the pipework is determined, the total heat loss per metre run can be calculated by dividing the temperature difference between the fluid and ambient air by the total resistance:

$$Q = \frac{\Delta t}{R_t} \text{ (W/m)} \tag{10.30}$$

Example 10.6

A pipe carries wet steam at 200°C through a building which has an ambient air temperature of 20°C. The pipe has an internal diameter of 53.5 mm, a wall thickness of 3.7 mm and is insulated to a thickness of 25 mm. The thermal conductivity of the pipe material is 46 W/m K and the thermal conductivity of the insulating material is 0.033 W/m K. Assuming that the inside and outside surface heat-transfer coefficients are 10,000 W/m^2 K and 10 W/m^2 K respectively, determine:

(i) The heat transfer per metre length of pipe.
(ii) The temperature of the outside surface of the insulation.
(iii) The heat loss from an uninsulated pipe, assuming that the external heat-transfer coefficient remains unchanged.

Solution

(i) *The total pipework resistance per metre length is:*

$$R_t = R_{si} + R_w + R_{ins} + R_{so}$$

and

$$R_{si} = \frac{1}{10,000 \times \pi \times 0.0535} = 0.00059 \text{ m K/W}$$

$$R_{so} = \frac{1}{10 \times \pi \times 0.1109} = 0.287 \text{ m K/W}$$

$$R_w = \frac{\ln(30.45/26.75)}{2 \times \pi \times 46} = 0.00045 \text{ m K/W}$$

$$R_{ins} = \frac{\ln(55.45/30.45)}{2 \times \pi \times 0.033} = 2.891 \text{ m K/W}$$

From the above calculation it can be seen that the resistance of the pipe wall is negligible compared with that of the insulation and the outside surface resistance. In addition the heat-transfer coefficient for the internal surface is very high and hence the internal surface resistance is negligible. Therefore, the total thermal resistance can be assumed to be:

$$R_t = R_{ins} + R_{so}$$
$$= 3.178 \text{ m K/W}$$

Therefore,

$$Q = \frac{(200 - 20)}{3.178} = 56.64 \text{ W/m}$$

(ii) *The surface temperature can be found by applying the following equation:*

$$\text{Temperature of the outside of the insulation} = t_a + (R_{so} \times Q)$$
$$= 20 + (0.287 \times 56.64) = 36.3°C$$

where t_a is the room air temperature (°C).

(iii) *For the uninsulated pipe*:

$$R_t = R_{si} + R_w + R_{so}$$
$$= 0.00059 + 0.00045 + 0.287 = 0.288 \text{ m K/W}$$

Therefore,

$$Q = \frac{(200 - 20)}{0.288} = 625 \text{ W/m}$$

As well as illustrating the mechanics of a pipework heat loss calculation, Example 10.6 illustrates the great benefit to be derived from insulation, since the 25 mm insulation layer reduced the heat loss from 625 to 56.6 W/m.

10.8.2 Economics of Pipework Insulation

It is well known that one of the simplest and most cost-effective ways of preventing energy wastage is to insulate pipework runs. Nevertheless it is not easy to determine to what extent pipework should be insulated. The capital cost of insulation increases with its thickness and the financial saving must be offset against the capital cost. The economic thickness of insulation should therefore be governed by the payback period that is required on the investment, as illustrated in Example 10.7.

Example 10.7

A steel pipe carries high pressure hot water at 120°C around a factory building. The owners of the factory propose to insulate the pipe using rock wool. Given the data below, determine the optimum thickness of the insulation and the simple payback period for that thickness.

Data:

Pipe outside diameter = 76.6 mm
Heat-transfer coefficient for outside surface insulation = 10 W/m² K
Thermal conductivity of insulation = 0.037 W/m K
Water temperature = 120°C
Temperature of air in factory = 15°C
Boiler efficiency = 70%
Unit price of gas = 1.52 p/kWh
Boiler operates for 2500 hours per annum

Insulation costs							
Thickness of insulation (mm)	[20]	[25]	[32]	[38]	[50]	[60]	[75]
Cost per metre length (£/m)	5.00	5.58	6.64	8.01	10.57	13.44	16.68

Assume that the write-off period for the insulation is 5 years.

Solution

Assuming that the thermal resistances of the pipe wall and of the inside surface of the pipe are both negligible, let

$$x = \text{thickness of insulation (mm)}$$

Now

$$R_{ins} = \frac{\ln(r_2/r_1)}{2\pi\lambda}$$

$$= \frac{\ln\left((38.3 + x)/38.3\right)}{2 \times \pi \times 0.037}$$

and

$$R_{so} = \frac{1}{h \times A}$$

$$= \frac{1}{10 \times \pi \times ((76.6 + 2x) \times 10^{-3})}$$

$$R_t = R_{ins} + R_{so}$$

and

$$Q = \frac{\Delta t}{R_t}$$

therefore

$$Q = \frac{(120 - 15)}{R_{ins} + R_{so}}$$

and

$$\text{Annual operating cost} = \frac{Q \times 2500 \times 1.52}{0.7 \times 100}$$

and

$$\text{Total annual cost} = \text{annual fuel cost} + \frac{\text{capital cost}}{\text{write-off period}}$$

The following table can be produced from the above equations:

Insulation thickness (mm)	Insulation resistance (m K/W)	External resistance (m K/W)	Heat loss (W/m)	Annual fuel cost (£/m)	Total annual cost (£/m)
0	0.00	0.42	252.68	13.72	13.72
20	1.81	0.27	50.47	2.74	3.74
25	2.16	0.25	43.52	2.36	3.48
32	2.61	0.23	36.99	2.01	3.34
38	2.96	0.21	33.09	1.80	3.40
50	3.59	0.18	27.83	1.51	3.62
60	4.05	0.16	24.90	1.35	4.04
75	4.67	0.14	21.85	1.19	4.52

It can be seen that the most economic thickness of insulation is 32 mm, since this has the lowest annual cost.

The payback period for the 32 mm insulation is:

$$\text{Payback period} = \frac{6.62}{(13.72 - 3.34)} = 0.638 \text{ years}$$

10.9 Boilers

Most heating systems, although not all, employ boilers to produce hot water or steam. Boiler efficiency therefore has an important influence on heating-related energy costs. The cost savings that can be achieved by improving overall boiler efficiency can be substantial. Essentially a boiler is a device in which a fossil fuel is burnt and the heat produced is transferred to water. The more effective this heat-transfer process, the more efficient the boiler. It is therefore important to maximize the heat transfer to the water and minimize boiler heat losses. Heat can be lost from boilers by a variety of methods, including flue gas losses, radiation losses and, in the case of steam boilers, blow-down losses. Although all these various losses have a significant effect on boiler energy consumption, the major reason for poor boiler performance occurs at the design stage, where the capacity of boilers is usually oversized and inappropriate boilers are often selected.

Boiler plant which is oversized will operate at part-load for most of the time, resulting in low seasonal efficiency and high operating costs. It has been estimated that a 15% increase in energy consumption can occur if a conventional boiler plant is oversized by 150% [17]. Boiler plant should be considered oversized if under the winter design condition the boilers are able to maintain an internal air temperature well above the design temperature (e.g. 21°C). Evidence of oversizing can be manifested in a number of ways: fuel bills may be higher than expected; excessive cycling of boiler plant may be experienced; and in installations equipped with modular boilers, a large proportion of the boilers may never be used.

Given that for much of the heating season external air temperatures are usually well above the winter design condition, it is important that any boiler installation be designed so that it operates efficiently at part-load. For most types of conventional boilers, efficiency falls dramatically below about 30% of rated capacity [18]. Large boilers are therefore at a disadvantage since for most of the time they will be operating well below their rated capacity. One simple way of overcoming this problem is to install a large number of small modular boilers with a sequence controller in preference to a few large boilers. This ensures that under part-load conditions, boilers which are always operating near their maximum efficiency will provide the bulk of the heating. With such a multi-boiler plant installation, it is wise to install a boiler sequence control system. This is a fully automatic microprocessor-controlled system which monitors and sequences on/off operations of boiler plant according to the demand for heat. This avoids running too many boilers on part-load and minimizes the number of boilers in operation at any one time.

Another technique which can be employed to ensure good part-load efficiencies is to use boilers with modulating burners. These burners modulate the fuel and air to provide a variable output from 20%–30% to 100%. With large modulating boilers it is possible to make substantial energy savings by installing variable speed drives on the combustion air fans. Variable speed drives reproduce the operating characteristics of fixed speed combustion air fans and adjustable dampers, whilst reducing the average electrical demand of the fan motor by approximately 60% [19].

10.9.1 Flue Gas Losses

All boilers require a minimum amount of air to ensure that complete combustion of the fuel takes place and that no carbon monoxide is produced. Yet, if too much air is added then heat is wasted in warming up the excess air, which then escapes through the flue. The amount of combustion air should therefore be limited to that necessary to ensure complete combustion of the fuel. In practice some excess air, around 15–25% for oil-fired boilers [19] and 15–30% for gas-fired boilers [20], is needed. The actual amount required to give the optimum boiler efficiency depends on the fuel used and the type of boiler and burner. If the air flow rate to a boiler is too low, then a proportion of the fuel will remain unburnt and running costs will increase. In the case of oil-fired plant, incomplete combustion will produce smoke which will be visible. For coal-fired plant, incomplete combustion results in unburnt carbon in the ash. It is therefore essential to maintain the correct fuel-to-air ratio at all times. With modern microprocessor-controlled burners, which are fitted to fuel valves and air dampers, it is possible to automatically select and maintain specific fuel-to-air ratios for a variety of fuels. These controllers continually monitor the level of oxygen in the flue gases, and alter the combustion air supply in order to maintain optimum conditions.

Flue gas losses are by far the greatest heat losses which occur from boilers. The flue gases contain considerable sensible heat and also latent heat which is 'bound up'

TABLE 10.19   Typical CO_2 and O_2 contents by volume expected in flue gas (dry basis) [18]

Fuel	Minimum fire		Full fire		
	CO_2 (%)	O_2 (%)	CO_2 (%)	O_2 (%)	CO (ppm)
Coal	11.0	8.5	14.0	5.0	2–500
Fuel oils	11.5	5.5	13.5	3.0	–
Butane	9.4	7.0	12.0	3.0	2–400
Propane	9.2	7.0	12.0	3.0	2–400
Natural gas	8.0	7.0	10.0	3.3	2–400

in water vapour. It is possible to determine the amount of heat which is being lost through the flue, by monitoring the presence of O_2 or CO_2 in the flue gases. If there is little excess air in the combustion gases, then the percentage of CO_2 will be high and the percentage of O_2 low. Conversely, if a large amount of excess air is present, the relationship will be reversed. In a typical gas-fired shell and tube boiler the flue gases should contain about 9–10% CO_2 and 3–5% O_2 [20], while for an oil-fired boiler the CO_2 content of the flue gases should be in the region of 13–14% [19]. Typical CO_2 and O_2 flue gas contents for efficient boiler operation are presented in Table 10.19.

With large boiler plant it is possible to increase boiler efficiency by preheating the combustion air. It has been estimated that the thermal efficiency of a boiler can be increased by approximately 1% if the temperature of the combustion air is raised by 20°C [19,20]. Any one of the following sources of heat can be utilized to preheat the boiler combustion air:

- Waste heat from the flue gases.
- Drawing high temperature air from the top of the boiler room.
- Recovering waste heat by drawing air over or through the boiler casing.

10.9.2   Other Heat Losses

With shell and tube boilers it is possible for the 'smoke' tubes to become fouled by soot and other deposits, resulting in a reduction in the amount of heat which is transferred from the hot flue gases to the water. This increases the temperature of the flue gases and results in greater flue gas losses. Boiler smoke tubes should therefore be cleaned regularly to minimize the flue gas temperature rise, since it has been estimated that a rise of 17°C in the flue gas temperature causes a decrease in efficiency of approximately 1% [19]. Boiler efficiency can also significantly be reduced by a build-up of scale on the water side of the smoke tubes. Water treatment should therefore be employed in order to prevent scale formation.

Heat can be lost through the surface casing of boilers. This is generally referred to as *radiation* loss, although it includes heat which is lost by convection. With modern boilers radiation losses are usually not greater than 1% of the maximum rating. On older boilers this figure may be as high as 10% where the insulation is in poor condition [19,20].

10.9.3 Boiler Blow-Down

With steam boilers it is necessary to eject a small proportion of the water regularly in order to remove sludge and to maintain acceptable levels of total dissolved solids. This process is called *blow-down* and it prevents scaling up of the tubes on the water side. Although necessary, blow-down represents a considerable energy loss and the level of blow-down should be kept to a minimum while still maintaining the recommended level of dissolved solids.

It is possible to recover waste heat from the blow-down process by collecting the flash steam which forms as the pressure falls through the blow-down valve. Because the condensate produced by the blow-down process is both hot and pure, with no dissolved solids, it can be added directly to the make-up water for the boiler, thus reducing energy consumption.

10.9.4 Condensing Boilers

Boiler flue gases are often in excess of 200°C and as such are a useful source of waste heat recovery. Heat exchangers can be installed in flues to recover both sensible and latent heat from the hot products of combustion. However, because of the corrosion problems associated with sulphur bearing fuels, such as fuel oil, flue gas heat recovery is generally only practised on gas-fired boilers. Gas-fired boilers which incorporate integral flue gas heat exchangers are known as *condensing boilers*. If used correctly, condensing boilers can achieve operating efficiencies in excess of 90% [18,21].

With a condensing boiler it is desirable to operate the system so that the return water temperature is as low as possible. This ensures that condensation of the flue gases occurs and that maximum heat recovery from flue gases is achieved. If a condensing boiler is used in conjunction with a weather compensating controller, the boiler will move into condensing mode during the milder part of the season, when return water temperatures are at their lowest. In this way, high efficiency is maintained under part-load conditions. In multiple boiler installations it is usually cost-effective to install only one condensing boiler. This should always be the lead boiler, since it exhibits the highest efficiencies. This ensures that good energy utilization will occur under part-load conditions.

References

[1]   Keating WR. The Eurowinter Group. Cold exposure and winter mortality from ischaemic heart disease, cerebrovascular disease, respiratory disease, and all causes in warm and cold regions of Europe. Lancet 1997;349:1341–46.
[2]   Forecasting the nation's health. Met Office Report, November; 2000.
[3]   Wilkinson P. Social and environmental determinants of excess winter deaths in England, 1986–1996. Report for the Joseph Rowntree Foundation, July; 2000.
[4]   Edholm OG. Man – hot and cold (Studies in Biology No. 97) (Chapter 1). London: Arnold; 1978.
[5]   CIBSE Guide A1, Environmental criteria for design; 1986.
[6]   Smith BJ, Phillips GM, Sweeney M. Environmental science (Chapter 2). Harlow: Longman Scientific and Technical; 1987.
[7]   CIBSE Guide A2, Weather and solar data; 1982.

[8] CIBSE Guide A3, Thermal properties of building structures; 1980.
[9] Smith BJ, Phillips GM, Sweeney M. Environmental science (Chapter 1). Harlow: Longman Scientific and Technical; 1987.
[10] CIBSE Guide A9, Estimation of plant capacity; 1983.
[11] Moss KJ. Energy management and operating costs in buildings (Chapter 1). London: E & FN Spon; 1997.
[12] CIBSE Guide B18, Owning and operating costs; 1986.
[13] Economic use of fired space heaters for industry and commerce, Fuel Efficiency Booklet 3. Department of the Environment; 1993.
[14] Enhancing the built environment. Pilkington Plc. website.
[15] CIBSE Guide B1, Heating; 1986.
[16] The economic thickness of insulation for hot pipes, Fuel Efficiency Booklet 8. Department of the Environment; 1994
[17] Hendrick R, Witte MJ, Leslie NP, Bassett WW. Furnace sizing criteria for energy-efficient set back strategies. ASHRAE Trans 1992;98:1239–46.
[18] Energy audits and surveys. CIBSE Applications Manual AM5; 1991.
[19] Economic use of oil-fired boiler plant, Fuel Efficiency Booklet 14. Department of the Environment; 1993.
[20] Economic use of gas-fired boiler plant, Fuel Efficiency Booklet 15. Department of the Environment; 1994.
[21] Condensing boilers. CIBSE Applications Manual AM3; 1989.

Bibliography

CIBSE Guide A1, Environmental criteria for design; 1986.
CIBSE Guide A2, Weather and solar data; 1982.
CIBSE Guide A3, Thermal properties of building structures; 1980.
CIBSE Guide A9, Estimation of plant capacity; 1983.
CIBSE Guide B1, Heating; 1986.
CIBSE Guide B18, Owning and operating costs; 1986.
Degree days, Fuel Efficiency Booklet 7. Department of the Environment; 1995.
Eastop TD, Croft DR. Energy efficiency for engineers and technologists (Chapters 4 and 5). Harlow: Longman Scientific & Technical; 1990.
Eastop TD, Watson WE. Mechanical services for buildings (Chapter 3). Harlow: Longman Scientific & Technical; 1992.
Edholm OG. Man – hot and cold (Studies in Biology No. 97) (Chapter 1). London: Arnold; 1978.
Economic use of fired space heaters for industry and commerce, Fuel Efficiency Booklet 3. Department of the Environment; 1993.
Economic use of oil-fired boiler plant, Fuel Efficiency Booklet 14. Department of the Environment; 1993.
Economic use of gas-fired boiler plant, Fuel Efficiency Booklet 15. Department of the Environment; 1994.
Levermore GJ. Building energy management systems (Chapter 10). London: E & FN Spon; 1992.
Moss KJ. Energy management and operating costs in buildings (Chapters 1 and 3). London: E & FN Spon; 1997.
Stoecker WF, Jones JW. Refrigeration and air conditioning (Chapters 2 and 4): McGraw-Hill International Editions; 1982.
The economic thickness of insulation for hot pipes, Fuel Efficiency Booklet 8. Department of the Environment; 1994.

CHAPTER 11

Waste Heat Recovery

In many applications there is the potential for recovering heat energy that would otherwise go to waste. This chapter describes various waste heat recovery technologies and examines the theoretical principles behind each.

11.1 Introduction

In many applications it is possible to greatly reduce energy costs by employing some form of waste heat recovery device. However, before investing in such technology it is important to first consider some generic issues:

- Is there a suitable waste heat source? If the answer to this question is 'yes', it is important to establish that the source is capable of supplying a sufficient 'quantity' of heat, and that the heat is of a good enough 'quality' to promote good heat transfer.
- Is there a market or use for the recovered waste heat? It is important to have a use for any waste heat which may be recovered. In many applications there may be no demand for the heat that is available, with the result that a large quantity of heat energy is dumped. In other situations there may be a long time lag between waste heat production and the demand for heat. Waste heat therefore cannot be utilized unless some form of thermal storage is adopted.
- Will the insertion of a heat recovery device actually save primary energy or reduce energy costs? Often the insertion of a heat exchanger increases the resistance of

the fluid streams, resulting in fan or pump energy consumption rising. Heat energy is therefore replaced by electrical energy, which may be produced at an efficiency of less than 35%.

- Will any investment in heat recovery technology be economic? Heat recovery devices can be expensive to install. It is, therefore, essential that the economic payback period be determined prior to any investment being undertaken.

Although the questions above may appear obvious, it is not uncommon to find cases where poor planning and analysis at the design stage has resulted in an installation where the impact of the heat recovery device is either minimal, or is even increasing energy costs. Consider the case of a heat exchanger installed in a warm exhaust air stream from a building. The insertion of the device causes the resistance of the air streams to rise, resulting in greater fan energy consumption. If the unit price of electricity is four times that of gas, then in order to just break even, the heat exchanger must recover four times the increase in electrical energy consumption, arising from the increased system resistance. Also, there may well be long periods when the external air temperature is such that little or no heat can be recovered. If, however, the fans run continuously then the increased electrical energy is being expended for little or no return. Given this, it is not surprising that many so-called 'energy recovery' systems, while appearing to save energy, are in fact increasing both primary energy consumption and energy costs.

If a strategic decision is made to invest in some form of heat recovery device, then the next logical step is to select the most appropriate system. There are a wide variety of heat recovery technologies, which can be divided into the following broad categories:

- *Recuperative heat exchangers*: where the two fluids involved in the heat exchange are separated at all times by a solid barrier.
- *Run-around coils*: where an independent circulating fluid is used to transport heat between the hot and cold streams.
- *Regenerative heat exchangers*: where hot and cold fluids pass alternately across a matrix of material.
- *Heat pumps*: where a vapour compression cycle is used to transfer heat between the hot and cold streams.

In addition to these, there are a few lesser-used technologies, such as heat pipes, which are discussed in Chapter 5.

11.2 Recuperative Heat Exchangers

In a recuperative heat exchanger the two fluids involved in the heat transfer are separated at all times by a solid barrier. This means that the mechanisms which control the heat transfer are convection and conduction. The thermal resistance of a heat exchanger can therefore be expressed as follows:

$$R = \frac{1}{U} = \frac{1}{h_i} + R_w + \frac{1}{h_o} + F_i + F_o \qquad (11.1)$$

where R is the thermal resistance of the heat exchanger (m² K/W), R_w is the thermal resistance of the separating wall (m² K/W), h_i and h_o are the heat transfer coefficient of internal and external surfaces (W/m² K), F_i and F_o are the internal and external fouling factors, and U is the overall heat transfer coefficient (i.e. U value) (W/m² K).

In short this can be written as:

$$\frac{1}{U_{dirty}} = \frac{1}{U_{clean}} + \text{Fouling factors} \tag{11.2}$$

In practice heat exchangers are often oversized so that even when fouled their performance still meets design requirements. The degree of oversizing is achieved by incorporating fouling factors into the sizing calculation.

Recuperative heat exchangers are the most common type of equipment used for waste heat recovery. They can only be used in applications where the hot and cold streams can be brought into close proximity with each other. Although the precise form of a heat exchanger may change with its particular application, there are three forms which are widely used:

(a) *Shell and tube heat exchanger*: Shell and tube heat exchangers consist of a bundle of tubes inside a cylindrical shell through which two fluids flow, one through the tubes and the other through the shell (as shown in Figure 11.1). Heat is exchanged by conduction through the tube walls. Baffles are often used to direct fluid around the heat exchanger and also to provide structural support for the tubes.

(b) *Plate heat exchanger*: Plate heat exchangers consist of a large number of thin metal plates (usually stainless steel but sometimes titanium or nickel), which are clamped tightly together and sealed with gaskets (see Figure 11.2). The thin plates are profiled so that 'flow ways' are created between the plates when they are packed together, and a very large surface area is created across which heat transfer can take place. Ports located at the corners of the individual plate separate the 'hot' and 'cold' fluid flows and direct them to alternate passages so that no intermixing

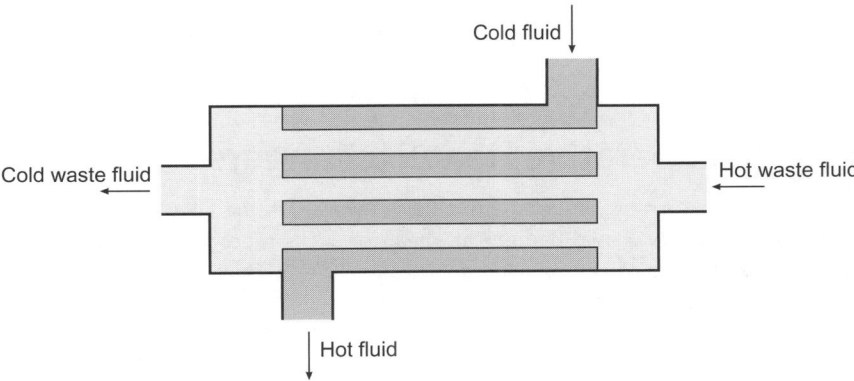

FIG 11.1 Shell and tube heat exchanger.

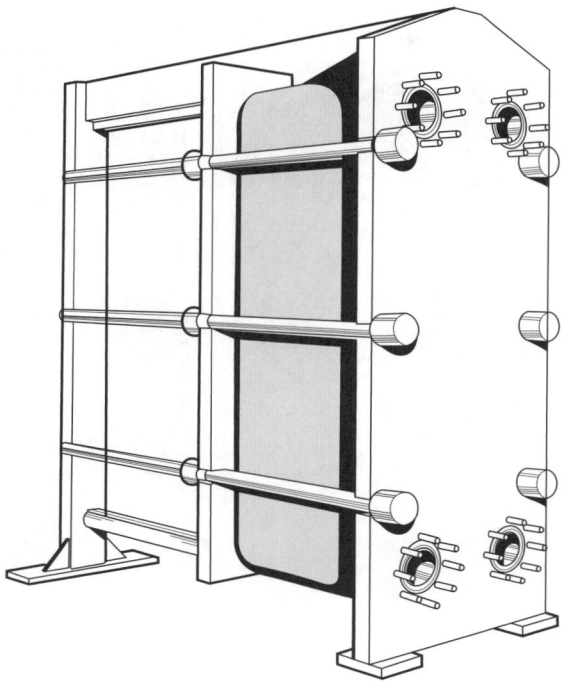

FIG 11.2 Plate heat exchanger.

of the fluids occurs. The whole exchanger experiences a counter-flow pattern. The maximum operating temperature is usually about 130°C if rubber sealing gaskets are fitted, but this can be extended to 200°C if compressed asbestos fibre seals are used [1]. Plate heat exchangers have become popular in recent years because they are extremely compact and can easily be expanded or contracted to accommodate future system modification.

(c) *Flat plate recuperator*: Flat plate recuperators consist of a series of metal (usually aluminium) plates separating 'hot' and 'cold' air or gas flows, sandwiched in a box-like structure (see Figure 11.3). The plates are sealed in order to prevent intermixing of the two fluid flows. They are often used in ducted air-conditioning installations to reclaim heat from the exhaust air stream, without any cross-contamination occurring.

11.3 Heat Exchanger Theory

The two most commonly used heat exchanger flow configurations are *counter flow* and *parallel flow*. These flow patterns are represented in Figures 11.4 and 11.5 respectively, along with their characteristic temperature profiles.

It should be noted that with the parallel flow configuration the 'hot' stream is always warmer than the 'cold' stream. With the counter-flow configuration it is possible for the

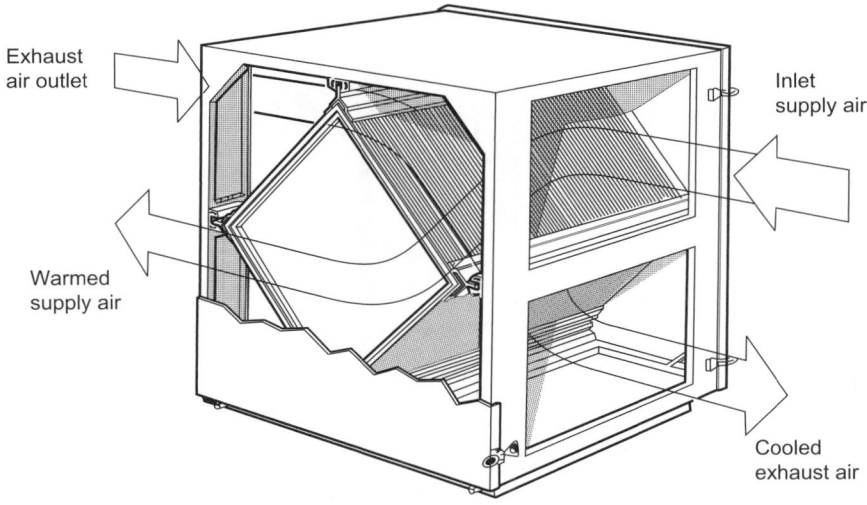

FIG 11.3 Flat plate recuperator.

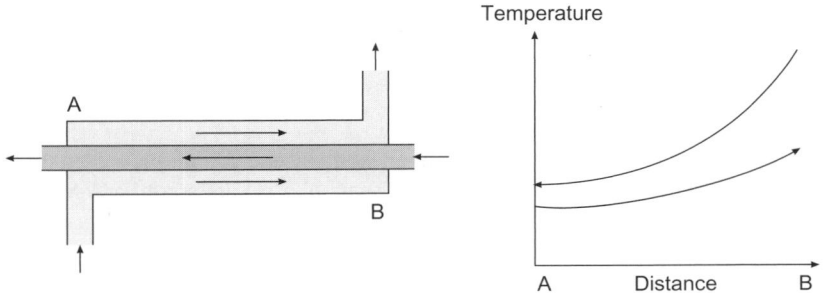

FIG 11.4 Counter-flow heat exchanger.

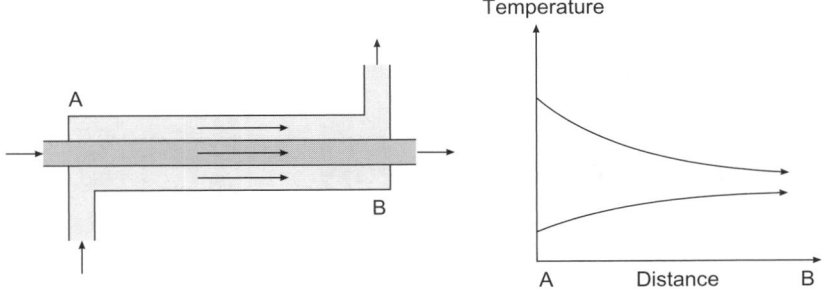

FIG 11.5 Parallel-flow heat exchanger.

outlet temperature of the cold fluid to be higher than the outlet temperature of the hot fluid.

The general equations which govern the heat transfer in recuperative heat exchangers are as follows:

$$Q = \dot{m}_h\, c_h(t_{h1} - t_{h2}) = \dot{m}_c\, c_c\, (t_{c1} - t_{c2}) \tag{11.3}$$

and

$$Q = UA_o(\text{LMTD})K \tag{11.4}$$

where Q is the rate of heat transfer (W), $\dot{m}_h$ is the mass flow rate of hot fluid (kg/s), $\dot{m}_c$ is the mass flow rate of cold fluid (kg/s), c_h is the specific heat of hot fluid (J/kg K), c_c is the specific heat of cold fluid (J/kg K), t_{h1} and t_{h2} are the inlet and outlet temperatures of hot fluid (°C), t_{c1} and t_{c2} are the outlet and inlet temperatures of cold fluid (°C), U is the overall heat transfer coefficient (i.e. U value) (W/m^2 K), A_o is the outside surface area of heat exchanger (m^2), LMTD is the logarithmic mean temperature difference (°C), and K is the constant which is dependent on the type of flow through the heat exchanger (e.g. $K = 1$ for counter flow and parallel flow, and is therefore often ignored).

The LMTD can be determined by:

$$\text{LMTD} = \frac{\Delta t_1 - \Delta t_2}{\ln (\Delta t_1/\Delta t_2)} \tag{11.5}$$

The following examples illustrate how the above equations can be used to design and analyse heat exchangers.

Example 11.1

A liquid waste stream has a flow rate of 3.5 kg/s and a temperature of 70°C, with a specific heat capacity of 4190 J/kg K. Heat recovered from the hot waste stream is used to preheat boiler make-up water. The flow rate of the make-up water is 2 kg/s, its temperature is 10°C and its specific heat capacity is 4190 J/kg K. The overall heat transfer coefficient of the heat exchanger is 800 W/m^2 K. If a make-up water exit temperature of 50°C is required, and assuming that there are no heat losses from the exchanger, determine:

  (i) The heat transfer rate.
 (ii) The exit temperature of the effluent.
(iii) The area of the heat exchanger required.

Solution
  (i) Now:

$$Q = \dot{m}_c\, c_c\, (t_{c1} - t_{c2})$$
$$= 2 \times 4190 \times (50 - 10)$$
$$= 335{,}200 \text{ W} = 335.2 \text{ kW}$$

(ii) Now

$$\dot{m}_h c_h(t_{h1} - t_{h2}) = \dot{m}_c c_c (t_{c1} - t_{c2})$$
$$3.5 \times 4190 \times (70 - t_{h2}) = 2 \times 4190 \times (50 - 10)$$
$$t_{h2} = 47.14°C$$

(iii) Now, because the water outlet temperature is above the outlet temperature of the effluent, a counter-flow heat exchanger is required:

$$\begin{aligned}
\text{LMTD} &= \frac{\Delta t_1 - \Delta t_2}{\ln (\Delta t_1/\Delta t_2)} \\
&= \frac{((70 - 50) - (47.14 - 10))}{\ln ((70 - 50)/(47.14 - 10))} \\
&= 27.69°C
\end{aligned}$$

Now

$$Q = UA(\text{LMTD})$$

therefore

$$A = \frac{335,200}{800 \times 27.69} = 15.13 \text{ m}^2$$

Example 11.2

Consider the *counter-flow* heat exchanger shown in Figure 11.6. Given the data below, determine the overall heat transfer rate for the heat exchanger.

Data:

Length of heat exchanger = 2 m
Internal radius of heat exchanger surface = 10 mm
External radius of heat exchanger surface = 11 mm
Thermal conductivity of heat exchanger surface = 386 W/m K

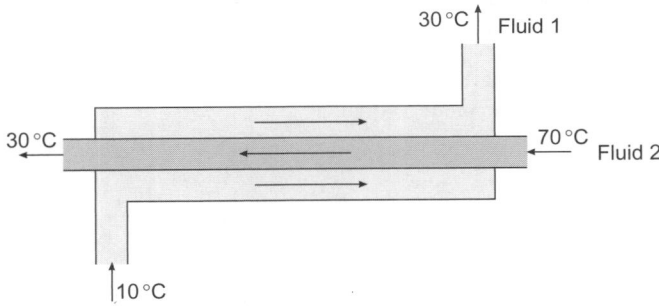

FIG 11.6 Heat exchanger.

Heat transfer coefficient of Fluid 1 $= 50 \text{W/m}^2 \text{K}$
Heat transfer coefficient of Fluid 2 $= 90 \text{W/m}^2 \text{K}$

Solution

By combining eqns (10.26) and (10.28) it can be shown that the total thermal resistance, R_t, of the heat exchanger is:

$$R_t = \frac{1}{h \cdot A_1} \times \frac{\ln(r_2/r_1)}{2\pi k \cdot l} \times \frac{1}{h \cdot A_2}$$

where k is the thermal conductivity of the pipe wall (W/m K), r_1 is the internal radius of the pipe (m), r_2 is the external radius of the pipe (m), l is the length of the pipe (m), h is the heat transfer coefficient (W/m^{2}K), and A_1 and A_2 are the external and internal surface areas (m^2).

And using eqn (10.30) the total heat transfer rate can be expressed as:

$$Q = \frac{\Delta t}{R_t} \text{ (W)}$$

Now:

$$A_1 = 2\pi \times 0.011 \times 2 = 0.138 \text{ m}^2$$

and

$$A_2 = 2\pi \times 0.01 \times 2 = 0.126 \text{ m}^2$$
$$R_t = \frac{1}{90 \times 0.126} \times \frac{\ln(0.011/0.01)}{2\pi \times 386 \times 2} \times \frac{1}{50 \times 0.138}$$

therefore

$$R_t = 0.233 \text{ W/K}$$

and

$$\text{LMTD} = \frac{(70 - 30) - (30 - 10)}{\ln[(70 - 30)/(30 - 10)]} = 28.85°\text{C}$$

therefore

$$Q = \frac{28.85}{0.233} = 123.8 \text{ W}$$

11.3.1 Number of Transfer Units (NTU) Concept

In some situations only the inlet temperatures and the flow rates of the *hot* and *cold* streams are known. Under these circumstances the use of the LMTD method results in a long and complex mathematical solution. To simplify such calculations the NTU method was developed [2,3].

NTU is defined as the ratio of the temperature change of one of the fluids divided by the mean driving force between the fluids, and can be expressed as:

For the hot fluid:

$$\text{NTU}_h = \frac{(t_{h1} - t_{h2})}{(\text{LMTD})K} = \frac{UA_o}{(\dot{m}c)_h} \tag{11.6}$$

For the cold fluid:

$$\text{NTU}_c = \frac{(t_{c1} - t_{c2})}{(\text{LMTD})K} = \frac{UA}{(\dot{m}c)_c} \tag{11.7}$$

(NB: For counter-flow and parallel-flow heat exchangers the K term can be ignored) Equations (11.6) and (11.7) are more commonly simplified to:

$$\text{NTU} = \frac{UA_o}{(\dot{m}c)_{min}} \tag{11.8}$$

where $(\dot{m}c)_{min}$ is the minimum thermal capacity (kW/K).

The ratio of the thermal capacities, R, is defined as:

$$R = \frac{(\dot{m}c)_{min}}{(\dot{m}c)_{max}} \tag{11.9}$$

If both fluids in the heat exchanger have the same thermal capacity then $R = 1$. At the other extreme when one of the fluids has an infinite thermal capacity, as in the case of an evaporating vapour, then $R = 0$.

Another useful concept is the *effectiveness*, E, of a heat exchanger. Effectiveness can be defined as the actual heat transfer divided by the maximum possible heat transfer across the heat exchanger, and can be expressed as:

$$E = \frac{Q}{Q_{max}} = \frac{Q}{(\dot{m}c)_{min}(t_{h\,max} - t_{c\,min})} \tag{11.10}$$

It is possible to derive the relationship between E, NTU and R for a variety of heat exchanger applications. The mathematical expressions for some of the more common applications are given below:

(i) Parallel flow:

$$E = \frac{1 - e^{[-\text{NTU}\,(1+R)]}}{1 + R} \tag{11.11}$$

(ii) Counter flow:

$$E = \frac{1 - e^{[-\text{NTU}\,(1-R)]}}{1 - R e^{[-\text{NTU}\,(1-R)]}}$$ (11.12)

If $R = 1$ then this expression simplifies to:

$$E = \frac{\text{NTU}}{1 + \text{NTU}}$$ (11.13)

(iii) Heat exchanger with condensing vapour of boiling liquid on one side:

$$E = 1 - e^{[-\text{NTU}]}$$ (11.14)

The NTU method for heat exchanger analysis is illustrated in Example 11.3.

Example 11.3

A contaminated water stream from a factory building has a temperature of 80°C, a flow rate of 6 kg/s and a specific heat capacity of 4.19 kJ/kg K. The incoming water supply to the manufacturing process is at 10°C and has a flow rate of 7 kg/s and a specific heat capacity of 4.19 kJ/kg K. It is proposed to install a counter-flow heat exchanger to recover the waste heat. If the heat exchanger has an overall area of 30 m² and an overall heat transfer coefficient of 800 W/m² K (assuming that there are no heat losses from the heat exchanger), determine:

 (i) The effectiveness of the heat exchanger.
 (ii) The heat transfer rate.
(iii) The exit temperature of the incoming water stream leaving the heat exchanger.

Solution
Now

$$(\dot{m}c)_{\text{min}} = 6 \times 4.19 = 25.14 \text{ kW/K}$$

and

$$(\dot{m}c)_{\text{max}} = 7 \times 4.19 = 29.33 \text{ kW/K}$$

therefore

$$R = \frac{25.14}{29.33} = 0.857$$

and

$$\text{NTU} = \frac{30 \times 800}{25.14 \times 1000} = 0.955$$

(i) Therefore:

$$E = \frac{1 - e^{[-0.955(1-0.857)]}}{1 - 0.857\, e^{[-0.955(1-0.857)]}}$$

$$E = 0.506$$

(ii) Now:

$$E = \frac{Q}{(\dot{m}c)_{min}(t_{h\,max} - t_{c\,min})}$$

therefore:

$$Q = 0.506 \times 25.14 \times [80 - 10] = 890.46 \text{ kW}$$

(iii) Therefore:

$$890.46 = 29.33 \times [t_{off} - 10]$$

therefore:

$$t_{off} = 40.4°C$$

11.4 Run-Around Coils

When two recuperative heat exchangers are linked together by a third fluid which transports heat between them, the system is known as a run-around coil. Run-around coils are often employed to recover waste heat from exhaust air streams and to preheat incoming supply air, thus avoiding the risk of cross-contamination between the two air streams. Such a system is shown in Figure 11.7. Run-around coils usually employ a glycol/water mixture as the working fluid which avoids the risk of freezing during the winter.

Run-around coils have the advantage that they can be used in applications where the two fluid streams are physically too far apart to use a recuperative heat exchanger.

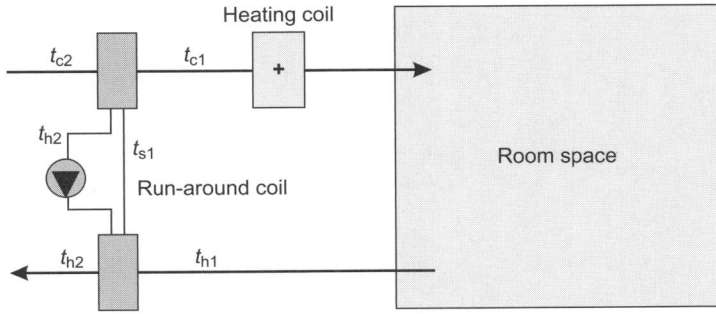

FIG 11.7 Run-around coil system.

Whilst this feature is usually considered advantageous it does result in increased energy consumption since a pump is introduced into the system, and may also result in heat loss from the secondary fluid. This makes it important to insulate the pipework circuit, otherwise the overall effectiveness of the system will become unacceptably low. Despite these drawbacks, when compared with many other methods of recovering waste heat, run-around coils are relatively inexpensive to install since they utilize standard air/water heating coils.

In the case of the system shown in Figure 11.7 the thermal capacity $(\dot{m}c)$ of the *cold* fluid is equal to that of the *hot* fluid since the two heat exchangers are identical. Therefore:

$$(\dot{m}c)_h = (\dot{m}c)_c = (\dot{m}c)_s \tag{11.15}$$

where $(\dot{m}c)_s$ is the thermal capacity of the secondary fluid (kW/K).

Consequently, it can be shown that:

$$t_{s1} = \frac{(t_{h1} + t_{c1})}{2}$$

and

$$t_{s2} = \frac{(t_{h2} + t_{c2})}{2}$$

where t_{s1} and t_{s2} are the flow and return temperatures of the secondary fluid (°C), t_{h1} and t_{h2} are the temperatures of the hot fluid stream before and after heat exchanger (°C), and t_{c2} and t_{c1} are the temperatures of the cold fluid stream before and after heat exchanger (°C).

Also, the overall heat transfer can be defined by

$$Q = (UA)_o \, (t_{h1} - t_{c1})$$

and

$$Q = (UA)_h \, (t_{h1} - t_{s1})$$
$$= (UA)_h \left(t_{h1} - \frac{(t_{h1} + t_{c1})}{2} \right)$$

where $(UA)_o$ is the product of U and A for the whole run-around coil (W/K), and $(UA)_h$ is the product of U and A for the heat exchanger in the hot stream (W/K).

Therefore:

$$(UA)_o \, (t_{h1} - t_{c1}) = (UA)_h \frac{(t_{h1} - t_{c1})}{2}$$

so

$$Q = \frac{(UA)_h \; (t_{h1} - t_{c1})}{2}$$

and since

$$Q = (\dot{m}c)_c \times (t_{c1} - t_{c2})$$

it can be shown that

$$Q = \frac{(UA)_h \; (t_{h1} - t_{c2})}{2 + [(UA)_h/(\dot{m}c)_c]} \qquad (11.16)$$

Example 11.4

A run-around coil is applied to a heating and ventilation system as shown in Figure 11.7. Air is supplied to the room space at 28°C and leaves at 20°C. The outside air temperature is −1°C. The supply air to the space has a mass flow rate of 3 kg/s and a mean specific heat capacity of 1.012 kJ/kg K. The specific heat of the secondary fluid is 3.6 kJ/kg K, and:

$$(UA)_c = (UA)_h = 5 \text{ kW/K}$$

Given this information, determine:

  (i)   The required mass flow rate of the secondary fluid.
 (ii)   The temperature of the air entering the supply air heating coil.
(iii)   The percentage energy saving achieved by using the run-around coil.

Solution
  (i) From eqn (11.15) it can be seen that:

$$(\dot{m}c)_c = (\dot{m}c)_s$$

therefore:

$$\dot{m}_s = \frac{3 \times 1.012}{3.6} = 0.843 \text{ kg/s}$$

 (ii) Now:

$$Q = \frac{(UA)_h \; (t_{h1} - t_{c2})}{2 + [(UA)_h/(\dot{m}c)_c]}$$

therefore:

$$Q = \frac{5 \times [20 - (-1)]}{2 + [5/(3 \times 1.012)]} = 28.79 \text{ kW}$$

and since

$$t_{c1} = t_{c2} + \frac{Q}{(\dot{m}c)_c}$$

therefore

$$t_{c1} = -1 + \frac{28.79}{(3 \times 1.012)} = 8.48°C$$

(iii) With run-around coil

$$Q = 3 \times 1.012 \times [28 - 8.48] = 59.263 \text{ kW}$$

Without run-around coil

$$Q = 3 \times 1.012 \times [28 - (-1)] = 88.044 \text{ kW}$$

therefore

$$\text{Percentage saving} = \frac{(88.044 - 59.263)}{88.044} \times 100 = 32.7\%$$

While it is relatively simple to derive an expression for the heat transfer of a run-around coil when the thermal capacities of the fluids are equal, it becomes much more complex when the thermal capacities of the two fluids are different, and the heat exchangers are also different. However, this problem can be overcome by using the NTU method.

It can be shown that for a run-around coil

$$\frac{1}{(UA)_o} = \frac{1}{(UA)_h} + \frac{1}{(UA)_c} \tag{11.17}$$

and from eqn (11.8)

$$\text{NTU} = \frac{UA_o}{(\dot{m}c)_{min}}$$

therefore

$$\text{NTU} = \frac{UA_h \times UA_c}{(\dot{m}c)_{min}(UA_h + UA_c)} \tag{11.18}$$

Example 11.5 illustrates how the NTU method can be applied to a run-around coil problem.

Example 11.5

It is intended that a run-around coil be installed to recover waste heat from a flue gas stream at 250°C, and to preheat a water stream at 10°C. The flue gas has a mass flow rate of 4 kg/s and that of the water is 2 kg/s. The individual heat exchangers used in the system are of a counter flow type. Given the following data determine:

(i) The overall effectiveness of the run-around coil.
(ii) The exit temperature of the water stream.

Data:

> Specific heat capacity of flue gas = 1.2 kJ/kg K
> Specific heat capacity of water = 4.19 kJ/kg K
> UA for the flue gas heat exchanger = 5 kW/K
> UA for the water heat exchanger = 18 kW/K

Solution

(i) Now

$$(\dot{m}c)_{min} = 4 \times 1.2 = 4.8 \text{ kW/K}$$

and

$$(\dot{m}c)_{max} = 2 \times 4.19 = 8.38 \text{ kW/K}$$

therefore

$$R = \frac{4.8}{8.38} = 0.573$$

and

$$NTU = \frac{5 \times 18}{4.8 \times (5 + 18)} = 0.815$$

and from eqn (11.13)

$$E = \frac{1 - e^{[-0.815(1-0.573)]}}{1 - 0.573e^{[-0.815(1-0.573)]}}$$

$$= 0.494$$

(ii) Now

$$E = \frac{Q}{(\dot{m}c)_{min}(t_{hmax} - t_{cmin})}$$

therefore

$$Q = 0.494 \times 4.8 \times [250 - 10] = 569.1 \text{ kW}$$

therefore

$$569.1 = 8.38 \times [t_{off} - 10]$$

therefore

$$t_{\text{off}} = 77.9°C$$

11.5 Regenerative Heat Exchangers

In a regenerative heat exchanger a matrix of material is alternately passed from a hot fluid to a cold fluid, so that heat is transferred between the two in a cyclical process. The most commonly used type of regenerative heat exchanger is the thermal wheel, which has a matrix of material mounted on a wheel, which slowly rotates at approximately 10 revolutions per minute, through hot and cold fluid streams (as shown in Figure 11.8). The major advantage of a thermal wheel is that there is a large surface area to volume ratio resulting in a relatively low cost per unit surface area.

The matrix material in a thermal wheel is usually an open-structured metal, such as knitted stainless steel or aluminium wire, or corrugated sheet aluminium or steel [1]. For use at higher temperatures honeycomb ceramic materials are used. Although thermal wheels are usually employed solely to recover sensible heat, it is possible to reclaim the enthalpy of vaporization of the moisture in the 'hot' stream passing through a thermal wheel. This is achieved by coating a non-metallic matrix with a hygroscopic or desiccant material such as lithium chloride [1].

Thermal wheels do have the major disadvantage that there is the possibility of cross-contamination between the air streams. This can be reduced considerably by ensuring that the cleaner of the two fluids is maintained at the highest pressure, and by using a purging device. Most thermal wheels incorporate a purge unit which allows a small

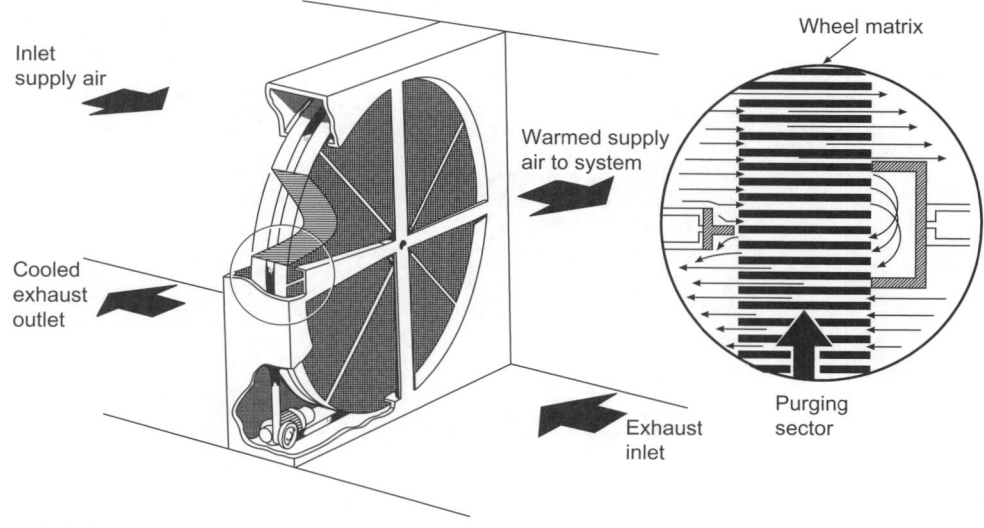

FIG 11.8 Thermal wheel.

proportion of the supply air to flush the contaminants from the wheel, thus keeping cross-contamination to a minimum (e.g. less than 0.04%) [1].

Thermal wheels are often used to recover heat from room ventilation systems such as that shown in Figure 11.9. In this type of application the thermal efficiency, η_t, can be defined by:

$$\eta_t = \frac{t_2 + t_1}{t_3 + t_1} \qquad (11.19)$$

Similarly the overall (total energy) efficiency, η_x, can be expressed as:

$$\eta_x = \frac{h_2 + h_1}{h_3 + h_1} \qquad (11.20)$$

where t_1, t_2 and t_3 are the air temperatures (°C), and h_1, h_2 and h_3 are the air enthalpies (°C).

In a similar manner to a recuperative heat exchanger it can be shown that for a thermal wheel the relationship between (UA) and (hA) is:

$$\frac{1}{(UA)_o} = \frac{1}{(hA)_h} + \frac{1}{(hA)_c} \qquad (11.21)$$

where $(UA)_o$ is the product of overall heat transfer coefficient and surface area of matrix, $(hA)_h$ is the product of heat transfer coefficient between the hot fluid and surface area of matrix, and $(hA)_c$ is the product of heat transfer coefficient between the cold fluid and surface area of matrix. Since the matrix area is constant, therefore:

$$U = \frac{h}{2} \qquad (11.22)$$

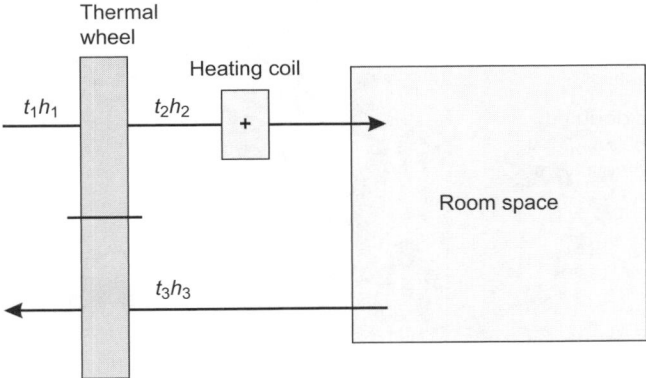

FIG 11.9 Thermal wheel application.

As with recuperative heat exchangers and run-around coils it is possible to use the NTU method to simplify the analysis of thermal wheels. Kays and London [4] derived the following empirical formula to describe the effectiveness of thermal wheels:

$$E = E_c \times \left(1 - \frac{1}{9[(\dot{m}c)_M/(\dot{m}c)_{min}]^{1.93}} \right) \tag{11.23}$$

where

$$(\dot{m}c)_M = N \cdot M \cdot c_M \tag{11.24}$$

N is the wheel revolutions per second, M is the mass of the matrix (kg), c_M is the specific heat capacity of matrix material (kJ/kg K), and

$$E_c = \frac{1 - e^{[-NTU(1-R)]}}{1 - Re^{[-NTU(1-R)]}} \quad \text{where} \quad R = (\dot{m}c)_{min}/(\dot{m}c)_{max}$$

or

$$E_c = \frac{NTU}{1 + NTU} \quad \text{when} \quad R = 1$$

Example 11.6

The exhaust air from a factory building is at a temperature of 35°C and has a flow rate of 6 kg/s and a specific heat capacity of 1.025 kJ/kg K. The incoming fresh air to the building is at −1°C and has a flow rate of 7 kg/s and a specific heat capacity of 1.025 kJ/kg K. It is proposed to insert a thermal wheel between the air streams to recover the sensible waste heat. Given the following information, determine:

 (i) The effectiveness of the thermal wheel.
 (ii) The heat transfer rate.
(iii) The exit temperature of the fresh air leaving the thermal wheel.
(iv) The exit temperature of the fresh air leaving the thermal wheel if its rotational speed is doubled.

Data:

>Wheel diameter = 1.2 m
>Wheel depth = 0.4 m
>Mass of wheel = 140 kg
>Surface area to volume ratio = 2500 m²/m³
>Specific heat of matrix material = 1.3 kJ/kg K
>Wheel speed = 8 rev/min
>Heat transfer coefficient for each air stream = 35 W/m² K

Solution

$$\text{Face area of wheel} = \frac{\pi \times 1.2^2}{4} = 1.12 \text{ m}^2$$
$$\text{Volume of wheel} = 1.13 \times 0.4 = 0.452 \text{ m}^3$$

(i) Now

$$A = 0.452 - 2500 = 1130 \text{ m}^2$$
$$(\dot{m}c)_{\min} = 6 \times 1.025 = 6.15 \text{ kW/K}$$
$$(\dot{m}c)_{\max} = 7 \times 1.025 = 7.175 \text{ kW/K}$$

therefore

$$R = \frac{6.15}{7.175} = 0.857$$

and from eqn (11.21)

$$U = \frac{h}{2} = \frac{35}{2} = 17.5 \text{ W/m}^2\text{K}$$

therefore

$$\text{NTU} = \frac{UA_o}{(\dot{m}c)_{\min}} = \frac{1130 \times 17.5}{6.15 \times 1000} = 3.215$$

therefore

$$E_c = \frac{1 - e^{[-3.215\,(1-0.857)]}}{1 - 0.857\,e^{[-3.215\,(1-0.857)]}} = 0.803$$

and

$$(\dot{m}c)_M = N \cdot M \cdot c_M = \frac{8}{60} \times 140 \times 1.3 = 24.27 \text{ kW/K}$$

therefore

$$E = 0.803 \times \left(1 - \frac{1}{9[24.27/6.15]^{1.93}}\right)$$
$$= 0.797$$

(ii) Now

$$E = \frac{Q}{(\dot{m}c)_{\min}\,(t_{h\max} - t_{c\min})}$$

therefore

$$Q = 0.797 \times 6.15 \times [35 - (-1)] = 176.46 \text{ kW}$$

(iii) Therefore

$$176.46 = 7.175 \times [t_{off} - (-1)]$$

therefore

$$t_{off} = 23.6°C$$

(iv) If $N = 2 \times 8 = 16$ rev/min, then

$$(\dot{m}c)_M = N \cdot M \cdot C_M = \frac{16}{60} \times 140 \times 1.3 = 48.53 \text{ kW/K}$$

therefore

$$E = 0.803 \times \left(1 - \frac{1}{9[48.53/6.15]^{1.93}}\right)$$
$$= 0.801$$

therefore

$$Q = 0.801 \times 6.15 \times [35 - (-1)] = 177.43 \text{ kW}$$

therefore

$$177.34 = 7.175 \times [t_{off} - (-1)]$$

therefore

$$t_{off} = 23.7°C$$

From this it can be seen that there is very little benefit to be gained from doubling the rotational speed of the thermal wheel.

11.6   Heat Pumps

A heat pump is essentially a vapour compression refrigeration machine which takes heat from a low temperature source such as air or water and upgrades it to be used at a higher temperature. Unlike a conventional refrigeration machine, the heat produced at the condenser is utilized and not wasted to the atmosphere. Figure 11.10 shows a simple vapour compression heat pump, together with the relevant pressure/enthalpy diagram.

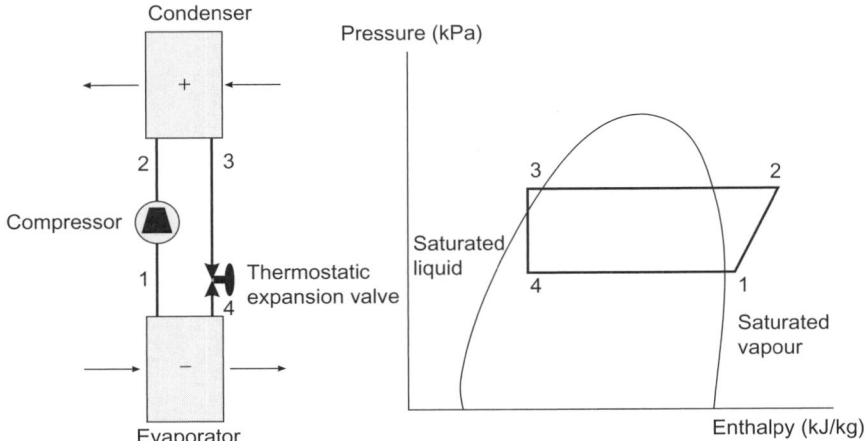

FIG 11.10 Vapour compression heat pump.

The performance of the vapour compression refrigeration cycle is quantified by the *coefficient of performance* (COP), which can be expressed as:

for a refrigeration machine:

$$COP_{ref} = \frac{\text{useful refrigeration output}}{\text{net work input}}$$

for a heat pump:

$$COP_{hp} = \frac{\text{useful heat rejected from cycle}}{\text{net work input}}$$

The COP of the vapour compression cycle is usually expressed in terms of a ratio of enthalpy differences; hence the COP of a refrigeration machine can be expressed as follows (referring to Figure 11.10):

$$COP_{ref} = \frac{h_1 - h_4}{h_2 - h_1} \qquad (11.25)$$

where

$$h = \text{specific enthalpy of refrigerant (kJ/kg)}$$

So, for a heat pump:

$$COP_{hp} = \frac{h_2 - h_3}{h_2 - h_1} \qquad (11.26)$$

From this it can be shown that:

$$COP_{hp} = COP_{ref} + 1$$

(11.27)

For an ideal heat pump the maximum possible COP is given by the Carnot cycle expression:

$$COP_{hp} = \frac{T_c}{T_c - T_e}$$

(11.28)

where T_e is the evaporating absolute temperature (K), and T_c is the condensing absolute temperature (K).

In practice the Carnot COP shown above can never be achieved, but the Carnot equation shows that the greater the difference between T_c and T_e the lower the COP of the heat pump. Heat pumps are therefore well suited to applications where the evaporating and condensing temperatures are close together, which is the case when recovering heat from exhaust air in heating and air-conditioning applications. As a result, heat pumps are often used in air-conditioning applications. They are also popular in applications where there is a need for both dehumidification and heating, such as in warehouses where the occurrence of a high humidity may cause condensation problems and result in the destruction of valuable stock.

Swimming pool buildings are particularly well suited to the application of heat pumps. In swimming pools the air leaving the pool hall is very humid and contains large amounts of latent heat bound up in the water vapour. Heat pumps are particularly well suited to recovering the enthalpy of vaporization from the moisture in the exhaust air. A typical example of the heat pump used in combination with a flat plate recuperator is shown in Figure 11.11. In this application sensible heat is taken from the swimming pool exhaust air by the flat plate recuperator and used to preheat the supply air stream. The evaporator of the heat pump then dehumidifies the exhaust air stream and recovers the latent heat bound up in the water vapour. The heat pump then rejects this heat (plus the 'work' input by the compressor) through the condenser, and thus heats the supply air to the pool.

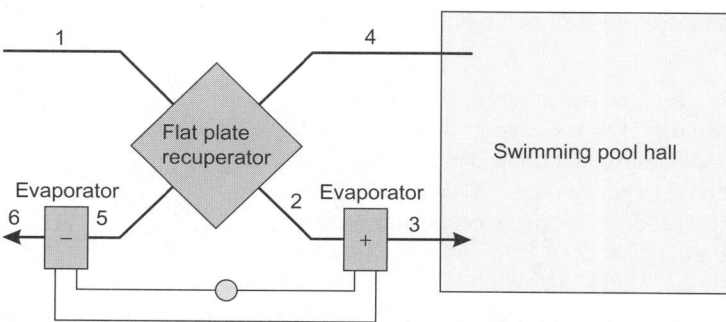

FIG 11.11 Heat recovery system for a swimming pool building.

Example 11.7

The heat pump, shown in Figure 11.11, operates on refrigerant HCFC 22. Given the following data, calculate:

(i) The COP of the heat pump.
(ii) The electrical energy consumed for each kW of heat produced.

Data:

  Condensing temperature = 50°C
  Evaporating temperature = 10°C
  Vapour temperature (leaving compressor) = 80°C
  Liquid temperature (leaving condenser) = 40°C
  Combined electrical and mechanical efficiency of motor = 90%

Solution

Using a pressure enthalpy chart (see Appendix 2), or by using thermodynamic tables for HCFC 22, it is possible to plot the refrigeration process as follows:

(i) Now

$$COP_{hp} = \frac{h_2 - h_3}{h_2 - h_1}$$

$$= \frac{346 - 150}{346 - 315} = 6.323$$

(ii) Electricity consumption per kW of heat produced $= \dfrac{1}{6.323 \times 0.9} = 0.176$ kW

Example 11.8

For the heat pump installation shown in Figure 11.11, calculate:

(i) The heat output of the heat pump.
(ii) The mass flow rate of refrigerant required in the heat pump circuit.
(iii) The power input required to the electric motor.
(iv) The specific enthalpy of the air leaving the evaporator coil.

Data:

  The mass flow rate of supply air = 6 kg/s
  Condition of air leaving pool hall = 29°C and 70% saturation
  Temperature of air supplied to pool hall = 34°C
  Outside air condition = −3°C and 100% saturation
  Effectiveness of flat plate recuperator = 0.7

Solution

Consider first the fresh outside air entering the system and passing through the flat plate recuperator. It enters the system at −3°C and 100% saturation; from a psychrometric chart (see Appendix 3) or from psychrometric tables, it can be determined that the moisture content of the incoming air stream is 0.0029 kg/kg (dry air) and its specific enthalpy is 4.2 kJ/kg.

Now

$$\text{The effectiveness of a flat plate recuperator} = \frac{\text{Heat transferred}}{\text{Max. theoretical heat transferred}}$$

Therefore, for the supply air stream, if the maximum theoretical heat transfer occurred, then it would be heated from $-1°C$ to $29°C$ at a constant moisture content of 0.0029 kg/kg. From a psychrometric chart or tables, the specific enthalpy of air at $29°C$ and 0.0029 kg/kg is 36.6 kJ/kg.

Therefore

The maximum theoretical heat transfer $= 36.6 - 4.2$.

Therefore

$$\text{Effectiveness} = \frac{\text{Heat transferred}}{(37.2 - 4.2)}$$

therefore

$$\text{Heat transferred } (h_2 - h_1) = 0.7\,(36.6 - 4.2) = 22.68 \text{ kJ/kg}$$

therefore

$$h_2 - 4.2 = 22.68 \text{ kJ/kg}$$
$$h_2 = 22.68 + 4.2 = 26.88 \text{ kJ/kg}$$

At a moisture content of 0.0029 kg/kg, h_2 equates to an air temperature of $19.3°C$. The heat pump condenser therefore has to raise the supply air temperature from $19.3°C$ to $34°C$, at which temperature the specific enthalpy is 41.6 kJ/kg.

(i) Therefore

$$Q_{cond} = \dot{m}_{air} \times (h_3 - h_2)$$
$$= 6 \times (41.6 - 26.88) = 88.32 \text{ kW}$$

(ii) From Example 11.7 it can be seen that for the condenser

$$Q_{cond} = \dot{m}_{ref} \times (346 - 150)$$

therefore

$$\dot{m}_{ref} = \frac{88.32}{346 - 150} = 0.451 \text{ kg/s}$$

(iii) Therefore

$$\text{Electric power input to compressor} = \frac{0.451\,(346 - 315)}{0.9} = 15.534 \text{ kW}$$

(iv) Considering now the exhaust air stream through the flat plate recuperator

$$Q_{\text{fpr}} = \dot{m}_{\text{air}} \times (h_2 - h_1) = \dot{m}_{\text{air}} \times (h_4 - h_5)$$

therefore

$$Q_{\text{fpr}} = 6 \times 22.68 = 136.08 \text{ kW}$$

Now, the air leaving the pool hall has a moisture content of 0.018 kg/kg and specific enthalpy (h_4) of 75.1 kJ/kg. Therefore:

$$h_5 = h_4 - \frac{Q_{\text{fpr}}}{\dot{m}_{\text{air}}}$$

therefore

$$h_5 = 75.1 - \frac{136.08}{6} = 52.42 \text{ kJ/kg}$$

and from Example 11.7:

$$Q_{\text{evap}} = 0.451 \times (315 - 150) = 74.415 \text{ kW}$$

and

$$Q_{\text{evap}} = \dot{m}_{\text{air}} \times (h_5 - h_6)$$

therefore

$$h_6 = 52.42 - \frac{74.414}{6} = 40.02 \text{ kJ/kg}$$

Many manufacturers produce machines which have the dual ability to act as both a refrigeration machine and a heat pump. These machines have twin condensers; an air cooled one for normal operation and a water cooled one for the heat pump mode. They are often installed in buildings and act as air-conditioning chillers. When operating in the heat pump mode the waste heat from the condenser is recovered and used to produce the domestic hot water for the building. This at first sight would appear to be a classic energy conservation measure. However, such 'energy-saving' measures should be treated with caution since in order to produce the domestic hot water it may be necessary to raise the condensing pressure considerably, with the result that the COP may be significantly reduced. When it is also considered that the unit price of electricity is usually 3 to 4 times that of gas, then the adoption of such a dual purpose machine may not be quite as advantageous as it appeared originally.

References

[1]　Cornforth JR. Combustion engineering and gas utilisation (Chapter 7). London: E & FN Spon; 1992.
[2]　Eastop TD, Croft DR. Energy efficiency for engineers and technologists (Chapter 5). Harlow: Longman Scientific and Technical; 1990.
[3]　Incropera FP, De Witt DP. Fundamentals of heat and mass transfer (Chapter 11). New York: John Wiley & Sons; 1990.
[4]　Kays WM, London AL. Compact heat exchangers. New York: McGraw-Hill; 1984.

Bibliography

Brookes G. Assessing the scope for heat recovery. In: Energy manager's workbook, 2. Cambridge: Energy Publications; 1985.

Cornforth JR. Combustion engineering and gas utilisation (Chapter 7). London: E & FN Spon; 1992.

Eastop TD, Croft DR. Energy efficiency for engineers and technologists (Chapter 5). Harlow: Longman Scientific and Technical; 1990.

McQuiston FC, Parker JD. Heating, ventilating, and air conditioning (Chapter 14). New York: John Wiley & Sons; 1994.

Ozisik MN. Heat transfer: a basic approach (Chapter 11). New York: McGraw-Hill; 1985.

Stoecker WF, Jones JW. Refrigeration and air conditioning (Chapter 2). 2nd ed. New York: McGraw-Hill; 1982.

Thumann A, Mehta DP. Handbook of energy engineering (Chapter 5). 4th ed. Lilburn, GA :The Fairmont Press (Prentice Hall); 1997.

CHAPTER 12

Combined Heat and Power

This chapter investigates the subject of combined heat and power (CHP). The general nature of CHP systems is discussed and the economic benefits appraised. In particular, CHP plant sizing strategies are evaluated and example design calculations presented.

12.1 The CHP Concept

From an energy point of view, the generation of electricity in thermal power stations is an extremely wasteful process. Most conventional thermal power stations exhibit efficiencies in the range 30–37% [1], while the newer combined cycle gas turbine stations still only achieve efficiencies in the region of 47% [1]. This means that over 50% of the primary energy consumed in the generation process is wasted and not converted into delivered electricity. This wasted energy is converted to heat which is ultimately rejected to the environment. The generation process also liberates considerable amounts of CO_2 into the atmosphere. It has been calculated that in the UK 0.43 kg of CO_2 is liberated for every 1 kWh of electrical energy delivered (2001 data) [2].

One easy way to appreciate the inefficiency of the electricity generation cycle is to consider the theoretical maximum efficiency of the process. The Carnot principle shows that the theoretical maximum thermal efficiency of any heat engine cycle can be determined by:

$$\eta_{carnot} = 1 - \frac{T_2}{T_1}$$

where T_1 is the maximum temperature available (K), and T_2 is the lowest temperature available (K).

For example, if the maximum temperature in a cycle is 1450 K and the cooling water minimum temperature is 285 K, then the maximum possible efficiency of the cycle is:

$$\eta_{carnot} = 1 - \frac{285}{1450} = 0.803 \text{ (or 80.3\%)}$$

The fact that this level of efficiency is not achieved in practice is due to the high degree of irreversibility in the process. Consequently, the efficiencies achieved in power stations are very much lower than the theoretical Carnot efficiency and are dependent on the type of prime mover used.

The low operating efficiencies achieved during the electricity generation process result in a great amount of energy being lost in the form of waste heat. Given the Earth's dwindling energy resources this is not a very satisfactory arrangement. It would be much better to collect the waste heat from the generation process and use it to heat buildings. By combining the *electrical generation* and *heat production* processes it is possible to produce a highly efficient system which makes good use of primary energy. It is the combination of the *electrical generation* and *heat production* processes which is the basis of the CHP, or *cogeneration*, concept. In a typical CHP installation, heat exchangers are used to reclaim waste heat from exhaust gases and other sources during the electricity generation process. In this way it is possible to achieve overall efficiencies in the region of 80%, if a system is correctly optimized [3].

CHP systems vary in size from large 'power stations' serving whole cities to small micro-CHP units serving individual buildings. The larger CHP systems tend to use gas or steam turbines, while smaller systems generally use internal combustion engines converted to run on natural gas. During the electricity generation process, waste heat is recovered from the exhaust gases, or used steam, and, in the case of micro-CHP systems, also from the engine jacket. Large cogeneration systems often use recovered heat to produce hot water for use in district heating schemes, while micro-CHP systems are generally used to heat single buildings.

CHP schemes enable electricity to be generated locally and eliminate much of the wastage of heat which normally occurs in conventional power plants. Through the use of CHP it is possible to:

•   Improve national energy efficiency and preserve non-renewable energy reserves. This is particularly important for nations which have limited fossil fuel resources and which are dependent on imported energy.

- Reduce the cost of transporting electrical energy. The transportation of electricity over long distances involves the construction of expensive transmission networks (consisting of cables, pylons, transformers and switchgear). The need for these is reduced by the use of locally based CHP schemes. Localized CHP schemes also save energy because they avert the need to transport electricity over long distances. There is a 4–8% energy loss during the transportation of electricity over long distances.
- Reduce the amount of atmospheric pollution produced, due to more efficient fuel conversion.

Although CHP has many potential benefits, there are a number of problems associated with it, which have inhibited its widespread use:

- CHP plant requires considerable capital expenditure. This necessitates a full financial appraisal of future energy demands, fuel prices and maintenance costs. Such an appraisal may only be accurate in the short term, with the result that organizations often 'play safe' and rely on conventional systems with which they are familiar.
- There must be a demand for the heat from any proposed CHP plant. Although in most applications it is possible to fully utilize the electricity produced by CHP plant, it is often much more difficult to utilize the heat which is produced. Most building types do not have the all-year-round demand for heat which is required to successfully employ a CHP plant. On the contrary many building types require cooling for large parts of the year.
- Backup plant is often required in CHP installations, in order to ensure security of supply of electricity and heat. This 'backup' plant adds to the capital cost of the installation.

Given the considerable capital expenditure associated with CHP schemes it is essential that any proposed CHP application be carefully evaluated to determine its suitability. It should be remembered with caution that there are many so-called *energy-saving* schemes which have proved to be expensive liabilities.

12.2 CHP System Efficiency

It is possible to illustrate the energy-saving merits of CHP systems by comparing the primary energy consumption of a typical micro-CHP plant with that consumed by a conventional system in which heat is produced in a boiler and electrical power is purchased from a utility company. Example 12.1 presents the energy balance for the two alternative systems.

Example 12.1

A building has an electrical power requirement of 80 kWe (i.e. 80 kW of electrical power) and a heat load of 122 kW. The owners of the building are considering installing a micro-CHP unit which utilizes an internal combustion engine converted to run on natural gas. Compare the primary energy consumption and unit energy costs of the CHP scheme with a conventional separate system.

Data:

> Efficiency of the conventional electricity supply process = 35%
> Efficiency of conventional boiler plant = 70%
> Mechanical efficiency of CHP unit = 32%
> Efficiency of CHP electricity generator = 95%
> Heat recovery efficiency of CHP unit = 68.16%
> Unit cost of gas = 0.9p/kWh
> Unit cost of electricity = 5.0p/kWh

Solution

The two options considered are as follows:

Option 1: Conventional system

$$\text{Primary fuel power input to generate electicity} = \frac{80}{0.35} = 228.6 \text{ kW}$$

and

$$\text{Power input to boilers} = \frac{122}{0.70} = 174.3 \text{ kW}$$

Therefore,

$$\text{Total primary power input} = 228.6 + 174.3 = 402.9 \text{ kW}$$

Therefore,

$$\text{Overall system efficiency} = \frac{80 + 122}{402.9} \times 100 = 50.1\%$$

and

$$\text{Energy cost for 1 hour's operation} = \frac{(80 \times 5.0) + (174.3 \times 0.9)}{100} = £5.57$$

Option 2: CHP system

$$\text{Fuel power input to CHP unit} = \frac{80}{0.32 \times 0.95} = 263.2 \text{ kW}$$

The waste heat produced by the CHP unit is passed through a heat exchanger with an efficiency of 68.16%, therefore:

$$\text{Recoverable heat power} = (263.2 \times (1 - 0.32)) \times 0.6816 = 122.0 \text{ kW}$$

Therefore,

$$\text{Overall system efficiency} = \frac{80 + 122}{263.2} \times 100 = 76.7\%$$

and

$$\text{Energy cost for 1 hour's operation} = (263.2 \times 0.9) = \text{£}2.37$$

Example 12.1 clearly shows that there are large potential energy cost savings to be gained through utilizing CHP in buildings.

12.3 CHP Systems

CHP systems can range from small 'micro' installations, designed to serve the needs of a single building, to large systems which satisfy the heating and electrical power requirements of whole towns. Micro-CHP systems utilizing internal combustion engines tend to be used in applications where electrical demand does not exceed 1 MWe. Gas turbines are popular on larger installations, while steam turbines are often used on the largest schemes.

12.3.1 Internal Combustion Engines

Internal combustion engines are often used to drive small micro-CHP systems. Mechanical power from this type of engine is used to drive a generator and heat is recovered from the engine exhaust, jacket water and lubricating oil. Micro-CHP units typically operate in the range 15 kWe to 1 MWe electrical output. Modified automotive derived engines are the most widely used systems up to 200 kWe electrical output, whereas more rugged stationary industrial engines are generally used for higher outputs [3]. The automotive engines used are generally modified lorry engines, which are converted to run on gas. These engines usually operate at a much slower and constant speed, typically 1500 rpm, than normal automotive engines. The engine life of a typical CHP prime mover is thus considerably longer than that of a typical automotive engine. Spark ignition gas engines tend to exhibit a heat-to-power ratio around 1.7:1 [3], whereas compression ignition diesel engines have heat-to-power ratios nearer 1:1.

12.3.2 Gas Turbines

Where a natural gas supply is available, gas turbines are often used as the prime mover for larger CHP systems. Gas turbines have a relatively low capital cost and are reliable. The peak-load mechanical efficiency of gas turbines is around 30%, which gives an optimum heat-to-power ratio of around 3:1 [4]. However, under part-load conditions efficiency can be substantially reduced. Gas turbines are usually fuelled by natural gas, but oil and pulverized coal have also been successfully employed.

A typical gas turbine CHP arrangement is shown in Figure 12.1. An air compressor, turbine and generator are mounted on a single shaft, with the turbine being the prime

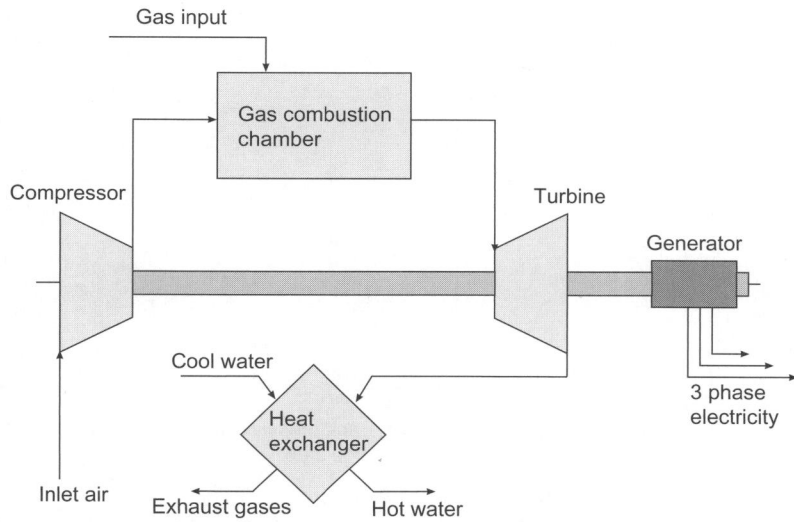

FIG 12.1 Schematic diagram of a gas turbine.

mover. Gas turbines employ an open cycle in which air is drawn into a compressor and compressed to a high pressure before being introduced into a combustion chamber where natural gas is burnt. On leaving the combustion chamber the pressurized combustion gases are forced at temperatures between 900°C and 1200°C [4] through a turbine, which in turn rotates a generator. On exiting the turbine, the hot combustion gases, at 450–550°C [4], pass through a heat exchanger to recover the waste heat.

12.3.3 Steam Turbines

Steam turbines are often used as the prime mover in larger CHP installations. Steam turbines can employ open or closed cycles, depending on whether or not the steam itself is used as the site-heating medium. In the closed system, high-pressure steam from a boiler is forced through a turbine, which in turn rotates a generator. Heat is then recovered from the steam by passing it through a condenser on its way back to the boiler. In open cycle systems the steam exiting the turbine is used directly to meet site-energy needs. The power produced by the steam turbine is therefore dependent on the extent to which the steam pressure is reduced through the turbine. The simplest open cycle arrangement is the *back-pressure* system, which employs a pressure regulator after the turbine, so that the steam is exhausted at the pressure required by the site. As the exhaust steam pressure is raised, so the temperature and heat output increase. However, this increase in heat output is at the expense of the power output, which reduces. By regulating the exhaust steam pressure it is possible to control the heat-to-power ratio of the CHP plant thus creating a very flexible system. Lower steam pressures can be used in the summer when less heat is required, resulting in higher electricity generating efficiencies. In winter when higher temperatures are required, steam pressure can be raised. Consequently, the heat-to-power ratio of steam turbine CHP schemes can be variable, ranging from 3:1 to as much as 12:1 [4].

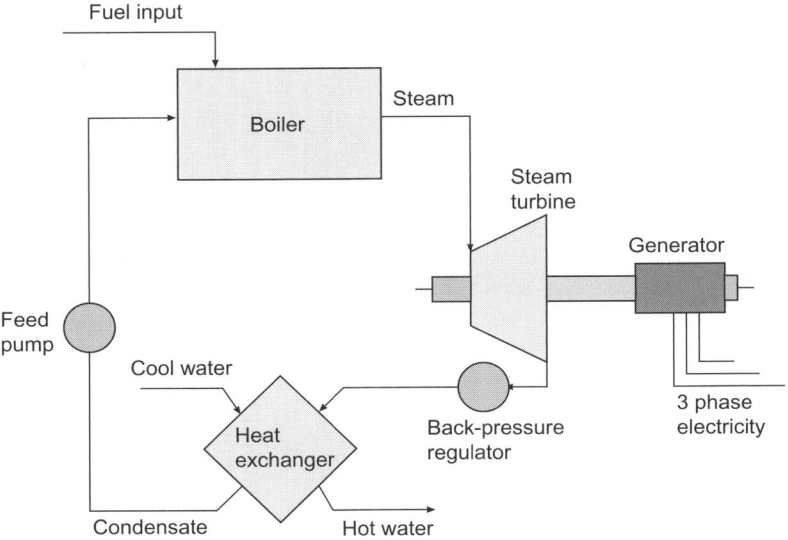

FIG 12.2 Schematic diagram of *back-pressure* steam turbine CHP system.

They are therefore best suited to schemes in which there is a high all-year-round heat requirement. A typical *back-pressure* steam turbine CHP arrangement is shown in Figure 12.2.

Because a boiler is employed to produce the steam to drive a turbine, a wide variety of fuels can be used, including refuse. Therefore, steam turbines are a good solution for *waste-to-energy* CHP schemes in which refuse is incinerated and the heat used to produce steam. In Scandinavia it is common practice to burn the waste products from the timber industry to produce steam in CHP schemes.

12.4 Micro-CHP Systems

Stand-alone micro-CHP units are a popular solution for many small- and medium-sized commercial applications. Micro-CHP units use an internal combustion engine as a prime mover and generally comprise an engine, an electricity generator, a heat recovery system, an exhaust and a control system (as shown in Figure 12.3).

In a micro-CHP system, optimum efficiency is achieved by maximizing the heat recovered from the engine and exhaust gases. In theory as much as 90% of the heat produced by the generation process can be recovered. Achieving this level of heat recovery requires the use of several heat exchangers, which makes the capital cost high. It is therefore more typical to recover around 50% of the fuel input as useful high-grade heat, with a further 10% recovered as low-grade heat [3]. The high-grade heat can be used to provide heating water in the region of 70–90°C and the low-grade heat to provide water at 30–40°C [3]. Most of the heat is recovered from the engine jacket, which has a temperature of approximately 120°C, while the rest is recovered from the

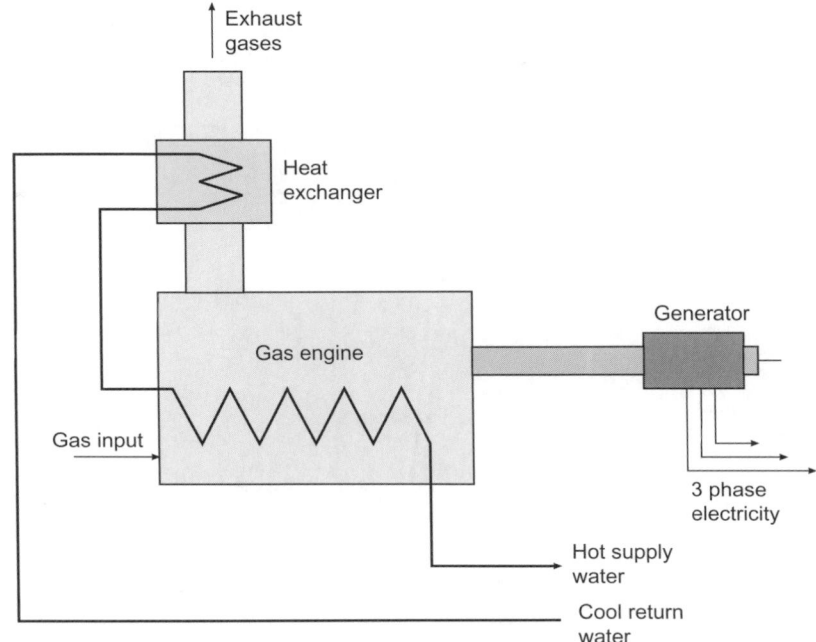

FIG 12.3 Schematic diagram of a micro-CHP unit.

exhaust gases, which can be at 650°C [4]. Both sensible and latent heat can be recovered from the exhaust gases.

Although most micro-CHP units provide low temperature hot water (LTHW) in the region 70–80°C, it is equally possible to provide medium temperature hot water (MTHW) (i.e. 90–120°C).

However, because of the higher water temperatures involved, heat recovery is reduced. Conversely, it is possible to increase heat recovery, and therefore the efficiency of a micro-CHP system, by reducing the hot water supply temperature to below 70°C. As most micro-CHP systems are required to produce domestic hot water (DHW), which must be stored at above 60°C to prevent the growth of *Legionella* spp., in practice the flow water temperature should be 70°C or above.

Micro-CHP units are often used in conjunction with boilers. In such systems the CHP unit should satisfy the base heating load, with the boilers only being used during periods of peak demand. This necessitates coupling the micro-CHP unit to the boilers, so that the two can work effectively together. In existing installations, where a CHP unit is replacing some old boilers, it is common practice to connect the CHP unit and boilers in series as this causes minimum interference to existing systems. In new installations, CHP units are often connected in parallel with boilers. Figure 12.4 illustrates both arrangements. No matter which arrangement, it is essential that the CHP unit operates as the lead 'boiler', as this maximizes its operating hours.

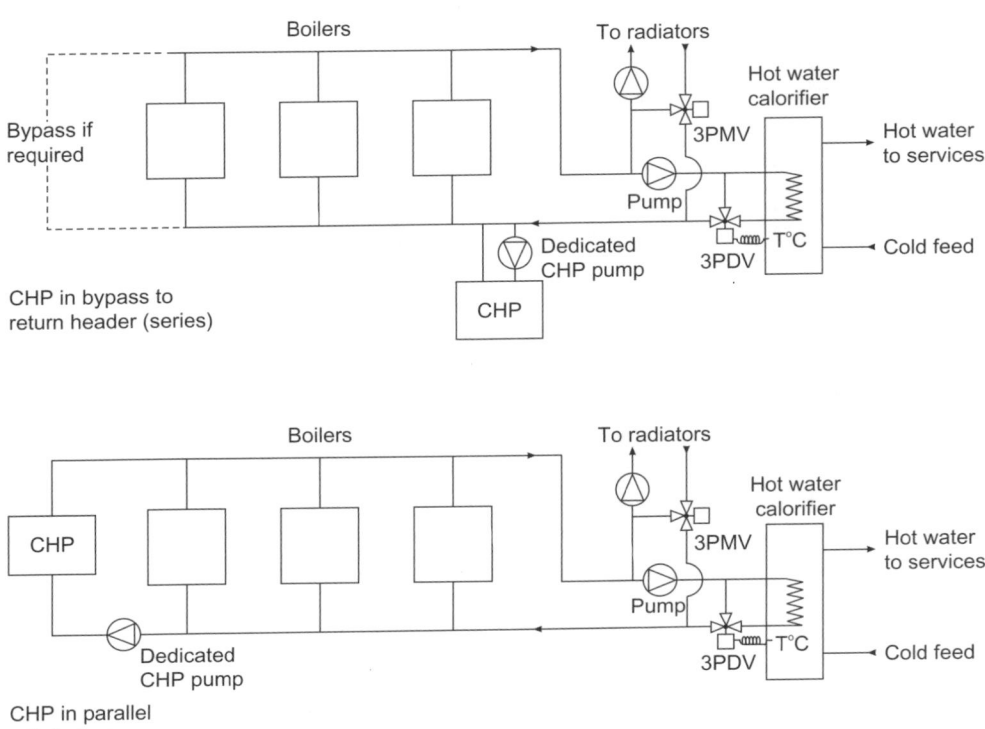

FIG 12.4 CHP piping arrangement. Crown copyright: reproduced with the permission of the Controller of Her Majesty's Stationery Office and the Queen's Printer for Scotland [3].

Many micro-CHP units incorporate a continuous monitoring facility as part of their control system. This enables building heat and power requirements to be monitored so that optimum performance of the plant is achieved. It also enables the system to be audited, so that the return on the capital investment can be calculated.

12.5 District Heating Schemes

Many larger CHP units are coupled to district heating schemes in which the pipework and pumping costs are dominant. In such schemes it is important to minimize both pipe diameters and water flow rates, by operating at a peak-flow water temperature of approximately 120°C, with a return water temperature of 70°C. This reduces both capital and operating costs. It is also common practice to vary supply water temperature with ambient air temperature so that system heat losses are minimized.

If LTHW is required in individual buildings on a district heating scheme, this can be achieved by installing remote heat exchangers in each building. This maintains hydraulic separation between the district heating water and the LTHW and makes the overall system safe and flexible. In Europe, variable temperature district heating schemes with heat exchangers are very popular.

12.6 CHP Applications

CHP systems are considered to be efficient users of primary energy because the waste heat produced by the generation process is utilized to satisfy heating requirements. If 'waste' heat cannot be utilized effectively, overall efficiency will drop dramatically. In simple terms, there is no point in installing a CHP system in an application which does not have an all-year-round demand for heat. CHP systems are therefore suitable for buildings such as leisure centres, swimming pools, hotels, hospitals and residential establishments, all of which have extensive DHW requirements for most or all of the year. Office buildings are generally thought to be unsuitable, since they frequently have a cooling load for much of the year and are only open during the day time. However, if the heat from a CHP unit is used to drive absorption refrigeration plant, then CHP can become a feasible option for office buildings.

Although the operational costs associated with CHP systems are low, the capital costs are high. It is therefore desirable to run a CHP unit for as long as possible in order to achieve the greatest return on the initial capital investment. It has been calculated that in order to achieve a simple payback of 3–4 years it is necessary to operate a CHP unit between 4500 and 6000 hours per year [3], which is equivalent to approximately 12.3–16.5 hours of operation for each day of the year. It is much better to undersize a CHP unit than to oversize it, since this will ensure that the unit runs continuously when in operation, with any shortfall in output being made up by backup boilers and bought-in electricity. It is therefore common practice to use the CHP unit to satisfy base heat load requirements. Ideally a CHP unit should be able to supply the entire summer heat load and a proportion of the winter load. Although it may be relatively small (possibly with a rated output of only 33–50% of the peak heating demand), it is possible to supply 60–90% of a building's annual heat requirement with a CHP unit because it supplies the base heat load.

In certain situations, where a CHP unit generates more electricity than can be consumed on site, it is possible to export power to the local utility company. This depends on the willingness of the utility company to purchase the electricity. It also requires the installation of an export meter. Therefore, for small-scale CHP installations it is not generally considered economic to export electricity. Micro-CHP units should therefore be sized so as not to exceed the base electrical load.

It is possible to use a CHP unit as a standby generator if so required. If used in this way its size will be governed by the required peak emergency electrical load. For normal operation it will be necessary to modulate down the output to match the reduced heat and power requirements, with the result that efficiency will be compromised. In such circumstances it may be more economical to install two smaller CHP units.

12.7 Operating and Capital Costs

The capital and installation costs of CHP plant can be significantly higher than those for conventional boiler plant. One significant cost which can easily be overlooked is the requirement of CHP systems to be synchronized in parallel with the local utility

TABLE 12.1   CHP installation and maintenance costs (1996 data) [5]

CHP engine size (kWe)	Installed capital cost (£/kWe)	Maintenance cost (p/kWhe)
45	1230	1.04
54	1170	1.02
90	1020	0.98
110	960	0.95
167	810	0.89
210	730	0.85
300	660	0.79
384	605	0.73
600	520	0.62

company's distribution grid, so that the grid and the CHP unit can work together to meet peak-site electrical demand. This involves the installation of expensive electrical switching equipment. In contrast to the capital costs, the operating costs associated with CHP are relatively low and comprise the fuel and maintenance costs. For micro-CHP units maintenance costs are generally in the range of 0.5–2.0p per kWhe of electricity generated [3], with the maintenance cost reducing for larger systems. Typical capital and maintenance costs for various-sized CHP units are shown in Table 12.1.

12.8 CHP Plant Sizing Strategies

In order to correctly size a CHP installation it is important to obtain as much accurate energy data as possible for the given application. Ideally these data should include:

- Monthly electricity and heat energy consumption data in kWh.
- Base- and peak-load demands (in kW) for both electricity and heat.
- The operational characteristics of the particular application.
- Unit cost data for electricity and gas (or oil).

Because it is important not to oversize a CHP plant it is advisable to undertake all the possible no-cost and low-cost energy efficiency measures before sizing the plant. This will avoid the CHP unit being oversized and should reduce the capital cost of the installation.

When determining the size of a CHP unit the most commonly used approach is to size the unit to meet the base heating load, as shown in Figure 12.5. This ensures that the CHP unit can run all year round, thus guaranteeing that the payback period on the initial capital investment is short. Backup boilers can then be used to meet the peak-load heating requirements. A CHP unit sized in this way usually generates less electricity than is required to meet the base electrical demand and therefore additional electrical energy must be purchased all year round from the local utility company. An alternative

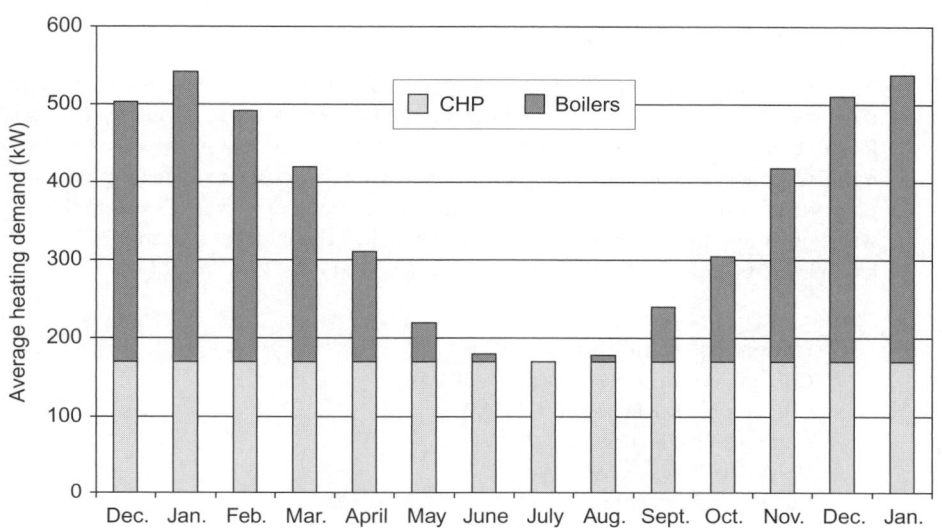

FIG 12.5 Base heat load sizing strategy for CHP plant.

approach is to size the CHP unit to meet the electrical base load. This usually means that for part of the year heat will have to be dumped because the heat produced by the CHP unit will exceed the base-load requirement. However, despite the dumping of heat this can be the most economic solution, since the unit cost of electricity can be as much as five times that of a unit of heat.

12.9 The Economics of CHP

For most of the small-scale CHP applications three factors dominate economic viability. These are:

- The capital cost of the installation.
- The potential number of operating hours per year.
- The relative costs of 'bought-in' electricity and gas (or fuel oil).

If any of these three variables are not favourable, then a particular CHP scheme may become non-viable. Given that fuel prices can be unstable, the last point is of particular importance. For example, if the unit cost of mains electricity should fall or the cost of gas rise, there will come a point when a particular CHP unit ceases to be economically viable. Other lesser factors which may influence the economic performance of a CHP scheme are:

- The heat-to-power ratio of the particular CHP plant.
- The difference in maintenance costs between a CHP scheme and a conventional scheme.
- The cost of having mains electricity as a backup system in case of breakdown or maintenance.

Given these costs, it is important to undertake a full economic appraisal of any proposed CHP scheme. Example 12.2 illustrates how a simple appraisal might be undertaken.

Example 12.2

An existing hotel building has an average electrical demand of 80 kWe and an average combined heating and hot water demand of 180 kW. The average annual load factor for the building is 0.75. The heating and hot water demand is currently served by two gas-fired boilers and mains electricity is bought in. It is proposed to install a micro-CHP plant which will run on gas and have a heat-to-power ratio of 1.7:1. The existing boilers will supplement the heat output from the CHP unit. If the initial cost of the CHP instal-lation is £76,000, determine the simple payback period.

Data:

Efficiency of existing boilers = 70%
CHP unit electric power output = 80 kWe
CHP unit gas power input = 286 kW
Unit price of electricity = 5.0p/kWh
Unit price of gas = 0.9p/kWh
Existing plant maintenance cost = £1000 per year
CHP scheme maintenance cost = £5000 per year

Solution

$$\text{Annual operating hours} = \text{load factor} \times \text{total hours per year}$$
$$= 0.75 \times 8760 = 6570 \text{ hours}$$

Considering the present scheme:

$$\text{Electricity cost} = \frac{80 \times 6570 \times 5.0}{100} = £26,28.00$$

$$\text{Gas cost} = \frac{180 \times 6570 \times 0.9}{0.7 \times 100} = £15,204.86$$

and

$$\text{Maintenance cost} = £1000.00$$

Therefore,

$$\text{Annual cost} = 26,280.00 + 15,204.86 + 1000.00$$
$$= £42,484.86$$

Considering the proposed CHP scheme:

$$\text{The average shortfall in CHP heat production} = 180 - (80 \times 1.7) = 44 \text{ kW}$$

Therefore,

$$\text{Annual CHP unit fuel cost} = \frac{286 \times 6570 \times 0.9}{100} = £16,911.18$$

$$\text{Annual boiler fuel cost} = \frac{44 \times 6570 \times 0.9}{0.7 \times 100} = £3,716.74$$

and

$$\text{Maintenance cost} = £5000.00$$

Therefore,

$$\text{Annual operating cost} = 16,911.18 + 3716.74 + 5000.00 = £25,627.92.$$

Now

$$\text{Payback} = \frac{\text{Capital cost}}{\text{Annual cost saving}}$$

Therefore,

$$\text{Payback} = \frac{76,000}{(42,484.86 - 25,627.92)}$$
$$= 4.51 \, \text{years}$$

While the analysis undertaken in Example 12.2 gives some indication of the economic viability of a CHP scheme, the method used is simplistic and has a number of inherent weaknesses. It assumes that the electrical and heating demands are constant at 80 kWe and 180 kW respectively. In reality this will not be the case. For long periods during the year demand will be higher than this, while at other times it will be lower. This means that during periods of high electrical demand (i.e. when the electrical demand exceeds 80 kWe), electricity will have to be purchased from the local utility company. However, during periods of low demand the CHP unit will be producing electricity and heat which cannot be utilized. As a result the analysis overestimates the potential cost savings achievable through using CHP.

A more sophisticated approach which overcomes some of the shortfalls described above is illustrated in Example 12.3.

Example 12.3

A new sports centre is to be built which will have a predicted annual heat load of 2,600,000 kWh and an annual electrical load of 830,000 kWhe. The peak winter heating and hot water demand is predicted to be 1000 kW and the base heat demand is 350 kW. The base electrical demand is 130 kWe. The sports centre plant will operate for 5130 hours per year. Given the following data, appraise the financial viability of three proposed schemes:

(a) Conventional scheme in which boilers produce all the heat, and electricity is purchased from a utility company.
(b) A CHP scheme in which the CHP plant is sized to meet the base electrical load.
(c) A CHP scheme in which the CHP plant is sized to meet the base heat load.

Data:

Efficiency of boilers = 70%
Mechanical efficiency of CHP unit = 30%
Efficiency of CHP electricity generator = 95%

Heat recovery efficiency of CHP unit = 70%
Unit cost of gas = 0.9p/kWh
Unit cost of electricity = 5.0p/kWh
Cost of maintaining boilers = 0.1p/kWh
CHP scheme maintenance cost = 0.9p/kWhe
Capital cost of boiler only scheme = £26.50 per kW
Capital cost of CHP scheme = £900 per kWe

Solution

(a) *Considering the conventional scheme*:

$$\text{Electricity cost} = \frac{830,000 \times 5.0}{100} = £41,500.00$$

$$\text{Gas cost} = \frac{2,600,000 \times 0.9}{0.7 \times 100} = £33,428.57$$

and

$$\text{Maintenance cost} = \frac{2,600,000 \times 0.1}{100} = £2600.00$$

Therefore

$$\text{Annual cost} = 41,500.00 + 33,428.57 + 2600.00 = £77,528.57$$

and

$$\text{Capital cost} = 26.50 \times 1000 = £26,500.00$$

(b) *Considering the CHP scheme, sized to meet the base electrical load*:

$$\text{Fuel power input to CHP unit} = \frac{130}{0.3 \times 0.95} = 456.14 \text{ kW}$$

The waste heat produced by the CHP unit is passed through a heat exchanger with an efficiency of 70%, therefore:

$$\text{Recoverable heat power} = (456.14 \times (1 - 0.3)) \times 0.70 = 223.51 \text{ kW}$$

Therefore,

$$\text{Annual electricity produced by CHP unit} = 130 \times 5130 = 666,900 \text{ kWhe}$$

and

$$\text{Annual heat produced by CHP unit} = 223.51 \times 5130 = 1,146,606.3 \text{ kWh}$$

Therefore,

$$\text{Annual CHP unit fuel cost} = \frac{454.14 \times 5130 \times 0.9}{100} = £21,059.98$$

$$\text{Annual boiler fuel cost} = \frac{(2,600,000 - 1,146,606.3) \times 0.9}{0.7 \times 100} = £18,686.49$$

$$\text{Annual cost of electricity purchased} \frac{(830,000 - 666,900) \times 5.0}{100} = £8155.00$$

and

$$\text{Maintenance cost} = \frac{0.9 \times 666,900}{100} = £6002.10$$

Therefore,

$$\text{Annual operating cost} = 21,059.98 + 18,686.49 + 8155.00 + 6002.10$$
$$= £53,903.57$$

and

$$\text{Capital cost of CHP scheme} = 900.00 \times 130 = £117,000.00$$

Therefore,

$$\text{Increased capital expenditure compared with scheme (a)} = 117,000.00 - 26,500.00$$
$$= £90,500.00$$

and

$$\text{Annual operating cost saving (compared with scheme (a))} = 77,528.57 - 53,903.57$$
$$= £23,625.00$$

Therefore,

$$\text{Payback on increased capital expenditure} = \frac{90,500.00}{23,625.00} = 3.8 \text{ years}$$

(c) *Considering the CHP scheme, sized to meet the base heat load*:

$$\text{Heat produced for each kWe of electrical power generated} = \frac{223.51}{130} = 1.719$$

Therefore, the heat-to-power ratio of the CHP unit is 1.719:1. Assuming that the CHP unit is sized to meet the base heat load of 350 kW, then:

$$\text{Electrical power output from CHP unit} = \frac{350}{1.719} = 203.61 \text{ kW}$$

Unfortunately, since the average electrical demand of the building is only 161.79 kWe, the CHP unit produces more electricity than can be consumed by the building.

Unless the electricity can be exported to the local utility company, the CHP unit will either have to be reduced in size, or else its output will have to be modulated down considerably.

If it is assumed that electricity can be exported at, say, 3.0p/kWhe, then:

$$\text{Annual revenue generated through exporting electricity} = \frac{(203.61 - 161.79) \times 5130 \times 3.0}{100}$$
$$= £6436.10$$

and

$$\text{Annual heat produced by CHP unit} = 350 \times 5130 = 1,795,500 \text{ kWh}$$
$$\text{Annual electricity produced by CHP unit} = 161.79 \times 5130 = 830,000 \text{ kWhe}$$

NB: The CHP unit provides all the electricity for the building.

$$\text{Fuel power input to CHP unit} = \frac{203.61}{0.3 \times 0.95} = 714.42 \text{ kW}$$

Therefore,

$$\text{Annual CHP unit fuel cost} = \frac{714.42 \times 5130 \times 0.9}{100} = £32,984.77$$
$$\text{Annual boiler fuel cost} = \frac{(2,600,000 - 1,795,500) \times 0.9}{0.7 \times 100} = £10,343.57$$

and

$$\text{Maintenance cost} = \frac{0.9 \times (203.61 \times 5130)}{100} = £9400.67$$

Therefore,

$$\text{Annual operating cost} = 32,984.77 + 10,343.57 + 9400.67 - 6436.10$$
$$= £46,292.91$$

and

$$\text{Capital cost of CHP scheme} = 900.00 \times 203.61 = £183,249.00$$

Therefore,

$$\text{Increased capital expenditure (compared with scheme (a))} = 183,249.00 - 26,500.00$$
$$= £156,749.00$$

and

$$\text{Annual operating cost saving (compared with scheme (a))} = 77,528.57 - 46,292.91$$
$$= £31,235.66$$

Therefore,

$$\text{Payback on increased capital expenditure} = \frac{156,749.00}{31,235.66} = 5.02 \text{ years}$$

Example 12.3 clearly demonstrates that both CHP schemes achieve substantial cost savings compared with the conventional scheme (a). However, it should be noted that although scheme (c), sized to meet the base heat load, produces the greatest annual cost savings, scheme (b) appears to be the more cost-effective of the two proposals. This is because:

- The capital cost of scheme (c) is much higher than that of scheme (b).
- Much of the electricity produced under scheme (c) is underutilized (i.e. exported for a relatively low return).

Example 12.3 therefore reinforces the conclusion that it is unwise to oversize a CHP plant and confirms that it is preferable to size the CHP plant to meet the electrical base load.

References

[1]   Beggs CB. A method for estimating the time-of-day carbon dioxide emissions per kWh of delivered electrical energy in England and Wales. Building Serv Eng Res Technol 1996;17(3):127–34.
[2]   Department of the Environment, Transport and the Regions. Environmental Reporting – Guidelines for Company Reporting on Greenhouse Gas Emissions, www.detr.gov.uk/environment/envrp/gas/05.htm, 8 May; 2001.
[3]   Department of the Environment. Guidance notes for the implementation of small scale packaged combined heat and power. Good Practice Guide 1; 1989.
[4]   Department of the Environment. Introduction to large-scale combined heat and power. Good Practice Guide 43; 1992.
[5]   Williams J, Griffiths T, Knight I. Sizing CHP for new hospitals. Building Serv J 1996;November:41–43.

Bibliography

Cost model: Combined heat and power system analysis. Building Serv J 1997;January:17–19.
Department of the Environment. Guidance notes for the implementation of small scale packaged combined heat and power. Good Practice Guide 1; 1989.
Department of the Environment. Introduction to large-scale combined heat and power. Good Practice Guide 43; 1992.
Eastop TD, Croft DR. Energy efficiency for engineers and technologists (Chapter 8). Harlow: Longman Scientific & Technical; 1990.
Williams J, Griffiths T, Knight I. Sizing CHP for new hospitals. Building Serv J 1996;November:41–43.

CHAPTER 13

Energy Efficient Air Conditioning and Mechanical Ventilation

Much energy is wasted in buildings through the use of inappropriate air-conditioning and mechanical ventilation systems. This situation has arisen because building designers are often ignorant of the issues associated with air conditioning and also because designers of air-conditioning systems are more interested in minimizing first costs rather than reducing overall energy consumption. There are, however, a number of new and innovative technologies, which have the potential to reduce energy consumption greatly. This chapter discusses the issues associated with the design of air-conditioning and mechanical ventilation systems, and introduces some of these new low energy technologies.

13.1 The Impact of Air Conditioning

Over the last 40 years or so, there has been a trend towards large deep plan buildings with highly insulated envelopes. This trend, coupled with the increased use of personal computers and the use of high illumination levels, has meant that many buildings overheat and thus require cooling for large parts of the year, even in countries which experience cool, temperate climates. Over the years boilers have steadily reduced in size and the use of air conditioning and mechanical ventilation has increased. When it is also considered that most of the Earth's population live in countries which have warm or hot climates, it is not difficult to appreciate that the provision of adequate cooling and ventilation is a much greater global issue than the provision of adequate heating. Unfortunately, many building designers are not fully aware of this simple fact, with the result that a great number of poorly designed buildings are erected, relying on large air-conditioning systems in order to maintain a tolerable internal environment.

The contribution of mechanical cooling towards overall global energy consumption should not be underestimated. In the UK alone, it has been estimated that approximately 10,000 GWh of electrical energy is consumed per annum by air-conditioning equipment [1]. This represents approximately 14% of all the electrical energy consumed in the commercial and public administration sectors in the UK. Of this figure, approximately 5853 GWh is consumed solely by refrigeration plant, the rest being consumed by fans, pumps and controls [2]. In the USA, the energy consumed by air-conditioning equipment is much higher. Indeed, in many of the southern states in the USA, electrical demand increases by 30–40% during the summer months solely due to the use of air-conditioning equipment [3]. As a result of this, the utility companies in the southern states of the USA have to install excess generating capacity to meet the summer peak, even though for most of the year this plant remains idle, which is clearly a very uneconomical situation. The problems faced by the electrical utilities in the USA are typical of many companies operating in warm climates throughout the world. In some countries, electrical demand is so high during the summer months that the authorities ration electricity by restricting the capacity of power cables which enter properties. In doing so they force building owners and users to utilize low energy design solutions.

It is a common misconception that most of the energy consumed by air-conditioning plant is associated with the operation of refrigeration machines. This is not the case. In reality much more energy is consumed by air-handling plant. A recent study of typical 'standard' air-conditioned office buildings in the UK found that refrigeration plant consumed 13% of total electricity consumption, while fans, pumps and controls consumed 26.5% of all the electrical energy consumed. In this type of office building approximately 35% of the total energy costs were spent on running the air-conditioning and mechanical ventilation systems [4]. A summary of the results of this study is presented in Table 13.1.

The environmental impact of air-conditioning equipment is considerable. Air conditioning is uniquely catastrophic from an environmental point of view, since it:

- Can contribute directly to atmospheric ozone depletion through the leakage of harmful refrigerants.
- Contributes directly to global warming through the leakage of refrigerants which are powerful greenhouse gases.
- Contributes to global warming by consuming large amounts of electricity and indirectly releases large quantities of CO_2 into the atmosphere.

A full discussion of the environmental problems associated with refrigerants is beyond the scope of this book. Nevertheless, a brief discussion of environmental matters is perhaps relevant here. Until recently, both CFCs and HCFCs were extensively used as refrigerants. Although CFCs and HCFCs are known to be potent greenhouse gases, they are much

TABLE 13.1 Energy consumption in various UK office buildings [4]

	Naturally ventilated cellular		Naturally ventilated open-plan		Air-conditioned standard		Air-conditioned prestige	
	Good practice (kWh/m^2)	Typical (kWh/m^2)	Good practice (kWh/m^2)	Typical (kWh/m^2)	Good practice (kWh/m^2)	Typical (kWh/m^2)	Good practice (kWh/m^2)	Typical (kWh/m^2)
Heating and hot water (gas or oil)	79	151	79	151	97	178	107	201
Mechanical cooling	0	0	1	2	14	31	21	41
Fans, pumps and controls	2	6	4	8	30	60	36	67
Humidification	0	0	0	0	8	18	12	23
Lighting	14	23	22	38	27	54	29	60
Office equipment	12	18	20	27	23	31	23	32
Catering (gas)	0	0	0	0	0	0	7	9
Catering (electricity)	2	3	3	5	5	6	13	15
Other electricity	3	4	4	5	7	8	13	15
Computer room (where applicable)	0	0	0	0	14	18	87	105
Total gas oil	79	151	79	151	97	178	114	210
Total electricity	33	54	54	85	128	226	234	358

more infamous for being potent ozone depletors. Indeed, it was the serious threat to the ozone layer which ended production of CFCs in 1995 under the Montreal Protocol [5]. Since then there has been heavy reliance on the use of HCFC-22 as an alternative to CFCs. While HCFC-22 is far more ozone friendly than CFC-11 or -12, it is still a potent greenhouse gas, having a global warming potential (GWP) of 1700 [6]. However, under the Montreal Protocol, HCFCs are also being phased out, with production due to cease completely by 2030 [7]. Consequently, the chemical manufacturers are currently developing a new generation of refrigerants, HFCs, to replace the old CFCs and HCFCs. Unfortunately, while HFCs are ozone benign they are still strong greenhouse gases. Notwithstanding this, the relative effect which refrigerants have on global warming is often overestimated. The contribution to global warming made by escaping refrigerants is far outweighed by the indirect CO_2 emissions resulting from the electrical consumption of refrigeration machines. This is graphically illustrated by Figure 13.1 which shows the relative contribution to global warming of associated CO_2 emissions compared with that of a variety of refrigerants [8].

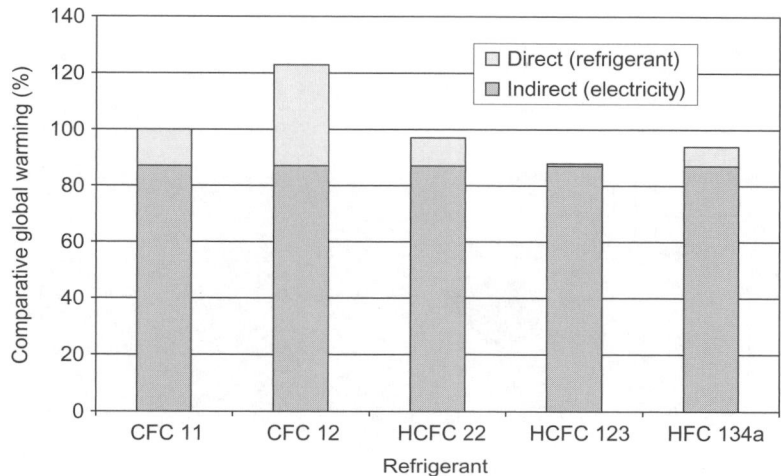

FIG 13.1   Comparison of the direct and indirect contribution of various refrigerant machine types towards global warming [8].

It can be seen from Figure 13.1 that the indirect contribution of air-conditioning equipment towards global warming is considerable. It has been estimated that in the UK alone, 4.2 million tonnes of CO_2 per annum are directly attributable to the use of air-conditioning refrigeration plant [2]. It is therefore not surprising that governments around the world are putting pressure on building designers to reduce or eliminate the need for mechanical cooling.

13.2   Air-Conditioning Systems

This chapter is not intended to be a text on the fundamentals of air-conditioning design, but rather a discussion of the application of air conditioning in buildings. Before discussing in detail the issues which affect the energy consumption of air-conditioning systems, it is necessary first to describe briefly the nature and operation of a generic air-conditioning installation. It should be noted that in this text, for ease of reference, the term *air conditioning* is used in its loosest sense to describe any system which employs refrigeration to cool air in buildings.

Figure 13.2 shows a simple air-conditioning system which illustrates many generic features. The system employs an air-handling unit (AHU) to blow air at a constant volume flow rate through ducts to a room space. Stale air is then removed from the room space via an extract duct using a return fan. In order to save energy, it is common practice to recirculate a large proportion (e.g. 70%) of the return air stream using mixing dampers located in the AHU. It is also common practice to propel air along the ducts at velocities in excess of 5 m/s. This ensures that ductwork sizes are kept to a minimum. Room space temperature is controlled by varying the temperature of the incoming supply air; in winter, air is supplied at a temperature higher than that of the room space, while in summer the air is supplied at a temperature lower than that of the room space.

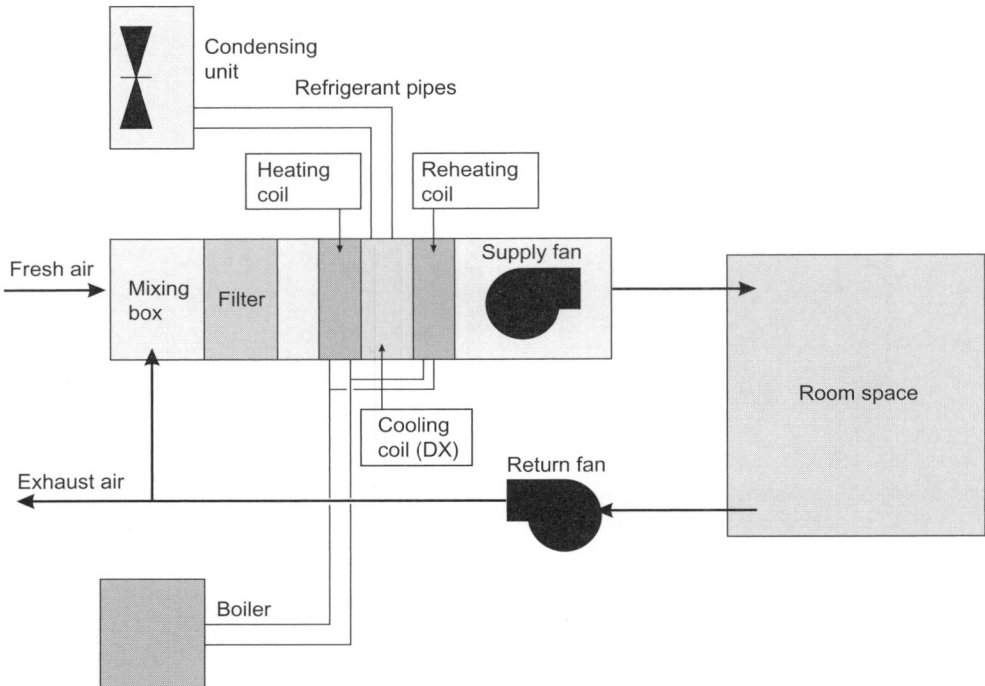

FIG 13.2   A simple ducted air-conditioning system with a direct expansion (DX) cooling coil.

In this way a comfortable environment can be maintained all year round in the room space.

The AHU in Figure 13.2 comprises:

- A mixing damper section to mix the incoming fresh air with recirculated air.
- A filter to clean the air.
- A heating coil (usually a hot water coil fed from a boiler but sometimes electric).
- A cooling coil to cool and dehumidify the air.
- A reheat coil to accurately control the air temperature and to compensate for any over-cooling by the cooling coil.
- A centrifugal fan to draw the air through the AHU and to push it through the ductwork.

In the case of the AHU shown in Figure 13.2, a direct expansion (DX) refrigeration coil is used to cool the supply air. This coil is the evaporator of a refrigeration system and contains liquid refrigerant which boils at a low temperature and pressure (e.g. at 5°C and 584 kPa) to become a low-pressure vapour. As liquid boils it draws large quantities of heat from the air stream and thus cools it. At the other end of the refrigerant pipes to the DX coil, a condensing unit is located which comprises a compressor, a condenser and a fan. The heat taken from the supply air stream by the DX coil is rejected at the condenser to the atmosphere.

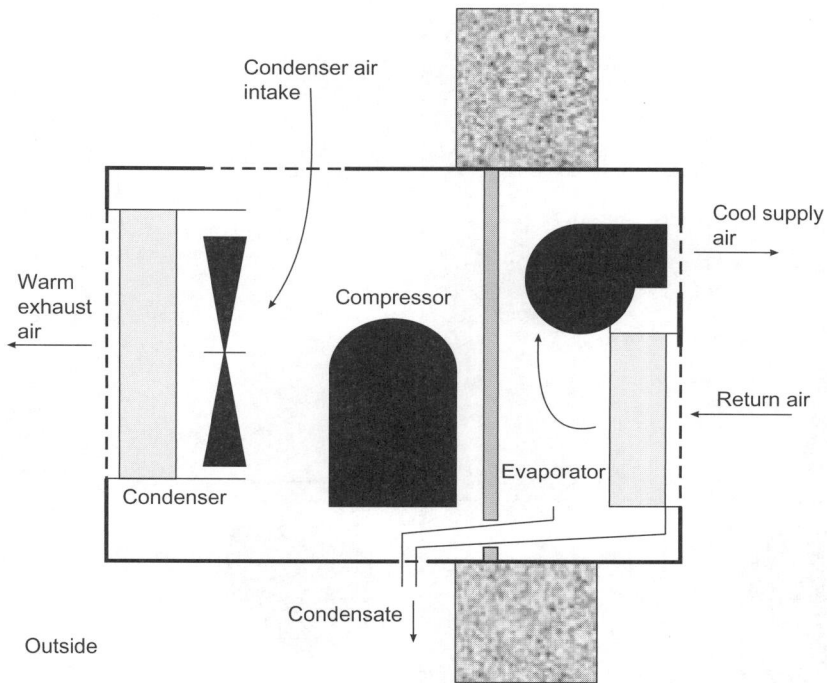

Condenser air intake

Cool supply air

Warm exhaust air

Compressor

Return air

Condenser

Evaporator

Condensate

Outside

FIG 13.3 A through-the-wall air-conditioning unit.

The system shown in Figure 13.2 is generic and is typical of many systems found throughout the world. There are, however, some variations which are worthy of note. In many applications in hot countries there is no requirement for heating, and so the heating coils are removed, leaving only the DX cooling coil. Similarly there may be no requirement to supply fresh air, in which case the filter and mixing dampers can be omitted. Common examples of such simple systems are the 'through-the-wall unit' (see Figure 13.3) and the 'split unit' systems (see Figure 13.4). These systems are inexpensive and easy to maintain, and not surprisingly, are very popular in many hot countries.

One of the major disadvantages of the systems described above is that in larger installations they require many condensing units to be placed on the outside of buildings. This can be both unsightly and impractical. So in many larger buildings, a superior solution is to install a centralized refrigeration machine, known as a chiller, to produce chilled water (e.g. at 7°C) which can then be pumped to a number of remote AHUs (see Figure 13.5). In this type of system, each AHU is fitted with a chilled water cooling coil instead of a DX coil. Chilled water cooling coils are superior to DX coils, because they facilitate closer control of the supply air temperature. Centralized chillers also have an environmental advantage over remote DX systems, insomuch as there are fewer refrigeration circuits to maintain, resulting in lower risk of refrigerant leaks. Chillers can utilize either air- or water-cooled condensers. Water-cooled condensers are more efficient than the air-cooled variety, but usually require a cooling tower, and are therefore a potential *Legionella pneumophila* hazard. For this reason, air-cooled chillers have

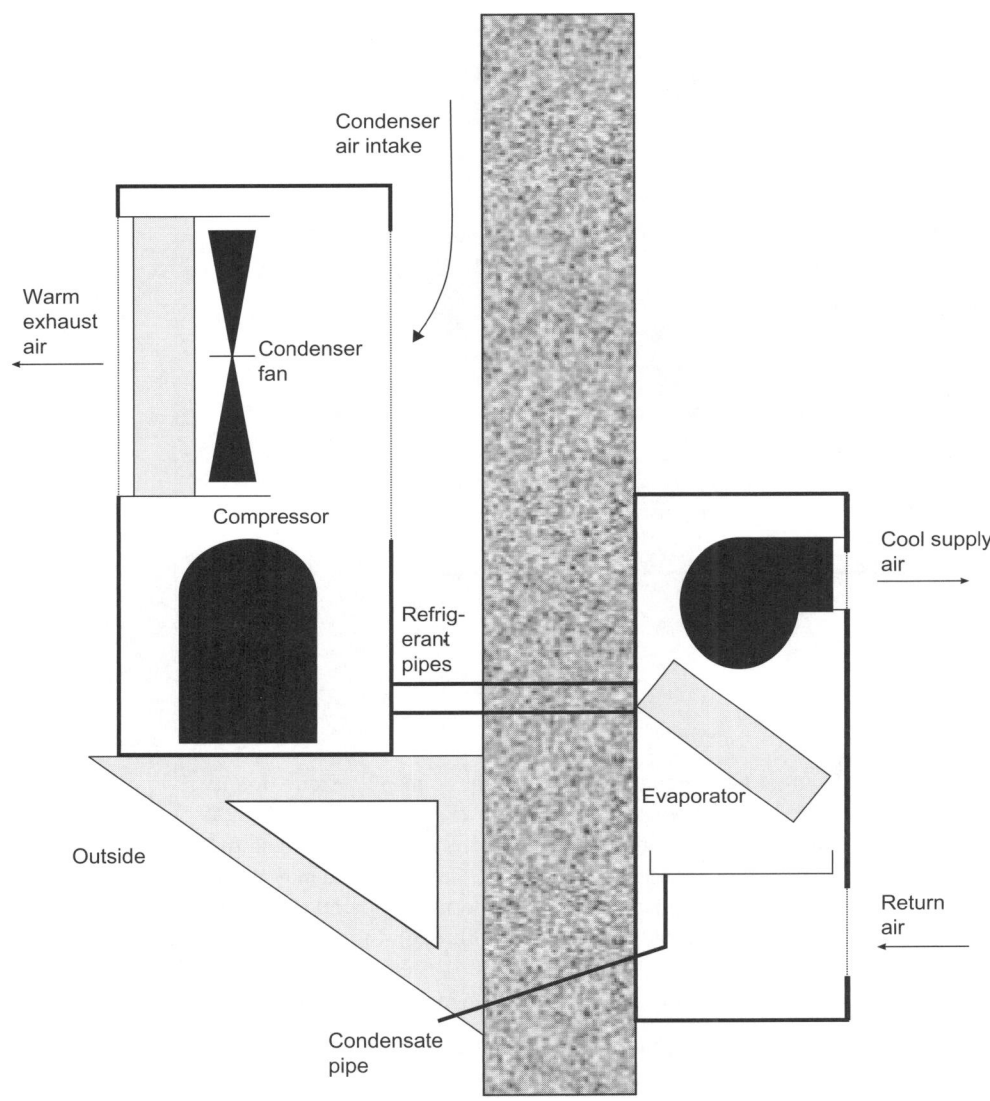

FIG 13.4 A split unit air-conditioning system.

become more popular than water-cooled chillers, because despite being less efficient they present no health hazard.

13.3 Refrigeration Systems

Most air-conditioning plant relies on some form of vapour compression refrigeration machine to remove heat from air. Figure 13.6 shows a schematic diagram of a simple,

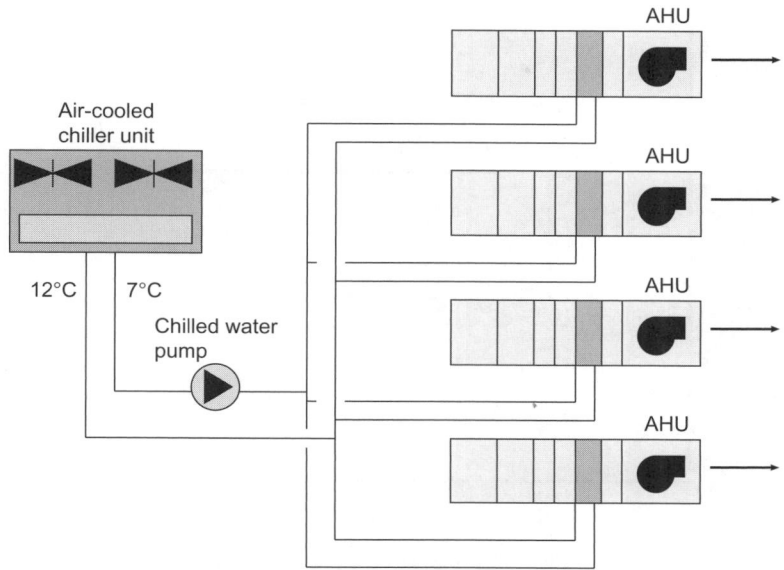

FIG 13.5 An air-cooled chiller system with multiple air-handling units.

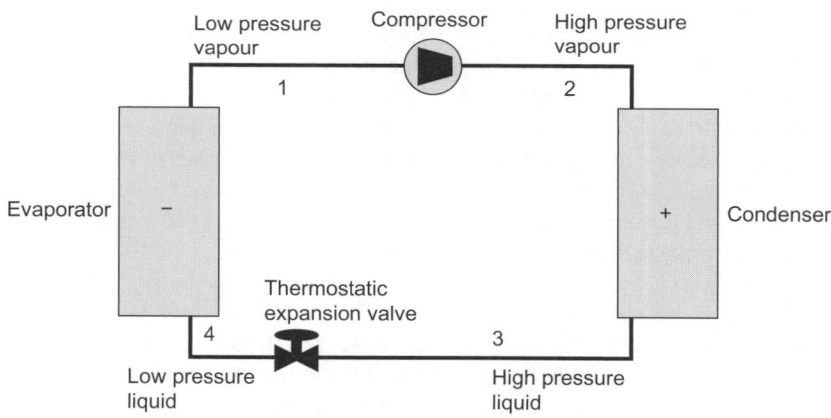

FIG 13.6 Vapour compression refrigeration cycles.

single-stage, vapour compression refrigeration system, similar to that found in many air-conditioning systems.

The vapour compression refrigeration cycle operates as follows:

1. Low-pressure liquid refrigerant in the evaporator boils to produce low-pressure vapour. The heat required to boil and vaporize the liquid within the evaporator is taken from an air or water stream passing over the outside of the evaporator.
2. After leaving the evaporator, the low-pressure refrigerant vapour enters the compressor where both its temperature and its pressure are raised by isentropic compression.

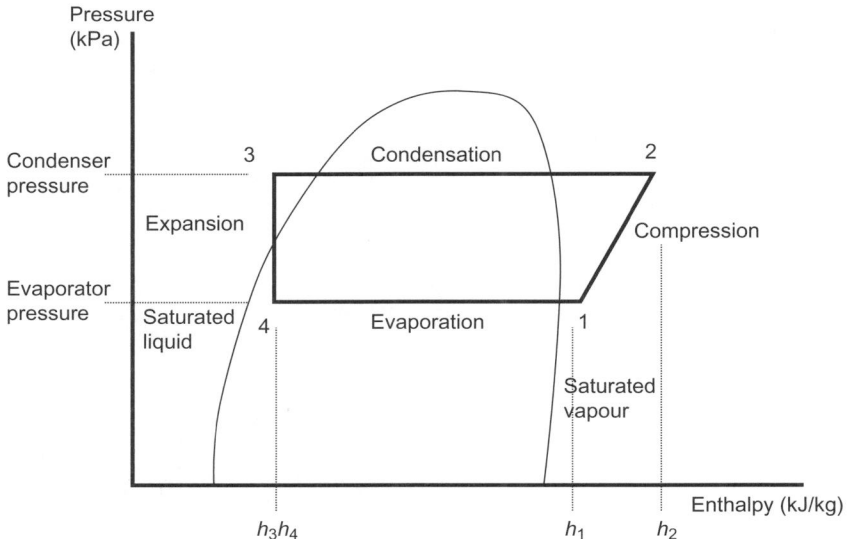

FIG 13.7 Pressure/enthalpy chart of vapour compression process.

3. The high-pressure refrigerant vapour then passes to the condenser where it is cooled and liquefied. The heat extracted in the condenser is released to the environment either directly by forcing air over the outside of the condenser, or indirectly using a secondary fluid, usually water, and a cooling tower.
4. The high-pressure liquid refrigerant then passes from the condenser to the expansion valve, where its pressure is lowered, and approximately 10% of the liquid 'flashes' (i.e. instantly turns from a liquid to a vapour) thus cooling the remainder of the liquid. The cooled low-pressure liquid then flows into the evaporator and the cycle begins all over again.

The boiling point of refrigerants varies with pressure. At low pressures, refrigerants boil at low temperatures (e.g. 2°C), while at much higher pressures the boiling point of the refrigerant is significantly raised (e.g. 35°C). In this way refrigerants can be vaporized and condensed at different temperatures, simply by altering system pressure. Since condensing and evaporating temperatures correspond to particular pressures, they are normally 'measured' using pressure gauges located before and after the compressor.

Figure 13.7 shows a plot of the vapour compression cycle on a pressure/enthalpy diagram. The refrigeration capacity of the system is the amount of cooling which the plant can achieve and is proportional to the length of the line between points 4 and 1. The power input to the system is through the compressor drive, and is represented by the line 1 to 2. Line 2 to 3 represents the heat rejection at the condenser. Line 3 to 4 represents the passage of the refrigerant through the expansion device and is a constant enthalpy process. It should be noted that the heat rejected by the condenser is equal to the total energy input at the evaporator and at the compressor. Note also that as the condensing pressure decreases, so too does the power input from the compressor.

The overall 'efficiency' of a vapour compression machine is normally described by the COP. The COP of a refrigeration machine is the ratio of the refrigeration capacity to the power input at the compressor. It can be expressed as (referring to Figure 13.7):

$$COP_{ref} = \frac{h_1 - h_4}{h_2 - h_1}$$
(13.1)

where h is the specific enthalpy of refrigerant (kJ/kg).

The higher the COP, the more efficient the refrigeration process. In the UK, refrigeration machines generally exhibit COPs in the range of 2.0–3.0 [2].

13.4   The Problems of the Traditional Design Approach

Having briefly discussed the nature of air-conditioning and refrigeration systems, the overall design of 'air-conditioned' buildings must now be considered. It is generally the case that in buildings the air-conditioning design is something of an afterthought. In many buildings the form and the envelope are designed in complete isolation from the mechanical services. Usually, air-conditioning engineers are required to design and install systems which fit unobtrusively into buildings (i.e. behind suspended ceilings); often these systems are required to overcome the environmental shortcomings of poor envelope design.

The traditional approach to air conditioning is to employ a constant volume flow rate system, similar to that described in Section 13.2. However, this design approach has a great many inherent weaknesses, which can loosely be categorized as:

- Weaknesses of the building design.
- Weaknesses of the refrigeration system.
- Weaknesses of the air system.

13.4.1   Building Design Weaknesses

Buildings have to function properly in a great many harsh environments around the world. In hot desert climates they are required to keep their occupants cool, while in polar regions keeping warm is the important issue. Buildings should therefore be designed so that the external envelope is the primary climate modifier, with the internal mechanical services simply fine-tuning the shortcomings of the envelope. This may seem an obvious statement, but clearly it is not one which is fully understood by many building designers. In Texas, which has a hot arid climate, there are many glass-clad office buildings. It would be intolerable to work in these buildings were it not for the use of very large air-conditioning systems to compensate for the inappropriate building envelope. This apparently ludicrous situation comes about for three specific reasons:

1.   Energy efficiency is often a low priority; minimizing the first cost is usually the prime consideration.

2. Design professionals often work in isolation from each other and have little understanding of building physics, or of how buildings function when occupied.
3. There is great incentive to maintain the status quo. Building services design engineers are usually paid a fee which is a fixed proportion of the total capital cost of the building services. Consequently, there is little incentive to reduce the capacity of the mechanical building services.

In order to avoid the creation of energy wasteful buildings, it is important that energy efficiency be at the forefront of the designer's mind. Critical decisions made at the design stage have huge ramifications on both capital and operating costs. If the envelope is a poor climate modifier then the building will experience high summer heat gains and high winter heat losses, necessitating the installation of large boilers and refrigeration chillers. These items of equipment may, however, only operate at peak load for a few hours per year, with the result that for most of the year they operate very inefficiently at part load. Conversely, if the building envelope successfully attenuates the winter and summertime peaks, then the plant sizes can be greatly reduced, resulting in the plant operating near its rated capacity for a much greater part of the year. Clearly, the latter situation is a much better utilization of capital expenditure than the former.

13.4.2 Refrigeration System Weaknesses

The strategy of installing refrigeration plant to meet the peak summertime cooling load of buildings often results in greatly oversized mechanical plant which operates inefficiently, at part load, for most of the year. It can also result in a greatly oversized electrical installation, since larger cables, transformers and switchgear must be installed to meet the peak refrigeration capacity. Not only does a system such as this have a high capital cost, it is also expensive to run since it uses peak-time electricity. In hot countries it may also incur high electrical demand related charges. Refrigeration chillers are often oversized because:

- System designers overestimate peak building heat gains to ensure that plant is not undersized.
- System designers make design assumptions which are widely inaccurate. For example, in most buildings the actual cooling load is much less than the design cooling load. This discrepancy primarily occurs because designers assume very high 'office equipment' heat gains, which in practice rarely materialize.
- Refrigeration chillers are often rated for hot climates such as that found in the USA. So when these machines are installed in a temperate climate location such as in the UK, their condensers are oversized and so they operate at part load even when under peak-load conditions.

The general oversizing of refrigeration machines results in very poor overall energy efficiencies. It has been estimated that of the refrigeration plant currently in operation in the UK, the average air-cooled chiller has a working gross COP of approximately 1.9, while water-cooled chillers exhibit an average gross COP of 3.0 [2]. These low figures are mainly due to the design of most of the refrigeration chillers used in the UK, namely machines which use thermostatic expansion valves and maintain a relatively fixed condensing pressure under part-load conditions. These machines display poor COPs under part-load conditions, which is unfortunate since for most of the year they operate in this state.

There are a number of alternative design strategies which can be used dramatically to reduce the size of refrigeration plant and improve operating costs. These are:

- The use of a solar defensive building envelope, incorporating features such as external shading and solar reflective glass to reduce the peak cooling load.
- The use of a thermally massive structure to absorb both internal and solar heat gains during peak periods.
- The use of night ventilation to purge the building structure of heat accumulated during the daytime.
- The use of ice thermal storage to shift some of the peak-time cooling load to the night-time.
- The use of a floating internal air temperature strategy, which allows internal temperatures to rise when conditions are exceptionally hot.

13.4.3   Air System Weaknesses

The strategy of using an *all-air* system to condition room air has the major disadvantage that it necessitates the transportation of large volumes of air and is thus inherently inefficient. It is generally the case that much larger volumes of supply air are required to sensibly cool room spaces than are required for the purpose of pure ventilation. Consequently, the provision of sensible cooling using an *all-air* system results in large fans and associated air-handling equipment, and also in large ceiling (or floor) voids to accommodate oversized ductwork. Although an expensive solution, resulting in increased energy and capital expenditure, all-air systems are still very popular, despite the existence of superior alternatives which use chilled water to perform the sensible cooling. One such alternative strategy is the use of chilled ceilings to perform sensible cooling, while reserving the ductwork system for ventilation purposes only. This strategy results in greatly reduced fan and ductwork sizes.

Another major drawback of the constant volume approach, described in Section 13.2, is that air duct and fan sizes are determined by the peak summertime condition which may only last for a few hours per year. For the rest of the year the fans push large volumes of air around needlessly, with the result that energy consumption on air handling is large. Many air-conditioning system designers argue that constant volume systems have the potential to provide large amounts of free cooling during the spring and autumn seasons. This unfortunately is a misconception since oversized fans consume such large quantities of electrical energy that any saving in refrigeration energy is wiped out. The evidence for this can be seen in Table 13.1, where in the air-conditioned buildings almost twice as much electrical energy is consumed by air-distribution systems compared with the refrigeration machines. One alternative strategy which overcomes this problem is to adopt a variable air volume system in which the quantity of the air handled reduces with the cooling load.

It is common practice in ducted air systems to size the main ducts assuming air velocities of 4–7 m/s. Designers use these relatively high air velocities in order to keep duct sizes to a minimum. Unfortunately, the use of such high air velocities results in large system resistances.

The fan power consumed in a ducted air system can be determined using eqn (13.2). Fan power,

$$W = \dot{v} \times \Delta P_{total} \tag{13.2}$$

where $\dot{v}$ is the volume flow rate of air discharged by the fan (m³/s), and ΔP_{total} is the total system pressure drop or resistance (Pa).

From eqn (13.2) it can be seen that there is a linear relationship between fan power and system resistance; the higher the system resistance, the higher the energy consumed by the fan. The system resistance is the sum of the system static pressure drop and the velocity pressure drop. The velocity pressure in particular strongly influences the pressure drop across ductwork bends and fittings. From eqn (13.3) it can be seen that the pressure drop across a ductwork fitting is a function of the square of the air velocity.

Pressure drop across ductwork fitting:

$$\Delta P = k \times (0.5\rho v^2) \tag{13.3}$$

where k is the velocity pressure loss factor for fitting, ρ is the density of air (kg/m³), v is the velocity of air (m/s), and $(0.5\ \rho v^2)$ is the velocity pressure (Pa).

Given eqns (13.2) and (13.3) it is not difficult to see that the use of high air velocities (i.e. in the region of 5 m/s) results in high fan powers and high energy consumption. However, if air velocities are reduced to approximately 1–2 m/s, as is the case in some *low energy* buildings, then fan energy consumption falls dramatically.

13.5 Alternative Approaches

The critique of the traditional approach to the design of air-conditioning systems presented in Section 13.4 highlights its many shortcomings and hints at a number of possible solutions. There are several alternative low energy strategies which may be employed to overcome the disadvantages of the conventional approach. Although interlinked, for ease of reference these alternative strategies can loosely be categorized as follows:

- Using passive solar defensive and natural ventilation measures to reduce the need for air conditioning;
- Splitting the sensible cooling and ventilation roles into two separate but complementary systems;
- Using low velocity and variable air volume flow systems;
- Using the thermal mass of buildings to absorb heat which can then be purged by a variety of ventilation techniques;
- Using thermal storage techniques to shift the peak cooling load to the night-time;
- Using displacement ventilation techniques;
- Using evaporative cooling; and
- Using desiccant cooling techniques.

Many of the energy conservation techniques listed above are discussed in detail in this chapter. Some of the techniques which relate specifically to building envelope design are specifically dealt with in Chapter 15.

13.6   Energy Efficient Refrigeration

Although a number of alternative cooling strategies are discussed in this chapter, there are still many applications which demand the use of conventional refrigeration plant. It is therefore necessary to understand the factors which influence the energy consumption of conventional vapour compression refrigeration machines. The major factors influencing energy performance are:

- The evaporating and condensing temperatures used.
- The type of refrigerant used.
- The type of compressor and condenser used.
- The defrost method used on the evaporator.
- The system controls.

Each of these factors can have a profound effect on overall energy consumption and are therefore worthy of further investigation.

13.6.1   Evaporators

The efficiency of vapour compression systems increases as the evaporating temperature increases. Generally, the higher the evaporating temperature used, the greater the system COP and the lower the energy consumption. It has been estimated that a rise in the evaporating temperature of 1°C results in an operating cost reduction of between 2% and 4% [9]. It is therefore desirable to maintain the evaporating temperatures as high as is practically possible. Maximum heat transfer across the evaporator should be achieved in order to prevent the evaporating temperature from dropping. In practice, this can be achieved by increasing the fluid flow across the evaporator, or by increasing its surface area. Also, in order to ensure high evaporating temperatures it is essential that good control of the system be maintained.

On air-cooling applications where the evaporator may be operating below 0°C the fin spacing must allow for ice build-up. In order to maintain an adequate airflow through the evaporator it is necessary to defrost the coil periodically. Defrosting techniques involve either the use of an electric heating element built into the coil or periodically reversing the refrigeration cycle so that the evaporator effectively becomes a hot condenser. While essential for the correct operation of the system, the defrost process can be a potential source of energy wastage. It is therefore important that the defrost operation only be initiated when absolutely necessary and that the defrost heat be evenly distributed over the whole of the fin block. Prolonged defrosting is energy wasteful and therefore the defrost cycle should be stopped as soon as possible. If not controlled and monitored properly defrost systems can needlessly waste large amounts of energy.

13.6.2 Condensers

Condensing temperature can have a dramatic influence on system COP, with lower condensing temperatures usually resulting in lower operating costs. It is estimated that a 1°C drop in condensing temperature reduces operating costs by approximately 2–4% [9]. However, if the condensing pressure fluctuates widely, problems can occur on machines which utilize thermostatic expansion valves. This is because such valves are unable to reliably control refrigerant flow at low pressure differentials. In order to overcome this problem, these machines often employ some form of condenser pressure control to raise the condenser pressure artificially. This results in unnecessarily high energy consumption, which could be avoided if electronic expansion devices were used instead.

There are three basic condenser systems commonly in use: air-cooled condensers, water-cooled condensers and evaporative condensers, each of which has its own peculiarities. Air-cooled condensers are by far the most popular heat rejection system. They generally comprise a fin and tube heat exchanger in which refrigerant vapour condenses. Air is forced over the heat exchanger by fans. Well-designed condensers should operate at a temperature no higher than 14°C above the ambient air temperature [10]. In larger air-cooled systems, condenser pressure is often controlled by switching off or slowing down fans. Although this practice is inefficient it does save on energy consumed by the condenser fans. One important advantage of air-cooled condensers is that they present no *Legionella pneumophila* risk.

Water-cooled condensers are much more compact than their air-cooled counterparts and comprise a shell-containing refrigerant, through which pass water-filled tubes. Secondary cooling water flows through these tubes to a cooling tower where the heat is finally rejected through an evaporative cooling process. In an efficient system, the temperature rise of the water passing through the condenser should be 5°C, with a difference of 5°C existing between the condensing temperature and the temperature of the water leaving the condenser [10].

Water-cooled systems are considerably more efficient than air-cooled systems, with the former requiring a cooling tower airflow rate of approximately 0.04–0.08 m³/s per kW of rejected heat and the latter requiring 0.14–0.2 m³/s to perform the same task [11]. However, there is a risk of *Legionella pneumophila* bacteria breeding in cooling towers, if they are not monitored and regularly treated with biocides. For this reason water-cooled condensers have become less popular in recent years.

Evaporative condensers are less popular than either air- or water-cooled condensers. They comprise refrigerant condensing tubes which are externally wet and over which air is forced. Evaporation of the water on the outside of the tubes increases the heat rejection rate and so this type of condenser is more efficient than its air-cooled counterpart. Evaporative condensers do, however, pose a *Legionella pneumophila* risk.

13.6.3 Compressors

The compressor is the only part of a vapour compression system which consumes energy. It is therefore important that the factors which influence compressor performance are well understood. The efficiency of a compressor can be expressed in several ways. In terms of overall energy consumption the most critical 'efficiency' is isentropic efficiency, which is defined as follows:

$$\text{Isentropic efficiency} = \frac{\text{ideal 'no loss' power input}}{\text{actual power input to shaft}} \times 100 \qquad (13.4)$$

It should be noted that isentropic efficiency does not take into account motor and drive inefficiencies, which must be allowed for when determining the overall efficiency of a compressor. With most types of compressors, particularly screw and centrifugal compressors, efficiencies fall dramatically under part-load operation. Compressor motor efficiency also decreases at part load. In general, therefore, part-load operation should be avoided if high efficiencies are to be maintained.

Part-load operation is the main reason for poor refrigeration plant efficiency. Many refrigeration machines spend less than 20% of the year operating at their nominal design condition. During the rest of the year they operate at part load, partly because of cooler ambient temperatures and partly because of reduced cooling duties. Unless these part-load conditions are properly allowed for at the design stage, it is likely that overall system COP will be poor. It is therefore important to select a compressor which exhibits good part-load efficiency. Multi-cylinder reciprocating compressors achieve reasonable part-load efficiencies because they are able to unload cylinders so that output is reduced in steps (e.g. 75%, 50% and 25%). Variable speed drives can also be used. These give good flexible control and can achieve reasonable efficiencies above 30% of full load [12].

13.6.4   Expansion Devices

In a refrigeration machine the expansion valve is used to reduce the pressure of the returning liquid refrigerant from the condensing pressure to the evaporating pressure. It also controls the flow of liquid refrigerant to the evaporator. It is therefore important that expansion valves be correctly selected and installed, since incorrect operation of the expansion valve can lead to reduced energy efficiency.

Thermostatic expansion valves are the most commonly used type of refrigerant regulation device. They regulate the flow of refrigerant through the system by opening and closing a small orifice using a 'needle' connected to a diaphragm (as shown in Figure 13.8). The diaphragm responds to pressure changes created inside a control phial which senses the temperature of the refrigerant leaving the evaporator. Both the phial and the valve contain refrigerant. As the load on the evaporator changes, so the temperature of the refrigerant leaving the evaporator also changes. The control phial senses these changes in temperature and automatically adjusts the refrigerant flow to accommodate the load changes.

The major disadvantage of thermostatic valves is that they cannot cope with large pressure differentials, such as those created when the condensing pressure is allowed to float with ambient air temperature. Thermostatic expansion valves tend to operate unsatisfactorily at less than 50% of their rated capacity [13]. Therefore, in refrigerating machines using thermostatic expansion valves it is often necessary to maintain an artificially high condensing temperature during conditions of low ambient temperature.

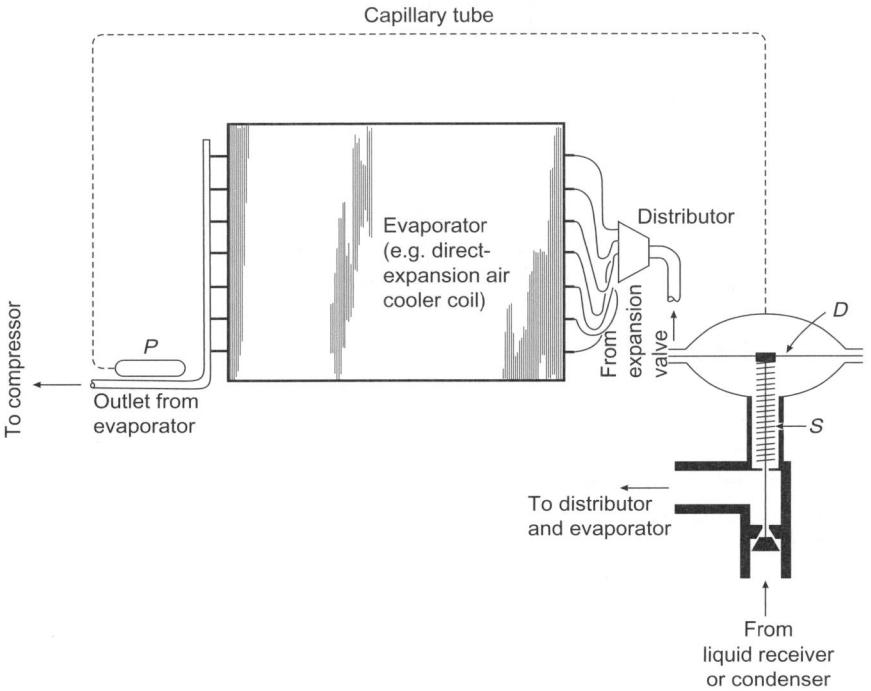

FIG 13.8 Thermostatic expansion device [11].

It can be seen from the discussion in Section 13.6.2 that if the condensing pressure is allowed to fall, the COP increases. Therefore, in theory, system efficiency should improve when ambient air temperature falls. Unfortunately, due to the operational characteristics of thermostatic expansion valves it is not possible to take advantage of this situation. Thermostatic expansion valves are therefore inherently inefficient. In recent years an alternative technology has arisen which overcomes this problem. By using electronic expansion valves it is possible to allow condensing pressures to drop while still maintaining a constant evaporating pressure. Unlike conventional thermostatic expansion valves, which operate on the degree of superheating in the evaporator, electronic expansion valves employ a microprocessor which constantly monitors the position of the valve, the temperature of the liquid in the evaporator, and the temperature of the vapour leaving the evaporator. They can therefore respond quickly to fluctuations in load and are not dependent on large differential pressures between the condenser and the evaporator. Consequently, it is possible under low ambient conditions to allow the condensing pressure to fall and the COP to improve.

13.6.5 Heat Recovery

Vapour compression refrigeration machines are simply a specific form of heat pump. This means that they reject large quantities of waste heat at the condenser. In many applications, through a little careful thought at the design stage, it is possible to utilize this waste heat profitably to reduce energy costs. In refrigeration installations heat can be recovered from:

- The compressor discharge gas, which is generally in the region 70–90°C, but can be as high as 150°C in some installations.
- The condenser, which is generally 10–30°C above ambient temperature.

High-quality waste heat can be recovered from the compressor discharge gas by using a desuperheater heat exchanger. This device recovers heat from the high temperature vapour before it reaches the condenser. At this point in the cycle the vapour is at its highest temperature and therefore the heat transfer is at its greatest. It is important to locate desuperheaters above condensers so that if any refrigerant vapour condenses, the liquid can safely drain away.

Heat may also be recovered at the condenser. However, because condensing temperatures should ideally be as low as possible, any heat recovered here will inevitably be at a relatively low temperature. The quality of this heat should, however, be sufficient to preheat domestic hot water. If higher condensing temperatures are envisaged as a result of any proposed heat recovery scheme, careful analysis should be undertaken to ensure that economic benefit will accrue. Remember, there are many so-called 'energy-saving' schemes in existence which have actually increased energy costs!

13.7   Splitting Sensible Cooling and Ventilation

When considering air conditioning, it is possible to save substantial amounts of energy by splitting up the sensible cooling and ventilation roles into two separate systems. This also enables fan and duct sizes to be greatly reduced. One commonly used method of separating these two roles is to use a fan coil system, which circulates chilled water through water/air heat exchangers (incorporating recirculation fans) located in room-mounted units. Although fan coils function well in many applications, they can take up valuable room space and also be noisy. In addition, they utilize recirculation fans which consume energy. A novel alternative approach is the use of passive chilled ceilings or beams, which comprise a cold surface mounted at high level within a room space. Chilled ceilings and beams perform room's sensible cooling and leave the ducted air system to perform the ventilation and latent cooling roles.

Chilled ceilings have a very slim profile and usually comprise a metal pipe coil bonded to a flat metal plate (as shown in Figure 13.9). They can be fixed directly to the soffit of a structural floor slab, thus eliminating the need for an expensive suspended ceiling. They are usually designed to have an average surface temperature of approximately 17°C, which can be achieved in practice by supplying low-grade chilled water at about 13°C. Because relatively high water temperatures are used it means that chiller evaporating temperatures can be high, resulting in very good refrigeration COPs being achieved.

The cooling power of chilled ceilings varies with the individual design used and the extent to which air turbulence occurs across the heat exchanger surface. In general an

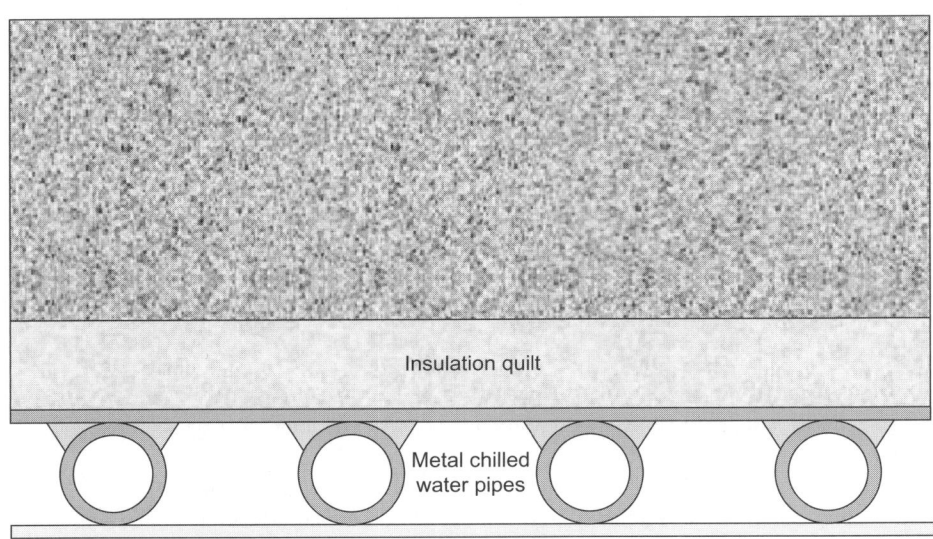

Insulation quilt

Metal chilled water pipes

Metal ceiling tile

FIG 13.9 Typical chilled ceiling.

output of approximately 50 W/m^2 is considered to be the maximum that can be obtained. This means that chilled ceilings are not suitable for applications which experience very high internal heat gains. Heat is transferred to the chilled ceiling by natural convection and radiation. Approximately 50% of the heat transfer occurs when warm air at the top of the room space comes into contact with the cool surface. The remaining heat transfer is by radiation from room occupants and other warm surfaces within the room space.

The radiative cooling capability of chilled ceilings is of particular importance and is worthy of further comment. At relative humidities below 70%, the thermal comfort of building occupants is primarily governed by room air temperature and room surface temperature. In order to assess and quantify relative thermal comfort, a number of thermal comfort indices have been developed. Although these comfort indices vary slightly from each other, they all seek to quantify the convective and radiative heat transfer to and from an occupant within a room space. The most widely used thermal comfort index in the UK is *dry resultant temperature*. Provided room air velocities are less than 0.1 m/s (which is usually the case), dry resultant temperature can be expressed as:

$$t_{res} = 0.5t_a + 0.5t_r \qquad (13.5)$$

where t_r the mean radiant temperature (°C), and t_a is the air temperature (°C).

Mean radiant temperature is the average surface temperature of all the surfaces 'seen' in a room space. It can be either measured indirectly using a globe thermometer or calculated from surface temperatures. For most cuboid-shaped rooms, the mean radiant temperature in the centre of the room can be expressed as:

$$t_r = \frac{\Sigma(A_s \cdot t_s)}{\Sigma A_s} \qquad (13.6)$$

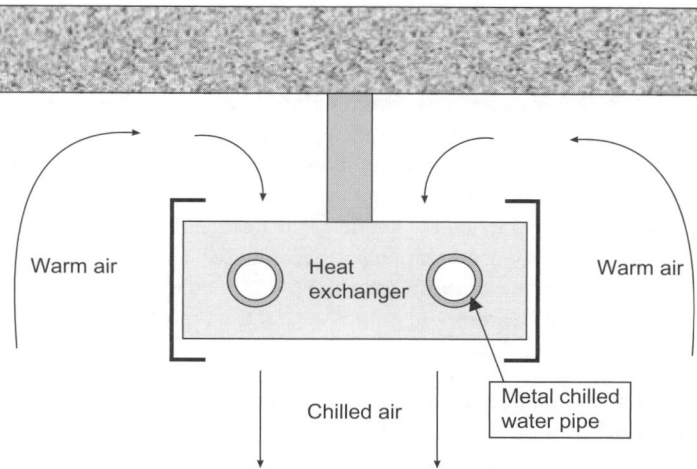

FIG 13.10 Typical chilled beam.

where A_s is the area of each component surface (m²), and t_s is the temperature of each component surface (°C).

By installing a large surface area of chilled ceiling at 17°C, it is possible to substantially reduce room mean radiant temperature. Consequently, air temperatures can be allowed to rise to, say, 23°C or 24°C without any deterioration in perceived comfort, with the result that energy can be saved.

A variation on the chilled ceiling theme is the passive chilled beam system (see Figure 13.10). Passive chilled beams work on a similar principle to chilled ceilings, but they achieve a much greater cooling output (e.g. 185 W/m²) and exhibit a much higher convective cooling component than chilled ceilings (e.g. approximately 85%). However, this can cause problems, since uncomfortable downdraughts can be created.

13.7.1 Ventilation

By utilizing chilled ceilings or beams, it is possible to free up ductwork systems to concentrate solely upon the ventilation and latent cooling tasks. Normally the fresh air requirement of room occupants is in the region 8–12 l/s per person. However, when using chilled ceilings or beams the ducted air ventilation system also has to perform all of the room latent cooling. In order to do this, it is common for the ventilation rate to be increased slightly to 18 l/s per person [14].

With chilled ceilings and beams it is important to ensure that the room air moisture content be maintained at a low level, otherwise condensation may occur on the cool surface and ultimately 'internal rain' may be formed. This makes it important to ensure that the incoming ventilation air is dehumidified, so that the room dew point temperature remains a few degrees below the surface temperature of the chilled ceilings. An ideal air condition for a room incorporating a chilled ceiling is 24°C and 40% relative humidity.

13.8   Fabric Thermal Storage

Although a full discussion of the role of fabric thermal storage is contained in Chapter 15, a few words on the subject are perhaps relevant here. The widespread use of suspended ceilings and carpets in buildings means that otherwise thermally heavyweight structures are converted into thermally lightweight ones. These low-admittance buildings are not able to absorb much heat and so surface temperatures tend to rise, with the result that there is a great need to get rid of the heat gains as they occur. This is one of the main reasons why air conditioning has become such an essential requirement of so many office buildings. By contrast, if the mass of the building structure is exposed, then a high-admittance environment is formed, and the thermal capacity of the structure can be utilized successfully to combat overheating.

The creation of a high-admittance environment by exposing thermal mass has implications on the comfort of occupants. It can be seen from the discussion in Section 13.7 that it is the dry resultant temperature and not the air temperature which is critical when establishing a comfortable environment. By exposing the 'mass' of a building it is possible to reduce the mean radiant temperature within the space, and thus the dry resultant temperature. So if an office building with openable windows and exposed concrete floor soffits has a mean radiant temperature of, for example, 20°C and the air temperature in the space is 28°C, then the perceived temperature (i.e. the dry resultant temperature) in the space will be only 24°C. While an internal air temperature of 28°C is generally considered unacceptable, a dry resultant temperature of 24°C will be perceived as tolerable on hot summer days.

In buildings which employ 'thermal mass' to control internal temperatures, it is common practice to expose concrete floor soffits to create a high-admittance environment, as can be seen in examples such as the Queens Building at De Montfort University [15] and the Elizabeth Fry Building at the University of East Anglia [16]. While it is possible to create a high-admittance environment by exposing concrete floor soffits, the structure needs to be purged periodically of heat absorbed over time, otherwise the mean radiant temperature of the room spaces will steadily rise until conditions become unacceptable. One effective method which can be employed to purge heat from the structure of buildings is night venting. Night venting involves passing cool outside air over or under the exposed surface of a concrete floor slab so that it is purged of the heat accumulated during the daytime. This can be done either by natural or mechanical means. At its most rudimentary, night venting may simply entail the opening of windows at night-time to induce cross-ventilation, while at its most sophisticated it may involve a dedicated mechanical night ventilation system and the use of floor voids.

When creating a night venting scheme it is important to ensure that good thermal coupling occurs between the air and the mass of the concrete floor, whilst at the same time ensuring that fan powers are kept to a minimum. One system which manages to achieve this is the Swedish Termodeck hollow concrete floor slab system (see Chapter 15). The Termodeck system has been used effectively in many locations, throughout northern Europe and in the UK [16,17], to produce buildings which are both thermally stable and energy efficient.

13.9   Ice Thermal Storage

In the exposed concrete soffit system described in Section 13.8, the cooling process is effectively 'load shifted' to the night-time by using a passive thermal storage technique. While this can be very effective, the system is limited to cool, temperate countries where night-time temperatures are low enough to purge accumulated heat. In hotter climates this strategy is impossible and so an alternative approach to load shifting is required. One alternative technology is ice thermal storage, which utilizes low cost night-time electricity to produce a 'cold store' for use during the daytime. The technique involves running refrigeration chillers during 'off-peak' hours to produce an ice store. During the daytime when electricity prices are high, the ice is melted to overcome building or process heat gains. The principal advantages of the system are as follows:

- Refrigeration energy costs can be significantly reduced, as a substantial portion of the cooling is undertaken using off-peak electricity.
- The capital cost of the refrigeration plant can be significantly reduced, if both the chillers and the store combine to satisfy the peak cooling load requirement.
- If an ice store is coupled with a conventional refrigeration plant, then it is possible to run the chiller constantly at 100% of its rated capacity and thus operate it in an efficient manner.
- If an ice store is coupled with an electronically controlled refrigeration plant, then it is possible to minimize the refrigeration energy expended. This is because the refrigeration plant will be running at night-time when ambient temperatures are low and so operating COPs will be high.
- Any electricity maximum demand charges incurred by the system will be significantly lower than those incurred by conventional refrigeration plant.
- By installing additional ice stores it is possible to increase the overall capacity of existing air-conditioning installations without purchasing new chillers or upgrading electrical systems.
- Ice storage systems enable CO_2 emissions to be reduced through load shifting [18] and can also reduce the quantity of refrigerant used.

Ice storage systems are generally associated with air-conditioned commercial or public buildings. However, ice storage systems have also been used successfully in process industries which experience large and predictable cooling loads. In this type of application it is often the case that a relatively small refrigeration machine can, over a long period of time, generate a large ice store. The ice store can then be melted over a relatively short period of time, to satisfy the peak cooling load. In this way small refrigeration machines can be used to satisfy very large cooling loads, with the result large capital savings can be made on refrigeration plant. In addition, capital cost savings can be made on electrical cables and switch gear, which is of particular importance for applications in remote locations.

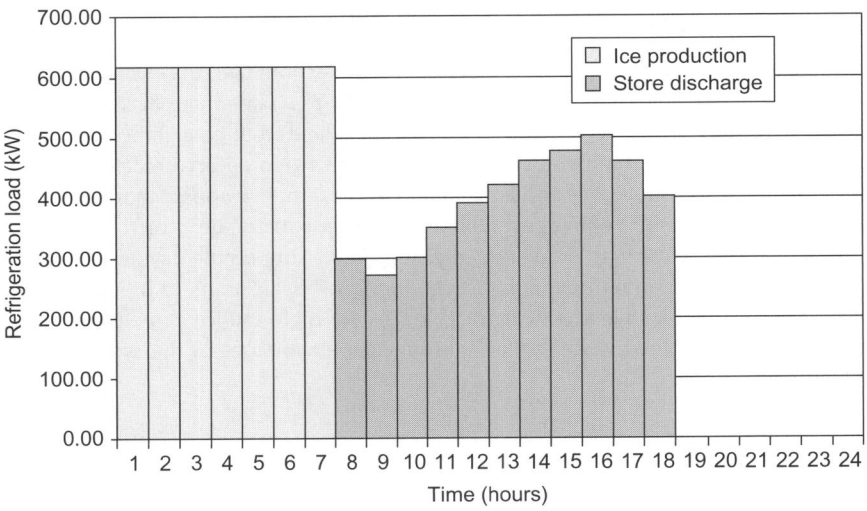

FIG 13.11 Full storage strategy.

13.9.1 Control Strategies

Ice thermal storage systems can be operated in a variety of ways, with the major control strategies being *full storage, partial storage* and *demand-limited storage.*

(a) *Full storage*: Under a *full storage* control strategy the total daytime cooling load is shifted to the night-time, with the chillers producing an ice store during the period when off-peak electricity charges apply. During the daytime the ice store is discharged to meet the building or process cooling load, as shown in Figure 13.11. While being the most effective of all the control strategies in terms of energy costs, *full storage* has the major drawback that the ice store and chiller plant required are much larger than for the other control strategies. Due to its prohibitively high capital cost *full storage* is rarely used.

(b) *Partial storage*: *Partial storage* is the collective term given to those ice storage control strategies which require both the chiller plant and the ice store to operate together to satisfy the daytime cooling load. During periods in which the building or industrial process experiences a cooling load, the ice store and the chiller plant work simultaneously to satisfy the cooling load. The advantage of *partial storage* is that both the store and the chiller plant are substantially smaller than would be the case for a *full storage* installation and thus the capital cost is lower. This makes *partial storage* a very popular option. The umbrella term partial storage can be sub-divided into two separate and distinct sub-strategies, namely *chiller priority* and *store priority*.

Under a *chiller priority* control strategy, the refrigeration plant runs continuously through both the ice production and the store discharge periods. During the daytime the refrigeration plant carries out the base-load cooling and the ice store is used to top up the refrigeration capacity of the chiller plant (see Figure 13.12), which would otherwise be unable to cope with the peak demand.

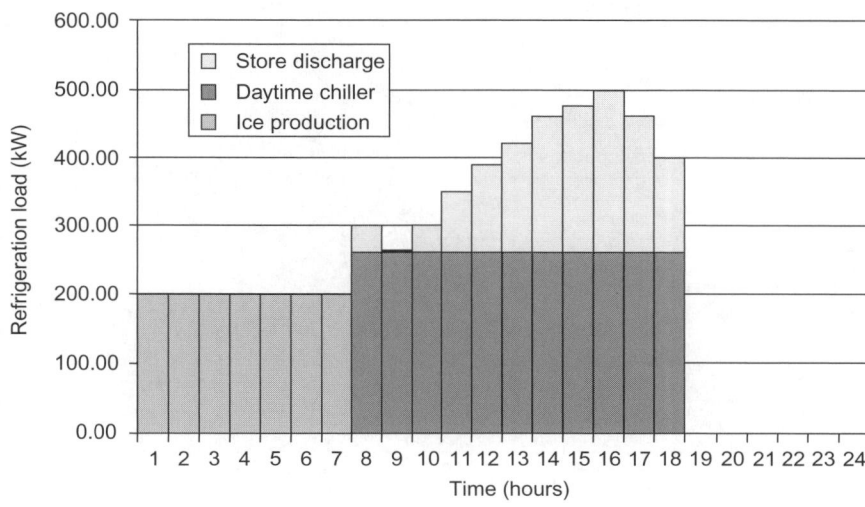

FIG 13.12 Chiller priority strategy.

Under a *chiller priority* strategy it is possible to achieve reductions in the region of 50% in chiller capacity when compared with a conventional refrigeration installation. The capital cost of installing an ice store can therefore be offset against the capital cost saving arising from the reduction in chiller capacity.

The philosophy behind the *store priority* control strategy is the opposite of the *chiller priority* strategy. Under a *store priority* strategy the ice store is given priority over the chiller during the daytime (see Figure 13.13). The objective of this strategy is to minimize the operation of the refrigeration plant during periods when electricity prices are high. The refrigeration chiller is only used to top up the refrigerating energy released by the ice store.

(c) *Demand-limited storage*: The object of a *demand-limited* control strategy is to limit peak electrical demand by shifting the cooling load out of periods in which the peak demand naturally occurs (see Figure 13.14). This greatly reduces the overall maximum demand of the installation and improves the overall load factor of the building, putting the operators in a stronger position when it comes to negotiating electricity supply contracts with the utility companies.

A *demand-limited* control strategy is particularly useful in situations where a utility company offers an electricity tariff which has either high unit charges or high demand charges for part of the daytime (e.g. from 12 am to 6 pm), as is often the case in hot countries during the summertime. Under these circumstances, during the period for which peak charges apply, the cooling load should be entirely satisfied by the refrigeration energy released from the ice store.

13.9.2 Ice Thermal Storage Systems

In broad terms, ice storage systems fall into two main categories, static systems and dynamic systems. Static systems have the general characteristic that ice is melted in the same location as it is generated. Unlike static systems where the ice remains in one

FIG 13.13 Store priority strategy.

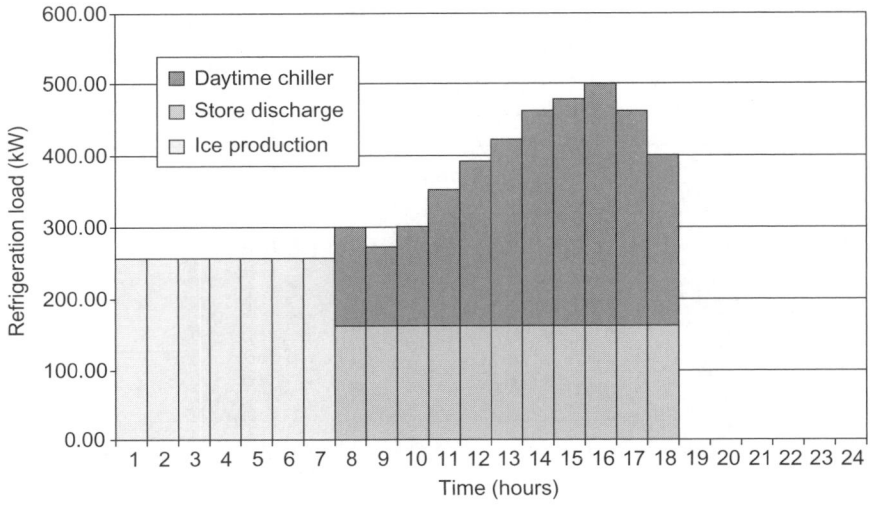

FIG 13.14 Demand-limiting strategy.

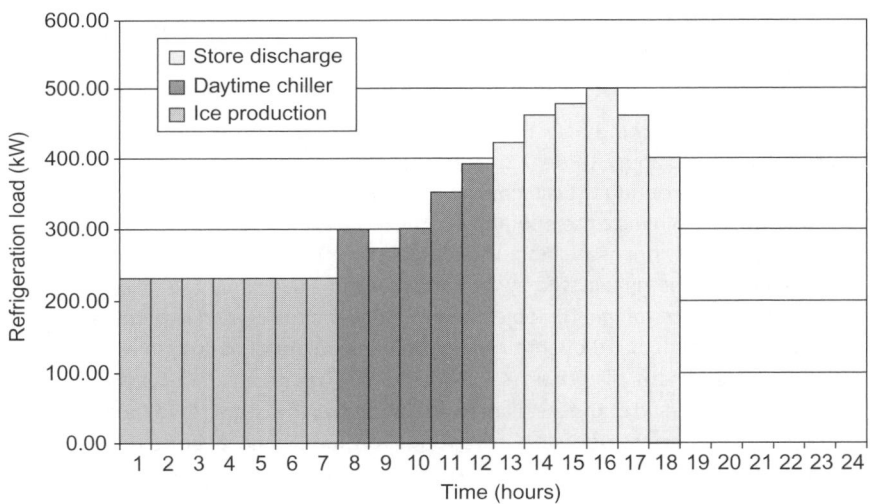

location throughout the entire operation of the installation, in dynamic systems the ice, once formed, is transported by some means to another location where it comes into contact with the working fluid, which is usually water.

The ice bank system shown in Figure 13.15 is typical of a static ice system. It consists of an insulated water storage tank, which contains a submerged bundle of small tubes. These tubes are evenly spaced within the tank volume, often in a spiral or serpentine form. During ice production a glycol/water solution at a sub-zero temperature is circulated through the tubes. This causes the water in the tank to freeze solid. During the discharge cycle, the ice is melted by the same glycol/water solution, this time circulating at a temperature above 0°C.

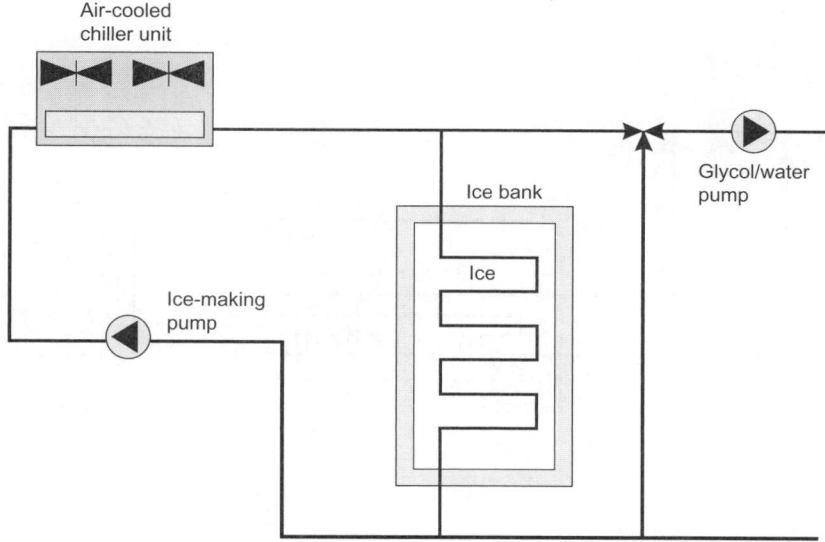

FIG 13.15 Ice bank system.

The most widely used dynamic system is the ice harvester. Ice harvesters have been used in the dairy industry for many years. They consist of an open insulated tank, above which a number of vertical refrigerant evaporator plates are located. Water is trickled over the surface of the plates so that it becomes frozen. Typically, within about 20 minutes an 8–10 mm thick layer of ice can be built up. The ice is harvested by removing it from the evaporator and allowing it to fall into the tank below. This process is achieved by interrupting the flow of liquid refrigerant through the evaporator plates and diverting hot discharge gas through them so that their surface temperature reaches approximately 5°C. A photoelectric switch can be used to stop ice production when the ice in the sump reaches the required level. To discharge the ice store, system water is circulated through the ice sump. A typical ice harvester installation is shown in Figure 13.16.

13.9.3 Sizing of Ice Storage Systems

The design calculations used to size ice storage systems depend on the precise control strategy which is adopted [19]. If a *chiller priority* control strategy is adopted then eqns (13.7)–(13.13) should be used. For a *store priority* strategy eqns (13.14)–(13.16) should be used:

$$Q_{st} + Q_{ch} = Q_j \qquad (13.7)$$

where Q_{st} is the refrigeration energy contained within the ice store (kWh), Q_{ch} is the refrigeration energy produced by chiller plant when operating in the daytime (kWh), and Q_j is the daily cooling load (energy) under design condition (kWh).

Under a *chiller priority* control strategy it is intended that the chiller plant should operate at full capacity throughout the daytime period. However, it is not always possible to

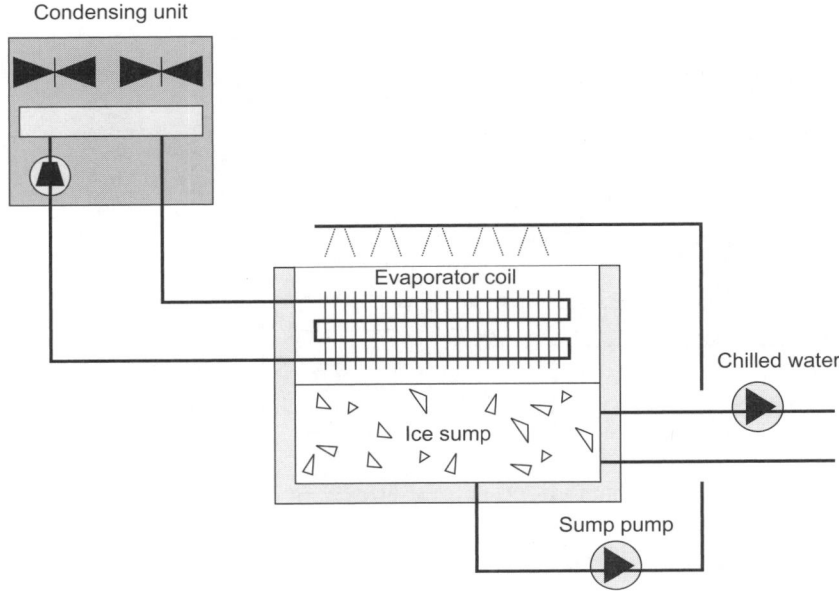

Condensing unit

Evaporator coil

Chilled water

Ice sump

Sump pump

FIG 13.16 Ice harvester system.

achieve this. A chiller plant will often operate at below its rated capacity for part of the daytime. Consequently, eqn (13.7) must be modified to accommodate this:

$$Q_{st} + Q_{ch} = Q_j + Q_u \qquad (13.8)$$

where Q_u is the unused chiller refrigeration energy (kWh).

The evaporating temperatures experienced by the refrigeration plant are much lower during the ice production than those experienced during daytime operation. Consequently, during the store-charging period the chiller plant will experience reduced refrigerating capacity. It can therefore be stated that:

$$Q_{ch} = P_r \cdot H \qquad (13.9)$$

and

$$Q_{st} = P_r \cdot k_r \cdot h \qquad (13.10)$$

where P_r is the rated duty of chiller under daytime operation (kW), k_r is the reduction factor for chiller producing ice, H is the duration of daytime chiller operation (hours), and h is the duration of ice production period (hours).

Therefore

$$Q_{st} + Q_{ch} = P_r \cdot (H + k_r \cdot h) \qquad (13.11)$$

By combining eqns (13.8) and (13.11) it can be shown that:

$$P_r = \frac{Q_j + Q_u}{H + k_r \cdot h} \tag{13.12}$$

By combining eqns (13.8) and (13.9) it can be shown that:

$$Q_{st} = Q_j + Q_u - H \cdot P_r \tag{13.13}$$

In order to derive the plant-sizing equations for a *store priority* control strategy, a slightly different approach is taken to that for the *chiller priority* equations. The concept of peak cooling load (P_m) is introduced. It can therefore be stated that:

$$Q_{st} + H \cdot P_r = H \cdot P_m - Q_v \tag{13.14}$$

where P_m is the peak cooling load experienced by building (kW), and Q_v is the unused ice storage capacity (kWh).

Therefore

$$Q_{st} = H \cdot P_m - Q_v - H \cdot P_r \tag{13.15}$$

By combining eqns (13.10) and (13.14) the following is produced:

$$P_r = \frac{H \cdot P_m - Q_v}{H + k_r \cdot h} \tag{13.16}$$

The process involved in sizing ice thermal storage systems is illustrated in Example 13.1.

Example 13.1

An office building has a peak daily cooling load of 5210 kWh, with a maximum instantaneous cooling duty of 620 kW. Given the following data:

(i) Determine the size of the ice store and chiller plant required for chiller priority, store priority and full storage control strategies, and for a conventional chiller-only system.
(ii) Determine the daily costs for the options outlined in (i) above.
(iii) Determine the system capital costs for the options outlined in (i) above.

Data:
Off-peak electricity period = 00.00–07.00 hours
Peak electricity period = 07.00–24.00 hours
Air-conditioning operation period = 08.00–18.00 hours
Daytime average COP = 3.00
Ice production COP = 2.25
Chiller capacity reduction factor for ice production = 0.75
Peak unit charge = 5.50p/kWh
Off-peak unit charge = 2.57p/kWh

Capital cost of ice storage = 25 £/kWh
Capital cost of refrigeration chiller = 240 £/kW
NB: Assume that there is no unused refrigeration energy or ice store capacity in the process.

Solution

(i) *Conventional chiller-only system*: There is no ice store so the chiller must have a refrigeration capacity of 620 kW.

Full storage control strategy: The chiller is not in operation during the daytime and so the ice store is required to satisfy all the daytime cooling load. Thus a large ice store is required to be built up over the 7-hour off-peak period. Therefore:

$$\text{Ice store capacity} = 5210 \text{ kWh}$$

and

$$\text{Nominal chiller duty} = \frac{5210}{7 \times 0.75} = 992.4 \text{ kW}$$

Chiller priority control strategy: The office air-conditioning system is operational for 10 hours.

Therefore:

$$\text{Nominal chiller duty} = \frac{5210}{10 + (0.75 \times 7)} = 341.6 \text{ kW}$$

and

$$\text{Store capacity} = 5210 - (10 \times 341.6) = 1793.6 \text{ kWh}$$

Store priority control strategy: The peak summertime cooling duty is 620 kW. Therefore:

$$\text{Nominal chiller duty} = \frac{10 \times 620}{10 + (0.75 \times 7)} = 406.6 \text{ kW}$$

and

$$\text{Store capacity} = (10 \times 620) - (10 \times 406.6) = 2134.4 \text{ kWh}$$

(ii) *Conventional chiller-only system*:

$$\text{Daily energy cost} = \frac{5210 \times 5.50}{3.0 \times 100} = £95.52$$

Full storage control strategy:

$$\text{Daily energy cost} = \frac{5210 \times 2.57}{2.25 \times 100} = £59.51$$

Chiller priority control strategy:

$$\text{Daily energy cost} = \frac{1793.6 \times 2.57}{2.25 \times 100} + \frac{(10 \times 341.6) \times 5.50}{3.0 \times 100}$$
$$= \pounds83.11$$

Store priority control strategy:

$$\text{Daily energy cost} = \frac{2134.4 \times 2.57}{2.25 \times 100} + \frac{(5210 - 2134.4) \times 5.50}{3.0 \times 100}$$
$$= \pounds80.77$$

(iii) *Conventional chiller-only system*:

$$\text{Capital cost of installation} = 620 \times 240 = \pounds148,800.00$$

Full storage control strategy:

$$\text{Capital cost of installation} = (992.4 \times 240) + (5210 \times 25) = \pounds368,426.00$$

Chiller priority control strategy:

$$\text{Capital cost of installation} = (341.6 \times 240) + (1793.6 \times 25) = \pounds126,824.00$$

Store priority control strategy:

$$\text{Capital cost of installation} = (406.6 \times 240) + (2134.4 \times 25) = \pounds150,944.00$$

Results summary:

	Conventional chiller-only system	Chiller priority	Store priority	Full storage
Chiller duty	620 kW	341.6 kW	406.6 kW	992.4 kW
Store capacity	n.a.	1793.6 kWh	2134.4 kWh	5210 kWh
Capital cost	£148,800	£126,824	£150,944	£368,426
Peak daily cost	£95.52	£83.11	£80.77	£59.51
Payback period[*]	n.a.	−4.85 years	0.40 years	16.71 years

[*]Indicative payback periods only, since calculated daily costs only apply to the peak summertime day.

From the results shown in Example 13.1 it can be seen that the initial choice of control strategy has a huge impact on the economic viability of any ice storage scheme. Given the inordinately large capital cost associated with *full storage* systems it is not surprising that these systems are rarely installed. The most popular strategy used is the *chiller priority* strategy which, as in the case in Example 13.1, can result in capital cost savings and a negative payback period.

13.10 Evaporative Cooling

So far, most of the cooling techniques discussed in this chapter have utilized the vapour compression refrigeration cycle to perform air cooling. There are, however, a number of alternative technologies, such as evaporative cooling and desiccant cooling, which can be utilized to perform air cooling. Direct evaporative cooling is perhaps the simplest of all the air-cooling techniques and is extremely energy efficient. It relies on an adiabatic heat exchange between air and water in which the air is both sensibly cooled and humidified. Most direct evaporative cooling systems comprise an open porous matrix over which water is trickled and through which air can pass (see Figure 13.17). As air passes over the wetted media, water evaporates and so the air becomes more humid. In order to evaporate, the water needs a 'package' of latent heat energy; this it takes from the air stream, with the result that the air is sensibly cooled. Figure 13.18 shows the evaporative cooling process on a psychrometric chart. It should be noted that the whole process is adiabatic and it follows the line of constant enthalpy on the psychrometric chart, which approximates to the line of constant wet-bulb temperature.

While direct evaporative coolers generally exhibit efficiencies of about 85% [20], their sensible cooling effectiveness depends very much on the dryness of the air entering the cooler. If the air is very dry, then a large amount of sensible cooling will be

FIG 13.17 A direct evaporative cooler.

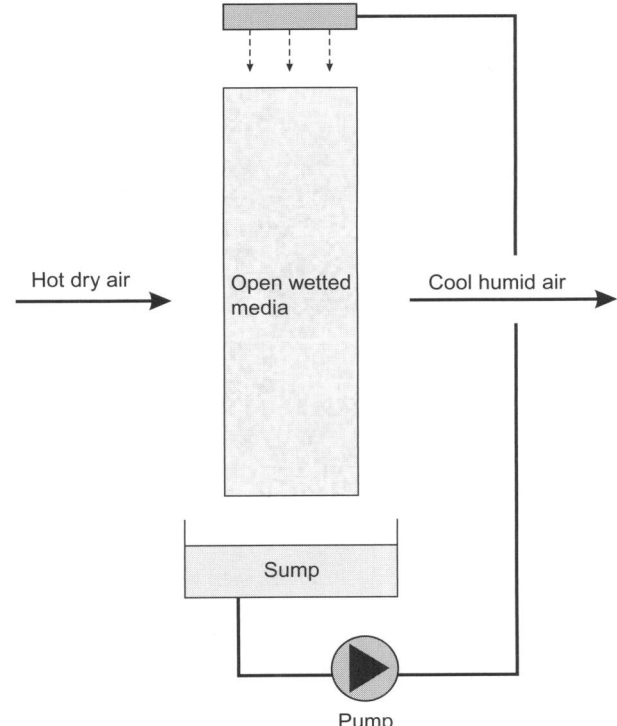

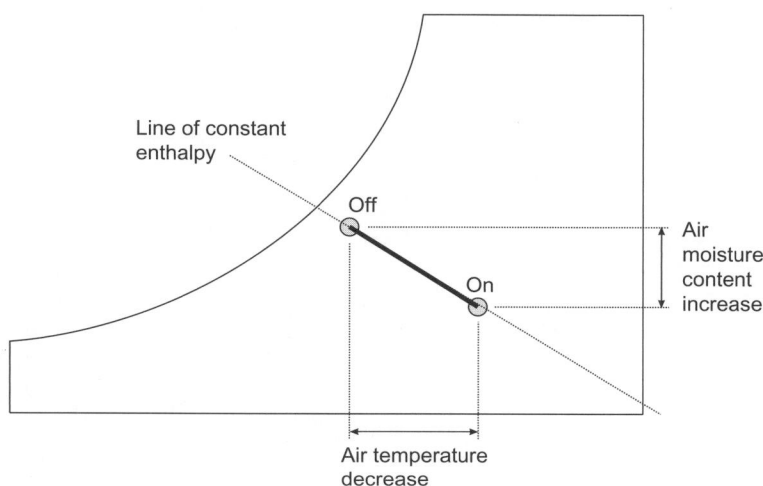

FIG 13.18   The direct evaporative cooling process.

achieved. Conversely, if the air has a high relative humidity, very little sensible cooling will be achieved. Not surprisingly, therefore, evaporative coolers have been used extensively for many years in hot arid countries, where they are often referred to as *desert coolers*. Direct evaporative cooling is very cost-effective and eliminates the need for any environmentally unfriendly refrigerants.

One major disadvantage of direct evaporative cooling is that it greatly raises the relative humidity and moisture content of the air entering the room space, which may ultimately cause discomfort to room occupants. This problem can be overcome by introducing a heat exchanger to create an *indirect* evaporative cooling system. With indirect systems it is standard practice to place an evaporative cooler in the room exhaust air stream coupled to a flat plate heat recuperator. By using this arrangement the cool but humid exhaust air stream can be used to sensibly cool the incoming fresh air supply stream. It should be noted that there is no moisture exchange between the two air streams and so the supply air remains relatively dry. Figure 13.19 shows the indirect evaporative cooling process on a psychrometric chart. Indirect evaporative coolers will usually achieve an effectiveness of at least 60% and can achieve effectiveness ratings as high as 85% [20].

13.11   Desiccant Cooling

Another alternative to the conventional vapour compression refrigeration cycle is to use a heat-driven cycle. It has long been understood that desiccant materials such as silicon can be used to dehumidify air. Such systems pass moist air over surfaces which are coated with a desiccant substance. As the moist air passes across these surfaces the desiccant material absorbs moisture from the air, thus dehumidifying the air stream. In order to drive off the moisture absorbed by the desiccant surface, the desiccant has to

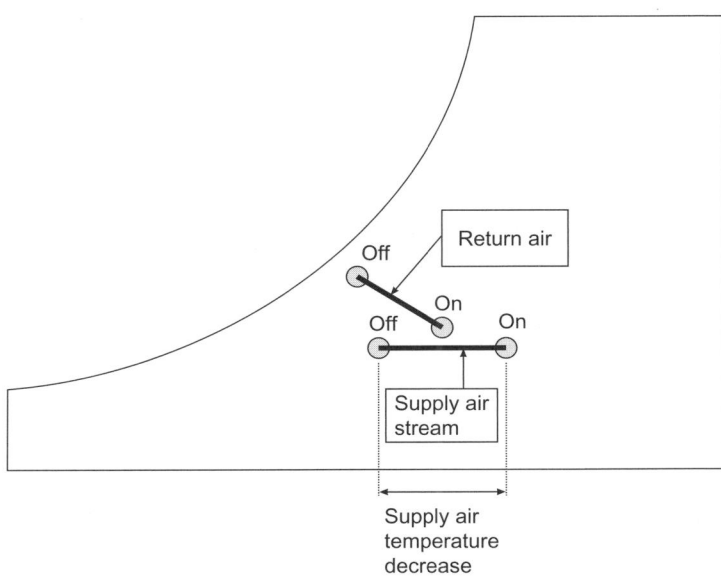

FIG 13.19 The indirect evaporative cooling process.

be physically moved into a hot dry air stream. In the case of the desiccant wheel system (one of the most commonly used desiccant systems) the moisture-laden section of the wheel rotates slowly at approximately 16 revolutions per hour from the moist air stream to the hot dry air stream where it is regenerated.

Recently desiccant cooling systems have been developed which combine a desiccant wheel with a thermal wheel in a single AHU to produce a system which is capable of heating, cooling and dehumidifying air with little or no need for conventional refrigeration [21]. Such systems have the potential to reduce both energy costs and environmental pollution when compared with conventional refrigeration systems. From an environmental point of view the desiccant cooling system has the advantage that electrical energy consumption is replaced by heat consumption, which produces much less CO_2.

A typical desiccant cooling AHU is shown in Figure 13.20. It comprises a thermal wheel and a desiccant wheel located in series. On the supply side, after the thermal wheel, a supplementary cooling coil or an evaporative cooler may be located if so required. A heating coil may also be located after the thermal wheel for use in winter if required. An evaporative cooler is located in the return air stream before the thermal wheel so that the heat transfer across the thermal wheel is increased. The desiccant cycle is an open heat-driven cycle; the 'driver' for the cycle is the regeneration heating coil located in the return air stream after the thermal wheel and before the desiccant wheel.

The psychrometric chart shown in Figure 13.21 illustrates the desiccant cooling and dehumidification process. During the summertime warm moist air at, for example, 26°C and 10.7 g/kg moisture content is drawn through the desiccant wheel so that it comes off at, say, 39°C and 7.3 g/kg moisture content. The psychrometric process line for the air passing

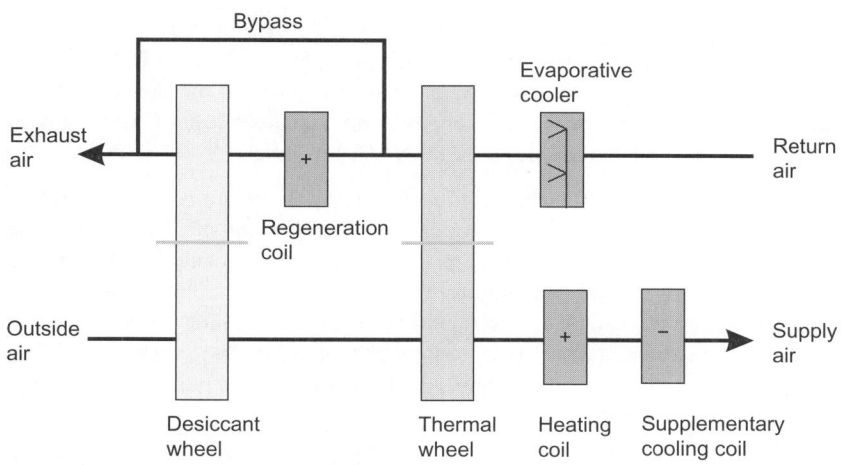

FIG 13.20 A typical desiccant cooling air-handling unit.

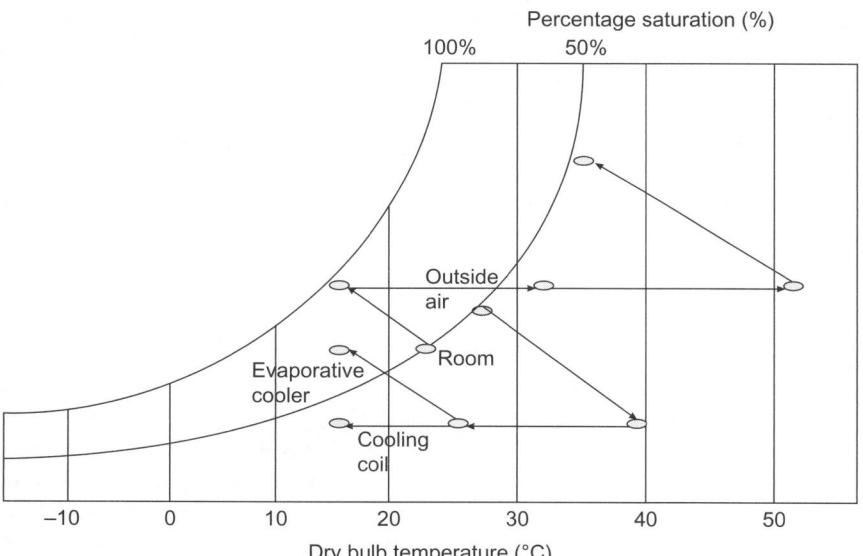

FIG 13.21 Desiccant system in cooling/dehumidification mode.

through the desiccant wheel on the supply side has a gradient approximately equal to that of a wintertime room ratio line of 0.6 on the psychrometric chart. The supply air stream then passes through the thermal wheel where it is sensibly cooled to, say, 23°C. The air then passes through a small DX or chilled water cooling coil where it is sensibly cooled to a supply condition of, say, 17°C and 7.3 g/kg moisture content. It should be noted that if humidity control is not required in the space, then the cooling coil may be replaced by an evaporative cooler with an adiabatic efficiency of approximately 85%, in which case air may be supplied to the room space at, say, 16.2°C and 10.2 g/kg moisture content.

On the return side, air from the room space at, for example, 22°C and 8.6 g/kg moisture content passes through an evaporative cooler so that it enters the thermal wheel at approximately 16.7°C and 10.8 g/kg moisture content. As the return air stream passes through the thermal wheel it is sensibly heated to approximately 33°C. The air stream is then heated up to approximately 55°C in order to regenerate the desiccant coil. It should be noted that in order to save energy, approximately 20% of the return air stream bypasses the regenerating coil and the desiccant wheel.

During the wintertime much of the heat for the supply air stream comes from recovered heat from the thermal wheel. Although the desiccant wheel could in theory be used as an additional heat exchanger, in practice it is not particularly effective due to its low rotational speed, and is therefore not normally used. Should further sensible heating be required this can be achieved either by locating a heating coil in the supply air stream after the thermal wheel, or by using radiators within the room space. In addition, an evaporative cooler on the supply side may be utilized to humidify the incoming air stream if so required.

It has been shown that the use of desiccant cooling can result in energy cost savings ranging from 14% to 50% depending on the application and cooling load [14]. Surprisingly, unlike conventional refrigeration systems, operating costs are at their lowest when desiccant cooling systems are operating under part load [14]. It is also worth noting that desiccant cooling systems are not well suited to applications in which low supply air temperatures are required. Desiccant cooling is best suited to those applications such as displacement ventilation, where supply air temperatures are close to the room air temperature. Although it is possible to make energy cost savings in 'all-air' applications, desiccant cooling systems are best applied to installations in which the bulk of the sensible cooling is performed by a water-based system, such as a chilled ceiling [14].

13.11.1   Solar Application of Desiccant Cooling

Being a heat-driven cycle, desiccant cooling affords an opportunity to utilize heat which might otherwise be wasted. It can therefore be coupled to solar collectors to produce a cooling system which, in theory, should be extremely environmentally friendly. However, the use of solar energy puts constraints on the application of desiccant cooling. For example, if the ratio of solar collectors to building floor area is 1:10, then the available heat (in a northern European application) to power the cycle will be in the region of 25–50 W/m^2, depending on the climate, type and orientation of the solar collectors [22]. Therefore, if this 'solar' heat is to be harnessed effectively, the desiccant cooling system must be applied in the correct fashion. The desiccant cooling cycle is an open cycle and as such it rejects moist air at a high temperature, which is unsuitable for recirculation. In fact, the greater the air volume flow rate supplied to the room space, the greater the fan power required and the heat energy consumed. Therefore, if desiccant cooling is used in an *all-air* application, the regeneration heat load is going to be very large, many times greater than the available solar energy. The bulk of the room's sensible cooling should therefore be carried out using a water-based system such as a chilled ceiling, with the desiccant AHU dehumidifying and 'tempering' the incoming fresh air. This strategy reduces the size of the AHU and its associated ductwork and enables the solar energy to make a significant contribution [22].

References

[1]   Grigg PF, John RW. Building services technologies to reduce greenhouse emissions. In: Proceeding of CIBSE National Conference, Canterbury, April; 1991. p. 231.

[2]   Calder K, Grigg PF. CO_2 impact of refrigeration used for air conditioning. BRE internal report; 1987.

[3]   Wendland RD. Storage to become rule, not exception. ASHRAE J 1987; May.

[4]   Energy use in offices. Energy Consumption Guide 19, Department of the Environment, Transport and the Regions; 1998.

[5]   The accelerated phase-out of class I ozone-depleting substances. United States Environmental Protection Agency; 1999.

[6]   Climate change: Intergovernmental Panel on Climate Change (IPCC) Second Assessment Report; 1995.

[7]   HCFC phase out schedule. United States Environmental Protection Agency; 1998.

[8]   Calm JM. Global warming impacts of chillers. IEA Heat Pump Centre Newsletter 1993;11(3):19–21.

[9]   Industrial refrigeration plant: Energy efficient operation and maintenance. Good Practice Guide 42, Department of the Environment; 1992.

[10] The economic use of refrigeration plant, Fuel Efficiency Booklet 11. Department of the Environment; 1994.

[11] Jones WP. Air conditioning engineering. London: Arnold; 1985.

[12] Energy efficient selection and operation of refrigeration compressors. Good Practice Guide 59, Department of the Environment; 1994.

[13] Dossat RJ. Principles of refrigeration. London: Wiley; 1981. p. 436.

[14] Beggs CB, Warwicker B. Desiccant cooling: Parametric energy study. Building Serv Eng Res Technol 1998;19(2):87–91.

[15] Bunn R. Learning curve. Building Serv J 1993;October:20–25.

[16] Standeven M, Cohen R, Bordass B, Leaman A. PROBE 14: Elizabeth Fry building. Building Serv J 1998;April:37–42.

[17] Bunn R. Cool desking. Building Serv J 1998;October:16–20.

[18] Beggs CB. Ice thermal storage: Impact on UK carbon dioxide emissions. Building Serv Eng Res Technol 1994;15(1):11–17.

[19] Beggs CB, Ward I. Ice storage: design study of the factors affecting installations. Building Serv Eng Res Technol 1992;13(2):49–59.

[20] Evaporative cooling applications. ASHRAE Applications Handbook (Chapter 50). ASHRAE; 1990.

[21] Busweiler U. Air conditioning with a combination of radiant cooling, displacement ventilation, and desiccant cooling. ASHRAE Trans 1993:503–10.

[22] Beggs CB, Halliday S. A theoretical evaluation of solar powered desiccant cooling in the United Kingdom. Building Serv Eng Res Technol 1999;20(3):113–17.

Bibliography

Beggs CB, Ward I. Ice storage: design study of the factors affecting installations. Building Serv Eng Res Technol 1992;13(2):49–59.

Beggs CB. Ice thermal storage: impact on UK carbon dioxide emissions. Building Serv Eng Res Technol 1994;15(1):11–17.

Beggs CB, Warwicker B. Desiccant cooling: parametric energy study. Building Serv Eng Res Technol 1998;19(2):87–91.

Beggs CB, Halliday S. A theoretical evaluation of solar powered desiccant cooling in the United Kingdom. Building Serv Eng Res Technol 1999;20(3):113–17.

Evaporative cooling applications. ASHRAE Applications Handbook (Chapter 50). ASHRAE; 1999.

Jones WP. Air conditioning engineering. London: Arnold; 1985.

Stoeker WF, Jones W. Refrigeration and air conditioning. New York: McGraw Hill; 1982.

CHAPTER 14

Energy Efficient Electrical Services

Much energy is needlessly wasted in buildings through neglect of electrical services. This chapter investigates energy-saving measures which can be applied specifically to electrical services in buildings. In particular, low energy lighting and the use of variable speed motor drives are discussed.

14.1   Introduction

Much energy is needlessly wasted in buildings through poor design and maintenance of electrical services. The energy that is wasted is of the worst kind, namely expensive electrical energy, which can be up to five times as expensive as the unit cost of heat. Unfortunately, excessive electrical energy consumption is all too often overlooked by misguided building designers, who focus on thermal energy consumption, which is relatively inexpensive. It has been shown that in a typical 'standard' air-conditioned office building in the UK, an average of £3.30 per m^2 (of floor area) per annum is spent running pumps and fans, and a further £2.97 per m^2 is spent on the lighting [1]. This compares with an average of only £1.78 per m^2 spent on heating, and £1.71 per m^2 spent on cooling [1]. These figures demonstrate that in the average office building much more money is spent on running fans, pumps and electric lighting than is spent on operating boilers or refrigeration plant. Yet there are a number of relatively simple technologies that can be applied to motor drives and luminaire installations to dramatically reduce energy costs. That energy costs in these areas can be greatly reduced is clear from the evidence of the UK office building study, which found that in *good practice* standard air-conditioned office buildings, only £1.65 per m^2 per year is spent running the pumps and fans, and only £1.48 per m^2 is spent on the lighting [1]. This equates in each case to energy cost reductions of about 50% when compared with typical air-conditioned office buildings.

14.2   Power Factor

Electric induction motors and fluorescent lamp fittings are classic examples of reactive (i.e. inductive) electrical loads. Reactive electrical loads are important because, unlike resistive loads such as incandescent light, they cause the current to become out of phase with the voltage (see Figure 14.1). This, in simple terms, means that items of equipment which are inductive in nature draw a larger current than would be anticipated by their useful power rating. Ultimately, it is the consumer who has to pay for this additional current.

The electrical power consumed by a resistive load can be determined by:

$$W = V \times 1 \tag{14.1}$$

where W is the power (W), V is the voltage (V), and I is the current (A).

Equation (14.1) defines the useful power consumed and applies to all types of resistive load where the current is in phase with the voltage. However, eqn (14.1) does not hold true for reactive loads, where the current lags behind the voltage, since reactive loads consume more power than can be usefully used. A reactive load, such as an induction motor, will therefore draw a larger current than would be anticipated by its useful

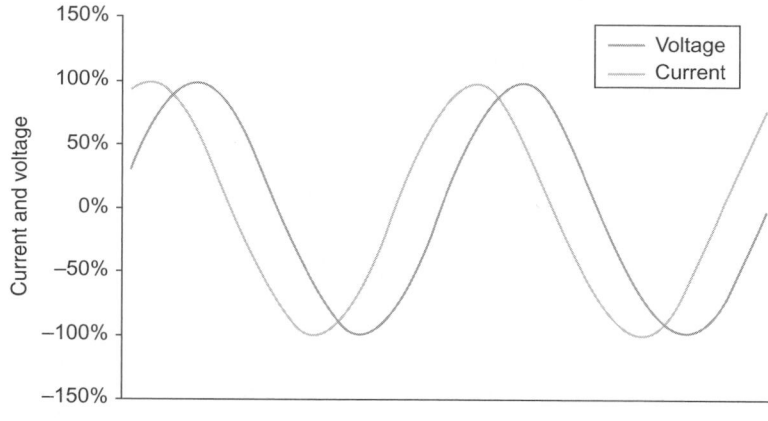

FIG 14.1 The effect of an inductive load on an electrical current and voltage.

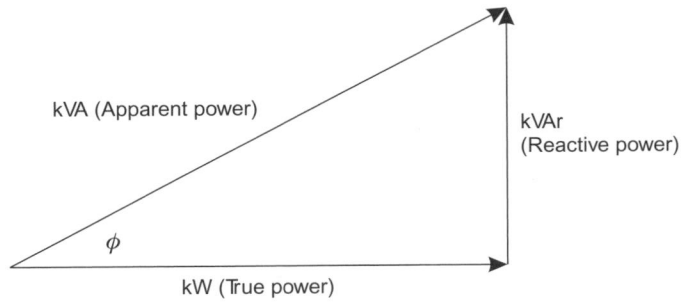

FIG 14.2 The relationship between kW, kVA and kVAr.

power rating. The reactive components of the load consume what is termed *reactive power*. In order to determine the apparent power consumed by a reactive load, the true power must be added vectorially to the reactive power, as shown in Figure 14.2.

It should be noted from Figure 14.2 that the reactive power is drawn at right angles to the true power. The apparent power is therefore a function of the true power consumed and the reactive power, and can be expressed as:

$$\text{Apparent power} = \frac{\text{True power}}{\cos\phi} \qquad (14.2)$$

where $\cos\phi$ is the power factor.

From Figure 14.2 and eqn (14.2) it is evident that when the current and voltage are in phase with each other (i.e. a resistive load), the apparent power is the same as the true power. When the two are out of phase (i.e. a reactive load) the apparent power consumed is always going to be greater than the true power. In order to differentiate between true and apparent power, true power is measured in watts (W) or kilowatts (kW), and apparent power is measured in volt amps (VA) or kilovolt amps (kVA). Similarly, reactive power is measured in volt amps reactive (VAr) or kilovolt amps reactive (kVAr). The ratio of true power to apparent power is known as the *power factor*. For a pure resistive load the power factor would be 1, and for a pure inductor the power factor would be 0:

$$\text{Power factor} = \frac{\text{True power}}{\text{Apparent power}} \qquad (14.3)$$

14.2.1 Effects of a Poor Power Factor

In many buildings and other installations the overall electrical load is heavily influenced by the presence of reactive loads such as induction motors and fluorescent tubes which create a lagging power factor. As a result, power factors of 0.7 or less are often experienced. Example 14.1 illustrates the impact of such a poor power factor.

Example 14.1

A 240V single-phase electric motor has a true power of 1.8 kW and exhibits a power factor of 0.7. Determine:

 (i)   The current required to drive the motor.
 (ii) The current required if the power factor was 1.

Solution

$$\text{True power (W)} = \text{Apparent power (VA)} \times \text{Power factor}$$

Therefore

$$\text{Current} = \frac{\text{Watts}}{\text{Volts} \times \text{Power factor}}$$

$$\text{(i) Current} = \frac{1800}{240 \times 0.7} = 10.71 \text{ A}$$

$$\text{(ii) Current} = \frac{1800}{240 \times 1} = 7.5 \text{ A}$$

Example 14.1 demonstrates that the lower the power factor, the greater the current required to provide the same useful power. The increased current required as a result of a poor power factor has the knock-on effect of increasing power losses. Because cables and other items of equipment have an electrical resistance, power is lost as heat when a current flows. The power (or I^2R) loss can be expressed as:

$$\text{Power loss} = I^2 \times R \qquad\qquad (14.4)$$

where I is the current (A), and R is the resistance (Ω).

It can be seen that for a circuit with a constant resistance, the greater the current, the greater the I^2R losses. In addition to increased currents and increased I^2R losses, a poor power factor has the knock-on effect that switchgear, cables and transformers all have to be increased in size. Example 14.2 illustrates this fact.

Example 14.2

A building is served by a 415V (line-to-line) three phase supply and has a true power load of 210 kW and a power factor of 0.7. Compare the installation with a similar one having a power factor of 1.

Solution

$$\text{Total current} = \frac{210,000}{415 \times 0.7 \times \sqrt{3}} \times 417.4 \text{ A}$$

If however, if the power factor was 1, then

$$\text{Total current} = \frac{210,000}{415 \times 1 \times \sqrt{3}} = 292.2 \text{ A}$$

TABLE 14.1   Impact of poor power factor

	Power factor = 0.7	Power factor = 1
Total current	417.4 A	292.2 A
Apparent power (kVA)	300 kVA	210 kVA
Switchgear rating	450 A	350 A
Transformer rating	400 kVA	300 kVA
Cable size	240 mm^2	150 mm^2

The impact of this reduction in current is shown in Table 14.1.

Examples 14.1 and 14.2 show that the lower the power factor the greater the current drawn and the greater the size of the infrastructure required. Therefore, if a consumer has a poor power factor the electricity utility company has to supply more 'electricity' than will be recorded as 'true power' in kW at the electricity meter. This means that the utility company will not be paid in full for all the electricity which it is supplying to the consumer. Utility companies overcome this problem by adopting one of two strategies:

Strategy 1: Installing meters and offering tariffs which record electricity consumption in kVA and not in kW.

Strategy 2: Using meters and tariffs which record electricity consumption in kW and levy an additional charge for the number of reactive power units (kVAr) consumed.

By using either approach a utility company can ensure that it receives the correct revenue for the electrical energy it supplies.

14.2.2   Power Factor Correction

The simplest way to correct a poor power factor is to minimize the problem in the first place. In many applications a poor power factor occurs as a result of the use of induction motors. Induction motors are commonplace in buildings and are used to drive fans and pumps. As such they are a necessity and cannot be avoided. The power factor of induction motors varies with the motor loading. Motors which may have a power factor of 0.8 at full load may have a power factor approaching 0.1 at low load, with the result that almost 90% of the total current drawn is reactive in nature [2]. Motors should therefore be selected with care, since an under-loaded large motor will exhibit a low power factor. The power factors exhibited by smaller motors are not as good as those of larger motors. Despite this, it is usually better to select a smaller motor than use an under-loaded large motor to perform the same job.

It is possible to correct a poor power factor by installing capacitors. The effect of capacitors on an alternating current is the opposite to that of a reactive load. They cause the current to lead the voltage. By installing capacitors into an electrical circuit it is possible to counteract the effect of any reactive load and correct a poor power factor. Power factor correcting capacitors can either be installed in a central bank before the main distribution panel, or mounted on individual items of equipment. It is generally considered better to correct the power factor for reactive loads at the item of equipment itself. This reduces the current drawn by the item of equipment and thus reduces the

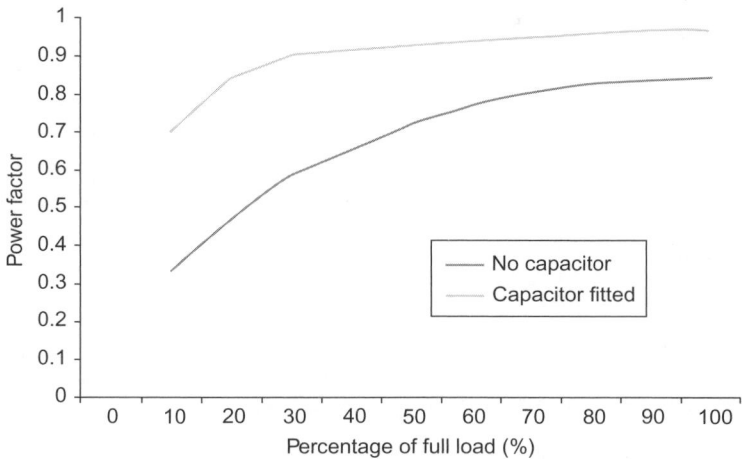

FIG 14.3 Impact of power factor correction on induction motors [2].

I^2R losses in all the wiring leading to the item of equipment. By fitting capacitors to an induction motor it is possible to greatly improve its power factor. An example of this is shown in Figure 14.3, where the introduction of capacitors results in the power factor being virtually constant with all loads over 50% of full load [2].

In large installations it may be more cost-effective to install a central bank of capacitors to correct power factor. It is possible to use banks of capacitors which automatically switch on and off in order to maintain an optimum power factor.

14.3   Electric Motors

Induction motors are widely used in many applications. Pumps, fans, compressors, escalators and lifts are all powered by motors of one type or another. Induction motors are therefore essential to the operation of most modern buildings. Furthermore, electric motors are often the most costly items of plant to run in many office buildings. It is therefore well worth understanding how induction motors use electrical energy and investigating possible energy-conservation measures.

All induction motors have inherent inefficiencies. These energy losses include [3]:

- Iron losses which are associated with the magnetic field created by the motor. They are voltage related and therefore constant for any given motor and independent of load.
- Copper losses (or I^2R losses) which are created by the resistance of the copper wires in the motor. The greater the resistance of the coil, the more heat is generated and the greater the power loss. These losses are proportional to the square of the load current.
- Friction losses which are constant for a given speed and independent of load.

These losses can be divided into those which vary with motor load and those which are constant whatever the load. When a motor is running at full load, the split between the two is about 70% and 30% respectively [3]. Under part load this split changes; at low load the current drawn is small and the I^2R losses are low. Consequently, the iron losses predominate and since they result from the consumption of reactive current, the

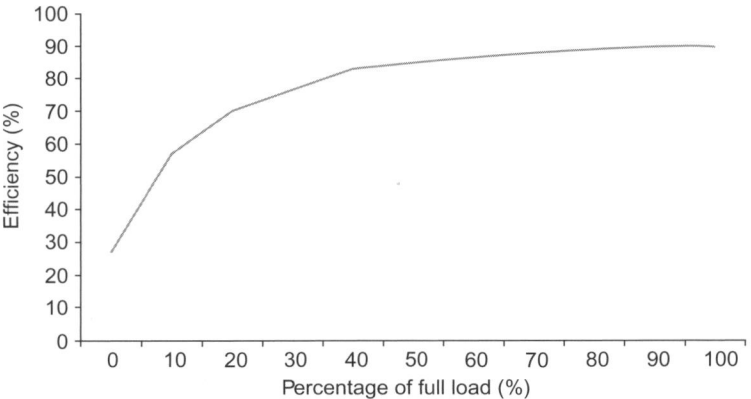

FIG 14.4 Relationship between motor loading and efficiency [2].

power factor is correspondingly low. Even at full load, induction motors exhibit a relatively poor power factor, typically around 0.8 [3].

14.3.1 Motor Sizing

Correct sizing of electric motors is critical to their efficient operation, since oversized motors tend to exhibit poor power factors and lower efficiencies. Depending on size and speed, a typical standard motor may have a full load efficiency between 55% and 95% [2]. Generally, the lower the speed, the lower the efficiency and the lower the power factor. Typically motors exhibit efficiencies which are reasonably constant down to approximately 75% full load. Thereafter they may lose approximately 5% down to 50% of full load, after which the efficiency falls rapidly (as shown in Figure 14.4) [2].

It can be seen from the performance curve in Figure 14.4 that it is possible to oversize a motor by up to 25% without seriously affecting its efficiency, provided that a motor is run at a relatively constant load. If the load fluctuates and rarely achieves 75% full load, then both the efficiency and the power factor of the motor will be adversely affected. In fact the power factor tends to fall off more rapidly than the efficiency under part-load conditions. Therefore, if motors are oversized, the need for power factor correction becomes greater. Oversizing of motors also increases the capital cost of the switchgear and wiring which serves the motor.

14.4 Variable Speed Drives (VSD)

Most induction motors used in buildings are fitted to fans or pumps. The traditional approach to pipework and ductwork systems has been to oversize pumps and fans at the design stage, and then to use commissioning valves and dampers to control the flow rate by increasing the system resistance. While mechanical constrictions are able to control the flow rate delivered by fans and pumps (see Figure 14.5), the constriction itself increases the system resistance and results in increased energy loss. This situation is highly undesirable and is one of the main reasons why the energy consumption associated with fans and pumps is so high in so many buildings [1]. An alternative approach to the use of valves and dampers is to control the flow rate by reducing the

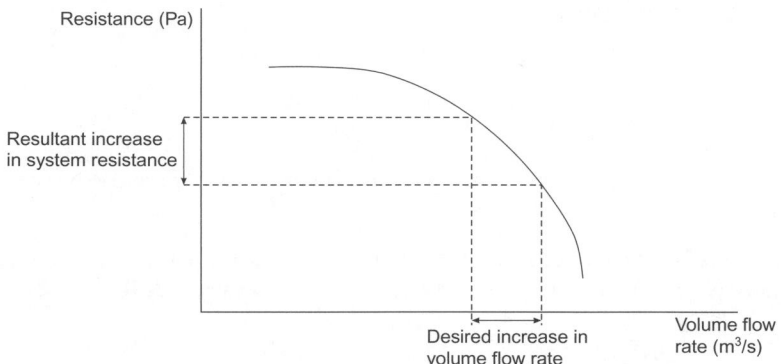

FIG 14.5 Impact of a volume control damper on system resistance.

speed of the fan or pump motor. This strategy results in considerable energy savings, as illustrated in Example 14.3.

Example 14.3

It is proposed to use a forward-curved centrifugal fan in a mechanical ventilation system. The fan is required to deliver a volume flow rate of 1.8 m³/s and the estimated system resistance is 500 Pa. However, the proposed fan delivers 2.06 m³/s against a resistance of 500 Pa while running at a speed of 1440 rpm. Determine the fan power input, if:

(a) A volume control damper is used to achieve a volume flow rate of 1.8 m³/s by increasing the total system resistance to 750 Pa.
(b) The fan speed is reduced in order to deliver 1.8 m³/s.

Solution

(a) Fan air power input:

$$W = \dot{v} \times P_t$$

where $\dot{v}$ is the air volume flow rate (m³/s), and P_t is the total system resistance (Pa).

Let W_1 be the fan power when delivering 2.06 m³/s against a resistance of 500 Pa, and W_2 be the fan power when delivering 1.8 m³/s against a resistance of 750 Pa.

Therefore

$$W_1 = 2.06 \times 500 = 1030 \text{ W}$$

and

$$W_2 = 1.8 \times 750 = 1350 \text{ W}$$

Therefore

$$\text{Increase in power consumption} = \frac{1350 - 1030}{1030} \times 100 = 31.1\%$$

(b) The fan laws state that:

$$\dot{v} \propto N$$

and

$$W \propto N^3$$

where $\dot{v}$ is the air volume flow rate (m³/s), N is the fan speed (rpm), and W is the fan air power input (W).

Let N_1 be the fan speed when delivering 2.06 m³/s against a resistance of 500 Pa, N_3 be the fan speed when delivering 1.8 m³/s, and W_3 be the fan power when delivering 1.8 m³/s.

Therefore

$$N_3 = 1440 \times \frac{1.8}{2.06} = 1258.3 \text{ rpm}$$

$$W_3 = 1030 \times \frac{1.8^3}{2.06^3} = 687.2 \text{ W}$$

Therefore

$$\begin{array}{c}\text{Reduction in power consumption} \\ (W_3 \text{ compared with } W_1)\end{array} = \frac{1030 - 687.2}{1030} \times 100 = 33.3\%$$

However

$$\begin{array}{c}\text{Reduction in power consumption} \\ (W_3 \text{ compared with } W_2)\end{array} = \frac{1350 - 687.2}{1350} \times 100 = 49.1\%$$

It can be seen from Example 14.3 that:

- The use of volume control dampers to regulate air flow significantly increases fan energy consumption. The precise magnitude of this increase will depend on the characteristics of the particular fan selected.
- Reducing the fan speed to regulate the air flow rate always results in fan energy savings.

The fan power savings which can be achieved through reducing fan speeds are considerable, especially when compared with the fan power increase which results from using volume control dampers. As a result there are great advantages to be gained, if fan and pump speeds can be controlled.

The energy savings achieved in Example 14.3 are indicative of the type of savings which can be achieved through the use of VSDs on fans and pumps. In most applications the potential for saving energy through the use of VSDs on pumps, fans and compressors is considerable. Most designers overestimate system resistances with the result that most pumps and fans are theoretically oversized before the actual fan or pump selection is undertaken. During the selection process, the cautious designer is unlikely to find a fan, or pump, which matches the theoretical 'calculated' specification and thus a larger one is selected which is sure to perform the required task. This strategy protects the system designer and ensures that he/she does not negligently undersize the fans or pumps. Unfortunately, it also ensures that the system is greatly oversized and that during the commissioning process, volume control dampers and dampers will have to be used to reduce the volume flow rate. Consequently, both the capital and future operating costs of the system are greatly increased. By using VSDs it is possible to ensure that even if fans and pumps are oversized, energy consumption will not be greatly increased. This makes the installation of VSDs one of the most cost-effective energy efficiency measures that can be taken. It has been estimated that for VSDs payback periods of less than 2 years are the norm [2].

In addition to the energy savings gained through using VSDs on constant flow systems, even greater savings can be made by employing VSDs on variable volume flow systems. When the load profiles and duty cycles of heating, air-conditioning and ventilation systems are examined in detail, it is found that most regularly operate well below their intended design specification. The main reason for this is that system designers are overcautious at the design stage. As a result, over-large constant volume flow rate, variable temperature systems are designed. While this approach works in practice, it means that pump and fan running costs are constant and high, no matter what the operating load. An alternative approach is to keep the temperature constant and vary the flow rate, so that pump and fan running costs reduce as the operating load reduces. The classic system which adopts this approach is the variable air volume (VAV) air-conditioning system, for which VSDs are ideally suited.

14.4.1   Principles of VSD Operation

Modern electronic VSD systems adjust the mains alternating current to regulate motor speed. Various electronic VSD systems are available. One of the most popular types is the *variable frequency drive*, which achieves speed control by varying the voltage and frequency output. Such drives regulate the voltage to the motor in proportion to the output frequency in order to ensure that the ratio of voltage to frequency remains relatively constant. Changes in motor speed are achieved by modulating the voltage and frequency to the motor. Figure 14.6 shows the basic components in a *variable frequency drive* VSD system.

Variable frequency drive systems comprise two main components, a rectifier and an inverter. The rectifier converts standard alternating current (ac) (e.g. 240 V and 50 Hz)

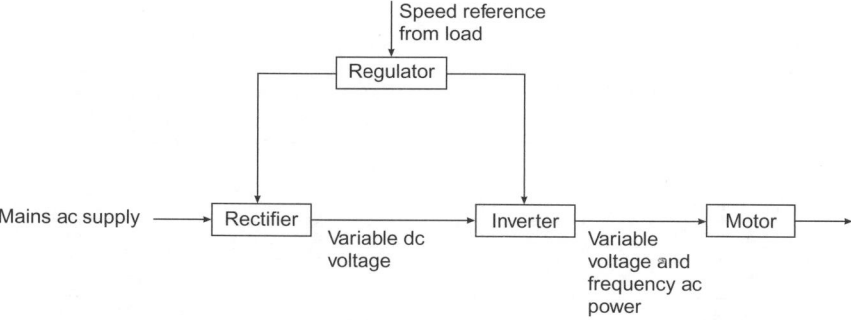

FIG 14.6 Components of a variable speed drive. Crown copyright: reproduced with the permission of the Controller of Her Majesty's Stationery Office and the Queen's Printer for Scotland [4].

to an adjustable direct current (dc), which is then fed to the inverter. The inverter comprises electronic switches which turn the dc power on and off to produce a pulsed ac power output. This can then be controlled to produce the required frequency and voltage. The switching characteristics of the inverter are modified by a regulator, so that the output frequency can be controlled.

The inverter is the critical part of a VSD system. One type of inverter currently in use is the pulse width modulated (PWM) inverter, which receives a fixed dc voltage from the rectifier and adjusts the output voltage and frequency. The PWM inverter produces a current waveform which approximates to the pure sine wave of mains ac supply.

14.5   Lighting Energy Consumption

The energy consumed by electric lighting in most building types is considerable. Table 14.2 shows the proportion of overall energy consumed by lighting for a variety of building types in the UK.

Although in many buildings the energy consumed by the heating system is often greater than that consumed by lighting, the energy costs associated with lighting are often considerably greater than those associated with the heating [1]. It is possible to achieve considerable energy cost savings through the careful design and maintenance of lighting schemes. On average, *good practice* 'standard' air-conditioned office buildings in the UK experience an annual lighting cost of £1.48 per m^2, which compares very favourably with the typical value of £2.97 per m^2 of floor space [1].

14.5.1   Daylighting

Although the focus of this chapter is on electrical services, daylighting is relevant to the subject of artificial lighting and so a short discussion is included here. The ability of daylighting to reduce lighting energy costs should not be underestimated. Daylight can make a substantial contribution to the lighting of buildings by reducing reliance on artificial lighting.

The major factors affecting the daylighting of an interior are the depth of the room, the size and location of windows, the glazing system and any external obstructions. These

TABLE 14.2   Typical energy consumption on lighting for various applications in the UK [5]

Building type	Typical percentage of energy consumed by lighting (%)
Banks	19
Factories	15
Hotels	9
Offices	16–20
Schools	9–12
Supermarkets	11

factors usually depend on decisions made at the initial design stage. Through appropriate planning at an early stage it is possible to produce a building which is energy efficient as well as having a pleasing internal appearance. Glazing can, however, impose severe constraints on the form and operation of a building. If poor design decisions are made concerning fenestration it is possible to create a building in which the occupants are uncomfortable, and in which energy consumption is high. Glazing should therefore be treated with care.

14.5.2 Lighting Definitions

Before discussing the factors which influence the energy consumption of artificial lighting schemes, it is important first to understand the terminology involved, and to appreciate how lighting schemes are designed. A full discussion of the subject of lighting design is, however, beyond the scope of this book.

When an incandescent lamp is switched on, it emits a luminous flux in all directions. The fundamental SI unit of luminous flux is the lumen (lm). It should be noted that the lumen is simply a measure of the quantity of *luminous flux*. It tells us nothing about the direction of the light. When a lamp is placed in a luminaire fitting with an integral reflector, the luminous flux from the lamp will be directed in one particular direction (e.g. downward in the case of a ceiling-mounted fitting). A certain number of lumens are therefore focused in a particular direction with a certain *luminous intensity*. Luminous intensity, as the term suggests, is the intensity of luminous flux in any given 3-dimensional angular direction and its SI unit is the candela (cd). 'Three-dimensional angular direction' is a difficult concept to define; but it is usually referred to as *solid angle*. It is the 3-dimensional equivalent of a 2-dimensional angle. The steradian is the SI unit of *solid angle* and is the 3-dimensional equivalent of the radian. The candela can therefore be defined as being a lumen per steradian. More precisely, one candela can be defined as the luminous intensity from a source producing light at 540,000,000 MHz and at a specific intensity of 1/683 W per steradian [6].

Lighting manufacturers use a system of polar diagrams to describe luminous intensity distribution from luminaire fittings. Figure 14.7 shows a typical polar diagram for a transverse section across a ceiling-mounted luminaire fitting. It should be noted that luminous intensity produced by the lamp is not the same in all directions. For example, while the intensity in a vertical direction is 112 cd per klm of lamp flux, the intensity at 40° to the vertical is only 88 cd per klm. Lighting manufacturers usually specify intensity in terms of cd per klm of installed lamp flux because it is often possible to use a variety of lamps in any particular luminaire fitting.

From a purely functional point of view, it is not so much the intensity of light coming from a light source (i.e. a luminaire fitting) that is important, but rather the amount of light that is falling on a particular surface. For example, a room may be illuminated only by spotlights which shine brightly on certain specific objects while leaving the rest of the room in relative darkness. If a person tries to read a book in a region of the room which is not well lit, they will experience difficulties. Although there may be a large luminous flux in the room, the problem is that very little of it is falling on the pages of the book. The person then experiences difficulties in reading. The amount of luminous

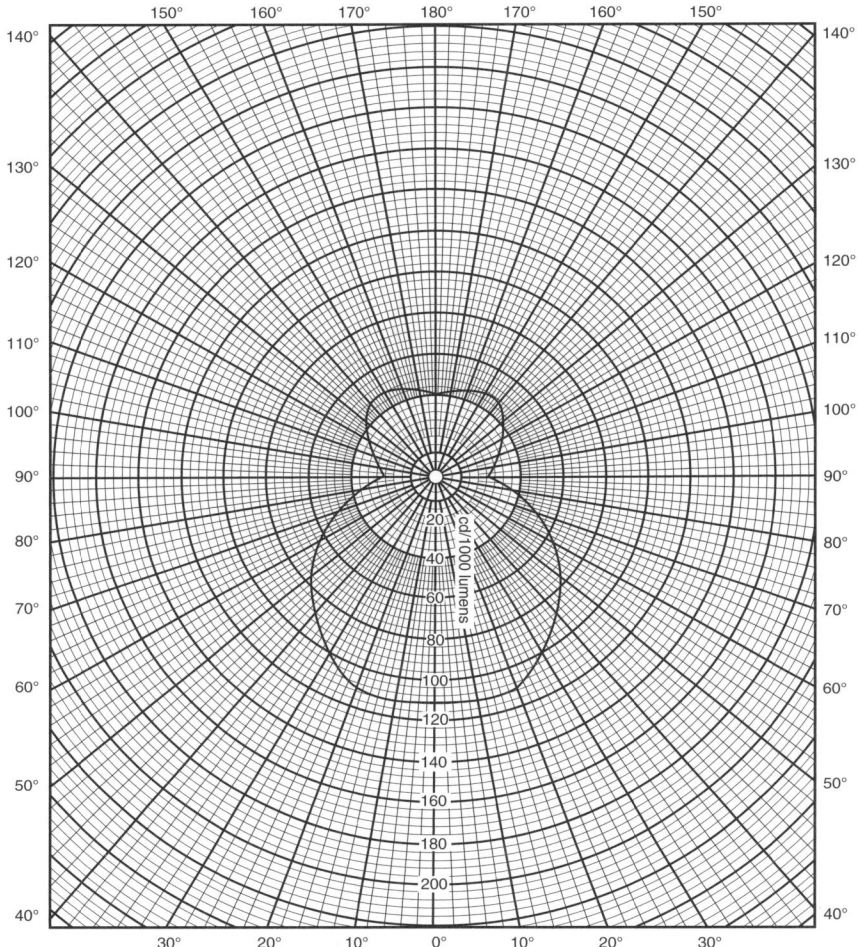

FIG 14.7 Polar intensity diagram. From Smith, Phillips and Sweeney (1987) *Environmental Science* © Longman Group Ltd, reprinted by permission of Pearson Education Ltd [6].

flux falling on a surface is therefore of great importance. It is referred to as *illuminance* and has the SI unit, the lux (lx). One lux is defined as a luminous flux of 1 lm falling on a surface having an area of 1 m². Artificial lighting schemes are usually specified as being capable of supplying a specified number of lux on a horizontal working plane. Generally, the more demanding the work, the higher the level of illuminance required.

Because light is a form of radiant energy, its ability to illuminate a surface (i.e. its illuminance) varies inversely with the square of the distance between the source and the surface. In simple terms, if the distance increases, the illuminance decreases by the square of the distance. This relationship is known as the inverse square law. Also, if a horizontal surface is illuminated from the side, so that the light hits the surface at an angle other than 90°, the available luminous flux is shared out over a larger surface area so that illuminance decreases. The angle at which light strikes a surface is therefore of importance. This fact can be combined with the inverse square law to produce the cosine law of illuminance, which can be expressed as

$$\text{Illuminance on a horizontal surface } E_h = \frac{I_\theta}{d^2} \times \cos\theta \qquad (14.5)$$

where θ is the angle at which light strikes the horizontal surface (i.e. angle from the vertical) (°), I_θ is the luminous intensity in direction θ (cd), and d is the distance of plane from light source (m).

Example 14.4 shows how the cosine law can be applied to the data contained in the polar diagram shown in Figure 14.7.

Example 14.4

Using the luminaire polar diagram shown in Figure 14.7, determine the illuminance on a horizontal surface. (Assume that the luminaire fitting contains two fluorescent tubes each with a luminous flux of 3200 lm.)

(i)   At a point (a) 3 m directly below the luminaire.
(ii) At a point (b) 2 m to the right of point (a).

Solution

(i)   From Figure 14.7 it can be seen that the luminous intensity in the vertical direction is 112 cd per klm of lamp flux. Therefore

$$\text{Luminous intensity in the vertical direction} = 112 \times (2 \times 3.2)$$
$$= 716.8 \text{ cd}$$

Therefore:

$$\text{Illuminance on a horizontal surface at point (a)} = \frac{716.8}{3^2} \times \cos\theta = 79.6 \text{ lx}$$

(ii) Considering point (b)

$$\tan\theta = \frac{2}{3} = 0.667$$

Therefore

$$\theta = 33.69°$$

and

$$d = \sqrt{(2^2 + 3^2)} = 3.606 \text{ m}$$

From Figure 14.7 it can be seen that the luminous intensity at 33.7° in the vertical is 96 cd per klm of lamp flux. Therefore

$$\text{Luminous intensity in the vertical direction} = 96 \times (2 \times 3.2)$$
$$= 614.4 \text{ cd}$$

Therefore

$$\text{Illuminance on a horizontal surface at point (b)} = \frac{614.4}{3.606^2} \times \cos 33.69 = 39.3 \text{ lx}$$

14.6 Artificial Lighting Design

The performance of an artificial lighting scheme is influenced by:

- The efficacy of the lamps (i.e. the light output per watt of electrical power consumed).
- The luminaire performance.
- The layout of the luminaire fittings.
- The surface reflectance of the decor and furnishing.
- The maintenance standards.

All these factors have to be allowed for when designing any lighting scheme. One method which is frequently used and which considers all these factors is the *lumen design method*. The lumen method enables regular lighting schemes to be designed quickly and easily, and so is particularly popular as a design method. The method enables the number of luminaires to be determined for any rectangular room space using eqn (14.6):

$$\text{Number of luminaire fitting required } n = \frac{E_{av} \times A}{\phi \times UF \times MF} \qquad (14.6)$$

where n is the number of luminaire fittings required, A is the area of working plane in room (i.e. room area) (m²), E_{av} is the average illuminance required on the working plane (lx), θ is the lighting design lumens per fitting (lm), UF is the utilization factor of luminaire fitting, and MF is the maintenance factor.

Each of the terms in eqn (14.6) corresponds with the list of factors outlined at the beginning of this section. However, in order to understand the relevance of each term, some explanation is required.

14.6.1 Average Illuminance (E_{av})

The required illuminance in a room depends on the nature of the tasks being undertaken in the space. Visual acuity improves at higher levels of illuminance. The more visually demanding the task, the higher the level of illuminance required on the working plane. The working plane is normally taken to be desk height. Table 14.3 shows appropriate levels of illuminance for a variety of activities and spaces.

TABLE 14.3   Required standard illuminances for various activities [7]

Standard maintained illuminance (lx)	Representative activities
50	Cable tunnels, indoor storage tanks, walkways
100	Corridors, changing rooms, bulk stores, auditoria
150	Loading bays, medical stores, switch rooms, plant rooms
200	Entrance foyers, monitoring automatic processes, casting concrete, turbine halls, dining rooms
300	Libraries, sports and assembly halls, teaching spaces, lecture theatres
500	General office spaces, engine assembly, kitchens, laboratories, retail shops
750	Drawing offices, meat inspection, chain stores
1000	General inspection, electronic assembly, gauge and tool rooms, supermarkets
1500	Fine work and inspection, hand tailoring, precision assembly
2000	Assembly of minute mechanisms, finished fabric inspection

14.6.2   Lighting Design Lumens (ρ)

The term *lighting design lumens* simply refers to the total lumen output of the lamps in a particular luminaire fitting. It should be noted that this is the lumen output when the lamps are new. It is also important to appreciate that lighting manufacturers produce luminaire fittings which might accommodate a variety of lamps, each of which will emit a different luminous flux. The type of lamp to be used in the luminaire should therefore be specified.

14.6.3   Utilization Factor (UF)

The UF can be expressed as:

$$UF = \frac{\text{Total flux reaching the working plane}}{\text{Total lamp flux}}$$

(14.7)

The UF takes into account both the direct luminous flux which reaches the working plane straight from the luminaire and the flux which reaches the working plane having been reflected from the walls and the ceiling. The UF is influenced by the nature of the luminaire used, the room surface reflectance and the room dimensions. Table 14.4 shows a typical set of UF data produced by a manufacturer for a particular luminaire fitting.

TABLE 14.4   Luminaire utilization factor

Room reflectance's ceiling (%) [wall %]	Room index					
	1.00	1.25	1.50	2.00	2.50	3.00
0.50 [50]	0.50	0.54	0.57	0.61	0.63	0.65
50 [30]	0.47	0.51	0.54	0.58	0.61	0.63
50 [10]	0.44	0.48	0.51	0.56	0.59	0.61

It should be noted that both the room surface reflectance and the room geometry are allowed for in Table 14.4. The room geometry is allowed for by the 'room index' which is expressed as:

$$\text{Room index} = \frac{L \times W}{H_m \times (L + W)}$$

(14.8)

where L is the length of room (m), W is the width of room (m), and H_m is the mounting height (i.e. height above working plane) (m).

14.6.4   Maintenance Factor (MF)

The effective light output from any luminaire decreases with time. This is because of a number of factors:

*   Lamp output decreases with time.
*   Luminaire reflectors and diffusers become dirty with time.
*   Room surfaces become dirty with time.

To compensate for this drop in luminaire output, an MF is introduced into the lumen design method. The MF also allows for the fact that periodically individual lamps fail and remain unattended for some period of time until they are replaced.

Both lamp survival and lamp output fall with time. Figure 14.8 shows output and survival characteristic curves for fluorescent and tungsten filament lamps. It can be seen that two types of lamps behave very differently. The lumen output of a fluorescent lamp falls by nearly 10% during the first 500 hours of operation [7]. Thereafter, the output decreases less rapidly. With a tungsten filament lamp the decrease in light output is much more gradual, although the lamp life is much shorter than that of a fluorescent tube.

The extent to which luminaire fittings become dirty depends very much on the type of fitting. For example, a ventilated luminaire, used in conjunction with an extract plenum, will cause dust and dirt from the room space to collect on the luminaire reflector with the result that it may quickly become dirty. Figure 14.9 shows how light output decreases with dirt deposition for a variety of luminaire types.

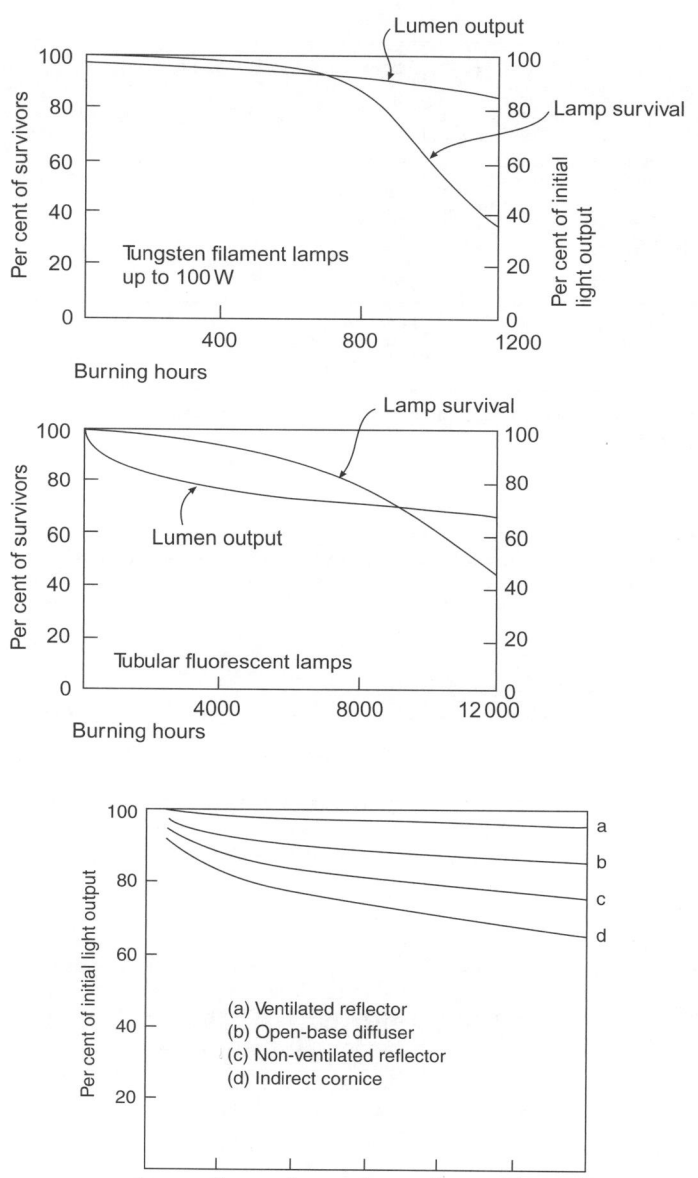

FIG 14.8 Lamp output and survival curves [7].

FIG 14.9 Fall in light output due to dirt deposition [7].

Tables 14.5, 14.6 and 14.7 are attempts to quantify the various factors associated with decreased luminaire output. Table 14.5 quantifies lamp performance over time in two ways, the *lumen maintenance factor* (LLMF) is the proportion of initial lamp lumens 'remaining' after a given time period, while the *lamp survival factor* (LSF) is the proportion of lamps surviving (i.e. lamps that have not failed) after a given time [8].

TABLE 14.5 Lamp lumen maintenance and survival factors

Lamp type	Factor	Operating hours		
		6000	10,000	12,000
Fluorescent (tri-phosphor)	LLMF	0.87	0.85	0.84
	LSF	0.99	0.85	0.75
Metal halide	LLMF	0.72	0.66	0.63
	LSF	0.91	0.83	0.77
Sodium (high pressure)	LLMF	0.91	0.88	0.87
	LSF	0.96	0.92	0.89

From Pritchard (1995) *Lighting* © Longman Group UK Ltd, reprinted by permission of Pearson Education Ltd [8].

TABLE 14.6 Luminaire maintenance factor (LMF)

Luminaire type	6 months cleaning interval			12 months cleaning interval			18 months cleaning interval		
	Clean	Normal	Dirty	Clean	Normal	Dirty	Clean	Normal	Dirty
Batten	0.95	0.92	0.88	0.93	0.98	0.83	0.91	0.87	0.80
Enclosed IP2X	0.92	0.87	0.83	0.88	0.82	0.77	0.85	0.79	*
Up-lighter	0.92	0.89	0.85	0.86	0.81	*	0.81	*	*

*Not recommended.
From Pritchard (1995) *Lighting* © Longman Group UK Ltd, reprinted by permission of Pearson Education Ltd [8].

TABLE 14.7 Room surface maintenance factor (RSMF)

Room index	Luminaire flux distribution	12 months cleaning interval			24 months cleaning interval		
		Clean	Normal	Dirty	Clean	Normal	Dirty
2.5–5.0	Direct	0.98	0.96	0.95	0.96	0.95	0.94
2.5–5.0	General	0.92	0.88	0.85	0.89	0.85	0.81
2.5–5.0	Indirect	0.88	0.82	0.77	0.84	0.77	0.70

From Pritchard (1995) *Lighting* © Longman Group UK Ltd, reprinted by permission of Pearson Education Ltd [8].

The *luminaire maintenance factor* (LMF) referred to in Table 14.6 quantifies the impact of various maintenance regimes on different luminaire types in a variety of environments.

The impact of various cleaning regimes on room surface reflectance is quantified in Table 14.7 by using a *room surface maintenance factor* (RSMF).

Example 14.5 shows how a realistic MF might be developed in practice.

Example 14.5

The lighting scheme in an office space comprises 60 batten-type luminaire fittings with fluorescent (tri-phosphor type) tubes. The lamps are changed in bulk every 6000 hours and the luminaire fittings and room surfaces are cleaned every 12 months. The cleanliness of the environment within the office space is normal and the luminous flux distribution from the luminaries is 'general' in nature. Determine a suitable maintenance factor for the installation.

Solution

From Table 14.5

$$LLMF = 0.87$$
$$LSF = 0.99$$

From Table 14.6

$$LMF = 0.98$$

From Table 14.7

$$RSMF = 0.88$$

Therefore

$$MF = 0.87 \times 0.99 \times 0.98 \times 0.88 = 0.74$$

When designing a lighting scheme it is important to ensure that the illuminance on the working plane is evenly distributed. If the luminaires are too far apart, gloomy patches will appear on the working plane. This makes it important not to exceed the *spacing to mounting height ratio* stated for the particular luminaire being used. The nominal spacing for luminaire fittings can be determined using eqn (14.9):

$$\text{Nominal spacing between fittings, } S = \sqrt{\frac{A}{n}} \qquad (14.9)$$

The process involved in the lumen design method is illustrated in Example 14.6.

Example 14.6

A $15 \times 9 \times 3\,m^3$ high office space is required to be illuminated to 500 lx. Given the following data, design a suitable artificial lighting layout for the space.

Data:
   Height of working plane = 800 mm
   Height of luminaire fittings above floor level = 3000 mm
   Design lumens per fitting = 8000 lm
   Maintenance factor = 75%

Ceiling reflectance factor = 50%
Wall reflectance factor = 50%

Maximum spacing to mounting height ratio = 1.2:1.0

Room reflectance's ceiling (%) [wall %]	Room index					
	1.00	**1.25**	**1.50**	**2.00**	**2.50**	**3.00**
50 [50]	0.50	0.54	0.57	0.61	0.63	0.65
50 [30]	0.47	0.51	0.54	0.58	0.61	0.63
50 [10]	0.44	0.48	0.51	0.56	0.59	0.61

Solution

Mounting height = 3.0 − 0.8 = 2.2 m

Using eqn (14.6)

$$\text{Room index} = \frac{15 \times 9}{2.2 \times (15 + 9)} = 2.56$$

Since the ceiling reflectance is 50%, the wall reflectance is 50% and the room index is 2.56. Therefore

$$UF = 0.632$$

Using eqn (14.6)

$$\text{Number of luminaire fitting required } n = \frac{500 \times (15 \times 9)}{8000 \times 0.632 \times 0.75} = 17.8$$

Since it is impossible to have 0.8 of a luminaire fitting, the number of luminaires required (n) must be 18.

Using eqn (14.9)

$$\text{Nominal spacing between fittings, } S = \sqrt{((15 \times 9)/18)} = 2.739 \text{ m}$$

Therefore

$$\text{Spacing:Mounting height} = 2.739{:}2.2 = 1.245{:}1.0$$

However, this spacing to mounting height ratio exceeds the maximum permissible ratio of 1.2:1.0. Therefore, it is necessary to increase the number of fittings to, say, 20.

Therefore

$$\text{Nominal spacing between fittings } S = \sqrt{((15 \times 9)/20)} = 2.598 \text{ m}$$

Therefore

Spacing:Mounting height 2.598 : 2.2 = 1.181 : 1.0

This spacing to mounting height ratio is acceptable. Therefore

Number of luminaire fittings required = 20

and

Suggested design layout: 4 rows of 5 fittings

14.7 Energy Efficient Lighting

The main factors which influence the energy consumption of lighting schemes are:

  (i) The light output per watt of electrical power consumed (i.e. lamp efficacy).
 (ii) Luminaire performance.
(iii) The number of luminaires and their location.
(iv) The reflectance of internal room surfaces.
 (v) Maintenance and procedure standards.
(vi) Duration of operation.
(vii) The switching and control techniques used.

While points (i) to (iv) above are concerned with the fundamental efficiency of any installation, points (v) to (vii) relate to the management and operation of the installation.

When considering the overall energy efficiency of luminaires it is helpful to look in isolation at the individual components which together make up the luminaire; namely the lamp, the control gear and the fitting.

14.7.1 Lamps

There are a wide variety of lamps which can be used in artificial lighting schemes. Fluorescent, tungsten filament, tungsten halogen, metal halide (MBI) and high-pressure sodium vapour (SON) are amongst the many lamp types in common use. Energy consumption varies greatly with the type of lamp used. Figure 14.10 shows comparative lamp efficacies for a variety of lamp types. Luminous efficacy is defined in lumens produced per watt of electricity consumed.

It can clearly be seen from Figure 14.10 that there is a wide variation in the luminous efficacy between the various lamp types. For example, compact fluorescent lamps have an efficacy of approximately 70 lm/W, while tungsten filament lamps exhibit an efficacy of approximately 10 lm/W. Clearly, the compact fluorescent lamp is a much more energy efficient option. It should also be noted that the luminous efficacy of any lamp type increases as power input is increased. While this increase may only be slight in some types of lamp (e.g. tungsten filament and tungsten halogen lamps), in others, such as high- and low-pressure sodium lamps (SON and SOX), the increase can be substantial.

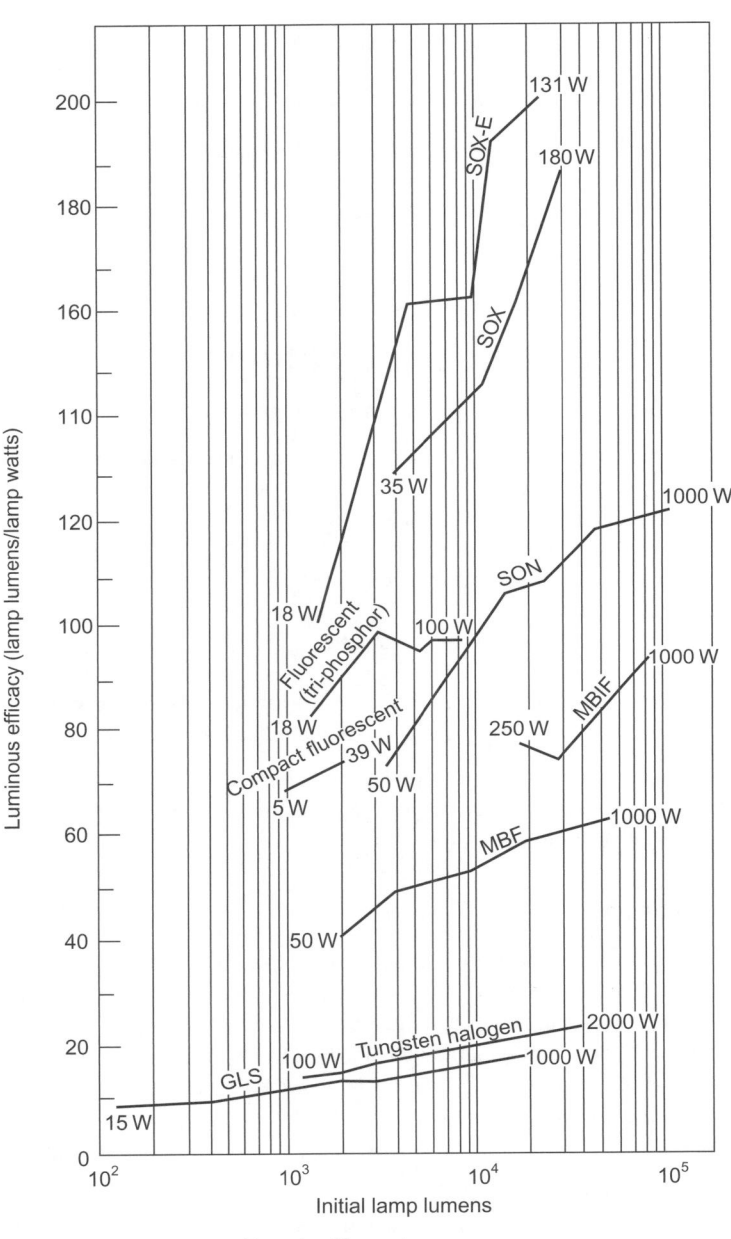

FIG 14.10 Efficacies of various lamps [9].

When designing new artificial lighting installations, it is important to install lamps which exhibit high efficacy. In older installations, it may be worth considering refurbishing existing luminaire fittings, so that they can incorporate newer more efficient lamp types. Refurbishment of older installations using modern equipment can often result in substantial energy savings as well as improved visual conditions. It is possible to improve older, less efficient, luminaires by replacing existing diffusers with modern reflector systems at relatively low cost. However, some changes can be considerably more expensive, such as replacement of the existing control gear to facilitate the use of low energy lamps.

Tungsten Filament Lamps
Although the use of tungsten filament lamps is widespread, they are particularly inefficient consumers of energy and should be avoided where possible. They have efficacies in the region of 8–15 lm/W [9], with most of the electrical energy being converted to heat, which can lead to space overheating problems. Lamp life is short, with most tungsten filaments burning out after approximately 1000 hours of use [7].

Compact Fluorescent Lamps
Because standard tungsten filament lamps exhibit such poor efficacies, compact fluorescent lamps were developed as a replacement. Where possible, tungsten lamps should be replaced by compact fluorescent lamps. These give comparable light output to tungsten lamps, but only consume approximately 20% of the power required by tungsten lamps [8]. As the rated life of the compact fluorescent lamps is in the region of 8000–12,000 hours, eight times longer than tungsten lamps, maintenance costs are greatly reduced, albeit at a higher initial cost.

Compact fluorescent lamps can be divided into two distinct categories: those with integral control gear and those which require separate gear. Since the life of control gear is generally longer than that of a fluorescent lamp, it is often better to install lamps with separate control gear, as this is more cost-effective. Lamps with integral control gear are more expensive, being specifically designed as a direct replacement for existing tungsten filament lamps. As with all discharge lamps, compact fluorescent lamps exhibit a poor factor, often as low as 0.5. However, this can be corrected by using capacitors.

Fluorescent Tubes
Fluorescent tubes are commonplace in most buildings and exhibit efficacies in the region of 80–100 lm/W [9]. Depending on the type of lamp and ballast used, they can last up to 18 times as long as tungsten filament lamps. In recent years the 26 mm diameter fluorescent tube has replaced the 38 mm diameter tubes as the standard for new installations. These slimmer lamps produce approximately the same light output as the larger diameter lamps, but consume around 8% less electricity [10].

Metal Halide Lamps
MBI lamps have become popular for a wide variety of applications and are available in a wide range of power ratings, 70–2000 W. They exhibit efficacies in the region of 70–100 lm/W, depending on their power rating [9]. MBI lamps are particularly popular in industrial applications.

High-Pressure Sodium Lamps

SON lamps have proved particularly useful for lighting large high bay areas, such as factories and warehouses, where their high efficacy (e.g. 70–120 lm/W) can produce a very energy efficient lighting scheme. They are also useful for exterior lighting, car parks and floodlighting. They are manufactured in a wide range of power ratings from 50 to 1000 W.

14.7.2 Control Gear

Because of their nature, all discharge lamps, such as fluorescent lamps, require control gear to operate, which comprises a starting device and ballast. A starting device is required to create the high potential difference between the lamp electrodes, so that an electrical discharge is promoted. Starters can be of a plug-in glow type, which should be replaced every second or third lamp change, or else should be of an electronic type. Ballast is necessary to control the current drawn by the lamp. If ballast were not installed, then the current would increase dramatically as the ionization process takes place with the result that damage would be caused to wiring and the fitting itself.

In addition to the lamp load, ballast consumes electricity. The type of ballast used therefore has an impact on overall energy consumption. Traditionally, ballast has come in the form of a wire-wound choke, comprising a copper wire wrapped around a metal core. Current flowing through the wire produces a magnetic field which dampens the growth of any further current, thus 'choking' the current to the desired level. While conventional wire-wound chokes work very well, they result in excess energy losses, typically in the region of 15–20% of total energy consumption. Recently new high-frequency electronic ballasts have been developed. These ballasts run at frequencies between 20 and 40 kHz [10], and can be fitted either with a rapid-start mechanism to facilitate instantaneous starting, or a 'soft-start' which prolongs the lamp life. High-frequency ballasts consume up to 30% less power than wire-wound chokes and have the additional benefit of increasing lamp life [10].

14.7.3 Lighting Controls

The appropriate use of lighting controls can result in substantial energy savings. These savings arise principally from better utilization of available daylight and from switching off electric lighting when a space is unoccupied. Therefore, when designing a lighting control strategy for any given application, it is important to understand the occupancy pattern in the space, since this will heavily influence the potential for energy savings.

There are four basic methods by which lighting installations can be controlled:

- Time-based control.
- Daylight-linked control.
- Occupancy-linked control.
- Localized switching.

Time signals may come from local solid-state switches or be derived from building management systems. These signals switch the lights on and off at set times. It is important to include local override so that lighting can be restored if the occupants need it.

Photoelectric cells can be used either simply to switch lighting on and off, or for dimming. They may be mounted either externally or internally. However, it is important to incorporate time delays into the control system to avoid repeated rapid switching caused, for example, by fast moving clouds. By using an internally mounted photoelectric dimming control system, it is possible to ensure that the sum of daylight and electric lighting always reaches the design level by sensing the total light in the controlled area and adjusting the output of the electric lighting accordingly. If daylight alone is able to meet the design requirements, then the electric lighting can be turned off. The energy-saving potential of dimming control is greater than a simple photoelectric switching system. Dimming control is also more likely to be acceptable to room occupants.

Occupancy-linked control can be achieved using infrared, acoustic, ultrasonic or micro-wave sensors, which detect either movement or noise in room spaces. These sensors switch lighting on when occupancy is detected, and off again after a set time period, when no occupancy movement is detected. They are designed to override manual switches and to prevent a situation where lighting is left on in unoccupied spaces. With this type of system it is important to incorporate a built-in time delay, since occupants often remain still or quiet for short periods and do not appreciate being plunged into darkness if not constantly moving around.

Localized switching should be used in applications which contain large spaces. Local switches give individual occupants control over their visual environment and also facilitate energy savings. By using localized switching it is possible to turn off artificial lighting in specific areas, while still operating it in other areas where it is required, a situation which is impossible if the lighting for an entire space is controlled from a single switch.

14.7.4 Maintenance

With the passage of time, luminaires and room surfaces get dirty, and lamp output decreases. Lamps also fail and need replacing. Consequently, the performance of all lighting installations decreases with time. It is therefore necessary to carry out regular maintenance in order to ensure that an installation is running efficiently. Simple cleaning of lamps and luminaires can substantially improve lighting performance. Therefore, at the design stage maintenance requirements should always be considered. Luminaires should be easily accessible for cleaning and lamp replacement. Bulk replacement of lamps should be planned, so that they are replaced at the end of their useful life, before light output deteriorates to an unacceptable level. The cleaning of lamps and luminaires should be planned on a similar basis. In order to minimize disruption to staff, planned cleaning and lamp replacement can take place during holiday periods.

References

[1] Energy use in offices. Energy Consumption Guide 19, Department of the Environment, Transport and the Regions; 1998.
[2] Economic use of electricity in industry, Fuel Efficiency Booklet 9. Department of the Environment; 1994.
[3] Guidance notes for reducing energy consumption costs of electric motor and drive systems. Good Practice Guide 2. Department of the Environment; 1995.

[4] Retrofitting AC variable speed drives. Good Practice Guide 14. Department of the Environment; 1994.

[5] Energy audits and surveys. CIBSE Applications Manual AM5; 1991.

[6] Smith BJ, Phillips GM, Sweeney M. Environmental science. Harlow: Longman Scientific and Technical; 1987 (chapter 8).

[7] CIBSE code for interior lighting; 1994.

[8] Pritchard DC. Lighting. 5th ed. Harlow: Longman Scientific and Technical; 1995 (chapter 7).

[9] Energy management and good lighting practices. Fuel Efficiency Booklet 12. Department of the Environment; 1993.

[10] Energy efficient lighting in buildings. Thermie Programme, Directorate-General for Energy. Commission of the European Communities; 1992.

Bibliography

Economic use of electricity in industry. Fuel Efficiency Booklet 9. Department of the Environment; 1994.

Energy efficient lighting in buildings. Thermie Programme, Directorate-General for Energy. Commission of the European Communities; 1992.

Energy management and good lighting practices. Fuel Efficiency Booklet 12. Department of the Environment; 1993.

Guidance notes for reducing energy consumption costs of electric motor and drive systems. Good Practice Guide 2. Department of the Environment; 1995.

Pritchard DC. Lighting. 5th ed. Harlow: Longman Scientific and Technical; 1995.

Retrofitting AC variable speed drives. Good Practice Guide 14. Department of the Environment; 1994.

CHAPTER 15

Passive Solar and Low Energy Building Design

This chapter deals with the use of passive techniques to control the environment within buildings. Through the use of passive solar strategies it is possible to produce an architecture which relies more on the building envelope, and less on the use of mechanical equipment as the primary climate modifier. In particular, the impact of passive environmental control strategies on the design and operation of buildings is discussed.

15.1 Introduction

Strictly speaking, the term *passive solar* refers to the harnessing of the sun's energy to heat, cool, ventilate and illuminate buildings without the use of mechanical equipment. As with so many artificial classifications it has become somewhat corrupted and now is a generic term for a design philosophy which seeks to produce low energy buildings which are sympathetic to the natural environment. A better term might therefore be *climate sympathetic architecture*, since buildings created by this design philosophy use their envelope as the primary climate modifier and relegate any mechanical plant that is required to a supplementary role. This is in contrast to the twentieth-century practice of erecting buildings with unsympathetic envelopes, thus creating a hostile internal environment, which can only be rectified by the use of extensive mechanical services. While the precise definition of the term *passive solar architecture* may be arguable, there is no doubt that its central aim is to produce low energy buildings which utilize relatively simple technologies. In such buildings the emphasis is on the envelope, with the result that passive solar buildings tend to have complex façades, which incorporate features such as external shading, opening windows and light shelves.

While it may be possible in certain applications and in some locations to rely totally on the sun's energy to provide a comfortable internal environment, in most passive solar buildings some mechanical plant is still required. This mechanical plant can be used either:

- to supplement the passive technologies as a secondary climate modifier or
- as a facilitator, which enables the passive technologies to perform in an optimum manner.

Most passive solar buildings are therefore in reality hybrids in which passive technologies are used in tandem with mechanical equipment to achieve a low energy solution. In recognition of this fact, a new term *mixed-mode* has come into being. Mixed-mode buildings are so called because they use a combination of natural ventilation and mechanical ventilation to achieve the desired cooling effect [1]. Mixed-mode strategies tend to provide solutions which are more flexible than those produced by pure passive strategies. They are therefore more suitable for use in speculative buildings where the final use of the building may not be known at the design stage.

Because passive solar buildings contain fewer moving parts compared with their mechanical counterparts, it is tempting to believe that *passive* buildings are simpler and easier to design. In fact nothing could be further from the truth. To create a good *passive* building, the designer must have a comprehensive knowledge and understanding of heat transfer and fluid mechanics. Unlike *mechanical* buildings, which use known and easily quantifiable system drivers such as boilers and fans, *passive* buildings use natural 'variables' as drivers, such as solar radiation and wind. This means that considerable analysis must be undertaken at the design stage to ensure that a robust design is produced (i.e. one which operates well under various meteorological conditions). If this is not done, considerable problems can arise and costly mistakes can be made. For example, a building heated purely by solar energy may become uncomfortably cool on days when there is heavy cloud. One major problem for designers is to predict, at the design stage, how passively controlled buildings will behave in practice. Failure to predict performance at the design stage can be a recipe for disaster. Therefore great care must be taken at the design stage. To assist in the design of passive buildings, engineers often use complex and powerful tools such as *computational fluid dynamics* (CFD) to predict accurately how such buildings will perform. However, the costs involved in using CFD are high and expertise is scarce. Indeed, in some applications the high cost of CFD analysis and the general lack of expertise in this field are major obstacles to the use of *passive techniques*.

15.2 Passive Solar Heating

Solar energy is the radiant heat source upon which all life ultimately depends. It is in plentiful supply, even in relatively northerly latitudes. Consider, for example, latitudes

45° north and 45° south (i.e. the respective latitudes of Minneapolis in the USA and Dunedin in New Zealand). At these latitudes the noontime solar intensity in mid-winter on south-facing vertical glazing is 595 W/m^2 [2]. Given that most of the Earth's population lives between these latitudes, it becomes clear that there is great world-wide potential for harnessing solar energy.

Passive solar heating techniques are particularly well suited to applications which experience both low winter air temperatures and clear skies. Under these conditions the abundant solar radiation available during the daytime can be collected and stored for use at night-time when heat is most required. Passive solar heating techniques have been successfully applied in North America on many small- and medium-sized buildings [3]. The headquarters building of the Rocky Mountain Institute in Colorado, USA, uses solar energy to provide its heating and hot water needs. Through the use of solar energy and a highly insulated envelope, the building manages to maintain an acceptable internal environment with virtually no conventional heating, despite experiencing outside air temperatures as low as 40°C [4]. Passive solar heating techniques have also been applied successfully in more northerly and cloudier climates. For example, St George's School in Wallasey, constructed in 1961, is an early example of one such building in the UK [4]. However, it is true to say that it is more difficult to utilize solar energy in the temperate and cloudy climates of northern Europe than it is in more southerly climates.

There are four basic approaches to passive solar heating: *direct gain* systems; *indirect gain* systems; *isolated gain* systems and *thermosiphon* systems [5,6]. All four techniques aim to store, in various ways, solar energy during the daytime for use at night-time when outside air temperatures are low. They all involve the use of high mass materials in the building fabric to store heat. In the *direct gain* system, solar radiation enters room spaces directly through large areas of south-facing glazing. In the *indirect gain* system, the solar radiation is intercepted by a high mass thermal storage element, which separates the room space from the south-facing glazing. The *isolated gain* system is a hybrid of the first two systems, which uses a separate sun space, such as a conservatory or atrium, to capture the solar energy. Finally, *thermosiphons* can be used to promote movement of warm air around buildings.

All solar heating systems rely on the use of large glazed areas to catch the sun's radiation. Glass transmits relatively short-wave solar radiation in the wavelength range 380–2500 nm, but blocks radiation at wavelengths exceeding 2500 nm. Although glass permits solar radiation to enter room spaces, it blocks much of the long-wave radiation which is emitted when the surfaces in the room become hot. This phenomenon is known as the *greenhouse effect* (which should not to be confused with the *greenhouse effect* associated with global warming) and it leads to heat build-up within room spaces. Due to the *greenhouse effect*, the temperature within room spaces rises until the heat losses by conduction and convection equal the heat gains by radiation.

As well as promoting the greenhouse effect within buildings, glazing also plays an important role in the self-regulation of solar heat gains. Glass transmits much more solar radiation when the angle of incidence is small, compared with when it is large. When the angle of incidence is large much of the incident solar radiation is reflected. This quality can be used to great effect by building designers. Consider the simple building shown

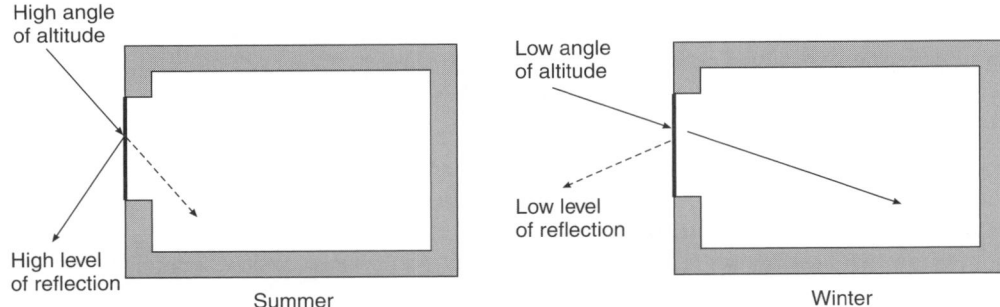

FIG 15.1 Solar reflection from glazing.

in Figure 15.1. In winter, when solar heat gains are most advantageous, the sun is low in the sky and the angle of incidence on the vertical glazing is small. This maximizes the solar transmission through the glass so that the sun's rays penetrate deep into the room space. Conversely, in summer, when solar heat gains are undesirable, the sun is high in the sky and the angle of incidence on the vertical glazing is large, with the result that much of the solar radiation is reflected. In addition, because the sun's angle of altitude is much higher in summer, vertical windows present a much smaller 'apparent' area to solar radiation in summer compared with winter (see Figure 15.2). As a result the solar intensity on vertical glazing is often much lower in summer than in winter. It should be noted that if horizontal roof lights are used the situation is reversed with the greatest solar heat gains being experienced during the summer months.

Most solar heating techniques rely on high mass materials to store heat. A variety of materials can be used to store solar energy; concrete, masonry blocks, water tanks and even rocks have all been used to fulfil this thermal storage role. Essentially, any material which has a high specific heat capacity and is a good conductor of heat can be used in this role.

15.2.1 Direct Gain Techniques

The utilization of direct solar gains is probably the simplest approach to passive solar heating. It involves using the actual living space within a building as the solar collector (as shown in Figure 15.3). To maximize the amount of solar radiation collected during the winter months, rooms should have large areas of south-facing glazing. Floors and walls of the rooms should be constructed from dense materials with a high thermal storage capacity. During the daytime, short-wave radiation is absorbed by the exposed high mass interior, while in the evening and at night-time heat is transferred from the warm room surfaces to the occupants and the air by radiation and convection. As well as facilitating thermal storage, during the daytime the exposed thermal mass absorbs heat and thus tempers the internal environment, so that overheating is prevented. In order to prevent conduction of the heat away from the high mass storage material, insulation material should always be placed between the dense interior and the outside. Although it is usual to use concrete or masonry blocks to achieve the thermal mass, it is possible to use water containers inside the building to store heat. However, these tend to be difficult to integrate into the overall building design.

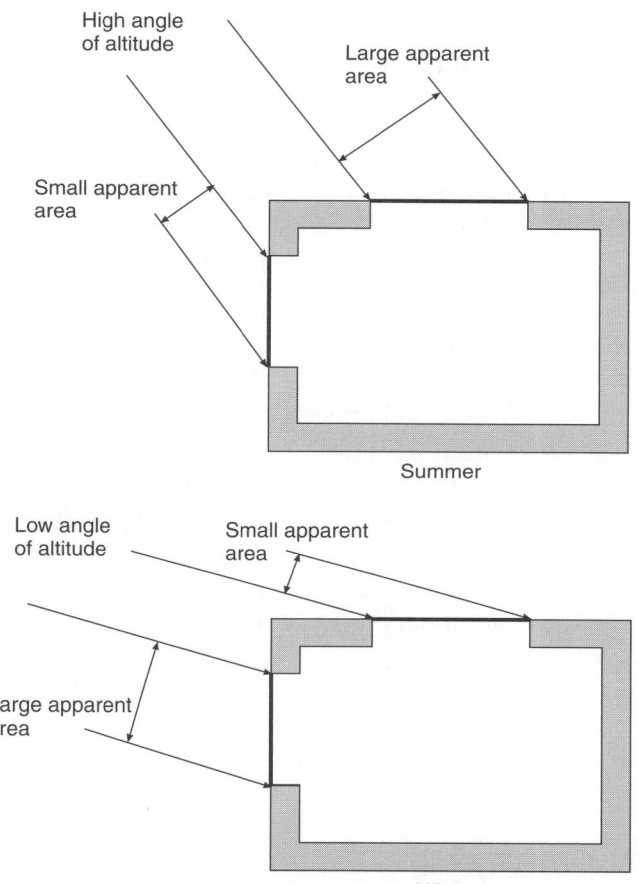

FIG 15.2 Solar angle and apparent area.

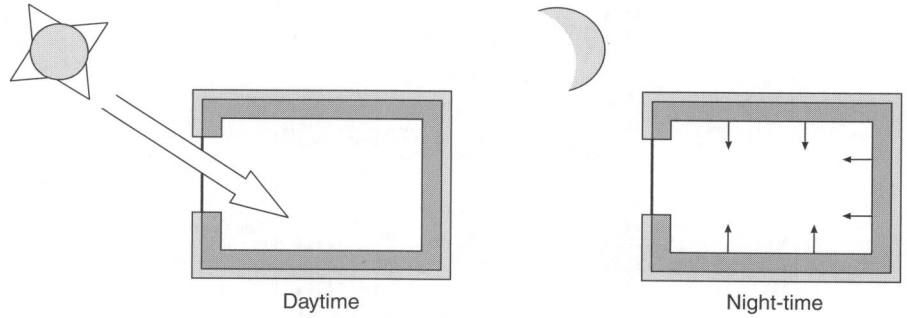

FIG 15.3 Direct gain solar heating.

15.2.2 Indirect Gain Techniques

In an *indirect gain* system, an element with high thermal mass is situated between the sun and the room space. Any solar energy striking the thermal mass is absorbed so that it heats up during the daytime. In the evening and at night-time heat is transferred to the rooms from the thermal mass by a combination of conduction, convection and radiation. Figure 15.4 illustrates the operation of one such indirect system, the Trombe wall, which comprises a masonry wall up to 600 mm thick, located directly behind a south-facing glass façade. The outward-facing surface of the masonry wall is usually painted black to maximize its absorption of solar radiation. During the daytime, solar radiation is absorbed by the masonry wall with the result that the air between the wall and the glass warms up. This causes the air to circulate through vents at the top and bottom of the wall and into the room space, thus warming it. At night the vents in the wall are sealed and the wall transfers heat energy by radiation and convection to the room space.

It is possible to increase the amount of solar radiation collected by a Trombe wall by placing a reflective surface directly on the ground in front of the façade. This material reflects solar radiation onto the thermal storage wall and thus increases its effectiveness.

Trombe walls work best in cold, clear climates which experience large amounts of solar radiation, such as those found at altitude in southern Europe. They are much less effective in northern European climates where cloud cover is often extensive in winter.

Another *indirect gain* technique, which has been used in the USA, is the solar roof pond. As well as providing passive heating in winter this system can also provide cooling in

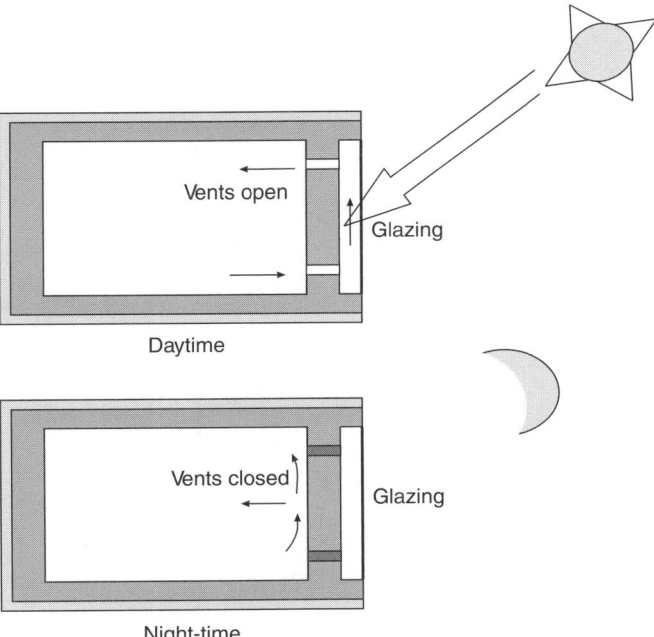

FIG 15.4 Trombe wall operation.

summer. It involves constructing a pond on a flat roof. In winter during the daytime the pond absorbs solar energy. At night the warm pond conducts heat through the roof structure and warms the rooms below by radiation. It is necessary at night in winter to cover the pond with movable insulation material. In summer, the pond can be used to provide passive cooling. Overnight the pond is cooled by exposing it to the night air and once cooled, the water mass is used to draw heat from the space below.

15.2.3   Isolated Gain Techniques

Isolated gain solar heating is essentially a hybrid of the direct and indirect gain systems and involves the construction of a separate sun room adjacent to a main living space. In the *isolated gain* system, solar radiation entering the sun room is retained in the thermal mass of the floor and the partition wall. Heat from the sun room then passes to the living space by conduction through the shared wall at the rear of the sun room and by convection through vents or doors in the shared wall. One classic example of an *isolated gain* system is the use of a south-facing glass conservatory on the side of a house. A typical isolated gain system is shown in Figure 15.5.

15.2.4   Thermosiphon Systems

If a flat solar collector containing water or air is placed below a heat exchanger, a thermosiphon will be created. As the fluid heats up in the solar collector it becomes less

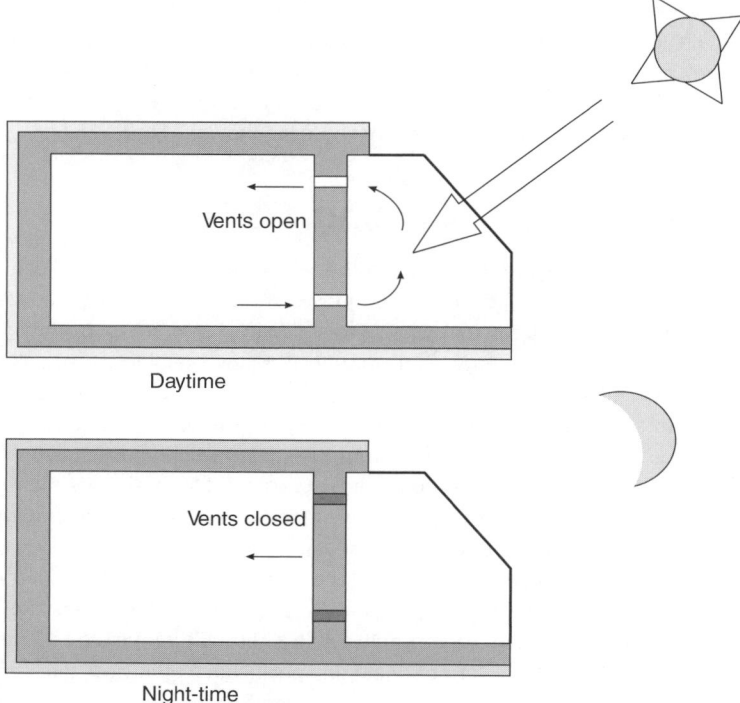

Daytime

Vents open

Night-time

Vents closed

FIG 15.5 Operation of an isolated gain system.

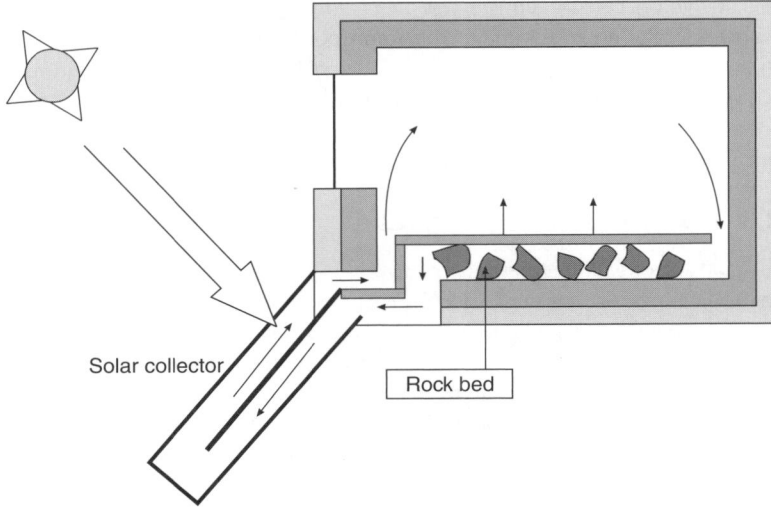

FIG 15.6 A thermosiphon system.

dense and more buoyant and thus rises to the heat exchanger. As the hot fluid travels through the heat exchanger it cools down and so drops to the solar collector below, where the whole process starts over again. It is possible to heat buildings passively by the use of a solar thermosiphon. In such a system the south-facing solar collectors are placed at a level lower than the room space. Warm air from the collectors is allowed to circulate around a floor void filled with rocks. During the daytime the hot air produced by the solar collectors is used to heat up the rocks and during the night-time the rocks give up their heat by convection to the room space (as shown in Figure 15.6).

15.3 Passive Solar Cooling

The term *passive solar cooling* is a very loose one, which can be used collectively to describe a variety of passive cooling techniques, some of which directly utilize solar energy. However, it is true to say that passive solar cooling has more to do with defending buildings against solar energy than utilizing it. Many buildings, especially large commercial buildings, experience overheating problems during the summer months. These problems often arise because of poor building envelope design. Rather than defending against solar gains, many buildings possess envelopes which actively promote the greenhouse effect, necessitating the installation of large air-conditioning systems. There are instead a wide variety of passive techniques which can be employed to prevent overheating, such as the use of solar shading and stack ventilation. However, in many buildings the use of these techniques alone is not enough to maintain a comfortable environment and so it is necessary to employ supplementary mechanical plant, to provide a mixed-mode solution. For example, while a naturally ventilated building may generally experience low levels of heat gain, in specific areas the heat gains may be high and so air conditioning may be required. It is therefore not uncommon to find 'low energy' buildings which exhibit both *passive* and *mechanical* characteristics.

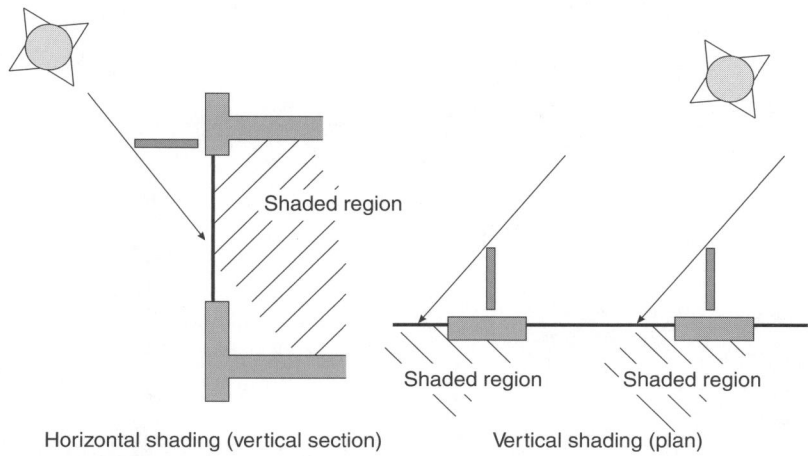

Horizontal shading (vertical section)   Vertical shading (plan)

FIG 15.7 External horizontal and vertical shading.

15.3.1 Shading Techniques

By far the best way of preventing overheating during the summer months, or indeed in any part of the year, is to employ adequate solar shading. It is far better to prevent solar radiation from entering a building than trying to deal with it once it has penetrated the building envelope. Shading techniques can broadly be classified as external, internal or mid-pane. External and, to a lesser extent, mid-pane shading techniques offer the best protection since they both prevent solar radiation from penetrating the building envelope. The use of internal shading measures, such as blinds, is much less effective, since although the blinds intercept the incoming solar radiation, they heat up and, in time, convect and radiate heat to the room space.

External shading can be extremely effective at preventing solar heat gains. By using external shades, such as fins, sails, balconies or even structural members, it is possible to achieve both a 'horizontal' and a 'vertical' shading effect (as shown in Figure 15.7). Vertical shading members, in particular, can be very useful since the sun moves through the sky in an arc from east to west and therefore for most of the time is not directly in front of any one window. However, external shading does have its downside. External shades and fins are exposed to the elements and therefore can deteriorate rapidly if not properly maintained. In addition, in city centre locations they can become colonized by pigeons.

Internal shading usually takes the form of horizontal, vertical or screen blinds which the building occupants can control. Although they are good at reducing instantaneous solar gains, they tend to warm up and emit heat into the room space. A compromise between external and internal shading is the use of blinds located in the air gap between the two panes of a double window (as shown in Figure 15.8). As the blinds warm up, heat is trapped in the window cavity and relatively little enters the room space. In some advanced window designs, the warm air produced in this cavity is vented either to outside or to the room space depending on whether additional heating or cooling is required (see Figure 15.8).

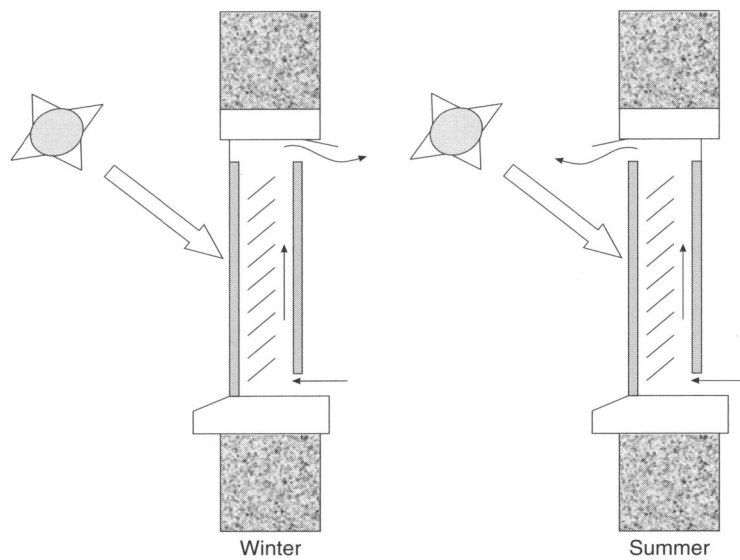

Winter   Summer

FIG 15.8 Mid-pane shading.

15.3.2 Solar Control Glazing

Figure 15.9 gives a breakdown of the component energy flows to and from a 6 mm clear float glass pane. It can be seen that approximately 78% of the incident solar radiation is transmitted directly through the glass, which explains why sunshine has such an instantaneous effect on the occupants of buildings. Approximately 7% of the incident radiation is reflected and the glass absorbs a further 15%. The heat which is absorbed warms up the glass and after a period of time the warm glass emits heat, both inwards and outwards, by radiation and convection.

It is possible to significantly reduce solar heat gains by using solar control glazing. This can be divided into two broad categories, solar absorbing and solar reflecting glass. Solar absorbing glass is body-tinted, typically bronze, grey, blue or green, using a variety of metal oxides. It works in a similar way to conventional sunglasses by reducing the overall transmission of solar radiation through the window. In doing so it also cuts down the transmission of light through the window. Solar absorbing glass exhibits much higher absorption properties than normal clear glass, with up to 70% absorption being achieved with bronze-tinted glass [7]. However, it should be noted that although much of the incident solar energy is absorbed, it is eventually re-emitted by the glass, with some of the re-emitted heat entering the interior of the building. Solar reflecting glass is, as the name suggests, highly reflective. The high reflection qualities of the glass are achieved by applying a thin layer of metal oxide to the external surface. Solar reflecting glass can be manufactured in a variety of colours, including silver, bronze, blue, green and grey. The mirrored surface of the glass reflects much of the solar radiation which falls on it and is more effective at cutting down the transmission of solar radiation than solar absorbing glass. It is important to note that this type of

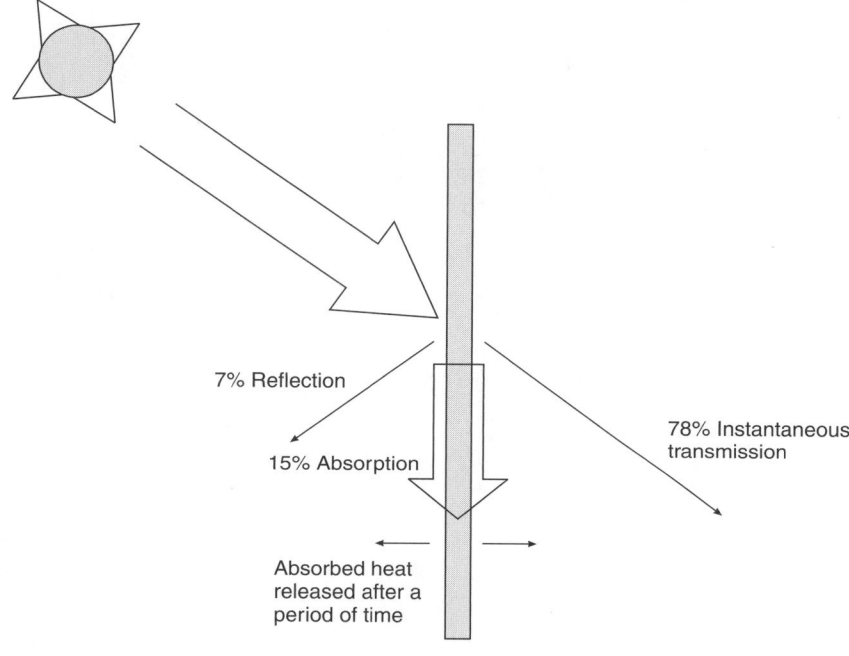

7% Reflection

15% Absorption

78% Instantaneous transmission

Absorbed heat released after a period of time

6 mm float glass

FIG 15.9 Radiation, reflection and absorption for 6 mm clear float glass.

glass reflects large quantities of solar radiation and that this can cause problems in surrounding buildings, which may overheat if care is not taken at the design stage.

15.3.3 Advanced Fenestration

One of the characteristics of many passive/mixed-mode buildings is the use of sophisticated fenestration systems to minimize solar heat gains. Windows in such buildings are often required to perform a number of different and sometimes conflicting tasks, including:

- Enabling daylight to enter the building
- Promoting natural ventilation
- Promoting solar heating
- Reducing solar heat gains
- Preventing the ingress of noise from outside
- Maintaining building security.

These tasks are usually achieved by installing complex window units, which incorporate some or all of the following features:

- Solar control glazing (e.g. solar reflecting or absorbing glass)
- External shading
- Internal or mid-pane blinds
- Openable windows or vents.

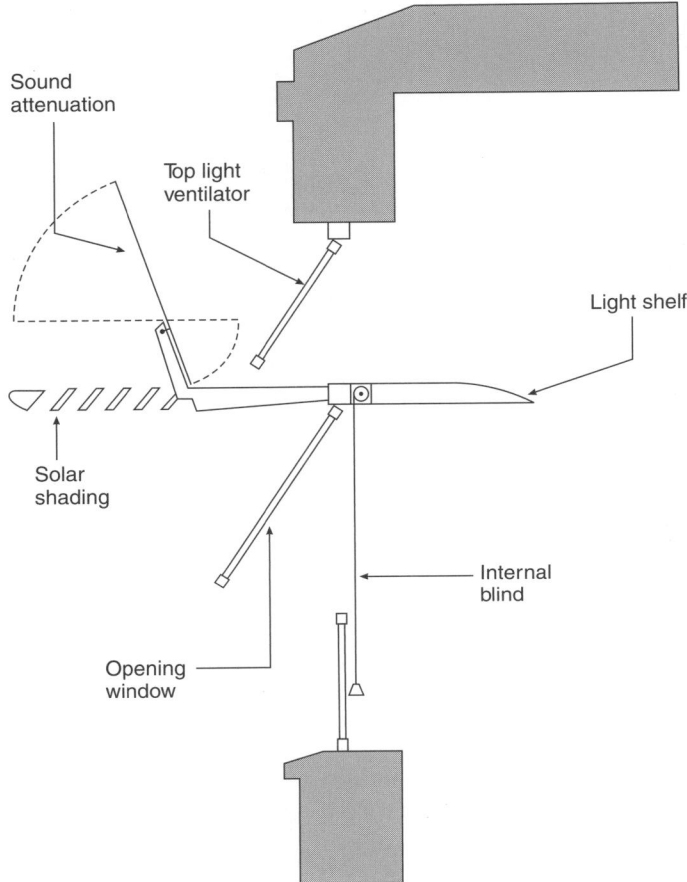

FIG 15.10 Typical advanced fenestration system.

In addition to the above features, many fenestration systems utilize light shelves to maximize daylight and minimize energy consumption on artificial lighting. Figure 15.10 shows a typical advanced fenestration system which might be found in a *passive* or *mixed-mode* building. Such fenestration systems are complex and resemble a 'Swiss army penknife'. It is important to appreciate the crucial role played by such windows. In many advanced naturally ventilated buildings the whole environmental control strategy is dependent on the successful operation of these complex windows. If for any reason they cannot be easily operated, the whole ventilation strategy becomes flawed and the internal environment may become uncomfortable.

15.3.4 Natural Ventilation

One of the key components of any *passive cooling* strategy is the use of natural ventilation, which can be divided into two basic strategies, cross-ventilation and buoyancy-driven (or stack) ventilation. Of the two strategies, stack ventilation is generally

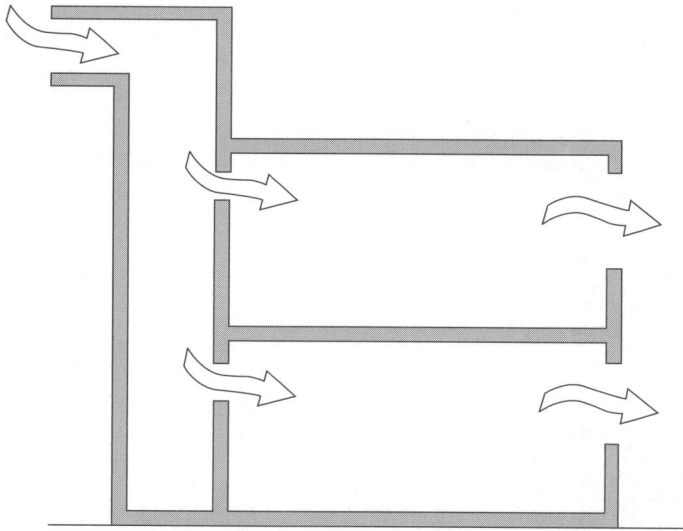

FIG 15.11 The use of a wind-scoop to produce cross-ventilation.

more predictable and more reliable than cross-ventilation. This is because, unlike cross-ventilation, stack ventilation is not dependent on wind speed or wind direction, both of which can be extremely variable. The use of stack ventilation is therefore more commonly found in passively controlled buildings than cross-ventilation.

Cross-ventilation occurs when openings are placed on opposite sides of a building, so that wind pressure pushes air through the room spaces. As air moves through a building it picks up heat and pollutants, and its temperature rises. This limits the width of room space which can effectively be cross-ventilated. It is recommended that plan width of a cross-ventilated space should not exceed five times the floor to ceiling height [10], which usually results in a maximum width of 14 m or 15 m. As a result of this, cross-ventilation tends to be restricted to buildings which have narrow plan widths.

Although cross-ventilation is normally achieved by opening windows, in hot desert countries, wind-scoops are often used (as shown in Figure 15.11). Wind-scoops capture the wind at high level and divert it through the occupied spaces in the building, thus cooling the interior. Wind-scoops can be particularly effective in regions where there is a dominant prevailing wind direction.

Stack ventilation relies on the fact that as air becomes warmer, its density decreases and it becomes more buoyant. As the name suggests, stack ventilation involves the creation of stacks or atria in buildings with vents at high level (as shown in Figure 15.12). As air becomes warmer due to internal and solar heat gains, it becomes more buoyant and thus rises up the stacks where it is exhausted at high level. In doing this a draught is created which draws in fresh air at low level to replace the warm air which has been displaced. Stack ventilation has the beauty of being self-regulating; when building heat gains are at their largest, the ventilation flow rate will be at its largest, due to the large buoyancy forces.

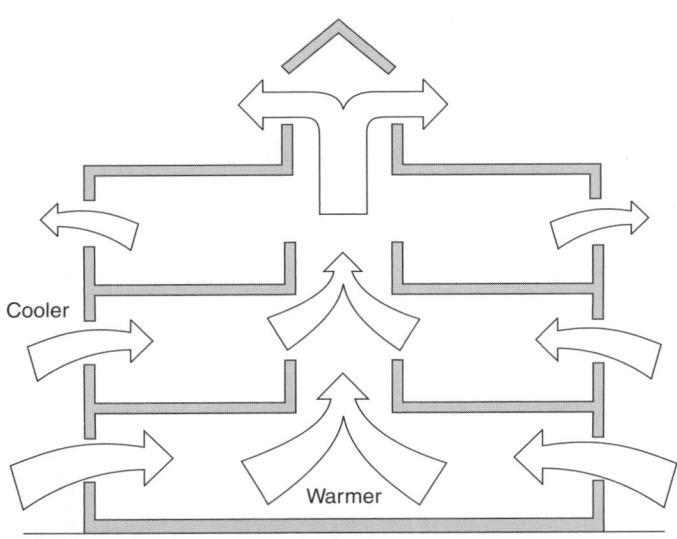

FIG 15.12 Stack ventilation.

The stack effect is driven by the pressure difference between air entering at low level and air leaving at high level. This can be calculated using eqn (15.1):

$$\text{Pressure difference, } \Delta P = gh(\rho_o - \rho_i) \tag{15.1}$$

where ΔP is the pressure difference between inlet and outlet (Pa), h is the height difference between inlet and outlet (m), ρ_i and ρ_o are the densities of air at inlet and outlet (kg/m³), and g is the acceleration due to gravity (i.e. 9.81 m/s²).

The density of air at any temperature can be determined using eqn (15.2):

$$\text{Density of air at temperature } t, \rho_t = 1.191 \times \frac{(273 + 20)}{(273 + t)} \tag{15.2}$$

where 1.191 kg/m³ is the density of air at 20°C. It can be seen from eqns (15.1) and (15.2) that the buoyancy force depends on the:

- Height difference between inlet and outlet vents.
- Temperature difference between the internal and external air.

The air volume flow rate drawn by the stack effect can be determined by:

$$V = C_d A_n \sqrt{[(2gh(\rho_o - \rho_t))/\rho_{av}]} \tag{15.3}$$

where V is the volume flow rate of air (m³/s), C_d is the coefficient of discharge of openings, A_n is the equivalent area of openings (m²), and ρ_{av} is the average density of air (kg/m³). The equivalent area of the openings (A_n) can be determined using eqn (15.4).

$$\frac{1}{(\Sigma A_n)^2} = \frac{1}{(\Sigma A_{in})^2} + \frac{1}{(\Sigma A_{out})^2} \tag{15.4}$$

where ΣA_{in} is the combined free area of inlet vents (m²), and ΣA_{out} is the combined free area of outlet vents (m²).

Example 15.1

A shopping mall is to be cooled using stack ventilation. The mall has vents at low level and in the roof. Given the below data, determine:

(i) The pressure difference driving the stack ventilation.
(ii) The ventilation air flow rate.
(iii) The cooling power produced by the stack ventilation.

Data:

    Free area of top vents = 12 m²
    Free area of lower vents = 6 m²
    Height difference between vents = 35 m
    Mean internal air temperature = 32°C
    External air temperature = 22°C
    Coefficient of discharge of openings is 0.61.

Solution

The equivalent area of openings is determined as follows:

$$\frac{1}{(\Sigma A_n)^2} = \frac{1}{6^2} + \frac{1}{12^2}$$

Therefore,

$$\Sigma A_n = 5.367 \ m^2$$

The density of air at 22°C is

$$\rho_{22} = 1.191 \times \frac{(273 + 20)}{(273 + 22)} = 1.183 \ kg/m^3$$

The density of air at 32°C is

$$\rho_{32} = 1.191 \times \frac{(273 + 20)}{(273 + 32)} = 1.144 \ kg/m^3$$

(i) The pressure difference can be determined by using eqn (15.1):

$$Pressure \ difference = 9.81 \times 35 \times (1.183 - 1.144) = 13.4 \ Pa$$

(ii) The volume flow rate can be determined by using eqn (15.3):

$$Volume \ flow \ rate = 0.61 \times 5.367 \times \sqrt{\frac{2 \times 13.4}{0.5 \times (1.183 + 1.144)}} = 15.71 \ m^3/s$$

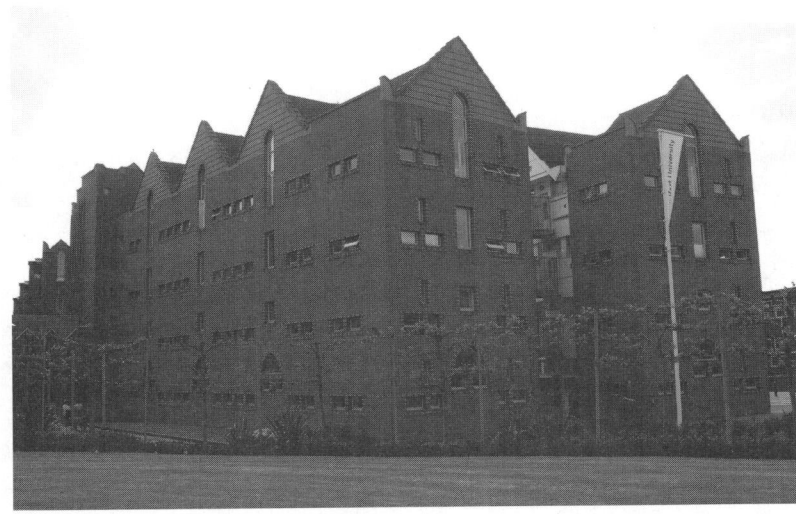

FIG 15.13 Queen's Building at De Montfort University, Leicester.

(iii)   Cooling power $= \dot{m} C_p (t_i - t_o)$

where $\dot{m}$ is the mass flow rate of air (kg/s), C_p is the specific heat capacity of air (i.e. 1.025 kJ/kg K), and t_i and t_o are the internal and external air temperatures (°C).

Therefore,

$$\text{Cooling power} = 15.71 \times [0.5 \times (1.183 + 1.144)] \times 1.025 \times (32 - 22) = 187.36 \text{ kW}$$

When employing stack ventilation it is important to remember that the stack effect diminishes the further up the building one goes, because the height difference reduces. The air inlet sizes must therefore increase as one travels up a building in order to maintain the same volume flow rate at each floor level. Because the stack effect diminishes towards the top of a building, it is often worth considering an alternative method of ventilation on upper floors.

15.3.5 Thermal Mass

During the 1990s in Europe and the UK a new generation of low energy buildings was constructed, which made extensive use of thermally massive surfaces. Two of the finest examples of these buildings are the Queen's Building at De Montfort University, Leicester [8,9] (see Figure 15.13) and the Elizabeth Fry Building at the University of East Anglia [10] (see Figure 15.14). These buildings use thermal mass as an integral part of their environmental control strategy to produce a thermally stable internal environment.

Thermal mass can be utilized in buildings to perform three separate, but interrelated, roles:

- Mass can be added to the building envelope to create thermal inertia, which damps down the extremes of the external environment.

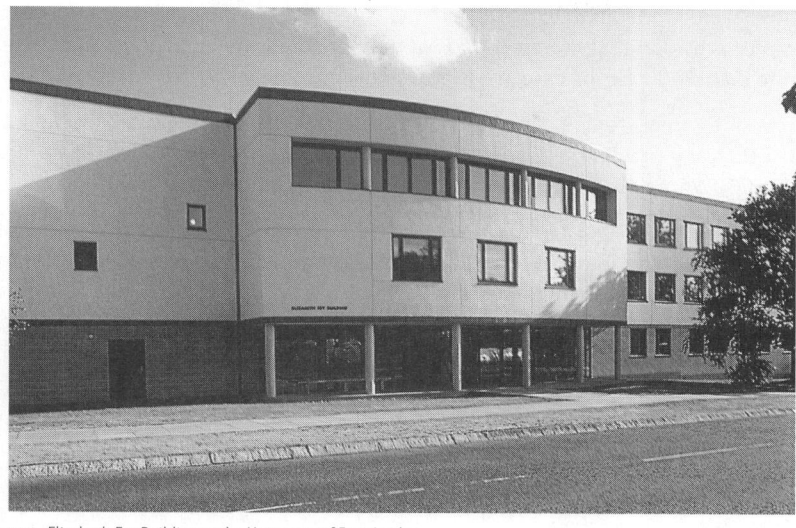

FIG 15.14 Elizabeth Fry Building at the University of East Anglia.

- Exposed mass can be added internally to create a high-admittance environment which is thermally stable.
- Mass can be added either separately or to the building structure to create a thermal store which can be used to cool buildings.

One unique feature of many 'high mass/low energy' buildings is their use of exposed mass to create a high-admittance internal environment. In most buildings the widespread use of suspended ceilings and carpets effectively converts otherwise thermally heavyweight structures into thermally lightweight ones, creating a low-admittance environment which is poor at absorbing heat energy. Surface temperatures tend to rise in such buildings, making it necessary to get rid of heat gains as they occur. This is one of the main reasons why air conditioning has become a requirement in so many office buildings. However, by exposing the mass of the building structure it is possible to form a high-admittance environment, which can successfully be utilized to combat overheating.

The creation of a high-admittance environment has implications on the comfort of occupants. It can be seen from the discussion in Sections 10.2 and 13.7 that it is the *dry resultant temperature* and not the air temperature which is critical to human comfort. Provided that room air velocities are less than 0.1 m/s, dry resultant temperature can be expressed as:

$$\text{Dry resultant temperature } t_{res} = 0.5t_a + 0.5t_r \qquad (15.5)$$

where t_r is the mean radiant temperature (°C), and t_a is the air temperature (°C).

By exposing the mass of the building structure it is possible to create a high-admittance environment and thus reduce the *mean radiant temperature* and the dry resultant temperature of the internal space. Given that the dry resultant temperature is the average of the sum of the air temperature and the mean radiant temperature, it is possible to allow the internal air temperature to rise in summer without any noticeable discomfort to the occupants, provided that the mean radiant temperature is maintained at a lower temperature than would be the case in a conventional building with suspended ceilings.

In terms of thermal storage capacity, floors are by far the single most important element within any building. A 50 mm deep 'skin' of exposed concrete can store in the region of 32 Wh/m^2 °C, giving it considerable potential to provide cooling, if utilized correctly.

Buildings with a high mass envelope are extremely good at reducing peak solar heat gains, because the mass increases the thermal inertia of the building. With heavy masonry walls the time lag between the incident solar radiation occurring on the external face and the heat being conducted to the interior is often in excess of 12 hours. The overall effect is therefore to dampen down the internal diurnal temperature range, thus minimizing peak heat gains. This results in a reduction in the required capacity of any air-conditioning plant which may have to be installed.

15.3.6 Night Venting

While the use of exposed concrete floor soffits may result in a high-admittance environment, problems can still arise if the structure is not periodically purged of heat. This is because the mean radiant temperature will steadily rise as the floors absorb more and more heat, until conditions become unacceptable. One effective low cost method by which heat can be purged from a building structure is by night venting. In terms of heat removal capability, ventilation is at its least effective during the daytime, when the difference in temperature between the interior of a building and the external ambient is small. In heavyweight buildings, night ventilation is much more beneficial, since the temperature differentials are much greater than during the daytime.

Therefore, with night venting it is possible to make the building structure cool, enabling the occupants and equipment to radiate heat to the exposed soffits of the floor slabs.

Night venting involves passing cool outside air over or under the exposed concrete floor slabs so that good heat transfer occurs. This can be done either by natural or by mechanical means. At its most rudimentary night venting may simply entail the opening of windows at night (see Figure 15.15), while a more sophisticated approach may involve a dedicated mechanical night ventilation system and the use of floor voids (see Figure 15.16). If floor voids are used in conjunction with a night venting scheme, then the cool slab can be used to pre-cool the supply air prior to its introduction to the room spaces. In addition, the use of a floor void allows displacement ventilation to be utilized.

15.3.7 Termodeck

When creating a night venting scheme it is important to ensure good thermal coupling between the air and the mass of the concrete floor, and also that fan powers are kept to a minimum. One system which achieves this objective well is the Swedish Termodeck hollow concrete floor slab system.

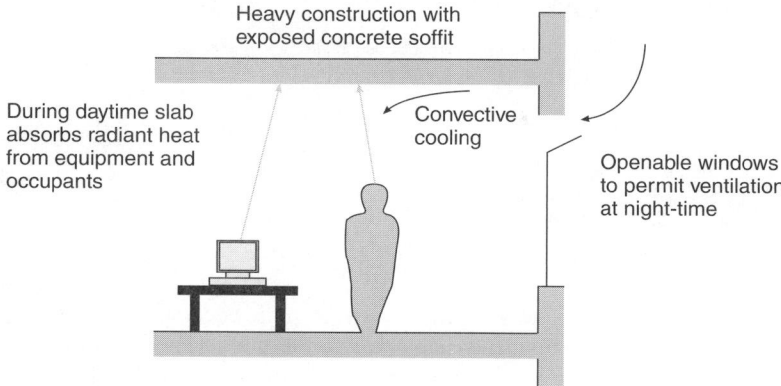

Heavy construction with exposed concrete soffit

During daytime slab absorbs radiant heat from equipment and occupants

Convective cooling

Openable windows to permit ventilation at night-time

FIG 15.15   Simple night venting scheme in which the windows are opened during the night.

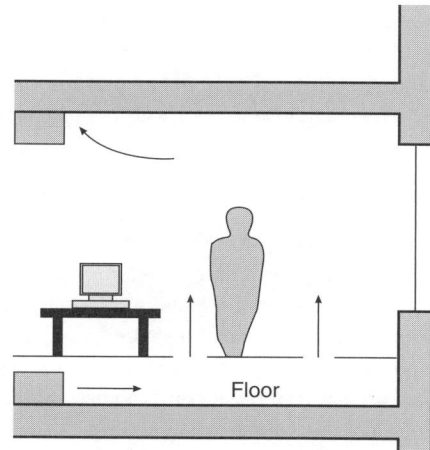

Floor

FIG 15.16   Night venting scheme where the ventilation air is introduced through floor void.

The Termodeck system has been used successfully in many locations throughout northern Europe and in the UK, notably in the Elizabeth Fry Building [10] and the Kimberlin Library Building at De Montfort University [11]. The Termodeck system ensures good thermal coupling between the air and the building mass by pushing ventilation air through the hollow cores in proprietary concrete floor slabs (as shown in Figure 15.17). By forming perpendicular coupling airways between the hollow cores, it is possible to form a 3 or 5 pass circuit through which supply air may pass, thus ensuring good heat transfer. During periods in which cooling is required, outside air at ambient temperature is blown through the hollow core slabs for almost 24 hours of the day. Overnight, the slab is cooled to approximately 18–20°C, so that during the daytime the incoming fresh air is pre-cooled by the slab before entering the room space. By exposing the soffit of the slab it is also possible to absorb heat radiated from occupants and equipment within the space.

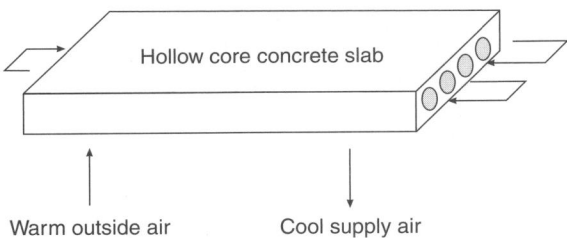

Warm outside air   Cool supply air

FIG 15.17 The Termodeck system.

The Termodeck system is particularly worthy of note because it produces buildings which are extremely thermally stable and comfortable without the need for any refrigeration. The example of the Elizabeth Fry Building illustrates this fact very well. In a study of low energy buildings in the UK [12], the performance of the Elizabeth Fry Building was outstanding. This building achieved the highest comfort score, while at the same time being one of the lowest consumers of energy; its electrical energy consumption in 1997 was only 61 kWh/m^2 and the normalized gas consumption for that year was 37 kWh/m^2 [10], which compares very favourably with the corresponding values of 128 kWh/m^2 and 97 kWh/m^2 set out in *Energy Consumption Guide 19* for good practice air-conditioned office buildings in the UK [13].

15.4 Building Form

The decision to utilize a passive environmental control strategy can put severe constraints on overall building form. For example, if natural ventilation is used to promote air movement, it will inevitably lead to the creation of a narrow plan building, unless atria or central ventilation stacks are used. This is because passive buildings are supposed to be climate responsive. Therefore the further an internal space is from an external surface, the less chance there is of harnessing the natural resources of the external environment. The use of a passive solar heating strategy also results in a narrow plan building, but with large areas of south-facing glazing. For this reason, passive solar heating schemes tend to be restricted to small- and medium-sized buildings. It is very difficult to use passive solar heating effectively on large deep plan buildings, not least because such buildings tend to overheat for large parts of the year and thus primarily need to be defended against solar heat gains.

Because larger commercial and public buildings generally experience overheating problems, when a passive strategy is applied to the design of these buildings it is usually a cooling/natural ventilation strategy rather than a solar heating one. This means that these so-called *advanced naturally ventilated* buildings all tend to utilize the same generic design strategies and technologies. Broadly speaking, these generic technologies/strategies are as follows:

- The use of a heavily insulated outer envelope.
- The use of carefully designed and often complex fenestration, which minimizes solar gains and building heat losses, whilst maximizing daylight penetration. It is also a requirement that the windows can be opened.

- The use of stacks or atria to promote stack ventilation.
- The use of night ventilation to purge the building structure of the heat accumulated during the daytime.
- The careful use of exposed building mass to dampen down swings in internal space temperature, and to promote radiant and convective cooling.

One of the characteristics of these advanced naturally ventilated buildings is that they often have complex façades with openable windows, vents, blinds, external shades and even light shelves. These façades incorporate advanced fenestration systems which have many moving parts and which are often controlled by a building management system (BMS). Such complex façades are necessary because the absence of internal mechanical services forces the external skin of the building to become the primary climate modifier and to perform a wide variety of tasks (e.g. daylighting, defending against solar radiation, ventilation and preventing the ingress of external noise). By creating a complex skin, the designers of such buildings are effectively distributing 'complexity' all around the building rather than concentrating it in a central plant room. This degree of complexity in the skin can have a considerable impact on both the performance of the occupants and the facilities management regime which must be adopted.

In contrast to advanced naturally ventilated buildings, the use of a mechanical ventilation system offers considerably more flexibility and enables deeper plans to be utilized. In this respect, the Termodeck system appears to offer great potential, as it facilitates good thermal coupling between the air and the building mass without the need for a particularly complex façade or an open plan interior.

The use of the generic passive technologies/strategies described above puts constraints on building design and dictates the building form. With larger buildings the use of natural ventilation often results in buildings which have atria. These buildings comprise a narrow rectangular plan wrapped around an atrium, which gives the appearance of a deep plan building. Vents in the top of the atrium are used to promote buoyancy-driven ventilation and air is drawn through vents or windows in the façade. As a result, passively cooled and ventilated buildings tend to look similar to each other, characterized by the use of atria or stacks and complex façade. Figures 15.18–15.21 show sections through four recently constructed passively cooled buildings in the UK: the Learning Resource Centre at Anglia Polytechnic University, Chelmsford; the Ionica Headquarters, Cambridge; the Inland Revenue Headquarters, Nottingham; and the School of Engineering, De Montfort University, Leicester.

It can be seen from the illustrations above that all four buildings exhibit many similarities. In the Anglia Polytechnic and Ionica buildings the designers have used atria to produce buoyancy-driven ventilation, whereas in the other two buildings purposely built stacks have been employed. Table 15.1 summarizes the features of all four buildings.

It should be noted that although some of the above buildings, especially the De Montfort building, do not appear to be narrow plan, from a ventilation point of view they are all narrow plan buildings. The practical maximum width of space which can be naturally ventilated is approximately 15 m. This dimension limits the form of the building to a narrow plan format. Nevertheless, by constructing a narrow plan rectangular

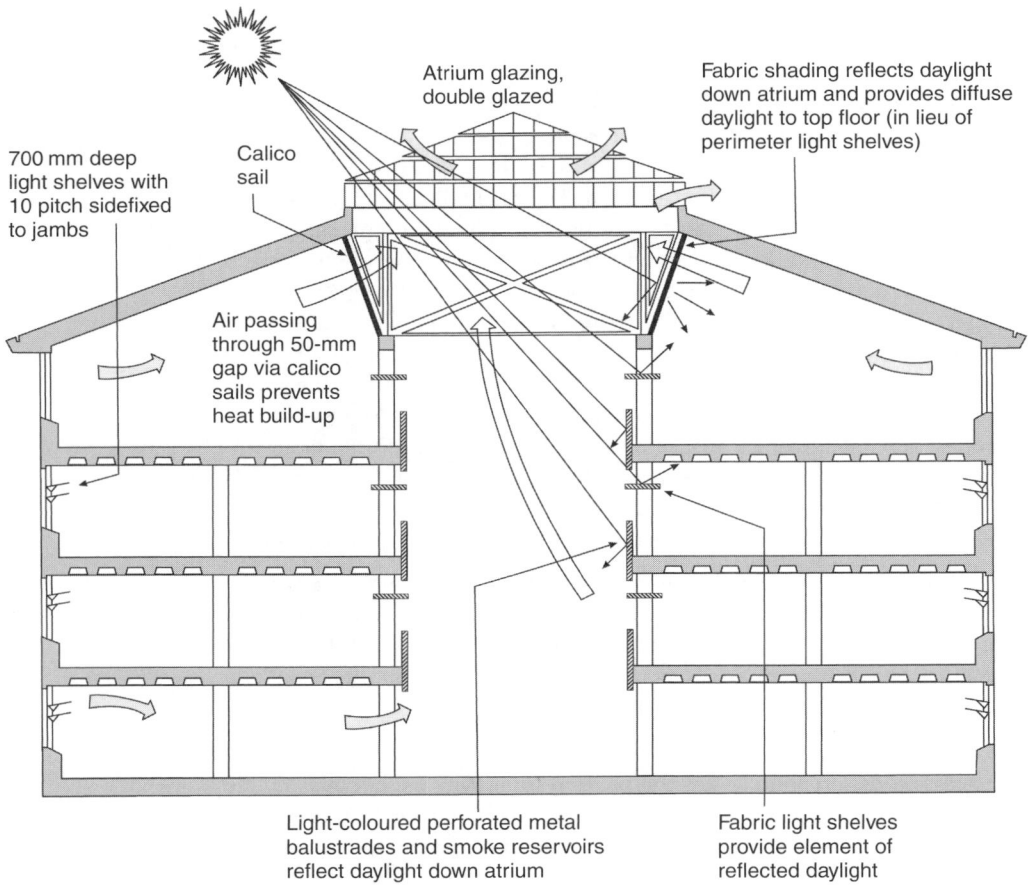

700 mm deep
light shelves with
10 pitch sidefixed
to jambs

Calico
sail

Atrium glazing,
double glazed

Fabric shading reflects daylight
down atrium and provides diffuse
daylight to top floor (in lieu of
perimeter light shelves)

Air passing
through 50-mm
gap via calico
sails prevents
heat build-up

Light-coloured perforated metal
balustrades and smoke reservoirs
reflect daylight down atrium

Fabric light shelves
provide element of
reflected daylight

FIG 15.18 Learning Resource Centre at Anglia Polytechnic University, Chelmsford [8].

building around an atrium, which is essentially a glass-covered courtyard, it is possible to achieve the appearance of a deep plan building. In the case of the De Montfort building, the deeper plan is achieved by putting ventilation stacks in the middle of the building.

15.5 Building Operation

The use of a passive environmental control strategy not only affects overall building form, it can also have a considerable impact on the operation of buildings and the performance of their occupants, especially if the building is large and naturally ventilated. By relying on a sophisticated envelope as the primary climate modifier and taking a minimalist approach to the mechanical building services, designers of such buildings need to be careful that they do not create an environment which hinders the performance of the occupants. Although designers may feel that they have produced a comfortable low energy building, the reality may be that it is detracting from the occupier's core business, rather than adding to it. With this in mind, it should be remembered that

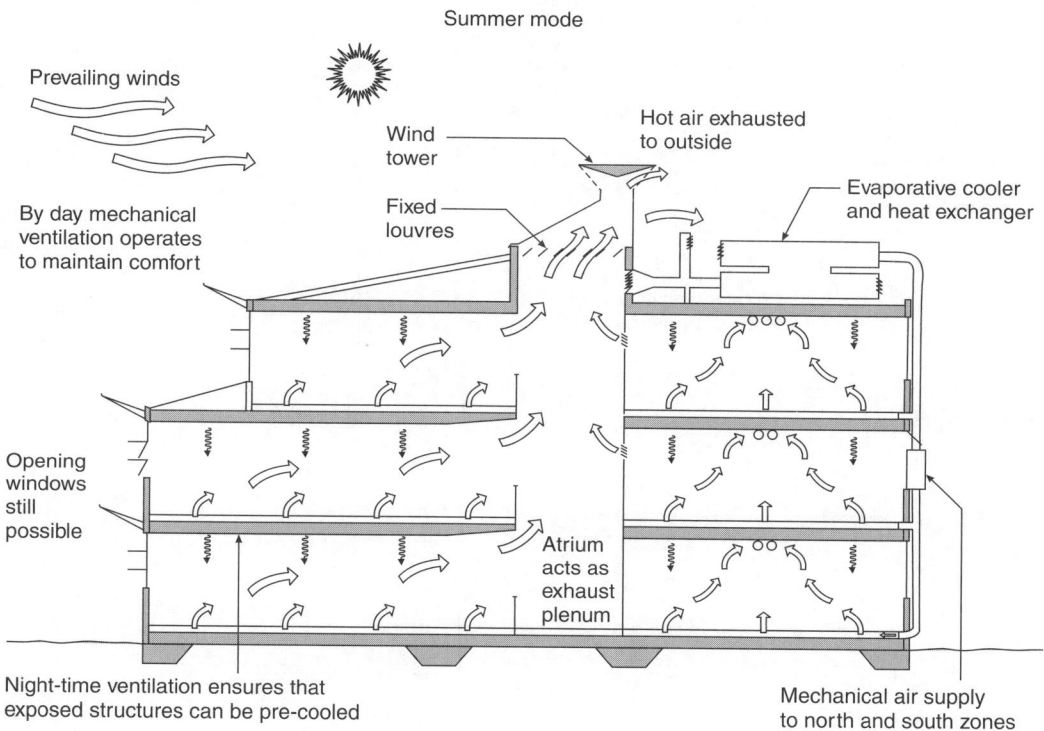

Summer mode

Prevailing winds

Wind tower

Hot air exhausted to outside

Evaporative cooler and heat exchanger

By day mechanical ventilation operates to maintain comfort

Fixed louvres

Opening windows still possible

Atrium acts as exhaust plenum

Night-time ventilation ensures that exposed structures can be pre-cooled

Mechanical air supply to north and south zones

FIG 15.19 Ionica Headquarters, Cambridge [8].

any property which gets a reputation for being uncomfortable, or unfit for its purpose, is unlikely to gain in value [14].

A study of prominent low energy buildings in the UK [12] found that higher levels of occupant satisfaction were easier to achieve in buildings which exhibited:

- A narrow plan form.
- Cellularization of working spaces.
- A high thermal mass.
- Stable and thermally comfortable conditions.
- Control of air infiltration.
- Openable windows close to users.
- A view out.
- Effective and clear controls.

Conversely, occupant satisfaction was harder to achieve in buildings which exhibited:

- A deep plan form.
- Open work areas.
- The presence of complex and unfamiliar technology.
- Situations where occupants had little control over their environment.
- High and intrusive noise levels.

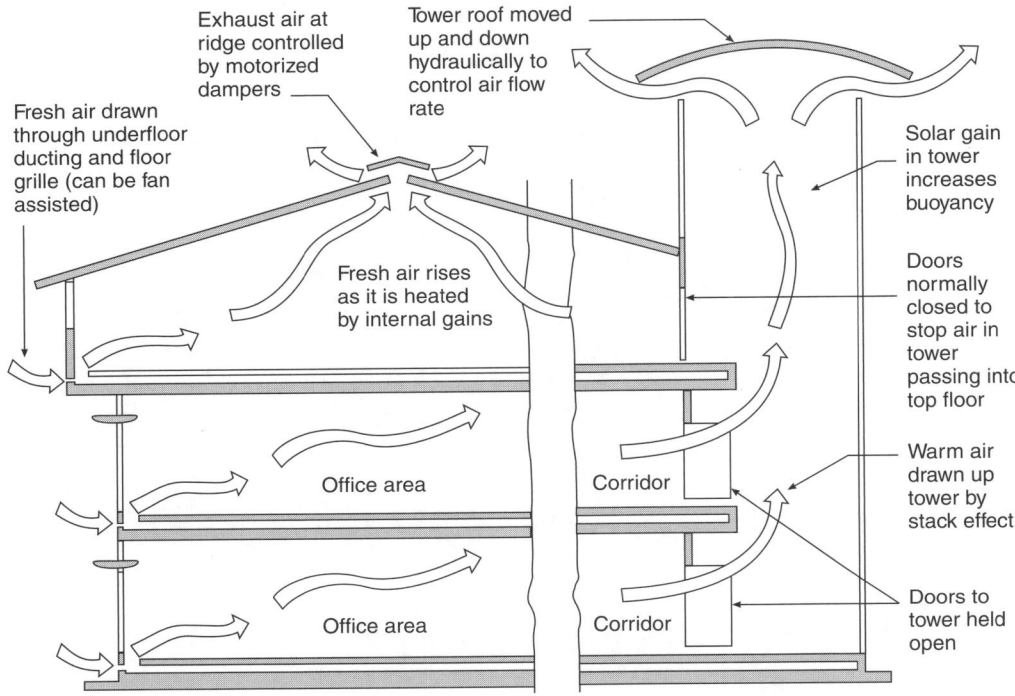

Exhaust air at ridge controlled by motorized dampers

Tower roof moved up and down hydraulically to control air flow rate

Fresh air drawn through underfloor ducting and floor grille (can be fan assisted)

Solar gain in tower increases buoyancy

Fresh air rises as it is heated by internal gains

Doors normally closed to stop air in tower passing into top floor

Office area

Corridor

Warm air drawn up tower by stack effect

Office area

Corridor

Doors to tower held open

FIG 15.20 Inland Revenue Headquarters, Nottingham [8].

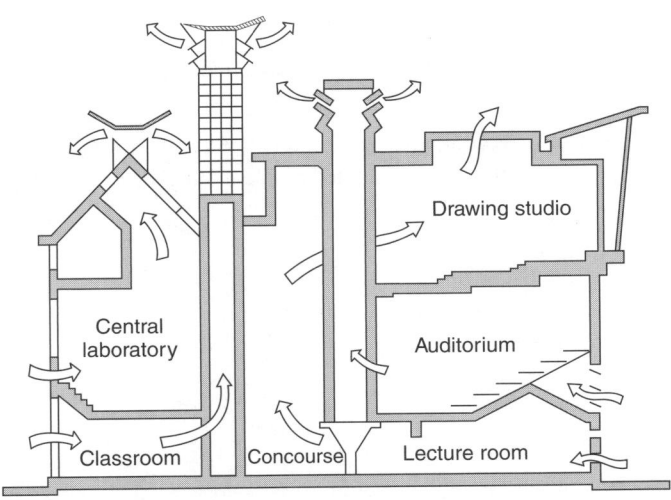

Drawing studio

Central laboratory

Auditorium

Classroom

Concourse

Lecture room

FIG 15.21 School of Engineering (Queen's Building), De Montfort University, Leicester [8].

Inspection of the above lists reveals a fairly consistent picture; in short, people prefer to work close to a window, which they can open, in a quiet cellular office space, which is thermally stable and comfortable. When these criteria are viewed in the context of passive buildings, a mixed picture emerges. Clearly, in some respects *passive* buildings are

TABLE 15.1   Summary of characteristics of sample buildings [8]

Building	Atrium or stacks	Complex windows with shading	Night venting	Exposed high mass soffits	Light shelves	Energy consumed per year (KWh/m²/year)
Anglia Polytechnic University	Atrium	Yes	Yes	Yes	Yes	82
Ionica Headquarters	Atrium	Yes	Yes	Yes	No	64
Inland Revenue Headquarters	Stacks	Yes	Yes	Yes	Yes	89
De Montfort University	Stacks	No	Yes	Yes	Yes	120

very positive since they tend to provide a high-admittance environment which is thermally stable and comfortable. In other respects they are not so beneficial. Many larger advanced naturally ventilated buildings have large open plan internal spaces because central atria or vent stacks are used. In these buildings many occupants are inevitably located some distance from the windows and therefore have little control over their environment. In addition, the use of large spaces and acoustically hard surfaces can lead to noise problems. Indeed, noise problems have been highlighted as a particular difficulty in advanced naturally ventilated buildings [12]. Given this, and the other reasons mentioned above, it is not surprising that some advanced naturally ventilated buildings display low levels of occupant comfort and productivity [12,15].

The complex nature of the fenestration required in advanced naturally ventilated buildings can be the cause of numerous problems and is therefore worthy of closer inspection. The issue of who has control over the opening of windows is of particular importance. In large naturally ventilated buildings, particularly those which require night ventilation, the function of the whole environmental control strategy can be impaired if, for any reason, certain windows are not opened. Consequently, BMS are often used to control the operation of windows, as the occupants cannot be relied upon to open the windows when required. This automatically brings the user into conflict with the BMS system with the result that occupants sitting near windows may be unable to shut the windows when they experience a draught, or conversely, open them when they feel too hot. If a BMS system is not used, issues of conflict can still arise when, for example, the occupants next to the windows may close them in situations where those requiring ventilation in the centre of the building need them to be open. The use of complex fenestration systems, with many moving parts, can also result in poor window sealing over a period of time, resulting in unwanted air infiltration.

From a maintenance point of view, complex fenestration can cause problems. The use of external shading and the numerous protruding and moving parts in these fenestration systems means that they are prone to mechanical damage and are difficult to clean. The manufacturers of these systems go to considerable effort to reduce potential cleaning difficulties, but it still remains true that from a facilities management point of view these systems need considerably more attention than conventional windows. A study by Kendrick and Martin has shown that the windows most suited for night venting and BMS system control (i.e. high level top hung and hopper windows) are the most difficult to clean from inside [16]. These advanced fenestration systems have important implications on the flexibility and day-to-day operation of the office space. They are required to be opened by the occupants and are designed to be cleaned from inside. Any desks, bookcases or benches against the external wall inhibit both the ability of the occupants to regulate their environment by opening windows, and the ability to clean and maintain the windows. Consequently, some facilities managers faced with this problem have opted for a 'furniture-free' zone next to the windows, or else have installed movable furniture next to the windows. While making the cleaning of windows easy, such a policy can hardly be considered to be designed to increase the comfort and productivity of building occupants. In addition, forcing the occupants away from the windows means that the potential daylighting zone is reduced and thus more people have to rely on artificial lighting, which in energy efficiency terms is very counterproductive.

Both developers and building tenants desire buildings which contain flexible space capable of being adapted to meet the evolving needs of organizations. This need for flexibility/adaptability has traditionally been resolved by designing deep open plan buildings. From a facilities management viewpoint the use of an advanced natural ventilation strategy imposes severe constraints on the flexibility of the working space. In particular, it is extremely difficult to partition off internal spaces in such buildings because:

- The insertion of full-height partitions may restrict or prevent air movement through the space, thus nullifying its environmental performance.
- It may be difficult to create an acceptable environment within any partitioned office spaces that are created. In a conventional office space it is possible to 'tap' into the nearest mechanical ventilation duct in the ceiling to serve a new space. In a naturally ventilated high mass building there may well be no ceiling and no mechanical ventilation services in the floor. This makes it difficult to adequately ventilate partitioned spaces.
- The lack of a suspended ceiling can lead to flexibility problems when repositioning luminaires.
- In many advanced high mass buildings the exposed floor soffits are formed by deeply recessed concrete floor beams. The geometry of these floor beams can create problems when erecting partitions.

Even if full-height partitions are not installed, the environmental performance of a naturally ventilated space may still be impaired by the insertion of high screens and furniture, which restrict the air flow and thus create 'dead' spots.

From the discussion above it is tempting to conclude that all *passive* and *mixed-mode* buildings result in operational difficulties. However, this is not the case. The example of the Elizabeth Fry Building, which utilizes the Termodeck system, clearly demonstrates that high mass *mixed-mode* buildings can be very successful. Of all the buildings surveyed in the UK study [12], it was the Elizabeth Fry Building which was outstanding. This building achieved the highest comfort score, while at the same time being one of the lowest consumers of energy. Of particular note is the fact that the building produced an extremely stable thermal environment and comfortable internal temperatures during summer without the need for any refrigeration, clearly demonstrating the success of the fabric thermal storage strategy. The reasons for its success are that the building:

- Is thermally stable and comfortable
- Has cellular work spaces
- Has a relatively narrow plan
- Is well sealed and has tight control over air infiltration
- Has windows which can be opened by the occupants.

These are all qualities which tend to promote user comfort and enhance productivity. When the Elizabeth Fry Building is compared with less successful advanced naturally ventilated buildings, it can be seen that its success lies in the fact that the Termodeck system is much more unobtrusive and flexible than the more rigid requirements of the naturally ventilated buildings. For example, the use of mechanical ventilation and hollow core slabs means that the façade of the building can be relatively simple, which frees up the windows so that they can be opened at will by the occupants without impairing the thermal performance of the building. The use of a mechanical ventilation system allows the internal space to be sub-divided into cellular rooms, something which is difficult to achieve in advanced naturally ventilated buildings. It also allows flexibility in the shape and form of the building. Unlike the advanced naturally ventilated buildings where 'complexity' is distributed around the skin of a building, the Termodeck system concentrates 'complexity' in a central plant room where it can easily be controlled and maintained.

References

[1]   Bordass WT, Entwistle MJ, Willis STP. Naturally ventilated and mixed-mode office buildings – opportunities and pitfalls. CIBSE National Conference, Brighton; 1994.
[2]   CIBSE Guide A2, Weather and solar data; 1982.
[3]   Hui HF, Fong T, Lai KW. Passive solar design in architecture. Hong Kong: The Hong Kong University; 1996.
[4]   Vale B, Vale R. Green architecture – design for a sustainable future. London: Thames and Hudson; 1991.
[5]   Mazria E. The passive solar energy book. Emmaus, PA: Rodale Press; 1979.
[6]   Lebens RM. Passive solar heating design. London: Applied Science Publishers; 1980.
[7]   Environmental control glasses, Pilkington.
[8]   Natural ventilation in non-domestic buildings. CIBSE Application Manual AM10; 1997.
[9]   Bunn R. Learning curve. Building Serv J 1993;October:20–25.
[10] Standeven M, Cohen R, Bordass B, Leaman A. PROBE 14: Elizabeth Fry building. Building Serv J 1998;April:37–42.
[11] Bunn R. Cool desking. Building Serv J 1998;October:16–20.
[12] Bordass W, Leaman A, Ruyssevelt P. PROBE strategic review: Report 4 – Strategic conclusions: Department of the Environment, Transport and the Regions; 1999 August.
[13] Energy use in offices. Energy Consumption Guide 19, Department of the Environment, Transport and the Regions; 1997.
[14] Beggs CB, Moodley K. Facilities management of passively controlled buildings. Facilities 1997;15(9/10):233–40. September/October.
[15] Leaman A. Comfort and joy. Building Serv J 1999;June:33–34.
[16] Kendrick C, Martin A. Refurbishment: The natural way. CIBSE J 1996;November:29.

Bibliography

Bordass W, Leaman A, Ruyssevelt P. PROBE strategic review: Report 4 – Strategic conclusions: Department of the Environment, Transport and the Regions; 1999 August.

Hill R, O'Keefe P, Snape C. The future of energy use (Chapter 7): Earthscan; 1995.

Natural ventilation in non-domestic buildings. CIBSE Application Manual AM10; 1997.

Vale B, Vale R. Green architecture – Design for a sustainable future. London: Thames and Hudson; 1991.

APPENDIX 1

Degree Days

A1.1 Heating Degree Days

The concept of *degree days* was first developed about 100 years ago for use in horticulture [1]. Nowadays, however, degree days are generally used to predict heating energy consumption in buildings. They provide building designers with a useful measure of the variation in outside temperature, which enables energy consumption to be related to prevailing weather conditions.

It is not difficult to appreciate that in a cold month such as January, a given building will consume more heating energy than in a warmer month such as March. This is because:

- the outside air temperature is likely to be colder during January than in March
- lower air temperatures are likely to persist for longer in January compared with that in March.

From this it can be seen that heat energy consumption relates both to the degree of coldness and the duration of that coldness. The degree day method allows for both these factors by setting a base outside air temperature, above which most domestic and commercial buildings do not require any heating. In the UK this base temperature is generally taken to be 15.5°C. If the average outside air temperature on any given day is below the base temperature, then heating will be required. However, the heat energy consumption in any given period is dependent not only on the magnitude of the temperature differential but also on its duration. For example, if an outside air temperature of 14.5°C prevails for 24 hours, then a deficit of 1°C will have been maintained for 1 day and 1 degree day will have been accrued. If the outside temperature remains at 14.5°C for each day of a week, then a total of 7 degree days will be accumulated. Similarly, if an outside air temperature of 10.5°C is maintained for 1 week then 35 degree days will be accumulated.

By summating the daily temperature deficits over any given month it is possible to calculate cumulative degree days for that particular month. Therefore, by monitoring daily outside air temperature, it is possible to produce tables of monthly heating degree days for various locations, which can be used by building designers and operators to estimate heating loads. For example, if a particular building experiences 346 heating degree days in January and only 286 in March, it is reasonable to assume that heating fuel consumption in January should be 1.21 times that for March.

Monthly and annual degree day figures are published in many sources. Table A1.1 shows 20-year average heating degree day data for the various geographical regions of the UK.

A1.2 Changing the Base Temperature

In the UK, degree day data are generally produced for a base temperature of 15.5°C. However, other countries may use different base temperatures. Indeed, in the UK the National Health Service uses an alternative base temperature of 18.5°C. It may therefore be necessary to convert data quoted at 15.5°C to another base temperature. This can be done with relative accuracy by using Hitchin's formula [1] below:

$$\text{Average degree days per day} = \frac{(t_b - t_o)}{1 - e^{-k(t_b - t_o)}}$$

where t_b is the base temperature (°C), t_o is the mean air temperature in the month (°C), and k is the constant.

The value of 'k' varies slightly with location and must be determined from 20-year weather data. However, a general k value of 0.71 can be assumed for most locations in the UK [1].

A1.3 Cooling Degree Days

Heating degree days are of considerable use when estimating and monitoring the energy consumption of non-air conditioned buildings. However, for air-conditioned buildings they are only of limited value. Consequently, the concept of the *cooling degree day* was developed.

TABLE A1.1 UK 20-year average heating degree day data to base 15.5°C [2]

Region	Jan	Feb	Mar	April	May	June	July	Aug	Sept	Oct	Nov	Dec	Average
Thames valley	346	322	286	205	120	51	22	25	54	130	242	312	2115
South eastern	368	344	312	233	150	74	39	44	82	160	267	334	2407
Southern	345	327	301	229	148	72	39	43	79	150	251	312	2296
South western	293	285	271	207	137	63	28	28	55	116	206	258	1947
Severn valley	321	305	280	201	128	56	24	27	61	138	237	300	2078
Midland	376	359	322	243	162	83	44	48	90	178	275	343	2523
West Pennines	361	340	312	230	144	75	38	39	78	157	267	328	2369
North western	375	345	323	245	167	90	50	56	96	171	284	341	2543
Borders	376	349	330	271	206	117	66	68	104	182	282	339	2690
North eastern	381	358	322	247	168	87	46	49	88	175	281	346	2548
East Pennines	372	352	313	232	154	78	42	44	81	165	272	341	2446
East Anglia	378	349	317	239	149	73	40	39	71	154	269	341	2419
West Scotland	383	352	328	246	170	94	58	64	111	188	299	352	2645
East Scotland	388	357	332	263	197	109	62	67	109	192	301	354	2731
North East Scotland	401	368	346	277	206	120	74	78	127	203	311	362	2873
Wales	330	320	307	240	170	92	49	45	77	145	235	294	2304
Northern Ireland	365	334	320	242	171	92	53	59	99	173	282	329	2519

Cooling degree days are defined as 'the mean number of degrees by which the outside temperature on a given day exceeds the base temperature, totalled for all the days in the period' [1].

There is, however, no general consensus on the base temperature that should be used for calculating cooling degree days and many users still use a 15.5°C base [1].

References

Degree days. Fuel Efficiency Booklet 7, Department of the Environment; 1993.
Energy audits and surveys. CIBSE Applications Manual AM5; 1991.

APPENDIX 2

Pressure–enthalpy diagram for R22

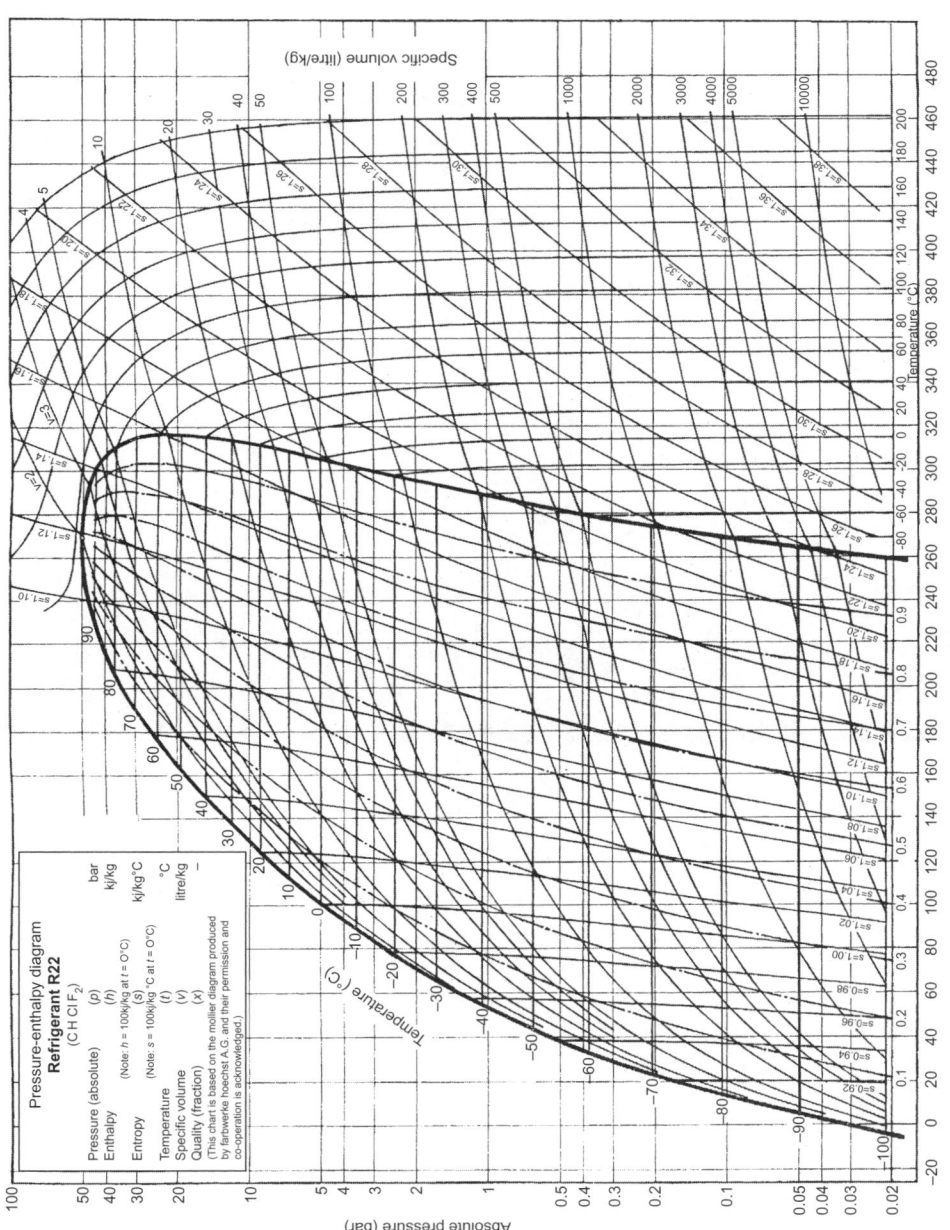

APPENDIX 3

CIBSE Psychrometric Chart

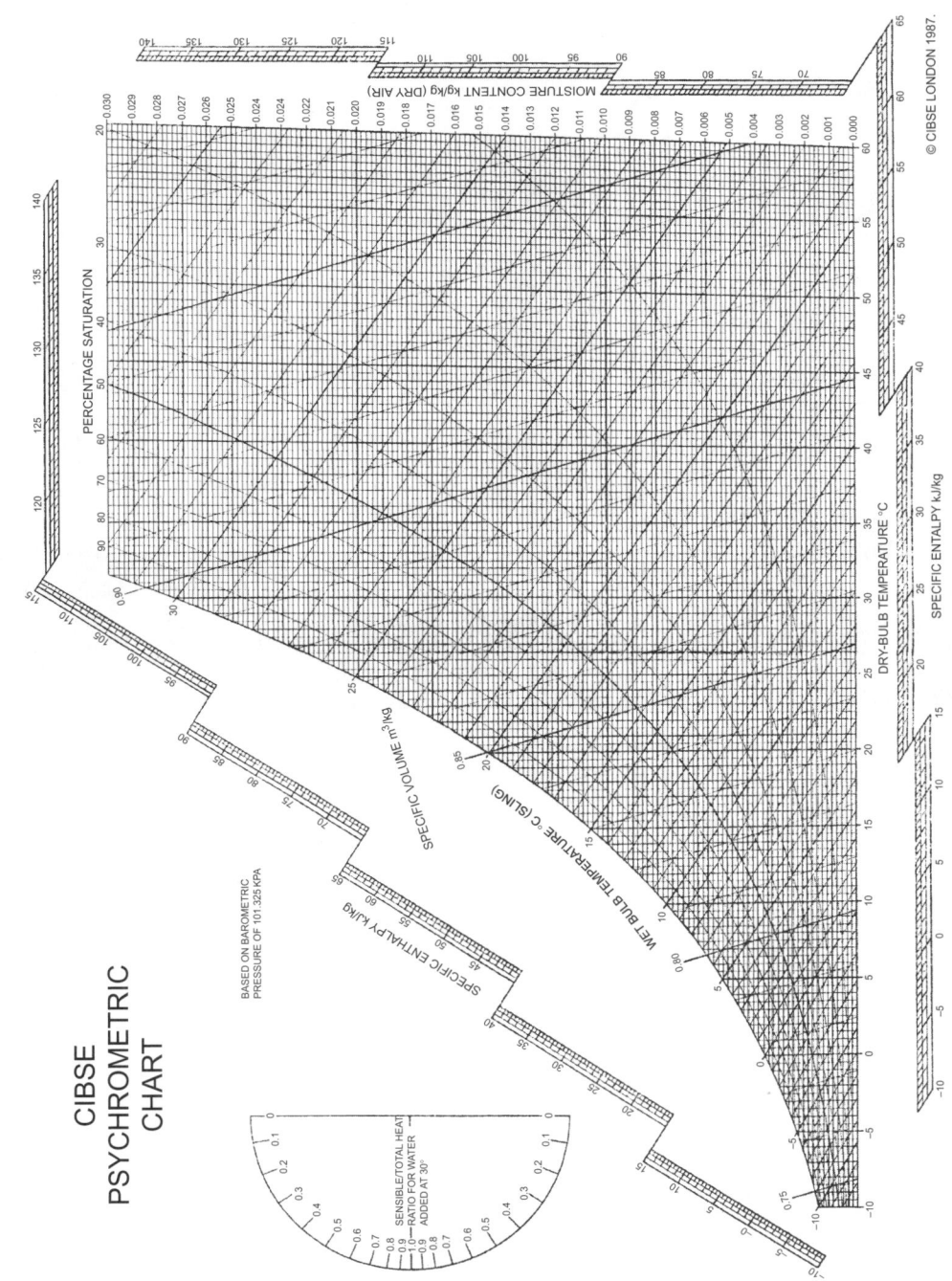

CIBSE
PSYCHROMETRIC
CHART

BASED ON BAROMETRIC
PRESSURE OF 101.325 KPA

© CIBSE LONDON 1987.

Index

Live/Advise
Anatomy & Physiology

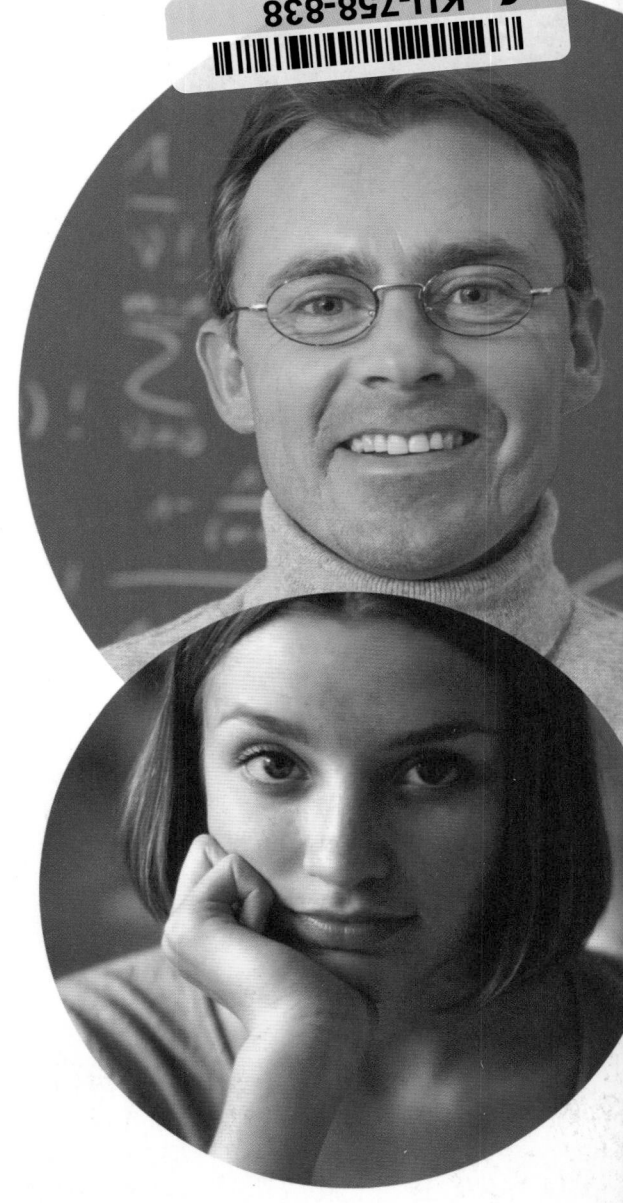

Lippincott Williams & Wilkins

offers online teaching advice and student tutoring with this textbook!

Instructors—this unique service will help you:

- generate classroom activities or discussion ideas
- provide information about the content of your adopted text or ancillary package
- evaluate lesson plans

To access the INSTRUCTOR portion of this service, visit http://thePoint.lww.com/LiveAdvise—and click on "Instructors"— the codes on this page are for STUDENT access only!

Students—here's what this service can do for you:

- answer questions outside of class—when your instructor is not available
- provide feedback on assignments before you turn them in
- help you study for tests

Student Login Instructions:

- Go to http://thePoint.lww.com/**Live**Advise and click the "Student" link
- Click the "How to set up a new account" link and follow the directions
- Once you access the **Live**Advise: **Anatomy & Physiology** page, enter the one-time use Username and Password from the scratch-off box on this page
- Create an original Username & Password. Remember to record this information and keep it in a safe place—you'll need it to gain access each time you log in to **Live**Advise: **Anatomy & Physiology**

Our **Live**Advise tutors are handpicked educators that are trained to help! They are very familiar with the textbook and ancillary package you are using in class. You can connect live with a tutor during certain hours of the week, or send e-mail style messages and receive a quick response—usually within 24 hours.

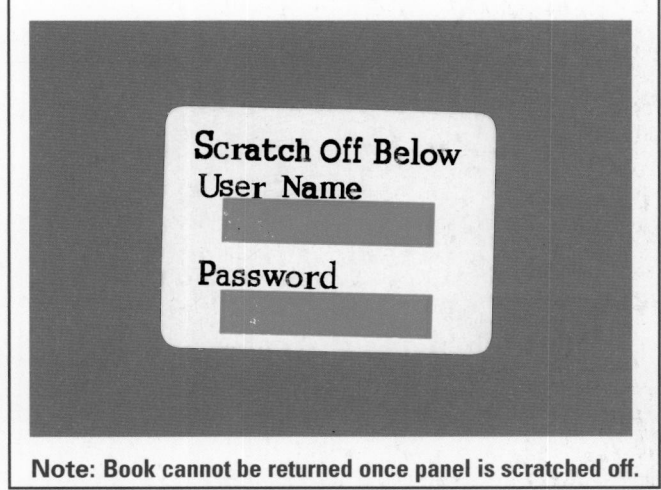

Scratch Off Below
User Name

Password

Note: Book cannot be returned once panel is scratched off.

Wolters Kluwer | Lippincott Williams & Wilkins
Health

Access to **LiveAdvise: **Anatomy & Physiology** is restricted to purchasers and adopters of the text. The code above is for student access only.*

MEMMLER'S

The Human Body in Health and Disease

11TH EDITION

MEMMLER'S
The Human Body in Health and Disease

11TH EDITION

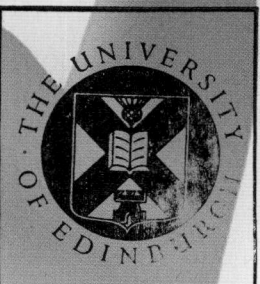
Barbara Janson Cohen

Jason James Taylor

(contributor)

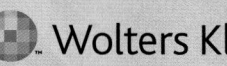 Wolters Kluwer | Lippincott Williams & Wilkins
Health

Philadelphia · Baltimore · New York · London
Buenos Aires · Hong Kong · Sydney · Tokyo

Senior Acquisitions Editor: David Troy
Developmental Editor: Dana Knighten
Managing Editor: Renee Thomas
Marketing Manager: Allison Noplock
Managing Editor, Production: Eve Malakoff-Klein
Designer: Doug Smock
Artist: Dragonfly Media Group
Compositor: Maryland Composition, Inc.
Printer: R.R. Donnelley

11th Edition
Copyright © 2009, 2005 Lippincott Williams & Wilkins, a Wolters Kluwer business.

351 West Camden Street   530 Walnut Street
Baltimore, MD 21201   Philadelphia, PA 19106

Printed in China

9 8 7 6 5 4 3 2 1

Library of Congress Cataloging-in-Publication Data

Cohen, Barbara J.
  Memmler's the human body in health and disease. — 11th ed. / Barbara Janson Cohen, Jason James Taylor.
     p. ; cm.
  Includes bibliographical references and index.
  ISBN 978-0-7817-6577-0 – 978-0-7817-9073-4 (pbk.)
  1. Human physiology. 2. Physiology, Pathological. 3. Human anatomy. I. Taylor, Jason J. II. Memmler, Ruth Lundeen. III. Title. IV. Title: Human body in health and disease.
  [DNLM: 1. Physiology. 2. Anatomy. 3. Pathology. QT 104 C678m 2009]
  QP34.5.M48 2009
  612--dc22
                                      2008013977

DISCLAIMER

Care has been taken to confirm the accuracy of the information present and to describe generally accepted practices. However, the authors, editors, and publisher are not responsible for errors or omissions or for any consequences from application of the information in this book and make no warranty, expressed or implied, with respect to the currency, completeness, or accuracy of the contents of the publication. Application of this information in a particular situation remains the professional responsibility of the practitioner; the clinical treatments described and recommended may not be considered absolute and universal recommendations.

The authors, editors, and publisher have exerted every effort to ensure that drug selection and dosage set forth in this text are in accordance with the current recommendations and practice at the time of publication. However, in view of ongoing research, changes in government regulations, and the constant flow of information relating to drug therapy and drug reactions, the reader is urged to check the package insert for each drug for any change in indications and dosage and for added warnings and precautions. This is particularly important when the recommended agent is a new or infrequently employed drug.

Some drugs and medical devices presented in this publication have Food and Drug Administration (FDA) clearance for limited use in restricted research settings. It is the responsibility of the health care provider to ascertain the FDA status of each drug or device planned for use in their clinical practice.

To purchase additional copies of this book, call our customer service department at (800) 638-3030 or fax orders to (301) 223-2320. International customers should call (301) 223-2300.

Visit Lippincott Williams & Wilkins on the Internet: http://www.lww.com. Lippincott Williams & Wilkins customer service representatives are available from 8:30 am to 6:00 pm, EST.

Preface

Memmler's *The Human Body in Health and Disease* is a textbook for introductory-level health professions and nursing students who need a basic understanding of anatomy and physiology, the interrelationships between structure and function, and the effects of disease on body systems.

Like preceding editions, the 11th edition remains true to Ruth Memmler's original vision. Designed for health professions and nursing students, the features and content specifically meet the needs of those who may be starting their health career preparation with little or no science background. This book's primary goals are:

- To provide the essential knowledge of human anatomy, physiology, and the effects of disease at an ideal level of detail and in language that is clear and understandable.

- To illustrate the concepts discussed with anatomic art that depicts the appropriate level of detail with accuracy, simplicity, and elegance and that is integrated seamlessly with the narrative.

- To incorporate the most recent scientific findings into the fundamental material on which Ruth Memmler's classic text is based.

- To include pedagogy designed to enhance interest in and understanding of the concepts presented.

- To teach the basic anatomic and medical terminology used in healthcare settings, preparing students to function efficiently in their chosen health career.

- To present an integrated teaching-learning package that includes all of the elements necessary for a successful learning experience.

This revision is the direct result of in-depth market feedback solicited to tell us what instructors and students at this level most need. We listened carefully to the feedback, and the results we obtained are integrated into many features of this book and into the ancillary package accompanying it. The text itself has been revised and updated where needed to improve organization of the material and to reflect current scientific thought. Because visual learning devices are so important to students at this level, this edition includes a new appendix with a series of dissection photographs. It also retains its extensive art program with updated versions of figures from previous editions. These features appear in an all-new design that makes the content more user-friendly and accessible than ever. The new ancillary package includes the innovative PASSport to Success for students as well as a com-prehensive package of instructor resources designed to provide instructors with maximum flexibility and efficiency.

Organization and Structure

Like previous editions, the 11th edition uses a body systems approach to the study of the normal human body and how disease affects it. The book is divided into seven units, grouping related information and body systems together as follows:

- Unit I, The Body as a Whole (Chapters 1–4), focuses on the body's organization, basic chemistry needed to understand body functions, cells and their functions, and tissues, glands, and membranes.

- Unit II, Disease and the First Line of Defense (Chapters 5 and 6), presents information on disease, organisms that produce disease, and the integumentary system, which is the body's first line of defense against injury and disease.

- Unit III, Movement and Support (Chapters 7 and 8), includes the skeletal and muscular systems.

- Unit IV, Coordination and Control (Chapters 9–12), focuses on the nervous system, the sensory system, and the endocrine system.

- Unit V, Circulation and Body Defense (Chapters 13–17), includes the blood, the heart and heart disease, blood vessels and circulation, the lymphatic system, and the immune system.

- Unit VI, Energy: Supply and Use (Chapters 18–22), includes the respiratory system; the digestive system; metabolism, nutrition, and temperature control; body fluids; and the urinary system.

- Unit VII, Perpetuation of Life (Chapters 23–25), covers the male and female reproductive systems, development and birth, and heredity and hereditary diseases.

The main Glossary defines the chapters' boldfaced terms. An additional Glossary of Word Parts is a reference tool that not only teaches basic medical and anatomic terminology but also helps students learn to recognize unfamiliar terms. Appendices include a variety of supplementary information that students will find useful as they work with the text, including the new dissection photograph appendix (Appendix 7) and answers to the Chapter Checkpoint questions and Zooming In illustration questions (Appendix 6) that are found in every chapter.

Pedagogic Features

Every chapter contains pedagogy that has been designed with the health professions and nursing student in mind

- **Learning Outcomes:** Chapter objectives on the first page of every chapter help the student organize and prioritize learning

- **Selected Key Terms:** List that accompanies the Learning Outcomes presents the most important terms covered in the chapter

- **Disease in Context (NEW to this edition):** Brief chapter-opening stories based on medical cases draw readers in by highlighting information in the chapters and showing how disease may affect the body's state of internal balance.

- **Chapter Checkpoints:** Brief questions at the end of main sections test and reinforce the student's recall of key information in that section. Answers are in Appendix 6.

- **"Zooming In" questions:** Questions with the figure legends test and reinforce the student's understanding of concepts depicted in the illustration. They are set in red to increase their visibility. Answers are in Appendix 6.

- **Phonetic pronunciations:** Easy-to-learn phonetic pronunciations are spelled out in the narrative, appearing in parentheses directly following many terms—no need for students to understand dictionary-style diacritical marks. (See the "Guide to Pronunciation" below.)

- **Special interest boxes:** Each chapter contains three special interest boxes focusing on topics that augment chapter content. The book includes five kinds of boxes altogether:

  - **Disease in Context Revisited (NEW to this edition):** Boxes that trace the outcome of the medical story that opens each chapter and show how the cases relate to material in the chapter and to others in the book.

  - **A Closer Look:** Provide additional in-depth scientific detail on topics in or related to the chapter.

  - **Clinical Perspective:** Focus on diseases and disorders relevant to the chapter, exploring what happens to the body when the normal structure-function relationship breaks down.

  - **Hot Topic:** Focus on current trends and research, reinforcing the link between anatomy and physiology and related news coverage that students may have seen.

  - **Health Maintenance:** Offer supplementary information on health and wellness issues.

- **Figures:** The art program includes full-color anatomic line art, some new or revised, with a level of detail that matches that of the narrative. Photomicrographs, radiographs, and other scans give students a preview of what they might see in real-world healthcare settings. Supplementary figures are available on the companion website as well as on the Student and Instructor Resource DVD-ROMs.

- **Tables:** The numerous tables in this edition summarize key concepts and information in an easy-to-review form. Additional summary tables are available on the companion website as well as on the Student and Instructor Resource DVD-ROMs.

- **Color figure and table numbers:** Figure and table numbers appear in color in the narrative, helping students quickly find their place after stopping to look at an illustration or table. Figure callouts appear in blue type, and table callouts, in red.

- **Word Anatomy:** This chart defines and illustrates the various word parts that appear in terms within the chapter. The prefixes, roots, and suffixes presented are grouped according to chapter headings so that students can find the relevant text. This learning tool helps students build vocabulary and promotes understanding of even unfamiliar terms based on a knowledge of common word parts.

- **Summary:** Outline-format summary provides a concise overview of chapter content, aiding in study and test preparation.

- **Questions for Study and Review:** Study questions have been thoroughly revised and organized hierarchically into three levels. (Note that answers appear on the Instructor's Resource DVD-Rom in the Instructor's Manual as well as on the Instructor's companion website):

  - **Building Understanding:** Includes fill-in-the-blank, matching, and multiple choice questions that test factual recall.

  - **Understanding Concepts:** Includes short-answer questions (define, describe, compare/contrast) that test and reinforce understanding of concepts.

  - **Conceptual Thinking:** : Includes short-essay questions that promote critical thinking skills. New in this edition are thought questions related to the Disease in Context case stories.

PASSport to Success for Students

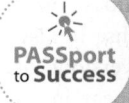 Look for this icon throughout the book for pertinent supplementary material on the companion website and student resource CD

The PASSport to Success is a practical system that lets students learn faster, remember more, and achieve success. Students discover their unique learning styles—visual, auditory, or kinesthetic—with a simple online assessment, then choose from a wealth of resources for each learning style including animations, 11 different types of online learning activities, an audio glossary, and other supplemental materials such as health professions career information, additional summary tables, additional images, study and test-taking tips, and a searchable online version of the text. Throughout the textbook, the graphic icon shown above alerts students to pertinent supplementary material.

The PASSport to Success is available on the DVD-Rom bound into this textbook as well as on the book's companion website at http://thePoint.lww.com/Memmler HumanBody11e. See the inside front cover of this text for the passcode you will need to gain access to the website, and see pages ix–xix for all details about the PASSport to Success and a complete listing of student resources.

Instructor Ancillary Package

All instructor resources are available to approved adopting instructors online at http://thePoint.lww.com/Memmler HumanBody11e as well as on the Instructor Resource DVD-Rom:

- **Print Instructor's Manual** includes the Instructor Resource DVD-Rom, and is also available in PDF format online.

- **Using the PASSport to Success in Your Course** provides practical tips for integrating this innovative approach.

- **Brownstone Test Generator** allows you to create customized exams from a bank of questions.

- **PowerPoint Presentations** include multiple choice and true/false questions for use with Student Response System technology.

- **Image Bank** includes labels-on and labels-off options.

- **Lesson Plans** are organized around the learning objectives and include lecture notes, in-class activities, and assignments, including student activities from the PASSport to Success.

- **Answers to Study Guide Questions** are the instructor's companions to the print student Study Guide.

- **Answers to Questions for Study and Review** match up with the quiz material found at the end of each chapter in the textbook.

- **Strategies for Effective Teaching** provide sound, tried-and-true advice for successful instruction.

- **LiveAdvise Tutoring Service** is available for instructors as well as students.

- **WebCT and Blackboard-ready Cartridge** allows you to integrate the ancillary materials into learning management systems.

Instructors also have access to all student ancillary assets, including the PASSport to Success, via thePoint website.

Guide to Pronunciation

The stressed syllable in each word is shown with capital letters. The vowel pronunciations are as follows:

Any vowel at the end of a syllable is given a long sound, as follows:

a as in say
e as in be
i as in nice
o as in go
u as in true

A vowel followed by a consonant and the letter e (as in rate) also is given a long pronunciation.

Any vowel followed by a consonant receives a short pronunciation, as follows:

a as in absent
e as in end
i as in bin
o as in not
u as in up

Summary

The 11th edition of *Memmler's The Human Body in Health and Disease* builds on the successes of the previous ten editions by offering clear, concise narrative into which accurate, aesthetically pleasing anatomic art has been woven. We have made every effort to respond thoughtfully and thoroughly to reviewers' and instructors' comments, offering the ideal level of detail for students preparing for a career in the health professions and nursing, the pedagogic features that best support it, and with the PASSport to Success, providing students with an integrated system for understanding and using their unique learning styles—and ultimately succeeding in the course. We hope you will agree that the 11th edition of *Memmler's* suits your educational needs.

Introducing... PASSport to Success

Succeed in anatomy and physiology with easy-to-use, multimedia tools that are tailored to your unique learning style.

Anatomy & Physiology may be the toughest course you ever *ace.*

You've probably heard horror stories from other students about learning A&P.

"It's challenging."
"Too much information, not enough time."
"Definitely the hardest class in the program."

It's true – anatomy and physiology is a tough subject. You will need to understand and remember the essentials of how the human body works – the organs, the systems, and the processes. Grasping this material is the foundation of your success, because you will use what you learn in this class throughout your coursework and your career.

There is no need to feel overwhelmed. You will succeed. Because you're about to discover something very important about yourself: your unique learning style.

How do you learn best? By seeing? By hearing? Or by doing?

Different people learn in different ways. Some students learn by reading. Others take in new information by listening to their instructors. You may prefer to write down notes. A simple self-assessment can tell you whether you're a visual, auditory, or kinesthetic learner.

When you understand the way that you process information most effectively, you can choose resources that fit your learning style.

The PASSport to Success is a practical system that lets you **learn faster**, **remember more**, and **achieve success**.

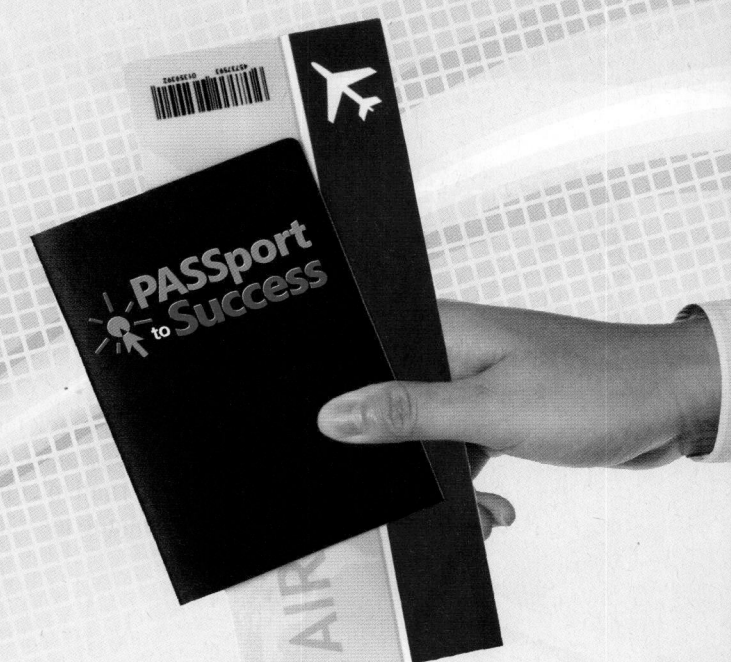

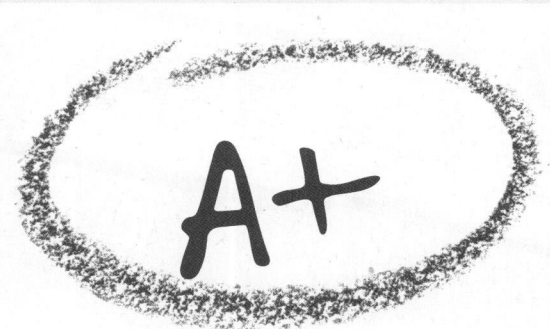

Your PASSport to Success begins now.
Turn the page for a snapshot of your journey!

→ → →

UNDERSTAND THE JOURNEY AHEAD

➤ Your fully illustrated textbook makes anatomy and physiology easy to understand with interactive study tools designed for your unique learning style.

DISCOVER YOUR LEARNING STYLE

➤ Enter your personal access code on *thePoint* website, complete the MyPowerLearning™ online learning styles assessment and print out your personal learning styles report.

What is your learning style?

🖋 **Visual?**

🖋 **Kinesthetic?**

🖋 **Auditory?**

PASSport to Success

USE YOUR TIME EFFECTIVELY

➢ Icons in the textbook, on the website, and on the CD-ROM guide you to visual, auditory and kinesthetic activities that will help you learn and succeed.

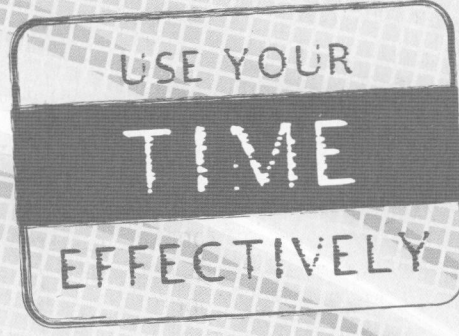

ACHIEVE ★ SUCCESS!

➢ Ace the exam and pass the course!

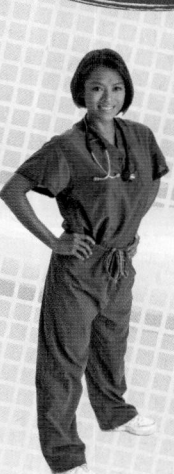

Turn the page to begin your tour!

→ → →

UNDERSTAND
THE JOURNEY AHEAD

Your journey begins with your textbook, *Memmler's The Human Body in Health and Disease*. Newly updated and fully illustrated, this easy-to-use textbook is filled with icons that guide you to resources and activities that are designed for your

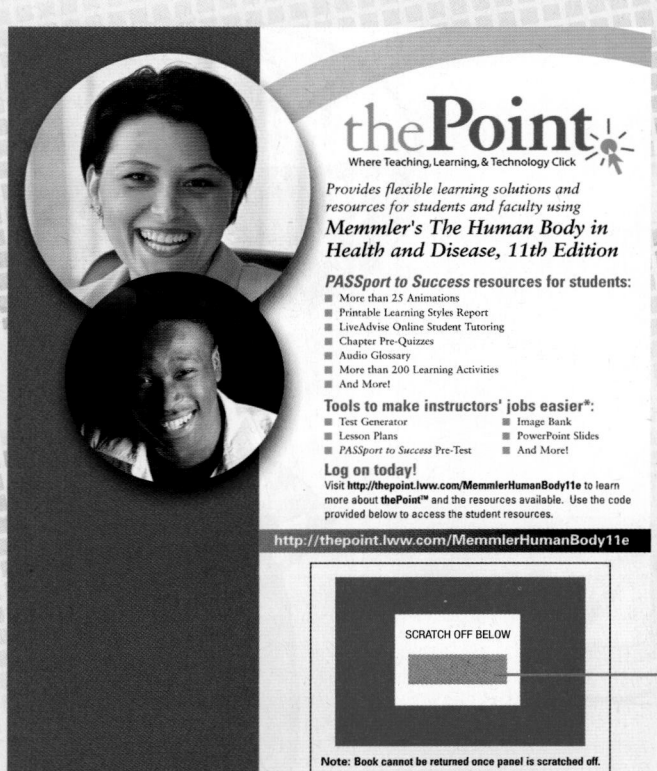

the Point
Where Teaching, Learning, & Technology Click

Provides flexible learning solutions and resources for students and faculty using
Memmler's The Human Body in Health and Disease, 11th Edition

PASSport to Success resources for students:
- More than 25 Animations
- Printable Learning Styles Report
- LiveAdvise Online Student Tutoring
- Chapter Pre-Quizzes
- Audio Glossary
- More than 200 Learning Activities
- And More!

Tools to make instructors' jobs easier*:
- Test Generator
- Lesson Plans
- PASSport to Success Pre-Test
- Image Bank
- PowerPoint Slides
- And More!

Log on today!
Visit http://thepoint.lww.com/MemmlerHumanBody11e to learn more about **thePoint™** and the resources available. Use the code provided below to access the student resources.

http://thepoint.lww.com/MemmlerHumanBody11e

SCRATCH OFF BELOW

Note: Book cannot be returned once panel is scratched off.

*The faculty resources are restricted to adopters of the text. Adopters have to be approved before accessing the faculty resources.

Wolters Kluwer | Lippincott Williams & Wilkins
Health

Inside the front cover of your textbook, you'll find your **personal access code**. Use it to log on to *thePoint* – the companion website for this textbook. On the website, you can search and sort learning activities by learning style and choose the ones that will help you understand the material quickly and efficiently.

Every chapter begins with a set of **Learning Outcomes** that explain what you need to learn, so you can focus your study time on the most important material.

Each chapter begins with **Disease in Context**, an interesting case story that uses a familiar, real-life scenario to illustrate key concepts in anatomy and physiology. Later in the chapter, the case story is revisited in more detail—improving your understanding and helping you remember the information.

CHAPTER

16

The Lymphatic System and Lymphoid Tissue

Learning Outcomes

After careful study of this chapter, you should be able to:

1. Define disease and list seven categories of disease
2. List seven predisposing causes of disease
3. Define terminology used in describing and treating disease
4. Define complementary and alternative medicine. Cite several alternative or complementary fields of practice
5. Explain methods by which microorganisms can be transmitted from one host to another
6. List four types of organisms studied in microbiology and give the characteristics of each
7. List some diseases caused by each type of microorganism
8. Define normal flora and explain the value of the normal flora
9. Describe the three types of bacteria according to shape
10. List several diseases in humans caused by worms
11. Give some reasons for the emergence and spread of microorganisms today
12. Describe several public health measures taken to prevent the spread of disease
13. Differentiate sterilization, disinfection, and antisepsis
14. Describe techniques included as part of standard precautions
15. List some antimicrobial agents and describe how they work
16. Describe several methods used to identify microorganisms in the laboratory
17. Show how word parts are used to build words related to disease (see Word Anatomy at the end of the chapter)

Selected Key Terms

The following terms and other boldface terms in the chapter are defined in the Glossary.

acute
antisepsis
asepsis
chronic
diagnosis
disease
disinfection
epidemic
etiology
helminth
microorganism
nosocomial infection
opportunistic infection
pathogen
pathophysiology
prion
prognosis
sign
spore
sterilization
symptom
syndrome
systemic
therapy
toxin
vector

PASSport to Success

Visit thePoint or see the Student Resource CD in the back of this book for definitions and pronunciations of key terms as well as a pretest for this chapter.

Disease in Context

Maria's Case: When Pathogens Attack

The man sharing the elevator with Maria Sanchez looked terrible — watery eyes, runny nose, and a sickly, run-down appearance. As the elevator opened and the man stepped toward the doors, he let out a loud sneeze. "Pardon me," he said, as the elevator closed behind him. If I get sick, I'd stay in bed, Maria thought. Maria didn't know it yet, but soon she would be.

The passenger left something behind when he exited the elevator. Microscopic droplets of mucus and water from his sneeze floated in the air. Inside each droplet were thousands of microorganisms, called viruses, capable of making Maria very sick. She inhaled several of these germ-laden droplets into her respiratory system as she waited for the elevator to reach her floor. Maria exited the elevator, unaware that her body had been invaded.

Maria's warm, moist environment for this microorganism. When a virus landed on the epithelial tissue lining her throat, protein spikes protruding from its surface fit snugly into receptors on an epithelial cell, stimulating endocytosis of the virus. Having successfully, the virus was inside the cell and ready to begin the second phase of its attack!

Shortly after entering the cell, the virus released its RNA, which was then transported into the cell's nucleus. Unable to recognize the viral RNA as foreign, the nucleus transcribed it into viral messenger RNA. Returning to the cytoplasm, this new RNA was translated into viral proteins at the ribosomes. Some of these proteins were combined with viral RNA to make new viruses. Others took over the machinery of the host cell to make more viral components.

Since entering the epithelial cell about 24 hours ago, the virus had successfully hijacked cellular RNA and protein synthesis. The cell had been turned into a virus-making factory! With the cell

readily exhausted, the next viruses that lined its cytoplasm exited to infect new cells. Although finally free of the pathogen, the cell lost its most resources left and Maria Sanchez's body has been invaded by the influenza virus. In this chapter's case, we'll learn more about viruses as well as other disease-producing organisms. Later in the case, we'll see how Maria's body is coping with its unwanted visitors.

Maria Sanchez's body has been invaded by the influenza virus. In this chapter, we'll learn more about viruses as well as other disease-producing organisms. Later in the case, we'll see how Maria's body is coping with its unwanted visitors.

When a virus landed on the epithelial tissue lining her throat, protein spikes protruding from its surface fit snugly into receptors on an epithelial cell, stimulating endocytosis of the virus. Having successfully "picked the lock" on the cell's plasma membrane, the virus was inside the cell and ready to begin the second phase of its attack! Maria Sanchez's body has been invaded by the influenza virus. In this chapter, we'll learn more about viruses as well as other disease-producing organisms. Later in the case, we'll see how Maria's body is coping with its unwanted visitors.

Shortly after entering the cell, the virus released its RNA, which was then transported into the cell's nucleus. Unable to recognize the viral RNA as foreign, the nucleus transcribed it into viral messenger RNA. Returning to the cytoplasm, this new RNA was translated into viral proteins at the ribosomes. Some of these proteins were combined with viral RNA to make new viruses. Others took over the machinery of the host cell to make more viral components.

Look for the **PASSport to Success** symbol throughout your textbook to locate additional resources and exercises that are designed for your learning style.

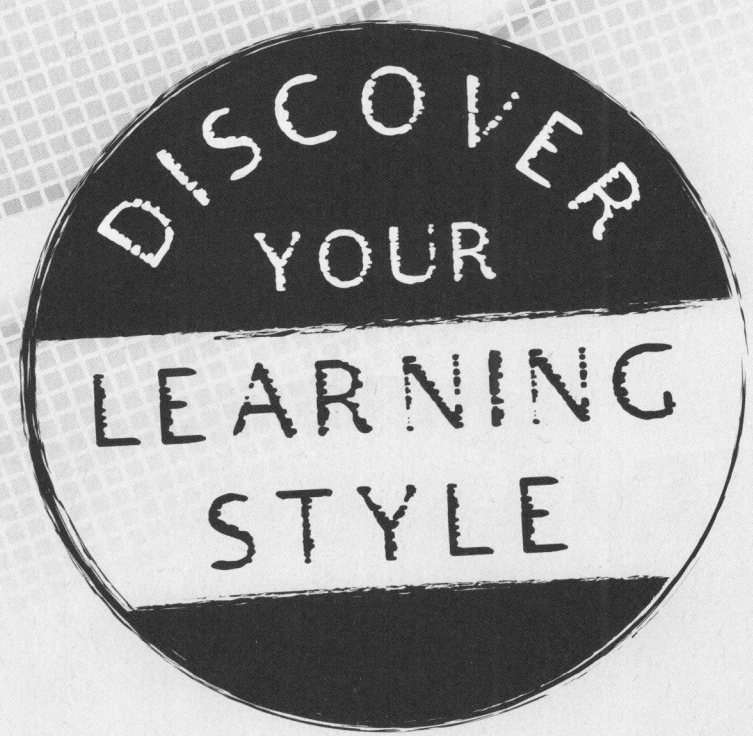

DISCOVER YOUR LEARNING STYLE

People learn in different ways. If you like to study animations, illustrations, and diagrams, you may be a visual learner. If you like to sound out new words or discuss material with other students, you may be an auditory learner. If you take a lot of notes during class and benefit from hands-on learning activities, you're probably a kinesthetic learner.

Most people have both a primary and a secondary learning style – and the PASSport to Success helps you identify both! Once you know how you learn best, you can choose learning activities that will help you master new material more efficiently.

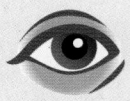 **Visual**

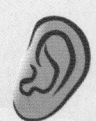 **Auditory**

 **Kinesthetic**

Take the Learning Styles Assessment

Discovering your learning style is easy – and fun! Here's how to begin:

1. Scratch off the personal access code inside the front cover of your textbook.

2. Log on to http://thePoint.lww.com/MemmlerHumanBody11e.

3. Click on "Student Resources" and then "PASSport to Success."

4. Once you are on the PASSport site, click on "MyPowerLearning."

5. Take the online self-assessment. *(Don't worry – There are no wrong answers!)*

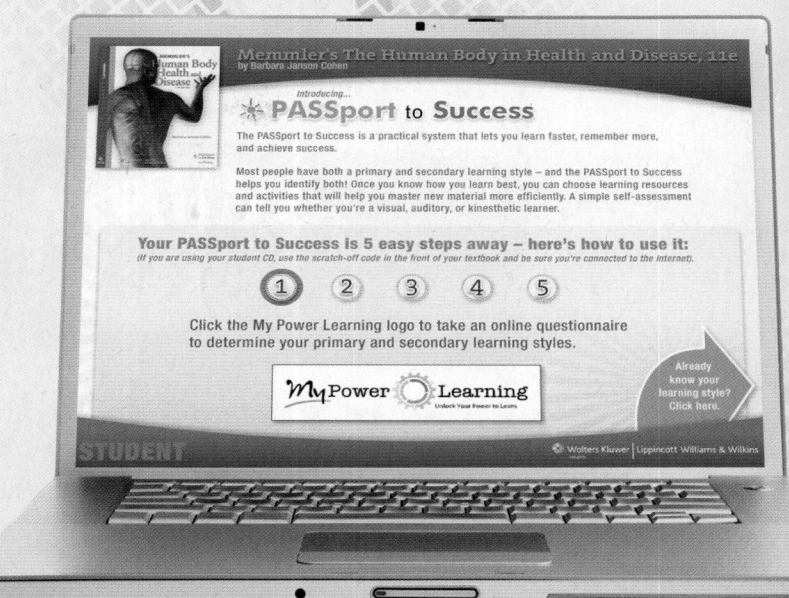

Read your custom report

Identifying your learning style is the first step to your academic success. In fact, many students say, "If I had known this in high school, my grades would have been so much better!" Your personal learning styles report not only reveals your primary and secondary learning styles, it also gives you tips and ideas to make the most of the resources that you'll find in the PASSport to Success.

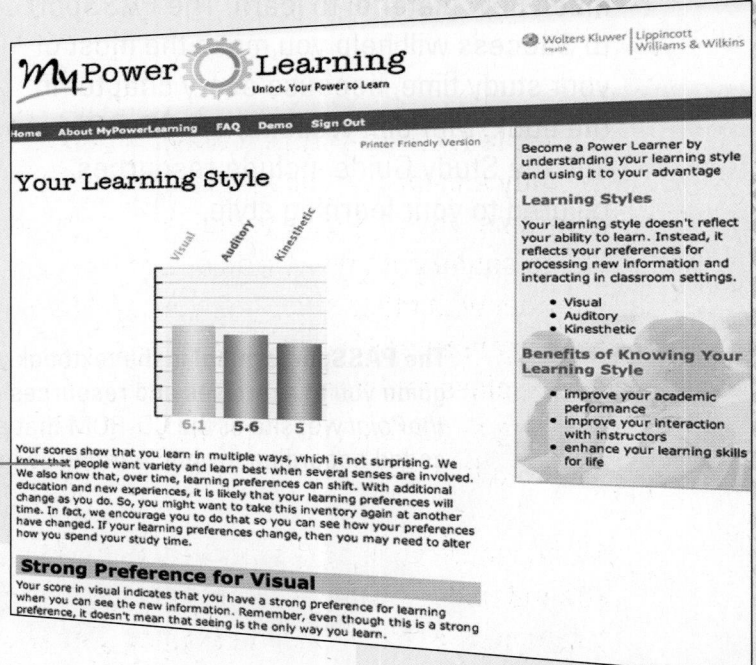

USE YOUR TIME EFFECTIVELY

Anatomy and physiology is a challenge for many students, because there is so much new material to learn. The PASSport to Success will help you make the most of your study time, because every chapter in the book, *thePoint* website, the CD-ROM and the Study Guide include resources tailored to your learning style.

The PASSport symbol in the textbook will guide you to exercises and resources on *thePoint* website or the CD-ROM that are coded according to your learning style.

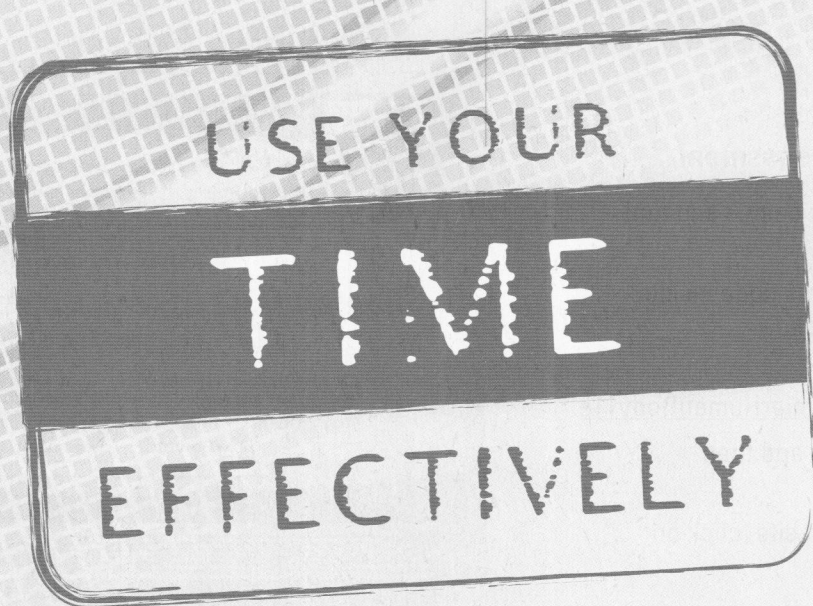

46   **Unit 1** The Body as a Whole

Box 3-2   Hot Topics

Proteomics: So Many Proteins, So Few Genes

To build the many different proteins that make up the body, cells rely on instructions encoded in the chromosomes' genes. Collectively, all the different genes on all the chromosomes make up the genome. Genes contain the instructions for making proteins, while the proteins themselves perform the body's functions.

Scientists are now studying the human proteome—all the proteins that can be expressed in a cell—to help them understand the proteins' structure and function. Unlike the genome, the proteome changes as the cell's activities and needs change. In 2003, after a decade of intense scientific activity, investigators mapped the entire human genome and realized that it contained only 35,000 genes, far fewer than initially expected. How could this relatively small number of genes code for several million proteins? They concluded that genes were not the whole story.

Gene transcription is only the b[...] thesis. In response to cell conditi[...] newly transcribed mRNA into sever[...] ribosome can use to build a differ[...] protein is built, enzymes can furthe[...] strands to produce several more [...] molecules help the newly formed [...] cise shapes and interact with each [...] more variations. Thus, while a gene[...] protein, modifications after gene tr[...] many more unique proteins. There [...] about the proteome, but scientis[...] search will lead to new technique[...] ing disease.

hours spends only about one hour in mitosis and the remaining time in interphase.

CHECKPOINT 3-10 ► What must happen to the DNA in a cell before mitosis can occur? During what stage in the life of a cell does this occur?

PASSport to Success Visit *thePoint* or see the Student Resource CD in the back of this book for a photomicrograph of a replicated chromosome.

Stages of Mitosis

Although mitosis is a continuous process, distinct changes can be seen in the dividing cell at four stages (Fig. 3-9).

■ In **prophase** (PRO-faze), the doubled strands of DNA return to their tightly wound spiral organization and become visible under the microscope as dark, thread-like chromosomes. The nucleus and the nuclear membrane begin to disappear. In the cytoplasm, the two centrioles move toward opposite ends of the cell and a spindle-shaped structure made of thin fibers begins to form between them.

■ In **metaphase** (MET-ah-faze), the chromosomes line up across the center (equator) of the cell attached to the spindle fibers.

■ As mitosis continues into t[...] membrane appears around [...] chromosomes, forming two [...]

Also during telophase, the [...] off to divide the cell. The midsec[...] eas becomes progressively smal[...] splits in two. There are now tw[...] cells, each with exactly the same [...] as was present in the parent ce[...] cells, skeletal muscle cells for ex[...] not divide following nuclear d[...] multiple mitoses, is a giant single[...] This pattern is extremely rare in [...]

During mitosis, all the organ[...] for the division process, tempor[...] cell divides, these organelles re[...] cell. Also at this time, the centr[...] preparation for the next cell divi[...]

Body cells differ in the rate [...] Some, such as nerve cells and mu[...] some point in development and [...] die. They remain in interphase. C[...] sperm cells, and skin cells, multi[...] destroyed by injury, disease, o[...] Cells that multiply slowly may b[...] tissue when injured, as in repair of a [...]

Immature cells that retain th[...] ture when necessary are known [...]

Whether you are a visual, auditory, or kinesthetic learner, you'll find plenty of activities that will help you absorb new information in ways that fit your learning style.

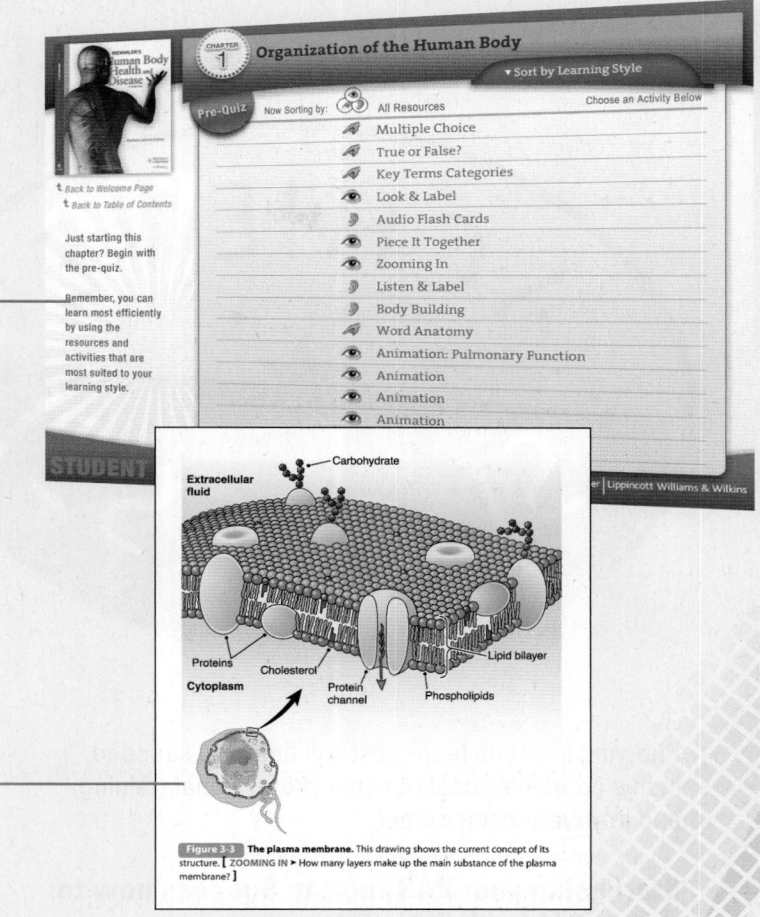

If you're a visual learner, you'll find dozens of illustrations and diagrams throughout your textbook, including an atlas with real dissection photos, as well as more than 25 animations online. You can also view additional activities, including zoom-in illustrations, look-and-label figures, and sectional diagrams on *thePoint* website and on the CD-ROM.

If you're a kinesthetic learner, you get more out of learning activities that let you work with your hands. As you go through your textbook, take notes and actively trace diagrams to take advantage of your touch-learning abilities. You'll also benefit from anatomy puzzles, exercises, and self-quizzes on *thePoint* website and the CD-ROM, as well as writing exercises and a look-and-label coloring atlas in the Study Guide.

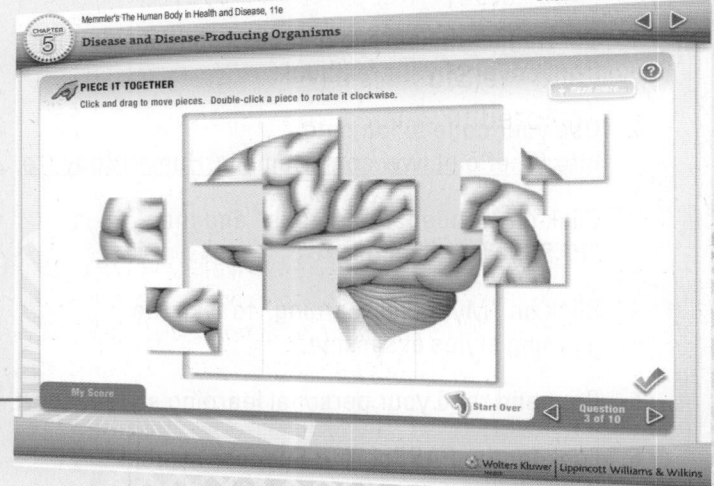

If you're an auditory learner, you may find it helpful to read aloud from your textbook. You'll benefit from in-class lectures and discussions about the material with your fellow students. In addition, you'll find audio flash cards, word anatomy exercises, and other resources on *thePoint* website and on the CD-ROM.

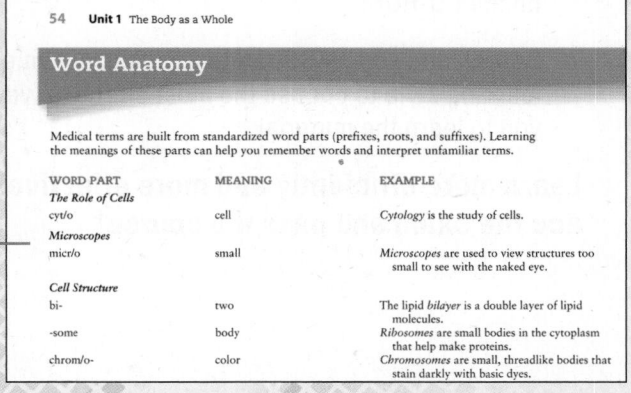

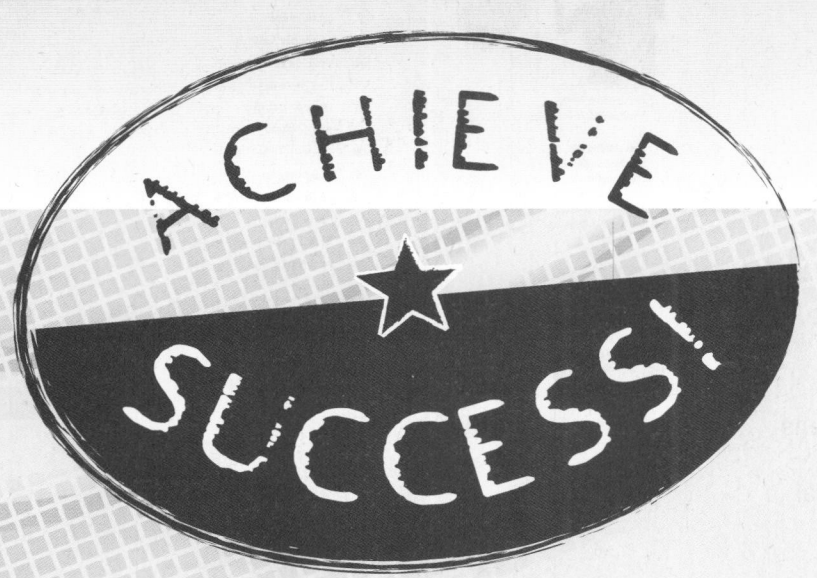

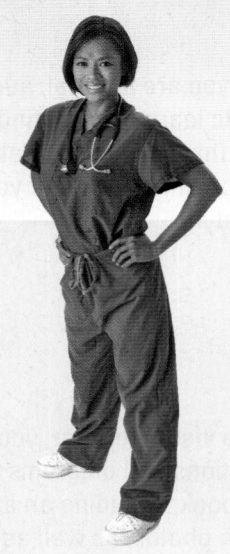

Knowing how you learn best will help you succeed in this course, throughout your professional training, and in your chosen career.

Start using your PASSport to Success now to ace anatomy and physiology:

1. Scratch off the personal access code inside the front cover of your textbook.

2. Use your code to log onto http://thePoint.lww.com/MemmlerHumanBody11e.

3. Click on "Student Resources" and then "PASSport to Success."

4. Click on "MyPowerLearning" to take the learning styles assessment.

5. Print and read your personal learning styles report.

6. Look for the PASSport to Success symbol throughout your textbook, which alerts you to resources and activities on *thePoint* website and on the CD-ROM.

7. Search and sort PASSport to Success activities by learning style to choose the most effective way for you to learn the material.

Learn more efficiently and more effectively, ace the exam and pass the course!

Your PASSport to Success includes:

✓ MyPowerLearning™ learning styles assessment
✓ Printable learning style report
✓ LiveAdvise one-to-one online student tutoring
✓ Chapter pre-quizzes
✓ More than 25 animations
✓ 11 different types of learning activities on *thePoint* website and your CD-ROM:
   • Multiple Choice
   • True or False?
   • Key Terms Categories
   • Fill-in-the-Blank
   • Look & Label
   • Audio Flash Cards
   • Word Anatomy
   • Piece It Together
   • Zooming In
   • Listen & Label
   • Body Building
✓ Audio glossary
✓ Supplementary images and tables
✓ Study and test-taking tips
✓ Career information boxes
✓ Answers to the textbook's Questions for Study and Review

Reviewers

We gratefully acknowledge the generous contributions of the reviewers whose names appear in the list that follows.

Kelsey Abrams
Student
Heritage High School
Littleton, Colorado

Diana Alagna
Instructor
Branford Hall Career Institute
Southington, Connecticut

Martin Alenduff
Instructor
Ivy Technical Community College
Columbus, Indiana

Christine Alger
Professor
SUNY at Stony Brook
Stony Brook, New York

Fara Amsalem
Instructor
International College
Naples, Florida

Darryl Anderson, MD
Medical Director
Medical Assisting Program
Plaza College
Jackson Heights, New York

Marty Arnson
Instructor
Gwinnett Area Technical Institute
Lawrenceville, Georgia

Judith Aronow
Instructor
Vermont Technical College
Randolph Center, Vermont

Dr. Joseph H. Balatbat
Vice-President of Academics Affairs
Sanford-Brown Institute
New York, New York

Gail A. Balser RN, BSN, MSN
Practical Nurse Instructor
Traviss Career Center
Lakeland, Florida

Kristen Blake-Bruzzini, PhD
Assistant Professor of Biology
College of Arts and Sciences
Maryville University
St. Louis, Missouri

Lynn Bolin
Instructor
Ohio Institute of Health Careers
Columbus, Ohio

Jackie Brittingham
Professor
Simpson College
Indianola, Iowa

Brendalyn Browner, RN, MSN
Assistant Department Chair, Nursing
Associate Professor
Georgia Perimeter College
Dunwoody, Georgia

Sheila Burcham
Instructor
Northwest Mississippi Community College
Senatobia, Mississippi

Naomi E. W. Carroll, PhD, RN
Professor, Health Information Technology
Austin Community College
Austin, Texas

Marianne Ciotti
Instructor
Lehigh Carbon Community College
Schnecksville, Pennsylvania

Sharon A. Coffey
Instructor
Huston Community College
Huston, Texas

W. Wade Cooper
Instructor
Shelton State Community College
Tuscaloosa, Alabama

Janie Corbitt, MLS, RN
Instructor, Allied Health Core
Central Georgia Technical College
Milledgeville, Georgia

Sarah Crum
Student
Lansdale School of Business
North Wales, Pennsylvania

Rachel J. Diehl, NR-CMA
Associate in Specialized Business Degree
Allied Health, Medical Assistant
Lansdale School of Business
North Wales, Pennsylvania

Georgiann Dudek
Instructor
Erie 2-Chautauqua-Cattaraugus BOCES
Angola, New York

Jason Egginton
Instructor
Sister Rosalind Schools and Clinics of
    Massage
St. Paul, Minnesota

Peter Embriano
Instructor
Fox Institute
West Hartford, Connecticut

Paul Enns, RN, BScN
Instructor
Assiniboine Community College
Brandon, Manitoba, Canada

Pamela A. Eugene, BAS, LRT, (R)
Associate Professor Health Sciences
Allied Health Division
Delgado Community College
New Orleans, Lousiana

Y. Everett
Student
Orlando Tech
Orlando, Florida

Janice H. Fortenberry, BS, MCS
Instructor of Human Anatomy and
    Physiology I and II
Science Division
Copiah-Lincoln Community College
Wesson, Mississippi

Rita Fulton, MS, MEd
Professor of Biology
Health Department
Belmont Technical College
St. Clairsville, Ohio

Carmen Gallien
Instructor
Louisiana Technical College
Louisiana

Mary Sue Gamroth
Instructor
Georgian College
Barrie, Ontario, Canada

David Gantt
Instructor
Georgia Campus - Philadelphia College
   of Osteopathic Medicine
Suwanne, Georgia

Rosalind Giles-Pereira, RN, BSN
Instructor
School of Health and Human Services
Camosun College
Victoria, British Columbia, Canada

Candace Gioia
Instructor
Pinellas Technical Education Center
Clearwater, Florida

Meredyth Given
Instructor
Pearl River Community College
Poplarville, Mississippi

Sabina Grigoryan
Student Practical Nurse
Nova Scotia Community College
Halifax, Nova Scotia, Canada

Michael J. Harman MS
Professor of Biology
Lone Star College - North Harris
Houston, Texas

William Havins
Instructor
Albuquerque Technical Vocational
   Institue
Albuquerque, New Mexico

Ann Henninger, PhD
Professor of Biology
Wartburg College
Waverly, Iowa

Liz Hoffman, MA Ed, CMA, (AAMA)
   CPT, (ASPT)
Associate Dean of Health Science
Baker College of Clinton Township
Clinton Township, Michigan

Kathleen Holbrook, CMT
Director/Instructor
Andrews & Holbrook Training Corp.
Latham, New York

Ladeen Hubbell
Instructor
Pearl River Community College
Poplarville, Mississippi

Atanas Ignatov, PhD
Associate Professor
Logan College of Chiropractic
Chesterfield, Missouri

Shakila Jalili
Practical Nursing student year 1
Akerley Campus, Nova Scotia
   Community College
Dartmouth, Nova Scotia, Canada

Linda M. Johnson, RN, MSN, MS
Nursing Instructor
City College of San Francisco
San Francisco, California

Ethel M. Jones, RN, EdS, DSN
Nursing Educator
H. Councill Trenholm State Technical
   College
Montgomery, Alabama

Jackie Jones
Instructor
Delgado Community College - City Park
New Orleans, Louisiana

Marie Kelley
Professor
Our Lady of the Lake College
Baton Rogue, Louisiana

Beverly Kirk
Instructor
Northeast Mississippi Community College
Booneville, Mississippi

Tom Kober
Instructor
Cincinnati State Technical and Community
   College
Cincinnati, Ohio

Megan Kowalski
Instructor
Northwest Business College - Chicago
Chicago, Illinois

Matthew A. Kreitzer, PhD
Associate Professor of Biology
Division of Natural Science and
   Mathematics
Indiana Wesleyan University
Marion, Indiana

Laura Latoza
Student
Orlando Tech
Orlando, Florida

Celinda Kay Leach
Division Chair for the School of Health
   Sciences
Ivy Tech Community College
Bloomington, Indiana

John J. Lepri, PhD
Associate Professor of Biology
The University of North Carolina at
   Greensboro
Greensboro, North Carolina

Connie Lieseke, CMA (AAMA), PBT,
   MLT(ASCP)
Medical Assisting Program Coordinator
Olympic College
Bremerton, Washington

Heather Longaphy
Student
Akerley Campus, Nova Scotia
   Community College
Dartmouth, Nova Scotia, Canada

Samuel T. Lopez, DPT
Associate Professor of Exercise Science
University of Nebraska at Kearney
Kearney, Nebraska

Charlene Mac Donnell
Student
Nova Scotia Community College
Dartmouth, Nova Scotia, Canada

Claire Maday-Travis
Instructor
The Salter School
Worcester, Massachusetts

Christel Marschall
Professor
Science Department
Lansing Community College
Lansing, Michigan

Wilsetta McClain
Department Chair
Coding and Phlebotomy
Baker College
Auburn Hills, Michigan

Katherine McCulloch
Instructor
Lincoln Technical Institute
Mount Laurel/Edison, New Jersey

Leanne McKinzey
Student
Centennial College
Toronto, Ontario, Canada

Nonna Morozova
Instructor
ASA College
Brooklyn/Manhattan, New York

Cora Newcomb, GCHE, ABD, MEd,
   PhD candidate
Professor
Medical Assistant Division
Technical College of the Lowcountry
Beaufort, South Carolina

David Newton
Professor
Dalton State College
Dalton, Georgia

Brian Nichols
Instructor
Lane Community College
Eugene, Oregon

Amy Obringer, PhD
Associate Professor of Biology
University of Saint Francis
Fort Wayne, Indiana

Eva Oltman, MEd, CPC, CMA
Professor/Division Chair of Allied Health
Jefferson Community and Technical College
Louisville, Kentucky

Stephen W. Perry, MS, MAR
Assistant Professor of Biology
Liberty University
Lynchburg, Virginia

Jennifer Pitcher
Student
Centennial College
Toronto, Ontario, Canada

Roberta L. Pohlman, PhD
Associate Professor of Biology
College of Science and Math
Wright State University
Dayton, Ohio

Merle D. Potter, NREMTP
EMS Educator/Flight Paramedic
Wyoming Medical Center/Wyoming Life
  Flight
Casper, Wyoming

Angela Powell
Student
Nova Scotia Community College
Dartmouth, Nova Scotia, Canada

Portia Resnick
Instructor
Somerset School of Massage Therapy
Piscataway, New Jersey

Holly Ressetar, PhD
Medical Course Coordinator
Department of Neurobiology and Anatomy
West Virginia University School of Medicine
Morgantown, West Virginia

Marshall Robb
Professor
William Woods University
Jefferson City/Columbia, Missouri

Kathy Sargent
Instructor
Ivy Tech Community College
Indianapolis, Indiana

Jenny Sarkovski
Student
Centennial College
Toronto, Ontario, Canada

Linda Scarborough, RN, CMA (AAMA),
  CPC, MSHA
Healthcare Management Technology
  Instructor
Lanier Technical College
Oakwood, Georgia

Rebecca Scheid
Instructor
Community College of Spokane
Spokane, Washington

Lorissa A. Sickmiller, BS, LMT,
  NCTMB
Instructor, Anatomy & Physiology
Institute of Therapeutic Massage
Ottawa, Ohio

Anne Simko, RN, BSN, MS
Department Head - LPN Program
Eli Whitney Technical School
Hamden, Connecticut

Alyssa Simonis
Student
Lansdale School of Business
North Wales, Pennsylvania

Richard Sims, MS
Adjunct Instructor of Biology
Jones County Jr. College
Ellisville, Mississippi

Doug Sizemore
Instructor
Bevill State Community College
Jasper, Alabama

Mitzie L. Sowell, PhD
Instructor
Pensacola Junior College
Pensacola, Florida

Amanda Smyth
Student
Lansdale School of Business
North Wales, Pennsylvania

Nita Stika, PhD, ABD
Professor
Concordia University Wisconsin
Mequon, Wisconsin

Kimberly Stone
Instructor
Heritage College
Denver, Colorado

Aleta Sullivan, PhD
Professor of Biology
Science, Mathematics and Business
  Department
Pearl River Community College
Poplarville, Mississippi

Eric L. Sun, PhD
Associate Dean and Professor of Biology
School of Arts and Sciences
Macon State College
Macon, Georgia

Tamara Thell
Instructor
Anoka Technical College
Anoka, Minnesota

Pamela Thinesen, MS
Biology Faculty
Century College
White Bear Lake, Minnesota

Anne Tiemann RN, MS
Associate Professor and Program Chair
Massage Therapy and Medical Assisting
McIntosh College
Dover, New Hampshire

Sandi Tschritter, BA, CPhT
Director, Pharmacy Technician Program
Spokane Community College
Spokane, Washington

Laura Travis
Instructor
Tennessee Technology Center at
  Dickson
Dickson, Tennessee

Judy K. Ward CMA(AAMA), PBT(ASCP),
  EMT-P
Medical Assisting Program Chair
School of Health Sciences
Ivy Tech Community College
Indianapolis, Indiana

Jamey Watson
Instructor
Lanier Technical College
Oakwood, Georgia

Henry C. Wormser, PhD
Professor of Medicinal Chemistry
Wayne State University
Eugene Applebaum College of Pharmacy
  and Health Sciences
Detroit, Michigan

Omyra M Vega, NRCMA
Associates in Allied Health
Lansdale School of Business
North Wales, Pennsylvania

Acknowledgments

It's on this page that I get to thank the many talented people who have helped in the preparation of this 11th edition of *Memmler's The Human Body in Health and Disease*. David Troy, Senior Acquisitions Editor, and Renee Thomas, Managing Editor, at Lippincott Williams and Wilkins, have guided this project with great dedication and skill from start to finish. Jason Taylor reviewed the entire manuscript and gave me much good advice on content and organization. He also wrote the Disease in Context case stories that enliven each chapter and unify the text. Kerry Hull reviewed the manuscript with a great eye for detail and a willingness to discuss any issue with us for as long as needed to reach a decision. Kerry also prepared the Study Guide and the Instructor's Manual with the aid of Molly Ward, Project Manager. Jennifer Clements, as always, advised on the art program and managed the electronic art files, helping to find illustrations when necessary.

My thanks to all the many reviewers, listed separately, who made such valuable and detailed comments on the text. Their insights and advice truly guided every aspect of this new edition.

Once again, thanks to Craig Durant and Dragonfly Media Group for executing any revisions needed to their brilliant drawings.

And as always, thanks to my husband Matthew, currently an instructor in anatomy and physiology, for his advice on and contributions to the text.

Barbara Janson Cohen

Brief Contents

Contents

UNIT

I

The Body as a Whole

This unit presents the basic levels of organization within the human body. Included is a description of the smallest units of life, called cells. Similar cells are grouped together as tissues, which are combined to form organs. Organs, in turn, work together in the various body systems, which together satisfy the needs of the entire organism. A short survey of chemistry, which deals with the composition of all matter and is important for the understanding of human physiology, is incorporated into this unit. These chapters prepare the student for the more detailed study of individual body systems in the units that follow.

CHAPTER 1

Organization of the Human Body

Learning Outcomes

After careful study of this chapter, you should be able to:

1. Define the terms *anatomy*, *physiology*, and *pathology*
2. Describe the organization of the body from chemicals to the whole organism
3. List 11 body systems and give the general function of each
4. Define *metabolism* and name the two phases of metabolism
5. Briefly explain the role of ATP in the body
6. Differentiate between extracellular and intracellular fluids
7. Define and give examples of homeostasis
8. Compare negative feedback and positive feedback
9. List and define the main directional terms for the body
10. List and define the three planes of division of the body
11. Name the subdivisions of the dorsal and ventral cavities
12. Name and locate the subdivisions of the abdomen
13. Name the basic units of length, weight, and volume in the metric system
14. Define the metric prefixes *kilo-*, *centi-*, *milli-*, and *micro-*
15. Show how word parts are used to build words related to the body's organization (see Word Anatomy at the end of the chapter)

Selected Key Terms

The following terms and other boldface terms in the chapter are defined in the Glossary

anabolism
anatomy
ATP
catabolism
cell
disease
dissect
feedback
gram
homeostasis
liter
metabolism
meter
organ
pathology
physiology
system
tissue

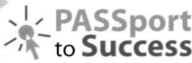

PASSport to Success

Visit *thePoint* or see the Student Resource CD in the back of this book for definitions and pronunciations of key terms as well as a pretest for this chapter.

Disease in Context

> ## Mike's Case: Emergency Care and Homeostatic Imbalance

"Location—Belle Grove Road. Single MVA. Male. Early 20s. Fire and police on scene," crackled the radio. "Medic 12. Respond channel 2."

"Medic 12 responding. En route to Belle Grove Road," Ed radioed back, while his partner, Samantha, flipped the switch for the lights and siren and hit the accelerator. The ambulance sped forward, weaving its way through traffic toward the car accident. When they arrived at the scene, police officers were directing traffic and a fire crew was at work on the vehicle. Samantha maneuvered the ambulance into position just as the crew breached the door of the crumpled minivan. Samantha and Ed grabbed their trauma bags and approached the wreck.

Ed bent down toward the injured man. "My name is Ed. I'm a paramedic. My partner and I are here to help you. I'm going to take a quick look at you, and then we're going to get you out of here."

Samantha inspected the vehicle. "Looks like the impact sent him up and over the steering wheel. Guessing from the cracked windshield, he may have a head injury. The steering column is bent, so I wouldn't rule out thorax or abdomen either."

"That fits with my initial assessment," replied Ed. "Patient's name is Mike. He's got forehead lacerations and he's disoriented. Chest seems fine, but his abdominal cavity could be a problem. There is significant bruising across the left lumbar and umbilical regions—probably from the steering wheel. When I palpated his upper left quadrant, it caused him considerable pain."

Samantha and Ed carefully immobilized Mike's cervical spine and, with the help of the fire crew, transferred him to a stretcher. Samantha started an IV of saline while Ed performed a detailed physical examination beginning cranially and working caudally. Mike's blood pressure was very low and his heart rate was very high—both signs of a cardiovascular emergency. In addition, he had become unresponsive to Ed's questions.

Ed shared his findings with Samantha while she placed an oxygen mask on Mike's nose and mouth. "He's hypotensive and has tachycardia. With the pain he reported earlier, signs are pointing to intraabdominal hemorrhage. We've got to get him to the trauma center right now."

Ed depends on his understanding of anatomy and physiology to help his patient and communicate with his partner. He suspects that Mike is bleeding internally, and that his heart is working hard to compensate for the drastic decrease in blood pressure. As we will see later, this homeostatic crisis must be reversed, or Mike's body systems will fail.

Studies of the normal structure and functions of the body are the basis for all medical sciences. It is only from understanding the normal that one can analyze what is going wrong in cases of disease. These studies give one an appreciation for the design and balance of the human body and for living organisms in general.

Studies of the Human Body

The scientific term for the study of body structure is **anatomy** (ah-NAT-o-me). The *–tomy* part of this word in Latin means "cutting," because a fundamental way to learn about the human body is to cut it apart, or **dissect** (dis-sekt) it. **Physiology** (fiz-e-OL-o-je) is the term for the study of how the body functions, and is based on a Latin term meaning "nature." Anatomy and physiology are closely related—that is, structure and function are intertwined. The stomach, for example, has a pouch-like shape because it stores food during digestion. The cells in the lining of the stomach are tightly packed to prevent strong digestive juices from harming underlying tissue. Anything that upsets the normal structure or working of the body is considered a **disease** and is studied as the science of **pathology** (pah-THOL-o-je).

Levels of Organization

All living things are organized from very simple levels to more complex levels (Fig. 1-1). Living matter is derived from simple chemicals. These chemicals are formed into the complex substances that make living **cells**—the basic units of all life. Specialized groups of cells form **tissues,** and tissues may function together as **organs.** Organs working together for the same general purpose make up the body **systems.** All of the systems work together to maintain the body as a whole organism.

CHECKPOINT **1-1** ➤ In studying the human body, one may concentrate on its structure or its function. What are these two studies called?

Body Systems

Most studies of the human body are organized according to the individual systems, as listed below, grouped according to their general functions.

■ Protection, support, and movement
  > The **integumentary** (in-teg-u-MEN-tar-e) **system.** The word *integument* (in-TEG-u-ment) means skin. The skin with its associated structures is considered a separate body system. The structures associated with the skin include the hair, the nails, and the sweat and oil glands.

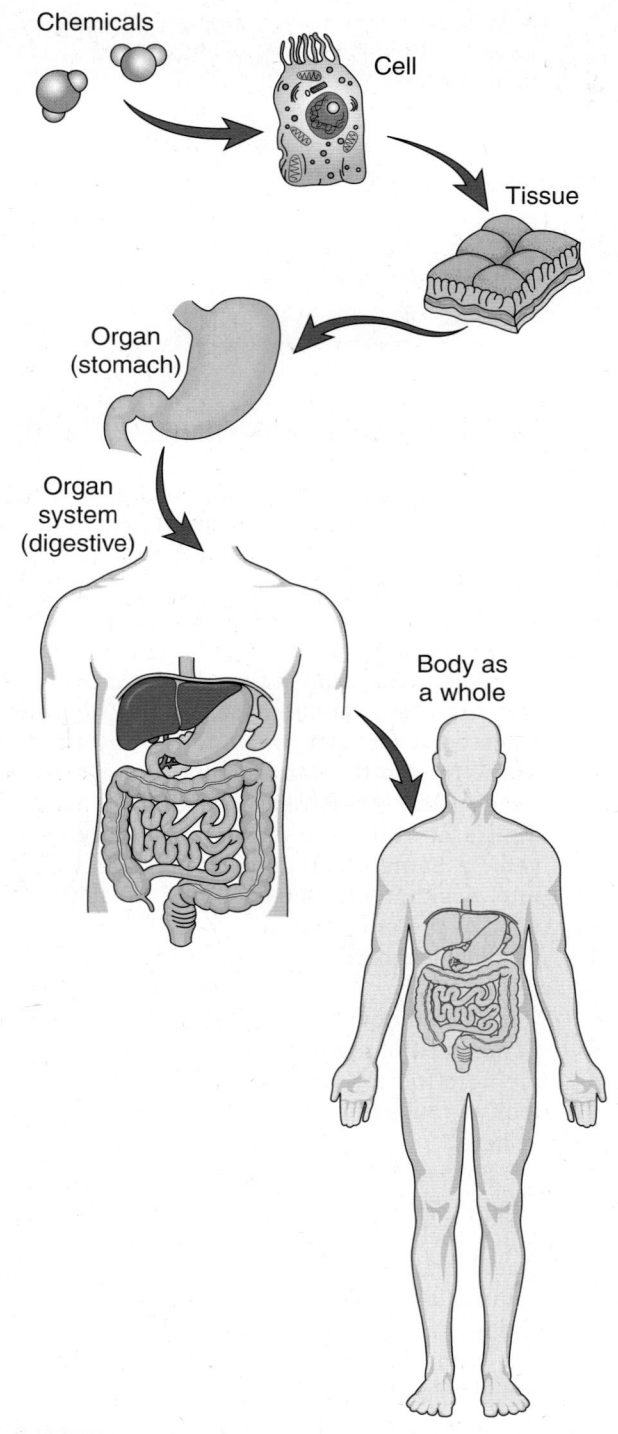

Figure 1-1 **Levels of organization.** The organ shown is the stomach, which is part of the digestive system.

  > The **skeletal system.** The basic framework of the body is a system of 206 bones and the joints between them, collectively known as the **skeleton.**
  > The **muscular system.** The muscles in this system are attached to the bones and produce movement of the skeleton. These skeletal muscles also give the

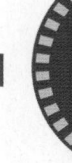

1

body structure, protect organs, and maintain posture. The two other types of muscles are smooth muscle, present in the walls of body organs, such as the stomach and intestine, and cardiac muscle, which makes up the wall of the heart.

■ Coordination and control

> The **nervous system.** The brain, the spinal cord, and the nerves make up this complex system by which the body is controlled and coordinated. The special sense organs (the eyes, ears, taste buds, and organs of smell), together with the receptors for pain, touch, and other generalized senses, receive stimuli from the outside world. These stimuli are converted into impulses that are transmitted to the brain. The brain directs the body's responses to these outside stimuli and also to stimuli that originate internally. Such higher functions as memory and reasoning also occur in the brain.

> The **endocrine** (EN-do-krin) **system.** The scattered organs known as endocrine glands are grouped together because they share a similar function. All produce special substances called hormones, which regulate such body activities as growth, food utilization within the cells, and reproduction. Examples of endocrine glands are the thyroid, pituitary, and adrenal glands.

■ Circulation

> The **cardiovascular system.** The heart and blood vessels make up the system that pumps blood to all the body tissues, bringing with it nutrients, oxygen, and other needed substances. This system then carries waste materials away from the tissues to points where they can be eliminated.

> The **lymphatic system.** Lymphatic vessels assist in circulation by bringing fluids from the tissues back to the blood. Lymphatic organs, such as the tonsils, thymus gland, and spleen, play a role in immunity, protecting against disease. The lymphatic system also aids in the absorption of digested fats through special vessels in the intestine. The fluid that circulates in the lymphatic system is called lymph. The lymphatic and cardiovascular systems together make up the circulatory system.

■ Nutrition and fluid balance

> The **respiratory system.** This system includes the lungs and the passages leading to and from the lungs. The respiratory system's purpose is to take in air and conduct it to the areas designed for gas exchange. Oxygen passes from the air into the blood and is carried to all tissues by the cardiovascular system. In like manner, carbon dioxide, a gaseous waste product, is taken by the circulation from the tissues back to the lungs to be expelled.

> The **digestive system.** This system is composed of all the organs that are involved with taking in nu-

trients (foods), converting them into a form that body cells can use, and absorbing them into the circulation. Organs of the digestive system include the mouth, esophagus, stomach, intestine, liver, and pancreas.

> The **urinary system.** The chief purpose of the urinary system is to rid the body of waste products and excess water. This system's main components are the kidneys, the ureters, the bladder, and the urethra. (Note that some waste products are also eliminated by the digestive and respiratory systems and by the skin.)

■ Production of offspring

> The **reproductive system.** This system includes the external sex organs and all related internal structures that are concerned with the production of offspring.

The number of systems may vary in different lists. Some, for example, show the sensory system as separate from the nervous system. Others have a separate entry for the immune system, which protects the body from foreign matter and invading organisms. The immune system is identified by its function rather than its structure and includes elements of both the cardiovascular and lymphatic systems. Bear in mind that even though the systems are studied as separate units, they are interrelated and must cooperate to maintain health.

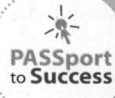

PASSport to Success Visit **thePoint** or see the Student Resource CD in the back of this book for a chart summarizing the body systems and their functions.

Metabolism and Its Regulation

All the life-sustaining reactions that occur within the body systems together make up **metabolism** (meh-TAB-o-lizm). Metabolism can be divided into two types of activities:

■ In **catabolism** (kah-TAB-o-lizm), complex substances are broken down into simpler compounds (Fig. 1-2). The breakdown of food yields simple chemical building blocks and energy to power cellular activities.

■ In **anabolism** (ah-NAB-o-lizm), simple compounds are used to manufacture materials needed for growth, function, and repair of tissues. Anabolism is the building phase of metabolism.

The energy obtained from the breakdown of nutrients is used to form a compound often described as the cell's "energy currency." It has the long name of **adenosine triphosphate** (ah-DEN-o-sene tri-FOS-fate), but is commonly abbreviated ATP. Chapter 20 has more information on metabolism and ATP.

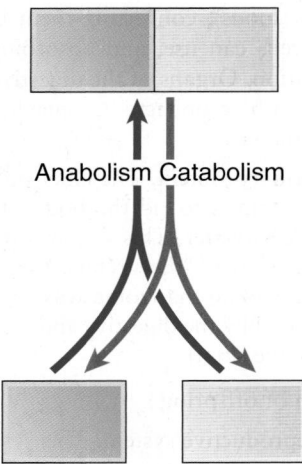

Anabolism Catabolism

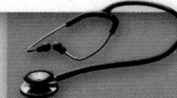 **Metabolism.** In catabolism substances are broken down into their building blocks. In anabolism simple components are built into more complex substances.

Homeostasis

Normal body function maintains a state of internal balance, an important characteristic of all living things. Such conditions as body temperature, the composition of body fluids, heart rate, respiration rate, and blood pressure must be kept within set limits to maintain health. (See Box 1-1, Homeostatic Imbalance: When Feedback Fails.) This steady state within the organism is called **homeostasis** (ho-me-o-STA-sis), which literally means "staying (stasis) the same (homeo)."

FLUID BALANCE Our bodies are composed of large amounts of fluids. The amount and composition of these fluids must be regulated at all times. One type of fluid bathes the cells, carries nutrient substances to and from the cells, and transports the nutrients into and out of the cells. This type is called **extracellular fluid** because it includes all body fluids outside the cells. Examples of extracellular fluids are blood, lymph, and the fluid between the cells in tissues. A second type of fluid, **intracellular fluid**, is contained within the cells. Extracellular and intracellular fluids account for about 60% of an adult's weight. Body fluids are discussed in more detail in Chapter 21.

FEEDBACK The main method for maintaining homeostasis is **feedback**, a control system based on information returning to a source. We are all accustomed to getting feedback about the results of our actions and using that information to regulate our behavior. Grades on tests and assignments, for example, may inspire us to work harder if they're not so great or "keep up the good work" if they are good.

Most feedback systems keep body conditions within a set normal range by reversing any upward or downward shift. This form of feedback is called **negative feedback**, because actions are reversed. A familiar example of negative feedback is the thermostat in a house (Fig. 1-3). When the house temperature falls, the thermostat triggers the furnace to turn on and increase the temperature; when the house temperature reaches an upper limit, the furnace is shut off. In the body, a center in the brain detects changes in temperature and starts mechanisms for cooling or

---

Box 1-1   **Clinical Perspectives**

Homeostatic Imbalance: When Feedback Fails

Each body structure contributes in some way to homeostasis, often through feedback mechanisms. The nervous and endocrine systems are particularly important in feedback. The nervous system's electrical signals react quickly to changes in homeostasis, while the endocrine system's chemical signals (hormones) react more slowly but over a longer time. Often both systems work together to maintain homeostasis.

As long as feedback keeps conditions within normal limits, the body remains healthy, but if feedback cannot maintain these conditions, the body enters a state of *homeostatic imbalance*. Moderate imbalance causes illness and disease, while severe imbalance causes death. At some level, all illnesses and diseases can be linked to homeostatic imbalance.

For example, feedback mechanisms closely monitor and maintain normal blood pressure. When blood pressure rises, negative feedback mechanisms lower it to normal limits. If these mechanisms fail, *hypertension* (high blood pressure) de-

velops. Hypertension further damages the cardiovascular system and, if untreated, may lead to death. With mild hypertension, lifestyle changes in diet, exercise, and stress management may lower blood pressure sufficiently, whereas severe hypertension often requires drug therapy. The various types of antihypertensive medication all help negative feedback mechanisms lower blood pressure.

Feedback mechanisms also regulate body temperature. When body temperature falls, negative feedback mechanisms raise it back to normal limits, but if these mechanisms fail and body temperature continues to drop, *hypothermia* develops. Its main effects are uncontrolled shivering, lack of coordination, decreased heart and respiratory rates, and, if left untreated, death. Cardiac surgeons use hypothermia to their advantage during open heart surgery. Cooling the body slows the heart and decreases its blood flow, helping to create a motionless and bloodless surgical field.

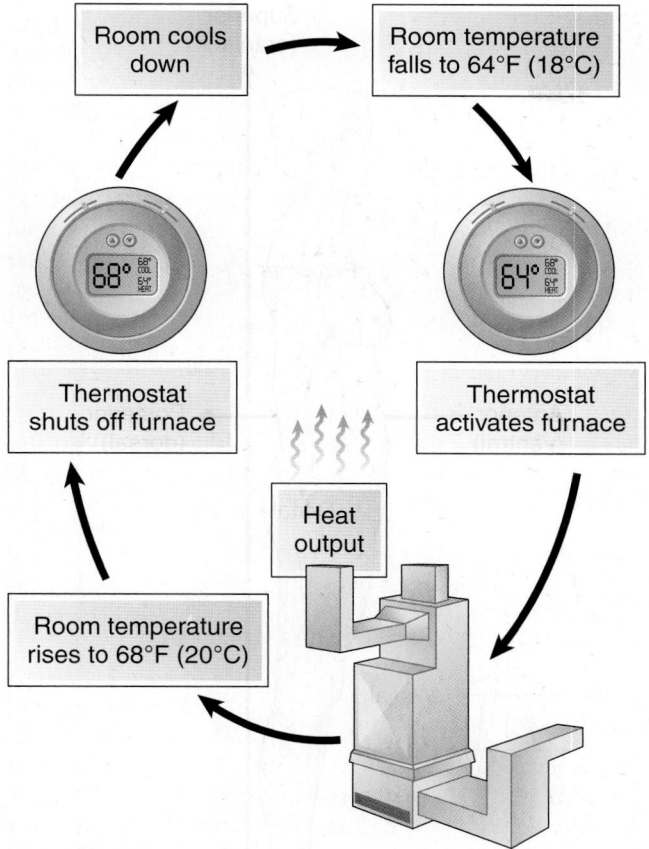

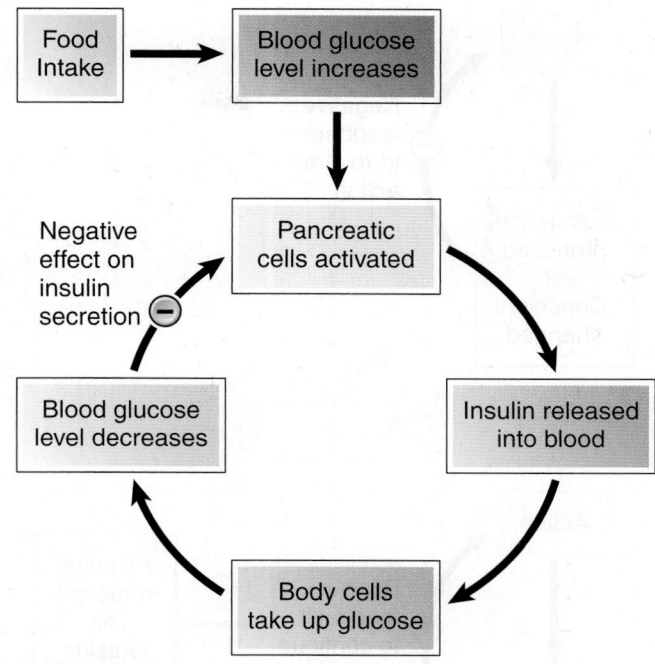

Figure 1-5 **Negative feedback in the endocrine system.** Glucose utilization regulates insulin production by means of negative feedback.

Figure 1-3 **Negative feedback.** A home thermostat illustrates how this type of feedback keeps temperature within a set range.

warming if the temperature is above or below the average set point of 37°C (98.6°F) (Fig. 1-4).

As another example, when glucose (a sugar) increases in the blood, the pancreas secretes insulin, which causes body cells to use more glucose. Increased uptake of glucose and the subsequent drop in blood sugar level serve as a signal to the pancreas to reduce insulin secretion (Fig. 1-5). As a result of insulin's action, the secretion of insulin is reversed. This type of self-regulating feedback loop is used in the endocrine system to maintain proper levels of hormones, as described in Chapter 12.

A few activities involve **positive feedback**, in which a given action promotes more of the same. The process of childbirth illustrates positive feedback. As the contractions of labor begin, the muscles of the uterus are stretched. The stretching sends nervous signals to the pituitary gland to release the hormone oxytocin into the blood. This hormone stimulates further contractions of the uterus. As contractions increase in force, the uterine muscles are stretched even more, causing further release of oxytocin. The escalating contractions and hormone release continue until the baby is born. In positive feedback, activity continues until the stimulus is removed or some outside force interrupts the activity. Positive and negative feedback are compared in Figure 1-6.

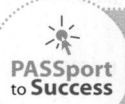

PASSport to Success Visit *thePoint* or see the Student Resource CD in the back of this book to view an animation on feedback.

The Effects of Aging

With age, changes occur gradually in all body systems. Some of these changes, such as wrinkles and gray hair, are obvious. Others, such as decreased kidney function, loss of bone mass, and formation of deposits within blood vessels, are not visible. However, they may make a person more subject to injury and disease. Changes due to aging will be described in chapters on the body systems.

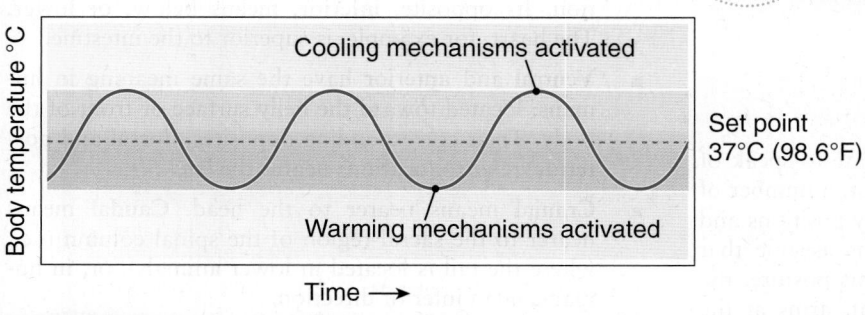

Figure 1-4 **Negative feedback and body temperature.** Body temperature is kept at a set point of 37°C by negative feedback acting on a center in the brain.

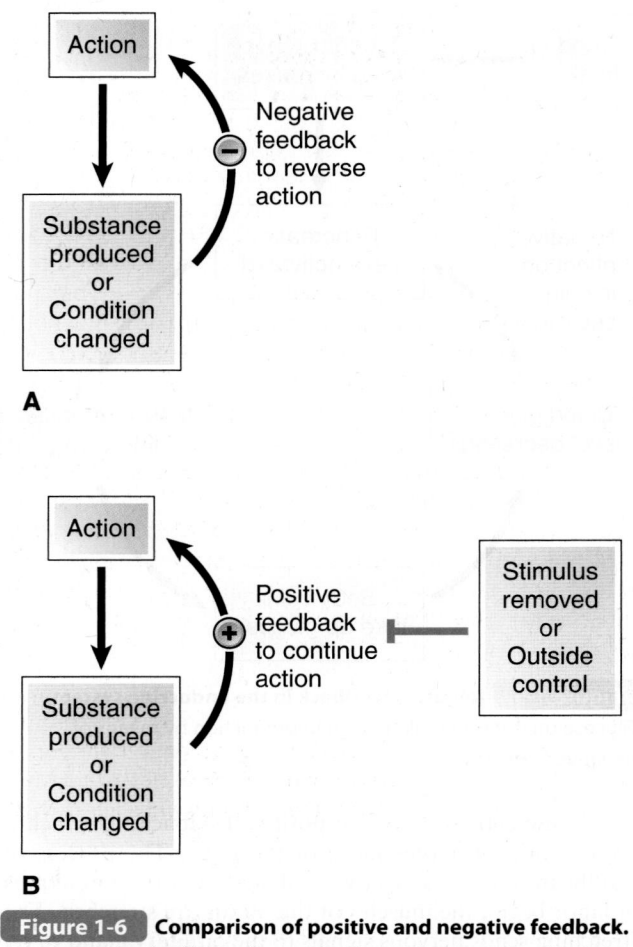

A

B

Figure 1-6 **Comparison of positive and negative feedback.**
(A) In negative feedback, the result of an action reverses the action.
(B) In positive feedback, the result of an action stimulates further
action. Positive feedback continues until the stimulus is removed or
an outside force stops the cycle.

CHECKPOINT 1-2 ➤ Metabolism is divided into a
breakdown phase and a building phase.
What are these two phases called?

CHECKPOINT 1-3 ➤ What type of system is used primarily
to maintain homeostasis?

Directions in the Body

Because it would be awkward and inaccurate to speak of
bandaging the "southwest part" of the chest, a number of
terms are used universally to designate body positions and
directions. For consistency, all descriptions assume that
the body is in the **anatomic position.** In this posture, the
subject is standing upright with face front, arms at the
sides with palms forward, and feet parallel, as shown in
Figure 1-7.

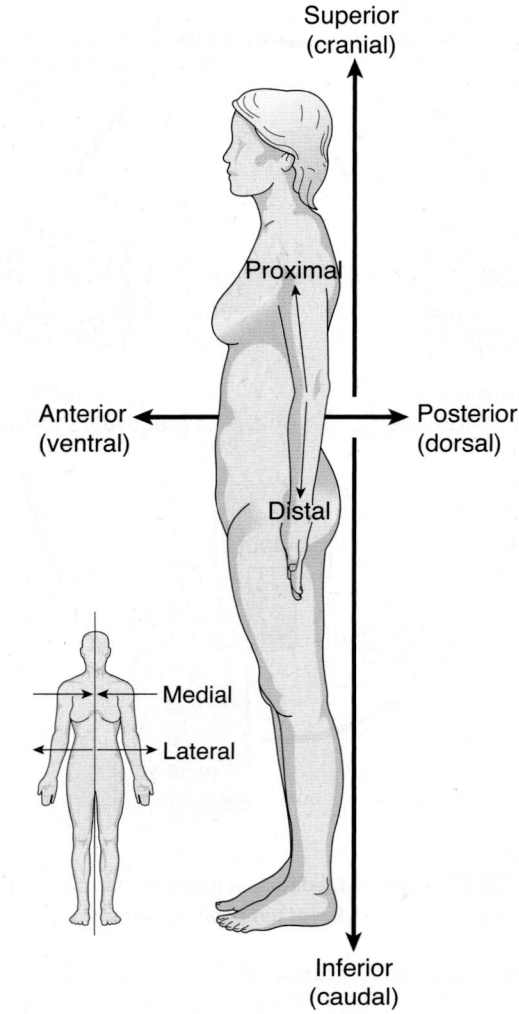

Figure 1-7 **Directional terms. [ZOOMING IN ➤** What is the
scientific name for the position in which the figures are standing? **]**

Directional Terms

The main terms for describing directions in the body are as
follows (see Fig. 1-7):

- **Superior** is a term meaning above, or in a higher position. Its opposite, **inferior,** means below, or lower.
  The heart, for example, is superior to the intestine.

- **Ventral** and **anterior** have the same meaning in humans: located toward the belly surface or front of the
  body. Their corresponding opposites, **dorsal** and **posterior,** refer to locations nearer the back.

- **Cranial** means nearer to the head. **Caudal** means
  nearer to the sacral region of the spinal column (i.e.,
  where the tail is located in lower animals), or, in humans, in an inferior direction.

- **Medial** means nearer to an imaginary plane that passes
  through the midline of the body, dividing it into left

and right portions. **Lateral**, its opposite, means farther away from the midline, toward the side.

■ **Proximal** means nearer the origin of a structure; **distal**, farther from that point. For example, the part of your thumb where it joins your hand is its proximal region; the tip of the thumb is its distal region.

Planes of Division

To visualize the various internal structures in relation to each other, anatomists can divide the body along three planes, each of which is a cut through the body in a different direction (Fig. 1-8).

■ The **frontal plane**. If the cut were made in line with the ears and then down the middle of the body, you would see an anterior, or ventral (front), section and a posterior, or dorsal (back), section. Another name for this plane is *coronal plane*.

■ The **sagittal** (SAJ-ih-tal) **plane**. If you were to cut the body in two from front to back, separating it into right and left portions, the sections you would see would be sagittal sections. A cut exactly down the midline of the body, separating it into equal right and left halves, is a **midsagittal** section.

■ The **transverse plane**. If the cut were made horizontally, across the other two planes, it would divide the body

into a superior (upper) part and an inferior (lower) part. A transverse plane is also called a *horizontal plane*.

TISSUE SECTIONS Some additional terms are used to describe sections (cuts) of tissues, as used to prepare them for study under the microscope (Fig. 1-9). A cross section (see figure) is a cut made perpendicular to the long axis of an organ, such as a cut made across a banana to give a small round slice. A longitudinal section is made parallel to the long axis, as in cutting a banana from tip to tip to make a slice for a banana split. An oblique section is made at an angle. The type of section used will determine what is seen under the microscope, as shown with a blood vessel in Figure 1-9.

These same terms are used for images taken by techniques such as computed tomography (CT) or magnetic resonance imaging (MRI). (See Box 1-2, Medical Imaging: Seeing Without Making a Cut.) In imaging studies, the term cross-section is used more generally to mean any two-dimensional view of an internal structure obtained by imaging, as shown in Figure 1-10.

CHECKPOINT **1-4** ➤ What are the three planes in which the body can be cut? What kind of a plane divides the body into two equal halves?

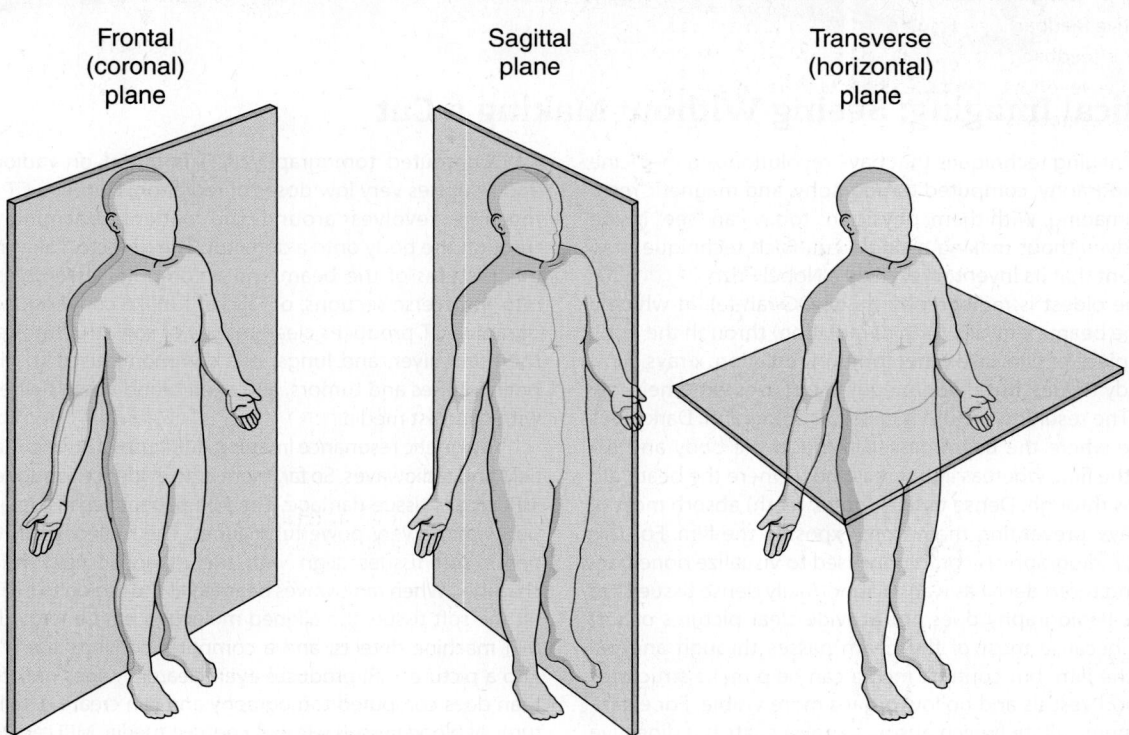

Figure 1-8 **Planes of division.** [ZOOMING IN ➤ Which plane divides the body into superior and inferior parts? Which plane divides the body into anterior and posterior parts?]

Frontal (coronal) plane   Sagittal plane   Transverse (horizontal) plane

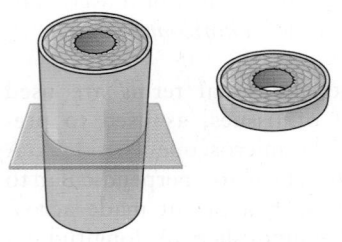
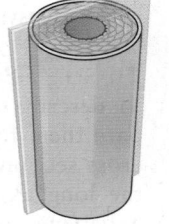
Cross section

Longitudinal section

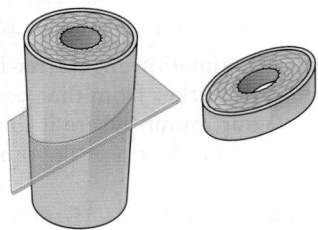
Oblique section

Figure 1-9 **Tissue sections.**

Body Cavities

Internally, the body is divided into a few large spaces, or **cavities**, which contain the organs. The two main cavities are the **dorsal cavity** and **ventral cavity** (Fig. 1-11).

Dorsal Cavity

The dorsal body cavity has two subdivisions: the **cranial cavity**, containing the brain, and the **spinal cavity (canal)**, enclosing the spinal cord. These two areas form one continuous space.

Ventral Cavity

The ventral cavity is much larger than the dorsal cavity. It has two main subdivisions, which are separated by the **diaphragm** (DI-ah-fram), a muscle used in breathing. The **thoracic** (tho-RAS-ik) **cavity** is located superior to (above) the diaphragm. Its contents include the heart, the lungs, and the large blood vessels that join the heart. The heart is contained in the pericardial cavity, formed by the pericardial sac; the lungs are in the pleural cavity, formed by the pleurae, the membranes that enclose the lungs (Fig. 1-12). The **mediastinum** (me-de-as-TI-num) is the space between the lungs, including the organs and vessels contained in that space.

Box 1-2 Hot Topics

Medical Imaging: Seeing Without Making a Cut

Three imaging techniques that have revolutionized medicine are radiography, computed tomography, and magnetic resonance imaging. With them, physicians today can "see" inside the body without making a single cut. Each technique is so important that its inventor received a Nobel Prize.

The oldest is radiography (ra-de-OG-rah-fe), in which a machine beams x-rays (a form of radiation) through the body onto a piece of film. Like other forms of radiation, x-rays damage body tissues, but modern equipment uses extremely low doses. The resulting picture is called a radiograph. Dark areas indicate where the beam passed through the body and exposed the film, whereas light areas show where the beam did not pass through. Dense tissues (bone, teeth) absorb most of the x-rays, preventing them from exposing the film. For this reason, radiography is commonly used to visualize bone fractures and tooth decay as well as abnormally dense tissues like tumors. Radiography does not provide clear pictures of soft tissues because most of the beam passes through and exposes the film, but contrast media can help make structures like blood vessels and hollow organs more visible. For example, barium sulfate (which absorbs x-rays) coats the digestive tract when ingested.

Computed tomography (CT) is based on radiography and also uses very low doses of radiation. During a CT scan, a machine revolves around the patient, beaming x-rays through the body onto a detector. The detector takes numerous pictures of the beam and a computer assembles them into transverse sections, or "slices." Unlike conventional radiography, CT produces clear images of soft structures such as the brain, liver, and lungs. It is commonly used to visualize brain injuries and tumors, and even blood vessels when used with contrast media.

Magnetic resonance imaging (MRI) uses a strong magnetic field and radiowaves. So far, there is no evidence to suggest that MRI causes tissue damage. The MRI patient lies inside a chamber within a very powerful magnet. The molecules in the patient's soft tissues align with the magnetic field inside the chamber. When radiowaves beamed at the region to be imaged hit the soft tissue, the aligned molecules emit energy that the MRI machine detects, and a computer converts these signals into a picture. MRI produces even clearer images of soft tissue than does computed tomography and can create detailed pictures of blood vessels without contrast media. MRI can visualize brain injuries and tumors that might be missed using CT.

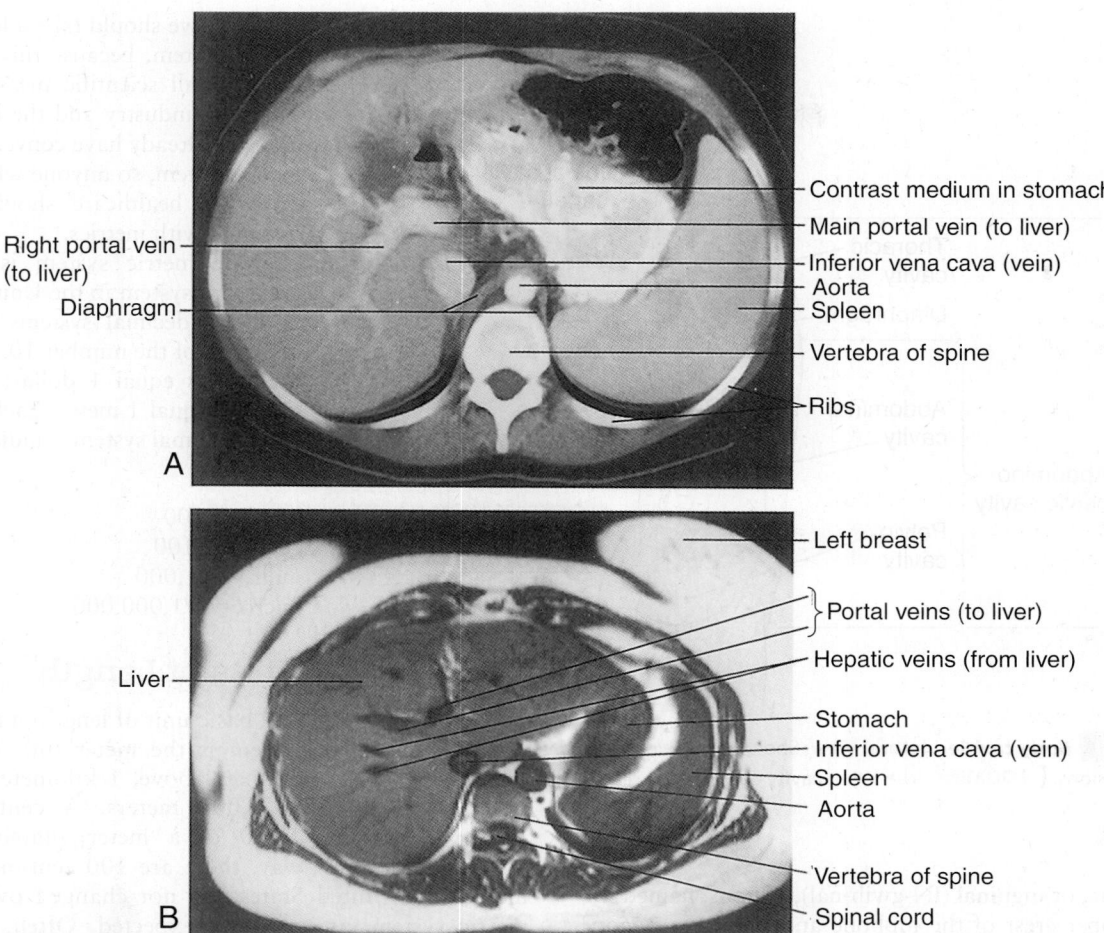

Right portal vein
(to liver)

Diaphragm

Contrast medium in stomach
Main portal vein (to liver)
Inferior vena cava (vein)
Aorta
Spleen
Vertebra of spine
Ribs

A

Left breast

Portal veins (to liver)

Hepatic veins (from liver)

Liver

Stomach
Inferior vena cava (vein)
Spleen
Aorta
Vertebra of spine
Spinal cord

B

Figure 1-10 **Cross-sections in imaging.** Images taken across the body through the liver and spleen by **(A)** computed tomography (CT) and **(B)** magnetic resonance imaging (MRI). (Reprinted with permission from Erkonen WE. *Radiology 101: Basics and Fundamentals of Imaging.* Philadelphia: Lippincott Williams & Wilkins, 1998.)

The **abdominopelvic** (ab-dom-ih-no-PEL-vik) **cavity** (see Fig. 1-11) is located inferior to (below) the diaphragm. This space is further subdivided into two regions. The superior portion, the **abdominal cavity**, contains the stomach, most of the intestine, the liver, the gallbladder, the pancreas, and the spleen. The inferior portion, set off by an imaginary line across the top of the hip bones, is the **pelvic cavity**. This cavity contains the urinary bladder, the rectum, and the internal parts of the reproductive system. See Appendix 7, Dissection Atlas, for a dissection photograph showing organs of the ventral cavity.

CHECKPOINT ▇▇ ➤ There are two main body cavities, one posterior and one anterior. Name these two cavities.

REGIONS OF THE ABDOMEN It is helpful to divide the abdomen for examination and reference into nine regions (Fig. 1-13).

The three central regions, from superior to inferior, are:

■ the **epigastric** (ep-ih-GAS-trik) **region,** located just inferior to the breastbone

■ the **umbilical** (um-BIL-ih-kal) **region** around the umbilicus (um-BIL-ih-kus), commonly called the *navel*

■ the **hypogastric** (hi-po-GAS-trik) **region,** the most inferior of all the midline regions

The regions on the right and left, from superior to inferior, are:

■ the **hypochondriac** (hi-po-KON-dre-ak) **regions,** just inferior to the ribs

■ the **lumbar regions,** which are on a level with the lumbar regions of the spine

CHECKPOINT ▇▇ ➤ Name the three central regions and the three left and right lateral regions of the abdomen.

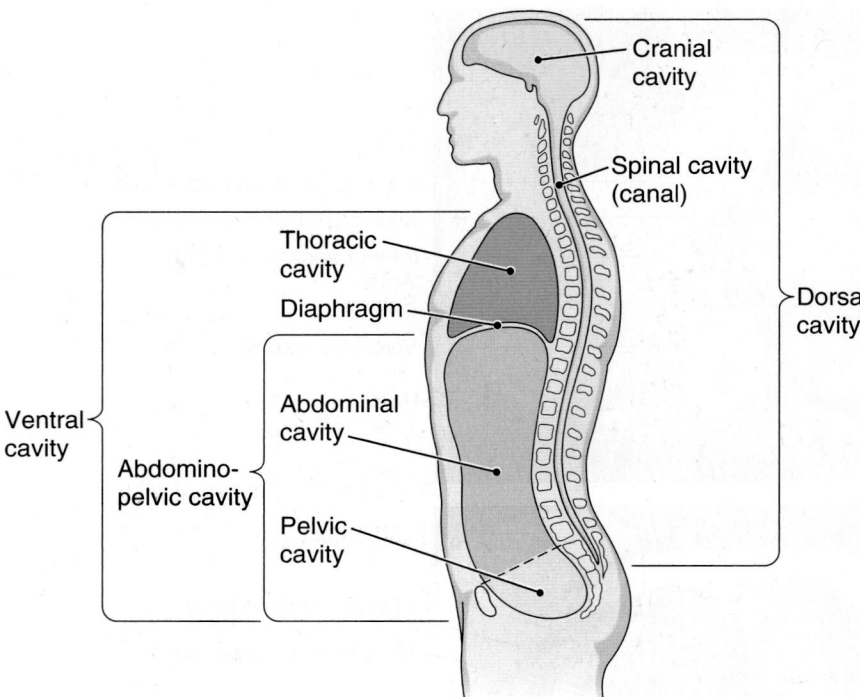

Figure 1-11 **Body cavities, lateral view.** Shown are the dorsal and ventral cavities with their subdivisions. [ZOOMING IN ➤ What cavity contains the diaphragm?]

■ the iliac, or **inguinal** (IN-gwih-nal), **regions**, named for the upper crest of the hipbone and the groin region, respectively

A simpler but less precise division into four quadrants is sometimes used. These regions are the right upper quadrant (RUQ), left upper quadrant (LUQ), right lower quadrant (RLQ), and left lower quadrant (LLQ) (Fig. 1-14).

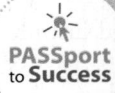

Visit **thePoint** or see the Student Resource CD in the back of this book for photographic versions of Figures 1-13 and 1-14, a list of the organs in each quadrant, and figures naming other body regions. Also see the Health Professions box, Health Information Technicians, for description of a profession that uses anatomic, physiologic, and medical terms.

The Metric System

Now that we have set the stage for further study of the body's structure and

function, we should take a look at the metric system, because this system is used for all scientific measurements. The drug industry and the healthcare industry already have converted to the metric system, so anyone who plans a career in healthcare should be acquainted with metrics.

The metric system is like the monetary system in the United States. Both are decimal systems based on multiples of the number 10. One hundred cents equal 1 dollar; 100 centimeters equal 1 meter. Each multiple in the decimal system is indicated by a prefix:

kilo = 1,000
centi = 1/100
milli = 1/1,000
micro = 1/1,000,000

Units of Length

The basic unit of length in the metric system is the **meter** (m). Using the prefixes above, 1 kilometer is equal to 1,000 meters. A centimeter is 1/100 of a meter; stated another way, there are 100 centimeters in 1 meter. The United States has not changed over to the metric system, as was once expected. Often, measurements on packages, bottles, and yard goods are now given according to both scales. In this text, equivalents in the more familiar units of inches and feet are included along with the metric units for comparison. There are 2.5 centimeters (cm) or 25 millimeters (mm) in 1 inch, as shown in Figure 1-15. Some equivalents that may help

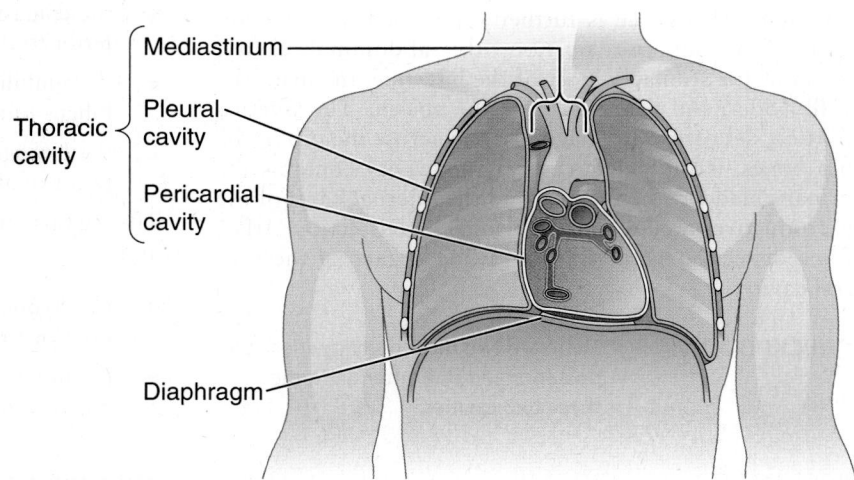

Figure 1-12 **The thoracic cavity.** Shown are the pericardial cavity, which contains the heart, and the pleural cavity, which contains the lungs.

1

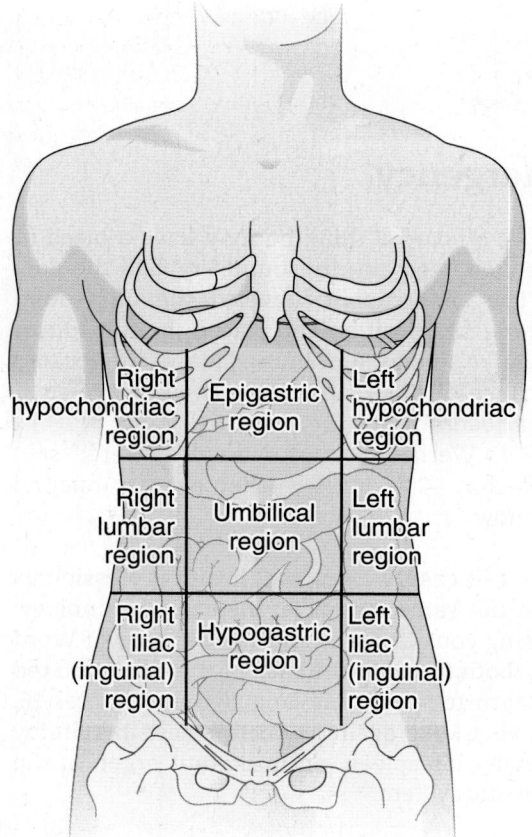

Figure 1-13 The nine regions of the abdomen.

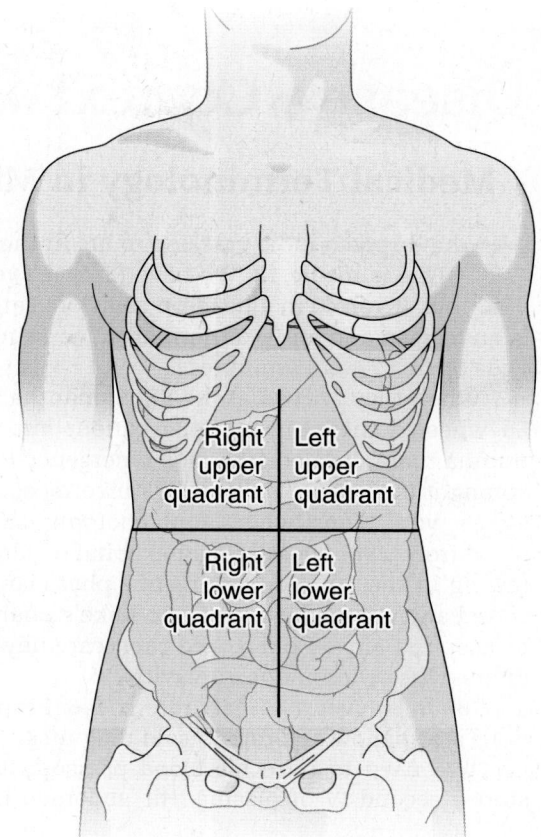

Figure 1-14 **Quadrants of the abdomen.** The organs within each quadrant are shown.

you to appreciate the size of various body parts are as follows:

> 1 mm = 0.04 inch, or 1 inch = 25 mm
> 1 cm = 0.4 inch, or 1 inch = 2.5 cm
> 1 m = 3.3 feet, or 1 foot = 30 cm

Units of Weight

The same prefixes used for linear measurements are used for weights and volumes. The **gram** (g) is the basic unit of weight. Thirty grams are about equal to 1 ounce and 1 kilogram to 2.2 pounds. Drug dosages are usually stated in grams or milligrams. One thousand milligrams equal 1 gram; a 500-milligram (mg) dose would be the equivalent of 0.5 gram (g), and 250 mg is equal to 0.25 g.

Units of Volume

The dosages of liquid medications are given in units of volume. The basic metric measurement for volume is the **liter** (L) (LE-ter). There are 1,000 milliliters (mL) in a liter. A liter is slightly greater than a quart, a liter being equal to 1.06 quarts. For smaller quantities, the milliliter is used most of the time. There are 5 mL in a teaspoon and 15 mL in a tablespoon. A fluid ounce contains 30 mL.

Temperature

The Celsius (centigrade) temperature scale, now in use by most countries and by scientists in this country, is discussed in Chapter 20.

A chart of all the common metric measurements and their equivalents is shown in Appendix 1. A Celsius-Fahrenheit temperature conversion scale appears in Appendix 2.

CHECKPOINT **1-7** ➤ Name the basic units of length, weight, and volume in the metric system.

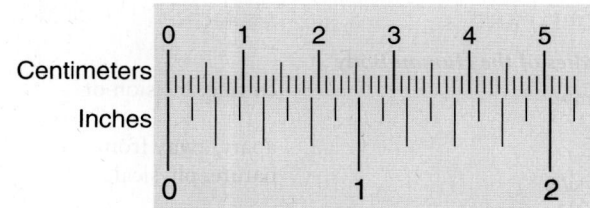

Figure 1-15 **Comparison of centimeters and inches.**

Disease in Context revisited

➤ Medical Terminology in Mike's Emergency

The dispatch radio crackled to life in the ER. "This is medic 12. We have Mike. 21 years old. Involved in a head-on collision. Patient is on oxygen and an IV of normal saline running wide open. ETA is 15 minutes."

When they arrived at the ER, Samantha and Ed wheeled their unconscious patient into the trauma room. Immediately, the emergency team sprang into action. The trauma nurse measured Mike's vital signs while a phlebotomist drew blood from a vein in Mike's antecubital region for testing in the lab. The emergency physician inserted an endotracheal tube into Mike's pharynx to keep his airway open, and then carefully examined his abdominopelvic cavity.

"BP is 80 over 40. Heart rate is 146. Respirations are shallow and rapid," said the nurse.

"We need to raise his blood pressure—let's start a second IV of plasma. His abdomen is as hard as a board. I think he may have a bleed in there—we need an ultrasound," replied the doctor. The sonographer wheeled the ultrasound machine into position and placed the transducer onto Mike's abdomen. Immediately, she located the cause of Mike's trauma—blood in the right upper quadrant.

"OK. We have a ruptured spleen here," said the doctor. "Call surgery—they need to operate right now."

In this case, we saw that health professionals speak the same language: medical terminology. By using your Glossary and the Glossary of Word Parts (both found at the back of this text), you too can learn to speak this language. In Chapter 16, we'll visit Mike again as doctors save his life by removing his spleen, an important organ of the lymphatic system.

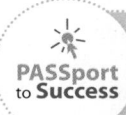

PASSport to Success

Interested in some of the health professions featured in this Disease in Context? Visit *thePoint* or see the Student Resource CD in the back of this book for more information on careers in the health professions.

Word Anatomy

Medical terms are built from standardized word parts (prefixes, roots, and suffixes). Learning the meanings of these parts can help you remember words and interpret unfamiliar terms.

WORD PART	MEANING	EXAMPLE
Studies of the Human Body		
-tomy	cutting, incision of	*Anatomy* can be revealed by making incisions in the body.
dis-	apart, away from	To *dissect* is to cut apart.
physi/o	nature, physical	*Physiology* is the study of how the body functions.
path/o	disease	*Pathology* is the study of disease.

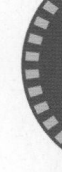

WORD PART	MEANING	EXAMPLE
Body Systems		
cata-	down	*Catabolism* is the breakdown of complex substances into simpler ones.
ana-	upward, again, back	*Anabolism* is the building up of simple compounds into more complex substances.
home/o-	same	*Homeostasis* is the steady state (sameness) within an organism.
stat	stand, stoppage, constancy	In *homeostasis*, "-stasis" refers to constancy.

Summary

I. **STUDIES OF THE HUMAN BODY**
  A. Anatomy—study of structure
  B. Physiology—study of function
  C. Pathology—study of disease
  D. Levels of organization—chemicals, cell, tissue, organ, organ system, whole organism

II. **BODY SYSTEMS**
  A. Integumentary system—skin and associated structures
  B. Skeletal system—support
  C. Muscular system—movement
  D. Nervous system—reception of stimuli and control of responses
  E. Endocrine system—production of hormones for regulation of growth, metabolism, and reproduction
  F. Cardiovascular system—movement of blood for transport
  G. Lymphatic system—aids in circulation, immunity, and absorption of digested fats
  H. Respiratory system—intake of oxygen and release of carbon dioxide
  I. Digestive system—intake, breakdown, and absorption of nutrients
  J. Urinary system—elimination of waste and water
  K. Reproductive system—production of offspring

III. **METABOLISM AND ITS REGULATION**
  A. Metabolism—all the chemical reactions needed to sustain life
    1. Catabolism—breakdown of complex substances into simpler substances; release of energy from nutrients
      a. ATP (adenosine triphosphate)—energy compound of cells
    2. Anabolism—building of body materials
  B. Homeostasis—steady state of body conditions
    1. Fluid balance
      a. Extracellular fluid—outside the cells
      b. Intracellular fluid—inside the cells
    2. Feedback—regulation by return of information within a system

      a. Negative feedback—reverses an action
      b. Positive feedback—promotes continued activity
  C. Effects of aging—changes in all systems

IV. **DIRECTIONS IN THE BODY**
  A. Anatomic position—upright, palms forward, face front, feet parallel
  B. Directional terms
    1. Superior—above or higher; inferior—below or lower
    2. Ventral (anterior)—toward belly or front surface; dorsal (posterior)—nearer to back surface
    3. Cranial—nearer to head; caudal—nearer to sacrum
    4. Medial—toward midline; lateral—toward side
    5. Proximal—nearer to point of origin; distal—farther from point of origin
  C. Planes of division
    1. Body divisions
      a. Sagittal—from front to back, dividing the body into left and right parts
        (1) Midsagittal—exactly down the midline
      b. Frontal (coronal)—from left to right, dividing the body into anterior and posterior parts
      c. Transverse—horizontally, dividing the body into superior and inferior parts
    2. Tissue sections
      a. Cross-section—perpendicular to long axis
      b. Transverse section—parallel to long axis
      c. Oblique section—at an angle

V. **BODY CAVITIES**
  A. Dorsal cavity—contains cranial and spinal cavities for brain and spinal cord
  B. Ventral cavity
    1. Thoracic—chest cavity
      a. Divided from abdominal cavity by diaphragm
      b. Contains heart and lungs

c. Mediastinum—space between lungs and the organs contained in that space
2. Abdominopelvic
   a. Abdominal—upper region containing stomach, most of intestine, pancreas, liver, spleen, and others
   b. Pelvic—lower region containing reproductive organs, urinary bladder, and rectum
   c. Nine regions of the abdomen
     (1) Central—epigastric, umbilical, hypogastric
     (2) Lateral (right and left)—hypochondriac, lumbar, iliac (inguinal)

d. Quadrants—abdomen divided into four regions

VI. **THE METRIC SYSTEM**—Based on multiples of 10
  A. Prefixes—indicate multiples of 10
    1. Kilo—1,000 times
    2. Centi—1/100th (0.01)
    3. Milli—1/1,000th (0.001)
    4. Micro—1/1,000,000 (0.000001)
  B. Units of length—meter is basic unit
  C. Units of weight—gram is basic unit
  D. Units of volume—liter is basic unit
  E. Temperature—measured in Celsius (centigrade) scale

Questions for Study and Review

BUILDING UNDERSTANDING

Fill in the blanks

1. Tissues may function together as _____.
2. Glands that produce hormones belong to the _____ system.
3. The eyes are located _____ to the nose.
4. Normal body function maintains a state of internal balance called _____.
5. The basic unit of volume in the metric system is the _____.

Matching > Match each numbered item with the most closely related lettered item.

___ **6.** One of two systems that control and coordinate other systems
___ **7.** The system that brings needed substances to the body tissues
___ **8.** The system that converts foods into a form that body cells can use
___ **9.** The cavity that contains the liver
___ **10.** The cavity that contains the urinary bladder

  a. nervous system
  b. abdominal cavity
  c. cardiovascular system
  d. pelvic cavity
  e. digestive system

Multiple Choice

___ **11.** The study of normal body structure is
  a. homeostasis
  b. anatomy
  c. physiology
  d. pathology

___ **12.** Fluids contained within cells are described as
  a. intracellular
  b. ventral
  c. extracellular
  d. dorsal

___ **13.** A type of feedback in which a given action promotes more of the same is called
  a. homeostasis
  b. biofeedback
  c. positive feedback
  d. negative feedback

___ **14.** The cavity that contains the mediastinum is the
  a. dorsal
  b. ventral
  c. abdominal
  d. pelvic

___ **15.** The foot is located _____ to the knee.
  a. superior
  b. inferior
  c. proximal
  d. distal

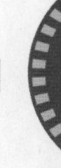

UNDERSTANDING CONCEPTS

16. Compare and contrast the studies of anatomy and physiology. Would it be wise to study one without the other?

17. List in sequence the levels of organization in the body from simplest to most complex. Give an example for each level.

18. Compare and contrast the anatomy and physiology of the nervous system with that of the endocrine system.

19. What is ATP? What type of metabolic activity releases the energy used to make ATP?

20. Compare and contrast intracellular and extracellular fluids.

21. Explain how an internal state of balance is maintained in the body.

22. List the subdivisions of the dorsal and ventral cavities. Name some organs found in each subdivision.

CONCEPTUAL THINKING

23. The human body is organized from very simple levels to more complex levels. With this in mind, describe why a disease at the chemical level can have an effect on organ system function.

24. In Mike's case, the paramedics and the emergency doctor suspected that Mike's hypotension and tachycardia both resulted from intraabdominal hemorrhage. Using your understanding of negative feedback, discuss why Mike's heart rate increased when his blood pressure decreased.

25. In Mike's case, the paramedics and emergency team injected several liters of saline and blood plasma into Mike's cardiovascular system. How might the addition of IV fluids stabilize Mike's blood pressure?

26. In Mike's case, the paramedics discovered bruising of the skin over Mike's left lumbar region and umbilical region. Mike also reported considerable pain in his upper left quadrant. Locate these regions on your own body and explain why it is important for health professionals to use medical terminology when describing the human body.

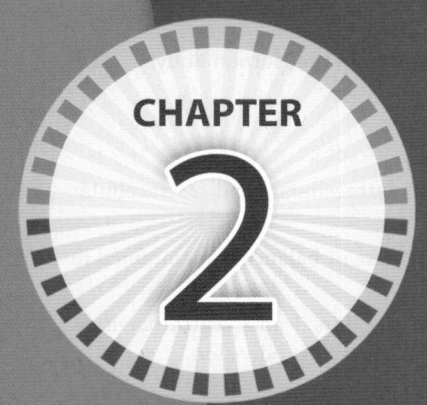

CHAPTER 2

Chemistry, Matter, and Life

Learning Outcomes

After careful study of this chapter, you should be able to:

1. Define an element
2. Describe the structure of an atom
3. Differentiate between molecules and compounds
4. Explain why water is so important to the body
5. Define *mixture*; list the three types of mixtures and give two examples of each
6. Differentiate between ionic and covalent bonds
7. Define an electrolyte
8. Define the terms *acid*, *base*, and *salt*
9. Explain how the numbers on the pH scale relate to acidity and basicity (alkalinity)
10. Define *buffer* and explain why buffers are important in the body
11. Define *radioactivity* and cite several examples of how radioactive substances are used in medicine
12. List three characteristics of organic compounds
13. Name the three main types of organic compounds and the building blocks of each
14. Define *enzyme*; describe how enzymes work
15. Show how word parts are used to build words related to chemistry, matter, and life (see Word Anatomy at the end of the chapter)

Selected Key Terms

The following terms and other boldface terms in the chapter are defined in the Glossary

acid
alkali
atom
base
buffer
carbohydrate
catalyst
chemistry
colloid
compound
denaturation
electrolyte
electron
element
enzyme
fat
ion
isotope
lipid
molecule
neutron
pH
protein
proton
radioactive
salt
solution
suspension
valence

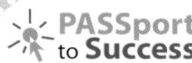

PASSport to Success

Visit *thePoint* or see the Student Resource CD in the back of this book for definitions and pronunciations of key terms as well as a pretest for this chapter.

Disease in Context

▶ Margaret's Case: Chemistry's Role in Health Science

"Ugghh," sighed Angela as she pulled into her parking spot. The heat wave was into its second week and she was getting tired of it. It was beginning to take its toll on the city too, especially on its young and old inhabitants. As Angela walked toward the hospital she thought back to yesterday's ICU shift. One particular elderly patient stood out in Angela's mind, probably because she reminded the nurse of her own grandmother.

The patient, Margaret Ringland, a 78-year-old widow, lived alone in her apartment on New York's Upper East Side. Yesterday, her niece, who comes every Monday to drop off some groceries, found Margaret collapsed on the floor, weak and confused. Her niece called 911, and Margaret was rushed to the emergency room. According to her medical chart, Margaret presented with flushed dry skin, a sticky oral cavity, and a furrowed tongue. She was confused and disoriented. She also had hypotension (low blood pressure) and tachycardia (an elevated heart rate). All were classic signs of dehydration, a severe deficiency of water. Without water, a compound composed of two hydrogen atoms covalently bonded to an oxygen atom (H_2O), Margaret's body was unable to perform essential metabolic processes and her tissues and organs were not in homeostatic balance. The central nervous system is particularly sensitive to changes in water volume, which accounted for Margaret's neurologic symptoms.

Although it was difficult to get a blood sample from Margaret's flattened veins, her blood work confirmed the initial diagnosis. Margaret's electrolyte levels were out of balance—especially her blood's sodium ion concentration, which was much too high, a condition called hypernatremia. Margaret's hematocrit was also higher than normal—a sign that the volume of water in her blood was too low. This decrease in blood volume was having serious consequences for her cardiovascular system. Margaret's blood pressure had dropped, which forced her heart to beat faster to ensure proper delivery of blood to her tissues.

The emergency team started an IV line in Margaret's antebrachium. An aqueous solution of 5% dextrose (another name for the carbohydrate monosaccharide called glucose) was delivered through the IV at a rate of 500 mL per hour. A catheter was also inserted into Margaret's urethra to allow for drainage of urine from her urinary bladder. Once stabilized, Margaret was moved to ICU for recovery.

Angela depends on her knowledge of chemistry to make sense of the signs and symptoms she observes in her patients. As you read Chapter 2, keep in mind that a firm understanding of the chemistry presented in this chapter will help you understand the anatomy and physiology of the cells, tissues, and organ systems discussed in subsequent chapters.

Greater understanding of living organisms has come to us through **chemistry,** the science that deals with the composition and properties of matter. Knowledge of chemistry and chemical changes helps us understand the normal and abnormal functioning of the body. The digestion of food in the intestinal tract, the production of urine by the kidneys, the regulation of breathing, and all other body activities involve the principles of chemistry. The many drugs used to treat diseases are chemicals. Chemistry is used for the development of drugs and for an understanding of their actions in the body.

To provide some insights into the importance of chemistry in the life sciences, this chapter briefly describes elements, atoms and molecules, compounds, and mixtures, which are fundamental forms of matter.

Elements

Matter is anything that takes up space, that is, the materials from which all of the universe is made. Elements are the substances that make up all matter. The food we eat, the atmosphere, water—everything around us, everything we can see and touch—is made of elements. There are 92 naturally occurring elements. (Twenty additional elements have been created in the laboratory.) Examples of elements include various gases, such as hydrogen, oxygen, and nitrogen; liquids, such as mercury used in barometers and other scientific instruments; and many solids, such as iron, aluminum, gold, silver, and zinc. Graphite (the so-called "lead" in a pencil), coal, charcoal, and diamonds are different forms of the element carbon.

Elements can be identified by their names or their chemical symbols, which are abbreviations of the modern or Latin names of the elements. Each element is also identified by its own number, which is based on the structure of its subunits, or atoms. The periodic table is a chart used by chemists to organize and describe the elements. Appendix 3 shows the periodic table and gives some information about how it is used. Table 2-1 lists some elements found in the human body along with their functions.

Atoms

The subunits of elements are **atoms.** These are the smallest complete units of matter. They cannot be broken down or changed into another form by ordinary chemical and physical means. These subunits are so small that millions of them could fit on the sharpened end of a pencil.

ATOMIC STRUCTURE Despite the fact that the atom is such a tiny particle, it has been carefully studied and has been found to have a definite structure. At the center of the atom is a nucleus, which contains positively charged electrical particles called **protons** (PRO-tonz) and noncharged particles called **neutrons** (NU-tronz). Together, the protons and neutrons contribute nearly all of the atom's weight.

In orbit outside the nucleus are **electrons** (e-LEK-tronz) (Fig. 2-1). These nearly weightless particles are negatively charged. It is the electrons that determine how the atom will react chemically. The protons and electrons of an atom always are equal in number, so that the atom as a whole is electrically neutral.

The **atomic number** of an element is equal to the number of protons that are present in the nucleus of each of its atoms. Because the number of protons is equal to the number of electrons, the atomic number also represents the

Table 2-1	Some Common Chemical Elements*	
Name	**Symbol**	**Function**
Oxygen	O	Part of water; needed to metabolize nutrients for energy
Carbon	C	Basis of all organic compounds; in carbon dioxide, the waste gas of metabolism
Hydrogen	H	Part of water; participates in energy metabolism, acid–base balance
Nitrogen	N	Present in all proteins, ATP (the energy compound), and nucleic acids (DNA and RNA)
Calcium	Ca	Builds bones and teeth; needed for muscle contraction, nerve impulse conduction, and blood clotting
Phosphorus	P	Active ingredient in the energy-storing compound ATP; builds bones and teeth; in cell membranes and nucleic acids
Potassium	K	Nerve impulse conduction; muscle contraction; water balance and acid–base balance
Sulfur	S	Part of many proteins
Sodium	Na	Active in water balance, nerve impulse conduction, and muscle contraction
Chlorine	Cl	Active in water balance and acid–base balance; found in stomach acid
Iron	Fe	Part of hemoglobin, the compound that carries oxygen in red blood cells

* *The elements are listed in decreasing order by weight in the body.*

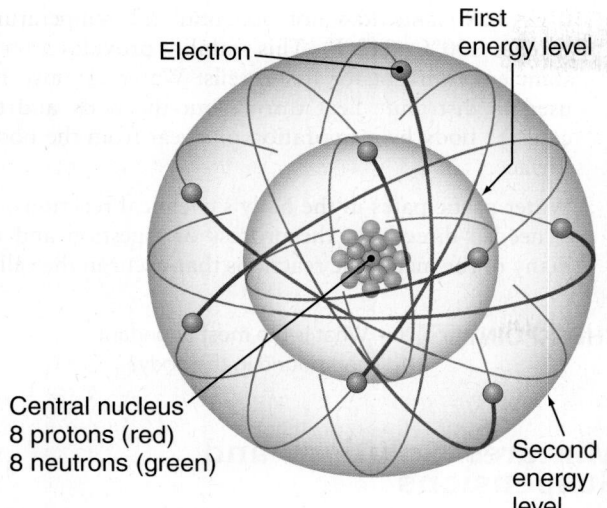

Figure 2-1 **Representation of the oxygen atom.** Eight protons and eight neutrons are tightly bound in the central nucleus. The eight electrons are in orbit around the nucleus, two at the first energy level and six at the second. [**ZOOMING IN** ➤ How does the number of protons in this atom compare with the number of electrons?]

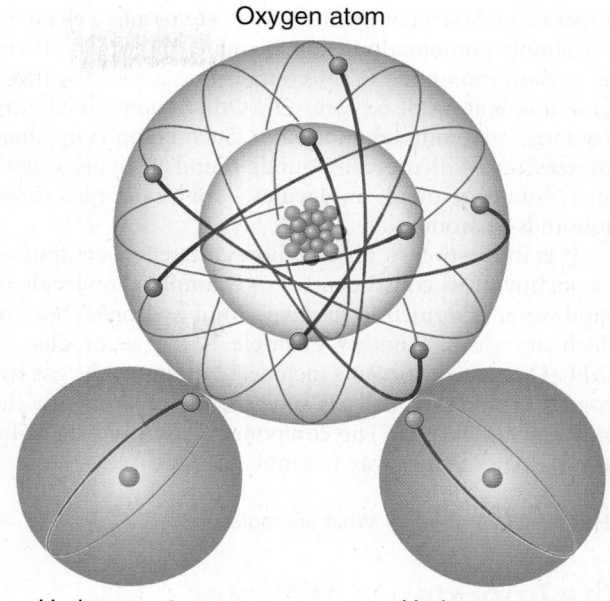

Figure 2-2 **Formation of water.** When oxygen reacts, two electrons are needed to complete the outermost energy level, as shown in this reaction with hydrogen to form water. [**ZOOMING IN** ➤ How many hydrogen atoms bond with an oxygen atom to form water?]

number of electrons whirling around the nucleus. Each element has a specific atomic number. No two elements share the same number. In Periodic Table of the Elements (see Appendix 3), the atomic number is located at the top of the box for each element.

The positively charged protons keep the negatively charged electrons in orbit around the nucleus by means of the opposite charges on the particles. Positively (+) charged protons attract negatively (−) charged electrons.

CHECKPOINT 2-1 ➤ What are atoms?

CHECKPOINT 2-2 ➤ What are three types of particles found in atoms?

ENERGY LEVELS An atom's electrons orbit at specific distances from the nucleus in regions called energy levels. The first energy level, the one closest to the nucleus, can hold only two electrons. The second energy level, the next in distance away from the nucleus, can hold eight electrons. More distant energy levels can hold more than eight electrons, but they are stable (nonreactive) when they have eight.

The electrons in the energy level farthest away from the nucleus give the atom its chemical characteristics. If the outermost energy level has more than four electrons but less than its capacity of eight, the atom normally completes this level by gaining electrons. In the process, it becomes negatively charged, because it has more electrons than protons. The oxygen atom illustrated in Figure 2-1 has six electrons in its second, or outermost, level. When oxygen enters into chemical reactions, it gains two electrons, as when it reacts with hydrogen to form water (Fig. 2-2). The oxygen atom then has two more electrons than protons. If the outermost

energy level has fewer than four electrons, the atom normally loses those electrons. In so doing, it becomes positively charged, because it now has more protons than electrons.

The number of electrons lost or gained by atoms of an element in chemical reactions is known as the **valence** of that element (from a Latin word that means "strength"). The outermost energy level, which determines the combining properties of the element, is the valence level. Valence is reported as a number with a + or − to indicate whether electrons are lost or gained in chemical reactions. Remember that electrons carry a negative charge, so when an atom gains electrons it becomes negatively charged and when an atom loses electrons it becomes positively charged. For example, the valence of oxygen, which gains two electrons in chemical reactions, is shown as O^{2-}.

Molecules and Compounds

A **molecule** (MOL-eh-kule) is formed when two or more atoms unite on the basis of their electron structures. A molecule can be made of like atoms—the oxygen molecule is made of two identical atoms—but more often a molecule is made of atoms of two or more different elements. For example, a molecule of water (H_2O) contains one atom of oxygen (O) and two atoms of hydrogen (H) (see Fig. 2-2).

Substances composed of two or more different elements are called **compounds**. Molecules are the smallest subunits of a compound. Each molecule of a compound contains the elements that make up that compound in the proper ratio. Some compounds are made of a few elements in a simple combination. For example, molecules of the gas carbon monoxide (CO) contain one atom of carbon (C) and one atom of oxygen (O). Other compounds have very large and complex molecules. Such complexity characterizes many of the compounds found in living organisms. Some protein molecules, for example, have thousands of atoms.

It is interesting to observe how different a compound is from any of its constituents. For example, a molecule of liquid water is formed from oxygen and hydrogen, both of which are gases. Another example is the sugar glucose ($C_6H_{12}O_6$). Its constituents include 12 atoms of the gas hydrogen, 6 atoms of the gas oxygen, and 6 atoms of the solid element carbon. The component gases and the solid carbon do not in any way resemble the glucose.

CHECKPOINT 2-3 ➤ What are molecules?

The Importance of Water

Water is the most abundant compound in the body. No plant or animal, including the human, can live very long without it. Water is of critical importance in all physiological processes in body tissues. A deficiency of water, or dehydration (de-hi-DRA-shun), can be a serious threat to health. Water carries substances to and from the cells and makes possible the essential processes of absorption, exchange, secretion, and excretion. What are some of the properties of water that make it such an ideal medium for living cells?

- Water can dissolve many different substances in large amounts. For this reason, it is called the **universal solvent**. Many of the body's necessary materials, such as gases, minerals, and nutrients, dissolve in water to be carried from place to place. Substances, such as salts, that mix with or dissolve in water are described as *hydrophilic* ("water-loving"); those, such as fats, that repel and do not dissolve in water are described as *hydrophobic* ("water-fearing").

- Water is stable as a liquid at ordinary temperatures. Water does not freeze until the temperature drops to 0°C (32°F) and does not boil until the temperature reaches 100°C (212°F). This stability provides a constant environment for living cells. Water can also be used to distribute heat throughout the body and to cool the body by evaporation of sweat from the body surface.

- Water participates in the body's chemical reactions. It is needed directly in the process of digestion and in many of the metabolic reactions that occur in the cells.

CHECKPOINT 2-4 ➤ What is the most abundant compound in the body?

Mixtures: Solutions and Suspensions

Not all elements or compounds combine chemically when brought together. The air we breathe every day is a mixture of gases, largely nitrogen, oxygen, and carbon dioxide, along with smaller percentages of other substances. The constituents in the air maintain their identity, although the proportions of each may vary. Blood plasma is also a mixture in which the various components maintain their identity. The many valuable compounds in the plasma remain separate entities with their own properties. Such combinations are called **mixtures**—blends of two or more substances (Table 2-2).

A mixture formed when one substance dissolves in another is called a **solution.** One example is salt water. In a solution, the component substances cannot be distinguished from each other and remain evenly distributed throughout; that is, the mixture is homogeneous (ho-mo-JE-ne-us). The dissolving substance, which in the body is water, is the **solvent.** The substance dissolved, salt in the case of salt water, is the **solute.** An **aqueous** (A-kwe-us) **solution** is one in which water is the solvent. Aqueous solutions of glucose, salts, or both of these together are used for intravenous fluid treatments.

In some mixtures, the substance distributed in the background material is not dissolved and will settle out unless the mixture is constantly shaken. This type of nonuniform, or heterogeneous (het-er-o-JE-ne-us), mixture is

Table 2-2	Mixtures	
Type	**Definition**	**Example**
Solution	Homogeneous mixture formed when one substance (solute) dissolves in another (solvent)	Table salt (NaCl) dissolved in water; table sugar (sucrose) dissolved in water
Suspension	Heterogeneous mixture in which one substance is dispersed in another but will settle out unless constantly mixed	Red blood cells in blood plasma; milk of magnesia
Colloid	Heterogeneous mixture in which the suspended material remains evenly distributed based on the small size and opposing charges of the particles	Blood plasma; cytosol

called a **suspension**. The particles in a suspension are separate from the material in which they are dispersed, and they settle out because they are large and heavy. Examples of suspensions are milk of magnesia, finger paints, and, in the body, red blood cells suspended in blood plasma.

One other type of mixture is important in body function. Some organic compounds form **colloids**, in which the molecules do not dissolve yet remain evenly distributed in the suspending material. The particles have electrical charges that repel each other, and the molecules are small enough to stay in suspension. The fluid that fills the cells (cytosol) is a colloidal suspension, as is blood plasma.

Many mixtures are complex, with properties of solutions, suspensions, and colloidal suspensions. Blood plasma has dissolved compounds, making it a solution. The red blood cells and other formed elements give blood the property of a suspension. The proteins in the plasma give it the property of a colloidal suspension. Chocolate milk also has all three properties.

CHECKPOINT `2-5` ➤ Both solutions and suspensions are types of mixtures. What is the difference between them?

Chemical Bonds

When discussing the structure of the atom, we mentioned the positively charged (+) protons that are located in the nucleus and the equal number of orbiting negatively charged (−) electrons that neutralize the protons (Fig. 2-3A). Atoms interact, however, to reach a stable number of electrons in the outermost energy level. These chemical interactions alter the neutrality of the atoms and also form a bond between them. In chemical reactions, electrons may be transferred from one atom to another or may be shared between atoms.

Ionic Bonds

When electrons are transferred from one atom to another, the type of bond formed is called an **ionic** (i-ON-ik) **bond**. The sodium atom, for example, tends to lose the single electron in its outermost shell (Fig. 2-3B), leaving an outermost shell with a stable number of electrons (8). Removal of a single electron from the sodium atom leaves one more proton than electrons, and the atom then has a single net positive charge. The sodium atom in this form is symbolized as Na^+. An atom or group of atoms with a positive or negative charge is called an **ion** (I-on). Any ion that is positively charged is a **cation** (CAT-i-on).

Alternately, atoms can gain electrons so that there are more electrons than protons. Chlorine, which has seven electrons in its outermost energy level, tends to gain one electron to fill the level to its capacity. Such an atom of chlorine is negatively charged (Cl^-) (see Fig. 2-3B). (Chemists refer to this charged form of chlorine as *chloride*.) Any negatively charged ion is an **anion** (AN-i-on).

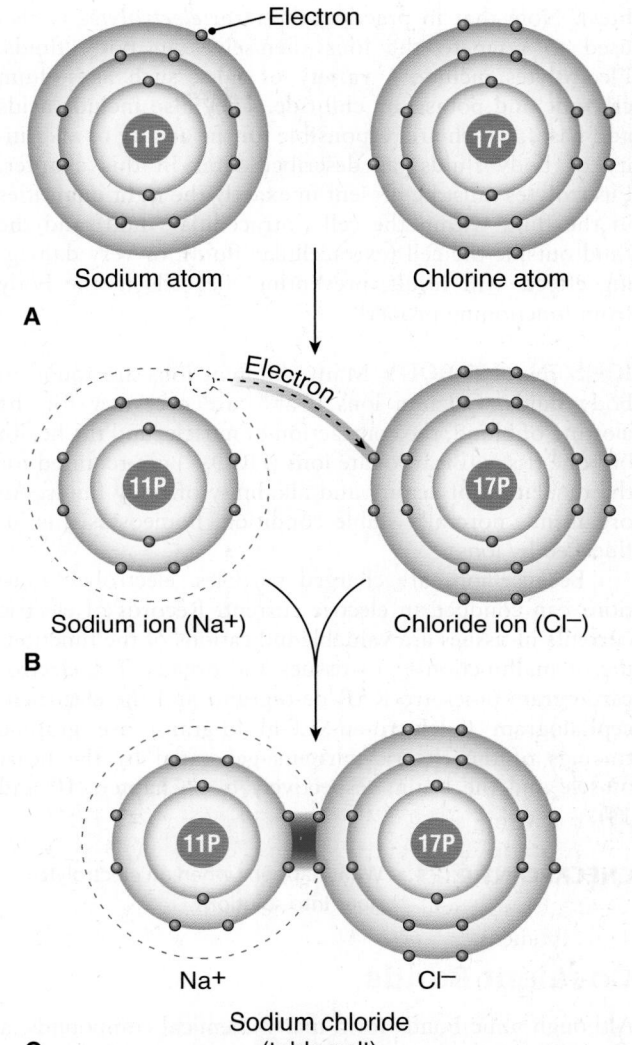

Figure 2-3 **Ionic bonding. (A)** A sodium atom has 11 protons and 11 electrons. A chlorine atom has 17 protons and 17 electrons. **(B)** A sodium atom gives up one electron to a chlorine atom in forming an ionic bond. The sodium atom now has 11 protons and 10 electrons, resulting in a positive charge of one. The chlorine becomes negatively charged by one, with 17 protons and 18 electrons. **(C)** The sodium ion (Na^+) is attracted to the chloride ion (Cl^-), forming the compound sodium chloride (table salt).

Let us imagine a sodium atom coming in contact with a chlorine atom. The chlorine atom gains an electron from the sodium atom, forming an ionic bond. The two newly formed ions (Na^+ and Cl^-), because of their opposite charges, attract each other to produce the compound sodium chloride, ordinary table salt (Fig. 2-3C).

ELECTROLYTES Ionically bonded substances, when they go into solution, separate into charged particles. Compounds formed by ionic bonds that release ions when they are in solution are called **electrolytes** (e-LEK-trolites). Note that in practice, the term *electrolytes* is also used to refer to the ions themselves in body fluids. Electrolytes include a variety of salts, such as sodium chloride and potassium chloride. They also include acids and bases, which are responsible for the acidity or alkalinity of body fluids, as described later in this chapter. Electrolytes must be present in exactly the right quantities in the fluid within the cell (intracellular fluid) and the fluid outside the cell (extracellular fluid), or very damaging effects will result, preventing the cells in the body from functioning properly.

IONS IN THE BODY Many different ions are found in body fluids. Calcium ions (Ca^{2+}) are necessary for the clotting of blood, the contraction of muscle, and the health of bone tissue. Bicarbonate ions (HCO_3^-) are required for the regulation of acidity and alkalinity of body fluids. An organism's normally stable condition, homeostasis, is influenced by ions.

Because ions are charged particles, electrolyte solutions can conduct an electric current. Records of electric currents in tissues are valuable indications of the functioning or malfunctioning of tissues and organs. The **electrocardiogram** (e-lek-tro-KAR-de-o-gram) and the **electroencephalogram** (e-lek-tro-en-SEF-ah-lo-gram) are graphic tracings of the electric currents generated by the heart muscle and the brain, respectively (see Chapters 10 and 14).

CHECKPOINT **2-6** ➤ What happens when an electrolyte goes into solution?

Covalent Bonds

Although ionic bonds form many chemical compounds, a much larger number of compounds are formed by another type of chemical bond. This bond involves not the exchange of electrons but a sharing of electrons between the atoms in the molecule and is called a **covalent bond**. This name comes from the prefix *co-*, meaning "together," and *valence*, referring to the electrons involved in chemical reactions between atoms. In a covalently bonded molecule, the valence electrons orbit around both of the atoms, making both of them stable. Covalent bonds may involve the sharing of one, two, or three pairs of electrons between atoms.

In some covalently bonded molecules, the electrons are equally shared, as in the case of a hydrogen molecule (H_2) and other molecules composed of identical atoms (Fig. 2-4). Electrons may also be shared equally in some molecules composed of different atoms, methane (CH_4), for example. If electrons are equally shared in forming a molecule, the electrical charges are evenly distributed around the atoms and the bond is described as a *nonpolar covalent bond*. That is, no part of the molecule is more negative or positive than any other part of the molecule. More commonly, the electrons are held closer to one atom than the other, as in the case of water (H_2O), shown in

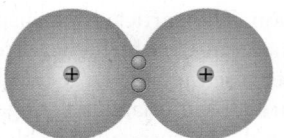

Hydrogen molecule (H₂)

Figure 2-4 **A nonpolar covalent bond.** The electrons involved in the bonding of a hydrogen molecule are equally shared between the two atoms of hydrogen. The electrons orbit evenly around the two. [ZOOMING IN ➤ How many electrons are needed to complete the energy level of each hydrogen atom?]

Figure 2-2. In a water molecule, the shared electrons are actually closer to the oxygen at any one time, making that region of the molecule more negative. Such bonds are called *polar covalent bonds*, because one part of the molecule is more negative and one part is more positive at any one time.

Anyone studying biological chemistry (biochemistry) is interested in covalent bonding because carbon, the element that is the basis of organic chemistry, forms covalent bonds with a wide variety of different elements. Thus, the compounds that are characteristic of living things are covalently bonded compounds. For a description of another type of bond, see Box 2-1, Hydrogen Bonds: Strength in Numbers.

CHECKPOINT **2-7** ➤ How is a covalent bond formed?

Compounds: Acids, Bases, and Salts

An **acid** is a chemical substance capable of donating a hydrogen ion (H^+) to another substance. A common example is hydrochloric acid, the acid found in stomach juices:

$$HCl \rightarrow H^+ + Cl^-$$
(hydrochloric acid) (hydrogen ion) (chloride ion)

A **base** is a chemical substance, usually containing a hydroxide ion (OH^-), that can accept a hydrogen ion. A base is also called an alkali (AL-kah-li). Sodium hydroxide, which releases hydroxide ion in solution, is an example of a base:

$$NaOH \rightarrow Na^+ + OH^-$$
(sodium hydroxide) (sodium ion) (hydroxide ion)

A reaction between an acid and a base produces a **salt**, such as sodium chloride:

$$HCl + NaOH \rightarrow NaCl + H_2O$$

The pH Scale

The greater the concentration of hydrogen ions in a solution, the greater the acidity of that solution. The greater the concentration of hydroxide ion (OH^-), the greater the basicity (alkalinity) of the solution. Based on changes in the

---

Box 2-1 A Closer Look

Hydrogen Bonds: Strength in Numbers

In contrast to ionic and covalent bonds, which hold atoms together, hydrogen bonds hold molecules together. Hydrogen bonds are much weaker than ionic or covalent bonds—in fact, they are more like "attractions" between molecules. While ionic and covalent bonds rely on electron transfer or sharing, hydrogen bonds form bridges between two molecules. A hydrogen bond forms when a slightly positive hydrogen atom in one molecule is attracted to a slightly negative atom in another molecule. Even though a single hydrogen bond is weak, many hydrogen bonds between two molecules can be strong.

Hydrogen bonds hold water molecules together, with the slightly positive hydrogen atom in one molecule attracted to a slightly negative oxygen atom in another. Many of water's unique properties come from its ability to form hydrogen bonds. For example, hydrogen bonds keep water liquid over a wide range of temperatures, which provides a constant environment for body cells.

Hydrogen bonds form not only between molecules but also within large molecules. Hydrogen bonds between regions of the same molecule cause it to fold and coil into a specific shape, as in the process that creates the precise

three-dimensional structure of proteins. Because a protein's structure determines its function in the body, hydrogen bonds are essential to protein activity.

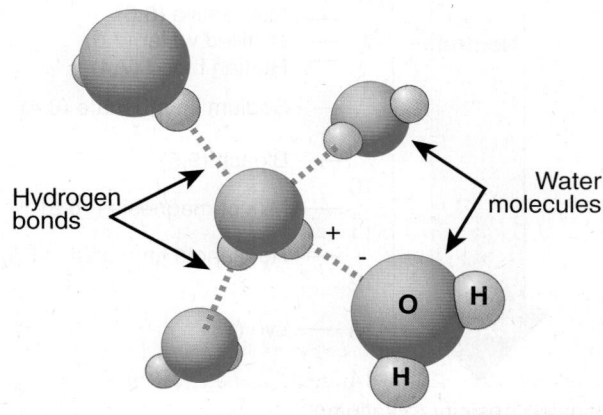

Hydrogen bonds. The bonds shown here are holding water molecules together.

---

balance of ions in solution, as the concentration of hydrogen ions increases, the concentration of hydroxide ions decreases. Conversely, as the concentration of hydroxide ions increases, the concentration of hydrogen ions decreases.

Acidity and alkalinity are indicated by pH units, which represent the relative concentrations of hydrogen and hydroxide ions in a solution. The pH units are listed on a scale from 0 to 14, with 0 being the most acidic and 14 being the most basic (Fig. 2-5). A pH of 7.0 is neutral. At pH 7.0 the solution has an equal number of hydrogen and hydroxide ions. Pure water has a pH of 7.0. Solutions that measure less than 7.0 are acidic; those that measure above 7.0 are alkaline (basic).

Because the pH scale is based on multiples of 10, each pH unit on the scale represents a 10-fold change in the number of hydrogen and hydroxide ions present. A solution registering 5.0 on the scale has 10 times the number of hydrogen ions as a solution that registers 6.0. The pH 5.0 solution also has one-tenth the number of hydroxide ions as the solution of pH 6.0. A solution registering 9.0 has one-tenth the number of hydrogen ions and 10 times the number of hydroxide ions as one registering 8.0. Thus, the lower the pH reading, the greater is the acidity, and the higher the pH, the greater is the alkalinity.

Blood and other body fluids are close to neutral but are slightly on the alkaline side, with a pH range of 7.35 to

7.45. Urine averages pH 6.0 but may range from 4.6 to 8.0 depending on body conditions and diet. Figure 2-5 shows the pH of some other common substances.

Because body fluids are on the alkaline side of neutral, the body may be in a relatively acidic state even if the pH does not drop below 7.0. For example, if the pH falls below 7.35 but is still greater than 7.0, one is described as being in an acidic state known as *acidosis*. Thus, within this narrow range, physiologic acidity differs from acidity as defined by the pH scale.

An increase in pH to readings greater than 7.45 is termed *alkalosis*. Any shifts in pH to readings above or below the normal range can be dangerous, even fatal.

Buffers

If a person is to remain healthy, a delicate balance must exist within the narrow limits of acidity and alkalinity of body fluids. This balanced chemical state is maintained in large part by **buffers**. Chemicals that serve as buffers form a system that prevents sharp changes in hydrogen ion concentration and thus maintains a relatively constant pH. Buffers are important in maintaining stability in the pH of body fluids. More information about body fluids, pH, and buffers can be found in Chapter 21.

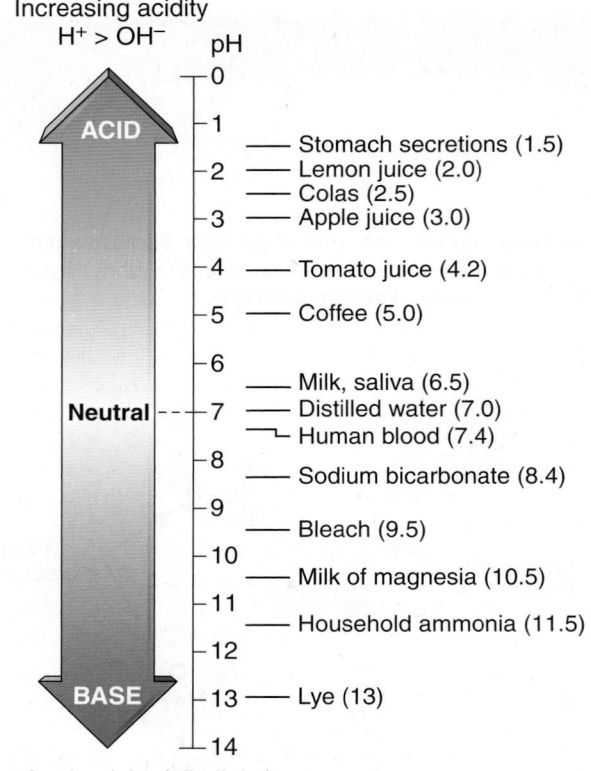

Increasing acidity
H⁺ > OH⁻

pH

ACID

—— Stomach secretions (1.5)
—— Lemon juice (2.0)
—— Colas (2.5)
—— Apple juice (3.0)

—— Tomato juice (4.2)

—— Coffee (5.0)

—— Milk, saliva (6.5)
Neutral — —— Distilled water (7.0)
—— Human blood (7.4)

—— Sodium bicarbonate (8.4)

—— Bleach (9.5)

—— Milk of magnesia (10.5)

—— Household ammonia (11.5)

BASE

—— Lye (13)

Increasing basicity (alkalinity)
OH⁻ > H⁺

Figure 2-5   **The pH scale.** Degree of acidity or alkalinity is shown in pH units. This scale also shows the pH of some common substances. [**ZOOMING IN ➤** What happens to the amount of hydroxide ion (OH⁻) present in a solution when the amount of hydrogen ion (H⁺) increases?]

CHECKPOINT 2-8 ➤ The pH scale is used to measure acidity and alkalinity of fluids. What number is neutral on the pH scale? What kind of compound measures lower than this number? Higher?

CHECKPOINT 2-9 ➤ What is a buffer?

Isotopes and Radioactivity

Elements may exist in several forms, each of which is called an **isotope** (I-so-tope). These forms are alike in their numbers of protons and electrons, but differ in their atomic weights because of differing numbers of neutrons in the nucleus. The most common form of oxygen, for example, has eight protons and eight neutrons in the nucleus, giving the atom an atomic weight of 16 atomic mass units (amu). But there are some isotopes of oxygen with only 6 or 7 neutrons in the nucleus and others with 9 to 11 neutrons. The isotopes of oxygen thus range in weight from 14 to 19 amu.

Some isotopes are stable and maintain constant characteristics. Others disintegrate (fall apart) and give off rays of atomic particles. Such isotopes are said to be **radioactive**. Radioactive elements may occur naturally, as is the case with isotopes of the very heavy elements radium and uranium. Others may be produced artificially by placing the atoms of lighter, nonradioactive elements in accelerators that smash their nuclei together.

Use of Radioactive Isotopes

The rays given off by some radioactive elements, also called *radioisotopes*, are used in the treatment of cancer because they have the ability to penetrate and destroy tissues. Radiation therapy is often given by means of machines that are able to release tumor-destroying particles. The sensitivity of the younger, dividing cells in a growing cancer allows selective destruction of these abnormal cells with minimal damage to normal tissues. Modern radiation instruments produce tremendous amounts of energy (in the multimillion electron-volt range) and yet can destroy deep-seated cancers without causing serious skin reactions.

In radiation treatment, a radioactive isotope, such as cobalt 60, is sealed in a stainless steel cylinder and mounted on an arm or crane. Beams of radioactivity are then directed through a porthole to the area to be treated. Implants containing radioactive isotopes in the form of needles, seeds, or tubes also are widely used in the treatment of different types of cancer.

In addition to its therapeutic values, irradiation is extensively used in diagnosis. X-rays penetrate tissues and produce an image of their interior on a photographic plate. Radioactive iodine and other "tracers" taken orally or injected into the bloodstream are used to diagnose abnormalities of certain body organs, such as the thyroid gland (see Box 2-2, Radioactive Tracers: Medicine Goes Nuclear). Rigid precautions must be followed by healthcare personnel to protect themselves and the patient when using radiation in diagnosis or therapy because the rays can destroy both healthy and diseased tissues.

CHECKPOINT 2-10 ➤ Some isotopes are stable; others break down to give off atomic particles. What word is used to describe isotopes that give off radiation?

Chemistry of Living Matter

Of the 92 elements that exist in nature, only 26 have been found in living organisms. Most of these are elements that are light in weight. Not all are present in large quantity. Hydrogen, oxygen, carbon, and nitrogen are the elements that make up about 96% of body weight (Fig. 2-6). Nine additional elements—calcium, sodium, potassium, phosphorus, sulfur, chlorine, magnesium, iron, and iodine—make up most of the remaining 4% of the body's elements. The remaining 13, including zinc, selenium, copper,

Box 2-2 Hot Topics

Radioactive Tracers: Medicine Goes Nuclear

Like radiography, computed tomography (CT), and magnetic resonance imaging (MRI), **nuclear medicine imaging** (NMI) offers a noninvasive way to look inside the body. An excellent diagnostic tool, NMI shows not only structural details but also provides information about body function. NMI can diagnose cancer, stroke, and heart disease earlier than techniques that provide only structural information.

NMI uses **radiotracers**, radioactive substances that specific organs absorb. For example, radioactive iodine is used to image the thyroid gland, which absorbs more iodine than any other organ. After a patient ingests, inhales, or is injected with a radiotracer, a device called a gamma camera detects the radiotracer in the organ under study and produces a picture, which is used in making a diagnosis. Radiotracers are broken down and eliminated through urine or feces, so they leave the body quickly. A patient's exposure to radiation in NMI is usually considerably lower than with x-ray or CT scan.

Three NMI techniques are **positron emission tomography** (PET), **bone scanning**, and the **thallium stress test**. PET is often used to evaluate brain activity by measuring the brain's use of radioactive glucose. PET scans can reveal brain tumors because tumor cells are often more metabolically active than normal cells and thus absorb more radiotracer. Bone scanning detects radiation from a radiotracer absorbed by bone tissue with an abnormally high metabolic rate, such as a bone tumor. The thallium stress test is used to diagnose heart disease. A nuclear medicine technologist injects the patient with radioactive thallium, and a gamma camera images the heart during exercise and then rest. When compared, the two sets of images help to evaluate blood flow to the working, or "stressed," heart.

cobalt, chromium, and others, are present in extremely small (trace) amounts totaling about 0.1% of body weight.

Organic Compounds

The chemical compounds that characterize living things are called **organic compounds**. All of these contain the element **carbon**. Because carbon can combine with a variety of different elements and can even bond to other carbon atoms to form long chains, most organic compounds consist of large, complex molecules. The starch found in potatoes, the fat in tissues, hormones, and many drugs are examples of organic compounds. These large molecules are often formed from simpler molecules called *building blocks*, which bond together in long chains.

The main types of organic compounds are carbohydrates, lipids, and proteins. (Another category, the nucleic acids, which are important in cellular functions, are discussed in Chapter 3.) All of these organic compounds contain carbon, hydrogen, and oxygen as their main ingredients.

Carbohydrates, lipids, and proteins, in addition to minerals and vitamins, must be taken in as part of a normal diet. These compounds are discussed further in Chapters 19 and 20.

CHECKPOINT 2-11 ➤ Where are organic compounds found?

CHECKPOINT 2-12 ➤ What element is the basis of organic chemistry?

CARBOHYDRATES The basic units of carbohydrates are simple sugars, or **monosaccharides** (mon-o-SAK-ah-rides) (Fig. 2-7A). **Glu-cose** (GLU-kose), a simple sugar that circulates in the blood as a nutrient for cells, is an example of a monosaccharide. Two simple sugars may be linked together to form a **disaccharide** (Fig. 2-7B), as represented by sucrose, or table sugar. More complex carbohydrates, or **polysaccharides** (Fig. 2-7C), consist of many simple sugars linked together with multiple side chains. Examples of polysaccharides are starch, which is manufactured in plant cells, and **glycogen** (GLI-ko-jen), a storage form of glucose found in liver cells and skeletal muscle cells. Carbohydrates in the form of sugars and starches are important dietary sources of energy.

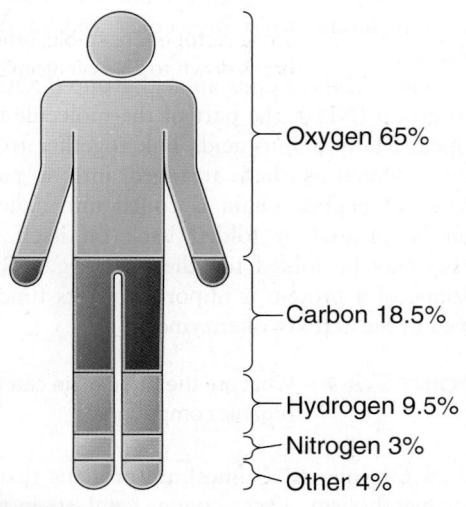

Oxygen 65%

Carbon 18.5%

Hydrogen 9.5%
Nitrogen 3%
Other 4%

Figure 2-6 The body's chemical composition by weight.

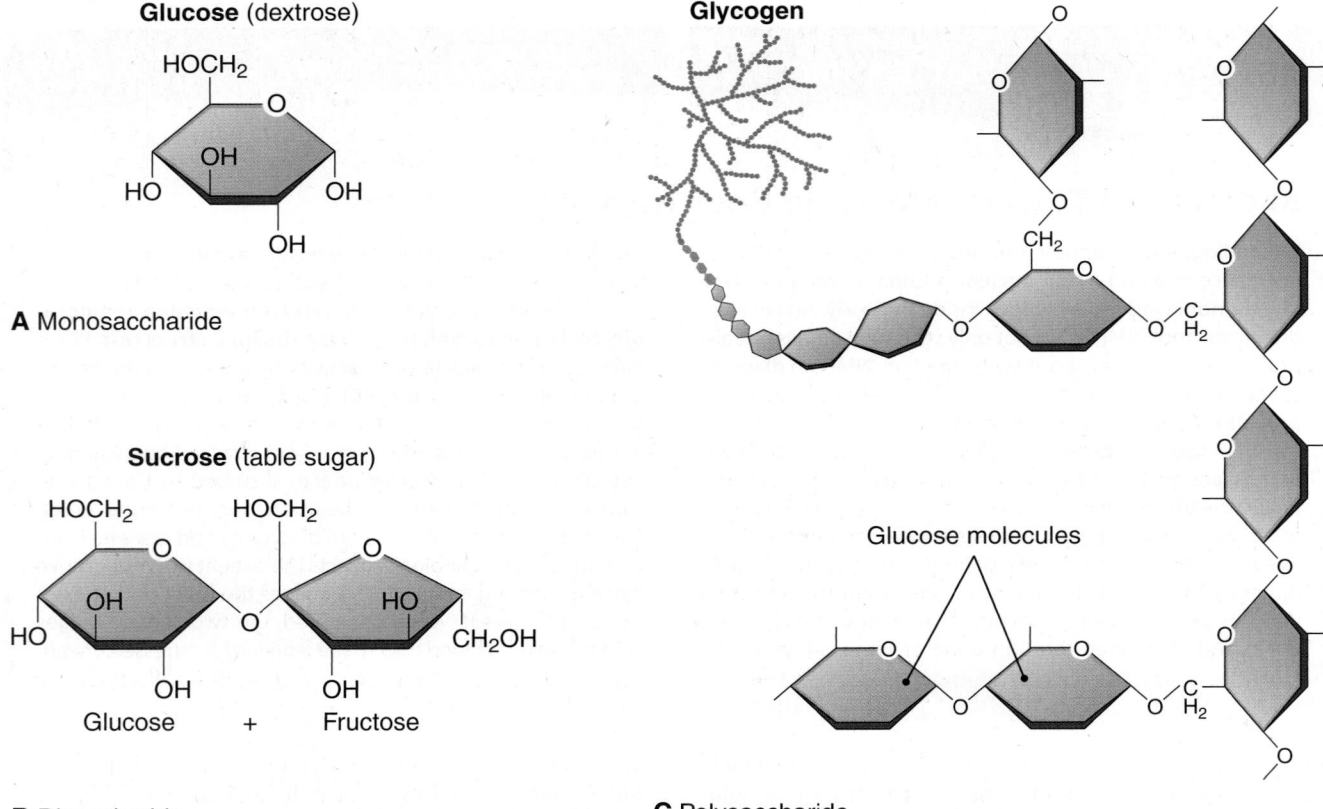

Glucose (dextrose)

A Monosaccharide

Sucrose (table sugar)

Glucose + Fructose

B Disaccharide

Glycogen

Glucose molecules

C Polysaccharide

Figure 2-7 **Examples of carbohydrates.** A monosaccharide **(A)** is a simple sugar. A disaccharide **(B)** consists of two simple sugars linked together, whereas a polysaccharide **(C)** consists of many simple sugars linked together in chains. [ZOOMING IN ➤ What are the building blocks of disaccharides and polysaccharides?]

LIPIDS **Lipids** are a class of organic compounds mainly found in the body as **fat**. Fats insulate the body and protect internal organs. In addition, fats are the main form in which energy is stored.

Simple fats are made from a substance called **glycerol** (GLIS-er-ol), commonly known as glycerin, in combination with fatty acids (Fig. 2-8A). One fatty acid is attached to each of the three carbon atoms in glycerol, so simple fats are described as **triglycerides** (tri-GLIS-er-ides). **Phospholipids** (fos-fo-LIP-ids) are complex lipids containing the element phosphorus. Among other functions, phospholipids make up a major part of the membrane around living cells. **Steroids** are lipids that contain rings of carbon atoms. They include **cholesterol** (ko-LES-ter-ol), another component of cell membranes (Fig. 2-8B); the steroid hormones, such as cortisol, produced by the adrenal gland; and the sex hormones, such as testosterone, produced by the testes, and estrogen and progesterone, produced by the ovaries.

PROTEINS All **proteins** (PRO-tenes) contain, in addition to carbon, hydrogen, and oxygen, the element **nitrogen** (NI-tro-jen). They may also contain sulfur or phosphorus. Proteins are the body's structural materials, found in muscle, bone, and connective tissue. They also make up the

pigments that give hair, eyes, and skin their color. It is protein that makes each individual physically distinct from others.

Proteins are composed of building blocks called **amino** (ah-ME-no) **acids** (Fig. 2-9A). Although there are only about 20 different amino acids found in the body, a vast number of proteins can be made by linking them together in different sized molecules and in different combinations.

Each amino acid contains an acid group (COOH) and an amino group (NH_2), the part of the molecule that has the nitrogen. Many amino acids link together to form a polypeptide, which is then arranged into a particular shape. The polypeptide chain is coiled into a helix and may then be pleated or folded back on itself. Several chains also may be folded together (see Fig. 2-9B). The overall shape of a protein is important to its function, as can be seen in the activity of enzymes.

CHECKPOINT 2-13 ➤ What are the three main categories of organic compounds?

ENZYMES **Enzymes** (EN-zimes) are proteins that are essential for metabolism. They serve as **catalysts** in the hundreds of reactions that take place within cells. Without

Glycerol

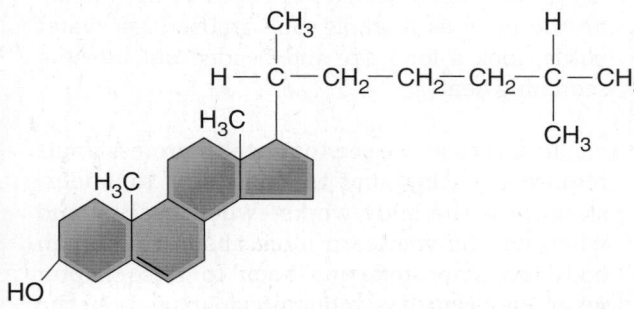

Fatty Acids

A   **Triglyceride (a simple fat)**

B   **Cholesterol (a steroid)**

Figure 2-8 **Lipids. (A)** A triglyceride, a simple fat, contains glycerol combined with three fatty acids. **(B)** Cholesterol is a type of steroid, a lipid that contains rings of carbon atoms. **[** ZOOMING IN ➤ How many carbon atoms are in glycerol? **]**

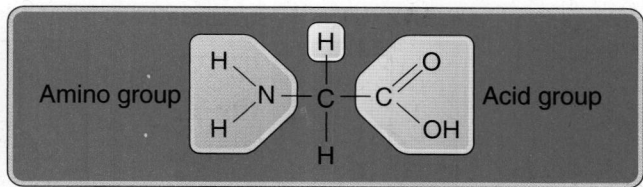

Simple amino acid

A

Coiled   Pleated   Folded

B

Figure 2-9 **Proteins. (A)** Amino acids are the building blocks of proteins. **(B)** Some shapes of proteins. **[** ZOOMING IN ➤ What part of an amino acid contains nitrogen? **]**

needed in very small amounts. Many of the vitamins and minerals required in the diet are parts of enzymes.

An enzyme's shape is important in its action. Its form must match the shape of the substrate or substrates the enzyme combines with in much the same way as a key fits a lock. This so-called "lock-and-key" mechanism is illustrated in Figure 2-10. Harsh conditions, such as extremes of temperature or pH, can alter an enzyme's shape and stop its action. The alteration of any protein so that it can no longer function is termed **denaturation**. Such an event is always harmful to the cells.

You can usually recognize the names of enzymes because, with few exceptions, they end with the suffix -*ase*. Examples are lipase, protease, and oxidase. The first part of the name usually refers to the substance acted on or the type of reaction in which the enzyme is involved.

CHECKPOINT **2-14** ➤ Enzymes are proteins that act as catalysts. What is a catalyst?

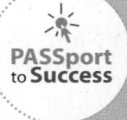 **PASSport to Success**   Visit *thePoint* or see the Student Resource CD in the back of this book to view an animation on enzymes. In addition, the Health Professions box, Pharmacists and Pharmacy Technicians, describes some professions that require knowledge of chemistry.

these catalysts, which increase the speed of chemical reactions, metabolism would not occur at a fast enough rate to sustain life. Because each enzyme works only on a specific substance, or **substrate**, and does only one specific chemical job, many different enzymes are needed. Like all catalysts, enzymes take part in reactions only temporarily; they are not used up or changed by the reaction. Therefore, they are

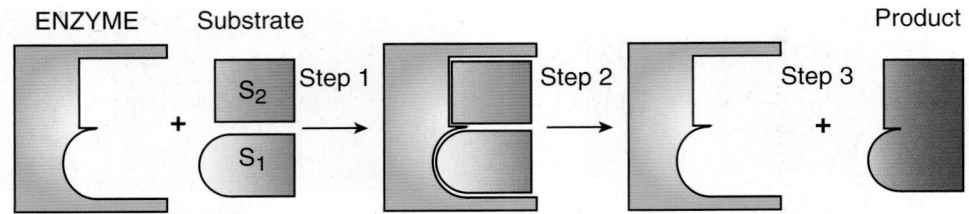

Figure 2-10 **Diagram of enzyme action.** The enzyme combines with substrate 1 (S_1) and substrate 2 (S_2). Once a new product is formed from the substrates, the enzyme is released unchanged. **[ZOOMING IN ➤** How does the shape of the enzyme before the reaction compare with its shape after the reaction? **]**

Disease in Context revisited

➤ Margaret: Back in Balance

"Good morning, Mrs. Ringland. How are you feeling today?" asked Angela.

"Much better, thank you," replied Margaret. "I'm so grateful that my niece found me when she did."

"I'm glad, too," said Angela. "With the heat wave we're having, dehydration can become a very serious problem. Older adults are particularly at risk of dehydration because with age there usually is a decrease in muscle protein, which contains a lot of water, and a relative increase in body fat, which does not. So, older adults don't have as much water reserve as younger adults. But," Angela continued as she flipped through Margaret's chart, "It looks like you are well on your way to a full recovery. Your electrolytes are back in balance. Your blood pressure is back to normal and your heart rate is good too. Your increased urine output tells me that your other organs are recovering as well."

"Does that mean I can get rid of this IV?" asked Margaret.

"Well, I'll check with your doctor first," replied Angela, "But, when you do have the IV removed, you will need to make sure that you drink plenty of fluids."

It was the end of another long shift and Angela was at her locker, changing into a pair of shorts and a T-shirt. As she closed her locker she thought of Margaret once again. It always amazed her that chemistry could have such a huge impact on the body as a whole. She grabbed her water bottle, took a long sip, and headed out into the scorching heat.

In this case, we see that health professionals require a background in chemistry to understand how the body works—when healthy and when not. As you learn more about the human body, consider referring back to this chapter when necessary. For more information about the elements that make up every single molecule within the body, see Appendix 3: Periodic Table of the Elements at the back of this book.

Word Anatomy

Medical terms are built from standardized word parts (prefixes, roots, and suffixes). Learning the meanings of these parts can help you remember words and interpret unfamiliar terms.

WORD PART	MEANING	EXAMPLE
Molecules and Compounds		
hydr/o	water	*Dehydration* is a deficiency of water.
phil	to like	*Hydrophilic* substances "like" water—they mix with or dissolve in it.
-phobia	fear	*Hydrophobic* substances "fear" water—they repel and do not dissolve in it.
hom/o-	same	*Homogeneous* mixtures are the same throughout.
heter/o-	different	*Heterogeneous* solutions are different (not uniform) throughout.
aqu/e	water	In an *aqueous* solution, water is the solvent.
Chemical Bonds		
co-	together	*Covalent* bonds form when atoms share electrons.
Chemistry of Living Matter		
sacchar/o	sugar	A *monosaccharide* consists of one simple sugar.
mon/o-	one	In *monosaccharide*, "mono-" refers to one.
di-	twice, double	A *disaccharide* consists of two simple sugars.
poly-	many	A *polysaccharide* consists of many simple sugars.
glyc/o	sugar, glucose, sweet	*Glycogen* is a storage form of glucose. It breaks down to release (generate) glucose.
tri-	three	*Triglycerides* have one fatty acid attached to each of three carbon atoms.
de-	remove	*Denaturation* of a protein removes its ability to function (changes its nature).
-ase	suffix used in naming enzymes	A *lipase* is an enzyme that acts on lipids.

Summary

I. ELEMENTS—Substances from which all matter is made
   A. Atoms—subunits of elements
      1. Atomic structure
         a. Protons—positively charged particles in the nucleus
         b. Neutrons—noncharged particles in the nucleus
         c. Electrons—negatively charged particles in energy levels around the nucleus
      2. Energy levels—orbits that hold electrons at specific distances from the nucleus

   a. Valence—number of electrons lost or gained in chemical reactions

II. MOLECULES AND COMPOUNDS
   A. Molecules—combinations of two or more atoms
   B. Compounds—substances composed of different elements
   C. The importance of water—solvent; stable; essential for metabolism
   D. Mixtures: solutions and suspensions
      1. Mixtures—blend of two or more substances
      2. Solution—substance (solute) remains evenly distributed in solvent (e.g., salt in water); homogeneous

3. Suspension—material settles out of mixture on standing (e.g., red cells in blood plasma); heterogeneous
4. Colloid—particles do not dissolve but remain suspended (e.g., cytosol)

III. **CHEMICAL BONDS**
   A. Ionic bonds—formed by transfer of electrons from one atom to another
      1. Electrolytes
         a. Ionically bonded substances
         b. Separate in solution into charged particles (ions); cation positive and anion negative
         c. Conduct electric current
      2. Ions in body fluids important for proper function
   B. Covalent bonds—formed by sharing of electrons between atoms
      1. Nonpolar—equal sharing of electrons (e.g., hydrogen gas, H_2)
      2. Polar—unequal sharing of electrons (e.g., water, H_2O)

IV. **COMPOUNDS: ACIDS, BASES AND SALTS**
   A. Acids—donate hydrogen ions
   B. Bases—accept hydrogen ions
   C. Salts—formed by reaction between acid and base
   D. The pH scale
      1. Measure of acidity or alkalinity of a solution
      2. Scale goes from 0 to 14
         a. 7 is neutral; below 7 is acidic; above 7 is alkaline (basic)
   E. Buffer—maintains constant pH of a solution

V. **ISOTOPES AND RADIOACTIVITY**
   A. Isotopes—forms of an element that differ in atomic weights (number of neutrons)
      1. Radioactive isotope gives off rays of atomic particles
   B. Use of radioactive isotopes
      2. Cancer therapy
      3. Diagnosis—tracers, x-rays

VI. **CHEMISTRY OF LIVING MATTER**
   A. Organic compounds—all contain carbon
      1. Carbohydrates (e.g., sugars, starches); made of simple sugars (monosaccharides)
      2. Lipids (e.g., fats, steroids); fats made of glycerol and fatty acids
      3. Proteins (e.g., structural materials, enzymes); made of amino acids
         a. Enzymes—organic catalysts

Questions for Study and Review

BUILDING UNDERSTANDING

Fill in the blanks

1. The basic units of elements are _____.
2. The atomic number is the number of_____ in an atom's nucleus.
3. A mixture of solute dissolved in solvent is called a(n) _____.
4. Blood has a pH of 7.35 to 7.45. Gastric juice has a pH of about 2.0. The more alkaline fluid is _____.
5. Proteins that catalyze metabolic reactions are called _____.

Matching > Match each numbered item with the most closely related lettered item.

___ 6. A simple carbohydrate such as glucose
___ 7. A complex carbohydrate such as glycogen
___ 8. An important component of cell membranes
___ 9. A hormone such as estrogen
___ 10. The basic building block of protein

   a. polysaccharide
   b. phospholipid
   c. steroid
   d. amino acid
   e. monosaccharide

Multiple Choice

___ 11. Red blood cells "floating" in plasma are an example of a mixture called a
   a. compound
   b. suspension
   c. colloid
   d. solution

___ 12. The most abundant compound in the body is
   a. carbohydrate
   b. protein
   c. lipid
   d. water

___ **13.** A compound that releases ions when it is in solution is called a(n)

  a. solvent
  b. electrolyte
  c. anion
  d. colloid

___ **14.** A chemical capable of donating hydrogen ions to other substances is called a(n)

  a. acid
  b. base
  c. salt
  d. catalyst

___ **15.** Organic compounds always contain the element

  a. oxygen
  b. carbon
  c. nitrogen
  d. phosphorus

UNDERSTANDING CONCEPTS

16. Compare and contrast the following terms:

  a. element and atom
  b. molecule and compound
  c. proton, neutron, and electron
  d. anion and cation
  e. ionic bond and covalent bond
  f. acid and base

17. What are some of the properties of water that make it an ideal medium for living cells?

18. Explain the importance of ions in the structure and function of the human body.

19. What is pH? Discuss the role of buffers in maintaining pH homeostasis in the body.

20. Compare and contrast carbohydrates and proteins.

21. Describe three different types of lipid.

22. Define the term *enzyme* and discuss the relationship between enzyme structure and enzyme function.

CONCEPTUAL THINKING

23. Based on your understanding of strong acids and bases, why does the body have to be kept at a close-to-neutral pH?

24. Why do we need enzymes, when usually heat is used to speed up chemical reactions?

25. In Margaret's case, she was hypotensive when she arrived at the hospital. Explain the link between dehydration and low blood pressure.

26. In Margaret's case, an aqueous solution of 5% dextrose was used to rehydrate her. Name the solution's solute and solvent.

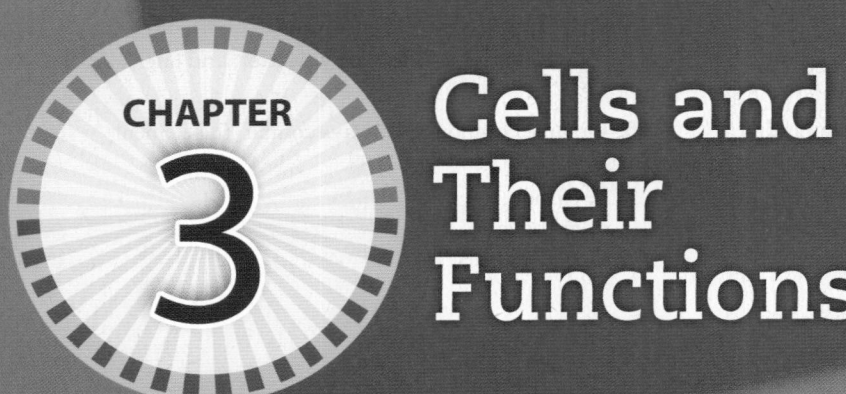

CHAPTER 3
Cells and Their Functions

Learning Outcomes

After careful study of this chapter, you should be able to:

1. List three types of microscopes used to study cells
2. Describe the function and composition of the plasma membrane
3. Describe the cytoplasm of the cell, including the name and function of the main organelles
4. Describe the composition, location, and function of the DNA in the cell
5. Compare the function of three types of RNA in the cells
6. Explain briefly how cells make proteins
7. Name and briefly describe the stages in mitosis
8. Define eight methods by which substances enter and leave cells
9. Explain what will happen if cells are placed in solutions with concentrations the same as or different from those of the cell fluids
10. Define *cancer*
11. List several risk factors for cancer
12. Show how word parts are used to build words related to cells and their functions (see Word Anatomy at the end of the chapter)

Selected Key Terms

The following terms and other boldface terms in the chapter are defined in the Glossary

active transport
cancer
chromosome
cytology
cytoplasm
diffusion
DNA
endocytosis
gene
interphase
isotonic
micrometer
microscope
mitochondria
mitosis
mutation
nucleotide
nucleus
organelle
osmosis
phagocytosis
plasma membrane
ribosome
RNA

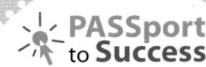

PASSport to Success

Visit *thePoint* or see the Student Resource CD in the back of this book for definitions and pronunciations of key terms as well as a pretest for this chapter.

Disease in Context

Jim's Case: Heart Disease from a Cell's Perspective

The buzzer sounded, signaling the end of the third quarter, and the Legal Eagles trailed by 10 points. Jim slammed the basketball down with disgust—he wasn't about to lose to a bunch of accountants. As usual, he'd have to step up his game to make up for the rest of the team.

Jim's attitude on the basketball court reflected his approach off the court. He worked long hours and had little patience for anyone who did not keep up with his grueling pace. By some accounts, Jim was a success—he was a partner in a large downtown law firm, he owned a big house, and he drove a fast car. However, his success came at a heavy cost. Jim's body wasn't keeping up with his lifestyle. He was overweight, out of shape, and had high blood pressure. The extra blood vessels needed to feed Jim's fat cells (called adipocytes) required his heart to pump harder to force blood through them. Since most cardiac muscle cells lack the ability to replicate themselves (a process called mitosis), they responded by synthesizing more contractile proteins. This allowed his cardiac muscle to contract with more force, but also resulted in thickening of the heart walls, which, in the long run, had actually decreased the efficiency of his heart.

Hypertension wasn't the only problem with Jim's cardiovascular system. Cholesterol from Jim's lipid-rich diet formed growths, called plaques, in the walls of many of his blood vessels. In his heart, fatty plaques bulged into the lumens of the coronary arteries, obstructing blood flow to his cardiac muscle cells. Over the years, Jim's coronary arteries compensated for his heart's lack of oxygen and nutrients by growing new vessel branches around the blockages—natural bypasses, made possible by mitosis, which reestablished blood flow to the muscle cells. At the best of times, Jim's heart received just enough oxygen and nutrients to pump adequate amounts of blood to his body's cells. Playing in the basketball game today, Jim had placed an unusually high demand on his heart, and it was having a difficult time keeping up.

The buzzer sounded again, signaling the start of the fourth quarter. With great effort, Jim won the jump ball, and his team began to move toward their opponents' basket. Jim was left behind at center court when he crumpled to the ground, clutching his chest, his cardiovascular system unable to meet the demands of his cardiac muscle. Jim was having a heart attack.

As we will see later, oxygen deficiency caused irreparable damage to Jim's cardiac muscle cells. When reading Chapter 3, keep in mind that events at the cellular level have ramifications for the structure and function of tissues, organs, and even the whole body.

The Role of Cells

The **cell** (sel) is the basic unit of all life. It is the simplest structure that shows all the characteristics of life, including organization, metabolism, responsiveness, homeostasis, growth, and reproduction. In fact, it is possible for a single cell to live independently of other cells. Examples of some free-living cells are microscopic organisms such as protozoa and bacteria, some of which produce disease. In a multicellular organism, cells make up all tissues. All the activities of the human body, which is composed of trillions of cells, result from the activities of individual cells. Cells produce all the materials manufactured within the body. The study of cells is **cytology** (si-TOL-o-je).

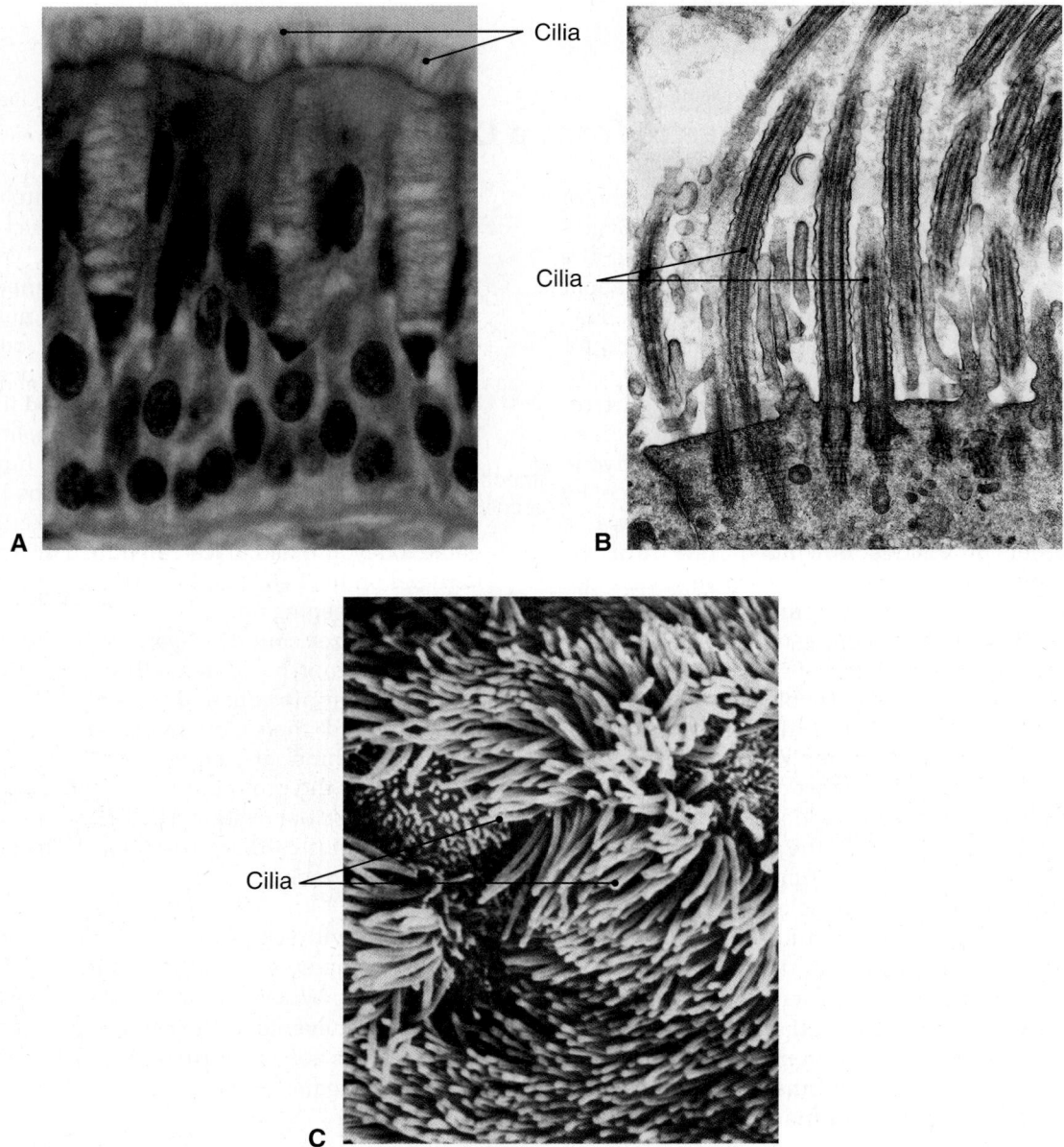

Figure 3-1   **Cilia photographed under three different microscopes. (A)** Cilia (hairlike projections) in cells lining the trachea under the highest magnification of a compound light microscope (1,000×). **(B)** Cilia in the bronchial lining viewed with a transmission electron microscope (TEM). Internal components are visible at this much higher magnification. **(C)** Cilia on cells lining an oviduct as seen with a scanning electron microscope (SEM) (7,000×). A three-dimensional view can be seen. (A, Reprinted with permission from Cormack DH. *Essential Histology*, 2nd ed. Philadelphia: Lippincott Williams & Wilkins, 2001; B, Reprinted with permission from Quinton P, Martinez R, eds. *Fluid and Electrolyte Transport in Exocrine Glands in Cystic Fibrosis*. San Francisco: San Francisco Press, 1982; C, Reprinted with permission from Hafez ESE. *Scanning Electron Microscopic Atlas of Mammalian Reproduction*. Tokyo: Igaku Shoin, 1975.) [**ZOOMING IN** ➤ Which microscope shows the most internal structure of the cilia? Which shows the cilia in three dimensions?]

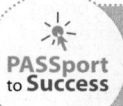

Visit **thePoint** or see the Student Resource CD in the back of this book for information on careers in cytotechnology, the clinical laboratory study of cells.

CHECKPOINT 3-1 ➤ The cell is the basic unit of life. What characteristics of life does it show?

Microscopes

The outlines of cells were first seen in dried plant tissue almost 350 years ago. Study of their internal structure, however, depended on improvements in the design of the **microscope**, a magnifying instrument needed to examine structures not visible with the naked eye. The single-lens microscope used in the late 17th century was later replaced by the **compound light microscope** most commonly used in laboratories today. This instrument, which can magnify an object up to 1,000 times, has two lenses and uses visible light for illumination. A much more powerful microscope, the **transmission electron microscope (TEM)**, uses an electron beam in place of visible light and can magnify an image up to 1 million times. Another type of microscope, the **scanning electron microscope (SEM)**, does not magnify as much (100,000×) and shows only surface features, but gives a three-dimensional view of an object. Figure 3-1 shows some cell structures viewed with each of these types of microscopes. The structures are cilia—short, hairlike projections from the cell that move nearby fluids. The metric unit used for microscopic measurements is the **micrometer** (MI-kro-me-ter), formerly called a micron. This unit is 1/1,000 of a millimeter and is symbolized with the Greek letter mu (μ), as μm.

Before scientists can examine cells and tissues under a microscope, they must usually color them with special dyes called **stains** to aid in viewing. These stains produce the variety of colors seen in pictures of cells and tissues taken under a microscope.

Cell Structure

Just as people may look different but still have certain features in common—two eyes, a nose, and a mouth, for example—all cells share certain characteristics. Refer to Figure 3-2 as we describe some of the parts that are

common to most animal cells. Table 3-1 summarizes information about the main cell parts.

CHECKPOINT 3-2 ➤ Name three types of microscopes.

Visit **thePoint** or see the Student Resource CD in the back of this book to view electron microscope pictures of the cell.

Plasma Membrane

The outer limit of the cell is the **plasma membrane**, formerly called the *cell membrane* (Fig. 3-3). The plasma membrane not only encloses the cell contents but also participates in many cellular activities, such as growth, reproduction, and interactions between cells, and is especially important in regulating what can enter and leave the cell. The main substance of this membrane is a double layer of lipid molecules, described as a bilayer. Because these lipids contain the element phosphorus, they are called **phospholipids**. Some molecules of cholesterol, another type of lipid, are located between the phospholipids. Cholesterol strengthens the membrane.

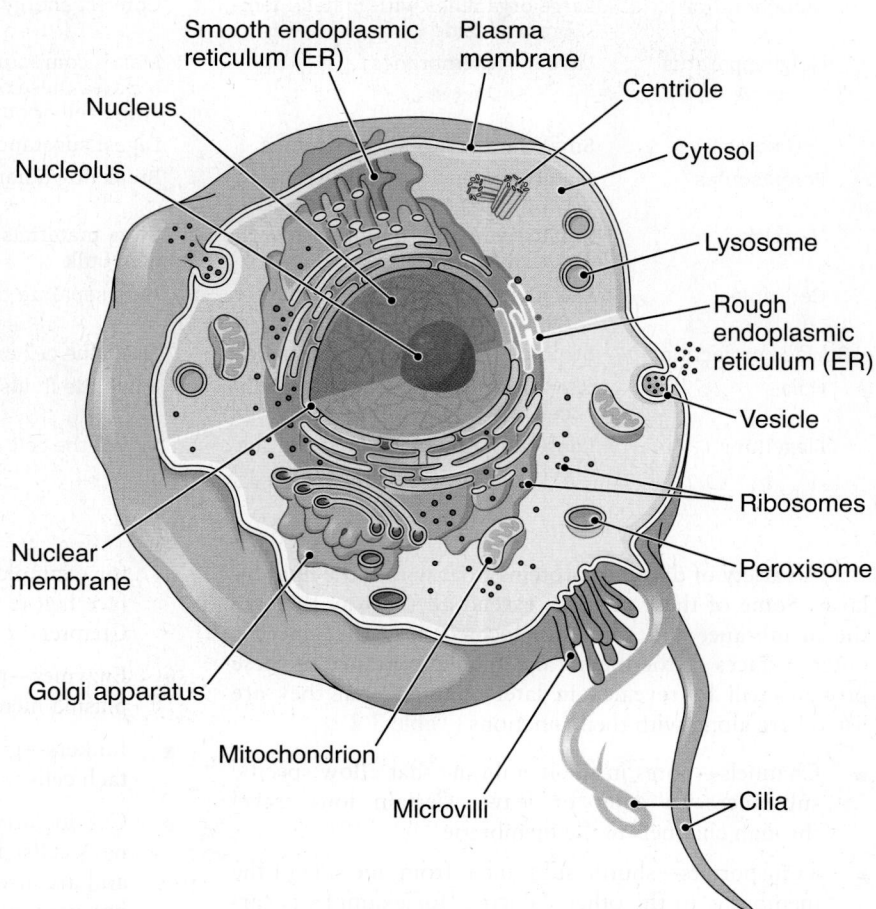

Figure 3-2 **A generalized animal cell, sectional view.** [ZOOMING IN ➤ What is attached to the ER to make it look rough? What is the liquid part of the cytoplasm called?]

Table 3-1	Cell Parts	
Name	**Description**	**Function**
Plasma membrane	Outer layer of the cell; composed mainly of lipids and proteins	Encloses the cell contents; regulates what enters and leaves the cell; participates in many activities, such as growth, reproduction, and interactions between cells
Microvilli	Short extensions of the cell membrane	Absorb materials into the cell
Nucleus	Large, dark-staining organelle near the center of the cell, composed of DNA and proteins	Contains the chromosomes, the hereditary units that direct all cellular activities
Nucleolus	Small body in the nucleus; composed of RNA, DNA, and protein	Makes ribosomes
Cytoplasm	Colloidal suspension that fills the cell from the nuclear membrane to the plasma membrane	Site of many cellular activities; consists of cytosol and organelles
Cytosol	The fluid portion of the cytoplasm	Surrounds the organelles
Endoplasmic reticulum (ER)	Network of membranes within the cytoplasm. Rough ER has ribosomes attached to it; smooth ER does not.	Rough ER sorts proteins and forms them into more complex compounds; smooth ER is involved with lipid synthesis
Ribosomes	Small bodies free in the cytoplasm or attached to the ER; composed of RNA and protein	Manufacture proteins
Mitochondria	Large organelles with folded membranes inside	Convert energy from nutrients into ATP
Golgi apparatus	Layers of membranes	Makes compounds containing proteins; sorts and prepares these compounds for transport to other parts of the cell or out of the cell
Lysosomes	Small sacs of digestive enzymes	Digest substances within the cell
Peroxisomes	Membrane-enclosed organelles containing enzymes	Break down harmful substances
Vesicles	Small membrane-bound sacs in the cytoplasm	Store materials and move materials into or out of the cell in bulk
Centrioles	Rod-shaped bodies (usually two) near the nucleus	Help separate the chromosomes during cell division
Surface projections	Structures that extend from the cell	Move the cell or the fluids around the cell
Cilia	Short, hairlike projections from the cell	Move the fluids around the cell
Flagellum	Long, whiplike extension from the cell	Moves the cell

A variety of different proteins float within the lipid bilayer. Some of these proteins extend all the way through the membrane, and some are located near the inner or outer surfaces of the membrane. The importance of these proteins will be revealed in later chapters, but they are listed here along with their functions (Table 3-2):

■ Channels—pores in the membrane that allow specific substances to enter or leave. Certain ions travel through channels in the membrane.

■ Transporters—shuttle substances from one side of the membrane to the other. Glucose, for example, is carried into cells using transporters.

■ Receptors—points of attachment for materials coming to the cell in the blood or tissue fluid. Some hormones,

for example, must attach to receptors on the cell surface before they can act upon the cell, as described in Chapter 12 on the endocrine system.

■ Enzymes—participate in reactions occurring at the plasma membrane.

■ Linkers—give structure to the membrane and help attach cells to each other.

■ Cell identity markers—proteins unique to an individual's cells. These are important in the immune system and are also a factor in transplantation of tissue from one person to another.

Carbohydrates are present in small amounts in the plasma membrane, combined either with proteins (glyco-

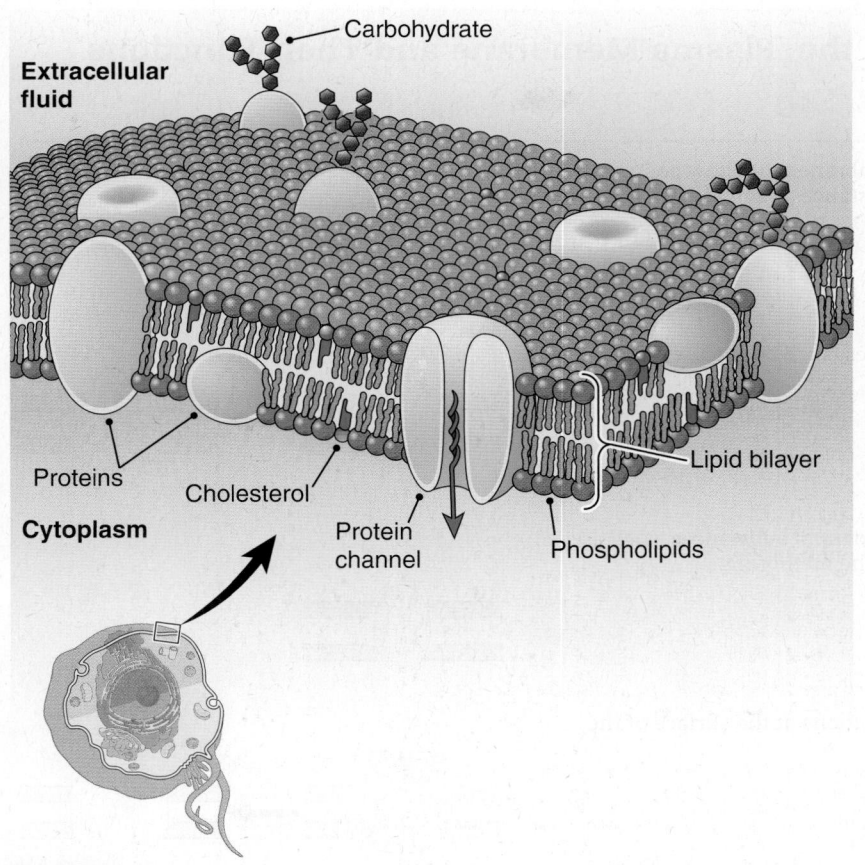

Extracellular fluid

Carbohydrate

Proteins

Cytoplasm

Cholesterol

Protein channel

Phospholipids

Lipid bilayer

Figure 3-3 **The plasma membrane.** This drawing shows the current concept of its structure. [**ZOOMING IN** ➤ How many layers make up the main substance of the plasma membrane?]

proteins) or with lipids (glycolipids). These carbohydrates help cells to recognize each other and to stick together.

In some cells, the plasma membrane is folded out into multiple small projections called microvilli (mi-kro-VIL-li). Microvilli increase the membrane's surface area, allowing for greater absorption of materials from the cell's environment, just as a sponge absorbs water. Microvilli are found on cells that line the small intestine, where they promote absorption of digested foods into the circulation. They are also found on kidney cells, where they reabsorb materials that have been filtered out of the blood.

CHECKPOINT 3-3 ➤ The outer limit of the cell is a complex membrane. What is the main substance of this membrane and what are three types of materials found within the membrane?

The Nucleus

Just as the body has different organs to carry out special functions, the cell contains specialized structures that perform different tasks. These structures are called **organelles,** which means "little organs." The largest of the organelles is the **nucleus** (NU-kle-us).

The nucleus is often called the *control center* of the cell because it contains the **chromosomes** (KRO-mo-somes), the threadlike units of heredity that are passed on from parents to their offspring. It is information contained in the chromosomes that governs all cellular activities, as described later in this chapter. Most of the time, the chromosomes are loosely distributed throughout the nucleus, giving that organelle a uniform, dark appearance when stained and examined under a microscope (see Fig. 3-2). When the cell is dividing, however, the chromosomes tighten into their visible threadlike forms.

Within the nucleus is a smaller globule called the **nucleolus** (nu-KLE-o-lus), which means "little nucleus." The job of the nucleolus is to assemble ribosomes, small bodies outside the nucleus that are involved in the manufacture of proteins.

The Cytoplasm

The remaining organelles are part of the **cytoplasm** (SI-to-plazm), the material that fills the cell from the nuclear membrane to the plasma membrane. The liquid part of the cytoplasm is the **cytosol,** a suspension of nutrients, minerals, enzymes, and other specialized materials in water. The main organelles are described here (see Table 3-1).

The **endoplasmic reticulum** (en-do-PLAS-mik re-TIK-u-lum) is a network of membranes located between the nuclear membrane and the plasma membrane. Its name literally means "network" (reticulum) "within the cytoplasm" (endoplasmic), but for ease, it is almost always called simply the **ER.** In some areas, the ER appears to have an even surface and is described as *smooth ER.* This type of ER is involved with the synthesis of lipids. In other areas, the ER has a gritty, uneven surface, causing it to be described as *rough ER.* The texture of rough ER comes from small bodies, called **ribosomes** (RI-bo-somz), attached to its surface. Ribosomes are necessary for the manufacture of proteins, as described later. They may be attached to the ER or be free in the cytoplasm.

CHECKPOINT 3-4 ➤ What are cell organelles?

CHECKPOINT 3-5 ➤ Why is the nucleus called the control center of the cell?

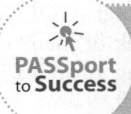

PASSport to Success

Visit ***thePoint*** or see the Student Resource CD in the back of this book to view an animation on the functions of proteins in the plasma membrane.

Table 3-2 Proteins in the Plasma Membrane and Their Functions

Type of Protein	Function	Illustration
Channels	Pores in the membrane that allow passage of specific substances, such as ions	
Transporters	Shuttle substances, such as glucose, across the membrane	
Receptors	Allow for attachment of substances, such as hormones, to the membrane	
Enzymes	Participate in reactions at the surface of the membrane	
Linkers	Give structure to the membrane and attach cells to other cells	
Cell identity markers	Proteins unique to a person's cells; important in the immune system and in transplantation of tissue from one person to another	

The **mitochondria** (mi-to-KON-dre-ah) are large organelles that are round or bean-shaped with folded membranes on the inside. Within the mitochondria, the energy from nutrients is converted to energy for the cell in the form of ATP. Mitochondria are the "power plants" of the cell. Active cells, such as muscle cells or sperm cells, need lots of energy and thus have large numbers of mitochondria.

Another organelle in a typical cell is the **Golgi** (GOL-je) **apparatus** (also called Golgi complex), a stack of membranous sacs involved in sorting and modifying proteins and then packaging them for export from the cell.

Several types of organelles appear as small sacs in the cytoplasm. These include **lysosomes** (LI-so-somz), which contain digestive enzymes. Lysosomes remove waste and foreign materials from the cell. They are also involved in destroying old and damaged cells as needed for repair and remodeling of tissue. **Peroxisomes** (per-OK-sih-somz) have enzymes that destroy harmful substances produced in metabolism (see Box 3-1, Lysosomes and Peroxisomes: Cellular Recycling). **Vesicles** (VES-ih-klz) are small, membrane-bound sacs used for storage. They can be used to move materials into or out of the cell, as described later.

Centrioles (SEN-tre-olz) are rod-shaped bodies near the nucleus that function in cell division. They help to organize the cell and divide the cell contents during this process.

Surface Organelles

Some cells have structures projecting from their surface that are used for motion. **Cilia** (SIL-e-ah) are small, hairlike projections that wave, creating movement of the fluids around the cell. For example, cells that line the passageways of the respiratory tract have cilia that move impurities out of the system. Ciliated cells in the female reproductive tract move the egg cell along the oviduct toward the uterus.

A long, whiplike extension from the cell is a **flagellum** (flah-JEL-lum). The only type of cell in the human body that has a flagellum is the male sperm cell. Each human sperm cell has a flagellum that propels it toward the egg in the female reproductive tract.

Cellular Diversity

Although all cells have some fundamental similarities, individual cells may vary widely in size, shape, and composition according to their function. The average cell size is 10 to 15 μm, but cells may range in size from the 7 μm of a red blood cell to the 200 μm or more in the length of a muscle cell.

Cell shape is related to cell function (Fig. 3-4). A neuron (nerve cell) has long fibers that transmit electrical energy from place to place in the nervous system. Cells in surface layers have a modified shape that covers and protects the tissue beneath. Red blood cells are small and round, which lets them slide through tiny blood vessels. They also have a thin outer membrane to allow for passage of gases into and out of the cell. As red blood cells mature, they lose the nucleus and most other organelles, making the greatest possible amount of space available to carry oxygen.

Aside from cilia and flagella, most human cells have all the organelles described above. These may vary in number, however. For example, cells producing lipids have lots of smooth ER. Cells that secrete proteins have lots of ribosomes and a prominent Golgi apparatus. All active cells have lots of mitochondria to manufacture the ATP needed for energy.

CHECKPOINT **3-6** ➤ What are the two types of organelles used for movement, and what do they look like?

Protein Synthesis

Because protein molecules play an indispensable part in the body's structure and function, we need to identify the cellular substances that direct protein production. As noted, the hereditary units that govern the cell are the chromosomes in the nucleus. Each chromosome in turn is divided into multiple subunits, called **genes** (Fig. 3-5). It is the genes that carry the messages for the development of particular inherited characteristics, such as brown eyes,

---

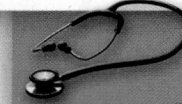

Box 3-1 Clinical Perspectives

Lysosomes and Peroxisomes: Cellular Recycling

Two organelles that play a vital role in cellular disposal and recycling are lysosomes and peroxisomes. **Lysosomes** contain enzymes that break down carbohydrates, lipids, proteins, and nucleic acids. These powerful enzymes must be kept within the lysosome because they would digest the cell if they escaped. In a process called **autophagy** (aw-TOF-ah-je), the cell uses lysosomes to safely recycle cellular structures, fusing with and digesting worn out organelles. The digested components then return to the cytoplasm for reuse. Lysosomes also break down foreign material, as when cells known as **phagocytes** (FAG-o-sites) engulf bacteria and then use lysosomes to destroy them. The cell may also use lysosomes to digest itself during **autolysis** (aw-TOL-ih-sis), a normal part of development. Cells that are no longer needed "self-destruct" by releasing lysosomal enzymes into their own cytoplasm.

Peroxisomes are small membranous sacs that resemble lysosomes but contain different kinds of enzymes. They break down toxic substances that may enter the cell, such as drugs and alcohol, but their most important function is to break down free radicals. These substances are byproducts of normal metabolic reactions but can kill the cell if not neutralized by peroxisomes.

Disease may result if either lysosomes or peroxisomes are unable to function. In Tay-Sachs disease, nerve cells' lysosomes lack an enzyme that breaks down certain kinds of lipids. These lipids build up inside the cells, causing malfunction that leads to brain injury, blindness, and death. Disease may also result if lysosomes or peroxisomes function when they should not. Some investigators believe this is the case in autoimmune diseases, in which the body develops an immune response to its own cells. Phagocytes engulf the cells and lysosomes destroy them. In addition, body cells themselves may self-destruct through autolysis. The joint disease rheumatoid arthritis is one such example.

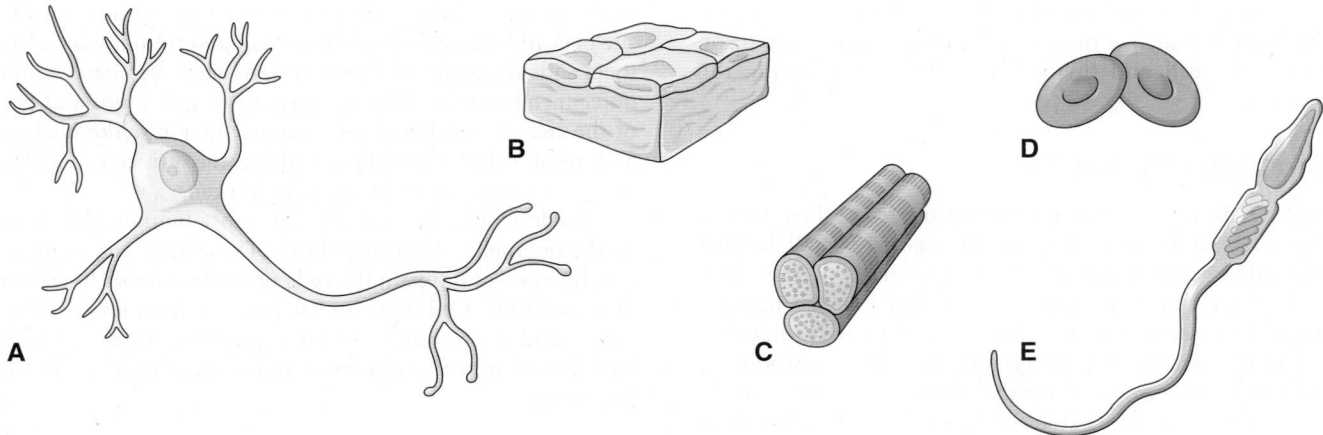

Figure 3-4 **Cellular diversity.** Cells vary in structure according to their functions. **(A)** A neuron has long extensions that pick up and transmit electrical impulses. **(B)** Epithelial cells cover and protect underlying tissue. **(C)** Muscle cells have fibers that produce contraction. **(D)** Red blood cells lose most organelles, which maximizes their oxygen-carrying capacity, and have a small, round shape that lets them slide through blood vessels. **(E)** A sperm cell is small and light and swims with a flagellum. [ZOOMING IN ➤ Which of the cells shown would best cover a large surface area?]

curly hair, or blood type, and they do so by directing protein manufacture in the cell.

Nucleic Acids: DNA and RNA

Genes are distinct segments of the complex organic chemical that makes up the chromosomes, a substance called **deoxyribonucleic** (de-ok-se-RI-bo-nu-kle-ik) **acid**, or **DNA**. DNA is composed of subunits called **nucleotides** (NU-kle-o-tides) (see Fig. 3-5). A related compound, **ribonucleic**

(RI-bo-nu-kle-ik) **acid**, or **RNA**, which participates in protein synthesis but is not part of the chromosomes, is also composed of nucleotides. There are four different nucleotides in DNA and four in RNA, but only three of these are common to both. Both DNA and RNA have nucleotides containing the components adenine (A), guanine (G), and cytosine (C), but DNA has one nucleotide containing thymine (T), whereas RNA has one containing uracil (U). Table 3-3 compares the structure and function of DNA and RNA.

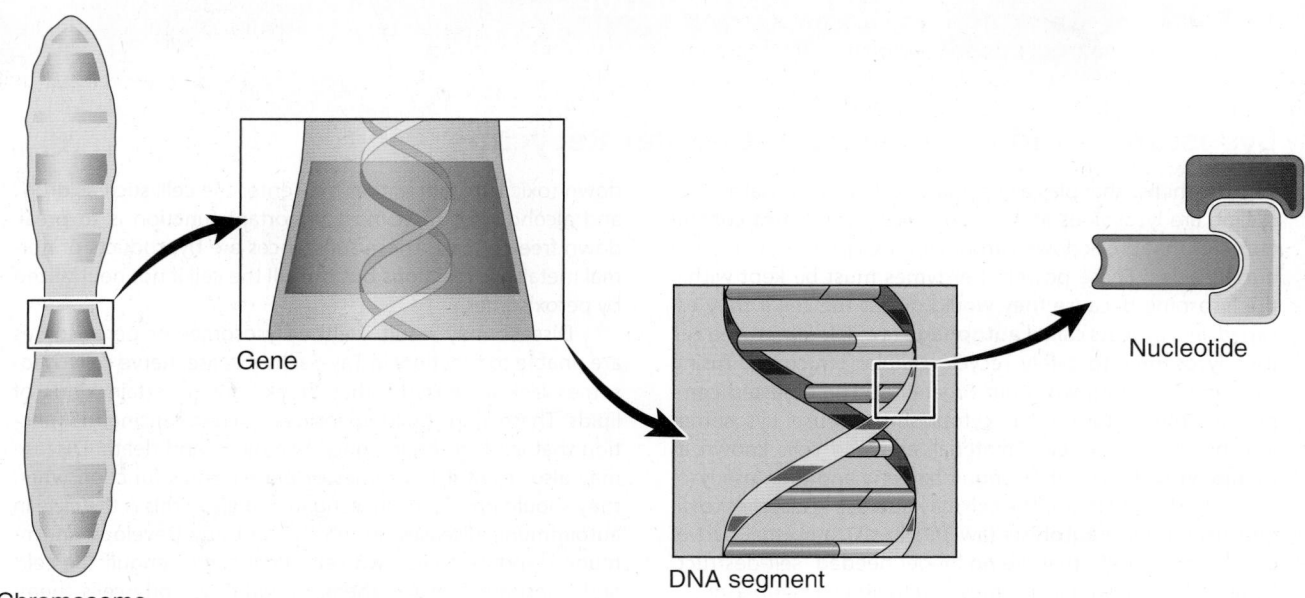

Chromosome

Gene

DNA segment

Nucleotide

Figure 3-5 **Subdivisions of a chromosome.** A gene is a distinct region of a chromosome. The entire chromosome is made of DNA. Nucleotides are the building blocks of DNA.

Table 3-3	Comparison of DNA and RNA	
	DNA	**RNA**
Location	Almost entirely in the nucleus	Almost entirely in the cytoplasm
Composition	Nucleotides contain adenine (A), guanine (G), cytosine (C), or thymine (T) Sugar: deoxyribose	Nucleotides contain adenine (A), guanine (G), cytosine (C), or uracil (U) Sugar: ribose
Structure	Double-stranded helix formed by nucleotide pairing A-T; G-C	Single strand
Function	Makes up the chromosomes, hereditary units that control all cell activities; divided into genes that carry the nucleotide codes for the manufacture of proteins	Manufacture proteins according to the nucleotide codes carried in the DNA; three types: messenger RNA (mRNA), ribosomal RNA (rRNA), and transfer RNA (tRNA)

Moving one step deeper into the structure of the nucleic acids, each nucleotide is composed of three units:

- A sugar, which in RNA is ribose and in DNA is deoxyribose (that is, a ribose with one less oxygen atom)
- A phosphorus-containing portion, or phosphate
- A nitrogen-containing portion known as a nitrogen base (the A, G, C, T, or U noted above)

The sugar and phosphate alternate to form a long chain to which the nitrogen bases are attached. It is variation in the nitrogen bases that accounts for the differences in the five different nucleotides.

DNA Most of the DNA in the cell is organized into chromosomes within the nucleus (a small amount of DNA is in the mitochondria located in the cytoplasm). Figure 3-6 shows a section of a chromosome and illustrates that the DNA exists as a double strand. Visualizing the complete molecule as a ladder, the sugar and phosphate units of the nucleotides make up the "side rails" of the ladder, and the nitrogen bases project from the side rails to make up the ladder's "steps." The two DNA strands are paired very specifically according to the identity of the nitrogen bases in the nucleotides. The adenine (A) nucleotide always pairs with the thymine (T) nucleotide; the guanine (G) nucleotide always pairs with the cytosine (C) nucleotide. The two strands of DNA are held together by weak bonds (hydrogen bonds; see Box 2-1). The doubled strands then coil into a spiral, giving DNA the descriptive name *double helix*.

The message of the DNA that makes up the individual genes is actually contained in the varying pattern of the four nucleotides along the strand. The nucleotides are like four letters in an alphabet that can be combined in different ways to make a variety of words. The words represent the amino acids used to make proteins, and a long string of words makes up a gene. Each gene thus codes for the building of amino acids into a specific cellular protein. Remember that all enzymes are proteins, and enzymes are

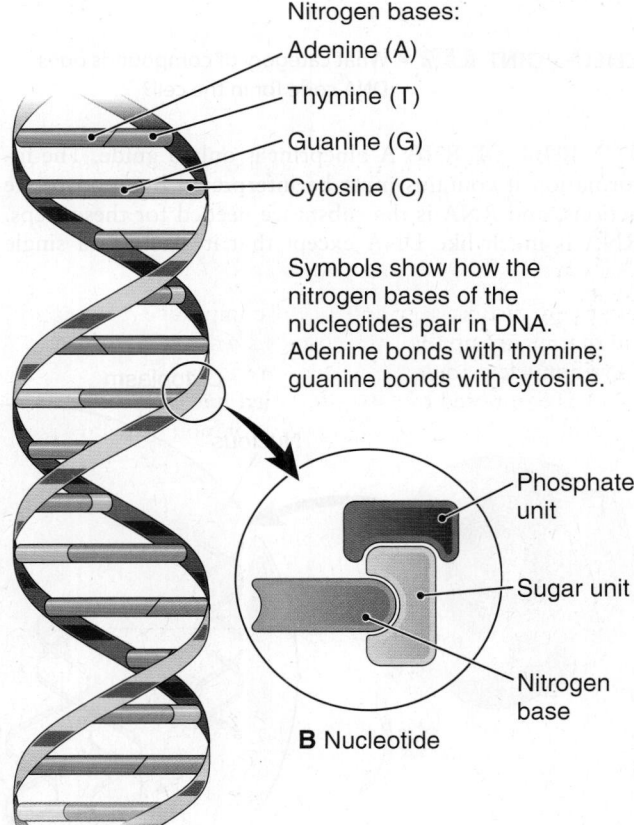

Nitrogen bases:
- Adenine (A)
- Thymine (T)
- Guanine (G)
- Cytosine (C)

Symbols show how the nitrogen bases of the nucleotides pair in DNA. Adenine bonds with thymine; guanine bonds with cytosine.

Phosphate unit

Sugar unit

Nitrogen base

B Nucleotide

A DNA

Figure 3-6 **Structure of DNA. (A)** This schematic representation of a chromosome segment shows the paired nucleic acid strands twisted into a double helix. **(B)** Each structural unit, or nucleotide, consists of a phosphate unit and a sugar unit attached to a nitrogen base. The sugar unit in DNA is deoxyribose. There are four different nucleotides in DNA. Their arrangement "spells out" the genetic instructions that control all activities of the cell. **[ZOOMING IN ➤** Two of the DNA nucleotides (A and G) are larger in size than the other two (T and C). How do the nucleotides pair up with regard to size? **]**

essential for all cellular reactions. DNA is thus the cell's master blueprint.

In light of observations on cellular diversity, you may wonder how different cells in the body can vary in appearance and function if they all have the same amount and same kind of DNA. The answer to this question is that only portions of the DNA in a given cell are active at any one time. In some cells, regions of the DNA can be switched on and off, under the influence of hormones, for example. However, as cells differentiate during development and become more specialized, regions of the DNA are permanently shut down, leading to the variations in the different cell types. Scientists now realize that the control of DNA action throughout the life of the cell is a very complex matter involving not only the DNA itself but proteins as well.

CHECKPOINT 3-7 ➤ What are the building blocks of nucleic acids?

CHECKPOINT 3-8 ➤ What category of compounds does DNA code for in the cell?

THE ROLE OF RNA A blueprint is only a guide. The information it contains must be interpreted by appropriate actions, and RNA is the substance needed for these steps. RNA is much like DNA except that it exists as a single strand of nucleotides and has the uracil (U) nucleotide instead of the thymine (T) nucleotide. Thus, when RNA pairs up with another molecule of nucleic acid to manufacture proteins, as explained below, adenine (A) bonds with uracil (U) in the RNA instead of thymine (T).

A detailed account of protein synthesis is beyond the scope of this book, but a highly simplified description and illustrations of the process are presented. The process begins with the transfer of information from DNA to RNA in the nucleus, a process known as *transcription* (Fig. 3-7). Before transcription begins, the DNA breaks its weak bonds and uncoils into single strands. Then a matching strand of RNA forms along one of the DNA strands by the process of nucleotide pairing. (For example, if the DNA strand reads CGAT, the corresponding mRNA will read GCUA. (Remember that RNA has U instead of T to bond with A.) When complete, this messenger RNA (mRNA) leaves the nucleus and travels to a ribosome in the cytoplasm (Fig. 3-8). Recall that ribosomes are the site of protein synthesis in the cell.

Ribosomes are composed of an RNA type called ribosomal RNA (rRNA) and also protein. At the ribosomes, the genetic message now contained within mRNA is decoded to build amino acids into the long chains that form proteins, a process termed *translation*. This final step requires a third RNA type, transfer RNA (tRNA), small molecules present in the cytoplasm (see Fig. 3-8).

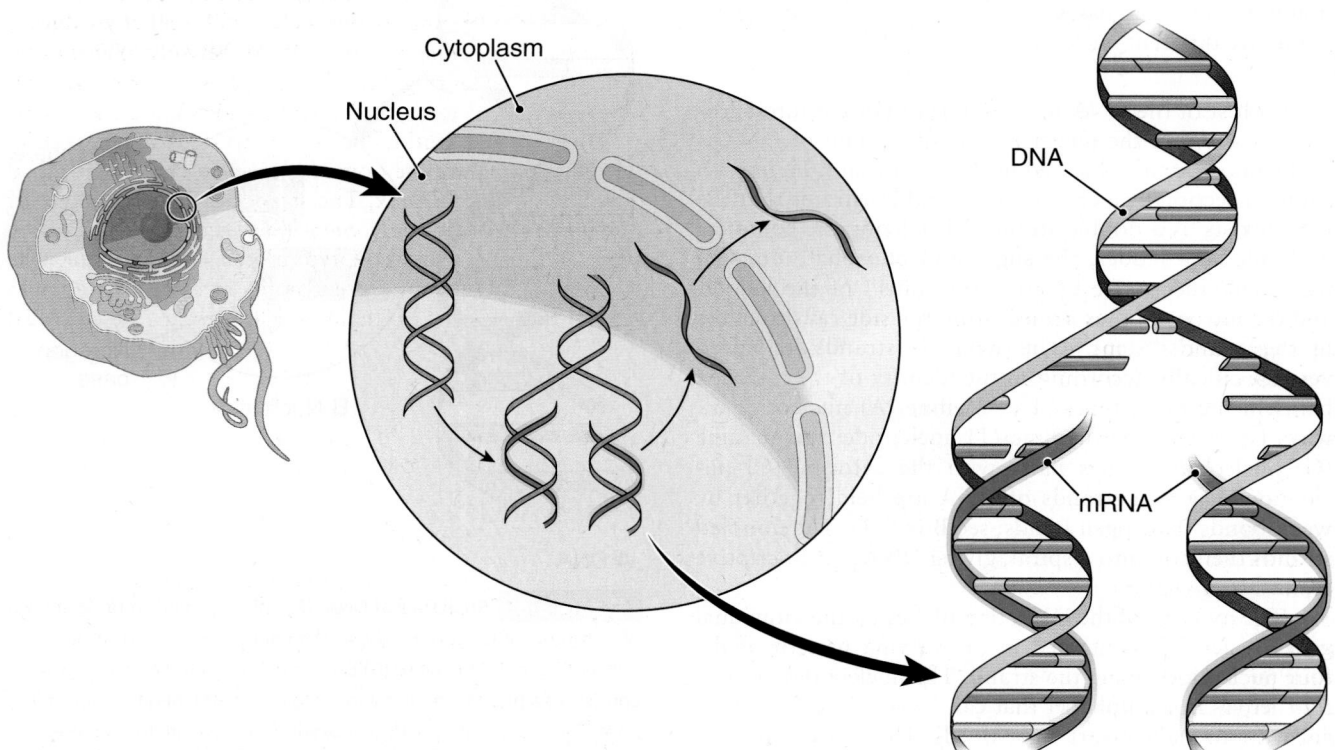

Figure 3-7 **Transcription.** In the first step of protein synthesis the DNA code is transcribed into messenger RNA (mRNA) by nucleotide base pairing. An enlarged view of the nucleic acids during transcription shows how mRNA forms according to the nucleotide pattern of the DNA. Note that adenine (A, red) in DNA bonds with uracil (U, brown) in RNA.

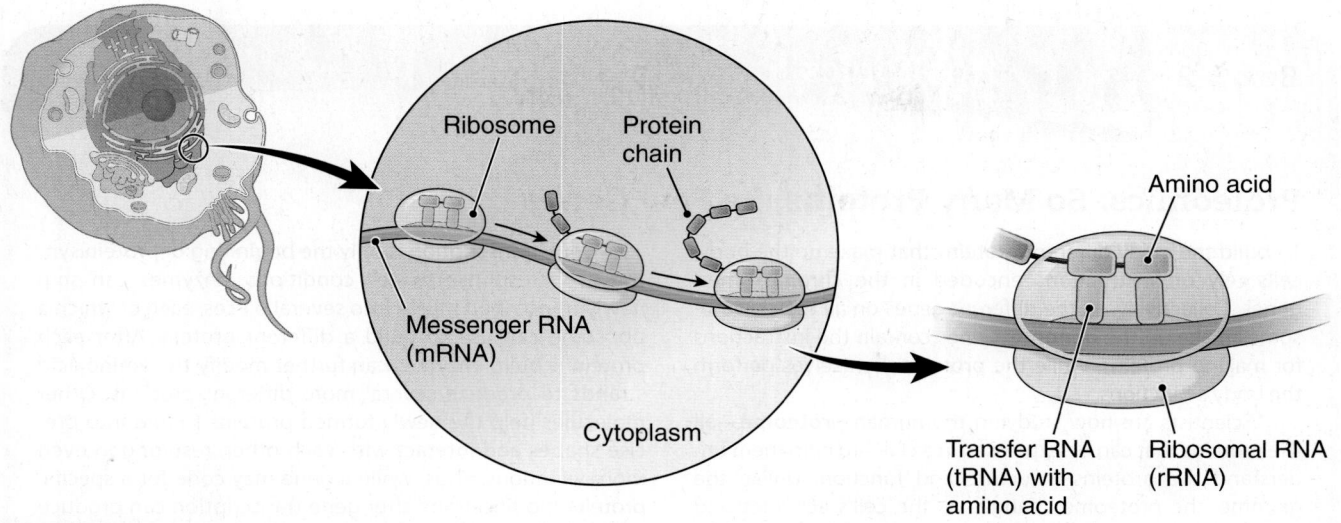

Figure 3-8 **Translation.** In protein synthesis, messenger RNA (mRNA) travels to the ribosomes in the cytoplasm. The information in the mRNA codes for the building of proteins from amino acids. Transfer RNA (tRNA) molecules bring amino acids to the ribosomes to build each protein.

Each transfer RNA carries a specific amino acid that can be added to a protein chain. A nucleotide code on each tRNA determines whether or not its amino acid will be added. After the amino acid chain is formed, it must be coiled and folded into the proper shape for that protein, as noted in Chapter 2. Table 3-4 summarizes information on the different types of RNA. Also see Box 3-2, Proteomics: So Many Proteins, So Few Genes.

CHECKPOINT **3-9** ➤ What three types of RNA are active in protein synthesis?

Cell Division

For growth, repair, and reproduction, cells must multiply to increase their numbers. The cells that form the sex cells (egg and sperm) divide by the process of *meiosis* (mi-O-sis), which cuts the chromosome number in half to prepare for union of the egg and sperm in fertilization. If not for this preliminary reduction, the number of chromosomes in the offspring would constantly double. The process of meiosis is discussed in Chapter 23. All other body cells, known as *somatic cells*, divide by the process of mitosis (mi-TO-sis). In this process, described later, each original parent cell becomes two identical daughter cells.

Before mitosis can occur, the genetic information (DNA) in the parent cell must be replicated (doubled), so that each of the two new daughter cells will receive a complete set of chromosomes. For example, a human cell that divides by mitosis must produce two cells with 46 chromosomes each, the same number of chromosomes that are present in the original parent cell. DNA replicates during **interphase**, the stage in the cell's life between one mitosis and the next. During this phase, DNA uncoils from its double-stranded form, and each strand takes on a matching strand of nucleotides according to the pattern of A-T, G-C pairing. There are now two strands, each identical to the original double helix. The strands are held together at a region called the *centromere* (SEN-tro-mere) until they separate during mitosis. A typical cell lives in interphase for most of its cycle and spends only a relatively short period in mitosis. For example, a cell reproducing every 20

Table 3-4	RNA
Types	**Function**
Messenger RNA (mRNA)	Is built on a strand of DNA in the nucleus and transcribes the nucleotide code; moves to cytoplasm and attaches to a ribosome
Ribosomal RNA (rRNA)	With protein makes up the ribosomes, the sites of protein synthesis in the cytoplasm; involved in the process of translating the genetic message into a protein
Transfer RNA (tRNA)	Works with other forms of RNA to translate the genetic code into protein; each molecule of tRNA carries an amino acid that can be used to build a protein at the ribosome

---

Box 3-2 · Hot Topics

Proteomics: So Many Proteins, So Few Genes

To build the many different proteins that make up the body, cells rely on instructions encoded in the chromosomes' genes. Collectively, all the different genes on all the chromosomes make up the **genome**. Genes contain the instructions for making proteins, while the proteins themselves perform the body's functions.

Scientists are now studying the human **proteome**—all the proteins that can be expressed in a cell—to help them understand the proteins' structure and function. Unlike the genome, the proteome changes as the cell's activities and needs change. In 2003, after a decade of intense scientific activity, investigators mapped the entire human genome and realized that it contained only 35,000 genes, far fewer than initially expected. How could this relatively small number of genes code for several million proteins? They concluded that genes were not the whole story.

Gene transcription is only the beginning of protein synthesis. In response to cell conditions, enzymes can snip newly transcribed mRNA into several pieces, each of which a ribosome can use to build a different protein. After each protein is built, enzymes can further modify the amino acid strands to produce several more different proteins. Other molecules help the newly formed proteins to fold into precise shapes and interact with each other, resulting in even more variations. Thus, while a gene may code for a specific protein, modifications after gene transcription can produce many more unique proteins. There is much left to discover about the proteome, but scientists hope that future research will lead to new techniques for detecting and treating disease.

---

hours spends only about one hour in mitosis and the remaining time in interphase.

CHECKPOINT **3-10** ➤ What must happen to the DNA in a cell before mitosis can occur? During what stage in the life of a cell does this occur?

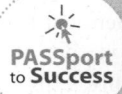
PASSport to Success Visit **thePoint** or see the Student Resource CD in the back of this book for a photomicrograph of a replicated chromosome.

Stages of Mitosis

Although mitosis is a continuous process, distinct changes can be seen in the dividing cell at four stages (Fig. 3-9).

- In **prophase** (PRO-faze), the doubled strands of DNA return to their tightly wound spiral organization and become visible under the microscope as dark, thread-like chromosomes. The nucleolus and the nuclear membrane begin to disappear. In the cytoplasm, the two centrioles move toward opposite ends of the cell and a spindle-shaped structure made of thin fibers begins to form between them.

- In **metaphase** (MET-ah-faze), the chromosomes line up across the center (equator) of the cell attached to the spindle fibers.

- In **anaphase** (AN-ah-faze), the centromere splits and the duplicated chromosomes separate and begin to move toward opposite ends of the cell.

- As mitosis continues into **telophase** (TEL-o-faze), a membrane appears around each group of separated chromosomes, forming two new nuclei.

Also during telophase, the plasma membrane pinches off to divide the cell. The midsection between the two areas becomes progressively smaller until, finally, the cell splits in two. There are now two new cells, or daughter cells, each with exactly the same kind and amount of DNA as was present in the parent cell. In just a few types of cells, skeletal muscle cells for example, the cell itself does not divide following nuclear division. The result, after multiple mitoses, is a giant single cell with multiple nuclei. This pattern is extremely rare in human cells.

During mitosis, all the organelles, except those needed for the division process, temporarily disappear. After the cell divides, these organelles reappear in each daughter cell. Also at this time, the centrioles usually replicate in preparation for the next cell division.

Body cells differ in the rate at which they reproduce. Some, such as nerve cells and muscle cells, stop dividing at some point in development and are not replaced if they die. They remain in interphase. Others, such as blood cells, sperm cells, and skin cells, multiply rapidly to replace cells destroyed by injury, disease, or natural wear-and-tear. Cells that multiply slowly may be triggered to divide when tissue is injured, as in repair of a bone fracture.

Immature cells that retain the ability to divide and mature when necessary are known as **stem cells** (see Box 4-1 in Chapter 4). All blood cells, for example, are produced from stem cells in the red bone marrow. Research has been done on stimulating stem cells to divide into various cell

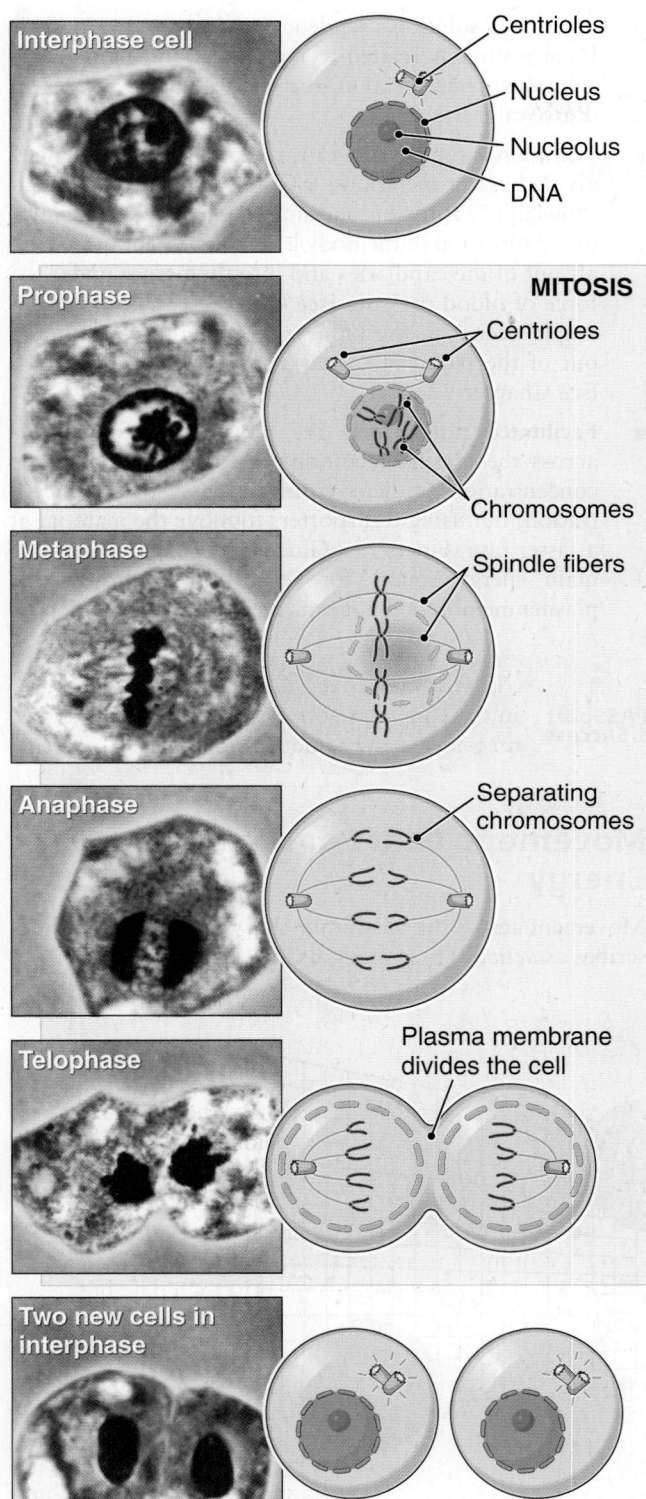

Figure 3-9 **The stages of mitosis.** When it is not dividing, the cell is in interphase. The cell shown is for illustration only. It is not a human cell, which has 46 chromosomes. (Photomicrographs reprinted with permission from Cormack DH. *Essential Histology*, 2nd ed. Philadelphia: Lippincott Williams & Wilkins, 2001.)

[**ZOOMING IN** ➤ If the original cell shown has 46 chromosomes, how many chromosomes will each new daughter cell have?]

Labels in figure:
- Interphase cell — Centrioles, Nucleus, Nucleolus, DNA
- Prophase — MITOSIS, Centrioles, Chromosomes
- Metaphase — Spindle fibers
- Anaphase — Separating chromosomes
- Telophase — Plasma membrane divides the cell
- Two new cells in interphase

types in the laboratory, but these studies have been controversial. Although it may be possible some day to use such cells to replace cells injured by disease, some people consider these studies unethical.

CHECKPOINT `3-11` ➤ What are the four stages of mitosis?

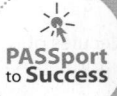

PASSport to Success Visit *thePoint* or see the Student Resource CD in the back of this book to view the animation *The Cell Cycle and Mitosis.*

Movement of Substances Across the Plasma Membrane

The plasma membrane serves as a barrier between the cell and its environment. Nevertheless, nutrients, oxygen, and many other substances needed by the cell must be taken in and waste products must be eliminated. Clearly, some substances can be exchanged between the cell and its environment through the plasma membrane. For this reason, the plasma membrane is described at a simple level as **semipermeable** (sem-e-PER-me-ah-bl). It is permeable, or passable, to some molecules but impassable to others. Some particles, proteins for example, are too large to travel through the membrane unaided.

The ability of a substance to travel through the membrane is based on several factors. Molecular size is the main factor that determines passage through the membrane, but solubility and electrical charge are also considerations. Water, a tiny molecule, is usually able to penetrate the membrane with ease. Nutrients, however, must be split into small molecules by digestion so that they can travel through the plasma membrane. For example, digestive enzymes convert sucrose (table sugar) to glucose and fructose, smaller molecules that enter the cell and serve as energy sources.

Various physical processes are involved in exchanges through the plasma membrane. One way of grouping these processes is according to whether they do or do not require cellular energy.

Movement That Does Not Require Cellular Energy

The adjective *passive* describes movement through the plasma membrane that does not require energy output by the cell. Passive mechanisms depend on the internal energy of the moving particles or the application of some outside source of energy. The methods include:

■ **Diffusion** is the constant movement of particles from a region of relatively higher concentration to one of lower concentration. Just as couples on a crowded dance floor spread out into all the available space to avoid hitting other dancers, diffusing substances spread throughout their available space until their concentration everywhere is the same—that is, they reach equilibrium (Fig. 3-10). This movement from higher to

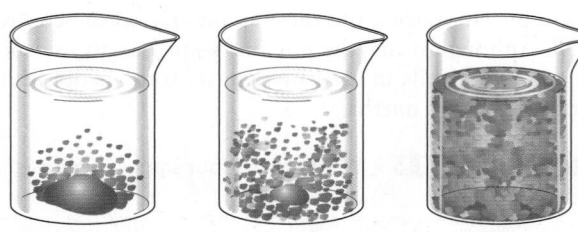

Figure 3-10 **Diffusion of a solid in a liquid.** The molecules of the solid tend to spread evenly throughout the liquid as they dissolve.

lower concentrations uses the particles' internal energy and does not require cellular energy, just as a sled will move from the top to the bottom of a snowy hill. The particles are said to follow their *concentration gradient* from higher concentration to lower concentration.

When substances diffuse through a membrane, such as the intact plasma membrane, passage is limited to those particles small enough to pass through spaces between molecules in the membrane, as shown with a large-scale example in Figure 3-11. In the body, soluble materials, such as nutrients, electrolytes, gases, and waste materials, are constantly moving into or out of the cells by diffusion.

■ **Osmosis** (os-MO-sis) is a special type of diffusion. The term applies specifically to the diffusion of water through a semipermeable membrane. The water molecules move, as expected, from an area where there are more of them to an area where there are fewer of them. That is, the solvent (the water molecules) moves from an area of lower *solute* concentration to an area of higher *solute* concentration (Fig. 3-12).

For a physiologist studying water's flow across membranes, as in exchange of fluids through capillaries in the circulation, it is helpful to know the direction in which water will flow and at what rate it will move. A measure of the force driving osmosis is called the *osmotic pressure*. This force can be measured, as illustrated in Figure 3-13, by applying enough pressure to the surface of a liquid to stop the inward flow of water by osmosis. The pressure needed to counteract osmosis is the osmotic pressure. In practice, the term osmotic pressure is used to

describe a solution's tendency to draw water in. This force is directly related to concentration: the higher a solutions' concentration, the greater is its tendency to draw water in.

■ **Filtration** is the passage of water and dissolved materials through a membrane as a result of a mechanical ("pushing") force on one side (Fig. 3-14). One example of filtration in the body is the movement of materials out of the capillaries and into the tissues under the force of blood pressure (see Chapter 15). Another example occurs in the kidneys as materials are filtered out of the blood in the first step of urine formation (see Chapter 22).

■ **Facilitated diffusion** is the movement of materials across the plasma membrane in the direction of the concentration gradient (from higher to lower concentration) but using transporters to move the material at a faster rate (Fig. 3-15). Glucose, the sugar that is the main energy source for cells, moves through the plasma membrane by means of facilitated diffusion.

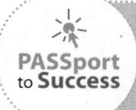 **PASSport to Success** Visit *thePoint* or see the Student Resource CD in the back of this book to view an animation on osmosis and osmotic pressure.

Movement That Requires Cellular Energy

Movement across the membrane that requires energy is describes as *active*. These methods include:

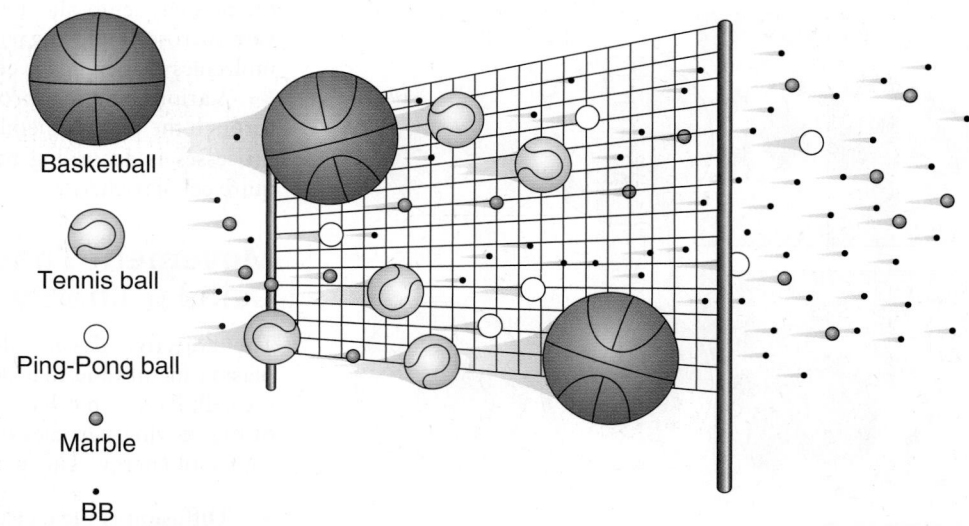

Figure 3-11 **Diffusion through a semipermeable membrane.** In this example, large objects (basketballs, tennis balls) cannot pass through the net, whereas the smaller ones (ping-pong balls, marbles, BBs) can. In the human body, large particles in the blood, such as proteins and blood cells, cannot pass through the walls of the capillaries, whereas small particles, such as nutrients, electrolytes, and gases, can. [ZOOMING IN ➤ If this picture represented diffusion in the body, what would the net be?]

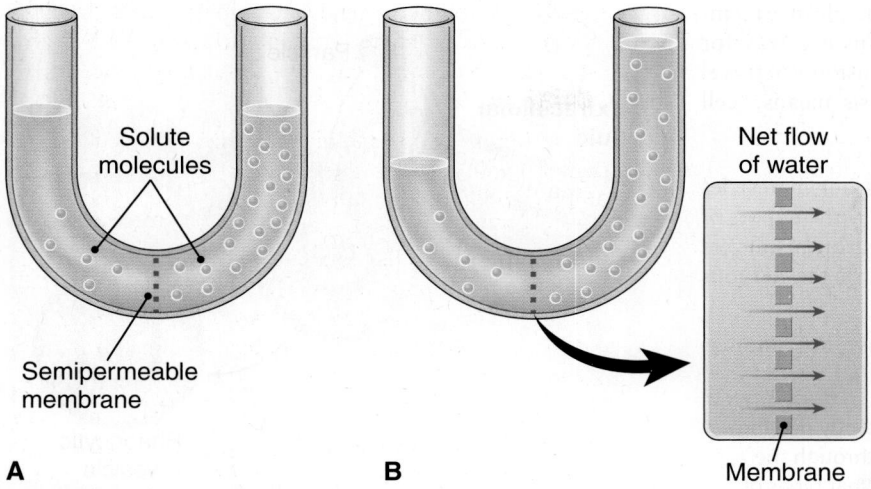

Figure 3-12 **A simple demonstration of osmosis.** Solute molecules are shown in yellow. All of the solvent (blue) is composed of water molecules. **(A)** Two solutions with different concentrations of solute are separated by a semipermeable membrane. Water can flow through the membrane, but the solute cannot. **(B)** Water flows into the more concentrated solution, raising the level of the liquid in that side. [ZOOMING IN ➤ What would happen in this system if the solute could pass through the membrane?]

■ **Active transport.** The plasma membrane has the ability to move small solute particles into or out of the cell opposite to the direction in which they would normally flow by diffusion. That is, the membrane moves them against the concentration gradient from an area where they are in relatively lower concentration to an area where they are in higher concentration. Because this movement goes against the natural flow of particles, it requires energy, just as getting a sled to the top

of a hill requires energy. It also requires proteins in the plasma membrane that act as **transporters** for the particles.

This process of active transport is one important function of the living cellular membrane. The nervous system and muscular system, for example, depend on the active transport of sodium, potassium, and calcium ions for proper function. The kidneys also carry out active transport in regulating the composition of urine. By means of active transport, the cell can take in what it needs from the surrounding fluids and remove materials from the cell. Because the plasma membrane can carry on active transport, the membrane is most accurately described, not as simply semipermeable, but as **selectively permeable**. It regulates what can enter and leave based on the needs of the cell.

There are several active methods for moving large quantities of material into or out of the cell. These methods are grouped together as **bulk transport**, because of the amounts of material moved, or **vesicular transport**, because small sacs, or vesicles, are needed for the processes.

■ **Endocytosis** (en-do-si-TO-sis) is a term that describes the bulk movement of materials into the cell. There are two examples:

> In **phagocytosis** (fag-o-si-TO-sis), relatively large particles are engulfed by the plasma membrane and moved into the cell (Fig. 3-16). Certain white blood cells carry out phagocytosis to rid the body of foreign material and dead cells. Material taken into a cell by phagocytosis is first enclosed in a vesicle made from the plasma membrane and is later destroyed by lysosomes.

 **PASSport to Success** Visit **thePoint** or see the Student Resource CD in the back of this book for an electron micrograph of pinocytosis.

Figure 3-13 **Osmotic pressure.** Osmotic pressure is the force needed to stop the flow of water by osmosis. Pressure on the surface of the fluid in side B counteracts the osmotic flow of water from side A to side B. [ZOOMING IN ➤ What would happen to osmotic pressure if the concentration of solute were increased on side B of this system?]

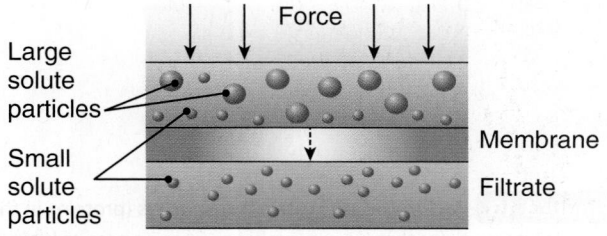

Figure 3-14 **Filtration.** A mechanical force pushes a substance through a membrane, although the membrane limits which particles can pass through based on size. The small particles go through the membrane and appear in the filtered solution (filtrate).

> In **pinocytosis** (pi-no-si-TO-sis), the plasma membrane engulfs droplets of fluid. This is a way for large protein molecules in suspension to travel into the cell. The word *pinocytosis* means "cell drinking."

■ In **exocytosis**, the cell moves materials out in vesicles (Fig. 3-17). One example of exocytosis is the export of neurotransmitters from neurons (neurotransmitters are chemicals that control the activity of the nervous system).

The transport methods described above are summarized in Table 3-5.

CHECKPOINT **3-12** ➤ Substances are constantly moving into and out of cells through the plasma membrane. What types of movement do not require cellular energy and what types of movement do require cellular energy?

How Osmosis Affects Cells

As stated earlier, water usually moves easily through the cell membrane. Therefore, for a normal fluid balance to be maintained, the fluid outside all cells must have the same concentration of dissolved substances (solutes) as the fluids inside the cells (Fig. 3-18). If not, water will move rapidly into or out of the cell by osmosis. Solutions with

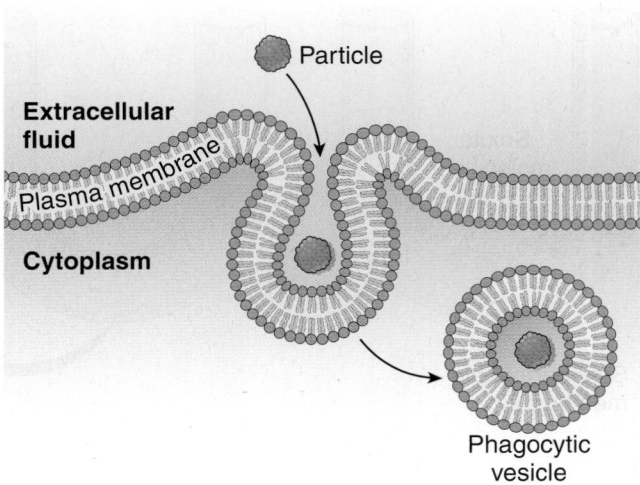

Figure 3-16 **Phagocytosis.** The plasma membrane encloses a particle from the extracellular fluid. The membrane then pinches off, forming a vesicle that carries the particle into the cytoplasm. **[ZOOMING IN ➤** What organelle would likely help to destroy a particle taken in by phagocytosis? **]**

concentrations equal to the concentration of the cytoplasm are described as **isotonic** (i-so-TON-ik). Tissue fluids and blood plasma are isotonic for body cells. Manufactured solutions that are isotonic for the cells and can thus be used to replace body fluids include 0.9% salt, or **normal saline**, and 5% dextrose (glucose).

A solution that is less concentrated than the intracellular fluid is described as **hypotonic**. Based on the principles of osmosis already explained, a cell placed in a hypotonic solution draws water in, swells, and may burst. When a red blood cell draws in water and bursts in this way, the cell is said to undergo **hemolysis** (he-MOL-ih-sis). If a cell is placed in a **hypertonic** solution, which is more concentrated than the cellular fluid, it loses water to the surrounding fluids and shrinks, a process termed **crenation** (kre-NA-shun) (see Fig. 3-18).

Fluid balance is an important facet of homeostasis and must be properly regulated for health. You can figure out in which direction water will move through the plasma membrane if you remember the saying "water follows salt," salt meaning any dissolved material (solute). The total amount and distribution of body fluids is discussed in Chapter 21. Table 3-6 summarizes the effects of different solution concentrations on cells.

Figure 3-15 **Facilitated diffusion.** Transporters (proteins in the plasma membrane) move solute particles through a membrane from an area of higher concentration to an area of lower concentration. **(A)** A solute particle enters the transporter. **(B)** The transporter changes shape. **(C)** The transporter releases the solute particle on the other side of the membrane. **[ZOOMING IN ➤** How would a change in the number of transporters affect a solute's movement by facilitated diffusion? **]**

3

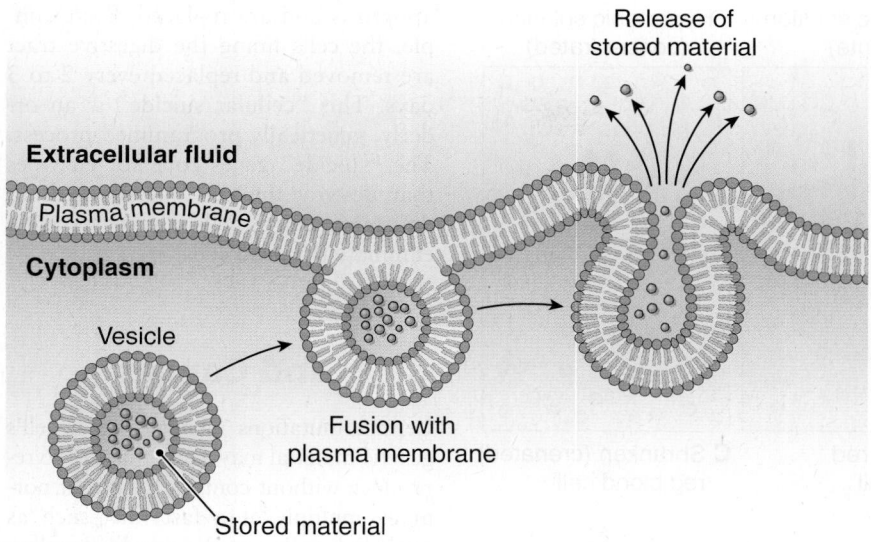

Figure 3-17 Exocytosis. A vesicle fuses with the plasma membrane then ruptures and releases its contents.

CHECKPOINT **3-13** ➤ The concentration of fluids in and around the cell is important in homeostasis. What term describes a fluid that is the same concentration as the fluid within the cell (intracellular fluid)? What type of fluid is less concentrated? More concentrated?

Cell Aging

As cells multiply throughout life, changes occur that may lead to their damage and death. Harmful substances known as *free radicals*, produced in the course of normal metabolism, can injure cells unless these materials are destroyed. Chapter 20 covers free radicals in more detail. Lysosomes may deteriorate as they age, releasing enzymes that can harm the cell. Alteration of the genes, or **mutation**, is a natural occurrence in the process of cell division and is increased by exposure to harmful substances and radiation in the environment. Mutations usually harm cells and may lead to cancer.

As a person ages, the overall activity of the body cells slows. One example of this change is the slowing down of repair processes. A bone fracture, for example, takes considerably longer to heal in an old person than in a young person.

Table 3-5	Membrane Transport	
Process	**Definition**	**Example**
Do not require cellular energy (passive)		
Diffusion	Random movement of particles with the concentration gradient (from higher concentration to lower concentration) until they reach equilibrium	Movement of nutrients, electrolytes, gases, wastes, and other soluble materials into and out of the cell
Osmosis	Diffusion of water through a semi-permeable membrane	Movement of water across the plasma membrane
Filtration	Movement of materials through a membrane under mechanical force	Movement of materials out of the blood under the force of blood pressure
Facilitated diffusion	Movement of materials across the plasma membrane along the concentration gradient using transporters to speed the process	Movement of glucose into the cells
Require cellular energy		
Active transport	Movement of materials through the plasma membrane against the concentration gradient using transporters	Transport of ions (e.g., Na^+, K^+, Ca^{2+}) in the nervous system and muscular system
Endocytosis	Transport of bulk amounts of materials into the cell using vesicles	Phagocytosis—intake of large particles, as when white blood cells take in waste materials; also pinocytosis—intake of fluid
Exocytosis	Transport of bulk amounts of materials out of the cell using vesicles	Release of neurotransmitters from neurons

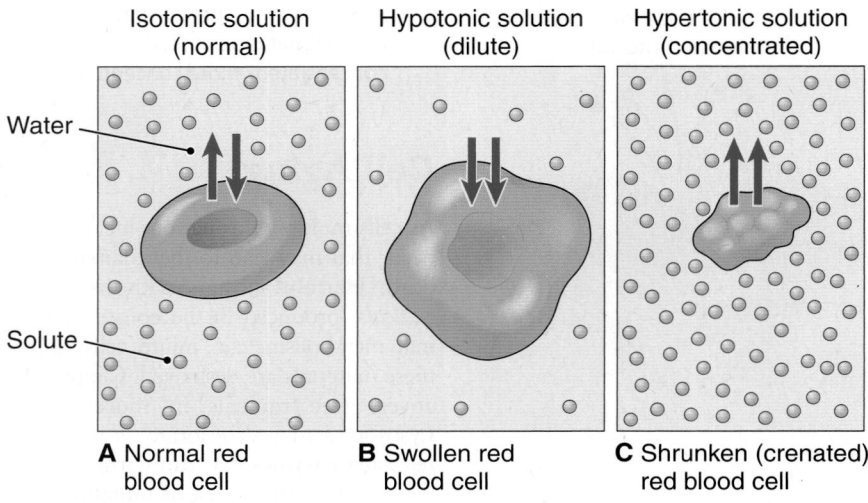

Isotonic solution (normal)

Hypotonic solution (dilute)

Hypertonic solution (concentrated)

Water

Solute

A Normal red blood cell

B Swollen red blood cell

C Shrunken (crenated) red blood cell

→ Direction of osmotic water movement

Figure 3-18 **The effect of osmosis on cells.** Water moves through a red blood cell membrane in solutions with three different concentrations of solute. **(A)** The isotonic (normal) solution has the same concentration as the cell fluid, and water moves into and out of the cell at the same rate. **(B)** A cell placed in a hypotonic (more dilute) solution draws water in, causing the cell to swell and perhaps undergo hemolysis (bursting). **(C)** The hypertonic (more concentrated) solution draws water out of the cell, causing it to shrink, an effect known as crenation. **[ZOOMING IN ➤** What would happen to red blood cells if blood lost through injury were replaced with pure water? **]**

One theory on aging holds that cells are preprogrammed to divide only a certain number of times before they die. Support for this idea comes from the fact that cells taken from a young person divide more times when grown in the laboratory than similar cells taken from an older individual. This programmed cell death, known as *apoptosis* (ah-pop-TO-sis), is a natural part of growth and remodeling before birth in the developing embryo. For example, apoptosis removes cells from the embryonic limb buds in the development of fingers and toes. Apoptosis also is needed in repair and remodeling of tissue throughout life. Cells subject to wear and tear regularly undergo

apoptosis and are replaced. For example, the cells lining the digestive tract are removed and replaced every 2 to 3 days. This "cellular suicide" is an orderly, genetically programmed process. The "suicide" genes code for enzymes that destroy the cell quickly without damaging nearby cells. Phagocytes then eliminate the dead cells.

Cells and Cancer

Certain mutations (changes) in a cell's genetic material may cause that cell to reproduce without control. Cells that normally multiply at a fast rate, such as epithelial cells, are more likely than slower-growing cells to undergo such transformations. If these altered cells do not die naturally or get destroyed by the immune system, they will continue to multiply and may spread (metastasize) to other tissues, producing **cancer.** Cancer cells form tumors, which interfere with normal functions, crowding out normal cells and robbing them of nutrients. There is more information on the various types of tumors in Chapter 4.

Cancer Risk Factors

The causes of cancer are complex, involving interactions between cellular factors and the environment. Because cancer may take a long time to develop, it is often difficult to identify its cause or causes. Certain forces increase the chances of developing the disease and are considered risk factors. These include the following:

■ **Heredity.** Certain types of cancer occur more frequently in some families than in others, indicating that

Table 3-6	Solutions and Their Effects on Cells		
Type of Solution	**Description**	**Examples**	**Effect on Cells**
Isotonic	Has the same concentration of dissolved substances as the fluid in the cell	0.9% salt (normal saline); 5% dextrose (glucose)	None; cell in equilibrium with its environment
Hypotonic	Has a lower concentration of dissolved substances than the fluid in the cell	Less than 0.9% salt or 5% dextrose	Cell takes in water, swells, and may burst; red blood cell undergoes hemolysis
Hypertonic	Has a higher concentration of dissolved substances than the fluid in the cell	Higher than 0.9% salt or 5% dextrose	Cell will lose water and shrink; cell undergoes crenation

3

Disease in Context revisited

▶ Jim's Trouble Continues with a Clot

Let's consider what was happening in Jim's body when he overexerted himself on the basketball court: his rapidly beating heart forced blood around a fatty plaque that bulged into the lumen of a coronary artery. Unable to resist the high pressure within the artery, the plaque ruptured and stimulated blood platelets to form a clot in the damaged vessel. Unfortunately for Jim, the clot prevented millions of cardiac muscle cells from receiving oxygen-rich blood. Without oxygen, the cells' mitochondria could not manufacture ATP; without ATP, the contractile proteins in the cells could not shorten. Within minutes, the cardiac muscle cells downstream from the clot stopped contracting, forcing Jim's heart into an irregular rhythm. This alteration dramatically decreased the volume of blood leaving his heart. Brain cells, called neurons, also depend on oxygen to manufacture ATP, and without adequate blood flow, they too began to shut down, causing Jim to lose consciousness.

Inside Jim's oxygen-starved cardiac muscle cells, lack of ATP had other serious consequences. Transporter proteins embedded in the cells' plasma membranes began to shut down. Without these transporters, the cells could not regulate their solute concentration. Quickly, the cells' cytoplasm became hypertonic to the surrounding tissue fluid. Following its osmotic gradient, extracellular water entered the affected cardiac muscle cells, causing them to burst and die. Jim is in big trouble.

In this case, we saw that events within Jim's cardiac muscle cells affected his whole body. Your understanding of cellular structure and function will help you to make sense of the structure and function of tissues, organs, and, ultimately, the entire body. Without immediate help, Jim's chances of survival are low. The case study in Chapter 14, The Heart and Heart Disease, will introduce you to some of the medical techniques that will save Jim's life.

---

there is some inherited predisposition to cancer development.

- **Chemicals.** Certain industrial and environmental chemicals are known to increase the risk of cancer. Any chemical that causes cancer is called a **carcinogen** (kar-SIN-o-jen). The most common carcinogens in our society are those present in cigarette smoke. Carcinogens are also present, both naturally and as additives, in foods. Certain drugs also may be carcinogenic.

- **Ionizing radiation.** Certain types of radiation can produce damage to cellular DNA that may lead to cancer. These include x-rays, rays from radioactive substances, and ultraviolet rays. For example, the ultravi-

olet rays received from sun exposure are very harmful to the skin.

- **Physical irritation.** Continued irritation, such as the contact of a hot pipe stem on the lip, increases cell division and thus increases the chance of mutation.

- **Diet.** It has been shown that diets high in fats and total calories are associated with an increased occurrence of certain cancers. A general lack of fiber and insufficient amounts of certain fruits and vegetables in the diet can leave one susceptible to cancers of the digestive tract.

- **Viruses** have been implicated in cancers of the liver, the blood (leukemias), lymphatic tissues (lymphomas), and the uterine cervix.

Word Anatomy

Medical terms are built from standardized word parts (prefixes, roots, and suffixes). Learning the meanings of these parts can help you remember words and interpret unfamiliar terms.

WORD PART	MEANING	EXAMPLE
The Role of Cells		
cyt/o	cell	*Cytology* is the study of cells.
Microscopes		
micr/o	small	*Microscopes* are used to view structures too small to see with the naked eye.
Cell Structure		
bi-	two	The lipid *bilayer* is a double layer of lipid molecules.
-some	body	*Ribosomes* are small bodies in the cytoplasm that help make proteins.
chrom/o-	color	*Chromosomes* are small, threadlike bodies that stain darkly with basic dyes.
end/o-	in, within	The *endoplasmic* reticulum is a membranous network within the cytoplasm.
lys/o	loosening, dissolving, separating	*Lysosomes* are small bodies (organelles) with enzymes that dissolve materials *(see also hemolysis).*
Cell Divisions		
inter-	between	*Interphase* is the stage between one cell division (mitosis) and the next.
pro-	before, in front of	*Prophase* is the first stage of mitosis.
meta-	change	*Metaphase* is the second stage of mitosis when the chromosomes change position and line up across the equator.
ana-	upward, back, again	In the *anaphase* stage of mitosis, chromosomes move to opposite sides of the cell.
tel/o-	end	*Telophase* is the last stage of mitosis.
semi-	partial, half	A *semipermeable* membrane lets some molecules pass through but not others.
phag/o	to eat, ingest	In *phagocytosis* the plasma membrane engulfs large particles and moves them into the cell.
pin/o	to drink	In *pinocytosis* the plasma membrane "drinks" (engulfs) droplets of fluid.
ex/o-	outside, out of, away from	In *exocytosis* the cell moves material out in vesicles.
iso-	same, equal	An *isotonic* solution has the same concentration as that of the cytoplasm.
hypo-	deficient, below, beneath	A *hypotonic* solution's concentration is lower than that of the cytoplasm.
hem/o	blood	*Hemolysis* is the destruction of red blood cells.
hyper-	above, over, excessive	A *hypertonic* solution's concentration is higher than that of the cytoplasm.
Cells and Cancer		
carcin/o	cancer, carcinoma	A *carcinogen* is a chemical that causes cancer.
-gen	agent that produces or originates	See preceding example.

Summary

3

I. **THE ROLE OF CELLS**
   A. Basic unit of life
   B. Show all characteristics of life—organization, metabolism, responsiveness, homeostasis, growth, reproduction

II. **MICROSCOPES**
   A. Types
      1. Compound light microscope
      2. Transmission electron microscope—magnifies up to 1 million times
      3. Scanning electron microscope—gives three-dimensional image
   B. Micrometer—metric unit commonly used for microscopic measurements (μm)
   C. Stains—dyes used to aid in viewing cells under the microscope

III. **CELL STRUCTURE**
   A. Plasma membrane—regulates what enters and leaves cell
      1. Phospholipid bilayer with proteins, carbohydrates, cholesterol
         a. Proteins—channels, transporters, receptors, enzymes, linkers, cell identity markers
   B. Nucleus
      1. Control center of the cell
      2. Contains the chromosomes (units of heredity)
      3. Contains the nucleolus, which manufactures ribosomes
   C. Cytoplasm—colloidal suspension that holds organelles
      1. Cytosol—liquid portion
      2. Organelles—structures that carry out special functions
         a. ER (endoplasmic reticulum), ribosomes, mitochondria, Golgi apparatus, lysosomes, peroxisomes, vesicles, centrioles
         b. Cilia, flagellum—surface organelles used for movement

IV. **PROTEIN SYNTHESIS**
   A. Nucleic acids—DNA and RNA
      1. Composed of nucleotides
         a. Each nucleotide has sugar, phosphate, nitrogen base
         b. Nitrogen bases vary, giving five nucleotides
      2. DNA
         a. Carries the genetic message
         b. Located almost entirely in the nucleus
         c. Composed of nucleotides containing adenine (A), guanine (G), cytosine (C), thymine (T)
         d. Double stranded by pairing of A-T, G-C, and wound into helix

   3. The role of RNA
      a. Single strand of nucleotides containing A, G, C, or uracil (U)
      b. Located in the cytoplasm
      c. Translates DNA message into proteins
      d. Three types
         (1) Messenger RNA (mRNA)—transcribes the message of the DNA
         (2) Ribosomal RNA (rRNA)—makes up the ribosomes, the site of protein synthesis
         (3) Transfer RNA (tRNA)—brings amino acids to be made into proteins

V. **CELL DIVISION**
   A. Meiosis—forms the sex cells (egg and sperm)
      1. Divides the chromosome number in half
   B. Mitosis—division of somatic (body) cells
      1. Chromosomes first replicate (double) during interphase
      2. Division of cell into two identical daughter cells
   C. Stages of mitosis—prophase, metaphase, anaphase, telophase

VI. **MOVEMENT OF SUBSTANCES ACROSS THE PLASMA MEMBRANE**
   A. Movement that does not require cellular energy (passive)
      1. Diffusion—molecules move from area of higher concentration to area of lower concentration
      2. Osmosis—diffusion of water through semipermeable membrane
         a. Osmotic pressure—measure of a solution's tendency to draw in water
      3. Filtration—movement of materials through plasma membrane under mechanical force
      4. Facilitated diffusion—movement of materials with aid of transporters in plasma membrane
   B. Movement that requires cellular energy (active)
      1. Active transport
         a. Movement of solute particles from area of lower concentration to area of higher concentration
         b. Requires transporters
      2. Endocytosis—movement of bulk amounts of material into the cell in vesicles
         a. Phagocytosis—engulfing of large particles
         b. Pinocytosis—intake of fluid droplets
      3. Exocytosis—movement of bulk amounts of materials out of the cell in vesicles
   C. How osmosis affects cells
      1. Isotonic solution—same concentration as cell fluids; cell remains the same

2. Hypotonic solution—lower concentration than cell fluids; cell swells and may undergo hemolysis (bursting)
3. Hypertonic solution—higher concentration than cell fluids; cell undergoes crenation (shrinking)

VII. CELL AGING
A. Mutations (changes) occur in genes
B. Slowing of cellular activity
C. Apoptosis—programmed cell death

VIII. CELLS AND CANCER .
A. Cancer
1. Uncontrolled growth of cells
2. Spread (metastasize) to other tissues
B. Cancer risk factors
1. Heredity
2. Chemicals—carcinogens
3. Ionizing radiation
4. Physical irritation
5. Diet
6. Viruses

Questions for Study and Review

BUILDING UNDERSTANDING

Fill in the blanks

1. The part of the cell that regulates what can enter or leave is the _____.

2. Distinct segments of DNA that code for specific proteins are called _____.

3. The cytosol and organelles make up the _____.

4. If Solution A has more solute and less water than Solution B, then Solution A is _____ to Solution B.

5. Mechanisms that require energy to move substances across the plasma membrane are called _____ transport mechanisms.

Matching > Match each numbered item with the most closely related lettered item.

___ **6.** DNA duplication takes place
___ **7.** DNA is tightly wound into chromosomes
___ **8.** Chromosomes line up along the cell's equator
___ **9.** Chromosomes separate and move toward opposite ends of the cell
___ **10.** Cell membrane pinches off, dividing the cell into two new daughter cells

a. metaphase
b. anaphase
c. telophase
d. interphase
e. prophase

Multiple Choice

___ **11.** The main component of the plasma membrane is
  a. phospholipid
  b. cholesterol
  c. carbohydrate
  d. protein

___ **12.** ATP is synthesized in the
  a. nucleus
  b. Golgi apparatus
  c. endoplasmic reticulum
  d. mitochondria

___ **13.** Transcription of the DNA strand TGAAC would produce an mRNA strand with the sequence
  a. CAGGU
  b. ACTTG

  c. CAGGT
  d. ACUUG

___ **14.** Somatic cells divide by the process called
  a. mitosis
  b. meiosis
  c. crenation
  d. hemolysis

___ **15.** Movement of solute from a region of high concentration to one of lower concentration is called
  a. exocytosis
  b. diffusion
  c. endocytosis
  d. osmosis

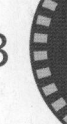

UNDERSTANDING CONCEPTS

16. List the components of the plasma membrane and state a function for each.

17. Compare and contrast the following cellular components:
    a. microvilli and cilia
    b. nucleus and nucleolus
    c. rough ER and smooth ER
    d. lysosome and peroxisome
    e. DNA and RNA
    f. chromosome and gene

18. Describe the role of each of the following in protein synthesis: DNA, nucleotide, RNA, ribosomes, rough ER, and Golgi apparatus.

19. List and define six methods by which materials cross the plasma membrane. Which of these requires cellular energy?

20. Why is the plasma membrane described as selectively permeable?

21. What will happen to a red blood cell placed in a 5.0% salt solution? In distilled water?

22. Discuss the link between genetic mutation and cancer. List six risk factors associated with cancer.

CONCEPTUAL THINKING

23. Cigarette smoke paralyzes the cilia of cells lining the respiratory tract. Explain the effects of this on respiratory system function.

24. In the Disease in Context case story, Jim's cardiac muscle cells adapted to his unhealthy lifestyle by synthesizing more contractile proteins. Beginning with events in the nucleus, describe the process of manufacturing a contractile protein.

25. In Jim's case, we saw that changes at the cellular level can ultimately affect the entire organism. Explain why this is so.

26. Kidney failure causes a buildup of waste and water in the blood. A procedure called hemodialysis removes these substances from the blood. During this procedure, the patient's blood passes by a semipermeable membrane within the dialysis machine. Waste and water from the blood diffuse across the membrane into dialysis fluid on the other side. Based on this information, compare the osmotic concentration of the blood with that of the dialysis fluid.

CHAPTER 4

Tissues, Glands, and Membranes

Learning Outcomes

After careful study of this chapter, you should be able to:

1. Name the four main groups of tissues and give the location and general characteristics of each
2. Describe the difference between exocrine and endocrine glands and give examples of each
3. Give examples of circulating, generalized, and structural connective tissues
4. Describe three types of epithelial membranes
5. List several types of connective tissue membranes
6. Explain the difference between benign and malignant tumors and give several examples of each type
7. List some signs of cancer
8. List six methods of diagnosing cancer
9. Describe three traditional methods of treating cancer
10. Show how word parts are used to build words related to tissues, glands, and membranes (see Word Anatomy at the end of the chapter)

Selected Key Terms

The following terms and other boldface terms in the chapter are defined in the Glossary

adipose
areolar
benign
cartilage
chemotherapy
collagen
endocrine
epithelium
exocrine
fascia
histology
malignant
matrix
membrane
metastasis
mucosa
myelin
neoplasm
neuroglia
neuron
parietal
serosa
staging
visceral

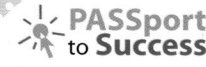

PASSport to Success

Visit *thePoint* or see the Student Resource CD in the back of this book for definitions and pronunciations of key terms as well as a pretest for this chapter.

Disease
in Context

➤ Ben's Case: How a Tissue Failure Affects the Entire Body

"Cough. Cough. Cough." Alison awoke with a start. *Not again*, she thought as she stumbled out of bed toward the baby's room. For the last few days, Alison's 2-year-old was sick with what appeared to be a nasty chest infection. This wasn't unusual for Ben—he had come down with several lung infections in the past and often seemed congested, but Alison had chalked this up to normal childhood illnesses. Lately though, Alison had become more worried, especially after taking Ben to their community center, where she noticed that he seemed smaller than the rest of the children his age and had trouble keeping up with them as they played in the gym. *I'll take him in to see the doctor tomorrow*, Alison thought as she sat down in the rocking chair beside Ben's crib and began patting his back.

At the medical center, Ben's doctor examined him carefully. Ben was smaller and weighed less than most boys his age, despite his mom's observation that he had a good appetite. His recurrent respiratory infections were also cause for worry. In addition, Alison reported that Ben had frequent bowel movement with stools that were often foul-smelling and greasy. The doctor's next question caught Alison off guard. "When you kiss your son,

does he taste saltier than what you might expect?" The doctor wasn't surprised when Alison answered yes. "I need to run a few more tests before I can make a diagnosis," he said. "In the meantime, let's start Ben on some oral antibiotics for his chest infection."

A few days later, Ben's doctor reviewed his chart and the lab test results. The sweat test revealed that Ben's sweat glands excreted abnormally high concentrations of salt. Chest and sinus radiography showed evidence of bacterial infection and thickening of the epithelial membrane lining Ben's respiratory passages. The blood test also indicated that Ben was deficient in several fat-soluble vitamins. With the evidence he had, the doctor was ready to make his diagnosis. Ben had cystic fibrosis.

Cystic fibrosis is caused by a mutation in a gene that codes for a channel protein in the plasma membrane of certain types of cells. Although the disease affects certain cells of only one of the four types of tissue (epithelium), its consequences are seen in many different organs and systems—especially the respiratory and digestive systems. We will learn more about the implications of this tissue disease later in the chapter.

Tissues are groups of cells similar in structure, arranged in a characteristic pattern, and specialized for the performance of specific tasks. The study of tissues is known as **histology** (his-TOL-o-je). This study shows that the form, arrangement, and composition of cells in different tissues account for their properties.

The tissues in our bodies might be compared with the different materials used to construct a building. Think for a moment of the great variety of building materials used according to need—wood, stone, steel, plaster, insulation, and others. Each of these has different properties, but together they contribute to the building as a whole. The same may be said of tissues. To read about the origin of the different tissues, see Box 4-1, Stem Cells: So Much Potential.

Tissue Classification

The four main tissue groups are the following:

- **Epithelial** (ep-ih-THE-le-al) **tissue** covers surfaces, lines cavities, and forms glands.
- **Connective tissue** supports and forms the framework of all parts of the body.
- **Muscle tissue** contracts and produces movement.
- **Nervous tissue** conducts nerve impulses.

This chapter concentrates mainly on epithelial and connective tissues; muscle and nervous tissues receive more attention in later chapters.

Epithelial Tissue

Epithelial tissue, or **epithelium** (ep-ih-THE-le-um), forms a protective covering for the body. It is the main tissue of the skin's outer layer. It also forms membranes, ducts, and the lining of body cavities and hollow organs, such as the organs of the digestive, respiratory, and urinary tracts.

Structure of Epithelial Tissue

Epithelial cells are tightly packed to better protect underlying tissue or form barriers between systems. The cells vary in shape and arrangement according to their function. Epithelial tissue is classified on the basis of these characteristics. In shape, the cells may be described as follows:

- **Squamous** (SKWA-mus)—flat and irregular
- **Cuboidal**—square
- **Columnar**—long and narrow

The cells may be arranged in a single layer, in which case it is described as **simple** (Fig. 4-1). Simple epithelium functions as a thin barrier through which materials can pass fairly easily. For example, simple epithelium allows for absorption of materials from the lining of the digestive tract into the blood and allows for passage of oxygen from the blood to body tissues. Areas subject to wear-and-tear that require protection are covered with epithelial cells in multiple layers, an arrangement described as **stratified** (Fig. 4-2). If the cells are staggered so that they appear to be in multiple layers but really are not, they are termed

---

Box 4-1   Hot Topics

Stem Cells: So Much Potential

At least 200 different types of cells are found in the human body, each with its own unique structure and function. All originate from unspecialized precursors called **stem cells**, which exhibit two important characteristics: they can divide repeatedly and have the potential to become specialized cells.

Stem cells come in two types. **Embryonic stem cells**, found in early embryos, are the source of all body cells and potentially can differentiate into any cell type. **Adult stem cells**, found in babies and children as well as adults, are stem cells that remain in the body after birth and can differentiate into only a few cell types. They assist with tissue growth and repair. For example, in red bone marrow, these cells differentiate into blood cells, whereas in the skin, they differentiate into new skin cells after a cut or scrape.

The potential healthcare applications of stem cell research are numerous. In the near future, stem cell transplants may be used to repair damaged tissues in treating illnesses such as diabetes, cancer, heart disease, Parkinson disease, and spinal cord injury. This research may also help explain how cells develop and why some cells develop abnormally, causing birth defects and cancer. Scientists may also use stem cells to test drugs before trying them on animals and humans.

But stem cell research is controversial. Some argue that it is unethical to use embryonic stem cells because they are obtained from aborted fetuses or fertilized eggs left over from in vitro fertilization. Others argue that these cells would be discarded anyway and have the potential to improve lives. A possible solution is the use of adult stem cells. However, adult stem cells are less abundant and lack embryonic stem cells' potential to differentiate, so more research is needed to make this a viable option.

pseudostratified. Terms for both shape and arrangement are used to describe epithelial tissue. Thus, a single layer of flat, irregular cells would be described as *simple squamous epithelium*, whereas tissue with many layers of these same cells would be described as *stratified squamous epithelium*.

Some organs, such as the urinary bladder, must vary a great deal in size as they work. These organs are lined with **transitional epithelium**, which is capable of great expansion but returns to its original form once tension is relaxed—as when, in this case, the urinary bladder is emptied.

Special Functions of Epithelial Tissue

Some epithelial tissues produce secretions, including **mucus** (MU-kus) (a clear, sticky fluid), digestive juices, sweat, and other substances. The air that we breathe passes over epithelium that lines the respiratory passageways. Mucus-secreting **goblet cells**, named for their shape, are scattered among the pseudostratified epithelial cells (Fig. 4-3A). The epithelial cells also have tiny hairlike projections called **cilia** (SIL-e-ah). Together, the mucus and the cilia help trap bits of dust and other foreign particles that could otherwise reach and damage the lungs. The digestive tract is lined with simple columnar epithelium that also contains goblet cells. They secrete mucus that protects the lining of the digestive organs (Fig. 4-3B).

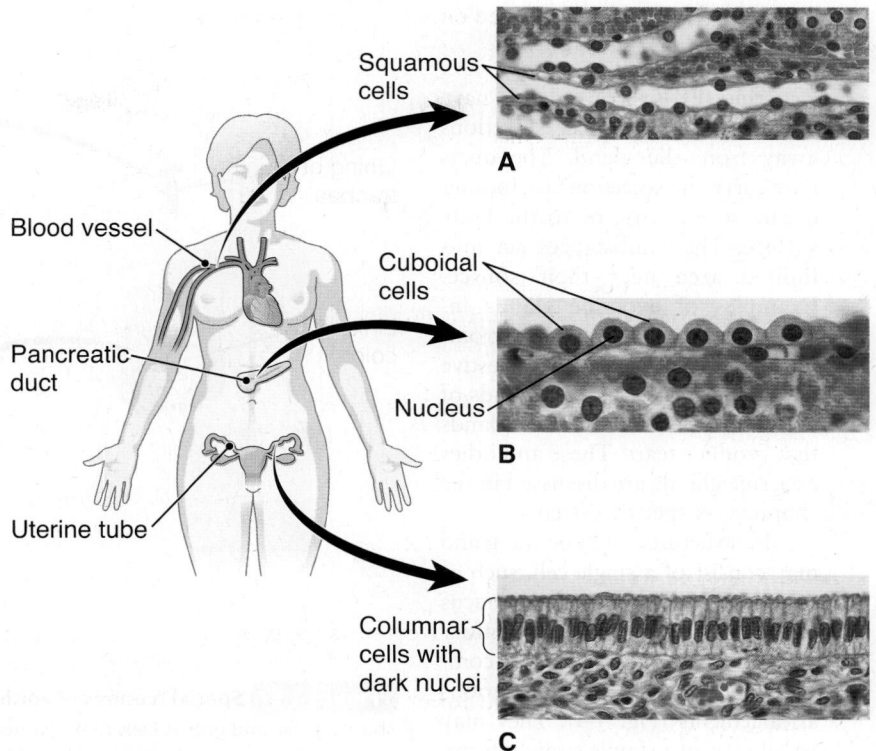

Figure 4-1 **Simple epithelial tissues. (A)** Simple squamous has flat, irregular cells with flat nuclei. **(B)** Cuboidal cells are square in shape with round nuclei. **(C)** Columnar cells are long and narrow with ovoid nuclei. (Reprinted with permission from Cormack DH. *Essential Histology*, 2nd ed. Philadelphia: Lippincott Williams & Wilkins, 2001.) [**ZOOMING IN** ➤ In how many layers are these epithelial cells?]

PASSport to Success Visit *thePoint* or see the Student Resource CD in the back of this book for a summary chart on epithelial tissue.

Epithelium repairs itself quickly after it is injured. In areas of the body subject to normal wear-and-tear, such as the skin, the inside of the mouth, and the lining of the intestinal tract, epithelial cells reproduce frequently, replacing damaged tissue. Certain areas of the epithelium that form the outer layer of the skin are capable of modifying themselves for greater strength whenever they are subjected to unusual wear-and-tear; the growth of calluses is a good example of this response.

Glands

The active cells of many glands are epithelial cells. A gland is an organ specialized to produce a substance that is sent out to other parts of the body. The gland manufactures these secretions from materials removed from the blood. Glands

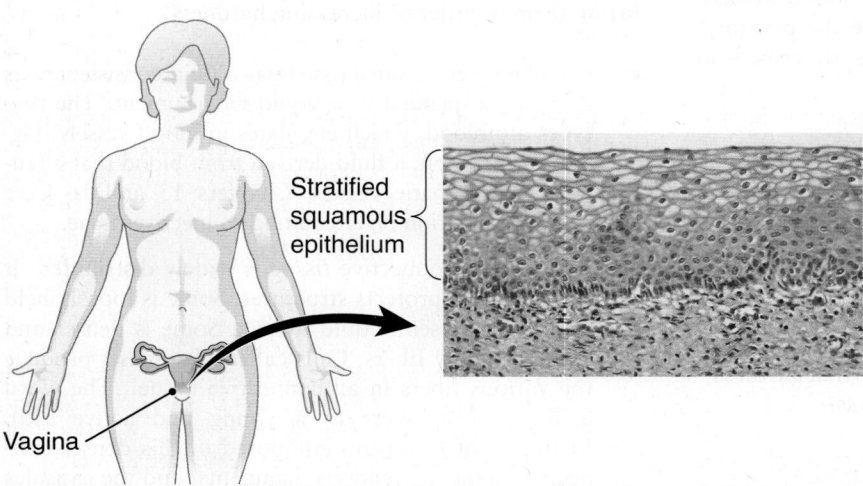

Figure 4-2 **Stratified squamous epithelium.** Cells are arranged in multiple layers. (Reprinted with permission from Cormack DH. *Essential Histology*, 2nd ed. Philadelphia: Lippincott Williams & Wilkins, 2001.)

are divided into two categories based on how they release their secretions:

- **Exocrine** (EK-so-krin) **glands** have ducts or tubes to carry secretions away from the gland. The ducts may carry the secretions to another organ, to a cavity, or to the body surface. These substances act in a limited area near their source. Examples of exocrine glands include the glands in the gastrointestinal tract that secrete digestive juices, the sebaceous (oil) glands of the skin, and the lacrimal glands that produce tears. These and other exocrine glands are discussed in the chapters on specific systems.

  In structure, an exocrine gland may consist of a single cell, such as the goblet cells that secrete mucus into the digestive and respiratory tracts. Most, however, are composed of multiple cells in various arrangements (Fig. 4-4). They may be tubular, in a simple straight form, or in a branched formation, as are found in the digestive tract. They may also be coiled, as are the sweat glands of the skin. They may be saclike, as are the sebaceous (oil) glands of the skin, or compound formations of tubes and sacs, as are the salivary glands in the mouth.

- **Endocrine** (EN-do-krin) **glands** secrete not through ducts, but directly into surrounding tissue fluid. Most often the secretions are then absorbed into the bloodstream, which carries them throughout the body. These secretions, called **hormones**, have effects on specific tissues known as the *target tissues*. Endocrine glands have an extensive network of blood vessels. These so-called *ductless glands* include the pituitary, thyroid, adrenal glands, and others described in greater detail in Chapter 12.

CHECKPOINT 4-1 ➤ Epithelium is classified according to cell shape. What are the three basic shapes?

CHECKPOINT 4-2 ➤ Glands are classified according to whether they secrete through ducts or secrete directly into surrounding fluid and the bloodstream. What are these two categories of glands?

Connective Tissue

The supporting fabric everywhere in the body is connective tissue. This is so extensive and widely distributed that

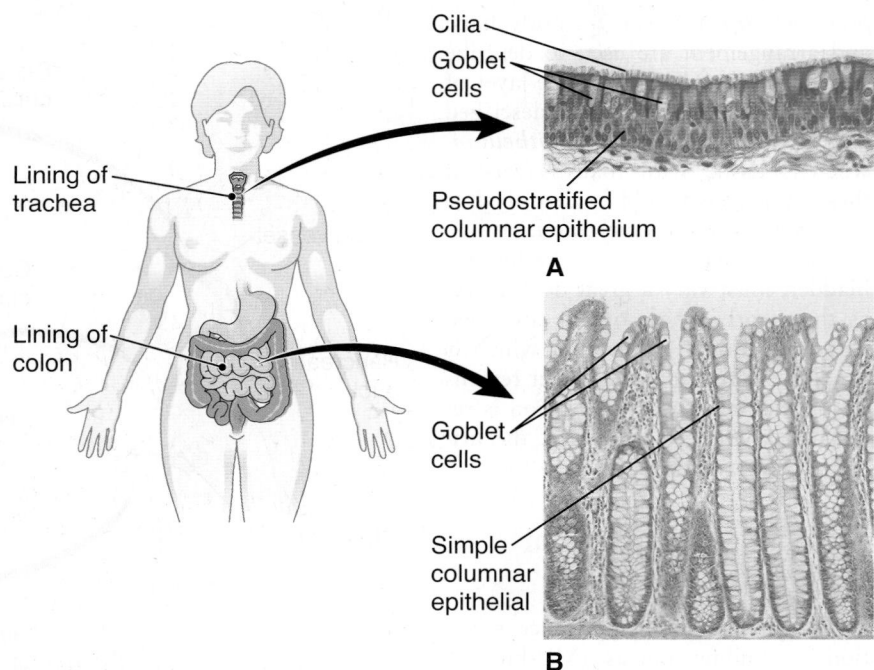

Figure 4-3 **Special features of epithelial tissues. (A)** The lining of the trachea showing cilia and goblet cells that secrete mucus. **(B)** The lining of the intestine showing goblet cells. (Reprinted with permission from Cormack DH. *Essential Histology*, 2nd ed. Philadelphia: Lippincott Williams & Wilkins, 2001.)

if we were able to dissolve all the tissues except connective tissue, we would still be able to recognize the entire body's contours. Connective tissue has large amounts of nonliving material between the cells. This intercellular background material or **matrix** (MA-trix) contains varying amounts of water, fibers, and hard minerals.

Histologists, specialists in the study of tissues, have numerous ways of classifying connective tissues based on their structure or function. Here we describe the different types according to their distribution and function, while listing them in order of increasing hardness.

- Circulating connective tissue has a fluid consistency; its cells are suspended in a liquid environment. The two types are blood, which circulates in blood vessels (Fig. 4-5), and lymph, a fluid derived from blood that circulates in lymphatic vessels. Chapters 13 and 16 have more information on circulating connective tissue.

- Generalized connective tissue is widely distributed. It supports and protects structures. Some is loosely held together in a semi-liquid matrix. Some is denser and contains many fibers. Cells called **fibroblasts** produce the various fibers in all connective tissue. (The word ending –*blast* refers to a young and active cell). Examples of structures composed of this denser connective tissue are tendons, ligaments, and the capsules (coverings) around some organs.

- Structural connective tissue is mainly associated with the skeleton. Examples are cartilage, which has a very

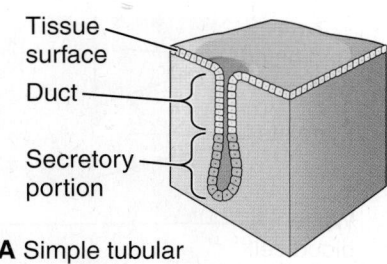

A Simple tubular

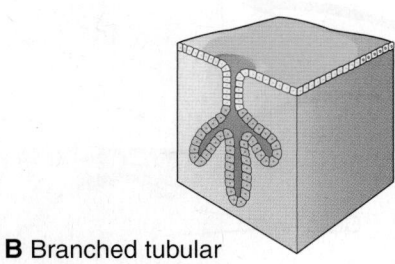

B Branched tubular

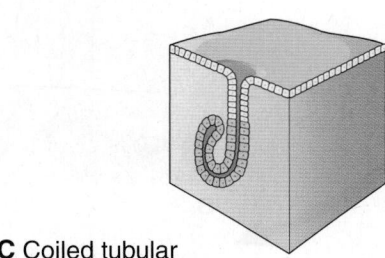

C Coiled tubular

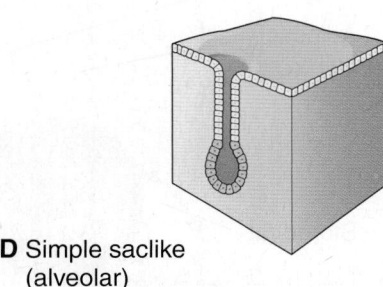

D Simple saclike (alveolar)

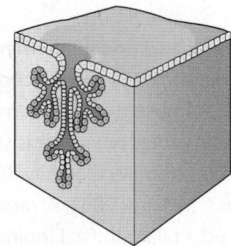

E Compound

Figure 4-4 **Some structural types of exocrine glands. (A)** Simple tubular, as found in the intestine. **(B)** Branched tubular, as found in the stomach. **(C)** Coiled tubular, such as the sweat glands of the skin. **(D)** Simple saclike (alveolar), such as the oil glands of the skin. **(E)** Compound, with tubes and sacs, such as the salivary glands.

firm consistency, and bone tissue, which is hardened by minerals in the matrix.

The generalized and structural connective tissues are described in greater detail below.

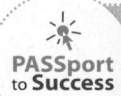

PASSport to Success Visit *thePoint* or see the Student Resource CD in the back of this book for a summary chart of the connective tissue types.

CHECKPOINT **4-3** ➤ Connective tissues vary according to the composition of the material that is between the cells. What is the general name for this intercellular material?

Generalized Connective Tissue

This tissue is found throughout the body and is less specific in function than other types. There are two forms: loose and dense.

Loose connective tissue, as the name implies, has a soft or semi-liquid consistency. The types are:

- **Areolar** (ah-RE-o-lar) **tissue** is named from a word that means "space" because of its open composition (see Fig. 4-5B). It contains cells and fibers in a soft, jellylike matrix. This tissue is found in membranes, around vessels and organs, between muscles, and under the skin. It is the most common type of connective tissue.

- **Adipose** (AD-ih-pose) **tissue** contains cells (adipocytes) that are able to store large amounts of fat (see Fig. 4-5C). The fat in this tissue is a reserve energy supply for the body. Adipose tissue is also a heat insulator, as in the underlying layers of the skin, and is protective padding for organs and joints.

Dense connective tissue is more firm and is characterized by the many fibers that give it strength and flexibility. The main type of fiber in this and other connective tissue is **collagen** (KOL-ah-jen), a flexible white protein. (See Box 4-2, Collagen: The Body's Scaffolding.) The different types vary in the main fibers they contain and how they are arranged:

- **Irregular dense connective tissue** has mostly collagenous fibers in random arrangement. This tissue makes up the fibrous membranes that cover various organs, as described later in this chapter. Particularly strong forms make up the tough capsules around certain organs, such as the kidney, the liver, and some glands.

- **Regular dense connective tissue** also has mostly collagenous fibers, but they are in a regular, parallel alignment like the strands of a cable. This tissue can pull in one direction. Examples are the cordlike **tendons**, which connect muscles to bones, and the **ligaments**, which connect bones to other bones (Fig. 4-6A).

- **Elastic connective tissue** has many elastic fibers that allow it to stretch and then return to its original length. This tissue appears in the vocal cords, the respiratory passageways, and the walls of blood vessels.

Structural Connective Tissue

The structural connective tissues are mainly associated with the skeleton and are stronger and more solid than all the other groups.

CARTILAGE Because of its strength and flexibility, cartilage is a structural material and provides reinforcement. It is also a shock absorber and a bearing surface that reduces friction between moving parts, as at joints. The cells that produce cartilage are **chondrocytes** (KON-dro-sites), a name derived from the word root *chondro*, meaning "cartilage" and the root *cyto*, meaning "cell." There are three forms of cartilage:

- **Hyaline** (HI-ah-lin) **cartilage** is the tough translucent material, popularly called gristle, that covers the ends of the long bones (see Fig. 4-6B). Hyaline cartilage also makes up the tip of the nose and reinforces the larynx ("voicebox") and the trachea ("windpipe").

- **Fibrocartilage** (fi-bro-KAR-tih-laj) is firm and rigid, and is found between vertebrae (segments) of the spine, at the anterior joint between the pubic bones of the hip, and in the knee joint.

- **Elastic cartilage** can spring back into shape after it is bent. An easy place to observe the properties of elastic cartilage is in the outer portion of the ear. It is also located in the larynx.

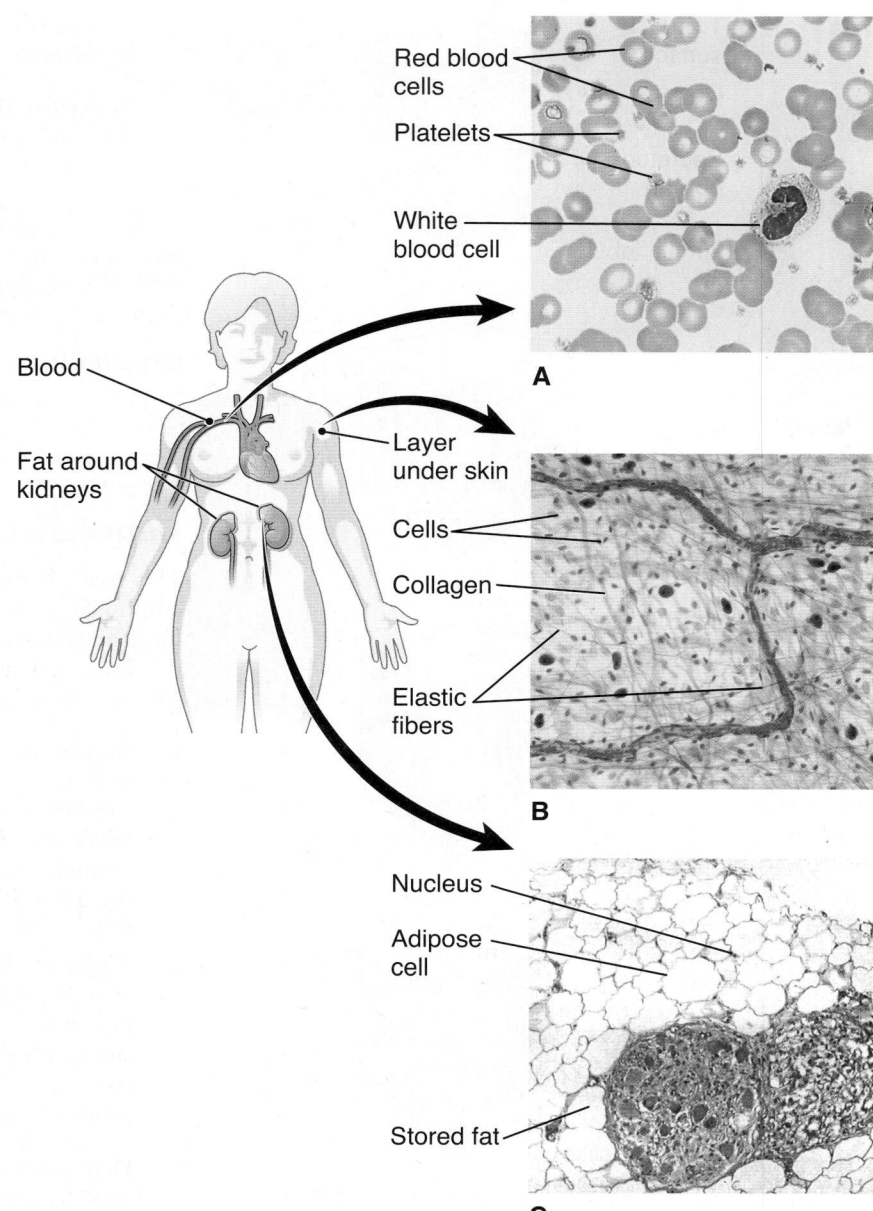

Figure 4-5 **Circulating and generalized (loose) connective tissue. (A)** Blood smear showing various blood cells in a liquid matrix. **(B)** Areolar connective tissue, a mixture of cells and fibers in a jellylike matrix. **(C)** Adipose tissue shown here surrounding dark-staining glandular tissue. The slide shows areas where fat is stored and nuclei at the edge of the cells. (A, reprinted with permission from McClatchey KD. *Clinical Laboratory Medicine*, 2nd ed. Baltimore: Lippincott Williams & Wilkins, 2001; B, reprinted with permission from Cormack DH. *Essential Histology*, 2nd ed. Philadelphia: Lippincott Williams & Wilkins, 2001; C, Reprinted with permission from Mills SE. *Histology for Pathologists*, 3rd ed. Philadelphia: Lippincott Williams & Wilkins, 2006.) [**ZOOMING IN** ➤ Which of these tissues has the most fibers? Which of these tissues is modified for storage?]

CHECKPOINT **4-4** ➤ Connective tissue is characterized by the presence of fibers. The main fibers in connective tissue are made of what protein?

BONE The tissue that composes bones, called **osseous** (OS-e-us) **tissue**, is much like cartilage in its cellular structure (see Fig. 4-6C). In fact, the skeleton of the fetus in the early stages of development is made almost entirely

4

Collagen: The Body's Scaffolding

The most abundant protein in the body, making up about 25% of total protein, is collagen. Its name, derived from a Greek word meaning "glue," reveals its role as the main structural protein in connective tissue.

Fibroblasts secrete collagen molecules into the surrounding matrix, where the molecules are then assembled into fibers. These fibers give the matrix its strength and its flexibility. Collagen fibers' high tensile strength makes them stronger than steel fibers of the same size, and their flexibility confers resilience on the tissues that contain them. For example, collagen in skin, bone, tendons, and ligaments resists pulling forces, whereas collagen found in joint cartilage and between vertebrae resists compression. Based on amino acid structure, there are at least 19 types of collagen, each of which imparts a different property to the connective tissue containing it.

The arrangement of collagen fibers in the matrix reveals much about the tissue's function. In the skin and membranes covering muscles and organs, collagen fibers are arranged irregularly, with fibers running in all directions. The result is a tissue that can resist stretching forces in many different directions. In tendons and ligaments, collagen fibers have a parallel arrangement, forming strong ropelike cords that can resist longitudinal pulling forces. In bone tissue, collagen fibers' meshlike arrangement promotes deposition of calcium salts into the tissue, which gives bone strength while also providing flexibility.

Collagen's varied properties are also evident in the preparation of a gelatin dessert. Gelatin is a collagen extract made by boiling animal bones and other connective tissue. It is a viscous liquid in hot water but forms a semisolid gel on cooling.

---

of cartilage. This tissue gradually becomes impregnated with salts of calcium and phosphorus that make bone characteristically solid and hard. The cells that form bone are called **osteoblasts** (OS-te-o-blasts), a name that combines the root for bone (*osteo*) with a root (*blast*) that means an immature cell. As these cells mature, they are referred to as **osteocytes** (OS-te-o-sites). Within the osseous tissue are nerves and blood vessels. A specialized type of tissue, the bone marrow, is enclosed within bones. The red bone marrow contained in certain regions produces blood cells. Chapter 7 has more information on bones.

CHECKPOINT **4-5** ➤ Connective tissue is the supportive and protective material found throughout the body. What are some examples of circulating, generalized, and structural connective tissue?

Muscle Tissue

Muscle tissue is designed to produce movement by contraction of its cells, which are called **muscle fibers** because most of them are long and threadlike. If a piece of well-cooked meat is pulled apart, small groups of these muscle fibers may be seen. Muscle tissue is usually classified as follows:

- **Skeletal muscle**, which works with tendons and bones to move the body (Fig. 4-7A). This type of tissue is described as **voluntary muscle** because it can be made to

contract by conscious thought. The cells in skeletal muscle are very large and are remarkable in having multiple nuclei and a pattern of dark and light banding described as **striations**. This type of muscle is also called striated muscle. Chapter 8 has more details on skeletal muscles.

- **Cardiac muscle**, which forms the bulk of the heart wall and is known also as **myocardium** (mi-o-KAR-de-um) (see Fig. 4-7B). This is the muscle that produces the regular contractions known as *heartbeats*. Cardiac muscle is described as **involuntary muscle** because it typically contracts independently of thought. Most of the time we are not aware of its actions at all. Cardiac muscle has branching cells and specialized membranes between the cells that appear as dark lines under the microscope. Their technical name is *intercalated* (in-TER-cal-a-ted) *disks*. The heart and cardiac muscle are discussed in Chapter 14.

- **Smooth muscle** is also involuntary muscle (see Fig. 4-7C). It forms the walls of the hollow organs in the ventral body cavities, including the stomach, intestines, gallbladder, and urinary bladder. Together these organs are known as viscera (VIS-eh-rah), so smooth muscle is sometimes referred to as *visceral muscle*. Smooth muscle is also found in the walls of many tubular structures, such as the blood vessels and the tubes that carry urine from the kidneys. A smooth muscle is attached to the base of each body hair. Contraction of these muscles causes the condition of the skin that we call *gooseflesh*. Smooth muscle cells are of a typical size and taper at each end. They are not striated and have only one nu-

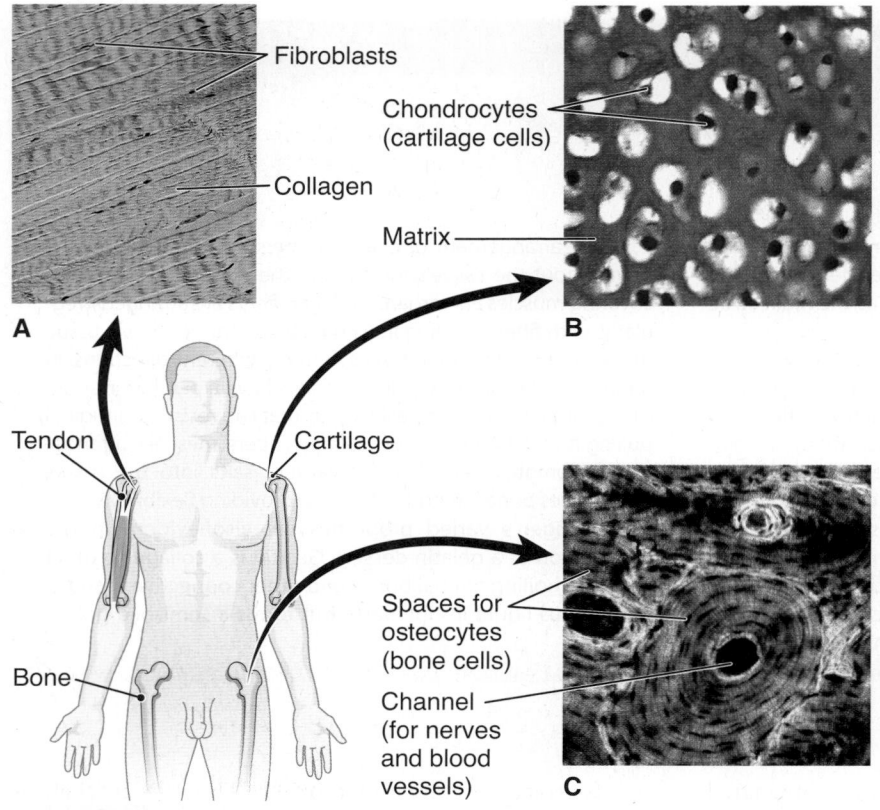

A

B

Fibroblasts

Chondrocytes
(cartilage cells)

Collagen

Matrix

Tendon

Cartilage

Bone

Spaces for
osteocytes
(bone cells)

Channel
(for nerves
and blood
vessels)

C

Figure 4-6 **Generalized (dense) and structural connective tissue. (A)** Fibrous connective tissue. In tendons and ligaments, collagenous fibers are arranged in the same direction. **(B)** In cartilage, the cells (chondrocytes) are enclosed in a firm matrix. **(C)** Bone is the hardest connective tissue. The cells (osteocytes) are within the hard matrix. (A and B, reprinted with permission from Mills SE. *Histology for Pathologists*, 3rd ed. Philadelphia: Lippincott Williams & Wilkins, 2006; C, reprinted with permission from Gartner LP, Hiatt JL. *Color Atlas of Histology*, 4th ed. Baltimore: Lippincott Williams & Wilkins, 2005.)

cleus per cell. Structures containing smooth muscle are discussed in the chapters on the various body systems.

Muscle tissue, like nervous tissue, repairs itself only with difficulty or not at all once an injury has been sustained. When injured, muscle tissue is frequently replaced with connective tissue.

CHECKPOINT 4-6 ➤ What are the three types of muscle tissue?

Nervous Tissue

The human body is made up of countless structures, each of which contributes to the action of the whole organism. This aggregation of structures might be compared to a large corporation. For all the workers in the corporation to coordinate their efforts, there must be some central control, such as the president or CEO. In the body, this central agent is the **brain** (Fig. 4-8A). Each body struc-

ture is in direct communication with the brain by means of its own set of "wires," called **nerves** (see Fig. 4-8B). Nerves from even the most remote parts of the body come together and feed into a great trunk cable called the **spinal cord,** which in turn leads into the central switchboard of the brain. Here, messages come in and orders go out 24 hours a day. Some nerves, the cranial nerves, connect directly with the brain and do not communicate with the spinal cord. This entire control system, including the brain, is made of nervous tissue.

The Neuron

The basic unit of nervous tissue is the **neuron** (NU-ron), or nerve cell (Fig. 4-8C). A neuron consists of a nerve cell body plus small branches from the cell called *fibers*. One type of fiber, the **dendrite** (DEN-drite), is generally short and forms tree-like branches. This type of fiber carries messages in the form of nerve impulses to the nerve cell body. A single fiber, the **axon** (AK-son), carries impulses away from the nerve cell body. Neurons may be quite long; their fibers can extend for several feet. A **nerve** is a bundle of such nerve cell fibers held together with connective tissue (see Fig. 4-8B).

Just as wires are insulated to keep them from being short-circuited, some axons are insulated and protected by a coating of material called **myelin** (MI-eh-lin). Groups of myelinated fibers form "white matter," named for the color of the myelin, which is much like fat in appearance and consistency.

Not all neurons have myelin, however; some axons are unmyelinated, as are all dendrites and all cell bodies. These areas appear gray in color. Because the outer layer of the brain has large collections of cell bodies and unmyelinated fibers, the brain is popularly termed *gray matter,* even though its interior is composed of white matter (see Fig. 4-8A).

Neuroglia

Nervous tissue is supported and protected by specialized cells known as **neuroglia** (nu-ROG-le-ah) or *glial* (GLI-al) *cells,* which are named from the Greek word *glia* meaning "glue." Some of these cells protect the brain from harmful substances; others get rid of foreign organisms and cellular debris; still others form the myelin sheath around axons. They do not, however, transmit nerve impulses.

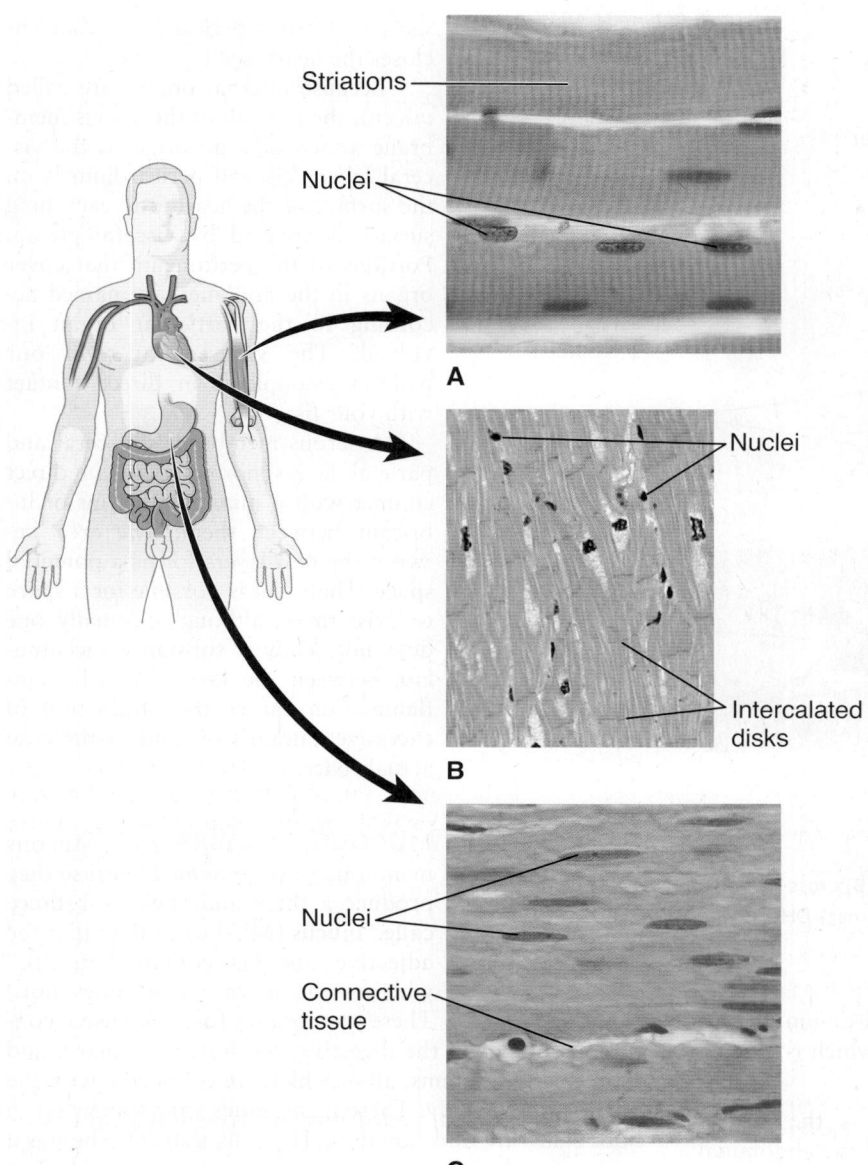

Striations

Nuclei

A

Nuclei

Intercalated
disks

B

Nuclei

Connective
tissue

C

Figure 4-7 **Muscle tissue. (A)** Skeletal muscle cells have bands (striations) and multiple nuclei. **(B)** Cardiac muscle makes up the wall of the heart. **(C)** Smooth muscle is found in soft body organs and in vessels. (A and C, reprinted with permission from Cormack DH. *Essential Histology*, 2nd ed. Philadelphia: Lippincott Williams & Wilkins, 2001; B, reprinted with permission from Gartner LP, Hiatt JL. *Color Atlas of Histology*, 4th ed. Baltimore: Lippincott Williams & Wilkins, 2005.)

A more detailed discussion of nervous tissue and the nervous system can be found in Chapters 9 and 10.

CHECKPOINT **4-7** ➤ What is the basic cellular unit of the nervous system and what is its function?

CHECKPOINT **4-8** ➤ What are the nonconducting support cells of the nervous system called?

Membranes

Membranes are thin sheets of tissue. Their properties vary: some are fragile, others tough; some are transparent, others opaque (i.e., they cannot be seen through). Membranes may cover a surface, may be a dividing partition, may line a hollow organ or body cavity, or may anchor an organ. They may contain cells that secrete lubricants to ease the movement of organs, such as the heart and lung, and the movement of joints. Epithelial membranes and connective tissue membranes are described below.

Epithelial Membranes

An **epithelial membrane** is so named because its outer surface is made of epithelium. Underneath, however, there is a layer of connective tissue that strengthens the membrane, and in some cases, there is a thin layer of smooth muscle under that. Epithelial membranes are made of closely packed active cells that manufacture lubricants and protect the deeper tissues from invasion by microorganisms. Epithelial membranes are of several types:

- **Serous** (SE-rus) **membranes** line the walls of body cavities and are folded back onto the surface of internal organs, forming their outermost layer.

- **Mucous** (MU-kus) **membranes** line tubes and other spaces that open to the outside of the body.

- The **cutaneous** (ku-TA-ne-us) **membrane**, commonly known as the **skin**, has an outer layer of epithelium. This membrane is complex and is discussed in detail in Chapter 6.

SEROUS MEMBRANES Serous membranes line the closed ventral body cavities and do not connect with the outside of the body. They secrete a thin, watery lubricant, known as serous fluid, that allows organs to move with a minimum of friction. The thin epithelium of serous membranes is a smooth, glistening kind of tissue called **mesothelium** (mes-o-THE-le-um). The membrane itself may be referred to as the **serosa** (se-RO-sah).

There are three serous membranes:

- The **pleurae** (PLU-re), or **pleuras** (PLU-rahs), line the thoracic cavity and cover each lung.

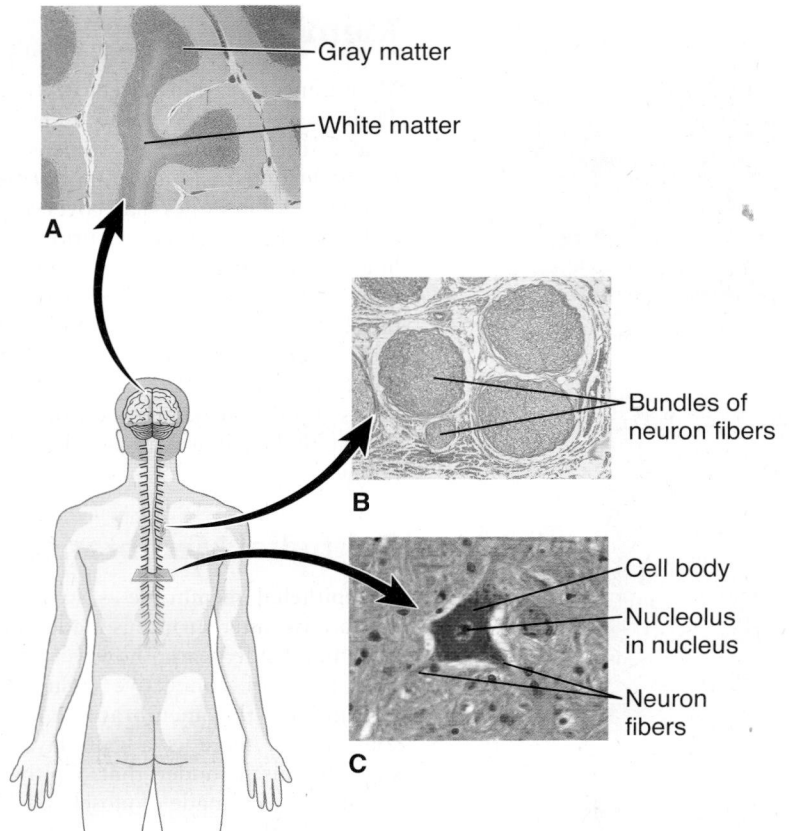

Gray matter

White matter

A

Bundles of neuron fibers

B

Cell body

Nucleolus in nucleus

Neuron fibers

C

Figure 4-8   **Nervous tissue. (A)** Brain tissue. **(B)** Cross-section of a nerve. **(C)** A neuron, or nerve cell. (Reprinted with permission from Cormack DH. *Essential Histology*, 2nd ed. Philadelphia: Lippincott Williams & Wilkins, 2001.)

- The **serous pericardium** (per-ih-KAR-de-um) forms part of a sac that encloses the heart, which is located in the chest between the lungs.

- The **peritoneum** (per-ih-to-NE-um) is the largest serous membrane. It lines the walls of the abdominal cavity, covers the abdominal organs, and forms supporting and protective structures within the abdomen (see Fig. 19-3 in Chapter 19).

Serous membranes are arranged so that one portion forms the lining of a closed cavity, while another part folds back to cover the surface of the organ contained in that cavity. The relationship between an organ and the serous membrane around it can be visualized by imagining your fist punching into a large, soft balloon (Fig. 4-9). Your fist is the organ and the serous membrane around it is in two layers, one against your fist and one folded back to form an outer layer. Although in two layers, each serous membrane is continuous.

The portion of the serous membrane attached to the wall of a cavity or sac is known as the **parietal** (pah-RI-eh-tal) **layer**; the word *parietal* refers to a wall. In the example above, the parietal layer is represented by the outermost layer of the balloon. Parietal pleura lines the thoracic (chest) cavity, and parietal pericardium lines the fibrous

sac (the fibrous pericardium) that encloses the heart (see Fig. 4-9).

Because internal organs are called *viscera*, the portion of the serous membrane attached to an organ is the **visceral layer**. Visceral pericardium is on the surface of the heart, and each lung surface is covered by visceral pleura. Portions of the peritoneum that cover organs in the abdomen are named according to the particular organ involved. The visceral layer in our balloon example is in direct contact with your fist.

A serous membrane's visceral and parietal layers normally are in direct contact with a minimal amount of lubricant between them. The area between the two layers forms a **potential space**. That is, it is *possible* for a space to exist there, although normally one does not. Only if substances accumulate between the layers, as when inflammation causes the production of excessive amounts of fluid, is there an actual space.

MUCOUS MEMBRANES Mucous membranes are so named because they produce a thick and sticky substance called **mucus** (MU-kus). (Note that the adjective *mucous* contains an "o," whereas the noun *mucus* does not.) These membranes form extensive continuous linings in the digestive, respiratory, urinary, and reproductive systems, all of which are connected with the outside of the body. These membranes vary somewhat in both structure and function. The cells that line the nasal cavities and the respiratory passageways are supplied with tiny, hairlike extensions called *cilia*, described in Chapter 3. The microscopic cilia move in waves that force secretions outward. In this way, foreign particles, such as bacteria, dust, and other impurities trapped in the sticky mucus, are prevented from entering the lungs and causing harm. Ciliated epithelium is also found in certain tubes of both the male and the female reproductive systems.

The mucous membranes that line the digestive tract have special functions. For example, the stomach's mucous membrane protects the deeper tissues from the action of powerful digestive juices. If for some reason a portion of this membrane is injured, these juices begin to digest a part of the stomach itself—as happens in cases of peptic ulcers. Mucous membranes located farther along in the digestive system are designed to absorb nutrients, which the blood then transports to all cells.

The noun **mucosa** (mu-KO-sah) refers to the mucous membrane of an organ.

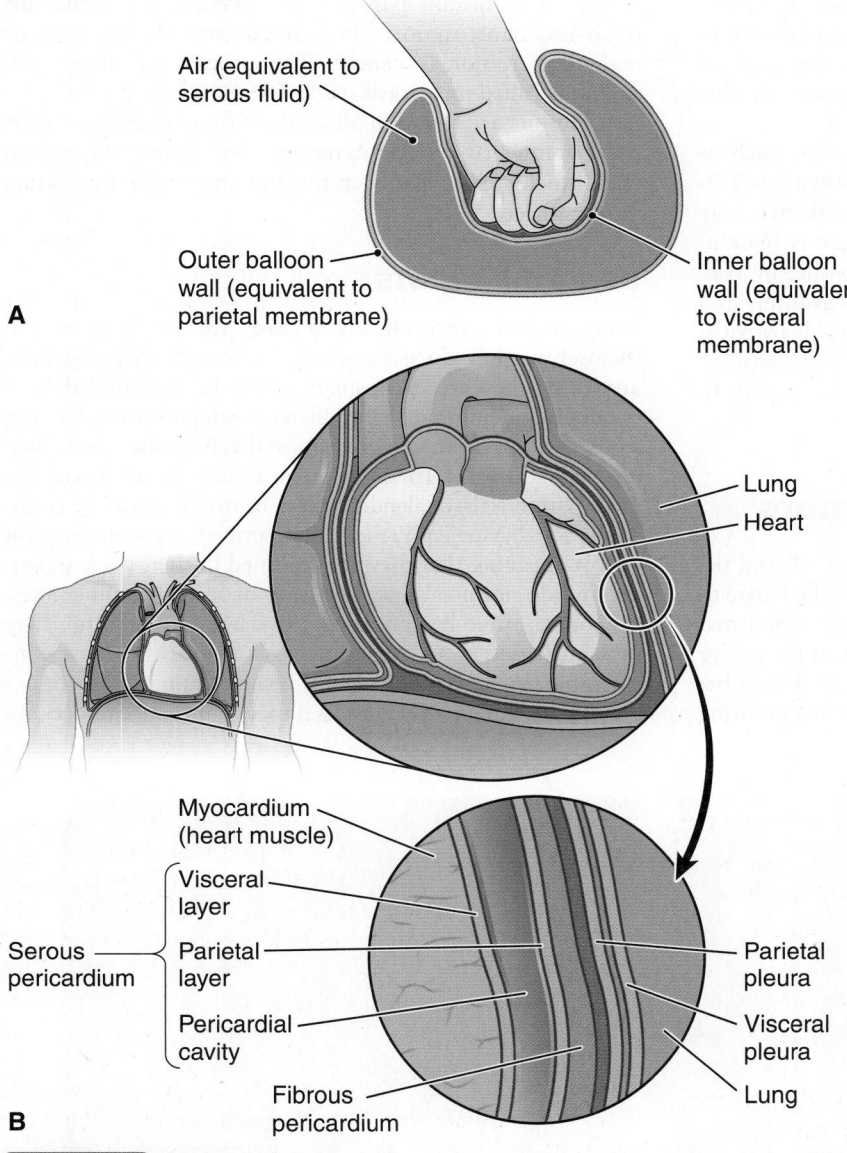

A

Air (equivalent to serous fluid)

Outer balloon wall (equivalent to parietal membrane)

Inner balloon wall (equivalent to visceral membrane)

Lung
Heart

Myocardium (heart muscle)

Visceral layer

Parietal layer

Pericardial cavity

Serous pericardium

Parietal pleura

Visceral pleura

Lung

Fibrous pericardium

B

Figure 4-9 **Organization of serous membranes. (A)** An organ fits into a serous membrane like a fist punching into a soft balloon. **(B)** The outer layer of a serous membrane is the parietal layer. The inner layer is the visceral layer. The fibrous pericardium reinforces the parietal pericardium.

CHECKPOINT **4-9** ► Epithelial membranes have an outer layer of epithelium. What are the three types of epithelial membranes?

Connective Tissue Membranes

The following list is an overview of membranes that consist of connective tissue with no epithelium. These membranes are described in greater detail in later chapters.

- **Synovial** (sin-O-ve-al) **membranes** are thin connective tissue membranes that line the joint cavities. They secrete a lubricating fluid that reduces friction between the ends of bones, thus permitting free movement of the joints. Synovial membranes also line small cushioning sacs near the joints called **bursae** (BUR-se).

- The **meninges** (men-IN-jeze) are several membranous layers covering the brain and the spinal cord.

Fascia (FASH-e-ah) refers to fibrous bands or sheets that support organs and hold them in place. Fascia is found in two regions:

- **Superficial fascia** is the continuous sheet of tissue that underlies the skin and contains adipose (fat) tissue that insulates the body and protects the skin. This tissue is also called *subcutaneous fascia* because it is located beneath the skin.

- **Deep fascia** covers, separates, and protects skeletal muscles.

Finally, there are membranes whose names all start with the prefix *peri-* because they are around organs:

- The **fibrous pericardium** (per-e-KAR-de-um) forms the cavity that encloses the heart, the pericardial cavity. This fibrous sac and the serous pericardial membranes described above are often described together as the pericardium (see Fig. 4-9B).

- The **periosteum** (per-e-OS-te-um) is the membrane around a bone.

- The **perichondrium** (per-e-KON-dre-um) is the membrane around cartilage.

Membranes and Disease

We are all familiar with a number of diseases that directly affect membranes. These range from the common cold, which is an inflammation of the nasal mucosa, to the sometimes fatal condition known as **peritonitis**, an infection of the peritoneum, which can follow rupture of the appendix and other mishaps in the abdominal region.

Although membranes usually help to prevent the spread of infection from one area of the body to another, they may sometimes act as pathways along which disease may travel. In general, epithelial membranes appear to have more resistance to infections than do layers made of connective tissue. Lowered resistance, however, may allow the transmission of infection along any membrane. For example, throat infections may travel along mucous membranes into other parts of the upper respiratory tract and even into the sinuses and the ears. In females, an infection may travel up the tubes and spaces of the reproductive system into the peritoneal cavity (see Fig. 23-14 in Chapter 23).

The connective tissue (or collagen) diseases, such as **systemic lupus erythematosus** (LU-pus er-ih-them-ah-TO-sus) (SLE) and **rheumatoid** (RU-mah-toyd) **arthritis**, may affect many parts of the body because collagen is the major intercellular protein in solid connective tissue. In SLE, serous membranes, such as the pleura, pericardium, and peritoneum, are often involved. In rheumatoid arthritis, the synovial membrane becomes inflamed and swollen, and the cartilage in the joints is gradually replaced with fibrous connective tissue.

Benign and Malignant Tumors

For a variety of reasons, the normal pattern of cell and tissue development may be broken by an uncontrolled growth of cells having no purpose in the body. Any abnormal growth of cells is called a **tumor**, or **neoplasm**. If the tumor is confined to a local area and does not spread, it is a **benign** (be-NINE) tumor. If the tumor spreads to neighboring

tissues or to distant parts of the body, it is a **malignant** (mah-LIG-nant) tumor. The general term for any type of malignant tumor is **cancer**. The process of tumor cell spread is called **metastasis** (meh-TAS-tah-sis).

Tumors are found in all kinds of tissue, but they occur most frequently in those tissues that repair themselves most quickly, specifically epithelium and connective tissue, in that order.

Benign Tumors

Benign tumors, theoretically at least, are not dangerous in themselves; they do not spread. Their cells stick together, and often they are encapsulated, that is, surrounded by a containing membrane. The cells in a benign tumor are very similar in appearance to the normal cells from which they are derived (Fig. 4-10A,B). Benign tumors grow as a single mass within a tissue, lending them neatly to complete surgical removal. Medically, they are described as growing *in situ* (SI-tu), meaning that they are confined to their place of origin and do not invade other tissues or spread to other sites. Of course, some benign tumors can be quite harmful; they may grow within an organ, increase in size, and cause considerable mechanical damage. A benign brain tumor, for example, can kill a person just as a malignant one can because

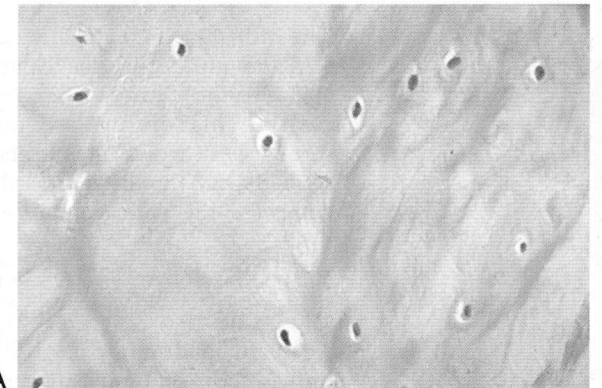

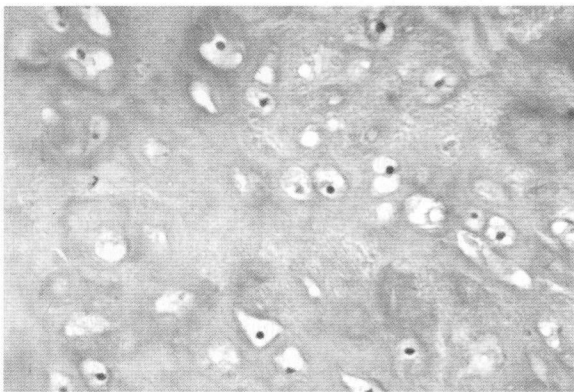

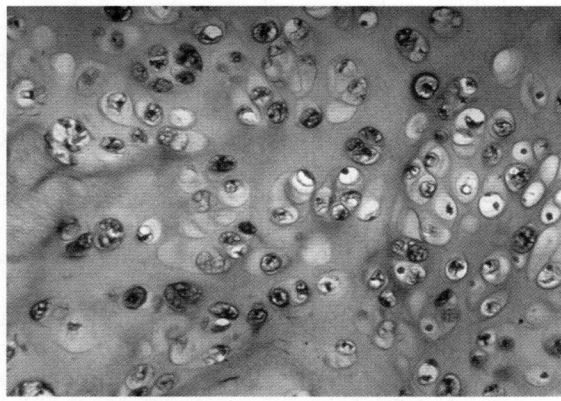

Figure 4-10 **Benign and malignant tumors. (A)** Normal cartilage. **(B)** A benign chondroma closely resembles normal cartilage. **(C)** Chondrosarcoma of bone. The tumor is composed of malignant chondrocytes, which have bizarre shapes and abnormal nuclei. (A and B, Reprinted with permission from Rubin E, Farber JL. *Pathology*, 3rd ed. Philadelphia: Lippincott Williams & Wilkins, 1999; C, Reprinted from Bullough PG, Vigorita VJ. *Atlas of Orthopaedic Pathology*. New York: Gower Medical Publishing, 1984. With permission from Elsevier.)

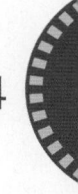

it grows in an enclosed area and compresses vital tissue. Some examples of benign tumors are given below (note that most of the names end in *-oma*, which means "tumor").

- **Papilloma** (pap-ih-LO-mah)—a tumor that grows in epithelium as a projecting mass. One example is a wart.

- **Adenoma** (ad-eh-NO-mah)—an epithelial tumor that grows in and about the glands (*adeno-* means "gland").

- **Lipoma** (lip-O-mah)—a connective tissue tumor originating in fatty (adipose) tissue.

- **Osteoma** (os-te-O-mah)—a connective tissue tumor that originates in the bones.

- **Myoma** (mi-O-mah)—a tumor of muscle tissue. Rare in voluntary muscle, it is common in some types of involuntary muscle, particularly in the uterus (womb). When found in the uterus, however, it is ordinarily called a *fibroid*.

- **Angioma** (an-je-O-mah)—a tumor that usually is composed of small blood or lymphatic vessels; an example is a birthmark.

- **Nevus** (NE-vus)—a small skin tumor that can appear in a variety of tissues. Some nevi are better known as moles; some are angiomas. Ordinarily, these tumors are harmless, but they can become malignant.

- **Chondroma** (kon-DRO-mah)—a tumor of cartilage cells that may remain within the cartilage or develop on the surface, as in the joints (see Fig. 4-10B).

Malignant Tumors

Malignant tumors, unlike benign tumors, can cause death no matter where they occur. Malignant cells are very different in appearance from their parent cells and are unable to function normally (see Fig. 4-10C). Malignant tumors, moreover, grow much more rapidly than benign tumors. The word *cancer* means "crab," and this is descriptive: a cancer sends out clawlike extensions into neighboring tissue. Cancer cells also spread by either the blood or the lymph (another circulating fluid), and when they arrive at other sites, they form new (secondary) growths, or **metastases** (meh-TAS-tah-seze).

Malignant tumors are classified into two main categories according to whether they originate in epithelial or connective tissue:

- **Carcinoma** (kar-sih-NO-mah). This type of cancer originates in epithelium and is by far the most common form of cancer. Usual sites of carcinoma are the skin, mouth, lung, breast, stomach, colon, prostate, and uterus. Carcinomas are usually spread by the lymphatic system (see Chapter 16).

- **Sarcoma** (sar-KO-mah). These are cancers of connective tissue and therefore may be found anywhere in the body. Their cells are usually spread by the blood, and they often form metastases in the lungs. The cells of a chondrosarcoma, a tumor that arises from cartilage cells, is shown in Figure 4-10C.

Cancers of the nervous system, lymphatic system, and blood are classified differently according to the cells in which they originate as well as other clinical features. A **neuroma** (nu-RO-mah) is a tumor that arises from a nerve. Because nervous tissue does not multiply throughout life, however, it is rarely involved in cancer. Usually, a nervous system tumor originates in the support (neuroglial) tissue of the brain or spinal cord and is called a **glioma** (gli-O-mah). A malignant neoplasm of lymphatic tissue is called a **lymphoma** (lim-FO-mah), and cancer of white blood cells is **leukemia** (lu-KE-me-ah).

CHECKPOINT 4-10 ➤ What is the difference between a benign and a malignant tumor?

Symptoms of Cancer

Everyone should be familiar with certain signs that may indicate early cancer and should report these signs for further investigation by their healthcare provider. Early symptoms may include unusual bleeding or discharge, persistent indigestion, chronic hoarseness or cough, changes in the color or size of moles, a sore that does not heal in a reasonable time, the presence of an unusual lump, and the presence of white patches inside the mouth or white spots on the tongue. Late symptoms of cancer include weight loss and pain. Many cancers are now diagnosed by routine screening tests that are part of the standard physical examination.

Diagnosis of Cancer

Improved methods of cancer detection lead to earlier and more successful treatment. These methods include the following:

- **Microscopic study** of tissue or cells removed from the body. **Biopsy** (BI-op-se) is the removal of living tissue for the purpose of microscopic examination. Specimens can be obtained by needle withdrawal (aspiration) of fluid; by a small punch, as of the skin; by an endoscope (lighted tube) introduced into a body cavity; or by surgical removal (excision). In some cases, fluids can be examined for signs of cancerous cells, as these cells often slough off into surrounding fluids. The most common example of this type of cytologic study is the Pap (Papanicolaou) test for cancer of the uterine cervix. Pleural or peritoneal fluids also may be studied for signs of cancerous cells.

- **Radiography** is the use of x-rays to obtain images of internal structures. A common application of this method is mammography, x-ray study of the breast. Radiologists can examine other structures such as the lungs, nervous system, and digestive system by this method, although they often need a contrast medium to show changes in soft tissues.

- **Ultrasound** (ultrasonography) is the use of reflected high-frequency sound waves to differentiate various kinds of tissue.

- **Computed tomography** (CT) is the use of x-rays to produce a cross-sectional picture of body parts, such as the brain (see Fig. 10-12A in Chapter 10).

- **Magnetic resonance imaging** (MRI) is the use of magnetic fields and radio waves to show changes in soft tissues.

- **Positron emission tomography** (PET) shows activity within an organ by computerized interpretation of the radiation emitted following administration of a radioactive substance, such as glucose. This method has been used to diagnose lung and brain tumors.

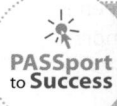 **PASSport to Success** Visit **thePoint** or see the Student Resource CD in the back of this book for information on careers in histotechnology—the laboratory study of tissues.

NEW METHODS OF DIAGNOSIS Tests for tumor markers are newer approaches to cancer diagnosis. Tumor markers are substances, such as hormones, enzymes, or other proteins, produced in greater than normal quantity by cancerous cells. Laboratories can detect these markers in cells or in body fluids, such as blood. The most widely used of these screenings is for PSA (prostate-specific antigen), a protein produced in large quantity by prostatic tumors. Some others are CA 125 in ovarian cancer, AFP (alpha-fetoprotein) in liver cancer, CEA (carcinoembryonic antigen) in digestive system and breast cancers, and CD antigens (proteins) in blood and lymphatic cancers. Although tumor markers are often produced in amounts too small to be detected early in the disease process, physicians can still use them to monitor treatment.

In some instances, cancer has been linked to changes in a person's genetic makeup. In these cases, a certain type of cancer would "run in families," and people could be genetically tested for a predisposition to that form of the disease. The clearest correlation between genetics and cancer has been established in a small percentage of breast cancers.

STAGING Oncologists (cancer specialists) use diagnostic studies for a process called staging, which is a procedure for establishing the extent of tumor spread, both at the original site and in other locations (metastases). **Staging** is important for selecting and evaluating therapy and for predicting the disease's outcome. The method commonly used for staging is the TNM system. These letters stand for primary tumor (T), regional lymph nodes (N), and distant metastases (M). Based on TNM results, a stage ranging in Roman numerals from I to IV in severity is assigned. Cancers of the blood, lymphatic system, and nervous system are evaluated by different methods.

Treatment of Cancer

Some standard cancer treatments are described first, followed by some newer approaches. Note that various treatment methods may be combined. For example, chemotherapy alone or with radiation therapy may precede surgery, or surgery may be performed before other treatment is given.

SURGERY Benign tumors usually can be removed completely by surgery. Malignant tumors cannot be treated so easily. If cancerous tissue is removed surgically, there is always the possibility that a few hidden cells will be left behind to resume tumor growth. If the cells have metastasized (spread) to distant locations, the predicted outcome is usually much less favorable.

The **laser** (LA-zer) is a device that produces a highly concentrated and intense beam of light. It is used to destroy tumors or as a cutting device for removing a tumorous growth. The laser's important advantages are its ability to coagulate blood and prevent bleeding and its capacity to direct a narrow beam of light accurately and attack harmful cells while avoiding normal cells.

Other methods for destroying cancerous tissue include electrosurgery, which uses high-frequency current; cryosurgery, which uses extreme cold generated by liquid nitrogen; and chemosurgery, which employs chemicals.

RADIATION Sometimes, surgery is preceded or followed by radiation. Radiation therapy is administered by x-ray machines or by the placement of small amounts of radioactive material within the involved organ. These materials can be in the form of needles, beads, seeds, or other devices. Some radioactive chemicals can be injected or taken orally. Radiation destroys the more rapidly dividing cancer cells while causing less damage to the more slowly dividing normal cells. A goal in radiation therapy is accurate focus of the radiation beam to reduce damage to normal body structures.

CHEMOTHERAPY Chemotherapy is a general term for treatment with drugs, but often the term is understood to mean the treatment of cancer with **antineoplastic** (an-ti-ne-o-PLAS-tik) **agents**. These agents are drugs that act selectively on actively growing cells, and they are most effective when used in combination. Certain types of leukemia, various cancers of the lymphatic system, and other forms of cancer often are treated effectively by this means. Researchers continue to develop new drugs and more effective drug combinations. Although antineoplastic agents are more toxic to tumor cells than to normal cells, they do also damage normal cells and must be administered under careful control by health professionals who understand the complications they may cause. Patients who receive these drugs, because of their weakened state, are subject to the development of opportunistic infections; that is, infections that develop in a person who has been weakened by disease.

NEWER APPROACHES TO CANCER TREATMENT The immune system constantly works to protect the body against abnormal and unwanted cells, a category that includes tumor cells. **Immunotherapy** involves the use of substances that stimulate the immune system as a whole or vaccines prepared specifically against a tumor to control growth. In certain types of breast cancer, antibodies have been used to block receptor sites for a factor that stimulates tumor growth.

Some cancers, such as those of the breast, testis, and prostate, are stimulated to grow more rapidly by hormones. Counteracting hormones or other chemicals that block receptors for the stimulants can be used to restrict tumor growth in these tissues.

For a tumor to establish itself, new blood vessels must develop and supply the rapidly growing cells with nutrients and oxygen. Some attempts have been made to block tumor growth by preventing this process of angiogenesis (growth of blood vessels).

CHECKPOINT 4-11 ➤ What are the three standard approaches to the treatment of cancer?

Tissues and Aging

With aging, tissues lose elasticity and collagen becomes less flexible. These changes affect the skin most noticeably, but internal changes occur as well. The blood vessels, for example, have a reduced capacity to expand. Less blood supply and lower metabolism slow the healing process. Tendons and ligaments stretch, causing a stooped posture and joint instability. Bones may lose calcium salts, becoming brittle and prone to fracture. With age,

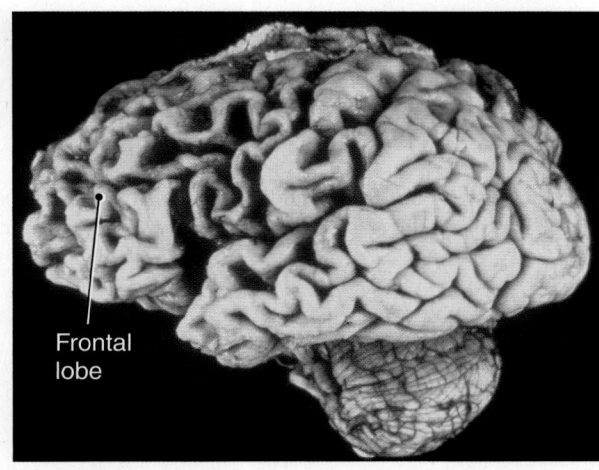

Figure 4-11 **Atrophy of the brain.** Brain tissue has thinned and larger spaces appear between sections of tissue, especially in the frontal lobe. (Reprinted with permission from Okazaki H, Scheithauer BW. *Atlas of Neuropathology.* New York: Gower Medical Publishing, 1988. By permission of the author.)

muscles and other tissues waste from loss of cells, a process termed *atrophy* (AT-ro-fe) (Fig. 4-11). Changes that apply to specific organs and systems are described in later chapters.

Disease in Context revisited

➤ Ben's Cystic Fibrosis

Ben's parents were shocked when the doctor diagnosed their 2-year-old with cystic fibrosis. Their immediate concern was, of course, for their son. The doctor reassured them that with proper treatment their son could lead a relatively normal life and that in the future, new therapies might even offer a cure. He asserted that they were not to blame for Ben's condition. Cystic fibrosis is an inherited disease—Ben's parents each carried a defective gene in their DNA and both had, by chance, passed copies to Ben. As a result, Ben was unable to synthesize a channel protein found in the plasma membranes of exocrine gland cells. Normally, this channel regulates the movement of chloride into the cell. Because the channels did not work in Ben's epithelial cells, chloride was trapped outside the cells. The negatively charged chloride ions attract positively charged sodium ions normally found in extracellular fluid. These two ions form the salt, sodium chloride, which is lost in high amounts in the sweat of individuals with cystic fibrosis.

Although the exact reason is still unclear, abnormal chloride channel function causes epithelial glands in many organs to produce thick, sticky mucus. In the lungs, this mucus causes difficulty breathing, inflammation, and bacterial infection. The thick mucus also decreases the ability of the large and small intestines to absorb nutrients, resulting in low weight gain, poor growth, and vitamin deficiencies. This problem is compounded by damage to the pancreas, preventing production of essential digestive enzymes.

During this case, we saw that a defective membrane channel in Ben's epithelial cells had wide-spread effects on his whole body. In later chapters, as you learn about the body's organs, remember that their structure and function are closely related to the condition of their constituent tissues. Cystic fibrosis is an inherited disease. The case study in Chapter 25, Heredity and Hereditary Diseases, will follow Alison as she learns more about Ben's condition.

Word Anatomy

Medical terms are built from standardized word parts (prefixes, roots, and suffixes). Learning the meanings of these parts can help you remember words and interpret unfamiliar terms.

WORD PART	MEANING	EXAMPLE
hist/o	tissue	*Histology* is the study of tissues.
Epithelial Tissue		
epi-	on, upon	*Epithelial* tissue covers body surfaces.
pseud/o-	false	*Pseudostratified* epithelium appears to be in multiple layers but is not.
Connective Tissue		
-blast	immature cell, early stage of cell	A *fibroblast* is a cell that produces fibers.
chondr/o	cartilage	A *chondrocyte* is a cartilage cell.
oss, osse/o	bone, bone tissue	*Osseous* tissue is bone tissue.
oste/o	bone, bone tissue	An *osteocyte* is a mature bone cell.
Muscle Tissue		
my/o	muscle	The *myocardium* is the heart muscle.
cardi/o	heart	See preceding example.
Nervous Tissue		
neur/o	nerve, nervous system	A *neuron* is a nerve cell.
Membranes		
pleur/o	side, rib	The *pleurae* are membranes that line the chest cavity.
peri-	around	The *peritoneum* wraps around the abdominal organs.
-itis	inflammation	*Peritonitis* is inflammation of the peritoneum.
arthr/o	joint	*Arthritis* is inflammation of a joint.
Benign and Malignant Tumors		
neo-	new	A *neoplasm* is an abnormal growth of new cells, a tumor.
mal-	bad, disordered, diseased, abnormal	A *malignant* tumor spreads to other parts of the body.
-oma	tumor, swelling	A *lipoma* is a tumor that originates in adipose (fatty) tissue.
onc/o	tumor	An *oncologist* is a specialist in cancer treatment.
papill/o	nipple	A *papilloma* is a projecting (nipple-like) tumor, such as a wart.
aden/o	gland	An *adenoma* is a tumor of a gland.
angi/o	vessel	An *angioma* is a tumor composed of small vessels.
leuk/o-	white, colorless	*Leukemia* is a cancer of white blood cells.
graph/o	writing, record	*Mammography* is x-ray imaging (radiography) of the breast (mamm/o).
ultra-	beyond	*Ultrasound* is high-frequency sound waves.
ant/i-	against	An *antineoplastic* agent is a drug active against cancer.

Summary

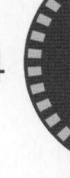

4

I. **TISSUE CLASSIFICATION**—epithelial tissue, connective tissue, muscle tissue, nervous tissue

II. **EPITHELIAL TISSUE**—covers surfaces; lines cavities, organs, and ducts
   A. Cells—squamous, cuboidal, columnar
   B. Arrangement—simple or stratified
   C. Special functions
      1. Produces secretions, e.g., mucus, digestive juices, sweat
      2. Filters impurities using cilia
   D. Glands—active cells are epithelial cells
      1. Exocrine
         a. Secrete through ducts
         b. Examples: digestive glands, tear glands, sweat and oil glands of skin
      2. Endocrine
         a. Secrete into body fluids and bloodstream
         b. Produce hormones

III. **CONNECTIVE TISSUE**—supports, binds, forms framework of body
   A. Circulating—fluid matrix; travels in vessels
      1. Blood
      2. Lymph
   B. Generalized—widely distributed; not specialized
      1. Loose—cells and fibers in semiliquid matrix
         a. Areolar—in membranes, around vessels and organs, under skin
         b. Adipose—stores fat; insulation, padding, energy reserve
      2. Dense—has many fibers (e.g. collagenous, elastic) made by fibroblasts
         a. Irregular—fibers not organized; in membranes, capsules
         b. Regular—fibers in parallel alignment; in tendons, ligaments
         c. Elastic—fibers can stretch and return to shape; in vocal cords, respiratory passageways, blood vessel walls
   C. Structural—mainly associated with skeleton
      1. Cartilage
         a. Strong and flexible
         b. Cushions and absorbs shock
         c. Produced by chondrocytes
         d. Types
            (1) Hyaline—covers ends of bones, makes up tip of nose, reinforces larynx and trachea
            (2) Fibrocartilage—in certain joints
            (3) Elastic—in outer ear, larynx
      2. Bone
         a. Matrix contains mineral salts

         b. Cells
            (1) Osteoblasts—produce bone
            (2) Osteocytes—mature bone cells

IV. **MUSCLE TISSUE**—contracts to produce movement
   A. Types
      1. Skeletal muscle—voluntary; moves skeleton
      2. Cardiac muscle—involuntary; forms main part of the heart
      3. Smooth muscle—involuntary; forms visceral organs

V. **NERVOUS TISSUE**
   A. Neuron—nerve cell
      1. Cell body—contains nucleus
      2. Dendrite—fiber carrying impulses toward cell body
      3. Axon—fiber carrying impulses away from cell body
         a. Myelin—fatty material that insulates some axons
            (1) Myelinated fibers—make up white matter
            (2) Unmyelinated cells and fibers—make up gray matter
   B. Neuroglia—support and protect nervous tissue

VI. **MEMBRANES**—thin sheets of tissue
   A. Epithelial membranes—outer layer epithelium
      1. Serous membrane—secretes watery fluid
         a. Parietal layer—lines body cavity
         b. Visceral layer—covers internal organs
         c. Examples—pleurae, pericardium, peritoneum
      2. Mucous membrane
         a. Secretes mucus
         b. Lines tube or space that opens to the outside (e.g., respiratory, digestive, reproductive tracts)
      3. Cutaneous membrane—skin
   B. Connective tissue membranes
      1. Synovial membrane—lines joint cavity
      2. Meninges—around brain and spinal cord
      3. Fascia—under skin and around muscles
      4. Pericardium—around heart; periosteum—around bone; perichondrium—around cartilage
   C. Membranes and disease—may confine infection, but may be route for spread

VII. **BENIGN AND MALIGNANT TUMORS**—tumor (neoplasm) results from uncontrolled growth of cells
   A. Benign tumor—localized
   B. Malignant tumor—invades tissue and metastasizes (spreads) to other locations
      1. Carcinoma—originates in epithelium
      2. Sarcoma—cancer of connective tissue

3. Others—cancers of nervous system, lymphatic system, blood
C. Symptoms of cancer—bleeding, persistent indigestion, hoarseness or cough, change in mole, lump, nonhealing sore, pain, weight loss
D. Diagnosis of cancer
1. Microscopic study (biopsy to obtain specimen), ultrasound, CT, MRI, PET
a. Also blood tests for markers, genetic tests

2. Staging—classification based on size of tumor and extent of invasion
E. Treatment of cancer
1. Surgical removal
2. Radiation
3. Chemotherapy—drugs
4. Others—immunotherapy, hormones, inhibitors of blood vessel formation
VIII. **TISSUES AND AGING**

Questions for Study and Review

BUILDING UNDERSTANDING

Fill in the blanks

1. A group of similar cells arranged in a characteristic pattern is called a(n) _____.
2. Glands that secrete their products directly into the blood are called _____ glands.
3. Tissue that supports and forms the framework of the body is called _____ tissue.

4. A tumor that is confined to a local area and does not spread is a(n) _____ tumor.
5. The removal of living tissue for the purpose of microscopic examination is called _____.

Matching > Match each numbered item with the most closely related lettered item.

____ 6. Membrane around the heart
____ 7. Membrane around each lung
____ 8. Membrane around bone
____ 9. Membrane around cartilage
____ 10. Membrane around abdominal organs

a. perichondrium
b. pericardium
c. peritoneum
d. periosteum
e. pleura

Multiple Choice

____ 11. Epithelium composed of a single layer of long and narrow cells is called
a. simple cuboidal epithelium
b. simple columnar epithelium
c. stratified cuboidal epithelium
d. stratified columnar epithelium

____ 12. Tendons and ligaments are examples of
a. areolar connective tissue
b. loose connective tissue
c. regular, dense connective tissue
d. cartilage

____ 13. A tissue composed of long striated cells with multiple nuclei is
a. smooth muscle tissue
b. cardiac muscle tissue
c. skeletal muscle tissue
d. nervous tissue

____ 14. A bundle of nerve cell fibers held together with connective tissue is called a(n)
a. dendrite
b. axon
c. nerve
d. myelin

____ 15. All of the following are types of epithelial membranes except
a. cutaneous membrane
b. mucous membrane
c. serous membrane
d. synovial membrane

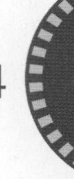

UNDERSTANDING CONCEPTS

16. Explain how epithelium is classified and discuss at least three functions of this tissue type.

17. Compare the structure and function of exocrine and endocrine glands and give two examples of each type.

18. Describe the functions of connective tissue. Name two kinds of fibers found in connective tissue and discuss how their presence affects tissue function.

19. Compare and contrast the three different types of muscle tissue.

20. Compare serous and mucous membranes.

21. Describe the difference between a benign tumor and a malignant tumor.

22. Define the term *cancer* and name some of its early symptoms. How is cancer diagnosed? How is it treated?

CONCEPTUAL THINKING

23. Prolonged exposure to cigarette smoke causes damage to ciliated epithelium that lines portions of the respiratory tract. Discuss the implications of this damage.

24. The middle ear is connected to the throat by a tube called the eustachian (auditory) tube. All are lined by a continuous mucous membrane. Using this information, describe why a throat infection (pharyngitis) may lead to an ear infection (otitis media).

25. In cystic fibrosis, the production of abnormally thick sticky mucus results in lung and digestive disorders. What are some of the normal functions of mucus in the body?

26. In Ben's case, an abnormal epithelial channel protein had widespread effects. Another hereditary disease, osteogenesis imperfecta, is characterized by abnormal collagen fiber synthesis. Which tissue type would be most affected by this disorder? List some possible symptoms of this disease.

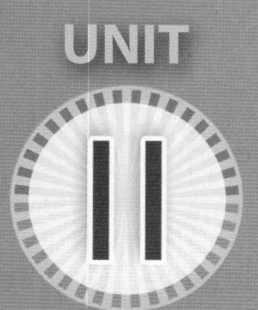

UNIT II

Disease and the First Line of Defense

➤ **Chapter 5**

Disease and Disease-Producing Organisms

➤ **Chapter 6**

The Skin in Health and Disease

The first chapter in this unit discusses deviation from the normal, which is the basis for disease. After a general discussion of different types of diseases, the chapter concentrates on infectious diseases and the organisms that cause them, including bacteria, viruses, fungi, protozoa, and worms. Other forms of disease are discussed in chapters on the individual body systems. The skin is the first defense against infections, organisms, and other sources of injury. The properties and functions of the skin are discussed in the second chapter of this unit.

CHAPTER 5

Disease and Disease-Producing Organisms

Learning Outcomes

After careful study of this chapter, you should be able to:

1. Define *disease* and list seven categories of disease
2. List seven predisposing causes of disease
3. Define terminology used in describing and treating disease
4. Define *complementary and alternative medicine*; cite several alternative or complementary fields of practice
5. Explain methods by which microorganisms can be transmitted from one host to another
6. List four types of organisms studied in microbiology and give the characteristics of each
7. List some diseases caused by each type of microorganism
8. Define *normal flora* and explain the value of the normal flora
9. Describe the three types of bacteria according to shape
10. List several diseases in humans caused by worms
11. Give some reasons for the emergence and spread of microorganisms today
12. Describe several public health measures taken to prevent the spread of disease
13. Differentiate *sterilization*, *disinfection*, and *antisepsis*
14. Describe techniques included as part of body substance precautions
15. List some antimicrobial agents and describe how they work
16. Describe several methods used to identify microorganisms in the laboratory
17. Show how word parts are used to build words related to disease (see Word Anatomy at the end of the chapter)

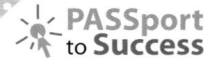

PASSport to Success

Visit *thePoint* or see the Student Resource CD in the back of this book for definitions and pronunciations of key terms as well as a pretest for this chapter.

Disease in Context

➤ Maria's Case: When Pathogens Attack

The man sharing the elevator with Maria Sanchez looked terrible—watery eyes, runny nose, and a sickly, run-down appearance. As the elevator opened and the man stepped toward the doors, he let out a loud sneeze. "Pardon me," he said, as the elevator closed behind him. *If I was that sick, I'd stay in bed*, Maria thought. Maria didn't know it yet, but soon she would be.

The passenger left something behind when he exited the elevator. Microscopic droplets of mucus and water from his sneeze floated in the air. Inside each droplet were thousands of microorganisms, called viruses, capable of making Maria very sick. She inhaled several of these germ-laden droplets into her respiratory system as she waited for the elevator to reach her floor. Maria exited the elevator unaware that her body had been invaded.

Maria's warm, moist respiratory tract was a perfect environment for this microorganism. When a virus landed on the epithelial tissue lining her throat, protein spikes protruding from its surface fit snugly into receptors on an epithelial cell, stimulating endocytosis of the virus. Having successfully "picked the lock" on the cell's plasma membrane, the virus was inside the cell and ready to begin the second phase of its attack!

Shortly after entering the cell, the virus released its RNA, which was then transported into the cell's nucleus. Unable to recognize the viral RNA as foreign, the nucleus transcribed it into viral messenger RNA. Returning to the cytoplasm, this new RNA was translated into viral proteins at the ribosomes. Some of these proteins were combined with viral RNA to make new viruses. Others took over the machinery of the host cell to make more viral components.

Since entering the epithelial cell about 24 hours ago, the virus had successfully hijacked cellular RNA and protein synthesis. The cell had been turned into a virus-making factory! With the cell nearly exhausted, the new viruses that filled its cytoplasm exited to infect new hosts. Although finally free of the pathogen, the cell had no more resources left and died.

Maria Sanchez' body has been invaded by the influenza virus. In this chapter, we'll learn more about viruses as well as other disease-producing organisms. Later in the case, we'll see how Maria's body is coping with its unwanted visitors.

Disease may be defined as abnormality of the structure or function of a part, organ, or system. The effects of a disease may be felt by a person or observed by others. Diseases may be of known or unknown causes and may show marked variation in severity and effects on an individual.

Categories of Disease

Diseases fall into a number of different, but often overlapping, categories. These include the following:

- **Infection.** Infectious organisms are believed to play a part in at least half of all human illnesses. Examples of diseases caused by infectious organisms are colds, acquired immunodeficiency syndrome (AIDS), "strep" throat, tuberculosis, and food poisoning. Microorganisms may also contribute to more complex disorders, for example, stomach ulcers and some forms of heart disease. Infectious diseases are discussed in this chapter. Other forms of illness mentioned below are discussed in later chapters.

- **Degenerative diseases.** These are disorders that involve tissue degeneration (breaking down) in any body system. Examples are muscular dystrophy, cirrhosis of the liver, Alzheimer disease, osteoporosis, and arthritis. Some of these disorders are hereditary; that is, they are passed on by parents through their reproductive cells. Others are due to infection, injury, substance abuse, or normal wear-and-tear. For some, such as multiple sclerosis, there is no known cause at present.

- **Nutritional disorders.** Most of us are familiar with diseases caused by a dietary lack of essential vitamins, minerals, proteins, or other substances required for health: scurvy due to a lack of vitamin C; beriberi due to a lack of thiamine; rickets due to a lack of calcium for bone development; kwashiorkor, a disease of children in underdeveloped countries caused by protein deficiency. This category also includes problems caused by excess intake of substances, such as alcohol, vitamins, minerals, or proteins, and the intake of too many calories leading to obesity (see Chapters 19 and 20).

- **Metabolic disorders.** These include any disruption of the reactions involved in cellular metabolism, such as diabetes, gout (a disorder of the joints), digestive disorders, and hereditary dysfunctions. Hormones regulate many metabolic reactions. Hormone-producing glands and the diseases caused by hormonal excess or deficiency are the subject of Chapter 12. Hereditary errors of metabolism result from genetic changes that affect enzymes. The basics of heredity are described in Chapter 25.

- **Immune disorders.** These relate to the system that protects us against infectious diseases (see Chapter 17). Some deficiencies in the immune system are inherited;

some, such as AIDS, are the result of infection. This category also includes allergies, in which the immune system is overactive, and autoimmune diseases, which occur when the immune system becomes active against one's own tissues. Examples of diseases that involve autoimmunity are rheumatoid arthritis, multiple sclerosis (MS), and systemic lupus erythematosus (SLE).

- **Neoplasms.** The word *neoplasm* means "new growth" and refers to cancer and other types of tumors. These were described in Chapter 4.

- **Psychiatric disorders.** Psychiatry is the medical field that specializes in the treatment of mental disorders. The brain and the nervous system as a whole are discussed in Chapters 9 and 10. Note, however, that it is often impossible to separate mental from physical factors in any discussion of disease.

Predisposing Causes of Disease

Other factors that enter into the production of a disease are known as **predisposing causes.** Although a predisposing cause may not in itself give rise to a disease, it increases the probability of a person's becoming ill. Examples of predisposing causes include the following:

- **Age.** Tissues degenerate with age, becoming less active and less capable of performing normal functions. Decline may be speeded by the normal wear-and-tear of life, by continuous infection, or by repeated minor injuries. Age may also be a factor in the incidence of specific diseases. For example, measles is more common in children than in adults. Other diseases may appear most commonly in young adults or people in middle years.

- **Gender.** Certain diseases are more characteristic of one gender than the other. Men are more susceptible to early heart disease, whereas women are more likely to develop adult onset diabetes and autoimmune diseases.

- **Heredity.** Some individuals inherit a "tendency" to acquire certain diseases—particularly diabetes, many allergies, and certain forms of cancer.

- **Living conditions and habits.** Individuals who habitually fail to get enough sleep or who pay little attention to diet and exercise are highly vulnerable to disease. The abuse of drugs, alcohol, and tobacco also can lower vitality and predispose to disease. Overcrowding and poor sanitation invite epidemics.

- **Emotional disturbance.** Some physical disturbances have their basis in emotional upsets, stress, and anxiety in daily living. Some headaches and so-called "nervous indigestion" are examples.

- **Physical and chemical damage.** Injuries that cause burns, cuts, fractures, or crushing damage to tissues predispose to infection and degeneration. Some chemicals that may be poisonous, carcinogenic, or otherwise injurious if present in excess are lead compounds (in paint), pesticides, solvents, carbon monoxide and other air pollutants, and a wide variety of other environmental toxins. Exposure to radiation is associated with an increased incidence of cancer. Many of the so-called "occupational diseases" are caused by exposure to harmful agents on the job. For example, inhalation of coal dust and other types of dusts or fibers has caused lung damage among miners. Metals or toxins may cause skin reactions, and exposure to pesticides and other agricultural chemicals has been associated with neurologic disorders and cancer.

- **Preexisting illness.** Any preexisting illness, especially a chronic disease such as high blood pressure or diabetes, increases one's chances of contracting another disease.

CHECKPOINT 5-1 ➤ What is disease?

CHECKPOINT 5-2 ➤ What is the definition of a predisposing cause of disease?

The Study of Disease

The modern approach to the study of disease emphasizes the close relationship of each disease's pathologic and physiologic aspects and the need to understand these fundamentals in treatment. The term used for this combined study in medical science is **pathophysiology.**

Underlying the basic medical sciences are the fundamental disciplines of physics and chemistry. Knowledge of these two sciences is essential to any real understanding of the life processes.

Disease Terminology

The study of the cause of any disease, or the theory of its origin, is **etiology** (e-te-OL-o-je). Diseases are often classified on the basis of severity and duration as follows:

- **Acute.** These diseases are relatively severe but usually last a short time.
- **Chronic.** These diseases are often less severe but are likely to be continuous or recurring for long periods.
- **Subacute.** These diseases are intermediate between acute and chronic, not being as severe as acute disorders nor as long lasting as chronic disorders.

A term used in describing a disease without known cause is **idiopathic** (id-e-o-PATH-ik), a word based on the Greek root *idio-* meaning "self-originating." These diseases are of unknown origin and as yet have no explanation. An **iatrogenic** (i-at-ro-JEN-ik) **disease** results from the adverse effects of treatment, including drug treatment and

surgery. The Greek root *iatro-* relates to a physician or to medicine.

Some health specialists study diseases in populations, a science known as **epidemiology** (ep-ih-de-me-OL-o-je). They collect information on a disease's geographical distribution and its tendency to appear in one gender, age group, or race more or less frequently than another. Some statistics they collect are:

- **Incidence,** the number of new disease cases appearing in a particular population during a specific time period
- **Prevalence,** the overall frequency of a disease in a given group, that is, the number of cases of a disease present in a given population during a specific period or at a particular time
- **Mortality rate,** the percentage of the population that dies from a given disease within a given time period

If many people in a given region acquire a certain disease at the same time, that disease is said to be **epidemic.** Epidemics of influenza, for example, occur periodically today, and epidemics of smallpox and bubonic plague occurred in earlier ages. If a given disease is found to a lesser extent but continuously in a particular region, the disease is **endemic** to that area. The common cold is endemic in human populations. A disease that is prevalent throughout an entire country or continent, or the whole world, is said to be **pandemic.** AIDS is now considered to be pandemic in certain areas of the globe (see Box 5-1).

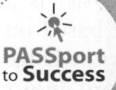
PASSport to Success   Visit **thePoint** or see the Student Resource CD in the back of this book to view a chart summarizing these and other terms related to disease.

CHECKPOINT 5-3 ➤ What two medical sciences are involved in any study of disease?

CHECKPOINT 5-4 ➤ What is a communicable disease?

Treatment and Prevention of Disease

To treat a patient, a physician must first make a **diagnosis** (di-ag-NO-sis), that is, reach a conclusion as to the nature or identity of the illness. To do this, the physician must know the **symptoms** (SIMP-toms), which are the disease conditions noted by the patient, and the **signs,** which are the evidence (objective manifestations) the physician or other healthcare professional can observe. Many diseases cause a variety of effects and involve more than one body system. A characteristic group of symptoms and signs that accompanies a disease is called a **syndrome** (SIN-drome). Some complex disorders even have "syndrome" in their names, such as Down syndrome, premenstrual syndrome, AIDS, and many others.

Box 5-1	A Closer Look

The CDC: Making People Safer and Healthier

The Centers for Disease Control and Prevention (CDC) in Atlanta, Georgia, is responsible for protecting and improving the health of the American public—at home and abroad. Established in 1946, the CDC has become a world leader in the fight against infectious disease, with an expanded role that now includes control and prevention of chronic diseases such as cancer, heart disease, and stroke. The CDC also works to protect the public from environmental hazards such as waterborne illnesses, weather emergencies, biologic and chemical terrorism, and dangers in the home and workplace. In addition, the CDC provides education to guide informed health and lifestyle decisions.

The CDC's stated goal is "healthy people in a healthy world—through prevention." During the 1940s, the newly created CDC joined state and local health officials in the fight against malaria. In the 1950s, it participated in the fight against polio, which has virtually been eliminated in the

United States and elsewhere. In the 1960s, the CDC joined the World Health Organization in efforts to eradicate small-pox worldwide, and in the 1970s, it identified the pathogen responsible for Legionnaires disease. In the 1980s, the CDC reported the first cases of AIDS and began intensive research on the disease, which continues today. During the 1990s, CDC researchers rapidly identified the strain of hantavirus that caused a serious and often fatal pulmonary disease in people in the southwestern U.S. and investigated an outbreak of deadly Ebola virus in Zaire. Currently, the CDC is working with laboratories throughout the U.S. to identify and control the organisms that cause West Nile disease and influenza.

The CDC employs about 8,500 people in state, federal, and foreign locations. They work in more than 170 occupations, including health information, laboratory science, and microbiology.

Frequently, the physician uses laboratory tests to help establish the diagnosis. Common methods used for diagnosis include imaging studies, blood tests, and study of tissues removed in biopsy. A **prognosis** (prog-NO-sis) is a prediction of the probable outcome of a disease based on the patient's condition and the physician's knowledge about the disease (*prognosis* is from the Greek word *gnosis* meaning "knowledge").

Nurses and other healthcare professionals play an extremely valuable role in the diagnostic process by observing closely for signs, collecting and organizing information from the patient about his or her symptoms, and then reporting this information to the physician. Once a patient's disorder is known, the physician prescribes a course of treatment, known as **therapy**. Treatment may include drugs, surgery, radiation, counseling, physical or occupational therapy, and many other measures, alone or in combinations. Specific measures in a course of treatment include those carried out by the nurse and other healthcare providers under the physician's orders.

Complementary and Alternative Medicine

The term *complementary and alternative medicine* (CAM) refers to methods of disease prevention or treatment that can be used along with or instead of traditional modern medical practices. Many of these nontraditional approaches have a long history in ancient philosophies and practices. Some examples of complementary and alternative practices are:

- **Naturopathy** (na-chur-OP-a-the), a philosophy of helping people to heal themselves by developing healthy lifestyles
- **Chiropractic** (ki-ro-PRAK-tik), a field that stresses manipulation to correct misalignment for treatment of musculoskeletal disorders
- **Acupuncture** (AK-u-punk-chur), an ancient Chinese method of inserting thin needles into the body at specific points to relieve pain or promote healing
- **Biofeedback** (bi-o-FEED-bak), which teaches people to control involuntary responses, such as heart rate and blood pressure, by means of electronic devices that monitor changes and feed information back to a person

Exercise, massage, yoga, meditation, nutritional counseling, and other health-promoting practices are also included under this heading.

The U.S. National Institutes of Health (NIH) has established the National Center for Complementary and Alternative Medicine (NCCAM) to study the value of these therapies.

HERBAL REMEDIES The use of plant-derived remedies has increased in industrialized countries in recent years. Many plant products are used as conventional drugs, but typically they are measured, purified, and often modified instead of being used in their natural state. Questions of purity, safety, dosage, and effectiveness have arisen in the use of herbal remedies as, to date, they have not been tested as rigorously as conventional drugs. The U.S. government does not test or regulate herbal remedies, and there are no requirements to report their adverse effects. There are, however, restrictions on the health claims that can be made by the manufacturers, and the U.S. Food and Drug Administration (FDA) can withdraw products from the market that cause unreasonable risk of harm at the recommended doses. The U.S. Office of Dietary Supplements (ODS) supports and coordinates research on herbal preparations.

Prevention of Disease

In recent years, physicians, nurses, and other healthcare workers have taken on increasing responsibilities in disease prevention. Throughout most of medical history, the physician's aim has been to cure patients of existing diseases. The modern concept of prevention, however, seeks to stop disease before it actually happens—to keep people well through the promotion of health. Areas of improvement include cessation of smoking, improved diet, weight control, and adequate exercise. A vast number of organizations exist for the purpose of promoting health, ranging from the World Health Organization (WHO) on an international level to local private, governmental, and community health programs. In the U.S., the Centers for Disease Control and Prevention (CDC) plays an important role in the study of disease (see Box 5-1). A rapidly growing responsibility of all people in health occupations is educating patients on the maintenance of total health, both physical and mental.

CHECKPOINT 5-5 ➤ A physician uses signs and symptoms to identify an illness. What is this identification called?

Infectious Disease

A predominant cause of disease in humans is the invasion of the body by disease-producing **microorganisms** (mi-kro-OR-gan-izms). The word *organism* means "anything having life"; *micro* means "very small." Thus, a microorganism is a tiny living thing, too small to be seen by the naked eye. Other terms for microorganism are *microbe* and, more popularly, *germ*. A microbe, or any other organism, that lives on or within a living **host** and at the host's expense is called a **parasite**.

Although most microorganisms are harmless to humans, and many are beneficial, a few types cause illness; that is, they are **pathogenic** (path-o-JEN-ic). Any disease-causing organism is a **pathogen** (PATH-o-jen). If the body is invaded by pathogens, with adverse effects, the condition is called an **infection**. If the infection is restricted to a relatively small area of the body, it is local; a generalized, or **systemic** (sis-TEM-ik), infection is one that affects the whole body. Systemic infections are usually spread by the blood.

An infection that takes hold because the host has been compromised (weakened) by disease is described as an **opportunistic infection**. For example, people with depressed immune systems, such as those with AIDS, become infected with organisms that are ordinarily harmless.

MODES OF TRANSMISSION A **communicable** disease is one that can be transmitted from one person to another; it is contagious or "catching." Organisms may be transmitted from an infected host to a new host by direct or indirect contact. For example, infected human hosts may transfer their microorganisms directly to other individuals by touching, shaking hands, kissing, or having sexual intercourse. Microorganisms may be transferred indirectly through touched objects, such as bedding, toys, food, and dishes.

The atmosphere is a carrier of microorganisms. Although microbes cannot fly, the dust in the air is alive with them. In close quarters, germ-laden droplets discharged by sneezing, coughing, and even normal conversation contaminate the atmosphere. Insects and other pests may deposit infectious material on food, skin, or clothing. Pathogens are also spread by such pests as rats, mice, fleas, lice, flies, and mosquitoes. Pets may be an indirect source of some infections.

An insect bite may introduce infectious organisms into the body. An insect or other animal that transmits a disease-causing organism from one host to another is termed a **vector** (VEK-tor). Crowded conditions and poor sanitation increase the spread of disease organisms by all of these mechanisms. (See Box 5-2, The Cold Facts about the Common Cold.)

PORTALS OF ENTRY AND EXIT There are several avenues through which microorganisms may enter the body: the skin, respiratory tract, and digestive system, as well as the urinary and reproductive systems. These portals of entry may also serve as exit routes, leading to the spread of infection. For example, discharges from the respiratory and intestinal tracts may spread infection through air, by contamination of hands, and by contamination of food and water supplies.

Control of infectious disease involves breaking the "chain of infection" by which microorganisms spread through a population. Microbial control is discussed later in this chapter.

> ☀ **PASSport to Success** Visit *thePoint* or see the Student Resource CD in the back of this book for a chart and illustrations pertaining to disease transmission.

CHECKPOINT 5-6 ➤ What is the relationship between a parasite and a host?

CHECKPOINT 5-7 ➤ What term describes any disease-causing organism?

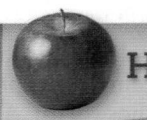

Box 5-2   **Health Maintenance**

The Cold Facts about the Common Cold

Every year, an estimated one billion Americans suffer from the symptoms of the common cold—runny nose, sneezing, coughing, and headache. Although most cases are mild and usually last about a week, colds are the leading cause of doctor visits and missed days at work and school.

Colds are caused by a viral infection of the mucous membranes of the upper respiratory tract. More than 200 different viruses are known to cause cold symptoms. While most colds occur in winter, scientists think that cold weather does not increase the risk of "catching" a cold; the incidence is probably higher in winter because people spend more time indoors, increasing the chances that the virus will spread from person to person.

Colds spread primarily from contact with a contaminated surface. When an infected person coughs or sneezes, small droplets of water filled with viral particles are propelled through the air. One unshielded sneeze may spread hundreds of thousands of viral particles several feet. Depending upon temperature and humidity, these particles may live as long as 3 to 6 hours, and others who touch the contaminated surface may pick up the particles on their hands.

To help prevent the transmission of cold viruses:

■ Avoid close contact with someone who is sneezing or coughing.
■ Wash hands frequently to remove any viral particles you may have picked up.
■ Avoid touching or rubbing your eyes, nose, or mouth with contaminated hands.
■ Clean contaminated surfaces with disinfectant.

There are currently no medically proven cures for the common cold and treatments only ease the symptoms. Because viruses cause the common cold, antibiotics are of no benefit. Getting plenty of rest and drinking lots of fluids are the best ways to speed recovery.

CHECKPOINT 5-8 ➤ What are some portals of entry and exit for microorganisms?

Microbiology—The Study of Microorganisms

Microorganisms are simple, usually single-cell, forms of life. The group includes bacteria, viruses, fungi, protozoa, and algae. The study of these microscopic organisms is **microbiology** (mi-kro-bi-OL-o-je). The organisms included in the study of microbiology along with their scientific specialties are listed here and summarized in Table 5-1:

■ **Bacteria** (bak-te-re-ah) are primitive, single-cell organisms that grow in a wide variety of environments. The study of bacteria, both beneficial and disease producing, is **bacteriology** (bak-te-re-OL-o-je). The group includes rickettsiae and chlamydiae, which are extremely small bacteria that multiply within living cells.

■ **Viruses** (VI-rus-es) are extremely small infectious agents that can multiply only within living cells. **Virology** (vi-ROL-o-je) is the study of viruses.

■ **Fungi** (FUN-ji) are a group that included yeasts and molds. **Mycology** (mi-KOL-o-je) is the study of fungi (the root *myco-* refers to a fungus).

■ **Protozoa** (pro-to-ZO-ah) are single-cell animals. Their study is **protozoology** (pro-to-zo-OL-o-je). Although the term *parasitology* (par-ah-si-TOL-o-je) is the study of parasites in general, in practice, it usually refers to the study of protozoa and worms (helminths).

■ **Algae** (AL-je) are very simple multicellular or single-cell aquatic plants. Their study is **algology** (al-GOL-o-je). These organisms rarely cause diseases and will not be described any further in this chapter.

Despite the fact that this discussion centers on pathogens, most microorganisms are harmless to humans and are actually essential to the continuation of all life on earth. Algae, single-cell plants, produce a large proportion of the oxygen we breathe, and they are food for aquatic animals. Through the actions of microorganisms, dead animals and plants are decomposed and transformed into substances that enrich the soil. Sewage is rendered harmless by microorganisms. Several bacterial groups transform atmospheric nitrogen into a form that plants can use, a process called *nitrogen fixation*. Farmers take advantage of this capacity by allowing a field to lie fallow (untilled) so that microorganisms can replenish the nitrogen in its soil. Certain bacteria and fungi produce the antibiotics that make our lives safer. Others produce the fermented products that make our lives more enjoyable, such as beer, wine, cheeses, and yogurt.

Normal Flora

We have a population of microorganisms that normally grows on and within our bodies. We live in balance with these organisms, which make up the **normal flora**. These

Table 5-1 Organisms Studied in Microbiology

Type of Organism	Name of Study	Characteristics of Organisms	Representative Examples
Bacteria	Bacteriology	Simple, single-cell organisms. Grow in many environments. Lack a true nucleus and most organelles.	Bacteria
Viruses	Virology	Composed of nucleic acid (DNA or RNA) and protein. Can reproduce only within living cells—obligate intracellular parasites.	Viruses
Fungi	Mycology	Very simple, non-green, plantlike organisms. Single-cell forms are yeasts; filamentous forms are molds.	Fungi
Protozoa	Protozoology	Single-cell, animal-like organisms.	Protozoa
Algae	Algology	Simple aquatic plants. Not parasitic.	Algae

populations are beneficial because they crowd out and prevent the growth of other harmful varieties of organisms. Some microorganisms that are normally harmless may become pathogenic if the normal flora are destroyed, as by the administration of antibiotics that act on a wide range of microorganisms.

CHECKPOINT 5-9 ➤ What are the categories of organisms studied in microbiology?

CHECKPOINT 5-10 ➤ What term refers to the microorganisms that normally live in or on the body?

Bacteria

Bacteria are single-cell organisms that are among the most primitive forms of life on earth. They are unique in that their genetic material is not enclosed in a membrane, that is, they do not have a true nucleus. They also lack most of the organelles found in plant and animal cells. They can be seen only with a microscope; from 10 to 1,000 bacteria (depending on the species) would, if lined up, span a pinhead. Staining of the cells with dyes helps make their structures more visible and reveals information about their properties.

Bacteria are found everywhere: in soil, in hot springs, in polar ice, and on and within plants and animals. Their requirements for water, nutrients, oxygen, temperature, and other factors vary widely according to species. Some are capable of carrying out photosynthesis, as do green plants; others must take in organic nutrients, as do animals. Some, described as **anaerobic** (an-air-O-bik), can grow in the absence of oxygen; others, called **aerobic** (air-O-bik), require oxygen. Other groups of bacteria are described as **facultative anaerobes**. These cells will use oxygen if it is present but are able to grow without oxygen if it is not available. *Escherichia coli*, an intestinal organism, is an example of a facultative anaerobe.

Some bacteria produce resistant forms, called **endospores**, that can tolerate long periods of dryness or other adverse conditions (Fig. 5-1). Because these endospores become airborne easily and are resistant to ordinary methods of disinfection, pathogenic organisms that form endospores are particularly dangerous. Note that it is common to shorten the name endospore to just "spore," but these structures are totally different in structure and purpose from the reproductive spores produced by fungi and plants. The organisms that cause tetanus, botulism (a deadly form of food poisoning), and anthrax are examples of spore-forming species.

Many types of bacteria are capable of swimming rapidly by means of threadlike appendages called **flagella** (flah-JEL-ah) (Fig. 5-2). Flagella may be located all around the cell, at one end, or at both ends. Short flagella-like structures called **pili** (PI-li) help bacteria to glide along solid surfaces. Pili also help to anchor bacteria to surfaces, such as to the surface of a liquid to get oxygen, and to attach bacteria to each other for exchange of genetic information in a process called *conjugation*.

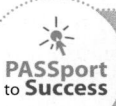
PASSport to Success Visit **thePoint** or see the Student Resource CD in the back of this book for an electron micrograph showing flagella and pili.

Bacteria comprise the largest group of pathogens. Not surprisingly, these pathogenic bacteria are most at home within the human body's "climate." When living conditions are suitable, the organisms reproduce by binary fission (simple cell division). Depending on the species and the growth conditions, cells can divide as rapidly as once every 20 minutes or as slowly as just once every 24 hours. When growing rapidly, populations can increase with unbeliev-

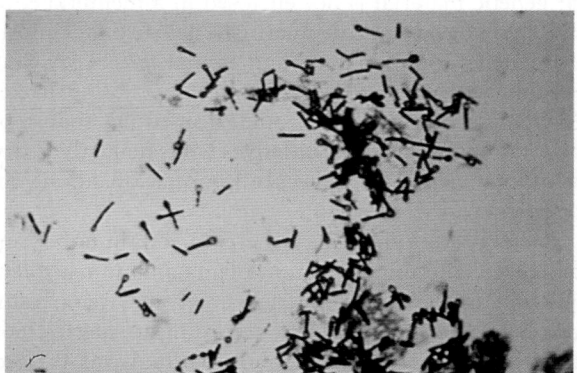
Figure 5-1 **Endospores.** These bacteria have endospores that are visible as clear enlargements at the ends of the cells. (Reprinted with permission from Koneman EW, Alien SD, Janda WM, et al. *Color Atlas and Textbook of Diagnostic Microbiology*, 5th ed. Philadelphia: Lippincott Williams & Wilkins, 1997.)

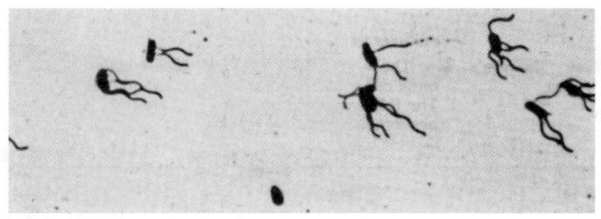
Figure 5-2 **Flagella.** Bacteria use these threadlike appendages to swim. (Reprinted with permission from Koneman EW, Alien SD, Janda WM, et al. *Color Atlas and Textbook of Diagnostic Microbiology*, 5th ed. Philadelphia: Lippincott Williams & Wilkins, 1997.)

able speed. Just 10 cells dividing at a rate of once every 20 minutes becomes a population of over 40,000 within 4 hours. Imagine this activity occurring in a wound or in a bowl of food left out at a picnic without refrigeration.

We have a number of natural defenses to protect our bodies against harmful microorganisms. These include physical barriers, such as the skin and mucous membranes, and the immune system, as described in Chapter 17. If bacteria succeed in overcoming these defenses, they can cause damage in two ways: by producing poisons, or **toxins**, and by entering the body tissues and growing within them. Table 1 in Appendix 5 lists some typical pathogenic bacteria and the diseases they cause.

CHECKPOINT 5-11 ➤ What are resistant forms of bacteria called?

SHAPE AND ARRANGEMENT OF BACTERIA There are so many different types of bacteria that their classification is complicated. For our purposes, a convenient and simple grouping is based on the shape and arrangement of these organisms as seen with a microscope:

- **Cocci** (KOK-si). These cells are round and are seen in characteristic arrangements (Fig. 5-3). Those that are in pairs are called **diplococci**. Those that are arranged in chains, like a string of beads, are called **streptococci**. A third group, seen in large clusters, is known as **staphylococci** (staf-ih-lo-KOK-si). Among the diseases caused by diplococci are gonorrhea and meningitis; streptococci and staphylococci are responsible for a wide variety of infections, including pneumonia, rheumatic fever, and scarlet fever.

- **Bacilli** (bah-SIL-i). These cells are straight, slender rods (Fig. 5-4), although some are cigar-shaped, with tapering ends. All endospore-forming bacteria are bacilli. Typical diseases caused by bacilli include tetanus, diphtheria, tuberculosis, typhoid fever, and Legionnaires disease.

- **Curved rods,** which includes several categories:
  - > **Vibrios** (VIB-re-oze) are short rods with a slight curvature, like a comma (Fig. 5-5A). Cholera is caused by a vibrio.

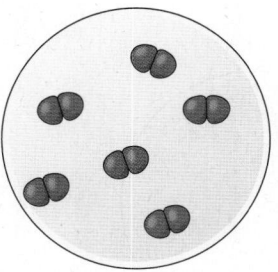
A Diplococci

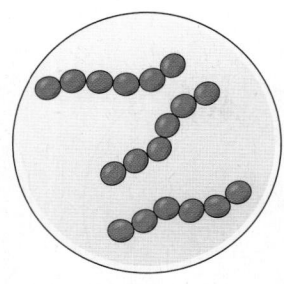
B Streptococci

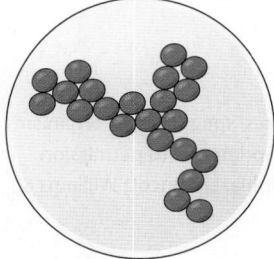
C Staphylococci

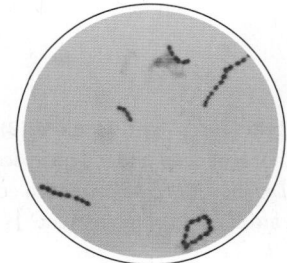
D Streptococci, photomicrograph

Figure 5-3 **Cocci, round bacteria (Gram stained). (A)** Diplococci , cocci in pairs. **(B)** Streptococci, cocci in chains. **(C)** Staphylococci, cocci in clusters. **(D)** Streptococci stained and viewed under a microscope. (D, Reprinted with permission from Koneman EW, Alien SD, Janda WM, et al. *Color Atlas and Textbook of Diagnostic Microbiology*, 5th ed. Philadelphia: Lippincott Williams & Wilkins, 1997.) [**ZOOMING IN** ➤ What word describes the shape and arrangement of the cells in D?]

> **Spirilla** (spi-RIL-a) are long and wavelike cells, resembling a corkscrew. The singular is *spirillum*.

> **Spirochetes** (SPI-ro-ketes) are similar to the spirilla, but are capable of waving and twisting motions (see Fig. 5-5B,C). One infection caused by a

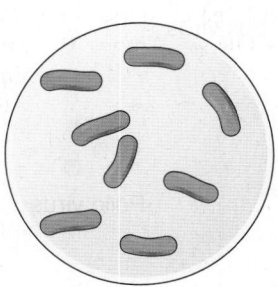
A Bacilli

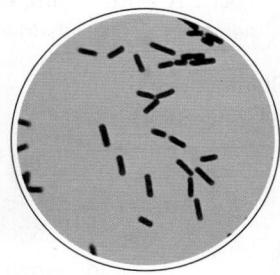
B Bacilli, photomicrograph

Figure 5-4 **Bacilli. (A)** Bacilli are rod-shaped bacteria. **(B)** Bacilli stained and viewed under a microscope. (B, Reprinted with permission from Koneman EW, Alien SD, Janda WM, et al. *Color Atlas and Textbook of Diagnostic Microbiology*, 5th ed. Philadelphia: Lippincott Williams & Wilkins, 1997.)

spirochete is syphilis. The syphilis spirochetes enter the body at the point of contact, usually through the genital skin or mucous membranes. They then travel into the bloodstream and set up a systemic infection. (See Table 1 in Appendix 5 for a summary of the three stages of syphilis.)

A spirochete is also responsible for Lyme disease, which has increased in the United States since it first appeared in the early 1960s. People who walk in or near woods are advised to wear white protective clothing that covers their ankles. They should examine their bodies for the freckle-sized ticks that carry the disease.

OTHER BACTERIA Members of the genus *Rickettsia* (rih-KET-se-ah) and the genus *Chlamydia* (klah-MID-e-ah) are classified as bacteria, although they are considerably smaller than other bacteria. These microorganisms can exist only inside living cells. Because they exist at the expense of their hosts, they are parasites; they are referred to as *obligate intracellular parasites* because they must grow within living cells.

The rickettsiae are the cause of several serious diseases in humans, such as typhus and Rocky Mountain spotted fever. In almost every instance, these organisms are transmitted through the bites of insects, such as lice, ticks, and fleas. A few common diseases caused by rickettsiae are listed in Table 1 in Appendix 5.

The chlamydiae are smaller than the rickettsiae. They are the causative organisms in trachoma (a serious eye infection that ultimately causes blindness), parrot fever or psittacosis, the sexually transmitted infection lymphogranuloma venereum, and some respiratory diseases (see Table 1 in Appendix 5).

NAMING BACTERIA As is common in naming higher plants and animals, the names of bacteria include a genus name, written with a capital letter, and a species name, written with a small letter, both names italicized. The genus or species names may be taken from the name of an organism's discoverer, as in *Escherichia*, named for Theodor Escherich, or *Rickettsia*, named for Howard T. Ricketts. Some other criteria are shape (e.g., genus *Staphylococcus*, *Bacillus*), the disease caused (e.g., *S. pneumoniae*, which causes pneumonia; *N. meningitidis*, the cause of meningitis), habitat (*S. epidermidis*, which grows on the skin), or growth characteristics. *S. pyogenes* produces pus, and colonies of *S. aureus*, based on the Latin word for gold, have a golden yellow color. More specific information is conveyed by adding names for subgroups such as type, subtype, strain, variety, etc.

CHECKPOINT 5-12 ➤ What are the three basic shapes of bacteria?

Viruses

Although bacteria seem small, they are enormous in comparison with **viruses** (Fig. 5-6). Viruses are comparable in

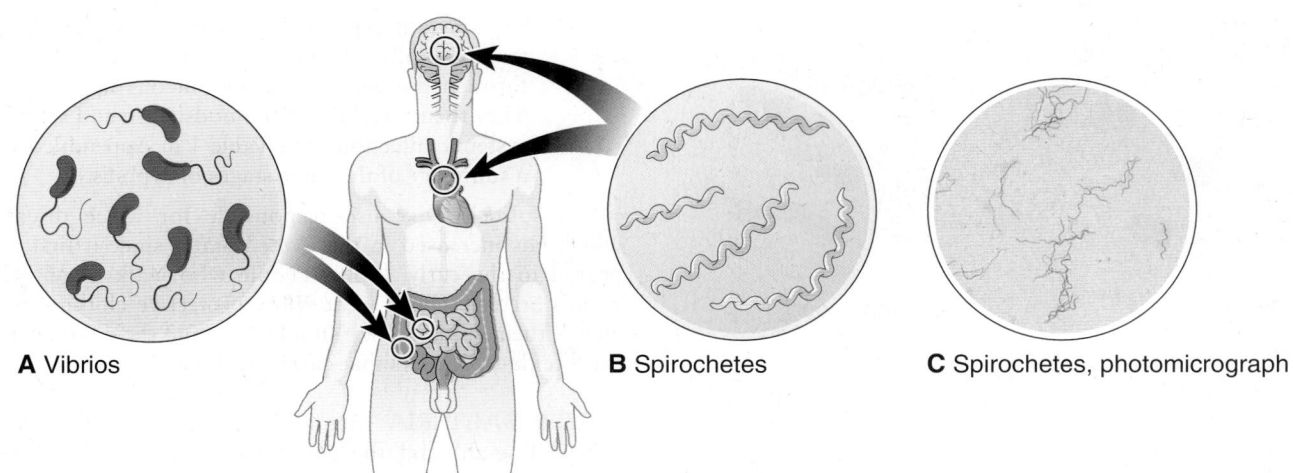

Figure 5-5 **Curved rods. (A)** Vibrios, comma-shaped organisms. A vibrio causes Asiatic cholera. **(B)** Spirochetes, spiral-shaped organisms that move with a twisting motion. A spirochete causes syphilis. **(C)** Spirochetes as seen under a microscope. (C, Reprinted with permission from Koneman EW, Alien SD, Janda WM, et al. *Color Atlas and Textbook of Diagnostic Microbiology*, 5th ed. Philadelphia: Lippincott Williams & Wilkins, 1997.) [**ZOOMING IN** ➤ What feature indicates that the cells in A are capable of movement?]

size to large molecules, but unlike other molecules, they contain genetic material and are able to reproduce. Viruses are so tiny that they are invisible with a light microscope; they can be seen only with an electron microscope. Because of their small size and the difficulties associated with growing them in the laboratory, viruses were not studied with much success until the middle of the 20th century.

Viruses have some of the fundamental properties of living matter, but they are not cellular, and they have no enzyme system. They consist of a nucleic acid core, either DNA or RNA, surrounded by a coat of protein (Fig. 5-7). Like the rickettsiae and the chlamydiae, they can grow only within living cells—they are obligate intracellular parasites. Unlike these other organisms, however, viruses are not susceptible to antibacterial agents (antibiotics) and must be treated with antiviral drugs.

Viruses are classified according to the type of nucleic acid they contain—DNA or RNA—and whether that nucleic acid is single stranded (ss) or double stranded (ds). They are further grouped according to the diseases they cause, of which there are a considerable number—measles, poliomyelitis, hepatitis, chickenpox, and the common cold, to name just a few. **AIDS** is a very serious viral disease discussed in Chapter 17. The virus that causes AIDS and other representative viruses are listed in Table 2 in Appendix 5.

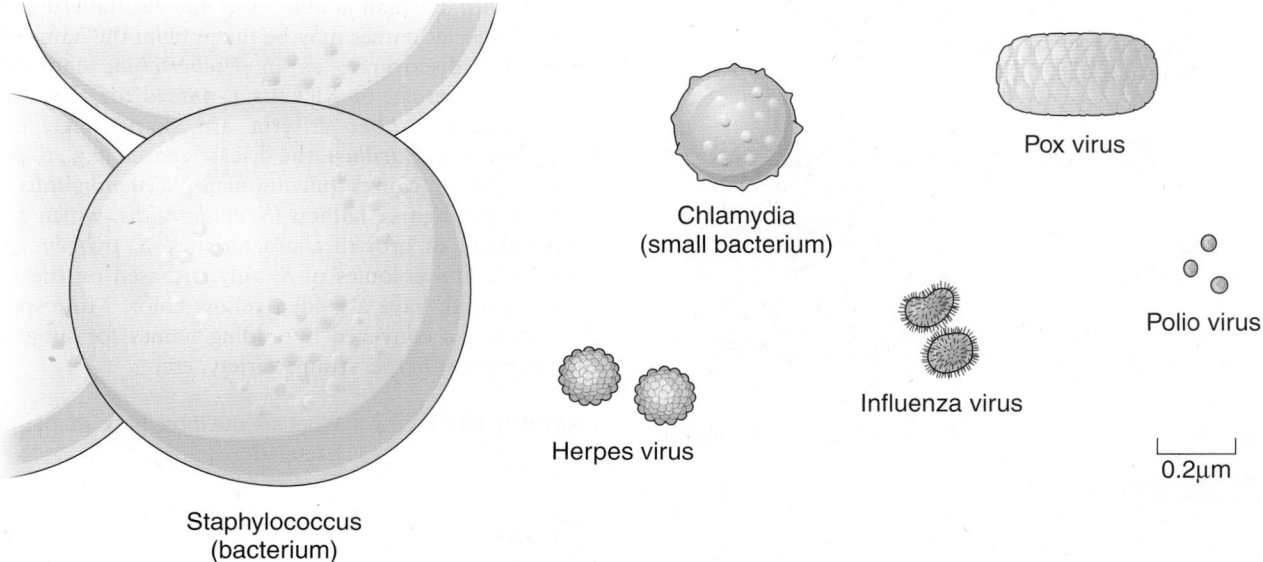

Figure 5-6 **Virus size comparison.** A chlamydia and a staphylococcus are shown for reference.

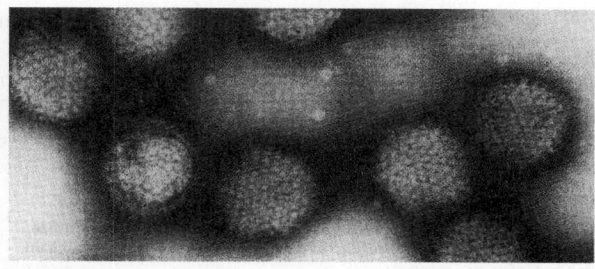

Figure 5-7 **Virus structure.** Note the regular arrangement of units in the protein coat. Magnified ×234,000. (Reprinted with permission from Koneman EW, Alien SD, Janda WM, et al. *Color Atlas and Textbook of Diagnostic Microbiology*, 5th ed. Philadelphia: Lippincott Williams & Wilkins, 1997.)

Viruses are named according to where they were isolated (Hanta, Ebola, West Nile), the symptoms they cause (yellow fever virus, which causes jaundice; hepatitis virus, which causes inflammation of the liver), the host (chickenpox, human immunodeficiency virus, swine influenza), or the vector that caries them (Colorado tick fever).

INFECTIOUS AGENTS SMALLER THAN VIRUSES

Viruses were considered the smallest known infectious agents until the discovery of two even smaller and simpler agents of disease. **Prions** (PRI-ons) are infectious particles composed solely of protein (the name comes from **prote**ina-ceous **in**fectious agent). Researchers have linked prions to several fatal diseases in humans and animals. They are very slow-growing and hard to destroy, producing spongy degeneration of brain tissue, described as *spongiform encephalopathy* (en-sef-ah-LOP-a-the). Some examples of diseases caused by prions are Creutzfeldt-Jacob disease (CJD) in humans; bovine spongiform encephalopathy (BSE), the so-called "mad cow disease," in cows, a variant of which affects humans; and scrapie in sheep. Some diseases caused by prions are described in Table 3 of Appendix 5.

Viroids (VI-royds), in contrast, are composed of RNA alone with no protein coat. They are also intracellular par-

asites, but so far, they have been linked only to diseases in plants.

CHECKPOINT 5-13 ➤ How do viruses differ from bacteria?

Fungi

The true **fungi** (FUN-ji) are a large group of simple plant-like organisms. Only a few types are pathogenic. Although fungi are much larger and more complicated than bacteria, they are a simple life form. They differ from the higher plants in that they lack the green pigment chlorophyll, which enables most plants to use the energy of sunlight to manufacture food. Like bacteria, fungi grow best in dark, damp places. Single-cell fungi are generally referred to as **yeasts**; the fuzzy, filamentous forms are called **molds** (Fig. 5-8). Molds reproduce in several ways, including by simple cell division and by production of multiple reproductive spores. Yeasts reproduce by simple cell division and can also form buds that pinch off as new cells. Familiar examples of fungi are mushrooms, puffballs, bread molds, and the yeasts used in baking and brewing.

FUNGAL DISEASES Diseases caused by fungi are called **mycotic** (mi-KOT-ik) infections (*myco-* means "fungus"). Examples of these are athlete's foot and ringworm. Common types of ringworm are *Tinea capitis* (TIN-e-ah KAP-ih-tis), which involves the scalp, and *Tinea corporis* (kor-PO-ris), which can grow on almost any nonhairy body surface.

One yeast-like fungus that may infect a weakened host is *Candida*. This is a normal inhabitant of the mouth and digestive tract that may produce skin lesions, an oral infection called *thrush*, digestive upset, or inflammation of the vaginal tract (vaginitis) as an opportunistic infection in a weakened host.

Although fungi cause few systemic diseases, some diseases they cause are very dangerous and may be difficult to cure. Pneumonia can result from the inhalation of fungal spores contained in dust particles. An atypical fungus,

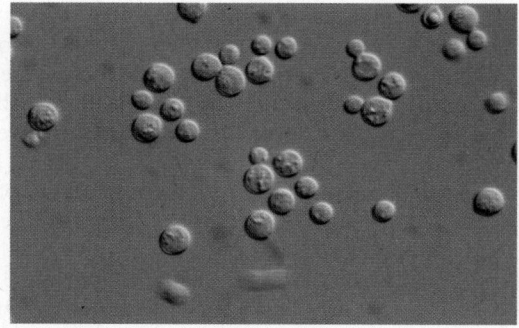

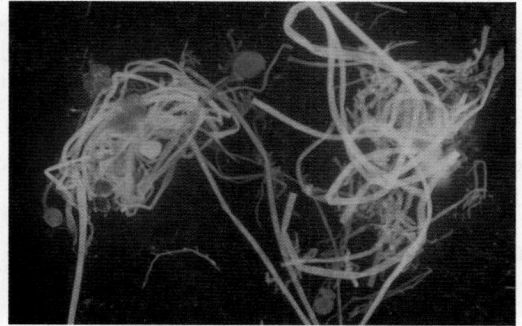

Figure 5-8 **Fungi. (A)** Yeasts. Some of these single-cell fungi are budding to form new cells **(B)** Molds, filamentous forms of fungi. (A, Reprinted with permission from LWW's Organism Central [CD-ROM for Windows]. Philadelphia: Lippincott Williams & Wilkins, 2001; B, Reprinted with permission from Koneman EW, Alien SD, Janda WM, et al. *Color Atlas and Textbook of Diagnostic Microbiology*, 5th ed. Philadelphia: Lippincott Williams & Wilkins, 1997.)

Pneumocystis jiroveci (formerly called *P. carinii*) causes a previously rare pneumonia known as PCP (*Pneumocystis* pneumonia) in people with AIDS and others with weakened immune systems. Table 4 in Appendix 5 lists typical fungal diseases.

Protozoa

With the **protozoa** (pro-to-ZO-ah), we come to the only group of microbes that can be described as animal-like. Although protozoa are also single-cell organisms, they are much larger than bacteria (Fig. 5-9).

Protozoa are found all over the world in the soil and in almost any body of water from moist grass to mud puddles to the sea. There are four main divisions of protozoa:

- **Amebas** (ah-ME-bas). An ameba (also spelled *amoeba*) is an irregular mass of cytoplasm that propels itself by extending part of its cell (a pseudopod, or "false foot") and then flowing into the extension. Amebic dysentery is caused by a pathogen of this group (see Fig. 5-9A,B).
- **Ciliates** (SIL-e-ates). This type of protozoon is covered with tiny hairs called cilia that produce a wave action to propel the organism.
- **Flagellates** (FLAJ-eh-lates). Long, whiplike filaments called flagella propel these organisms. One of this group, a **trypanosome** (tri-PAN-o-some), causes African sleeping sickness, which is spread by the tsetse fly (see Fig. 5-9C,D). *Giardia* is a flagellated protozoon that contaminates water supplies throughout the world. It infects the intestinal tract, causing diarrhea. The disease, giardiasis, is the most common waterborne disease in the United States.
- **Sporozoa** (spor-o-ZO-ah) are also known as **apicomplexans** (ap-i-kom-PLEK-sans). Unlike other protozoa, sporozoa cannot propel themselves. They are obligate parasites, unable to grow outside a host. Members of the genus *Plasmodium* (plaz-MO-de-um) cause malaria (see Fig. 5-9E,F). These protozoa, carried by a mosquito vector, cause much serious illness in the tropics, resulting in over 1 million deaths each year. The sporozoon *Cryptosporidium* is an opportunistic pathogen that causes severe and prolonged diarrhea in people suffering from AIDS and others with an inadequate immune system.

Table 5 in Appendix 5 presents a list of typical pathogenic protozoa with the diseases they cause.

CHECKPOINT **5-14** ➤ What group of microorganisms is most animal-like?

Parasitic Worms

Many species of worms, also referred to as **helminths**, are parasites with human hosts. The study of worms, particularly parasitic worms, is called **helminthology** (hel-min-THOL-o-je). Whereas invasion by any form of organism is usually called an *infection*, the presence of parasitic worms in the body also can be termed an *infestation* (Fig. 5-10). Although worms themselves can be seen with the naked eye, one needs a microscope to see their eggs or larval forms.

Roundworms

Many human parasitic worms are classified as roundworms, and the large worm **ascaris** (AS-kah-ris) is one of the most common (see Fig. 5-10A). This worm is prevalent in many parts of Asia, where it is found mostly in larval form. In the United States, it is found most frequently among children (ages 4 to 12 years) in rural areas with warm climates.

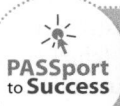

PASSport to Success — Visit **thePoint** or see the Student Resource CD in the back of this book to see photographs of roundworms.

Ascaris is a long, white-yellow worm pointed at both ends. It may infest the lungs or the intestines, producing intestinal obstruction if present in large numbers. The eggs produced by the adult worms are deposited with feces (excreta) in the soil. These eggs are very resistant; they can live in soil during either freezing or hot, dry weather and cannot be destroyed even by strong antiseptics. New worms develop within the eggs and later reach the digestive system of a host by means of contaminated food. Ascaris infestation may be diagnosed by a routine stool examination.

Another fairly common infestation, particularly in children, is the seat worm, or **pinworm** (*Enterobius vermicularis*), which is also hard to control and eliminate. The worms average 12 mm (somewhat less than 1/2 inch) in length and live in the large intestine. The adult female moves outside the vicinity of the anus to lay its thousands of eggs. A child's fingers often transfer these eggs from the itching anal area to the mouth. In the digestive system of the host, the eggs develop to form new adult worms, and thus a new infestation is begun. A child also may infect others by this means. In addition, pinworm eggs that are expelled from the body constitute a hazard because they may live in the external environment for several months. Patience and every precaution, with careful attention to medical instructions, are necessary to get rid of the worms. It is essential to wash the hands, keep the fingernails clean, and avoid finger sucking.

Hookworms are parasites that live in the small intestine. They are dangerous because they suck blood from the host, causing such a severe anemia (blood deficiency) that the victim becomes sluggish, both physically and mentally. Most victims become susceptible to various chronic infections because of extremely reduced resistance following continuous blood loss.

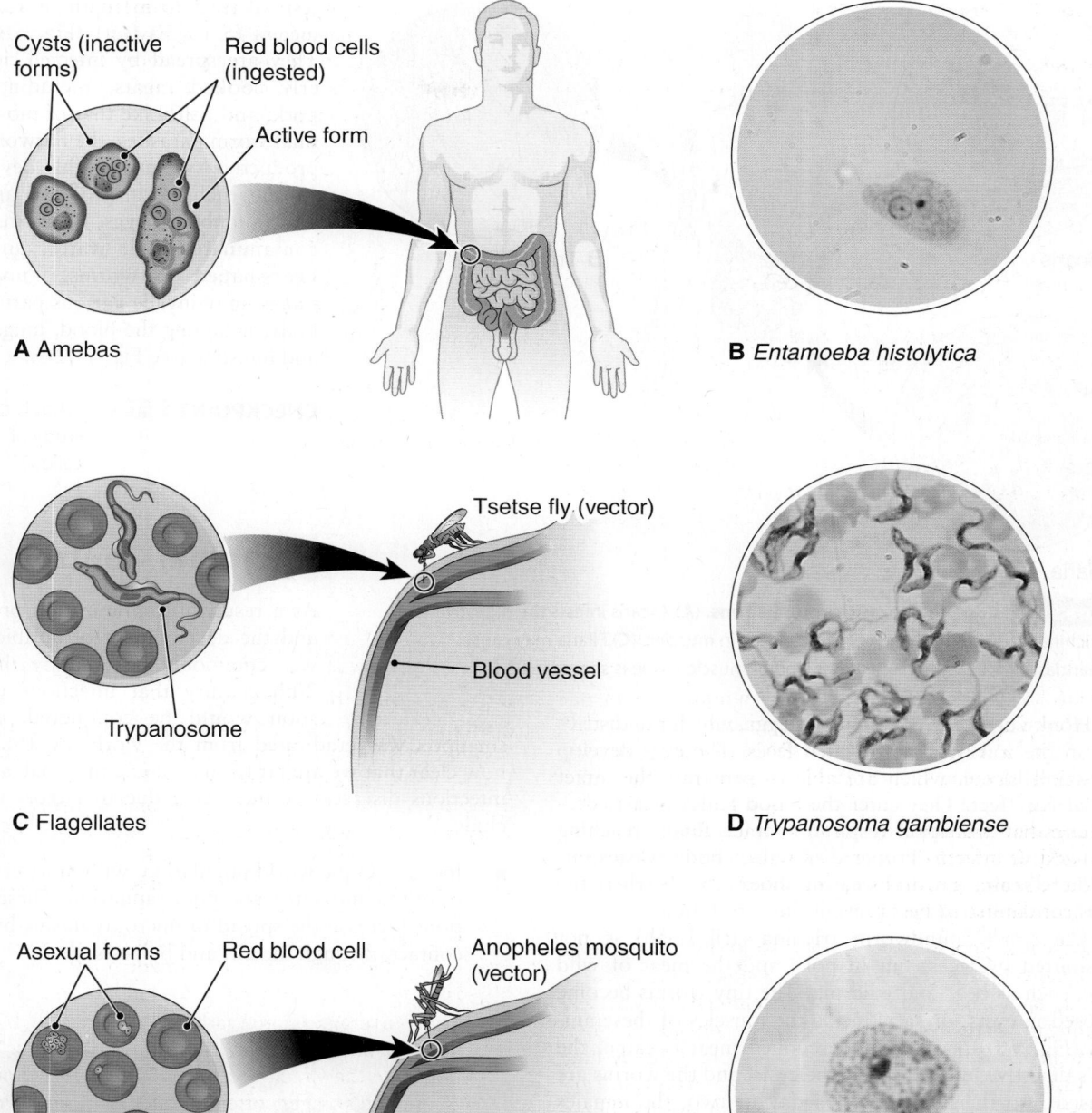

Figure 5-9 **Some parasitic protozoa. (A)** Amebas. **(B)** *Entamoeba histolytica*, cause of amebic dysentery, seen under the microscope. **(C)** Flagellates. Trypanosomes cause African sleeping sickness. **(D)** Trypansomes in a blood sample seen under the microscope. **(E)** Sporozoa. *Plasmodium vivax* causes malaria. **(F)** An enlarged red blood cell with a single parasite seen under the microscope. (B, D, F, Reprinted with permission from Koneman EW, Alien SD, Janda WM, et al. *Color Atlas and Textbook of Diagnostic Microbiology,* 5th ed. Philadelphia: Lippincott Williams & Wilkins, 1997.) **[ZOOMING IN ➤** Why are the parasites in E described as intracellular? What is the role of the vectors shown in C and E? **]**

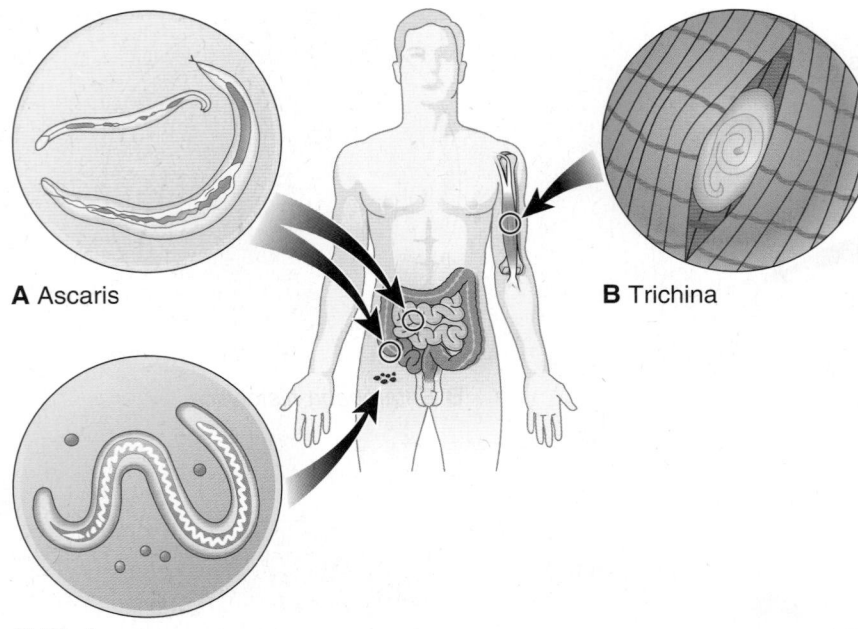

A Ascaris

B Trichina

C Filaria

Figure 5-10 **Common parasitic roundworms. (A)** Ascaris infests the digestive tract. **(B)** Trichina is transmitted in meat and encysts in muscles. **(C)** Filaria may cause elephantiasis. **[ZOOMING IN ➤** What kind of muscle tissue is shown in B? **]**

Hookworms lay thousands of eggs, which are distributed in the soil by contaminated feces. The eggs develop into small larvae, which are able to penetrate the intact skin of bare feet. They enter the blood and are carried to the lungs and the upper respiratory tract, finally reaching the digestive system. Proper disposal of body wastes, attention to sanitation, and wearing shoes in areas where the soil is contaminated best prevent this infestation.

The small roundworm **trichina** (trik-I-nah) is not transmitted by feces, but in pork and the meat of wild game, such as bear and wild pig. The tiny worms become enclosed in cysts, or sacs, inside the muscles of these animals (Fig. 5-10B). If the undercooked meat is eaten, the host's digestive juices dissolve the cysts, and the worms are released into the intestine. In a day or two, the females mate and lay eggs. When the larvae emerge, they travel to the host's muscles, where they again become encysted. This disease is **trichinosis** (trik-ih-NO-sis).

Biting insects, such as flies and mosquitoes, transmit the tiny, threadlike filaria worm that causes **filariasis** (fil-ah-RI-ah-sis) (see Fig. 5-10C). The worms grow in large numbers, causing various disturbances. If they clog the lymphatic vessels, a condition called **elephantiasis** (el-eh-fan-TI-ah-sis) results, in which the lower extremities, the scrotum, the breasts and other areas may become tremendously enlarged (Fig. 5-11). Filariasis is most common in tropical and subtropical lands, such as southern Asia and many of the South Pacific islands.

Flatworms

Some flatworms resemble long ribbons, whereas others have the shape of a leaf. Tapeworms may grow in the in-

testinal tract to a length of 1.5 to 15 meters (5 to 50 feet) (Fig. 5-12A,B). They are spread by infected, improperly cooked meats, including beef, pork, and fish. Like that of most intestinal worm parasites, the flatworm's reproductive system is highly developed, so that each worm produces an enormous number of eggs, which may then contaminate food, water, and soil. Leaf-shaped flatworms, known as *flukes*, may invade various parts of the body, including the blood, lungs, liver, and intestine (see Fig. 5-12C).

CHECKPOINT 5-15 ➤ What is the study of worms called?

Microbial Control

As a result of immunization programs and the development of antibiotics, it was commonly believed by the mid-20th century that infectious diseases soon would be conquered. Indeed, smallpox was eradicated from the world by 1980. It is now clear that we are far from reaching this goal, and that infectious diseases are increasing due to factors that include:

- Increase in the world population, with more crowding of people into cities and poor sanitation. These conditions increase the spread of microorganisms by direct contact, through the air, and by pests.

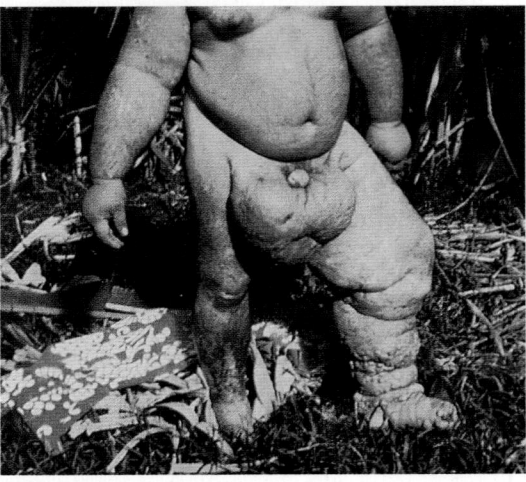

Figure 5-11 **Filariasis.** The photo shows massive enlargement (elephantiasis) of the scrotum and left leg. (Reprinted with permission from Rubin E, Farber JL. Pathology, 3rd ed. Philadelphia: Lippincott Williams & Wilkins, 1999.)

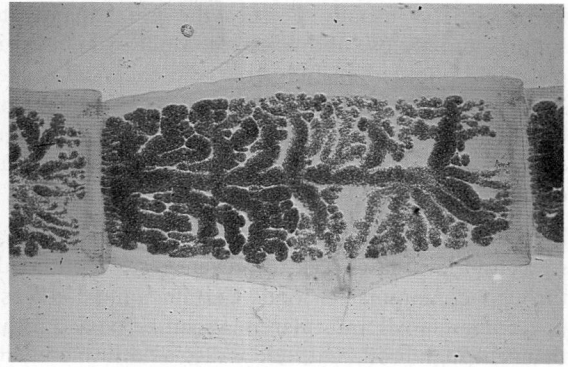

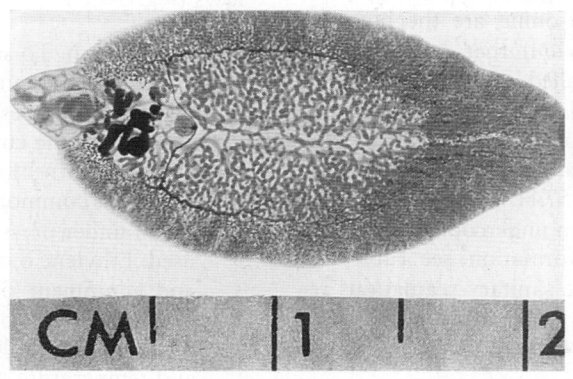

Figure 5-12 **Flatworms. (A)** Tapeworms can measure more than 30 feet in length. The arrow shows the headlike attachment point. **(B)** Segments of a tapeworm. **(C)** A fluke. (Reprinted with permission from Koneman EW, Alien SD, Janda WM, et al. *Color Atlas and Textbook of Diagnostic Microbiology*, 5th ed. Philadelphia: Lippincott Williams & Wilkins, 1997.)

- Disruption of animal habitats, with more contact between humans and animals, allowing the spread of animal pathogens to human hosts. Some organisms that have made this shift include HIV, the cause of AIDS, which originated in chimpanzees; West Nile virus from birds; severe acute respiratory syndrome (SARS), which probably came from a small wild mammal used for food; and various strains of influenza.

- Increased travel, especially air travel, which can spread an infectious organism throughout the globe in a day. SARS spread rapidly from China to other countries in the spring of 2003.

- Medical advances that keep people alive longer, but in a debilitated state, subject to opportunistic infections.

- Changes in food handling that allow foods to be stored, processed, and shipped long distances on a large scale, sometimes with inadequate oversight.

Because of their huge variety and adaptability, there is scarcely a place on earth that is naturally free of microorganisms. One exception is the interior of normal body tissue. However, body surfaces and passageways leading to the outside, such as the mouth, throat, nasal cavities, and large intestine, harbor an abundance of both harmless and potentially pathogenic microbes. If a person's natural defenses are sound, he or she may harbor many microbes

safely. If that person's resistance becomes lowered, however, an infection can result. Although many vaccines are available to protect against disease, inhabitants in poor areas may not have access to them. Lack of immunization in combination with lowered resistance due to poor nutrition and disease create a susceptible host.

Microbes and Public Health

All societies establish and enforce measures designed to protect the health of their populations. Most of these practices are concerned with preventing the spread of infectious organisms. A few examples of fundamental public health considerations are listed below:

- **Sewage and garbage disposal.** In times past, when people disposed of the household "slops" by simply throwing them out the window, great epidemics were inevitable. Modern practice is to divert sewage into a processing plant in which harmless microbes are put to work destroying the pathogens. The resulting noninfectious "sludge" makes excellent fertilizer.

- **Water purification.** Drinking water that has become polluted with untreated sewage may be contaminated with such dangerous pathogens as typhoid bacilli, polio and hepatitis viruses, and dysentery amebas. A filtering process usually purifies the municipal water supply, and a close and constant watch is kept on its microbial population. Industrial and chemical wastes, such as asbestos fibers, acids and detergents from homes and from industry, and pesticides used in agriculture, complicate the problem of obtaining pure drinking water.

- **Prevention of food contamination.** Various national, state, and local laws seek to prevent disease outbreaks through contaminated food. Certain animal diseases (e.g., tuberculosis and tularemia) can be passed to humans through food, and food is also a natural breeding place for many dangerous pathogens. Some of the organisms that cause food poisoning are the botulism bacillus (*Clostridium botulinum*) that grows in improperly canned foods, so-called *staph* (*Staphylococcus aureus*), and species of *Salmonella* transmitted in eggs, poultry, and dairy products. In recent years, a variety of the normally harmless intestinal bacillus *Escherichia coli* (*E. coli* 0157:H7) has caused outbreaks of food poisoning from undercooked meat and from produce. For further information, see Table 1 in Appendix 5. Most cities have sanitary regulations requiring, among other things, compulsory periodic inspection of food-handling establishments.

- **Milk pasteurization.** Milk is rendered free of pathogens by pasteurization, a process in which the milk is heated to 63°C (145°F) for 30 minutes and then cooled rapidly before being packaged. Sometimes, slightly higher temperatures are used for a much shorter time with satisfactory results. The entire pasteurization process, including the cooling and packing, is accomplished in a closed system, without any exposure to air. Pasteurized milk still contains microbes, but no harmful ones. Pasteurization is also used to preserve other beverages and dairy products.

Aseptic Methods

In the practice of medicine, surgery, nursing, and other health fields, specialized procedures are followed to reduce or eliminate the growth of pathogenic organisms. The term *sepsis* refers to the presence of pathogenic organisms (or their toxins) in the blood or tissues; **asepsis** (a-SEP-sis) is its opposite—a condition in which no pathogens are present. Procedures that are designed to kill, remove, or prevent the growth of microbes are called *aseptic methods*.

There are several terms designating aseptic practices. These are often confused with one another. Some of the more commonly used terms and their definitions are as follows (Fig. 5-13):

- **Sterilization.** To sterilize an object means to kill *every* living microorganism on it. In operating rooms and delivery rooms especially, staff members keep sterile as much of the environment as possible, including the clothing worn by personnel and the instruments used. The most common sterilization method is by means of steam under pressure in an **autoclave**. Dry heat is also used. Ethylene oxide, a gas, is used to sterilize supplies and equipment that are not able to withstand high temperatures. Most pathogens can be killed by exposure to boiling water for 4 minutes. However, the time and temperature required to ensure the destruction of all spore-forming organisms in sterilization are much greater than those required to kill most pathogens.

- **Disinfection.** Disinfection refers to any measure that kills all pathogens (except spores) but does not necessarily kill all harmless microbes. Most **disinfectants** (disinfecting agents) are chemicals that can be applied directly to nonliving surfaces. Examples are chlorine compounds, such as household bleach, phenol compounds, and mercury compounds. Commercial disinfectant products contain more than one chemical

Sterilization	Disinfection	Antisepsis
Autoclave	Examples: Chlorine bleach Ammonia Phenol	Examples: Alcohol Hydrogen peroxide Antibacterial soap

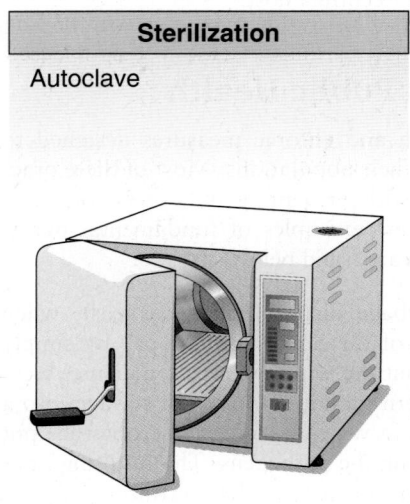 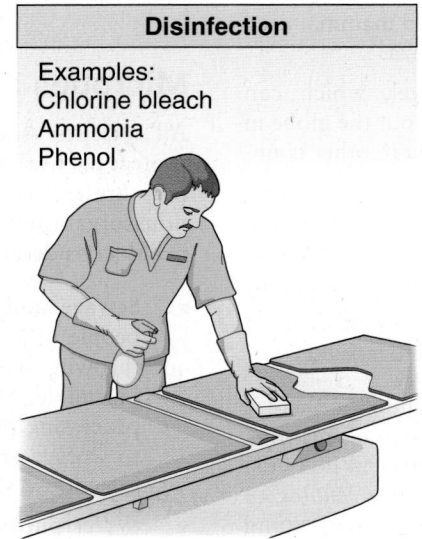 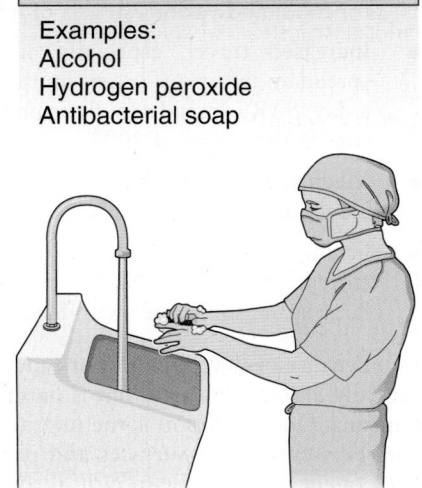

Figure 5-13 **Aseptic methods.**

agent in order to kill a variety of organisms. Two other terms for bacteria-killing agents, synonymous with disinfectant, are **bactericide** and **germicide**, agents that kill bacteria and germs.

- **Antisepsis.** This term refers to any process in which pathogens are not necessarily killed but are prevented from multiplying, a state called **bacteriostasis** (bak-te-re-o-STA-sis) (*stasis* means "steady state"). **Antiseptics** are less powerful than disinfectants and are safe to use on living tissues. Examples are alcohol, organic iodine solutions, and hydrogen peroxide.

Infection Control Techniques

In the 1980s, concern about the spread of blood-borne infections, such as hepatitis B and HIV, led to the development of isolation and barrier techniques for the handling of blood and other body fluids that might contain blood. These *universal precautions* have now been extended to include all potentially infective body substances and are entitled *body substance precautions* or *body substance isolation*. According to guidelines established by the CDC (Centers for Disease Control and Prevention), healthcare personnel must use barriers for any contact with moist body substances, mucous membranes, or nonintact skin, whether or not blood is visible and regardless of the patient's diagnosis. Gloves must be worn for each patient contact and changed if necessary during care. Protective coverings such as a mask, eye protection, face shield, or fluid-repellent gown should be worn during procedures that may generate sprays of blood or body fluids. Soiled linen, trash, and other waste must be treated as if contaminated and disposed of properly. Needles and other sharp instruments must be handled safely and disposed of in puncture-proof containers. To avoid the risk of needlestick injuries, **needles are not recapped**. In circumstances when it is necessary to recap, the needle should be slipped into the cap with one hand or by using a recapping device.

Additional isolation precautions are instituted for infections that are spread by airborne routes, such as tuberculosis, measles (rubeola), and SARS; for those spread by droplets or direct contact; and for infections involving antibiotic-resistant organisms. These measures may include keeping a patient in a private room and limiting visitor contact, filtering circulating air, and having health personnel wear protective clothing.

HANDWASHING Handwashing is the single most important measure for preventing the spread of infection in all settings. Thorough washing promptly after patient contact and after contact with any body secretions is of utmost importance in infection control. Standard precautions include handwashing after glove removal due to the rapid multiplication of normal flora inside the gloves. Gloves are not considered a substitute for handwashing because they may have small defects, they may be torn, or hands may become contaminated when the gloves are removed.

OSHA The Occupational Safety and Health Administration (OSHA) is a U.S. government agency that establishes minimum health and safety standards for workers. The agency has issued regulations for protection against infectious materials based on the CDC guidelines and has enforced these regulations. Employers at healthcare facilities must provide workers with the equipment and supplies needed to prevent their exposure to infectious materials.

CHECKPOINT 5-16 ➤ Aseptic practices are intended to eliminate pathogens. What are the three levels of asepsis?

CHECKPOINT 5-17 ➤ What is the single most important measure for preventing the spread of infection?

Antimicrobial Agents

Antimicrobial (antiinfective) agents are drugs that act to kill or inhibit infectious microorganisms. These include antibacterial, antiviral, antifungal, and antiparasitic substances, which interfere with vital metabolic processes that the infecting agents need to survive and reproduce. A drug that acts on intestinal worms is an anthelmintic (ant-hel-MIN-tik) agent or vermifuge (VER-mih-fuj). The term *antibiotic*, in its most general sense, refers to any substance that acts against a living organism, but the term has come to be used only for drugs that act against bacteria.

ANTIBIOTICS (ANTIBACTERIAL AGENTS) An **antibiotic** is a substance produced by living cells that has the power to kill or arrest the growth of bacteria. Most antibiotics are derived from fungi (molds) and soil bacteria. Penicillin, the first widely used antibiotic, is made from a common blue mold, *Penicillium*. Often, the drugs derived from penicillin can be recognized by the ending *-cillin* in the name. Other fungi that produce a large number of antibiotics are members of the group *Cephalosporium*. The soil bacteria *Streptomyces* produce some frequently used antibiotics. These drug names often end in *-mycetin*.

The development of antibiotics has been of incalculable benefit to humanity. Since the time that penicillin saved many lives on the battlefields of World War II in the 1940s, antibiotics have been considered miracle drugs. Enthusiasm for their use, however, has given rise to some undesirable effects.

One danger of antibiotic use is the development of opportunistic infections. As noted, there is a normal flora of microorganisms in the body that competes with pathogens. Antibiotics, especially those that kill a wide variety of bacteria (broad-spectrum antibiotics), eliminate these competitors and allow pathogens to thrive. For example, antibiotics often destroy the normal flora of the vaginal tract and allow a troublesome yeast infection to develop.

The widespread use of antibiotics has resulted in the natural selection of pathogens that are resistant to these medications. Under some circumstances, bacteria can even transfer genes for resistance directly from one cell to another. Some strains of common organisms, such as streptococci, staphylococci, pneumococci, *E. coli*, and tuberculosis are now resistant to most antibiotics (see Appendix 5 for diseases caused by these microorganisms).

The prevalence of antibiotic-resistant pathogens is a serious problem in hospitals today. These organisms cause infections that do not respond to drugs. In the United States, about 5% of acute care hospital patients contract one or more such infections. Patients who are elderly or severely debilitated are most susceptible to these **nosocomial** (nos-o-KO-me-al) (hospital-acquired) infections (the word *nosocomial* comes from a Greek word for hospital). Some strains currently causing nosocomial infections are methicillin-resistant *Staphylococcus aureus* (MRSA) and vancomycin-resistant enterococci (VRE).

When taking antibiotics, it is important to complete the entire course of treatment to guarantee the destruction of all pathogens. If not, the more resistant cells will be able to survive treatment and grow out in great numbers, leading to the development of strains that do not respond to that antibiotic. Also, patients should not press physicians to prescribe antibiotics when they will do no good, as for the treatment of viral infections such as colds and flu.

Pharmaceutical companies may be able to find new antibiotics. Also, using these drugs in combinations may help to eliminate all the bacteria causing an infection. We may be able to reverse the trend toward resistance by using these drugs with more care. Large quantities of antibiotics are now used in agriculture to control disease among farm animals and increase productivity. Some people now shop for meats that are free of antibiotics. There is some evidence that susceptibility to a given drug will reappear when a bacterial population is no longer exposed to it.

CHECKPOINT `5-18` ➤ What is an antibiotic?

ANTIVIRAL AGENTS There are not many effective antiviral drugs, and each one has a limited range of action. These agents function to:

- block removal of the protein coat of the virus after it enters a cell, as in treatment of influenza A virus.

- block production of viral nucleic acid, as does the drug AZT (zidovudine). The reverse transcriptase inhibitors used to treat HIV infections block the enzyme needed for viral RNA to function in the host cell.

- block enzymes that are needed to assemble and release new virus particles, as does the drug indinavir, a so-called *protease inhibitor*, used to treat HIV infection.

Note that viruses mutate rapidly to become resistant to these drugs, and none can eliminate latent (temporarily inactive) infections. In treating AIDS, the drugs are commonly used in combinations.

Laboratory Identification of Pathogens

The nurse, physician, or laboratory worker often obtains specimens from patients to identify bacteria and other organisms. Specimens most frequently studied are blood, spinal fluid, feces, urine, and sputum, along with swabbings from other areas. Swabs are used to collect specimens from the nose, throat, eyes, and cervix as well as from ulcers or other infected areas. The healthcare worker must label each specimen completely and accurately with the patient's name, appropriate identification, source of the specimen, physician's name, the date, and time. He or she must then deliver it to the laboratory promptly.

Bacterial Isolations and Tests

In the lab, bacterial cells are grown out in cultures using substances called **media**, such as nutrient broth or agar, that the bacteria can use as food. Individual organisms are then isolated, that is, separated from other cells in the specimen, usually by streaking the cultures over the surface of a solid medium. The isolated cells then multiply to form separate colonies (clones) on the surface of the medium (Fig. 5-14). The laboratory technicians then perform a variety of tests to identify the organism or organisms obtained from the specimen. At this time, the organism is usually tested for sensitivity to various antibiotics that might be used to treat the infection. This whole procedure is described as a culture and sensitivity (C & S).

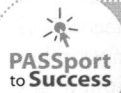

PASSport to Success   Visit **thePoint** or see the Student Resource CD in the back of this book for more information on careers in medical technology.

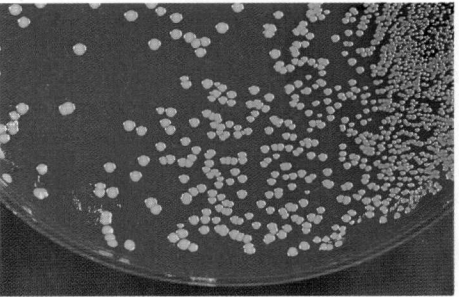

Figure 5-14   **Isolated colonies of bacteria growing on a solid medium.** Each colony contains all the offspring of a single cell. (Reprinted with permission from Koneman EW, Alien SD, Janda WM, et al. *Color Atlas and Textbook of Diagnostic Microbiology*, 5th ed. Philadelphia: Lippincott Williams & Wilkins, 1997.)

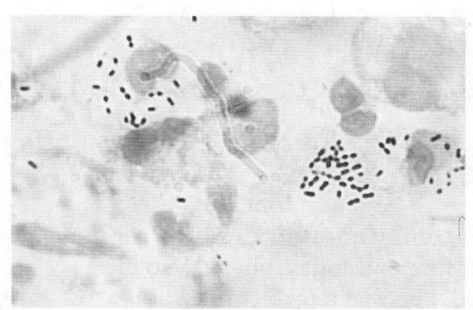 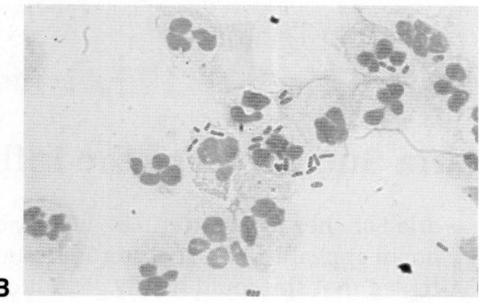

A   **B**

Figure 5-15 **Gram's stained bacteria. (A)** Gram-positive diplococci. **(B)** Gram-negative bacilli among white blood cells in a urine sediment. (Reprinted with permission from Koneman EW, Alien SD, Janda WM, et al. *Color Atlas and Textbook of Diagnostic Microbiology*, 5th ed. Philadelphia: Lippincott Williams & Wilkins, 1997.)

5

Staining Techniques

One of the most frequently used methods for beginning the process of identification involves examining the cells under the microscope. To make the cells visible under the microscope, they must first be stained with colored dyes (stains), which are applied to a thin smear of the culture on a glass slide. The most commonly used staining procedure is known as the **Gram's stain** (Fig. 5-15). A bluish purple dye (such as crystal violet) is applied, and then a weak iodine solution is added. This causes a colorfast combination within certain organisms, so that washing with alcohol does not remove the dye. These bacteria are said to be *Gram positive* and appear bluish purple under the microscope (Fig. 5-15A). Examples are the pathogenic staphylococci and streptococci; the cocci that cause certain types of pneumonia; and the bacilli that produce diphtheria, tetanus, and anthrax. Other organisms are said to be *Gram negative* because the coloring can be removed from them with a solvent. These are then stained for visibility, usually with a red dye (see Fig. 5-15B). Examples of gram-negative organisms are the diplococci that cause gonorrhea and epidemic meningitis and the bacilli that produce typhoid fever, pneumonia, and one type of dysentery. The colon bacillus (*E. coli*) normally found in the intestine is also Gram negative, as is the cholera vibrio. Can you tell which of the organisms in Figure 5-3 are Gram positive and which are Gram negative?

Another stain used to identify organisms is the **acid-fast stain**. After being stained with a reddish dye (carbolfuchsin), the smear is treated with acid. Most bacteria quickly lose their stain upon application of the acid, but the organisms that cause tuberculosis and other acid-fast cells retain the red stain. The negative cells are then stained with a different dye, usually a blue one.

A few organisms, such as the spirochetes of syphilis and the rickettsiae, do not stain with any of the commonly used dyes. Special techniques must be used to identify these organisms.

Other Methods of Identification

In addition to the various staining procedures, laboratory techniques for identifying bacteria include:

- observing the cultures' growth characteristics in liquid and solid medium.
- studying the cells' oxygen requirements.
- observing the ability of the bacteria to utilize (ferment) various carbohydrates (sugars).
- analyzing reactions to various test chemicals.
- studying the bacteria by serologic (immunologic) tests based on the antigen–antibody reaction (see Chapter 17).

Laboratories now use modern techniques of genetic analysis to identify organisms based on their nucleic acids. They use the polymerase chain reaction (PCR) to make multiple copies of an organism's unique DNA or RNA sequences. These sequences are then identified by so-called "genetic fingerprinting" methods. Genetic tests are faster and cheaper than standard culturing procedures and can be used directly on a patient specimen. Scientists have used PCR to identify the infectious agent for diseases such as AIDS, hepatitis, and Lyme disease, and for identifying the pathogens that cause emerging diseases such as West Nile disease and severe acute respiratory syndrome (SARS). Epidemiologists use PCR to identify the source and monitor the spread of infections in a population, because it can identify individuals infected with the same strain of an organism.

CHECKPOINT **5-19** ➤ One way of identifying microorganisms is to examine them under a microscope. Before examination, the cells are colored so they can be seen. What are the dyes used to color the cells called?

Disease in Context revisited

➤ Maria Succumbs to the Influenza Virus

Maria Sanchez looked terrible—watery eyes, runny nose, and a sickly, run-down appearance. Just yesterday, she felt fine. But today, she was so fatigued that she could hardly get out of bed. She had a fever, chills, and a cough that left her throat aching. Maria was certainly feeling the effects of the influenza virus that had invaded the epithelial lining of her respiratory tract about 3 days ago.

Many of Maria's local symptoms were due to the virus. Her watery eyes and runny nose were the result of extracellular fluid leaking from holes in the mucous membrane lining her respiratory tract—holes left from the death and shedding of millions of epithelial cells! Without these ciliated cells, Maria wasn't able to move the extra fluid up and out of her respiratory tract, so she periodically coughed in an effort to do so. Maria's systemic symptoms were due, in large part, to her body's counter-attack against the virus. Since viruses work most efficiently at near-normal body temperature, her fever actually slowed viral replication. Her fatigue helped beat the virus too. By staying in bed, her body was able to conserve energy that her immune system could use to fight the virus. In a few days, that system would beat the virus and she would make a complete recovery.

During this case, we saw that the influenza virus that invaded Maria's body is designed to hijack her epithelial cells and force them to make new viruses. Maria's body is also well-designed to combat the virus. In Chapter 17, Body Defenses, Immunity, and Vaccines, we'll revisit Maria again and learn how immunization can help protect Maria from influenza in the future.

Word Anatomy

Medical terms are built from standardized word parts (prefixes, roots, and suffixes). Learning the meanings of these parts can help you remember words and interpret unfamiliar terms.

WORD PART	MEANING	EXAMPLE
Categories of Disease		
psych/o	mind	The medical field of *psychiatry* specializes in treatment of mental disorders.
pre-	before	A *predisposing* cause enters into production of disease.
Study of Disease		
idio-	self, separate, distinct	An *idiopathic* disease has no known cause; it is "self-originating."
iatro	physician, medicine	An *iatrogenic* disease results from the adverse effects of treatment.
pan-	all	A *pandemic* disease is prevalent throughout an entire country, continent, or the world.
syn-	together	A *syndrome* is a group of symptoms and signs that together characterize a disease.
chir/o	hand	*Chiropractic* treatment involves use of the hands for manipulation to correct misalignment of the body.
Infectious Disease		
myc/o	fungus	*Mycology* is the study of fungi.
aer/o	air, gas	An *aerobic* organism requires air (oxygen) to grow.
an-	absent, deficient, lack of	An *anaerobic* organism does not require air (oxygen) to grow.
tox/o	poison	Bacteria can harm the body by producing *toxins*.
diplo-	double	*Diplococci* are round bacteria arranged in pairs.
strepto-	chain	*Streptococci* are round bacteria arranged in chains.
staphylo-	grapelike cluster	*Staphylococci* are bacteria in clusters.
py/o	pus	The species name *pyogenes* indicates that an organism produces pus.
Microbial Control		
septic	poison, rot, decay	*Aseptic* methods are used to kill or prevent the growth of microorganisms.
–cide	kill or destroy	A *bactericide* is an agent that kills bacteria.

5

Summary

I. **CATEGORIES OF DISEASE**—infection, degenerative disease, nutritional disorders, metabolic disorders, immune disorders, neoplasms, psychiatric disorders
   A. Predisposing causes of disease—age, gender, heredity, living conditions and habits, emotional disturbance, physical and chemical damage, preexisting illness

II. **THE STUDY OF DISEASE**—pathophysiology
   A. Disease terminology
      1. Etiology—study of origin or causation
      2. Terms related to severity and duration
         a. Acute—severe, of short duration
         b. Chronic—less severe, of long duration
         c. Subacute—intermediate, between acute and chronic
      3. Idiopathic—of unknown cause
      4. Iatrogenic—results from adverse effects of treatment
      5. Epidemiology—study of diseases in populations
         a. Statistics
            (1) Incidence—number of new cases in a population during specific time
            (2) Prevalence—number of cases in a population at a given time
            (3) Mortality rate—percentage of the population that dies from disease within a given period
         b. Categories
            (1) Epidemic—widespread in a given region
            (2) Endemic—found at lesser level but continuously in a population
            (3) Pandemic—prevalent throughout an entire country or the world

III. **TREATMENT AND PREVENTION OF DISEASE**
   A. Diagnosis—determination of the nature of the illness
      1. Symptom—change in body function felt by the patient
      2. Sign—change in body function observable by others
      3. Syndrome—group of signs and symptoms that characterize a disease
   B. Prognosis—prediction of probable outcome of disease
   C. Therapy—course of treatment
   D. Complementary and alternative medicine (CAM)—methods of disease prevention or treatment used along with or instead of traditional modern medical practices—e.g. naturopathy, chiropractic, acupuncture, biofeedback
      1. Herbal remedies—plant products

   E. Prevention of disease—removal of potential causes of disease

IV. **INFECTIOUS DISEASE**
   A. Parasite—organism that lives on or within a host at host's expense
   B. Pathogen—disease-causing organism
   C. Infection—invasion by pathogens with adverse effects
      1. Local—small area
      2. Systemic—generalized; usually spread by blood
   D. Opportunistic infection—takes hold in a weakened host
   E. Communicable infection—can be spread from person to person; is contagious
   F. Modes of transmission
      1. Direct contact
      2. Indirect—touched objects, air, pests
         a. Vector—animal that transfers organisms from host to host
      3. Portals of entry and exit—skin, respiratory, digestive, urinary, and reproductive systems

V. **MICROBIOLOGY—THE STUDY OF MICROORGANISMS**
   A. Normal flora—population of microorganisms normally growing on and within the body
   B. Bacteria
      1. Some features
         a. Oxygen requirements—aerobic, anaerobic, facultative anaerobes
         b. Endospores—resistant forms
         c. Flagella—used for swimming
         d. Pili—short, threadlike; used for attachment
      2. Shape and arrangement
         a. Cocci—round
            (1) Diplococci—pairs
            (2) Streptococci—chains
            (3) Staphylococci—clusters
         b. Bacilli—straight rods; some produce endospores
         c. Curved rods
            (1) Vibrios—comma shaped
            (2) Spirilla—corkscrew or wavy
            (3) Spirochetes—flexible spirals
      3. Other bacteria—obligate intracellular parasites
         a. Rickettsiae
         b. Chlamydiae
   C. Viruses
      1. Contain only nucleic acid and protein
      2. Obligate intracellular parasites
      3. Infectious agents smaller than viruses
         a. Prions—contain only protein; cause slow-growing brain diseases

  b. Viroids—contain only RNA
D. Fungi—simple, plantlike organisms
  1. Yeasts—single cell
  2. Molds—filamentous
E. Protozoa—single-cell, animal-like organisms
  1. Amebas—dysentery
  2. Ciliates
  3. Flagellates—African sleeping sickness, giardiasis
  4. Sporozoa (apicomplexans)—malaria, *Cryptosporidium* infection

VI. PARASITIC WORMS (HELMINTHS)
A. Roundworms
  1. Ascaris
  2. Pinworms
  3. Hookworms
  4. Trichina—transmitted in undercooked meat
  5. Filaria—causes filariasis (elephantiasis)
B. Flatworms
  1. Tapeworms
  2. Flukes

VII. MICROBIAL CONTROL
A. Emergence and spread of microorganisms—factors related to population growth, technology
B. Microbes and public health
  1. Sewage and garbage disposal
  2. Water purification
  3. Prevention of food contamination
  4. Milk pasteurization
C. Aseptic methods
  1. Sterilization—killing of all organisms
  2. Disinfection—destruction of all pathogens (except endospores); bactericidal
  3. Antisepsis—pathogens killed or prevented from multiplying (bacteriostasis); safe for living tissue

D. Infection control techniques
  1. Body substance precautions (body substance isolation)
   a. Assume all body fluids potentially infective
   b. Barriers—gloves, masks, eye protection, gowns
   c. Handwashing stressed
   d. OSHA—Occupational Safety and Health Administration
E. Antimicrobial agents—interfere with essential metabolism
  1. Antibiotics—antibacterial agents
   a. Disadvantages—opportunistic infections, bacterial resistance, nosocomial (hospital-acquired) infections
  2. Antivirals—block removal of protein coat, production of nucleic acid, assembly and release of new virus

VIII. LABORATORY IDENTIFICATION OF PATHOGENS
A. Collection of specimens; accurate labeling and prompt delivery to lab
B. Bacterial isolations and tests
C. Staining techniques (e.g., Gram's, acid-fast)
D. Other methods of identification
  1. Growth characteristics
  2. Oxygen requirements
  3. Fermentation
  4. Reactions to test chemicals
  5. Serologic (immunologic) tests
  6. Genetic analysis
   a. PCR (polymerase chain reaction) duplicates unique nucleic acids
   b. Segments identified for a genetic "fingerprint"

Questions for Study and Review

BUILDING UNDERSTANDING

Fill in the blanks

1. An inadequate diet may result in _____ disorders such as scurvy or rickets.

2. The study of the cause of any disease or the theory of its origin is _____.

3. A(n) _____ infection attacks an individual already weakened by disease.

4. Mycotic infections are caused by _____.

5. Certain molds and soil bacteria produce bacteria-killing substances called _____.

Matching > Match each numbered item with the most closely related lettered item.

____ **6.** Organisms that cause pneumonia, diphtheria, and syphilis

____ **7.** Organisms that cause AIDS, hepatitis, and the common cold

____ **8.** Organisms that cause athlete's foot, ringworm, and thrush

____ **9.** Organisms that cause amebic dysentery, giardiasis, and malaria

____ **10.** Organisms that cause pinworm, trichinosis, and filariasis

a. protozoa

b. helminths

c. viruses

d. fungi

e. bacteria

Multiple Choice

____ **11.** The incidence of early heart disease is higher in men than women. A predisposing cause of this disease appears to be

a. age
b. gender
c. heredity
d. living conditions and habits

____ **12.** A syndrome is defined as a

a. disease accompanied by a characteristic group of signs and symptoms
b. widespread disease
c. disease that is neither acute nor chronic
d. communicable disease

____ **13.** Structures that allow some bacteria to move along solid surfaces are called

a. endospores
b. flagella
c. pili
d. vibrios

____ **14.** Which of the following protozoa are obligate parasites?

a. amebas
b. flagellates
c. sporozoa
d. ciliates

____ **15.** An antibiotic should be prescribed only for a

a. fungal infection
b. viral infection
c. parasitic infection
d. bacterial infection

UNDERSTANDING CONCEPTS

16. Explain the difference between the terms in each of the following pairs:

a. acute and chronic
b. epidemic and endemic
c. symptom and sign
d. host and parasite
e. pathogen and vector

17. List five portals that pathogens may use to enter or exit the body.

18. Classify bacteria into three groups based on oxygen requirements and three groups based on shape.

19. How do rickettsiae and chlamydiae differ from other bacteria in size and living habits? Name some diseases caused by rickettsiae and chlamydiae.

20. What is the difference between a virus and a prion?

21. Explain how an infectious disease can emerge and spread across the country and the world. Name some public health measures that can prevent disease outbreaks.

22. Why are standard precautions followed? What measures are included in the use of standard precautions?

CONCEPTUAL THINKING

23. While you are on a work-exchange program in the tropics, a cholera epidemic sweeps through the area where you are staying. Of the 1,000 people living in the area, 100 people contract cholera and 10 die of it in 1 month. What is the percentage incidence and mortality rate of cholera during that time? What precautions could you take to lessen your risk of contracting this bacterial disease?

24. Mr. Baker is in the hospital with severe burns to more than half of his body. His chart calls for close adherence to aseptic methods. Describe three procedures used in healthcare facilities to ensure asepsis. What kind of infection is Mr. Baker at increased risk of contracting during his long recovery in the hospital?

25. While working in the lab, you are given the job of identifying bacteria cultured from a patient's sputum sample. You smear a sample of the bacteria onto a glass slide and Gram's stain it. Microscopic examination reveals bluish purple cells arranged in chains. What do you think the bacteria could be? What disease could the patient have? What kind of drug therapy may be prescribed?

26. In Maria's case, what was the virus' portal of entry? To prevent Maria from spreading the virus to other people, what infection control technique would you suggest?

5

CHAPTER 6

The Skin in Health and Disease

Learning Outcomes

After careful study of this chapter, you should be able to:

1. Name and describe the layers of the skin
2. Describe the subcutaneous tissue
3. Give the location and function of the accessory structures of the skin
4. List the main functions of the skin
5. Summarize the information to be gained by observation of the skin
6. List the main disorders of the skin
7. Show how word parts are used to build words related to the skin (see Word Anatomy at the end of the chapter)

Selected Key Terms

The following terms and other boldface terms in the chapter are defined in the Glossary

alopecia
arrector pili
cicatrix
dermatitis
dermis
epidermis
erythema
exfoliation
integument
keloid
keratin
lesion
melanin
scar
sebaceous
sebum
stratum
subcutaneous
sudoriferous

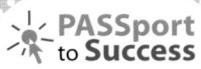

PASSport to Success

Visit *thePoint* or see the Student Resource CD in the back of this book for definitions and pronunciations of key terms as well as a pretest for this chapter.

Disease in Context

➤ Paul's Case: Sun-Damaged Skin

"Wait a minute," Paul said to his reflection in the mirror as he trimmed his goatee after shaving. He had noticed a small nodule to the side of his left nostril. The lump was mostly pink with a pearly-white border, and painless to the touch. *I haven't seen that before. Probably just a pimple, or maybe a small cyst*, Paul thought, although he couldn't help thinking back to the many hours he had spent as a kid sailing competitively at the seashore. *I know sun exposure isn't great for your skin, even dangerous, and I wasn't real careful about wearing sunscreen. Even if I did, it would have washed off anyway while I was sailing*, he rationalized. Paul finished his trimming and decided the lump was probably nothing.

Despite his attempts to forget about the lump, Paul was concerned. Over the next several days he showed the small, rounded mass to several people to get their opinions. No one had an answer when he asked, "What do you think this is?" When several weeks produced no change, except maybe a little depression in the center of the mass, worry led him to make an appointment with a dermatologist.

"Well Paul, I'm not sure. It could be nothing, but we better look a little closer," said Dr. Nielsen. "It could be benign, but we have to be sure that it's not a small skin cancer. This is a very common site for such a lesion. Basal cell and squamous cell carcinomas arise from the underlying epithelial cells of the skin, especially in sun-exposed areas. UV rays from the sun can damage DNA, causing the cells to divide more rapidly than normal, resulting in an abnormal growth. Basal cell and squamous cell carcinomas are the most common forms of cancer but are usually completely treatable. We'll remove this and send it to the pathology lab to see what's going on." Paul left Dr. Nielsen's office with a small bandage over the site of excision, some ointment to apply, and instructions to call the office in 3 days.

Paul's dermatologist suspects that Paul may have skin cancer—a disease affecting the integumentary system. In this chapter, we'll learn that skin is just one part of the system. Later in the chapter, we'll revisit Paul and learn the final diagnosis of that lump on his nose.

The skin is the one system that can be inspected in its entirety without requiring surgery or special equipment. The skin not only gives clues to its own health but also reflects the health of other body systems. Although the skin may be viewed simply as a membrane enveloping the body, it is far more complex than the other epithelial membranes described in Chapter 4.

The skin is associated with accessory structures, also known as appendages, which include glands, hair, and nails. Together with blood vessels, nerves, and sensory organs, the skin and its associated structures form the **integumentary** (in-teg-u-MEN-tar-e) **system.** This name is from the word integument (in-TEG-u-ment), which means "covering." The term cutaneous (ku-TA-ne-us) also refers to the skin. The functions of this system are discussed later in the chapter after a description of its structure.

> **PASSport to Success**
> Visit *thePoint* or see the Student Resource CD in the back of this book for a summary chart of skin structures.

Structure of the Skin

The skin consists of two layers (Fig. 6-1):

- The **epidermis** (ep-ih-DER-mis), the outermost portion, which itself is subdivided into thin layers called **strata** (STRA-tah) (sing. stratum). The epidermis is composed entirely of epithelial cells and contains no blood vessels.

- The **dermis,** or true skin, has a framework of connective tissue and contains many blood vessels, nerve endings, and glands.

Figure 6-2 is a photograph of the skin as seen through a microscope showing the layers and some accessory structures.

Epidermis

The epidermis is the surface portion of the skin, the outermost cells of which are constantly lost through wear and tear. Because there are no blood vessels in the epidermis,

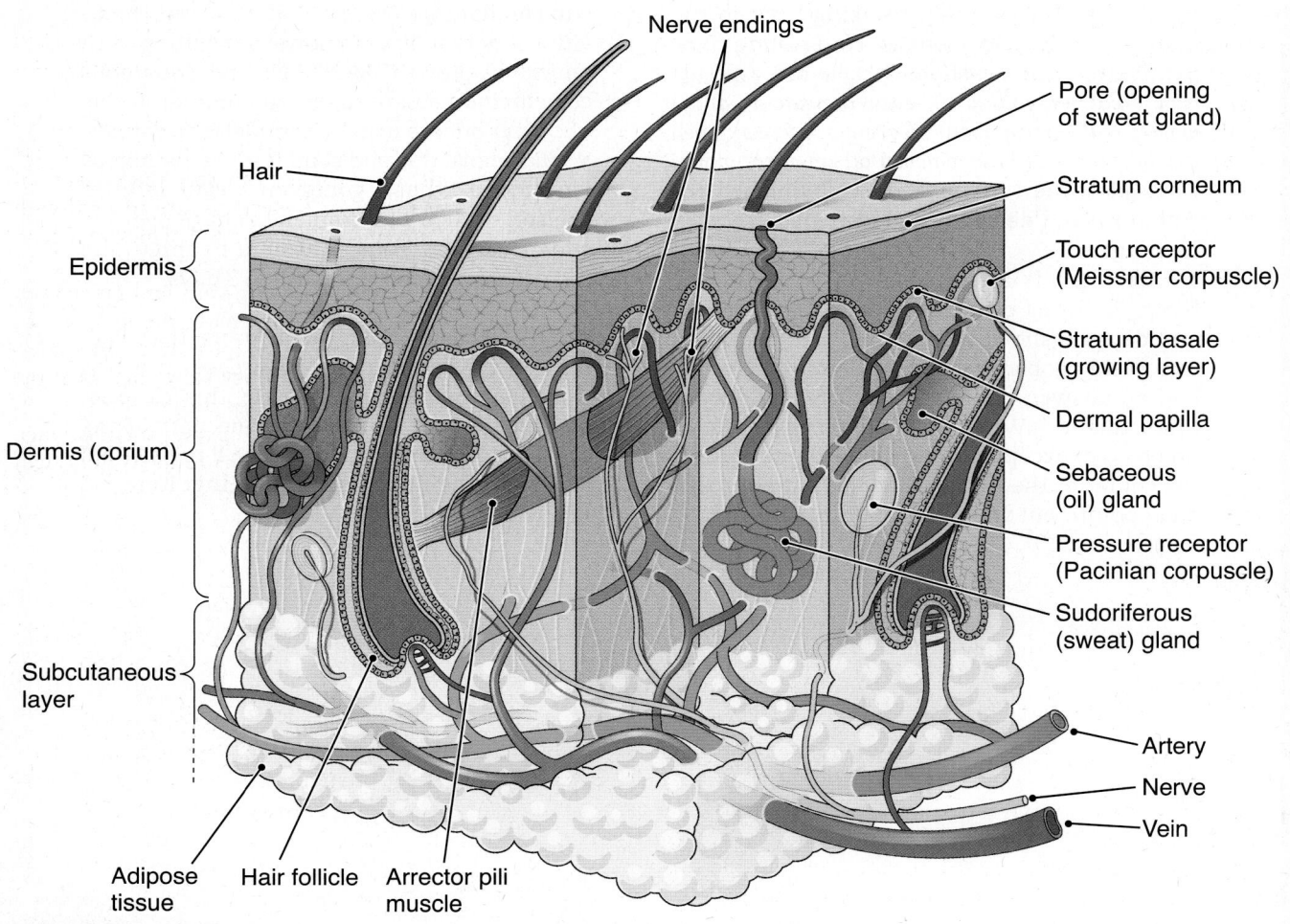

Nerve endings

Hair

Epidermis

Dermis (corium)

Subcutaneous layer

Adipose tissue

Hair follicle

Arrector pili muscle

Pore (opening of sweat gland)

Stratum corneum

Touch receptor (Meissner corpuscle)

Stratum basale (growing layer)

Dermal papilla

Sebaceous (oil) gland

Pressure receptor (Pacinian corpuscle)

Sudoriferous (sweat) gland

Artery

Nerve

Vein

Figure 6-1 **Cross-section of the skin.**

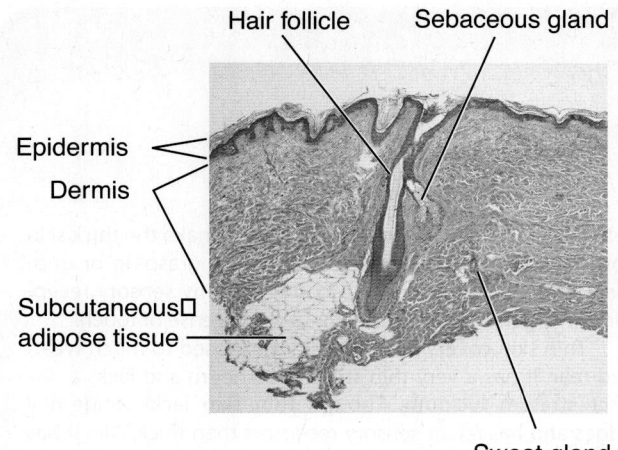

Hair follicle   Sebaceous gland

Epidermis

Dermis

Subcutaneous☐
adipose tissue

Sweat gland

Figure 6-2 **Microscopic view of thin skin.** Tissue layers and some accessory structures are labeled. (Reprinted with permission from Cormack DH. *Essential Histology*, 2nd ed. Philadelphia: Lippincott Williams & Wilkins, 2001.)

the cells must be nourished by capillaries in the underlying dermis. New epidermal cells are produced in the deepest layer, which is closest to the dermis. The cells in this layer, the **stratum basale** (bas-A-le), or **stratum germinativum** (jer-min-a-TI-vum), are constantly dividing and producing daughter cells, which are then pushed upward toward the skin's surface. As the epidermal cells die from the gradual loss of nourishment, they undergo changes. Mainly, their cytoplasm is replaced by large amounts of a protein called **keratin** (KER-ah-tin), which thickens and protects the skin (Fig. 6-3).

By the time epidermal cells approach the surface, they have become flat, filled with keratin, and horny, forming the uppermost layer of the epidermis, the **stratum corneum**

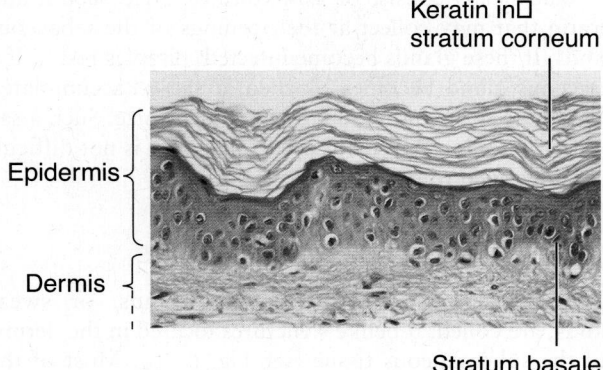

Keratin in☐
stratum corneum

Epidermis

Dermis

Stratum basale

Figure 6-3 **Upper portion of the skin.** Layers of keratin in the stratum corneum are visible at the surface. Below are layers of stratified squamous epithelium making up the remainder of the epidermis. (Reprinted with permission from Cormack DH. *Essential Histology*, 2nd ed. Philadelphia: Lippincott Williams & Wilkins, 2001.)

(KOR-ne-um). The stratum corneum is a protective layer and is more prominent in thick skin than in thin skin. Cells at the surface are constantly being lost and replaced from below, especially in areas of the skin that are subject to wear and tear, as on the scalp, face, soles of the feet, and palms of the hands. Although this process of **exfoliation** (eks-fo-le-A-shun) occurs naturally at all times, many cosmetics companies sell products to promote exfoliation, presumably to "enliven" and "refresh" the skin.

Between the stratum basale and the stratum corneum there are additional layers of stratified epithelium that vary in number and quantity depending on the skin's thickness.

Cells in the deepest layer of the epidermis produce **melanin** (MEL-ah-nin), a dark pigment that colors the skin and protects it from the harmful rays of sunlight. The cells that produce this pigment are the **melanocytes** (MEL-ah-no-sites). Irregular patches of melanin are called freckles.

Dermis

The **dermis**, the so-called "true skin," has a framework of elastic connective tissue and is well supplied with blood vessels and nerves. Because of its elasticity, the skin can stretch, even dramatically as in pregnancy, with little damage. Most of the skin's accessory structures, including the sweat glands, the oil glands, and the hair, are located in the dermis and may extend into the subcutaneous layer under the skin.

The thickness of the dermis also varies in different areas. Some places, such as the soles of the feet and the palms of the hands, are covered with very thick layers of skin, whereas others, such as the eyelids, are covered with very thin and delicate layers. (See Box 6-1, Thick and Thin Skin: Getting a Grip on Their Differences.)

Portions of the dermis extend upward into the epidermis, allowing blood vessels to get closer to the surface cells (see Figs. 6-1 and 6-2). These extensions, or **dermal papillae**, can be seen on the surface of thick skin, such as at the tips of the fingers and toes. Here they form a distinct pattern of ridges that help to prevent slipping, such as when grasping an object. The unchanging patterns of the ridges are determined by heredity. Because they are unique to each person, fingerprints and footprints can be used for identification.

CHECKPOINT **6-1** ▶ The skin and all its associated structures comprise a body system. What is the name of this system?

CHECKPOINT **6-2** ▶ The skin itself is composed of two layers. Moving from the superficial to the deeper layer, what are the names of these two layers?

Subcutaneous Layer

The dermis rests on the **subcutaneous** (sub-ku-TA-ne-us) **layer**, sometimes referred to as the hypodermis or the su-

Box 6-1 A Closer Look

Thick and Thin Skin: Getting a Grip on Their Differences

The skin is the largest organ in the body, weighing about 4 kg. Though it appears uniform in structure and function, its thickness in fact varies, from less than 1 mm covering the eyelids to more than 5 mm on the upper back. Many of the functional differences between skin regions reflect the thickness of the epidermis and not the skin's overall thickness. Based on epidermal thickness, skin can be categorized as **thick** (about 1 mm deep) or **thin** (about 0.1 mm deep).

Areas of the body exposed to significant wear-and-tear (the palms, fingertips, and bottoms of the feet and toes) are covered with thick skin. It is composed of a thick stratum corneum and an extra layer not found in thin skin, the stratum lucidum, both of which make thick skin resistant to abrasion. Thick skin is also characterized by epidermal ridges (e.g., fingerprints) and numerous sweat glands, but lacks hair and

sebaceous (oil) glands. These adaptations make the thick skin covering the hands and feet effective for grasping or gripping. Thick skin's dermis also contains many sensory receptors, giving the hands and feet a superior sense of touch.

Thin skin covers body areas not exposed to much wear-and-tear. It has a very thin stratum corneum and lacks a distinct stratum lucidum. Though thin skin lacks epidermal ridges and has fewer sensory receptors than thick skin, it has several specializations that thick skin does not. Thin skin is covered with hair, which may help prevent heat loss from the body. In fact, hair is most densely distributed in skin that covers regions of great heat loss—the head, axillae (armpits), and groin. Thin skin also contains numerous sebaceous glands, making it supple and free of cracks that might let infectious organisms enter.

---

perficial fascia (see Fig. 6-1). This layer connects the skin to the surface muscles. It consists of loose connective tissue and large amounts of adipose (fat) tissue. The fat serves as insulation and as a reserve energy supply. Continuous bundles of elastic fibers connect the subcutaneous tissue with the dermis, so there is no clear boundary between the two.

The blood vessels that supply the skin with nutrients and oxygen and help to regulate body temperature run through the subcutaneous layer. This tissue is also rich in nerves and nerve endings, including those that supply nerve impulses to and from the dermis and epidermis. The thickness of the subcutaneous layer varies in different parts of the body; it is thinnest on the eyelids and thickest on the abdomen.

CHECKPOINT **6-3** ➤ What is the composition of the subcutaneous layer?

Accessory Structures of the Skin

The integumentary system includes some structures associated with the skin—glands, hair, and nails—that not only protect the skin itself but have some more generalized functions as well.

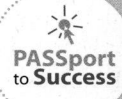

PASSport to Success Visit **thePoint** or see the Student Resource CD in the back of this book for a summary of the skin's accessory structures.

Sebaceous (Oil) Glands

The **sebaceous** (se-BA-shus) **glands** are saclike in structure, and their oily secretion, **sebum** (SE-bum), lubricates the skin and hair and prevents drying. The ducts of the sebaceous glands open into the hair follicles (Fig. 6-4A).

Babies are born with a covering produced by these glands that resembles cream cheese; this secretion is called the **vernix caseosa** (VER-niks ka-se-O-sah), which literally means "cheesy varnish." Modified sebaceous glands, **meibomian** (mi-BO-me-an) **glands**, are associated with the eyelashes and produce a secretion that lubricates the eyes.

Blackheads consist of a mixture of dried sebum and keratin that may collect at the openings of the sebaceous glands. If these glands become infected, pimples result. If a sebaceous gland becomes blocked, a sac of accumulated sebum may form and gradually increase in size. Such a sac is referred to as a **sebaceous cyst**. Usually, it is not difficult to remove such tumorlike cysts by surgery.

Sudoriferous (Sweat) Glands

The **sudoriferous** (su-do-RIF-er-us) **glands**, or sweat glands, are coiled, tubelike structures located in the dermis and the subcutaneous tissue (see Fig. 6-4B). Most of the sudoriferous glands function to cool the body. They release sweat, or perspiration, that draws heat from the skin as the moisture evaporates at the surface. These **eccrine** (EK-rin) type sweat glands are distributed throughout the skin. Each gland has a secretory portion and an excretory tube that extends directly to the surface and opens at a pore (see also Fig. 6-1). Because sweat contains small

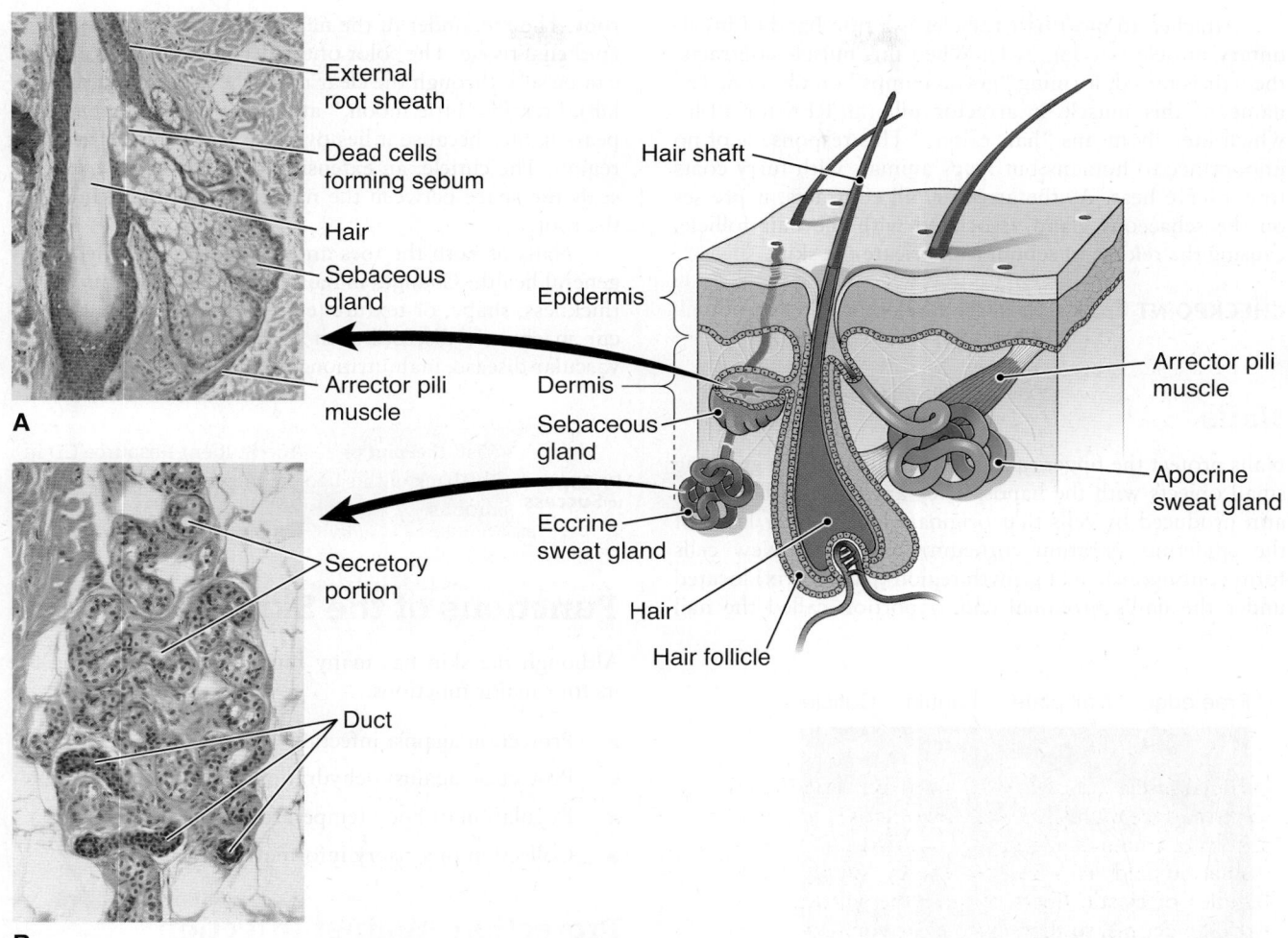

A

B

External root sheath

Dead cells forming sebum

Hair

Sebaceous gland

Arrector pili muscle

Secretory portion

Duct

Hair shaft

Epidermis

Dermis

Sebaceous gland

Eccrine sweat gland

Hair

Hair follicle

Arrector pili muscle

Apocrine sweat gland

Figure 6-4 **Portion of skin showing associated glands and hair. (A)** A sebaceous (oil) gland and its associated hair follicle. **(B)** An eccrine (temperature-regulating) sweat gland. (A and B, Reprinted with permission from Cormack DH. *Essential Histology*, 2nd ed. Philadelphia: Lippincott Williams & Wilkins, 2001.) **[ZOOMING IN ➤** How do the sebaceous glands and apocrine sweat glands secrete to the outside? What kind of epithelium makes up the sweat glands? **]**

amounts of dissolved salts and other wastes in addition to water, these glands also serve a minor excretory function.

Present in smaller number, the **apocrine** (AP-o-krin) sweat glands are located mainly in the armpits (axillae) and groin area. These glands become active at puberty and release their secretions through the hair follicles in response to emotional stress and sexual stimulation. The apocrine glands release some cellular material in their secretions. Body odor develops from the action of bacteria in breaking down these organic cellular materials.

Several types of glands associated with the skin are modified sweat glands. These are the **ceruminous** (seh-RU-min-us) **glands** in the ear canal that produce ear wax, or **cerumen**; the **ciliary** (SIL-e-er-e) **glands** at the edges of the eyelids; and the **mammary glands**.

CHECKPOINT **6-4** ➤ Some skin glands produce an oily secretion called sebum. What is the name of these glands?

CHECKPOINT **6-5** ➤ What is the scientific name for the sweat glands?

Hair

Almost all of the body is covered with hair, which in most areas is soft and fine. Hairless regions are the palms of the hands, soles of the feet, lips, nipples, and parts of the external genital areas. Hair is composed mainly of keratin and is not living. Each hair develops, however, from living cells located in a bulb at the base of the **hair follicle**, a sheath of epithelial and connective tissue that encloses the hair (see Fig. 6-4). Melanocytes in this growth region add pigment to the developing hair. Different shades of melanin produce the various hair colors we see in the population. The part of the hair that projects above the skin is the **shaft**; the portion below the skin is the **root** of the hair.

Attached to most hair follicles is a thin band of involuntary muscle (see Fig. 6-1). When this muscle contracts, the hair is raised, forming "goose bumps" on the skin. The name of this muscle is **arrector pili** (ah-REK-tor PI-li), which literally means "hair raiser." This response is of no importance to humans but helps animals with furry coats to conserve heat. As the arrector pili contracts, it presses on the sebaceous gland associated with the hair follicle, causing the release of sebum to lubricate the skin.

CHECKPOINT **6-6** ➤ Each hair develops within a sheath. What is this sheath called?

Nails

Nails protect the fingers and toes and also help in grasping small objects with the hands. They are made of hard keratin produced by cells that originate in the outer layer of the epidermis (stratum corneum) (Fig. 6-5). New cells form continuously in a growth region (nail matrix) located under the nail's proximal end, a portion called the **nail**

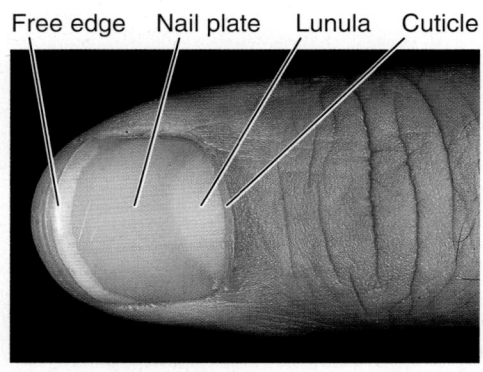

A

Free edge | Nail plate | Lunula | Cuticle

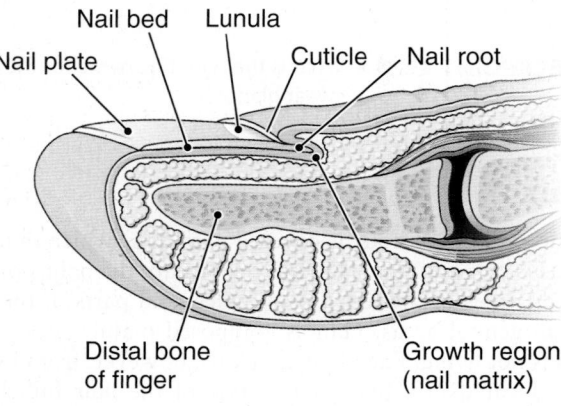

B

Nail bed | Lunula
Nail plate
Cuticle | Nail root
Distal bone of finger
Growth region (nail matrix)

Figure 6-5 **Nail structure. (A)** Photograph of a nail, superior view. **(B)** Midsagittal section of a fingertip. (A, Reprinted with permission from Bickley LS. *Bates' Guide to Physical Examination and History Taking*, 8th ed. Philadelphia: Lippincott Williams & Wilkins, 2003.)

root. The remainder of the **nail plate** rests on a **nail bed** of epithelial tissue. The color of the dermis below the nail bed can be seen through the clear nail. The pale **lunula** (LU-nu-lah), literally "little moon," at the nail's proximal end appears lighter because it lies over the nail's thicker growing region. The **cuticle**, an extension of the stratum corneum, seals the space between the nail plate and the skin above the root.

Nails of both the toes and the fingers are affected by general health. Changes in nails, including abnormal color, thickness, shape, or texture (e.g., grooves or splitting), occur in chronic diseases such as heart disease, peripheral vascular disease, malnutrition, and anemia.

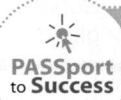

PASSport to Success

Visit *thePoint* or see the Student Resource CD in the back of this book to view some of these conditions.

Functions of the Skin

Although the skin has many functions, the following are its four major functions:

- Protection against infection
- Protection against dehydration (drying)
- Regulation of body temperature
- Collection of sensory information

Protection Against Infection

Intact skin forms a primary barrier against invasion of pathogens. The cells of the stratum corneum form a tight interlocking pattern that resists penetration. The surface cells are constantly shed, thus mechanically removing pathogens. Rupture of this barrier, as in cases of wounds or burns, invites infection of deep tissues. The skin also protects against bacterial toxins (poisons) and some harmful chemicals in the environment.

Protection Against Dehydration

Both keratin in the epidermis and the oily sebum released to the skin's surface from the sebaceous glands help to waterproof the skin and prevent water loss by evaporation.

Regulation of Body Temperature

Both the loss of excess heat and protection from cold are important functions of the skin. Indeed, most of the skin's blood flow is concerned with temperature regulation. In cold conditions, vessels in the skin constrict (become narrower) to reduce blood flow to the surface and diminish heat loss. The skin may become visibly pale under these conditions. Special vessels that directly connect arteries and veins in the skin of the ears, nose, and other exposed locations provide the volume of blood flow needed to prevent freezing.

To cool the body, the skin forms a large surface for radiating body heat to the surrounding air. When the blood vessels dilate (widen), more blood is brought to the surface so that heat can be dissipated.

The other mechanism for cooling the body involves the sweat glands, as noted above. The evaporation of perspiration draws heat from the skin. A person feels uncomfortable on a hot and humid day because water does not evaporate as readily from the skin into the surrounding air. A dehumidifier makes one more comfortable even when the temperature remains high.

As is the case with so many body functions, temperature regulation is complex and involves other areas, including certain centers in the brain.

Collection of Sensory Information

Because of its many nerve endings and other special receptors, the skin may be regarded as one of the body's chief sensory organs. Free nerve endings detect pain and moderate changes in temperature. Other types of sensory receptors in the skin respond to light touch and deep pressure. Figure 6-1 shows some free nerve endings, a touch receptor (Meissner corpuscle), and a deep pressure receptor (Pacinian corpuscle) in a section of skin.

Many of the reflexes that make it possible for humans to adjust themselves to the environment begin as sensory impulses from the skin. As elsewhere in the body, the skin works with the brain and the spinal cord to accomplish these important functions.

Other Activities of the Skin

Substances can be absorbed through the skin in limited amounts. Some drugs—for example, estrogens, other steroids, anesthetics, and medications to control motion sickness—can be absorbed from patches placed on the skin. (See Box 6-2, Medication Patches: No Bitter Pill to Swallow.) Most medicated ointments used on the skin, however, are for the treatment of local conditions only. Even medication injected into the subcutaneous tissues is absorbed very slowly.

There is also a minimal amount of excretion through the skin. Water and electrolytes (salts) are excreted in sweat (perspiration). Some nitrogen-containing wastes are eliminated through the skin, but even in disease, the amount of waste products excreted by the skin is small.

Vitamin D needed for the development and maintenance of bone tissue is manufactured in the skin under the effects of ultraviolet radiation in sunlight.

Note that the human skin does not "breathe." The pores of the epidermis serve only as outlets for perspiration from the sweat glands and sebum (oil) from the sebaceous glands. They are not used for exchange of gases.

CHECKPOINT **6-7** ➤ What two mechanisms are used to regulate temperature through the skin?

6

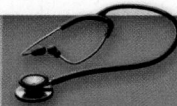

Box 6-2 **Clinical Perspectives**

Medication Patches: No Bitter Pill to Swallow

For most people, pills are a convenient way to take medication, but for others, they have drawbacks. Pills must be taken at regular intervals to ensure consistent dosing, and they must be digested and absorbed into the bloodstream before they can begin to work. For those who have difficulty swallowing or digesting pills, **transdermal (TD) patches** offer an effective alternative to oral medications.

TD patches deliver a consistent dose of medication that diffuses at a constant rate through the skin into the bloodstream. There is no daily schedule to follow, nothing to swallow, and no stomach upset. TD patches can also deliver medication to unconscious patients, who would otherwise require intravenous drug delivery. TD patches are used in hormone replacement therapy, to treat heart disease, to manage pain, and to suppress motion sickness. Nicotine patches are also used as part of programs to quit smoking.

TD patches must be used carefully. Drug diffusion through the skin takes time, so it is important to know how long the patch must be in place before it is effective. It is also important to know how long the medication's effects take to disappear after the patch is removed. Because the body continues to absorb what has already diffused into the skin, removing the patch does not entirely remove the medicine. Also, increased heat may elevate drug absorption to dangerous levels.

A recent advance in TD drug delivery is **iontophoresis**. Based on the principle that like charges repel each other, this method uses a mild electrical current to move ionic drugs through the skin. A small electrical device attached to the patch uses positive current to "push" positively charged drug molecules through the skin, and a negative current to push negatively charged ones. Even though very low levels of electricity are used, people with pacemakers should not use iontophoretic patches. Another disadvantage is that they can move only ionic drugs through the skin.

Observation of the Skin

What can the skin tell you? What do its color, texture, and other attributes indicate? Is there any damage? Much can be learned by an astute observer. In fact, the first indication of a serious systemic disease (such as syphilis) may be a skin disorder.

Color

The color of the skin depends on a number of factors, including the following:

- Amount of pigment in the epidermis
- Quantity of blood circulating in the surface blood vessels
- Composition of the circulating blood, including:
  > Quantity of oxygen
  > Concentration of hemoglobin
  > Presence of bile, silver compounds, or other chemicals

PIGMENT The skin's main pigment, as we have noted, is called **melanin**. This pigment is also found in the hair, the middle coat of the eyeball, the iris of the eye, and certain tumors. Melanin is common to all races, but darker people have a much larger quantity in their tissues. The melanin in the skin helps to protect against the sun's damaging ultraviolet radiation. Thus, skin that is exposed to the sun shows a normal increase in this pigment, a response we call tanning.

Sometimes, there are abnormal increases in the quantity of melanin, which may occur either in localized areas or over the entire body surface. For example, diffuse spots of pigmentation may be characteristic of some endocrine disorders. In **albinism** (AL-bih-nizm), a hereditary disorder that affects melanin production, there is lack of pigment in the skin, hair, and eyes.

Another pigment that imparts color to the skin is carotene, a pigment obtained from carrots and other orange and yellow vegetables. Carotene is stored in fatty tissue and skin. Also visible is hemoglobin, the pigment that gives blood its color, which can be seen through the vessels in the dermis.

DISCOLORATION Pallor (PAL-or) is paleness of the skin, often caused by reduced blood flow or by reduction in hemoglobin, as occurs in cases of anemia. Pallor is most easily noted in the lips, nail beds, and mucous membranes. **Flushing** is redness of the skin, often related to fever. Signs of flushing are most noticeable in the face and neck.

When there is not enough oxygen in circulating blood, the skin may take on a bluish discoloration termed **cyanosis** (si-ah-NO-sis) (Fig. 6-6A). This is a symptom of heart failure and of breathing problems, such as asthma or respiratory obstruction.

A yellowish discoloration of the skin may be caused by excessive amounts of bile pigments, mainly bilirubin (BIL-ih-ru-bin), in the blood (Fig. 6-6B). (Bile is a substance produced by the liver that aids in fat digestion; see Chapter 19.) This condition, called **jaundice** (JAWN-dis) (from the French word for "yellow"), may be a symptom of certain disorders, including:

- A tumor pressing on the common bile duct or a stone within the duct, either of which would obstruct bile flow into the small intestine
- Inflammation of the liver (hepatitis), commonly caused by a virus
- Certain blood diseases in which red blood cells are rapidly destroyed (hemolyzed)
- Immaturity of the liver. Neonatal (newborn) jaundice occurs when the liver is not yet capable of processing bilirubin (bile pigment). Most such cases correct themselves without treatment in about a week, but this form of jaundice may be treated by exposure to special fluorescent light that helps the body to eliminate bilirubin.

Another possible cause of a yellowish skin discoloration is the excessive intake of carrots and other deeply colored vegetables. This condition is known as **carotenemia** (kar-o-te-NE-me-ah).

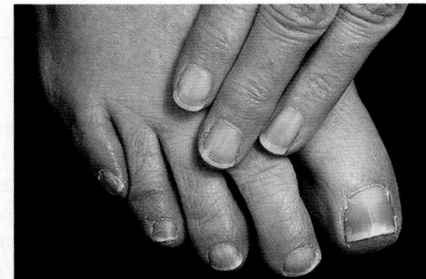 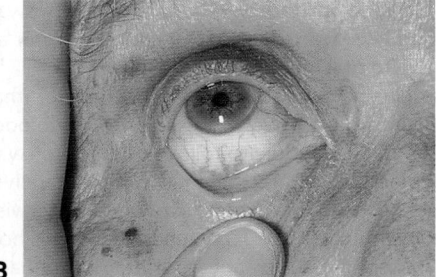

Figure 6-6 **Discoloration of the skin. (A)** Cyanosis is a bluish discoloration caused by lack of oxygen. It is seen here in the toes as compared to normal fingertips. **(B)** Jaundice is a yellowish discoloration caused by bile pigments in the blood. (Reprinted with permission from Bickley LS. *Bates' Guide to Physical Examination and History Taking*, 8th ed. Philadelphia: Lippincott Williams & Wilkins, 2003.) [**ZOOMING IN** ➤ What color is associated with cyanosis? What color is associated with jaundice?]

Certain types of chronic poisoning may cause gray or brown discoloration of the skin. A peculiar bronze cast is present in Addison disease (malfunction of the adrenal gland). Many other disorders cause skin discoloration, but their discussion is beyond the scope of this chapter.

CHECKPOINT 6-8 ➤ What are some pigments that impart color to the skin?

Lesions

A **lesion** (LE-zhun) is any wound or local damage to tissue. In examining the skin for lesions, it is important to make note of their type, arrangement, and location. Lesions may be flat or raised or may extend below the skin's surface.

SURFACE LESIONS A surface lesion is often called a **rash** or, if raised, an **eruption** (e-RUP-shun). Skin rashes may be localized, as in diaper rash, or generalized, as in measles and other systemic infections. Often, these lesions are accompanied by **erythema** (er-eh-THE-mah), or redness of the skin. The following are some terms used to describe surface skin lesions:

- **Macule** (MAK-ule)—a spot that is neither raised nor depressed. Macules are typical of measles and descriptive of freckles (Fig. 6-7A).

- **Papule** (PAP-ule)—a firm, raised area, as in some stages of chickenpox and in the second stage of syphilis (see Fig. 6-7B). A pimple is a papule. A large firm papule is called a **nodule** (NOD-ule).

- **Vesicle** (VES-ih-kl)—a blister or small fluid-filled sac as seen in chickenpox or shingles eruptions (see Fig. 6-7C). Another term for a vesicle is a **bulla** (BUL-ah).

- **Pustule** (PUS-tule)—a vesicle filled with pus. Pustules may develop if vesicles become infected (see Fig. 6-7D).

DEEPER LESIONS A deeper skin lesion may develop from a surface lesion or may be caused by **trauma** (TRAW-mah), that is, a wound or injury. Because such breaks may be followed by infection, wounds should be cared for to prevent the entrance of pathogens and toxins into deeper tissues and body fluids. Deeper injuries to the skin include the following:

- **Excoriation** (eks-ko-re-A-shun)—a scratch into the skin

- **Laceration** (las-er-A-shun)—a rough, jagged wound made by tearing of the skin

- **Ulcer** (UL-ser)—a sore associated with disintegration and death of tissue (Fig. 6-8A)

- **Fissure** (FISH-ure)—a crack in the skin. Athlete's foot, for example, can produce fissures. Tongue fissures may be normal variations in the tongue's surface (see Fig. 6-8B), but may also appear on the lips or tongue as a result of injury or disease.

CHECKPOINT 6-9 ➤ What is a lesion?

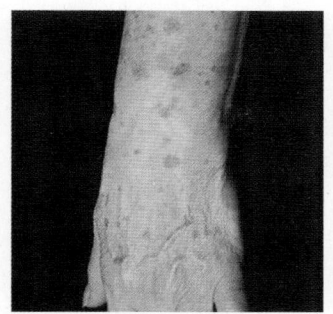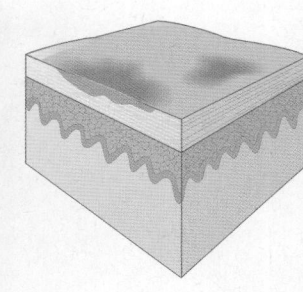

A Macule

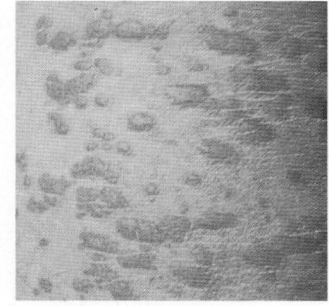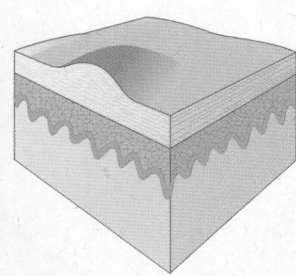

B Papule

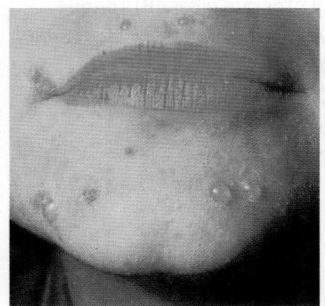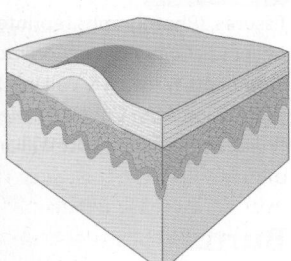

C Vesicle

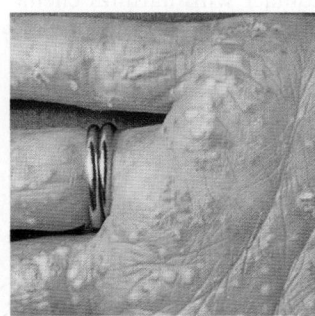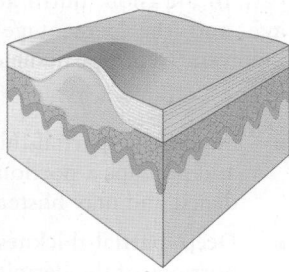

D Pustule

Figure 6-7 **Surface lesions. (A)** Macules on the dorsal surface of the hand, wrist, and forearm. **(B)** Papules on the knee. **(C)** Vesicles on the chin. **(D)** Pustules on the palm. (Photographs reprinted with permission from Bickley LS. *Bates' Guide to Physical Examination and History Taking*, 8th ed. Philadelphia: Lippincott Williams & Wilkins, 2003. Line drawings reprinted with permission from Cohen BJ. *Medical Terminology*, 5th ed. Philadelphia: Lippincott Williams & Wilkins, 2008.)

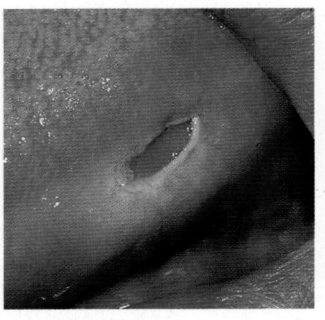
A Ulcer

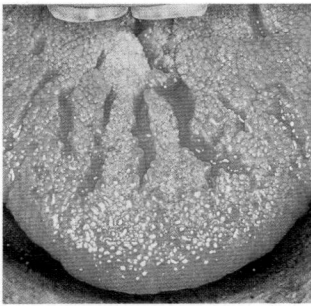
B Fissures

Figure 6-8   **Deeper lesions. (A)** Tongue ulcer. **(B)** Tongue fissures. (Photographs reprinted with permission from Langlais RP, Miller CS. *Color Atlas of Common Oral Diseases*, 3rd ed. Philadelphia: Lippincott Williams & Wilkins, 2002. Line drawings reprinted with permission from Cohen BJ. *Medical Terminology*, 5th ed. Philadelphia: Lippincott Williams & Wilkins, 2008.)

Burns

Most burns are caused by contact with hot objects, explosions, or scalding with hot liquids. They may also be caused by electrical injuries, contact with harmful chemicals, or abrasion. Burns are assessed by the depth of damage and the percentage of body surface area (BSA) involved. Depth of tissue destruction is categorized as follows:

- **Superficial partial-thickness**—involves the epidermis and perhaps a portion of the dermis. The tissue is reddened and may blister, as in cases of sunburn.

- **Deep partial-thickness**—involves the epidermis and portions of the dermis. The tissue is blistered and broken, with a weeping surface. Causes include scalding and exposure to flame.

- **Full-thickness**—involves the full skin and sometimes subcutaneous tissue and underlying tissues as well. The tissue is broken, dry and pale, or charred. These injuries may require skin grafting and may result in loss of digits or limbs.

The above classification replaces an older system of ranking burns as first-, second-, and third-degree according to the depth of tissue damage.

The amount of body surface area involved in a burn may be estimated by using the **rule of nines**, in which surface areas are assigned percentages in multiples of nine (Fig. 6-9). The more accurate Lund and Browder method divides the body into small areas and estimates the proportion of BSA that each contributes.

Infection is a common complication of burns, because the skin, a major defense against invasion of microorganisms, is damaged. Respiratory complications may be caused by inhalation of smoke and toxic chemicals, and circulatory problems may result from loss of fluids and electrolytes. Treatment of burns includes respiratory care, administration of fluids, wound care, and pain control. Patients must be monitored for circulatory complications, infections, and signs of posttraumatic stress.

SUNBURN Sunlight can cause chemical and biologic changes in the skin. On exposure, the skin first becomes reddened (erythematous) and then may become swollen and blistered. Sunlight can cause severe burns that result in serious illness.

Excessive exposure to the ultraviolet (UV) radiation in sunlight causes genetic mutations in skin cells that interfere with repair mechanisms and may lead to cancer. It also causes premature skin aging involving wrinkling, discoloration ("age spots" or "liver spots") and a "leathery" texture. Note that radiation exposure in tanning booths is no safer than sun tanning.

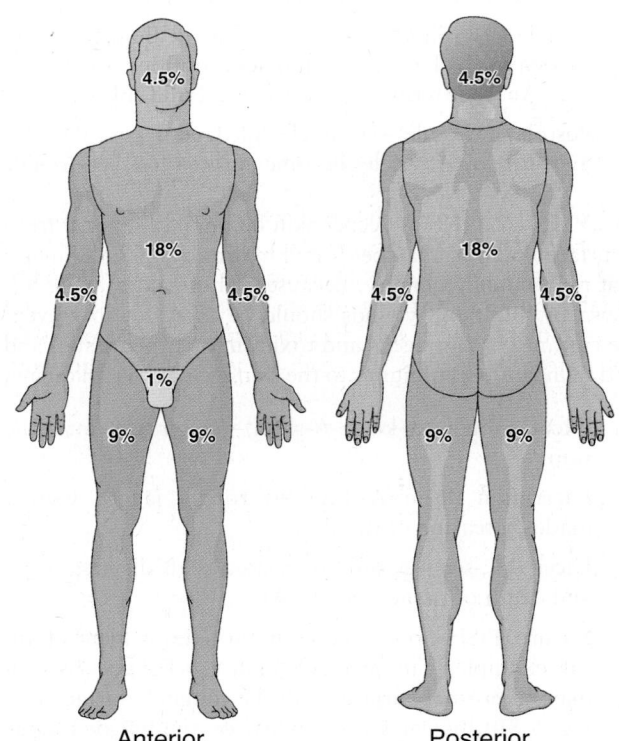

Anterior   Posterior

Figure 6-9   **The rule of nines.** This method is used to estimate percentages of body surface area (BSA) in treatment of burns.

Disease in Context revisited

▶ Squamous Cell Carcinoma

Paul was edgy during the 3 days before he called back at the dermatologist's office. *What if I have skin cancer? Even if it's treatable, I may have a scar—and right smack in the center of my face!* Finally, he made the call, and learned from Dr. Nielsen that he did indeed have a small squamous cell carcinoma.

"I recommend that you consult Dr. Morris, a local surgeon who specializes in a procedure that guarantees the removal of all abnormal cells," the dermatologist advised. "Mohs surgery is done in stages, with the surgeon first removing just the visible lesion and then checking microscopically to be sure that the margins of the excised tissue are free of cancerous cells. If not, additional tissue is removed by degrees until the margins are clean."

Fortunately, Dr. Morris had to repeat the procedure only once after the first pathology examination to be sure of success. Paul left reassured after several hours. Dr. Morris was confident that Paul was safe from the cancer and that scarring would be minimal. "Let's make an appointment

for a follow-up visit when I'll remove the stitches and you can see for yourself," he said.

That evening Paul described his day to his wife and told of his additional instructions. "I need to see my regular dermatologist every 6 months now, as I may be prone to these types of carcinomas." Paul can't undo earlier damage, but he can prevent further insult to his skin by wearing sunscreen outdoors and reapplying it often. The doctor also advised him to cover up in the sun and avoid times of high sun intensity. "Come to think of it," Paul said to his wife, "that's good advice for you too!"

In this case, we saw the carcinogenic effect of sun damage on the integumentary system. (To review the topics of neoplasms and malignancy, refer back to Chapters 3 and 4.) Unfortunately for Paul, the effects of years of sun damage are not limited to his skin. In Chapter 11, *The Sensory System*, we'll learn how sun exposure can affect other systems as well.

Tissue Repair

True tissue regeneration after injury can occur only in areas that have actively dividing cells or cells that can be triggered to divide by injury. Specifically, these tissues are the epithelial and connective tissues. Even among the connective tissues, repair occurs more slowly in tissues that are not very active metabolically, in cartilage for example. Muscle tissue and nervous tissue, which stop dividing early in life, generally do not restore themselves, although some types can carry out minimal regeneration. When muscle and nervous tissues are injured, they are generally replaced by connective tissue.

Repair of a skin wound or lesion begins after blood has clotted and a scab has formed at the surface to protect underlying tissue. From damaged capillaries, new vessels branch and grow into the injured tissue. Fibroblasts (fiber-producing cells) manufacture collagen to close the gap made by the wound. A large wound requires extensive growth of new connective tissue, which develops from within the wound. This new tissue forms a **scar**, also called a **cicatrix** (SIK-ah-triks).

After the upper layer of epithelium has regenerated, the scab is released. The underlying scar tissue may then continue to show at the surface as a white line. Scar tissue is strong but is not as flexible as normal tissue and does

not function like the tissue it replaces. Suturing (sewing) the edges of a clean wound together, as is done in the case of operative wounds, decreases the amount of connective tissue needed for repair and thus reduces the size of the resulting scar.

Excess collagen production in the formation of a scar may result in the development of **keloids** (KE-loyds), tumorlike masses or sharply raised areas on the skin surface. These are not dangerous but may be removed for the sake of appearance.

Wound healing is affected by:

- Nutrition—A complete and balanced diet will provide the nutrients needed for cell regeneration. All required vitamins and minerals are important, but especially vitamins A and C, which are needed for collagen.

- Blood supply—The blood brings oxygen and nutrients to the tissues and also carries away waste materials and toxins (poisons) that might form during the healing process. White blood cells attack invading bacteria at the site of the injury. Poor circulation, as occurs in cases of diabetes, for example, will delay wound healing.

- Infection—Contamination prolongs inflammation and interferes with the formation of materials needed for wound repair.

■ Age—Healing is generally slower among the elderly due to a slower rate of cell replacement. The elderly also may have a lowered immune response to infection.

CHECKPOINT 6-10 ➤ What two categories of tissues repair themselves most easily?

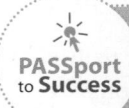

Visit *thePoint* or see the Student Resource CD in the back of this book to view an animation on wound healing.

Effects of Aging on the Integumentary System

As people age, wrinkles, or crow's feet, develop around the eyes and mouth owing to the loss of fat and collagen in the underlying tissues. The dermis becomes thinner, and the skin may become transparent and lose its elasticity, an effect sometimes called "parchment skin." Pigment formation decreases with age. However, there may be localized areas of extra pigmentation in the skin with the formation of brown spots ("liver spots"), especially on areas exposed to the sun (e.g., the back of the hands). Circulation to the dermis decreases, so white skin looks paler.

The hair does not replace itself as rapidly as before and thus becomes thinner on the scalp and elsewhere on the body. Decreased melanin production leads to gray or white hair. Hair texture changes as the hair shaft becomes less dense, and hair, like the skin, becomes drier as sebum production decreases.

The sweat glands decrease in number, so there is less output of perspiration and lowered ability to withstand heat. The elderly are also more sensitive to cold because of less fat in the skin and poor circulation. The fingernails may flake, become brittle, or develop ridges, and toenails may become discolored or abnormally thickened.

Care of the Skin

The most important factors in caring for the skin are those that ensure good general health. Proper nutrition and adequate circulation are vital to skin maintenance. Regular cleansing removes dirt and dead skin debris and sustains the slightly acid environment that inhibits bacterial growth. Careful hand washing with soap and water, with attention to the under-nail areas, is a simple measure that reduces the spread of disease.

The skin needs protection from continued exposure to sunlight to prevent premature aging and cancerous changes. Appropriate applications of sunscreens before and during time spent in the sun, especially after swimming, can prevent skin damage. Limiting sun exposure during midday and covering up with protective clothing are also important.

Skin Disorders

Skin disorders range from simple superficial nuisances, such as acne and rashes, to more deep-seated problems that may lead to systemic disease.

Dermatitis

Dermatosis (der-mah-TO-sis) is a general term referring to any skin disease. Inflammation of the skin is called **dermatitis** (der-mah-TI-tis). It may be caused by many kinds of irritants, such as the oil of poison oak or poison ivy plants, detergents, and strong acids, alkalis, or other chemicals. Prompt removal of the irritant is the most effective method of prevention and treatment. A thorough cleansing as soon as possible after contact with plant oils may prevent the development of itching eruptions.

ATOPIC DERMATITIS Atopic dermatitis (ah-TOP-ik der-mah-TI-tis) or **eczema** (EK-ze-mah) is characterized by intense itching and skin inflammation (Fig. 6-10). The affected areas show redness (erythema), blisters (vesicles), pimplelike lesions (papules), and scaling and crusting of the skin surface. Scratching (excoriation) of the skin can lead to a secondary bacterial infection. Atopic dermatitis commonly first occurs in early childhood, with the recurrence of acute episodes throughout life. The skin may be excessively sensitive to many soaps, detergents, rough fabrics, or perspiration. The person with atopic dermatitis may also be subject to allergic disorders, such as hay fever, asthma, and food allergies.

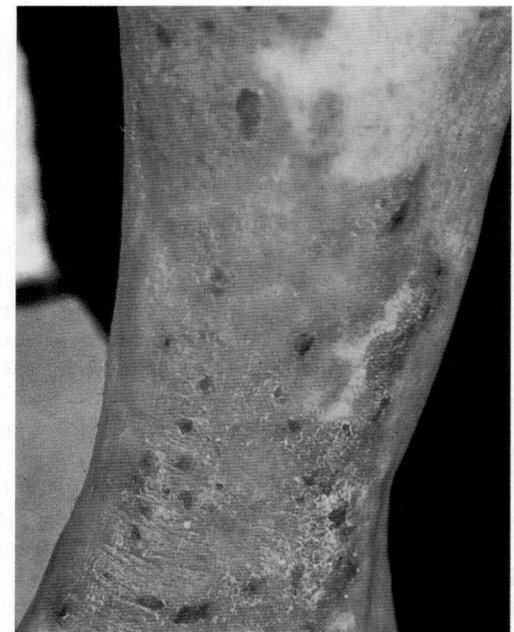

Figure 6-10 **Atopic dermatitis (eczema).** Scratches (excoriation) are visible in the photo. (Reprinted with permission from Bickley LS. *Bates' Guide to Physical Examination and History Taking*, 8th ed. Philadelphia: Lippincott Williams & Wilkins, 2003.)

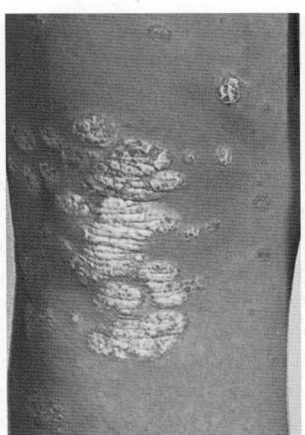

Figure 6-11 **Psoriasis.** Silvery surface scales are visible. (Reprinted with permission from Bickley LS. *Bates' Guide to Physical Examination and History Taking*, 8th ed. Philadelphia: Lippincott Williams & Wilkins, 2003.)

Psoriasis

Psoriasis (so-RI-ah-sis) is a chronic overgrowth of the epidermis leading to large, sharply outlined, red (erythematous), flat areas (plaques) covered with silvery scales (Fig. 6-11). The cause of this chronic, recurrent skin disease is unknown, but there is sometimes a hereditary pattern, and an immune disorder may be involved. Psoriasis is treated with topical corticosteroids and exposure to ultraviolet (UV) light.

CHECKPOINT 6-11 ➤ What is the difference between dermatosis and dermatitis?

Cancer

Skin cancer is the most common form of cancer in the United States. Exposure to sunlight predisposes to development of skin cancer, which, in the United States, is most common among people who have fair skin and who live in the Southwest, where exposure to the sun is consistent and may be intense.

Basal cell and squamous cell carcinomas arise in the epidermis and generally appear on the face, neck, and hands (Fig. 6-12A,B). Early detection and treatment in these cases usually results in cure, although squamous cell carcinoma is the more likely to metastasize.

Melanoma (mel-ah-NO-mah) is a malignant tumor of melanocytes (melanin-forming cells). This type of cancer originates in a **nevus** (NE-vus), a mole or birthmark, anywhere in the body (see Fig. 6-12C). Unlike a normal mole, which has an evenly round shape and well-defined border, a melanoma may show irregularity in shape. Other signs of melanoma are a change in color or uneven color and increase in size of a mole. A predisposing factor for melanoma is severe, blistering sunburn, although these cancers can appear in areas not sun-exposed, such as the soles of the feet, between fingers and toes, and in mucous membranes.

CHECKPOINT 6-12 ➤ What is the name for a cancer of the skin's pigment-producing cells?

Acne and Other Skin Infections

Acne (AK-ne) is a disease of the sebaceous (oil) glands connected with the hair follicles. The common type, called **acne vulgaris** (vul-GA-ris), is found most often in people between the ages of 14 and 25 years. The infection takes the form of pimples, which generally surround blackheads. Acne is usually most severe at adolescence, when certain endocrine glands that control sebaceous secretions are particularly active.

IMPETIGO Impetigo (im-peh-TI-go) is an acute contagious disease of staphylococcal or streptococcal origin that may be serious enough to cause death in newborn infants. It takes the form of blisterlike lesions that become filled with pus and contain millions of virulent bacteria. It is found most frequently among poor and undernourished children. Affected people may reinfect themselves or infect others.

VIRAL INFECTIONS One virus that involves the skin is **herpes** (HER-peze) **simplex virus**, which causes the forma-

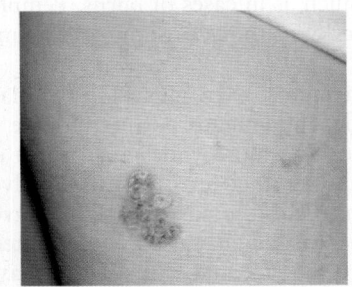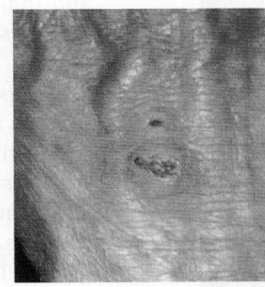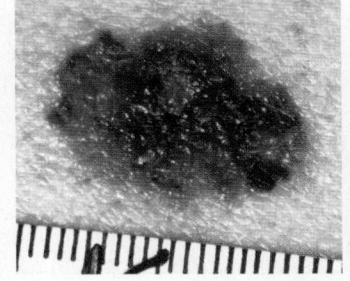

Figure 6-12 **Skin cancer. (A)** Basal cell carcinoma. **(B)** Squamous cell carcinoma. **(C)** Malignant melanoma. (A, Reprinted with permission from Goodheart HP. *Goodheart's Photoguide of Common Skin Disorders; Diagnosis and Management*, 2nd ed. Philadelphia: Lippincott Williams & Wilkins, 2003; B, Reprinted with permission from Bickley LS. *Bates' Guide to Physical Examination and History Taking*, 8th ed. Philadelphia: Lippincott Williams & Wilkins, 2003; C, Reprinted with permission from Rubin E, Farber JL. *Pathology*, 3rd ed. Philadelphia: Lippincott Williams & Wilkins, 1999.)

tion of watery vesicles (cold sores, fever blisters) on the skin and mucous membranes. Type I herpes causes lesions around the nose and mouth; type II is responsible for genital infections (see Table 2 in Appendix 5).

Shingles (herpes zoster) is seen in adults and is caused by the same virus that causes chickenpox (varicella). Infection follows nerve pathways, producing small lesions on the skin. Vesicular lesions may be noted along the course of a nerve. Pain, increased sensitivity, and itching are common symptoms that usually last longer than a year. Prompt treatment with antiviral drugs decreases the disease's severity.

A **wart**, or **verruca** (veh-RU-kah), is a small tumor caused by a virus of the human papillomavirus (HPV) group. Warts may appear anywhere on the body, including the genital region and the soles of the feet (plantar wart). They can be removed by chemical treatment or surgery. Usually benign, warts have been associated with cancer, especially in the case of genital warts and cancer of the cervix (neck of the uterus).

FUNGAL INFECTIONS Fungi are non-green, plantlike microorganisms that may cause surface infections of the skin. These superficial mycotic (fungal) infections, commonly known as tinea or ringworm, may appear on the face, body, scalp, hands, or feet (Fig. 6-13). When on the foot, the condition is usually called **athlete's foot**, as fungal growth is promoted by the dampness of perspiration. Fungal nail infections commonly result from wearing false nails or acrylic nails, as fungal growth is promoted by the moisture that accumulates under the artificial nails.

Fungal infections are difficult to treat. Topical antifungal agents may be effective, but often the patient must take an oral antifungal drug.

CHECKPOINT 6-13 ➤ What are some viruses that affect the skin?

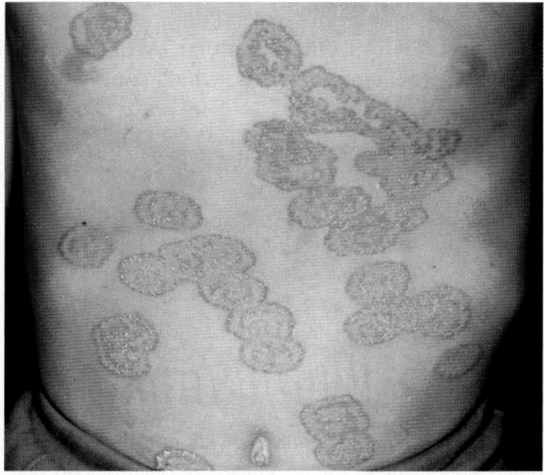

Figure 6-13 **Tinea (ringworm) of the body.** (Reprinted with permission from Hall JC. *Sauer's Manual of Skin Diseases*, 8th ed. Philadelphia: Lippincott Williams & Wilkins, 1999.)

CHECKPOINT 6-14 ➤ What causes tinea or ringworm infections?

Alopecia (Baldness)

Alopecia (al-o-PE-she-ah), or baldness, may be caused by a number of factors. The most common type, known as male pattern baldness, is an expression of heredity and aging; it is influenced by male sex hormones. Topical applications of the drug minoxidil (used as an oral medication to control blood pressure) have produced hair growth in this type of baldness. Alopecia also may result from a systemic disease, such as uncontrolled diabetes, thyroid disease, or malnutrition. In such cases, control of the disease results in regrowth of hair. An expanding list of drugs has been linked with baldness, including the chemotherapeutic drugs used in treating neoplasms.

Allergy and Other Immune Disorders

Allergy, also known as hypersensitivity, is an unfavorable immune response to a substance that is normally harmless to most people (see Chapter 17). Foods, drugs, cosmetics, and a variety of industrial substances can provoke allergic responses in some people. Often the skin is involved in such responses, showing inflammation, rashes, vesicles, or other forms of eruptions, usually accompanied by severe **pruritus** (pru-RI-tus), or itching.

Urticaria (ur-tih-KA-re-ah), or hives, is an allergic reaction characterized by the temporary appearance of elevated red patches known as *wheals*.

AUTOIMMUNE DISORDERS An autoimmune disease results from an immune reaction to one's own tissues. The following diseases that involve the skin are believed to be caused, at least in part, by autoimmune reactions.

Pemphigus (PEM-fi-gus) is characterized by the formation of blisters, or bullae (BUL-e) in the skin and mucous membranes caused by a separation of epidermal cells from underlying tissue layers. Rupture of these lesions leaves deeper areas of the skin unprotected from infection and fluid loss, much as in cases of burns. Pemphigus is fatal unless treated by methods to suppress the immune system.

Lupus erythematosus (LU-pus er-ih-the-mah-TO-sus) (LE) is a chronic, inflammatory, autoimmune disease of connective tissue. The more widespread form of the disease, systemic lupus erythematosus (SLE), involves the skin and other organs. The discoid form (DLE) involves only the skin. It is seen as rough, raised, violet-tinted papules, usually limited to the face and scalp. There may also be a butterfly-shaped rash across the nose and cheeks, described as a malar (cheekbone) rash. The skin lesions of lupus are worsened by exposure to sunlight's ultraviolet radiation. SLE is more prevalent in women than in men and has a higher incidence among Asians and African Americans than in other populations.

Scleroderma is a disease of unknown cause that involves overproduction of collagen with thickening and tightening of the skin. Sweat glands and hair follicles are also involved. A very early sign of scleroderma is numbness, pain, and tingling on exposure to cold caused by constriction of blood vessels in the fingers and toes. Skin symptoms first appear on the forearms and around the mouth. Internal organs become involved in a diffuse form of scleroderma called progressive systemic sclerosis (PSS).

Pressure Ulcers

Pressure ulcers are skin lesions that appear where the body rests on skin that covers bony projections, such as the spine, heel, elbow, or hip. The pressure interrupts circulation leading to ulceration and death of tissue. Poor general health, malnutrition, age, obesity, and infection contribute to the development of pressure ulcers.

Lesions first appear as redness of the skin. If ignored, they may penetrate the skin and underlying muscle, extending even to bone and requiring months to heal.

Pads or mattresses to relieve pressure, regular cleansing and drying of the skin, frequent change in position, and good nutrition help to prevent pressure ulcers. Prevention of pressure ulcer by these methods is far easier than treatment of an established ulcer.

Other terms for pressure ulcers are *decubitus ulcer* and *bedsore*. Both of these terms refer to lying down, although pressure ulcers may appear in anyone with limited movement, not only those who are confined to bed.

CHECKPOINT 6-15 ➤ What are several autoimmune disorders that involve the skin?

PASSport to Success

Visit *thePoint* or see the Student Resource CD in the back of this book for an illustration of systemic lupus erythematosus. Observation and care of the skin are important in nursing as well as other healthcare professions. These resources also have information on nursing careers.

Word Anatomy

Medical terms are built from standardized word parts (prefixes, roots, and suffixes). Learning the meanings of these parts can help you remember words and interpret unfamiliar terms.

WORD PART	MEANING	EXAMPLE
Structure of the Skin		
derm/o	skin	The *epidermis* is the outermost layer of the skin.
corne/o	horny	The stratum *corneum* is the outermost thickened, horny layer of the skin.
melan/o	dark, black	A *melanocyte* is a cell that produces the dark pigment melanin.
sub-	under, below	The *subcutaneous* layer is under the skin.
Accessory Structures of the Skin		
ap/o-	separation from, derivation from	The *apocrine* sweat glands release some cellular material in their secretions.
pil/o	hair	The *arrector pili* muscle raises the hair to produce "goose bumps."
Observation of the Skin		
alb/i	white	*Albinism* is a condition associated with a lack of pigment, so the skin appears white.
-ism	state of	See preceding example.
cyan/o	blue	*Cyanosis* is a bluish discoloration of the skin caused by lack of oxygen.
-sis	condition, process	See preceding example.
bili	bile	*Bilirubin* is a pigment found in bile.

WORD PART	MEANING	EXAMPLE
Observation of the Skin		
-emia	condition of blood	In *carotenemia*, vegetable pigments, as from carrots, appear in the blood and give color to the skin.
eryth	red	*Erythema* is redness of the skin.
Skin Disorders		
dermat/o	skin	*Dermatosis* is any skin disease.
scler/o	hard	*Scleroderma* is associated with a hardening of the skin.

Summary

I. **STRUCTURE OF THE SKIN**
   A. Epidermis—surface layer of the skin
      1. Stratum basale (stratum germinativum)
         a. Produces new cells
         b. Melanocytes produce melanin—dark pigment
      2. Stratum corneum
         a. Surface layer of dead cells
         b. Contain keratin
   B. Dermis (true skin)
      1. Deeper layer of the skin
      2. Has blood vessels and accessory structures
   C. Subcutaneous layer
      1. Under the skin
      2. Made of connective tissue and adipose (fat) tissue

II. **ACCESSORY STRUCTURES OF THE SKIN**
   A. Sebaceous (oil) glands
      1. Release sebum—lubricates skin and hair
   B. Sudoriferous (sweat) glands
      1. Eccrine type
         a. Control body temperature
         b. Widely distributed
         c. Vent directly to surface
      2. Apocrine type
         a. Respond to stress
         b. In armpit and groin
         c. Excrete through hair follicle
   C. Hair
      1. Develop in hair follicle (sheath)
      2. Active cells at base of follicle
   D. Nails
      1. Grow from nail matrix at proximal end

III. **FUNCTIONS OF THE SKIN**
   A. Protection against infection—barrier
   B. Protection against dehydration—keratin and sebum waterproof skin
   C. Regulation of body temperature—blood supply and sweat glands
   D. Collection of sensory information—receptors in skin
   E. Other activities of the skin—absorption, excretion, manufacture of vitamin D

IV. **OBSERVATION OF THE SKIN**
   A. Color
      1. Pigment—mainly melanin, also carotene, hemoglobin
      2. Discoloration—pallor, flushing, cyanosis, jaundice, poisoning
   B. Lesions—wound or local damage
      1. Surface lesions (rash, eruption)
         a. Macule (spot), papule (firm, raised), vesicle (blister), pustule (pus-filled)
      2. Deeper lesions
         b. excoriation (scratch), laceration (tear), ulcer (sore), fissure (crack)
   C. Burns
      1. Evaluated by depth of damage and amount of body surface area (BSA) involved
      2. Sunburn—risk factor in skin cancer and causes premature skin aging

V. **TISSUE REPAIR**
      1. Requires actively dividing cells
      2. Easiest in epithelial and connective tissue
      3. Fibrous material forms scar (cicatrix)
      4. Influenced by nutrition, blood supply, infection, age

VI. **EFFECTS OF AGING ON THE INTEGUMENTARY SYSTEM**

VII. **CARE OF THE SKIN**
   A. Good nutrition
   B. Cleansing
   C. Sun protection

VIII. **SKIN DISORDERS**
   A. Dermatitis—inflammation
      1. Atopic dermatitis (eczema)
   B. Psoriasis
   C. Cancer
      1. Basal cell carcinoma
      2. Squamous cell carcinoma
      3. Melanoma—cancer of melanocytes
   D. Acne and other skin infections
      1. Acne—disease of sebaceous glands related to increased endocrine secretions

2. Impetigo—infectious disease of infants and children
3. Viral infections—herpes viruses, shingles, human papilloma virus
4. Fungal (mycotic) infections—tinea (ringworm)

E. Alopecia—baldness

F. Allergy and other immune disorders
  1. Allergy—hypersensitivity
     a. Urticaria (hives)
  2. Autoimmune disorders—pemphigus, lupus erythematosus, scleroderma
G. Pressure ulcers (decubitus ulcer, bedsore)
  1. Caused by pressure on skin over bone

Questions for Study and Review

6

BUILDING UNDERSTANDING

Fill in the blanks

1. Cells of the stratum corneum contain large amounts of a protein called _____.
2. Sweat glands located in the axillae and groin are called _____ sweat glands.
3. The name of the muscle that raises the hair is _____.
4. A dark-colored pigment that protects the skin from ultraviolet light is called _____.
5. A medical term that means "scar" is _____.

Matching > Match each numbered item with the most closely related lettered item.

___ **6.** Skin sensitivity characterized by intense itching and inflammation

___ **7.** A viral infection that follows nerve pathways, producing small lesions on the overlying skin

___ **8.** Severe itching of the skin

___ **9.** Allergic reaction characterized by the appearance of wheals

___ **10.** Chronic skin disease characterized by red flat areas covered with silvery scales

a. urticaria
b. pruritis
c. shingles
d. psoriasis
e. eczema

Multiple Choice

___ **11.** The epidermis is _____ to the dermis.
  a. superficial
  b. deep
  c. lateral
  d. medial

___ **12.** Acne is an infection of a
  a. sudoriferous gland
  b. sebaceous gland
  c. ceruminous gland
  d. meibomian gland

___ **13.** The medical term for baldness is
  a. alopecia
  b. pemphigus
  c. verruca
  d. dermatitis

___ **14.** Accumulation of bile pigments in the blood causes
  a. pallor
  b. cyanosis
  c. jaundice
  d. carotenemia

___ **15.** Basal cell and squamous cell carcinomas are cancers of
  a. epidermal cells
  b. dermal cells
  c. melanocytes
  d. subcutaneous fat

UNDERSTANDING CONCEPTS

16. Compare and contrast the epidermis, dermis, and hypodermis. How are the outermost cells of the epidermis replaced?

17. What are the four most important functions of the skin?

18. Describe the location and function of the two types of skin glands.

19. Describe the events associated with skin wound healing.

20. What changes may occur in the skin with age?

21. What is the difference between the terms *dermatosis* and *dermatitis*? List examples of irritants that can cause dermatitis.

22. Discuss some ways to prevent and control athlete's foot.

23. What is a decubitus ulcer? List the two best measures for preventing decubitus ulcer.

CONCEPTUAL THINKING

24. Skin is the largest organ in your body. Explain why it is an organ.

25. Remember Mr. Baker from the last chapter? He sustained full-thickness burns to his legs while lighting a fire with gasoline. After Mr. Baker is informed that he will require skin grafting, he asks you why his own skin won't heal by itself. How would you answer his question? Using the rule of nines, estimate Mr. Baker's percentage of body surface area burned.

26. In Paul's case, sun damage caused skin cancer. Which layer of skin was damaged? Why is this layer most likely to become cancerous?

Movement and Support

III

This unit deals with the skeletal and muscular systems, which work together to execute movement and to support and protect vital organs. It covers the additional functions of the skeletal system in housing the blood-forming tissue and storing some minerals. The chapter on muscles describes the characteristics of all types of muscles and then concentrates on the muscles that are attached to the skeleton and how they function. The main skeletal muscles are named and located and their actions are described.

CHAPTER 7

The Skeleton: Bones and Joints

Learning Outcomes

After careful study of this chapter, you should be able to:

1. List the functions of bones
2. Describe the structure of a long bone
3. Differentiate between compact bone and spongy bone with respect to structure and location
4. Differentiate between red and yellow marrow with respect to function and location
5. Name the three different types of cells in bone and describe the functions of each
6. Explain how a long bone grows
7. Name and describe various markings found on bones
8. List the bones in the axial skeleton
9. Explain the purpose of the infant fontanels
10. Describe the normal curves of the spine and explain their purpose
11. List the bones in the appendicular skeleton
12. Compare the structure of the female pelvis and the male pelvis
13. Describe five types of bone disorders
14. Name and describe eight types of fractures
15. Describe how the skeleton changes with age
16. Describe the three types of joints
17. Describe the structure of a synovial joint and give six examples of synovial joints
18. Demonstrate six types of movement that occur at synovial joints
19. Describe four types of arthritis
20. List some causes of backache
21. Describe methods used to correct diseased joints
22. Show how word parts are used to build words related to the skeleton (see Word Anatomy at the end of the chapter)

Selected Key Terms

The following terms and other boldface terms in the chapter are defined in the Glossary

amphiarthrosis
arthritis
arthroscope
arthroplasty
bursa
circumduction
diaphysis
diarthrosis
endosteum
epiphysis
fontanel
joint
osteoblast
osteoclast
osteocyte
osteon
osteopenia
osteoporosis
periosteum
resorption
skeleton
synarthrosis
synovial

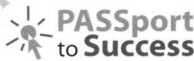

PASSport to Success

Visit *thePoint* or see the Student Resource CD in the back of this book for definitions and pronunciations of key terms as well as a pretest for this chapter.

Disease in Context

➤ Reggie's Case: A Footballer's Fractured Femur

"Donnelly throws deep for a touchdown. Wilson makes a beautiful catch! Ooh, a nasty hit from number 34." The crowd roared their approval for the wide receiver. On the ground, Reggie Wilson knew that something was wrong with his hip. In fact, he thought he had actually heard the bone break! It didn't take long for the coaches and medical staff to realize that Reggie needed help. And it didn't take long for the ambulance to get him to the trauma center closest to the stadium.

At the hospital, the emergency team examined Reggie. His injured leg appeared shorter than the other and was adducted and laterally rotated—all signs of a hip fracture. An x-ray confirmed the team's suspicions: Reggie had sustained an intertrochanteric fracture of his right femur. He would need surgery, but luckily for Reggie, the fracture line extended from the greater trochanter to the lesser trochanter and didn't involve the femoral neck. This meant that the blood supply to the femoral head was not in danger, so the surgery would be more straightforward.

In the operating room, the surgical team applied traction to Reggie's right leg, pulling on it to reposition the broken ends of his proximal femur back into anatomic position (verified with another x-ray). Then, the orthopedic surgeon made an incision beginning at the tip of the greater trochanter and continuing distally along the lateral thigh through the skin, subcutaneous fat, and vastus lateralis muscle. After exposing the proximal femur, the surgeon drilled a hole and installed a titanium screw through the greater trochanter, neck, and into the femoral head. He then positioned a titanium plate over the screw and fastened it to the femoral shaft with four more screws. Confident that the broken ends of the femur were firmly held together, the surgeon closed the wound with sutures and skin staples. Reggie was then wheeled into the recovery room.

The surgical team successfully realigned the fractured ends of Reggie's femur. Now Reggie's body will begin the healing process. In this chapter we'll learn more about bones and joints. Later in the chapter we'll see how Reggie's skeletal system is repairing itself.

The skeleton is the strong framework on which the body is constructed. Much like the frame of a building, the skeleton must be strong enough to support and protect all the body structures. Bone tissue is the most dense form of the connective tissues described in Chapter 4. Bones work with muscles to produce movement at the joints. The bones and joints, together with supporting connective tissue, form the skeletal system. See Appendix 7: Dissection Atlas for pictures of a complete human skeleton, both anterior and posterior views. You can refer to these pictures as you study this chapter.

Bones

Bones have a number of functions, several of which are not evident in looking at the skeleton:

- To serve as a firm framework for the entire body
- To protect such delicate structures as the brain and the spinal cord
- To work as levers with attached muscles to produce movement
- To store calcium salts, which may be resorbed into the blood if calcium is needed
- To produce blood cells (in the red marrow)

Bone Structure

The complete bony framework of the body, known as the **skeleton** (Fig. 7-1), consists of 206 bones. It is divided into a central portion, the axial skeleton, and the extremities, which make up the appendicular skeleton. The individual bones in these two divisions will be described in detail later in this chapter. The bones of the skeleton can be of several different shapes. They may be flat (ribs, cranium), short (carpals of wrist, tarsals of ankle), or irregular (vertebrae, facial bones). The most familiar shape, however, is the **long bone,** the type of bone that makes up almost all of the skeleton of the arms and legs. The long narrow shaft of this type of bone is called the **diaphysis** (di-AF-ih-sis). At the center of the diaphysis is a **medullary** (MED-u-lar-e) **cavity,** which contains bone marrow. The long bone also has two irregular ends, a proximal and a distal **epiphysis** (eh-PIF-ih-sis) (Fig. 7-2).

BONE TISSUE Bones are not lifeless. Even though the spaces between the cells of bone tissue are permeated with stony deposits of calcium salts, the bone cells themselves are very much alive. Bones are organs, with their own system of blood vessels, lymphatic vessels, and nerves.

There are two types of bone tissue, also known as **osseous** (OS-e-us) **tissue.** One type is **compact bone,** which is hard and dense (Fig. 7-3). This tissue makes up the main shaft of a long bone and the outer layer of other bones. The cells in this type of bone are located in rings of bone

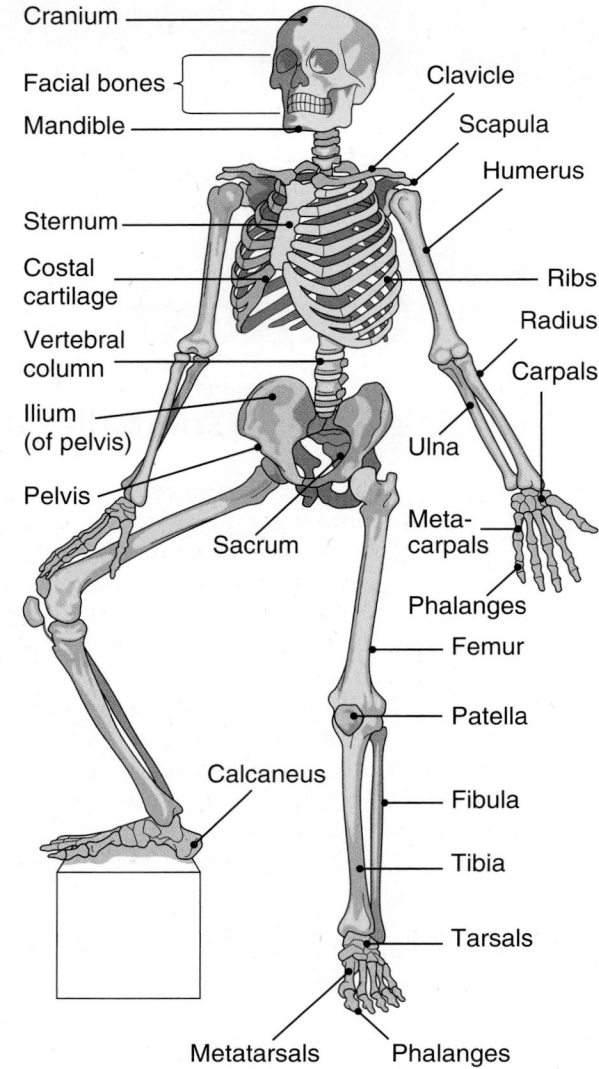

Cranium
Facial bones
Mandible
Sternum
Costal cartilage
Vertebral column
Ilium (of pelvis)
Pelvis
Sacrum
Calcaneus
Metatarsals
Clavicle
Scapula
Humerus
Ribs
Radius
Carpals
Ulna
Meta-carpals
Phalanges
Femur
Patella
Fibula
Tibia
Tarsals
Phalanges

Figure 7-1 **The skeleton.** The axial skeleton is shown in yellow; the appendicular, in blue.

tissue around a central **haversian** (ha-VER-shan) **canal** containing nerves and blood vessels. The bone cells live in spaces (lacunae) between the rings and extend out into many small radiating channels so that they can be in contact with nearby cells. Each ringlike unit with its central canal makes up a **haversian system,** also known as an **osteon** (OS-te-on) (see Fig. 7-3B). Forming a channel across the bone, from one side of the shaft to the other, are many **perforating** (Volkmann) **canals,** which also house blood vessels and nerves.

The second type of bone tissue, called **spongy bone,** or **cancellous bone,** has more spaces than compact bone. It is made of a meshwork of small, bony plates filled with red marrow. Spongy bone is found at the epiphyses (ends) of the long bones and at the center of other bones. Figure 7-4 shows a photograph of both compact and spongy tissue in a bone section.

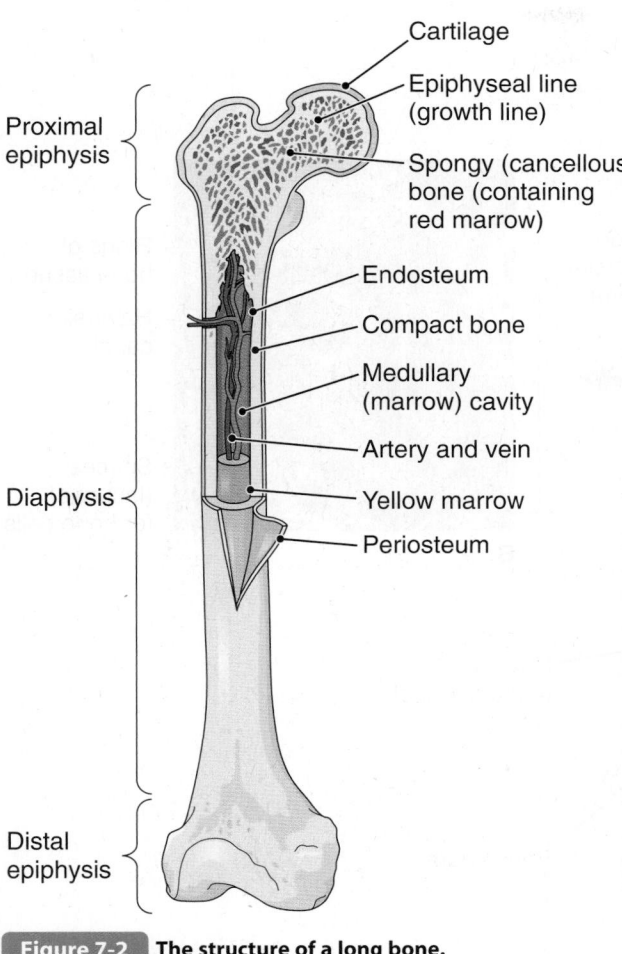

Proximal epiphysis

Cartilage

Epiphyseal line (growth line)

Spongy (cancellous) bone (containing red marrow)

Endosteum

Compact bone

Medullary (marrow) cavity

Artery and vein

Yellow marrow

Periosteum

Diaphysis

Distal epiphysis

Figure 7-2   **The structure of a long bone.**

CHECKPOINT **7-1** ➤ A long bone has a long, narrow shaft and two irregular ends. What are the scientific names for the shaft and the ends of a long bone?

CHECKPOINT **7-2** ➤ What are the two types of osseous (bone) tissue and where is each type found?

BONE MARROW Bones contain two kinds of marrow. **Red marrow** is found at the ends of the long bones and at the center of other bones (see Fig. 7-2). Red bone marrow manufactures blood cells. **Yellow marrow** is found chiefly in the central cavities of the long bones. Yellow marrow is composed largely of fat.

BONE MEMBRANES Bones are covered on the outside (except at the joint region) by a membrane called the **periosteum** (per-e-OS-te-um) (see Fig. 7-2). This membrane's inner layer contains cells (osteoblasts) that are essential in bone formation, not only during growth but also in the repair of injuries. Blood vessels and lymphatic vessels in the periosteum play an important role in the nourishment of bone tissue. Nerve fibers in the periosteum make their

presence known when one suffers a fracture, or when one receives a blow, such as on the shinbone. A thinner membrane, the **endosteum** (en-DOS-te-um), lines the bone's marrow cavity; it too contains cells that aid in the growth and repair of bone tissue.

Bone Growth and Repair

During early development, the embryonic skeleton is at first composed almost entirely of cartilage. (Portions of the skull develop from fibrous connective tissue.) The conversion of cartilage to bone, a process known as **ossification,** begins during the second and third months of embryonic life. At this time, bone-building cells, called **osteoblasts** (OS-te-o-blasts), become active. First, they begin to manufacture the **matrix,** which is the material located between the cells. This intercellular substance contains large quantities of **collagen,** a fibrous protein that gives the tissue strength and resilience. Then, with the help of enzymes, calcium compounds are deposited within the matrix.

Once this intercellular material has hardened, the cells remain enclosed within the lacunae (small spaces) in the matrix. These cells, now known as **osteocytes** (OS-te-o-sites), are still living and continue to maintain the existing bone matrix, but they do not produce new bone tissue. When bone has to be remodeled or repaired later in life, new osteoblasts develop from stem cells in the endosteum and periosteum.

One other cell type found in bone develops from a type of white blood cell (monocyte). These large, multinucleated **osteoclasts** (OS-te-o-klasts) are responsible for the process of **resorption,** which is the breakdown of bone tissue. Resorption is necessary for bone remodeling and repair, as occurs during growth and after injury. Bone tissue is also resorbed when its stored minerals are needed by the body.

Both the formation and resorption of bone tissue are regulated by hormones. Vitamin D promotes calcium absorption from the intestine. Other hormones involved in these processes are produced by glands in the neck. Calcitonin from the thyroid gland promotes the uptake of calcium by bone tissue. Parathyroid hormone (PTH) from the parathyroid glands at the posterior of the thyroid causes bone resorption and release of calcium into the blood. These hormones are discussed more fully in Chapter 12.

CHECKPOINT **7-3** ➤ What are the three types of cells found in bone and what is the role of each?

FORMATION OF A LONG BONE In a long bone, the transformation of cartilage into bone begins at the center of the shaft during fetal development. Around the time of birth, secondary bone-forming centers, or **epiphyseal** (ep-ih-FIZ-e-al) **plates,** develop across the ends of the bones (see Figs. 7-2 and 7-4). The long bones continue to grow in length at these centers by calcification of new cartilage

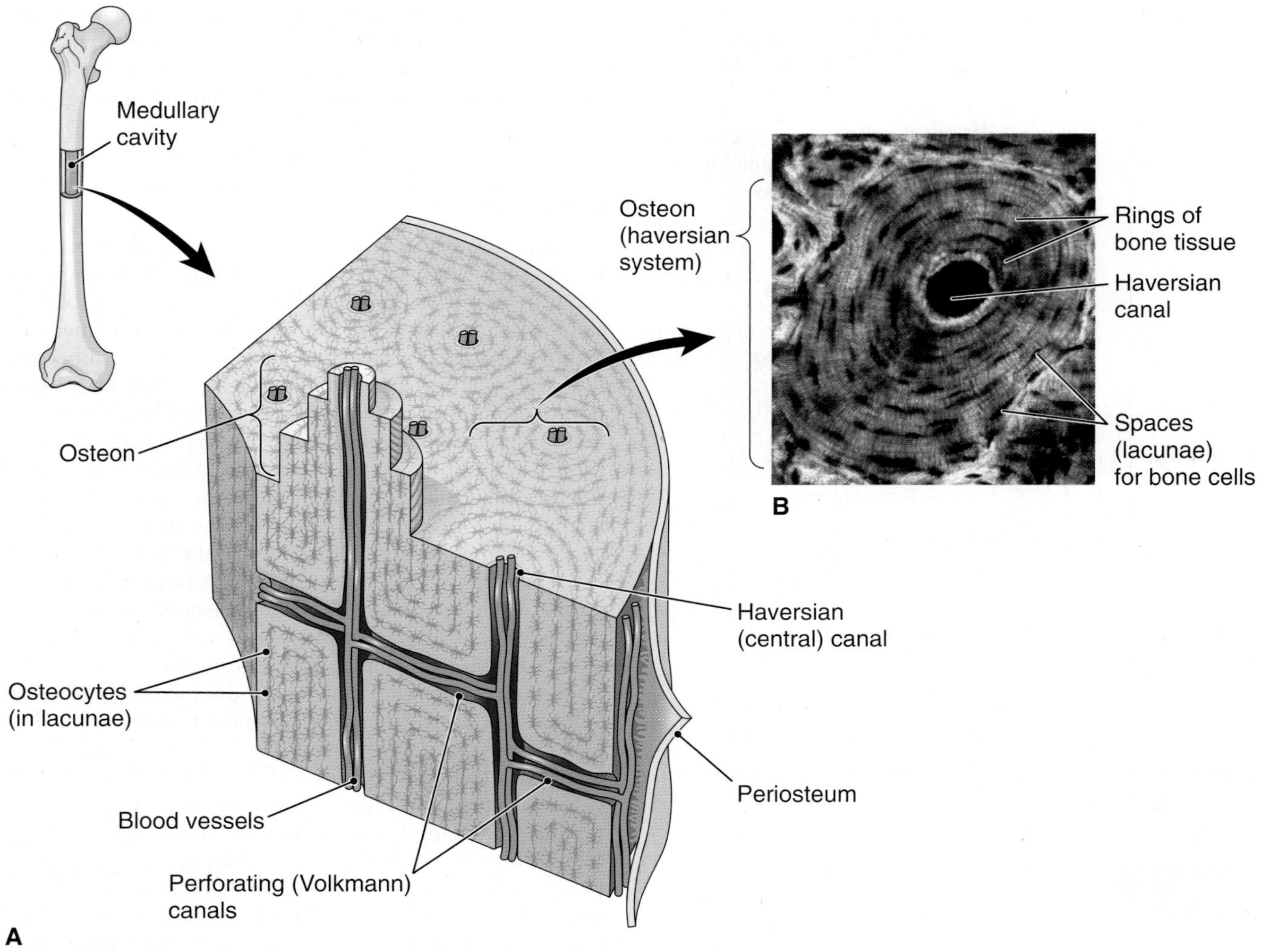

Medullary
cavity

Osteon
(haversian
system)

Osteon

Osteocytes
(in lacunae)

Blood vessels

Perforating (Volkmann)
canals

A

Rings of
bone tissue

Haversian
canal

Spaces
(lacunae)
for bone cells

B

Haversian
(central) canal

Periosteum

Figure 7-3   **Compact bone tissue. (A)** This section shows osteocytes (bone cells) within osteons (haversian systems). It also shows the canals that penetrate the tissue. **(B)** Microscopic view of compact bone in cross section (×300) showing a complete osteon. In living tissue, osteocytes (bone cells) reside in spaces (lacunae) and extend out into channels that radiate from these spaces. (B, Reprinted with permission from Gartner LP, Hiatt JL. *Color Atlas of Histology*, 4th ed. Baltimore: Lippincott Williams & Wilkins, 2005.)

through childhood and into the late teens. Finally, by the late teens or early 20s, the bones stop growing in length. Each epiphyseal plate hardens and can be seen in x-ray films as a thin line, the epiphyseal line, across the end of the bone. Physicians can judge a bone's future growth by the appearance of these lines on x-ray films.

As a bone grows in length, the shaft is remodeled so that it grows wider as the central marrow cavity increases in size. Thus, alterations in a bone's shape result from the addition of bone tissue to some surfaces and its resorption from others.

The processes of bone resorption and bone formation continue throughout life, more actively in some places than in others, as bones are subjected to wear-and-tear or injuries. The bones of small children are relatively pliable because they contain a larger proportion of cartilage and are undergoing active bone formation. In elderly people, there is a slowing of bone tissue renewal. As a result, the bones are weaker and more fragile. Elderly people also have a de-

creased ability to form the protein framework on which calcium salts are deposited. Fractures in elderly people heal more slowly because of these decreases in bone metabolism.

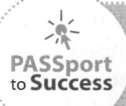

Visit **thePoint** or see the Student Resource CD in the back of this book to view the animation *Bone Growth*, showing the growth process in a long bone.

CHECKPOINT 7-4 ➤ As the embryonic skeleton is converted from cartilage to bone, the intercellular matrix becomes hardened. What compounds are deposited in the matrix to harden it?

CHECKPOINT 7-5 ➤ After birth, long bones continue to grow in length at secondary centers. What are these centers called?

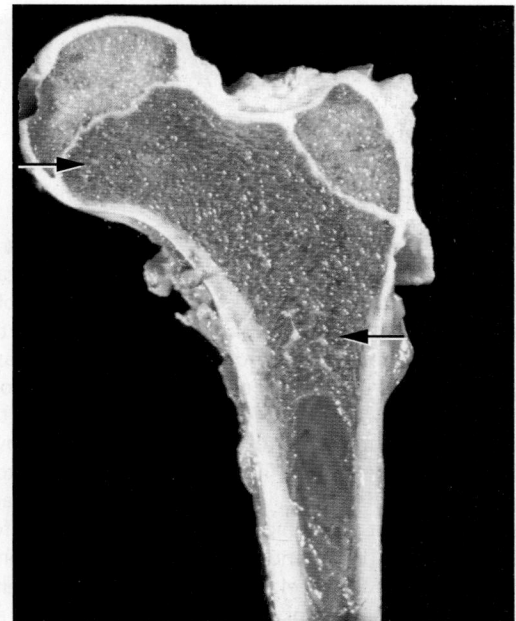

Figure 7-4 **Bone tissue, longitudinal section.** The epiphysis (end) of this long bone has an outer layer of compact bone. The remainder of the tissue is spongy (cancellous) bone, shown by the arrows. Transverse growth lines are also visible. (Reprinted with permission from Rubin R, Strayer DS. *Rubin's Pathology: Clinicopathologic Foundations of Medicine,* 5th ed. Baltimore: Lippincott Williams & Wilkins, 2007.)

Bone Markings

In addition to their general shape, bones have other distinguishing features, or **bone markings**. These markings include raised areas and depressions, which help to form joints or serve as points for muscle attachments, and various holes, which allow the passage of nerves and blood vessels. Some of these identifying features are described next.

PROJECTIONS
- **Head**—a rounded, knoblike end separated from the rest of the bone by a slender region, the neck.
- **Process**—a large projection of a bone, such as the superior part of the ulna in the forearm that creates the elbow.
- **Condyle** (KON-dile)—a rounded projection; a small projection above a condyle is an epicondyle.
- **Crest**—a distinct border or ridge, often rough, such as over the top of the hip bone.
- **Spine**—a sharp projection from the surface of a bone, such as the spine of the scapula (shoulder blade).

DEPRESSIONS OR HOLES
- **Foramen** (fo-RA-men)—a hole that allows a vessel or a nerve to pass through or between bones. The plural is foramina (fo-RAM-ih-nah).

- **Sinus** (SI-nus)—an air space found in some skull bones.
- **Fossa** (FOS-sah)—a depression on a bone surface. The plural is fossae (FOS-se).
- **Meatus** (me-A-tus)—a short channel or passageway, such as the channel in the temporal bone of the skull that leads to the inner ear.

Examples of these and other markings can be seen on the bones illustrated in this chapter. To find out how these markings can be used in healthcare, see Box 7-1, Landmarking: Seeing with Your Fingers.

CHECKPOINT **7-6** ➤ Bones have a number of projections, depressions, and holes. What are some functions of these markings?

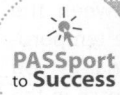 **PASSport to Success** Visit **thePoint** or see the Student Resource CD in the back of this book to view bone markings on an illustration of a whole skeleton.

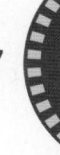

Bones of the Axial Skeleton

The skeleton may be divided into two main groups of bones (see Fig. 7-1):

- The **axial** (AK-se-al) **skeleton** consists of 80 bones and includes the bony framework of the head and the trunk.
- The **appendicular** (ap-en-DIK-u-lar) **skeleton** consists of 126 bones and forms the framework for the **extremities** (limbs) and for the shoulders and hips.

We describe the axial skeleton first and then proceed to the appendicular skeleton. Table 7-1 provides an outline of all the bones included in this discussion.

Framework of the Skull

The bony framework of the head, called the **skull**, is subdivided into two parts: the cranium and the facial portion. Refer to Figures 7-5 through 7-8, which show different views of the skull, as you study the following descriptions. Color-coding of the bones will aid in identification as the skull is seen from different positions.

CRANIUM This rounded chamber that encloses the brain is composed of eight distinct cranial bones.

- The **frontal bone** forms the forehead, the anterior of the skull's roof, and the roof of the eye orbit (socket). The **frontal sinuses** (air spaces) communicate with the nasal cavities (see Figs. 7-7 and 7-8). These sinuses and others near the nose are described as **paranasal sinuses**.

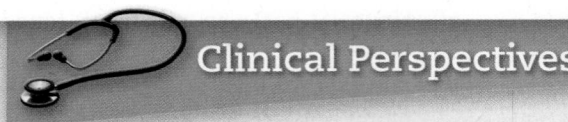

Box 7-1   Clinical Perspectives

Landmarking: Seeing with Your Fingers

Most body structures lie beneath the skin, hidden from direct view except in dissection. A technique called **landmarking** allows healthcare providers to locate hidden structures simply and easily. Bony prominences, or landmarks, can be palpated (felt) beneath the skin to serve as reference points for locating other internal structures. Landmarking is used during physical examinations and surgeries, when giving injections, and for many other clinical procedures. The lower tip of the sternum, the xiphoid process, is a reference point in the administration of cardiopulmonary resuscitation (CPR).

Practice landmarking by feeling for some of the other bony prominences. You can feel the joint between the mandible and the temporal bone of the skull (the temporomandibular joint, or TMJ) anterior to the ear canal as you move your lower jaw up and down. Feel for the notch in the sternum (breast bone) between the clavicles (collar bones).

Approximately 4 cm below this notch you will feel a bump called the sternal angle. This prominence is an important landmark because its location marks where the trachea splits to deliver air to both lungs. Move your fingers lateral to the sternal angle to palpate the second ribs, important landmarks for locating the heart and lungs. Feel for the most lateral bony prominence of the shoulder, the acromion process of the scapula (shoulder blade). Two to three fingerbreadths down from this point is the correct injection site into the deltoid muscle of the shoulder. Place your hands on your hips and palpate the iliac crest of the hip bone. Move your hands forward until you reach the anterior end of the crest, the anterior superior iliac spine (ASIS). Feel for the part of the bony pelvis that you sit on. This is the ischial tuberosity. It and the ASIS are important landmarks for locating safe injection sites in the gluteal region.

- The two **parietal** (pah-RI-eh-tal) bones form most of the top and the side walls of the cranium.

- The two **temporal bones** form part of the sides and some of the base of the skull. Each one contains **mastoid sinuses** as well as the ear canal, the eardrum, and the ear's entire middle and internal portions. The **mastoid process** of the temporal bone projects downward immediately behind the external part of the ear. It contains the mastoid air cells and is a place for muscle attachment.

- The **ethmoid** (ETH-moyd) **bone** is a light, fragile bone located between the eyes (see Fig. 7-7). It forms a part of the eye orbit's medial wall, a small portion of the cranial floor, and most of the nasal cavity roof. It contains several air spaces, comprising some of the paranasal sinuses. A thin, platelike, downward extension of this bone (the perpendicular plate) forms much of the nasal septum, a midline partition in the nose (see Fig. 7-5A).

- The **sphenoid** (SFE-noyd) **bone,** when seen from a superior view, resembles a bat with its wings extended. It lies at the base of the skull anterior to the temporal bones and forms part of the eye socket. The sphenoid contains a saddlelike depression, the **sella turcica** (SEL-ah TUR-sih-ka), that holds and protects the pituitary gland (see Fig. 7-7).

- The **occipital** (ok-SIP-ih-tal) **bone** forms the skull's posterior and a part of its base. The **foramen magnum**, located at the base of the occipital bone, is a large opening through which the spinal cord communicates with the brain (see Figs. 7-6 and 7-7).

Uniting the skull bones is a type of flat, immovable joint known as a **suture** (SU-chur) (see Fig. 7-5). Some of the most prominent cranial sutures are these:

- The coronal (ko-RO-nal) suture joins the frontal bone with the two parietal bones along the coronal plane.

- The squamous (SKWA-mus) suture joins the temporal bone to the parietal bone on the cranium's lateral surface (named because it is in a flat portion of the skull).

- The lambdoid (LAM-doyd) suture joins the occipital bone with the parietal bones in the posterior cranium (named because it resembles the Greek letter lambda).

- The sagittal (SAJ-ih-tal) suture joins the two parietal bones along the superior midline of the cranium, along the sagittal plane (see Fig. 7-5C).

FACIAL BONES The facial portion of the skull is composed of 14 bones (see Fig. 7-5):

- The **mandible** (MAN-dih-bl), or lower jaw bone, is the skull's only movable bone.

- The two **maxillae** (mak-SIL-e) fuse in the midline to form the upper jaw bone, including the anterior part of the hard palate (roof of the mouth). Each maxilla contains a large air space, called the **maxillary sinus**, that communicates with the nasal cavity.

- The two **zygomatic** (zi-go-MAT-ik) **bones,** one on each side, form the prominences of the cheeks.

- Two slender **nasal bones** lie side by side, forming the bridge of the nose.

Table 7-1	Bones of the Skeleton	
Region	**Bones**	**Description**
Axial Skeleton		
Skull		
Cranium	Cranial bones (8)	Chamber enclosing the brain; houses the ear and forms part of the eye socket
Facial portion	Facial bones (14)	Form the face and chambers for sensory organs
Hyoid		U-shaped bone under lower jaw; used for muscle attachments
Ossicles	Ear bones (3)	Transmit sound waves in inner ear
Trunk		
Vertebral column	Vertebrae (26)	Enclose the spinal cord
Thorax	Sternum	Anterior bone of the thorax
	Ribs (12 pair)	Enclose the organs of the thorax
Appendicular Skeleton		
Upper division		
Shoulder girdle	Clavicle	Anterior; between sternum and scapula
	Scapula	Posterior; anchors muscles that move arm
Upper extremity	Humerus	Proximal arm bone
	Ulna	Medial bone of forearm
	Radius	Lateral bone of forearm
	Carpals (8)	Wrist bones
	Metacarpals (5)	Bones of palm
	Phalanges (14)	Bones of fingers
Lower division		
Pelvis	Os coxae (2)	Join sacrum and coccyx of vertebral column to form the bony pelvis
Lower extremity	Femur	Thigh bone
	Patella	Kneecap
	Tibia	Medial bone of leg
	Fibula	Lateral bone of leg
	Tarsal bones (7)	Ankle bones
	Metatarsals (5)	Bones of instep
	Phalanges (14)	Bones of toes

7

- The two **lacrimal** (LAK-rih-mal) **bones,** each about the size of a fingernail, form the anterior medial wall of each orbital cavity.

- The **vomer** (VO-mer), shaped like the blade of a plow, forms the inferior part of the nasal septum (see Fig. 7-5A).

- The paired **palatine** (PAL-ah-tine) **bones** form the posterior part of the hard palate (see Figs. 7-6 and 7-8).

- The two **inferior nasal conchae** (KON-ke) extend horizontally along the lateral wall (side) of the nasal cavities. The paired superior and middle conchae are part of the ethmoid bone (see Figs. 7-5A and 7-8).

In addition to the cranial and facial bones, there are three tiny bones, or **ossicles** (OS-sik-ls), in each middle ear (see Chapter 11) and, just below the mandible (lower jaw), a single horseshoe, or U-shaped, bone called the **hyoid** (HI-oyd) **bone,** to which the tongue and other muscles are attached (see Fig. 7-5B).

Openings in the base of the skull provide spaces for the entrance and exit of many blood vessels, nerves, and other structures. Bone projections and depressions (fossae) provide for muscle attachment. Some portions protect delicate structures, for example, the eye orbit and the part of the temporal bone that encloses the inner ear. The sinuses provide lightness and serve as resonating chambers for the voice (which is why your voice sounds better to you as you are speaking than it sounds when you hear it played back as a recording).

INFANT SKULL The infant's skull has areas in which the bone formation is incomplete, leaving so-called soft spots, properly called **fontanels** (fon-tah-NELS) (Fig. 7-9). These flexible regions allow the skull to compress and change shape during the birth process. They also allow for rapid

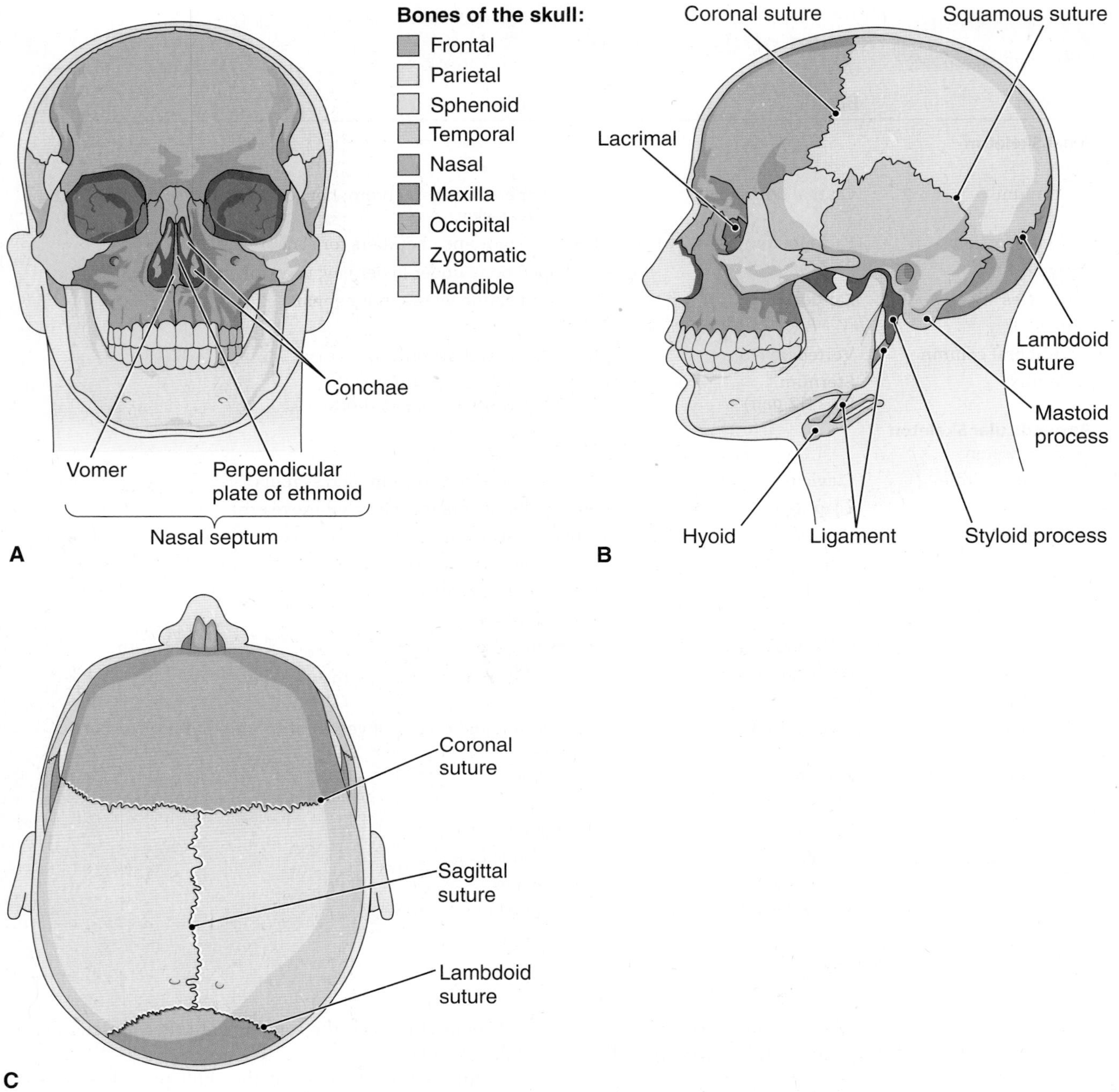

Bones of the skull:
- ☐ Frontal
- ☐ Parietal
- ☐ Sphenoid
- ☐ Temporal
- ☐ Nasal
- ☐ Maxilla
- ☐ Occipital
- ☐ Zygomatic
- ☐ Mandible

A — Anterior view labels: Conchae, Vomer, Perpendicular plate of ethmoid, Nasal septum

B — Left lateral view labels: Coronal suture, Squamous suture, Lacrimal, Lambdoid suture, Mastoid process, Hyoid, Ligament, Styloid process

C — Superior view labels: Coronal suture, Sagittal suture, Lambdoid suture

Figure 7-5   **The skull. (A)** Anterior view. **(B)** Left lateral view. **(C)** Superior view. [ZOOMING IN ➤ What type of joint is between the bones of the skull?]

brain growth during infancy. Although there are a number of fontanels, the largest and most recognizable is near the front of the skull at the junction of the two parietal bones and the frontal bone. This anterior fontanel usually does not close until the child is about 18 months old.

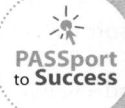

Visit **thePoint** or see the Student Resource CD in the back of this book for supplementary pictures of the anterior and posterior head and neck.

Framework of the Trunk

The bones of the trunk include the spine, or **vertebral** (VER-teh-bral), **column**, and the bones of the chest, or **thorax** (THO-raks).

VERTEBRAL COLUMN This bony sheath for the spinal cord is made of a series of irregularly shaped bones. These number 33 or 34 in the child, but because of fusions that occur later in the lower part of the spine, there usually are

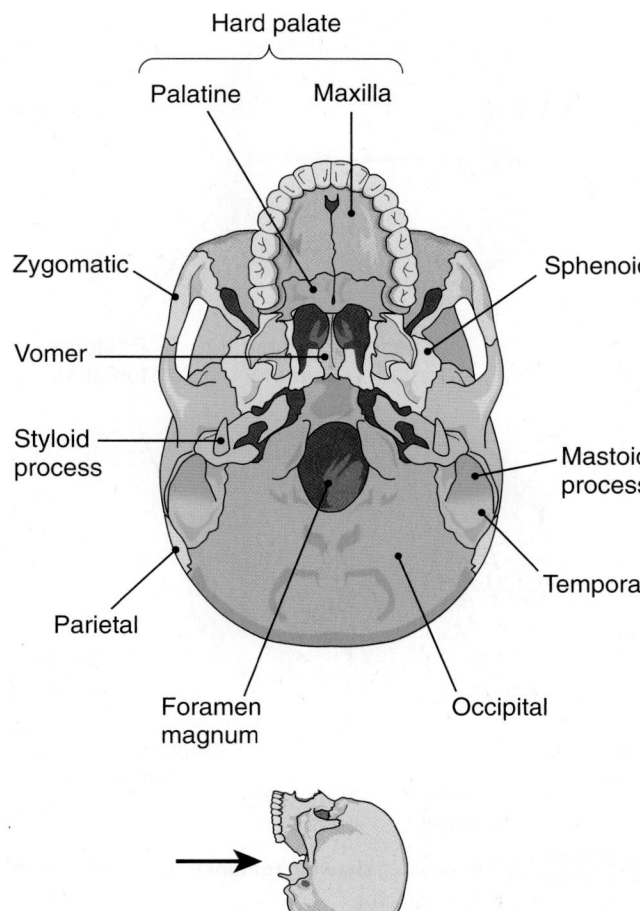

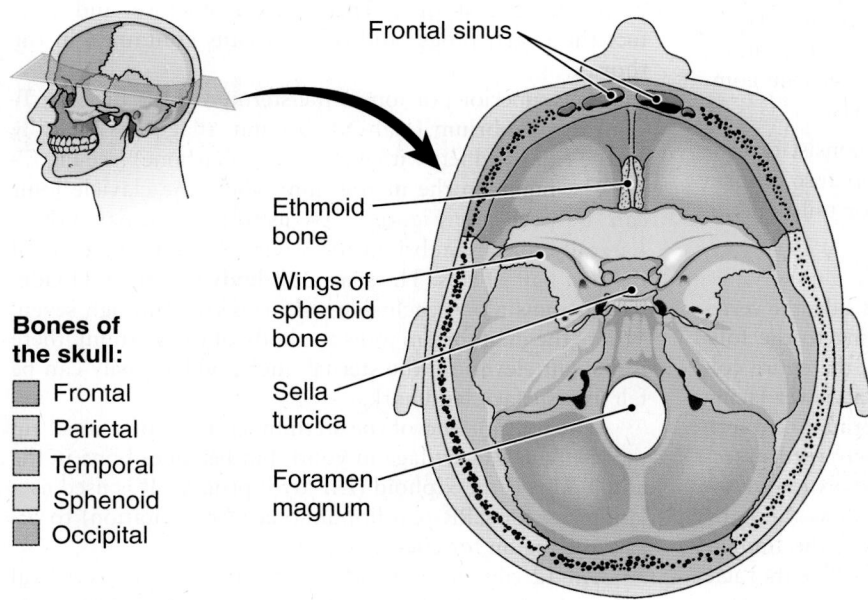

Bones of the skull:

- ▣ Frontal
- ▢ Parietal
- ▢ Temporal
- ▢ Sphenoid
- ▢ Occipital

Figure 7-7 **Floor of cranium, superior view.** The internal surfaces of some of the cranial bones are visible. **[ZOOMING IN ➤** What is a foramen? **]**

just 26 separate bones in the adult spinal column. Figures 7-10 and 7-11 show the vertebral column from lateral and anterior views.

The **vertebrae** (VER-teh-bre) have a drum-shaped **body** (centrum) located anteriorly (toward the front) that serves as the weight-bearing part; disks of cartilage between the vertebral bodies absorb shock and provide flexibility (see Fig. 7-11). In the center of each vertebra is a large hole, or foramen. When all the vertebrae are linked in series by strong connective tissue bands (ligaments), these spaces form the spinal canal, a bony cylinder that protects the spinal cord. Projecting posteriorly (toward the back) from the bony arch that encircles the spinal cord is the **spinous process**, which usually can be felt just under the skin of the back. Projecting laterally is a **transverse process** on each side. These processes are attachment points for muscles. When viewed from a lateral aspect, one can see that the vertebral column has a series of **intervertebral foramina**, formed between the vertebrae as they join together, through which spinal nerves emerge from the spinal cord (see Fig. 7-10).

The bones of the vertebral column are named and numbered from superior to inferior and according to location. There are five groups:

- The **cervical** (SER-vih-kal) **vertebrae**, seven in number (C1 to C7), are located in the neck (see Fig. 7-11). The first vertebra, called the **atlas**, supports the head (Fig. 7-12). (This vertebra is named for the mythologic character who was able to support the world in his hands.) When one nods the head, the skull rocks on the atlas at the occipital bone. The second cervical vertebra, the **axis** (see Fig. 7-12), serves as a pivot when the head is turned from side to side. It has an upright toothlike part, the **dens**, that projects into the atlas as a pivot point. The absence of a body in these vertebrae allows for the extra movement. Only the cervical vertebrae have a hole in the transverse process on each side (see Fig. 7-11). These **transverse foramina** accommodate blood vessels and nerves that supply the neck and head.

- The **thoracic vertebrae**, 12 in number (T1 to T12), are located in the chest. They are larger and stronger than the cervical vertebrae and each has a longer spinous process that points downward (see Fig. 7-11). The posterior ends of the 12 pairs of ribs are attached to these vertebrae.

- The **lumbar vertebrae**, five in number (L1 to L5), are located in the small of the back. They are larger and heavier than the vertebrae superior to them and can support more weight (see Fig. 7-11). All of their processes are shorter and thicker.

7

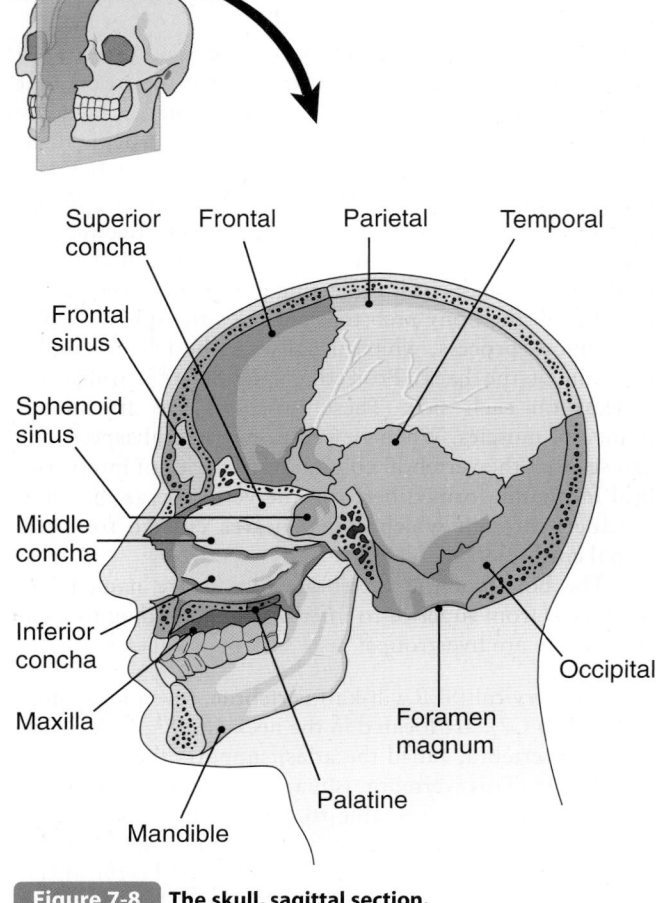

Superior concha — Frontal — Parietal — Temporal

Frontal sinus

Sphenoid sinus

Middle concha

Inferior concha

Maxilla

Mandible

Palatine

Foramen magnum

Occipital

Figure 7-8 The skull, sagittal section.

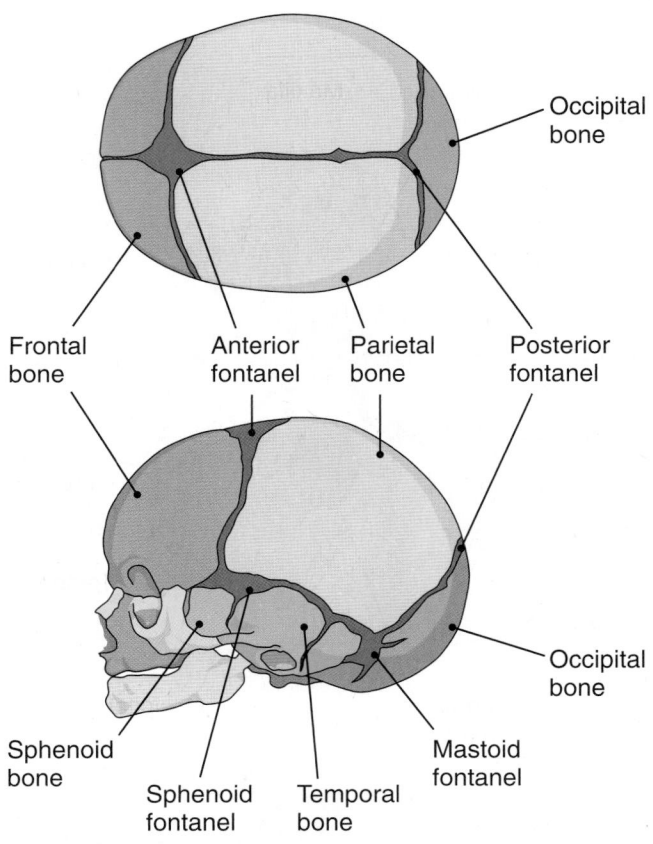

Occipital bone

Frontal bone — Anterior fontanel — Parietal bone — Posterior fontanel

Sphenoid bone — Sphenoid fontanel — Temporal bone — Mastoid fontanel

Occipital bone

Figure 7-9 Infant skull, showing fontanels. [ZOOMING IN ➤ Which is the largest fontanel?]

- The **sacral** (SA-kral) **vertebrae** are five separate bones in the child. They eventually fuse to form a single bone, called the **sacrum** (SA-krum), in the adult. Wedged between the two hip bones, the sacrum completes the posterior part of the bony pelvis.

- The **coccygeal** (kok-SIJ-e-al) **vertebrae** consist of four or five tiny bones in the child. These later fuse to form a single bone, the **coccyx** (KOK-siks), or tail bone, in the adult.

Curves of the Spine When viewed from the side, the vertebral column shows four curves, corresponding to the four vertebral groups (see Fig. 7-10). In the fetus, the entire column is concave forward (curves away from a viewer facing the fetus), as seen in Figure 7-13. This is the primary curve.

When an infant begins to assume an erect posture, secondary curves develop. These curves are convex (curve toward the viewer). The cervical curve appears as the baby holds its head up at about 3 months of age; the lumbar curve appears when the child begins to walk. The thoracic and sacral curves remain the two primary curves. These curves of the vertebral column provide some of the resilience and spring so essential in balance and movement.

THORAX The bones of the thorax form a cone-shaped cage (Fig. 7-14). Twelve pairs of **ribs** form the bars of this cage, completed anteriorly by the **sternum** (STER-num), or breastbone. These bones enclose and protect the heart, lungs, and other organs contained in the thorax.

The superior portion of the sternum is the broadly T-shaped **manubrium** (mah-NU-bre-um) that joins laterally on the right and left with a clavicle (collarbone) (see Fig. 7-1). The point on the manubrium where the clavicle joins can be seen on Figure 7-14 as the clavicular notch. Laterally, the manubrium joins with the anterior ends of the first pair of ribs. The sternum's **body** is long and blade-like. It joins along each side with ribs two through seven. Where the manubrium joins the body of the sternum, there is a slight elevation, the **sternal angle**, which easily can be felt as a surface landmark.

The inferior end of the sternum consists of a small tip that is made of cartilage in youth but becomes bone in the adult. This is the **xiphoid** (ZIF-oyd) **process**. It is used as a landmark for CPR (cardiopulmonary resuscitation) to locate the region for chest compression.

All 12 ribs on each side are attached to the vertebral column posteriorly. However, variations in the anterior attachment of these slender, curved bones have led to the following classification:

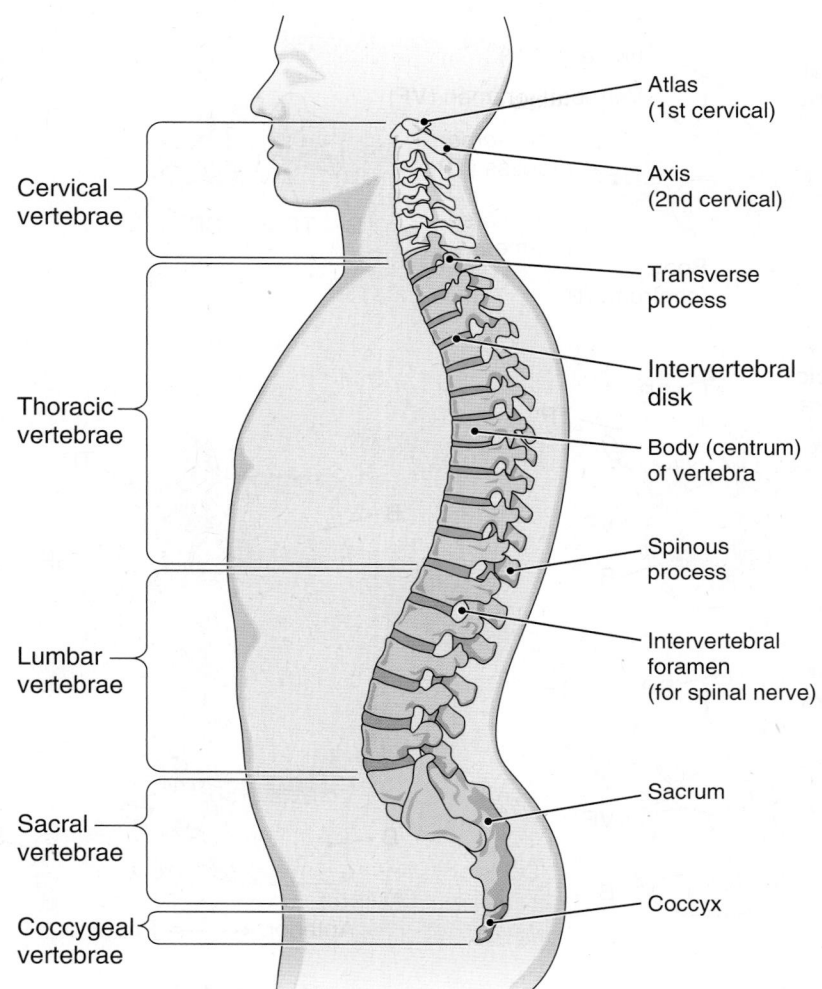

Atlas
(1st cervical)

Axis
(2nd cervical)

Transverse
process

Intervertebral
disk

Body (centrum)
of vertebra

Spinous
process

Intervertebral
foramen
(for spinal nerve)

Sacrum

Coccyx

Cervical
vertebrae

Thoracic
vertebrae

Lumbar
vertebrae

Sacral
vertebrae

Coccygeal
vertebrae

Figure 7-10 **Vertebral column, left lateral view. [ZOOMING IN ➤ From an anterior view, which group(s) of vertebrae form a convex curve? Which group(s) form a concave curve?]**

- **True ribs,** the first seven pairs, are those that attach directly to the sternum by means of individual extensions called **costal** (KOS-tal) **cartilages.**

- **False ribs** are the remaining five pairs. Of these, the 8th, 9th, and 10th pairs attach to the cartilage of the rib above. The last two pairs have no anterior attachment at all and are known as **floating ribs.**

The spaces between the ribs, called **intercostal spaces,** contain muscles, blood vessels, and nerves.

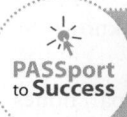 **PASSport to Success** Visit **thePoint** or see the Student Resource CD in the back of this book for additional pictures of the skeleton of the torso.

CHECKPOINT 7-7 ➤ The axial skeleton consists of the bones of the skull and the trunk. What bones make up the skeleton of the trunk?

CHECKPOINT 7-8 ➤ What are the five regions of the vertebral column?

Bones of the Appendicular Skeleton

The appendicular skeleton may be considered in two divisions: upper and lower. The upper division on each side includes the shoulder, the arm (between the shoulder and the elbow), the forearm (between the elbow and the wrist), the wrist, the hand, and the fingers. The lower division includes the hip (part of the pelvic girdle), the thigh (between the hip and the knee), the leg (between the knee and the ankle), the ankle, the foot, and the toes.

The Upper Division of the Appendicular Skeleton

The bones of the upper division may be divided into two groups, the shoulder girdle and the upper extremity.

THE SHOULDER GIRDLE The shoulder girdle consists of two bones (Fig. 7-15):

- The **clavicle** (KLAV-ih-kl), or collarbone, is a slender bone with two shallow curves. It joins the sternum anteriorly and the scapula laterally and helps to support the shoulder. Because it often receives the full force of falls on outstretched arms or of blows to the shoulder, it is the most frequently broken bone.

- The **scapula** (SKAP-u-lah), or shoulder blade, is shown from anterior and posterior views in Figure 7-15. The **spine** of the scapula is the posterior raised ridge that can be felt behind the shoulder in the upper portion of the back. Muscles that move the arm attach to fossae (depressions), known as the **supraspinous fossa** and the **infraspinous fossa,** superior and inferior to the scapular spine. The **acromion** (ah-KRO-me-on) is the process that joins the clavicle. This can be felt as the highest point of the shoulder. Below the acromion there is a shallow socket, the **glenoid cavity,** that forms a ball-and-socket joint with the arm bone (humerus). Medial to the glenoid cavity is the **coracoid** (KOR-ah-koyd) **process,** to which muscles attach.

7

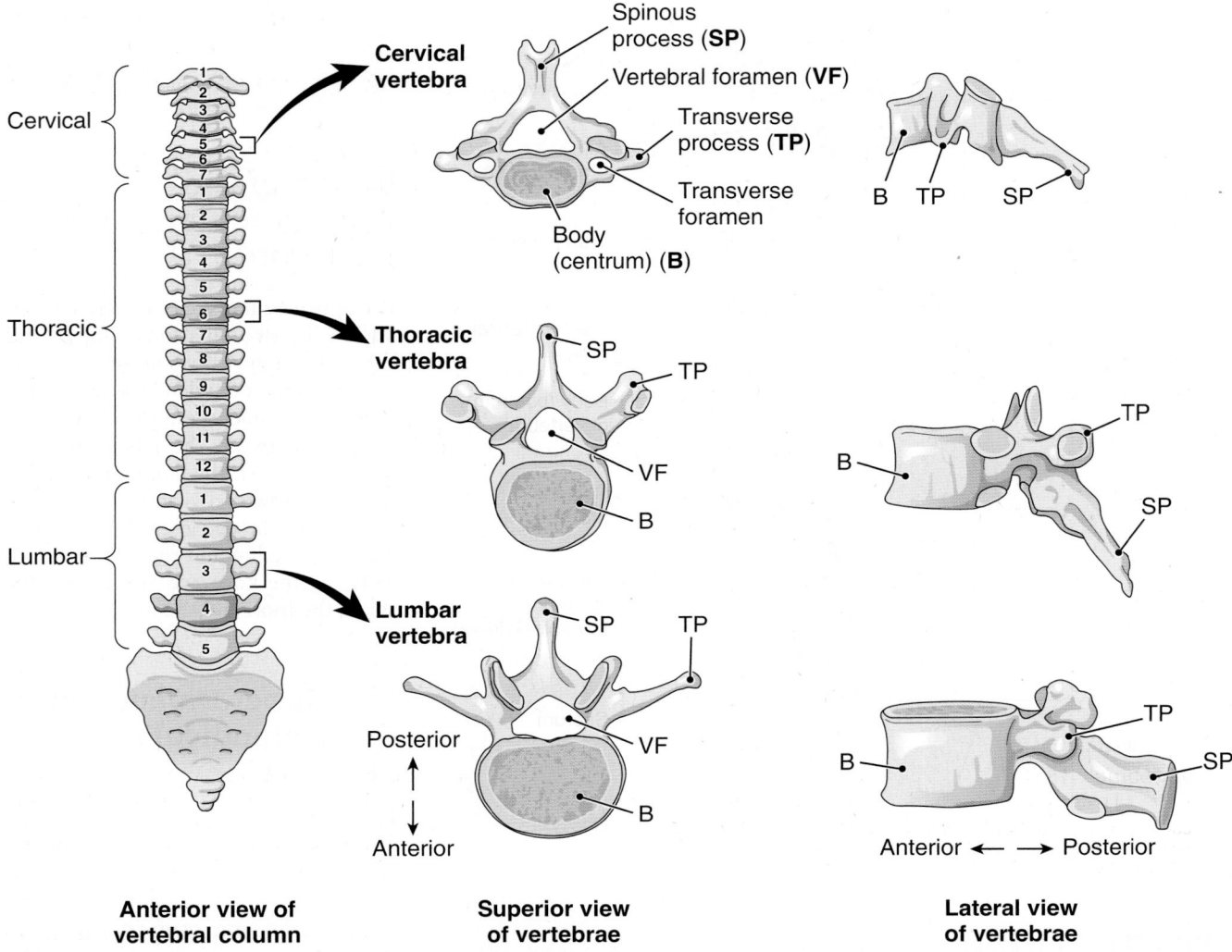

Anterior view of vertebral column   **Superior view of vertebrae**   **Lateral view of vertebrae**

Figure 7-11 **The vertebral column and vertebrae.**

THE UPPER EXTREMITY The upper extremity is also referred to as the upper limb, or simply the arm, although technically, the arm is only the region between the shoulder and the elbow. The region between the elbow and wrist is the forearm. The upper extremity consists of the following bones:

- The proximal bone is the **humerus** (HU-mer-us), or arm bone (Fig. 7-16). The head of the humerus forms a joint with the glenoid cavity of the scapula. The distal end has a projection on each side, the medial and lateral **epicondyles** (ep-ih-KON-diles), to which tendons attach, and a pulley-shaped midportion, the **trochlea** (TROK-le-ah), that forms a joint with the ulna of the forearm.

- The forearm bones are the **ulna** (UL-nah) and the **radius** (RA-de-us). In the anatomic position, the ulna lies on the medial side of the forearm in line with the little finger, and the radius lies laterally, above the thumb (Fig. 7-17). When the forearm is supine, with the palm

up or forward, the two bones are parallel; when the forearm is prone, with the palm down or back, the distal end of the radius rotates around the ulna so that the shafts of the two bones are crossed (Fig. 7-18). In this position, a distal projection (styloid process) of the ulna shows at the outside of the wrist.

- The proximal end of the ulna has the large **olecranon** (o-LEK-rah-non) that forms the point of the elbow (see Fig. 7-17). The trochlea of the distal humerus fits into the ulna's deep **trochlear notch**, allowing a hinge action at the elbow joint. This ulnar depression, because of its deep half-moon shape, is also known as the semilunar notch (Fig. 7-19).

- The wrist contains eight small **carpal** (KAR-pal) **bones** arranged in two rows of four each. The names of these eight different bones are given in Figure 7-20.

- Five **metacarpal bones** are the framework for the palm of each hand. Their rounded distal ends form the knuckles.

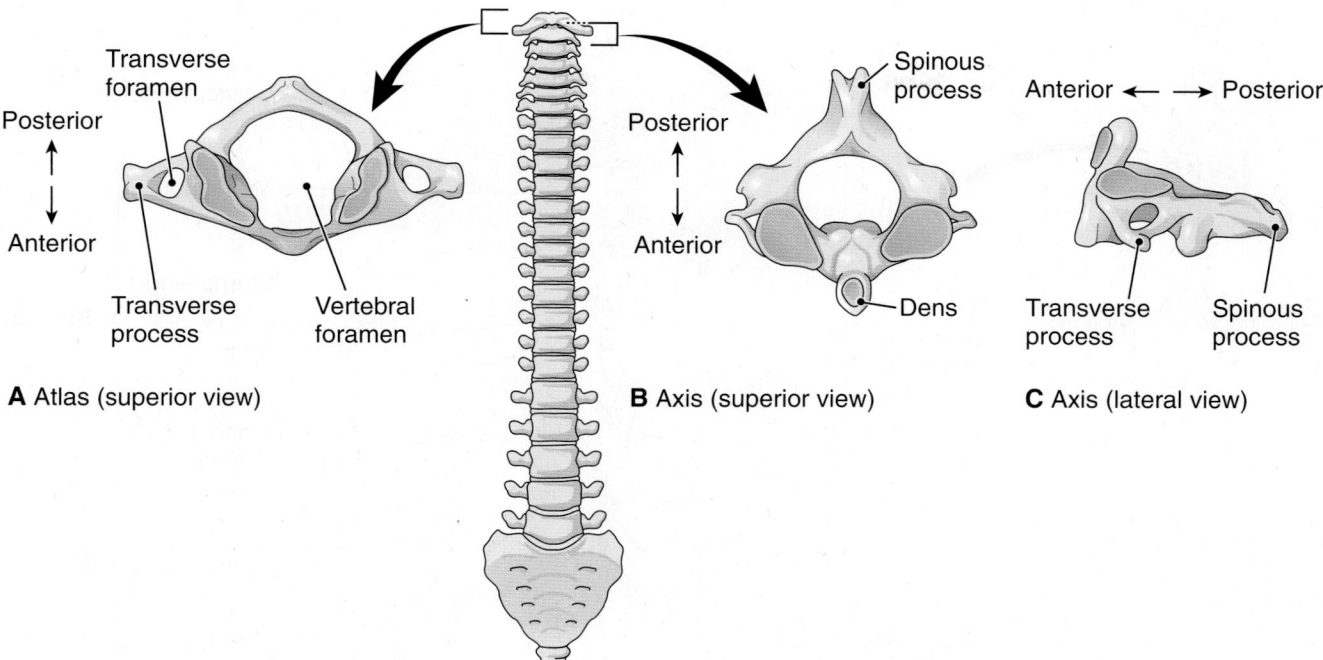

Figure 7-12 **The first two cervical vertebrae. (A)** The atlas (1st cervical vertebra), superior view. **(B)** The axis (2nd cervical vertebra), superior view. **(C)** The axis, lateral view.

- There are 14 **phalanges** (fah-LAN-jeze), or finger bones, in each hand, two for the thumb and three for each finger. Each of these bones is called a **phalanx** (FA-lanx). They are identified as the first, or proximal, which is attached to a metacarpal; the second, or

middle; and the third, or distal. Note that the thumb has only two phalanges, a proximal and a distal (see Fig. 7-20).

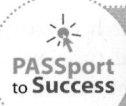

Visit **thePoint** or see the Student Resource CD in the back of this book for additional pictures of the upper extremity skeleton.

The Lower Division of the Appendicular Skeleton

The bones of the lower division also fall into two groups, the pelvis and the lower extremity.

THE PELVIC BONES The hip bone, or **os coxae**, begins its development as three separate bones that later fuse (Fig. 7-21). These individual bones are:

- The **ilium** (IL-e-um) forms the upper, flared portion. The **iliac** (IL-e-ak) **crest** is the curved rim along the ilium's superior border. It can be felt just below the waist. At either end of the crest are two bony projections. The most prominent of these is the **anterior superior iliac spine**, which is often used as a surface landmark in diagnosis and treatment.

- The **ischium** (IS-ke-um) is the lowest and strongest part. The **ischial** (IS-ke-al) **spine** at the posterior of the pelvic outlet is used as a reference point during childbirth to indicate the progress of the presenting

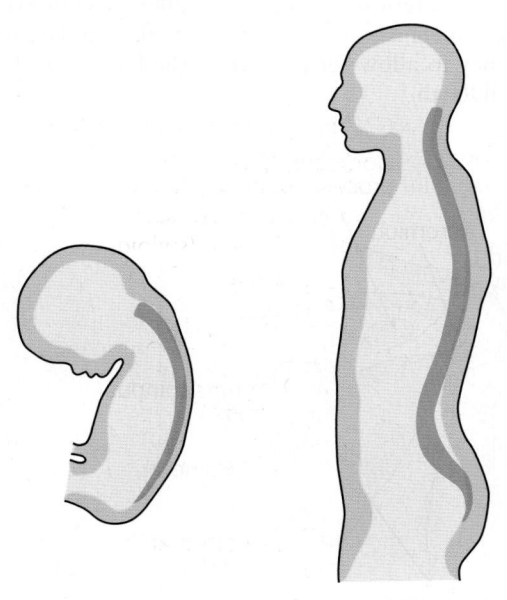

Fetus   Adult

Figure 7-13 **Curves of the spine.** Compare the fetus *(left)* with the adult *(right)*.

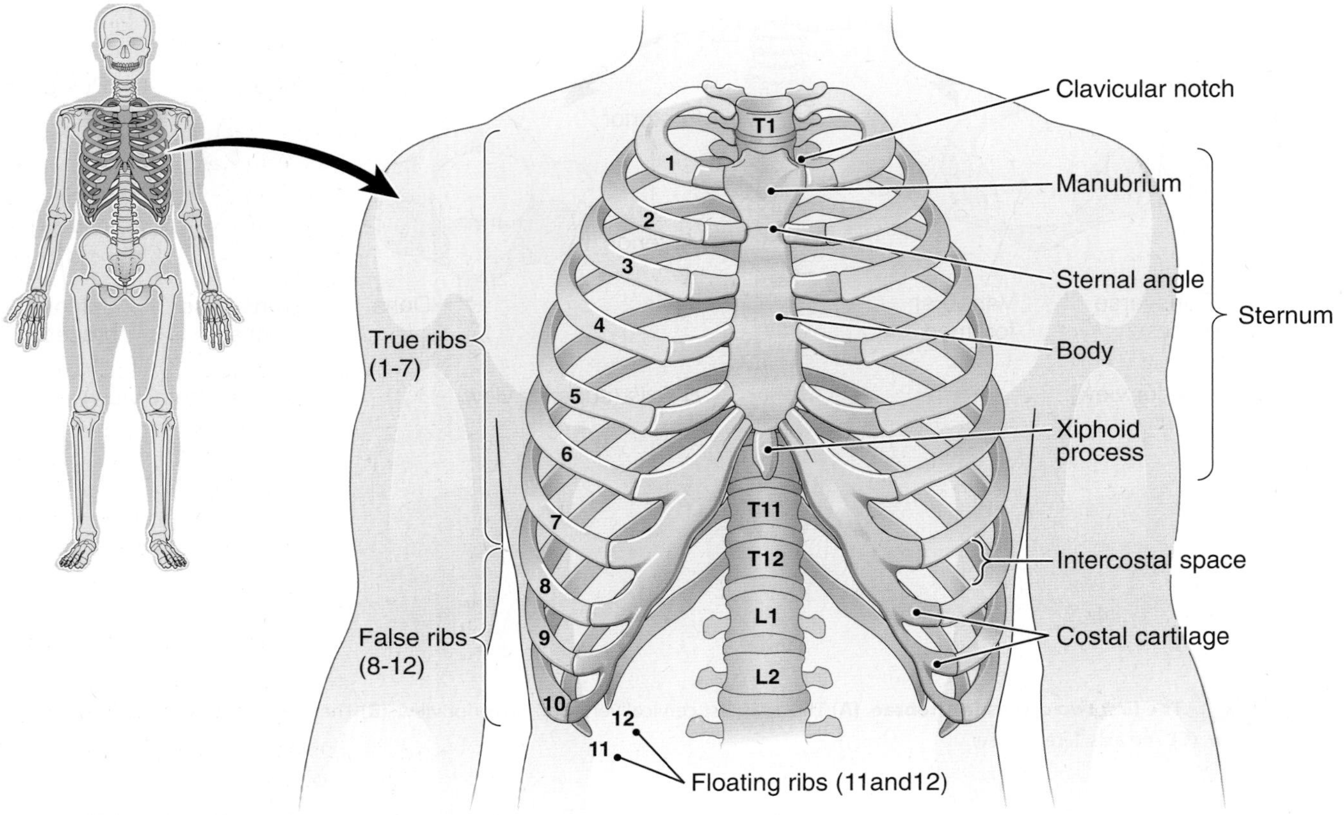

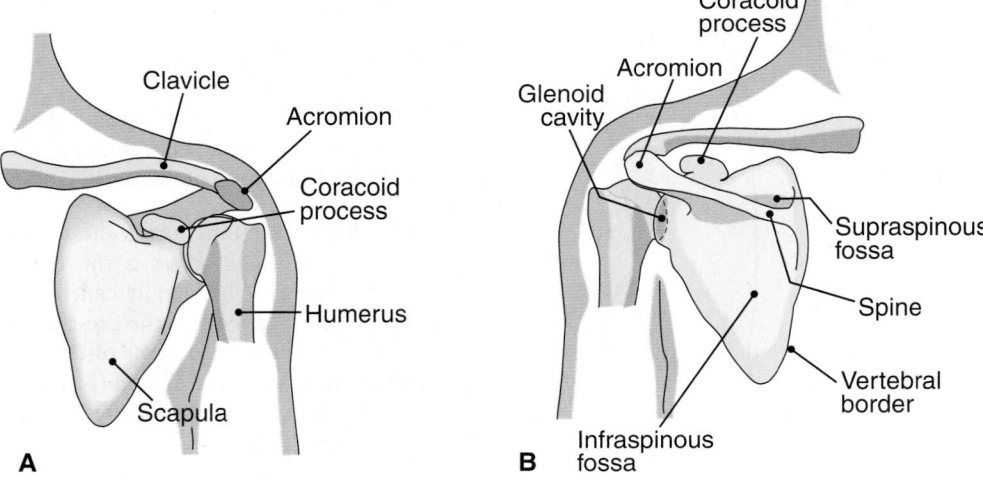

True ribs
(1-7)

False ribs
(8-12)

Clavicular notch
Manubrium
Sternal angle
Sternum
Body
Xiphoid
process
Intercostal space
Costal cartilage
Floating ribs (11and12)

Figure 7-14 **Bones of the thorax, anterior view.** The first 7 pairs of ribs are the true ribs; pairs 8 through 12 are the false ribs, of which the last 2 pairs are also called floating ribs. **[ZOOMING IN ➤** To what bones do the costal cartilages attach? **]**

part (usually the baby's head) down the birth canal. Just inferior to this spine is the large **ischial tuberosity**, which helps support the trunk's weight when a person sits down. One is sometimes aware of this ischial projection when sitting on a hard surface for a while.

■ The **pubis** (PU-bis) forms the anterior part of the os coxae. The joint formed by the union of the two hip bones anteriorly is called the **pubic symphysis** (SIM-fih-sis). This joint becomes more flexible late in pregnancy to allow for passage of the baby's head during childbirth.

Clavicle
Acromion
Coracoid
process
Humerus
Scapula
A

Coracoid
process
Acromion
Glenoid
cavity
Supraspinous
fossa
Spine
Vertebral
border
Infraspinous
fossa
B

Figure 7-15 **The shoulder girdle and scapula. (A)** Bones of the shoulder girdle, left anterior view. **(B)** Left scapula, posterior view. **[ZOOMING IN ➤** What does the prefix *supra* mean? What does the prefix *infra* mean? **]**

The largest foramina in the entire body are found near the anterior of each hip bone on either side of the pubic symphysis. Each opening is partially covered by a membrane and is called an **obturator** (OB-tu-ra-tor) **foramen** (see Fig. 7-21).

The two ossa coxae join in forming the pelvis, a strong bony girdle completed posteriorly by the sacrum and coccyx of the spine. The pelvis supports the trunk and the organs in the lower abdomen, or pelvic cavity, including the urinary bladder, the internal reproductive organs, and parts of the intestine.

The female pelvis is adapted for pregnancy and childbirth (Fig. 7-22). Some ways in which the female pelvis differs from that of the male are:

- It is lighter in weight.
- The ilia are wider and more flared.
- The pubic arch, the anterior angle between the pubic bones, is wider.
- The pelvic opening is wider and more rounded.
- The lower diameter, the pelvic outlet, is larger.
- The sacrum and coccyx are shorter and less curved.

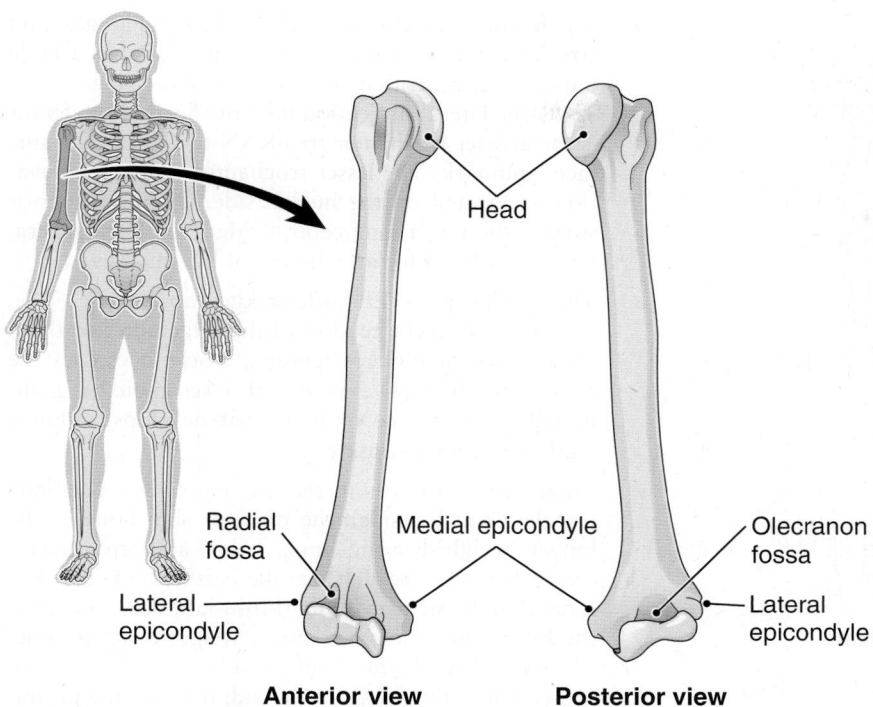

Anterior view   **Posterior view**

Figure 7-16   **The right humerus.**

Portions of all three pelvic bones contribute to the formation of the **acetabulum** (as-eh-TAB-u-lum), the deep socket that holds the head of the femur (thigh bone) to form the hip joint.

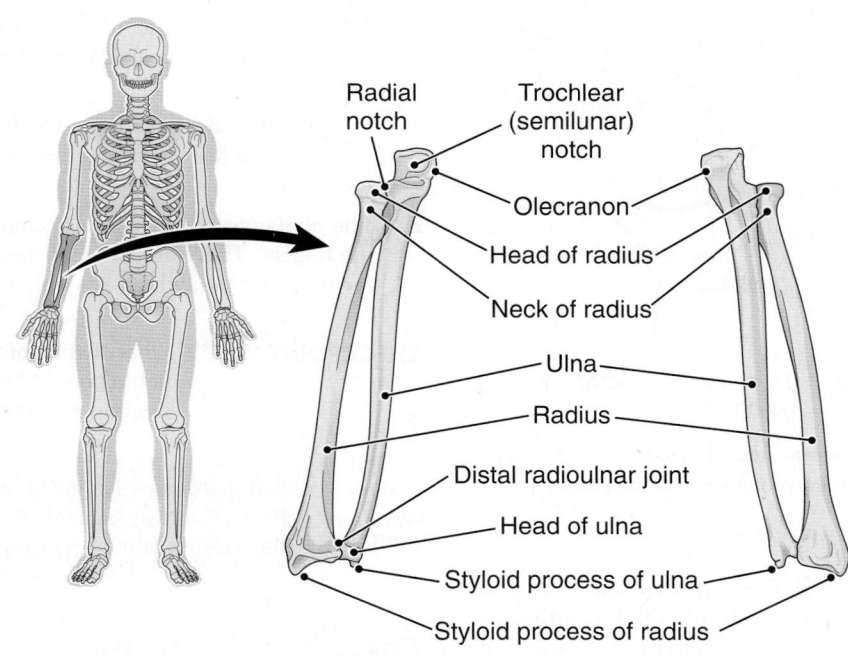

Anterior view   **Posterior view**

Figure 7-17   **Radius and ulna of the right forearm. [ZOOMING IN ➤** What is the lateral bone of the forearm? **]**

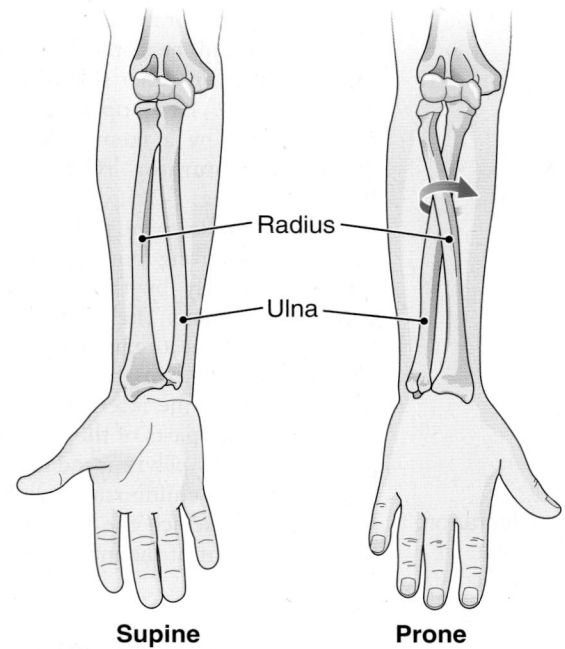

Figure 7-18 **Movements of the forearm.** When the palm is supine (facing up or forward), the radius and ulna are parallel. When the palm is prone (facing down or to the rear), the radius crosses over the ulna.

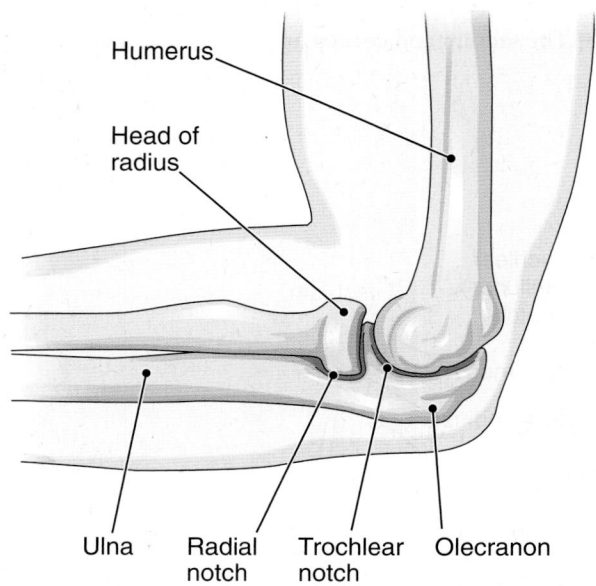

Figure 7-19 **Left elbow, lateral view.** [ZOOMING IN ➤ What part of what bone forms the bony prominence of the elbow?]

THE LOWER EXTREMITY The lower extremity is also referred to as the lower limb, or simply the leg, although technically the leg is only the region between the knee and the ankle. The portion of the extremity between the hip and the knee is the thigh. The lower extremity consists of the following bones:

- The **femur** (FE-mer), the thigh bone, is the longest and strongest bone in the body. Proximally, it has a large ball-shaped head that joins the os coxae (Fig. 7-23). The large lateral projection near the head of the femur is the **greater trochanter** (tro-KAN-ter), used as a surface landmark. The **lesser trochanter**, a smaller elevation, is located on the medial side. On the posterior surface there is a long central ridge, the **linea aspera**, which is a point for attachment of hip muscles.

- The **patella** (pah-TEL-lah), or kneecap (see Fig. 7-1), is embedded in the tendon of the large anterior thigh muscle, the quadriceps femoris, where it crosses the knee joint. It is an example of a **sesamoid** (SES-ah-moyd) **bone**, a type of bone that develops within a tendon or a joint capsule.

- There are two bones in the leg (Fig. 7-24). Medially (on the great toe side), the **tibia**, or shin bone, is the longer, weight-bearing bone. It has a sharp anterior crest that can be felt at the surface of the leg. Laterally, the slender **fibula** (FIB-u-lah) does not reach the knee joint; thus, it is not a weight-bearing bone. The **medial malleolus** (mal-LE-o-lus) is a downward projection at the tibia's distal end; it forms the prominence on the inner aspect of the ankle. The **lateral malleolus**, at the fibula's distal end, forms the prominence on the outer aspect of the ankle. Most people think of these projections as their "ankle bones," whereas, in truth, they are features of the tibia and fibula.

- The structure of the foot is similar to that of the hand. However, the foot supports the body's weight, so it is stronger and less mobile than the hand. There are seven **tarsal bones** associated with the ankle and foot. These are named and illustrated in Figure 7-25. The largest of these is the **calcaneus** (kal-KA-ne-us), or heel bone.

- Five **metatarsal bones** form the framework of the instep, and the heads of these bones form the ball of the foot (see Fig. 7-25).

- The **phalanges** of the toes are counterparts of those in the fingers. There are three of these in each toe except for the great toe, which has only two.

CHECKPOINT **7-9** ➤ What division of the skeleton consists of the bones of the shoulder girdle, hip, and extremities?

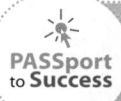

PASSport to Success

Visit **thePoint** or see the Student Resource CD in the back of this book for additional pictures of the skeleton of the pelvis and lower extremity.

Disorders of Bone

Bone disorders include metabolic diseases, in which there is a lack of normal bone formation or excess loss of bone

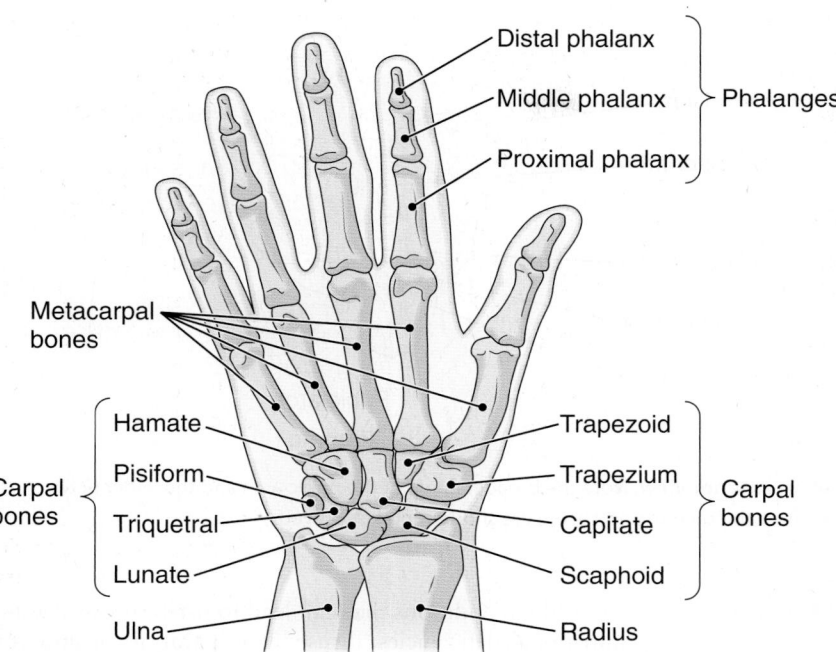

Figure 7-20   **Bones of the right hand, anterior view.**

Metabolic Disorders

Osteoporosis (os-te-o-po-RO-sis) is a disorder of bone formation in which there is a lack of normal calcium salt deposits and a decrease in bone protein. There is an increased breakdown of bone tissue without an increase in the deposit of new bone by osteoblasts (Fig. 7-26). The bones thus become fragile and break easily, most often involving the spine, pelvis, and long bones.

Although everyone loses bone tissue with age, this loss is most apparent in postmenopausal women, presumably because of decline in estrogen. The early stages of bone loss involve a reduction in bone density to below average levels, a condition known as **osteopenia** (os-te-o-PE-ne-ah). Several treatments for osteopenia are available, but medical experts are not in agreement about when treatment should be given and what that treatment should be. Hormone replacement therapy (HRT) is now in question because long-term studies have cast doubt on the safety and effectiveness of the most commonly used form of the drugs. Nonhormonal medications are available to reduce bone resorption and even promote the development of new bone tissue. With regard to nondrug measures, an increase in calcium intake throughout life delays the onset and decreases the severity of this disorder. Weight-bearing exercises, such as weight lifting and brisk walking, are also important to stimulate

tissue; tumors; infections; and structural problems, such as malformation or fractures. Many bone disorders can be diagnosed by x-ray studies.

> **PASSport to Success**
> Visit **thePoint** or see the Student Resource CD in the back of this book for information on careers in radiology.

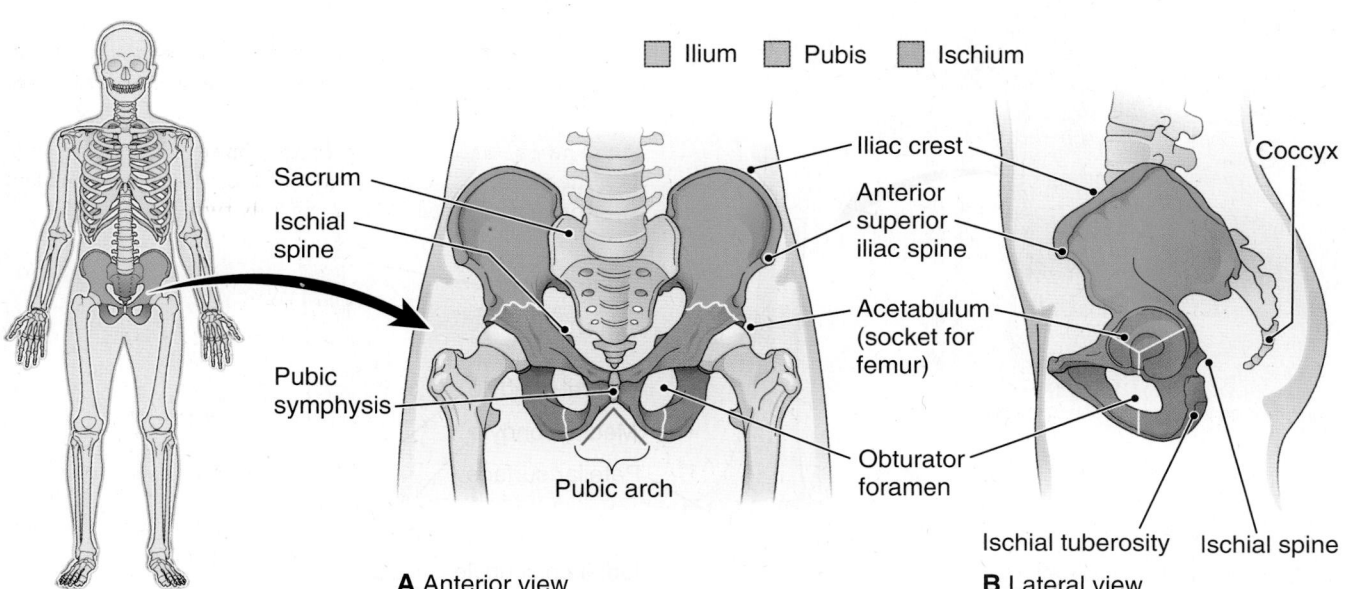

Figure 7-21   **The pelvic bones. (A)** Anterior view. **(B)** Lateral view; shows joining of the three pelvic bones to form the acetabulum.
[ZOOMING IN ► What bone is nicknamed the "sit bone"? **]**

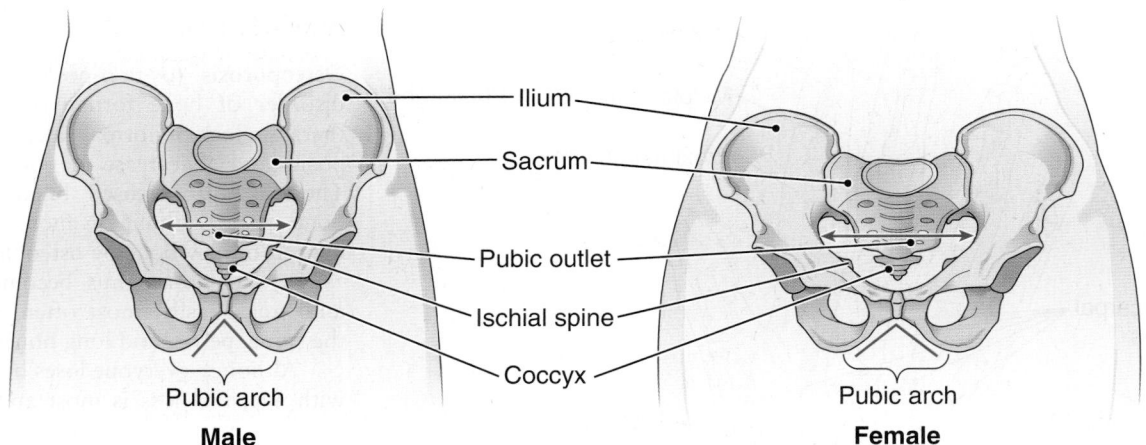

Figure 7-22 **Comparison of male and female pelvis, anterior view.** Note the broader angle of the pubic arch and the wider pelvic outlet in the female. Also, the ilia are wider and more flared; the sacrum and coccyx are shorter and less curved.

growth of bone tissue. (See Box 7-2, Three Steps Toward a Strong and Healthy Skeleton.)

Changes in bone can be followed with radiographic bone mineral density (BMD) tests to determine possible loss of bone mass. However, there is no clear correlation between bone density alone and fracture risk among post-menopausal women.

Other conditions that can lead to osteoporosis include nutritional deficiencies; disuse, as in paralysis or immobilization in a cast; and excess steroids from the adrenal gland.

Abnormal calcium metabolism may cause various bone disorders. In one of these, called Paget disease, or **osteitis deformans** (os-te-I-tis de-FOR-mans), the bones un-

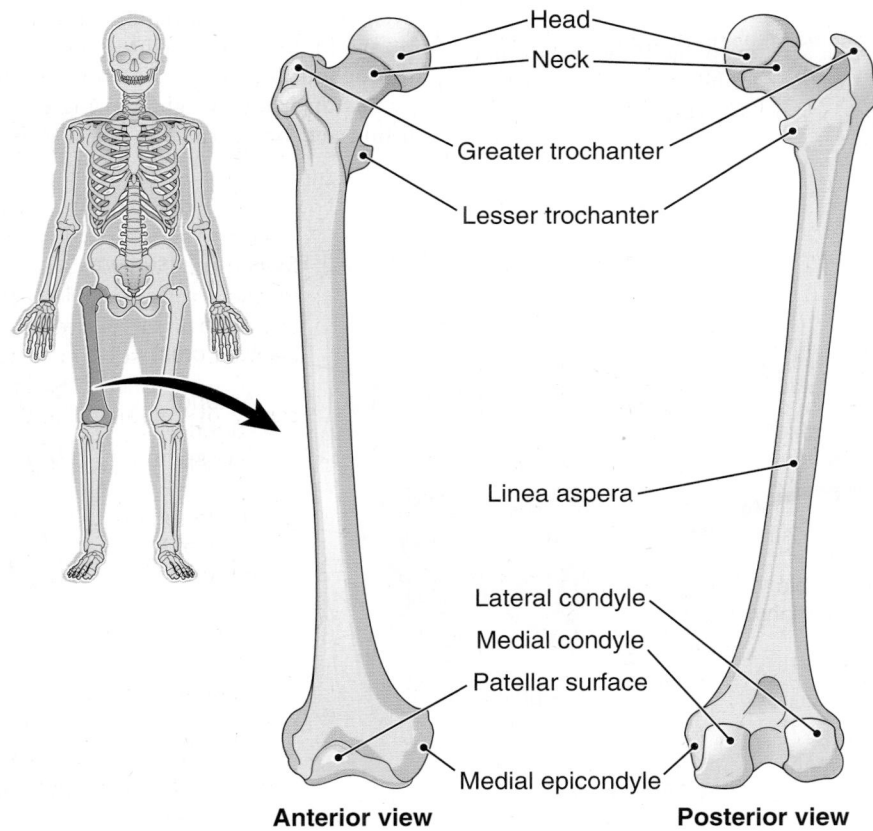

Figure 7-23 **The right femur (thigh bone).**

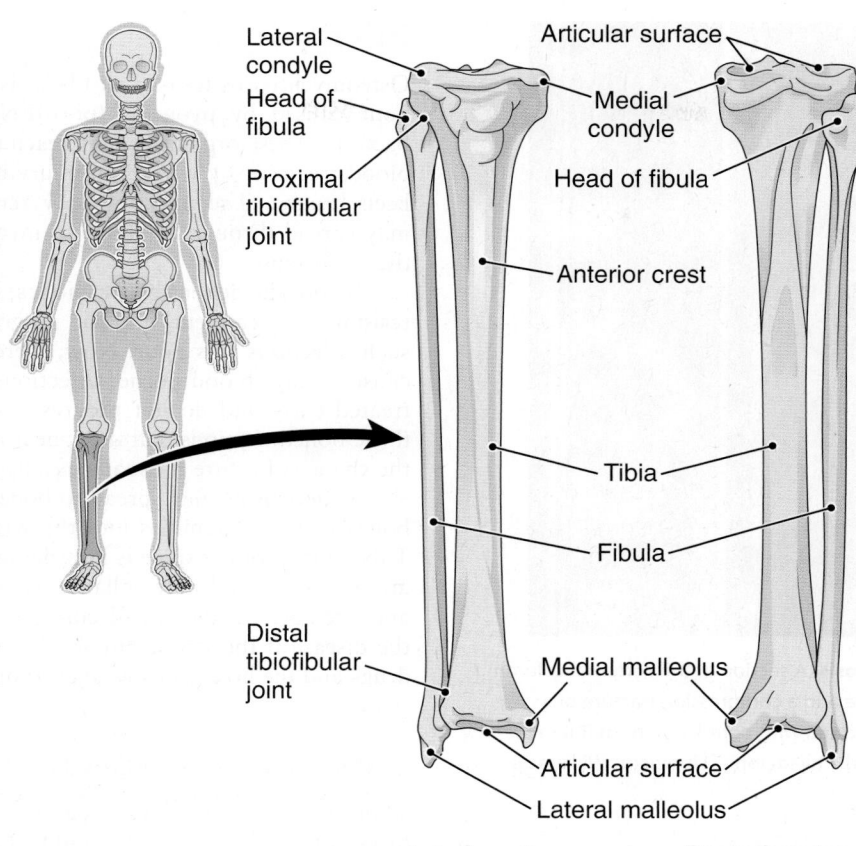

Lateral condyle
Head of fibula
Proximal tibiofibular joint
Articular surface
Medial condyle
Head of fibula
Anterior crest
Tibia
Fibula
Distal tibiofibular joint
Medial malleolus
Articular surface
Lateral malleolus

Anterior view   **Posterior view**

Figure 7-24 **Tibia and fibula of the right leg.** [ZOOMING IN ➤ What is the medial bone of the leg?]

dergo periods of calcium loss followed by periods of excessive deposition of calcium salts. As a result, the bones become deformed. Cause and cure are not known at the present time. The bones also can become decalcified owing to the effect of a tumor of the parathyroid gland (see Chapter 12).

In **osteomalacia** (os-te-o-mah-LA-she-ah) bone tissue softens due to lack of calcium salt formation. Possible causes include vitamin D deficiency, renal disorders, liver disease, and certain intestinal disorders. When osteomalacia occurs in children, the disease is known as **rickets**. The disorder is usually caused by a deficiency of vitamin D and was common among children in past centuries who had poor diets and inadequate exposure to sunlight. Rickets affects the bones and their growth plates, causing the skeleton to remain soft and become distorted.

Tumors

Tumors, or neoplasms, that develop in bone tissue may be benign, as is the case with certain cysts, or they may be malignant, as are **osteosarcomas** and **chondrosarcomas.** Osteosarcoma most commonly occurs in a young person in a bone's growing region, especially around the knee. Chondrosarcoma arises in cartilage and

Fibula
Lateral malleous
Tarsal bones
Cuboid
Cuneiforms
Tibia
Medial malleolus
Talus
Calcaneus
Navicular
Tarsal bones
Metatarsal bones
Phalanges

Figure 7-25 **Bones of the right foot.** [ZOOMING IN ➤ Which tarsal bone is the heel bone?]

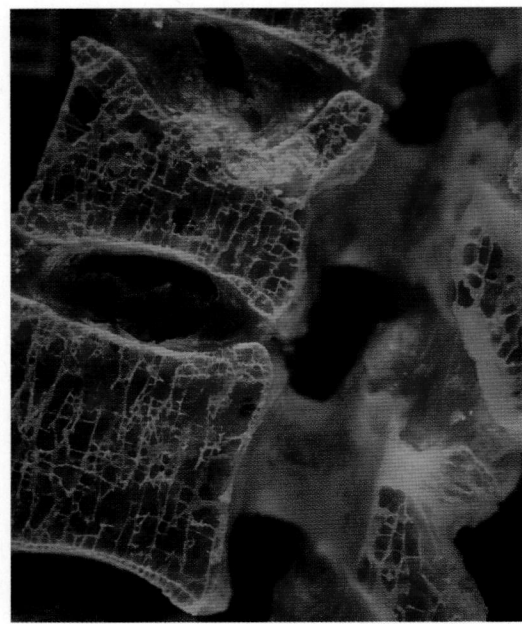

Figure 7-26 **Osteoporosis.** A section of the vertebral column showing loss of bone tissue and a compression fracture of a vertebral body (top). (Reprinted with permission from Rubin E, Farber JL. *Pathology*, 3rd ed. Philadelphia: Lippincott Williams & Wilkins, 1999.)

usually appears in midlife. In older people, tumors at other sites often metastasize (spread) to bones, most commonly to the spine.

Infection

Osteomyelitis (os-te-o-mi-eh-LI-tis) is an inflammation of bone caused by **pyogenic** (pi-o-JEN-ik) (pus-producing) bacteria. These organisms may reach the bone through the bloodstream or by way of an injury in which the skin has been broken. The infection may remain localized, or it may spread through the bone to involve the marrow and the periosteum.

Before the advent of antibiotics, bone infections were resistant to treatment, and the prognosis for people with such infections was poor. Now, there are fewer cases because many blood-borne infections are prevented or treated early and do not progress to affect the bones. If those bone infections that do appear are treated promptly, the chance of a cure is usually excellent.

Tuberculosis may spread to bones, especially the long bones of the extremities and the wrist and ankle bones. Tuberculosis of the spine is **Pott disease**. Infected vertebrae are weakened and may collapse, causing pain, deformity, and pressure on the spinal cord. Antibiotics can control the disease if the strains involved are not resistant to the drugs and the host is not weakened by other diseases.

Structural Disorders

Abnormalities of the spinal curves are known as **curvatures of the spine** (Fig. 7-27) and include:

■ **Kyphosis** (ki-FO-sis), an exaggeration of the thoracic curve, commonly referred to as "hunchback"

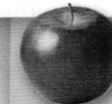

Box 7-2   **Health Maintenance**

Three Steps Toward a Strong and Healthy Skeleton

The skeleton is the body's framework. It supports and protects internal organs, helps to produce movement, and manufactures blood cells. Bone also stores nearly all of the body's calcium, releasing it into the blood when needed for processes such as nerve transmission, muscle contraction, and blood clotting. Proper nutrition, exercise, and a healthy lifestyle can help the skeleton perform all these essential roles.

A well-balanced diet supplies the nutrients and energy needed for strong, healthy bones. Calcium and phosphorus confer strength and rigidity. Protein supplies the amino acids needed to make collagen, which gives bone tissue flexibility, and vitamin C helps stimulate collagen synthesis. Foods rich in both calcium and phosphorus include dairy products, fish, beans, and leafy green vegetables. Meat is an excellent source of protein, whereas citrus fruits are rich in vitamin C. Vitamin D helps the digestive system absorb calcium into the

bloodstream, making it available for bone. Foods rich in vitamin D include fish, liver, and eggs.

When body fluids become too acidic, bone releases calcium and phosphate and is weakened. Both magnesium and potassium help regulate the pH of body fluids, with magnesium also helping bone absorb calcium. Foods rich in magnesium and potassium include beans, potatoes, and leafy green vegetables. Bananas and dairy products are high in potassium.

Like muscle, bone becomes weakened with disuse. Consistent exercise promotes a stronger, denser skeleton by stimulating bone to absorb more calcium and phosphate from the blood, reducing the risk of osteoporosis. A healthy lifestyle also includes avoiding smoking and excessive alcohol consumption, both of which decrease bone calcium and inhibit bone growth. High levels of caffeine in the diet may also rob the skeleton of calcium.

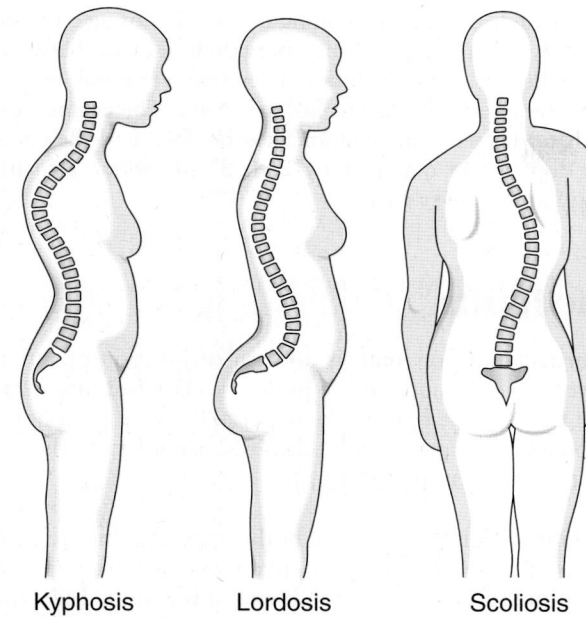

Kyphosis Lordosis Scoliosis

Figure 7-27 **Abnormalities of the spinal curves.**

Cleft palate is a congenital deformity in which there is an opening in the roof of the mouth owing to faulty union of the maxillary bones. An infant born with this defect has difficulty nursing because the mouth communicates with the nasal cavity above, and the baby therefore sucks in air rather than milk. Surgery is usually performed to correct the condition.

Flatfoot is a common disorder in which the tendons and ligaments that support the foot's long arch are weakened and the curve of the arch flattens (see Fig. 7-25). This arch normally helps to absorb shock and distribute body weight and aids in walking. Flatfoot may be brought on by excess weight or poor posture and may also result from a hereditary failure of arch formation. It may cause difficulty or pain in walking. An arch support may be helpful in treating flatfoot.

Fractures

A **fracture** is a break in a bone, usually caused by trauma (Fig. 7-28). Almost any bone can be fractured with sufficient force. Such injuries may be classified as follows:

- **Lordosis** (lor-DO-sis), an excessive lumbar curve, commonly known as "swayback"
- **Scoliosis** (sko-le-O-sis), a lateral curvature of the vertebral column

Scoliosis is the most common of these disorders. In extreme cases, it may cause compression of internal organs. Scoliosis occurs in the rapid growth period of the teens, more often in girls than in boys. Early discovery and treatment produce good results.

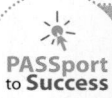
PASSport to Success

Visit **thePoint** or see the Student Resource CD in the back of this book for pictures of scoliosis and other spinal curvatures.

- **Closed fracture**—a simple bone fracture with no open wound
- **Open fracture**—a broken bone protrudes through the skin or an external wound leads to a broken bone
- **Greenstick fracture**—one side of the bone is broken and the other is bent. These are most common in children.
- **Impacted fracture**—the broken ends of the bone are jammed into each other
- **Comminuted** (KOM-ih-nu-ted) **fracture**—there is more than one fracture line and the bone is splintered or crushed
- **Spiral fracture**—the bone has been twisted apart. These are relatively common in skiing accidents.
- **Transverse fracture**—the fracture goes straight across the bone

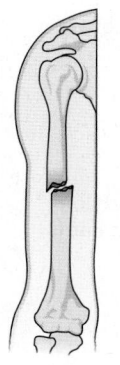 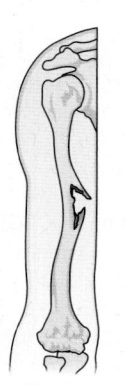 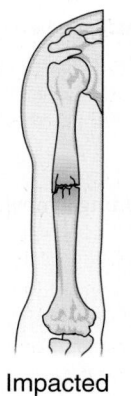 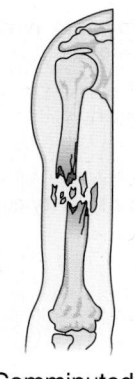 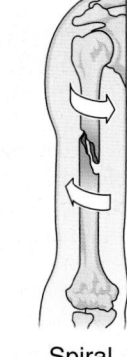 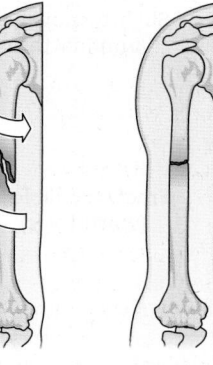 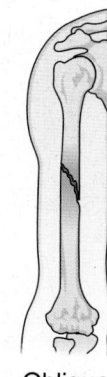

Closed Open Greenstick Impacted Comminuted Spiral Transverse Oblique

Figure 7-28 **Types of fractures.**

- **Oblique fracture**—the break occurs at an angle across the bone

The most important step in first aid care of fractures is to prevent movement of the affected parts. Protection by simple splinting after careful evaluation of the situation, leaving as much as possible "as is," and a call for expert help are usually the safest measures. People who have back injuries may be spared serious spinal cord damage if they are carefully and correctly moved on a firm board or door. If trained paramedics or rescue personnel can reach the scene, untrained people should follow a "hands off" rule. If there is no external bleeding, covering the victim with blankets may help combat shock. First aid should always be immediately directed toward the control of hemorrhage.

Skeletal Changes in the Aging

The aging process includes significant changes in all connective tissues, including bone. There is a loss of calcium salts and a decrease in the amount of protein formed in bone tissue. The reduction of collagen in bone and in tendons, ligaments, and skin contributes to the stiffness so often experienced by older people. Muscle tissue is also lost throughout adult life. Thus, there is a tendency to decrease the exercise that is so important to the maintenance of bone tissue.

Changes in the vertebral column with age lead to a loss in height. Approximately 1.2 cm (about 0.5 inches) are lost each 20 years beginning at 40 years of age, owing primarily to a thinning of the intervertebral disks (between the bodies of the vertebrae). Even the vertebral bodies themselves may lose height in later years. The costal (rib) cartilages become calcified and less flexible, and the chest may decrease in diameter by 2 to 3 cm (about 1 inch), mostly in the lower part.

The Joints

An **articulation**, or **joint**, is an area of junction or union between two or more bones. Joints are classified into three main types on the basis of the material between the adjoining bones. They may also be classified according to the degree of movement permitted (Table 7-2):

- **Fibrous joint.** The bones in this type of joint are held together by fibrous connective tissue. An example is a **suture** (SU-chur) between bones of the skull. This type of joint is immovable and is termed a **synarthrosis** (sin-ar-THRO-sis).

- **Cartilaginous joint.** The bones in this type of joint are connected by cartilage. Examples are the joint between the pubic bones of the pelvis—the pubic symphysis—and the joints between the bodies of the vertebrae. This type of joint is slightly movable and is termed an **amphiarthrosis** (am-fe-ar-THRO-sis).

Table 7-2	Joints		
Type	**Movement**	**Material Between the Bones**	**Examples**
Fibrous	Immovable (synarthrosis)	No joint cavity; fibrous connective tissue between bones	Sutures between skull bones
Cartilaginous	Slightly movable (amphiarthrosis)	No joint cavity; cartilage between bones	Pubic symphysis; joints between vertebral bodies
Synovial	Freely movable (diarthrosis)	Joint cavity containing synovial fluid	Gliding, hinge, pivot, condyloid, saddle, ball-and-socket joints

- **Synovial** (sin-O-ve-al) **joint.** The bones in this type of joint have a potential space between them called the **joint cavity,** which contains a small amount of thick, colorless fluid. This lubricant, **synovial fluid,** resembles uncooked egg white (*ov* is the root, meaning "egg") and is secreted by the membrane that lines the joint cavity. The synovial joint is freely movable and is termed a **diarthrosis** (di-ar-THRO-sis). Most joints are synovial joints; they are described in more detail next.

CHECKPOINT 7-10 ➤ What are the three types of joints classified according to the type of material between the adjoining bones?

More About Synovial Joints

The bones in freely movable joints are held together by **ligaments,** bands of fibrous connective tissue. Additional ligaments reinforce and help stabilize the joints at various points (Fig. 7-29A). Also, for strength and protection, there is a **joint capsule** of connective tissue that encloses each joint and is continuous with the periosteum of the bones (see Fig. 7-29B). The bone surfaces in freely movable joints are protected by a smooth layer of hyaline cartilage called the **articular** (ar-TIK-u-lar) **cartilage** (see Fig. 7-29B). Some complex joints may have cartilage between the bones that acts as a cushion, such as the crescent-shaped **medial meniscus** (meh-NIS-kus) and lateral meniscus in the knee joint (Fig. 7-30). Fat may also appear as padding around a joint.

Near some joints are small sacs called **bursae** (BER-se), which are filled with synovial fluid (see Fig. 7-30). These lie in areas subject to stress and help ease movement over and around the joints. Inflammation of a bursa, as a result of injury or irritation, is called **bursitis.**

TYPES OF SYNOVIAL JOINTS
Synovial joints are classified according to the types of movement they allow, as described and illustrated in Table 7-3. Listed in order of increasing range of motion, they are:

- Gliding joint
- Hinge joint
- Pivot joint
- Condyloid joint
- Saddle joint
- Ball-and-socket joint

MOVEMENT AT SYNOVIAL JOINTS The chief function of the freely movable joints is to allow for changes of position and so provide for motion. These movements are named to describe changes in the positions of body parts (Fig. 7-31). For example, there are four kinds of angular movement, or movement that changes the angle between bones, as listed on the following page:

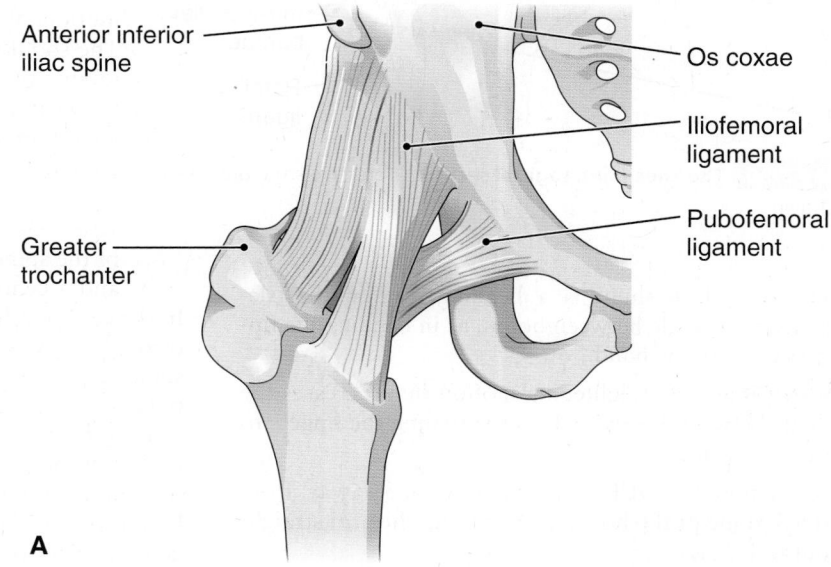

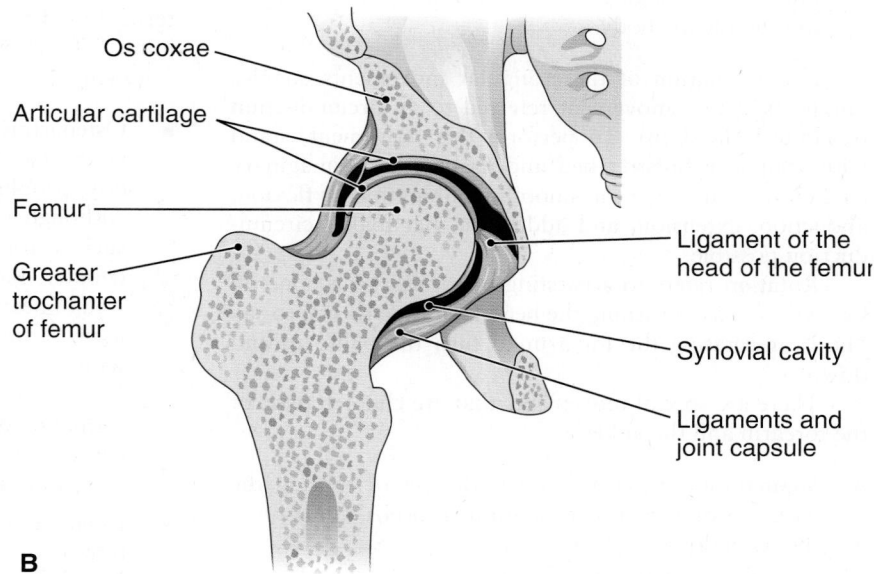

Figure 7-29 **Structure of a synovial joint. (A)** Anterior view of the hip joint showing ligaments that reinforce and stabilize the joint. **(B)** Frontal section through right hip joint showing protective structures.

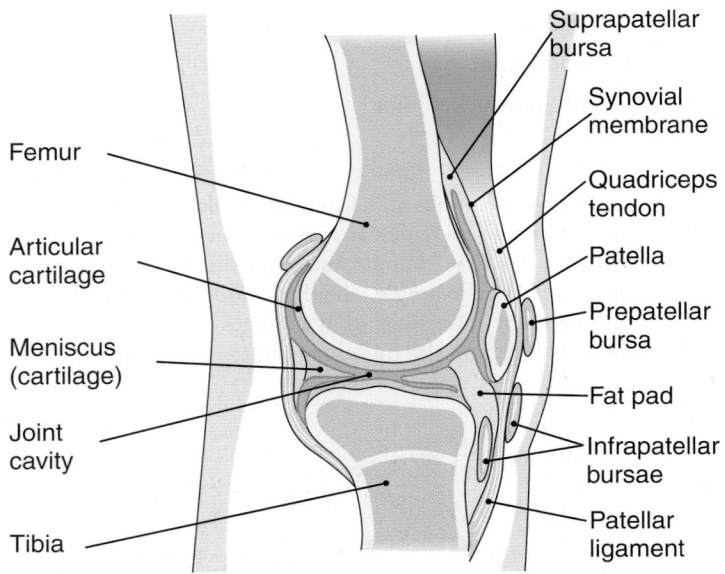

Labels (clockwise): Suprapatellar bursa, Synovial membrane, Quadriceps tendon, Patella, Prepatellar bursa, Fat pad, Infrapatellar bursae, Patellar ligament, Tibia, Joint cavity, Meniscus (cartilage), Articular cartilage, Femur

Figure 7-30 **The knee joint, sagittal section.** Protective structures are also shown.

- **Flexion** (FLEK-shun) is a bending motion that decreases the angle between bones, as in bending the fingers to close the hand.

- **Extension** is a straightening motion that increases the angle between bones, as in straightening the fingers to open the hand.

- **Abduction** (ab-DUK-shun) is movement away from the midline of the body, as in moving the arm straight out to the side.

- **Adduction** is movement toward the midline of the body, as in bringing the arm back to its original position beside the body.

A combination of these angular movements enables one to execute a movement referred to as **circumduction** (ser-kum-DUK-shun). To perform this movement, stand with your arm outstretched and draw a large imaginary circle in the air. Note the smooth combination of flexion, abduction, extension, and adduction that makes circumduction possible.

Rotation refers to a twisting or turning of a bone on its own axis, as in turning the head from side to side to say "no," or rotating the forearm to turn the palm up and down.

There are special movements that are characteristic of the forearm and the ankle:

- **Supination** (su-pin-A-shun) is the act of turning the palm up or forward; **pronation** (pro-NA-shun) turns the palm down or backward.

- **Inversion** (in-VER-zhun) is the act of turning the sole inward, so that it faces the opposite foot; **eversion** (e-VER-zhun) turns the sole outward, away from the body.

- In **dorsiflexion** (dor-sih-FLEK-shun), the foot is bent upward at the ankle, narrowing the angle between the leg and the top of the foot; in **plantar flexion**, the toes point downward, as in toe dancing, flexing the arch of the foot.

CHECKPOINT **7-11** ➤ What is the most freely movable type of joint?

Disorders of Joints

Joints are subject to certain mechanical disorders. A **dislocation** is a derangement of the joint parts. Ball-and-socket joints, which have the widest range of motion, also have the greatest tendency to dislocate. The shoulder joint is the most frequently dislocated joint in the body. A **sprain** is the wrenching of a joint with rupture or tearing of the ligaments. There may also be injuries to the cartilage within the joint, most commonly in the knee joint.

HERNIATED DISK The disks between the vertebrae of the spine consist of an outer ring of fibrocartilage and a central mass known as the nucleus pulposus. In the case of a **herniated disk**, this central mass protrudes through a weakened outer cartilaginous ring into the spinal canal (Fig. 7-32). The herniated or "slipped" disk puts pressure on the spinal cord or spinal nerves, often causing back spasms or pain along the sciatic nerve that travels through the leg, a pain known as sciatica. It is sometimes necessary to remove the disk and fuse the vertebrae involved. Newer techniques make it possible for surgeons to remove only a specific portion of the disk.

ARTHRITIS The most common type of joint disorder is termed **arthritis**, which means "inflammation of the joints." There are different kinds of arthritis, including the following:

- **Osteoarthritis** (os-te-o-arth-RI-tis), also known as degenerative joint disease (DJD), usually occurs in elderly people as a result of normal wear and tear. Although it appears to be a natural result of aging, such factors as obesity and repeated trauma can contribute. Osteoarthritis occurs mostly in joints used in weight bearing, such as the hips, knees, and spinal column. It involves degeneration of the joint cartilage, with growth of new bone at the edges of the joints (Fig. 7-33). Degenerative changes include bone spur formation at the edges of the articular surfaces, thickening of the synovial membrane, atrophy of the cartilage, and calcification of the ligaments.

- **Rheumatoid arthritis** is a crippling condition characterized by joint swelling in the hands, the feet, and elsewhere as a result of inflammation and overgrowth of the synovial membranes and other joint tissues. The articular cartilage is gradually destroyed, and the joint cavity develops adhesions—that is, the surfaces tend

Table 7-3	Synovial Joints	
Type of Joint	**Type of Movement**	**Examples**
Gliding joint	Bone surfaces slide over one another	Joints in the wrist and ankles (Figs. 7-20 and 7-25)
Hinge joint	Allows movement in one direction, changing the angle of the bones at the joint	Elbow joint; joints between phalanges of fingers and toes (Figs. 7-19, 7-20, and 7-25)
Pivot joint	Allows rotation around the length of the bone	Joint between the first and second cervical vertebrae; joint at proximal ends of the radius and ulna (Figs. 7-10 and 7-19)
Condyloid joint	Allows movement in two directions	Joint between the metacarpal and the first phalanx of the finger (knuckle) (Fig. 7-20); joint between the occipital bone of the skull and the first cervical vertebra (atlas) (Fig. 7-10)
Saddle joint	Like a condyloid joint, but with deeper articulating surfaces	Joint between the wrist and the metacarpal bone of the thumb (Fig. 7-20)
Ball-and-socket joint	Allows movement in many directions around a central point. Gives the greatest freedom of movement	Shoulder joint and hip joint (Figs. 7-15 and 7-29)

to stick together—so that the joints stiffen and ultimately become useless. The exact cause of rheumatoid arthritis is uncertain. However, the disease shares many characteristics of autoimmune disorders, in which antibodies are produced that attack the body's own tissues. The role of inherited susceptibility is clear. Treatment includes rest, appropriate exercise, and medications to reduce pain and swelling. Removal of specific antibodies from the blood and administration of drugs to suppress abnormal antibody production have been successful.

■ **Septic (infectious) arthritis** arises when bacteria spread to involve joint tissue, usually by way of the bloodstream. Bacteria introduced during invasive medical procedures, illegal drug injections, or by other means can settle in joints. A variety of organisms are commonly involved, including *Streptococcus, Staphylococcus,* and *Neisseria* species. The joints and the bones themselves are subject to attack by the tuberculosis organism, and the result may be gradual bone destruction near the joint.

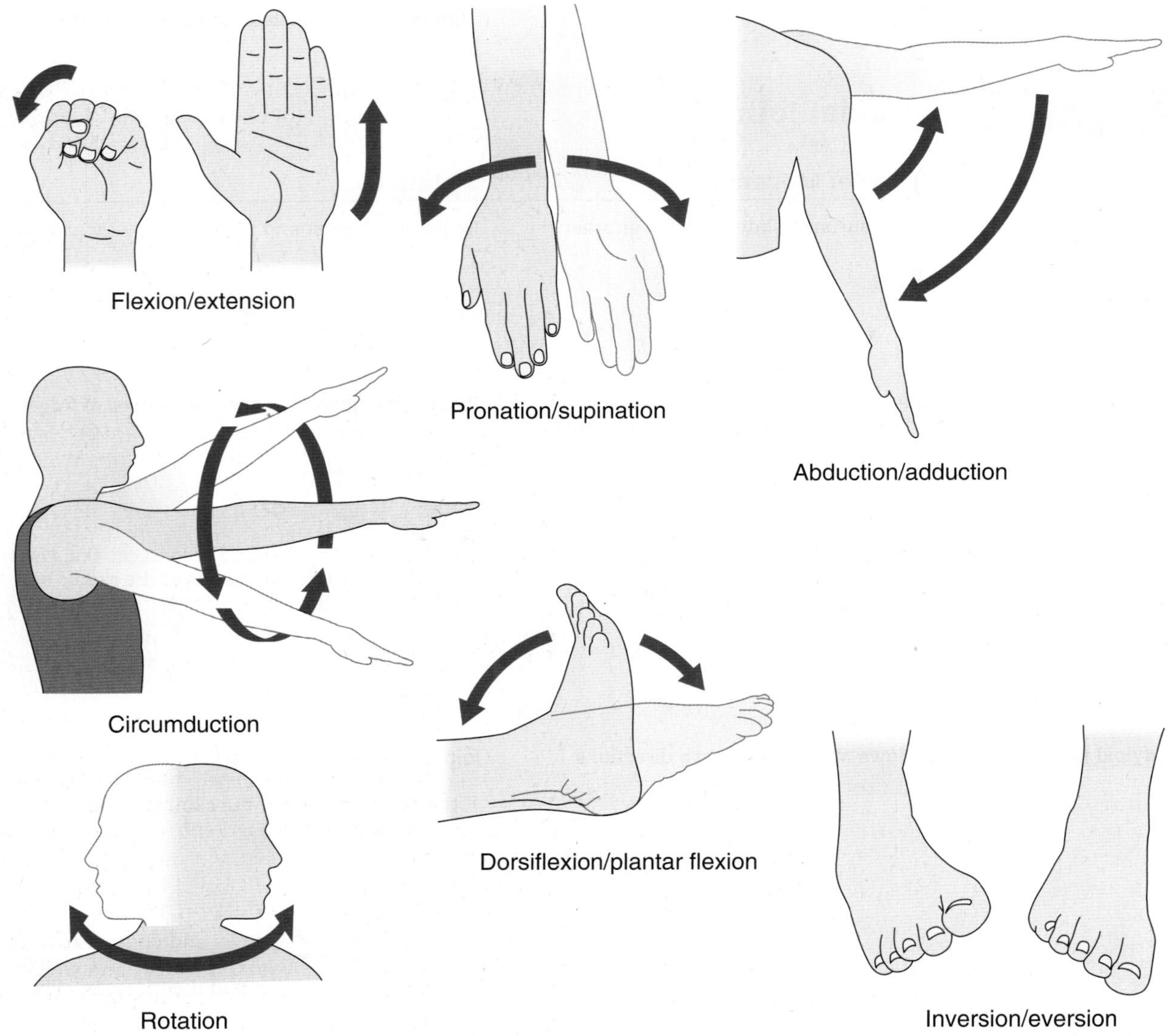

Flexion/extension

Pronation/supination

Abduction/adduction

Circumduction

Dorsiflexion/plantar flexion

Rotation

Inversion/eversion

Figure 7-31 **Movements at synovial joints.**

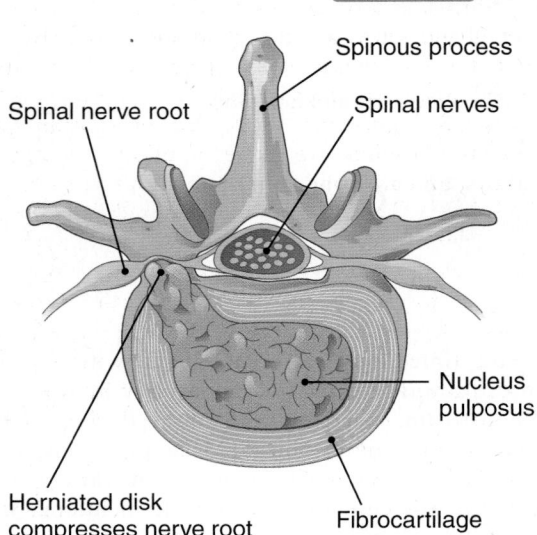

Spinous process

Spinal nerve root

Spinal nerves

Nucleus pulposus

Herniated disk compresses nerve root

Fibrocartilage

Figure 7-32 **Herniated disk.** The central portion (nucleus pulposus) of an intervertebral disk protrudes through the outer rim of cartilage to put pressure on a spinal nerve. (Reprinted with permission from Cohen BJ. *Medical Terminology*, 5th ed. Philadelphia: Lippincott Williams & Wilkins, 2008.)

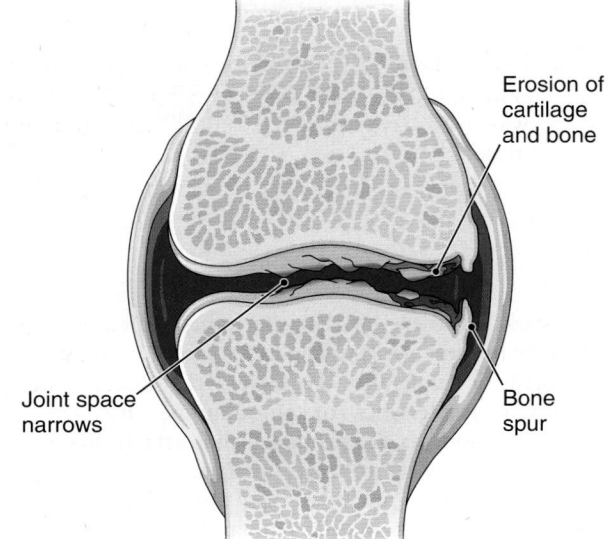

Erosion of cartilage and bone

Joint space narrows

Bone spur

Figure 7-33 **Joint changes in osteoarthritis (DJD).** The left side shows early changes with breakdown of cartilage and narrowing of the joint space. The right side shows progression of the disease with loss of cartilage and formation of bone spurs.

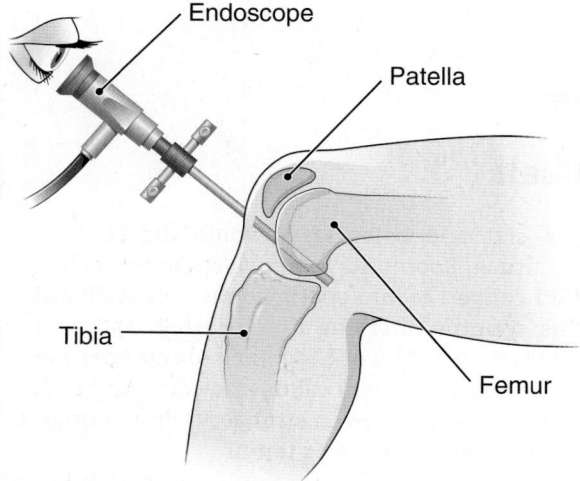

Endoscope

Patella

Tibia

Femur

- **Gout** is a kind of arthritis caused by a metabolic disturbance. One product of metabolism is uric acid, which normally is excreted in the urine. If there happens to be an overproduction of uric acid, or for some reason not enough is excreted, the accumulated uric acid forms crystals that are deposited as masses around the joints and in other areas. As a result, the joints become inflamed and extremely painful. Any joint can be involved, but the one most commonly affected is the big toe. Most gout sufferers are men past middle life.

BACKACHE Backache is another common complaint. Some of its causes are listed below:

- Diseases of the vertebrae, such as infections or tumors, and in older people, osteoarthritis or bone atrophy (wasting away) following long illnesses and lack of exercise.

- Disorders of the intervertebral disks, especially those in the lower lumbar region. Pain may be very severe, with muscle spasms and the extension of symptoms along the course of the sciatic nerve in the leg.

- Abnormalities of the lower vertebrae or of the ligaments and other supporting structures.

- Disorders involving abdominopelvic organs or those in the space behind the peritoneum (such as the kidney). Variations in the position of the uterus are seldom a cause.

- Strains on the lumbosacral joint (where the lumbar region joins the sacrum) or strains on the sacroiliac joint (where the sacrum joins the ilium of the pelvis).

Backache can be prevented by attention to proper movement and good posture. It is most important that the back itself not be used for lifting. A weight to be lifted should be brought close to the body and then the legs should do the actual lifting. An adequate exercise program and control of body weight are also important.

CHECKPOINT 7-12 ➤ What is the most common type of joint disorder?

Joint Repair

Physicians can examine injured joints from outside and even repair them surgically with a lighted instrument known as an **arthroscope** (AR-thro-skope), a type of endoscope (Fig. 7-34). Using arthroscopic techniques, orthopedic surgeons (specialists in the treatment of musculoskeletal disorders) can repair or replace ligaments and remove or reshape cartilage with minimal invasion. Abnormal amounts of fluid that accumulate in a joint cavity as a result of injury can be drained by a tapping procedure called **arthrocentesis** (ar-thro-sen-TE-sis).

If joint degeneration is severe, and conservative therapies, such as medication, physical therapy, and weight loss have failed, a joint replacement or **arthroplasty** (AR-thro-plas-te) may be required. Millions of such surgeries have been performed successfully to restore function in cases of injury, arthritis, and other chronic degenerative bone diseases. Hips and knees are the joints most commonly replaced, but surgeons can also replace shoulder, elbow, wrist, hand, ankle, and foot joints.

The strong, non-toxic, and corrosion-resistant prosthetic (artificial) joints are made of plastic, ceramic, or metal alloys, and are bonded in place with screws or glue. Some are designed to promote bone growth into them to aid in attachment. Computer-controlled machines now produce individualized joints. Until recently, arthroplasty was rarely performed on young people because prosthetic joints had a lifespan of only about 10 years. Current methods have increased this range to 20 years or more, so arthroplasties will require fewer replacements.

7

Disease in Context revisited

►Reggie's Fracture Begins to Heal Itself

"So, Doc, what's the chance my leg's going to heal up enough to play football again?" asked Reggie. "Well," replied the doctor, "It's going to take some time before you're catching footballs again, but once your hip heals, it will be better than new."

The surgeon knew that even before the surgery to realign its broken ends, Reggie's femur had already begun to heal itself. Immediately after the injury occurred on the football field, a blood clot formed around the fracture. A day or two later, chemical messengers within the clot would stimulate blood vessels from the periosteum and endosteum to invade the clot, bringing connective tissue cells with them. Over the next several weeks, fibroblasts and chondroblasts in the clot would secrete collagen and cartilage, converting it into a soft callus. Meanwhile, macrophages would remove the remains of the blood clot and osteoclasts would digest dead bone tissue. Soon after, osteoblasts in the callus would convert it into spongy bone called a hard callus. Months after the injury, osteoclasts and osteoblasts would work together to remodel the outer layers of the hard callus into compact bone, resulting in a repair even stronger than the original bone tissue in Reggie's femur.

During this case, we saw how fractured bones are repaired using screws and plates. We also saw that the body has its own "orthopedic surgeons"—cells like osteoblasts and osteoclasts, which can engineer a bone repair that is even stronger than the original. Although Reggie's skeletal system is beginning to repair itself, he is not out of danger yet. In Chapter 15, a blood clot puts Reggie's life in jeopardy.

Word Anatomy

Medical terms are built from standardized word parts (prefixes, roots, and suffixes). Learning the meanings of these parts can help you remember words and interpret unfamiliar terms.

WORD PART	MEANING	EXAMPLE
Bones		
dia-	through, between	The *diaphysis*, or shaft, of a long bone is between the two ends, or epiphyses.
oss, osse/o	bone, bone tissue	*Osseous* tissue is another name for bone tissue.
oste/o	bone, bone tissue	The *periosteum* is the fibrous membrane around a bone.
-clast	break	An *osteoclast* breaks down bone in the process of resorption.
Bones of the Axial Skeleton		
para-	near	The *paranasal* sinuses are near the nose.
pariet/o	wall	The *parietal* bones form the side walls of the skull.
cost/o	rib	*Intercostal* spaces are located between the ribs.
Bones of the Appendicular Skeleton		
supra-	above, superior	The *supraspinous* fossa is a depression superior to the spine of the scapula.
infra-	below, inferior	The *infraspinous* fossa is a depression inferior to the spine of the scapula.
meta-	near, beyond	The *metacarpal* bones of the palm are near and distal to the carpal bones of the wrist.

WORD PART	MEANING	EXAMPLE
Disorders of Bone		
-penia	lack of	In *osteopenia*, there is a lack of bone density.
-malacia	softening	*Osteomalacia* is a softening of bone tissue.
The Joints		
arthr/o	joint, articulation	A *synarthrosis* is an immovable joint, such as a suture.
amphi-	on both sides, around, double	An *amphiarthrosis* is a slightly movable joint.
ab-	away from	*Abduction* is movement away from the midline of the body.
ad-	toward, added to	*Adduction* is movement toward the midline of the body.
circum-	around	*Circumduction* is movement around a joint in a circle.

Summary

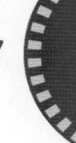

7

I. **BONES**
   A. Main functions
      1. Serve as body framework
      2. Protect organs
      3. Serve as levers for movement
      4. Store calcium salts
      5. Form blood cells
   B. Bone structure
      1. Long bone
         a. Diaphysis—shaft
         b. Epiphysis—end
      2. Bone tissue
         a. Compact—in shaft of long bones; outside of other bones
         b. Spongy (cancellous)—in end of long bones; center of other bones
      3. Bone marrow
         a. Red—in spongy bone
         b. Yellow—in central cavity of long bones
      4. Bone membranes—contain bone-forming cells
         a. Periosteum—covers bone
         b. Endosteum—lines marrow cavity
   C. Bone growth and repair
      1. Bone cells
         a. Osteoblasts—bone-forming cells
         b. Osteocytes—mature bone cells that maintain bone
         c. Osteoclasts—cells that break down (resorb) bone; derived from monocytes, types of white blood cells
      2. Formation of a long bone—begins in center of shaft and continues at epiphyseal plate
   D. Bone markings
      1. Projections—head, process, condyle, crest, spine
      2. Depressions and holes—foramen, sinus, fossa, meatus

II. **BONES OF THE AXIAL SKELETON**
   A. Framework of the skull
      1. Cranium—frontal, parietal, temporal, ethmoid, sphenoid, occipital
      2. Facial bones—mandible, maxilla, zygomatic, nasal, lacrimal, vomer, palatine, inferior nasal conchae
      3. Other—ossicles (of ear), hyoid
      4. Infant skull—fontanels (soft spots)
   B. Framework of the trunk
      1. Vertebral column—divisions: cervical, thoracic, lumbar, sacral, coccygeal
         a. Curves
            (1) Thoracic and sacral—concave, primary
            (2) Cervical and lumbar—convex, secondary
      2. Thorax
         a. Sternum—manubrium, body, xiphoid process
         b. Ribs
            (1) True—first seven pairs
            (2) False—remaining five pairs, including two floating ribs

III. **BONES OF THE APPENDICULAR SKELETON**
   A. Upper division
      1. Shoulder girdle—clavicle, scapula
      2. Upper extremity—humerus, ulna, radius, carpals, metacarpals, phalanges
   B. Lower division
      1. Pelvic bones—os coxae (hip bone): ilium, ischium, pubis
         a. Female pelvis lighter, wider, more rounded than male
      2. Lower extremity—femur, patella, tibia, fibula, tarsals, metatarsals, phalanges

IV. **DISORDERS OF BONE**
   A. Metabolic—osteoporosis, osteopenia, osteitis deformans, osteomalacia, rickets

B. Tumors
C. Infection—osteomyelitis, tuberculosis (in spine is called Pott disease)
D. Structural disorders—curvature of the spine, cleft palate, flat foot
E. Fractures—closed, open, greenstick, impacted, comminuted, spiral, transverse, oblique
F. Changes in aging—loss of calcium salts, decreased collagen production, thinning of intervertebral disks, loss of flexibility

V. **THE JOINTS (ARTICULATIONS)**
A. Kinds of joints
1. Fibrous—immovable (synarthrosis)
2. Cartilaginous—slightly movable (amphiarthrosis)
3. Synovial—freely movable (diarthrosis)
B. More about synovial joints
1. Structure of synovial joints
a. Joint cavity—contains synovial fluid
b. Ligaments—hold joint together
c. Joint capsule—strengthens and protects joint
d. Articular cartilage—covers ends of bones
e. Bursae—fluid-filled sacs near joints; cushion and protect joints and surrounding tissue
2. Types of synovial joints—gliding, hinge, pivot, condyloid, saddle, ball-and-socket
3. Movement at synovial joints
a. Angular—flexion, extension, abduction, adduction
b. Circular—circumduction, rotation
c. Special at forearm—supination, pronation
d. Special at ankle—inversion, eversion, dorsiflexion, plantar flexion
C. Disorders of Joints
1. Dislocations and sprains
2. Herniated disk—central portion of intervertebral disk projects through outer cartilage
3. Arthritis—osteoarthritis, rheumatoid arthritis, infectious arthritis, gout
4. Backache
D. Joint repair
1. Arthroscope—endoscope used to examine and repair joints
2. Arthroplasty—joint replacement

Questions for Study and Review

BUILDING UNDERSTANDING

Fill in the blanks

1. The shaft of a long bone is called the _____.

2. The structural unit of compact bone is the _____.

3. Red bone marrow manufactures _____.

4. Bones are covered by a connective tissue membrane called _____.

5. Bone matrix is produced by _____.

Matching > Match each numbered item with the most closely related lettered item.

___ **6.** A rounded bony projection

___ **7.** A sharp bony prominence

___ **8.** A hole through bone

___ **9.** A bony depression

___ **10.** An air-filled bony cavity

a. condyle

b. foramen

c. fossa

d. sinus

e. spine

Multiple Choice

___ **11.** On which of the following bones would the mastoid process be found?
    a. occipital bone
    b. femur
    c. temporal bone
    d. humerus

___ **12.** An abnormal exaggeration of the thoracic curve is called
    a. kyphosis
    b. lordosis
    c. osteitis deformans
    d. Pott disease

___ **13.** A splintered or crushed bone with multiple fractures is classified as having a(n) _____ fracture.

    a. open
    b. impacted
    c. comminuted
    d. greenstick

___ **14.** A joint that is freely moveable is called a(n) _____ joint.

    a. arthrotic
    b. amphiarthrotic
    c. diarthrotic
    d. synarthrotic

___ **15.** Which of the following synovial joints describes the hip?

    a. gliding
    b. hinge
    c. pivot
    d. ball-and-socket

UNDERSTANDING CONCEPTS

16. List five functions of bone and describe how a long bone's structure enables it to carry out each of these functions.

17. Explain the differences between the terms in each of the following pairs:

    a. osteoblast and osteocyte
    b. periosteum and endosteum
    c. compact bone and spongy bone
    d. epiphysis and diaphysis
    e. axial skeleton and appendicular skeleton

18. Discuss the process of long bone formation during fetal development and childhood. What role does resorption play in bone formation?

19. Name the bones of the:

    a. cranium and face
    b. thoracic cavity, vertebral column, and pelvis
    c. upper and lower limbs

20. Compare and contrast osteoporosis, osteomalacia, and osteomyelitis.

21. Name three effects of aging on the skeletal system.

22. What are the similarities and differences between osteoarthritis, rheumatoid arthritis, and gout?

23. Differentiate between the terms in each of the following pairs:

    a. flexion and extension
    b. abduction and adduction
    c. supination and pronation
    d. inversion and eversion
    e. circumduction and rotation
    f. dorsiflexion and plantar flexion

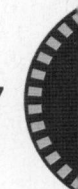

7

CONCEPTUAL THINKING

24. The vertebral bodies are much larger in the lower back than the neck. What is the functional significance of this structural difference?

25. Nine-year-old Alek is admitted to the emergency room with a closed fracture of the right femur. Radiography reveals that the fracture crosses the distal epiphyseal plate. What concerns should Alek's healthcare team have about the location of his injury?

26. In the case story, Reggie presented with three typical signs of hip fracture—shortening, adduction, and lateral rotation of the affected limb. What causes these signs? (HINT—the skeleton is part of the musculoskeletal system.)

27. In Reggie's case, he fractured the proximal end of his right femur, an integral component of his hip. Name the joint disorders that Reggie is more at risk of in (a) the short term, and (b) the long term.

CHAPTER 8

The Muscular System

Learning Outcomes

After careful study of this chapter, you should be able to:

1. Compare the three types of muscle tissue
2. Describe three functions of skeletal muscle
3. Briefly describe how skeletal muscles contract
4. List the substances needed in muscle contraction and describe the function of each
5. Define the term *oxygen debt*
6. Describe three compounds stored in muscle that are needed to generate energy in highly active muscle cells
7. Cite the effects of exercise on muscles
8. Compare isotonic and isometric contractions
9. Explain how muscles work in pairs to produce movement
10. Compare the workings of muscles and bones to lever systems
11. Explain how muscles are named
12. Name some of the major muscles in each muscle group and describe the main function of each
13. Describe how muscles change with age
14. List the major muscular disorders
15. Show how word parts are used to build words related to the muscular system (see Word Anatomy at the end of the chapter)

Selected Key Terms

The following terms and other boldface terms in the chapter are defined in the Glossary

acetylcholine
actin
antagonist
bursitis
fascicle
glycogen
insertion
lactic acid
motor unit
myalgia
myoglobin
myosin
neuromuscular junction
neurotransmitter
origin
oxygen debt
prime mover
spasm
synapse
synergist
tendon
tonus

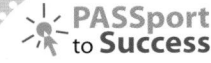

PASSport to Success

Visit *thePoint* or see the Student Resource CD in the back of this book for definitions and pronunciations of key terms as well as a pretest for this chapter.

Disease in Context

Sue's Case: A Muscle Mystery

Dr. Mathews glanced at his patient's chart as he stepped into the consulting room to see her. Sue Pritchard was 26 years old, white, and, according to her medical history, relatively healthy. "Hi Sue. It's been a while since your last visit. What can I do for you today?" asked the doctor.

"I'm probably making a mountain out of a molehill," Sue replied. "But, I've been having some odd symptoms that got me worried. For the last couple of weeks I've noticed that my right hand is getting weak. Just the other day, I had barely enough strength to hold my coffee cup! On top of that, I've had trouble walking. I haven't fallen down or anything, but I feel like I'm off balance."

Based on Sue's description of her symptoms, Dr. Mathews initially suspected a problem with her muscular system. He checked her hand strength and verified that her right hand was weaker than her left—unusual since she was right-handed. He compared both of Sue's arms and observed slight atrophy of the flexor muscles in her right forearm. He tested several of her reflexes and noted that the responses in her biceps brachii and quadriceps femoris muscles were exaggerated in her right limbs. He had Sue do a few simple coordination tests like touching her nose and standing on one foot. As in the previous tests, Sue seemed to have more difficulty with right-sided tasks than left. "Have you had any pain or tingling in your arms or legs lately?" the doctor asked.

"Yes!" answered Sue. "In fact, last night I had a cramp in my right leg that was so painful I had to get out of bed and walk it off. And, my fingertips have been tingling on and off for the last few days too."

Dr. Mathews quickly recognized that Sue's problem was not just limited to her muscular system. It also appeared that her nervous system was involved.

Dr. Mathews' knowledge of the structure and function of the muscular system helps him to diagnose medical conditions. In this chapter you will learn about muscle tissue and the connection it has with nervous tissue. Later in the chapter, we'll find out more about Sue's condition.

Types of Muscle

There are three kinds of muscle tissue: smooth, cardiac, and skeletal muscle, as introduced in Chapter 4. After a brief description of all three types (Table 8-1), this chapter concentrates on skeletal muscle, which has been studied the most.

Smooth Muscle

Smooth muscle makes up the walls of the hollow body organs as well as those of the blood vessels and respiratory passageways. It moves involuntarily and produces the wave-like motions of peristalsis that move substances through a system. Smooth muscle can also regulate the diameter of an opening, such as the central opening of blood vessels, or produce contractions of hollow organs, such as the uterus. Smooth muscle fibers (cells) are tapered at each end and have a single, central nucleus. The cells appear smooth under the microscope because they do not contain the visible bands, or **striations**, that are seen in the other types of muscle cells. Smooth muscle may contract in response to a nerve impulse, hormonal stimulation, stretching, and other stimuli. The muscle contracts and relaxes slowly and can remain contracted for a long time.

Cardiac Muscle

Cardiac muscle, also involuntary, makes up the heart's wall and creates the pulsing action of that organ. The cells of cardiac muscle are striated, like those of skeletal muscle. They differ in having one nucleus per cell and branching interconnections. The membranes between the cells are specialized to allow electrical impulses to travel rapidly through them, so that contractions can be better coordinated. These membranes appear as dark lines between the cells (see Table 8-1) and are called intercalated (in-TER-kah-la-ted) disks, because they are "inserted between" the cells. The electrical impulses that produce cardiac muscle contractions are generated within the muscle itself but can be modified by nervous stimuli and hormones.

Skeletal Muscle

When viewed under the microscope, skeletal muscle cells appear heavily striated. The arrangement of protein threads within the cell that produces these striations is described later. The cells are very long and cylindrical and have multiple nuclei per cell. During development, the nuclei of these cells divide repeatedly by mitosis without division of the cell contents, resulting in a large, multinucleated cell. Such cells can contract as a large unit when stimulated. The nervous system stimulates skeletal muscle to contract, and the tissue usually contracts and relaxes rapidly. Because it is under conscious control, skeletal muscle is described as voluntary.

Skeletal muscle is so named because most of these muscles are attached to bones and produce movement at the joints. There are a few exceptions. The muscles of the abdominal wall, for example, are partly attached to other muscles, and the muscles of facial expression are attached to the skin. Skeletal muscles constitute the largest amount of the body's muscle tissue, making up about 40% of the total body weight. This muscular system is composed of more than 600 individual skeletal muscles. Although each one is a distinct structure, muscles usually act in groups to execute body movements.

Table 8-1	Comparison of the Different Types of Muscle		
	Smooth	**Cardiac**	**Skeletal**
Location	Wall of hollow organs, vessels, respiratory passageways	Wall of heart	Attached to bones
Cell characteristics	Tapered at each end, branching networks, nonstriated	Branching networks; special membranes (intercalated disks) between cells; single nucleus; lightly striated	Long and cylindrical; multinucleated; heavily striated
Control	Involuntary	Involuntary	Voluntary
Action	Produces peristalsis; contracts and relaxes slowly; may sustain contraction	Pumps blood out of heart; self-excitatory but influenced by nervous system and hormones	Produces movement at joints; stimulated by nervous system; contracts and relaxes rapidly

CHECKPOINT **8-1** ➤ What are the three types of muscle?

The Muscular System

The three primary functions of skeletal muscles are:

- Movement of the skeleton. Muscles are attached to bones and contract to change the position of the bones at a joint.

- Maintenance of posture. A steady partial contraction of muscle, known as **muscle tone**, keeps the body in position. Some of the muscles involved in maintaining posture are the large muscles of the thighs, back, neck, and shoulders as well as the abdominal muscles.

- Generation of heat. Muscles generate most of the heat needed to keep the body at 37°C (98.6°F). Heat is a natural by-product of muscle cell metabolism. When we are cold, muscles can boost their heat output by the rapid small contractions we know of as shivering.

CHECKPOINT **8-2** ➤ What are the three main functions of skeletal muscle?

Structure of a Muscle

In forming whole muscles, individual muscle fibers are arranged in bundles, or **fascicles** (FAS-ih-kls), held to-gether by fibrous connective tissue (Fig. 8-1, Table 8-2). The deepest layer of this connective tissue, the **endomysium** (en-do-MIS-e-um) surrounds the individual fibers in the fascicles. Around each fascicle is a connective tissue layer known as the **perimysium** (per-ih-MIS-e-um). The entire muscle is then encased in a tough connective tissue sheath, the **epimysium** (ep-ih-MIS-e-um), which forms the innermost layer of the **deep fascia**, the tough, fibrous sheath that encloses a muscle. (Note that all these layers are named with prefixes that describe their position added to the root *my/o*, meaning "muscle.") All of these support-ing tissues merge to form the **tendon**, the band of connec-tive tissue that attaches a muscle to a bone (see Fig. 8-1).

Muscle Cells in Action

Nerve impulses coming from the brain and the spinal cord stimulate skeletal muscle fibers (see Chapter 9). Because these impulses are traveling away from the central nervous system (CNS), they are described as **motor** impulses (as contrasted to sensory impulses traveling toward the CNS), and the neurons (nerve cells) that carry these impulses are described as motor neurons. As the neuron contacts the muscle, its axon (fiber) branches to supply from a few to hundreds of individual muscle cells, or in some cases more than 1,000 (Fig. 8-2).

A single neuron and all the muscle fibers it stimulates comprise a **motor unit**. Small motor units are used in fine coordination, as in movements of the eye. Larger motor

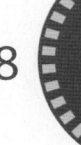

8

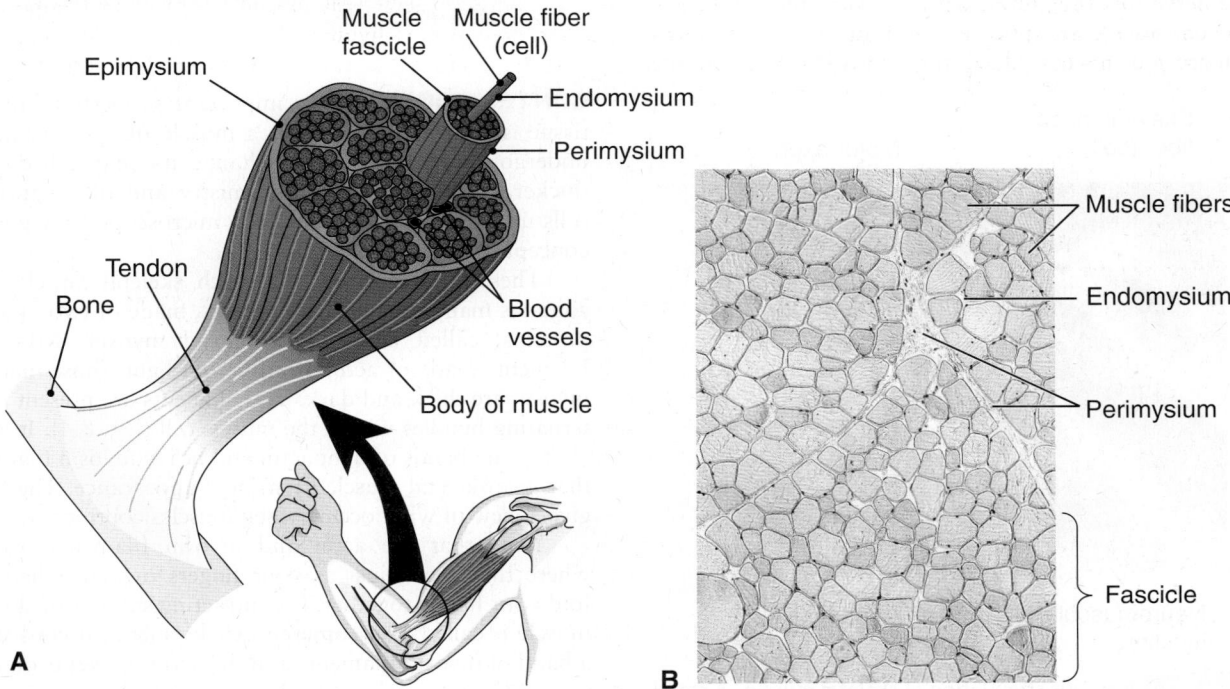

A

B

Figure 8-1 **Structure of a skeletal muscle. (A)** Structure of a muscle showing the tendon that attaches it to a bone. **(B)** Muscle tissue seen under a microscope. Portions of several fascicles are shown with connective tissue coverings. (B, Reprinted with permission from Gartner LP, Hiatt JL. *Color Atlas of Histology*, 3rd ed. Philadelphia: Lippincott Williams & Wilkins, 2000.) **[ZOOMING IN ➤** What is the innermost layer of connective tissue in a muscle? What layer of connective tissue surrounds a fascicle of muscle fibers? **]**

Table 8-2	Connective Tissue Layers in Skeletal Muscle	
Name of Layer	**Location**	
Endomysium	Around each individual muscle fiber	
Perimysium	Around fascicles (bundles) of muscle fibers	
Epimysium	Around entire muscle; forms the innermost layer of the deep fascia	

units are used for maintaining posture or for broad movements, such as walking or swinging a tennis racquet.

THE NEUROMUSCULAR JUNCTION The point at which a nerve fiber contacts a muscle cell is called the **neuromuscular junction** (NMJ) (Fig. 8-3). It is here that a chemical classified as a **neurotransmitter** is released from the neuron to stimulate the muscle fiber. The specific neurotransmitter released here is **acetylcholine** (as-e-til-KO-lene), abbreviated ACh, which is found elsewhere in the body as well. A great deal is known about the events that occur at this junction, and this information is important in understanding muscle action.

The neuromuscular junction is an example of a **synapse** (SIN-aps), a point of communication between cells. Between the cells there is a tiny space, the **synaptic cleft**, across which the neurotransmitter must travel. Until its release, the neurotransmitter is stored in tiny membranous sacs, called vesicles, in the nerve fiber's endings. Once released, the neurotransmitter crosses the synaptic cleft and attaches to receptors, which are proteins embedded in the muscle cell membrane.

The membrane forms multiple folds at this point that increase surface area and hold a maximum number of receptors. The muscle cell's receiving membrane is known as the **motor end plate**.

Muscle fibers, like nerve cells, show the property of **excitability**; that is, they are able to transmit electrical current along the plasma membrane. When the muscle is stimulated at the neuromuscular junction, an electrical impulse is generated that spreads rapidly along the muscle cell membrane. This spreading wave of electrical current is called the **action potential** because it calls the muscle cell into action. Chapter 9 provides more information on synapses and the action potential.

CHECKPOINT **8-3** ➤ Muscles are activated by the nervous system. What is the name of the special synapse where a nerve cell makes contact with a muscle cell?

CHECKPOINT **8-4** ➤ What neurotransmitter is involved in the stimulation of skeletal muscle cells?

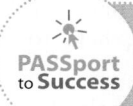
PASSport to Success
Visit **thePoint** or see the Student Resource CD in the back of this book for the animation *The Neuromuscular Junction and Neurotransmitters.*

CONTRACTION Another important property of muscle tissue is **contractility**. This is a muscle fiber's capacity to undergo shortening and to change its shape, becoming thicker. Studies of muscle chemistry and observation of cells under the powerful electron microscope have given a concept of how muscle cells work.

These studies reveal that each skeletal muscle fiber contains many threads, or filaments, made of two kinds of proteins, called **actin** (AK-tin) and **myosin** (MI-o-sin). Filaments made of actin are thin and light; those made of myosin are thick and dark. The filaments are present in alternating bundles within the muscle cell (Fig. 8-4). It is the alternating bands of light actin and heavy myosin filaments that give skeletal muscle its striated appearance. They also give a view of what occurs when muscles contract.

Note that the actin and myosin filaments overlap where they meet, just as your fingers overlap when you fold your hands together. A contracting subunit of skeletal muscle is called a **sarcomere** (SAR-ko-mere). It consists of a band of myosin filaments and the actin filaments on each side of them (see Fig. 8-4). In movement, the myosin filaments "latch on" to the actin filaments in their overlapping region by means of many paddlelike extensions called myosin heads. In this way, the myosin heads form attachments between the actin and myosin filaments that are described as cross-bridges. Using the energy of ATP for

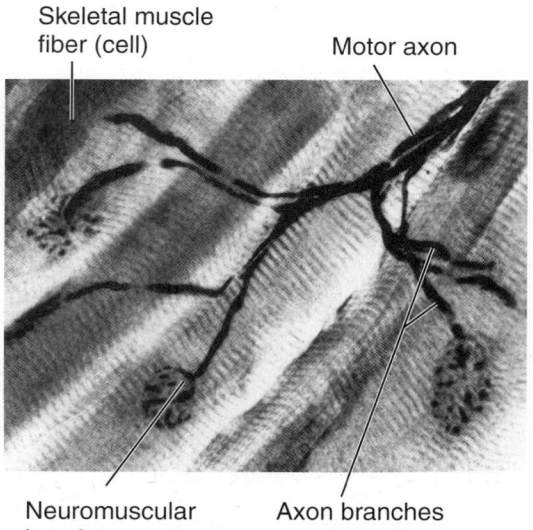

Skeletal muscle fiber (cell)

Motor axon

Neuromuscular junction

Axon branches

Figure 8-2 **Nervous stimulation of skeletal muscle.** A motor axon branches to stimulate multiple muscle fibers (cells). The point of contact between the neuron and the muscle cell is the neuromuscular junction. (Reprinted with permission from Cormack DH. *Essential Histology*, 2nd ed. Philadelphia: Lippincott Williams & Wilkins, 2001.)

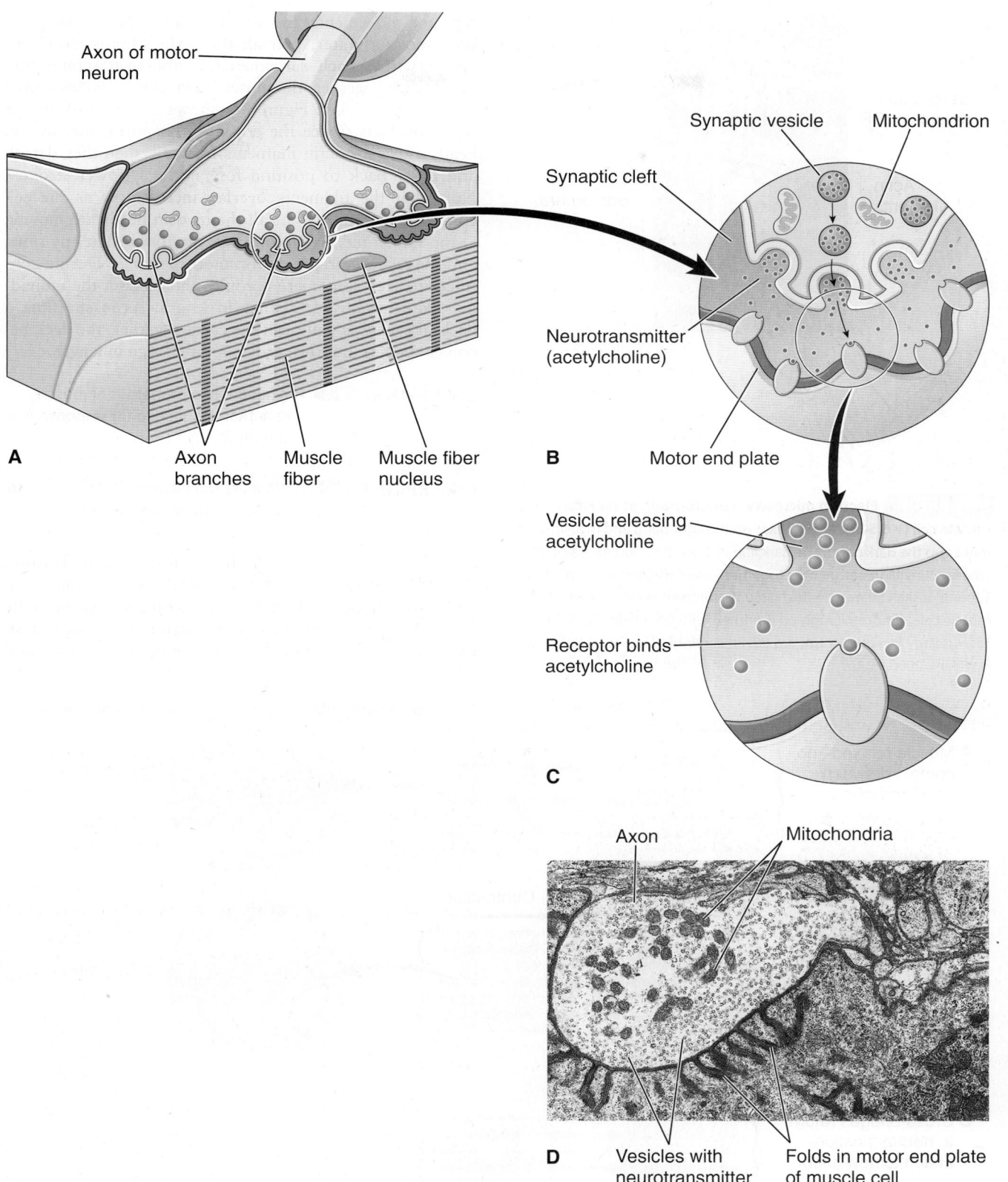

Figure 8-3 **Neuromuscular junction (NMJ).** **(A)** The branched end of a motor neuron makes contact with the membrane of a muscle fiber (cell). **(B)** Enlarged view of the NMJ showing release of neurotransmitter (acetylcholine) into the synaptic cleft. **(C)** Acetylcholine attaches to receptors in the motor end plate, whose folds increase surface area. **(D)** Electron microscope photograph of the neuromuscular junction. (D, Courtesy of A. Sima.)

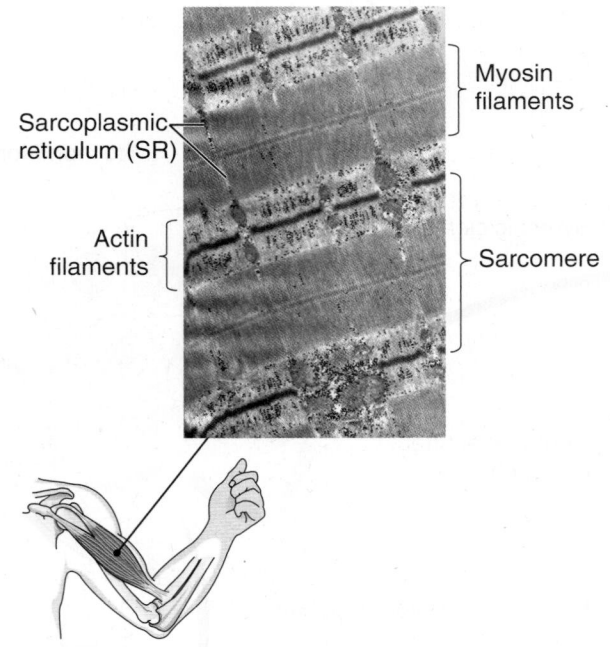

Figure 8-4 **Electron microscope photograph of skeletal muscle cell (×6,500).** Actin makes up the light band and myosin makes up the dark band. The dark line in the actin band marks points where actin filaments are held together. A sarcomere is a contracting subunit of skeletal muscle. The sarcoplasmic reticulum is the ER of muscle cells. (Photomicrograph reprinted with permission from Mills SE. *Histology for Pathologists*, 3rd ed. Philadelphia: Lippincott Williams & Wilkins, 2006.)

repeated movements, the myosin heads, like the oars of a boat moving water, pull all the actin strands closer together within each sarcomere. As the overlapping filaments slide together, the muscle fiber contracts, becoming shorter and thicker. Figure 8-5 shows a section of muscle as it contracts. Once the cross-bridges form, the myosin heads move the actin filaments forward, then they detach and move back to position for another "power stroke." Note that the filaments overlap increasingly as the cell contracts. (In reality, not all the myosin heads are moving at the same time. About one half are forward at any time, and the rest are preparing for another swing.) During contraction, each sarcomere becomes shorter, but the individual filaments do not change in length. As in shuffling a deck of cards, as you push the cards together, the deck becomes smaller, but the cards do not change in length.

CHECKPOINT **8-5** ➤ What are two properties of muscle cells that are needed for response to a stimulus?

CHECKPOINT **8-6** ➤ What are the filaments that interact to produce muscle contraction?

THE ROLE OF CALCIUM In addition to actin, myosin, and ATP, calcium is needed for muscle contraction. It enables cross-bridges to form between actin and myosin so the sliding filament action can begin. When muscles are at rest, two additional proteins called **troponin** (tro-PO-nin) and

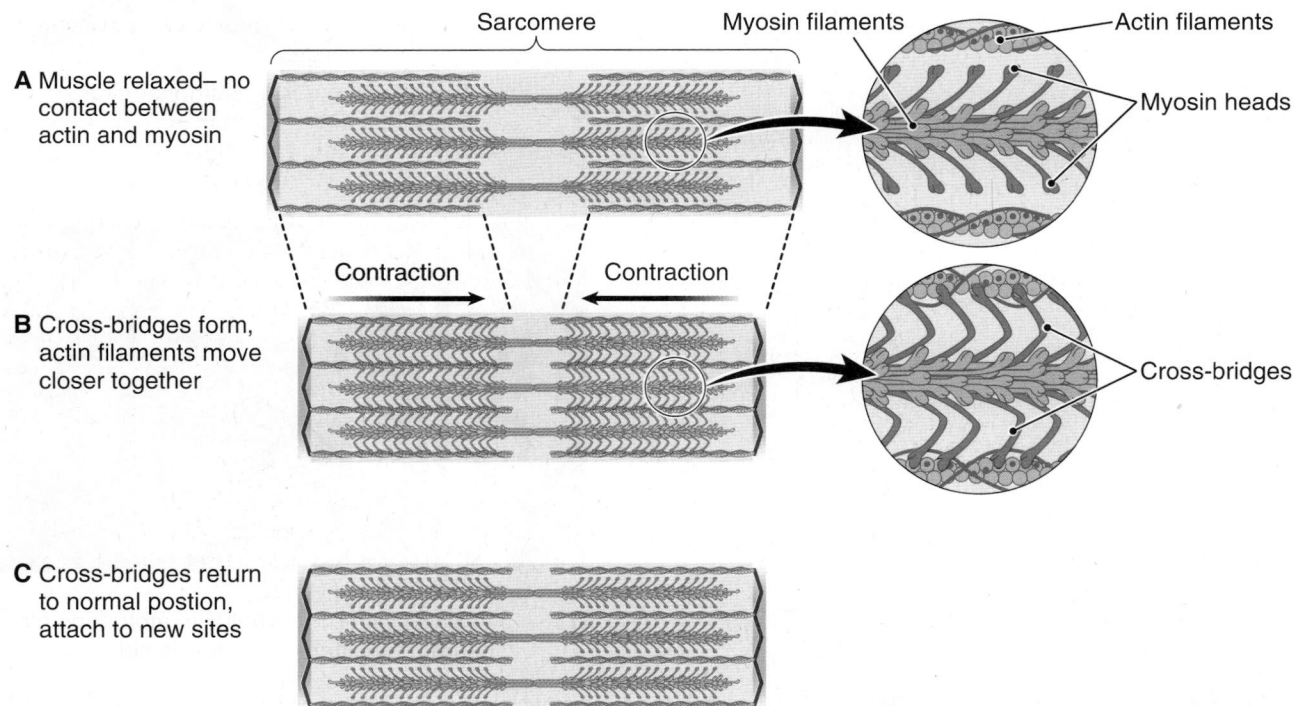

Figure 8-5 **Sliding filament mechanism of skeletal muscle contraction.** **(A)** Muscle is relaxed and there is no contact between the actin and myosin filaments. **(B)** Cross-bridges form and the actin filaments are moved closer together as the muscle fiber contracts. **(C)** The cross-bridges return to their original position and attach to new sites to prepare for another pull on the actin filaments and further contraction. [**ZOOMING IN** ➤ Do the actin or myosin filaments change in length as contraction proceeds?]

tropomyosin (tro-po-MI-o-sin) block the sites on actin filaments where cross-bridges can form (Fig. 8-6). When calcium attaches to the troponin, these proteins move aside, uncovering the binding sites. In resting muscles, the calcium is not available because it is stored within the cell's endoplasmic reticulum, which, in muscle cells, is called the **sarcoplasmic reticulum (SR)**. Calcium is released into the cytoplasm only when the cell is stimulated by a nerve fiber. Muscles relax when nervous stimulation stops and the calcium is then pumped back into the SR, ready for the next contraction.

A summary of the events in a muscle contraction is as follows:

1. Acetylcholine (ACh) is released from a neuron ending into the synaptic cleft at the neuromuscular junction.

2. ACh binds to the muscle's motor end plate and produces an action potential.

3. The action potential travels to the sarcoplasmic reticulum (SR).

4. The sarcoplasmic reticulum releases calcium into the cytoplasm.

5. Calcium shifts troponin and tropomyosin so that binding sites on actin are exposed.

6. Myosin heads bind to actin, forming cross-bridges.

7. Myosin heads pull actin filaments together within the sarcomeres and the cell shortens.

8. ATP is used to detach myosin heads and move them back to position for another "power stroke."

9. Muscle relaxes when stimulation ends and the calcium is pumped back into the sarcoplasmic reticulum.

Box 8-1, Muscle Contraction and Energy, has additional details on skeletal muscle contraction.

Energy Sources

As noted earlier, all muscle contraction requires energy in the form of ATP. The source of this energy is the oxidation (commonly called "burning") of nutrients within the cells.

To produce ATP, muscle cells must have an adequate supply of oxygen and glucose or other usable nutrient. The circulating blood constantly brings these substances to the cells, but muscle cells also store a small reserve supply of each to be used when needed, during vigorous exercise, for example. The following are compounds that store oxygen, energy, or nutrients in muscle cells:

- **Myoglobin** (mi-o-GLO-bin) stores additional oxygen. This compound is similar to the blood's hemoglobin but is located specifically in muscle cells, as indicated by the root *my/o* in its name.

- **Glycogen** (GLI-ko-jen) stores additional glucose. It is a polysaccharide made of multiple glucose molecules and it can be broken down into glucose when needed by the muscle cells.

- **Creatine** (KRE-ah-tin) **phosphate** stores energy. It is a compound similar to ATP, in that it has a high energy bond that releases energy when it is broken. This energy is used to make ATP for muscle contraction when the muscle cell has used up its ATP.

CHECKPOINT 8-7 ➤ What mineral is needed to allow actin and myosin to interact?

CHECKPOINT 8-8 ➤ Muscle cells obtain energy for contraction from the oxidation of nutrients. What compound is formed in oxidation that supplies the energy for contraction?

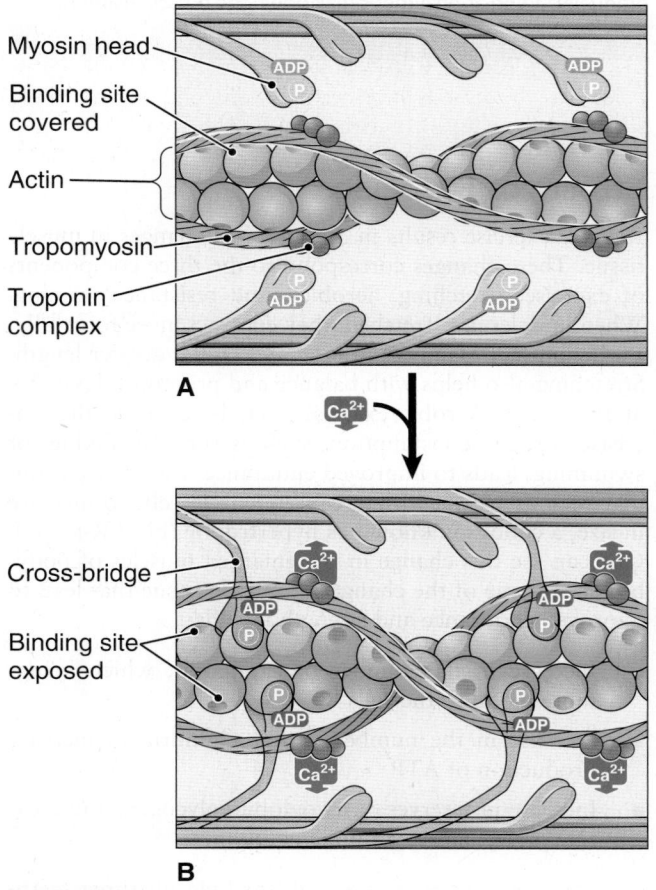

Figure 8-6   Role of calcium in muscle contraction. (A) Troponin and tropomyosin cover the binding sites where cross-bridges can form between actin and myosin. **(B)** Calcium shifts troponin and tropomyosin away from binding sites so cross-bridges can form.

Labels in figure (A): Myosin head; Binding site covered; Actin; Tropomyosin; Troponin complex. Labels in figure (B): Cross-bridge; Binding site exposed.

OXYGEN CONSUMPTION During most activities of daily life, the tissues receive adequate oxygen, and muscles can function aerobically. During strenuous activity, however, a person may not be able to breathe in oxygen rapidly enough to meet the needs of the hard-working muscles. At first, the myoglobin, glycogen, and creatine

Box 8-1   A Closer Look

Muscle Contraction and Energy

When we think of muscle contraction, we might imagine a runner's rippling muscles. But muscle contraction actually occurs at a microscopic level within the sarcomere's working parts: the thick and thin filaments.

Thick filaments are composed of many myosin molecules, each shaped like two golf clubs twisted together with the myosin heads projecting away from the sarcomere's center (see Fig. 8-6). Each myosin head can bind ATP and convert it into ADP and a phosphate molecule, which remain bound. The chemical energy released during this reaction charges the myosin head, enabling it to do work.

Thin filaments' actin molecules are twisted together like two strands of beads. Each "bead" has a myosin-binding site, but the two regulatory proteins, troponin and tropomyosin, cover the binding sites when the muscle is at rest. When calcium shifts these proteins away from the binding sites, the following cycle of events occurs:

1. The charged myosin heads attach to the actin molecules and form cross-bridges between the thick and thin filaments.
2. Using their stored energy, the myosin heads pull the thin filaments to the center of the sarcomere, releasing the ADP and phosphate molecules.
3. New ATP molecules bind to the myosin heads, causing them to detach from actin and breaking the cross-bridges.
4. The myosin heads convert ATP into ADP and phosphate, which recharges them.

After death, muscles enter a stage of rigidity known as rigor mortis. This phenomenon illustrates ATP's crucial role in muscle contraction. Shortly after death, muscle cells begin to degrade. Calcium escapes into the cytoplasm, and the muscle filaments slide together. Metabolism has ceased, however, and there is no ATP to disengage the filaments, so they remain locked in a contracted state. Rigor mortis lasts about 24 hours, gradually fading as enzymes break down the muscle filaments.

phosphate stored in the tissues meet the increased demands, but continual exercise depletes these stores.

For a short time, glucose may be used anaerobically, that is, without the benefit of oxygen. This anaerobic process generates ATP rapidly and permits greater magnitude of activity than would otherwise be possible, as, for example, allowing sprinting instead of jogging. However, anaerobic metabolism is inefficient; it does not produce as much ATP as does metabolism in the presence of oxygen. Also, an organic acid called **lactic acid** accumulates in the cells when this alternate metabolic pathway is used. Anaerobic metabolism can continue only until the buildup of lactic acid causes the muscles to fatigue.

Muscles operating anaerobically are in a state of **oxygen debt**. After stopping exercise, a person must continue to take in extra oxygen by continued rapid breathing (panting) until the debt is paid in full. That is, enough oxygen must be taken in to convert the lactic acid to other substances that can be metabolized further. In addition, the glycogen, myoglobin, and creatine phosphate that are stored in the cells must be replenished. The time after strenuous exercise during which extra oxygen is needed is known as the period of recovery oxygen consumption.

CHECKPOINT 8-9 ➤ When muscles work without oxygen, a compound is produced that causes muscle fatigue. What is the name of this compound?

Effects of Exercise

Regular exercise results in a number of changes in muscle tissue. These changes correspond to the three components of exercise: stretching, aerobics, and resistance training. When muscles are stretched, they contract more forcefully, as the internal filaments can interact over a greater length. Stretching also helps with balance and promotes flexibility at the joints. Aerobic exercise, that is, exercise that increases oxygen consumption, such as running, biking, or swimming, leads to improved endurance. Resistance training, such as weight lifting, causes muscle cells to increase in size, a condition known as hypertrophy (hi-PER-tro-fe). One can see this change in the enlarged muscles of bodybuilders. Some of the changes in muscle tissue that lead to improved endurance and strength include:

- Increase in the number of capillaries, which brings more blood to the cells
- Increase in the number of mitochondria to increase production of ATP
- Increase in reserves of myoglobin, glycogen, and creatine phosphate to promote endurance

An exercise program should include all three methods—stretching, aerobic exercise, and resistance training—with periods of warm-up and cool-down before and after working out. This type of varied program is described as cross-training or interval training.

In addition to affecting muscle tissue itself, exercise causes some systemic changes. The **vasodilation** (vas-o-di-LA-shun), or widening of blood vessel diameter, that occurs during exercise allows blood to flow more easily to muscle tissue. With continued work, more blood is pumped back to the heart. The heart's temporarily increased load strengthens the myocardium and improves its circulation. With exercise training, the heart's chambers gradually enlarge to accommodate more blood. A trained athlete's resting heart rate is lower than the average rate because the heart can function more efficiently.

Regular exercise also improves breathing and respiratory efficiency. Circulation in the capillaries surrounding the alveoli (air sacs) is increased, and this brings about enhanced gas exchange. The more efficient distribution and use of oxygen delays the onset of oxygen debt. Even moderate regular exercise has the additional benefits of weight control, strengthening of the bones, decreased blood pressure, and decreased risk of heart attacks. The effects of exercise on the body are studied in the fields of sports medicine and exercise physiology. Box 8-2, Anabolic Steroids: Winning at All Costs?, has information on how steroids affect muscles.

Types of Muscle Contractions

Muscle **tone** refers to a muscle's partially contracted state that is normal even when the muscle is not in use. The maintenance of this tone, or **tonus** (TO-nus), is due to the action of the nervous system in keeping the muscles in a constant state of readiness for action. Muscles that are little used soon become flabby, weak, and lacking in tone.

In addition to the partial contractions that are responsible for muscle tone, there are two other types of contractions on which the body depends:

- In **isotonic** (i-so-TON-ik) **contractions,** the tone or tension within the muscle remains the same but the muscle as a whole shortens, producing movement; that is, work is accomplished. Lifting weights, walking, running, or any other activity in which the muscles become shorter and thicker (forming bulges) are isotonic contractions.

- In **isometric** (i-so-MET-rik) **contractions,** there is no change in muscle length but there is a great increase in muscle tension. Pushing against an immovable force produces an isometric contraction. For example, if you push the palms of your hands hard against each other, there is no movement, but you can feel the increased tension in your arm muscles.

Most body movements involve a combination of both isotonic and isometric contractions. When walking, for example, some muscles contract isotonically to propel the body forward, but at the same time, other muscles are contracting isometrically to keep your body in position.

The Mechanics of Muscle Movement

Most muscles have two or more points of attachment to the skeleton. The muscle is attached to a bone at each end by means of a cordlike extension called a **tendon** (Fig. 8-7). All of the connective tissue within and around the muscle merges to form the tendon, which then attaches directly to the bone's periosteum (see Fig. 8-1). In some instances, a broad sheet called an **aponeurosis** (ap-o-nu-RO-sis) may attach muscles to bones or to other muscles.

In moving the bones, one end of a muscle is attached to a more freely movable part of the skeleton, and the other end is attached to a relatively stable part. The less

8

Box 8-2	Hot Topics

Anabolic Steroids: Winning at All Costs?

Anabolic steroids mimic the effects of the male sex hormone testosterone by promoting metabolism and stimulating growth. These drugs are legally prescribed to promote muscle regeneration and prevent atrophy from disuse after surgery. However, athletes also purchase them illegally, using them to increase muscle size and strength and improve endurance.

When steroids are used illegally to enhance athletic performance, the doses needed are large enough to cause serious side effects. They increase blood cholesterol levels, which may lead to atherosclerosis, heart disease, kidney failure, and stroke. Steroids damage the liver, making it more susceptible to disease and cancer, and suppress the immune system, increasing the risk of infection and cancer. In men, steroids cause impotence, testicular atrophy, low sperm count, infertility, and the development of female sex characteristics such as breasts (gynecomastia). In women, steroids disrupt ovulation and menstruation and produce male sex characteristics such as breast atrophy, enlargement of the clitoris, increased body hair, and deepening of the voice. In both sexes steroids increase the risk for baldness and, especially in men, cause mood swings, depression, and violence.

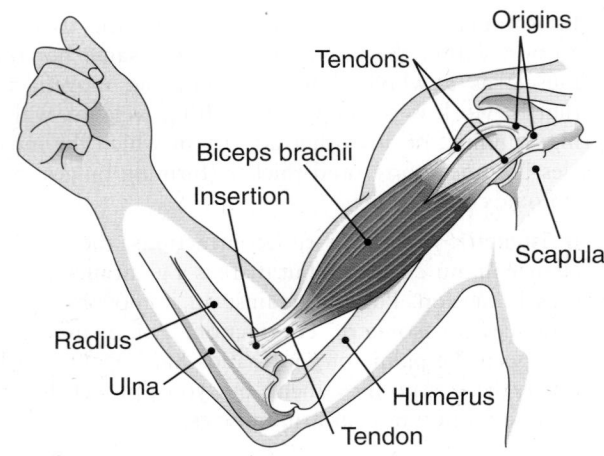

Figure 8-7 **Muscle attachments to bones.** Three attachments are shown—two origins and one insertion.
[**ZOOMING IN** ➤ Does contraction of the biceps brachii produce flexion or extension at the elbow?**]**

movable (more fixed) attachment is called the **origin;** the attachment to the body part that the muscle puts into action is called the **insertion.** When a muscle contracts, it pulls on both attachment points, bringing the more movable insertion closer to the origin and thereby causing movement of the body part. Figure 8-7 shows the action of the biceps brachii (in the upper arm) in flexing the arm at the elbow. The insertion on the radius of the forearm is brought toward the origin at the scapula of the shoulder girdle.

CHECKPOINT **8-10** ➤ Muscles are attached to bones by means of tendons: one attached to a less movable part of the skeleton, and one attached to a movable part. What are the names of these two attachment points?

Muscles Work Together

Many of the skeletal muscles function in pairs. A movement is performed by a muscle called the **prime mover;** the muscle that produces an opposite movement to that of the prime mover is known as the **antagonist.** Clearly, for any given movement, the antagonist must relax when the prime mover contracts. For example, when the biceps brachii at the front of the arm contracts to flex the arm, the triceps brachii at the back must relax; when the triceps brachii contracts to extend the arm, the biceps brachii must relax. In addition to prime movers and antagonists, there are also muscles that steady body parts or assist prime movers. These "helping" muscles are called **synergists** (SIN-er-jists), because they work with the prime movers to accomplish a movement.

As the muscles work together, actions are coordinated to accomplish many complex movements. Note that during development, the nervous system must gradually begin to coordinate our movements. A child learning to walk or to write, for example, may use muscles unnecessarily at first or fail to use appropriate muscles when needed.

CHECKPOINT **8-11** ➤ Muscles work together to produce movement. What is the name of the muscle that produces a movement as compared with the muscle that produces an opposite movement?

Levers and Body Mechanics

Proper body mechanics help conserve energy and ensure freedom from strain and fatigue; conversely, such ailments as lower back pain—a common complaint—can be traced to poor body mechanics. Body mechanics have special significance to healthcare workers, who frequently must move patients and handle cumbersome equipment. Maintaining the body segments in correct alignment also affects the vital organs that are supported by the skeleton.

If you have had a course in physics, recall your study of levers. A lever is simply a rigid bar that moves about a fixed pivot point, the fulcrum. There are three classes of levers, which differ only in the location of the fulcrum (F), the effort (E), or force, and the resistance (R), the weight or load. In a first-class lever, the fulcrum is located between the resistance and the effort; a see-saw or a scissors is an example of this class (Fig. 8-8). The second-class lever has the resistance located between the fulcrum and the effort; a wheelbarrow or a mattress lifted at one end is an illustration of this class (Fig. 8-8B). In the third-class lever, the effort is between the resistance and the fulcrum. A forceps or a tweezers is an example of this type of lever. The effort is applied in the tool's center, between the fulcrum, where the pieces join, and the resistance at the tip.

The musculoskeletal system can be considered a system of levers, in which the bone is the lever, the joint is the fulcrum, and the force is applied by a muscle. An example of a first-class lever in the body is using the muscles at the back of the neck to lift the head at the joint between the skull's occipital bone and the first cervical vertebra (atlas) (see Fig. 8-8). A second-class lever is exemplified by raising your weight to the ball of your foot (the fulcrum) using the calf muscles.

However, there are very few examples of first- and second-class levers in the body. Most lever systems in the body are of the third-class type. A muscle usually inserts over a joint and exerts force between the fulcrum and the resistance. That is, the fulcrum is behind both the point of effort and the weight. As shown in Figure 8-8C, when the biceps brachii flexes the forearm at the elbow, the muscle exerts its force at its insertion on the radius. The weight of the hand and forearm creates the resistance, and the fulcrum is the elbow joint, which is behind the point of effort.

By understanding and applying knowledge of levers to body mechanics, the healthcare worker can improve his or her skill in carrying out numerous clinical maneuvers and procedures.

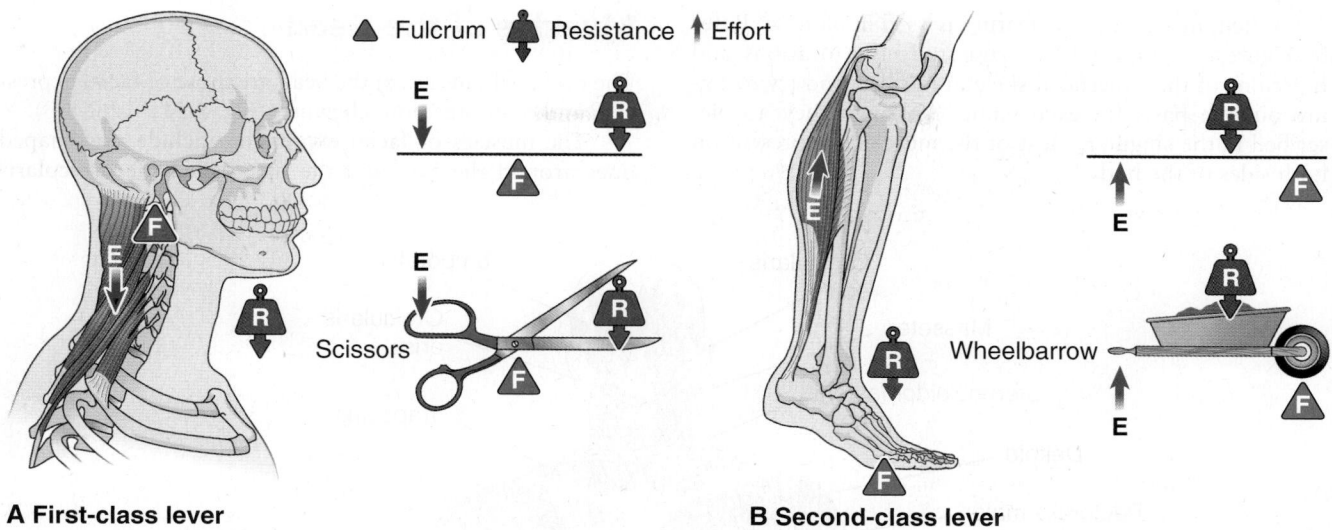

A First-class lever

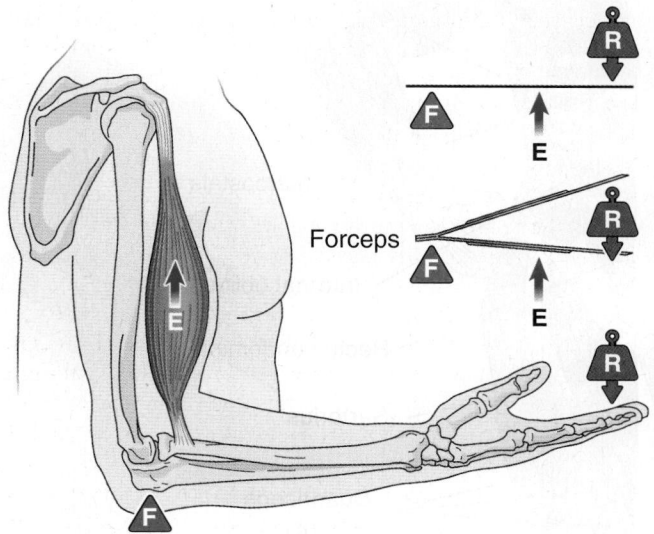

B Second-class lever

C Third-class lever

Figure 8-8 **Levers.** Three classes of levers are shown along with tools and anatomic examples that illustrate each type. R, resistance (weight); E, effort (force); F, fulcrum (pivot point).

CHECKPOINT **8-12** ➤ Muscles and bones work together as lever systems. Of the three classes of levers, which one represents the action of most muscles?

Skeletal Muscle Groups

The study of muscles is made simpler by grouping them according to body regions. Knowing how muscles are named can also help in remembering them. A number of different characteristics are used in naming muscles, including the following:

- Location, named for a nearby bone, for example, or for position, such as lateral, medial, internal, or external
- Size, using terms such as maximus, major, minor, longus, or brevis
- Shape, such as circular (orbicularis), triangular (deltoid), or trapezoid (trapezius)
- Direction of fibers, including straight (rectus) or angled (oblique)
- Number of heads (attachment points), as indicated by the suffix -ceps, as in biceps, triceps, and quadriceps
- Action, as in flexor, extensor, adductor, abductor, or levator

Often, more than one feature is used in naming. Refer to Figures 8-9 and 8-10 as you study the locations and functions of the superficial skeletal muscles and try to figure out the basis for each name. Although they are described in the singular, most of the muscles are present on both sides of the body.

Muscles of the Head

The principal muscles of the head are those of facial expression and of mastication (chewing) (Fig. 8-11, Table 8-3).

The muscles of facial expression include ring-shaped ones around the eyes and the lips, called the **orbicularis**

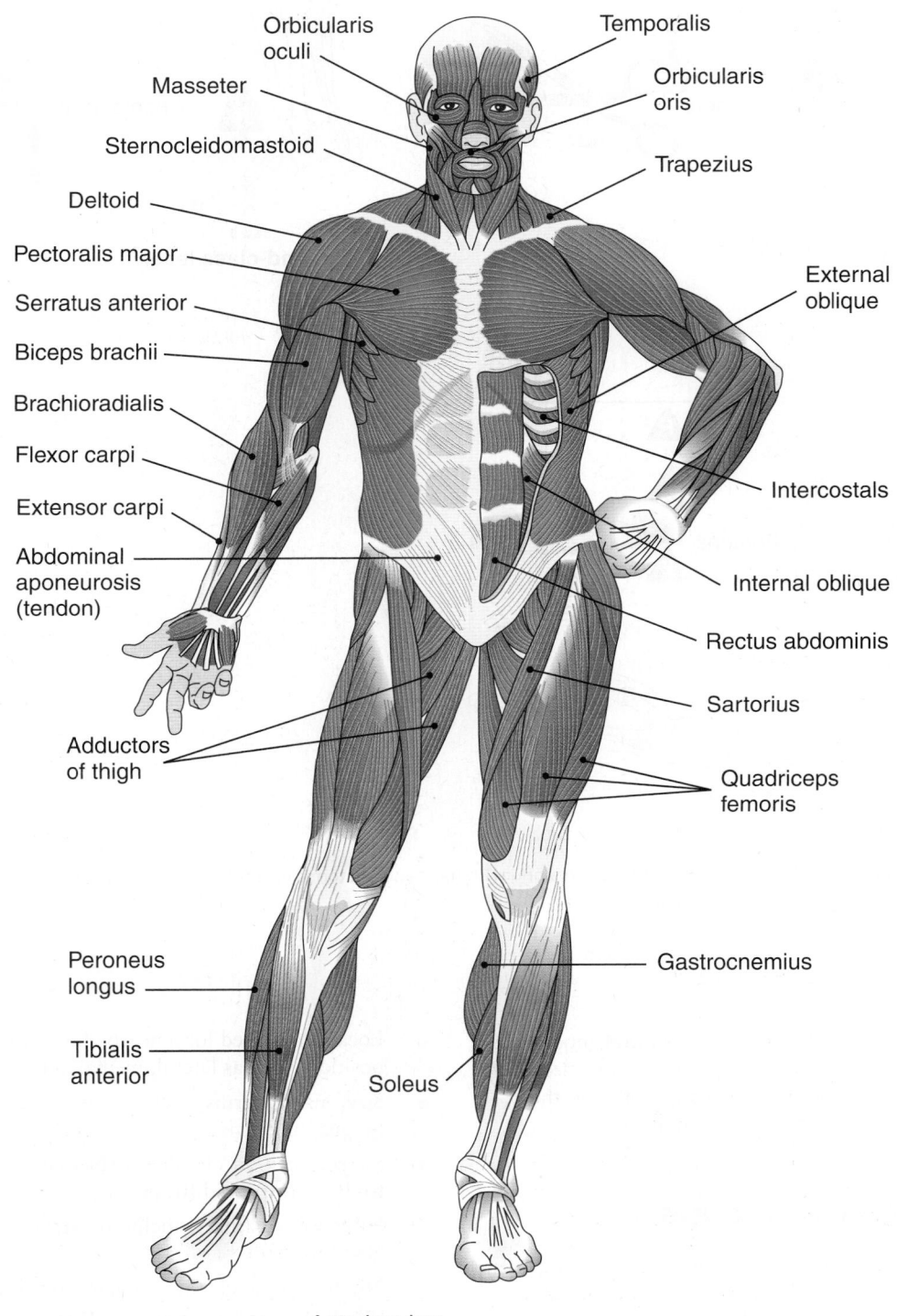

Orbicularis oculi

Masseter

Sternocleidomastoid

Deltoid

Pectoralis major

Serratus anterior

Biceps brachii

Brachioradialis

Flexor carpi

Extensor carpi

Abdominal aponeurosis (tendon)

Adductors of thigh

Peroneus longus

Tibialis anterior

Temporalis

Orbicularis oris

Trapezius

External oblique

Intercostals

Internal oblique

Rectus abdominis

Sartorius

Quadriceps femoris

Gastrocnemius

Soleus

Anterior view

Figure 8-9 **Superficial muscles, anterior view.** Associated structure is labeled in parentheses.

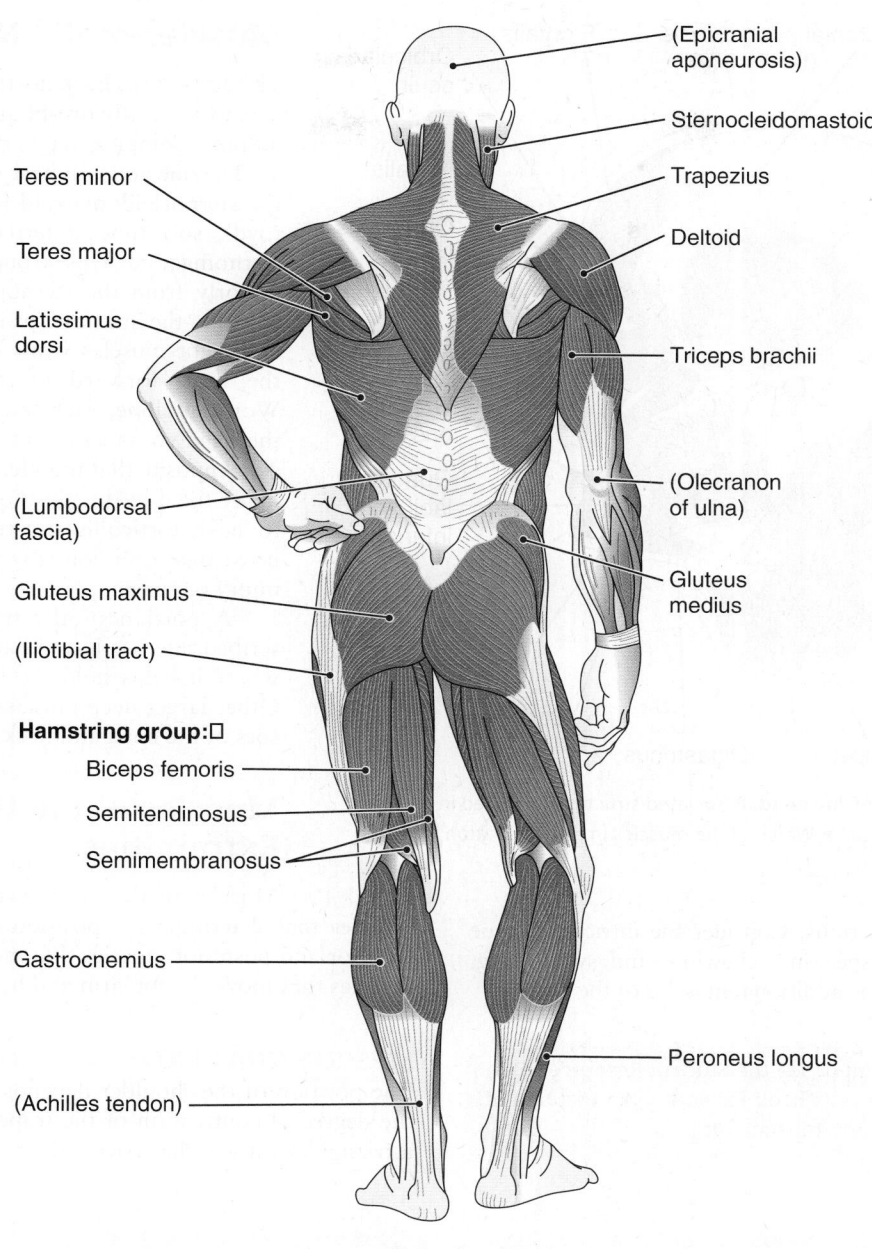

Teres minor

Teres major

Latissimus dorsi

(Lumbodorsal fascia)

Gluteus maximus

(Iliotibial tract)

Hamstring group:

Biceps femoris

Semitendinosus

Semimembranosus

Gastrocnemius

(Achilles tendon)

(Epicranial aponeurosis)

Sternocleidomastoid

Trapezius

Deltoid

Triceps brachii

(Olecranon of ulna)

Gluteus medius

Peroneus longus

Posterior view

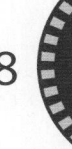

8

Figure 8-10 **Superficial muscles, posterior view.** Associated structures are labeled in parentheses.

(or-bik-u-LAH-ris) **muscles** because of their shape (think of "orbit"). The muscle surrounding each eye is called the **orbicularis oculi** (OK-u-li), whereas the lip muscle is the **orbicularis oris**. These muscles, of course, all have antagonists. For example, the **levator palpebrae** (PAL-pe-bre) **superioris**, or lifter of the upper eyelid, is the antagonist for the orbicularis oculi.

One of the largest muscles of expression forms the fleshy part of the cheek and is called the **buccinator** (BUK-se-na-tor). Used in whistling or blowing, it is sometimes referred to as the trumpeter's muscle. You can readily think of other muscles of facial expression: for instance, the an-

tagonists of the orbicularis oris can produce a smile, a sneer, or a grimace. There are a number of scalp muscles that lift the eyebrows or draw them together into a frown.

There are four pairs of mastication (chewing) muscles, all of which insert on and move the mandible. The largest are the **temporalis** (TEM-po-ral-is), which is superior to the ear, and the **masseter** (mas-SE-ter) at the angle of the jaw.

The tongue has two muscle groups. The first group, called the **intrinsic muscles**, is located entirely within the tongue. The second group, the **extrinsic muscles**, originates outside the tongue. It is because of these many muscles that the tongue has such remarkable flexibility and can perform

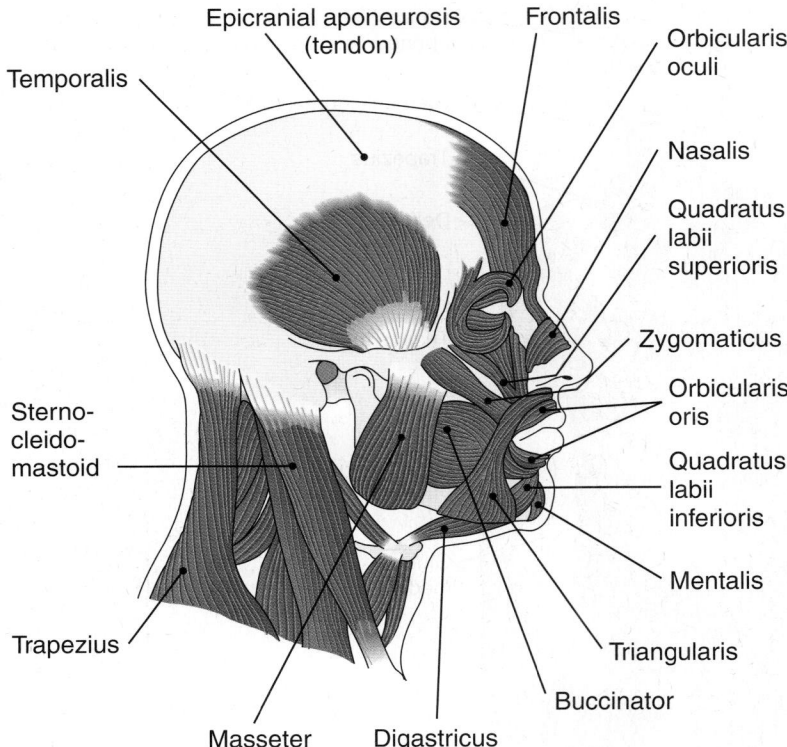

Figure 8-11 **Muscles of the head.** Associated structure is labeled in parentheses. [ZOOMING IN ➤ Which of the muscles in this illustration is named for a bone it is near?]

so many different functions. Consider the intricate tongue motions involved in speaking, chewing, and swallowing. Figure 8-11 shows some additional muscles of the face.

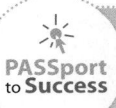
PASSport to Success   Visit **thePoint** or see the Student Resource CD in the back of this book for additional pictures of head and neck musculature.

Muscles of the Neck

The neck muscles tend to be ribbonlike and extend vertically or obliquely in several layers and in a complex manner (Fig. 8-11, Table 8-3). The one you will hear of most frequently is the **sternocleidomastoid** (ster-no-kli-do-MAS-toyd), sometimes referred to simply as the sternomastoid. This strong muscle extends superiorly from the sternum across the lateral neck to the mastoid process. When the left and right muscles work together, they bring the head forward on the chest (flexion). Working alone, each muscle tilts and rotates the head so as to orient the face toward the side opposite that muscle. If the head is abnormally fixed in this position, the person is said to have **torticollis** (tor-tih-KOL-is), or wryneck; this condition may be caused by muscle injury or spasm.

A portion of the trapezius muscle (described later) is located at the posterior neck, where it helps hold the head up (extension). Other larger deep muscles are the chief extensors of the head and neck.

Muscles of the Upper Extremities

Muscles of the upper extremities include the muscles that determine the position of the shoulder, the anterior and posterior muscles that move the arm, and the muscles that move the forearm and hand.

MUSCLES THAT MOVE THE SHOULDER AND ARM
The position of the shoulder depends to a large extent on the degree of contraction of the **trapezius** (trah-PE-ze-us), a triangular muscle that covers the posterior neck and ex-

Table 8-3	**Muscles of the Head and Neck***	
Name	Location	Function
Orbicularis oculi	Encircles eyelid	Closes eye
Levator palpebrae superioris (deep muscle; not shown)	Posterior orbit to upper eyelid	Opens eye
Orbicularis oris	Encircles mouth	Closes lips
Buccinator	Fleshy part of cheek	Flattens cheek; helps in eating, whistling, and blowing wind instruments
Temporalis	Above and near ear	Closes jaw
Masseter	At angle of jaw	Closes jaw
Sternocleidomastoid	Along lateral neck, to mastoid process	Flexes head; rotates head toward opposite side from muscle

These and other muscles of the face are shown in Figure 8–11.

tends across the posterior shoulder to insert on the clavicle and scapula (Fig. 8-10, Table 8-4). The trapezius muscles enable one to raise the shoulders and pull them back. The superior portion of each trapezius can also extend the head and turn it from side to side.

The **latissimus** (lah-TIS-ih-mus) **dorsi** is the wide muscle of the back and lateral trunk. It originates from the vertebral spine in the middle and lower back and covers the inferior half of the thoracic region, forming the posterior portion of the axilla (armpit). The fibers of each muscle converge to a tendon that inserts on the humerus. The latissimus dorsi powerfully extends the arm, bringing it down forcibly as, for example, in swimming.

A large **pectoralis** (pek-to-RAL-is) **major** is located on either side of the superior chest (see Fig. 8-9). This muscle arises from the sternum, the upper ribs, and the clavicle and forms the anterior "wall" of the axilla; it inserts on the superior humerus. The pectoralis major flexes and adducts the arm, pulling it across the chest.

The **serratus** (ser-RA-tus) **anterior** is below the axilla, on the lateral chest. It originates on the upper eight or nine ribs on the lateral and anterior thorax and inserts in the scapula on the side toward the vertebrae. The serratus anterior moves the scapula forward when, for example, one is pushing something. It also aids in raising the arm above the horizontal level.

The **deltoid** covers the shoulder joint and is responsible for the roundness of the upper arm just inferior to the shoulder (see Figs. 8-9 and 8-10). This muscle is named for its triangular shape, which resembles the Greek letter delta. The deltoid is often used as an injection site. Arising from the shoulder girdle (clavicle and scapula), the deltoid fibers converge to insert on the lateral surface of the humerus. Contraction of this muscle abducts the arm, raising it laterally to the horizontal position.

The shoulder joint allows for a very wide range of movement. This freedom of movement is possible because the humerus fits into a shallow socket, the scapula's glenoid cavity. This joint requires the support of four deep muscles and their tendons, which compose the **rotator cuff**. The four muscles are the supraspinatus, infraspinatus, teres minor, and subscapularis, known together as SITS, based on the first letters of their names. In certain activities, such as swinging a golf club, playing tennis, or pitching a baseball, the rotator cuff muscles may be injured, even torn, and may require surgery for repair.

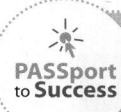 **PASSport to Success** Visit **thePoint** or see the Student Resource CD in the back of this book for additional pictures of muscles that move the shoulder and arm and also the muscles of the rotator cuff.

Table 8-4	Muscles of the Upper Extremities*	
Name	**Location**	**Function**
Trapezius	Posterior neck and upper back, to clavicle and scapula	Raises shoulder and pulls it back; extends head
Latissimus dorsi	Middle and lower back, to humerus	Extends and adducts arm behind back
Pectoralis major	Superior, anterior chest, to humerus	Flexes and adducts arm across chest; pulls shoulder forward and downward
Serratus anterior	Inferior to axilla on lateral chest, to scapula	Moves scapula forward; aids in raising arm, punching, or reaching forward
Deltoid	Covers shoulder joint, to lateral humerus	Abducts arm
Biceps brachii	Anterior arm along humerus, to radius	Flexes forearm at the elbow and supinates hand
Brachialis	Posterior to biceps brachii; inserts at anterior elbow joint	Main flexor of forearm
Brachioradialis	Lateral forearm from distal end of humerus to distal end of radius	Flexes forearm at the elbow
Triceps brachii	Posterior arm, to ulna	Extends forearm to straighten upper extremity
Flexor carpi group	Anterior forearm, to hand	Flexes hand
Extensor carpi group	Posterior forearm, to hand	Extends hand
Flexor digitorum group	Anterior forearm, to fingers	Flexes fingers
Extensor digitorum group	Posterior forearm, to fingers	Extends fingers

*These and other muscles of the upper extremities are shown in Figures 8–9, 8–10, and 8–12.

MUSCLES THAT MOVE THE FOREARM AND HAND

The **biceps brachii** (BRA-ke-i), located at the anterior arm along the humerus, is the muscle you usually display when you want to "flex your muscles" to show your strength (Fig. 8-12A). It inserts on the radius and flexes the forearm. It is a supinator of the hand. The **brachialis** (bra-ke-AL-is) lies deep to the biceps brachii and inserts distally over the anterior elbow joint. It flexes the forearm in all positions, sustains flexion, and steadies the slow extension of the forearm.

Another forearm flexor at the elbow is the **brachioradialis** (bra-ke-o-ra-de-A-lis), a prominent forearm muscle that originates at the distal humerus and inserts on the distal radius.

The **triceps brachii**, located on the posterior arm, inserts on the olecranon of the ulna (Fig. 8-12B). It is used to straighten the arm, as in lowering a weight from an arm curl. It is also important in pushing because it converts the arm and forearm into a sturdy rod.

Most of the muscles that move the hand and fingers originate from the radius and the ulna (see Fig. 8-12).

Some of them insert on the carpal bones of the wrist, whereas others have long tendons that cross the wrist and insert on bones of the hand and the fingers.

The **flexor carpi** and the **extensor carpi muscles** are responsible for many hand movements. Muscles that produce finger movements are the several **flexor digitorum** (dij-e-TO-rum) and the **extensor digitorum muscles**. The names of these muscles may include bones they are near, their action, or their length, for example, longus for long and brevis for short.

Special muscle groups in the fleshy parts of the hand execute the intricate movements that can be performed with the thumb and the fingers. The thumb's freedom of movement has been one of humankind's most useful capacities.

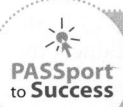

PASSport to Success Visit *thePoint* or see the Student Resource CD in the back of this book for additional pictures of the muscles that move the forearm and hand.

Muscles of the Trunk

The trunk muscles include the muscles involved in breathing, the thin muscle layers of the abdomen, and the muscles of the pelvic floor. The following discussion also includes the deep muscles of the back that support and move the vertebral column.

MUSCLES OF RESPIRATION The most important muscle involved in the act of breathing is the **diaphragm**. This dome-shaped muscle forms the partition between the thoracic cavity above and the abdominal cavity below (Fig. 8-13). When the diaphragm contracts, the central dome-shaped portion is pulled downward, thus enlarging the thoracic cavity from top to bottom.

The **intercostal muscles** are attached to and fill the spaces between the ribs. The external and internal intercostals run at angles in opposite directions. Contraction of the intercostal muscles elevates the ribs, thus enlarging the thoracic cavity from side to side and from anterior to posterior. The mechanics of breathing are described in Chapter 18.

CHECKPOINT 8-13 ➤ What muscle is most important in breathing?

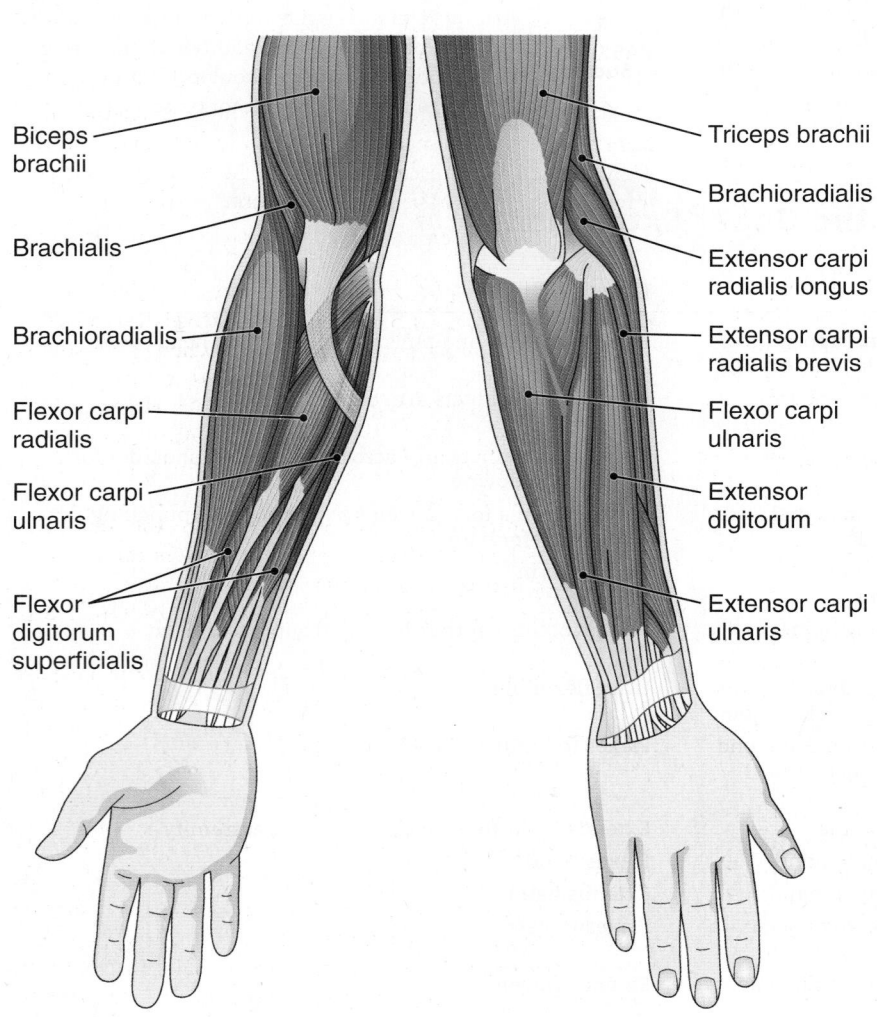

Biceps brachii

Brachialis

Brachioradialis

Flexor carpi radialis

Flexor carpi ulnaris

Flexor digitorum superficialis

Triceps brachii

Brachioradialis

Extensor carpi radialis longus

Extensor carpi radialis brevis

Flexor carpi ulnaris

Extensor digitorum

Extensor carpi ulnaris

A Anterior view   **B** Posterior view

Figure 8-12 **Muscles that move the forearm and hand.**

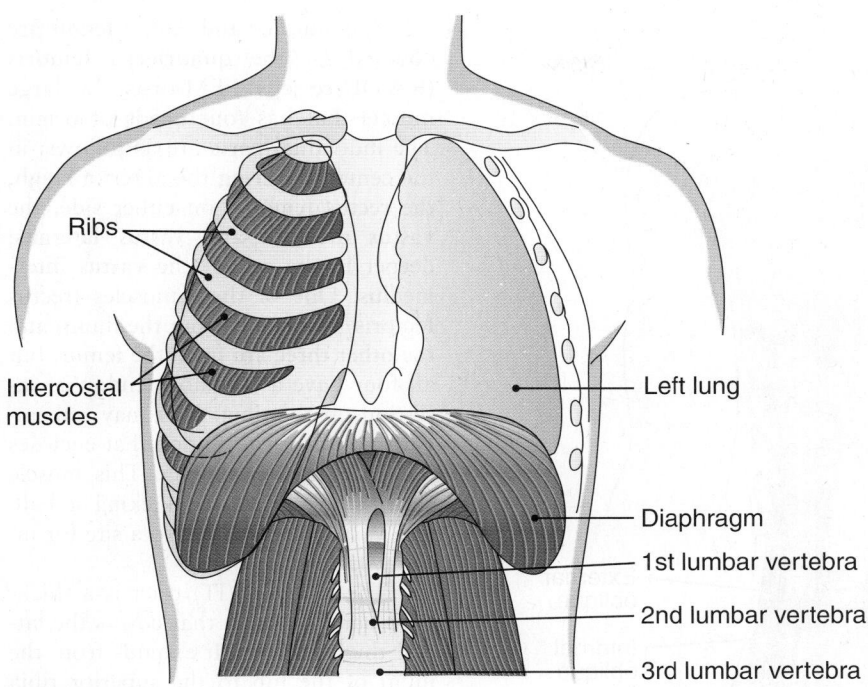

Ribs

Intercostal
muscles

Left lung

Diaphragm

1st lumbar vertebra

2nd lumbar vertebra

3rd lumbar vertebra

Figure 8-13 **Muscles of respiration.** Associated structures are also shown.

MUSCLES OF THE ABDOMEN AND PELVIS The abdominal wall has three muscle layers that extend from the back (dorsally) and around the sides (laterally) to the front (ventrally) (Fig. 8-14, Table 8-5). They are the **external oblique** on the exterior, the **internal oblique** in the middle, and the **transversus abdominis**, the innermost. The connective tissue from these muscles extends anteriorly and encloses the vertical **rectus abdominis** of the anterior abdominal wall. The fibers of these muscles, as well as their connective tissue extensions (aponeuroses), run in different directions, resembling the layers in plywood and resulting in a strong abdominal wall. The midline meeting of the aponeuroses forms a whitish area called the **linea alba** (LIN-e-ah AL-ba), which is an important abdominal landmark. It extends from the tip of the sternum to the pubic joint (see Fig. 8-14).

These four pairs of abdominal muscles act together to protect the internal organs and compress the abdominal cavity, as in coughing, emptying the bladder (urination) and bowel (defecation), sneezing, vomiting, and childbirth (labor). The two oblique muscles and the rectus abdominis help bend the trunk forward and sideways.

The pelvic floor, or **perineum** (per-ih-NE-um), has its own form of diaphragm, shaped somewhat like a shallow dish. One of the principal muscles of this pelvic diaphragm is the **levator ani** (le-VA-tor A-ni), which acts on the rectum and thus aids in defecation. The superficial and deep muscles of the female perineum are shown in Figure 8-15 along with some associated structures.

CHECKPOINT **8-14** ▶ What structural feature gives strength to the muscles of the abdominal wall?

DEEP MUSCLES OF THE BACK The deep muscles of the back, which act on the vertebral column itself, are thick vertical masses that lie under the trapezius and latissimus dorsi. The **erector spinae** muscles make up a large group located between the sacrum and the skull. These muscles extend the spine and maintain the vertebral column in an erect posture. The muscles can be strained in lifting heavy objects if the spine is flexed while lifting. One should bend at the hip and knee instead and use the thigh and buttock muscles to help in lifting.

Deeper muscles in the lumbar area extend the vertebral column in that region. These deep back muscles are not shown in the illustrations.

Muscles of the Lower Extremities

The muscles in the lower extremities, among the longest and strongest muscles in the body, are specialized for locomotion and balance. They include the muscles that move the thigh and leg and those that control movement of the foot.

MUSCLES THAT MOVE THE THIGH AND LEG The **gluteus maximus** (GLU-te-us MAK-sim-us), which forms much of the buttock's fleshy part, is relatively large in humans because of its support function when a person is standing erect (Fig. 8-10, Table 8-6). This muscle extends the thigh and is important in walking and running. The **gluteus medius**, which is partially covered by the gluteus maximus, abducts the thigh. It is one of the sites used for intramuscular injections.

The **iliopsoas** (il-e-o-SO-as) arises from the ilium and the bodies of the lumbar vertebrae; it crosses the anterior hip joint to insert on the femur (Fig. 8-16A). It is a powerful thigh flexor and helps keep the trunk from falling backward when one is standing erect.

The **adductor muscles** are located on the medial part of the thigh. They arise from the pubis and ischium and insert on the femur. These strong muscles press the thighs together, as in grasping a saddle between the knees when riding a horse. They include the **adductor longus** and **adductor magnus**.

The **sartorius** (sar-TO-re-us) is a long, narrow muscle that begins at the iliac spine, winds downward and medially across the entire thigh, and ends on the tibia's superior medial surface. It is called the tailor's muscle because it is used in crossing the legs in the manner of tailors, who in days gone by sat cross-legged on the floor. The **gracilis** (grah-SIL-is) extends from the pubic bone to the medial tibia. It adducts the thigh at the hip and flexes the leg at the knee.

8

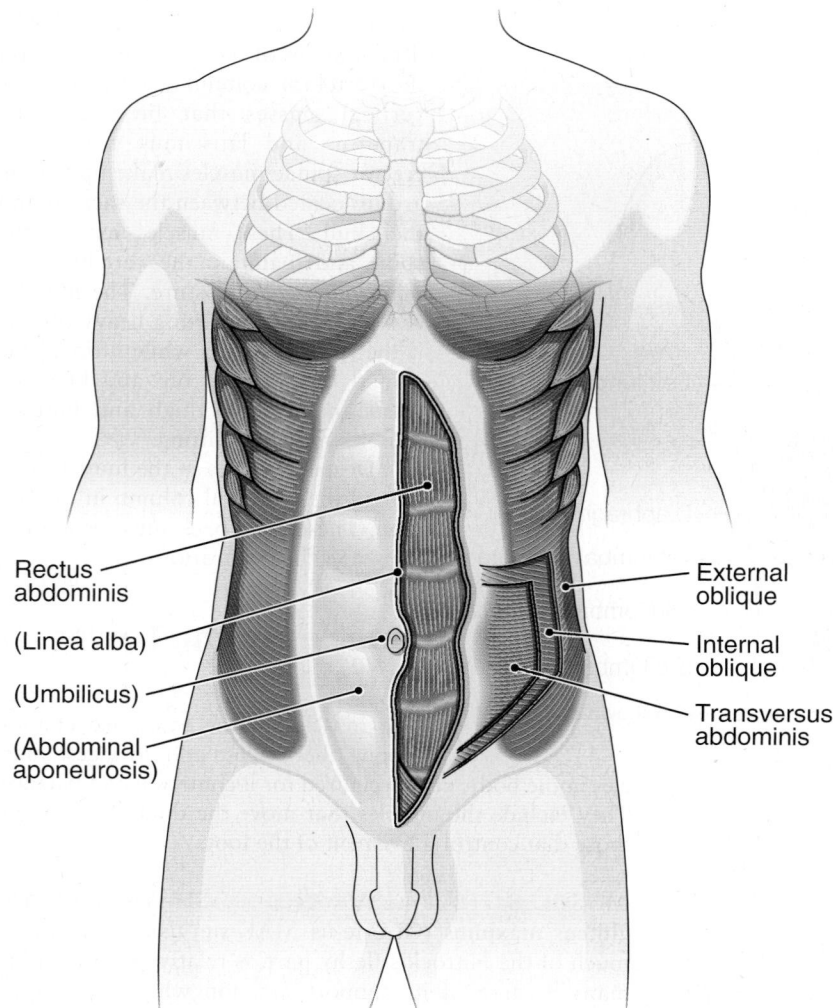

Rectus abdominis

(Linea alba)

(Umbilicus)

(Abdominal aponeurosis)

External oblique

Internal oblique

Transversus abdominis

Figure 8-14 **Muscles of the abdominal wall.** Surface tissue is removed on the right side to show deeper muscles. Associated structures are labeled in parentheses.

The anterior and lateral femur are covered by the **quadriceps femoris** (KWOD-re-seps FEM-or-is), a large muscle that has four heads of origin. The individual parts are as follows: in the center, covering the anterior thigh, the **rectus femoris**; on either side, the **vastus medialis** and **vastus lateralis**; deeper in the center, the **vastus intermedius**. One of these muscles (rectus femoris) originates from the ilium, and the other three are from the femur, but all four have a common tendon of insertion on the tibia. You may remember that this is the tendon that encloses the knee cap, or patella. This muscle extends the leg, as in kicking a ball. The vastus lateralis is also a site for intramuscular injections.

The iliotibial (IT) tract is a thickened band of fascia that covers the lateral thigh muscles. It extends from the ilium of the hip to the superior tibia and reinforces the fascia of the thigh (fascia lata) (see Fig. 8-16).

The **hamstring muscles** are located in the posterior part of the thigh (see Fig. 8-16B). Their tendons can be felt behind the knee as they descend to insert on the tibia and fibula. The hamstrings flex the leg on the thigh, as in kneeling. Individually, moving from lateral to medial position, they are the **biceps femoris**, the **semimembranosus**, and the **semitendinosus**. The name of this muscle group refers to the tendons at the posterior of the knee by which these muscles insert on the leg.

Table 8-5	Muscles of the Trunk*	
Name	Location	Function
Diaphragm	Dome-shaped partition between thoracic and abdominal cavities	Dome descends to enlarge thoracic cavity from top to bottom
Intercostals	Between ribs	Elevate ribs and enlarge thoracic cavity

Muscles of abdominal wall:
  External oblique
  Internal oblique
  Transversus abdominis
  Rectus abdominis
	Anterolateral abdominal wall	Compress abdominal cavity and expel substances from body; flex spinal column

Levator ani	Pelvic floor	Aids defecation
Erector spinae (deep; not shown)	Group of deep vertical muscles between the sacrum and skull	Extends vertebral column to produce erect posture

*These and other muscles of the trunk are shown in Figures 8–13, 8–14, and 8–15.

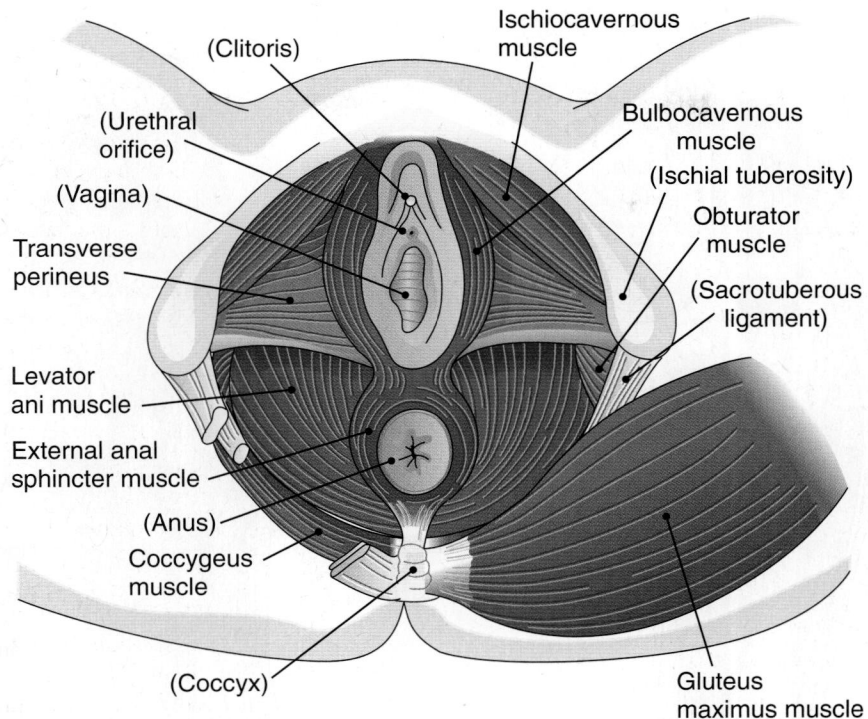

(Clitoris)

(Urethral orifice)

(Vagina)

Transverse perineus

Levator ani muscle

External anal sphincter muscle

(Anus)

Coccygeus muscle

(Coccyx)

Ischiocavernous muscle

Bulbocavernous muscle

(Ischial tuberosity)

Obturator muscle

(Sacrotuberous ligament)

Gluteus maximus muscle

Figure 8-15 **Muscles of the female perineum (pelvic floor).** Associated structures are labeled in parentheses.

8

Table 8-6   Muscles of the Lower Extremities*

Name	Location	Function
Gluteus maximus	Superficial buttock, to femur	Extends thigh
Gluteus medius	Deep buttock, to femur	Abducts thigh
Iliopsoas	Crosses anterior hip joint, to femur	Flexes thigh
Adductor group (e.g., adductor longus, adductor magnus)	Medial thigh, to femur	Adducts thigh
Sartorius	Winds down thigh, ilium to tibia	Flexes thigh and leg (to sit cross-legged)
Gracilis	Pubic bone to medial surface of tibia	Adducts thigh at hip; flexes leg at knee
Quadriceps femoris: Rectus femoris Vastus medialis Vastus lateralis Vastus intermedius (deep; not shown)	Anterior thigh, to tibia	Extends leg
Hamstring group: Biceps femoris Semimembranosus Semitendinosus	Posterior thigh, to tibia and fibula	Flexes leg
Gastrocnemius	Calf of leg, to calcaneus, inserting by the Achilles tendon	Plantar flexes foot at ankle (as in tiptoeing)
Soleus	Posterior leg deep to gastrocnemius	Plantar flexes foot at ankle
Tibialis anterior	Anterior and lateral shin, to foot	Dorsiflexes foot (as in walking on heels); inverts foot (sole inward)
Peroneus longus	Lateral leg, to foot	Everts foot (sole outward)
Flexor digitorum group	Posterior leg and foot to inferior surface of toe bones	Flexes toes
Extensor digitorum group	Anterior surface of leg bones to superior surface of toe bones	Extends toes

*These and other muscles of the lower extremities are shown in *Figures 8–16 and 8–17*.

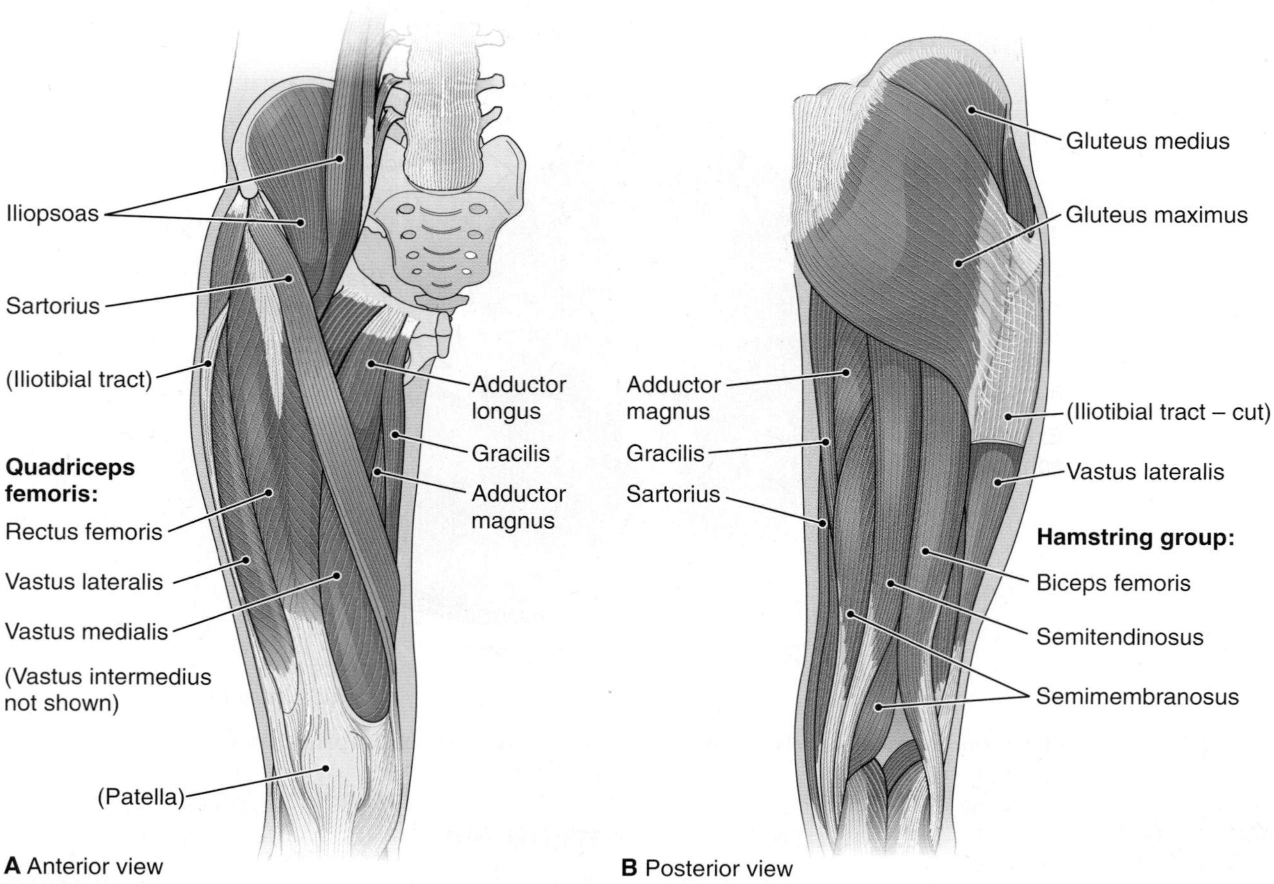

Iliopsoas

Sartorius

(Iliotibial tract)

Quadriceps femoris:

Rectus femoris

Vastus lateralis

Vastus medialis

(Vastus intermedius not shown)

(Patella)

Adductor longus

Gracilis

Adductor magnus

A Anterior view

Gluteus medius

Gluteus maximus

Adductor magnus

Gracilis

Sartorius

(Iliotibial tract – cut)

Vastus lateralis

Hamstring group:

Biceps femoris

Semitendinosus

Semimembranosus

B Posterior view

Figure 8-16 **Muscles of the thigh.** Associated structures are labeled in parentheses.

MUSCLES THAT MOVE THE FOOT The **gastrocnemius** (gas-trok-NE-me-us) is the chief muscle of the calf of the leg (its name means "belly of the leg") (Fig. 8-17). It has been called the toe dancer's muscle because it is used in standing on tiptoe. It ends near the heel in a prominent cord called the **Achilles tendon** (see Fig. 8-17B), which attaches to the calcaneus (heel bone). The Achilles tendon is the largest tendon in the body. According to Greek mythology, the region above the heel was the only place that Achilles was vulnerable, and if the Achilles tendon is cut, it is impossible to walk. The soleus (SO-le-us) is a flat muscle deep to the gastrocnemius. It also inserts by means of the Achilles tendon and, like the gastrocnemius, flexes the foot at the ankle.

Another leg muscle that acts on the foot is the **tibialis** (tib-e-A-lis) **anterior**, located on the anterior region of the leg (see Fig. 8-17A). This muscle performs the opposite function of the gastrocnemius. Walking on the heels uses the tibialis anterior to raise the rest of the foot off the ground (dorsiflexion). This muscle is also responsible for inversion of the foot. The muscle for the foot's eversion is the **peroneus** (per-o-NE-us) **longus**, also called the fibularis longus, located on the lateral leg. This muscle's long tendon crosses under the foot, forming a sling that supports the transverse (metatarsal) arch.

The toes, like the fingers, are provided with flexor and extensor muscles. The tendons of the extensor muscles are located in the superior part of the foot and insert on the superior surface of the phalanges (toe bones). The flexor digitorum tendons cross the sole of the foot and insert on the undersurface of the phalanges.

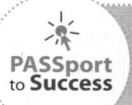 **PASSport to Success** Visit **thePoint** or see the Student Resource CD in the back of this book for additional pictures of the muscles that move the lower extremity.

Effects of Aging on Muscles

Beginning at about 40 years of age, there is a gradual loss of muscle cells with a resulting decrease in the size of each individual muscle. There is also a loss of power, notably in the extensor muscles, such as the large sacrospinalis near the vertebral column. This causes the "bent over" appearance of a hunchback (kyphosis), which in women is often referred to as the *dowager's hump*. Sometimes, there is a tendency to bend (flex) the hips and knees. In addition to causing the previously noted changes in the vertebral column (see Chapter 7), these effects on the extensor muscles

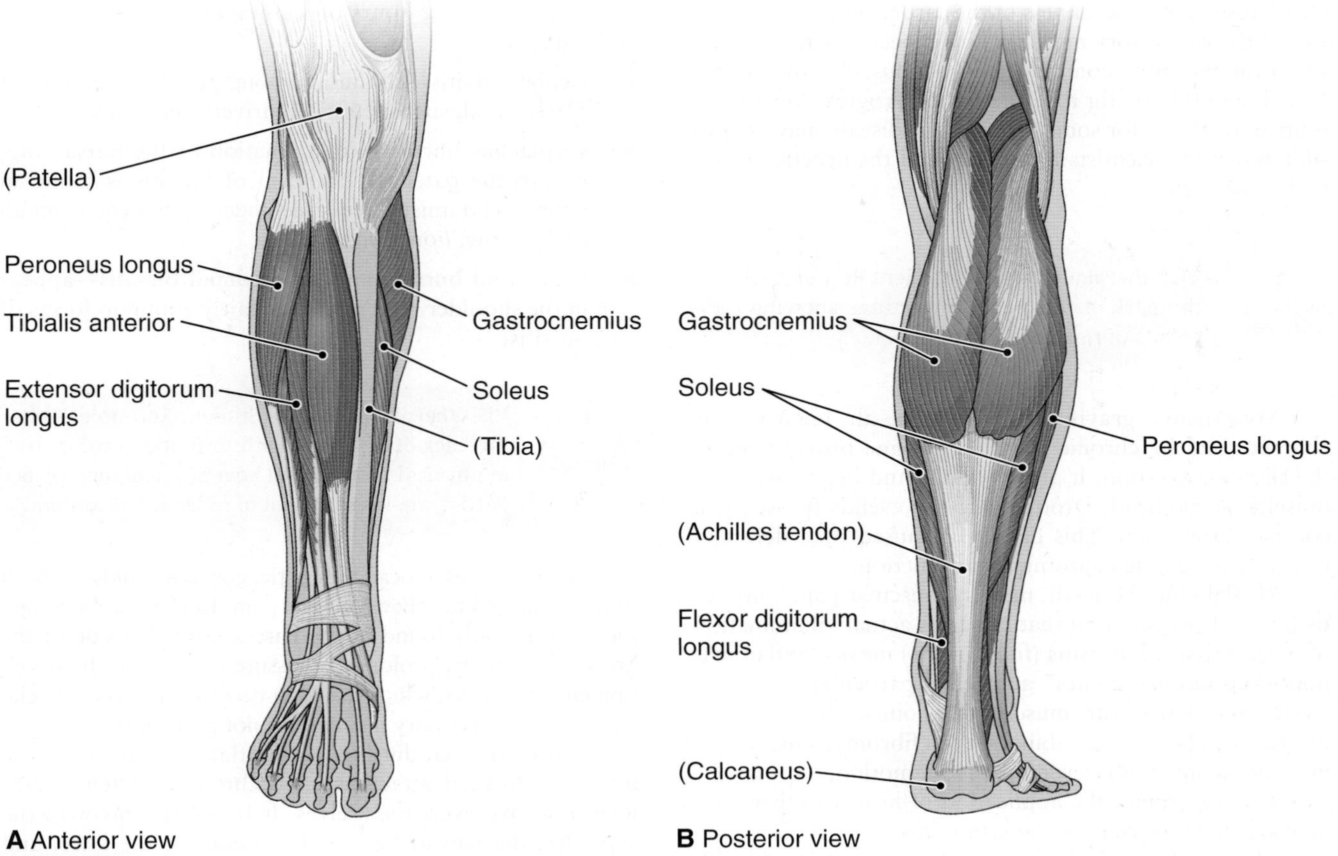

(Patella)

Peroneus longus

Tibialis anterior

Extensor digitorum longus

Gastrocnemius

Soleus

(Tibia)

A Anterior view

Gastrocnemius

Soleus

Peroneus longus

(Achilles tendon)

Flexor digitorum longus

(Calcaneus)

B Posterior view

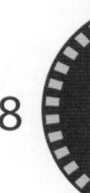

8

Figure 8-17 **Muscles that move the foot.** Associated structures are labeled in parentheses.

result in a further decrease in the elderly person's height. Activity and exercise throughout life delay and decrease these undesirable effects of aging. Even among the elderly, resistance exercise, such as weight lifting, increases muscle strength and function.

Muscular Disorders

A **spasm** is a sudden and involuntary muscular contraction, which is always painful. A spasm of the visceral muscles is called **colic**, a good example of which is the intestinal muscle spasm often referred to as a *bellyache*. Spasms also occur in the skeletal muscles. If the spasms occur in a series, the condition may be called a **seizure** or **convulsion**.

Cramps are strong, painful muscle contractions, especially of the leg and foot. They are most likely to follow unusually strenuous activity. Cramps that occur during sleep or rest are called *recumbency cramps*.

Strains are common muscle injuries caused by overuse or overstretching. With strains, there is pain, stiffness, and swelling, most commonly in the lower back or neck. The elbow or shoulder may also be affected. Charley horse is soreness and stiffness in a muscle caused by strain, usually referring to strain of the thigh's quadriceps muscle. The

term *Charley horse* comes from the practice of using Charley as a name for old lame horses that were kept around for family use when they were no longer able to do hard work.

Sprains are more severe than strains and involve tearing of the ligaments around a joint, usually as a result of abnormal or excessive joint movement. In severe cases, the ligament can actually tear away from its bone. The ankle is a common site of sprains, as when the ankle is "turned," that is, the foot is turned inward and body weight forces excessive inversion at the joint. The knee is another common site of this type of injury. The pain and swelling accompanying a sprain can be reduced by the immediate application of ice packs, which constrict some of the smaller blood vessels and reduce internal bleeding.

Atrophy (AT-ro-fe) is a wasting or decrease in the size of a muscle when it cannot be used, such as when an extremity must be placed in a cast after a fracture.

Diseases of Muscles

Muscular dystrophy (DIS-tro-fe) is a group of disorders in which there is deterioration of muscles that still have intact nerve function. These disorders all progress at different rates. The most common type, which is found most frequently in male children, causes weakness and paralysis.

Death results from weakness of the cardiac muscle or paralysis of the respiratory muscles. Life expectancy is about 20 years for the most common type of muscular dystrophy, and about 40 years for the other types. Progress toward definitive treatment for some forms of the disease may be possible now that scientists have identified the genetic defects that cause them.

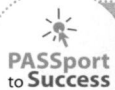 **PASSport to Success** Visit *thePoint* or see the Student Resource CD in the back of this book for pictures showing the effects of muscular dystrophy.

Myasthenia gravis (mi-as-THE-ne-ah GRA-vis) is characterized by chronic muscular fatigue brought on by the slightest exertion. It affects adults and begins with the muscles of the head. Drooping of the eyelids (ptosis) is a common early sign. This disease is caused by a defect in transmission at the neuromuscular junction.

Myalgia (mi-AL-je-ah) means "muscular pain"; **myositis** (mi-o-SI-tis) is a term that indicates actual inflammation of muscle tissue. **Fibrositis** (fi-bro-SI-tis) means "inflammation of connective tissues" and refers particularly to those tissues associated with muscles and joints. Usually, these disorders appear in combination as **fibromyositis**, which may be acute, with severe pain on motion, or may be chronic. Sometimes, the application of heat, together with massage and rest, relieves the symptoms.

Fibromyalgia syndrome (FMS) is associated with widespread muscle aches, tenderness, and stiffness along with fatigue and sleep disorders. FMS is difficult to diagnose, and there is no known cause, but it may be an autoimmune disease, in which the immune system reacts to one's own tissues. Treatment may include a controlled exercise program and treatment with pain relievers, muscle relaxants, or antidepressants.

Disorders of Associated Structures

Bursitis is inflammation of a bursa, a fluid-filled sac that minimizes friction between tissues and bone. Some bursae communicate with joints; others are closely related to muscles. Sometimes, bursae develop spontaneously in response to prolonged friction. Bursitis can be very painful, with swelling and limitation of motion. Some examples of bursitis are listed below:

- **Olecranon bursitis**—inflammation of the bursa over the point of the elbow (olecranon). Another name for the disorder is student's elbow, as it can be caused by long hours of leaning on the elbows while studying.

- **Ischial bursitis**—common among people who must sit a great deal, such as taxicab drivers and truckers

- **Prepatellar bursitis**—inflammation of the bursa anterior to the patella. This form of bursitis is found in people who must often kneel, hence the name from an earlier time, *housemaid's knee*.

- **Subdeltoid bursitis** and **subacromial bursitis**—appear in the shoulder region and are fairly common forms of bursitis.

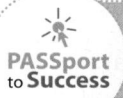 **PASSport to Success** Visit *thePoint* or see the Student Resource CD in the back of this book for information on careers in physical therapy and how physical therapists participate in treatment of muscular disorders.

In some cases a local anesthetic, corticosteroids, or both may be injected to relieve bursitis pain. **Bunions** are enlargements commonly found at the base and medial side of the great toe. Usually, prolonged pressure has caused the development of a bursa, which has then become inflamed. Special shoes may be necessary if surgery is not performed.

Tendinitis (ten-din-I-tis), an inflammation of muscle tendons and their attachments, occurs most often in athletes who overexert themselves. It frequently involves the shoulder, the hamstring muscle tendons at the knee, and the Achilles tendon near the heel. **Tenosynovitis** (ten-o-sin-o-VI-tis), which involves the synovial sheath that encloses tendons, is found most often in women in their 40s after an injury or surgery. It may involve swelling and severe pain with activity.

Shinsplints is experienced as pain and soreness along the tibia ("shin bone") from stress injury of structures in the leg. Some causes of shinsplints are tendinitis at the insertion of the tibialis anterior muscle, sometimes with inflammation of the tibial periosteum, and even stress fracture of the tibia itself. Shinsplints commonly occurs in runners, especially when they run on hard surfaces without adequate shoe support.

Carpal tunnel syndrome involves the tendons of the flexor muscles of the fingers as well as the nerves supplying the hand and fingers. Numbness and weakness of the hand is caused by pressure on the median nerve as it passes through a tunnel formed by the carpal bones of the wrist. Carpal tunnel syndrome is one of the most common repetitive-use disorders. It affects many workers who use their hands and fingers strenuously, such as factory workers, keyboard operators, and musicians.

Disease in Context revisited

> Sue's Multiple Sclerosis

Having finished the physical examination of his patient, Dr. Mathews thought carefully about what he had discovered. Sue, a 26-year-old white female, presented with muscle weakness, atrophy, and abnormal reflexes localized to the right side of her body. At first, it seemed likely that Sue was suffering from a muscular system disorder. Muscular dystrophy is characterized by muscle deterioration and weakness, but the doctor knew that the disease is genetic and its effects appear during childhood. Myasthenia gravis, a disorder of the neuromuscular junction, is also characterized by muscle weakness and appears during adulthood. But, it usually begins affecting muscles of the head, not the limbs. Fibromyalgia syndrome affects adults and is associated with widespread muscle aches. This didn't seem to fit either because Sue's disorder was localized to her right side.

It was Sue's report of pain and tingling in her right limbs that provided the last clue Dr. Mathews needed to make his diagnosis. Sue probably had a disorder of the nervous system called multiple sclerosis. The disease is characterized by both muscular and nervous symptoms, which first appear in adults and are sometimes localized to one side of the body. After explaining his findings to Sue, Dr. Mathews ordered an MRI of her brain and spinal cord and referred her to a neurologist for further treatment.

During this case, Dr. Mathews examined Sue's muscular system. He quickly realized that Sue's symptoms suggested that she had a nervous system disorder. The case study in Chapter 9, The Nervous System: The Spinal Cord and Spinal Nerves, will follow Sue as she learns more about multiple sclerosis.

Word Anatomy

Medical terms are built from standardized word parts (prefixes, roots, and suffixes). Learning the meanings of these parts can help you remember words and interpret unfamiliar terms.

WORD PART	MEANING	EXAMPLE
The Muscular System		
my/o	muscle	The *endomysium* is the deepest layer of connective tissue around muscle cells.
sarc/o	flesh	A *sarcomere* is a contracting subunit of skeletal muscle.
troph/o	nutrition, nurture	Muscles undergo *hypertrophy*, an increase in size, under the effects of resistance training.
vas/o	vessel	*Vasodilation* (widening) of the blood vessels in muscle tissue during exercise brings more blood into the tissue.
iso-	same, equal	In an *isotonic* contraction, muscle tone remains the same, but the muscle shortens.
ton/o	tone, tension	See preceding example.
metr/o	measure	In an *isometric* contraction, muscle length remains the same, but muscle tension increases.
The Mechanics of Muscle Movement		
brachi/o	arm	The biceps *brachii* and triceps *brachii* are in the arm.
erg/o	work	*Synergists* are muscles that work together.

WORD PART	MEANING	EXAMPLE
Skeletal Muscle Groups		
quadr/i	four	The *quadriceps* muscle group consists of four muscles.
Muscular Disorders		
a-	absent, lack of	*Atrophy* is a wasting of muscle as a result of disuse (lack of nourishment).
dys-	disordered, difficult	In muscular *dystrophy*, there is deterioration of muscles.
sthen/o	strength	*Myasthenia* gravis is characterized by muscular fatigue (lack of strength).
-algia	pain	*Myalgia* is muscular pain.

Summary

I. **TYPES OF MUSCLE**
   A. Smooth muscle
      1. In walls of hollow organs, vessels, and respiratory passageways
      2. Cells tapered, single nucleus, nonstriated
      3. Involuntary, produces peristalsis, contracts and relaxes slowly
   B. Cardiac muscle
      1. Muscle of heart wall
      2. Cells branch, single nucleus, lightly striated
      3. Involuntary, self-excitatory
   C. Skeletal muscle
      1. Most attached to bones and move skeleton
      2. Cells long, cylindrical; multiple nuclei, heavily striated
      3. Voluntary, contracts and relaxes rapidly

II. **MUSCULAR SYSTEM**
   A. Functions
      1. Movement of skeleton
      2. Maintenance of posture
      3. Generation of heat
   B. Structure of a muscle
      1. Held by connective tissue
         a. Endomysium around individual fibers
         b. Perimysium around fascicles (bundles)
         c. Epimysium around whole muscle
   C. Muscle cells in action
      1. Neuromuscular junction (NMJ)
         a. Point where nerve fiber stimulates muscle cell
         b. Neurotransmitter is acetylcholine (ACh)
            (1) Generates an action potential
         c. Motor end plate—membrane of muscle cell at NMJ
      2. Contraction—sliding together of filaments to shorten muscle
         a. Actin—thin and light
         b. Myosin—thick and dark with projecting heads

      3. Role of calcium—uncovers binding sites so cross-bridges can form between actin and myosin
   D. Energy sources
      1. ATP—supplies energy
         a. Myoglobin—stores oxygen
         b. Glycogen—stores glucose
         c. Creatine phosphate—stores energy
      2. Oxygen consumption
         a. Oxygen debt—develops during strenuous exercise
            (1) Anaerobic metabolism
            (2) Yields lactic acid—causes muscle fatigue
         b. Recovery oxygen consumption
            (1) Removes lactic acid
            (2) Replenishes reserved compounds
   E. Effects of exercise
      1. Changes in structure and function of muscle cells
      2. Vasodilation brings blood to tissues
      3. Heart strengthened
      4. Breathing improved
   F. Types of muscle contractions
      1. Tonus—partially contracted state
      2. Isotonic contractions—muscle shortens to produce movement
      3. Isometric contractions—tension increases, but muscle does not shorten

III. **MECHANICS OF MUSCLE MOVEMENT**
   A. Attachments of skeletal muscles
      1. Tendon—cord of connective tissue that attaches muscle to bone
         a. Origin—attached to more fixed part
         b. Insertion—attached to moving part
      2. Aponeurosis—broad band of connective tissue that attaches muscle to bone or other muscle
   B. Muscles work together
      1. Prime mover—performs movement

2. Antagonist—produces opposite movement
3. Synergist—steadies body parts and assists prime mover
C. Levers and body mechanics—muscles function with skeleton as lever systems
   1. Components
      a. Lever—bone
      b. Fulcrum—joint
      c. Force—muscle contraction
   2. Most muscles work as third-class levers (fulcrum-effort-weight)

IV. **SKELETAL MUSCLE GROUPS**
A. Naming of muscles—location, size, shape, direction of fibers, number of heads, action
B. Muscles of the head
C. Muscles of the neck
D. Muscles of the upper extremities
   1. Muscles that move the shoulder and arm
   2. Muscles that move the forearm and hand
E. Muscles of the trunk
   1. Muscles of respiration
   2. Muscles of the abdomen and pelvis

3. Deep muscles of the back
F. Muscles of the lower extremities
   1. Muscles that move the thigh and leg
   2. Muscles that move the foot

V. **EFFECTS OF AGING ON MUSCLES**
A. Decrease in size of muscles
B. Weakening of muscles, especially extensors

VI. **MUSCULAR DISORDERS**
A. Spasms and injuries
   1. Spasm—sudden painful contraction
   2. Strains—overuse injuries
   3. Sprains—tearing of ligament
   4. Atrophy—wasting
B. Diseases of muscles
   1. Muscular dystrophy—group of disorders
   2. Myasthenia gravis
   3. Myalgia, myositis, fibromyositis
   4. Fibromyalgia syndrome (FMS)—generalized disturbance of unknown cause
C. Disorders of associated structures—bursitis, bunions, tendinitis, shinsplints, carpal tunnel syndrome

8

Questions for Study and Review

BUILDING UNDERSTANDING

Fill in the blanks

1. Individual muscle fibers are arranged in bundles called _____.

2. The point at which a nerve fiber contacts a muscle cell is called the _____.

3. A contraction in which there is no change in muscle length but there is a great increase in muscle tension is _____.

4. A term that means "muscular pain" is _____.

5. A disease characterized by chronic muscular fatigue due to defects in neuromuscular transmission is called _____.

Matching > Match each numbered item with the most closely related lettered item.

___ **6.** Extends vertebral column to produce erect posture

___ **7.** Elevates ribs and enlarges thoracic cavity

___ **8.** Flattens cheeks

___ **9.** Aids in defecation

___ **10.** Closes eye

a. levator ani

b. buccinator

c. orbicularis oris

d. erector spinae

e. intercostal muscles

Multiple Choice

___ **11.** From superficial to deep, the correct order of muscle structure is

a. deep fascia, epimysium, perimysium, and endomysium

b. epimysium, perimysium, endomysium, and deep fascia

c. deep fascia, endomysium, perimysium, and epimysium

d. endomysium, perimysium, epimysium, and deep fascia

___ **12.** The function of calcium ions in skeletal muscle contraction is to

    a. bind to receptors on the motor end plate to stimulate muscle contraction

    b. cause a pH change in the cytoplasm to trigger muscle contraction

    c. bind to the myosin binding sites on actin so that myosin will have something to attach to

    d. bind to regulatory proteins so that the myosin binding sites on the actin can be exposed

___ **13.** A broad flat extension that attaches muscle to bone is called a(n)

    a. tendon

    b. fascicle

    c. aponeurosis

    d. motor end plate

___ **14.** Seizures or convulsions are examples of

    a. strains

    b. fibrositis

    c. myositis

    d. spasms

___ **15.** A disease associated with widespread muscle aches, tenderness, and stiffness and with no known cause is

    a. muscular dystrophy

    b. fibromyalgia

    c. myositis

    d. bursitis

UNDERSTANDING CONCEPTS

16. Compare smooth, cardiac, and skeletal muscle with respect to location, structure, and function. Briefly explain how each type of muscle is specialized for its function.

17. Describe three substances stored in skeletal muscle cells that are used to manufacture a constant supply of ATP.

18. Name and describe muscle(s) that

    a. open and close the eye

    b. close the jaw

    c. flex and extend the head

    d. flex and extend the forearm

    e. flex and extend the hand and fingers

    f. flex and extend the leg

    g. flex and extend the foot and toes

19. During a Cesarean section, a transverse incision is made through the abdominal wall. Name the muscles incised and state their functions.

20. What effect does aging have on muscles? What can be done to resist these effects?

21. Define *atrophy* and give one cause.

22. What are muscular dystrophies, and what are some of their effects?

23. Describe bursitis and its several forms.

CONCEPTUAL THINKING

24. Recall that the neurotransmitter acetylcholine initiates skeletal muscle contraction. Normally, acetylcholine is broken down shortly after its release into the synaptic cleft by the enzyme acetylcholinesterase. Many insecticides contain chemicals called organophosphates, which interfere with acetylcholinesterase activity. Based on this information, what could happen to an individual exposed to high concentrations of organophosphates?

25. Margo recently began "working out" and jogs three times a week. After her jog she is breathless and her muscles ache. From your understanding of muscle physiology, describe what has happened inside of Margo's skeletal muscle cells. How do Margo's muscles recover from this? If Margo continues to exercise, what changes would you expect to occur in her muscles?

26. Alfred suffered a mild stroke, leaving him partially paralyzed on his left side. Physical therapy was ordered to prevent left-sided atrophy. Prescribe some exercises for Alfred's shoulder and thigh.

27. In Sue's case, her disorder prevents motor impulses from arriving at neuromuscular junctions. With this in mind, explain why one of her symptoms is muscle atrophy.

Two chapters in this unit describe the nervous system and some of its many parts and complex functions. The organs of special sense and other sensory receptors are described in a separate chapter. The last chapter in this unit discusses hormones and the organs that produce them. Working with the nervous system, these hormones play an important role in coordination and control.

CHAPTER 9

The Nervous System: The Spinal Cord and Spinal Nerves

Learning Outcomes

After careful study of this chapter, you should be able to:

1. Describe the organization of the nervous system according to structure and function
2. Describe the structure of a neuron
3. Describe how neuron fibers are built into a nerve
4. Explain the purpose of neuroglia
5. Diagram and describe the steps in an action potential
6. Briefly describe the transmission of a nerve impulse
7. Explain the role of myelin in nerve conduction
8. Briefly describe transmission at a synapse
9. Define *neurotransmitter* and give several examples of neurotransmitters
10. Describe the distribution of gray and white matter in the spinal cord
11. List the components of a reflex arc
12. Define a simple reflex and give several examples of reflexes
13. Describe and name the spinal nerves and three of their main plexuses
14. Compare the location and functions of the sympathetic and parasympathetic nervous systems
15. Explain the role of cellular receptors in the action of neurotransmitters
16. Describe several disorders of the spinal cord and of the spinal nerves
17. Show how word parts are used to build words related to the nervous system (see Word Anatomy at the end of the chapter)

Selected Key Terms

The following terms and other boldface terms in the chapter are defined in the Glossary

acetylcholine
action potential
afferent
autonomic nervous system
axon
dendrite
effector
efferent
epinephrine
ganglion
interneuron
motor
nerve
nerve impulse
neuritis
neuroglia
neurotransmitter
parasympathetic nervous system
plexus
receptor
reflex
sensory
somatic nervous system
sympathetic nervous system
synapse
tract

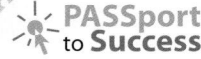

PASSport to Success

Visit *thePoint* or see the Student Resource CD in the back of this book for definitions and pronunciations of key terms as well as a pretest for this chapter.

Disease in Context

► Sue's Second Case: The Importance of Myelin

Dr. Jensen glanced at her patient's chart as she stepped into the consulting room to see her. Sue Pritchard was 26 years old, white, and had been referred to her by Sue's family physician. According to her chart, Sue had presented with motor and sensory deficits, which led her doctor to suspect she had multiple sclerosis (MS). In addition to the referral, her doctor had ordered a magnetic resonance image (MRI) of her brain and spinal cord. "Hi Sue. My name is Dr. Jensen. I'm a neurologist, which means I specialize in the diagnosis and treatment of nervous system disorders like MS. Let's start with a few tests to determine how well your brain and spinal cord communicate with the rest of your body. Then, we'll take a look at your MRI results."

Using a reflex hammer, Dr. Jensen tapped on the tendons of several muscles in Sue's arms and legs to elicit stretch reflexes. She observed abnormal responses—a typical sign of damage to the parts of the spinal cord that control reflexes. The doctor also detected muscle weakness in Sue's limbs—an indication of damage to the descending tracts of white matter in the spinal cord, which carry motor nerve impulses from the brain to skeletal muscle. In addition, the neurologist discovered that Sue's sense of touch was impaired—an indication of damage to the spinal cord's ascending tracts, which carry sensory impulses from receptors in the skin to the brain. Dr. Jensen had discovered that Sue exhibited several of the most common clinical signs of MS.

After the physical examination, Dr. Jensen showed Sue the results of the MRI scan done earlier. "Here's the MRI of your spinal cord. You can see that it is surrounded by bones called vertebrae, which protect it from injury. The nervous tissue making up the spinal cord is organized into two regions—this inner region called gray matter, and this outer one called white matter. If you look closely at the white matter, you can see several damaged areas, which we call lesions. They are causing many of your symptoms because they prevent your spinal cord from transmitting impulses between your brain and the rest of your body. These lesions, or scleroses, are what give multiple sclerosis its name."

The clinical and diagnostic evidence shows that Sue has multiple sclerosis—a disease of neurons in the central nervous system (CNS). In this chapter, we'll learn more about neurons and the spinal cord, one part of the CNS.

Role of the Nervous System

No body system is capable of functioning alone. All are interdependent and work together as one unit to maintain normal conditions, termed *homeostasis*. The nervous system serves as the chief coordinating agency for all systems. Conditions both within and outside the body are constantly changing. The nervous system must detect and respond to these changes (known as *stimuli*) so that the body can adapt itself to new conditions. The nervous system can be compared with a large corporation, in which market researchers (sensory receptors) feed information into middle management (the spinal cord), who then transmit information to the chief executive officer, or CEO (the brain). The CEO organizes and interprets the information and then sends directions out to workers (effectors) who carry out appropriate actions for the good of the company. In this process, memos and e-mails, like the nerves, carry information throughout the system.

Although all parts of the nervous system work in coordination, portions may be grouped together on the basis of either structure or function.

Structural Divisions

The anatomic, or structural, divisions of the nervous system are as follows (Fig. 9-1):

- The **central nervous system** (CNS) includes the brain and spinal cord.
- The **peripheral** (per-IF-er-al) **nervous system** (PNS) is made up of all the nerves outside the CNS. It includes all the **cranial nerves** that carry impulses to and from the brain and all the **spinal nerves** that carry messages to and from the spinal cord.

The CNS and PNS together include all of the nervous tissue in the body.

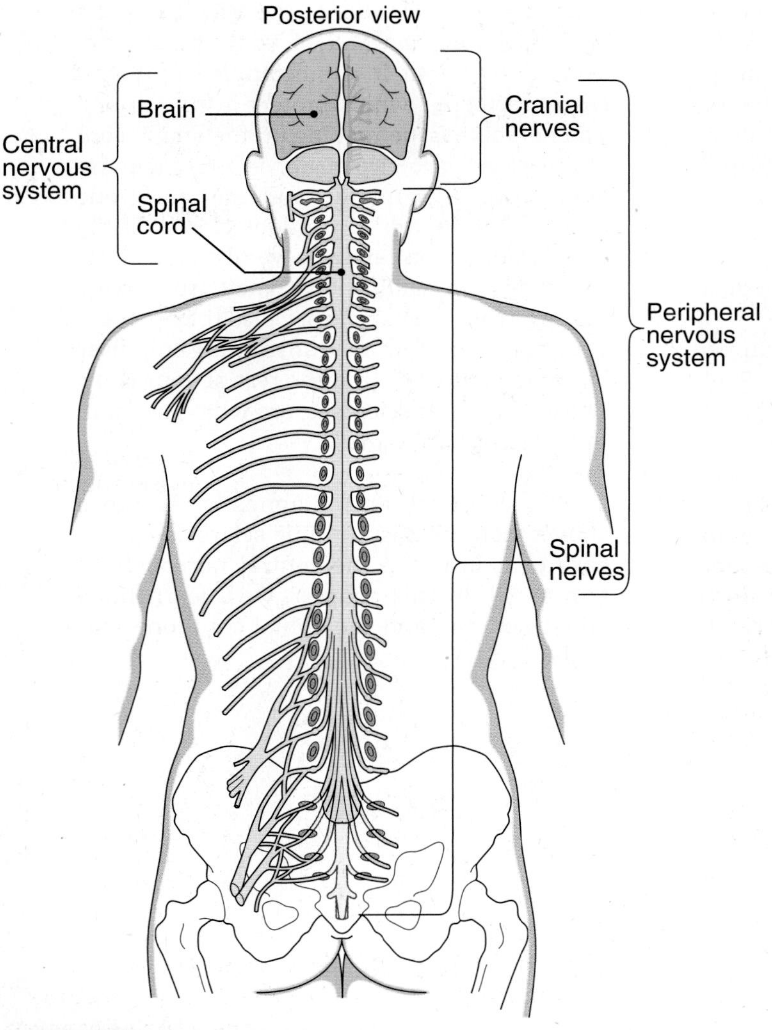

Functional Divisions

Functionally, the nervous system is divided according to whether control is voluntary or involuntary and according to what type of tissue is stimulated (Table 9-1). Any tissue or organ that carries out a nervous system command is called an **effector**, all of which are muscles or glands.

The **somatic nervous system** is controlled voluntarily (by conscious will), and all its effectors are skeletal muscles (described in Chapter 8). The nervous system's involuntary division is called the **autonomic nervous system** (ANS), making reference to its automatic activity. It is also called the **visceral nervous system** because it controls smooth muscle, cardiac muscle, and glands, which make up most of the soft body organs, the viscera.

The ANS is further subdivided into a **sympathetic nervous system** and a **parasympathetic nervous system** based on organization and how each affects specific organs. The ANS is described later in this chapter.

Although these divisions are helpful for study purposes, the lines that divide the nervous system according to function are not as distinct as those that classify the system structurally. For example, the diaphragm, a skeletal muscle, typically functions in breathing without conscious thought. In addition, we have certain rapid reflex responses involving skeletal muscles—drawing the hand away from a hot stove, for example—that do not involve the brain. In contrast, people can be trained to consciously control involuntary functions, such as blood pressure, heart rate, and breathing rate, by techniques known as *biofeedback*.

Figure 9-1 Anatomic divisions of the nervous system.

Table 9-1	Functional Divisions of the Nervous System		
		Characteristics	
Division	Control	Effectors	Subdivisions
Somatic nervous system	Voluntary	Skeletal muscle	None
Autonomic nervous system	Involuntary	Smooth muscle, cardiac muscle, and glands	Sympathetic and parasympathetic systems

CHECKPOINT 9-1 ➤ What are the two divisions of the nervous system based on structure?

CHECKPOINT 9-2 ➤ The nervous system can be divided functionally into two divisions based on type of control and effectors. What division is voluntary and controls skeletal muscle, and what division is involuntary and controls involuntary muscles and glands?

Neurons and Their Functions

The functional cells of the nervous system are highly specialized cells called **neurons** (Fig. 9-2). These cells have a unique structure related to their function.

Structure of a Neuron

The main portion of each neuron, the cell body, contains the nucleus and other organelles typically found in cells. A distinguishing feature of the neurons, however, are the long, threadlike fibers that extend out from the cell body and carry impulses across the cell (Fig. 9-3). There are two kinds of fibers: dendrites and axons.

- **Dendrites** are neuron fibers that conduct impulses *to* the cell body. Most dendrites have a highly branched, treelike appearance (see Fig. 9-2). In fact, the name comes from a Greek word meaning "tree." Dendrites function as **receptors** in the nervous system. That is, they receive the stimulus that begins a neural pathway. In Chapter 11, we describe how the dendrites of the sensory system may be modified to respond to a specific type of stimulus.

- **Axons** (AK-sons) are neuron fibers that conduct impulses *away from* the cell body (see Fig. 9-2). These impulses may be delivered to another neuron, to a muscle, or to a gland. An axon is a single fiber, which may be quite long, but it may give off branches and its ending is branched.

THE MYELIN SHEATH Some axons are covered with a fatty material called **myelin** that insulates and protects the fiber (see Fig. 9-2). In the PNS, this covering is produced by

specialized protective cells called **Schwann** (shvahn) **cells** that wrap around the axon like a jelly roll depositing layers of myelin (Fig. 9-4). When the sheath is complete, small

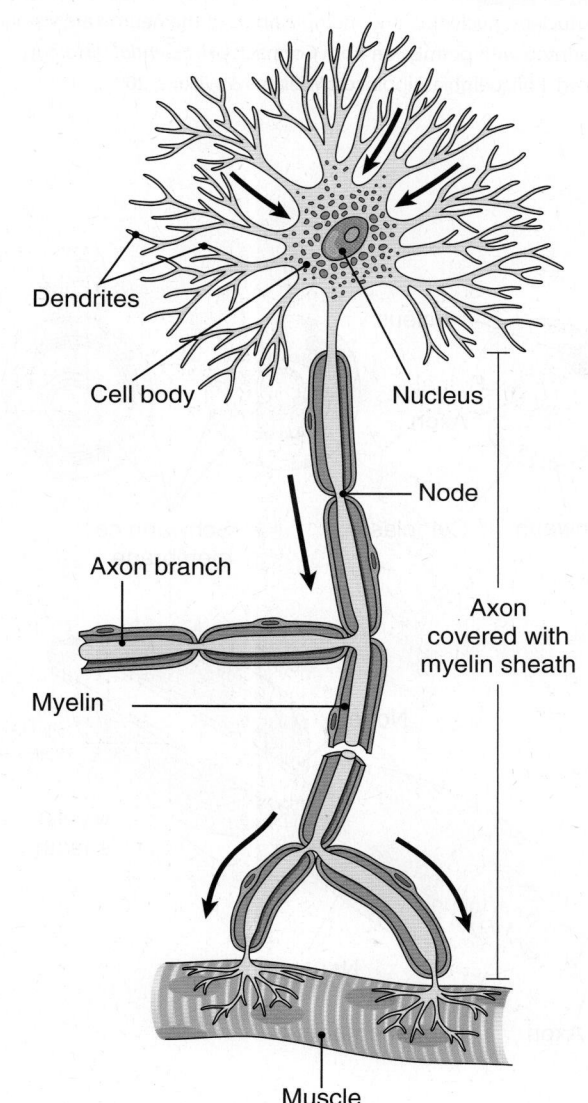

Figure 9-2 **Diagram of a motor neuron.** The break in the axon denotes length. The arrows show the direction of the nerve impulse. [**ZOOMING IN** ➤ Is the neuron shown here a sensory or a motor neuron?]

Dendrites
Cell body
Nucleus
Node
Axon branch
Axon covered with myelin sheath
Myelin
Muscle

9

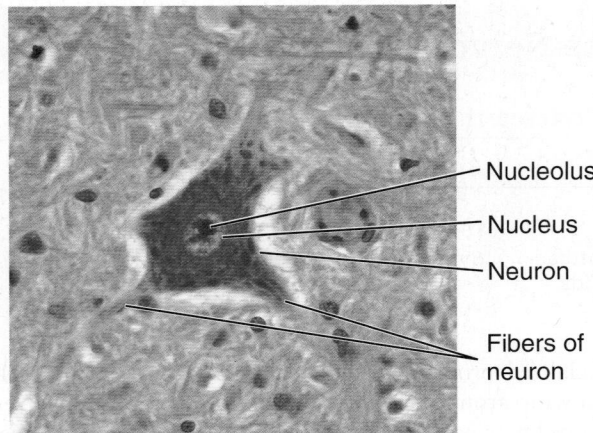

Figure 9-3 **A typical neuron as seen under the microscope.**
The nucleus, nucleolus, and multiple fibers of the neuron are visible.
(Reprinted with permission from Cormack DH. *Essential Histology*,
2nd ed. Philadelphia: Lippincott Williams & Wilkins, 2001.)

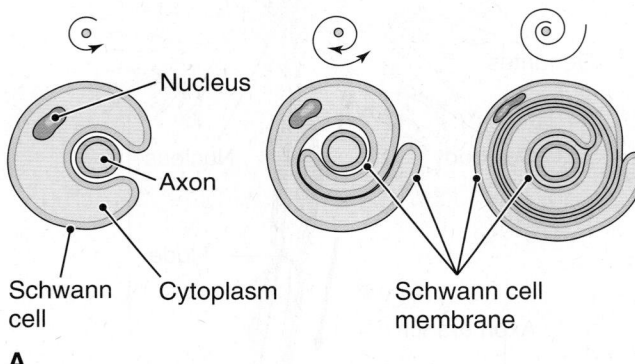

A

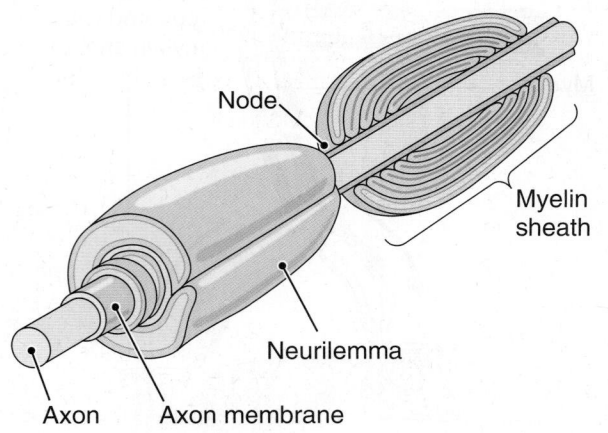

B

Figure 9-4 **Formation of a myelin sheath. (A)** Schwann cells
wrap around the axon, creating a myelin coating. **(B)** The
outermost layer of the Schwann cell forms the neurilemma. Spaces
between the cells are the nodes (of Ranvier).

spaces remain between the individual cells. These tiny gaps,
called **nodes** (originally, nodes of Ranvier), are important
in speeding nerve impulse conduction.

The Schwann cells' outermost membranes form a thin
coating known as the **neurilemma** (nu-rih-LEM-mah). This
covering is a part of the mechanism by which some peripheral nerves repair themselves when injured. Under some circumstances, damaged nerve cell fibers may regenerate by
growing into the sleeve formed by the neurilemma. Cells of
the brain and the spinal cord are myelinated, not by
Schwann cells, but by other types of protective cells. As a
result, they have no neurilemma. If they are injured, the
damage is permanent. Even in the peripheral nerves, however, repair is a slow and uncertain process.

Myelinated axons, because of myelin's color, are
called **white fibers** and are found in the **white matter** of the
brain and spinal cord as well as most nerves throughout
the body. The fibers and cell bodies of the **gray matter** are
not covered with myelin.

CHECKPOINT **9-3** ➤ The neuron, the functional unit of the
nervous system, has long fibers
extending from the cell body. What is
the name of the fiber that carries
impulses toward the cell body and
what is the name of the fiber that
carries impulses away from the cell
body?

CHECKPOINT **9-4** ➤ Myelin is a substance that covers and
protects some axons. What color
describes myelinated fibers, and what
color describes the nervous system's
unmyelinated tissue?

Types of Neurons

The job of neurons in the PNS is to relay information constantly either to or from the CNS. Neurons that conduct
impulses *to* the spinal cord and brain are described as **sensory neurons**, also called **afferent neurons**. Those cells that
carry impulses *from* the CNS out to muscles and glands
are **motor neurons**, also called **efferent neurons**. Neurons
that relay information within the CNS are **interneurons**,
also called *central* or *association neurons*.

Nerves and Tracts

Everywhere in the nervous system, neuron fibers are collected into bundles of varying size (Fig. 9-5). A fiber bundle located within the PNS is a **nerve**. A similar grouping,
but located within the CNS, is a **tract**. Tracts are located
both in the brain and in the spinal cord, where they conduct impulses to and from the brain.

A nerve or tract can be compared to an electric cable
made up of many wires. The "wires," the nerve cell fibers,
in a nerve or tract are bound together with connective tis-

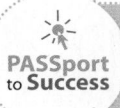

Figure 9-5 **Cross section of a nerve as seen under the microscope (×132).** Two fascicles (subdivisions) are shown. Perineurium (P) surrounds each fascicle. Epineurium (Ep) is around the entire nerve. Individual axons (Ax) are covered with a myelin sheath (MS), around which is the endoneurium (En) (inset). (Reprinted with permission from Gartner LP, Hiatt JL. *Color Atlas of Histology*, 3rd ed. Philadelphia: Lippincott Williams & Wilkins, 2000.)

sue, just like muscle fibers in a muscle. As in muscles, the individual fibers are organized into subdivisions called *fascicles*. The names of the connective tissue layers are similar to their names in muscles, but the root *neur/o*, meaning "nerve" is substituted for the muscle root *my/o*, as follows:

- Endoneurium is around an individual fiber.
- Perineurium is around a fascicle.
- Epineurium is around the whole nerve.

A nerve may contain all sensory fibers, all motor fibers, or a combination of both types of fibers. A few of the cranial nerves contain only sensory fibers conducting impulses toward the brain. These are described as **sensory (afferent) nerves**. A few of the cranial nerves contain only motor fibers conducting impulses away from the brain and these are classified as **motor (efferent) nerves**. However, most of the cranial nerves and *all* of the spinal nerves contain both sensory *and* motor fibers and are referred to as **mixed nerves**. Note that in a mixed nerve, impulses may be traveling in two directions (toward or away from the CNS), but each individual fiber in the nerve is carrying im-

pulses in one direction only. Think of the nerve as a large highway. Traffic may be going north and south, for example, but each car is going forward in only one direction.

CHECKPOINT 9-5 ➤ Nerves are bundles of neuron fibers in the PNS. These nerves may be carrying impulses either toward or away from the CNS. What name is given to nerves that convey impulses toward the CNS, and what name is given to nerves that transport away from the CNS?

Neuroglia

In addition to conducting tissue, the nervous system contains cells that support and protect the neurons. Collectively, these cells are called **neuroglia** (nu-ROG-le-ah) or **glial** (GLI-al) **cells**, from a Greek word meaning "glue." There are different types of neuroglia, each with specialized functions, some of which are the following:

- Protect and nourish nervous tissue
- Support nervous tissue and bind it to other structures
- Aid in repair of cells
- Act as phagocytes to remove pathogens and impurities
- Regulate the composition of fluids around and between cells

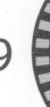

Neuroglia appear throughout the central and peripheral nervous systems. The Schwann cells that produce the myelin sheath in the peripheral nervous system are one type of neuroglia. Another example is shown in Figure 9-6. These cells are astrocytes, named for their star-like appearance. In the brain they attach to capillaries (small blood vessels) to help protect the brain from harmful substances.

Unlike neurons, neuroglia continue to multiply throughout life. Because of their capacity to reproduce, most tumors of the nervous system are tumors of neuroglial tissue and not of nervous tissue itself.

CHECKPOINT 9-6 ➤ The nervous system's nonconducting cells protect, nourish, and support the neurons. What are these cells called?

PASSport to Success Visit *thePoint* or see the Student Resource CD in the back of this book for a summary of the different neuroglial types.

The Nervous System at Work

The nervous system works by means of electrical impulses sent along neuron fibers and transmitted from cell to cell at highly specialized junctions.

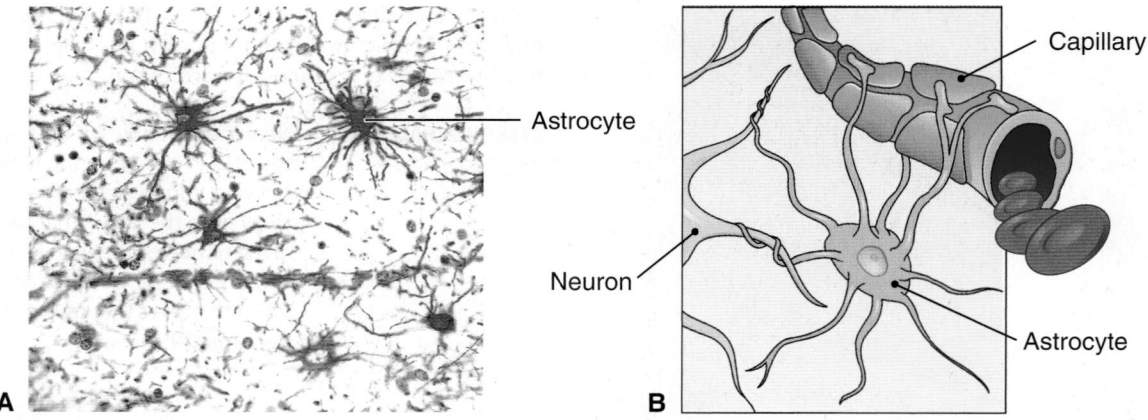

Figure 9-6 **Examples of neuroglia. (A)** Astrocytes in the white matter of the brain. **(B)** Astrocytes attach to capillaries and help to protect the brain from harmful substances. (A, reprinted with permission from Mills SE. *Histology for Pathologists*, 3rd ed. Philadelphia: Lippincott Williams & Wilkins, 2006; B, modified with permission from McConnell TH. *The Nature of Disease: Pathology for the Health Professions*. Baltimore: Lippincott Williams & Wilkins, 2006.)

The Nerve Impulse

The mechanics of nerve impulse conduction are complex but can be compared to the spread of an electric current along a wire. What follows is a brief description of the electrical changes that occur as a resting neuron is stimulated and transmits a nerve impulse.

The plasma membrane of an unstimulated (resting) neuron carries an electrical charge, or **potential**. This resting potential is maintained by ions (charged particles) concentrated on either side of the membrane. At rest, the inside of the membrane is negative as compared with the outside. In this state, the membrane is said to be *polarized*. As in a battery, the separation of charges on either side of the membrane creates a possibility (potential) for generating energy. If there is a way for the charges to move toward each other, electricity (a nerve impulse) will be generated.

A **nerve impulse** starts with a local reversal in the membrane potential caused by changes in the ion concentrations on either side. This sudden electrical change at the membrane is called an **action potential**, as described in Chapter 8 on the muscles. A simple description of the events in an action potential is as follows (Fig. 9-7):

- The resting state. In addition to an electrical difference on the two sides of the plasma membrane at rest, there is also a slight difference in the concentration of ions on either side. At rest, sodium ions (Na^+) are a little more concentrated at the outside of the membrane. At the same time, potassium ions (K^+) are a little more concentrated at the inside of the membrane.

- Depolarization. A stimulus of adequate force, such as electrical, chemical or mechanical energy, causes specific channels in the membrane to open and allow Na^+ ions to flow into the cell. (Remember that substances flow by diffusion from an area where they are in higher concentration to an area where they are in lower concentration.) As these positive ions enter, they raise the charge on the inside of the membrane, a change known as **depolarization** (see Fig. 9-7).

- Repolarization. In the next step of the action potential, K^+ channels open to allow K^+ to leave the cell. As the electrical charge returns to its resting value, the membrane is under-

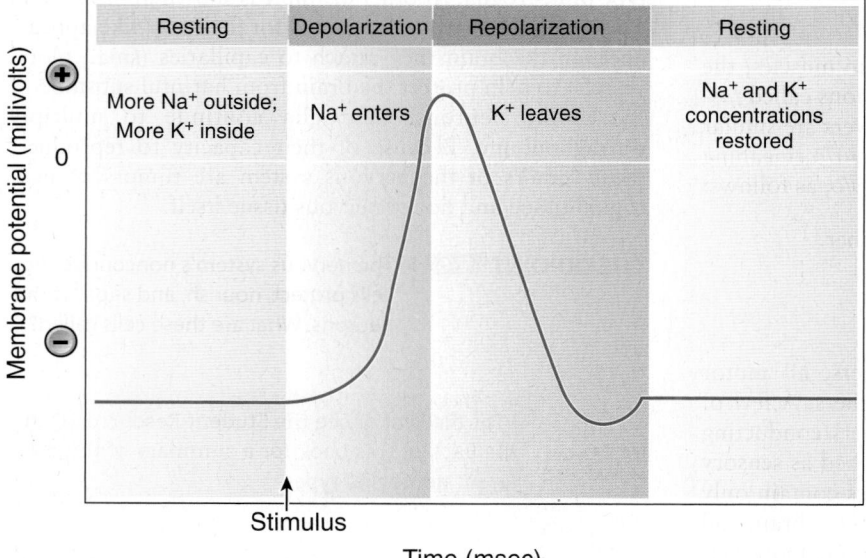

Figure 9-7 **The action potential.** In depolarization, Na^+ membrane channels open and Na^+ enters the cell. In repolarization, K^+ membrane channels open and K^+ leaves the cell. During the resting stage, the Na^+/K^+ pump returns ion concentrations to their original concentrations so the membrane can be stimulated again.

going **repolarization**. At the same time that the membrane is repolarizing, the cell uses active transport to move Na$^+$ and K$^+$ back to their original concentrations on either side of the membrane. This movement of ions through the plasma membrane against the concentration gradient requires transporters and energy from ATP. As Na$^+$ is transported to the outside of the cell and K$^+$ is transported to the inside of the cell, their concentration gradients are restored so that another action potential can occur. This transport mechanism is described as the **sodium–potassium pump** or Na$^+$–K$^+$ pump.

The action potential occurs rapidly—in less than one thousandth of a second, an is followed by a rapid return to the resting state. However, this local electrical change in the membrane stimulates an action potential at an adjacent point along the membrane (Fig. 9-8). In scientific terms, the channels in the membrane are "voltage dependent," that is, they respond to an electrical stimulus. And so, the action potential spreads along the membrane as a wave of electrical current. The spreading action potential is the nerve impulse, and in fact, the term *action potential* is used to mean the nerve impulse. A stimulus is any force that can start an action potential by opening membrane channels and allowing Na$^+$ to enter the cell.

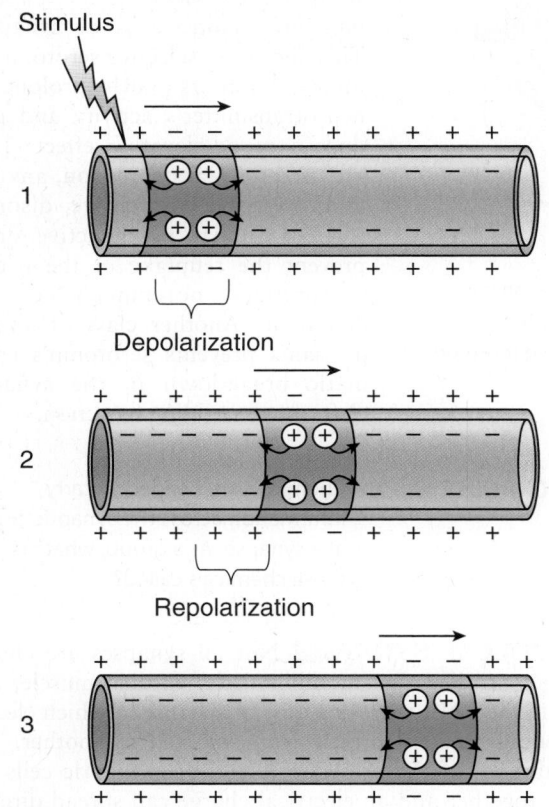

Figure 9-8 A nerve impulse. From a point of stimulation, a wave of depolarization followed by repolarization travels along the membrane of a neuron. This spreading action potential is a nerve impulse.

THE ROLE OF MYELIN IN CONDUCTION As previously noted, some axons are coated with the fatty material myelin. If a fiber is not myelinated, the action potential spreads continuously along the cell's membrane (see Fig. 9-4). When myelin is present on an axon, however, it insulates the fiber against the spread of current. This would appear to slow or stop conduction along these fibers, but in fact, the myelin sheath speeds conduction. The reason is that the action potential must "jump" like a spark from node (space) to node along the sheath (see Fig. 9-3), and this type of conduction, called **saltatory** (SAL-tah-to-re) **conduction**, is actually faster than continuous conduction.

CHECKPOINT 9-7 ➤ An action potential occurs in two stages. In the first stage, the charge on the membrane reverses, and in the second stage, it returns to the resting state. What are the names of these two stages?

CHECKPOINT 9-8 ➤ What ions are involved in generating an action potential?

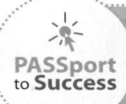

PASSport to Success Visit *thePoint* or see the Student Resource CD in the back of this book for animations *The Synapse and the Nerve Impulse* and *The Myelin Sheath*.

The Synapse

Neurons do not work alone; impulses must be transferred between neurons to convey information within the nervous system. The point of junction for transmitting the nerve impulse is the **synapse** (SIN-aps), a term that comes from a Greek word meaning "to clasp" (Fig. 9-9). At a synapse, transmission of an impulse usually occurs from the axon of one cell, the **presynaptic cell**, to the dendrite of another cell, the **postsynaptic cell**.

As described in Chapter 8, information must be passed from one cell to another at the synapse across a tiny gap between the cells, the **synaptic cleft**. Information usually crosses this gap in the form of a chemical known as a **neurotransmitter**. While the cells at a synapse are at rest, the neurotransmitter is stored in many small vesicles (sacs) within the enlarged axon endings, usually called *end-bulbs* or *terminal knobs*, but known by several other names as well.

When a nerve impulse traveling along a neuron membrane reaches the end of the presynaptic axon, some of these vesicles fuse with the membrane and release their neurotransmitter into the synaptic cleft (an example of exocytosis, as described in Chapter 3). The neurotransmitter then acts as a chemical signal to the postsynaptic cell.

On the postsynaptic receiving membrane, usually that of a dendrite, but sometimes another cell part, there are special sites, or **receptors**, ready to pick up and respond to specific neurotransmitters. Receptors in the postsynaptic cell's membrane influence how or if that cell will respond to a given neurotransmitter.

9

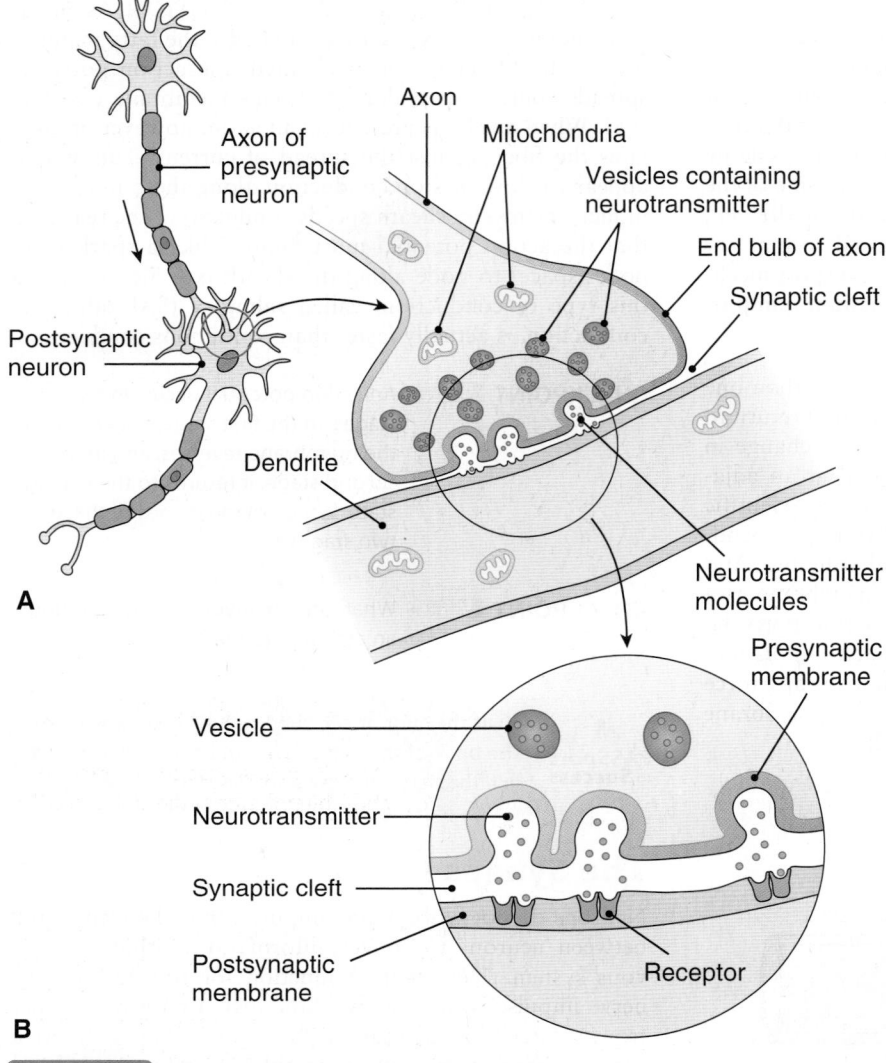

Axon of presynaptic neuron

Postsynaptic neuron

Dendrite

Axon

Mitochondria

Vesicles containing neurotransmitter

End bulb of axon

Synaptic cleft

Neurotransmitter molecules

A

Presynaptic membrane

Vesicle

Neurotransmitter

Synaptic cleft

Postsynaptic membrane

Receptor

B

Figure 9-9 **A synapse. (A)** The end-bulb of the presynaptic (transmitting) axon has vesicles containing neurotransmitter, which is released into the synaptic cleft to the membrane of the postsynaptic (receiving) cell. **(B)** Close-up of a synapse showing receptors for neurotransmitter in the postsynaptic cell membrane.

or a single cell may be stimulated by a number of different axons (Fig. 9-10). The cell's response is based on the total effects of all the neurotransmitters it receives at any one time.

After its release into the synaptic cleft, the neurotransmitter may be removed by several methods:

- It may slowly diffuse away from the synapse.
- It may be destroyed rapidly by enzymes in the synaptic cleft.
- It may be taken back into the presynaptic cell to be used again, a process known as *reuptake.*

The method of removal helps determine how long a neurotransmitter will act.

Many drugs that act on the mind, substances known as *psychoactive drugs*, function by affecting neurotransmitter activity in the brain. Prozac, for example, increases the level of the neurotransmitter serotonin by blocking its reuptake into presynaptic cells at synapses. This and other selective serotonin reuptake inhibitors (SSRIs) prolong the neurotransmitter's activity and produce a mood-elevating effect. They are used to treat depression, anxiety, and obsessive-compulsive disorder (OCD). Similar psychoactive drugs prevent the reuptake of the neurotransmitters norepinephrine and dopamine. Another class of antidepressants prevents serotonin's enzymatic breakdown in the synaptic cleft, thus extending its action.

NEUROTRANSMITTERS Although there are many known neurotransmitters, the main ones are epinephrine (ep-ih-NEF-rin), also called **adrenaline**; a related compound, **norepinephrine** (nor-ep-ih-NEF-rin), or **noradrenaline**; and **acetylcholine** (as-e-til-KO-lene). Acetylcholine (ACh) is the neurotransmitter released at the neuromuscular junction, the synapse between a neuron and a muscle cell. All three of the above neurotransmitters function in the ANS.

It is common to think of neurotransmitters as stimulating the cells they reach; in fact, they have been described as such in this discussion. Note, however, that some of these chemicals inhibit the postsynaptic cell and keep it from reacting, as will be demonstrated later in discussions of the autonomic nervous system.

The connections between neurons can be quite complex. One cell can branch to stimulate many receiving cells,

CHECKPOINT **9-9** ➤ Chemicals are needed to carry information across the synaptic cleft at a synapse. As a group, what are all these chemicals called?

ELECTRICAL SYNAPSES Not all synapses are chemically controlled. In smooth muscle, cardiac muscle, and also in the CNS, there is a type of synapse in which electrical energy travels directly from one cell to another. The membranes of the presynaptic and postsynaptic cells are close together and an electrical charge can spread directly between them. These electrical synapses allow more rapid and more coordinated communication. In the heart, for example, it is important that large groups of cells contract together for effective pumping action.

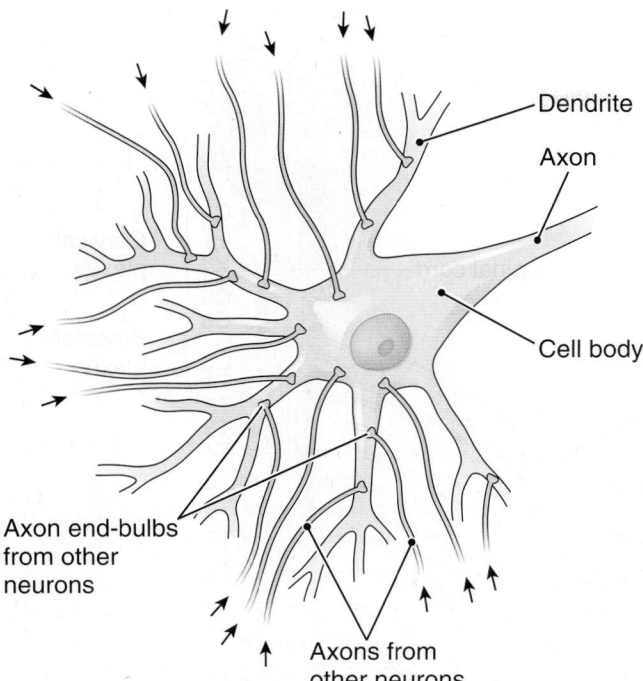

Dendrite

Axon

Cell body

Axon end-bulbs
from other
neurons

Axons from
other neurons

Figure 9-10 **The effects of neurotransmitters on a neuron.** A single neuron is stimulated by axons of many other neurons. The cell responds according to the total of all the excitatory and inhibitory neurotransmitters it receives.

The Spinal Cord

The spinal cord is the link between the peripheral nervous system and the brain. It also helps to coordinate impulses within the CNS. The spinal cord is contained in and protected by the vertebrae, which fit together to form a continuous tube extending from the occipital bone to the coccyx (Fig. 9-11). In the embryo, the spinal cord occupies the entire spinal canal, extending down into the tail portion of the vertebral column. The bony column grows much more rapidly than the nervous tissue of the cord, however, and eventually, the end of the spinal cord no longer reaches the lower part of the spinal canal. This disparity in growth continues to increase, so that in adults, the spinal cord ends in the region just below the area to which the last rib attaches (between the first and second lumbar vertebrae).

Structure of the Spinal Cord

The spinal cord has a small, irregularly shaped internal section of gray matter (unmyelinated tissue) surrounded by a larger area of white matter (myelinated axons) (Fig. 9-12). The internal gray matter is arranged so that a column of gray matter extends up and down dorsally, one on each side; another column is found in the ventral region on each side. These two pairs of columns, called the **dorsal horns** and **ventral horns**, give the gray matter an H-shaped appearance in cross-section. The bridge of gray matter that

connects the right and left horns is the **gray commissure** (KOM-ih-shure). In the center of the gray commissure is a small channel, the **central canal**, that contains cerebrospinal fluid, the liquid that circulates around the brain and spinal cord. A narrow groove, the **posterior median sulcus** (SUL-kus), divides the right and left portions of the posterior white matter. A deeper groove, the **anterior median fissure** (FISH-ure), separates the right and left portions of the anterior white matter.

ASCENDING AND DESCENDING TRACTS The spinal cord is the pathway for sensory and motor impulses traveling to and from the brain. These impulses are carried in the thousands of myelinated axons in the white matter of the spinal cord, which are subdivided into tracts (groups of fibers). Sensory (afferent) impulses entering the spinal cord are transmitted toward the brain in **ascending tracts** of the white matter. Motor (efferent) impulses traveling from the brain are carried in **descending tracts** toward the peripheral nervous system.

CHECKPOINT **9-10** ➤ The spinal cord contains both gray and white matter. How is this tissue arranged in the spinal cord?

CHECKPOINT **9-11** ➤ What is the purpose of the tracts in the white matter of the spinal cord?

The Reflex Arc

The nervous system receives, interprets, and acts on both external and internal stimuli. The spinal cord is a relay center for coordinating neural pathways. A complete pathway through the nervous system from stimulus to response is termed a **reflex arc** (Fig. 9-13). This is the nervous system's basic functional pathway. The fundamental parts of a reflex arc are the following (Table 9-2):

1. **Receptor**—the end of a dendrite or some specialized receptor cell, as in a special sense organ, that detects a stimulus

2. **Sensory neuron**, or afferent neuron—a cell that transmits impulses toward the CNS. Sensory impulses enter the dorsal horn of the spinal cord's gray matter.

3. **Central nervous system**—where impulses are coordinated and a response is organized. One or more interneurons may carry impulses to and from the brain, may function within the brain, or may distribute impulses to different regions of the spinal cord. Almost every response involves connecting neurons in the CNS.

4. **Motor neuron**, or efferent neuron—a cell that carries impulses away from the CNS. Motor impulses leave the cord through the ventral horn of the spinal cord's gray matter.

5. **Effector**—a muscle or a gland outside the CNS that carries out a response

9

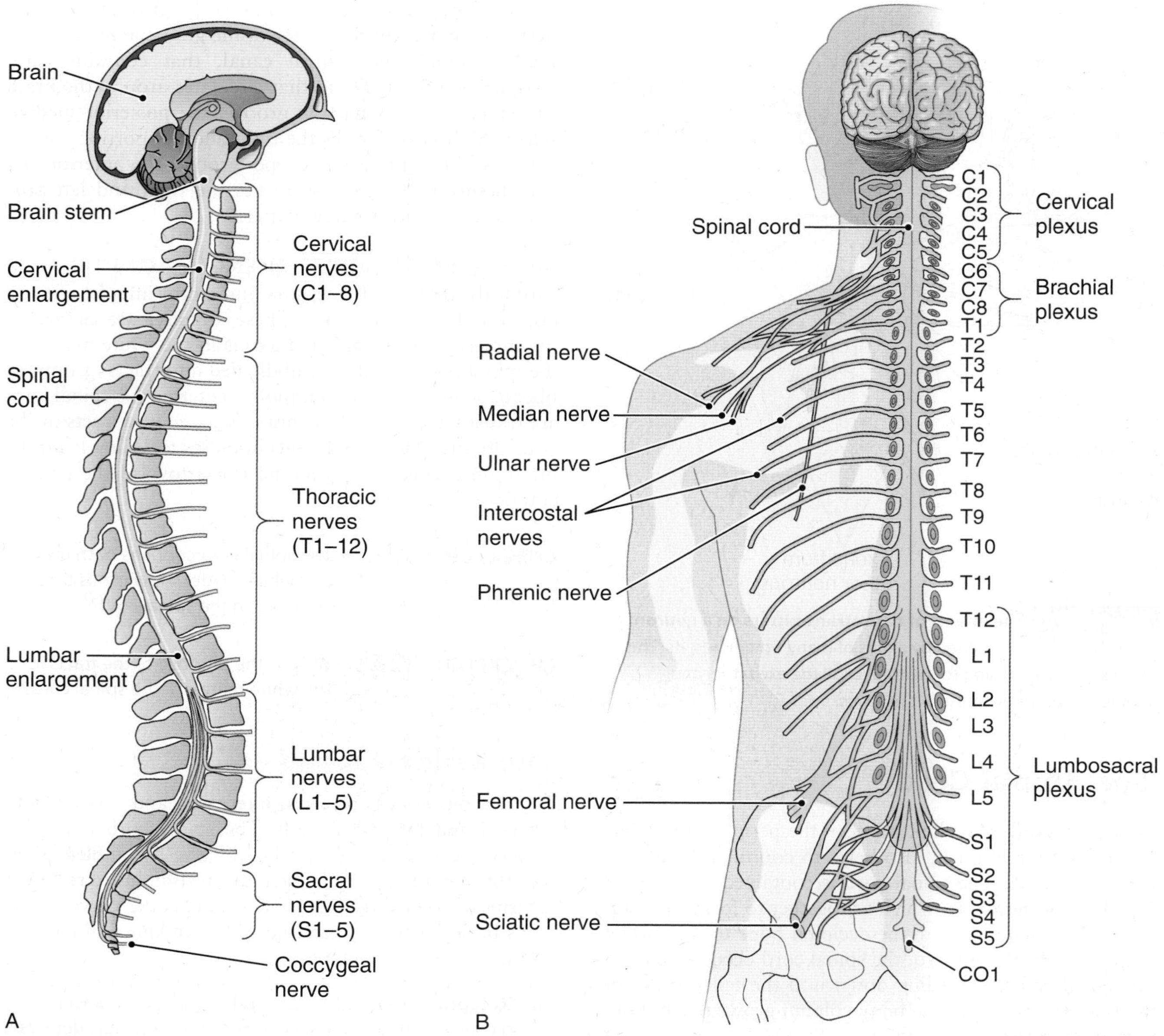

Brain

Brain stem

Cervical enlargement

Spinal cord

Lumbar enlargement

Cervical nerves (C1–8)

Thoracic nerves (T1–12)

Lumbar nerves (L1–5)

Sacral nerves (S1–5)

Coccygeal nerve

A

Spinal cord

Radial nerve

Median nerve

Ulnar nerve

Intercostal nerves

Phrenic nerve

Femoral nerve

Sciatic nerve

C1
C2
C3
C4
C5
C6
C7
C8
T1
T2
T3
T4
T5
T6
T7
T8
T9
T10
T11
T12
L1
L2
L3
L4
L5
S1
S2
S3
S4
S5
CO1

Cervical plexus

Brachial plexus

Lumbosacral plexus

B

Figure 9-11 **Spinal cord and spinal nerves.** Nerve plexuses (networks) are shown. **(A)** Lateral view. **(B)** Posterior view. **[ZOOMING IN ➤** Is the spinal cord the same length as the spinal column? How does the number of cervical vertebrae compare to the number of cervical spinal nerves? **]**

At its simplest, a reflex arc can involve just two neurons, one sensory and one motor, with a synapse in the CNS. Few reflex arcs require only this minimal number of neurons. (The knee-jerk reflex described below is one of the few examples in humans.) Most reflex arcs involve many more, even hundreds, of connecting neurons within the CNS. The many intricate patterns that make the nervous system so responsive and adaptable also make it difficult to study, and investigation of the nervous system is one of the most active areas of research today.

CHECKPOINT **9-12** ➤ What name is given to a pathway through the nervous system from a stimulus to an effector?

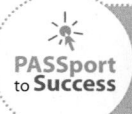

Visit *thePoint* or see the Student Resource CD in the back of this book to view the animation *The Reflex Arc.*

REFLEX ACTIVITIES Although reflex pathways may be quite complex, a **simple reflex** is a rapid, uncomplicated, and automatic response involving very few neurons. Reflexes are specific; a given stimulus always produces the same response. When you fling out an arm or leg to catch your balance, withdraw from a painful stimulus, or blink to avoid an object approaching your eyes, you are experiencing reflex behavior. A simple reflex arc that passes

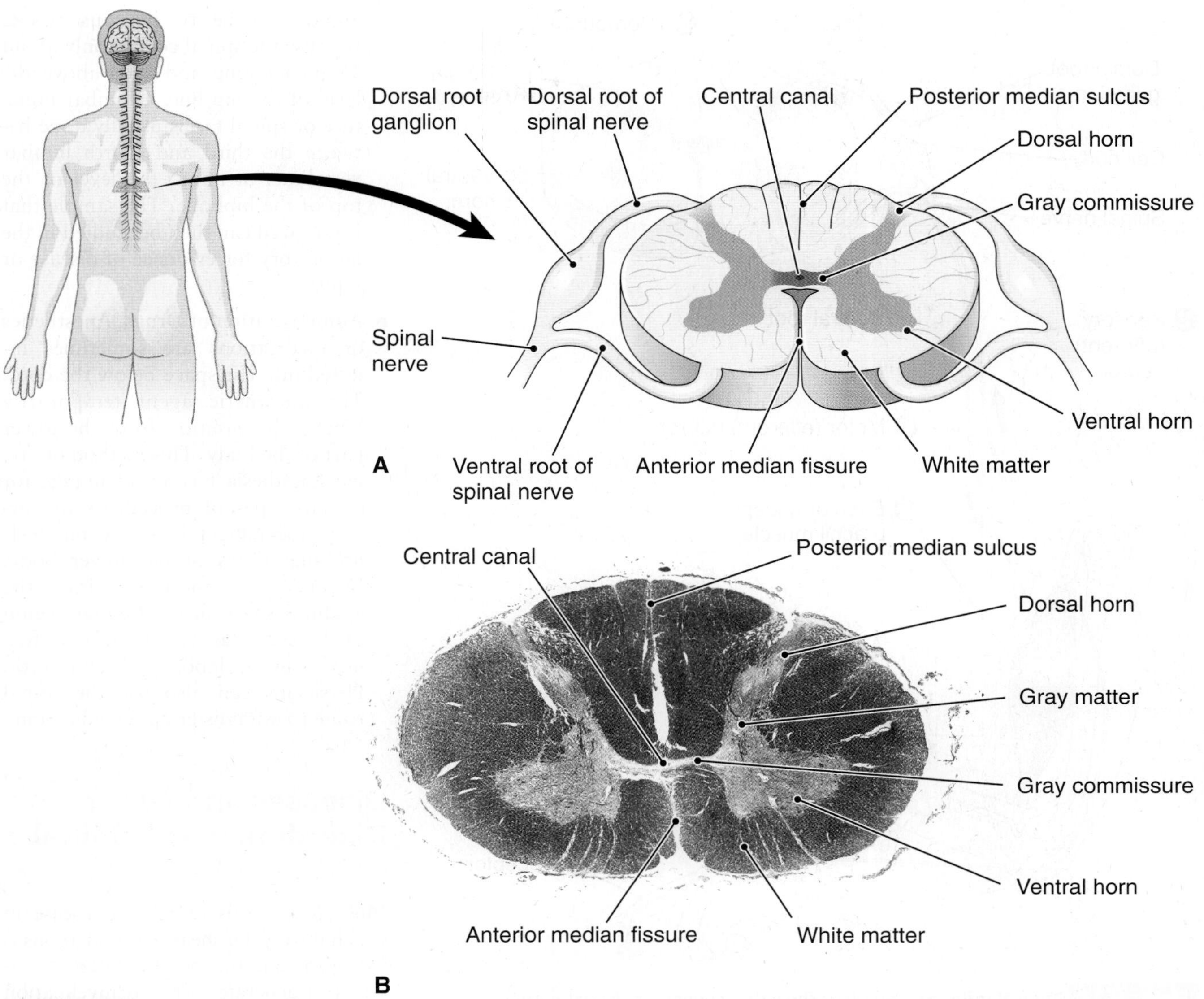

Dorsal root ganglion

Dorsal root of spinal nerve

Central canal

Posterior median sulcus

Dorsal horn

Gray commissure

Spinal nerve

Ventral horn

A Ventral root of spinal nerve

Anterior median fissure

White matter

Central canal

Posterior median sulcus

Dorsal horn

Gray matter

Gray commissure

Ventral horn

Anterior median fissure

White matter

B

Figure 9-12 **The spinal cord. (A)** Cross section of the spinal cord showing the organization of the gray and white matter. The roots of the spinal nerves are also shown. **(B)** Microscopic view of the spinal cord in cross section (×5). (B, Reprinted with permission from Mills SE. *Histology for Pathologists*, 3rd ed. Philadelphia: Lippincott Williams & Wilkins, 2006.)

through the spinal cord alone and does not involve the brain is termed a **spinal reflex**. Returning to our opening corporation analogy, it's as if middle management makes a decision independently, without involving the CEO.

The **stretch reflex**, in which a muscle is stretched and responds by contracting, is one example of a spinal reflex. If you tap the tendon below the kneecap (the patellar tendon), the muscle of the anterior thigh (quadriceps femoris) contracts, eliciting the knee-jerk reflex (Fig. 9-14).

Such stretch reflexes may be evoked by appropriate tapping of most large muscles (such as the triceps brachii in the arm and the gastrocnemius in the calf of the leg). Because reflexes are simple and predictable, they are used in physical examinations to test the condition of the nervous system.

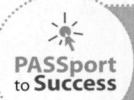

Visit **thePoint** or see the Student Resource CD in the back of this book for an illustration of the following spinal cord procedures.

Medical Procedures Involving the Spinal Cord

- Lumbar Puncture. It is sometimes necessary to remove a small amount of cerebrospinal fluid (CSF) from the nervous system for testing. CSF is the fluid that circulates in and around the brain and spinal cord. This fluid is taken from the space below the spinal cord to

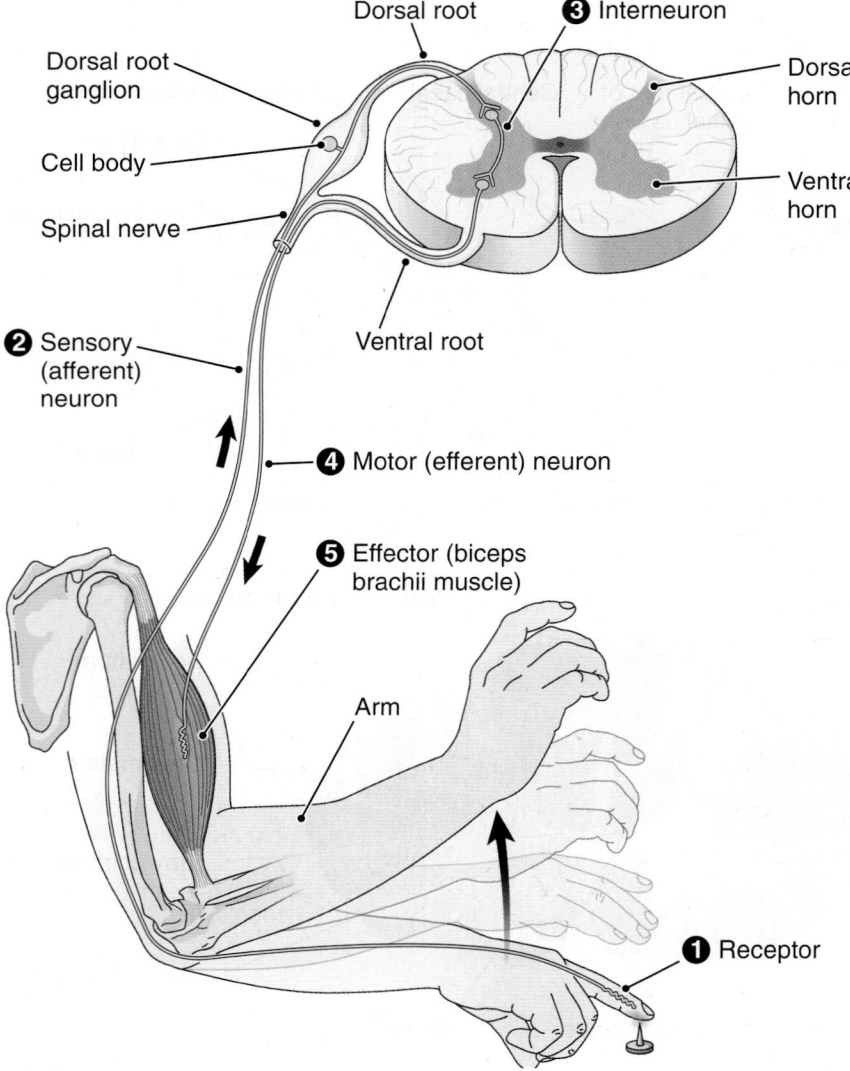

Dorsal root

❸ Interneuron

Dorsal root ganglion

Cell body

Spinal nerve

Dorsal horn

Ventral horn

Ventral root

❷ Sensory (afferent) neuron

❹ Motor (efferent) neuron

❺ Effector (biceps brachii muscle)

Arm

❶ Receptor

Figure 9-13 **Typical reflex arc.** Numbers show the sequence in the pathway of impulses through the spinal cord (*solid arrows*). Contraction of the biceps brachii results in flexion of the arm at the elbow. [ZOOMING IN ► Is this a somatic or an autonomic reflex arc? What type of neuron is located between the sensory and motor neuron in the CNS?]

Table 9-2	Components of a Reflex Arc
Component	**Function**
Receptor	End of a dendrite or specialized cell that responds to a stimulus
Sensory neuron	Transmits a nerve impulse toward the CNS
Central nervous system	Coordinates sensory impulses and organizes a response. Usually requires interneurons
Motor neuron	Carries impulses away from the CNS toward the effector, a muscle or a gland
Effector	A muscle or gland outside the CNS that carries out a response

avoid damage to nervous tissue. Because the spinal cord is only about 18 inches long and ends above the level of the hip line, a lumbar puncture or spinal tap is usually done between the third and fourth lumbar vertebrae, at about the level of the top of the hipbone. The sample that is removed can then be studied in the laboratory for evidence of disease or injury.

■ Administration of Drugs. Anesthetics or medications are sometimes injected into the space below the cord. The anesthetic agent temporarily blocks all sensation from the lower part of the body. This method of giving anesthesia has an advantage for certain types of procedures or surgery; the patient is awake but feels nothing in his or her lower body. Injection of anesthetic into the epidural space in the lumbar region of the spine (an "epidural") is often used during labor and childbirth. Physicians can also use the spinal route to administer pain medication.

Diseases and Other Disorders of the Spinal Cord

Multiple sclerosis (MS) is a disease in which the myelin sheath around axons is damaged and the neuron fibers themselves degenerate. This demyelination process slows the speed of nerve impulse conduction and disrupts nervous system communication. Both the spinal cord and the brain are affected. Although scientists do not completely understand the cause of MS, there is strong evidence that it involves an attack on the myelin sheath by a person's own immune system, a situation described as *autoimmunity*. Genetic makeup, in combination with environmental factors, may trigger MS. Some research suggests that a prior viral or bacterial infection, even one that occurred many years before, may set off the disease.

MS is the most common chronic CNS disease of young adults in the United States. The disease affects women about twice as often as men, and it is more common in temperate climates and in people of northern

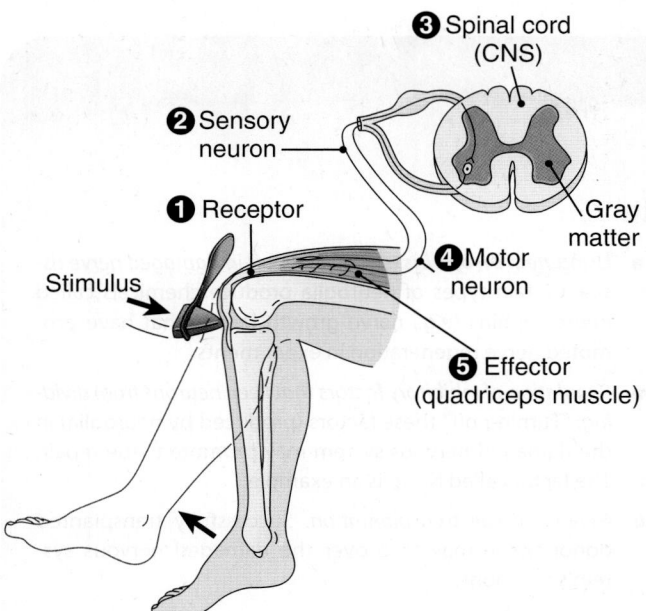

❸ Spinal cord (CNS)

❷ Sensory neuron

❶ Receptor

Stimulus

Gray matter

❹ Motor neuron

❺ Effector (quadriceps muscle)

Figure 9-14 **The patellar (knee-jerk) reflex.** Numbers indicate the sequence of a reflex arc. [**ZOOMING IN** ➤ How many total neurons are involved in this spinal reflex? What neurotransmitter is released at the synapse shown by number 5?]

European ancestry. MS progresses at different rates depending on the individual, and it may be marked by episodes of relapse and remission. At this point, no cure has been found for MS, but drugs that stop the autoimmune response and drugs that relieve MS symptoms are currently under study.

Amyotrophic (ah-mi-o-TROF-ik) **lateral sclerosis** is a nervous system disorder in which motor neurons are destroyed. The progressive destruction causes muscle atrophy and loss of motor control until finally the affected person is unable to swallow or talk.

Poliomyelitis (po-le-o-mi-eh-LI-tis) ("polio") is a viral disease of the nervous system that occurs most commonly in children. Polio is spread by ingestion of water contaminated with feces containing the virus. Infection of the gastrointestinal tract leads to passage of the virus into the blood, from which it spreads to the CNS. Poliovirus tends to multiply in the spinal cord's motor neurons, leading to paralysis, including paralysis of the breathing muscles.

Polio has been virtually eliminated in many countries through the use of vaccines against the disease—first the injected Salk vaccine developed in 1954, followed by the Sabin oral vaccine. A goal of the World Health Organization (WHO) is the total eradication of polio by worldwide vaccination programs, and several philanthropic organizations have joined in this effort.

TUMORS Tumors that affect the spinal cord commonly arise in the support tissue in and around the cord. They are frequently tumors of the nerve sheaths, the meninges, or neuroglia. Symptoms are caused by pressure on the cord

and the roots of the spinal nerves. These include pain, numbness, weakness, and loss of function. Spinal cord tumors are diagnosed by magnetic resonance imaging (MRI) or other imaging techniques, and treatment is by surgery and radiation.

INJURIES Spinal cord injuries may result from wounds, fracture or dislocation of the vertebrae, herniation of intervertebral disks, or tumors. The most common causes of accidental injury to the cord are motor vehicle accidents; falls; sports injuries, especially diving accidents; and job-related injuries. Spinal cord injuries are more common in the young adult age group and many are related to alcohol or drug use.

Cord damage may cause paralysis or loss of sensation in structures supplied by nerves below the level of injury. Different degrees of loss are named using the root *-plegia*, meaning "paralysis," for example:

- Monoplegia (mon-o-PLE-je-ah)- paralysis of one limb
- Diplegia (di-PLE-je-ah)- paralysis of both upper or both lower limbs
- Paraplegia (par-ah-PLE-je-ah)- paralysis of both lower limbs
- Hemiplegia (hem-e-PLE-je-ah)- paralysis of one side of the body
- Tetraplegia (tet-rah-PLE-je-ah) or quadriplegia (kwah-drih-PLE-je-ah)- paralysis of all four limbs

Box 9-1, Spinal Cord Injury: Crossing the Divide, contains information on treatment of these injuries.

The Spinal Nerves

There are 31 pairs of spinal nerves, each pair numbered according to the level of the spinal cord from which it arises (see Fig. 9-11). Note that the nerves that arise near the end of the cord travel in a group within the spinal canal until each exits from its appropriate intervertebral foramen. Each nerve is attached to the spinal cord by two roots: the **dorsal root** and the **ventral root** (see Fig. 9-12). On each dorsal root is a marked swelling of gray matter called the **dorsal root ganglion**, which contains the cell bodies of the sensory neurons. A **ganglion** (GANG-le-on) is any collection of nerve cell bodies located outside the CNS. Fibers from sensory receptors throughout the body lead to the dorsal roots and these dorsal root ganglia.

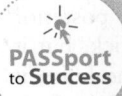

PASSport to Success

Visit *thePoint* or see the Student Resource CD in the back of this book for an illustration of the spinal nerves at the end of the spinal cord.

A spinal nerve's ventral root contains motor (efferent) fibers that supply muscles and glands (effectors). The cell bodies of these neurons are located in the cord's ventral gray matter (ventral horns). Because the dorsal (sensory)

9

Box 9-1   **Hot Topics**

Spinal Cord Injury: Crossing the Divide

Approximately 11,000 new cases of spinal cord injury occur each year in the United States, the majority involving males ages 16 to 30. Because neurons show little, if any, capacity to repair themselves, spinal cord injuries almost always result in a loss of sensory or motor function (or both), and therapy has focused on injury management rather than cure. However, scientists are investigating four improved treatment approaches:

- *Minimizing spinal cord trauma after injury.* Intravenous injection of the steroid methylprednisolone shortly after injury reduces swelling at the site of injury and improves recovery.

- *Using **neurotrophins** to induce repair in damaged nerve tissue.* Certain types of neuroglia produce chemicals called neurotrophins (e.g., nerve growth factor) that have promoted nerve regeneration in experiments.

- *Regulation of inhibitory factors that keep neurons from dividing.* "Turning off" these factors (produced by neuroglia) in the damaged nervous system may promote tissue repair. The factor called Nogo is an example.

- *Nervous tissue transplantation.* Successfully transplanted donor tissue may take over the damaged nervous system's functions.

---

and ventral (motor) roots combine to form the spinal nerve, all spinal nerves are mixed nerves.

Branches of the Spinal Nerves

Each spinal nerve continues only a short distance away from the spinal cord and then branches into small posterior divisions and larger anterior divisions. The larger anterior branches interlace to form networks called **plexuses** (PLEK-sus-eze), which then distribute branches to the body parts (see Fig. 9-11). The three main plexuses are described as follows:

- The **cervical plexus** supplies motor impulses to the neck muscles and receives sensory impulses from the neck and the back of the head. The phrenic nerve, which activates the diaphragm, arises from this plexus.

- The **brachial** (BRA-ke-al) **plexus** sends numerous branches to the shoulder, arm, forearm, wrist, and hand. The radial nerve emerges from the brachial plexus.

- The **lumbosacral** (lum-bo-SA-kral) **plexus** supplies nerves to the pelvis and legs. The largest branch in this plexus is the **sciatic** (si-AT-ik) **nerve**, which leaves the dorsal part of the pelvis, passes beneath the gluteus maximus muscle, and extends down the posterior thigh. At its beginning, it is nearly 1 inch thick, but it soon branches to the thigh muscles; near the knee, it forms two subdivisions that supply the leg and the foot.

DERMATOMES Sensory neurons from all over the skin, except for the skin of the face and scalp, feed information into the spinal cord through the spinal nerves. The skin surface can be mapped into distinct regions that are supplied by a single spinal nerve. Each of these regions is called a **dermatome** (DER-mah-tome) (Fig. 9-15).

Sensation from a given dermatome is carried over its corresponding spinal nerve. This information can be used to identify the spinal nerve or spinal segment that is involved in an injury, as sensation from its corresponding skin surface will be altered. In some areas, the dermatomes are not absolutely distinct. Some dermatomes may share a nerve supply with neighboring regions. For this reason, it is necessary to numb several adjacent dermatomes to achieve successful anesthesia.

CHECKPOINT `9-13` ➤ How many pairs of spinal nerves are there?

Disorders of the Spinal Nerves

Peripheral neuritis (nu-RI-tis), or peripheral neuropathy, is the degeneration of nerves supplying the distal areas of the extremities. It affects both sensory and motor function, causing symptoms of pain and paralysis. Causes include chronic intoxication (alcohol, lead, drugs), infectious diseases (meningitis), metabolic diseases (diabetes, gout), or nutritional diseases (vitamin deficiency, starvation). Identification and treatment of the underlying disorder is most important. Because peripheral neuritis is a symptom rather than a disease, a complete physical examination may be needed to establish its cause.

Sciatica (si-AT-ih-kah) is a form of peripheral neuritis characterized by severe pain along the sciatic nerve and its branches. The most common causes of this disorder are

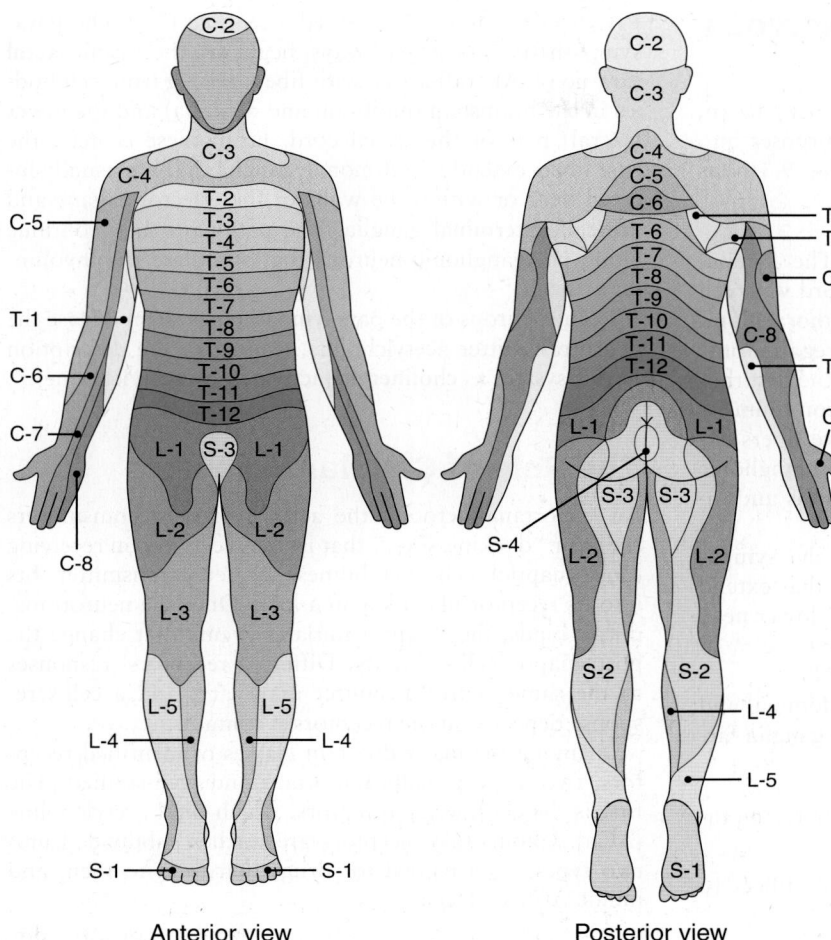

Anterior view   Posterior view

Figure 9-15 **Dermatomes.** A dermatome is a region of the skin supplied by a single spinal nerve. [**ZOOMING IN** ➤ Which spinal nerves carry impulses from the skin of the toes? From the anterior hand and fingers?]

rupture of a disk between the lower lumbar vertebrae and arthritis of the lower spinal column.

Herpes zoster, commonly known as *shingles*, is characterized by numerous blisters along the course of certain nerves, most commonly the intercostal nerves, which are branches of the thoracic spinal nerves in the waist area. Shingles is caused by a reactivation of a prior chickenpox virus infection and involves an attack on the sensory cell bodies inside the spinal ganglia. Initial symptoms include fever and pain, followed in 2 to 4 weeks by the appearance of vesicles (fluid-filled skin lesions). The drainage from these vesicles contains highly contagious liquid. The neuralgic pains may persist for years and can be distressing. This infection may also involve the first branch of the fifth cranial nerve and cause pain in the eyeball and surrounding tissues. Early treatment of a recurrent attack with antiviral drugs may reduce the neuralgia.

Guillain-Barré syndrome (ge-YAN bar-RA) is classified as a polyneuropathy (pol-e-nu-ROP-a-the), that is, a

disorder involving many nerves. There is progressive muscle weakness caused by loss of myelin, with numbness and paralysis, which may involve the breathing muscles. Sometimes the autonomic nervous system is involved, resulting in problems with involuntary functions. The cause of Guillain-Barré syndrome is not known, but it often follows an infection, usually a viral infection. It may result from an abnormal immune response to one's own nerve tissue. Most people recover completely from the disease with time, but recovery may take months or even years.

PASSport to **Success**

Occupational therapists often help to care for people with nervous system disorders. Visit **thePoint** or see the Student Resource CD in the back of this book for more information about this career.

The Autonomic Nervous System (ANS)

The autonomic (visceral) nervous system regulates the action of the glands, the smooth muscles of hollow organs and vessels, and the heart muscle. These actions are carried on automatically; whenever a change occurs that calls for a regulatory adjustment, it is made without conscious awareness.

Most ANS studies concentrate on the motor (efferent) portion of the system. All autonomic pathways contain two motor neurons connecting the spinal cord with the effector organ. The two neurons synapse in ganglia that serve as relay stations along the way. The first neuron, the preganglionic neuron, extends from the spinal cord to the ganglion. The second neuron, the postganglionic neuron, travels from the ganglion to the effector. This differs from the voluntary (somatic) nervous system, in which each motor nerve fiber extends all the way from the spinal cord to the skeletal muscle with no intervening synapse. Some of the autonomic fibers are within the spinal nerves; some are within the cranial nerves (see Chapter 10).

CHECKPOINT 9-14 ➤ How many neurons are there in each motor pathway of the ANS?

9

Divisions of the Autonomic Nervous System

The ANS motor neurons are arranged in a distinct pattern, which has led to their separation for study purposes into **sympathetic** and **parasympathetic** divisions (Fig. 9-16), as described below and summarized in Table 9-3.

SYMPATHETIC NERVOUS SYSTEM The sympathetic motor neurons originate in the spinal cord with cell bodies in the thoracic and lumbar regions, the **thoracolumbar** (tho-rah-ko-LUM-bar) area. These preganglionic fibers arise from the spinal cord at the level of the first thoracic spinal nerve down to the level of the second lumbar spinal nerve. From this part of the cord, nerve fibers extend to ganglia where they synapse with postganglionic neurons, the fibers of which extend to the glands and involuntary muscle tissues.

Many of the sympathetic ganglia form the **sympathetic chains**, two cordlike strands of ganglia that extend along either side of the spinal column from the lower neck to the upper abdominal region. (Note that Figure 9-16 shows only one side for each division of the ANS.)

In addition, the nerves that supply the abdominal and pelvic organs synapse in three single **collateral ganglia** farther from the spinal cord. These are the:

- Celiac ganglion, which sends fibers mainly to the digestive organs

- Superior mesenteric ganglion, which sends fibers to the large and small intestines

- Inferior mesenteric ganglion, which sends fibers to the distal large intestine and organs of the urinary and reproductive systems

The postganglionic neurons of the sympathetic system, with few exceptions, act on their effectors by releasing the neurotransmitter epinephrine (adrenaline) and the related compound norepinephrine (noradrenaline). This system is therefore described as **adrenergic**, which means "activated by adrenaline."

PARASYMPATHETIC NERVOUS SYSTEM The parasympathetic motor pathways begin in the **craniosacral** (kra-ne-o-SAK-ral) areas, with fibers arising from cell bodies in the brainstem (midbrain and medulla) and the lower (sacral) part of the spinal cord. From these centers, the first fibers extend to autonomic ganglia that are usually located near or within the walls of the effector organs and are called **terminal ganglia**. The pathways then continue along postganglionic neurons that stimulate the involuntary tissues.

The neurons of the parasympathetic system release the neurotransmitter acetylcholine, leading to the description of this system as **cholinergic** (activated by acetylcholine).

The Role of Cellular Receptors

An important factor in the actions of neurotransmitters are their "docking sites," that is, the receptors on receiving (postsynaptic) cell membranes. A neurotransmitter fits into its receptor like a key in a lock. Once the neurotransmitter binds, the receptor initiates events that change the postsynaptic cell's activity. Different receptors' responses to the same neurotransmitter may vary, and a cell's response depends on the receptors it contains.

Among the many different classes of identified receptors, two are especially important and well-studied. The first is the cholinergic receptors, which bind acetylcholine (ACh). Cholinergic receptors are further subdivided into two types, each named for drugs that bind to them and mimic ACh's effects:

- Nicotinic receptors (which bind nicotine) are found on skeletal muscle cells and stimulate muscle contraction when ACh is present.

- Muscarinic receptors (which bind muscarine, a poison) are found on effector cells of the parasympathetic nervous system. ACh can either stimulate or inhibit muscarinic receptors depending on the effector organ. For example, ACh stimulates digestive organs but inhibits the heart.

Table 9-3	Divisions of the Autonomic Nervous System	
Characteristics	**Divisions**	
	Sympathetic nervous system	**Parasympathetic nervous system**
Origin of fibers	Thoracic and lumbar regions of the spinal cord; thoracolumbar	Brain stem and sacral regions of the spinal cord; craniosacral
Location of ganglia	Sympathetic chains and three single collateral ganglia (celiac, superior mesenteric, inferior mesenteric)	Terminal ganglia in or near the effector organ
Neurotransmitter (see Table 9–4)	Adrenaline and noradrenaline; adrenergic	Acetylcholine; cholinergic
Effects	Response to stress; fight-or-flight response	Reverses fight-or-flight (stress) response; stimulates some activities

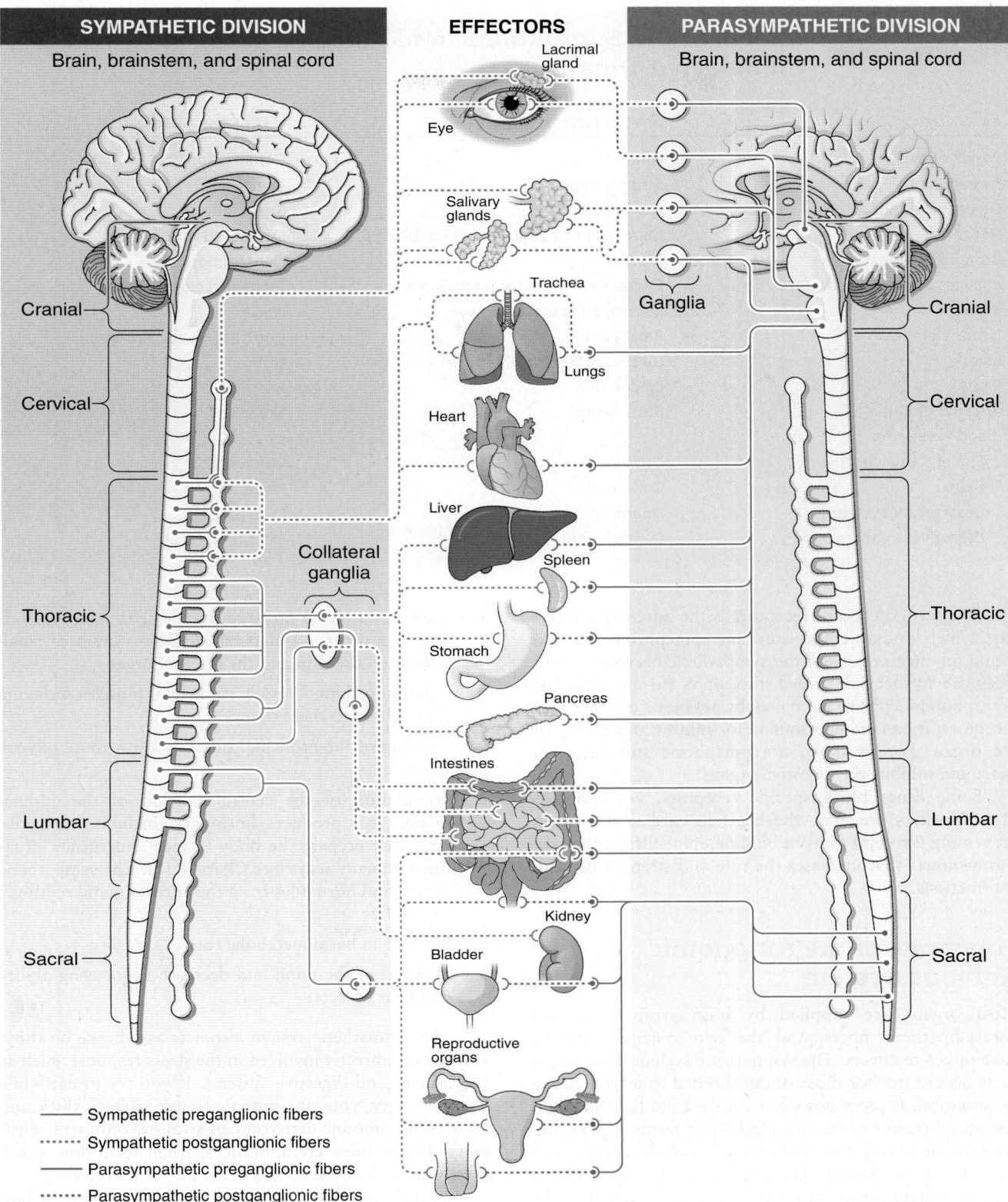

SYMPATHETIC DIVISION

Brain, brainstem, and spinal cord

EFFECTORS

PARASYMPATHETIC DIVISION

Brain, brainstem, and spinal cord

Cranial

Cervical

Thoracic

Lumbar

Sacral

Collateral ganglia

Lacrimal gland

Eye

Salivary glands

Ganglia

Trachea

Lungs

Heart

Liver

Spleen

Stomach

Pancreas

Intestines

Kidney

Bladder

Reproductive organs

Cranial

Cervical

Thoracic

Lumbar

Sacral

— Sympathetic preganglionic fibers
⋯⋯ Sympathetic postganglionic fibers
— Parasympathetic preganglionic fibers
⋯⋯ Parasympathetic postganglionic fibers

Figure 9-16 **Autonomic nervous system.** The diagram shows only one side of the body for each division. [**ZOOMING IN ➤** Which division of the autonomic nervous system has ganglia closer to the effector organ?]

9

Table 9-4	Effects of the Sympathetic and Parasympathetic Systems on Selected Organs	
Effector	**Sympathetic system**	**Parasympathetic system**
Pupils of eye	Dilation	Constriction
Sweat glands	Stimulation	None
Digestive glands	Inhibition	Stimulation
Heart	Increased rate and strength of beat	Decreased rate of beat
Bronchi of lungs	Dilation	Constriction
Muscles of digestive system	Decreased contraction (peristalsis)	Increased contraction
Kidneys	Decreased activity	None
Urinary bladder	Relaxation	Contraction and emptying
Liver	Increased release of glucose	None
Penis	Ejaculation	Erection
Adrenal medulla	Stimulation	None
Blood vessels to:		
Skeletal muscles	Dilation	Constriction
Skin	Constriction	None
Respiratory system	Dilation	Constriction
Digestive organs	Constriction	Dilation

The second class of receptors is the adrenergic receptors, which bind norepinephrine and epinephrine. They are found on effector cells of the sympathetic nervous system. They are further subdivided into alpha (α) and beta (β). When norepinephrine (or epinephrine) binds to adrenergic receptors, it can either stimulate or inhibit, depending on the organ. For example, norepinephrine stimulates the heart and inhibits the digestive organs.

Some drugs block specific receptors. For example, "beta-blockers" regulate the heart in cardiac disease by preventing β receptors from binding epinephrine, the neurotransmitter that increases the rate and strength of heart contractions.

Functions of the Autonomic Nervous System

Most organs are supplied by both sympathetic and parasympathetic fibers, and the two systems generally have opposite effects. The sympathetic system tends to act as an accelerator for those organs needed to meet a stressful situation. It promotes what is called the **fight-or-flight response** because in the most primitive terms, the person must decide to stay and "fight it out" with the enemy or to run away from danger. The times when the sympathetic nervous system comes into play can be summarized by the four Es, that is, times of emergency, excitement, embarrassment, and exercise. If you think of what happens to a person who is in any of these situations, you can easily remember the effects of the sympathetic nervous system:

- Increase in the rate and force of heart contractions

- Increase in blood pressure due partly to the more effective heartbeat and partly to constriction of small arteries in the skin and the internal organs

- Dilation of blood vessels to skeletal muscles, bringing more blood to these tissues

- Dilation of the bronchial tubes to allow more oxygen to enter

- Stimulation of the central portion of the adrenal gland. This produces hormones, including epinephrine, that prepare the body to meet emergency situations in many ways (see Chapter 12). The sympathetic nerves and hormones from the adrenal gland reinforce each other

- Increase in basal metabolic rate

- Dilation of the pupil and decrease in focusing ability (for near objects)

The sympathetic system also acts as a brake on those systems not directly involved in the stress response, such as the urinary and digestive systems. If you try to eat while you are angry, you may note that your saliva is thick and so small in amount that you can swallow only with difficulty. Under these circumstances, when food does reach the stomach, it seems to stay there longer than usual.

The parasympathetic system normally acts as a balance for the sympathetic system once a crisis has passed. It is the "rest and digest" system. It causes constriction of the pupils, slowing of the heart rate, and constriction of the bronchial tubes. However, the parasympathetic nervous system also stimulates certain activities needed for maintenance of homeostasis. Among other actions, it promotes

Disease in Context revisited

➤ Sue Learns About Her MS

"Sue, I can't really answer the question of why you developed multiple sclerosis," Dr. Jensen explained to her patient. "There is evidence that the disease has a genetic component but the environment, and perhaps even a virus, might be involved. We do know that multiple sclerosis affects women more frequently than men, and is more prevalent in areas like the northern United States and Canada. We also know that MS is an autoimmune disease. Normally, immune cells travel through the brain and spinal cord looking for pathogens. In multiple sclerosis, the immune cells make a mistake and cause inflammation in healthy nervous tissue. This inflammatory response damages neuroglial cells called oligodendrocytes. These cells form the myelin sheath that covers and insulates the axons of neurons much like the plastic covering on an electrical wire does. When the oligodendrocytes are damaged, they are unable to make this myelin sheath and the axons can't properly transmit nerve impulses. Right now, it appears that the largest areas of demyelination are in the white matter tracts of your spinal cord."

"Is there a medication I can take to stop the disease?" asked Sue.

"Unfortunately," replied the doctor, "there isn't a cure for MS yet. But, we can slow down the disease's progress using anti-inflammatory drugs and interferons to decrease the inflammation and depress the immune response."

During this case we saw that neurons carrying information to and from the central nervous system require myelin sheaths. Inflammation and subsequent damage of the myelin sheath in diseases like multiple sclerosis have profound effects on sensory and motor function. For more information about the inflammatory response and interferon, see Chapter 17. We'll visit Sue one last time in Chapter 24, Development and Birth, and learn how she copes with her disease while pregnant.

the formation and release of urine and activity of the digestive tract. Saliva, for example, flows more easily and profusely under its effects. These stimulatory actions are summarized by the acronym SLUDD: salivation, lacrimation (tear formation), urination, digestion, defecation.

Most body organs receive both sympathetic and parasympathetic stimulation, the effects of the two systems on a given organ generally being opposite. Table 9-4 shows some of the actions of these two systems.

CHECKPOINT **9-15** ➤ Which division of the ANS stimulates a stress response, and which division reverses the stress response?

Word Anatomy

Medical terms are built from standardized word parts (prefixes, roots, and suffixes). Learning the meanings of these parts can help you remember words and interpret unfamiliar terms.

WORD PART	MEANING	EXAMPLE
Role of the Nervous System		
soma-	body	The *somatic* nervous system controls skeletal muscles that move the body.
aut/o	self	The *autonomic* nervous system is automatically controlled and is involuntary.

WORD PART	MEANING	EXAMPLE
neur/i	nerve, nervous tissue	The *neurilemma* is the outer membrane of the myelin sheath around an axon.
-lemma	sheath	See preceding example.

The Nervous System at Work

de-	remove	*Depolarization* removes the charge on the plasma membrane of a cell.
re-	again, back	*Repolarization* restores the charge on the plasma membrane of a cell.
post-	after	The *postsynaptic* cell is located after the synapse and receives neurotransmitter from the presynaptic cell.

The Spinal Cord

myel/o	spinal cord	*Poliomyelitis* is an infectious disease that involves the spinal cord and other parts of the CNS.
-plegia	paralysis	*Monoplegia* is paralysis of one limb.
para-	beyond	*Paraplegia* is paralysis of both lower limbs.
hemi-	half	*Hemiplegia* is paralysis of one side of the body.
tetra-	four	*Tetraplegia* is paralysis of all four limbs.

Summary

I. ROLE OF THE NERVOUS SYSTEM
  A. Structural divisions—anatomic
    1. Central nervous system (CNS)—brain and spinal cord
    2. Peripheral nervous system (PNS)—spinal and cranial nerves
  B. Functional divisions—physiologic
    1. Somatic nervous system—voluntary; supplies skeletal muscles
    2. Autonomic (visceral) nervous system—involuntary; supplies smooth muscle, cardiac muscle, glands

II. NEURONS AND THEIR FUNCTIONS
  A. Structure of a neuron
    1. Cell body
    2. Cell fibers
      a. Dendrite—carries impulses to cell body
      b. Axon—carries impulses away from cell body
    3. Myelin sheath
      a. Covers and protects some axons
      b. Speeds conduction
      c. Made by Schwann cells in PNS; other cells in CNS
        (1) Neurilemma—outermost layer of Schwann cell; aids axon repair
      d. White matter—myelinated tissue; gray matter—unmyelinated tissue

  B. Types of neurons
    1. Sensory (afferent)—carry impulses toward CNS
    2. Motor (efferent)—carry impulses away from CNS
    3. Interneurons—in CNS
  C. Nerves and tracts—bundles of neuron fibers
    1. Nerve—in peripheral nervous system
      a. Held together by connective tissue
        (1) Endoneurium—around a single fiber
        (2) Perineurium—around each fascicle
        (3) Epineurium—around whole nerve
      b. Types of nerves
        (1) Sensory (afferent) nerve—contains only fibers that carry impulses toward the CNS (from a receptor)
        (2) Motor (efferent) nerve—contains only fibers that carry impulses away from the CNS (to an effector)
        (3) Mixed nerve—contains both sensory and motor fibers
    2. Tract—in central nervous system

III. NEUROGLIA
  A. Nonconducting cells
  B. Protect and support nervous tissue

IV. THE NERVOUS SYSTEM AT WORK
  A. Nerve impulse
    1. Potential—electrical charge on the plasma membrane of neuron

2. Action potential
   a. Depolarization—reversal of charge
   b. Repolarization—return to normal
   c. Involves changes in concentrations of Na$^+$ and K$^+$
3. Nerve impulse—spread of action potential along membrane
4. Myelin sheath speeds conduction

B. Synapse—junction between neurons
   1. Nerve impulse transmitted from presynaptic neuron to postsynaptic neuron
   2. Neurotransmitter—carries impulse across synapse
   3. Receptors—in postsynaptic membrane; pick up neurotransmitters
   4. Neurotransmitter removed by diffusion, destruction by enzyme, return to presynaptic cell (reuptake)
   5. Electrical synapses—in smooth muscle, cardiac muscle, CNS

V. **SPINAL CORD**
   A. Location
      1. In vertebral column
      2. Ends between first and second lumbar vertebrae
   B. Structure of the spinal cord
      1. H-shaped area of gray matter
      2. White matter around gray matter
         a. Ascending tracts—carry impulses toward brain
         b. Descending tracts—carry impulses away from brain
   C. Reflex arc—pathway through the nervous system
      1. Components
         a. Receptor—detects stimulus
         b. Sensory neuron—receptor to CNS
         c. Central neuron—in CNS
         d. Motor neuron—CNS to effector
         e. Effector—muscle or gland that responds
      2. Reflex activities—simple reflex is rapid, automatic response using few neurons
         a. Examples—stretch reflex, eye blink, withdrawal reflex
         b. Spinal reflex—coordinated in spinal cord
   D. Medical procedures involving the spinal cord
      a. Lumbar puncture
      b. Administration of drugs
   E. Diseases and other disorders of the spinal cord
      1. Diseases—multiple sclerosis, amyotrophic lateral sclerosis, poliomyelitis

2. Tumors
3. Injuries

VI. **SPINAL NERVES—31 PAIRS**
   A. Roots
      1. Dorsal (sensory)
      2. Ventral (motor)
   B. Mixed nerves—combine sensory and motor fibers
   C. Branches of the spinal nerves
      1. Plexuses—networks formed by anterior branches
         a. Cervical plexus
         b. Brachial plexus
         c. Lumbosacral plexus
      2. Dermatome—region of the skin supplied by a single spinal nerve
   D. Disorders of the spinal nerves—peripheral neuritis, sciatica, herpes zoster, Guillain-Barré

VII. **AUTONOMIC NERVOUS SYSTEM (VISCERAL NERVOUS SYSTEM)**
   A. Characteristics
      1. Involuntary
      2. Controls glands, smooth muscle, heart (cardiac) muscle
      3. Two motor neurons (preganglionic and postganglionic)
   B. Divisions of the autonomic nervous system
      1. Sympathetic nervous system
         a. Thoracolumbar
         b. Adrenergic—uses adrenaline
         c. Synapses in sympathetic chains and three collateral ganglia (celiac, superior mesenteric, inferior mesenteric)
      2. Parasympathetic system
         a. Craniosacral
         b. Cholinergic—uses acetylcholine
         c. Synapses in terminal ganglia in or near effector organs
   C. Cellular receptors
      1. Affect neurotransmitter's action
      2. Types
         a. Cholinergic—bind ACh
         b. Adrenergic—bind norepinephrine and epinephrine
   D. Functions of the autonomic nervous system
      1. Divisions
         a. Sympathetic—stimulates fight-or-flight (stress) response
         b. Parasympathetic—returns body to normal
      2. Usually have opposite effects on an organ

9

Questions for Study and Review

BUILDING UNDERSTANDING

Fill in the blanks

1. The brain and spinal cord make up the _____ nervous system.

2. Action potentials are conducted away from the neuron cell body by the _____.

3. During an action potential, the flow of Na$^+$ into the cell causes _____.

4. In the spinal cord, sensory information travels in _____ tracts.

5. With few exceptions, the sympathetic nervous system uses the neurotransmitter _____ to act on effector organs.

Matching > Match each numbered item with the most closely related lettered item.

___ **6.** Cells that carry impulses from the CNS

___ **7.** Cells that carry impulses to the CNS

___ **8.** Cells that carry impulses within the CNS

___ **9.** Cells that detect a stimulus

___ **10.** Cells that carry out a response to a stimulus

   a. receptors

   b. effectors

   c. sensory neurons

   d. motor neurons

   e. interneurons

Multiple Choice

___ **11.** Skeletal muscles are voluntarily controlled by the
   a. central nervous system
   b. somatic nervous system
   c. parasympathetic nervous system
   d. sympathetic nervous system

___ **12.** The cells involved in most nervous system tumors are called
   a. motor neurons
   b. sensory neurons
   c. interneurons
   d. neuroglia

___ **13.** The correct order of synaptic transmission is
   a. postsynaptic neuron, synapse, and presynaptic neuron
   b. presynaptic neuron, synapse, and postsynaptic neuron
   c. presynaptic neuron, postsynaptic neuron, and synapse
   d. postsynaptic neuron, presynaptic neuron, and synapse

___ **14.** Afferent nerve fibers enter the part of the spinal cord called the
   a. dorsal horn
   b. ventral horn
   c. gray commissure
   d. central canal

___ **15.** The "fight-or-flight" response is promoted by the
   a. sympathetic nervous system
   b. parasympathetic nervous system
   c. somatic nervous system
   d. reflex arc

UNDERSTANDING CONCEPTS

16. Differentiate between the terms in each of the following pairs:

    a. neurons and neuroglia
    b. vesicle and receptor
    c. gray matter and white matter
    d. nerve and tract

17. Describe an action potential. How does conduction along a myelinated fiber differ from conduction along an unmyelinated fiber?

18. Discuss the structure and function of the spinal cord.

19. Explain the reflex arc using stepping on a tack as an example.

20. Describe the anatomy of a spinal nerve. How many pairs of spinal nerves are there?

21. Define a *plexus*. Name the three main spinal nerve plexuses.

22. Compare and contrast multiple sclerosis and Guillain-Barré syndrome.

23. Differentiate between the functions of the sympathetic and parasympathetic divisions of the autonomic nervous system.

CONCEPTUAL THINKING

24. Clinical depression is associated with abnormal serotonin levels. Medications that block the removal of this neurotransmitter from the synapse can control the disorder. Based on this information, is clinical depression associated with increased or decreased levels of serotonin? Explain your answer.

25. Mr. Hayward visits his dentist for a root canal and is given Novocaine, a local anesthetic, at the beginning of the procedure. Novocaine reduces membrane permeability to Na^+. What effect does this have on action potential?

26. In Sue's case, her symptoms were caused by demyelination in her central nervous system. Would her symptoms be the same or different if her spinal nerves were involved? Explain why.

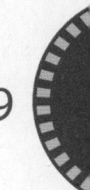

9

CHAPTER 10

The Nervous System: The Brain and Cranial Nerves

Learning Outcomes

After careful study of this chapter, you should be able to:

1. Give the location and functions of the four main divisions of the brain
2. Name and describe the three meninges
3. Cite the function of cerebrospinal fluid and describe where and how this fluid is formed
4. Name and locate the lobes of the cerebral hemispheres
5. Cite one function of the cerebral cortex in each lobe of the cerebrum
6. Name two divisions of the diencephalon and cite the functions of each
7. Locate the three subdivisions of the brain stem and give the functions of each
8. Describe the cerebellum and cite its functions
9. Name some techniques used to study the brain
10. Cite the names and functions of the 12 cranial nerves
11. List some disorders that involve the brain, its associated structures, or the cranial nerves
12. Show how word parts are used to build words related to the nervous system (see Word Anatomy at the end of the chapter)

Selected Key Terms

The following terms and other boldface terms in the chapter are defined in the Glossary

aphasia
brain stem
cerebellum
cerebral cortex
cerebrospinal fluid (CSF)
cerebrum
concussion
diencephalon
electroencephalograph (EEG)
gyrus (pl. gyri)
hematoma
hypothalamus
medulla oblongata
meninges
midbrain
pons
stroke
sulcus (pl. sulci)
thalamus
ventricle

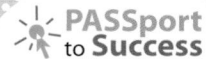

PASSport to Success

Visit *thePoint* or see the Student Resource CD in the back of this book for definitions and pronunciations of key terms as well as a pretest for this chapter.

Disease in Context

> Frank's Case: Blood Clot in the Brain

Ross loved his job as a physiotherapist. He especially enjoyed his current position at the hospital where he was a member of the brain injury team. His responsibility was to design and implement rehabilitation programs for patients recovering from brain injury.

When Ross arrived at work there was a new medical chart waiting for him at his desk. He opened it and scanned its contents. Yesterday evening, Frank Carter, a 68-year-old African American, was transported by ambulance to the emergency room. According to Frank's wife, he had collapsed suddenly in their living room. Worried that he was having a heart attack, she called 911. At the hospital, Frank appeared confused and disoriented. His speech was slurred and he had difficulty forming words. He reported double-vision, dizziness, and a severe headache. He had a history of high blood pressure and, according to his wife, had smoked a pack of cigarettes per day

for most of his adult life. The emergency room physician examined Frank and noted muscle weakness and a diminished sense of touch on the right side of his face and arm. Based upon his neurological findings, the physician ordered an emergency CT scan of Frank's brain. The results of the scan indicated that there was a blood clot blocking Frank's left middle cerebral artery, preventing blood flow to his left cerebral hemisphere. Frank wasn't having a heart attack—he was having a stroke. The emergency physician administered tissue plasminogen activator (tPA) to dissolve the clot and restore blood flow to his brain.

Frank's neurological symptoms are due to a lack of blood flow to a part of his brain called the cerebrum. In this chapter we'll learn about the structure and function of the brain. We'll also revisit Frank and look at Ross' assessment of his stroke symptoms.

The Brain

The brain occupies the cranial cavity and is covered by membranes, fluid, and the skull bones. Although the brain's various regions communicate and function together, the brain may be divided into distinct areas for ease of study (Fig. 10-1, Table 10-1):

- The **cerebrum** (SER-e-brum) is the largest part of the brain. It is divided into right and left **cerebral** (SER-e-bral) **hemispheres** by a deep groove called the **longitudinal fissure** (Fig. 10-2). Each hemisphere is further subdivided into lobes.

- The **diencephalon** (di-en-SEF-ah-lon) is the area between the cerebral hemispheres and the brain stem. It includes the thalamus and the hypothalamus.

- The **brain stem** connects the cerebrum and diencephalon with the spinal cord. The superior portion of the brain stem is the **midbrain.** Inferior to the midbrain is the **pons** (ponz), followed by the **medulla oblongata** (meh-DUL-lah ob-long-GAH-tah). The pons connects the midbrain with the medulla, whereas the medulla connects the brain with the spinal cord through a large opening in the base of the skull (foramen magnum).

- The **cerebellum** (ser-eh-BEL-um) is located immediately below the posterior part of the cerebral hemispheres and is connected with the cerebrum, brain stem, and spinal cord by means of the pons. The word *cerebellum* means "little brain."

Each of these divisions is described in greater detail later in this chapter.

CHECKPOINT **10-1** ➤ What are the main divisions of the brain?

Protective Structures of the Brain and Spinal Cord

The **meninges** (men-IN-jez) are three layers of connective tissue that surround both the brain and spinal cord to form a complete enclosure (Fig. 10-3). The outermost of these membranes, the **dura mater** (DU-rah MA-ter), is the thickest and toughest of the meninges. (*Mater* is from the Latin meaning "mother," referring to the protective function of the meninges; *dura* means "hard.") Around the brain, the dura mater is in two layers, and the outer layer is fused to the cranial bones. In certain places, these two layers separate to provide venous channels, called **dural sinuses,** for the drainage of blood coming from the brain tissue.

The middle layer of the meninges is the **arachnoid** (ah-RAK-noyd). This membrane is loosely attached to the

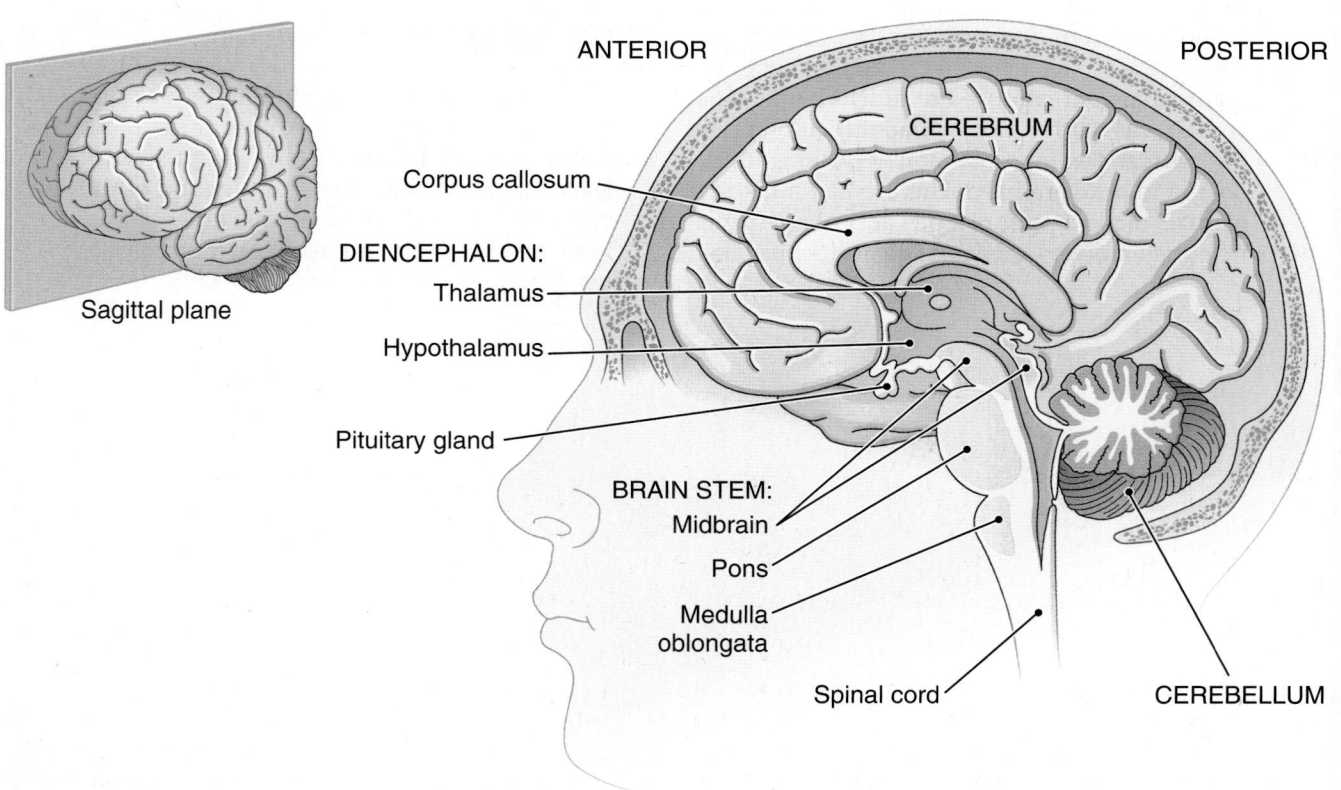

ANTERIOR   POSTERIOR

CEREBRUM

Corpus callosum

DIENCEPHALON:
   Thalamus
   Hypothalamus

Pituitary gland

BRAIN STEM:
   Midbrain
   Pons
   Medulla oblongata

Spinal cord   CEREBELLUM

Sagittal plane

Figure 10-1 **Brain, sagittal section.** Main divisions are shown.

Table 10-1	Organization of the Brain

Division	Description	Functions
Cerebrum	Largest and uppermost portion of the brain. Divided into two hemispheres, each subdivided into lobes	Cortex (outer layer) is site for conscious thought, memory, reasoning, and abstract mental functions, all localized within specific lobes
Diencephalon	Between the cerebrum and the brain stem. Contains the thalamus and hypothalamus	Thalamus sorts and redirects sensory input. Hypothalamus maintains homeostasis, controls autonomic nervous system and pituitary gland
Brain stem	Anterior region below the cerebrum	Connects cerebrum and diencephalon with spinal cord
Midbrain	Below the center of the cerebrum	Has reflex centers concerned with vision and hearing. Connects cerebrum with lower portions of the brain
Pons	Anterior to the cerebellum	Connects cerebellum with other portions of the brain. Helps to regulate respiration
Medulla oblongata	Between the pons and the spinal cord	Links the brain with the spinal cord. Has centers for control of vital functions, such as respiration and the heartbeat
Cerebellum	Below the posterior portion of the cerebrum. Divided into two hemispheres	Coordinates voluntary muscles. Maintains balance and muscle tone

10

deepest of the meninges by weblike fibers, allowing a space for the movement of cerebrospinal fluid (CSF) between the two membranes. (The arachnoid is named from the Latin word for spider because of its weblike appearance).

The innermost layer around the brain, the **pia mater** (PI-ah MA-ter), is attached to the nervous tissue of the brain and spinal cord and follows all the contours of these structures (see Fig. 10-3). It is made of a delicate connec-

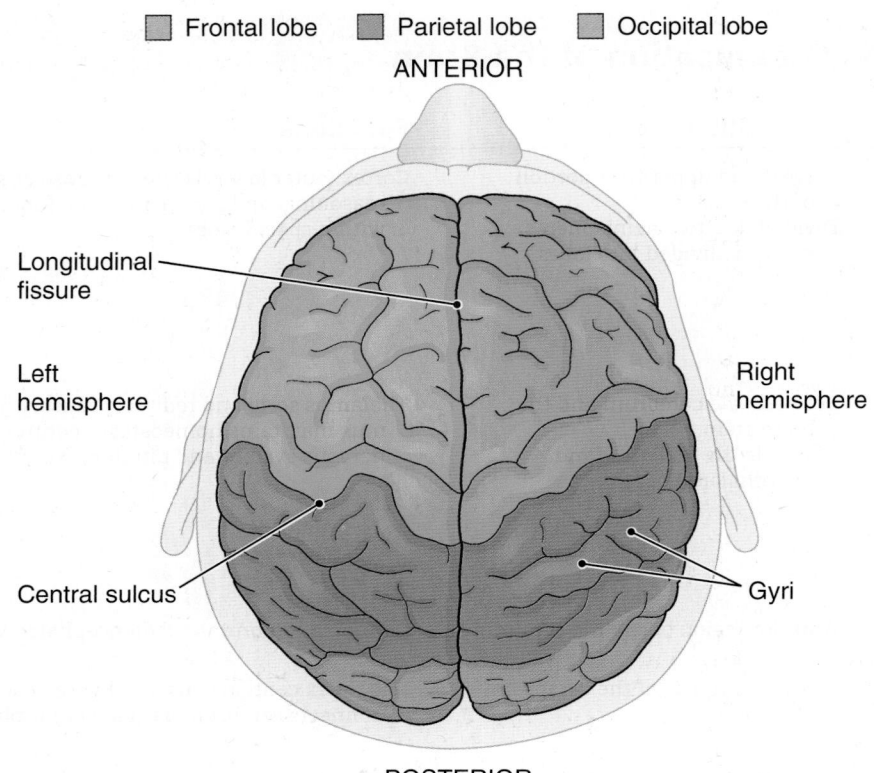

Figure 10-2 **External surface of the brain, superior view.** The division into two hemispheres and into lobes is visible.

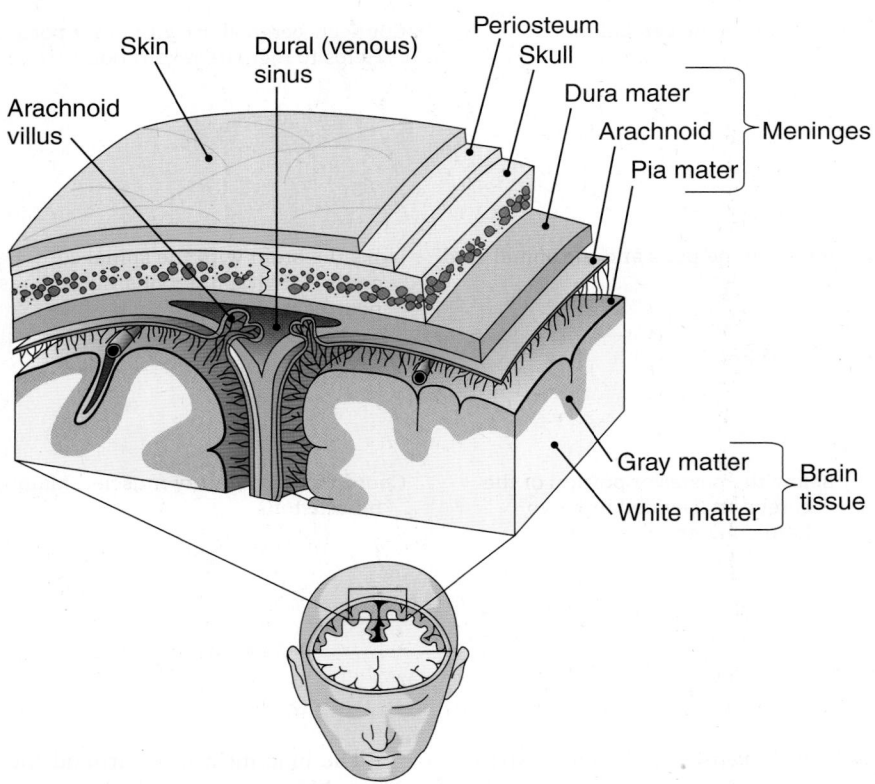

Figure 10-3 **Frontal (coronal) section of the top of the head.** The meninges and related parts are shown. [**ZOOMING IN** ➤ What is located in the spaces where the dura mater divides into two layers?]

tive tissue (*pia* meaning "tender" or "soft"). The pia mater holds blood vessels that supply nutrients and oxygen to the brain and spinal cord.

CHECKPOINT 10-2 ➤ The meninges are protective membranes around the brain and spinal cord. What are the names of the three layers of the meninges from the outermost to the innermost?

Cerebrospinal Fluid

Cerebrospinal (ser-e-bro-SPI-nal) **fluid** is a clear liquid that circulates in and around the brain and spinal cord (Fig. 10-4). The function of the CSF is to support nervous tissue and to cushion shocks that would otherwise injure these delicate structures. This fluid also carries nutrients to the cells and transports waste products from the cells.

CSF flows freely through passageways in and around the brain and spinal cord and finally flows out into the subarachnoid space of the meninges. Much of the fluid then returns to the blood through projections called *arachnoid villi* in the dural sinuses (see Figs. 10-3 and 10-4).

VENTRICLES CSF forms in four spaces within the brain called **ventricles** (VEN-trih-klz) (Fig. 10-5). A vascular network in each ventricle, the **choroid** (KOR-oyd) **plexus**, forms CSF by filtration of the blood and by cellular secretion.

The four ventricles that produce CSF extend somewhat irregularly into the various parts of the brain. The largest are the lateral ventricles in the two cerebral hemispheres. Their extensions into the lobes of the cerebrum are called **horns**. These paired ventricles communicate with a midline space, the third ventricle, by means of openings called **interventricular foramina** (fo-RAM-in-ah). The third ventricle is surrounded by the diencephalon. Continuing down from the third ventricle, a small canal, the **cerebral aqueduct**, extends through the midbrain into the fourth ventricle, which is located between the brain stem and the cerebellum. This ventricle is continuous with the central canal of the spinal cord. In the roof of the fourth ventricle are three openings that allow the escape of CSF to the area that surrounds the brain and spinal cord.

Box 10-1, The Blood–Brain Barrier: Access Denied, presents information on protecting the brain.

CHECKPOINT 10-3 ➤ In addition to the meninges, CSF helps to support and protect the brain and spinal cord. Where is CSF produced?

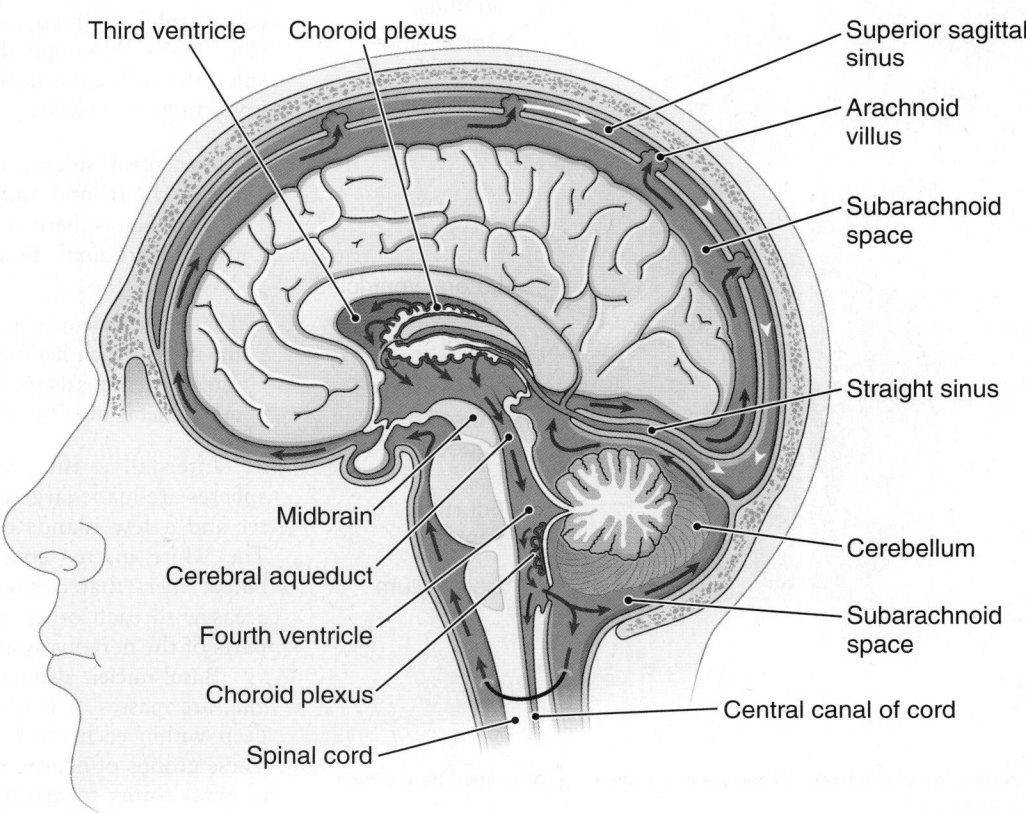

Figure 10-4 **Flow of cerebrospinal fluid (CSF).** Black arrows show the flow of CSF from the choroid plexuses and back to the blood in dural sinuses; white arrows show the flow of blood. (The actual passageways through which the CSF flows are narrower than those shown here, which have been enlarged for visibility.) [**ZOOMING IN** ➤ Which ventricle is continuous with the central canal of the spinal cord?]

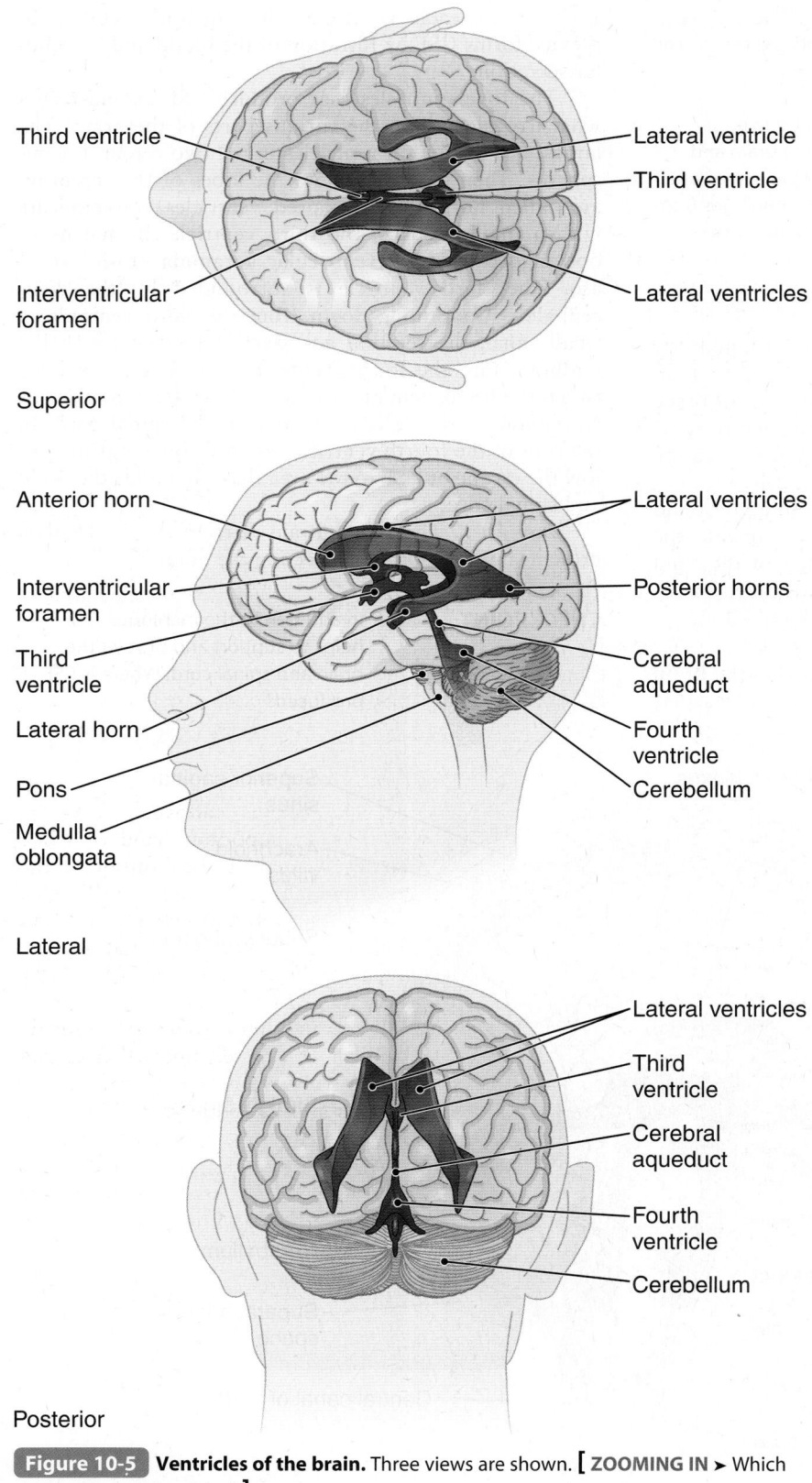

Superior

Lateral

Posterior

Figure 10-5 **Ventricles of the brain.** Three views are shown. [**ZOOMING IN** ➤ Which are the largest ventricles?]

The Cerebral Hemispheres

Each cerebral hemisphere is divided into four visible **lobes** named for the overlying cranial bones. These are the frontal, parietal, temporal, and occipital lobes (Fig. 10-6). In addition, there is a small fifth lobe deep within each hemisphere that cannot be seen from the surface. Not much is known about this lobe, which is called the **insula** (IN-su-lah).

The outer nervous tissue of the cerebral hemispheres is gray matter that makes up the **cerebral cortex** (see Fig. 10-3). This thin layer of gray matter (2–4 mm thick) is the most highly evolved portion of the brain and is responsible for conscious thought, reasoning, and abstract mental functions. Specific functions are localized in the cortex of the different lobes, as described in greater detail later.

The cortex is arranged in folds forming elevated portions known as **gyri** (JI-ri), singular *gyrus*. These raised areas are separated by shallow grooves called **sulci** (SUL-si), singular *sulcus* (Fig. 10-7). Although there are many sulci, the following two are especially important landmarks:

- The **central sulcus**, which lies between the frontal and parietal lobes of each hemisphere at right angles to the longitudinal fissure (see Figs. 10-2 and 10-6)

- The **lateral sulcus**, which curves along the side of each hemisphere and separates the temporal lobe from the frontal and parietal lobes (see Fig. 10-6)

Internally, the cerebral hemispheres are made largely of white matter and a few islands of gray matter. The white matter consists of myelinated fibers that connect the cortical areas with each other and with other parts of the nervous system.

Basal nuclei, also called **basal ganglia**, are masses of gray matter located deep within each cerebral hemisphere. These groups of neurons work with the cerebral cortex to regulate body movement and the muscles of facial expression. The neurons of the basal nuclei secrete the neurotransmitter **dopamine** (DO-pah-mene).

Box 10-1 A Closer Look

The Blood–Brain Barrier: Access Denied

Neurons in the central nervous system (CNS) function properly only if the composition of the extracellular fluid bathing them is carefully regulated. The semipermeable blood–brain barrier helps maintain this stable environment by allowing some substances to cross it while blocking others. Whereas it allows glucose, amino acids, and some electrolytes to cross, it prevents passage of hormones, drugs, neurotransmitters, and other substances that might adversely affect the brain.

Structural features of CNS capillaries create this barrier. In most parts of the body, capillaries are lined with simple squamous epithelial cells that are loosely attached to each other. The small spaces between cells let materials move between the bloodstream and the tissues. In CNS capillaries, the simple squamous epithelial cells are joined by tight junctions that limit passage of materials between them. Astrocytes—specialized neuroglial cells that wrap around capillaries and limit their permeability—also contribute to this barrier.

The blood–brain barrier excludes pathogens, although some viruses, including poliovirus and herpesvirus, can bypass it by traveling along peripheral nerves into the CNS. Some streptococci also can breach the tight junctions. Disease processes, such as hypertension, ischemia (lack of blood supply), and inflammation, can increase the blood-brain barrier's permeability.

The blood–brain barrier is an obstacle to delivering drugs to the brain. Some antibiotics can cross it, whereas others cannot. Neurotransmitters also pose problems. In Parkinson disease, the neurotransmitter dopamine is deficient in the brain. Dopamine itself will not cross the barrier, but a related compound, L-dopa, will. L-dopa crosses the blood-brain barrier and is then converted to dopamine. Mixing a drug with a concentrated sugar solution and injecting it into the bloodstream is another effective delivery method. The solution's high osmotic pressure causes water to osmose out of capillary cells, shrinking them and opening tight junctions through which the drug can pass.

□ Frontal lobe □ Parietal lobe □ Temporal lobe □ Occipital lobe

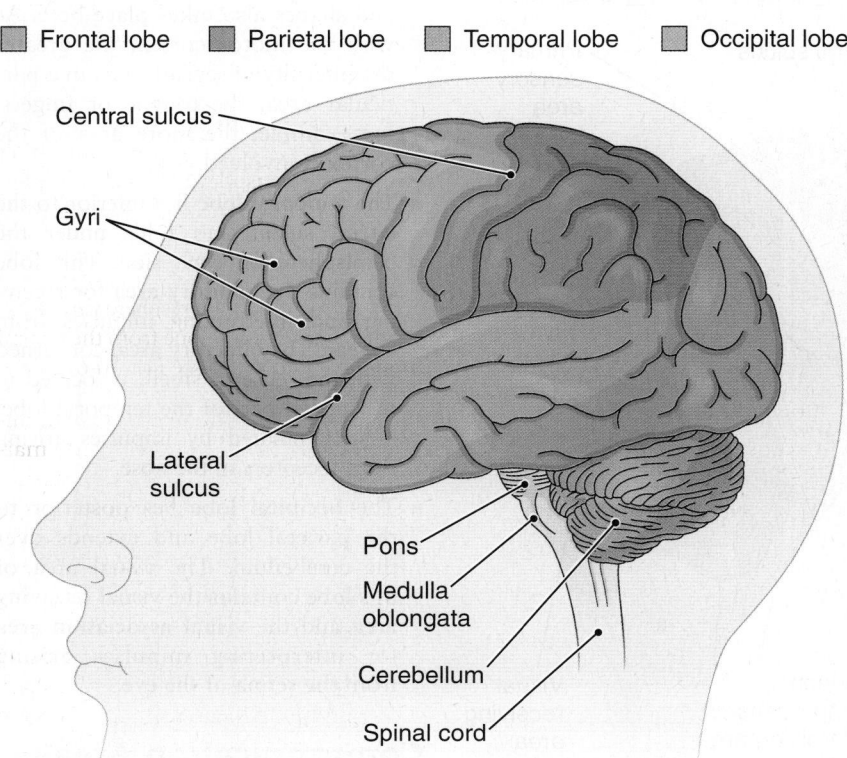

Figure 10-6 **External surface of the brain, lateral view.** The lobes and surface features of the cerebrum are visible. [**ZOOMING IN** ➤ What structure separates the frontal from the parietal lobe?]

The **corpus callosum** (kah-LO-sum) is an important band of white matter located at the bottom of the longitudinal fissure (see Fig. 10-1). This band is a bridge between the right and left hemispheres, permitting impulses to cross from one side of the brain to the other.

The **internal capsule** is a compact band of myelinated fibers that carries impulses between the cerebral hemispheres and the brain stem. The vertical fibers that make up the internal capsule travel between the thalamus and some of the basal nuclei on each side and then radiate toward the cerebral cortex.

CHECKPOINT 10-4 ➤ What are the four surface lobes of each cerebral hemisphere?

Functions of the Cerebral Cortex

It is within the cerebral cortex, the layer of gray matter that forms the surface of

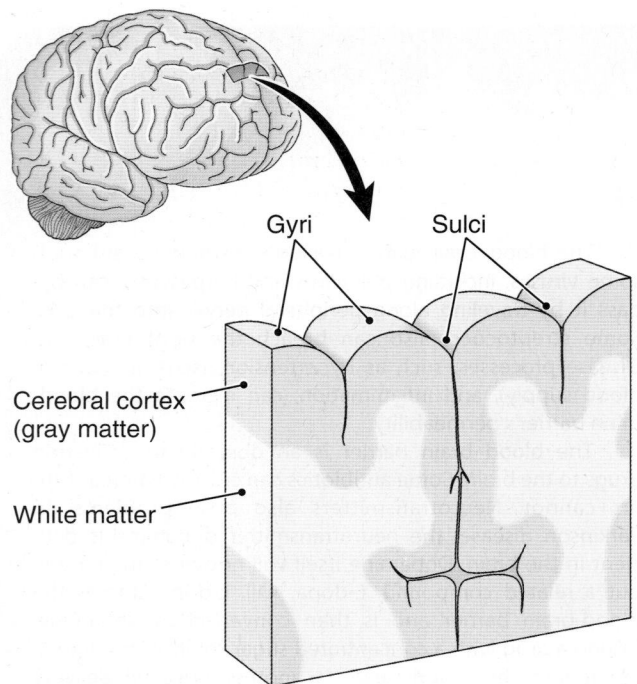

Gyri   Sulci

Cerebral cortex (gray matter)

White matter

Figure 10-7 **Section of the cerebrum.** Labels point out surface features, the cerebral cortex, and the white matter. **[ZOOMING IN ➤** How is the cortex provided with increased surface area? **]**

■ Frontal lobe   ■ Parietal lobe   ■ Temporal lobe   ■ Occipital lobe

Primary motor area

Central sulcus

Primary sensory area

Written speech area

Motor speech (Broca) area

Auditory receiving area

Auditory association area

Speech comprehension (Wernicke) area

Visual receiving area

Figure 10-8 **Functional areas of the cerebral cortex. [ZOOMING IN ➤** What cortical area is posterior to the central sulcus? What area is anterior to the central sulcus? **]**

each cerebral hemisphere, that nerve impulses are received and analyzed. These activities form the basis of knowledge. The brain "stores" information, much of which can be recalled on demand by means of the phenomenon called *memory*. It is in the cerebral cortex that thought processes such as association, judgment, and discrimination take place. Conscious deliberation and voluntary actions also arise from the cerebral cortex.

Although the various brain areas act in coordination to produce behavior, particular functions are localized in the cortex of each lobe (Fig. 10-8). Some of these are described below:

■ The **frontal lobe,** which is relatively larger in humans than in any other organism, lies anterior to the central sulcus. The gyrus just anterior to the central sulcus in this lobe contains a **primary motor area,** which provides conscious control of skeletal muscles. Note that the more detailed the action, the greater the amount of cortical tissue involved (Fig. 10-9). The frontal lobe also contains two areas important in speech (the speech centers are discussed later).

■ The **parietal lobe** occupies the superior part of each hemisphere and lies posterior to the central sulcus. The gyrus just behind the central sulcus in this lobe contains the **primary sensory area,** where impulses from the skin, such as touch, pain, and temperature, are interpreted. The estimation of distances, sizes, and shapes also takes place here. As with the motor cortex, the greater the intensity of sensation from a particular area, the tongue or fingers, for example, the more area of the cortex is involved.

■ The **temporal lobe** lies inferior to the lateral sulcus and folds under the hemisphere on each side. This lobe contains the **auditory area** for receiving and interpreting impulses from the ear. The **olfactory area,** concerned with the sense of smell, is located in the medial part of the temporal lobe; it is stimulated by impulses arising from receptors in the nose.

■ The **occipital lobe** lies posterior to the parietal lobe and extends over the cerebellum. The visual area of this lobe contains the **visual receiving area** and the **visual association area** for interpreting impulses arising from the retina of the eye.

Communication Areas

The ability to communicate by written and verbal means is an interesting example of how areas of the cerebral cor-

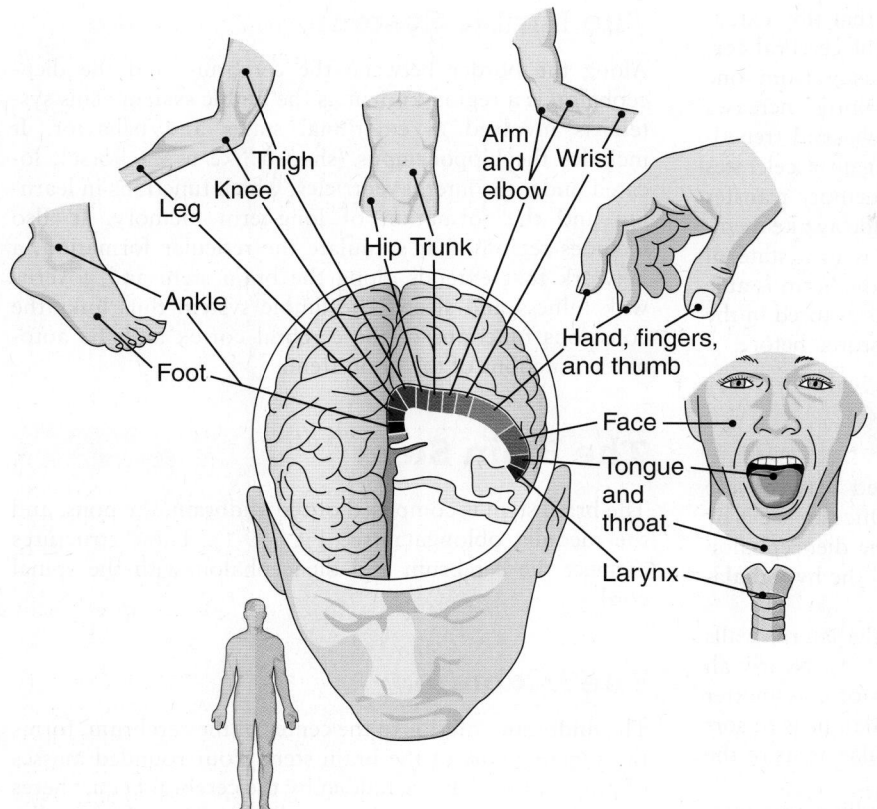

Figure 10-9 **Motor areas of the cerebral cortex (frontal lobe).** The amount of cortex involved in control of a body part is proportional to the degree of coordination needed in movement. The small figure indicates that control is contralateral. The right hemisphere controls the left side of the body and the left hemisphere controls the right side of the body.

tongue, the soft palate, and the larynx are controlled here, in a region named the **motor speech area**, or **Broca** (bro-KAH) **area** (see Fig. 10-8). A person who suffers damage to this area may have difficulty in producing speech (motor aphasia). Similarly, the written speech center lies anterior to the cortical area that controls the arm and hand muscles. The ability to write words is usually one of the last phases in the development of learning words and their meanings.

■ The **visual areas** of the occipital cortex are also involved in communication. Here, visual images of language are received. The visual area that lies anterior to the receiving cortex then interprets these visual impulses as words. The ability to read with understanding also develops in this area. You might *see* writing in the Japanese language, for example, but this would involve only the visual receiving area in the occipital lobe unless you could also *understand* the words.

There is a functional relation among areas of the brain. Many neurons must work together to enable a person to receive, interpret, and respond to verbal and written messages as well as to touch (tactile stimulus) and other sensory stimuli.

tex are interrelated (see Fig. 10-8). The development and use of these areas are closely connected with the learning process.

■ The **auditory areas** lie in the temporal lobe. One of these areas, the **auditory receiving area**, detects sound impulses transmitted from the environment, whereas the surrounding area, the **auditory association area**, interprets the sounds. Another region of the auditory cortex, the **speech comprehension area**, or **Wernicke** (VER-nih-ke) **area**, functions in speech recognition and the meaning of words. Someone who suffers damage in this region of the brain, as by a stroke, will have difficulty in understanding the meaning of speech. The beginnings of language are learned by hearing; thus, the auditory areas for understanding sounds are near the auditory receiving area of the cortex. Babies often appear to understand what is being said long before they do any talking themselves. It is usually several years before children learn to read or write words.

■ The **motor areas** for spoken and written communication lie anterior to the most inferior part of the frontal lobe's motor cortex. The speech muscles in the

CHECKPOINT **10-5** ➤ Higher functions of the brain occur in a thin layer of gray matter on the surface of the cerebral hemispheres. What is the name of this outer layer of gray matter?

Memory and the Learning Process

Memory is the mental faculty for recalling ideas. In the initial stage of the memory process, sensory signals (e.g., visual, auditory) are retained for a very short time, perhaps only fractions of a second. Nevertheless, they can be used for further processing. **Short-term memory** refers to the retention of bits of information for a few seconds or perhaps a few minutes, after which the information is lost unless reinforced. **Long-term memory** refers to the storage of information that can be recalled at a later time. There is a tendency for a memory to become more fixed the more often a person repeats the remembered experience; thus, short-term memory signals can lead to long-term memories. Furthermore, the more often a memory is recalled, the more indelible it becomes; such a memory can be so deeply fixed in the brain that it can be recalled immediately.

Careful anatomic studies have shown that tiny extensions called *fibrils* form at the synapses in the cerebral cortex, enabling impulses to travel more easily from one neuron to another. The number of these fibrils increases with age. Physiologic studies show that rehearsal (repetition) of the same information again and again accelerates and potentiates the degree of short-term memory transfer into long-term memory. A person who is wide awake memorizes far better than does a person who is in a state of mental fatigue. It has also been noted that the brain is able to organize information so that new ideas are stored in the same areas in which similar ones had been stored before.

The Diencephalon

The **diencephalon**, or interbrain, is located between the cerebral hemispheres and the brain stem. One can see it by cutting into the brain's central section. The diencephalon includes the **thalamus** (THAL-ah-mus) and the **hypothalamus** (Fig. 10-10).

The two parts of the thalamus form the lateral walls of the third ventricle (see Figs. 10-1 and 10-5). Nearly all sensory impulses travel through the masses of gray matter that form the thalamus. The role of the thalamus is to sort out the impulses and direct them to particular areas of the cerebral cortex.

The hypothalamus is located in the midline area inferior to the thalamus and forms the floor of the third ventricle. It helps to maintain homeostasis by controlling body temperature, water balance, sleep, appetite, and some emotions, such as fear and pleasure. Both the sympathetic and parasympathetic divisions of the autonomic nervous system are under hypothalamic control, as is the pituitary gland. The hypothalamus thus influences the heartbeat, the contraction and relaxation of blood vessels, hormone secretion, and other vital body functions.

CHECKPOINT **10-6** ➤ What are the two main portions of the diencephalon and what do they do?

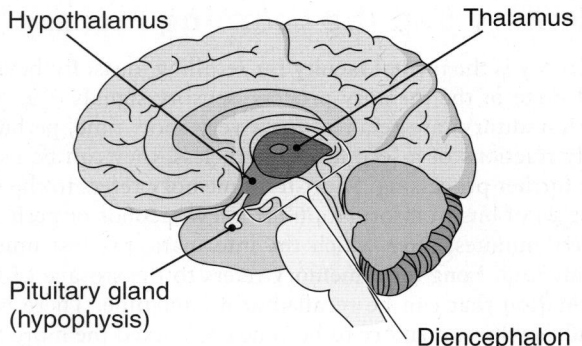

Hypothalamus

Thalamus

Pituitary gland (hypophysis)

Diencephalon

Figure 10-10 **Regions of the diencephalon.** The figure shows the relationship among the thalamus, hypothalamus, and pituitary gland (hypophysis). [**ZOOMING IN** ➤ To what part of the brain is the pituitary gland attached?]

The Limbic System

Along the border between the cerebrum and the diencephalon is a region known as the **limbic system**. This system is involved in emotional states and behavior. It includes the **hippocampus** (shaped like a sea horse), located under the lateral ventricles, which functions in learning and the formation of long-term memory. It also includes regions that stimulate the **reticular formation**, a network that extends along the brain stem and governs wakefulness and sleep. The limbic system thus links the conscious functions of the cerebral cortex and the automatic functions of the brain stem.

The Brain Stem

The brain stem is composed of the midbrain, the pons, and the medulla oblongata (see Fig. 10-1). These structures connect the cerebrum and diencephalon with the spinal cord.

The Midbrain

The **midbrain**, inferior to the center of the cerebrum, forms the superior part of the brain stem. Four rounded masses of gray matter that are hidden by the cerebral hemispheres form the superior part of the midbrain. These four bodies act as centers for certain reflexes involving the eye and the ear, for example, moving the eyes in order to track an image or to read. The white matter at the anterior of the midbrain conducts impulses between the higher centers of the cerebrum and the lower centers of the pons, medulla, cerebellum, and spinal cord. Cranial nerves III and IV originate from the midbrain.

The Pons

The **pons** lies between the midbrain and the medulla, anterior to the cerebellum (see Fig. 10-1). It is composed largely of myelinated nerve fibers, which connect the two halves of the cerebellum with the brain stem as well as with the cerebrum above and the spinal cord below. (Its name means "bridge.")

The pons is an important connecting link between the cerebellum and the rest of the nervous system, and it contains nerve fibers that carry impulses to and from the centers located above and below it. Certain reflex (involuntary) actions, such as some of those regulating respiration, are integrated in the pons. Cranial nerves V through VIII originate from the pons.

The Medulla Oblongata

The **medulla oblongata** of the brain stem is located between the pons and the spinal cord (see Fig. 10-1). It appears white externally because, like the pons, it contains many myelinated nerve fibers. Internally, it contains collections of cell bodies (gray matter) called **nuclei,** or *centers.* Among these are vital centers, such as the following:

- The **respiratory center** controls the muscles of respiration in response to chemical and other stimuli.

- The **cardiac center** helps regulate the rate and force of the heartbeat.

- The **vasomotor** (vas-o-MO-tor) **center** regulates the contraction of smooth muscle in the blood vessel walls and thus controls blood flow and blood pressure.

The ascending sensory fibers that carry messages through the spinal cord up to the brain travel through the medulla, as do descending motor fibers. These groups of fibers form tracts (bundles) and are grouped together according to function.

The motor fibers from the motor cortex of the cerebral hemispheres extend down through the medulla, and most of them cross from one side to the other (decussate) while going through this part of the brain. The crossing of motor fibers in the medulla results in contralateral control—the right cerebral hemisphere controls muscles in the left side of the body and the left cerebral hemisphere controls muscles in the right side of the body, a characteristic termed *contralateral* (opposite side) *control.*

The medulla is an important reflex center; here, certain neurons end, and impulses are relayed to other neurons. The last four pairs of cranial nerves (IX through XII) are connected with the medulla.

CHECKPOINT **10-7** ➤ What are the three subdivisions of the brain stem?

The Cerebellum

The **cerebellum** is made up of three parts: the middle portion (vermis) and two lateral hemispheres, the left and right (Fig. 10-11). Like the cerebral hemispheres, the cerebellum has an outer area of gray matter and an inner portion that is largely white matter. However, the white matter is distributed in a treelike pattern. The functions of the cerebellum are as follows:

- Help coordinate voluntary muscles to ensure smooth, orderly function. Disease of the cerebellum causes muscular jerkiness and tremors.

- Help maintain balance in standing, walking, and sitting as well as during more strenuous activities. Messages from the internal ear and from sensory receptors in tendons and muscles aid the cerebellum.

- Help maintain muscle tone so that all muscle fibers are slightly tensed and ready to produce changes in position as quickly as necessary.

CHECKPOINT **10-8** ➤ What are some functions of the cerebellum?

Brain Studies

Some of the imaging techniques used to study the brain are described in Box 1-2, Medical Imaging: Seeing Without Making a Cut, in Chapter 1. These techniques include:

- CT (computed tomography) scan, which provides photographs of the bone, soft tissue, and cavities of the brain (Fig. 10-12A). Anatomic lesions, such as tumors or scar tissue accumulations, are readily seen.

- MRI (magnetic resonance imaging), which gives more views of the brain than CT and may reveal tumors, scar tissue, and hemorrhaging not shown by CT (see Fig. 10-12B).

- PET (positron emission tomography), which visualizes the brain in action (see Fig. 10-12C).

The Electroencephalograph

The interactions of the brain's billions of nerve cells give rise to measurable electric currents. These may be recorded using an instrument called the **electroencephalograph** (e-lek-tro-en-SEF-ah-lo-graf). Electrodes placed on the head pick up the electrical signals produced as the brain functions. These signals are then amplified and recorded to produce the tracings, or brain waves, of an electroencephalogram (EEG).

The electroencephalograph is used to study sleep patterns, to diagnose disease, such as epilepsy, to locate tumors, to study the effects of drugs, and to determine brain death. Figure 10-13 shows some typical normal and abnormal tracings.

Disorders of the Brain and Associated Structures

Infection and other factors can cause inflammation of the brain and its protective structures. **Meningitis** (men-in-JI-tis) is an inflammation of the meninges, the coverings of the brain and spinal cord. It is usually caused by bacteria that enter through the ear, nose, or throat, or are carried by the blood. In many cases, an injury, invasive procedure, septicemia (blood infection), or an adjoining infection allows the entry of pathogenic organisms. One of these organisms, the meningococcus (*Neisseria meningitidis*) is responsible for epidemics of meningitis among people living in close quarters. Other causative bacteria are *Haemophilus influenzae* (Hib), *Streptococcus pneumoniae,* and *Escherichia coli.* Some viruses, including the mumps virus, can cause meningitis, but usually produce mild forms of the disease that require no treatment.

Headache, stiff neck, nausea, and vomiting are common symptoms of meningitis. Diagnosis is by lumbar puncture and examination of the CSF for pathogens and white blood cells (pus). In cases of bacterial meningitis, early treatment with antibiotics can have good results.

10

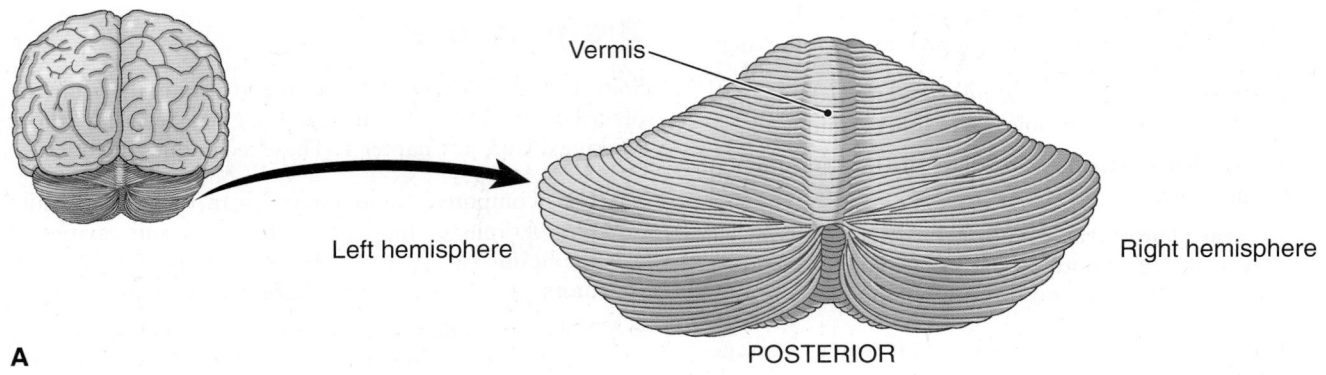

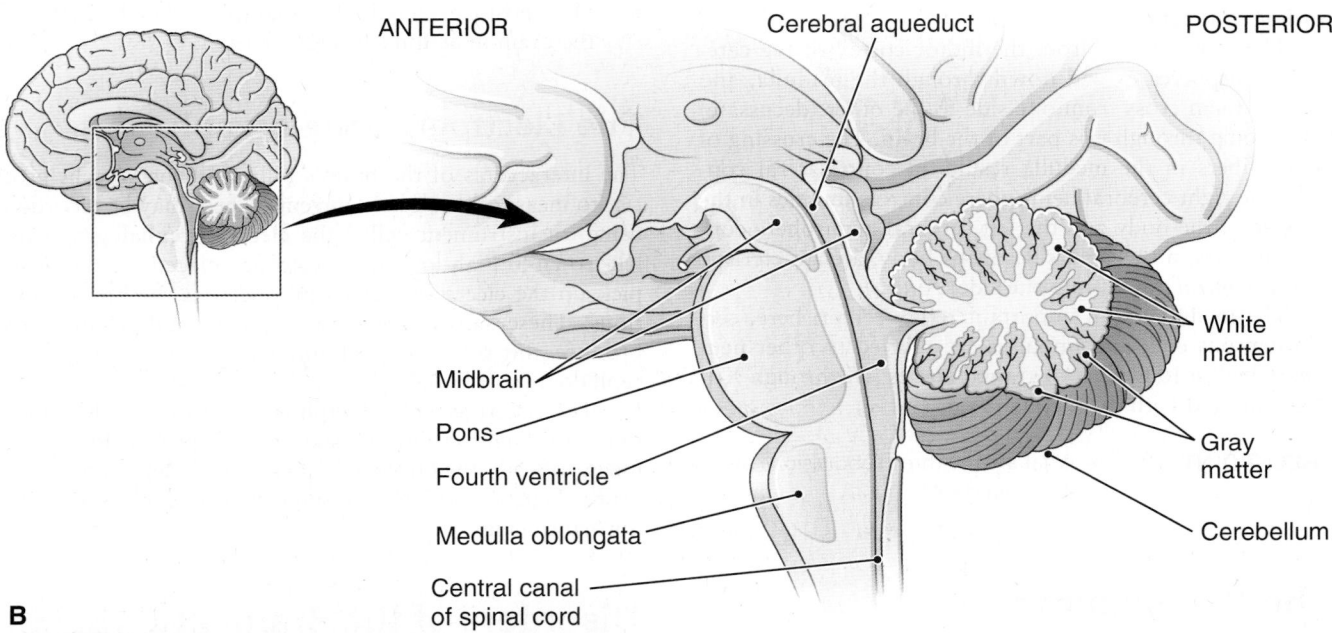

Figure 10-11 **The cerebellum. (A)** Posterior view showing the two hemispheres. **(B)** Midsagittal section showing the distribution of gray and white matter. The three parts of the brain stem (midbrain, pons, and medulla oblongata) are also labeled.

Untreated cases have a high death rate. Vaccines are available against some of the bacteria that cause meningitis.

Inflammation of the brain is termed **encephalitis** (en-sef-ah-LI-tis), based on the scientific name for the brain, which is *encephalon*. Infectious agents that cause encephalitis include poliovirus, rabies virus, HIV (the cause of AIDS), insect-borne viruses, such as West Nile virus, and, rarely, the viruses that cause chickenpox and measles. Less frequently, exposure to toxic substances or reactions to certain viral vaccines can cause encephalitis. Brain swelling and diffuse nerve cell destruction accompany invasion of the brain by lymphocytes (white blood cells) in cases of encephalitis. Typical symptoms include fever, vomiting, and coma.

Hydrocephalus

An abnormal accumulation of CSF within the brain is termed **hydrocephalus** (hi-dro-SEF-ah-lus) (Fig. 10-14). It may result either from overproduction or impaired drainage of the fluid. As CSF accumulates in the ventricles or its transport channels, mounting pressure can squeeze the brain against the skull and destroy brain tissue. Possible causes include congenital malformations present during development, tumors, inflammation, or hemorrhage.

Hydrocephalus is more common in infants than in adults. Because the skull's fontanels have not closed in the developing infant, the cranium itself can become greatly enlarged. In contrast, in the adult, cranial enlargement cannot occur, so that even a slight increase in fluid results in symp-

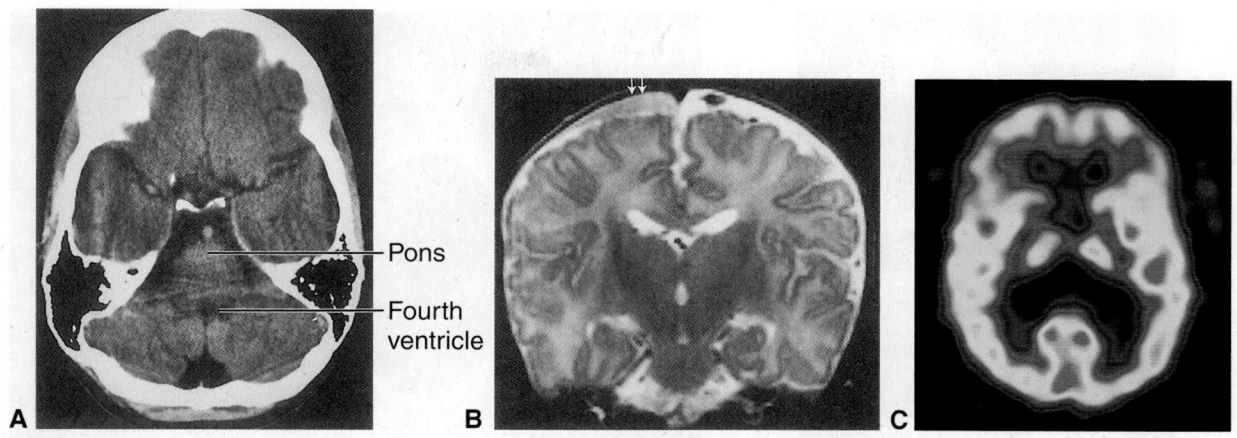

Figure 10-12 **Imaging the brain. (A)** CT scan of a normal adult brain at the level of the fourth ventricle. **(B)** MRI of the brain showing a point of injury (arrows). **(C)** PET scan. (A and B, reprinted with permission from Erkonen WE. *Radiology 101*. Philadelphia: Lippincott Williams & Wilkins, 1998; C, Courtesy of Newport Diagnostic Center, Newport Beach, CA.)

toms of increased pressure within the skull and brain damage. Treatment of hydrocephalus involves the creation of a shunt (bypass) to drain excess CSF from the brain.

Stroke and Other Brain Disorders

Stroke, or **cerebrovascular** (ser-e-bro-VAS-ku-lar) **accident** (CVA), is by far the most common kind of brain disorder. The most common cause is a blood clot that blocks blood flow to an area of brain tissue. Another frequent cause is the rupture of a blood vessel resulting in **cerebral hemorrhage** (HEM-eh-rij) and destruction of

brain tissue. Stroke is most common among people older than 40 years of age and those with arterial wall damage, diabetes, or hypertension (high blood pressure). Smoking and excess alcohol consumption also increase the risk of stroke. Restoring blood flow to the affected area can reduce long-term damage. This can be done surgically or by administration of clot-dissolving medication, usually followed by medication to reduce brain swelling and minimize further damage.

A stroke's effect depends on the location of the artery and the extent of the involvement. Damage to the internal capsule's white matter in the inferior part of the cerebrum

10

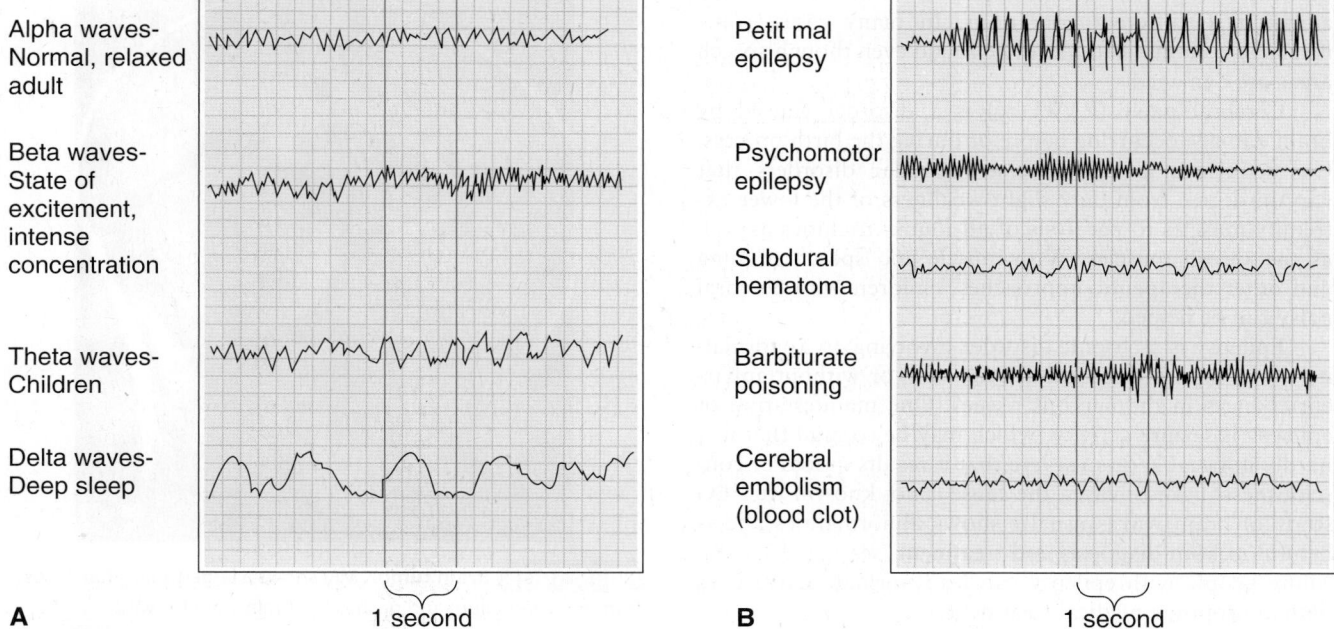

Figure 10-13 **Electroencephalography. (A)** Normal brain waves. **(B)** Abnormal brain waves.

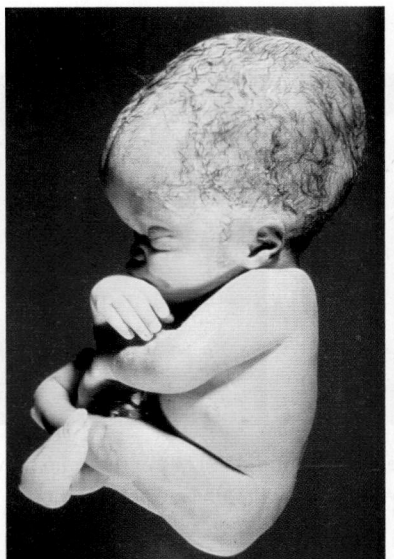

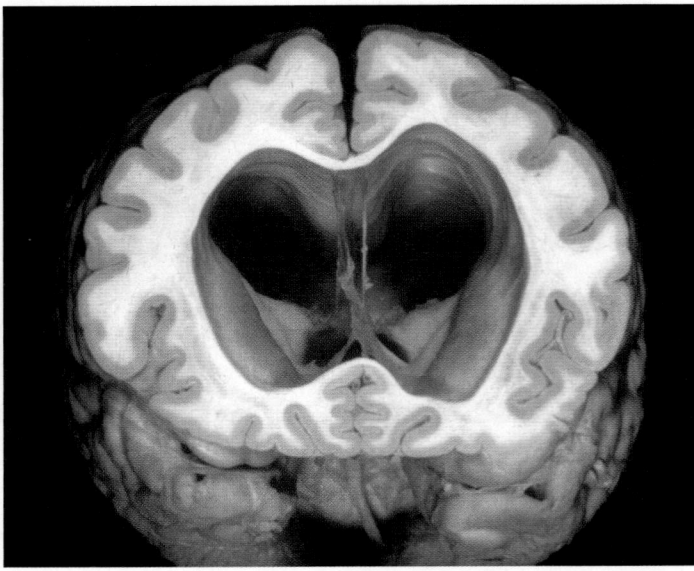

A **B**

Figure 10-14 **Hydrocephalus. (A)** Congenital hydrocephalus causing pronounced enlargement of the head. **(B)** Coronal section of the brain showing marked enlargement of the lateral ventricles caused by a tumor that obstructed the flow of CSF. (Reprinted with permission from Rubin E, Farber JL. *Pathology*, 3rd ed. Philadelphia: Lippincott Williams & Wilkins, 1999.)

may cause extensive paralysis of the side opposite the affected area.

One possible aftereffect of stroke or other brain injury is **aphasia** (ah-FA-ze-ah), a loss or defect in language communication. Losses may involve the ability to speak or write (expressive aphasia) or to understand written or spoken language (receptive aphasia). The type of aphasia present depends on what part of the brain is affected. The lesion that causes aphasia in the right-handed person is likely to be in the left cerebral hemisphere.

Often, much can be done for stroke victims by care and retraining. The brain has tremendous reserves for adapting to different conditions. In many cases, some means of communication can be found even though speech areas are damaged.

Cerebral palsy (PAWL-ze) is a disorder caused by brain damage occurring before or during the birth process. Characteristics include diverse muscular disorders that vary in degree from only slight weakness of the lower extremity muscles to paralysis of all four extremities as well as the speech muscles. With muscle and speech training and other therapeutic approaches, children with cerebral palsy can be helped.

Epilepsy is a chronic disorder involving an abnormality of the brain's electrical activity with or without apparent changes in the nervous tissues. One manifestation of epilepsy is seizure activity, which may be so mild that it is hardly noticeable or so severe that it results in loss of consciousness. In most cases, the cause is not known. An EEG study of brain waves usually shows abnormalities and is helpful in both diagnosis and treatment (see Fig. 10-13B). Many people with epilepsy can lead normal, active lives with appropriate medical treatment.

Tumors of the brain may develop in people of any age but are somewhat more common in young and middle-aged

adults than in other groups (Fig. 10-15). Most brain tumors originate from the neuroglia (support tissue of the brain) and are called **gliomas** (gli-O-mas). Such tumors tend not to metastasize (spread to other areas), but they nevertheless can do harm by compressing brain tissue. The symptoms produced depend on the type of tumor, its location, and its degree of destructiveness. Involvement of the cerebrum's frontal portion often causes mental symptoms, such as changes in personality and in levels of consciousness.

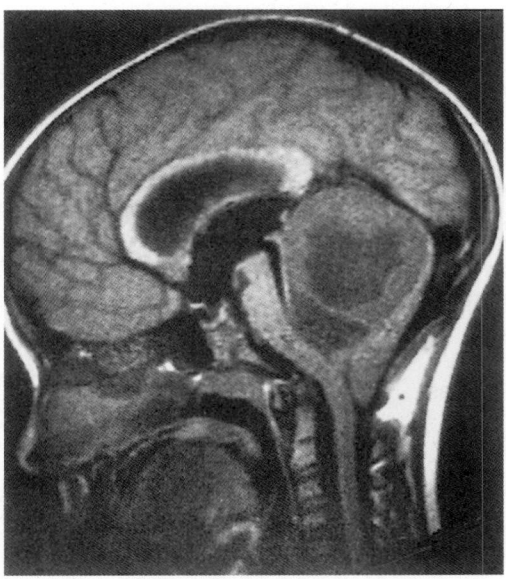

Figure 10-15 **Brain tumor.** MRI shows a large tumor that arises from the cerebellum and pushes the brain stem forward. (Reprinted with permission from Erkonen WE. *Radiology 101*. Philadelphia: Lippincott Williams & Wilkins, 1998.)

Early surgery and radiation therapy offer hope of cure in some cases. The blood-brain barrier, however, limits the effectiveness of injected chemotherapeutic agents (see Box 10-1). A newer approach to chemotherapy for brain tumors is to implant timed-release drugs into a tumor site at the time of surgery.

CHECKPOINT 10-9 ➤ What is the common term for cerebrovascular accident (CVA)?

CHECKPOINT 10-10 ➤ What type of cells are commonly involved in brain tumors?

 **PASSport to Success**
Visit **thePoint** or see the Student Resource CD in the back of this book to view the animation *Stroke*, which illustrates this disorder.

Injury

A common result of head trauma is bleeding into or around the meninges (Fig. 10-16). Damage to an artery from a skull fracture, usually on the side of the head, may result in bleeding between the dura mater and the skull, an **epidural hematoma** (he-mah-TO-mah). The rapidly accumulating blood puts pressure on blood vessels and interrupts blood flow to the brain. Symptoms include headache, partial paralysis, dilated pupils, and coma. If the pressure is not relieved within a day or two, death results.

A tear in the wall of a dural sinus causes a **subdural hematoma**. This often results from a blow to the front or back of the head that separates the dura from the arachnoid, as occurs when the moving head hits a stationary object. Blood gradually accumulates in the subdural space, putting pressure on the brain and causing headache, weakness, and confusion. Death results from continued bleeding. Bleeding into the brain tissue itself results in an intracerebral hematoma.

Cerebral **concussion** (kon-CUSH-on) results from a blow to the head or from sudden movement of the brain against the skull, as in violent shaking. The effects include loss of consciousness, headache, dizziness, vomiting, and even paralysis and impaired brain function. These vary in length and severity with the degree of damage.

Frequent observations of level of consciousness, pupil response, and extremity reflexes are important in the patient with a head injury (see Box 10-2, Brain Injury: A Heads-Up).

Degenerative Diseases

Alzheimer (ALZ-hi-mer) **disease** is a brain disorder resulting from an unexplained degeneration of the cerebral cortex and hippocampus (Fig. 10-17). The disorder develops gradually and eventually causes severe intellectual impairment with mood changes and confusion. Memory loss, especially for recent events, is a common early symptom. Dangers associated with Alzheimer disease are injury, infection, malnutrition, and inhalation of food or fluids into the lungs. Changes in the brain occur many years before noticeable signs of the disease appear. These changes include the development of amyloid, an abnormal protein, and a tangling of neuron fibers that prevents communication between cells.

At present, there is no cure, but several drugs have been developed that can delay the progression of early disease. In some tests, herbal extracts of *Ginkgo biloba*, the hormone estrogen, vitamin E, antiinflammatory drugs, and calcium channel blockers (drugs used primarily to regulate the heartbeat) have shown some signs of preventing or delaying the disease. Drugs also can control some of its physical and behavioral effects. Stress reduction is an important part of patient care.

Multi-infarct dementia (de-MEN-she-ah) represents the accumulation of brain damage resulting from chronic ischemia (is-KE-me-ah) (lack of blood supply), such as would be caused by a series of small strokes. There is a stepwise deterioration of function. People with multi-infarct dementia are troubled by progressive loss of memory, judgment, and cognitive function. Many people older than 80 years of age have some evidence of this disorder.

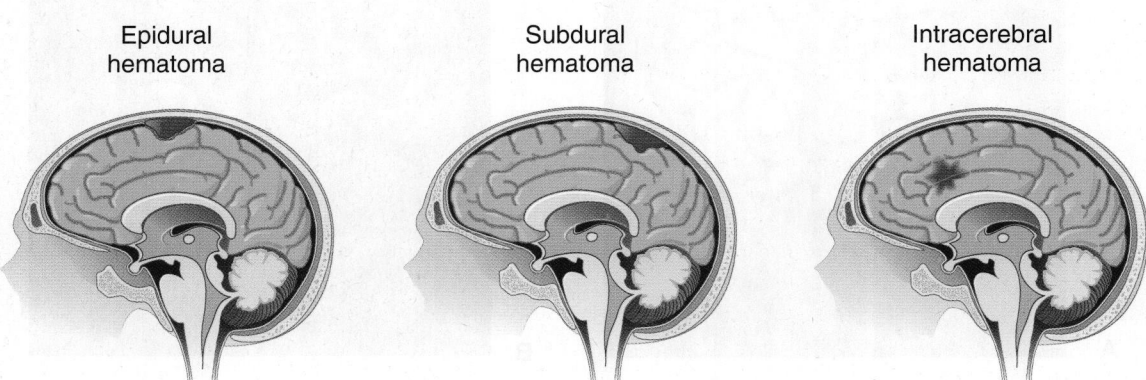

Epidural hematoma   Subdural hematoma   Intracerebral hematoma

Figure 10-16 **Hematomas.** Compare the locations of epidural, subdural, and intracerebral hematomas. (Reprinted with permission from Cohen BJ. *Medical Terminology*, 4th ed. Philadelphia: Lippincott Williams & Wilkins, 2004.)

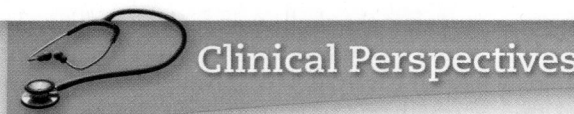

Box 10-2   Clinical Perspectives

Brain Injury: A Heads-Up

Traumatic brain injury is a leading cause of death and disability in the United States. Each year, approximately 1.5 million Americans sustain a brain injury, of whom about 50,000 will die and 80,000 will suffer long-term or permanent disability. The leading causes of traumatic brain injury are motor vehicle accidents, gunshot wounds, and falls. Other causes include shaken baby syndrome (caused by violent shaking of an infant or toddler) and second impact syndrome (when a second head injury occurs before the first has fully healed).

Brain damage occurs either from penetrating head trauma or acceleration-deceleration events where a head in motion suddenly comes to a stop. Nervous tissue, blood vessels, and possibly the meninges may be bruised, torn, lacerated, or ruptured, which may lead to swelling, hemorrhage, and hematoma. The best protection from brain injury is to prevent it. The following is a list of safety tips:

- Always wear a seat belt and secure children in approved car seats.

- Never drive after using alcohol or drugs or ride with an impaired driver.

- Always wear a helmet during activities such as biking, motorcycling, in-line skating, horseback riding, football, ice hockey, and batting and running bases in baseball and softball.

- Inspect playground equipment and supervise children using it. Never swing children around to play "airplane," nor vigorously bounce or shake them.

- Allow adequate time for healing after a head injury before resuming potentially dangerous activities.

- Prevent falls by using a nonslip bathtub or shower mat and using a step stool to reach objects on high shelves. Use a safety gate at the bottom and top of stairs to protect young children (and adults with dementia or other disorienting conditions).

- Keep unloaded firearms in a locked cabinet or safe and store bullets in a separate location.

For more information, contact the Brain Injury Association of America.

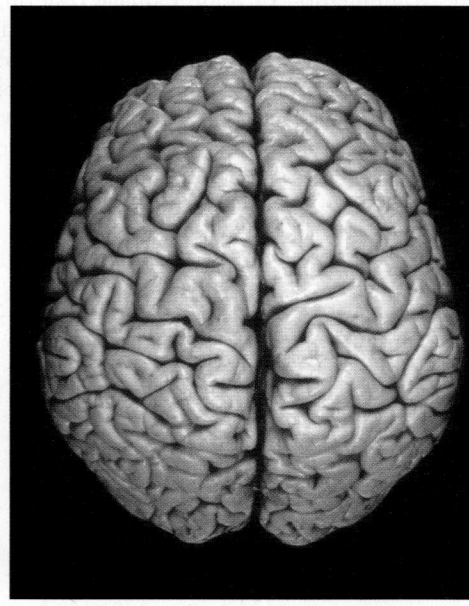

A

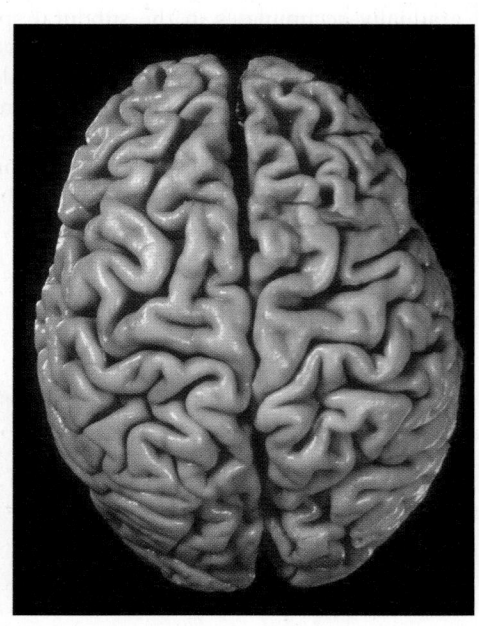

B

Figure 10-17 **Effects of Alzheimer disease. (A)** Normal brain. **(B)** Brain of a patient with Alzheimer disease shows atrophy of the cortex with narrow gyri and enlarged sulci. (Reprinted with permission from Rubin E, Farber JL. *Pathology*, 3rd ed. Philadelphia: Lippincott Williams & Wilkins, 1999.)

Parkinson disease is a progressive neurologic condition characterized by tremors, rigidity of limbs and joints, slow movement, and impaired balance. The disease usually arises from cell death in a part of the brain, the substantia nigra, that produces the neurotransmitter dopamine. The lack of dopamine results in overactivity of the basal nuclei, brain areas that control voluntary movement. The average age of onset is 55 years. Similar changes, together known as *parkinsonism*, may result from encephalitis or other brain diseases, exposure to certain toxins, or repeated head injury, as may occur in boxing.

The main therapy for Parkinson disease is administration of L-dopa, a substance that is capable of entering the brain and converting to dopamine (see Box 10-1). Drugs are now available that mimic the effects of dopamine, prevent its breakdown, or increase the effectiveness of L-dopa. Other approaches to treatment include implanting fetal cells that can do the missing cells' job and implanting a device that electrically stimulates the brain to control symptoms of Parkinson disease.

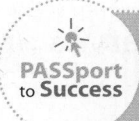

PASSport to Success

Speech therapists help to treat patients with language or communication problems from any cause. Visit *thePoint* or see the Student Resource CD in the back of this book for more information on this career.

Cranial Nerves

There are 12 pairs of cranial nerves (in this discussion, when a cranial nerve is identified, a pair is meant). They are numbered, usually in Roman numerals, according to their connection with the brain, beginning anteriorly and proceeding posteriorly (Fig. 10-18). Except for the first two pairs, all the cranial nerves arise from the brain stem. The first 9 pairs and the 12th pair supply structures in the head.

From a functional viewpoint, we may think of cranial nerve messages as belonging to one of four categories:

- **Special sensory impulses,** such as those for smell, taste, vision, and hearing, located in special sense organs in the head.
- **General sensory impulses,** such as those for pain, touch, temperature, deep muscle sense, pressure, and vibrations. These impulses come from receptors that are widely distributed throughout the body.
- **Somatic motor impulses** resulting in voluntary control of skeletal muscles.
- **Visceral motor impulses** producing involuntary control of glands and involuntary muscles (cardiac and smooth muscle). These motor pathways are part of the autonomic nervous system, parasympathetic division.

Names and Functions of the Cranial Nerves

A few of the cranial nerves (I, II, and VIII) contain only sensory fibers; some (III, IV, VI, XI, and XII) contain all or mostly motor fibers. The remainder (V, VII, IX, and X) contain both sensory and motor fibers; they are known as *mixed nerves*. All 12 nerves are listed below and summarized in Table 10-2:

I. The **olfactory nerve** carries smell impulses from receptors in the nasal mucosa to the brain.

II. The **optic nerve** carries visual impulses from the eye to the brain.

III. The **oculomotor nerve** is concerned with the contraction of most of the eye muscles.

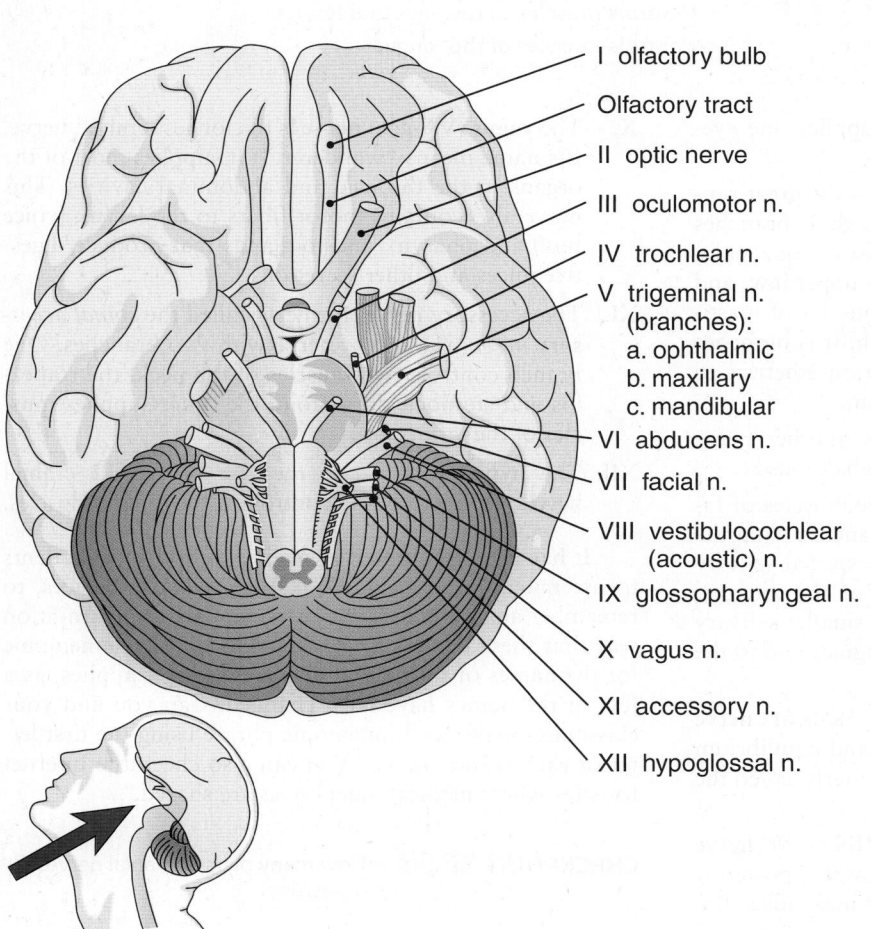

I olfactory bulb
Olfactory tract
II optic nerve
III oculomotor n.
IV trochlear n.
V trigeminal n.
(branches):
a. ophthalmic
b. maxillary
c. mandibular
VI abducens n.
VII facial n.
VIII vestibulocochlear (acoustic) n.
IX glossopharyngeal n.
X vagus n.
XI accessory n.
XII hypoglossal n.

Figure 10-18 **Cranial nerves.** The 12 pairs of cranial nerves are seen from the base of the brain.

Table 10-2	The Cranial Nerves and Their Functions	

Nerve (Roman numeral designation)	Name	Function
I	Olfactory	Carries impulses for the sense of smell toward the brain
II	Optic	Carries visual impulses from the eye to the brain
III	Oculomotor	Controls contraction of eye muscles
IV	Trochlear	Supplies one eyeball muscle
V	Trigeminal	Carries sensory impulses from eye, upper jaw, and lower jaw toward the brain
VI	Abducens	Controls an eyeball muscle
VII	Facial	Controls muscles of facial expression; carries sensation of taste; stimulates small salivary glands and lacrimal (tear) gland
VIII	Vestibulocochlear	Carries sensory impulses for hearing and equilibrium from the inner ear toward the brain
IX	Glossopharyngeal	Carries sensory impulses from tongue and pharynx (throat); controls swallowing muscles and stimulates the parotid salivary gland
X	Vagus	Supplies most of the organs in the thoracic and abdominal cavities; carries motor impulses to the larynx (voice box) and pharynx
XI	Accessory	Controls muscles in the neck and larynx
XII	Hypoglossal	Controls muscles of the tongue

IV. The **trochlear** (TROK-le-ar) **nerve** supplies one eyeball muscle.

V. The **trigeminal** (tri-JEM-in-al) **nerve** is the great sensory nerve of the face and head. It has three branches that transport general sense impulses (e.g., pain, touch, temperature) from the eye, the upper jaw, and the lower jaw. Motor fibers to the muscles of mastication (chewing) join the third branch. It is branches of the trigeminal nerve that a dentist anesthetizes to work on the teeth without causing pain.

VI. The **abducens** (ab-DU-senz) **nerve** is another nerve sending controlling impulses to an eyeball muscle.

VII. The **facial nerve** is largely motor. The muscles of facial expression are all supplied by branches from the facial nerve. This nerve also includes special sensory fibers for taste (anterior two-thirds of the tongue), and it contains secretory fibers to the smaller salivary glands (the submandibular and sublingual) and to the lacrimal (tear) gland.

VIII. The **vestibulocochlear** (ves-tib-u-lo-KOK-le-ar) **nerve** carries sensory impulses for hearing and equilibrium from the inner ear. This nerve was formerly called the auditory or acoustic nerve.

IX. The **glossopharyngeal** (glos-o-fah-RIN-je-al) **nerve** contains general sensory fibers from the posterior tongue and the pharynx (throat). This nerve also contains sensory fibers for taste from the posterior third of the tongue, secretory fibers that supply the largest salivary gland (parotid), and motor nerve fibers to control the swallowing muscles in the pharynx.

X. The **vagus** (VA-gus) **nerve** is the longest cranial nerve. (Its name means "wanderer.") It supplies most of the organs in the thoracic and abdominal cavities. This nerve also contains motor fibers to the larynx (voice box) and pharynx and to glands that produce digestive juices and other secretions.

XI. The **accessory nerve** (formerly called the *spinal accessory nerve*) is a motor nerve with two branches. One branch controls two muscles of the neck, the trapezius and sternocleidomastoid; the other supplies muscles of the larynx.

XII. The **hypoglossal nerve**, the last of the 12 cranial nerves, carries impulses controlling the tongue muscles.

It has been traditional in medical schools for students to use mnemonics (ne-MON-iks), or memory devices, to remember anatomic lists. As an aside, part of the tradition was that these devices be bawdy. The original mnemonic for the names of the cranial nerves no longer applies, as a few of the names have been changed. Can you and your classmates make up a mnemonic phrase using the first letter of each cranial nerve? You can also check the Internet for sites where medical mnemonics are shared.

CHECKPOINT 10-11 ➤ How many pairs of cranial nerves are there?

CHECKPOINT 10-12 ➤ The cranial nerves are classified as being sensory, motor, or mixed. What is a mixed nerve?

Disorders Involving the Cranial Nerves

Destruction of optic nerve (II) fibers may result from increased pressure of the eye's fluid on the nerves, as occurs in glaucoma, from the effect of poisons, and from some infections. Certain medications, when used in high doses over long periods, can damage the branch of the vestibulocochlear nerve responsible for hearing.

Injury to a nerve that contains motor fibers causes paralysis of the muscles supplied by these fibers. The oculomotor nerve (III) may be damaged by certain infections or various poisonous substances. Because this nerve supplies so many muscles connected with the eye, including the levator, which raises the eyelid, injury to it causes a paralysis that usually interferes with eye function.

Bell palsy is a facial paralysis caused by damage to the facial nerve (VII), usually on one side of the face. This injury results in facial distortion because of one-sided paralysis of the muscles of facial expression.

Neuralgia (nu-RAL-je-ah) in general means "nerve pain." A severe spasmodic pain affecting the fifth cranial nerve is known as **trigeminal neuralgia** or **tic douloureux** (tik du-lu-RU) (from French, meaning "painful twitch"). At first, the pain comes at relatively long intervals, but as time goes on, intervals between episodes usually shorten while pain durations lengthen. Treatments include microsurgery and high-frequency current.

Aging of the Nervous System

The nervous system is one of the first systems to develop in the embryo. By the beginning of the third week of development, the rudiments of the central nervous system have appeared. Beginning with maturity, the nervous system begins to undergo changes. The brain begins to decrease in size and weight due to a loss of cells, especially in the cerebral cortex, accompanied by decreases in synapses and neurotransmitters. The speed of processing information decreases, and movements are slowed. Memory diminishes, especially for recent events. Changes in the vascular system throughout the body with a narrowing of the arteries (atherosclerosis) reduce the brain's blood flow. Vascular degeneration increases the likelihood of stroke.

Much individual variation is possible, however, with regard to location and severity of changes. Although age might make it harder to acquire new skills, tests have shown that practice enhances skill retention. As with other body systems, the nervous system has vast reserves, and most elderly people are able to cope with life's demands.

Disease in Context revisited

▶ Frank's Stroke Recovery

"Good morning Mr. Carter. My name is Ross Baker and I'm a physiotherapist with the Brain Injury Team. My job is to assist your stroke recovery by helping you regain your strength, balance, and coordination. Before we continue, may I test your muscular and sensory functions?"

With Frank's permission, the physiotherapist began his assessment. He noted hemiplegia (muscle paralysis) in Frank's right arm and leg. Stroke damage to the primary motor area in the frontal lobe of Frank's *left* cerebral hemisphere had caused motor deficits in his *right* limbs. Loss of contralateral control is typical in stroke patients because most motor fibers from the cerebral cortex cross over (decussate) from one side of the medulla oblongata to the other before continuing down the spinal cord in descending tracts. For Frank, this meant that motor information from his damaged left cerebral hemisphere was not reaching the skeletal muscles of his right limbs.

The physiotherapist also noted a diminished sense of touch (hypesthesia) on Frank's right side, which suggested that the stroke had damaged the left parietal lobe's primary sensory area as well. Like motor deficits, contralateral sensory deficits are typical in stroke patients because sensory fibers that enter one side of the spinal cord immediately cross over to the opposite side before continuing up the cord in ascending pathways. As a result, sensory information from Frank's right side was not processed in his left cerebral cortex.

Ross used his understanding of brain and spinal cord anatomy to make sense of Frank's symptoms. Based on his assessment of Frank's motor and sensory deficits, Ross will devise and implement a rehabilitation plan for him. Other allied health professionals like occupational and speech therapists will also help Frank recover from his stroke. See *thePoint* or see the Student Resource CD in the back of this book for more information on these and other health professions careers.

Word Anatomy

Medical terms are built from standardized word parts (prefixes, roots, and suffixes). Learning the meanings of these parts can help you remember words and interpret unfamiliar terms.

WORD PART	MEANING	EXAMPLE
Protective Structures of the Brain and Spinal Cord		
cerebr/o	brain	*Cerebrospinal* fluid circulates around the brain and spinal cord.
chori/o	membrane	The *choroid* plexus is the vascular membrane in the ventricle that produces CSF.
gyr/o	circle	A *gyrus* is a circular raised area on the surface of the brain.
encephal/o	brain	The *diencephalon* is the part of the brain located between the cerebral hemispheres and the brain stem.
contra-	opposed, against	The cerebral cortex has *contralateral* control of motor function.
later/o	lateral, side	See preceding example.
Brain Studies		
tom/o	cut	*Tomography* is a method for viewing sections as if cut through the body.
Disorders of the Brain and Associated Structures		
cephal/o	head	*Hydrocephalus* is the accumulation of fluid within the brain.
-rhage	bursting forth	A cerebral *hemorrhage* is a sudden bursting forth of blood in the brain.
phasia	speech, ability to talk	*Aphasia* is a loss or defect in language communication.
Cranial Nerves		
gloss/o	tongue	The *hypoglossal* nerve controls muscles of the tongue.

Summary

I. **THE BRAIN**
   A. Main parts—cerebrum, diencephalon, brain stem, cerebellum

II. **PROTECTIVE STRUCTURES OF THE BRAIN AND SPINAL CORD**
   A. Meninges
      1. Dura mater—tough outermost layer
      2. Arachnoid—weblike middle layer
      3. Pia mater—vascular innermost layer
   B. Cerebrospinal fluid (CSF)
      1. Circulates around and within brain and spinal cord
      2. Cushions and protects
      3. Ventricles—four spaces within brain where CSF is produced
         a. Choroid plexus—vascular network in ventricle that produces CSF

III. **THE CEREBRAL HEMISPHERES**
   A. Structure
      1. Two hemispheres
      2. Lobes—frontal, parietal, temporal, occipital, insula
      3. Cortex—outer layer of gray matter
         a. In gyri (folds) and sulci (grooves)
         b. Specialized functions—interpretation, memory, conscious thought, judgment, voluntary actions
      4. Basal nuclei (ganglia)—regulate movement and facial expression
      5. Corpus callosum—band of white matter connecting cerebral hemispheres
      6. Internal capsule—connects each cerebral hemisphere to lower parts of brain
   B. Functions of the cerebral cortex
   C. Communication areas
   D. Memory and the learning process

IV. **DIENCEPHALON**—Area between cerebral hemispheres and brain stem
   A. Thalamus—directs sensory impulses to cortex
   B. Hypothalamus—maintains homeostasis, controls pituitary
   C. Limbic system
      1. Contains parts of cerebrum and diencephalon
      2. Controls emotion and behavior

V. **BRAIN STEM**
   A. Midbrain—involved in eye and ear reflexes
   B. Pons—connecting link for other divisions
   C. Medulla oblongata
      1. Connects with spinal cord

   2. Contains vital centers for respiration, heart rate, vasomotor activity

VI. **THE CEREBELLUM**—Regulates coordination, balance, muscle tone

VII. **BRAIN STUDIES**
   A. Imaging—computed tomography (CT), magnetic resonance imaging (MRI), positron emission tomography (PET)
   B. Electroencephalograph (EEG)—measures electrical waves produced as brain functions

VIII. **DISORDERS OF THE BRAIN AND ASSOCIATED STRUCTURES**
   A. Inflammation
      1. Meningitis—inflammation of the meninges
      2. Encephalitis—inflammation of the brain
   B. Hydrocephalus—abnormal accumulation of CSF
   C. Stroke and other brain disorders
      1. Cerebrovascular accident (CVA); stroke
         a. Causes—cerebral hemorrhage, blood clot
         b. Effects—paralysis, aphasia
      2. Cerebral palsy—cause is brain damage before or during birth
      3. Epilepsy—characterized by seizures
      4. Tumors—usually involve neuroglia (gliomas)
   D. Injury
      1. Often results in hematoma—accumulation of blood
      2. Concussion—caused by sudden blow
   E. Degenerative diseases
      1. Alzheimer disease—degeneration of cerebral cortex and hippocampus
      2. Multi-infarct dementia—caused by many small strokes
      3. Parkinson disease—deficiency of neurotransmitter dopamine

IX. **CRANIAL NERVES**
   A. 12 pairs attached to brain
   B. Functions
      1. Carry special and general sensory impulses
      2. Carry somatic and visceral motor impulses
   C. Types
      1. Sensory (I, II, VIII)
      2. Motor (III, IV, VI, XI, XII)
      3. Mixed (V, VII, IX, X)
   D. Disorders involving the cranial nerves
      1. Bell palsy—facial paralysis (cranial nerve VII)
      2. Trigeminal neuralgia—pain in cranial nerve V

X. **AGING OF THE NERVOUS SYSTEM**

10

Questions for Study and Review

BUILDING UNDERSTANDING

Fill in the blanks

1. The thickest and toughest layer of the meninges is the _____.

2. The third and fourth ventricles are connected by a small canal called the _____.

3. The muscles of speech are controlled by a region named _____.

4. Inflammation of the brain is termed _____.

5. The cells responsible for most brain tumors are _____.

Matching > Match each numbered item with the most closely related lettered item.

___ 6. The sensory nerve of the face

___ 7. The motor nerve of the muscles of facial expression

___ 8. The sensory nerve for hearing and equilibrium

___ 9. The motor nerve for swallowing

___ 10. The motor nerve for digestion

    a. trigeminal nerve

    b. facial nerve

    c. vestibulocochlear nerve

    d. glossopharyngeal nerve

    e. vagus nerve

Multiple Choice

___ 11. The cerebrum is divided into left and right hemispheres by the
    a. central sulcus
    b. lateral sulcus
    c. longitudinal fissure
    d. insula

___ 12. The primary sensory area interprets all of the following sensations except
    a. vision
    b. pain
    c. touch
    d. temperature

___ 13. An abnormal accumulation of CSF within the brain is called
    a. cerebral hemorrhage
    b. subdural hematoma
    c. hemiplegia
    d. hydrocephalus

___ 14. Tremors, limb rigidity, slow movement, and impaired balance are signs of
    a. meningitis
    b. Bell palsy
    c. Alzheimer disease
    d. Parkinson disease

___ 15. Pain messages are classified as
    a. special sensory impulses
    b. general sensory impulses
    c. somatic motor impulses
    d. visceral motor impulses

UNDERSTANDING CONCEPTS

16. Briefly describe the effects of injury to the following brain areas:
    a. cerebrum
    b. diencephalon
    c. brain stem
    d. cerebellum

17. A neurosurgeon has drilled a hole through her patient's skull and is preparing to remove a cerebral glioma. List, in order, the membranes she must cut through to reach the cerebral cortex.

18. Compare and contrast the functions of the following structures:
    a. frontal lobe and parietal lobe
    b. temporal lobe and occipital lobe
    c. thalamus and hypothalamus

19. What is the function of the limbic system? Describe the effect of damage to the hippocampus.

20. Compare and contrast the following nervous system disorders:
    a. meningitis and encephalitis
    b. epidural hematoma and subdural hematoma
    c. Alzheimer disease and multi-infarct dementia
    d. Bell palsy and trigeminal neuralgia

21. Describe Parkinson disease and therapies used to treat it.

22. The term cerebellum means "little cerebrum." Why is this an appropriate term?

23. Make a table of the 12 cranial nerves and their functions. According to your table, which ones are sensory, motor, or mixed?

CONCEPTUAL THINKING

24. The parents of Molly R. (2-month-old Caucasian female) are informed that their daughter requires a shunt to drain excess CSF from her brain. What disorder does Molly have? How would you explain this disorder to her parents? What would happen to Molly if the shunt was not put in place?

25. In the case story, Frank suffered a stroke. How would you explain the term "stroke" to his family? Why

were many of his symptoms isolated to the right side of his body?

26. In Frank's case, stroke damage was isolated to his cerebrum. Some strokes, though, can affect the brain stem. Why is damage to this part of the brain life-threatening?

10

CHAPTER 11

The Sensory System

Learning Outcomes

After careful study of this chapter, you should be able to:

1. Describe the function of the sensory system
2. Differentiate between the special and general senses and give examples of each
3. Describe the structure of the eye
4. List and describe the structures that protect the eye
5. Define *refraction* and list the refractive parts of the eye
6. Differentiate between the rods and the cones of the eye
7. Compare the functions of the extrinsic and intrinsic muscles of the eye
8. Describe the nerve supply to the eye
9. Describe the three divisions of the ear
10. Describe the receptor for hearing and explain how it functions
11. Compare static and dynamic equilibrium and describe the location and function of these receptors
12. Explain the function of proprioceptors
13. List several methods for treatment of pain
14. Describe sensory adaptation and explain its value
15. List some disorders of the sensory system
16. Show how word parts are used to build words related to the sensory system (see Word Anatomy at the end of the chapter)

Selected Key Terms

The following terms and other boldface terms in the chapter are defined in the Glossary

accommodation
cataract
choroid
cochlea
conjunctiva
convergence
cornea
glaucoma
gustation
lacrimal apparatus
lens (crystalline lens)
olfaction
organ of Corti
ossicle
proprioceptor
refraction
retina
sclera
semicircular canal
sensory adaptation
sensory receptor
tympanic membrane
vestibule
vitreous body

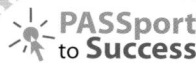

PASSport to **Success**

Visit *thePoint* or see the Student Resource CD in the back of this book for definitions and pronunciations of key terms as well as a pretest for this chapter.

Disease in Context

➤ Paul's Second Case: Seeing More of the Sun's Effects

Paul glanced once again at the postcard sitting on his entranceway table as he arrived home in the evening. He knew it said he was due for a checkup with his ophthalmologist, but after his run-in with skin cancer six months earlier, he was in no hurry to see the inside of a medical office. *Well, it's just routine, and I may need a slight change in my prescription, so I'll make the call*, he thought.

At the office, Dr. Gilbert greeted Paul and asked how he was feeling in general and if he thought there had been any change in his vision. "My vision sometimes seems a little blurry, especially when my eyes are tired, but no major changes," Paul replied. Dr. Gilbert proceeded with the eye exam, testing his visual acuity and checking on his astigmatism.

"You're right; not much change," said the ophthalmologist. "But, we'll give you a new prescription for your glasses. At 42, you're a little young for presbyopia—far-sightedness that develops with age—but we'll do the routine check for glaucoma. I know your father developed that condition, and it does have a hereditary factor." The doctor dilated Paul's eyes with drops and examined the fundus of each eye with an ophthalmoscope. In answer to Paul's query, he explained that in this way he could examine the health of the retina and the optic nerve and also look at the vessels at the back of the eye for any signs of diabetes or circulatory problems. In addition, he used a tonometer to test for glaucoma, a condition that can damage the eye with high fluid pressure. "I need to check on another patient," he told Paul. "Then I'll be back to explain what I've found. Just sit in the waiting room for a few minutes, please."

Dr. Gilbert uses his knowledge of the structure and function of the eye to diagnose medical conditions. In this chapter, you will learn about the eye and other sensory system organs. As well, we'll examine the consequences of Paul's sun-loving youth on his eyes and vision.

The Senses

The sensory system protects a person by detecting changes in the environment. An environmental change becomes a *stimulus* when it initiates a nerve impulse, which then travels to the central nervous system (CNS) by way of a sensory (afferent) neuron. A stimulus becomes a sensation—something we experience—only when a specialized area of the cerebral cortex interprets the nerve impulse received. Many stimuli arrive from the external environment and are detected at or near the body surface. Others, such as stimuli from the viscera, originate internally and help to maintain homeostasis.

Sensory Receptors

The part of the nervous system that detects a stimulus is the **sensory receptor**. In structure, a sensory receptor may be one of the following:

- The free dendrite of a sensory neuron, such as the receptors for pain and temperature
- A modified ending, or **end-organ**, on the dendrite of an afferent neuron, such as those for touch
- A specialized cell associated with an afferent neuron, such as the rods and cones of the eye's retina and the receptors in the other special sense organs

Receptors can be classified according to the type of stimulus to which they respond:

- Chemoreceptors, such as receptors for taste and smell, detect chemicals in solution.
- Photoreceptors, located in the retina of the eye, respond to light.
- Thermoreceptors detect change in temperature. Many of these receptors are located in the skin.
- Mechanoreceptors respond to movement, such as stretch, pressure, or vibration. These include pressure receptors in the skin, receptors that monitor body position, and the receptors of hearing and equilibrium in the ear, which are activated by the movement of cilia on specialized receptor cells.

Any receptor must receive a stimulus of adequate intensity, that is, at least a **threshold stimulus**, in order to respond and generate a nerve impulse.

Special and General Senses

Another way of classifying the senses is according to the distribution of their receptors. A **special sense** is localized in a special sense organ; a **general sense** is widely distributed throughout the body.

- **Special senses**
  - > **Vision** from receptors in the eye
  - > **Hearing** from receptors in the internal ear
  - > **Equilibrium** from receptors in the internal ear
  - > **Taste** from receptors in the tongue
  - > **Smell** from receptors in the upper nasal cavities
- **General senses**
  - > **Pressure, temperature, pain,** and **touch** from receptors in the skin and internal organs
  - > Sense of **position** from receptors in the muscles, tendons, and joints

The Eye and Vision

In the embryo, the eye develops as an outpocketing of the brain. It is a delicate organ, protected by a number of structures:

- The skull bones form the walls of the eye orbit (cavity) and protect the posterior part of the eyeball.
- The upper and lower eyelids aid in protecting the eye's anterior portion (Fig. 11-1). The eyelids can be closed to keep harmful materials out of the eye, and blinking helps to lubricate the eye. A muscle, the levator palpebrae, is attached to the upper eyelid. When this muscle contracts, it keeps the eye open. If the muscle becomes weaker with age, the eyelids may droop and interfere with vision, a condition called *ptosis*.
- The eyelashes and eyebrow help to keep foreign matter out of the eye.
- A thin membrane, the **conjunctiva** (kon-junk-TI-vah), lines the inner surface of the eyelids and covers the visible portion of the white of the eye (sclera). Cells

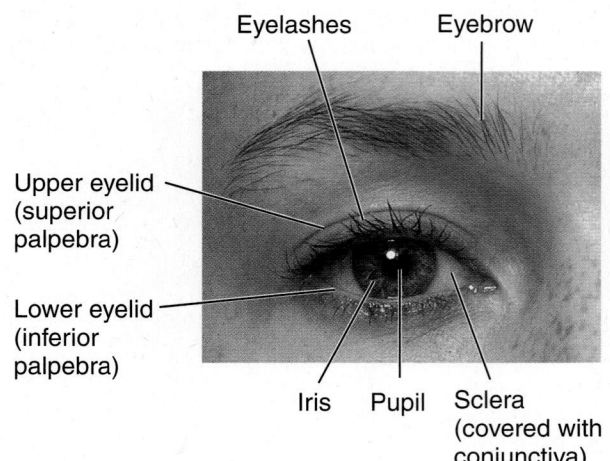

Figure 11-1 **The eye's protective structures.** (Reprinted with permission from Bickley LS. *Bates' Guide to Physical Examination and History Taking*, 8th ed. Philadelphia: Lippincott Williams & Wilkins, 2003.)

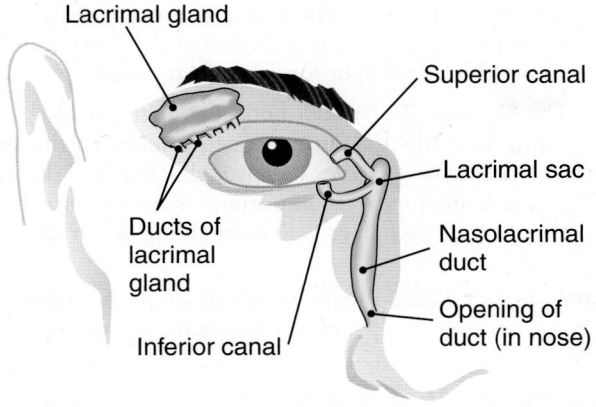

Figure 11-2 **The lacrimal apparatus.** The lacrimal (tear) gland and its associated ducts are shown.

Lacrimal gland

Superior canal

Lacrimal sac

Nasolacrimal duct

Opening of duct (in nose)

Inferior canal

Ducts of lacrimal gland

within the conjunctiva produce mucus that aids in lubricating the eye. Where the conjunctiva folds back from the eyelid to the eye's anterior surface, a sac is formed. The lower portion of the conjunctival sac can be used to instill medication drops. With age, the conjunctiva often thins and dries, resulting in inflammation and enlarged blood vessels.

- Tears, produced by the **lacrimal** (LAK-rih-mal) **glands** (Fig. 11-2), lubricate the eye and contain an enzyme that protects against infection. As tears flow across the eye from the lacrimal gland, located in the orbit's upper lateral part, they carry away small particles that may have entered the eye. The tears then flow into ducts near the eye's nasal corner where they drain into the nose by way of the **nasolacrimal** (na-zo-LAK-rih-

mal) **duct** (see Fig. 11-2). An excess of tears causes a "runny nose"; a greater overproduction of them results in the tears spilling onto the cheeks. With age, the lacrimal glands produce less secretion, but tears still may overflow onto the cheek if the nasolacrimal ducts become plugged.

PASSport to Success Visit **thePoint** or see the Student Resource CD in the back of this book for an image of *ptosis*.

CHECKPOINT 11-1 ➤ What are some structures that protect the eye?

Coats of the Eyeball

The eyeball has three separate coats, or tunics (Fig. 11-3).

1. The outermost tunic, called the **sclera** (SKLE-rah), is made of tough connective tissue. It is commonly referred to as the *white of the eye*. It appears white because of the collagen it contains and because it has no blood vessels to add color. (Reddened or "bloodshot" eyes result from inflammation and swelling of blood vessels in the conjunctiva).

2. The second tunic of the eyeball is the **choroid** (KO-royd). This coat is composed of a delicate network of connective tissue interlaced with many blood vessels. It also contains much dark brown pigment. The choroid may be compared to the dull black lining of a camera in that it prevents incoming light rays from scattering and reflecting off the eye's inner surface. The blood vessels at the posterior, or fundus, of the eye can reveal signs of disease, and visualization of these vessels with an **ophthalmoscope** (of-THAL-mo-skope) is an important part of a medical examination.

3. The innermost tunic, the **retina** (RET-ih-nah), is the eye's actual receptor layer. It contains light-sensitive cells known as **rods** and **cones**, which generate the nerve impulses associated with vision.

CHECKPOINT 11-2 ➤ What are the names of the tunics of the eyeball?

Pathway of Light Rays and Refraction

As light rays pass through the eye toward the retina, they travel through a

Figure 11-3 **The eye.** Note the three tunics, the refractive parts of the eye (cornea, aqueous humor, lens, vitreous body), and other structures involved in vision.

Tunics — Sclera, Choroid, Retina

Fovea centralis

Vitreous body

Optic nerve

Optic disk (blind spot)

Suspensory ligaments

Aqueous humor

Cornea

Pupil

Iris

Lens

Ciliary muscle

Conjunctival sac

11

series of transparent, colorless parts described below and seen in Figure 11-3. On the way, they undergo a process known as **refraction**, which is the bending of light rays as they pass from one substance to another substance of different density. (For a simple demonstration of refraction, place a spoon into a glass of water and observe how the handle appears to bend at the surface of the water.) Because of refraction, light from a very large area can be focused on a very small area of the retina. The eye's transparent refracting parts are listed here, according to the pathway of light traveling from exterior to interior:

1. The **cornea** (KOR-ne-ah) is an anterior continuation of the sclera, but it is transparent and colorless, whereas the rest of the sclera is opaque and white. The cornea is referred to frequently as the *window* of the eye. It bulges forward slightly and is the main refracting structure of the eye. The cornea has no blood vessels; it is nourished by the fluids that constantly wash over it.

2. The **aqueous** (A-kwe-us) **humor**, a watery fluid that fills much of the eyeball anterior to the lens, helps maintain the cornea's slight forward curve. The aqueous humor is constantly produced and drained from the eye.

3. The **lens**, technically called the *crystalline lens*, is a clear, circular structure made of a firm, elastic material. The lens has two bulging surfaces and is thus de-

scribed as biconvex. The lens is important in light refraction because it is elastic and its thickness can be adjusted to focus light for near or far vision.

4. The **vitreous** (VIT-re-us) **body** is a soft jellylike substance that fills the entire space posterior to the lens (the adjective *vitreous* means "glasslike"). Like the aqueous humor, it is important in maintaining the shape of the eyeball as well as in aiding in refraction.

CHECKPOINT 11-3 ➤ What are the structures that refract light as it passes through the eye?

Function of the Retina

The retina has a complex structure with multiple layers of cells (Fig. 11-4). The deepest layer is a pigmented layer just anterior to the choroid. Next are the rods and cones, the receptor cells of the eye, named for their shape. Details on how these two types of cells differ are presented in Table 11-1. Anterior to the rods and cones are connecting neurons that carry impulses toward the optic nerve.

The rods are highly sensitive to light and thus function in dim light, but they do not provide a sharp image. They are more numerous than the cones and are distributed more toward the periphery (anterior portion) of the retina. (If you visualize the retina as the inside of a bowl, the rods would be located toward the bowl's lip). When you enter into dim light, such as a darkened movie theater, you cannot see for a short period. It is during this time that the rods are beginning to function, a change that is described as **dark adaptation**. When you are able to see again, images are blurred and appear only in shades of gray, because the rods are unable to differentiate colors.

The cones function in bright light, are sensitive to color, and give sharp images. The cones are localized at the retinal center, especially in a tiny depressed area near the optic nerve that is called the **fovea centralis** (FO-ve-ah sen-TRA-lis) (Fig. 11-5; see also Fig. 11-3). (Note that *fovea* is a general term for a pit or depression.) Because this area contains the highest concentration of cones, it is the point of sharpest vision. The fovea is contained within a yellowish spot, the **macula lutea** (MAK-u-lah LU-te-ah), an area that may show degenerative changes with age.

There are three types of cones, each sensitive to either red, green, or blue light. Color blindness results from a lack of retinal cones. People who completely lack cones are totally colorblind; those who lack one type of cone

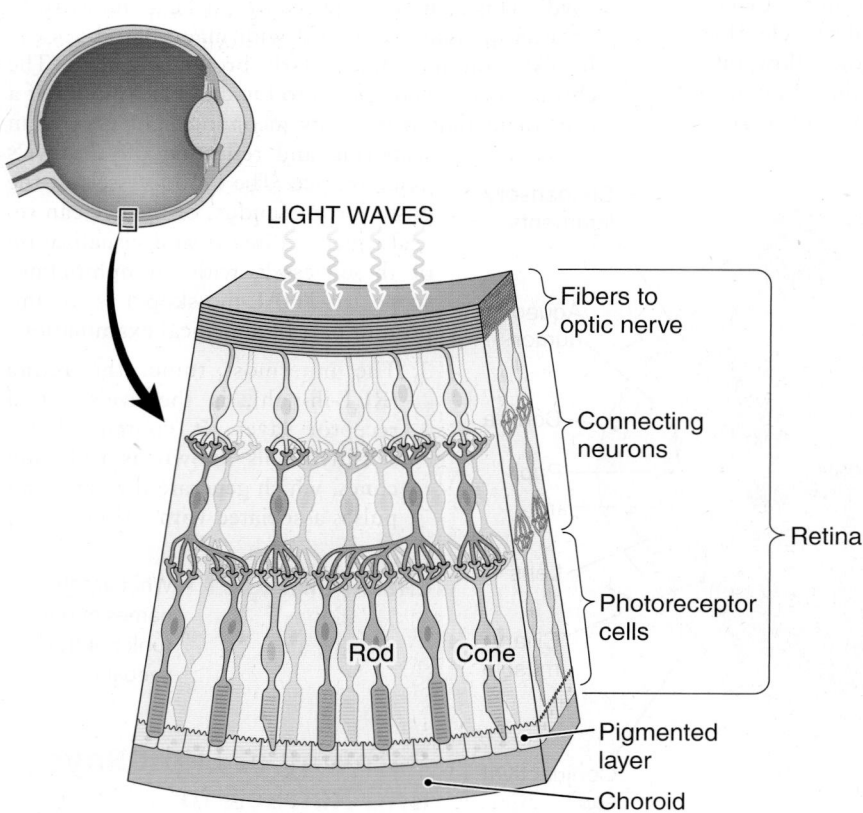

LIGHT WAVES

Fibers to optic nerve

Connecting neurons

Retina

Photoreceptor cells

Rod   Cone

Pigmented layer

Choroid

Figure 11-4 **Structure of the retina.** Rods and cones form a deep layer of the retina, near the choroid. Connecting neurons carry visual impulses toward the optic nerve.

Table 11-1	Comparison of the Rods and Cones of the Retina	
Characteristic	**Rods**	**Cones**
Shape	Cylindrical	Flask shaped
Number	About 120 million in each retina	About 6 million in each retina
Distribution	Toward the periphery (anterior) of the retina	Concentrated at the center of the retina
Stimulus	Dim light	Bright light
Visual acuity (sharpness)	Low	High
Pigments	Rhodopsin (visual purple)	Pigments sensitive to red, green, or blue
Color perception	None; shades of gray	Respond to color

are partially color blind. This disorder, because of its pattern of inheritance, occurs almost exclusively in males.

The rods and cones function by means of pigments that are sensitive to light. The rod pigment is **rhodopsin** (ro-DOP-sin), or visual purple. Vitamin A is needed for manufacture of these pigments. If a person is lacking in vitamin A, and thus rhodopsin, he or she may have difficulty seeing in dim light because the light is inadequate to activate the rods; this condition is termed **night blindness**. Nerve impulses from the rods and cones flow into sensory neurons that eventually merge to form the optic nerve (cranial nerve II) at the eye's posterior (see Figs. 11-3 and 11-5). The impulses travel to the visual center in the brain's occipital cortex.

When an **ophthalmologist** (of-thal-MOL-o-jist), a physician who specializes in treatment of the eye, examines the retina with an ophthalmoscope, he or she can see abnormalities in the retina and in the retinal blood vessels. Some of these changes may signal more widespread diseases that affect the eye, such as diabetes and high blood pressure (hypertension).

CHECKPOINT 11-4 ➤ What are the receptor cells of the retina?

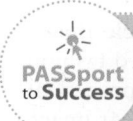

PASSport to Success
Visit **thePoint** or see the Student Resource CD in the back of this book to view the animation *The Retina*, which illustrates the structure and function of this visual receptor.

Muscles of the Eye

Two groups of muscles are associated with the eye. Both groups are important in adjusting the eye so that a clear image can form on the retina.

THE EXTRINSIC MUSCLES The voluntary muscles attached to the eyeball's outer surface are the **extrinsic** (eks-TRIN-sik) **muscles**. The six ribbonlike extrinsic muscles connected with each eye originate on the orbital bones and insert on the surface of the sclera (Fig. 11-6). They are named

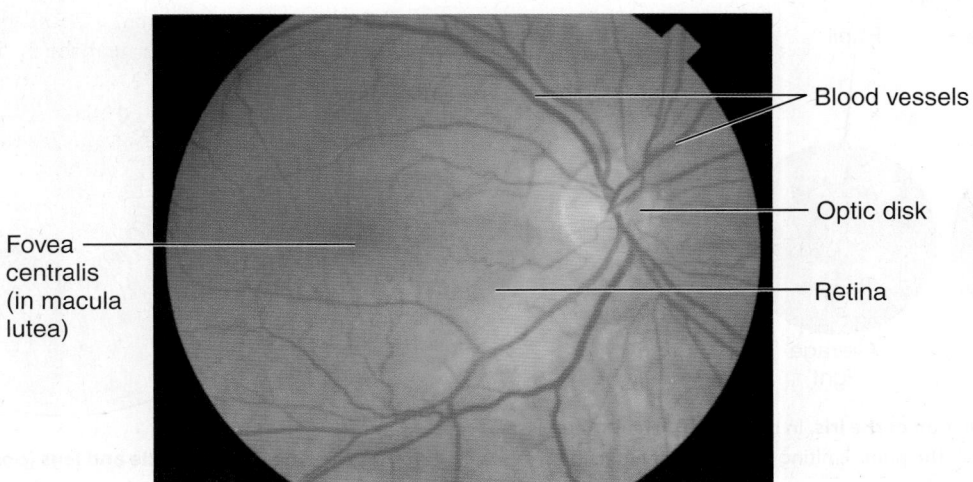

Figure 11-5 **The fundus (back) of the eye as seen through an ophthalmoscope.** (Reprinted with permission from Moore KL, Dalley AF. *Clinically Oriented Anatomy*, 4th ed. Baltimore: Lippincott Williams & Wilkins, 1999.)

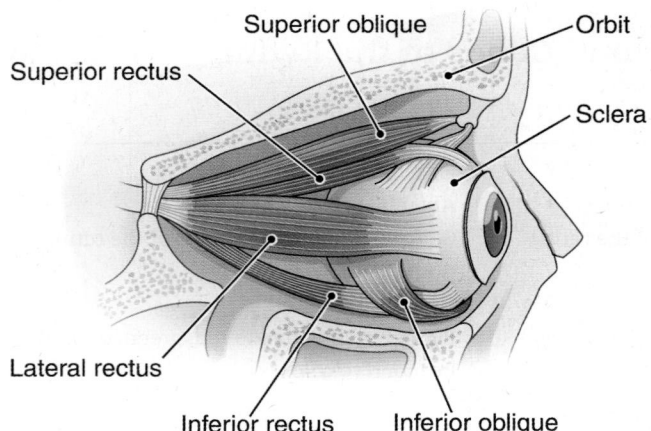

Figure 11-6 **Extrinsic muscles of the eye.** The medial rectus is not shown. [**ZOOMING IN** ➤ What characteristics are used in naming the extrinsic eye muscles?]

for their location and the direction of the muscle fibers. These muscles pull on the eyeball in a coordinated fashion so that both eyes center on one visual field. This process of **convergence** is necessary to the formation of a clear image on the retina. Having the image come from a slightly different angle from each retina is believed to be important for three-dimensional (stereoscopic) vision, a characteristic of primates.

CHECKPOINT **11-5** ➤ What is the function of the extrinsic muscles of the eye?

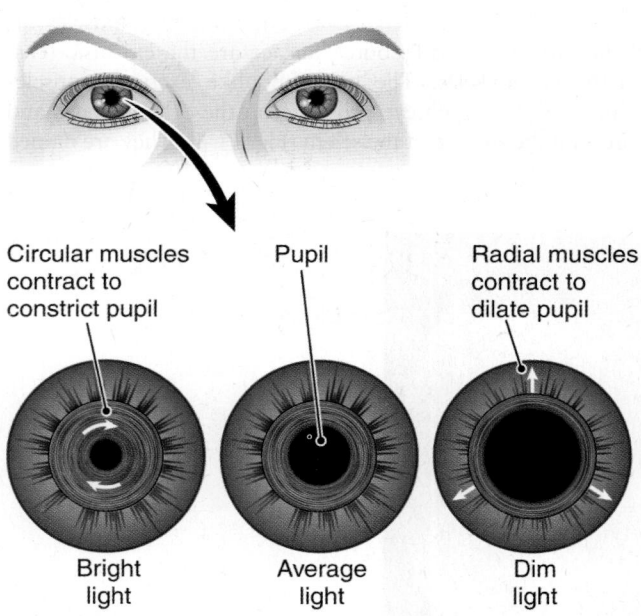

Figure 11-7 **Function of the iris.** In bright light, circular muscles contract and constrict the pupil, limiting the light that enters the eye. In dim light, the radial muscles contract and dilate the pupil, allowing more light to enter the eye. [**ZOOMING IN** ➤ What muscles of the iris contract to make the pupil smaller? Larger?]

THE INTRINSIC MUSCLES The involuntary muscles located within the eyeball are the **intrinsic** (in-TRIN-sik) **muscles.** They form two circular structures within the eye, the iris and the ciliary muscle.

The **iris** (I-ris), the colored or pigmented part of the eye, is composed of two sets of muscle fibers that govern the size of the iris's central opening, the **pupil** (PU-pil) (Fig. 11-7). One set of fibers is arranged in a circular fashion, and the other set extends radially like the spokes of a wheel. The iris regulates the amount of light entering the eye. In bright light, the iris's circular muscle fibers contract, reducing the size of the pupil. This narrowing is termed *constriction*. In contrast, in dim light, the radial muscles contract, pulling the opening outward and enlarging it. This enlargement of the pupil is known as *dilation*.

The **ciliary** (SIL-e-ar-e) **muscle** is shaped somewhat like a flattened ring with a central hole the size of the iris's outer edge. This muscle holds the lens in place by means of filaments, called **suspensory ligaments,** that project from the ciliary muscle to the edge of the lens around its entire circumference (Fig. 11-8). The ciliary muscle controls the lens' shape to allow for vision at near and far distances. This process of **accommodation** occurs as follows.

The light rays from a close object diverge (separate) more than do the light rays from a distant object (Fig. 11-9). Thus, when viewing something close, the lens must become more rounded to bend the light rays more and focus them on the retina. When the ciliary muscle is relaxed, tension on the suspensory ligaments keeps the lens in a more

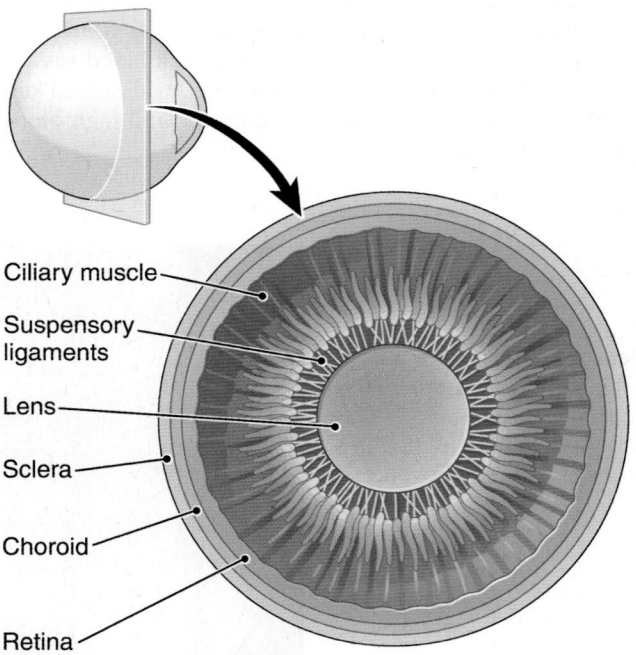

Figure 11-8 **The ciliary muscle and lens (posterior view).** Contraction of the ciliary muscle relaxes tension on the suspensory ligaments, allowing the lens to become more round for near vision. [**ZOOMING IN** ➤ What structures hold the lens in place?]

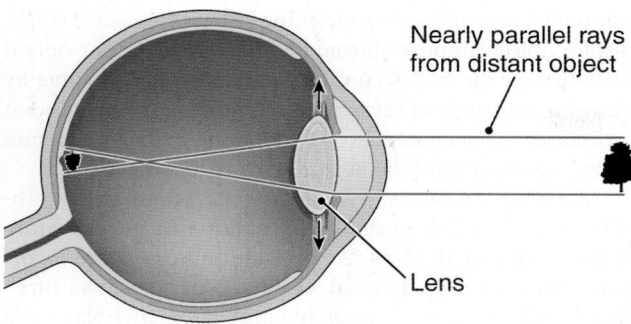

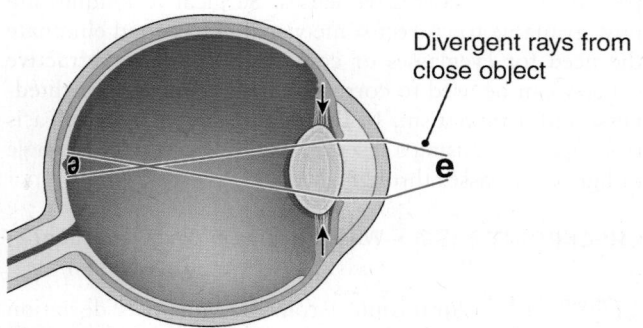

Nearly parallel rays from distant object

Lens

Divergent rays from close object

Figure 11-9 **Accommodation for near vision.** When viewing a close object, the lens must become more rounded to focus light rays on the retina.

flattened shape. For close vision, the ciliary muscle contracts, which draws the ciliary ring forward and relaxes tension on the suspensory ligaments. The elastic lens then recoils and becomes thicker, in much the same way that a rubber band thickens when the pull on it is released. When the ciliary muscle relaxes again, the lens flattens. These actions change the lens' refractive power to accommodate for near and far vision.

In young people, the lens is elastic, and therefore its thickness can be readily adjusted according to the need for near or distance vision. With aging, the lens loses elasticity and therefore its ability to accommodate for near vision. It becomes difficult to focus clearly on close objects, a condition called **presbyopia** (pres-be-O-pe-ah), which literally means "old eye."

CHECKPOINT **11-6** ➤ What is the function of the iris?

CHECKPOINT **11-7** ➤ What is the function of the ciliary muscle?

Nerve Supply to the Eye

Two sensory nerves supply the eye (Fig. 11-10):

- The **optic nerve** (cranial nerve II) carries visual impulses from the retinal rods and cones to the brain.
- The **ophthalmic** (of-THAL-mik) **branch of the trigeminal nerve** (cranial nerve V) carries impulses of pain, touch, and temperature from the eye and surrounding parts to the brain.

The optic nerve arises from the retina a little toward the medial or nasal side of the eye. There are no retinal rods and cones in the area of the optic nerve. Consequently, no image can form on the retina at this point, which is known as the blind spot or **optic disk** (see Figs. 11-3 and 11-5).

The optic nerve transmits impulses from the retina to the thalamus (part of the diencephalon), from which they are directed to the occipital cortex. Note that the light rays passing through the eye are actually overrefracted (bent) so that an image falls on the retina upside down and backward (see Fig. 11-9). It is the job of the brain's visual centers to reverse the images.

Three nerves carry motor impulses to the eyeball muscles:

- The oculomotor nerve (cranial nerve III) is the largest; it supplies voluntary and involuntary motor impulses to all but two eye muscles.
- The trochlear nerve (cranial nerve IV) supplies the superior oblique extrinsic eye muscle (see Fig. 11-6).

11

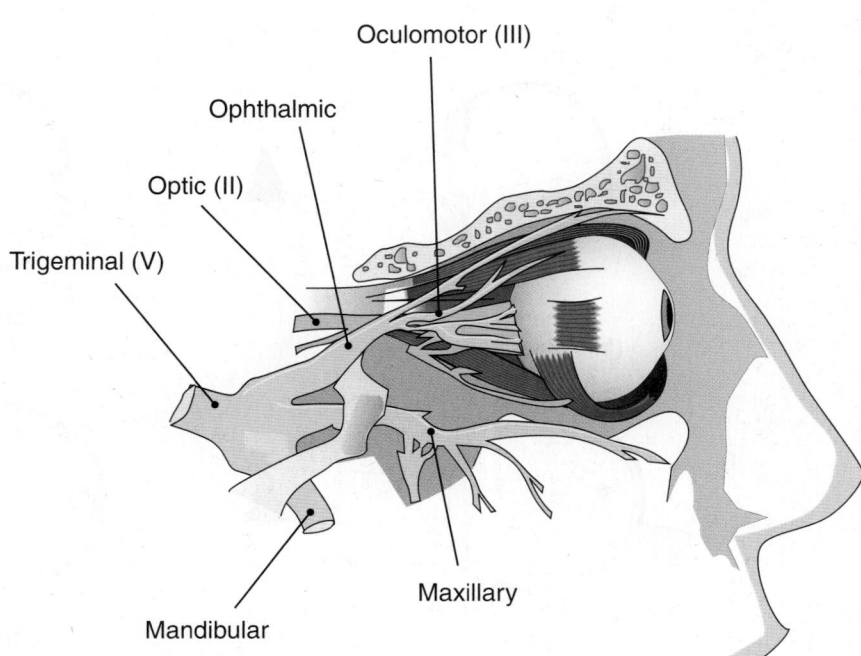

Oculomotor (III)

Ophthalmic

Optic (II)

Trigeminal (V)

Maxillary

Mandibular

Figure 11-10 **Nerves of the eye.** [ZOOMING IN ➤ Which of the nerves shown moves the eye?]

- The abducens nerve (cranial nerve VI) supplies the lateral rectus extrinsic eye muscle.

To summarize, the steps in vision are:

1. Light refracts.
2. The muscles of the iris adjust the pupil.
3. The ciliary muscle adjusts the lens (accommodation).
4. The extrinsic eye muscles produce convergence.
5. Light stimulates retinal receptor cells (rods and cones).
6. The optic nerve transmits impulses to the brain.
7. The occipital lobe cortex interprets the impulses.

CHECKPOINT 11-8 ➤ What is cranial nerve II and what does it do?

Errors of Refraction and Other Eye Disorders

Hyperopia (hi-per-O-pe-ah), or farsightedness, usually results from an abnormally short eyeball (Fig. 11-11A). In this situation, light rays focus behind the retina because they cannot bend sharply enough to focus on the retina. The lens can thicken only to a given limit to accommodate for near vision. If the need for refraction exceeds this limit, a person must move an object away from the eye to see it clearly. Glasses with convex lenses that increase light refraction can correct for hyperopia.

Myopia (mi-O-pe-ah), or nearsightedness, is another eye defect related to development. In this case, the eyeball is too long or the cornea bends the light rays too sharply, so

that the focal point is in front of the retina (see Fig. 11-11B). Distant objects appear blurred and may appear clear only if brought near the eye. A concave lens corrects for myopia by widening the angle of refraction and moving the focal point backward. Nearsightedness in a young person becomes worse each year until the person reaches his or her 20s.

Another common visual defect, **astigmatism** (ah-STIG-mah-tizm), is caused by irregularity in the curvature of the cornea or the lens. As a result, light rays are incorrectly bent, causing blurred vision. Astigmatism is often found in combination with hyperopia or myopia, so a careful eye examination is needed to obtain an accurate prescription for corrective lenses. Surgical techniques are now available to correct some visual defects and eliminate the need for eyeglasses or contact lenses. Such refractive surgery can be used to correct nearsightedness, farsightedness, and astigmatism. In these procedures, the cornea is reshaped, often using a laser, to change the refractive angle of light as it passes through.

CHECKPOINT 11-9 ➤ What are some errors of refraction?

STRABISMUS Strabismus (strah-BIZ-mus) is a deviation of the eye that results from lack of eyeball muscle coordination. That is, the two eyes do not work together. In **convergent strabismus**, the eye deviates toward the nasal side, or medially. This disorder gives an appearance of being cross-eyed. In **divergent strabismus**, the affected eye deviates laterally.

If these disorders are not corrected early, the transmission and interpretation of visual impulses from the affected eye to the brain is decreased. The brain does not develop ways to "see" images from the eye. Loss of vision in a

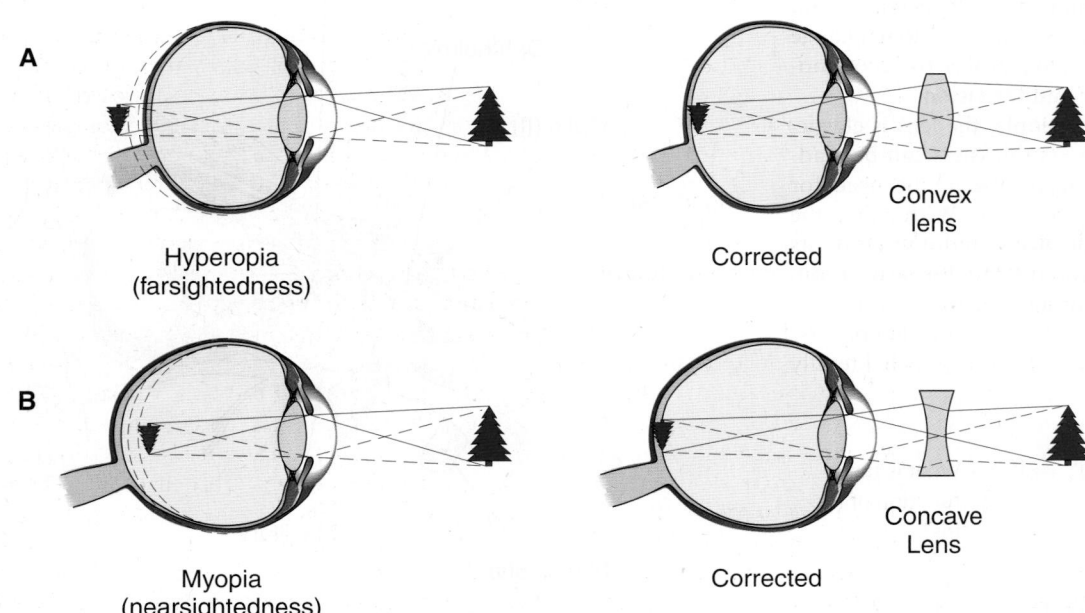

A Hyperopia
(farsightedness)

Convex
lens
Corrected

B Myopia
(nearsightedness)

Concave
Lens
Corrected

Figure 11-11 **Errors of refraction. (A)** Hyperopia (farsightedness). **(B)** Myopia (nearsightedness). A convex lens corrects for hyperopia; a concave lens corrects for myopia, as shown in the right column of the figure.

healthy eye because it cannot work properly with the other eye is termed **amblyopia** (am-ble-O-pe-ah). Care by an ophthalmologist as soon as the condition is detected may result in restoration of muscle balance. In some cases, eye exercises, eye glasses, and patching of one eye correct the defect. In other cases, surgery is required to alter muscle action.

INFECTIONS Inflammation of the conjunctiva is called **conjunctivitis** (kon-junk-tih-VI-tis). It may be acute or chronic and may be caused by a variety of irritants and pathogens. "Pinkeye" is a highly contagious acute conjunctivitis that is usually caused by cocci or bacilli. Sometimes, irritants such as wind and excessive glare cause an inflammation, which may in turn lead to susceptibility to bacterial infection.

Inclusion conjunctivitis is an acute eye infection caused by *Chlamydia trachomatis* (klah-MID-e-ah trah-KO-mah-tis). This same organism causes a sexually transmitted reproductive tract infection. In underdeveloped countries where this eye infection appears in chronic form, it is known as **trachoma** (trah-KO-mah). If not treated, scarring of the conjunctiva and cornea can cause blindness. The use of antibiotics and proper hygiene to prevent reinfection has reduced the incidence of blindness from this disorder in many parts of the world.

An acute eye infection of the newborn, caused by organisms acquired during passage through the birth canal, is called **ophthalmia neonatorum** (of-THAL-me-ah ne-o-na-TO-rum). The usual cause is gonococcus, chlamydia, or some other sexually transmitted organism. Preventive doses of an appropriate antiseptic or antibiotic solution are routinely administered into a newborn's conjunctiva just after birth.

The iris, choroid coat, ciliary body, and other parts of the eyeball may become infected by various organisms. Such disorders are likely to be serious; fortunately, they are not common. Syphilis spirochetes, tubercle bacilli, and a variety of cocci may cause these painful infections. They may follow a sinus infection, tonsillitis, conjunctivitis, or other disorder in which the infecting agent can spread from nearby structures. An ophthalmologist is trained to diagnose and treat these conditions.

INJURIES The most common eye injury is a laceration or scratch of the cornea caused by a foreign body. Injuries caused by foreign objects or by infection may result in corneal scar formation, leaving an area of opacity through which light rays cannot pass. If such an injury involves the central area anterior to the pupil, blindness may result.

Because the cornea lacks blood vessels, a person can receive a corneal transplant without danger of rejection. Eye banks store corneas obtained from donors, and corneal transplantation is a fairly common procedure.

Severe traumatic eye injuries, such as penetration of deeper structures, may not be subject to surgical repair. In such cases, an operation to remove the eyeball, a procedure called **enucleation** (e-nu-kle-A-shun), is performed.

It is important to prevent infection in cases of eye injury. Even a tiny scratch can become so seriously infected that blindness may result. Injuries by pieces of glass and other sharp objects are a frequent cause of eye damage. The incidence of accidents involving the eye has been greatly reduced by the use of protective goggles.

CATARACT A **cataract** is an opacity (cloudiness) of the lens or the lens' outer covering. An early cataract causes a gradual loss of visual acuity (sharpness). An untreated cataract leads to complete vision loss. Surgical removal of the lens followed by implantation of an artificial lens is a highly successful procedure for restoring vision. Although the cause of cataracts is not known, age is a factor, as is excess exposure to ultraviolet rays. Diseases such as diabetes, as well as certain medications, are known to accelerate cataract development.

GLAUCOMA **Glaucoma** is a condition characterized by excess pressure of the aqueous humor. This fluid is produced constantly from the blood, and after circulation in the eye, it is reabsorbed into the bloodstream. Interference with this fluid's normal reentry into the bloodstream leads to an increase in pressure inside the eyeball.

The most common type of glaucoma usually progresses rather slowly, with vague visual disturbances being the only symptom. In most cases, the aqueous humor's high pressure causes destruction of some optic nerve fibers before the person is aware of visual change. Many glaucoma cases are diagnosed by the measurement of pressure in the eye, which should be part of a routine eye examination for people older than 35 years or for those with a family history of glaucoma. Early diagnosis and continuous treatment with medications to reduce pressure frequently result in the preservation of vision.

DISORDERS INVOLVING THE RETINA Diabetes as a cause of blindness is increasing in the United States. In **diabetic retinopathy** (ret-in-OP-ah-the), the retina is damaged by blood vessel hemorrhages and growth of new vessels. Other eye disorders directly related to diabetes include optic atrophy, in which the optic nerve fibers die; cataracts, which occur earlier and with greater frequency among diabetics than among nondiabetics; and retinal detachment.

In cases of **retinal detachment,** the retina separates from the underlying choroid layer as a result of trauma or an accumulation of fluid or tissue between the layers. This disorder may develop slowly or may occur suddenly. If it is left untreated, complete detachment can occur, resulting in blindness. Surgical treatment includes a sort of "spot welding" with an electric current or a weak laser beam. A series of pinpoint scars (connective tissue) develops to reattach the retina.

Macular degeneration is another leading cause of blindness. This name refers to the macula lutea, the yellow area of the retina that contains the fovea centralis. Changes in this area distort the center of the visual field. In one form of macular degeneration, material accumulates on the retina, causing gradual vision loss. In another form, abnormal blood vessels grow under the retina, causing it to detach. Laser surgery may stop the growth of these vessels and delay vision

11

loss. Factors contributing to macular degeneration are smoking, exposure to sunlight, and a high cholesterol diet. Some forms are known to be hereditary. Box 11-1, Eye Surgery: A Glimpse of the Cutting Edge, provides information on new methods of treating eye disorders.

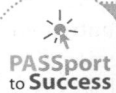

PASSport to Success   Visit *thePoint* or see the Student Resource CD in the back of this book for illustrations of the eye disorders described and also cataract surgery.

The Ear

The ear is the sense organ for both hearing and equilibrium (Fig. 11-12). It is divided into three main sections:

- The **outer ear** includes an outer projection and a canal ending at a membrane.
- The **middle ear** is an air space containing three small bones.
- The **inner ear** is the most complex and contains the sensory receptors for hearing and equilibrium.

The Outer Ear

The external portion of the ear consists of a visible projecting portion, the **pinna** (PIN-nah), also called the **auricle** (AW-rih-kl), and the **external auditory canal**, or **meatus** (me-A-tus), that leads into the ear's deeper parts. The pinna directs sound waves into the ear, but it is probably of little importance in humans. The external auditory canal extends medially from the pinna for about 2.5 cm or more, depending on which wall of the canal is measured. The skin lining this tube is thin and, in the first part of the canal, contains many wax-producing **ceruminous** (seh-RU-mih-nus) **glands.** The wax, or **cerumen** (seh-RU-men), may become dried and impacted in the canal and must then be removed. The same kinds of disorders that involve the skin elsewhere—atopic dermatitis, boils, and other infections—may also affect the skin of the external auditory canal.

The **tympanic** (tim-PAN-ik) **membrane,** or eardrum, is at the end of the external auditory canal. It is a boundary between this canal and the middle ear cavity, and it vibrates freely as sound waves enter the ear.

The Middle Ear and Ossicles

The middle ear cavity is a small, flattened space that contains three small bones, or **ossicles** (OS-ih-klz) (see Fig. 11-12). The three ossicles are joined in such a way that they amplify the sound waves received by the tympanic membrane as they transmit the sounds to the inner ear. The first bone is shaped like a hammer and is called the **malleus** (MAL-e-us) (Fig. 11-13). The handlelike part of the malleus is attached to the tympanic membrane, whereas the headlike part is connected to the second bone, the **incus** (ING-kus). The incus is shaped like an anvil, an

---

Box 11-1   Hot Topics

Eye Surgery: A Glimpse of the Cutting Edge

Cataracts, glaucoma, and refractive errors are the most common eye disorders affecting Americans. In the past, cataract and glaucoma treatments concentrated on managing the diseases. Refractive errors were corrected using eyeglasses and, more recently, contact lenses. Today, laser and microsurgical techniques can remove cataracts, reduce glaucoma, and allow people with refractive errors to put their eyeglasses and contacts away. These cutting-edge procedures include:

- *Laser in situ keratomileusis (LASIK)* to correct refractive errors. During this procedure, a laser reshapes the cornea to allow light to refract directly on the retina, rather than in front of or behind it. A microkeratome (surgical knife) is used to cut a flap in the cornea's outer layer. A computer-controlled laser sculpts the middle layer of the cornea and then the flap is replaced. The procedure takes only a few minutes and patients recover their vision quickly and usually with little postoperative pain.

- *Laser trabeculoplasty* to treat glaucoma. This procedure uses a laser to help drain fluid from the eye and lower intraocular pressure. The laser is aimed at drainage canals located between the cornea and iris and makes several burns that are believed to open the canals and allow fluid to drain better. The procedure is typically painless and takes only a few minutes.

- *Phacoemulsification* to remove cataracts. During this surgical procedure, a very small incision (approximately 3 mm long) is made through the sclera near the cornea's outer edge. An ultrasonic probe is inserted through this opening and into the center of the lens. The probe uses sound waves to emulsify the lens' central core, which is then suctioned out. Then, an artificial lens is permanently implanted in the lens capsule. The procedure is typically painless, although the patient may feel some discomfort for 1 to 2 days afterward.

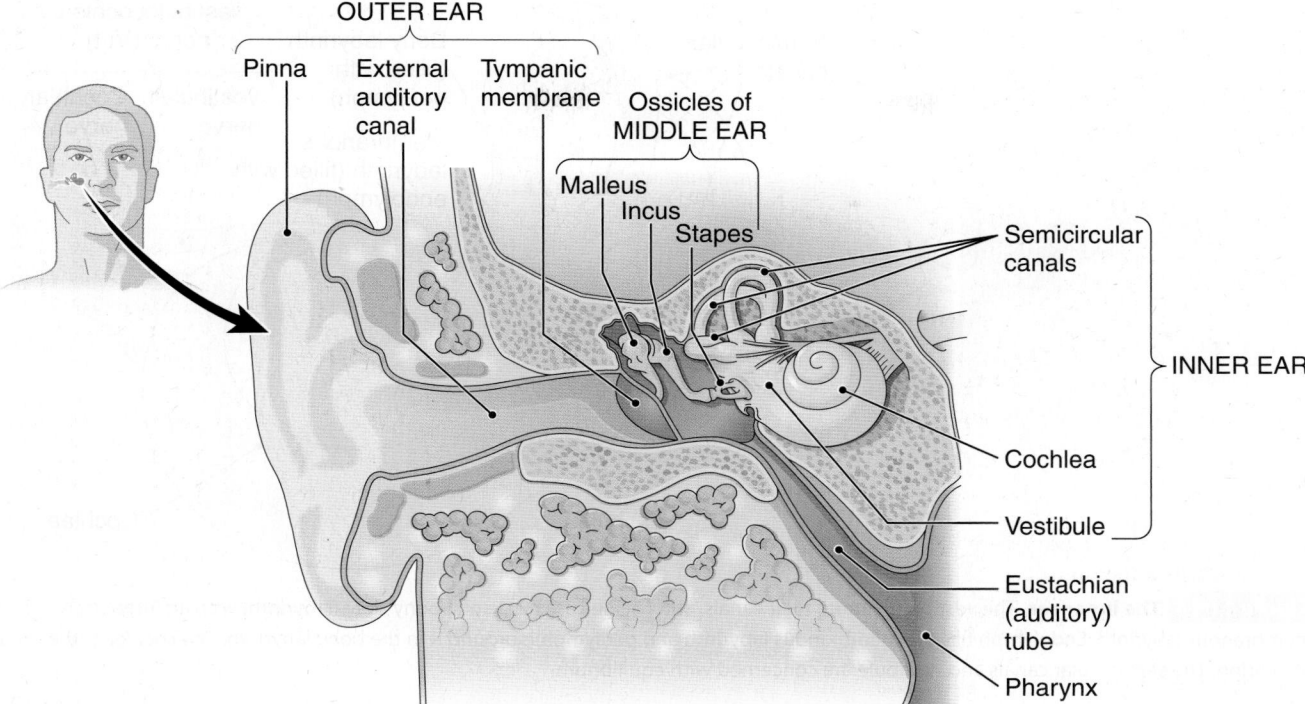

Pinna

External auditory canal

Tympanic membrane

Ossicles of MIDDLE EAR

Malleus

Incus

Stapes

Semicircular canals

INNER EAR

Cochlea

Vestibule

Eustachian (auditory) tube

Pharynx

Figure 11-12 **The ear.** Structures in the outer, middle, and inner divisions are shown.

iron block used in shaping metal, as is used by a black-smith. The innermost ossicle is shaped somewhat like the stirrup of a saddle and is called the **stapes** (STA-peze). The base of the stapes is in contact with the inner ear.

CHECKPOINT **11-10** ► What are the ossicles of the ear and what do they do?

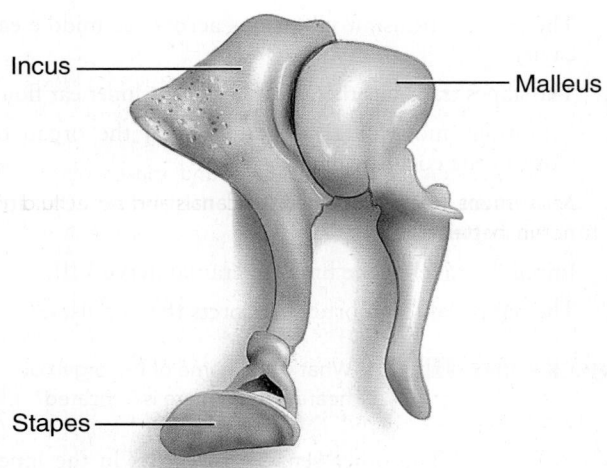

Incus

Malleus

Stapes

Figure 11-13 **The ossicles of the middle ear.** The handle of the malleus is in contact with the tympanic membrane, and the headlike part with the incus. The base of the stapes is in contact with the inner ear (×30). (Image provided by Anatomical Chart Co.)

THE EUSTACHIAN TUBE The **eustachian** (u-STA-shun) **tube** (auditory tube) connects the middle ear cavity with the throat, or pharynx (FAR-inks) (see Fig. 11-12). This tube opens to allow pressure to equalize on the two sides of the tympanic membrane. A valve that closes the tube can be forced open by swallowing hard, yawning, or blowing with the nose and mouth sealed, as one often does when experiencing pain from pressure changes in an airplane.

The mucous membrane of the pharynx is continuous through the eustachian tube into the middle ear cavity. At the posterior of the middle ear cavity is an opening into the mastoid air cells, which are spaces inside the temporal bone's mastoid process (see Fig. 7-5B).

The Inner Ear

The ear's most complicated and important part is the internal portion, which is described as a *labyrinth* (LAB-ih-rinth) because it has a complex mazelike construction. It consists of three separate areas containing sensory receptors. The skeleton of the inner ear is called the **bony labyrinth** (Fig. 11-14). It has three divisions:

- The **vestibule** consists of two bony chambers that contain some of the receptors for equilibrium.

- The **semicircular canals** are three projecting bony tubes located toward the posterior. Areas at the bases of the semicircular canals also contain receptors for equilibrium.

11

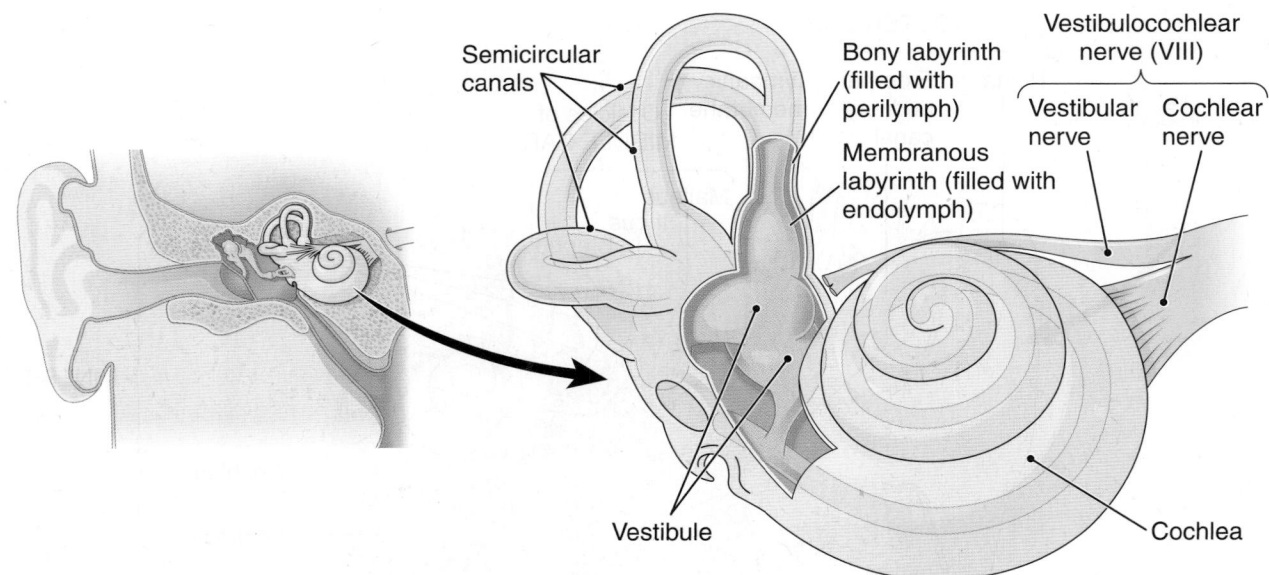

Figure 11-14 **The inner ear.** The vestibule, semicircular canals, and cochlea are made of a bony shell (labyrinth) with an interior membranous labyrinth. Endolymph fills the membranous labyrinth and perilymph is around it in the bony labyrinth. The cochlea is the organ of hearing. The semicircular canals and vestibule are concerned with equilibrium.

■　The **cochlea** (KOK-le-ah) is coiled like a snail shell and is located toward the anterior. It contains the receptors for hearing.

All three divisions of the bony labyrinth contain a fluid called **perilymph** (PER-e-limf).

Within the bony labyrinth is an exact replica of this bony shell made of membrane, much like an inner tube within a tire. The tubes and chambers of this **membranous labyrinth** are filled with a fluid called **endolymph** (EN-do-limf) (see Fig. 11-14). The endolymph is within the membranous labyrinth, and the perilymph surrounds it. These fluids are important to the sensory functions of the inner ear.

HEARING The organ of hearing, called the **organ of Corti** (KOR-te), consists of ciliated receptor cells located inside the membranous cochlea, or **cochlear duct** (Fig. 11-15). Sound waves enter the external auditory canal and cause vibrations in the tympanic membrane. The ossicles amplify these vibrations and finally transmit them from the stapes to a membrane covering the **oval window** of the inner ear.

As the sound waves move through the fluids in these chambers, they set up vibrations in the cochlear duct. As a result, the tiny, hairlike cilia on the receptor cells (hair cells) begin to move back and forth against the **tectorial membrane** above them. (The membrane is named from a Latin word that means "roof.") This motion sets up nerve impulses that travel to the brain in the **cochlear nerve**, a branch of the eighth cranial nerve (formerly called the *auditory* or *acoustic nerve*). Sound waves ultimately leave the ear through another membrane-covered space in the bony labyrinth, the **round window**.

Hearing receptors respond to both the pitch (tone) of sound and its intensity (loudness). The various pitches stimulate different regions of the organ of Corti. Receptors detect higher-pitched sounds near the base of the cochlea and lower-pitched sounds near the top. Loud sounds stimulate more cells and produce more vibrations, sending more nerve impulses to the brain. Exposure to loud noises, such as very loud music, jet plane noise, or industrial noises, can damage the receptors for particular pitches of sound and lead to hearing loss for those tones.

The steps in hearing are:

1. Sound waves enter the external auditory canal.

2. The tympanic membrane vibrates.

3. The ossicles transmit vibrations across the middle ear cavity.

4. The stapes transmits the vibrations to the inner ear fluid.

5. Vibrations move cilia on hair cells of the organ of Corti in the cochlear duct.

6. Movement against the tectorial membrane generates nerve impulses.

7. Impulses travel to the brain in cranial nerve VIII.

8. The temporal lobe cortex interprets the impulses.

CHECKPOINT **11-11** ➤ What is the name of the organ of hearing and where is it located?

EQUILIBRIUM The other sensory receptors in the inner ear are those related to equilibrium (balance). They are located in the vestibule and the semicircular canals. Receptors for the sense of equilibrium are also ciliated cells or hair cells. As the head moves, a shift in the position of the cilia within the thick fluid around them generates a nerve impulse.

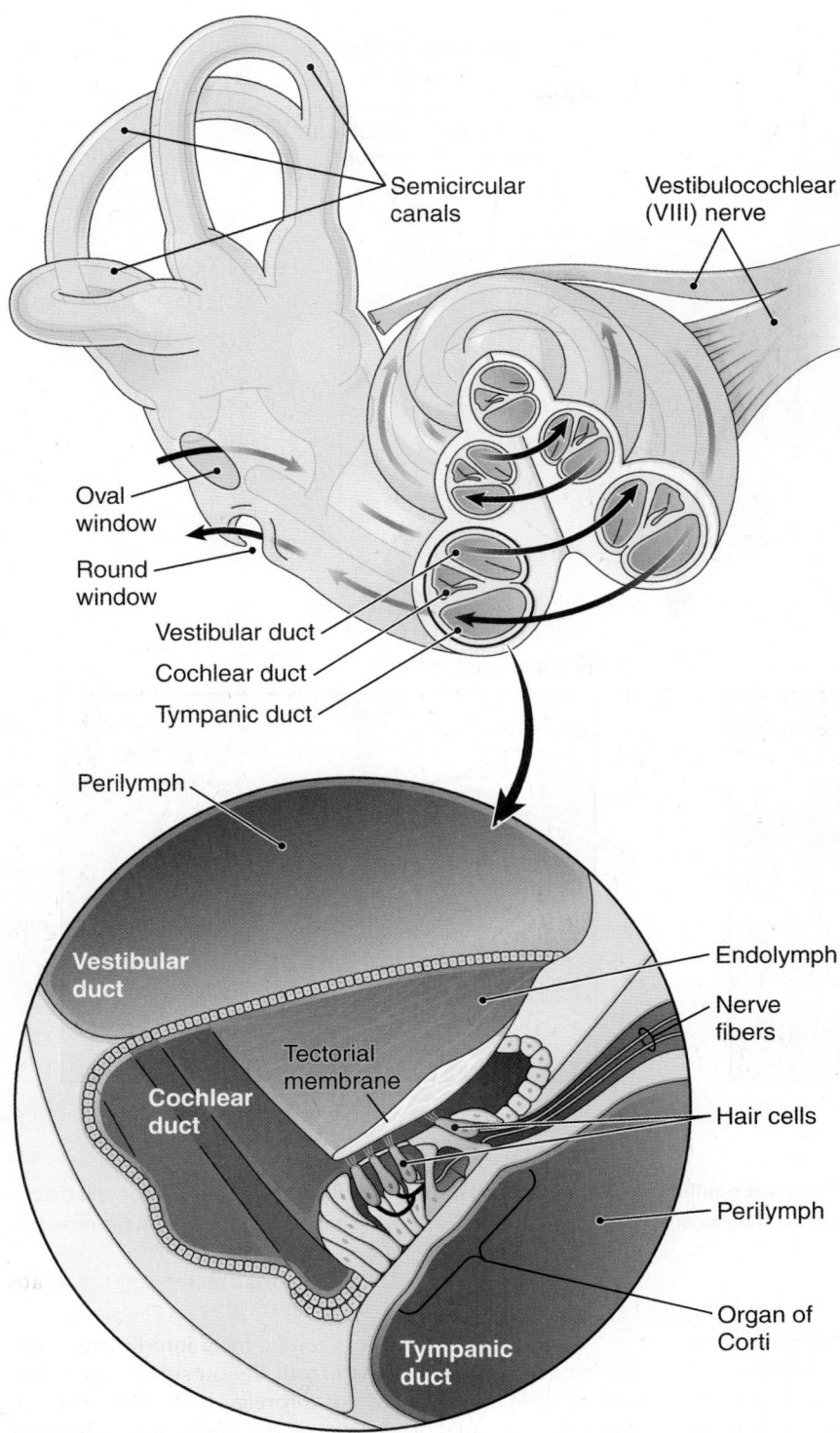

Figure 11-15 **Cochlea and the organ of Corti.** The arrows show the direction of sound waves in the cochlea.

Labels in figure: Semicircular canals · Vestibulocochlear (VIII) nerve · Oval window · Round window · Vestibular duct · Cochlear duct · Tympanic duct · Perilymph · Vestibular duct · Cochlear duct · Tectorial membrane · Tympanic duct · Endolymph · Nerve fibers · Hair cells · Perilymph · Organ of Corti

CHECKPOINT 11-12 ➤ Where are the receptors for equilibrium located?

Receptors located in the vestibule's two small chambers sense the position of the head or the position of the body when moving in a straight line, as in a moving vehicle or when tilting the head. This form of equilibrium is termed **static equilibrium**. Each receptor is called a **macula**. (There is also a macula in the eye, but *macula* is a general term that means "spot.") The fluid above the hair cells contains small crystals of calcium carbonate, called **otoliths** (O-to-liths), which add drag to the fluid around the receptor cells and increase the effect of gravity's pull (Fig. 11-16). Similar devices that help in balance are found in lower animals, such as fish and crustaceans.

The receptors for **dynamic equilibrium** function when the body is spinning or moving in different directions. The receptors, called **cristae** (KRIS-te), are located at the bases of the semicircular canals (Fig. 11-17). It's easy to remember what these receptors do, because the semicircular canals go off in different directions.

Nerve fibers from the vestibule and from the semicircular canals form the **vestibular** (ves-TIB-u-lar) **nerve**, which joins the cochlear nerve to form the vestibulocochlear nerve, the eighth cranial nerve.

CHECKPOINT 11-13 ➤ What are the two types of equilibrium?

Otitis and Other Disorders of the Ear

Infection and inflammation of the middle ear cavity, **otitis media** (o-TI-tis ME-de-ah), is relatively common. A variety of bacteria and viruses may cause otitis media, and it is a frequent complication of measles, influenza, and other infections, especially those of the pharynx. Pathogens are transmitted from the pharynx to the middle ear most often in children, partly because the eustachian tube is relatively short and horizontal in the child; in the adult, the tube is longer and tends to slant down toward the pharynx. Antibiotic drugs have reduced complications and have caused a marked reduction in the amount of surgery done to drain middle ear infections. In some cases, however, pressure from pus or exudate in the middle ear can be relieved only by cutting the tympanic membrane, a procedure called a **myringotomy** (mir-in-GOT-o-me). Placement of a **tympanostomy**

11

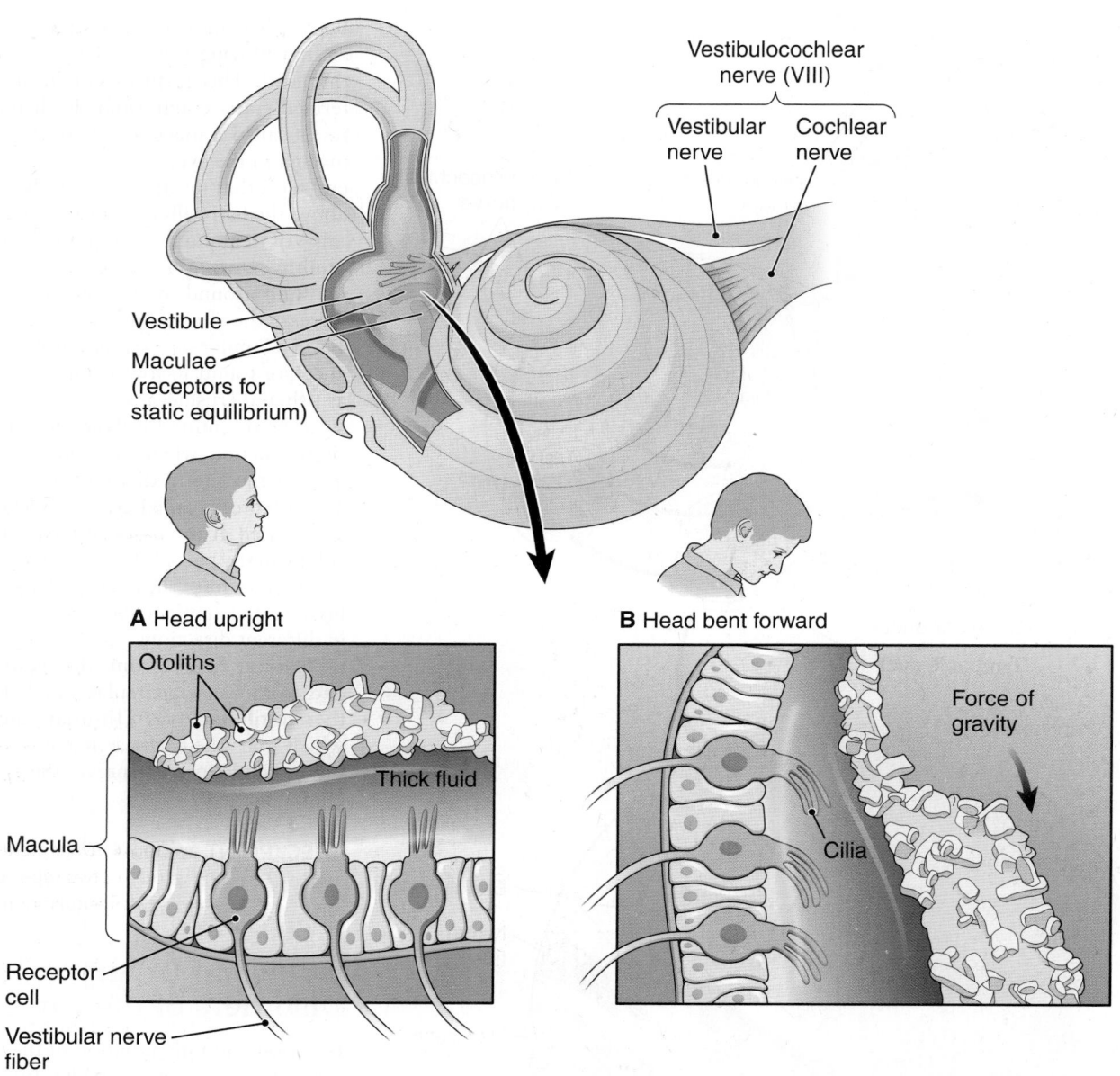

A Head upright

B Head bent forward

Figure 11-16 **Action of the receptors (maculae) for static equilibrium.** As the head moves, the thick fluid above the receptor cells (hair cells), weighted with otoliths, pulls on the cells' cilia, generating a nerve impulse. [**ZOOMING IN** ➤ What happens to the cilia on the receptor cells when the fluid around them moves?]

(tim-pan-OS-to-me) **tube** in the eardrum allows pressure to equalize and prevents further damage to the eardrum.

Otitis externa is inflammation of the external auditory canal. Infections in this area may be caused by a fungus or bacterium. They are most common among those living in hot climates and among swimmers, leading to the alternate name "swimmer's ear."

HEARING LOSS Another disorder of the ear is hearing loss, which may be partial or complete. When the loss is complete, the condition is called **deafness**. The two main types of hearing loss are **conductive hearing loss** and **sensorineural hearing loss**.

Conductive hearing loss results from interference with the passage of sound waves from the outside to the inner ear. In this condition, wax or a foreign body may obstruct the external canal. Blockage of the eustachian tube prevents the equalization of air pressure on both sides of the tympanic membrane, thereby decreasing the membrane's ability to vibrate. Another cause of conductive hearing loss is damage to the tympanic membrane and ossicles resulting from chronic otitis media or from **otosclerosis** (o-to-skle-RO-sis), a hereditary bone disorder that prevents normal vibration of the stapes. Surgical removal of the diseased stapes and its replacement with an artificial device allows sound conduction from the ossicles to the cochlea.

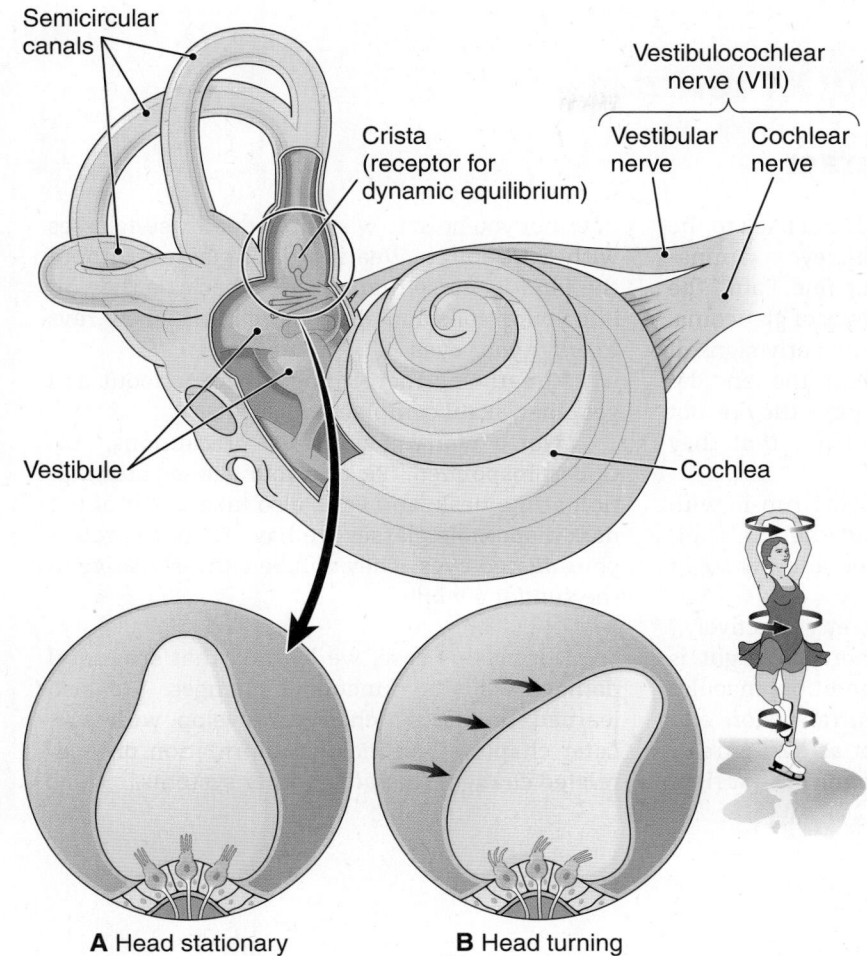

A Head stationary   **B** Head turning

Figure 11-17 **Action of the receptors (cristae) for dynamic equilibrium.** As the body spins or moves in different directions, the cilia bend as the head changes position, generating nerve impulses.

Sensorineural hearing loss may involve the cochlea, the vestibulocochlear nerve, or the brain areas concerned with hearing. It may result from prolonged exposure to loud noises, from the long-term use of certain drugs, or from exposure to various infections and toxins. People with severe hearing loss that originates in the inner ear may benefit from a cochlear implant. This prosthetic device stimulates the cochlear nerve directly, bypassing the receptor cells, and may restore hearing for medium to loud sounds.

> **PASSport to Success** Visit *thePoint* or see the Student Resource CD in the back of this book for information on how audiologists help to treat hearing disorders.

Presbycusis (pres-be-KU-sis) is a slowly progressive hearing loss that often accompanies aging. The condition involves gradual atrophy of the sensory receptors and cochlear nerve fibers. The affected person may experience

a sense of isolation and depression, and may need psychological help. Because the ability to hear high-pitched sounds is usually lost first, it is important to address elderly people in clear, low-pitched tones.

Other Special Sense Organs

The sense organs of taste and smell are designed to respond to chemical stimuli.

Sense of Taste

The sense of taste, or **gustation** (gus-TA-shun), involves receptors in the tongue and two different nerves that carry taste impulses to the brain (Fig. 11-18). The taste receptors, known as **taste buds**, are located along the edges of small, depressed areas called **fissures**. Taste buds are stimulated only if the substance to be tasted is in solution or dissolves in the fluids of the mouth. Receptors for four basic tastes are localized in different regions, forming a "taste map" of the tongue (see Fig. 11-18B):

- **Sweet** tastes are most acutely experienced at the tip of the tongue (hence the popularity of lollipops and ice cream cones).

- **Salty** tastes are most acute at the anterior sides of the tongue.

- **Sour** tastes are most effectively detected by the taste buds located laterally on the tongue.

- **Bitter** tastes are detected at the tongue's posterior part.

Taste maps vary among people, but in each person certain tongue regions are more sensitive to a specific basic taste. Other tastes are a combination of these four with additional smell sensations. More recently, researchers have identified some other tastes besides these basic four: water, alkaline (basic), and metallic. Another is umami (u-MOM-e), a pungent or savory taste based on a response to the amino acid glutamate. Glutamate is found in MSG (monosodium glutamate), a flavor enhancer used in Asian food. Water taste receptors are mainly in the throat and may help to regulate water balance.

The nerves of taste include the facial and the glossopharyngeal cranial nerves (VII and IX). The interpretation of taste impulses is probably accomplished by the brain's lower frontal cortex, although there may be no sharply separate gustatory center.

11

Disease in Context revisited

➤ Early Signs of Cataract

Dr. Gilbert's assistant called Paul back to the consultation room after his eye examination. "You seem to be doing fine, Paul," the ophthalmologist reported. "No signs of glaucoma. I am a little concerned about some early signs of cataract, though. These opacities of the lens develop with age in most people, and they're not hereditary, but there's firm evidence that they are influenced by sun exposure."

"Yikes!" Paul exploded. "Another run-in with the sun! I've already heard about the sun's unfriendly rays with my skin cancer, and I thought that's where it would end."

"Cataracts can be dealt with pretty effectively," said Dr. Gilbert, "but there's more. Sunlight is also a factor in a more serious condition, macular degeneration, which affects central vision and can lead to blindness. That's not as easily treatable at present. I don't see any signs of that right now, but you need to wear good quality sunglasses with a UV filter. Wearing dark glasses without the filter is worse than nothing, because they dilate your pupils and allow more harmful UV rays to enter your eyes."

"Great! One more thing to worry about as I get older," Paul complained.

"Not a worry if you take precautions," Dr. Gilbert responded. "Pick up your glasses prescription at the desk, and Paul, also take a pair of the dark disposable glasses we have there to protect your dilated eyes. They will be extra-sensitive to the sun for a while."

During this case, we learned that structural damage leads to functional changes. We also learned that some changes develop with age. Later chapters will include information on age-related changes that affect other systems.

Sense of Smell

The importance of the sense of smell, or **olfaction** (ol-FAK-shun), is often underestimated. This sense helps to detect gases and other harmful substances in the environment and helps to warn of spoiled food. Smells can trigger memories and other psychological responses. Smell is also important in sexual behavior.

The receptors for smell are located in the epithelium of the nasal cavity's superior region (see Fig. 11-18). Again, the chemicals detected must be in solution in the fluids that line the nose. Because these receptors are high in the nasal cavity, one must "sniff" to bring odors upward in the nose.

The impulses from the smell receptors are carried by the olfactory nerve (I), which leads directly to the olfactory center in the brain's temporal cortex. The interpretation of smell is closely related to the sense of taste, but a greater variety of dissolved chemicals can be detected by smell than by taste. The smell of foods is just as important in stimulating appetite and the flow of digestive juices as is the sense of taste. When one has a cold, food often seems tasteless and unappetizing because nasal congestion reduces the ability to smell the food.

The olfactory receptors deteriorate with age and food may become less appealing. It is important when presenting food to elderly people that the food look inviting so as to stimulate their appetites.

CHECKPOINT 11-14 ➤ What are the special senses that respond to chemical stimuli?

The General Senses

Unlike the special sensory receptors, which are localized within specific sense organs, limited to a relatively small area, the general sensory receptors are scattered throughout the body. These include receptors for touch, pressure, heat, cold, position, and pain (Fig. 11-19).

Sense of Touch

The touch receptors, **tactile** (TAK-til) **corpuscles**, are found mostly in the dermis of the skin and around hair follicles. Touch sensitivity varies with the number of touch receptors in different areas. They are especially numerous and close together in the tips of the fingers and the toes. The lips and the tip of the tongue also contain many of these receptors and are very sensitive to touch. Other areas, such as the back of the hand and the back of the neck, have fewer receptors and are less sensitive to touch. Also included in this category are receptors in the walls of the large arteries that monitor blood pressure. Known as **baroreceptors** (bar-o-re-SEP-torz), these receptors trigger responses that control blood pressure as the vessels stretch (see Chapter 15).

Sense of Temperature

The temperature receptors are **free nerve endings**, receptors that are not enclosed in capsules but are merely branchings of nerve fibers. Temperature receptors are widely distributed in the skin, and there are separate receptors for heat and cold. A warm object stimulates only the heat receptors, and a cool object affects only the cold receptors. Internally, there are temperature receptors in the brain's hypothalamus, which help to adjust body temperature according to the temperature of the circulating blood.

Sense of Position

Receptors located in muscles, tendons, and joints relay impulses that aid in judging one's position and changes in the locations of body parts in relation to each other. They also inform the brain of the amount of muscle contraction and tendon tension. These rather widespread receptors, known as **proprioceptors** (pro-pre-o-SEP-tors), are aided in this function by the internal ear's equilibrium receptors.

Information received by these receptors is needed for the coordination of muscles and is important in such activities as walking, running, and many more complicated skills, such as playing a musical instrument. They help to provide a sense of body movement, known as **kinesthesia** (kin-es-THE-ze-ah). Proprioceptors play an important part in maintaining muscle tone and good posture. They also help to assess the weight of an object to be lifted so that the right amount of muscle force is used.

The nerve fibers that carry impulses from these receptors enter the spinal cord and ascend to the brain in the posterior part of the cord. The cerebellum is a main coordinating center for these impulses.

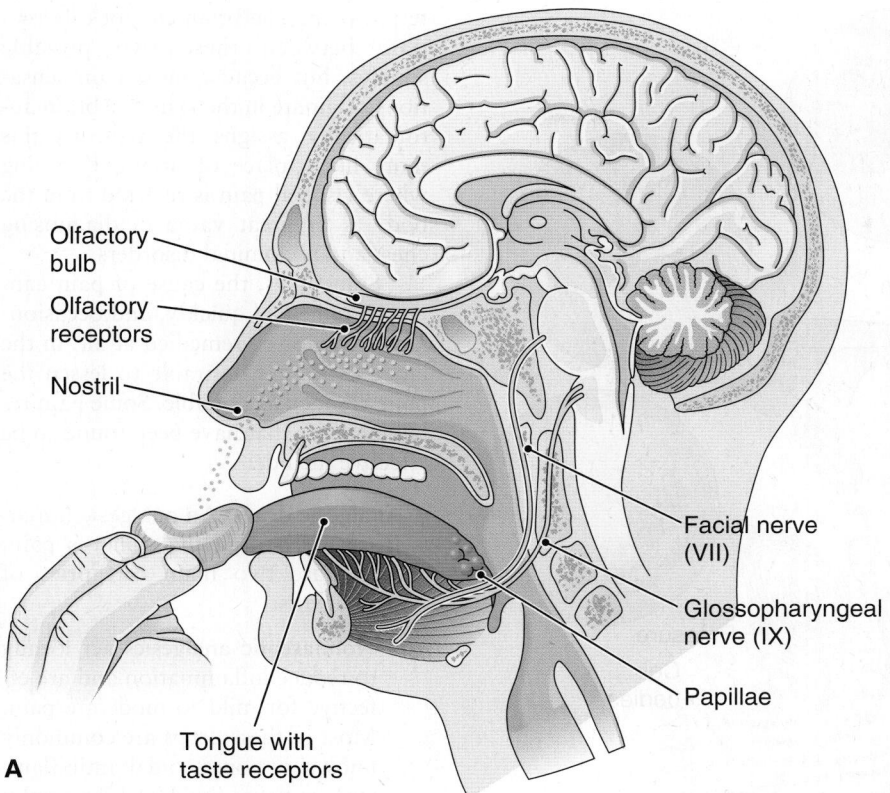

TASTE ZONES:
Sweet   Salty   Sour   Bitter

B

Figure 11-18 **Special senses that respond to chemicals. (A)** Organs of taste (gustation) and smell (olfaction). **(B)** A taste map of the tongue.

Olfactory bulb
Olfactory receptors
Nostril
Facial nerve (VII)
Glossopharyngeal nerve (IX)
Papillae
Tongue with taste receptors
A

Sense of Pressure

Even when the skin is anesthetized, it can still respond to pressure stimuli. These sensory end-organs for deep pressure are located in the subcutaneous tissues beneath the skin and also near joints, muscles, and other deep tissues. They are sometimes referred to as *receptors for deep touch.*

CHECKPOINT **11-15** ➤ What are examples of general senses?

CHECKPOINT **11-16** ➤ What are proprioceptors and where are they located?

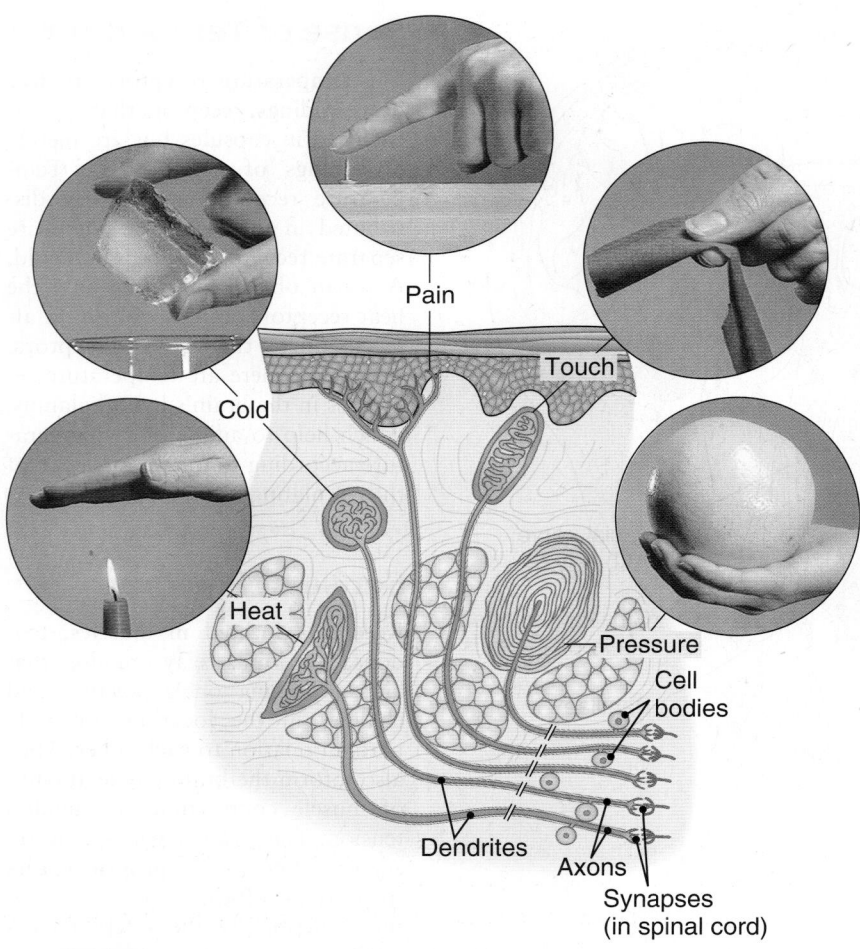

Pain

Touch

Cold

Heat

Pressure

Cell bodies

Dendrites

Axons

Synapses (in spinal cord)

Figure 11-19 **Sensory receptors in the skin.** Synapses are in the spinal cord.

Sense of Pain

Pain is the most important protective sense. The receptors for pain are widely distributed free nerve endings. They are found in the skin, muscles, and joints and to a lesser extent in most internal organs (including the blood vessels and viscera). Two pathways transmit pain to the CNS. One is for acute, sharp pain, and the other is for slow, chronic pain. Thus, a single strong stimulus produces the immediate sharp pain, followed in a second or so by the slow, diffuse, burning pain that increases in severity with time.

Referred pain is pain that is felt in an outer part of the body, particularly the skin, but actually originates in an internal organ located nearby. Liver and gallbladder disease often cause referred pain in the skin over the right shoulder. Spasm of the coronary arteries that supply the heart may cause pain in the left shoulder and arm. Infection of the appendix is felt as pain of the skin covering the lower right abdominal quadrant.

Apparently, some neurons in the spinal cord have the twofold duty of conducting impulses from visceral pain receptors in the chest and abdomen and from somatic pain receptors in neighboring areas of the skin, resulting in re-

ferred pain. The brain cannot differentiate between these two possible sources, but because most pain sensations originate in the skin, the brain automatically assigns the pain to this more likely place of origin. Knowing where visceral pain is referred to in the body is of great value in diagnosing chest and abdominal disorders.

Sometimes, the cause of pain cannot be remedied quickly, and occasionally it cannot be remedied at all. In the latter case, it is desirable to lessen the pain as much as possible. Some pain relief methods that have been found to be effective include:

- **Analgesic drugs.** An analgesic (an-al-JE-zik) is a drug that relieves pain. There are two main categories of such agents:

  - > **Nonnarcotic analgesics** act locally to reduce inflammation and are effective for mild to moderate pain. Most of these drugs are commonly known as nonsteroidal antiinflammatory drugs (NSAIDs). Examples are ibuprofen (i-bu-PRO-fen) and naproxen (na-PROK-sen).

  - > **Narcotics** act on the CNS to alter the perception and response to pain. Effective for severe pain, narcotics are administered by varied methods, including orally and by intramuscular injection. They are also effectively administered into the space surrounding the spinal cord. An example of a narcotic drug is morphine.

- > **Anesthetics.** Although most commonly used to prevent pain during surgery, anesthetic injections are also used to relieve certain types of chronic pain.

- > **Endorphins** (en-DOR-fins) are released naturally from certain brain regions and are associated with pain control. Massage, acupressure, and electric stimulation are among the techniques that are thought to activate this system of natural pain relief.

- > **Applications of heat or cold** can be a simple but effective means of pain relief, either alone or in combination with medications. Care must be taken to avoid injury caused by excessive heat or cold.

- > **Relaxation or distraction techniques** include several methods that reduce pain perception in the CNS. Relaxation techniques counteract the fight-or-flight response to pain and complement other pain-control methods.

Sensory Adaptation

When sensory receptors are exposed to a continuous stimulus, receptors often adjust themselves so that the sensation becomes less acute. The term for this phenomenon is **sensory adaptation**. For example, if you immerse your hand in very warm water, it may be uncomfortable; however, if you leave your hand there, soon the water will feel less hot (even if it has not cooled appreciably).

Receptors adapt at different rates. Those for warmth, cold, and light pressure adapt rapidly. In contrast, those for pain do not adapt. In fact, the sensations from the slow pain fibers tend to increase over time. This variation in receptors allows us to save energy by not responding to unimportant stimuli while always heeding the warnings of pain.

Word Anatomy

Medical terms are built from standardized word parts (prefixes, roots, and suffixes). Learning the meanings of these parts can help you remember words and interpret unfamiliar terms.

WORD PART	MEANING	EXAMPLE
The Eye and Vision		
ophthalm/o	eye	An *ophthalmologist* is a physician who specializes in treatment of the eye.
-scope	instrument for examination	An *ophthalmoscope* is an instrument used to examine the posterior of the eye.
lute/o	yellow	The macula *lutea* is a yellowish spot in the retina that contains the fovea centralis.
presby-	old	*Presbyopia* is farsightedness that occurs with age.
-opia	disorder of the eye or vision	*Hyperopia* is farsightedness.
ambly/o	dimness	*Amblyopia* is poor vision in a healthy eye that cannot work properly with the other eye.
e-	out	*Enucleation* is removal of the eyeball.
The Ear		
tympan/o	drum	The *tympanic* membrane is the eardrum.
equi-	equal	*Equilibrium* is balance (*equi-* combined with the Latin word *libra* meaning "balance").
ot/o	ear	*Otitis* is inflammation of the ear.
lith	stone	*Otoliths* are small crystals in the inner ear that aid in static equilibrium.
myring/o	tympanic membrane	*Myringotomy* is a cutting of the tympanic membrane to relieve pressure.
-stomy	creation of an opening between two structures	A *tympanostomy* tube creates a passageway through the tympanic membrane.
-cusis	hearing	*Presbycusis* is hearing loss associated with age.

11

WORD PART	MEANING	EXAMPLE
The General Senses		
propri/o-	own	*Proprioception* is perception of one's own body position.
kine	movement	*Kinesthesia* is a sense of body movement.
-esthesia	sensation	*Anesthesia* is loss of sensation, as of pain.
-alges/i	pain	An *analgesic* is a drug that relieves pain.
narc/o	stupor	A *narcotic* is a drug that alters the perception of pain.

Summary

I. **THE SENSES**
   A. Protect by detecting changes (stimuli) in the environment
   B. Sensory receptors—detect stimuli
      1. Structural types
         a. Free dendrite
         b. End-organ—modified dendrite
         c. Specialized cell—in special sense organs
      2. Types based on stimulus
         a. Chemoreceptors—respond to chemicals
         b. Thermoreceptors—respond to temperature
         c. Photoreceptors—respond to light
         d. Mechanoreceptors—respond to movement
   C. Special and general senses
      1. Special senses—vision, hearing, equilibrium, taste, smell
      2. General senses—touch, pressure, temperature, position, pain

II. **THE EYE AND VISION**
   A. Protection of the eyeball—bony orbit, eyelid, eyelashes, conjunctiva, lacrimal glands (produce tears)
   B. Coats of the eyeball
      1. Sclera—white of the eye
         a. Cornea—anterior
      2. Choroid—pigmented; contains blood vessels
      3. Retina—receptor layer
   C. Pathway of light rays and refraction
      1. Refraction—bending of light rays as they pass through substances of different density
      2. Refracting parts—cornea, aqueous humor, lens, vitreous body
   D. Function of the retina
      1. Cells
         a. Rods—cannot detect color; function in dim light
         b. Cones—detect color; function in bright light
      2. Pigments—sensitive to light; rod pigment is rhodopsin

   E. Muscles of the eye
      1. Extrinsic muscles—six move each eyeball
      2. Intrinsic muscles
         a. Iris—colored ring around pupil; regulates the amount of light entering the eye
         b. Ciliary muscle—regulates the thickness of the lens to accommodate for near vision
   F. Nerve supply to the eye
      1. Sensory nerves
         a. Optic nerve (II)—carries impulses from retina to brain
         b. Ophthalmic branch of trigeminal (V)
      2. Motor nerves—move eyeball
         a. Oculomotor (III), trochlear (IV), abducens (VI)
   G. Errors of refraction and other eye disorders
      1. Errors of refraction—hyperopia (farsightedness), myopia (nearsightedness), astigmatism
      2. Strabismus—deviation
      3. Infections—conjunctivitis, trachoma, ophthalmia neonatorum
      4. Injuries
      5. Cataract—opacity of the lens
      6. Glaucoma—damage caused by increased pressure
      7. Retinal disorders—retinopathy, retinal detachment, macular degeneration

III. **THE EAR**
   A. Outer ear—pinna, auditory canal (meatus), tympanic membrane (eardrum)
   B. Middle ear and ossicles
      1. Ossicles—malleus, incus, stapes
      2. Eustachian tube—connects middle ear with pharynx to equalize pressure
   C. Inner ear
      1. Bony labyrinth—contains perilymph
      2. Membranous labyrinth—contains endolymph
      3. Divisions
         a. Cochlea—contains receptors for hearing (organ of Corti)

b. Vestibule—contains receptors for static equilibrium (maculae)

c. Semicircular canals—contain receptors for dynamic equilibrium (cristae)

4. Receptor (hair) cells function by movement of cilia

5. Nerve—vestibulocochlear (auditory) nerve (VIII)

D. Disorders of the ear

1. Otitis (infection)—otitis media, otitis externa

2. Hearing loss

a. conductive

b. sensorineural

IV. OTHER SPECIAL SENSE ORGANS

A. Sense of taste (gustation)

1. Receptors—taste buds on tongue

2. Basic tastes—sweet, salty, sour, bitter

3. Nerves—facial (VII) and glossopharyngeal (IX)

B. Sense of smell (olfaction)

1. Receptors—in upper part of nasal cavity

2. Nerve—olfactory nerve (I)

V. GENERAL SENSES

A. Sense of touch—tactile corpuscles

B. Sense of pressure—receptors in skin deep tissue, large arteries

C. Sense of temperature—receptors are free nerve endings

D. Sense of position (proprioception)—receptors are proprioceptors in muscles, tendons, joints

1. Kinesthesia—sense of movement

E. Sense of pain—receptors are free nerve endings

1. Referred pain—originates internally but felt at surface

2. Relief of pain—analgesic drugs, anesthetics, endorphins, heat, cold, relaxation and distraction techniques

VI. SENSORY ADAPTATION

A. Adjustment of receptors so that sensation becomes less acute

B. Receptors adapt at different rates; pain receptors do not adapt

Questions for Study and Review

11

BUILDING UNDERSTANDING

Fill in the blanks

1. The part of the nervous system that detects a stimulus is the _____.

2. The bending of light rays as they pass from air to fluid is called _____.

3. Nerve impulses are carried from the ear to the brain by the _____ nerve.

4. Information about the position of the knee joint is provided by _____.

5. A receptor's ability to decrease its sensitivity to a continuous stimulus is called _____.

Matching > Match each numbered item with the most closely related lettered item.

___ **6.** Slowly progressive hearing loss

___ **7.** Irregularity in the curvature of the cornea or lens

___ **8.** Deviation of the eye due to lack of coordination of the eyeball muscles

___ **9.** Increased pressure inside the eyeball

___ **10.** Loss of vision in a healthy eye because it cannot work properly with the other eye

a. glaucoma

b. amblyopia

c. presbycusis

d. astigmatism

e. strabismus

Multiple Choice

___ **11.** All of the following are special senses except
   a. smell
   b. taste
   c. equilibrium
   d. pain

___ **12.** From superficial to deep, the order of the eyeball's tunics is
   a. retina, choroid, and sclera
   b. sclera, retina, and choroid
   c. choroid, retina, and sclera
   d. sclera, choroid, and retina

___ **13.** The part of the eye most responsible for light refraction is the
   a. cornea
   b. lens
   c. vitreous body
   d. retina

___ **14.** Information from the retina is carried to the brain by the
   a. ophthalmic nerve
   b. optic nerve
   c. oculomotor nerve
   d. abducens nerve

___ **15.** Receptors in the vestibule sense
   a. muscle tension
   b. sound
   c. light
   d. equilibrium

UNDERSTANDING CONCEPTS

16. Differentiate between the terms in each of the following pairs:
   a. special sense and general sense
   b. aqueous humor and vitreous body
   c. rods and cones
   d. endolymph and perilymph
   e. static and dynamic equilibrium

17. Trace the path of a light ray from the outside of the eye to the retina.

18. Define *convergence* and *accommodation* and describe several disorders associated with them.

19. List in order the structures that sound waves pass through in traveling through the ear to the receptors for hearing.

20. Compare and contrast conductive hearing loss and sensorineural hearing loss.

21. Name the four basic tastes. Where are the taste receptors? Name the nerves of taste.

22. Trace the pathway of a nerve impulse from the olfactory receptors to the olfactory center in the brain.

23. Name several types of pain-relieving drugs. Describe several methods for relieving pain that do not involve drugs.

CONCEPTUAL THINKING

24. Maria M., a 4-year-old female, is taken to see the pediatrician because of a severe earache. Examination reveals that the tympanic membrane is red and bulging outward toward the external auditory canal. What disorder does Maria have? Why is the incidence of this disorder higher in children than in adults? What treatment options are available to Maria?

25. You and a friend have just finished riding the roller coaster at the amusement park. As you walk away from the ride, your friend stumbles and comments that the ride has affected her balance. How do you explain this?

26. In the case story, Paul discovered he might be developing an age-related eye disorder. What is a cataract? What are some other age-related disorders of the sensory system?

11

CHAPTER 12

The Endocrine System: Glands and Hormones

Learning Outcomes

After careful study of this chapter, you should be able to:

1. Compare the effects of the nervous system and the endocrine system in controlling the body
2. Describe the functions of hormones
3. Discuss the chemical composition of hormones
4. Explain how hormones are regulated
5. Identify the glands of the endocrine system on a diagram
6. List the hormones produced by each endocrine gland and describe the effects of each on the body
7. Describe how the hypothalamus controls the anterior and posterior pituitary
8. Describe the effects of hyposecretion and hypersecretion of the various hormones
9. List tissues other than the endocrine glands that produce hormones
10. List some medical uses of hormones
11. Explain how the endocrine system responds to stress
12. Show how word parts are used to build words related to the endocrine system (see Word Anatomy at the end of the chapter)

Disease in Context

▶ Becky's Case: When an Endocrine Organ Fails

Becky stumbled down the stairs, wiping the sleep from her eyes, and hoping that Max hadn't finished all the pancakes that she could smell from the kitchen. "How was your sleep last night?" asked Becky's mother, who slid a plate across the table toward her. "Awful," sighed Becky, drowning her pancakes in a lake of syrup. "I woke up a bunch of times to go to the bathroom."

"Were you actually able to make it this time?" chimed Becky's little brother. Becky wished Max hadn't brought *that* up. She hoped he wasn't blabbing to his friends that she was wetting the bed again. "You know, if you didn't drink so much, you wouldn't have to pee so much," explained Max, as his sister gulped down her third glass of orange juice. Becky ate her pancakes and pretended that she didn't care about Max's comment. But, he was right. She was so thirsty—and hungry!

It was a long day when the bell finally rang and Becky boarded the bus for the ride home. Math class had been a disaster because she couldn't concentrate. During gym she was tired and had a stomach ache. And, she had to keep asking for permission to go to the bathroom! Now, she was exhausted and her head hurt. During breakfast, her mom mentioned she would make an appointment for Becky to see her doctor. Now, Becky thought that was a good idea.

Later that week, Becky's pediatrician weighed her, measured her height, and asked her a bunch of questions. "So, let me see if I've got this right, Becky," said Dr. Carter. "For the past week or so, you've felt lethargic and nauseated and had a headache. You've been really thirsty and have needed to urinate frequently. You've also been really hungry. You've had some difficulty concentrating at school and have even felt fatigued when playing sports." Becky wasn't too sure what lethargic meant, but other than that he seemed to have gotten the facts right. So, Becky nodded her head yes.

Turning to Becky's mother, Dr. Carter said, "Checking her chart, it appears that she's lost several pounds since her last appointment—despite her appetite. I'm going to order a urine test and blood test. I'd like to see what her glucose levels are." Becky didn't enjoy the tests one bit. Having to pee in a cup was gross and as for the blood test, that was the worst!

A few days later, Dr. Carter called Becky's mother. "The urinalysis was positive for glucose and ketones, suggesting that Becky is not metabolizing glucose correctly. Her blood test revealed that she's hyperglycemic. In other words, her blood sugar is too high. We need to run a few more tests, but my diagnosis so far is that Becky has type 1 diabetes mellitus and needs insulin."

Dr. Carter suspects that Becky's pancreas, an important endocrine organ, does not produce sufficient amounts of the hormone insulin. Without insulin, Becky's cells cannot convert glucose into energy. As we will see later, Dr. Carter's diagnosis has a dramatic effect on Becky's health.

The endocrine system consists of a group of glands that produces regulatory chemicals called **hormones**. The endocrine system and the nervous system work together to control and coordinate all other body systems. The nervous system controls such rapid actions as muscle movement and intestinal activity by means of electrical and chemical stimuli. The effects of the endocrine system occur more slowly and over a longer period. They involve chemical stimuli only, and these chemical messengers have widespread effects on the body.

Although the nervous and endocrine systems differ in some respects, the two systems are closely related. For example, the activity of the pituitary gland, which in turn regulates other glands, is controlled by the brain's hypothalamus. The connections between the nervous system and the endocrine system enable endocrine function to adjust to the demands of a changing environment.

Hormones

Hormones are chemical messengers that have specific regulatory effects on certain cells or organs. Hormones from the endocrine glands are released, not through ducts, but directly into surrounding tissue fluids. Most then diffuse into the bloodstream, which carries them throughout the body. They regulate growth, metabolism, reproduction, and behavior. Some hormones affect many tissues, for example, growth hormone, thyroid hormone, and insulin. Others affect only specific tissues. For example, one pituitary hormone, thyroid-stimulating hormone (TSH), acts only on the thyroid gland; another, adrenocorticotropic hormone (ACTH), stimulates only the outer portion of the adrenal gland. Others act more locally, close to where they are secreted.

The specific tissue acted on by each hormone is the **target tissue**. The cells that make up these tissues have **receptors** in the plasma membrane or within the cytoplasm to which the hormone attaches. Once a hormone binds to a receptor on or in a target cell, it affects cell activities, regulating the manufacture of proteins, changing the permeability of the membrane, or affecting metabolic reactions.

Hormone Chemistry

Chemically, hormones fall into two main categories:

- **Amino acid compounds.** These hormones are proteins or related compounds also made of amino acids. All hormones except those of the adrenal cortex and the sex glands fall into this category.

- **Lipids.** These hormones are made of fatty acids. Most are **steroids**, derived from cholesterol. Steroid hormones are produced by the adrenal cortex and the sex glands. They can be recognized by the ending *–one*, as in progesterone, testosterone. Prostaglandins, described later in this chapter, are also in the lipid category.

CHECKPOINT 12-1 ➤ What are hormones and what are some effects of hormones?

Hormone Regulation

The amount of each hormone that is secreted is normally kept within a specific range. Negative feedback, described in Chapter 1, is the method most commonly used to regulate these levels. In negative feedback, the hormone itself (or the result of its action) controls further hormone secretion. Each endocrine gland tends to oversecrete its hormone, exerting more effect on the target tissue. When the target tissue becomes too active, there is a negative effect on the endocrine gland, which then decreases its secretory activity.

We can use as an example the secretion of thyroid hormones (Fig. 12-1). As described in more detail later in the chapter, a pituitary hormone, called *thyroid-stimulating hormone* (TSH), triggers hormone secretion from the thyroid gland located in the neck. As blood levels of these hormones rise under the effects of TSH, they act as negative feedback messengers to inhibit TSH release from the pituitary. With less TSH, the thyroid releases less hormone and blood levels drop. When hormone levels fall below the normal range, the pituitary can again begin to release TSH. This is a typical example of the kind of self-regulating system that keeps hormone levels within a set normal range.

Less commonly, some hormones are produced in response to positive feedback. In this case, response to a hormone promotes further hormone release. Examples are the action of oxytocin during labor, as described in Chapter 1, and the release of some hormones in the menstrual cycle, as described in Chapter 23.

Hormone release may fall into a rhythmic pattern. Hormones of the adrenal cortex follow a 24-hour cycle related to a person's sleeping pattern, with the secretion level greatest just before arising and least at bedtime. Hormones of the female menstrual cycle follow a monthly pattern.

CHECKPOINT 12-2 ➤ Hormone levels are normally kept within a specific range. What is the most common method used to regulate secretion of hormones?

The Endocrine Glands and Their Hormones

The remainder of this chapter deals with hormones and the tissues that produce them. Refer to Figure 12-2 to locate each of the endocrine glands as you study them. Table 12-1 summarizes the information on the endocrine glands and their hormones. Each section of the chapter also includes information on the effects of a hormone's hypersecretion (oversecretion) or hyposecretion (undersecretion), summarized in Table 12-2.

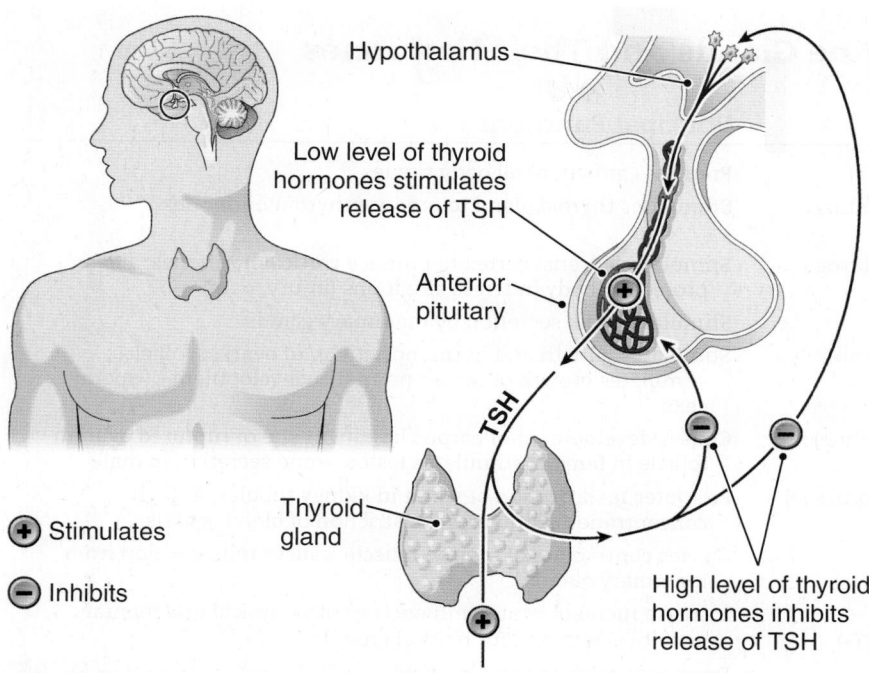

Figure 12-1 **Negative feedback control of thyroid hormones.** The anterior pituitary releases thyroid-stimulating hormone (TSH) when the blood level of thyroid hormones is low. A high level of thyroid hormones inhibits release of TSH and thyroid hormone levels fall.

Although most of the discussion centers on the endocrine glands, it is important to note that many tissues—other than the endocrine glands—also secrete hormones. That is, they produce substances that act on other tissues, usually at some distance from where they are produced. These tissues include the brain, digestive organs, and kidney. Some of these other tissues will be discussed later in the chapter.

The Pituitary

The **pituitary** (pih-TU-ih-tar-e), or **hypophysis** (hi-POF-ih-sis), is a small gland about the size of a cherry. It is located in a saddlelike depression of the sphenoid bone just posterior to the point where the optic nerves cross. It is surrounded by bone except where it connects with the brain's hypothalamus by a stalk called the **infundibulum** (in-fun-DIB-u-lum). The gland is divided into two parts, the **anterior lobe** and the **posterior lobe** (Fig. 12-3).

The pituitary is often called the *master gland* because it releases hormones that affect the working of other glands, such as the thyroid, gonads (ovaries and testes), and adrenal glands. (Hormones that stimulate other glands may be recognized by the ending *-tropin*, as in *thyrotropin*, which means "acting on the thyroid gland.") However, the pituitary itself is controlled by the hypothalamus, by means of secretions and nerve impulses sent to the pituitary through the infundibulum (see Fig. 12-3).

CONTROL OF THE PITUITARY

The hormones produced in the anterior pituitary are not released until chemical messengers called **releasing hormones** arrive from the hypothalamus. These releasing hormones travel to the anterior pituitary by way of a special type of circulatory pathway called a **portal system**. By this circulatory "detour," some of the blood that leaves the hypothalamus travels to capillaries in the anterior pituitary before returning to the heart. As the blood circulates through the capillaries, it delivers the hormones that stimulate the release of anterior pituitary secretions. Hypothalamic releasing hormones are indicated with the

12

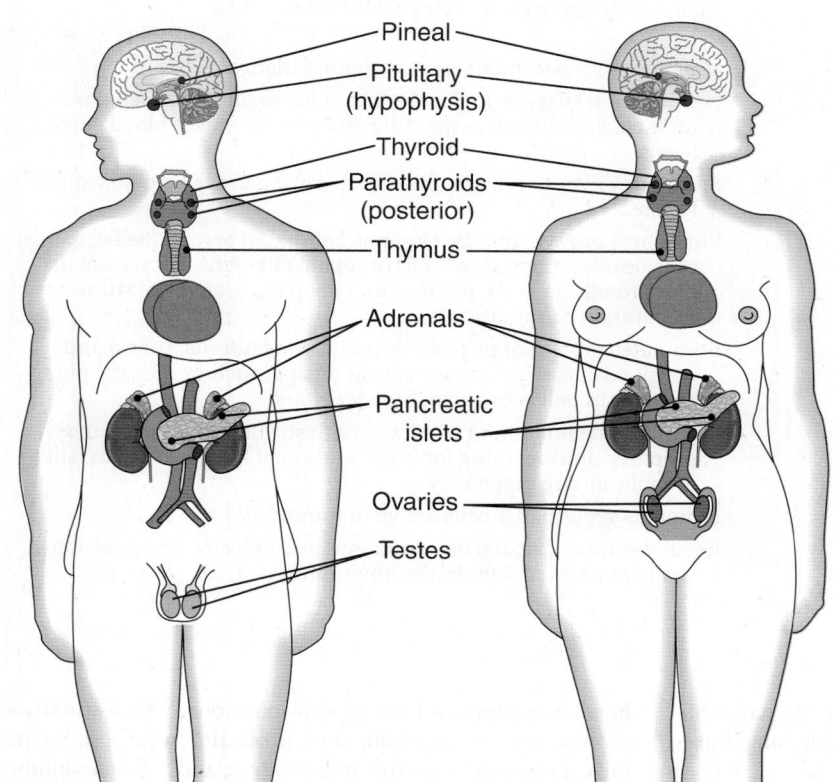

Figure 12-2 **The endocrine glands.**

| Table 12-1 | | The Endocrine Glands and Their Hormones |

Gland	Hormone	Principal Functions
Anterior pituitary	GH (growth hormone)	Promotes growth of all body tissues
	TSH (thyroid-stimulating hormone)	Stimulates thyroid gland to produce thyroid hormones
	ACTH (adrenocorticotropic hormone)	Stimulates adrenal cortex to produce cortical hormones; aids in protecting body in stress situations (injury, pain)
	PRL (prolactin)	Stimulates milk secretion by mammary glands
	FSH (follicle-stimulating hormone)	Stimulates growth and hormone activity of ovarian follicles; stimulates growth of testes; promotes development of sperm cells
	LH (luteinizing hormone)	Causes development of corpus luteum at site of ruptured ovarian follicle in female; stimulates testosterone secretion in male
Posterior pituitary	ADH (antidiuretic hormone)	Promotes reabsorption of water in kidney tubules; at high concentration stimulates constriction of blood vessels
	Oxytocin	Causes contraction of uterine muscle; causes milk ejection from mammary glands
Thyroid	Thyroxine (T_4) and triiodothyronine (T_3)	Increase metabolic rate, influencing both physical and mental activities; required for normal growth
	Calcitonin	Decreases calcium level in blood
Parathyroids	PTH (parathyroid hormone)	Regulates exchange of calcium between blood and bones; increases calcium level in blood
Adrenal medulla	Epinephrine and norepinephrine	Increases blood pressure and heart rate; activates cells influenced by sympathetic nervous system plus many not affected by sympathetic nerves
Adrenal cortex	Cortisol (95% of glucocorticoids)	Aids in metabolism of carbohydrates, proteins, and fats; active during stress
	Aldosterone (95% of mineralocorticoids)	Aids in regulating electrolytes and water balance
	Sex hormones	May influence secondary sexual characteristics
Pancreatic islets	Insulin	Needed for transport of glucose into cells; required for cellular metabolism of foods, especially glucose; decreases blood sugar levels
	Glucagon	Stimulates liver to release glucose, thereby increasing blood sugar levels
Testes	Testosterone	Stimulates growth and development of sexual organs (testes, penis) plus development of secondary sexual characteristics, such as hair growth on body and face and deepening of voice; stimulates maturation of sperm cells
Ovaries	Estrogens (e.g., estradiol)	Stimulates growth of primary sexual organs (uterus, tubes) and development of secondary sexual organs, such as breasts, plus changes in pelvis to ovoid, broader shape
	Progesterone	Stimulates development of secretory tissue of mammary glands; prepares uterine lining for implantation of fertilized ovum; aids in maintaining pregnancy
Thymus	Thymosin	Promotes growth of T cells active in immunity
Pineal	Melatonin	Regulates mood, sexual development, and daily cycles in response to the amount of light in the environment

abbreviation *RH* added to an abbreviation for the name of the hormone stimulated. For example, the releasing hormone that controls growth hormone is GH-RH.

Two anterior pituitary hormones are also regulated by inhibiting hormones (IH) from the hypothalamus. Inhibiting hormones suppress both growth hormone, which stimulates growth and metabolism, and prolactin, which stimulates milk production in the mammary glands. These inhibiting hormones are abbreviated GH-IH (growth hormone-inhibiting hormone) and PIH (prolactin-inhibiting hormone).

Table 12-2	Disorders Associated with Endocrine Dysfunction	
Hormone	**Effects of Hypersecretion**	**Effects of Hyposecretion**
Growth hormone	Gigantism (children), acromegaly (adults)	Dwarfism (children)
Antidiuretic hormone	Syndrome of inappropriate antidiuretic hormone (SIADH)	Diabetes insipidus
Aldosterone	Aldosteronism	Addison disease
Cortisol	Cushing syndrome	Addison disease
Thyroid hormone	Graves disease, thyrotoxicosis	Infantile hypothyroidism in children; myxedema in adults
Insulin	Hypoglycemia	Diabetes mellitus; hyperglycemia
Parathyroid hormone	Bone degeneration	Tetany (muscle spasms)

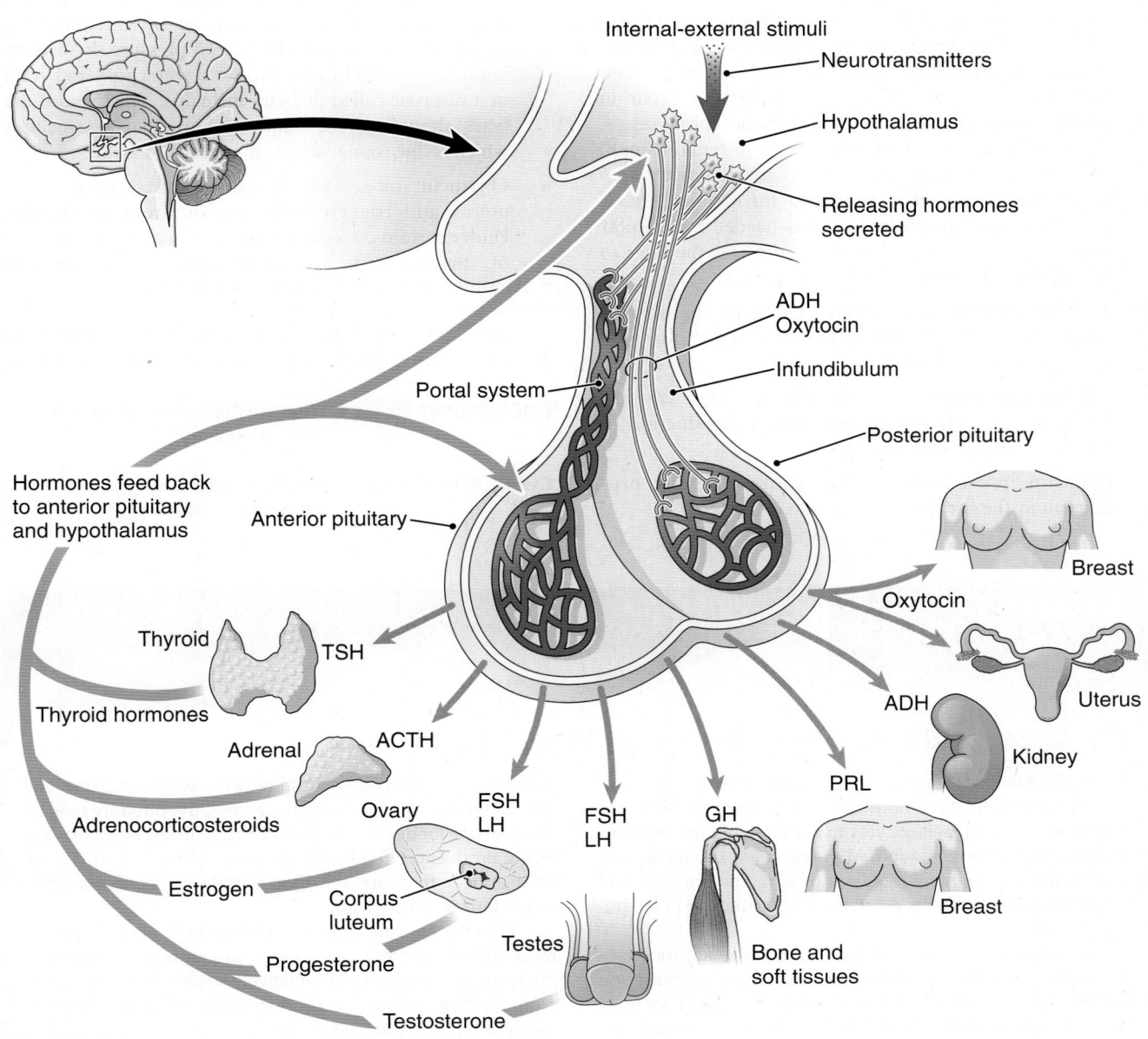

Figure 12-3 **The hypothalamus, pituitary gland, and target tissues.** Arrows indicate the hormones' target tissues and feedback pathways. [**ZOOMING IN** ➤ What two structures does the infundibulum connect?]

The two hormones of the posterior pituitary (antidiuretic hormone, or ADH, and oxytocin) are actually produced in the hypothalamus and stored in the posterior pituitary. Their release is controlled by nerve impulses that travel over pathways (tracts) between the hypothalamus and the posterior pituitary.

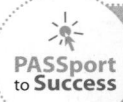

Visit **thePoint** or see the Student Resource CD in the back of this book for more details and illustrations of the disorders in Table 12-2.

CHECKPOINT `12-3` ➤ What part of the brain controls the pituitary?

ANTERIOR LOBE HORMONES

- **Growth hormone (GH)**, or **somatotropin** (so-mah-to-TRO-pin), acts directly on most body tissues, promoting protein manufacture that is essential for growth. GH causes increases in size and height to occur in youth, before the closure of long bone epiphyses. A young person with a GH deficiency will remain small, though well proportioned, unless treated with adequate hormone. GH is produced throughout life. It stimulates protein synthesis and is needed for cellular maintenance and repair. It also stimulates the liver to release fatty acids for energy in time of stress.

- **Thyroid-stimulating hormone** (TSH), or **thyrotropin** (thi-ro-TRO-pin), stimulates the thyroid gland to produce thyroid hormones.

- **Adrenocorticotropic** (ad-re-no-kor-tih-ko-TRO-pik) **hormone** (**ACTH**) stimulates hormone production in the cortex of the adrenal glands.

- **Prolactin** (pro-LAK-tin) (**PRL**) stimulates milk production in the breasts.

- **Follicle-stimulating hormone (FSH)** stimulates the development of eggs in the ovaries and sperm cells in the testes.

- **Luteinizing** (LU-te-in-i-zing) **hormone** (**LH**) causes ovulation in females and sex hormone secretion in both males and females.

FSH and LH are classified as **gonadotropins** (gon-ah-do-TRO-pinz), hormones that act on the gonads to regulate growth, development, and reproductive function in both males and females.

POSTERIOR LOBE HORMONES

- **Antidiuretic** (an-ti-di-u-RET-ik) **hormone** (**ADH**) promotes the reabsorption of water from the kidney tubules and thus decreases water excretion. Large amounts of this hormone cause contraction of smooth muscle in blood vessel walls and raise blood pressure. Inadequate amounts of ADH cause excessive water loss and result in a disorder called **diabetes insipidus**. This type of diabetes should not be confused with diabetes mellitus, which is due to inadequate amounts of insulin.

- **Oxytocin** (ok-se-TO-sin) causes contractions of the uterus and triggers milk ejection from the breasts. Under certain circumstances, commercial preparations of this hormone are administered during or after childbirth to cause uterine contraction.

Box 12-1 offers information on melanocyte-stimulating hormone, another hormone produced in the pituitary gland.

CHECKPOINT `12-4` ➤ What are the hormones from the anterior pituitary?

CHECKPOINT `12-5` ➤ What hormones are released from the posterior pituitary?

Box 12-1 A Closer Look

Melanocyte-Stimulating Hormone: More Than a Tan?

In amphibians, reptiles, and certain other animals, melanocyte-stimulating hormone (MSH) darkens skin and hair by stimulating melanocytes to manufacture the pigment melanin. In humans, though, MSH levels are usually so low that its role as a primary regulator of skin pigmentation and hair color is questionable. What, then, is its function in the human body?

Recent research suggests that MSH is probably more important as a neurotransmitter in the brain than as a hormone in the rest of the body. When the pituitary gland secretes ACTH, it secretes MSH as well. This is so because pituitary cells do not produce ACTH directly but produce a large precursor

molecule, proopiomelanocortin (POMC), which enzymes cut into ACTH and MSH. In Addison disease, the pituitary tries to compensate for decreased glucocorticoid levels by increasing POMC production. The resulting increased levels of ACTH and MSH appear to cause the blotchy skin pigmentation that characterizes the disease.

MSH's other roles include helping the brain to regulate food intake, fertility, and even the immune response. Interestingly, despite MSH's relatively small role in regulating pigmentation, women do produce more MSH during pregnancy and often have darker skin.

TUMORS OF THE PITUITARY The effects of pituitary tumors depend on the cell types in the excess tissue. Some of these tumors contain an excessive number of the cells that produce growth hormone. A person who develops such a tumor in childhood will grow to an abnormally tall stature, a condition called **gigantism** (ji-GAN-tizm) (see Table 12-2). Although people with this condition are large, they are usually very weak.

If the GH-producing cells become overactive in the adult, a disorder known as **acromegaly** (ak-ro-MEG-ah-le) develops. In acromegaly, the bones of the face, hands, and feet widen. The fingers resemble a spatula, and the face takes on a coarse appearance: the nose widens, the lower jaw protrudes, and the forehead bones may bulge. Multiple body systems may be affected by acromegaly, including the cardiovascular and nervous systems.

Tumors may destroy the pituitary's secreting tissues so that signs of underactivity develop. Patients with this condition often become obese and sluggish and may exhibit signs of underactivity of other endocrine glands that are controlled by the pituitary, such as the ovaries, testes, or thyroid. Pituitary tumors also may involve the optic nerves and cause blindness.

Evidence of tumor formation in the pituitary gland may be obtained by radiographic examinations of the skull. The pressure of the tumor distorts the sella turcica, the saddlelike space in the sphenoid bone that holds the pituitary. Physicians also use computed tomography (CT) and magnetic resonance imaging (MRI) scans to diagnose pituitary abnormalities.

The Thyroid Gland

The **thyroid**, located in the neck, is the largest of the endocrine glands (Fig. 12-4). The thyroid has two roughly oval lateral lobes on either side of the larynx (voice box) connected by a narrow band called an **isthmus** (IS-mus). A connective tissue capsule encloses the entire gland.

HORMONES OF THE THYROID GLAND The thyroid produces two hormones that regulate metabolism. The

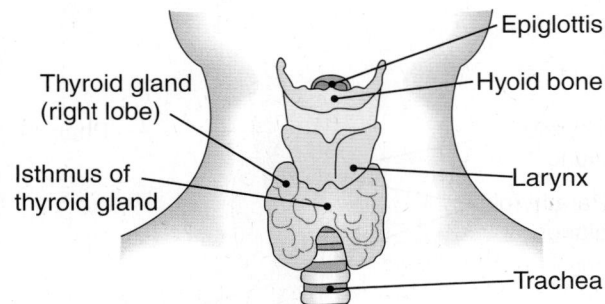

Figure 12-4 **Thyroid gland (anterior view).** The two lobes and isthmus of the thyroid are shown in relation to other structures in the throat. The epiglottis is a cartilage of the larynx. [**ZOOMING IN** ➤ What structure is superior to the thyroid? Inferior to the thyroid?]

principal hormone is **thyroxine** (thi-ROK-sin), which is symbolized as T$_4$, based on the four iodine atoms in each molecule. The other hormone, which contains three atoms of iodine, is **triiodothyronine** (tri-i-o-do-THI-ro-nene), or T$_3$. These hormones function to increase the metabolic rate in body cells. In particular, they increase energy metabolism and protein metabolism. Both thyroid hormones and growth hormone are needed for normal growth.

The thyroid gland needs an adequate iodine supply to produce its hormones. Iodine deficiency is rare now because of widespread availability of this mineral in iodized salt, vegetables, seafood, dairy products, and processed foods.

Another hormone produced by the thyroid gland is **calcitonin** (kal-sih-TO-nin), which is active in calcium metabolism. Calcitonin lowers the amount of calcium circulating in the blood by promoting the deposit of calcium in bone tissue. Calcitonin works with parathyroid hormone and with vitamin D to regulate calcium metabolism, as described below.

DISORDERS OF THE THYROID GLAND A **goiter** (GOY-ter) is an enlargement of the thyroid gland, which may or may not be associated with overproduction of hormone. A **simple goiter** is the uniform overgrowth of the thyroid gland, with a smooth surface appearance. An **adenomatous** (ad-eh-NO-mah-tus), or **nodular, goiter** is an irregular-appearing goiter accompanied by tumor formation.

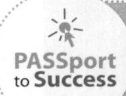

PASSport to Success

Visit **thePoint** or see the Student Resource CD in the back of this book for a goiter illustration.

For various reasons, the thyroid gland may become either underactive or overactive. Thyroid underactivity, known as **hypothyroidism** (hi-po-THI-royd-izm), shows up as two characteristic states related to age:

- **Infantile hypothyroidism** is a condition resulting from hypothyroidism in infants and children. The usual cause is a failure of the thyroid gland to form during fetal development (congenital hypothyroidism). The infant suffers lack of physical growth and lack of mental development. Early and continuous treatment with replacement hormone can alter the outlook of this disease. By state law, all newborns are tested for hypothyroidism in the U.S.

- **Myxedema** (mik-seh-DE-mah) results from thyroid atrophy (wasting) in the adult. The patient becomes sluggish both mentally and physically and often feels cold. The hair becomes dry and the skin becomes dry and waxy. The tissues of the face swell. Because thyroid hormone can be administered orally, the patient with myxedema regains health easily, although treatment must be maintained throughout life.

Hyperthyroidism is the opposite of hypothyroidism, that is, overactivity of the thyroid gland with excessive hormone secretion. A common form of hyperthyroidism is **Graves disease**, which is characterized by a goiter, a strained appearance of the face, intense nervousness, weight loss, a rapid pulse, sweating, tremors, and an abnormally quick metabolism. Another characteristic symptom is protrusion (bulging) of the eyes, known as **exophthalmos** (ek-sof-THAL-mos), which is caused by swelling of the tissue behind the eyes (Fig. 12-5). Treatment of hyperthyroidism may take the following forms:

- Suppression of hormone production with medication
- Destruction of thyroid tissue with radioactive iodine
- Surgical removal of part of the thyroid gland

An exaggerated form of hyperthyroidism with a sudden onset is called a **thyroid storm**. Untreated, it is usually fatal, but with appropriate care, most affected people can be saved.

Thyroiditis (thi-royd-I-tis) is a general term meaning inflammation of the thyroid. The cause may be infection or autoimmunity, that is, abnormal production of antibodies to the thyroid gland. **Hashimoto disease** is an autoimmune thyroiditis that may be hereditary and may also involve excess intake of iodine. The disease results in thyroid enlargement (goiter) and hypothyroidism. It is treated with thyroid hormone replacement and, in some cases, surgery.

CHECKPOINT 12-6 ➤ What is the effect of thyroid hormones on cells?

TESTS OF THYROID FUNCTION The most frequently used thyroid function tests are blood tests that measure the uptake of radioactive iodine added to a blood sample. These very sensitive tests are used to detect abnormal thyroid function and to monitor response to drug therapy. A test for the level of thyroid-stimulating hormone (from the pituitary) is frequently done at the same time. Further testing involves giving a person oral radioactive iodine and measuring the amount and distribution of radiation that accumulates in the thyroid gland.

The Parathyroid Glands

The four tiny **parathyroid glands** are embedded in the thyroid's posterior capsule (Fig. 12-6). The secretion of these glands, **parathyroid hormone** (**PTH**), promotes calcium release from bone tissue, thus increasing the amount of calcium circulating in the bloodstream. PTH also causes the kidney to conserve calcium. Low PTH, as may be caused by removal of the parathyroids, results in muscle spasms known as *tetany*.

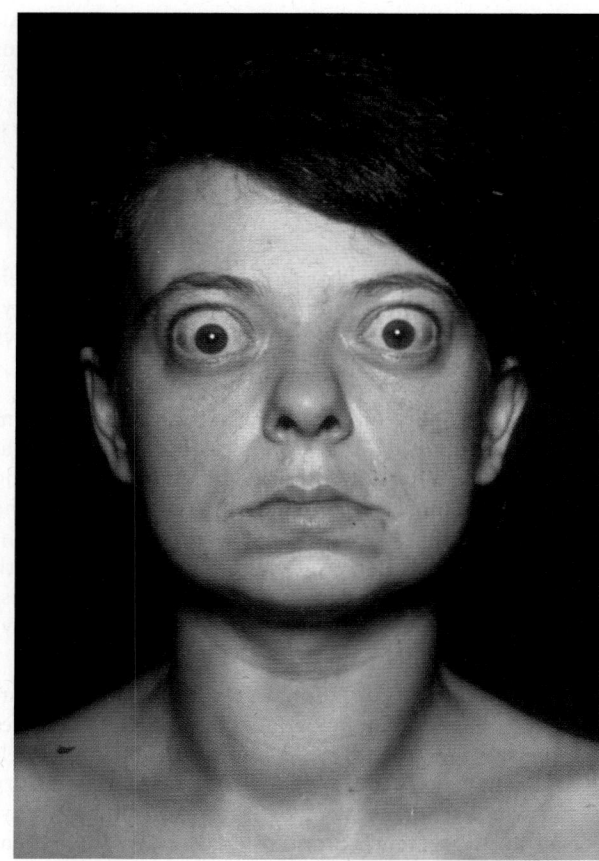

Figure 12-5 **Graves disease showing goiter and exophthalmos.** Goiter is enlargement of the thyroid; exophthalmos is bulging of the eyes. (Sandoz Pharmaceutical Corporation.)

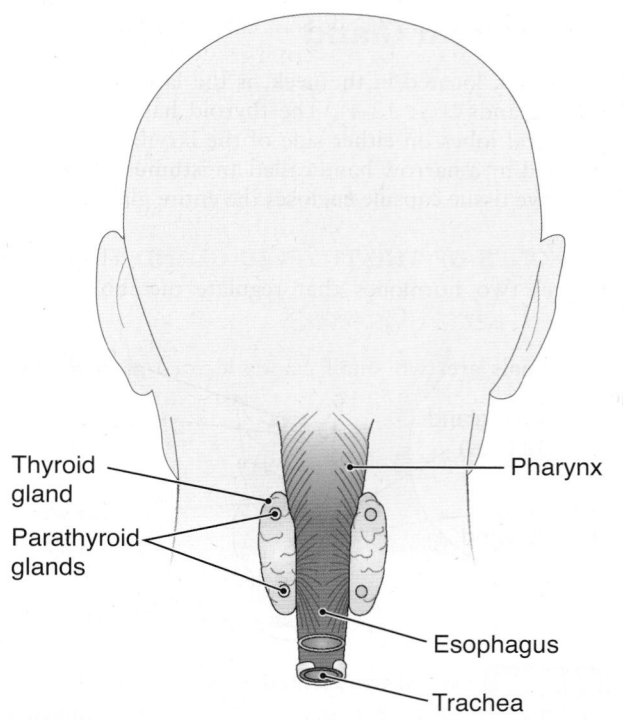

Figure 12-6 **Parathyroid glands (posterior view).** The four small parathyroid glands are embedded in the posterior surface of the thyroid.

Thyroid gland
Parathyroid glands
Pharynx
Esophagus
Trachea

PTH works with calcitonin from the thyroid gland to regulate calcium metabolism. These hormone levels are controlled by negative feedback based on the amount of calcium in the blood. When calcium is high, calcitonin is produced; when calcium is low, PTH is produced.

CALCIUM METABOLISM Calcium balance is required not only for the health of bones and teeth but also for the proper function of the nervous system and muscles. One other hormone is needed for calcium balance in addition to calcitonin and PTH. This is **calcitriol** (kal-sih-TRI-ol), technically called dihydroxycholecalciferol (di-hi-drok-se-ko-le-kal-SIF-eh-rol), the active form of vitamin D. Calcitriol is produced by modification of vitamin D in the liver and then the kidney. It increases intestinal absorption of calcium to raise blood calcium levels.

Calcitonin, PTH, and calcitriol work together to regulate the amount of calcium in the blood and provide calcium for bone maintenance and other functions.

DISORDERS OF THE PARATHYROID GLANDS
Inadequate production of parathyroid hormone, as a result of removal or damage to the parathyroid glands, for example, causes a series of muscle contractions involving particularly the hands and face. These spasms result from a low concentration of blood calcium, and the condition is called **tetany** (TET-ah-ne). This low calcium tetany should not be confused with the infection called *tetanus* (lockjaw).

In contrast, if there is excess production of PTH, as may happen in parathyroid tumors, calcium is removed from its normal storage place in the bones and released into the bloodstream. The loss of calcium from the bones leads to fragile bones that fracture easily. Because the kidneys ultimately excrete the calcium, kidney stone formation is common in such cases.

CHECKPOINT 12-7 ➤ What mineral is regulated by calcitonin and parathyroid hormone (PTH)?

The Adrenal Glands

The **adrenals** are two small glands located atop the kidneys. Each adrenal gland has two parts that act as separate glands. The inner area is called the **medulla,** and the outer portion is called the **cortex** (Fig. 12-7).

HORMONES FROM THE ADRENAL MEDULLA The hormones of the adrenal medulla are released in response to stimulation by the sympathetic nervous system. The principal hormone produced by the medulla is **epinephrine,** also called **adrenaline.** Another hormone released from the adrenal medulla, **norepinephrine** (noradrenaline), is closely related chemically and is similar in its actions to epinephrine. These two hormones are referred to as the *fight-or-flight hormones* because of their effects during emergency situations. We have already learned about these hormones in studying the autonomic nervous system.

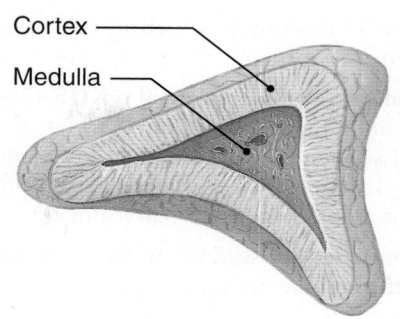

Figure 12-7 **The adrenal gland.** The medulla secretes epinephrine and norepinephrine. The cortex secretes steroid hormones. (Reprinted with permission from Gartner LP, Hiatt JL. *Color Atlas of Histology*, 3rd ed. Philadelphia: Lippincott Williams & Wilkins, 2000.) **[ZOOMING IN** ➤ What is the outer region of the adrenal gland called? The inner region? **]**

When released from nerve endings instead of being released directly into the bloodstream, they function as neurotransmitters. Some of their effects are as follows:

- Stimulation of the involuntary muscle in the walls of the arterioles, causing these muscles to contract and blood pressure to rise accordingly
- Conversion of glycogen stored in the liver into glucose. The glucose pours into the blood and travels throughout the body, allowing the voluntary muscles and other tissues to do an extraordinary amount of work
- Increase in the heart rate
- Increase in the metabolic rate of body cells
- Dilation of the bronchioles, through relaxation of the smooth muscle in their walls

CHECKPOINT 12-8 ➤ The main hormone from the adrenal medulla also functions as a neurotransmitter in the sympathetic nervous system. What is the name of this hormone?

HORMONES FROM THE ADRENAL CORTEX There are three main groups of hormones secreted by the adrenal cortex:

- **Glucocorticoids** (glu-ko-KOR-tih-koyds) maintain the body's carbohydrate reserve by stimulating the liver to convert amino acids into glucose (sugar) instead of protein. The production of these hormones increases in times of stress to aid the body in responding to unfavorable conditions. They raise the level of nutrients in the blood, not only glucose, but also amino acids from tissue proteins and fatty acids from fats stored in adipose tissue. Glucocorticoids also have the ability to suppress the inflammatory response and are often administered as medication for this purpose. The major

12

hormone of this group is **cortisol**, which is also called *hydrocortisone*.

- **Mineralocorticoids** (min-er-al-o-KOR-tih-koyds) are important in the regulation of electrolyte balance. They control sodium reabsorption and potassium secretion by the kidney tubules. The major hormone of this group is **aldosterone** (al-DOS-ter-one).

- **Sex hormones** are secreted in small amounts, having little effect on the body.

DISORDERS OF THE ADRENAL CORTEX Hypofunction of the adrenal cortex gives rise to a condition known as **Addison disease**, a disease characterized chiefly by muscle atrophy (loss of tissue), weakness, skin pigmentation, and disturbances in salt and water balance.

Hypersecretion of cortisol results in a condition known as **Cushing syndrome**, the symptoms of which include obesity with a round ("moon") face, thin skin that bruises easily, muscle weakness, bone loss, and elevated blood sugar. Use of steroid drugs also may produce these symptoms. If aldosterone is secreted in excess, as a result of hyperfunction of the adrenal cortex, the condition is termed *aldosteronism*.

Adrenal gland tumors give rise to a wide range of symptoms resulting from an excess or a deficiency of the hormones secreted.

CHECKPOINT 12-9 ➤ What three categories of hormones are released by the adrenal cortex?

CHECKPOINT 12-10 ➤ What effect does cortisol have on glucose levels in the blood?

The Pancreas and Its Hormones

Scattered throughout the **pancreas** are small groups of specialized cells called **islets** (I-lets), also known as **islets of Langerhans** (LAHNG-er-hanz) (Fig. 12-8). These cells make up the endocrine portion of the pancreas. The cells surrounding the islets secrete digestive juices. They make up the exocrine portion of the pancreas, which is independent of the islets and secretes through ducts into the small intestine (see Chapter 19).

The most important hormone secreted by the islets is **insulin** (IN-su-lin), which is produced by beta (β) cells. Insulin is active in the transport of glucose across plasma membranes, thus increasing cellular glucose uptake. Once inside a cell, glucose is metabolized for energy. Insulin also increases the rate at which the liver takes up glucose and converts it to glycogen and the rate at which the liver changes excess glucose into fatty acids, which can then be converted to fats and stored in adipose tissue. Through these actions, insulin has the effect of lowering the blood sugar level. Insulin has other metabolic effects as well. It promotes the cellular uptake of amino acids and stimulates their manufacture into proteins.

A second islet hormone, produced by alpha (α) cells, is **glucagon** (GLU-kah-gon), which works with insulin to reg-

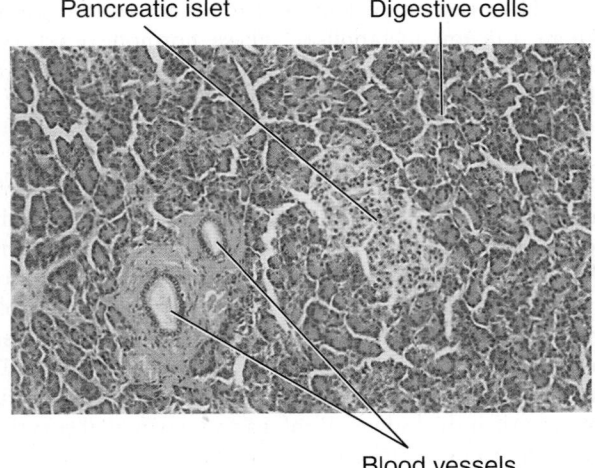

Pancreatic islet   Digestive cells

Blood vessels

Figure 12-8 **Microscopic view of pancreatic cells.** Light-staining islet cells are visible among the many cells that produce digestive juices. (Courtesy of Dana Morse Bittus and B. J. Cohen.)

ulate blood sugar levels. Glucagon causes the liver to release stored glucose into the bloodstream. It also increases the rate at which glucose is made from proteins in the liver. In these two ways, glucagon increases blood sugar.

CHECKPOINT 12-11 ➤ What two hormones produced by the islets of the pancreas act to regulate glucose levels in the blood?

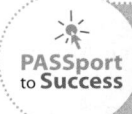

PASSport to Success

Visit *thePoint* or see the Student Resource CD in the back of this book for a flow chart showing the relationship between pancreatic hormones and sugar metabolism.

DIABETES MELLITUS When the pancreatic islet cells fail to produce enough insulin or body cells do not respond to the insulin, glucose is not available to the cells for energy. Instead, the sugar remains in the blood, a symptom called **hyperglycemia** (hi-per-gli-SE-me-ah). The excess sugar then must be removed by the kidneys and excreted in the urine. This condition, **diabetes mellitus** (di-ah-BE-teze mel-LI-tus), is the most common endocrine disorder. Diabetes mellitus is named for Greek words that mean "siphon," based on the high output of urine, and "honey" because of the urine's sweetness. It is this form of diabetes (in contrast to diabetes insipidus) that is meant when the term *diabetes* is used alone.

Diabetes is divided into two main types:

- Type 1 diabetes mellitus (T1DM) is less common but more severe. This disease usually appears before the age of 30 years and is brought on by an autoimmune (self) destruction of the insulin-producing β cells in the islets. People with T1DM need close monitoring of blood sugar levels and insulin injections.

■ Type 2 diabetes mellitus (T2DM) characteristically occurs in adults, although the incidence has gone up considerably in the United States in recent years among younger people. It is typically associated with overweight in both adults and children. These people retain the ability to secrete varying amounts of insulin, depending on the disease's severity. However, the ability of their body cells to respond to the hormone is diminished. This disease usually can be controlled with diet, oral medication to increase insulin production and improve its effectiveness, and weight reduction for the obese patient. Treatment with injectable insulin may be necessary with age and during illness or other stress.

Metabolic syndrome (also called syndrome X or insulin resistance syndrome) is related to T2DM and describes a state of hyperglycemia and obesity caused by insulin resistance in association with some metabolic disorders, including high levels of plasma triglycerides (fats), low levels of high-density lipoproteins (HDLs, the healthy form of cholesterol), and hypertension (high blood pressure). These factors together increase the risk of heart disease, stroke, and diabetes. Metabolic syndrome is treated with weight loss, exercise, improved diet, drugs to lower blood pressure and cholesterol, and drugs to decrease insulin resistance.

> **PASSport to Success**
> Visit **thePoint** or see the Student Resource CD in the back of this book for an illustration on the effects of metabolic syndrome.

Diabetes that develops during pregnancy is termed *gestational diabetes*. This form of diabetes usually disappears after childbirth, although it may be a sign that diabetes mellitus will develop later in life. Gestational diabetes usually affects women with a family history of diabetes, those who are obese, or those who are of older age. Diagnosis and treatment are important because of a high risk of complications for both the mother and the fetus.

Diabetes may also develop in association with other disorders, including pancreatic disease or other endocrine disorders. Viral infections, toxic chemicals in the environment, and drugs may also be involved.

Typical signs of diabetes are excess thirst (polydipsia), excess urination (polyuria), and excess eating (polyphagia), all brought on by high glucose in the blood and abnormal metabolism. The disease is diagnosed by measuring blood glucose levels with or without fasting and by monitoring blood glucose levels after oral administration of glucose (oral glucose tolerance test). Categories of impaired fasting blood glucose (IFG) and impaired glucose tolerance (IGT) are stages between a normal response to glucose and diabetes.

Uncontrolled diabetes is also associated with many long-term complications, including the following:

■ Abnormal fat metabolism. Low insulin levels result in the release of more fatty acids from adipose cells. The liver converts the fatty acids into phospholipids and cholesterol, resulting in high blood levels of fats and the accelerated development of atherosclerosis (arterial degeneration).

■ Damage to arteries, including those of the retina (diabetic retinopathy) and heart. Capillaries, such as those in the kidney, are often damaged as well.

■ Damage to peripheral nerves, with accompanying pain and loss of sensation. Damage to the autonomic nervous system can result in poor stomach emptying.

■ Decreased transport of amino acids, the building blocks of proteins. This may explain the weakness and poor tissue repair seen in people who have been diabetic for many years. It may also explain the reduced resistance to infection noted in diabetic patients.

Careful management of diabetes can reduce the severity of long-term complications. Patients must follow their prescribed diet consistently, take medication as ordered, eat at regular times, and follow a regular program of exercise. Patients on insulin must test their blood sugar regularly. These tests have traditionally been done on blood obtained by a finger prick, but new devices are available that can read the blood glucose level through the skin and even warn of a significant change. A test for long-term glucose control measures average blood glucose during the previous 2 to 3 months based on glucose bound to hemoglobin (HbA_{1c}) in red blood cells.

A need for insulin requires multiple injections during the day. An alternate method for insulin administration is by means of a pump that provides an around-the-clock supply. The insulin is placed in a device that then injects it into the subcutaneous tissues of the abdomen. People taking insulin injections are subject to episodes of low blood sugar and should carry notification of their disease.

Methods of administering insulin by pills or capsules, inhaler spray, or skin patches are still in the experimental stage. Researchers are also studying the possibility of transplanting the pancreas or islet cells to take over for failed cells in people with diabetes.

CHECKPOINT 12-12 ➤ What hormone is low or ineffective in cases of diabetes mellitus?

The Sex Glands

The sex glands, the female ovaries and the male testes, not only produce the sex cells but also are important endocrine organs. The hormones produced by these organs are needed in the development of the sexual characteristics, which usually appear in the early teens, and for the maintenance of the reproductive organs once full development has been attained. Those features that typify a male or female other than the structures directly concerned with reproduction are termed **secondary sex characteristics**. They include a deep voice and facial and body hair in males, and wider hips, breast development, and a greater ratio of fat to muscle in females.

HORMONES OF THE SEX GLANDS All male sex hormones are classified as **androgens** (AN-dro-jens). The main androgen produced by the testes is testosterone (tes-TOS-ter-one).

In the female, the hormones that most nearly parallel testosterone in their actions are the **estrogens** (ES-tro-jens), produced by the ovaries. Estrogens contribute to the development of the female secondary sex characteristics and stimulate mammary gland development, the onset of menstruation, and the development and functioning of the reproductive organs.

The other hormone produced by the ovaries, called **progesterone** (pro-JES-ter-one), assists in the normal development of pregnancy (gestation). All the sex hormones are discussed in more detail in Chapter 23.

CHECKPOINT 12-13 ► In addition to controlling reproduction, sex hormones confer certain features associated with male and female gender. What are these features called as a group?

The Thymus Gland

The **thymus gland** is a mass of lymphoid tissue that lies in the upper part of the chest superior to the heart. This gland is important in the development of immunity. Its hormone, **thymosin** (THI-mo-sin), assists in the maturation of certain white blood cells known as T cells (T lymphocytes) after they have left the thymus gland and taken up residence in lymph nodes throughout the body.

The Pineal Gland

The **pineal** (PIN-e-al) **gland** is a small, flattened, cone-shaped structure located posterior to the midbrain and connected to the roof of the third ventricle (see Fig. 12-2).

The pineal produces the hormone **melatonin** (mel-ah-TO-nin) during dark periods. Little hormone is produced during daylight hours. This pattern of hormone secretion influences the regulation of sleep–wake cycles. (See also Box 12-2, Seasonal Affective Disorder.) Melatonin also appears to delay the onset of puberty.

Other Hormone-Producing Tissues

Originally, the word *hormone* applied to the secretions of the endocrine glands only. The term now includes various body substances that have regulatory actions, either locally or at a distance from where they are produced. Many body tissues produce substances that regulate the local environment. Some of these other hormone-producing organs are the following:

- The stomach secretes a hormone that stimulates its own digestive activity.

- The small intestine secretes hormones that stimulate the production of digestive juices and help regulate the digestive process.

- The kidneys produce a hormone called **erythropoietin** (e-rith-ro-POY-eh-tin), which stimulates red blood cell production in the bone marrow. This hormone is produced when there is a decreased oxygen supply in the blood.

- The brain, as noted, secretes releasing hormones and release-inhibiting hormones that control the anterior pituitary, as well as ADH and oxytocin that are released from the posterior pituitary.

- The atria (upper chambers) of the heart produce a substance called **atrial natriuretic** (na-tre-u-RET-ik) **peptide** (**ANP**) in response to their increased filling

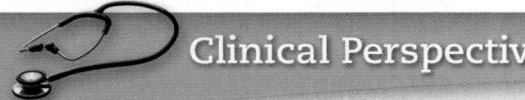

Box 12-2   Clinical Perspectives

Seasonal Affective Disorder: Seeing the Light

We all sense that long dark days make us blue and sap our motivation. Are these learned responses or is there a physical basis for them? Studies have shown that the amount of light in the environment does have a physical effect on behavior. Evidence that light alters mood comes from people who are intensely affected by the dark days of winter—people who suffer from **seasonal affective disorder**, aptly abbreviated SAD. When days shorten, these people feel sleepy, depressed, and anxious. They tend to overeat, especially carbohydrates. Research suggests that SAD has a genetic basis and may be associated with decreased levels of serotonin.

As light strikes the retina of the eye, it sends impulses that decrease the amount of melatonin produced by the pineal gland in the brain. Because melatonin depresses mood, the final effect of light is to elevate mood. Daily exposure to bright lights has been found to improve the mood of most people with SAD. Exposure for 15 minutes after rising in the morning may be enough, but some people require longer sessions both morning and evening. Other aids include aerobic exercise, stress management techniques, and antidepressant medications.

with blood. ANP increases sodium excretion by the kidneys and lowers blood pressure.

■ The **placenta** (plah-SEN-tah) produces several hormones during pregnancy. These cause changes in the uterine lining and, later in pregnancy, help to prepare the breasts for lactation. Pregnancy tests are based on the presence of placental hormones.

Prostaglandins

Prostaglandins (pros-tah-GLAN-dins) are a group of local hormones made by most body tissues. Their name comes from the fact that they were first discovered in male prostate glands. Prostaglandins are produced, act, and are rapidly inactivated in or close to their sites of origin. A bewildering array of functions has been ascribed to these substances. Some prostaglandins cause constriction of blood vessels, bronchial tubes, and the intestine, whereas others cause dilation of these same structures. Prostaglandins are active in promoting inflammation; certain antiinflammatory drugs, such as aspirin, act by blocking prostaglandin production. Some prostaglandins have been used to induce labor or abortion and have been recommended as possible contraceptive agents.

Overproduction of prostaglandins by the uterine lining (endometrium) can cause painful cramps of the uterine muscle. Treatment with prostaglandin inhibitors has been successful in some cases. Much has been written about these substances, and extensive research on them continues.

CHECKPOINT 12-14 ➤ What are some organs other than the endocrine glands that produce hormones?

Hormones and Treatment

Hormones used for medical treatment are obtained from several different sources. Some are extracted from animal tissues. Some hormones and hormonelike substances are available in synthetic form, meaning that they are manufactured in commercial laboratories. A few hormones are produced by the genetic engineering technique of recombinant DNA. In this method, a gene for the cellular manufacture of a given product is introduced in the laboratory into the common bacterium *Escherichia coli*. The organisms are then grown in quantity, and the desired substance is harvested and purified.

A few examples of natural and synthetic hormones used in treatment are:

■ **Growth hormone** is used for the treatment of children with a deficiency of this hormone. It is also used to strengthen bones and build body mass in the elderly. Adequate supplies are available from recombinant DNA techniques.

■ **Insulin** is used in the treatment of diabetes mellitus. Pharmaceutical companies now produce "human" insulin by recombinant DNA methods.

■ **Adrenal steroids**, primarily the glucocorticoids, are used for the relief of inflammation in such diseases as rheumatoid arthritis, lupus erythematosus, asthma, and cerebral edema; for immunosuppression after organ transplantation; and for relief of symptoms associated with circulatory shock.

■ **Epinephrine** (adrenaline) has many uses, including stimulation of the heart muscle when rapid response is required, treatment of asthmatic attacks by relaxation of the small bronchial tubes, and treatment of the acute allergic reaction called **anaphylaxis** (an-ah-fi-LAK-sis).

■ **Thyroid hormones** are used in the treatment of hypothyroid conditions (infantile hypothyroidism and myxedema) and as replacement therapy after surgical removal of the thyroid gland.

■ **Oxytocin** is used to cause uterine contractions and induce labor.

■ **Androgens**, including testosterone and androsterone, are used in severe chronic illness to aid tissue building and promote healing.

■ **Estrogen and progesterone** are used as oral contraceptives (birth control pills; "the pill"). They are highly effective in preventing pregnancy. Occasionally, they give rise to unpleasant side effects, such as nausea. More rarely, they cause serious complications, such as thrombosis (blood clots) or hypertension (high blood pressure). These adverse side effects are more common among women who smoke. Any woman taking birth control pills should have a yearly medical examination.

Estrogen and progesterone preparations have been used to treat symptoms associated with menopause and protect against adverse changes that occur after menopause. Recent studies on the most popular form of these hormones have raised questions about their benefits and revealed some risks associated with their use. This issue is still under study.

Hormones and Stress

Stress in the form of physical injury, disease, emotional anxiety, and even pleasure calls forth a specific physiologic response that involves both the nervous system and the endocrine system. The nervous system response, the "fight-or-flight" response, is mediated by parts of the brain, especially the hypothalamus, and by the sympathetic nervous system, which releases epinephrine. During stress, the hypothalamus also triggers the release of ACTH from the anterior pituitary. The hormones released from the adrenal cortex as a result of ACTH stimulation raise the levels of glucose and other nutrients in the blood and inhibit

12

inflammation. Growth hormone, thyroid hormones, sex hormones, and insulin are also released.

These hormones help the body meet stressful situations. Unchecked, however, they are harmful and may lead to such stress-related disorders as high blood pressure, heart disease, ulcers, insomnia, back pain, and headaches. Cortisones decrease the immune response, leaving the body more susceptible to infection.

Although no one would enjoy a life totally free of stress in the form of stimulation and challenge, unmanaged stress, or "distress," has negative physical effects. For this reason, techniques such as biofeedback and meditation to control stress are useful. The simple measures of setting priorities, getting adequate periods of relaxation, and getting regular physical exercise are important in maintaining total health.

CHECKPOINT **12-15** ➤ What are some hormones released in time of stress?

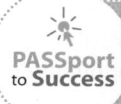
Visit **thePoint** or see the Student Resource CD in the back of this book for information on careers in exercise and fitness.

Aging and the Endocrine System

Some of the changes associated with aging, such as loss of muscle and bone tissue, can be linked to changes in the endocrine system. The main clinical conditions associated with the endocrine system involve the pancreas and the thyroid.

Many elderly people develop type 2 diabetes mellitus as a result of decreased insulin secretion, which is made worse by poor diet, inactivity, and increased body fat. Some elderly people also show the effects of decreased thyroid hormone secretion.

Sex hormones decline during the middle-age years in both males and females. These changes come from decreased activity of the gonads but also involve the more basic level of the pituitary gland and the secretion of gonadotropic hormones. Decrease in bone mass leading to osteoporosis is one result of these declines. With age, there is also a decrease in growth hormone levels and diminished activity of the adrenal cortex.

Thus far, the only commonly applied treatment for endocrine failure associated with age has been sex hormone replacement therapy for women at menopause. This supplementation has shown some beneficial effects on mucous membranes, the cardiovascular system, bone mass, and mental function.

Disease in Context revisited

➤ Becky's New "Normal"

Becky stumbled down the stairs wiping the sleep from her eyes as she made her way to the kitchen, hoping that Max hadn't finished all the pancakes that she could smell from down the hallway. "Good morning, sleepy-head," greeted her mother as she handed Becky the glucose monitor and lancet. "How was your sleep last night?"

"Great," yawned Becky as she lanced the side of her finger and squeezed a tiny drop of blood onto the monitor's test strip. After a few seconds, the monitor beeped and displayed her blood glucose concentration. "I'm normal," said Becky, half-expecting a wise-crack from her little brother, but he kept on eating.

Since Dr. Carter's diagnosis, Becky had been getting used to her new "normal." It wasn't easy being diabetic. She had to be really careful about what she ate and when. She had to measure her glucose before meals and inject herself with insulin after. Monitoring her glucose wasn't too bad, but Becky didn't think she would ever get used to the needles. She was also a little worried about what the kids at school were saying about her and her disease. One unexpected benefit was that Max seemed to have a new-found respect for her and her ability to inject herself. "What a weirdo!" she thought as she carefully poured a little bit of syrup on her pancakes.

During this case, we saw that the lack of the hormone insulin had widespread effects on Becky's whole body. In later chapters, we will learn more about the endocrine system's role in regulating body function. We'll also check on how Becky is managing her diabetes in Chapter 20: Metabolism, Nutrition, and Body Temperature.

Word Anatomy

Medical terms are built from standardized word parts (prefixes, roots, and suffixes). Learning the meanings of these parts can help you remember words and interpret unfamiliar terms.

WORD PART	MEANING	EXAMPLE
The Endocrine Glands and Their Hormones		
trop/o	acting on, influencing	*Somatotropin* stimulates growth in most body tissues.
cortic/o	cortex	*Adrenocorticotropic* hormone acts on the adrenal cortex.
lact/o	milk	*Prolactin* stimulates milk production in the breasts.
ur/o	urine	*Antidiuretic* hormone promotes reabsorption of water in the kidneys and decreases excretion of urine.
oxy	sharp, acute	*Oxytocin* stimulates uterine contractions during labor.
toc/o	labor	See preceding example.
acr/o	end, extremity	*Acromegaly* causes enlargement of hands and feet.
-megaly	enlargement	See preceding example.
myx/o	mucus	In *myxedema*, the skin takes on a swollen, waxy appearance.
edem	swelling	See preceding example.
ren/o	kidney	The *adrenal* glands are near (ad-) the kidneys.
nephr/o	kidney	*Epinephrine* is another name for adrenaline.
insul/o	pancreatic islet, island	*Insulin* is a hormone produced by the pancreatic islets.
glyc/o	sugar, glucose	*Hyperglycemia* is high blood sugar.
andr/o	male	An *androgen* is any male sex hormone.
Other Hormone-Producing Tissues		
-poiesis	making, forming	*Erythropoietin* is a hormone from the kidneys that stimulates production of red blood cells.
natri	sodium (*L. natrium*)	Atrial *natriuretic* peptide stimulates release of sodium in the urine.

Summary

I. **HORMONES**
    A. Functions of hormones
        1. Affect other cells or organs—target tissue
        2. Widespread effects on growth, metabolism, reproduction
        3. Bind to receptors on target cells
    B. Hormone chemistry
        1. Amino acid compounds—proteins and related compounds
        2. Lipids—made from fatty acids
            a. Steroids

            (1) Derived from cholesterol
            (2) Produced by adrenal cortex and sex glands
            b. Prostaglandins
    C. Regulation of hormones—mainly negative feedback

II. **ENDOCRINE GLANDS AND THEIR HORMONES**
    A. Pituitary
        1. Regulated by hypothalamus
            a. Anterior pituitary
                (1) Releasing hormones (RH) sent through portal system

(2) Inhibiting hormones for GH and PRL
    b. Posterior pituitary
        (1) Stores hormones made by hypothalamus
        (2) Released by nervous stimulation
    2. Anterior lobe hormones
        a. Growth hormone (GH)—stimulates growth, tissue repair
        b. Thyroid-stimulating hormone (TSH)
        c. Adrenocorticotropic hormone (ACTH)—acts on cortex of adrenal gland
        d. Prolactin (PRL)—stimulates milk production in mammary glands
        e. Follicle-stimulating hormone (FSH)—acts on gonads
        f. Luteinizing hormone (LH)—acts on gonads
    3. Posterior lobe hormones
        a. Antidiuretic hormone (ADH)—promotes reabsorption of water in the kidneys
        b. Oxytocin—stimulates uterine contractions
    4. Pituitary tumors—may cause underactivity or overactivity of pituitary
B. Thyroid gland
    1. Hormones of the thyroid gland
        a. Thyroxine (T4) and triiodothyronine (T3) increase metabolic rate
        b. Calcitonin—decreases blood calcium levels
    2. Disorders of the thyroid gland
        a. Goiter—enlarged thyroid
        b. Hypothyroidism—causes infantile hypothyroidism or myxedema
        c. Hyperthyroidism—e.g., Graves disease
        d. Thyroiditis—inflammation of thyroid; e.g., Hashimoto thyroiditis
    3. Thyroid function tests—radioactive iodine used
C. Parathyroid glands—secrete parathyroid hormone (PTH), which increases blood calcium levels
    1. Calcium metabolism
    2. Disorders of the parathyroid glands
D. Adrenal glands
    1. Hormones of adrenal medulla (inner region)
        a. Epinephrine and norepinephrine—act as neurotransmitters
    2. Hormones of adrenal cortex (outer region)
        a. Glucocorticoids—released during stress to raise nutrients in blood; e.g., cortisol
        b. Mineralocorticoids—regulate water and electrolyte balance; e.g., aldosterone
        c. Sex hormones—produced in small amounts
    3. Disorders of the adrenal cortex
E. Pancreas—islet cells of pancreas secrete hormones
    1. Insulin
        a. Lowers blood glucose
        b. Lack or poor cellular response causes diabetes mellitus
            (1) Type 1 (T1DM)—autoimmune disease that requires insulin
            (2) Type 2 (T2DM)—usually controlled with diet, exercise, weight loss

            (3) Gestational—occurs curing pregnancy
    2. Glucagon
        a. Raises blood glucose
F. Sex glands—needed for reproduction and development of secondary sex characteristics
    1. Testes—secrete testosterone
    2. Ovaries—secrete estrogen and progesterone
G. Thymus gland—secretes thymosin, which aids in development of T lymphocytes
H. Pineal gland—secretes melatonin
    1. Regulates sexual development and sleep–wake cycles
    2. Controlled by environmental light

III. **OTHER HORMONE-PRODUCING TISSUES**
A. Stomach and small intestine—secrete hormones that regulate digestion
B. Kidneys—secrete erythropoietin, which increases production of red blood cells
C. Brain—releasing and inhibiting hormones, ADH, oxytocin
D. Atria of heart—ANP causes loss of sodium by kidney and lowers blood pressure
E. Placenta—secretes hormones that maintain pregnancy and prepare breasts for lactation
F. Prostaglandins—produced by cells throughout body; have varied effects

IV. **HORMONES AND TREATMENT**
A. Growth hormone—treatment of deficiency in children, in elderly for bone strength and body mass
B. Insulin—treatment of diabetes mellitus
C. Steroids—reduction of inflammation, suppression of immunity
D. Epinephrine—treatment of asthma, anaphylaxis, shock
E. Thyroid hormone—treatment of hypothyroidism
F. Oxytocin—contraction of uterine muscle
G. Androgens—promote healing
H. Estrogen and progesterone—contraception, symptoms of menopause

V. **HORMONES AND STRESS**
A. Body's response to stress involves nervous and endocrine systems, hormones
B. Fight-or-flight response mediated by brain: hypothalamus, sympathetic nervous system
C. Hormones help body to meet stressful situations
D. Unmanaged stress can be harmful; stress management techniques help maintain overall health

VI. **AGING AND THE ENDOCRINE SYSTEM**
A. Aging-associated changes linked with endocrine system changes—loss of muscle and bone tissue
B. Main clinical conditions associated with endocrine system involve pancreas, thyroid
    1. Type 2 diabetes mellitus
    2. Decline in sex hormones in males and females
        a. Decreased bone mass—osteoporosis
C. Sex hormone replacement therapy for women at menopause—only common treatment for age-associated endocrine failure

Questions for Study and Review

BUILDING UNDERSTANDING

Fill in the blanks

1. Chemical messengers carried by the blood are called _____.

2. The part of the brain that regulates endocrine activity is the _____.

3. Red blood cell production in the bone marrow is stimulated by _____.

4. A hormone produced by the heart is _____.

5. Local hormones active in promoting inflammation are _____.

Matching > Match each numbered item with the most closely related lettered item.

___ **6.** A disorder caused by overproduction of growth hormone in the adult.

___ **7.** A disorder caused by underproduction of parathyroid hormone.

___ **8.** A disorder caused by overproduction of insulin.

___ **9.** A disorder caused by overproduction of growth hormone in the child.

___ **10.** A disorder caused by underproduction of antidiuretic hormone.

a. hypoglycemia

b. gigantism

c. tetany

d. diabetes insipidus

e. acromegaly

Multiple Choice

___ **11.** A target tissue responds to a hormone only if it has the appropriate
  a. amino acid
  b. transporter
  c. ion channel
  d. receptor

___ **12.** Uterine contractions and milk ejection are promoted by
  a. prolactin
  b. oxytocin
  c. estrogen
  d. luteinizing hormone

___ **13.** The principal hormone that increases the metabolic rate in body cells is
  a. thyroxine
  b. triiodothyronine
  c. aldosterone
  d. progesterone

___ **14.** Epinephrine and norepinephrine are released by the
  a. adrenal cortex
  b. adrenal medulla
  c. kidneys
  d. pancreas

___ **15.** Sleep-wake cycles are regulated by the
  a. pituitary
  b. thyroid
  c. thymus
  d. pineal

12

UNDERSTANDING CONCEPTS

16. With regard to regulation, what are the main differences between the nervous system and the endocrine system?

17. Explain how the hypothalamus and pituitary gland regulate certain endocrine glands. Use the thyroid as an example.

18. Name the two divisions of the pituitary gland. List the hormones released from each division and describe the effects of each.

19. Compare and contrast the following hormones:
a. calcitonin and parathyroid hormone
b. cortisol and aldosterone
c. insulin and glucagon
d. testosterone and estrogen

CONCEPTUAL THINKING

24. In the case story, Dr. Carter noted that Becky presented with the three cardinal signs of type 1 diabetes mellitus. What are they? What causes them?

25. How is type 1 diabetes mellitus similar to starvation?

20. Describe the anatomy of the following endocrine glands:
a. thyroid
b. pancreas
c. adrenals

21. Compare and contrast the following diseases:
a. myxedema and Graves disease
b. type 1 diabetes and type 2 diabetes
c. Addison disease and Cushing syndrome

22. Name the hormone released by the thymus gland; by the pineal body. What are the effects of each?

23. List several hormones released during stress. What is the relationship between prolonged stress and disease?

26. Mr. Jefferson has rheumatoid arthritis, which is being treated with glucocorticoids. During a recent checkup, his doctor notices that Mr. Jefferson's face is "puffy" and his arms are bruised. Why does the doctor decide to lower his patient's glucocorticoid dosage?

UNIT V

Circulation and Body Defense

The chapters in this unit discuss the systems that move materials through the body. The blood is the main transport medium. It circulates through the cardiovascular system, consisting of the heart and the blood vessels. The lymphatic system, in addition to other functions, helps to balance body fluids by bringing substances from the tissues back to the heart. Components of the blood and the lymphatic system are involved in body defenses against infection as part of the immune system.

CHAPTER 13

The Blood

Learning Outcomes

After careful study of this chapter, you should be able to:

1. List the functions of the blood
2. List the main ingredients in plasma
3. Describe the formation of blood cells
4. Name and describe the three types of formed elements in the blood and give the function of each
5. Characterize the five types of leukocytes
6. Define *hemostasis* and cite three steps in hemostasis
7. Briefly describe the steps in blood clotting
8. Define *blood type* and explain the relation between blood type and transfusions
9. List the possible reasons for transfusions of whole blood and blood components
10. Define *anemia* and list the causes of anemia
11. Define *leukemia* and name the two types of leukemia
12. Describe several forms of clotting disorders
13. Specify the tests used to study blood
14. Show how word parts are used to build words related to the blood (see Word Anatomy at the end of the chapter)

Selected Key Terms

The following terms and other boldface terms in the chapter are defined in the Glossary

agglutination
anemia
antigen
antiserum
centrifuge
coagulation
cryoprecipitate
erythrocyte
fibrin
hematocrit
hemoglobin
hemolysis
hemorrhage
hemostasis
leukemia
leukocyte
megakaryocyte
plasma
platelet (thrombocyte)
serum
thrombocytopenia
transfusion

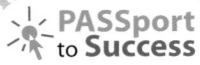

PASSport to Success

Visit *thePoint* or see the Student Resource CD in the back of this book for definitions and pronunciations of key terms as well as a pretest for this chapter.

Disease
in Context

> ## Cole's Case: A Hemoglobin Abnormality

Both baby Cole and his mother Jada were resting comfortably in the maternity ward. Although Cole was only a few hours old, he had already been bathed, fed, and thoroughly examined by a pediatrician. As part of the hospital's routine neonatal procedures, a sample of Cole's blood was collected and sent to the hematology laboratory.

When Cole's blood sample arrived in the laboratory, a technologist divided it into several portions for analysis. First, she tested for Cole's blood type. When she added anti-B serum to his blood, the erythrocytes in the sample clumped together. There was no reaction to the anti-A serum. Since the antibodies in the sera showed only B antigens on the red blood cells, the medical laboratory technologist knew that Cole's blood was type B. Next, she performed a blood cell count using an automated machine. Cole's platelet count was normal, suggesting that he did not suffer from thrombocytopenia, the most common clotting disorder. His leukocyte count

was normal too, signifying that his immune system was healthy. His erythrocyte count was also within normal limits, indicating that his red bone marrow (the site of erythrocyte production) was functioning as well. As required by many hospitals in the United States, the technologist screened Cole's blood for the presence of abnormal hemoglobin in his erythrocytes. When the test result came back positive for abnormal hemoglobin, the technologist requested that a blood sample be drawn from both of Cole's parents. She needed to run some more sensitive blood tests to determine whether or not the infant suffered from sickle cell disease.

The medical laboratory technologist performed several tests on Cole's blood. In this chapter, you will study blood and learn about its constituents and functions. Later, we'll find out more about Cole's abnormal hemoglobin.

The circulating blood is of fundamental importance in maintaining homeostasis. This life-giving fluid brings nutrients and oxygen to the cells and carries away waste. The heart pumps blood continuously through a closed system of vessels. The heart and blood vessels are described in Chapters 14 and 15.

Blood is classified as a connective tissue because it consists of cells suspended in an intercellular background material, or matrix. Blood cells share many characteristics of origination and development with other connective tissues. However, blood differs from other connective tissues in that its cells are not fixed in position; instead, they move freely in the plasma, the blood's liquid portion.

Whole blood is a viscous (thick) fluid that varies in color from bright scarlet to dark red, depending on how much oxygen it is carrying. (It is customary in drawings to color blood high in oxygen as red and blood low in oxygen as blue.) The blood volume accounts for approximately 8% of total body weight. The actual quantity of circulating blood differs with a person's size; the average adult male, weighing 70 kg (154 pounds), has about 5 liters (5.2 quarts) of blood.

Functions of the Blood

The circulating blood serves the body in three ways: transportation, regulation, and protection.

Transportation

- **Gases.** Oxygen from inhaled air diffuses into the blood through thin membranes in the lungs and is carried by the circulation to all body tissues. Carbon dioxide, a waste product of cell metabolism, is carried from the tissues to the lungs, where it is breathed out.

- **Nutrients.** The blood transports nutrients and other needed substances, such as electrolytes (salts) and vitamins, to the cells. These materials enter the blood from the digestive system or are released into the blood from body reserves.

- **Waste.** The blood transports the waste products from the cells to sites where they are removed. For example, the kidney removes excess water, acid, electrolytes, and urea (a nitrogen-containing waste). The liver removes blood pigments, hormones, and drugs, and the lungs eliminate carbon dioxide.

- **Hormones.** The blood carries hormones from their sites of origin to the organs they affect.

Regulation

- **pH.** Buffers in the blood help keep the pH of body fluids steady at about 7.4. (The actual range of blood pH is 7.35 to 7.45.) Recall that pH is a measure of a solution's acidity or alkalinity. At an average pH of 7.4, blood is slightly alkaline (basic).

- **Fluid balance.** The blood regulates the amount of fluid in the tissues by means of substances (mainly proteins) that maintain the proper osmotic pressure. Recall that osmotic pressure is related to the concentration of dissolved and suspended materials in a solution. Proper osmotic pressure is needed for fluid balance, as described in Chapter 15.

- **Heat.** The blood transports heat that is generated in the muscles to other parts of the body, thus aiding in the regulation of body temperature.

Protection

- **Disease.** The blood is important in defense against disease. It carries the cells and antibodies of the immune system that protect against pathogens.

- **Blood loss.** The blood contains factors that protect against blood loss from the site of an injury. The process of blood coagulation, needed to prevent blood loss, is described later in this chapter.

CHECKPOINT 13-1 ➤ What are some substances transported in the blood?

CHECKPOINT 13-2 ➤ What is the pH range of the blood?

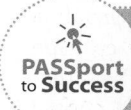 **PASSport to Success**   Visit *thePoint* or see the Student Resource CD in the back of this book for information on careers in hematology, the study of blood.

Blood Constituents

The blood is divided into two main components (Fig. 13-1). The liquid portion is the **plasma**. The **formed elements,** which include cells and cell fragments, fall into three categories, as follows:

- **Erythrocytes** (eh-RITH-ro-sites), from *erythro,* meaning "red," are the red blood cells, which transport oxygen.

- **Leukocytes** (LU-ko-sites), from *leuko,* meaning "white," are the several types of white blood cells, which protect against infection.

- **Platelets,** also called **thrombocytes** (THROM-bo-sites), are cell fragments that participate in blood clotting.

Table 13-1 summarizes information on the different types of formed elements. Figure 13-2 shows all the categories of formed elements in a blood smear, that is, a blood sample spread thinly over the surface of a glass slide, as viewed under a microscope.

CHECKPOINT 13-3 ➤ What are the two main components of blood?

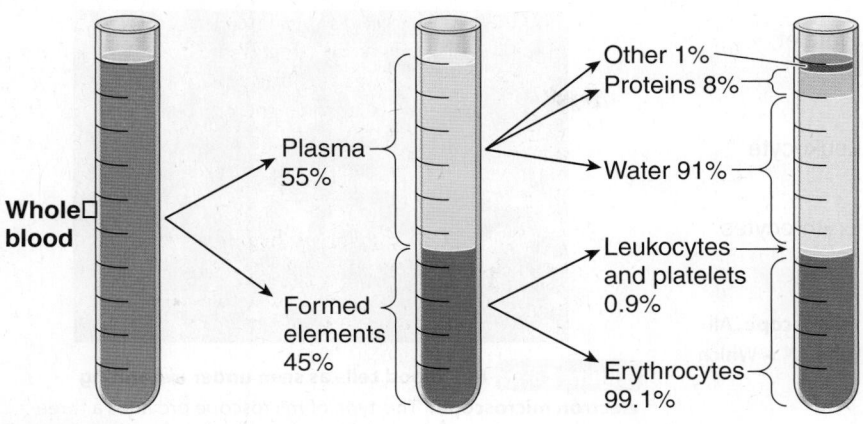

Figure 13-1 **Composition of whole blood.** Percentages show the relative proportions of the different components of plasma and formed elements.

Blood Plasma

About 55% of the total blood volume is plasma. The plasma itself is 91% water. Many different substances, dissolved or suspended in the water, make up the other 9% by weight (see Fig. 13-1). The plasma content may vary somewhat because substances are removed and added as the blood circulates to and from the tissues. However, the body tends to maintain a fairly constant level of most substances. For example, the level of glucose, a simple sugar, is maintained at a remarkably constant level of about one-tenth of one percent (0.1%) in solution.

After water, the next largest percentage (about 8%) of material in the plasma is **protein**. The plasma proteins include the following:

- **Albumin** (al-BU-min), the most abundant protein in plasma, is important for maintaining the blood's osmotic pressure. This protein is manufactured in the liver.

- **Clotting factors**, necessary for blood coagulation, are also manufactured in the liver.

- **Antibodies** combat infection. Antibodies are made by certain white blood cells.

- **Complement** consists of a group of enzymes that helps antibodies in their fight against pathogens (see Chapter 17).

The remaining 1% of the plasma consists of nutrients, electrolytes, and other materials that must be transported. With regard to the nutrients, the principal carbohydrate found in the plasma is glucose. This simple sugar is absorbed from digested foods in the intestine. It is also stored as glycogen in the liver and skeletal muscles; this glucose can be released as needed to supply energy. Amino acids, the products of protein digestion, also circulate in the plasma. Lipids constitute a small percentage of blood plasma. Lipid components include fats, cholesterol, and lipoproteins, which are proteins bound to cholesterol.

The electrolytes in the plasma appear primarily as chloride, carbonate, or phosphate salts of sodium, potassium, calcium, and magnesium. These salts have a variety of functions, including the formation of bone (calcium and phosphorus), the production of certain hormones (such as iodine for the production of thyroid hormones), and the maintenance of the acid–base balance (such as sodium and potassium carbonates and phosphates present in buffers).

Other materials transported in plasma include vitamins, hormones, waste products, drugs, and dissolved gases, primarily oxygen and carbon dioxide.

13

Table 13-1	Formed Elements of Blood		
Formed Element	**Number per μL of Blood**	**Description**	**Function**
Erythrocyte (red blood cell)	5 million	Tiny (7 μm diameter), biconcave disk without nucleus (anuclear)	Carries oxygen bound to hemoglobin; also carries some carbon dioxide and buffers blood
Leukocyte (white blood cell)	5,000 to 10,000	Larger than red cell with prominent nucleus that may be segmented (granulocyte) or unsegmented (agranulocyte); vary in staining properties	Protects against pathogens; destroys foreign matter and debris; some are active in the immune system; located in blood, tissues, and lymphatic system
Platelet	150,000 to 450,000	Fragment of large cell (megakaryocyte)	Hemostasis; forms a platelet plug and starts blood clot-

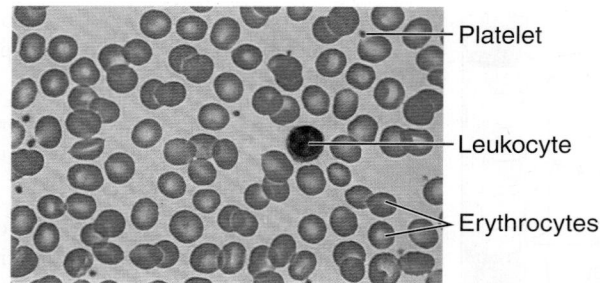

Platelet

Leukocyte

Erythrocytes

Figure 13-2 **Blood cells as viewed under the microscope.** All three types of formed elements are visible. [ZOOMING IN ➤ Which cells are the most numerous in the blood?]

CHECKPOINT 13-4 ➤ Next to water, what is the most abundant type of substance in plasma?

The Formed Elements

All of the blood's formed elements are produced in red bone marrow, which is located in the ends of long bones and in the inner mass of all other bones. The ancestors of all the blood cells are called **hematopoietic** (blood-forming) **stem cells**. These cells have the potential to develop into any of the blood cell types produced within the red bone marrow.

In comparison with other cells, most blood cells are short lived. The need for constant blood cell replacement means that normal activity of the red bone marrow is absolutely essential to life.

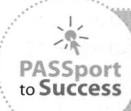

PASSport to Success

Visit **thePoint** or see the Student Resource CD in the back of this book for a chart detailing the development of all the formed elements.

CHECKPOINT 13-5 ➤ Where do blood cells form?

CHECKPOINT 13-6 ➤ What type of cell gives rise to all blood cells?

ERYTHROCYTES Erythrocytes, the red blood cells (RBCs, or red cells), measure about 7 μm in diameter. They are disk-shaped bodies with a depression on both sides. This biconcave shape creates a central area that is thinner than the edges (Fig. 13-3). Erythrocytes are different from other cells in that the mature form found in the circulating blood lacks a nucleus (is anuclear) and also lacks most of the other organelles commonly found in cells. As red cells mature, these components are lost, providing more space for the cells to carry oxygen. This vital gas is bound in the red cells to **hemoglobin** (he-mo-GLO-bin), a protein that contains iron (see Box 13-1,

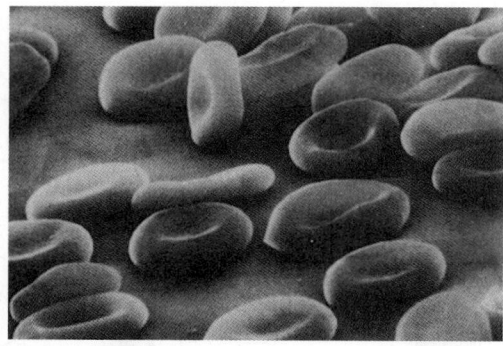

Figure 13-3 **Red blood cells as seen under a scanning electron microscope.** This type of microscope provides a three-dimensional view of the cells. [ZOOMING IN ➤ Why are these cells described as biconcave?]

Hemoglobin: Door-to-Door Oxygen Delivery). Hemoglobin, combined with oxygen, gives the blood its characteristic red color. The more oxygen carried by the hemoglobin, the brighter is the blood's red color. Therefore, the blood that goes from the lungs to the tissues is a bright red because it carries a great supply of oxygen; in contrast, the blood that returns to the lungs is a much darker red because it has given up much of its oxygen to the tissues.

Hemoglobin has two lesser functions in addition to the transport of oxygen. Hemoglobin that has given up its oxygen is able to carry hydrogen ions. In this way, hemoglobin acts as a buffer and plays an important role in acid–base balance (see Chapter 21). Hemoglobin also carries some carbon dioxide from the tissues to the lungs for elimination. The carbon dioxide is bound to a different part of the molecule than the part that holds oxygen, so that it does not interfere with oxygen transport.

Hemoglobin's ability to carry oxygen can be blocked by carbon monoxide. This odorless and colorless but harmful gas combines with hemoglobin to form a stable compound that can severely restrict the erythrocytes' ability to carry oxygen. Carbon monoxide is a byproduct of the incomplete burning of fuels, such as gasoline and other petroleum products and coal, wood, and other carbon-containing materials. It also occurs in cigarette smoke and automobile exhaust.

Erythrocytes are by far the most numerous of the blood cells, averaging from 4.5 to 5 million per microliter (μL or mcL) of blood. (A microliter is one millionth of a liter.) Because mature red cells have no nucleus and cannot divide, they must be replaced constantly. After leaving the bone marrow, they circulate in the bloodstream for about 120 days before their membranes deteriorate and they are destroyed by the liver and spleen. Red cell production is stimulated by the hormone **erythropoietin** (eh-rith-ro-POY-eh-tin) (**EPO**), which is released from the kidney in response to decreased oxygen. Constant red cell production requires an adequate supply of nutrients, particularly protein, the B vitamins B_{12} and folic acid, required for the production of DNA, and the minerals iron and copper for

Box 13-1	A Closer Look

Hemoglobin: Door-to-Door Oxygen Delivery

The hemoglobin molecule is a protein made of four amino acid chains (the globin part of the molecule), each of which holds an iron-containing heme group. Each of the four hemes can bind one molecule of oxygen.

Hemoglobin allows the blood to carry much more oxygen than it could were the oxygen simply dissolved in the plasma. A red blood cell contains about 250 million hemoglobins, each capable of binding four molecules of oxygen. So, a single red blood cell can carry about one billion oxygen molecules! Hemoglobin reversibly binds oxygen, picking it up in the lungs and releasing it in the body tissues. Active cells need more oxygen and also generate heat and acidity. These changing conditions promote the release of oxygen from hemoglobin into metabolically active tissues.

Immature red blood cells (erythroblasts) produce hemoglobin as they mature into erythrocytes in the red bone marrow. When the liver and spleen destroy old erythrocytes they break down the released hemoglobin. Some of its components are recycled, and the remainder leaves the body as a brown fecal pigment called stercobilin. In spite of some conservation, dietary protein and iron are still essential to maintain hemoglobin supplies.

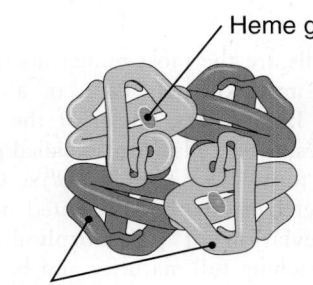

Hemoglobin. This protein in red blood cells consists of four amino acid chains (globins), each with an oxygen-binding heme group.

the production of hemoglobin. Vitamin C is also important for the proper absorption of iron from the small intestine.

CHECKPOINT 13-7 ➤ Red cells are modified to carry a maximum amount of hemoglobin. What is the main function of hemoglobin?

LEUKOCYTES The **leukocytes**, or white blood cells (WBCs, or white cells), are different from the erythrocytes in appearance, quantity, and function. The cells themselves are round, but they contain prominent nuclei of varying shapes and sizes. Occurring at a concentration of 5,000 to 10,000 per microliter (μL) of blood, leukocytes are outnumbered by red cells by about 700 to 1. Although the red cells have a definite color, the leukocytes are colorless.

The different types of white cells are identified by their size, the shape of the nucleus, and the appearance of granules in the cytoplasm when the cells are stained. The stain commonly used for blood is Wright stain, which is a mixture of dyes that differentiates the various blood cells. The "granules" in the white cells are actually lysosomes and other secretory vesicles. They are present in all white blood cells, but they are more easily stained and more visible in some cells than in others. The relative percentage of the different types of leukocytes is a valuable clue in arriving at a medical diagnosis (Table 13-2).

The granular leukocytes, or **granulocytes** (GRAN-u-lo-sites), are so named because they show visible granules

13

Table 13-2	Leukocytes (White Blood Cells)	
Cell Type	Relative Percentage (Adult)	Function
Granulocytes		
Neutrophils	54%–62%	Phagocytosis
Eosinophils	1%–3%	Allergic reactions; defense against parasites
Basophils	<1%	Allergic reactions; inflammatory reactions
Agranulocytes		
Lymphocytes	25%–38%	Immunity (T cells and B cells)
Monocytes	3%–7%	Phagocytosis

in the cytoplasm when stained (see Fig. 13-4A–C). Each has a very distinctive, highly segmented nucleus. The different types of granulocytes are named for the type of dyes they take up when stained. They include the following:

- **Neutrophils** (NU-tro-fils) stain with either acidic or basic dyes and show lavender granules.

- **Eosinophils** (e-o-SIN-o-fils) stain with acidic dyes (eosin is one) and have beadlike, bright pink granules.

- **Basophils** (BA-so-fils) stain with basic dyes and have large, dark blue granules that often obscure the nucleus.

The neutrophils are the most numerous of the white cells, constituting approximately 60% of all leukocytes (see Table 13-2). Because the nuclei of the neutrophils have various shapes, these cells are also called **polymorphs** (meaning "many forms") or simply *polys*. Other nicknames are *segs*, referring to the segmented nucleus, and *PMNs*, an abbreviation of **poly**morphonuclear neutrophils. Before reaching full maturity and becoming segmented, a neutrophil's nucleus looks like a thick, curved band (Fig. 13-5). An increase in the number of these **band cells** (also called *stab* or *staff cells*) is a sign of infection and active neutrophil production.

The eosinophils and basophils make up a small percentage of the white cells but increase in number during allergic reactions.

The agranular leukocytes, or **agranulocytes**, are so named because they lack easily visible granules (see Fig. 13-4D,E). Their nuclei are round or curved and are not segmented. There are two types of agranular leukocytes:

- **Lymphocytes** (LIM-fo-sites) are the second most numerous of the white cells. Although lymphocytes originate in the red bone marrow, they develop to maturity in lymphoid tissue and can multiply in this tissue as well (see Chapter 16). They circulate in the lymphatic system and are active in immunity.

- **Monocytes** (MON-o-sites) are the largest in size. They average about 5% of the leukocytes.

Function of Leukocytes Leukocytes clear the body of foreign material and cellular debris. Most importantly, they destroy pathogens that may invade the body. Neutrophils and monocytes engage in **phagocytosis** (fag-o-si-TO-sis), the engulfing of foreign matter (Fig. 13-6). Whenever pathogens enter the tissues, as through a wound, phagocytes are attracted to the area. They squeeze between the cells of the capillary walls and proceed by ameboid (ah-ME-boyd), or amebalike, motion to the area of infection where they engulf the invaders. Lysosomes in the cytoplasm then digest the foreign organisms and the cells eliminate the waste products.

When foreign organisms invade, the bone marrow and lymphoid tissue go into emergency production of white cells, and their number increases enormously as a result.

Granulocytes

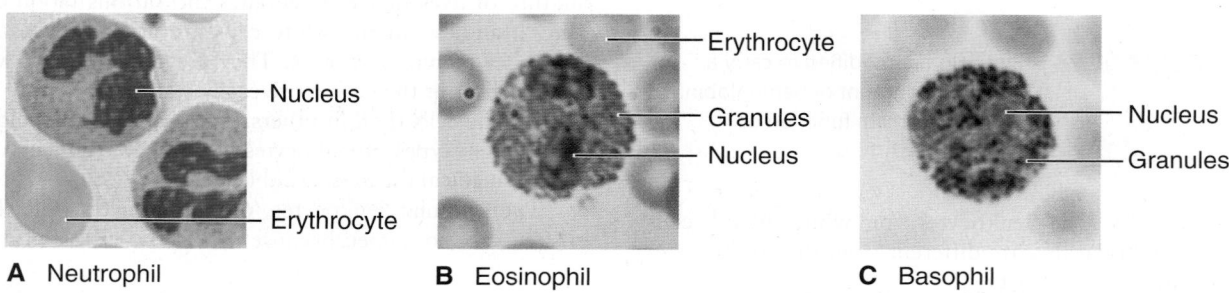

A Neutrophil   **B** Eosinophil   **C** Basophil

Agranulocytes

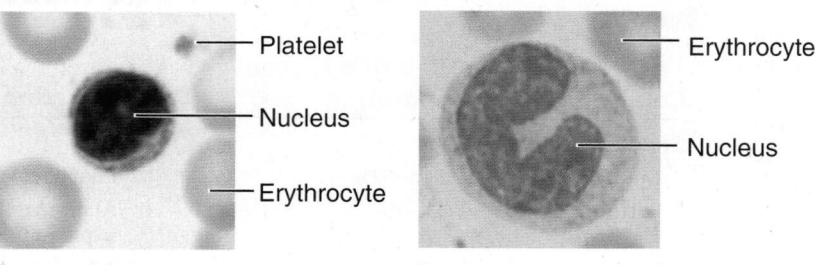

D Lymphocyte   **E** Monocyte

Figure 13-4 **Granulocytes (A-C) and agranulocytes (D,E). (A)** The neutrophil has a large, segmented nucleus. **(B)** The eosinophil has many bright pink-staining granules. **(C)** The basophil has large dark blue-staining granules. **(D)** The lymphocyte has a large undivided nucleus. **(E)** The monocyte is the largest of the leukocytes. [**ZOOMING IN** ➤ Which group of leukocytes has segmented nuclei? Which specific type of leukocyte is largest in size? Smallest in size?]

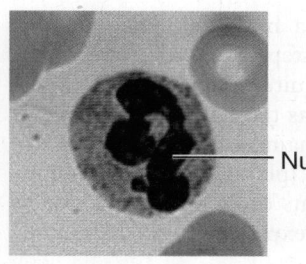

Nucleus

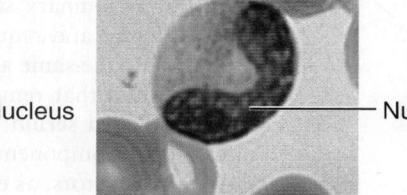

Nucleus

A Mature neutrophil

B Band cell
(immature neutrophil)

Figure 13-5 **Stages in neutrophil development.** **(A)** A mature neutrophil has a segmented nucleus. **(B)** An immature neutrophil is called a band cell because the nucleus is shaped like a thick, curved band. (×1325) (Reprinted with permission from Gartner LP, Hiatt JL. *Color Atlas of Histology*, 3rd ed. Philadelphia: Lippincott Williams & Wilkins, 2000.)

Detection of an abnormally large number of white cells in the blood is an indication of infection. In battling pathogens, leukocytes themselves may be destroyed. A mixture of dead and living bacteria, together with dead and living leukocytes, forms **pus.** A collection of pus localized in one area is known as an **abscess.**

Some monocytes enter the tissues, enlarge, and mature into **macrophages** (MAK-ro-faj-ez), which are highly active in disposing of invaders and foreign material. Although most circulating lymphocytes live only 6 to 8 hours, those that enter the tissues may survive for longer periods—days, months, or even years.

CHECKPOINT **13-8** ➤ What are the types of granular leukocytes? Of agranular leukocytes?

CHECKPOINT **13-9** ➤ What is the most important function of leukocytes?

Some lymphocytes become **plasma cells,** active in the production of circulating antibodies needed for immunity. The activities of the various white cells are further discussed in Chapter 17.

PLATELETS The **blood platelets** (thrombocytes) are the smallest of all the formed elements (Fig. 13-7A). These tiny structures are not cells in themselves but rather fragments constantly released from giant bone marrow cells called **megakaryocytes** (meg-ah-KAR-e-o-sites) (Fig. 13-7B). Platelets do not have nuclei or DNA, but they do contain active enzymes and mitochondria. The number of platelets in the circulating blood has been estimated to range from 150,000 to 450,000 per μL. They have a lifespan of about 10 days.

Platelets are essential to blood **coagulation** (clotting). When blood comes in contact with any tissue other than the smooth lining of the blood vessels, as in the case of injury, the platelets stick together and form a plug that seals the wound. The platelets then release chemicals that participate in the formation of a clot to stop blood loss. More details on these reactions follow.

CHECKPOINT **13-10** ➤ What is the function of blood platelets?

Hemostasis

Hemostasis (he-mo-STA-sis) is the process that prevents blood loss from the circulation when a blood vessel is ruptured by an injury. Events in hemostasis include the following:

1. **Contraction** of the smooth muscles in the blood vessel wall. This reduces blood flow and loss from the defect

13

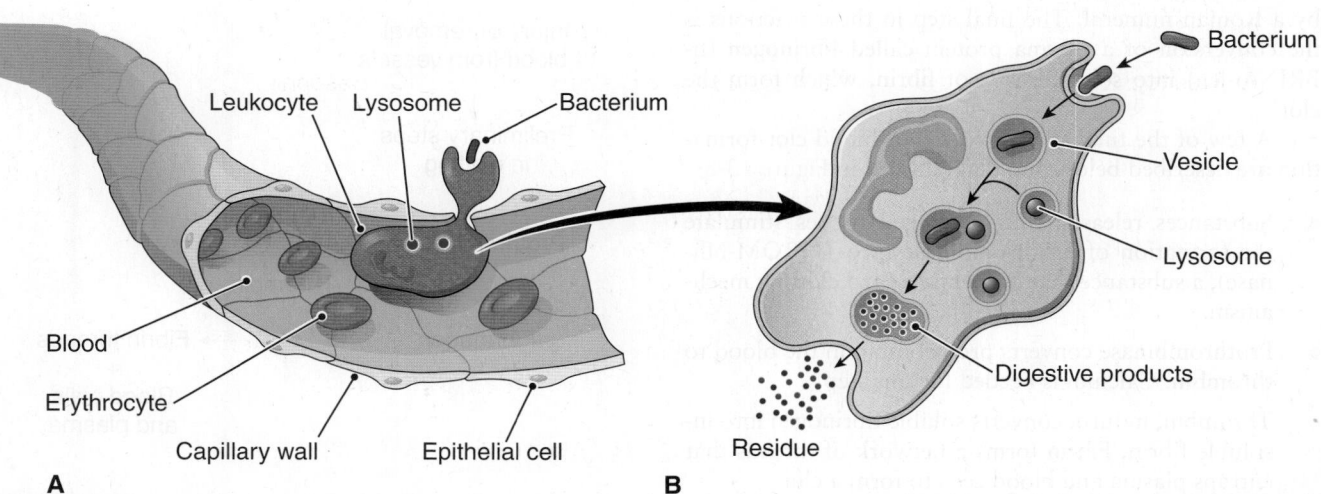

Figure 13-6 **Phagocytosis.** **(A)** A phagocytic leukocyte (white blood cell) squeezes through a capillary wall in the region of an infection and engulfs a bacterium. **(B)** The bacterium is enclosed in a vesicle and digested by a lysosome. [**ZOOMING IN** ➤ What type of epithelium makes up the capillary wall?]

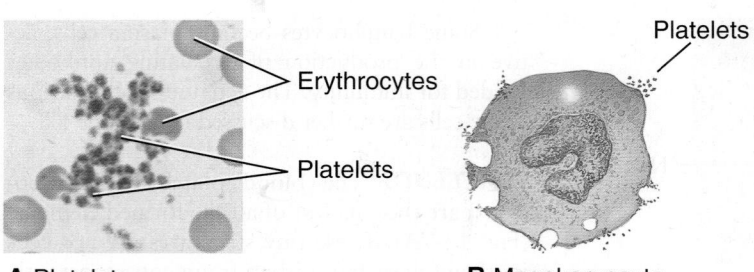

A Platelets

B Megakaryocyte

Platelets

Erythrocytes

Platelets

Platelets

Figure 13-7 **Platelets (thrombocytes).** **(A)** Platelets in a blood smear. **(B)** A megakaryocyte releases platelets. (B, Reprinted with permission from Gartner LP, Hiatt JL. *Color Atlas of Histology*, 3rd ed. Philadelphia: Lippincott Williams & Wilkins, 2000.)

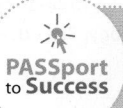

in the vessel. The term for this reduction in a vessel's diameter is *vasoconstriction*.

2. Formation of a **platelet plug.** Activated platelets become sticky and adhere to the defect to form a temporary plug.

3. Formation of a **blood clot** (coagulation).

Blood Clotting

The many substances necessary for blood clotting, or coagulation, are normally inactive in the bloodstream. A balance is maintained between compounds that promote clotting, known as **procoagulants**, and those that prevent clotting, known as **anticoagulants**. In addition, there are chemicals in the circulation that dissolve any unnecessary and potentially harmful clots that may form. Under normal conditions, the substances that prevent clotting prevail. When an injury occurs, however, the procoagulants are activated, and a clot is formed.

The clotting process is a well-controlled series of separate events involving 12 different factors, each designated by a Roman numeral. The final step in these reactions is the conversion of a plasma protein called **fibrinogen** (fi-BRIN-o-jen) into solid threads of **fibrin**, which form the clot.

A few of the final steps involved in blood clot formation are described below and diagrammed in Figure 13-8:

- Substances released from damaged tissues stimulate the formation of **prothrombinase** (pro-THROM-bih-nase), a substance that triggers the final clotting mechanism.

- Prothrombinase converts prothrombin in the blood to **thrombin.** Calcium is needed for this step.

- Thrombin, in turn, converts soluble fibrinogen into insoluble fibrin. **Fibrin** forms a network of threads that entraps plasma and blood cells to form a clot.

Blood clotting occurs in response to injury. Blood also clots when it comes into contact with some surface other than the lining of a blood vessel, for example, a glass or

plastic tube used for a blood specimen. In this case, the preliminary steps of clotting are somewhat different and require more time, but the final steps are the same as those described above.

The fluid that remains after clotting has occurred is called **serum** (plural, *sera*). Serum contains all the components of blood plasma *except* the clotting factors, as expressed in the formula:

Plasma = serum + clotting factors

Several methods used to measure the body's ability to coagulate blood are described later in this chapter.

> **PASSport to Success** Visit *thePoint* or see the Student Resource CD in the back of this book for a summary diagram and an animation on hemostasis.

CHECKPOINT 13-11 ➤ What happens when fibrinogen converts to fibrin?

Blood Types

If for some reason the amount of blood in the body is severely reduced, through **hemorrhage** (HEM-eh-rij) (excessive bleeding) or disease, the body cells suffer from lack of oxygen and nutrients. One possible measure to take in such an emergency is to administer blood from another person into the veins of the patient, a procedure called **transfusion.** Care must be taken in transferring blood from one person to another, however, because the patient's plasma may contain substances, called *antibodies* or *agglutinins*, that can cause the red cells of the donor's blood to

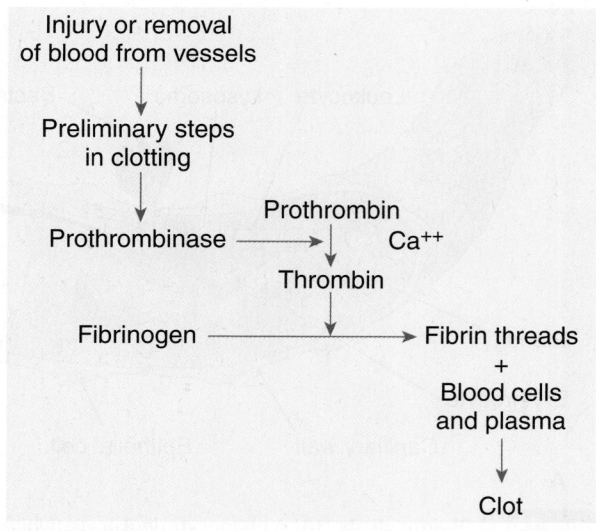

Figure 13-8 **Final steps in blood clot formation.** [ZOOMING IN ➤ What material in the blood forms a clot?]

rupture and release their hemoglobin. Such cells are said to be **hemolyzed** (HE-mo-lized), and the resulting condition can be dangerous.

Certain proteins, called **antigens** (AN-ti-jens) or *agglutinogens*, on the surface of the red cells cause these incompatibility reactions. There are many types of such proteins, but only two groups are particularly likely to cause a transfusion reaction, the so-called A and B antigens and the Rh factor.

The ABO Blood Type Group

There are four blood types involving the A and B antigens: A, B, AB, and O (Table 13-3). These letters indicate the type of antigen present on the red cells. If only the A antigen is present, the person has type A blood; if only the B antigen is present, he or she has type B blood. Type AB red cells have both antigens, and type O have neither. Of course no one has antibodies to his or her own blood type antigens, or their plasma would destroy their own cells. Each person does, however, develop antibodies that react with the AB antigens he or she is lacking. (The reason for the development of these antibodies is not totally understood, because people usually develop antibodies only when they have been exposed to an antigen.) It is these antibodies in the patient's plasma that can react with antigens on the donor's red cells to cause a transfusion reaction.

TESTING FOR BLOOD TYPE Blood sera containing antibodies to the A or B antigens are used to test for blood type. These antisera are prepared in animals using either the A or the B antigens to induce a response. Blood serum containing antibodies that can agglutinate and destroy red cells with A antigen is called **anti-A serum**; blood serum containing antibodies that can destroy red cells with B antigen is called **anti-B serum**. When combined with a blood sample in the laboratory, each antiserum causes the corresponding red cells to clump together in a process known as **agglutination** (ah-glu-tih-NA-shun). The blood's agglutination pattern when mixed *separately* with these two sera reveals its blood type (Fig. 13-9). Type A reacts with anti-A serum only; type B reacts with anti-B serum only. Type AB agglutinates with both, and type O agglutinates with neither A nor B.

A blood specimen from any person who has had a prior blood transfusion or a pregnancy is tested further for

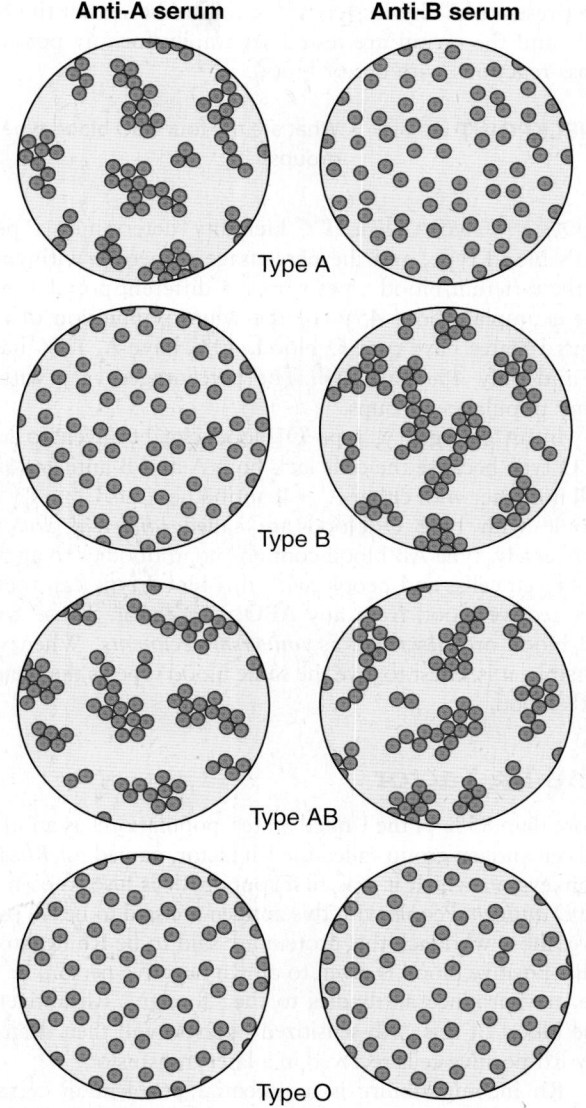

Anti-A serum   **Anti-B serum**

Type A

Type B

Type AB

Type O

Figure 13-9 **Blood typing.** Labels at the top of each column denote the kind of antiserum added to the blood samples. Anti-A serum agglutinates (causes to clump) red cells in type A blood, but anti-B serum does not. Anti-B serum agglutinates red cells in type B blood, but anti-A serum does not. Both sera agglutinate type AB blood cells, and neither serum agglutinates type O blood. [**ZOOMING IN ►** Can you tell from these reactions whether these cells are Rh positive or Rh negative?]

13

Table 13-3		The ABO Blood Group System			
Blood Type	Red Blood Cell Antigen	Reacts with Antiserum	Plasma Antibodies	Can Take From	Can Donate To
A	A	Anti-A	Anti-B	A, O	A, AB
B	B	Anti-B	Anti-A	B, O	B, AB
AB	A, B	Anti-A, Anti-B	None	AB, A, B, O	AB
O	None	None	Anti-A, Anti-B	O	O, A, B, AB

the presence of any less common antibodies. Both the red cells and the serum are tested separately for any possible cross-reactions with donor blood.

CHECKPOINT 13-12 ➤ What are the four ABO blood type groups?

BLOOD COMPATIBILITY Heredity determines a person's blood type, and the percentage of people with each of the different blood types varies in different populations. For example, about 45% of the white population of the United States have type O blood, 40% have A, 11% have B, and only 4% have AB. The percentages vary within other population groups.

In an emergency, type O blood can be given to any ABO type because the cells lack both A and B antigens and will not react with either A or B antibodies (see Table 13-3). People with type O blood are called *universal donors*. Conversely, type AB blood contains no antibodies to agglutinate red cells, and people with this blood type can therefore receive blood from any ABO type donor. Those with AB blood are described as *universal recipients*. Whenever possible, it is safest to give the same blood type as the recipient's blood.

The Rh Factor

More than 85% of the United States' population has another red cell antigen group called the **Rh factor**, named for *Rh*esus monkeys, in which it was first found. Rh is also known as the *D antigen*. People with this antigen are said to be **Rh positive**; those who lack this protein are said to be **Rh negative**. If Rh-positive blood is given to an Rh-negative person, he or she may produce antibodies to the "foreign" Rh antigens. The blood of this "Rh-sensitized" person will then destroy any Rh-positive cells received in a later transfusion.

Rh incompatibility is a potential problem in certain pregnancies. A mother who is Rh negative may develop antibodies to the Rh protein of an Rh-positive fetus (the fetus having inherited this factor from the father). Red cells from the fetus that enter the mother's circulation during pregnancy and childbirth evoke the response. In a subsequent pregnancy with an Rh-positive fetus, some of the anti-Rh antibodies may pass from the mother's blood into the blood of her fetus and destroy the fetus's red cells. This condition is called **hemolytic disease of the newborn** (HDN). An older name is *erythroblastosis fetalis*. HDN is now prevented by administration of immune globulin $Rh_o(D)$, trade name RhoGAM, to the mother during pregnancy and shortly after delivery. These preformed antibodies clear the mother's circulation of Rh antigens and prevent stimulation of an immune response. In many cases, a baby born with HDN could be saved by a transfusion that replaces much of the baby's blood with Rh-negative blood.

CHECKPOINT 13-13 ➤ What are the blood antigens most often involved in incompatibility reactions?

Uses of Blood and Blood Components

Blood can be packaged and kept in blood banks for emergencies. To keep the blood from clotting, a solution such as citrate-phosphate-dextrose-adenine (CPDA-1) is added. The blood may then be stored for up to 35 days. The blood supplies in the bank are dated with an expiration date to prevent the use of blood in which red cells may have disintegrated. Blood banks usually have all types of blood and blood products available. It is important that there be an extra supply of type O, Rh-negative blood because in an emergency this type can be used for any patient. It is normal procedure to test the recipient and give blood of the same type.

A person can donate his or her own blood before undergoing elective (planned) surgery to be used during surgery if needed. This practice eliminates the possibility of incompatibility and of disease transfer as well. Such **autologous** (aw-TOL-o-gus) (self-originating) blood is stored in a blood bank only until the surgery is completed.

Whole Blood Transfusions

The transfer of whole human blood from a healthy person to a patient is often a life-saving process. Whole blood transfusions may be used for any condition in which there is loss of a large volume of blood, for example:

- In the treatment of massive hemorrhage from serious mechanical injuries

- For blood loss during internal bleeding, as from bleeding ulcers

- During or after an operation that causes considerable blood loss

- For blood replacement in the treatment of hemolytic disease of the newborn

Caution and careful evaluation of the need for a blood transfusion is the rule, however, because of the risk for transfusion reactions and the transmission of viral diseases, particularly hepatitis.

Use of Blood Components

Most often, when some blood ingredient is needed, it is not whole blood but a blood component that is given. Blood can be broken down into its various parts, which may be used for different purposes.

A common method for separating the blood plasma from the formed elements is by use of a **centrifuge** (SEN-trih-fuje), a machine that spins in a circle at high speed to separate a mixture's components according to density. When a container of blood is spun rapidly, all the blood's formed elements are pulled into a clump at the bottom of the container. They are thus separated from the plasma, which is less dense. The formed elements may be further separated and used for specific purposes, for example, packed red cells alone or platelets alone.

Blood losses to the donor can be minimized if the blood is removed, the desired components are separated, and the remainder is returned to the donor. The general term for this procedure is **hemapheresis** (hem-ah-fer-E-sis) (from the Greek word *apheresis* meaning "removal") If the plasma is removed and the formed elements returned to the donor, the procedure is called **plasmapheresis** (plas-mah-fer-E-sis).

USE OF PLASMA Blood plasma alone may be given in an emergency to replace blood volume and prevent circulatory failure (shock). Plasma is especially useful when blood typing and the use of whole blood are not possible, such as in natural disasters or in emergency rescues. Because the red cells have been removed from the plasma, there are no incompatibility problems; plasma can be given to anyone. Plasma separated from the cellular elements is usually further separated by chemical means into various components, such as plasma protein fraction, serum albumin, immune serum, and clotting factors.

The packaged plasma that is currently available is actually plasma protein fraction. Further separation yields serum albumin that is available in solutions of 5% or 25% concentration. In addition to its use in treatment of circulatory shock, these solutions are given when plasma proteins are deficient. They increase the blood's osmotic pressure and thus draw fluids back into circulation. The use of plasma proteins and serum albumin has increased because these blood components can be treated with heat to prevent transmission of viral diseases.

In emergency situations healthcare workers may administer fluids known as *plasma expanders*. These are cell-free isotonic solutions used to maintain blood fluid volume to prevent circulatory shock.

Fresh plasma may be frozen and saved. When frozen plasma is thawed, a white precipitate called **cryoprecipitate** (kri-o-pre-SIP-ih-tate) forms in the bottom of the container. Plasma frozen when it is less than 6 hours old contains all the factors needed for clotting. Cryoprecipitate is especially rich in clotting factor VIII and fibrinogen. These components may be given when there is a special need for these factors.

The plasma's gamma globulin fraction contains antibodies produced by lymphocytes when they come in contact with foreign agents, such as bacteria and viruses. Antibodies play an important role in the immune system (see Chapter 17). Commercially prepared immune sera are available for administration to patients in immediate need of antibodies, such as infants born to mothers with active hepatitis.

CHECKPOINT **13-14** ► How is blood commonly separated into its component parts?

Blood Disorders

Abnormalities involving the blood may be divided into three groups:

- **Anemia** (ah-NE-me-ah), a disorder in which there is an abnormally low level of hemoglobin or red cells in the blood and thus impaired delivery of oxygen to the tissues.

- **Leukemia** (lu-KE-me-ah), a neoplastic blood disease characterized by an increase in the number of white cells.

- **Clotting disorders**, conditions characterized by an abnormal tendency to bleed because of a breakdown in the body's clotting mechanism.

Anemia

Anemia may result from loss of red cells, as through excessive bleeding (hemorrhage), or from conditions that cause the cells to hemolyze (rupture). In other cases, bone marrow failure or nutritional deficiencies impede the production of red cells or hemoglobin.

 **PASSport to Success** Visit *thePoint* or see the Student Resource CD in the back of this book for summary diagrams of the erythrocyte life cycle and causes of anemia.

EXCESSIVE LOSS OR DESTRUCTION OF RED CELLS Red cells may form properly but be lost through injury or destroyed after they are formed.

Hemorrhagic anemia Hemorrhagic loss of red cells may be sudden and acute or gradual and chronic. The average adult has about 5 liters of blood. If a person loses as much as 2 liters suddenly, death usually results. If the loss is gradual, however, over a period of weeks, or months, the body can compensate and withstand the loss of as much as 4 or 5 liters. Possible causes of chronic blood loss include bleeding ulcers, excessive menstrual flow, and bleeding hemorrhoids (piles). If the cause of the blood loss can be corrected, the body is usually able to restore the blood to normal. This process can take as long as 6 months, and until the blood returns to normal, the affected person may have **hemorrhagic** (hem-eh-RAJ-ik) **anemia**.

Hemolytic anemia Anemia caused by excessive red cell destruction is called **hemolytic** (he-mo-LIH-tik) **anemia**. The spleen, along with the liver, normally destroys old red cells. Occasionally, an overactive spleen destroys the cells too rapidly, causing anemia. Infections may also cause red cell loss. For example, the malarial parasite multiplies in and destroys red cells, and certain bacteria, particularly streptococci, produce a toxin that causes hemolysis.

Certain inherited diseases that cause the production of abnormal hemoglobin may also result in hemolytic anemia. The hemoglobin in normal adult cells is of the A type and is designated *HbA*. In the inherited disease **sickle cell anemia**, the hemoglobin in many of the red cells is abnormal (HbS). When these cells give up their oxygen to the tissues, they are transformed from the normal disk shape into a sickle shape (Fig. 13-10). These sickle cells are fragile

13

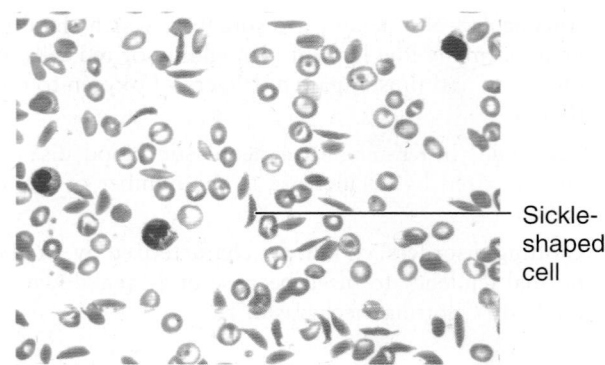

Sickle-shaped cell

Figure 13-10 **A blood smear in sickle cell anemia.** Abnormal cells take on a crescent (sickle) shape when they give up oxygen. (Reprinted with permission from Rubin R, Strayer DS. *Rubin's Pathology: Clinicopathologic Foundations of Medicine*, 5th ed. Baltimore: Lippincott Williams & Wilkins, 2007.) [ZOOMING IN ➤ What kind of cell is in the upper left corner of this picture? What are the small dark bodies between the cells?]

and tend to break easily. Because of their odd shape, they also tend to become tangled in masses that can block smaller blood vessels. When obstruction occurs, there may be severe joint swelling and pain, especially in the fingers and toes, as well as abdominal pain. This aspect of sickle cell anemia is referred to as *sickle cell crisis.*

Sickle cell anemia occurs almost exclusively in black people. About 8% of African Americans have one of the genes for the abnormal hemoglobin and are said to have the **sickle cell trait.** It is only when the involved gene is transmitted from both parents that the clinical disease appears. About 1% of African Americans have two of these genes and thus have **sickle cell disease.** One drug has been found to reduce the frequency of painful crisis in certain adults. Hydroxyurea causes the body to make some hemoglobin of an alternate form (fetal hemoglobin) so that the red cells are not as susceptible to sickling. People taking hydroxyurea require blood tests every 2 weeks to assess for drug-induced bone marrow suppression.

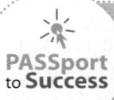

PASSport to Success

Visit **thePoint** or see the Student Resource CD in the back of this book for a figure explaining and illustrating sickle cell disease in greater detail.

IMPAIRED PRODUCTION OF RED CELLS OR HEMOGLOBIN Many factors can interfere with normal red cell production. Anemia that results from a deficiency of some nutrient is referred to as *nutritional anemia*. These conditions may arise from a deficiency of the specific nutrient in the diet, from an inability to absorb the nutrient, or from drugs that interfere with the body's use of the nutrient.

Deficiency Anemia The most common nutritional anemia is **iron-deficiency anemia.** Iron is an essential constituent of hemoglobin. The average diet usually provides enough iron to meet the needs of the adult male, but this diet often is inadequate to meet the needs of growing children and women of childbearing age.

A diet deficient in proteins or vitamins can also result in anemia. Folic acid, one of the B complex vitamins, is necessary for blood cell production. Folic acid deficiency anemia occurs in people with alcoholism, in elderly people on poor diets, and in infants or others suffering from intestinal disorders that interfere with the absorption of this water-soluble vitamin.

Pernicious (per-NISH-us) **anemia** is characterized by a deficiency of vitamin B_{12}, a substance essential for proper red cell formation. The cause is a permanent deficiency of **intrinsic factor**, a gastric juice secretion that is responsible for vitamin B_{12} absorption from the intestine. Neglected pernicious anemia can bring about deterioration in the nervous system, causing difficulty in walking, weakness and stiffness in the extremities, mental changes, and permanent damage to the spinal cord. Early treatment, including the intramuscular injection of vitamin B_{12} and attention to a prescribed diet, ensures an excellent outlook. This treatment must be kept up for the rest of the patient's life to maintain good health.

Thalassemia (thal-ah-SE-me-ah) includes a group of hereditary blood deficiencies in which hemoglobin is normal but is not produced in adequate amounts. To compound the problem, erythrocytes may be destroyed in the bone marrow before they mature. The red cells are small and pale, as in iron deficiency anemia, but instead of having low iron reserves, these patients absorb too much iron from the digestive tract and have excess iron in the blood and bone marrow. Forms of thalassemia may vary from causing chronic, lifelong anemia to premature death. The two mains types are α (alpha) and β (beta), according to the part of the hemoglobin molecule affected. Severe β thalassemia is also called *Cooley anemia.* Thalassemia is found mostly in populations of Mediterranean descent (the name comes from the Greek word for "sea").

Bone Marrow Suppression Bone marrow suppression or failure also leads to decreased red cell production. One type of bone marrow failure, **aplastic** (a-PLAS-tik) **anemia,** may be caused by a variety of physical and chemical agents. Chemical substances that injure the bone marrow include certain prescribed drugs and toxic agents such as gold compounds, arsenic, and benzene. Physical agents that may injure the marrow include x-rays, atomic radiation, radium, and radioactive phosphorus.

The damaged bone marrow fails to produce either red or white cells, so that the anemia is accompanied by **leukopenia** (lu-ko-PE-ne-ah), a drop in the number of white cells. Removal of the toxic agent, followed by blood transfusions until the marrow is able to resume its activity, may result in recovery. Bone marrow transplantations have also been successful.

Bone marrow suppression also may develop in patients with certain chronic diseases, such as cancer, kidney or liver disorders, and rheumatoid arthritis. Some medications are now available to stimulate bone marrow production of specific types of blood cells. The hormone EPO made by recombinant methods (genetic engineering) can be given in cases of severe anemia to stimulate red cell production.

CHECKPOINT 13-15 ➤ What is anemia?

Leukemia

Leukemia is a neoplastic disease of blood-forming tissue. It is characterized by an enormous increase in the number of white cells. Although the cells are high in number, they are incompetent and cannot perform their normal jobs. They also crowd out the other blood cells.

As noted earlier, the white cells have two main sources: red marrow, also called *myeloid tissue,* and lymphoid tissue. If this wild proliferation of white cells stems from cancer of the bone marrow, the condition is called **myelogenous** (mi-eh-LOJ-en-us) **leukemia.** When the cancer arises in the lymphoid tissue, so that most of the abnormal cells are lymphocytes, the condition is called **lymphocytic** (lim-fo-SIT-ik) **leukemia.** Both types of leukemia appear in acute and chronic forms.

> **PASSport to Success**
> Visit *thePoint* or see the Student Resource CD in the back of this book for micrographs of leukemic blood.

The cause of leukemia is unknown. Both inborn factors and various environmental agents have been implicated. Among the latter are chemicals (such as benzene), x-rays, radioactive substances, and viruses.

Patients with leukemia exhibit the general symptoms of anemia because the white cells overwhelm the red cells. In addition, they have a tendency to bleed easily, owing to a lack of platelets. White cell failure lowers immunity, resulting in frequent infections. The spleen is greatly enlarged, and several other organs may be increased in size because of internal accumulation of white cells. Treatment consists of x-ray therapy and chemotherapy (drug treatment), but the disease is malignant and thus may be fatal. With new chemotherapeutic methods, the outlook is improving, and many patients survive for years.

A bone marrow transplant can sometimes restore the normal hematopoietic stem cells destroyed along with abnormal cells in leukemia treatment. Hematologists also use the procedure to treat sickle cell anemia, thalassemia, aplastic anemia, and some immune disorders. Most patients receive allogenic transplants of cells from a close relative's bone marrow. It is important that the donor marrow match the recipient's marrow as closely as possible to avoid rejection, so potential donors undergo blood tests to determine compatibility. Sometimes the patient's own bone marrow can be harvested, treated, and replaced in an autologous transplant, which eliminates rejection. After intravenous delivery of the transplant, the donor stem cells travel to the recipient's bone marrow where they begin to produce new blood cells. Recovery time is long,

and during this period the patient is very susceptible to infection, but bone marrow transplants improve survival rates for patients with leukemia and certain other blood disorders.

CHECKPOINT 13-16 ➤ What is leukemia?

Clotting Disorders

Most clotting disorders involve a disruption of the coagulation process, which brings about abnormal bleeding. Alternately, the disturbance may originate with excess clotting.

Hemophilia (he-mo-FIL-e-ah) is a rare hereditary bleeding disorder, a disease that influenced history by its occurrence in some Russian and Western European royal families. All forms of hemophilia are characterized by a deficiency of a specific clotting factor, most commonly factor VIII. In those with hemophilia, any injury may cause excess bruising and serious abnormal bleeding. There is also spontaneous internal bleeding, especially in the digestive tract, brain, and other soft tissues. Bleeding into the joints, a common effect of hemophilia, is not only painful, but can lead to serious disability if untreated. The needed clotting factors are now available in purified concentrated form for treatment in cases of injury, preparation for surgery, or abnormal bleeding. Cryoprecipitate contains factor VIII, and clotting factors are also produced by recombinant (genetic engineering) methods.

Von Willebrand disease is another hereditary clotting disorder. It involves a shortage of von Willebrand factor, a plasma component that helps platelets to adhere (stick) to damaged tissue and also carries clotting factor VIII. This disorder is treated by administration of the appropriate clotting factor. In mild cases, a drug similar to the hormone ADH may work to prevent bleeding by raising the level of von Willebrand factor in the blood.

The most common clotting disorder is a deficient number of circulating platelets (thrombocytes). The condition, called **thrombocytopenia** (throm-bo-si-to-PE-ne-ah), results in hemorrhage in the skin or mucous membranes. The decrease in platelets may result from their decreased production or increased destruction. There are several possible causes of thrombocytopenia, including diseases of the red bone marrow, liver disorders, and various drug toxicities. When a drug causes the disorder, its withdrawal leads to immediate recovery.

Disseminated intravascular coagulation (DIC) is a serious clotting disorder involving excessive coagulation. This disease occurs in cases of tissue damage caused by massive burns, trauma, certain acute infections, cancer, and some disorders of childbirth. During the progress of DIC, platelets and various clotting factors are used up faster than they can be produced, and serious hemorrhaging may result.

CHECKPOINT 13-17 ➤ What blood components are low in cases of thrombocytopenia?

13

Disease in Context revisited

➤ Sickle Cell Anemia

Dr. Kepron, a pediatric hematologist, carefully read Cole Armstrong's medical chart. Cole, now 2 days old, was positive for the presence of Hemoglobin S. Blood tests from his parents, Jada and Darryl, confirmed Cole's diagnosis—sickle cell anemia.

Later that afternoon, Dr. Kepron met with Cole's parents. "Cole has been diagnosed with sickle cell anemia," explained the doctor. "The disease is caused by a mutation in the gene that directs the manufacture of a blood protein called hemoglobin." Dr. Kepron told Darryl and Jada that they each carried two versions of the gene, one normal and one abnormal, but they did not express the disease because the normal gene masked the effect of the abnormal one. Cole had inherited a copy of the abnormal hemoglobin gene from each of his parents and thus expressed the disease.

"Hemoglobin is found in red blood cells," continued the doctor. "It's the protein that transports oxygen from the lungs to other tissues in the body. Normally, the red blood cells are round and flexible, which lets them bend and twist as they pass through the narrow capillaries in the body. Cole's abnormal hemoglobin causes the red blood cells to become stiff and sickle-shaped. As a result, the cells can become stuck in the capillaries, blocking blood flow and the delivery of oxygen to tissues and organs. I'm going to work with you to manage Cole's disease—if we monitor him carefully we should be able to minimize organ and tissue damage."

During this case we saw that sickle cell anemia is an inherited disease. To learn more about heredity and hereditary diseases, see Chapter 25.

Blood Studies

Many kinds of studies can be done on blood, and some of these have become a standard part of a routine physical examination. The tests included in a **complete blood count (CBC)** are shown in Appendix 4-2. Machines that are able to perform several tests at the same time have largely replaced manual procedures, particularly in large institutions. Standard blood tests are listed in Tables 2 and 3 of Appendix 4.

The Hematocrit

The **hematocrit** (he-MAT-o-krit) (Hct), the volume percentage of red cells in whole blood, is determined by spinning a blood sample in a high-speed centrifuge for 3 to 5 minutes to separate the cellular elements from the plasma (Fig. 13-11).

The hematocrit is expressed as the volume of packed red cells per unit volume of whole blood. For example, "hematocrit, 38%" in a laboratory report means that the patient has 38 mL red cells per dL (100 mL) of blood; red cells comprise 38% of the total blood volume. For adult men, the normal range is 42% to 54%, whereas for adult women the range is slightly lower, 36% to 46%. These normal ranges, like all normal ranges for humans, may vary depending on the method used and the interpretation of the results by an individual laboratory. Hematocrit values much below or much above these figures point to an abnormality requiring further study.

Hemoglobin Tests

A sufficient amount of hemoglobin in red cells is required for adequate oxygen delivery to the tissues. To measure its level, the hemoglobin is released from the red cells, and the color of the blood is compared with a known color scale.

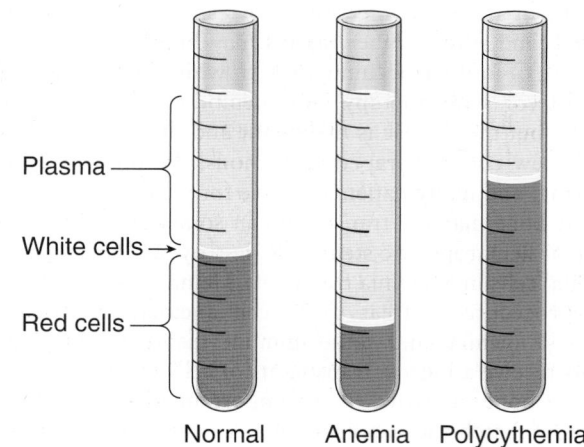

Plasma

White cells →

Red cells

Normal   Anemia   Polycythemia

Figure 13-11   Hematocrit. The tube on the left shows a normal hematocrit. The middle tube shows that the percentage of red blood cells is low, indicating anemia. The tube on the right shows an excessively high percentage of red cells, as seen in polycythemia. (Reprinted with permission from Cohen BJ. *Medical Terminology*, 4th ed. Philadelphia: Lippincott Williams & Wilkins, 2004.)

Hemoglobin (Hb) is expressed in grams per dL of whole blood. Normal hemoglobin concentrations for adult males range from 14 to 17 g per 100 mL blood. Values for adult women are in a somewhat lower range, at 12 to 15 g per 100 mL blood. The hemoglobin reading can also be expressed as a percentage of a given standard, usually the average male normal of 15.6 g Hb/dL. Thus, a reading of 90% would mean 90% of 15.6 or 14 g Hb/dL. A decrease in hemoglobin to below normal levels signifies anemia.

Normal and abnormal types of hemoglobin can be separated and measured by the process of **electrophoresis** (e-lek-tro-fo-RE-sis). In this procedure, an electric current is passed through the liquid that contains the hemoglobin to separate different components based on their electrical charge. This test is useful in the diagnosis of sickle cell anemia and other disorders caused by abnormal types of hemoglobin.

Blood Cell Counts

Most laboratories use automated methods for obtaining the data for blood counts. Visual counts are sometimes done using a **hemocytometer** (he-mo-si-TOM-eh-ter), a ruled slide used to count the cells in a given volume of blood under the microscope.

RED CELL COUNTS The normal red cell count varies from 4.5 to 5.5 million cells per μL (mcL) of blood. An increase in the red cell count is called **polycythemia** (pol-e-si-THE-me-ah). People who live at high altitudes develop polycythemia, as do patients with the disease **polycythemia** (pol-e-si-THE-me-ah) **vera**, a disorder of the bone marrow.

WHITE CELL COUNTS The leukocyte count varies from 5,000 to 10,000 cells per μL of blood. In **leukopenia**, the white count is below 5,000 cells per μL. This condition indicates depressed bone marrow or a bone marrow neoplasm. In **leukocytosis** (lu-ko-si-TO-sis), the white cell count exceeds 10,000 cells per μL. This condition is characteristic of most bacterial infections. It may also occur after hemorrhage, in cases of gout (a type of arthritis), and in uremia, the presence of nitrogenous waste in the blood as a result of kidney disease.

PLATELET COUNTS It is difficult to count platelets visually because they are so small. Laboratories can obtain more accurate counts with automated methods. These counts are necessary for the evaluation of platelet loss (thrombocytopenia) such as occurs after radiation therapy or cancer chemotherapy. The normal platelet count ranges from 150,000 to 450,000 per μL of blood, but counts may fall to 100,000 or less without causing serious bleeding problems. If a count is very low, a platelet transfusion may be given.

The Blood Slide (Smear)

In addition to the above tests, a CBC includes the examination of a stained blood slide (see Fig. 13-2). In this procedure, a drop of blood is spread thinly and evenly over a glass slide, and a special stain (Wright) is applied to differentiate the otherwise colorless white cells. The slide is then studied under the microscope. The red cells are examined for abnormalities in size, color, or shape and for variations in the percentage of immature forms, known as reticulocytes (see Box 13-2 to learn about reticulocytes and how their counts are used to diagnose disease). The number of platelets is estimated. Parasites, such as the malarial organism and others, may be found. In addition, a **differential white count** is done. This is an estimation of the percentage of each white cell type in the smear. Because each type has a specific function, changes in their proportions can be a valuable diagnostic aid (see Table 13-2).

CHECKPOINT 13-18 ➤ The hematocrit is a common blood test. What is a hematocrit?

Blood Chemistry Tests

Batteries of tests on blood serum are often done by machine. One machine, the Sequential Multiple Analyzer (SMA), can run some 20 tests per minute. Tests for electrolytes, such as sodium, potassium, chloride, and bicarbonate, may be performed at the same time along with tests for blood glucose, and nitrogenous waste products, such as blood urea nitrogen (BUN), and **creatinine** (kre-AT-in-in).

Other tests check for enzymes. Increased levels of **CK** (creatine kinase), **LDH** (lactic dehydrogenase), and other enzymes indicate tissue damage, such as damage that may occur in heart disease. An excess of **alkaline phosphatase** (FOS-fah-tase) could indicate a liver disorder or metastatic cancer involving bone (see Table 3 in Appendix 4).

Blood can be tested for amounts of lipids, such as cholesterol, triglycerides (fats), and lipoproteins, or for amounts of plasma proteins. These tests help to diagnose and evaluate diseases. For example, the presence of more than the normal amount of glucose in the blood indicates unregulated diabetes mellitus. The list of blood chemistry tests is extensive and is constantly increasing. We may now obtain values for various hormones, vitamins, antibodies, and toxic or therapeutic drug levels.

Coagulation Studies

Before surgery and during treatment of certain diseases, hemophilia for example, it is important to know that coagulation will take place within normal time limits. Because clotting is a complex process involving many reactants, a delay may result from a number of different causes, including lack of certain hormonelike substances, calcium salts, or vitamin K. The amounts of the various clotting factors are evaluated by percentage to aid in the diagnosis and treatment of bleeding disorders.

Additional tests for coagulation include tests for bleeding time, clotting time, capillary strength, and platelet function.

13

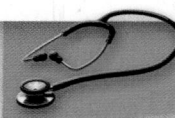

Box 13-2   Clinical Perspectives

Counting Reticulocytes to Diagnose Disease

As erythrocytes mature in the red bone marrow, they go through a series of stages in which they lose their nucleus and most other organelles, maximizing the space available to hold hemoglobin. In one of the last stages of development, small numbers of ribosomes and some rough endoplasmic reticulum remain in the cell and appear as a network, or reticulum, when stained. Cells at this stage are called **reticulocytes**. Reticulocytes leave the red bone marrow and enter the bloodstream where they become fully mature erythrocytes in about 24 to 48 hours. The average number of red cells maturing through the reticulocyte stage at any given time is about 1% to 2%. Changes in these numbers can be used in diagnosing certain blood disorders.

When erythrocytes are lost or destroyed, as from chronic bleeding or some form of hemolytic anemia, red blood cell production is "stepped up" to compensate for the loss. Greater numbers of reticulocytes are then released into the blood before reaching full maturity, and counts increase above normal. On the other hand, a decrease in the number of circulating reticulocytes suggests a problem with red blood cell production, as in cases of deficiency anemias or suppression of bone marrow activity.

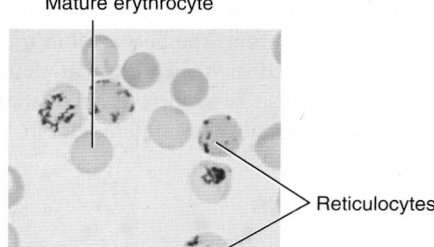

Reticulocytes. Some ribosomes and rough ER appear as a network in a late stage of erythrocyte development. (Reprinted with permission from Cormack DH. *Essential Histology*, 2nd ed. Philadelphia: Lippincott Williams & Wilkins, 2001.)

Bone Marrow Biopsy

A special needle is used to obtain a small sample of red marrow from the sternum, sacrum, or iliac crest in a procedure called a **bone marrow biopsy**. If marrow is taken from the sternum, the procedure may be referred to as a **sternal puncture**. Examination of the cells gives valuable information that can aid in the diagnosis of bone marrow disorders, including leukemia and certain kinds of anemia.

Word Anatomy

Medical terms are built from standardized word parts (prefixes, roots, and suffixes). Learning the meanings of these parts can help you remember words and interpret unfamiliar terms.

WORD PART	MEANING	EXAMPLE
Blood Constituents		
erythr/o	red, red blood cell	An *erythrocyte* is a red blood cell.
leuk/o	white, colorless	A *leukocyte* is a white blood cell.
thromb/o	blood clot	A *thrombocyte* is a cell fragment that is active in blood clotting.
hemat/o	blood	*Hematopoietic* stem cells form (-poiesis) all of the blood cells.
hemo	blood	*Hemoglobin* is a protein the carries oxygen in the blood.

WORD PART	MEANING	EXAMPLE
morph/o	shape	The nuclei of *polymorphs* have many shapes.
lymph/o	lymph, lymphatic system	*Lymphocytes* are white blood cells that circulate in the lymphatic system.
mon/o	single, one	A *monocyte* has a single, unsegmented nucleus.
phag/o	eat, ingest	Certain leukocytes take in foreign matter by the process of *phagocytosis*.
macr/o	large	A *macrophage* takes in large amounts of foreign matter by phagocytosis.
kary/o	nucleus	A *megakaryocyte* has a very large nucleus.

Hemostasis

-gen	producing, originating	*Fibrinogen* converts to fibrin in the formation of a blood clot.
pro-	before, in front of	Prothrombinase is an enzyme (-ase) that converts *pro-thrombin* to thrombin.

Blood Types

-lysis	loosening, dissolving, separating	A recipient's antibodies to donated red cells can cause *hemolysis* of the cells.

Uses of Blood and Blood Components

cry/o	cold	*Cryoprecipitate* forms when blood plasma is frozen and then thawed.

Blood Disorders

–emia (from –hemia)	blood	*Anemia* is a lack (an-) of red cells or hemoglobin.
–penia	lack of	*Leukopenia* is a lack of white cells.

Summary

13

I. **FUNCTIONS OF THE BLOOD**
   A. Transportation—of oxygen, carbon dioxide, nutrients, minerals, vitamins, hormones, waste
   B. Regulation—of pH, fluid balance, body temperature
   C. Protection—against foreign organisms, blood loss

II. **BLOOD CONSTITUENTS**
   A. Plasma—liquid component
      1. Water—main ingredient
      2. Proteins—albumin, clotting factors, antibodies, complement
      3. Nutrients—carbohydrates, lipids, amino acids
      4. Electrolytes (minerals)
      5. Waste products
      6. Gases—oxygen and carbon dioxide
      7. Hormones and other materials
   B. The formed elements—produced in red bone marrow from hematopoietic stem cells
      1. Erythrocytes (red cells)—carry oxygen bound to hemoglobin
      2. Leukocytes (white cells)—destroy invading organisms and remove waste
         a. Granulocytes—neutrophils (polymorphs, segs, PMNs), eosinophils, basophils
         b. Agranulocytes—lymphocytes, monocytes
      3. Platelets (thrombocytes)
         a. Fragments of megakaryocytes
         b. Participate in blood clotting

III. **HEMOSTASIS—PREVENTION OF BLOOD LOSS**
   A. Steps
      1. Contraction of blood vessels
      2. Formation of platelet plug
      3. Formation of blood clot
   B. Blood Clotting
      1. Regulators
         a. Procoagulants—promote clotting

b.   Anticoagulants—prevent clotting
2.   12 clotting factors
3.   Final steps in blood clotting
   a.   Prothrombinase converts prothrombin to thrombin
   b.   Thrombin converts fibrinogen to solid threads of fibrin
   c.   Threads form clot
4.   Serum—fluid that remains after blood has clotted

IV.   **BLOOD TYPES**
  A.   ABO blood type group—types A, B, AB, and O
    1.   Tested by mixing blood sample with antisera to different antigens
    2.   Incompatible transfusions cause destruction of donor red cells
  B.   Rh factor—positive or negative

V.   **USES OF BLOOD AND BLOOD COMPONENTS**
  A.   Blood banks—store blood
    1.   Autologous blood—donated for a person's own use
  B.   Whole blood transfusions—used only to replace large blood losses
  C.   Use of blood components—formed elements separated by centrifugation
  D.   Use of plasma
    1.   Protein fractions
    2.   Cryoprecipitate—obtained by freezing; contains clotting factors
    3.   Gamma globulin—contains antibodies

VI.   **BLOOD DISORDERS**
  A.   Anemia—lack of hemoglobin or red cells

    1.   Loss or destruction of cells
      a.   Hemorrhage
      b.   Hemolysis (e.g., sickle cell anemia)
    2.   Impaired production of cells
      a.   Deficiency anemia (e.g., nutritional anemia, thalassemia)
      b.   Pernicious anemia
      c.   Bone marrow suppression
  B.   Leukemia—excess production of white cells
    1.   Myelogenous leukemia—cancer of bone marrow
    2.   Lymphocytic leukemia—cancer of lymphoid tissue
  C.   Clotting disorders
    1.   Hemophilia, von Willebrand disease—hereditary lack of clotting factors
    2.   Thrombocytopenia—lack of platelets
    3.   Disseminated intravascular coagulation (DIC)

VII.   **BLOOD STUDIES**
  A.   Hematocrit—measures percentage of packed red cells in whole blood
  B.   Hemoglobin tests—color test, electrophoresis
  C.   Blood cell counts
  D.   Blood slide (smear)
  E.   Blood chemistry tests—electrolytes, waste products, enzymes, glucose, hormones
  F.   Coagulation studies—clotting factor assays, bleeding time, clotting time, capillary strength, platelet function
  G.   Bone marrow biopsy

Questions for Study and Review

BUILDING UNDERSTANDING

Fill in the blanks

1.   The liquid portion of blood is called _____.
2.   The ancestors of all blood cells are called _____cells.
3.   Platelets are produced by certain giant cells called _____.
4.   Some monocytes enter the tissues and mature into phagocytic cells called _____.
5.   Erythrocytes have a lifespan of approximately _____ days.

Matching ▸ Match each numbered item with the most closely related lettered item.

____   **6.** an increased erythrocyte count
____   **7.** a decreased erythrocyte count
____   **8.** an increased leukocyte count
____   **9.** a decreased leukocyte count
____   **10.** a decreased platelet count

a. thrombocytopenia

b. anemia

c. leukopenia

d. leukocytosis

e. polycythemia

Multiple choice

____ **11.** Red blood cells transport oxygen that is bound to
  a. erythropoietin
  b. complement
  c. hemoglobin
  d. thrombin

____ **12.** All of the following are granulocytes except
  a. lymphocytes
  b. neutrophils
  c. eosinophils
  d. basophils

____ **13.** Antibodies are produced by
  a. erythrocytes
  b. macrophages
  c. plasma cells
  d. band cells

____ **14.** The correct sequence of hemostatic events is
  a. vessel contraction, plug formation, blood clot
  b. blood clot, plug formation, vessel contraction
  c. plug formation, blood clot, vessel contraction
  d. vessel contraction, blood clot, plug formation

____ **15.** If one wanted to measure the number of eosinophils in a blood sample, he or she would conduct the following test:
  a. hematocrit
  b. electrophoresis
  c. complete blood cell count
  d. differential white blood cell count

UNDERSTANDING CONCEPTS

16. List the three main functions of blood. What is the average volume of circulating blood in the body?

17. Compare and contrast the following:
  a. formed elements and plasma
  b. erythrocyte and leukocyte
  c. hemorrhage and transfusion
  d. hemapheresis and plasmapheresis

18. List four main types of proteins in blood plasma and state their functions. What are some other substances carried in blood plasma?

19. Describe the structure and function of erythrocytes. State the normal blood cell count for erythrocytes.

20. Construct a chart that compares the structure and function of the five types of leukocytes. State the normal blood cell count for leukocytes.

21. Diagram the three final steps in blood clot formation.

22. Name the four blood types in the ABO system. What antigens and antibodies (if any) are found in each type?

23. Compare and contrast the following disease conditions:
  a. hemolytic anemia and aplastic anemia
  b. myelogenous leukemia and lymphocytic leukemia
  c. hemophilia and von Willebrand disease

CONCEPTUAL THINKING

24. J. Regan, a 40-year-old firefighter, has just had his annual physical. He is in excellent health, except for his red blood cell count, which is elevated. How might Mr. Regan's job explain his polycythemia?

25. If leukemia is associated with an elevated white blood cell count, why is it also associated with an increased risk of infection?

26. In Cole's case, he was diagnosed with sickle cell disease. Increased risk of infection is one consequence of the disease. Explain why a hemoglobin abnormality increases the risk of infection.

13

CHAPTER 14

The Heart and Heart Disease

Learning Outcomes

After careful study of this chapter, you should be able to:

1. Describe the three layers of the heart wall
2. Describe the structure of the pericardium and cite its functions
3. Compare the functions of the right and left sides of the heart
4. Name the four chambers of the heart and compare their functions
5. Name the valves at the entrance and exit of each ventricle and cite the function of the valves
6. Briefly describe blood circulation through the myocardium
7. Briefly describe the cardiac cycle
8. Name and locate the components of the heart's conduction system
9. Explain the effects of the autonomic nervous system on the heart rate
10. List and define several terms that describe variations in heart rates
11. Explain what produces the two main heart sounds
12. Describe several common types of heart disease
13. List five actions that can be taken to minimize the risk of heart disease
14. Briefly describe four methods for studying the heart
15. Describe several approaches to the treatment of heart disease
16. Show how word parts are used to build words related to the heart (see Word Anatomy at the end of the chapter)

Selected Key Terms

The following terms and other boldface terms in the chapter are defined in the Glossary

arrhythmia
atherosclerosis
atrium
bradycardia
coronary
coronary thrombosis
diastole
echocardiograph
electrocardiograph
endocardium
epicardium
fibrillation
infarct
ischemia
murmur
myocardium
pacemaker
pericardium
plaque
septum
stenosis
systole
tachycardia
valve
ventricle

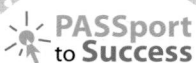

PASSport to Success

Visit *thePoint* or see the Student Resource CD in the back of this book for definitions and pronunciations of key terms as well as a pretest for this chapter.

Disease in Context

Jim's Second Case: A Coronary Emergency

The emergency room's dispatch radio echoed from the triage desk. "This is Medic 5 en route with Jim, a 46-year-old Caucasian male. Suspected acute myocardial infarction while playing basketball. Cardiopulmonary resuscitation was initiated on scene. Patient was defibrillated in ambulance twice. Portable ECG indicates S-T interval depression and an inverted T wave. Patient is receiving oxygen through nasal cannulae. ETA approximately 10 minutes."

When Jim arrived at the ER, the emergency team rushed to stabilize him. A trauma nurse measured Jim's vital signs—he was hypertensive with tachycardia—while another inserted an IV needle into Jim's arm and placed an oxygen mask over his nose and mouth. Meanwhile, a phlebotomist drew blood from Jim's other arm for testing in the lab. A cardiology technician attached ECG leads to Jim's chest and began to record his cardiac muscle's electrical activity. The emergency doctor looked at the printout from the electrocardiograph and confirmed that Jim was having a heart attack. The doctor knew that one or more of the coronary arteries feed-ing Jim's heart muscle was blocked with a thrombus (blood clot). He administered several medications in an attempt to restore blood flow to the heart and minimize myocardial damage. Aspirin, which prevents platelets from adhering to each other, was given to inhibit the formation of any more thrombi. Nitroglycerin, a potent vasodilator, was given to widen Jim's coronary arteries and thus increase blood flow to the heart. Morphine was given to manage Jim's pain and lower his cardiac output in order to reduce the heart's workload. Lastly, tissue plasminogen activator was administered to dissolve the thrombi present in Jim's coronary arteries.

Thanks to the quick action of the paramedics and emergency team, Jim was resting comfortably in the intensive care unit a few hours after thrombolytic treatment—he was lucky to be alive! Later in the chapter, we'll visit Jim again and learn how cardiac surgeons repair coronary arteries to prevent future infarctions.

Circulation and the Heart

The next two chapters investigate how the blood delivers oxygen and nutrients to the cells and carries away the waste products of cellular metabolism. The continuous one-way circuit of blood through the blood vessels is known as the **circulation**. The prime mover that propels blood throughout the body is the **heart**. This chapter examines the heart's structure and function as a foundation for the detailed discussion of blood vessels that follows.

The heart's importance has been recognized for centuries. Strokes (the contractions) of this pump average about 72 per minute and are carried on unceasingly for a whole lifetime. The beating of the heart is affected by the emotions, which may explain the frequent references to it in song and poetry. However, the heart's vital functions and its disorders are of more practical concern.

Location of the Heart

The heart is slightly bigger than a person's fist. This organ is located between the lungs in the center and a bit to the left of the body's midline (Fig. 14-1). It occupies most of the mediastinum, the central region of the thorax. The heart's **apex**, the pointed, inferior portion, is directed toward the left. The broad, superior **base** is the area of attachment for the large vessels carrying blood into and out of the heart. See Appendix 7 for a dissection photograph of the heart in position in the thorax.

Structure of the Heart

The heart is a hollow organ, with walls formed of three different layers. Just as a warm coat might have a smooth lining, a thick and bulky interlining, and an outer layer of a third fabric, so the heart wall has three tissue layers (Fig. 14-2, Table 14-1). Starting with the innermost layer, these are as follows:

- The **endocardium** (en-do-KAR-de-um) is a thin, smooth layer of epithelial cells that lines the heart's interior. The endocardium provides a smooth surface for easy flow as blood travels through the heart. Extensions of this membrane cover the flaps (cusps) of the heart valves.

- The **myocardium** (mi-o-KAR-de-um), the heart muscle, is the thickest layer and pumps blood through the vessels. Cardiac muscle's unique structure is described in more detail next.

- The **epicardium** (ep-ih-KAR-de-um) is a serous membrane that forms the thin, outermost layer of the heart wall.

The Pericardium

The **pericardium** (per-ih-KAR-de-um) is the sac that encloses the heart (Fig. 14-2, Table 14-2). The formation of the pericardial sac was described and illustrated in Chapter 4 under a discussion of membranes (see Fig. 4-9). This sac's outermost and heaviest layer is the fibrous pericardium. Connective tissue anchors this pericardial layer to the diaphragm, located inferiorly; the sternum, located anteriorly; and to other structures surrounding the heart, thus holding the heart in place. A serous membrane lines this fibrous sac and folds back at the base to cover the heart's surface. Anatomically, the outer layer of this serous membrane is called the parietal layer, and the inner layer is the visceral layer, also known as the epicardium, as previously noted. A thin film of fluid between these two layers reduces friction as the heart moves within the pericardium. Normally the visceral and parietal layers are very close together, but fluid may accumulate in the region between them, the pericardial cavity, under certain disease conditions.

Special Features of the Myocardium

Cardiac muscle cells are lightly striated (striped) based on alternating actin and myosin filaments, as seen in skeletal muscle cells (see Chapter 8). Unlike skeletal muscle cells, however, cardiac muscle cells have a single nucleus instead of multiple nuclei. Also, cardiac muscle tissue is involuntarily controlled. There are specialized partitions between cardiac muscle cells that show faintly under a microscope (Fig. 14-3). These **intercalated** (in-TER-cah-la-ted) **disks** are actually modified plasma

Thyroid gland
Trachea
Base of heart
Right lung
Left lung
Ribs (cut)
Diaphragm   Pericardium   Apex of heart

Figure 14-1 **The heart in position in the thorax (anterior view). [ZOOMING IN ▸** Why is the left lung smaller than the right lung? **]**

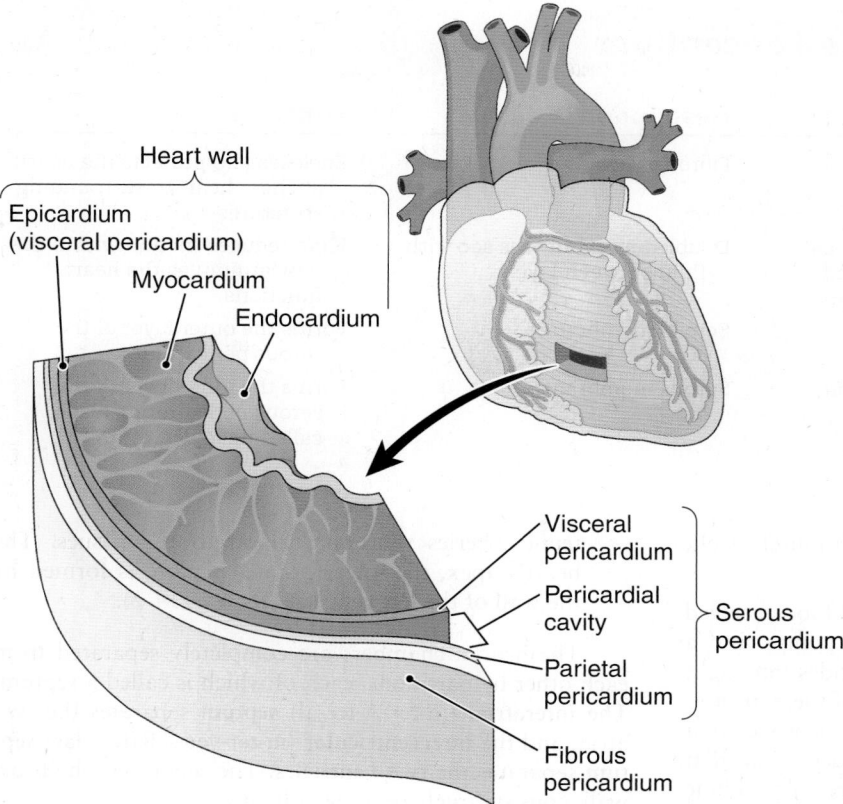

Figure 14-2 **Layers of the heart wall and pericardium.** The serous pericardium covers the heart and lines the fibrous pericardium. [ZOOMING IN ➤ Which layer of the heart wall is the thickest?]

Another feature of cardiac muscle tissue is the branching of the muscle fibers (cells). These fibers are interwoven so that the stimulation that causes the contraction of one fiber results in the contraction of a whole group. The intercalated disks and the branching cellular networks allow cardiac muscle cells to contract in a coordinated manner.

Divisions of the Heart

Healthcare professionals often refer to the *right heart* and the *left heart*, because the human heart is really a double pump (Fig. 14-4). The right side pumps blood low in oxygen to the lungs through the **pulmonary circuit**. The left side pumps oxygenated blood to the remainder of the body through the **systemic circuit**. Each side of the heart is divided into two chambers. See Appendix 7 for a photograph of the human heart showing the chambers and the vessels that connect to the heart.

FOUR CHAMBERS The upper chambers on the right and left sides, the **atria** (A-tre-ah), are mainly blood-receiving chambers (Fig. 14-5, Table 14-3). The lower chambers on the right and left side, the **ventricles** (VEN-trih-klz) are forceful pumps. The chambers, listed in the order in which blood flows through them, are as follows:

membranes that firmly attach adjacent cells to each other but allow for rapid transfer of electrical impulses between them. The adjective *intercalated* is from Latin and means "inserted between."

CHECKPOINT 14-1 ➤ What are the names of the innermost, middle, and outermost layers of the heart?

CHECKPOINT 14-2 ➤ What is the name of the sac that encloses the heart?

1. The **right atrium** (A-tre-um) is a thin-walled chamber that receives the blood returning from the body tissues. This blood, which is low in oxygen, is carried in veins, the blood vessels leading back to the heart. The superior vena cava brings blood from the head, chest, and arms; the inferior vena cava delivers blood from the trunk and legs. A third vessel that opens into the

Table 14-1	Layers of the Heart Wall		
Layer	Location	Description	Function
Endocardium	Innermost layer of the heart wall	Thin, smooth layer of epithelial cells	Lines the interior of the chambers and covers the heart valves
Myocardium	Middle layer of the heart wall	Thick layer of cardiac muscle	Contracts to pump blood into the arteries
Epicardium	Outermost layer of the heart wall	Thin serous membrane	Covers the heart and forms the visceral layer of the serous pericardium

Table 14-2	**Layers of the Pericardium**		
Layer	**Location**	**Description**	**Function**
Fibrous pericardium	Outermost layer	Fibrous sac	Encloses and protects the heart; anchors heart to surrounding structures
Serous pericardium	Between the fibrous pericardium and the myocardium	Doubled membranous sac with fluid between layers	Fluid reduces friction within the pericardium as the heart functions
Parietal layer	Lines the fibrous pericardium	Serous membrane	Forms the outer layer of the serous pericardium
Visceral layer	Surface of the heart	Serous membrane	Forms the inner layer of the serous pericardium; also called the epicardium

right atrium brings blood from the heart muscle itself, as described later in this chapter.

2. The **right ventricle** pumps the venous blood received from the right atrium to the lungs. It pumps into a large pulmonary trunk, which then divides into right and left pulmonary arteries. Branches of these arteries carry blood to the lungs. An artery is a vessel that takes blood from the heart to the tissues. Note that the pulmonary arteries in Figure 14-5 are colored blue because they are carrying deoxygenated blood, unlike other arteries, which carry oxygenated blood.

3. The **left atrium** receives blood high in oxygen content as it returns from the lungs in pulmonary veins. Note that the pulmonary veins in Figure 14-5 are colored red because they are carrying oxygenated blood, unlike other veins, which carry deoxygenated blood.

4. The **left ventricle**, which is the chamber with the thickest wall, pumps oxygenated blood to all parts of the body. This blood goes first into the aorta (a-OR-tah), the largest artery, and then into the branching sys-

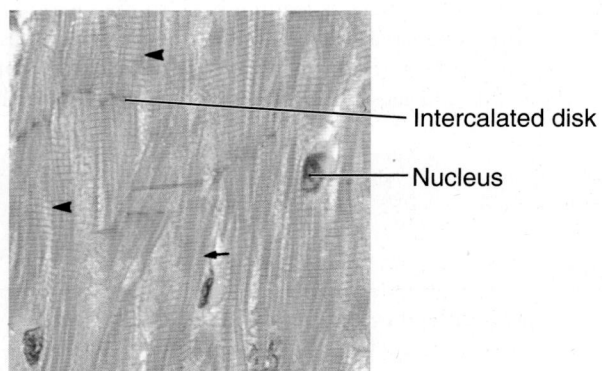

Figure 14-3 **Cardiac muscle tissue viewed under the microscope (×540).** The sample shows light striations (arrowheads), intercalated disks, and branching fibers (arrow). (Reprinted with permission from Gartner LP, Hiatt JL. *Color Atlas of Histology*, 3rd ed. Philadelphia: Lippincott Williams & Wilkins, 2000.)

temic arteries that take blood to the tissues. The heart's apex, the lower pointed region, is formed by the wall of the left ventricle (see Fig. 14-2).

The heart's chambers are completely separated from each other by partitions, each of which is called a **septum**. The **interatrial** (in-ter-A-tre-al) **septum** separates the two atria, and the **interventricular** (in-ter-ven-TRIK-u-lar) **septum** separates the two ventricles. The septa, like the heart wall, consist largely of myocardium.

CHECKPOINT 14-3 ➤ The heart is divided into four chambers. What is the upper receiving chamber on each side called? What is the lower pumping chamber called?

FOUR VALVES One-way valves that direct blood flow through the heart are located at the entrance and exit of each ventricle (Fig. 14-6, Table 14-4). The entrance valves are the **atrioventricular** (a-tre-o-ven-TRIK-u-lar) **(AV) valves**, so named because they are between the atria and ventricles. The exit valves are the **semilunar** (sem-e-LU-nar) **valves**, so named because each flap of these valves resembles a half-moon. Each valve has a specific name, as follows:

- The **right atrioventricular (AV) valve** is also known as the **tricuspid** (tri-KUS-pid) **valve** because it has three cusps, or flaps, that open and close. When this valve is open, blood flows freely from the right atrium into the right ventricle. When the right ventricle begins to contract, however, the valve is closed by blood squeezed backward against the cusps. With the valve closed, blood cannot return to the right atrium but must flow forward into the pulmonary arterial trunk.

- The **left atrioventricular (AV) valve** is the bicuspid valve, but it is commonly referred to as the **mitral** (MI-tral) **valve** (named for a miter, the pointed, two-sided hat worn by bishops). It has two heavy cusps that permit blood to flow freely from the left atrium into the left ventricle. The cusps close when the left ventricle begins to contract; this closure prevents blood from returning to the left atrium and ensures the forward flow of blood into the aorta. Both the right and left AV valves are attached by means of thin fibrous threads to columnar muscles, called *papillary muscles*, in the walls of the ventricles. The function of these threads, called the **chordae tendineae** (KOR-de ten-DIN-e-e) (see Fig. 14-6), is to stabilize the valve flaps when the ventricles contract so that the blood's force will not push them up into the atria. In this manner, they help to prevent a backflow of blood when the heart beats.

■ The **pulmonary** (PUL-mon-ar-e) **valve**, also called the *pulmonic valve*, is a semilunar valve located between the right ventricle and the pulmonary trunk that leads to the lungs. As soon as the right ventricle begins to relax from a contraction, pressure in that chamber drops. The higher pressure in the pulmonary artery, described as *back pressure*, closes the valve and prevents blood from returning to the ventricle.

■ The **aortic** (a-OR-tik) **valve** is a semilunar valve located between the left ventricle and the aorta. After contraction of the left ventricle, back pressure closes the aortic valve and prevents the back flow of blood from the aorta into the ventricle.

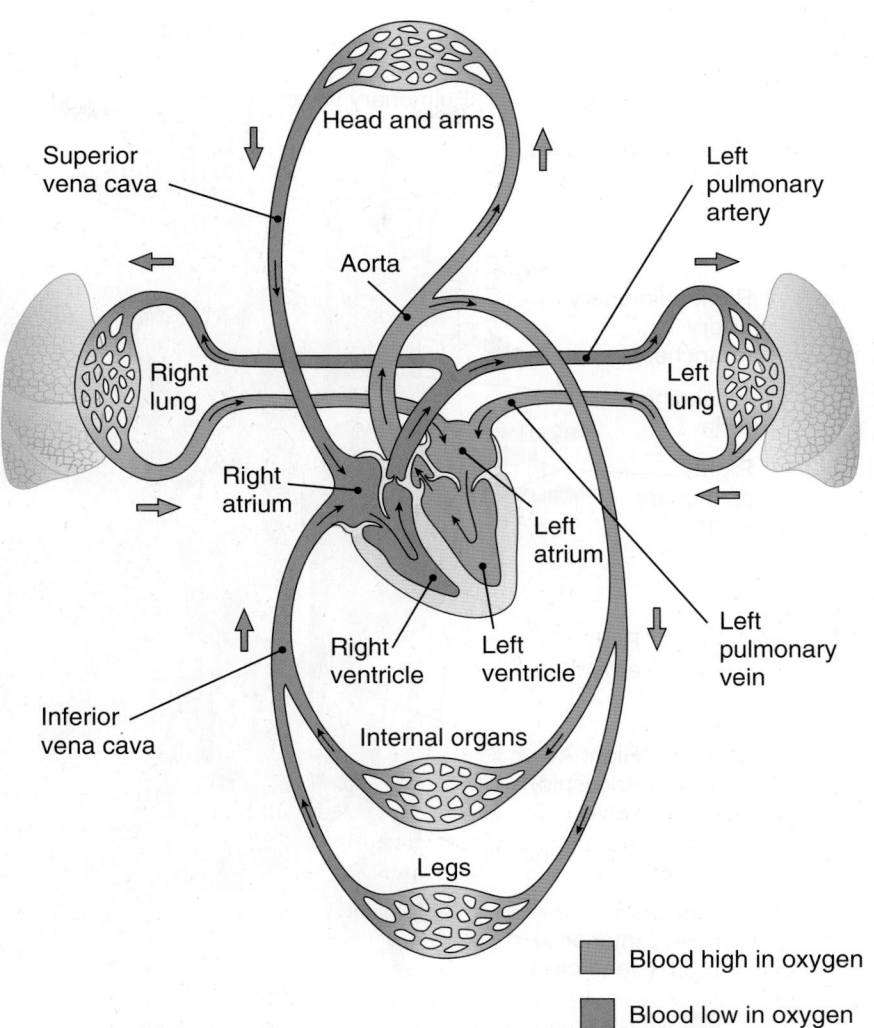

Figure 14-4 **The heart as a double pump.** The right side of the heart pumps blood through the pulmonary circuit to the lungs to be oxygenated; the left side of the heart pumps blood through the systemic circuit to all other parts of the body. [ZOOMING IN ▸ What vessel carries blood into the systemic circuit?]

Figure 14-7 traces a drop of blood as it completes a full circuit through the heart's chambers. Note that blood passes through the heart twice in making a trip from the heart's right side through the pulmonary circuit to the lungs and back to the heart's left side to start on its way through the systemic circuit. Although Figure 14-7 follows the path of a single drop of blood in sequence through the heart, the heart's two sides function in unison to pump blood through both circuits at the same time.

PASSport to Success Visit *thePoint* or see the Student Resource CD in the back of this book for a detailed picture of the chordae tendineae and for the animations *Blood Circulation* and *The Cardiac Cycle*.

CHECKPOINT 14-4 ▸ What is the purpose of valves in the heart?

Blood Supply to the Myocardium

Only the endocardium comes into contact with the blood that flows through the heart chambers. Therefore, the myocardium must have its own blood vessels to provide oxygen and nourishment and to remove waste products. Together, these blood vessels provide the **coronary** (KOR-o-na-re) **circulation**. The main arteries that supply blood to the heart muscle are the right and left coronary arteries (Fig. 14-8), named because they encircle the heart like a crown. These arteries, which are the first to branch off the aorta, arise just above the cusps of the aortic valve and branch to all regions of the heart muscle. They receive blood when the heart relaxes because the aortic valve must be closed to expose the entrance to these vessels (Fig. 14-9). After passing through capillaries in the myocardium, blood drains into a system of cardiac veins that brings blood back toward the right atrium. Blood finally collects

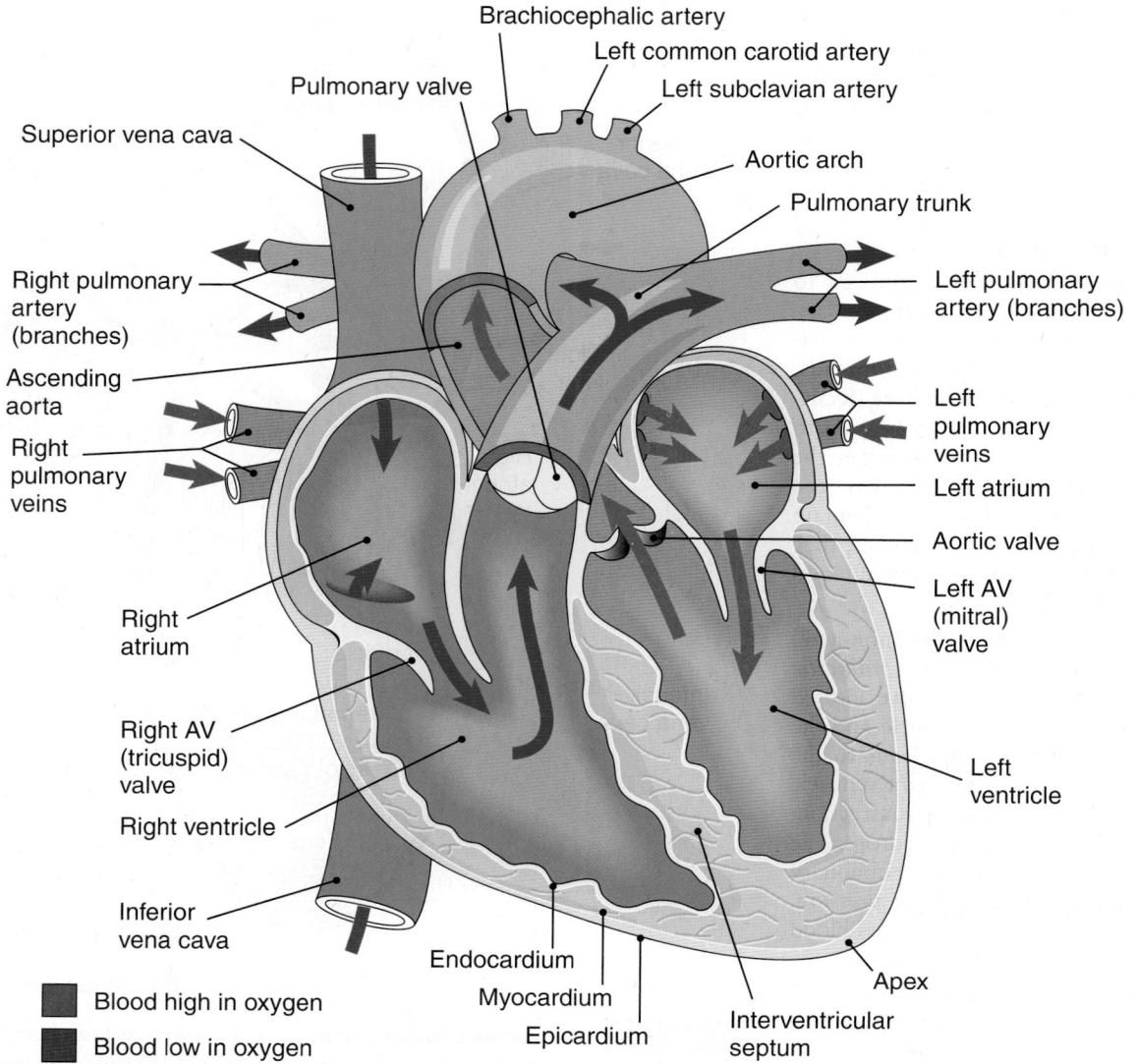

Figure 14-5 **The heart and great vessels.** The abbreviation AV means atrioventricular. [**ZOOMING IN ➤** Which heart chamber has the thickest wall?]

Table 14-3	Chambers of the Heart	
Chamber	**Location**	**Function**
Right atrium	Upper right chamber	Receives blood from the venae cavae and the coronary sinus; pumps blood into the right ventricle
Right ventricle	Lower right chamber	Receives blood from the right atrium and pumps blood into the pulmonary trunk; branches carry blood to the lungs to be oxygenated
Left atrium	Upper left chamber	Receives oxygenated blood coming back to the heart from the lungs in the pulmonary veins; pumps blood into the left ventricle
Left ventricle	Lower left chamber	Receives blood from the left atrium and pumps blood into the aorta to be carried to tissues in the systemic circuit

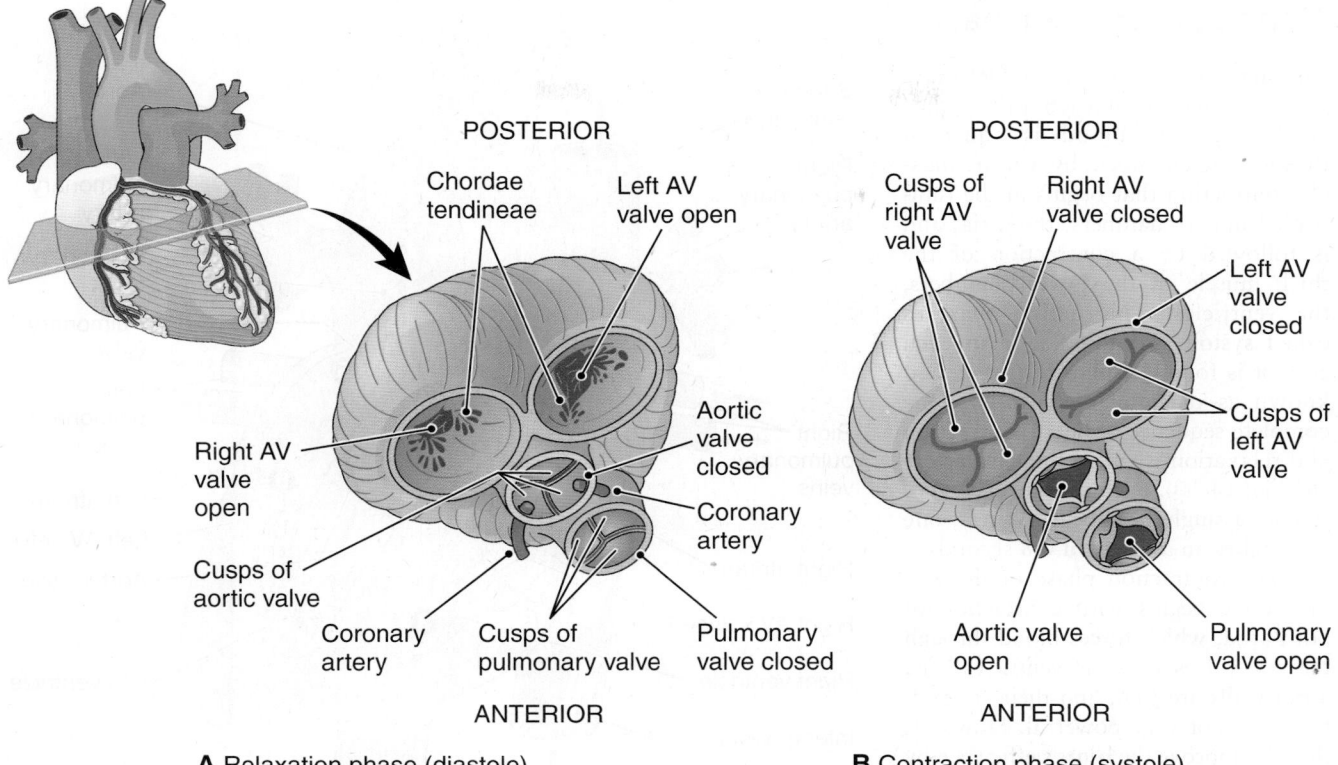

A Relaxation phase (diastole)   **B** Contraction phase (systole)

Figure 14-6 **Valves of the heart (superior view from anterior, atria removed).** **(A)** When the heart is relaxed (diastole), the AV valves are open and blood flows freely from the atria to the ventricles. The pulmonary and aortic valves are closed. **(B)** When the ventricles contract, the AV valves close and blood pumped out of the ventricles opens the pulmonary and aortic valves. [ZOOMING IN ➤ How many cusps does the right AV valve have? The left?]

in the **coronary sinus,** a dilated vein that opens into the right atrium near the inferior vena cava (see Fig. 14-8).

CHECKPOINT 14-5 ➤ The myocardium must have its own vascular system to supply it with blood. What name is given to this blood supply to the myocardium?

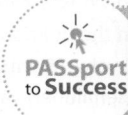 **PASSport to Success**   Visit **thePoint** or see the Student Resource CD in the back of this book for the animation *Myocardial Blood Flow.*

14

Table 14-4		**Valves of the Heart**	
Valve	**Location**	**Description**	**Function**
Right AV valve	Between the right atrium and right ventricle	Valve with three cusps; tricuspid valve	Prevents blood from flowing back up into the right atrium when the right ventricle contracts (systole)
Left AV valve	Between the left atrium and left ventricle	Valve with two cusps; bicuspid or mitral valve	Prevents blood from flowing back up into the left atrium when the left ventricle contracts (systole)
Pulmonary semi-lunar valve	At the entrance to the pulmonary trunk	Valve with three half-moon shaped cusps	Prevents blood from flowing back into the right ventricle when the right ventricle relaxes (diastole)
Aortic semilunar valve	At the entrance to the aorta	Valve with three half-moon shaped cusps	Prevents blood from flowing back into the left ventricle when the left ventricle relaxes (diastole)

Function of the Heart

Although the heart's right and left sides are separated from each other, they work together. Blood is squeezed through the chambers by a heart muscle contraction that begins in the thin-walled upper chambers, the atria, and is followed by a contraction of the thick muscle of the lower chambers, the ventricles. This active phase is called **systole** (SIS-to-le), and in each case, it is followed by a resting period known as **diastole** (di-AS-to-le). One complete sequence of heart contraction and relaxation is called the **cardiac cycle** (Fig. 14-10). Each cardiac cycle represents a single heartbeat. At rest, one cycle takes an average of 0.8 seconds.

The contraction phase of the cardiac cycle begins with contraction of both atria, which forces blood through the AV valves into the ventricles. The atrial walls are thin, and their contractions are not very powerful. However, they do improve the heart's efficiency by forcing blood into the ventricles before these lower chambers contract. Atrial contraction is completed at the time ventricular contraction begins. Thus, a resting phase (diastole) begins in the atria at the same time that a contraction (systole) begins in the ventricles.

After the ventricles have contracted, all chambers are relaxed for a short period as they fill with blood. Then another cycle begins with an atrial contraction followed by a ventricular contraction. Although both upper and lower chambers have a systolic and diastolic phase in each cardiac cycle, discussions of heart function usually refer to these phases as they occur in the ventricles, because these chambers contract more forcefully and drive blood into the arteries.

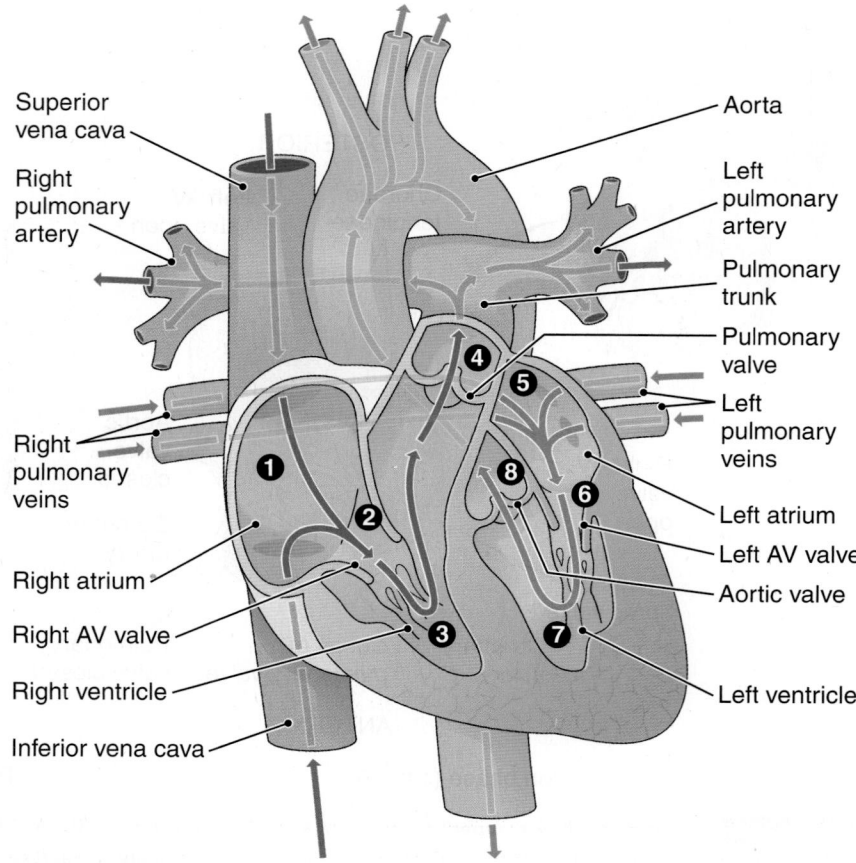

Figure 14-7 **Pathway of blood through the heart.** Blood from the systemic circuit enters the right atrium (1) through the superior and inferior venae cavae, flows through the right AV (tricuspid) valve (2), and enters the right ventricle (3). The right ventricle pumps the blood through the pulmonary (semilunar) valve (4) into the pulmonary trunk, which divides to carry blood to the lungs in the pulmonary circuit. Blood returns from the lungs in the pulmonary veins, enters the left atrium (5), and flows through the left AV (mitral) valve (6) into the left ventricle (7). The left ventricle pumps the blood through the aortic (semilunar) valve (8) into the aorta, which carries blood into the systemic circuit.

Cardiac Output

A unique property of heart muscle is its ability to adjust the strength of contraction to the amount of blood received. When the heart chamber is filled and the wall stretched (within limits), the contraction is strong. As less blood enters the heart, contractions become less forceful. Thus, as more blood enters the heart, as occurs during exercise, the muscle contracts with greater strength to push the larger volume of blood out into the blood vessels (see Box 14-1, Cardiac Reserve).

The volume of blood pumped by each ventricle in 1 minute is termed the **cardiac output** (CO). It is the product of the **stroke volume** (SV)—the volume of blood ejected from the ventricle with each beat—and the **heart rate** (HR)—the number of times the heart beats per minute. To summarize:

$$CO = HR \times SV$$

CHECKPOINT 14-6 ➤ The cardiac cycle consists of an alternating pattern of contraction and relaxation. What name is given to the contraction phase? To the relaxation phase?

CHECKPOINT 14-7 ➤ Cardiac output is the amount of blood pumped by each ventricle in 1 minute. What two factors determine cardiac output?

The Heart's Conduction System

Like other muscles, the heart muscle is stimulated to contract by a wave of electrical energy that passes along the cells. This

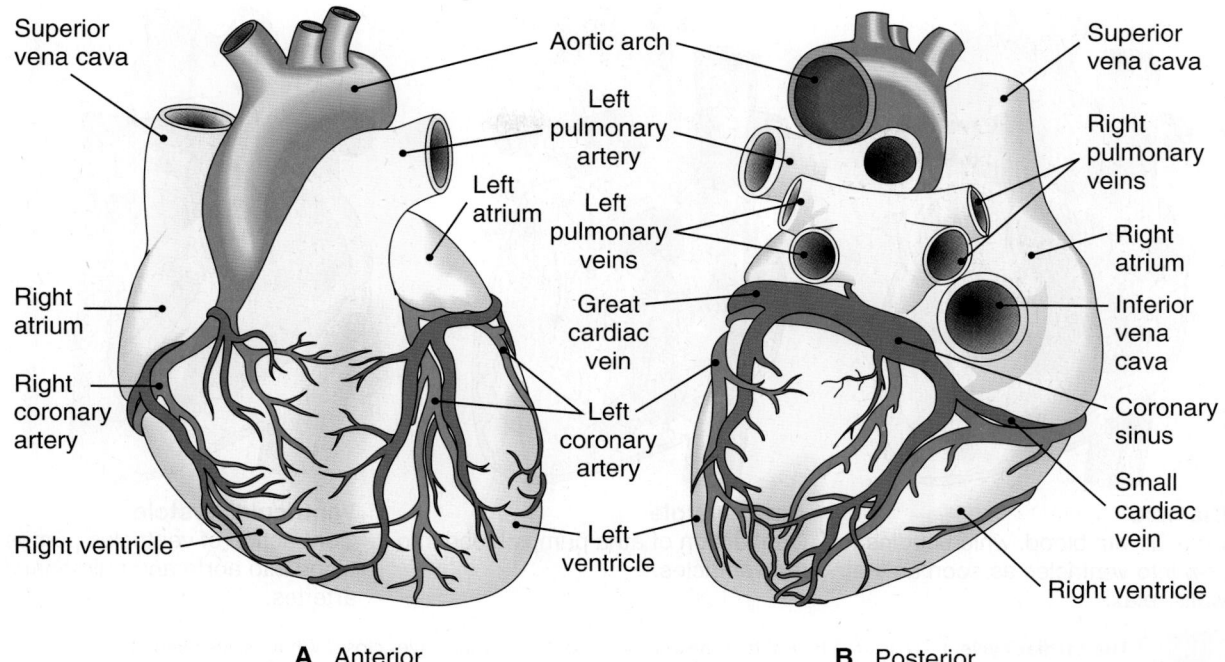

Figure 14-8 **Blood vessels that supply the myocardium.** Coronary arteries and cardiac veins are shown. **(A)** Anterior view. **(B)** Posterior view.

action potential is generated by specialized tissue within the heart and spreads over structures that form the heart's conduction system (Fig. 14-11). Two of these structures are tissue masses called **nodes,** and the remainder consists of specialized fibers that branch through the myocardium.

The **sinoatrial (SA) node** is located in the upper wall of the right atrium in a small depression described as a sinus.

This node initiates the heartbeats by generating an action potential at regular intervals. Because the SA node sets the rate of heart contractions, it is commonly called the **pacemaker.** The second node, located in the interatrial septum at the bottom of the right atrium, is called the **atrioventricular (AV) node.**

The **atrioventricular bundle,** also known as the **bundle of His,** is located at the top of the interventricular septum. It

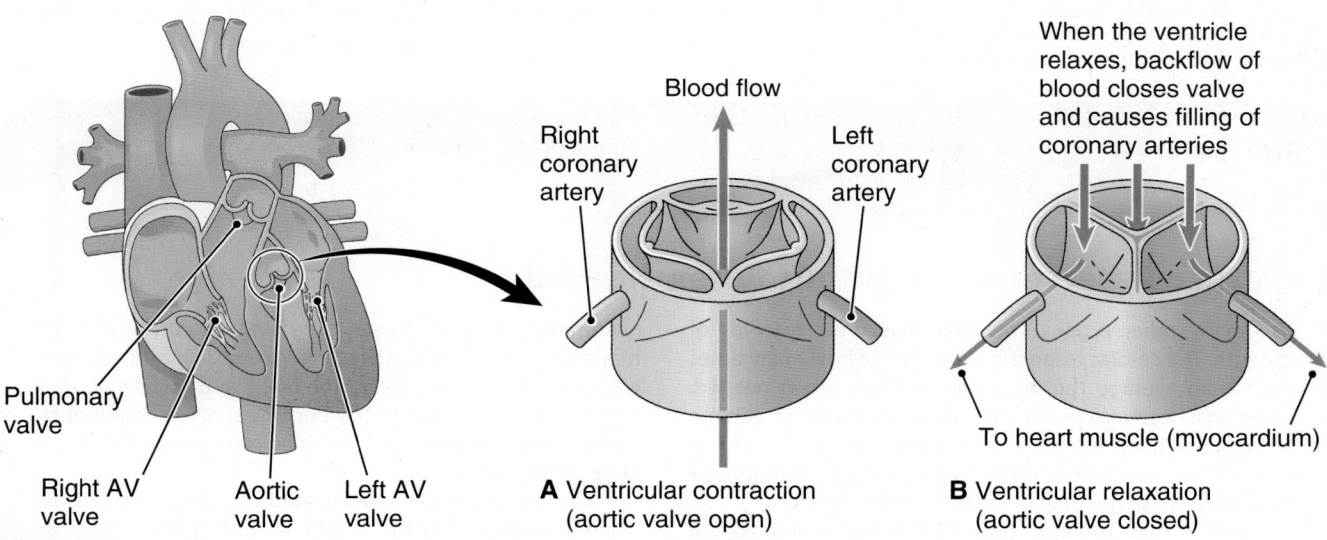

Figure 14-9 **Opening of coronary arteries in the aortic valve (anterior view).** **(A)** When the left ventricle contracts, the aortic valve opens. The valve cusps prevent filling of the coronary arteries. **(B)** When the left ventricle relaxes, backflow of blood closes the aortic valve and the coronary arteries fill. (Modified with permission from Moore KL, Dalley AF. *Clinically Oriented Anatomy,* 4th ed. Baltimore: Lippincott Williams & Wilkins, 1999.)

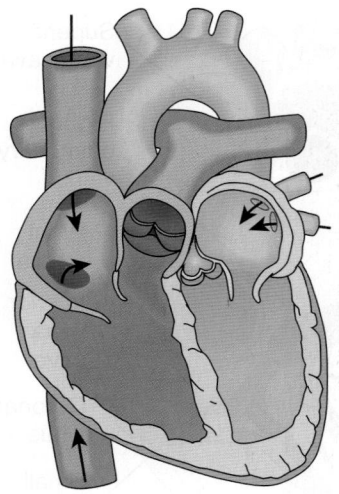

Diastole
Atria fill with blood, which begins to flow into ventricles as soon as their walls relax.

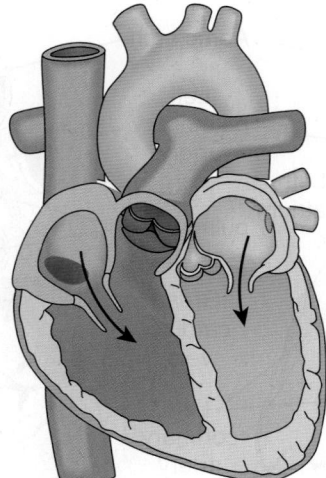

Atrial systole
Contraction of atria pumps blood into the ventricles.

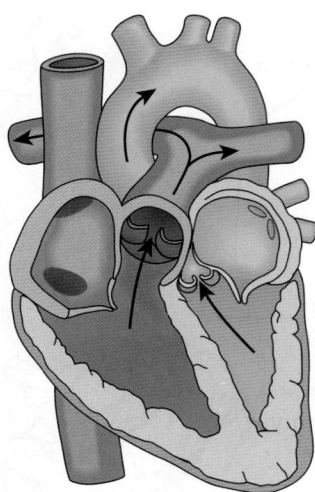

Ventricular systole
Contraction of ventricles pumps blood into aorta and pulmonary arteries.

Figure 14-10 **The cardiac cycle.** [ZOOMING IN ➤ When the ventricles contract, what valves close? What valves open?]

has branches that extend to all parts of the ventricular walls. Fibers travel first down both sides of the interventricular septum in groups called the right and left bundle branches. Smaller **Purkinje** (pur-KIN-je) **fibers**, also called *conduction myofibers*, then travel in a branching network throughout the myocardium of the ventricles. Intercalated disks allow the rapid flow of impulses throughout the heart muscle.

THE CONDUCTION PATHWAY The order in which impulses travel through the heart is as follows:

1. The sinoatrial node generates the electrical impulse that begins the heartbeat (see Fig. 14-11).

2. The excitation wave travels throughout the muscle of each atrium, causing the atria to contract. At the same time, impulses also travel directly to the AV node by means of fibers in the wall of the atrium that make up the **internodal pathways**.

3. The atrioventricular node is stimulated. A relatively slower rate of conduction through the AV node allows time for the atria to contract and complete the filling of the ventricles before the ventricles contract.

4. The excitation wave travels rapidly through the bundle of His and then throughout the ventricular walls by means of the bundle branches and Purkinje fibers.

Box 14-1 A Closer Look

Cardiac Reserve: Extra Output When Needed

Like many other organs, the heart has great reserves of strength. The cardiac reserve is a measure of how many times more than average the heart can produce when needed. Based on a heart rate of 75 beats/minute and a stroke volume of 70 mL/beat, the average cardiac output for an adult at rest is about 5 L/minute. This means that at rest, the heart pumps the equivalent of the total blood volume each minute.

During mild exercise, this volume might double and even double again during strenuous exercise. For most people the cardiac reserve is 4 to 5 times the resting output. This increase is achieved by an increase in either stroke volume,

heart rate, or both. In athletes exercising vigorously, the ratio may reach 6 to 7 times the resting volume. In contrast, those with heart disease may have little or no cardiac reserve. They may be fine at rest but quickly become short of breath or fatigued when exercising or even when carrying out the simple tasks of daily living.

Cardiac reserve can be evaluated using an exercise stress test that measures cardiac output while the patient walks on a treadmill or pedals an exercise bicycle. The exercise becomes more and more strenuous until the patient's peak cardiac output (cardiac reserve) is reached.

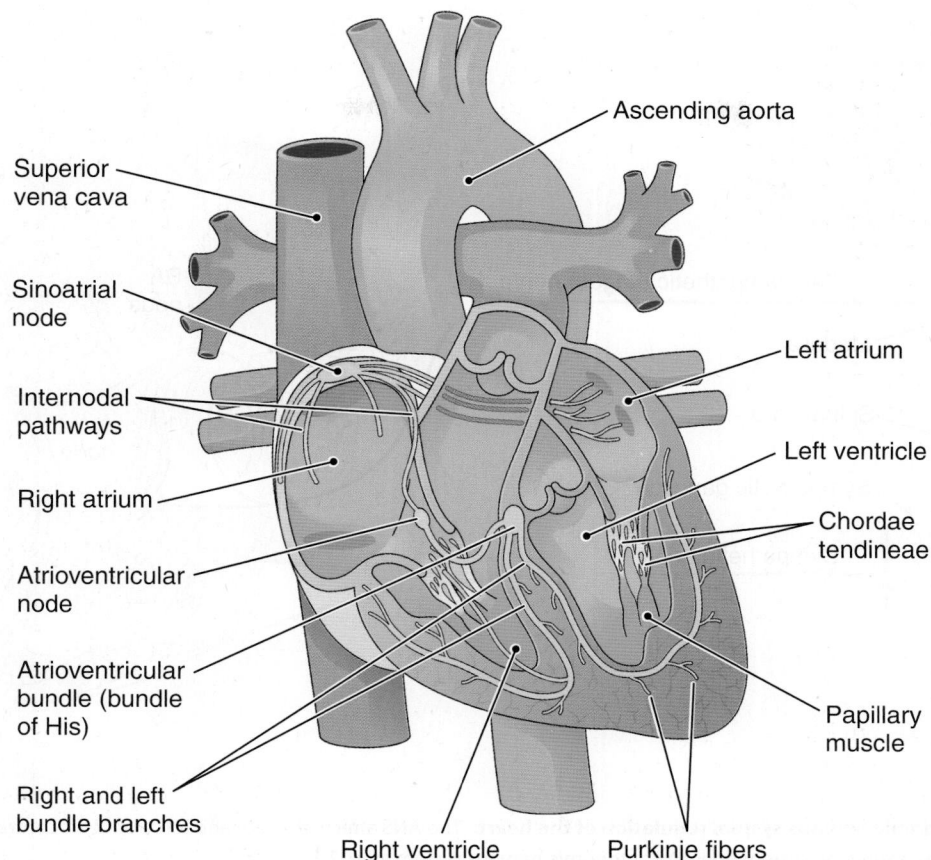

Superior
vena cava

Sinoatrial
node

Internodal
pathways

Right atrium

Atrioventricular
node

Atrioventricular
bundle (bundle
of His)

Right and left
bundle branches

Ascending aorta

Left atrium

Left ventricle

Chordae
tendineae

Papillary
muscle

Right ventricle   Purkinje fibers

Figure 14-11 **Conduction system of the heart.** The sinoatrial (SA) node, the atrioventricular (AV) node, and specialized fibers conduct the electrical energy that stimulates the heart muscle to contract. **[ZOOMING IN ➤** What parts of the conduction system do the internodal pathways connect? **]**

The entire ventricular musculature contracts almost at the same time.

A normal heart rhythm originating at the SA node is termed a **sinus rhythm**. As a safety measure, a region of the conduction system other than the SA node can generate a heartbeat if the SA node fails, but it does so at a slower rate.

CHECKPOINT **14-8** ➤ The heartbeat is started by a small mass of tissue in the upper right atrium. This structure is commonly called the pacemaker, but what is its scientific name?

Control of the Heart Rate

Although the heart's fundamental beat originates within the heart itself, the heart rate can be influenced by the nervous system, hormones, and other factors in the internal environment.

The autonomic nervous system (ANS) plays a major role in modifying the heart rate according to need (Fig. 14-12). Sympathetic nervous system stimulation increases

the heart rate in response to increased activity. During a fight-or-flight response, the sympathetic nerves can boost the cardiac output two to three times the resting value. Sympathetic fibers increase the contraction rate by stimulating the SA and AV nodes. They also increase the contraction force by acting directly on the fibers of the myocardium. These actions translate into increased cardiac output. Parasympathetic stimulation decreases the heart rate to restore homeostasis. The parasympathetic nerve that supplies the heart is the vagus nerve (cranial nerve X). It slows the heart rate by acting on the SA and AV nodes.

These ANS influences allow the heart to meet changing needs rapidly. The heart rate is also affected by substances circulating in the blood, including hormones, ions, and drugs. Regular exercise strengthens the heart and increases the amount of blood ejected with each beat. Consequently, the body's circulatory needs at rest can be met with a lower heart rate. Trained athletes usually have a low resting heart rate.

VARIATIONS IN HEART RATES

■ **Bradycardia** (brad-e-KAR-de-ah) is a relatively slow heart rate of less than 60 beats/minute. During rest and sleep, the heart may beat less than 60

14

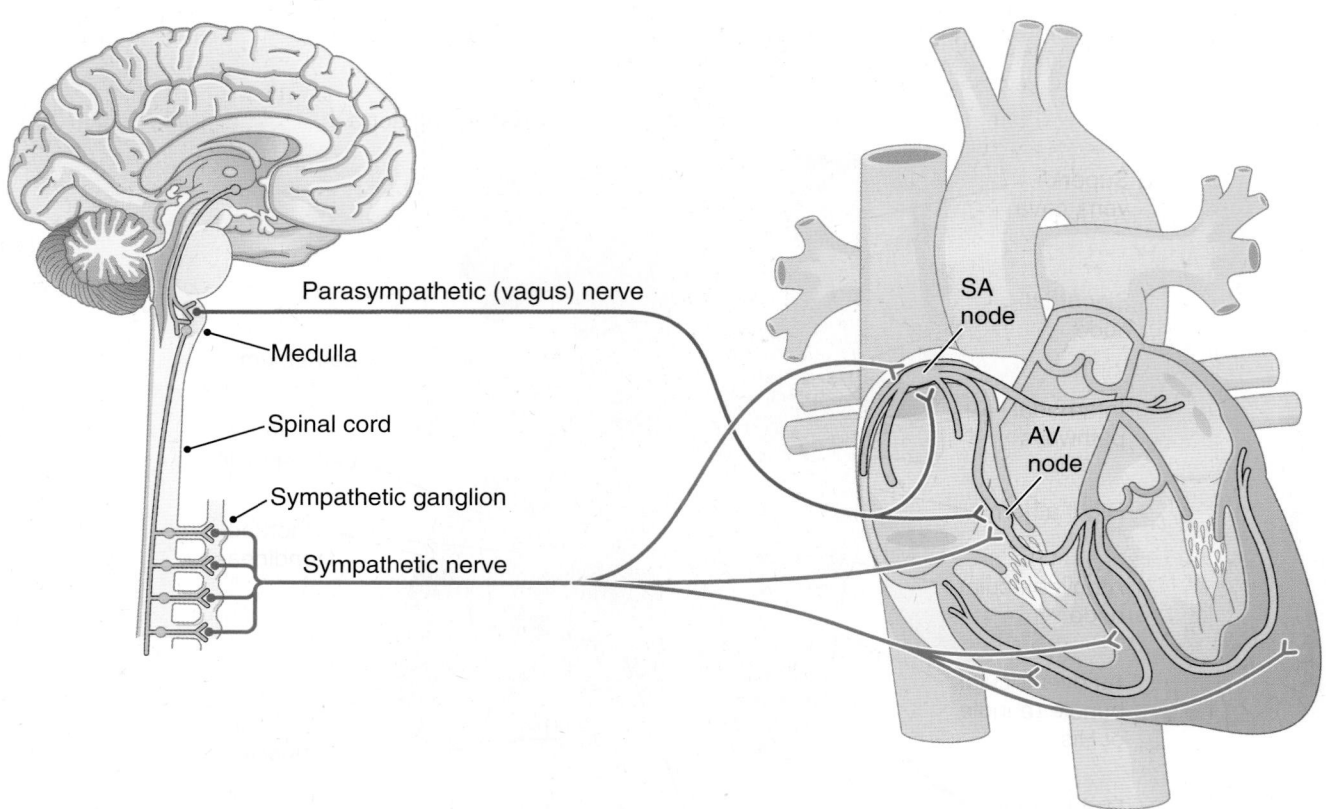

Figure 14-12 **Autonomic nervous system regulation of the heart.** The ANS affects the rate and force of heart contractions. [ZOOMING IN ➤ What parts of the conduction system does the autonomic nervous system affect?]

beats/minute, but the rate usually does not fall below 50 beats/minute.

■ **Tachycardia** (tak-e-KAR-de-ah) refers to a heart rate of more than 100 beats/minute. Tachycardia is normal during exercise or stress but may also occur under abnormal conditions.

■ **Sinus arrhythmia** (ah-RITH-me-ah) is a regular variation in heart rate caused by changes in the rate and depth of breathing. It is a normal phenomenon.

■ **Premature beat,** also called *extrasystole,* is a beat that comes before the expected normal beat. In healthy people, premature beats may be initiated by caffeine, nicotine, or psychological stresses. They are also common in people with heart disease.

Heart Sounds

The normal heart sounds are usually described by the syllables "lub" and "dup." The first heart sound (S_1), the "lub," is a longer, lower-pitched sound that occurs at the start of ventricular systole. It is probably caused by a combination of events, mainly closure of the atrioventricular valves. This action causes vibrations in the blood passing through the valves and in the tissue surrounding the valves. The second heart sound (S_2), the "dup," is shorter and sharper. It occurs at the beginning of ventricular relaxation and is caused largely by sudden closure of the semilunar valves.

MURMURS An abnormal sound is called a **murmur** and is usually due to faulty valve action. For example, if a valve fails to close tightly and blood leaks back, a murmur is heard. Another condition giving rise to an abnormal sound is the narrowing (stenosis) of a valve opening.

The many conditions that can cause abnormal heart sounds include congenital (birth) defects, disease, and physiologic variations. An abnormal sound caused by any structural change in the heart or the vessels connected with the heart is called an **organic murmur.** Certain normal sounds heard while the heart is working may also be described as murmurs, such as the sound heard during rapid filling of the ventricles. To differentiate these from abnormal sounds, they are more properly called **functional murmurs.**

CHECKPOINT 14-9 ➤ What system exerts the main influence on the rate and strength of heart contractions?

CHECKPOINT 14-10 ➤ What is a heart murmur?

Heart Disease

Diseases of the heart and circulatory system are the most common causes of death in industrialized countries. Few people escape having some damage to the heart and blood vessels in a lifetime.

Classifications of Heart Disease

There are many ways of classifying heart disease. The heart's anatomy forms the basis for one grouping of heart pathology:

- **Endocarditis** (en-do-kar-DI-tis) means "inflammation of the heart's lining." Endocarditis may involve the lining of the chambers, but the term most commonly refers to inflammation of the endocardium covering the valves and valvular disease.
- **Myocarditis** (mi-o-kar-DI-tis) is inflammation of heart muscle.
- **Pericarditis** (per-ih-kar-DI-tis) refers to inflammation of the serous membrane on the heart surface as well as that lining the pericardial sac.

These inflammatory diseases are often caused by infection, but may also be secondary to other types of respiratory or systemic diseases.

Another classification of heart disease is based on causative factors:

- **Congenital heart disease** is a condition present at birth.
- **Rheumatic** (ru-MAT-ik) **heart disease** originates with an attack of rheumatic fever in childhood or in youth.
- **Coronary artery disease** involves the walls of the blood vessels that supply the heart muscle.
- **Heart failure** is caused by deterioration of the heart tissues and is frequently the result of long-standing disorders, such as high blood pressure.

Congenital Heart Disease

Congenital heart diseases often are the result of defects in fetal development. Two of these disorders represent the abnormal persistence of structures that are part of the normal fetal circulation (Fig. 14-13A). Because the lungs are not used until a child is born, the fetus has some adaptations that allow blood to bypass the lungs. The fetal heart has a small hole, the **foramen ovale** (for-A-men o-VAL-e), in the

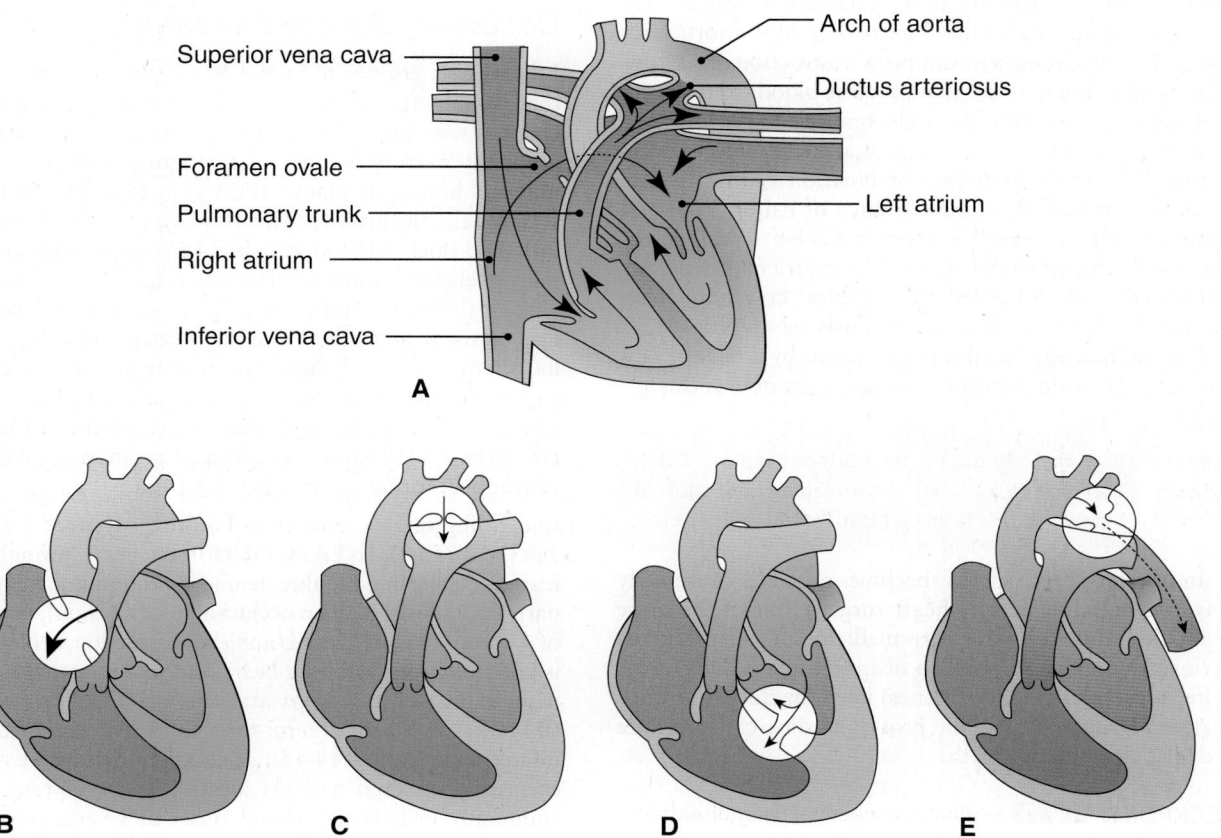

Figure 14-13 **Congenital heart defects.** **(A)** Normal fetal heart showing the foramen ovale and ductus arteriosus. **(B)** Persistence of the foramen ovale results in an atrial septal defect. **(C)** Persistence of the ductus arteriosus (patent ductus arteriosus) forces blood back into the pulmonary artery. **(D)** A ventricular septal defect. **(E)** Coarctation of the aorta restricts outward blood flow in the aorta. (Reprinted with permission from Porth CM. Pathophysiology, 7th ed. Philadelphia: Lippincott Williams & Wilkins, 2004.)

14

septum between the right and left atria. This opening allows some blood to flow directly from the right atrium into the left atrium, thus bypassing the lungs. Failure of the foramen ovale to close is one cause of an abnormal opening known as an **atrial septal defect** (see Fig. 14-13B).

The **ductus arteriosus** (ar-te-re-O-sus) in the fetus is a small blood vessel that connects the pulmonary artery and the aorta so that some blood headed toward the lungs will enter the aorta instead. The ductus arteriosus normally closes on its own once the lungs are in use. Persistence of the vessel after birth is described as **patent** (open) **ductus arteriosus** (see Fig. 14-13C).

The most common single congenital heart defect is a hole in the septum between the two ventricles, a disorder known as **ventricular septal defect** (see Fig. 14-13D).

In each of the above defects, part of the heart's left side output goes back to the lungs instead of out to the body. A small defect remaining from the foramen ovale or a small patent ductus may cause no difficulty and is often not diagnosed until an adult is examined for other cardiac problems. More serious defects greatly increase the left ventricle's work and may lead to heart failure. In addition, ventricular septal defect creates high blood pressure in the lungs, which damages lung tissue.

Other congenital defects that tax the heart involve restriction of outward blood flow. **Coarctation** (ko-ark-TA-shun) **of the aorta** is a localized narrowing of the aortic arch (see Fig. 14-13E). Another example is obstruction or narrowing of the pulmonary trunk that prevents blood from passing in sufficient quantity from the right ventricle to the lungs.

In many cases, several congenital heart defects occur together. The most common combination is that of four specific defects known as the **tetralogy of Fallot** (FAH-yo): pulmonary artery stenosis; interventricular septal defect; aortic displacement to the right; right ventricular hypertrophy (size increase). So-called "blue babies" commonly have this disorder. The blueness, or **cyanosis** (si-ah-NO-sis), of the skin and mucous membranes is caused by a relative lack of oxygen. (See Chapter 18 for other causes of cyanosis.)

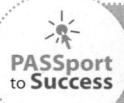

Visit **thePoint** or see the Student Resource CD in the back of this book for a tetralogy of Fallot diagram.

In recent years, it has become possible to remedy many congenital defects by heart surgery, one of the more spectacular advances in modern medicine. A patent ductus arteriosus may also respond to drug treatment. During fetal life, prostaglandins (hormones) keep the ductus arteriosus open. Drugs that inhibit prostaglandins can promote the duct's closing after birth.

CHECKPOINT 14-11 ➤ What is congenital heart disease?

Rheumatic Heart Disease

A certain type of streptococcal infection, the type that causes "strep throat," is indirectly responsible for rheumatic fever and rheumatic heart disease. The toxin produced by these streptococci causes a normal immune response. However, in some cases, the initial infection may be followed some 2 to 4 weeks later by rheumatic fever, a generalized inflammatory disorder with marked swelling of the joints. The antibodies formed to combat the toxin are believed to cause this disease. These antibodies may also attack the heart valves, producing a condition known as *rheumatic endocarditis*. The heart valves, particularly the mitral valve, become inflamed, and the normally flexible valve cusps thicken and harden. The mitral valve may not open sufficiently (mitral stenosis) to allow enough blood into the ventricle or may not close effectively, allowing blood to return to the left atrium (mitral regurgitation). Either condition interferes with blood flow from the left atrium into the left ventricle, causing pulmonary congestion, an important characteristic of mitral heart disease. The incidence of rheumatic heart disease has declined with antibiotic treatment of streptococcal infections. However, children who do not receive adequate diagnosis and treatment are subject to developing the disease.

CHECKPOINT 14-12 ➤ What types of organisms cause rheumatic fever?

Coronary Artery Disease

Like vessels elsewhere in the body, the coronary arteries that supply the heart muscle can undergo degenerative changes with time. The lumen (space) inside the vessel may gradually narrow because of a progressive deposit of fatty material known as **plaque** (PLAK) in the lining of the vessels, usually the arteries. This process, called **atherosclerosis** (ath-er-o-skleh-RO-sis), causes thickening and hardening of the vessels with a loss of elasticity (Fig. 14-14). The *athero* part of the name means "gruel," because of the porridge-like material that adheres to the vessel walls. The vessels' narrowing leads to **ischemia** (is-KE-me-ah), a lack of blood supply to the areas fed by those arteries. Degenerative changes in the arterial wall also may cause the inside vascular surface to become roughened, promoting blood clot (thrombus) formation (see Fig. 14-14C).

MYOCARDIAL INFARCTION In the heart, thrombus formation results in a life-threatening condition known as **coronary thrombosis**. Sudden **occlusion** (ok-LU-zhun), or closure, of a coronary vessel with complete obstruction of blood flow is commonly known as a *heart attack*. Because the area of tissue damaged in a heart attack is described as an **infarct** (IN-farkt), the medical term for a heart attack is **myocardial infarction** (MI) (Fig. 14-15). The oxygen-deprived tissue will eventually undergo necrosis (death). The symptoms of MI commonly include the abrupt onset of severe, constricting chest pain that may radiate to the left arm, back, neck, or jaw. Patients may experience shortness of breath, sweating, nausea, vomiting, or pain in the epigastric region, which can be mistaken for indigestion. They may feel weak, restless, or anxious and the skin may be pale, cool, and moist.

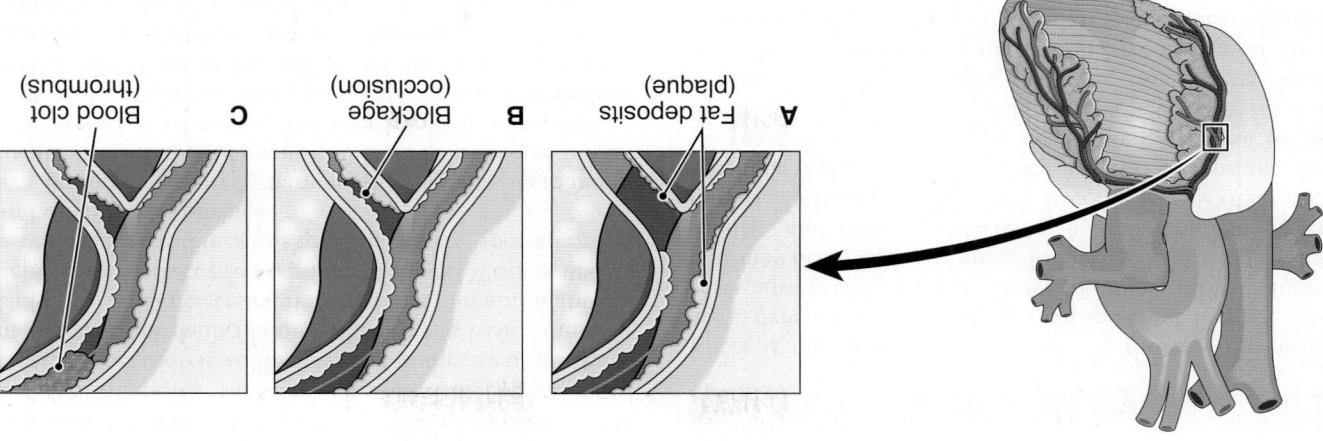

Figure 14-14 Coronary atherosclerosis. **(A)** Fat deposits (plaque) narrow an artery, leading to ischemia (lack of blood supply). **(B)** Plaque causes blockage (occlusion) of a vessel. **(C)** Formation of a blood clot (thrombus) in a vessel leads to myocardial infarction (MI).

A Fat deposits (plaque)

B Blockage (occlusion)

C Blood clot (thrombus)

ANGINA PECTORIS Inadequate blood flow to the heart muscle causes a characteristic discomfort, called angina pectoris (an-JI-nah PEK-to-ris), felt in the region of the heart and in the left arm and shoulder. Angina pectoris may be accompanied by a feeling of suffocation and a general sensation of forthcoming doom. Coronary artery disease is a common cause of angina pectoris, although the condition has other causes as well.

ABNORMALITIES OF HEART RHYTHM Coronary artery disease or myocardial infarction often results in an abnormal rhythm of the heartbeat, or **arrhythmia** (ah-RITH-me-ah). Extremely rapid but coordinated contractions, numbering up to 300 per minute, are described as **flutter.** An episode of rapid, wild, and uncoordinated heart muscle contractions is called **fibrillation** (fih-brih-LA-shun), which may involve the atria only or both the atria and the ventricles. Ventricular fibrillation is a serious disorder because there is no effective heartbeat. It must be corrected by a **defibrillator,** a device that generates a strong electrical current to discharge all the cardiac muscle cells at once, allowing a normal rhythm to resume.

An interruption of electric impulses in the heart's conduction system is called **heart block.** The seriousness of this condition depends on how completely the impulses are blocked. It may result in independent beating of the chambers if the ventricles respond to a second pacemaker.

TREATMENT OF HEART ATTACKS The death rate for heart attacks is high when treatment is delayed. Initial

PASSport to Success Visit thePoint or see the Student Resource CD in the back of this book for an illustration of the clinical signs of MI.

vessel. Complete and prolonged lack of blood to any part of the myocardium results in tissue necrosis and weakening of the heart wall.

MI is diagnosed by electrocardiography (ECG) and assays for specific substances in the blood. **Creatine kinase** (CK) is an enzyme normal to muscle cells. It is released in increased amounts when any muscle tissue is damaged. The form of CK specific to cardiac muscle cells is creatine kinase MB (CK-MB). Troponin (Tn) is a protein that regulates muscle cell contraction (see Chapter 8). Increased plasma levels, in particular the forms TnT and TnI, indicate MI.

The outcome of a myocardial infarction depends largely on the extent and location of the damage. Many people die within the first hour after onset of symptoms, but prompt, aggressive treatment can improve outcomes. Medical personnel make immediate efforts to relieve chest pain, stabilize the heart rhythm, and reopen the blocked

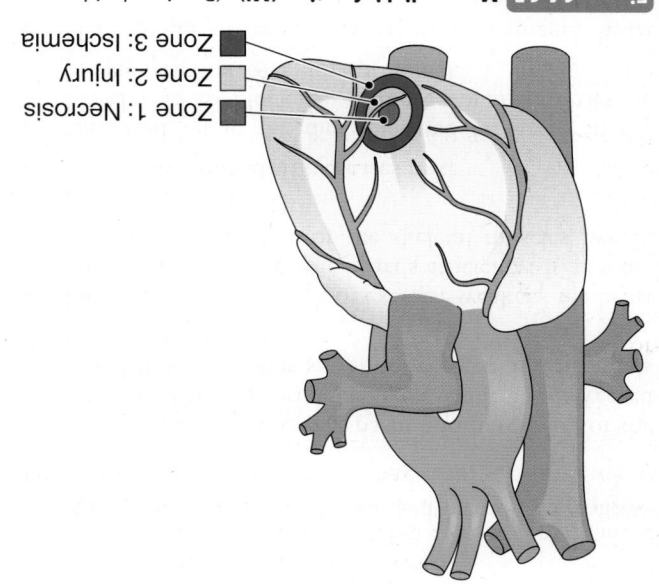

Zone 1: Necrosis
Zone 2: Injury
Zone 3: Ischemia

Figure 14-15 Myocardial infarction (MI). (Reprinted with permission from Cohen BJ. *Medical Terminology,* 5th ed. Philadelphia: Lippincott Williams & Wilkins, 2008.)

treatment involves cardiopulmonary resuscitation (CPR) and defibrillation at the scene when needed. The American Heart Association is adding training in the use of the **automated external defibrillator (AED)** to the basic course in CPR. The AED detects fatal arrhythmia and automatically delivers the correct preprogrammed shock. Work is underway to place machines in shopping centers, sports venues, and other public settings.

Prompt transport by paramedics who are able to monitor the heart and give emergency drugs helps people to survive and reach a hospital. The next step is to restore blood flow to the ischemic areas by administering **thrombolytic** (throm-bo-LIT-ik) **drugs,** which act to dissolve the clots blocking the coronary arteries. Therapy must be given promptly to prevent permanent heart muscle damage. In many cases, a pulmonary artery catheter (tube) is put in place to monitor cardiac function and response to medication. Supportive care includes treatment of chest pain with intravenous (IV) morphine. Healthcare workers monitor heart rhythm and give medications to maintain a functional rhythm. Oxygen is given to improve heart muscle function. Some patients require surgery, such as angioplasty to reopen vessels or a vascular graft to bypass damaged vessels; others may need an artificial pacemaker to maintain a normal heart rhythm.

Recovery from a heart attack and resumption of a normal lifestyle is often possible if the patient follows his or her prescribed drug therapy plan and takes steps to reduce cardiac risk factors.

CHECKPOINT 14-13 ► Narrowing or blockage of the vessels that supply the heart muscle causes coronary artery disease. What degenerative process commonly causes narrowing of these vessels?

Heart Failure

Heart failure is a condition in which the heart is unable to pump sufficient blood to supply the tissues with oxygen and nutrients. The heart's chambers enlarge to contain more blood than the stretched fibers are able to pump. Blood backs up into the lungs, increasing blood pressure in the lungs. The ventricular muscles do not get enough blood, decreasing their ability to contract. Additional mechanisms cause the retention of fluid, leading to the name *congestive heart failure* (CHF). In an attempt to increase blood flow, the nervous system increases constriction of the blood vessels, increasing blood pressure. Soon there is a fluid accumulation in the lungs, liver, abdomen, and legs. People can live with compensated heart failure by attention to diet, drug therapy, and a balance of activity and rest.

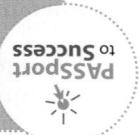

PASSport to Success

Visit **thePoint** or see the Student Resource CD in the back of this book for an illustration of the clinical effects of congestive heart failure and for the animation Heart Failure.

The Heart in the Elderly

There is much individual variation in the way the heart ages, depending on heredity, environmental factors, diseases, and personal habits. However, some of the changes that may occur with age are as follows. The heart becomes smaller, and there is a decrease in the strength of heart muscle contraction. The valves become less flexible, and incomplete closure may produce an audible murmur. By 70 years of age, the cardiac output may decrease by as much as 35%. Damage within the conduction system can produce abnormal rhythms, including extra beats, rapid atrial beats, and slowing of ventricular contraction rate. Temporary failure of the conduction system (heart block) can cause periodic loss of consciousness. Because of the decrease in the heart's reserve strength, elderly people are often limited in their ability to respond to physical or emotional stress.

Prevention of Heart Disease

Prevention of heart ailments is based on identification of cardiovascular risk factors and modification of those factors that can be changed. Risk factors that cannot be modified include the following:

- Age. The risk of heart disease increases with age.
- Gender. Until middle age, men have greater risk than women. Women older than 50 years or past menopause have risk equal to that of males.
- Heredity. Those with immediate family members with heart disease are at greater risk.
- Body type, particularly the hereditary tendency to deposit fat in the abdomen or on the chest surface, increases risk.

Risk factors that can be changed include the following:

- Smoking, which leads to spasm and hardening of the arteries. These arterial changes result in decreased blood flow and poor supply of oxygen and nutrients to the heart muscle.
- Physical inactivity. Lack of exercise weakens the heart muscle and decreases the heart's efficiency. It also decreases the efficiency of the skeletal muscles, which further taxes the heart.
- Weight over the ideal increases risk.
- Saturated fat in the diet. Elevated fat levels in the blood lead to blockage of the coronary arteries by plaque (see Box 14-2, Lipoproteins).
- High blood pressure (hypertension) damages heart muscle.
- Diabetes and gout. Both diseases cause damage to small blood vessels.

Heart Studies

Experienced listeners can gain much information about the heart using a stethoscope (STETH-o-skope). This relatively simple instrument is used to convey sounds from within the patient's body to an examiner's ear.

The electrocardiograph (ECG or EKG) is used to record electrical changes produced as the heart muscle contracts. (The abbreviation EKG comes from the German spelling of the word.) The ECG may reveal certain myocardial injuries. Electrodes (leads) placed on the skin surface pick up electrical activity, and the ECG tracing, or electrocardiogram, represents this activity as waves. The P wave represents the activity of the atria; the QRS and T waves represent the activity of the ventricles (Fig. 14-16). Changes in the waves and the intervals between them are used to diagnose heart damage and arrhythmias.

Many people with heart disease undergo catheterization (kath-eh-ter-i-ZA-shun). In right heart catheterization, an extremely thin tube (catheter) is passed through the veins of the right arm or right groin and then into the right side of heart. A fluoroscope (flu-OR-o-scope), an instrument for examining deep structures with x-rays, is used to show the route taken by the catheter. The tube is passed all the way through the pulmonary valve into the large lung arteries. Blood samples are obtained along the way for testing, and pressure readings are taken.

In left heart catheterization, a catheter is passed through an artery in the left groin or arm to the heart. The cardiologist can then inject dye into the coronary arteries to map vascular damage. The tube may also be passed through the aortic valve into the left ventricle for studies of pressure and volume in that chamber.

Ultrasound consists of sound waves generated at a frequency above the human ear's range of sensitivity. In echocardiography (ek-o-kar-de-OG-rah-fe), also known as

Efforts to prevent heart disease should include having regular physical examinations and minimizing the controllable risk factors.

Figure 14-16 Normal ECG tracing. The tracing shows a single cardiac cycle. [**ZOOMING IN ▸** What is the length of the cardiac cycle shown in this diagram?]

Box 14-2 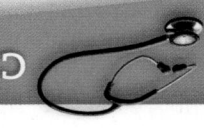 Clinical Perspectives

Lipoproteins: What's the Big DL?

Although cholesterol has received a lot of bad press in recent years, it is a necessary substance in the body. It is found in bile salts needed for digestion of fats, in hormones, and in the cell's plasma membrane. However, high levels of cholesterol in the blood have been associated with atherosclerosis and heart disease.

It now appears that the total amount of blood cholesterol is not as important as the form in which it occurs. Cholesterol is transported in the blood in combination with other lipids and with protein, forming compounds called lipoproteins. These compounds are distinguished by their relative density. High-density lipoprotein (HDL) is about one-half protein, whereas low-density lipoprotein (LDL) has a higher proportion of cholesterol and less protein. VLDLs, or very-low-density lipoproteins, are substances that are converted to LDLs.

LDLs carry cholesterol from the liver to the tissues, making it available for membrane or hormone synthesis. HDLs remove cholesterol from the tissues, such as the arterial walls, and carry it back to the liver for reuse or disposal. Thus, high levels of HDLs indicate efficient removal of arterial plaques, whereas high levels of LDLs suggest that arteries will become clogged.

Diet is an important factor in regulating lipoprotein levels. Saturated fatty acids (found primarily in animal fats) raise LDL levels, while unsaturated fatty acids (found in most vegetable oils) lower LDL levels and stimulate cholesterol excretion. Thus, a diet lower in saturated fat and higher in unsaturated fat may reduce the risk of atherosclerosis and heart disease. Other factors that affect lipoprotein levels include cigarette smoking, coffee drinking, and stress, which raise LDL levels, and exercise, which lowers LDL levels.

CHECKPOINT 14-14 ▶ What do ECG and EKG stand for?

Treatment of Heart Disease

Heart specialists employ medical and surgical approaches, often in combination, in treating heart disease.

Medications

One of the oldest drugs for heart treatment, and still the most important drug for many patients, is **digitalis** (dij-ih-TAL-is). This agent, which slows and strengthens heart muscle contractions, is obtained from the leaf of the fox-glove, a plant originally found growing wild in many parts of Europe. Foxglove is now cultivated to ensure a steady supply of digitalis for medical purposes.

Several forms of **nitroglycerin** are used to relieve angina pectoris. This drug dilates (widens) the vessels in the coronary circulation and improves the heart's blood supply.

Beta-adrenergic blocking agents ("beta-blockers") control sympathetic stimulation of the heart. They reduce the rate and strength of heart contractions, thus reducing the heart's oxygen demand. Propranolol is one example. **Antiarrhythmic agents** (e.g., quinidine) are used to regulate the rate and rhythm of the heartbeat. *Slow calcium-channel blockers* aid in the treatment of coronary heart disease and hypertension by several mechanisms. They may dilate vessels, control the force of heart contractions, or regulate conduction through the atrioventricular node. Their actions are based on the fact that calcium ions must enter muscle cells before contraction can occur.

Anticoagulants (an-ti-ko-AG-u-lants) are valuable drugs for some heart patients. They may be used to prevent clot formation in patients with damage to heart valves or blood vessels or in patients who have had a myocardial in-

faction. **Aspirin** (AS-pir-in), chemically known as acetyl-salicylic (a-SE-til-sal-ih-SIL-ik) acid (ASA), is an inexpensive and time-tested drug for pain and inflammation that reduces blood clotting by interfering with platelet activity. A small daily dose of aspirin is recommended for patients with angina pectoris, those who have suffered a myocardial infarction, and those who have undergone surgery to open or bypass narrowed coronary arteries. It is contraindicated for people with bleeding disorders or gastric ulcers, because aspirin irritates the stomach lining.

Correction of Arrhythmias

If the SA node fails to generate a normal heartbeat or there is some failure in the cardiac conduction system, an electric, battery-operated artificial **pacemaker** can be employed (Fig. 14-17). This device, implanted under the skin, supplies regular impulses to stimulate the heartbeat. The implantation site is usually in the left chest area. A pacing wire (lead) from the pacemaker is then passed into the heart and lodged in the heart. The lead may be fixed in an atrium or a ventricle (usually on the right side). A dual chamber pacemaker has a lead in each chamber to coordinate beats between the atrium and ventricle; others can be set to stimulate a beat only when the heart fails to do so on its own. Another type of pacemaker adjusts its pacing rate

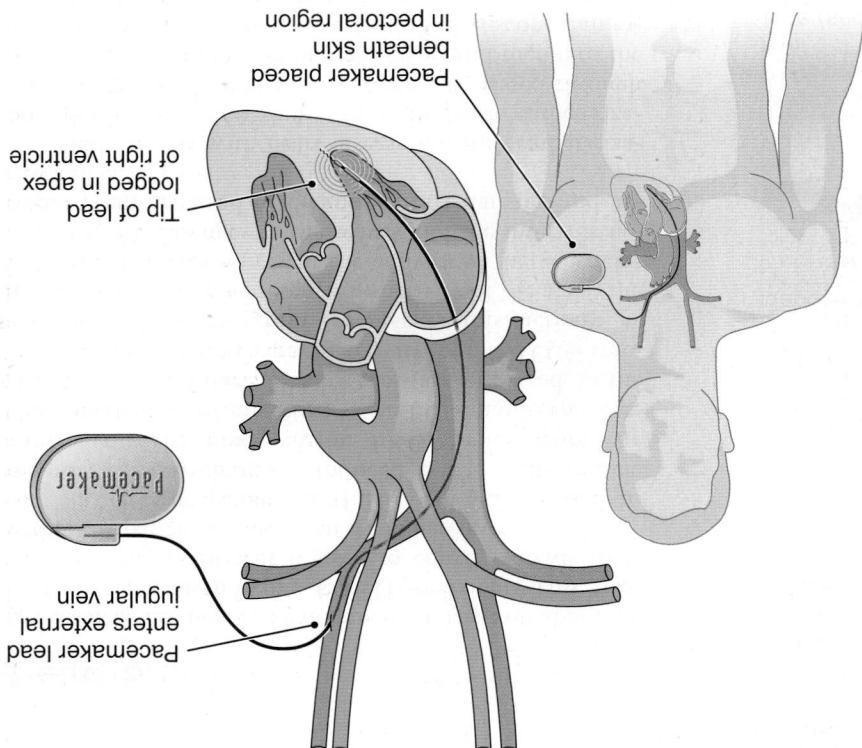

Figure 14-17 **Placement of an artificial pacemaker.** The lead is placed in an atrium or ventricle (usually on the right side). A dual chamber pacemaker has leads in both chambers. (Reprinted with permission from Cohen BJ. *Medical Terminology*, 5th ed. Philadelphia: Lippincott Williams & Wilkins, 2008.)

Labels: Pacemaker lead enters external jugular vein; Tip of lead lodged in apex of right ventricle; Pacemaker placed beneath skin in pectoral region; Pacemaker

ultrasound cardiography, high-frequency sound waves are sent to the heart from a small instrument on the chest surface. The ultrasound waves bounce off the heart and are recorded as they return, showing the heart in action. Movement of the echoes is traced on an electronic instrument called an *oscilloscope* and recorded on film. (The same principle is employed by submarines to detect ships.) The method is safe and painless, and it does not use x-rays. It provides information on the size and shape of heart structures, on cardiac function, and on possible heart defects.

in response to changing activity, as during exercise. This rather simple device has saved many people whose hearts cannot beat effectively alone. In an emergency, a similar stimulus can be supplied to the heart muscle through electrodes placed externally on the chest wall.

In cases of chronic ventricular fibrillation, a battery-powered device can be implanted in the chest to restore a normal rhythm. The device detects a rapid abnormal rhythm and delivers a direct shock to the heart. The restoration of a normal heartbeat either by electric shock or drugs, is called *cardioversion*, and this device is known as an implantable cardioverter-defibrillator (ICD). A lead wire from the defibrillator is placed in the right ventricle through the pulmonary artery. In cases of severe tachycardia, tissue that is causing the disturbance can be destroyed (ablated) by surgery or catheterization.

Heart Surgery

The heart-lung machine makes possible many operations on the heart and other thoracic organs. There are several types of machines in use, all of which serve as temporary substitutes for the patient's heart and lungs. The machine siphons off the blood from the large vessels entering the heart on the right side, so that no blood passes through the heart and lungs. While in the machine, the blood is oxygenated, and carbon dioxide is removed chemically. The blood is also "defoamed," or rid of air bubbles, which could fatally obstruct blood vessels. The machine then pumps the processed blood back into the general circulation through a large artery. Modern advances have enabled cardiac surgeons to perform certain procedures without bypassing the circulation, partially immobilizing the heart while it continues to beat.

Coronary artery bypass graft (CABG) to relieve obstruction in the coronary arteries is a common and often successful treatment (Fig. 14-18). While the damaged coronary arteries remain in place, healthy segments of blood vessels from other parts of the patient's body are grafted onto the vessels to bypass any obstructions. Usually, parts of the saphenous vein (a superficial vein in the leg) or the mammary artery in the chest are used.

Sometimes, as many as six or seven segments are required to establish an adequate blood supply. The mortality associated with this operation is low, and most patients are able to return to a nearly normal lifestyle after recovery from the surgery. The effectiveness of this procedure diminishes over a period of years, however, owing to blockage of the replacement vessels.

Less invasive surgical procedures include the technique of **angioplasty** (AN-je-o-plas-te), which is used to open restricted arteries in the heart and other areas of the body. In coronary angioplasty, a fluoroscope is used to guide a catheter with a balloon to the affected area (Fig. 14-19). There, the balloon is inflated to break up the blockage in the coronary artery, thus restoring effective circulation to the heart muscle. To prevent repeated blockage, a small tube called a **stent** may be inserted in the vessel to keep it open (Fig. 14-20). Modern stents are coated with drugs that prevent reocclusion.

Diseased valves may become so deformed and scarred from endocarditis that they are ineffective and often obstructive. In most cases, there is so much damage that **valve replacement** is the best treatment. Substitute valves made of a variety of natural and artificial materials have been used successfully.

The news media have given considerable attention to the **surgical transplantation** of human hearts and sometimes of lungs and hearts together. This surgery is done in specialized centers and is available to some patients with degenerative heart disease who are otherwise in good health. Tissues of the recently deceased donor and of the recipient must be as closely matched as possible to avoid rejection.

Efforts to replace a damaged heart with a completely artificial heart have not met with long-term success so far. There are devices available, however, to assist a damaged heart in pumping during recovery from heart attack or while a patient is awaiting a donor heart. The ventricular assist device (VAD) draws blood from a ventricle and pumps it into the aorta (on the left) or the pulmonary artery (on the right). Medical researchers are also testing a fully implantable artificial heart to use for the same purpose.

CHECKPOINT 14-15 ➤ What technique is used to open a restricted coronary artery with a balloon catheter?

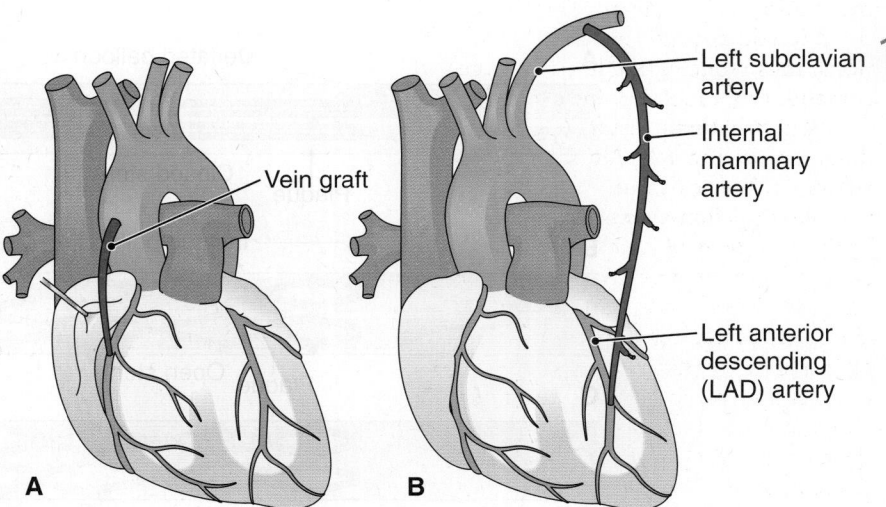

Figure 14-18 **Coronary artery bypass graft (CABG). (A)** This graft uses a segment of the saphenous vein to carry blood from the aorta to a part of the right coronary artery that is distal to the occlusion. **(B)** The mammary artery is grafted to bypass an obstruction in the left anterior descending (LAD) artery. (Reprinted with permission from Cohen BJ. *Medical Terminology*, 5th ed. Philadelphia: Lippincott Williams & Wilkins, 2008.)

Labels: Left subclavian artery; Internal mammary artery; Left anterior descending (LAD) artery; Vein graft

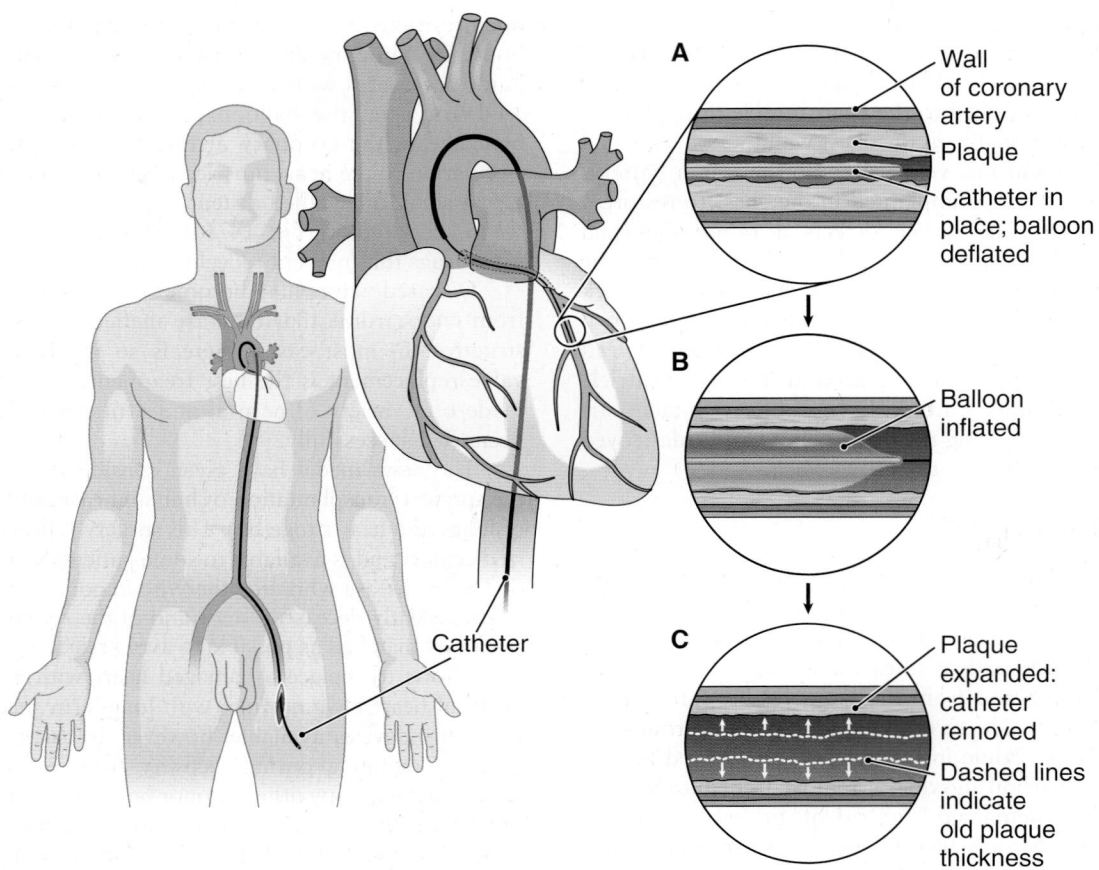

Figure 14-19 **Coronary angioplasty (PTCA).** **(A)** A guide catheter is threaded into the coronary artery. **(B)** A balloon catheter is inserted through the occlusion and inflated. **(C)** The balloon is inflated and deflated until plaque is flattened and the vessel is opened. (Reprinted with permission from Cohen BJ. *Medical Terminology*, 5th ed. Philadelphia: Lippincott Williams & Wilkins, 2008.)

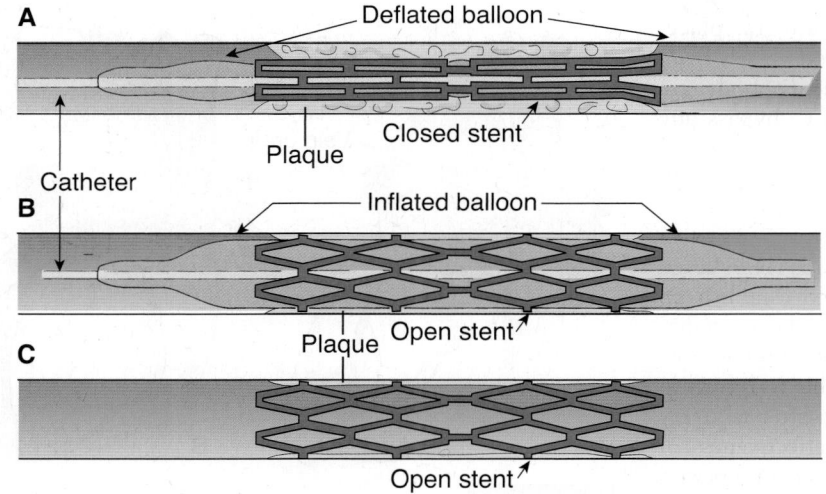

Figure 14-20 **Arterial Stent. (A)** Stent closed, before balloon inflation. **(B)** Stent open, balloon inflated. The stent will remain expanded after balloon is deflated and removed. **(C)** Stent open, balloon removed. (Reprinted with permission from Cohen BJ. *Medical Terminology*, 5th ed. Philadelphia: Lippincott Williams & Wilkins, 2008.)

Disease in Context revisited

▶ Jim's Heart Surgery

Several weeks after his heart attack, Jim was back in the hospital for his coronary bypass surgery. Even though his cardiologist had fully explained the procedure to him, Jim was still nervous—in a couple of hours a surgeon would literally have Jim's heart in his hands!

Jim was brought to the operating room and given general anesthesia. While the cardiac surgeon sawed through Jim's sternum, the saphenous vein was harvested from Jim's leg. Having split the sternum and retracted the ribs, the cardiac surgeon made an incision through the tough fibrous pericardium surrounding Jim's heart. Next, the surgeon inserted a cannula into Jim's right atrium and another one into his aorta. The doctor connected the cannulae to the heart-lung machine and stopped Jim's heart from beating. Now, venous blood from Jim's right atrium flowed through the heart-lung machine where it was oxygenated before being pumped into Jim's aorta. Then, the surgeon prepared the left coronary artery for bypass. He made a small incision through the arterial wall and carefully sutured the cut end of the harvested vein to the opening. Next, he sutured the other end of the vein to a small opening that he made in the aorta, bypassing the occluded portion of the coronary artery. He repeated this procedure two more times in different parts of Jim's obstructed coronary arteries—giving Jim a "triple bypass." The surgeon disconnected Jim from the heart-lung machine and restarted his heart. Blood flowed through the vein grafts to Jim's myocardium, bypassing the diseased parts of Jim's coronary arteries. Jim's surgery was a success!

Although this chapter concentrates on medical terms related to the heart, Jim's case also contains terminology about blood vessels. In Chapter 15, Blood Vessels and Blood Circulation, you will examine these terms in more detail.

Word Anatomy

Medical terms are built from standardized word parts (prefixes, roots, and suffixes). Learning the meanings of these parts can help you remember words and interpret unfamiliar terms.

WORD PART	MEANING	EXAMPLE
Structure of the Heart		
cardi/o	heart	The *myocardium* is the heart muscle.
pulmon/o	lung	The *pulmonary* circuit carries blood to the lungs.
Function of the Heart		
sin/o	sinus	The *sinoatrial* node is in a space (sinus) in the wall of the right atrium.
brady-	slow	*Bradycardia* is a slow heart rate.
tachy-	rapid	*Tachycardia* is a rapid heart rate.
Heart Disease		
cyan/o	blue	*Cyanosis* is a bluish discoloration of the skin due to lack of oxygen.
sten/o	narrowing, closure	*Stenosis* is a narrowing of a structure, such as a valve.
scler/o	hard	In *atherosclerosis*, vessels harden with fatty, gruel-like (ather/o) material that deposits on vessel walls.

14

WORD PART	MEANING	EXAMPLE
isch-	suppression	Narrowing of blood vessels leads to ischemia, a lack of blood (-emia) supply to tissues.

Heart Studies

| steth/o | chest | A *stethoscope* is used to listen to body sounds, such as those heard through the wall of the chest. |

Treatment of Heart Disease

| angi/o | vessel | *Angioplasty* is used to reshape vessels that are narrowed by disease. |
| -plasty | molding, surgical formation | See preceding example. |

Summary

I. **CIRCULATION AND THE HEART**
   A. Heart contractions drive blood through the blood vessels
   B. Location of the heart
      1. In mediastinum
      2. Slightly left of the midline; apex pointed toward left

II. **STRUCTURE OF THE HEART**
   A. Layers
      1. Endocardium—thin inner layer of epithelium
      2. Myocardium—thick muscle layer
      3. Epicardium—thin outer layer of serous membrane
         a. Also called visceral pericardium
   B. Pericardium
      1. Sac that encloses the heart
      2. Outer layer fibrous
      3. Inner layers—parietal and visceral serous membranes
   C. Special features of myocardium
      1. Lightly striated
      2. Intercalated disks
      3. Branching of fibers
   D. Divisions of the heart
      1. Two sides divided by septa
      2. Four chambers
         a. Atria—left and right receiving chambers
         b. Ventricles—left and right pumping chambers
      3. Four valves—prevent backflow of blood
         a. Right atrioventricular (AV) valve—tricuspid
         b. Left atrioventricular valve—mitral or bicuspid
         c. Pulmonary (semilunar) valve—at entrance to pulmonary artery

   d. Aortic (semilunar) valve—at entrance to aorta
   E. Blood supply to the myocardium
      1. Coronary arteries—first branches of aorta; fill when heart relaxes
      2. Coronary sinus—collects venous blood from heart and empties into right atrium

III. **FUNCTION OF THE HEART**
   A. Cardiac cycle
      1. Diastole—relaxation phase
      2. Systole—contraction phase
   B. Cardiac output
      1. Definition—volume pumped by each ventricle per minute
      2. Stroke volume—amount pumped with each beat
      3. Heart rate—number of beats per minute
   C. Heart's conduction system
      1. Sinoatrial node (pacemaker)—at top of right atrium
      2. Atrioventricular node—between atria and ventricles
      3. Atrioventricular bundle (bundle of His)—at top of interventricular septum
         a. Bundle branches—right and left, on either side of septum
         b. Purkinje fibers—branch through myocardium of ventricles
   D. Control of the heart rate
      1. Autonomic nervous system
         a. Sympathetic system—speeds heart rate
         b. Parasympathetic system—slows heart rate through vagus nerve
      2. Others—hormones, ions, drugs
      3. Variations in heart rates
         a. Bradycardia—slower rate than normal; less than 60 beats/minute

b. Tachycardia—faster rate than normal; more than 100 beats/minute

c. Sinus arrhythmia—related to breathing changes

d. Premature beat—extrasystole

E. Heart sounds

  1. Normal

    a. S$_1$ ("lub")—occurs at closing of atrioventricular valves

    b. S$_2$ ("dup")—occurs at closing of semilunar valves

  2. Abnormal—murmur

IV. **HEART DISEASE**

A. Classification of heart disease

  1. Anatomic classification—endocarditis, myocarditis, pericarditis

  2. Causal classification

B. Congenital heart diseases—present at birth

  1. Failure of fetal lung bypasses to close

    a. Atrial septal defect

    b. Patent ductus arteriosus

  2. Ventricular septal defect

  3. Narrowing of aorta or pulmonary artery

  4. Tetralogy of Fallot

C. Rheumatic heart disease—results from a type of streptococcal infection

  1. Mitral stenosis—valve cusps do not open

  2. Mitral regurgitation—valve cusps do not close

D. Coronary artery disease

  1. Characteristics

    a. Atherosclerosis—thickening and hardening of arteries with plaque

    b. Ischemia—lack of blood to area fed by blocked arteries

    c. Coronary occlusion—closure of coronary arteries, as by a thrombus (clot)

    d. Infarct—area of damaged tissue

    e. Angina pectoris—pain caused by lack of blood to heart muscle

    f. Abnormal rhythm—arrhythmia

      (1) Flutter—rapid, coordinated beats

      (2) Fibrillation—rapid, uncoordinated contractions of heart muscle

      (3) Heart block—interruption of electric conduction

  2. Diagnosis

    a. ECG

    b. Substances in blood—creatine kinase MB, troponin

3. Treatment of heart attacks—CPR, defibrillation, thrombolytic drugs, monitoring, good health habits

E. Heart failure—due to hypertension, disease, malnutrition, anemia, age

V. **THE HEART IN THE ELDERLY**

A. Individual variations in how heart ages

B. Common variations include:

  1. Decrease in heart size, strength of muscle contraction, flexibility of values, cardiac output

  2. Abnormal rhythms, temporary failure of conduction system

VI. **PREVENTION OF HEART DISEASE**

A. Risk factors

B. Preventive measures—physical examination, proper diet, quitting smoking, regular exercise, control of chronic illness

VII. **HEART STUDIES**

A. Stethoscope—used to listen to heart sounds

B. Electrocardiograph (ECG, EKG)—records electrical activity as waves

C. Catheterization—thin tube inserted into heart for blood samples, pressure readings, and other tests

D. Fluoroscope—examines deep tissue with x-rays; used to guide catheter

E. Echocardiography—uses ultrasound to record pictures of heart in action

VIII. **TREATMENT OF HEART DISEASE**

A. Medications—examples are digitalis, nitroglycerin, beta-adrenergic blocking agents, antiarrhythmic agents, slow channel calcium-channel blockers, anticoagulants

B. Correction of arrhythmia

  1. Artificial pacemakers—electronic devices implanted under skin to regulate heartbeat

  2. Implantable cardioverter-defibrillator (ICD)

  3. Destruction of abnormal tissue

C. Heart surgery

  1. Bypass—vessels grafted to detour blood around blockage

  2. Angioplasty—balloon catheter used to open blocked arteries

    a. Stents used to keep vessels open

  3. Valve replacement

  4. Heart transplantation

  5. Ventricular assist devices

  6. Artificial hearts

14

Questions for Study and Review

BUILDING UNDERSTANDING

Fill in the blanks

1. The central thoracic region that contains the heart is the _____.

2. The layer of the heart responsible for pumping blood is called the_____.

3. The heart beat is initiated by electrical impulses from the_____.

4. Lack of blood to a tissue fed by blocked arteries is called _____.

5. Pain caused by lack of blood to heart muscle is called _____.

Matching > Match each numbered item with the most closely related lettered item.

___ 6. receives deoxygenated blood from the body

___ 7. receives oxygenated blood from the lungs

___ 8. sends deoxygenated blood to the lungs

___ 9. sends oxygenated blood to the body

a. right atrium

b. left atrium

c. right ventricle

d. left ventricle

Multiple choice

___ 10. Rapid transfer of electrical signals between cardiac muscle cells is promoted by

  a. the striated nature of the cells
  b. branching of the cells
  c. the abundance of mitochondria within the cells
  d. intercalated disks between the cells

___ 11. The upper chambers of the heart are separated by the

  a. intercalated disk
  b. interatrial septum
  c. interventricular septum
  d. ductus arteriosus

___ 12. One complete sequence of heart contraction and relaxation is called the

  a. systole
  b. diastole
  c. cardiac cycle
  d. cardiac output

___ 13. A medication that reduces the rate and strength of heart contractions by lowering sympathetic tone is called a(n)

  a. anticoagulant
  b. antiarrhythmic agent
  c. slow calcium-channel blocker
  d. beta-adrenergic blocking agent

___ 14. The ductus arteriosus shunts blood away from the

  a. lungs and towards the aorta
  b. lungs and towards the superior vena cava
  c. aorta and towards the lungs
  d. away from the superior vena cava and towards the lungs

___ 15. A regular variation in heart rate due to changes in the rate and depth of breathing is called a

  a. murmur
  b. cyanosis
  c. sinus arrhythmia
  d. stent

UNDERSTANDING CONCEPTS

16. Differentiate between the terms in each of the following pairs:

   a. pulmonary and systemic circuit
   b. coronary artery and coronary sinus
   c. serous pericardium and fibrous pericardium
   d. systole and diastole

17. Explain the purpose of the four heart valves and describe their structure and location. What prevents the valves from opening backwards?

18. Trace a drop of blood from the superior vena cava to the lungs and then from the lungs to the aorta.

19. Describe the order in which electrical impulses travel through the heart. What is an interruption of these impulses in the heart's conduction system called?

20. Compare the effects of the sympathetic and parasympathetic nervous systems on heart function.

21. Compare and contrast the following disease conditions:

   a. endocarditis and pericarditis
   b. tachycardia and bradycardia
   c. functional murmur and organic murmur
   d. flutter and fibrillation
   e. atrial and ventricular septal defect

22. What part does infection play in rheumatic heart disease?

23. List some age-related changes to the heart.

CONCEPTUAL THINKING

24. In the case story, Jim suffered a massive myocardial infarction. What can Jim do to lower his risk of having it happen again? What risk factors can he not change? Apply your knowledge of these factors to your own life or the life of someone you know.

25. Three-month-old Hannah R. is brought to the doctor by her parents. They have noticed that when she cries she becomes breathless and turns blue. The doctor examines Hannah and notices that she is lethargic, small for her age, and has a loud mitral valve murmur. With this information, explain the cause of Hannah's symptoms.

14

CHAPTER 15

Blood Vessels and Blood Circulation

Learning Outcomes

After careful study of this chapter, you should be able to:

1. Differentiate among the five types of blood vessels with regard to structure and function
2. Compare the pulmonary and systemic circuits relative to location and function
3. Name the four sections of the aorta and list the main branches of each section
4. Define *anastomosis*, cite its function, and give several examples
5. Compare superficial and deep veins and give examples of each type
6. Name the main vessels that drain into the superior and inferior venae cavae
7. Define *venous sinus* and give several examples of venous sinuses
8. Describe the structure and function of the hepatic portal system
9. Explain the forces that affect exchange across the capillary wall
10. Describe the factors that regulate blood flow
11. Define *pulse* and list factors that affect pulse rate
12. List the factors that affect blood pressure
13. Explain how blood pressure is commonly measured
14. List reasons why hypertension should be controlled
15. List some disorders that involve the blood vessels
16. List steps in first aid for hemorrhage
17. List four types of shock
18. Show how word parts are used to build words related to the blood vessels and circulation (see Word Anatomy at the end of the chapter)

Selected Key Terms

The following terms and other boldface terms in the chapter are defined in the Glossary

anastomosis
aneurysm
aorta
arteriole
artery
atherosclerosis
baroreceptor
capillary
embolus
endarterectomy
endothelium
hemorrhage
hypertension
hypotension
ischemia
phlebitis
pulse
shock
sinusoid
sphygmomanometer
thrombus
varicose vein
vasoconstriction
vasodilation
vein
vena cava
venous sinus
venule

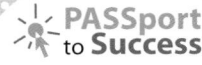

PASSport to Success

Visit *thePoint* or see the Student Resource CD in the back of this book for definitions and pronunciations of key terms as well as a pretest for this chapter.

Disease in Context

> ## Reggie's Second Case: Embolytic Emergency

"And now, news from the Sports Desk. Yesterday, wide receiver Reggie Wilson was side-lined with a femoral fracture. Team doctors don't expect him to return until later in the season." Reggie pressed the off button on the hospital's television remote and closed his eyes for a moment. The last 24 hours had been a whirlwind—first the injury, then the surgery, and now the prospect of a long road to recovery. *Well, I've made it through tough situations before,* Reggie thought as he fell asleep.

Inside Reggie's thigh, his femur was beginning to repair itself, but a more dangerous situation lurked in the femoral vein that lay beside the fractured bone. During the accident, the vein's thin inner wall had been injured. Even though Reggie had received heparin (an anticoagulant) after his surgery, blood platelets had adhered to the damaged vein and formed a tiny clot on the inner lining of the vessel. Now that Reggie's thigh was immobile, blood flowed much more slowly through the femoral vein. This venous stasis allowed more and more platelets to stick together at the site of the clot until finally his vein was completely obstructed. Reggie had developed deep vein thrombosis. Blood continued to flow into Reggie's thigh through his femoral artery, but now, it could not flow out through the vein. Reggie's thigh began to swell and turn red because of the build up of blood within it. Although still asleep, Reggie felt some discomfort from the swelling in his leg and shifted his weight to relieve it. That slight movement caused a small piece of the clot to break away from the thrombus and be carried away toward his heart. Now, Reggie had developed an embolism!

A blood clot is traveling through Reggie's systemic veins toward his heart and lungs. In this chapter, we'll examine the important role the vascular system plays in carrying blood to and from the tissues. Later in the chapter, we'll see how Reggie's medical team manages his new emergency.

The blood vessels, together with the four chambers of the heart, form a closed system in which blood is carried to and from the tissues. Although whole blood does not leave the vessels, components of the plasma and tissue fluids can be exchanged through the walls of the tiniest vessels, the capillaries.

The vascular system is easier to understand if you refer to the appropriate illustrations in this chapter as the vessels are described. When this information is added to what you already know about the blood and the heart, a picture of the cardiovascular system as a whole will emerge.

Blood Vessels

Blood vessels may be divided into five groups, named below according to the sequence of blood flow from the heart:

1. Arteries carry blood away from the heart and toward the tissues. The heart's ventricles pump blood into the arteries.

2. **Arterioles** (ar-TE-re-olz) are small subdivisions of the arteries. They carry blood into the capillaries.

3. **Capillaries** are tiny, thin-walled vessels that allow for exchanges between systems. These exchanges occur between the blood and the body cells and between the blood and the air in the lung tissues. The capillaries connect the arterioles and venules.

4. **Venules** (VEN-ulz) are small vessels that receive blood from the capillaries and begin its transport back toward the heart.

5. **Veins** are vessels formed by the merger of venules. They continue the transport of blood until it is returned to the heart

CHECKPOINT **15-1** ➤ What are the five types of blood vessels?

Blood Circuits

The vessels together may be subdivided into two groups, or circuits: pulmonary and systemic. Figure 15-1 diagrams blood flow in a closed system and the vessels in these two circuits. The true anatomic relation of these circuits to the heart is shown in Chapter 14, Figure 14-4.

THE PULMONARY CIRCUIT The **pulmonary circuit** delivers blood to the lungs, where carbon dioxide is eliminated and oxygen is replenished. The pulmonary vessels that carry blood to and from the lungs include the following:

1. The pulmonary trunk and its arterial branches, which carry blood from the right ventricle to the lungs

2. The capillaries in the lungs, through which gases are exchanged

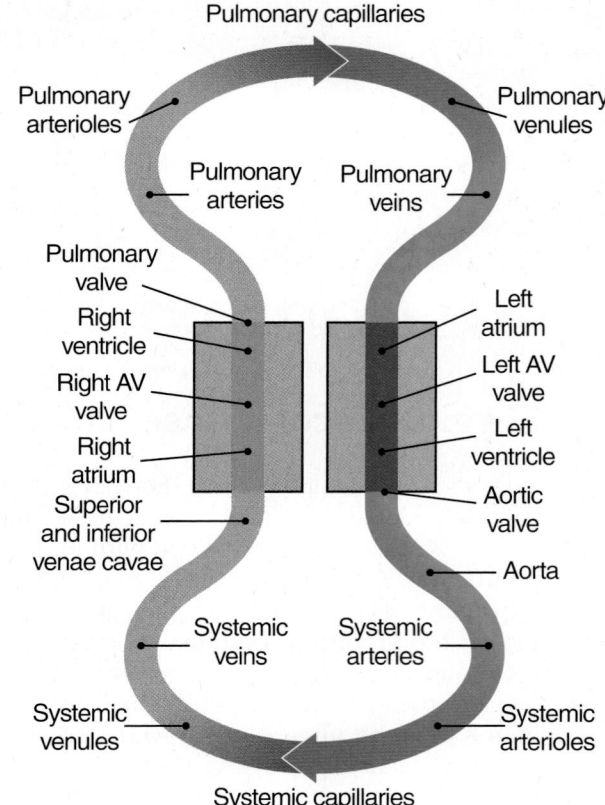

Figure 15-1 **Blood flow in a closed system of vessels.** Oxygen content changes as blood flows through the capillaries. [ZOOMING IN ➤ Judging from color coding, which vessels pick up oxygen? Which vessels release oxygen?]

3. The pulmonary veins, which carry blood back to the left atrium

The pulmonary vessels differ from those in the systemic circuit in that the pulmonary arteries carry blood that is *low* in oxygen, and the pulmonary veins carry blood that is *high* in oxygen. All the remaining arteries carry highly oxygenated blood, and all remaining veins carry blood that is low in oxygen.

THE SYSTEMIC CIRCUIT The **systemic** (sis-TEM-ik) **circuit** serves the rest of the body. These vessels supply nutrients and oxygen to all the tissues and carry waste materials away from the tissues for disposal. The systemic vessels include the following:

1. The **aorta** (a-OR-tah), which receives blood from the left ventricle and then branches into the systemic arteries carrying blood to the tissues

2. The systemic capillaries, through which materials are exchanged

3. The systemic veins, which carry blood back toward the heart. The venous blood flows into the right atrium of the heart through the superior vena cava and inferior vena cava.

CHECKPOINT 15-2 ➤ What are the two blood circuits and what areas does each serve?

Vessel Structure

The arteries have thick walls because they must be strong enough to receive blood pumped under pressure from the heart's ventricles (Fig. 15-2). The three tunics (coats) of the arteries resemble the three tissue layers of the heart. Named from internal to external, they are:

1. The innermost membrane of simple, flat epithelial cells makes up the **endothelium** (en-do-THE-le-um), forming a smooth surface over which the blood flows easily.
2. The middle and thickest layer is made of smooth (involuntary) muscle, which is under the control of the autonomic nervous system.
3. An outer tunic is made of a supporting connective tissue.

Elastic tissue between the layers of the arterial wall allows these vessels to stretch when receiving blood and then return to their original size. The amount of elastic tissue diminishes as the arteries branch and become smaller.

The small subdivisions of the arteries, the arterioles, have thinner walls in which there is little elastic connective tissue but relatively more smooth muscle. The autonomic nervous system controls this involuntary muscle. The vessels become narrower (constrict) when the muscle contracts and widen (dilate) when the muscle relaxes. In this manner, the arterioles regulate the amount of blood that enters the various tissues at a given time. Change in the diameter of the arterioles is also a major factor in blood pressure control.

The microscopic capillaries that connect arterioles and venules have the thinnest walls of any vessels: one cell layer. The capillary walls are transparent and are made of smooth, squamous epithelial cells that are a continuation of the arterial lining. The thinness of these walls allows for exchanges between the blood and the body cells and between the lung tissue and the outside air. The capillary boundaries are the most important center of activity for the entire circulatory system. Their function is explained later in this chapter (see also Box 15-1, Capillaries).

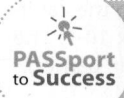

PASSport to Success

Visit **thePoint** or see the Student Resource CD in the back of this book for micrographs of capillaries in longitudinal and cross sections.

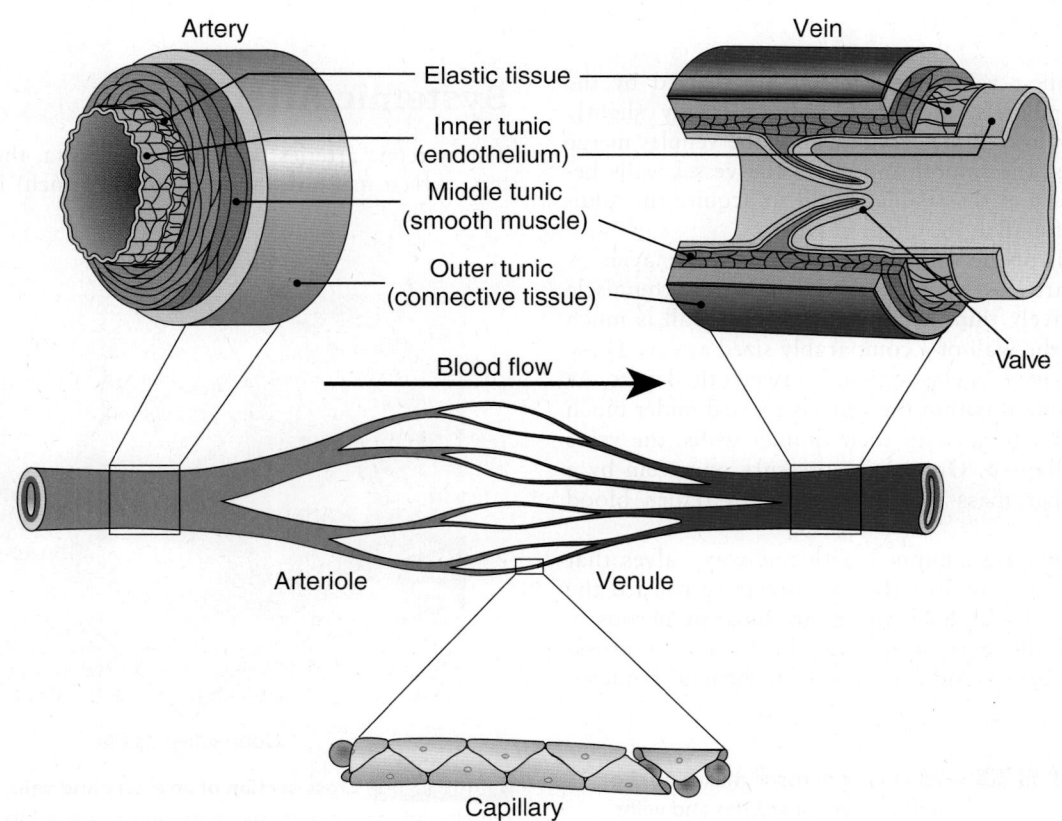

Figure 15-2 **Sections of small blood vessels.** Drawings show the thick wall of an artery, the thin wall of a vein, and the single-layered wall of a capillary. A venous valve also is shown. The arrow indicates the direction of blood flow. [**ZOOMING IN** ➤ Which vessels have valves that control blood flow?]

Box 15-1 | **A Closer Look**

Capillaries: The Body's Free Trade Zones

The exchange of substances between body cells and the blood occurs along about 50,000 miles (80,000 kilometers) of capillaries. Exchange rates vary because, based on their structure, different types of capillaries vary in permeability.

Continuous capillaries are the most common type and are found in muscle, connective tissue, the lungs, and the central nervous system (CNS). These capillaries are composed of a continuous layer of endothelial cells. Adjacent cells are loosely attached to each other, with small openings called intercellular clefts between them. Although continuous capillaries are the least permeable, water and small molecules can diffuse easily through their walls. Large molecules, such as plasma proteins and blood cells, cannot. In certain body regions, like the CNS, adjacent endothelial cells are joined tightly together, making the capillaries impermeable to many substances (see Box 10-1, The Blood-Brain Barrier, in Chapter 10 on the blood-brain barrier).

Fenestrated (FEN-es-tra-ted) capillaries are much more permeable than continuous capillaries, because they have many holes, or fenestrations, in the endothelium. These sieve-like capillaries are permeable to water and solutes as large as peptides. In the digestive tract, fenestrated capillaries permit rapid absorption of water and nutrients into the bloodstream. In the kidneys, they permit rapid filtration of blood plasma, the first step in urine formation.

Discontinuous capillaries, or sinusoids, are the most permeable. In addition to fenestrations, they have large spaces between endothelial cells that allow the exchange of water, large solutes, such as plasma proteins, and even blood cells. Sinusoids are found in the liver and red bone marrow, for example. Albumin, clotting factors, and other proteins formed in the liver enter the bloodstream through sinusoids. In red bone marrow, newly formed blood cells travel through sinusoids to join the bloodstream.

The smallest veins, the venules, are formed by the union of capillaries, and their walls are only slightly thicker than those of the capillaries. As the venules merge to form veins, the smooth muscle in the vessel walls becomes thicker and the venules begin to acquire the additional layers found in the larger vessels.

The walls of the veins have the same three layers as those of the arteries. However, the middle smooth muscle tunic is relatively thin in the veins. A vein wall is much thinner than the wall of a comparably sized artery. These vessels also have less elastic tissue between the layers. As a result, the blood within the veins is carried under much lower pressure. Because of their thinner walls, the veins are easily collapsed. Only slight pressure on a vein by a tumor or other mass may interfere with return blood flow.

Most veins are equipped with one-way valves that permit blood to flow in only one direction: toward the heart (see Fig. 15-2). Such valves are most numerous in the veins of the extremities. Figure 15-3 is a cross-section of an artery and a vein as seen through a microscope.

CHECKPOINT **15-3** ➤ What type of tissue makes up the middle layer of arteries and veins, and how is this tissue controlled?

CHECKPOINT **15-4** ➤ How many cell layers make up the wall of a capillary?

Systemic Arteries

The systemic arteries begin with the aorta, the largest artery, which measures about 2.5 cm (1 inch) in diameter.

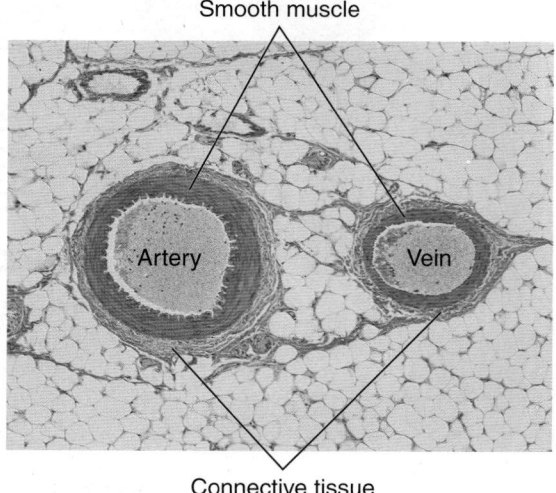

Figure 15-3 **Cross-section of an artery and vein.** The smooth muscle and connective tissue of the vessels are visible in this photomicrograph. (Reprinted with permission from Cormack DH. *Essential Histology*, 2nd ed. Philadelphia: Lippincott Williams & Wilkins, 2001.) [**ZOOMING IN** ➤ Which type of vessel shown has a thicker wall?]

This vessel receives blood from the left ventricle, then travels downward through the body, branching to all organs. (See Appendix 7 for a dissection photograph showing the major arteries of the trunk.)

The Aorta and Its Parts

The aorta ascends toward the right from the left ventricle. Then it curves posteriorly and to the left. It continues downward posterior to the heart and just anterior to the vertebral column, through the diaphragm, and into the abdomen (Figs. 15-4 and 15-5). The aorta is one continuous artery, but it may be divided into sections:

1. The **ascending aorta** is near the heart and inside the pericardial sac.

2. The **aortic arch** curves from the right to the left and also extends posteriorly.

3. The **thoracic aorta** lies just anterior to the vertebral column posterior to the heart and in the space behind the pleura.

4. The **abdominal aorta** is the longest section of the aorta, spanning the abdominal cavity.

The thoracic and abdominal aorta together make up the descending aorta.

BRANCHES OF THE ASCENDING AORTA AND AORTIC ARCH The aorta's first, or ascending, part has two branches near the heart, called the **left** and **right coronary arteries**, which supply the heart muscle. These form a crown around the heart's base and give off branches to all parts of the myocardium.

The aortic arch, located immediately beyond the ascending aorta, divides into three large branches.

1. The **brachiocephalic** (brak-e-o-seh-FAL-ik) **artery** is a short vessel that supplies the arm and the head on the right side. After extending upward somewhat less than 5 cm (2 inches), it divides into the **right subclavian** (sub-KLA-ve-an) **artery**, which extends under the right clavicle (collar bone) and supplies the right upper extremity (arm), and the **right common carotid** (kah-ROT-id) **artery**, which supplies the right side of the neck, head, and brain. Note that the brachiocephalic artery is unpaired.

2. The **left common carotid artery** extends upward from the highest part of the aortic arch. It supplies the left side of the neck and the head.

3. The **left subclavian artery** extends under the left clavicle and supplies the left upper extremity. This is the aortic arch's last branch.

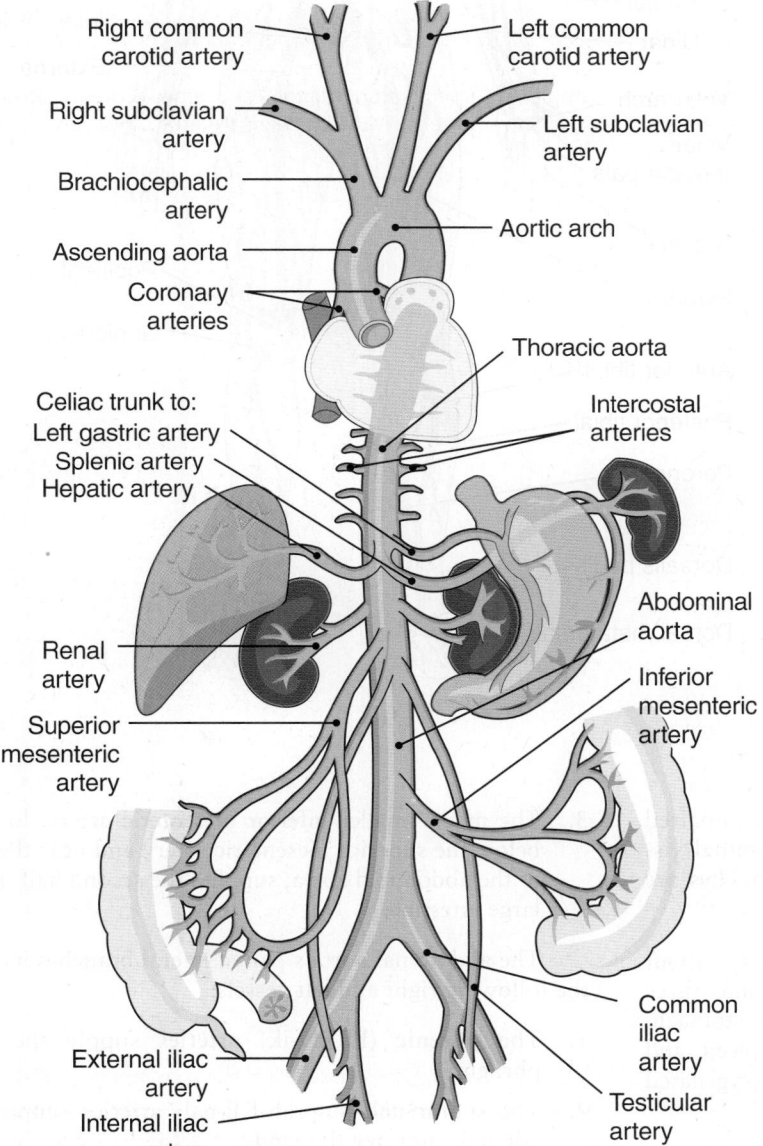

Right common carotid artery
Right subclavian artery
Brachiocephalic artery
Ascending aorta
Coronary arteries
Left common carotid artery
Left subclavian artery
Aortic arch
Thoracic aorta
Celiac trunk to:
Left gastric artery
Splenic artery
Hepatic artery
Intercostal arteries
Renal artery
Superior mesenteric artery
Abdominal aorta
Inferior mesenteric artery
External iliac artery
Internal iliac artery
Common iliac artery
Testicular artery

Figure 15-4 **The aorta and its branches.** [ZOOMING IN ➤ How many brachiocephalic arteries are there?]

BRANCHES OF THE DESCENDING AORTA The thoracic aorta supplies branches to the chest wall and **esophagus** (e-SOF-ah-gus), the bronchi (subdivisions of the trachea), and their treelike subdivisions in the lungs. There are usually 9 to 10 pairs of **intercostal** (in-ter-KOS-tal) **arteries** that extend between the ribs, sending branches to the muscles and other structures of the chest wall.

The abdominal aorta has unpaired branches extending anteriorly

15

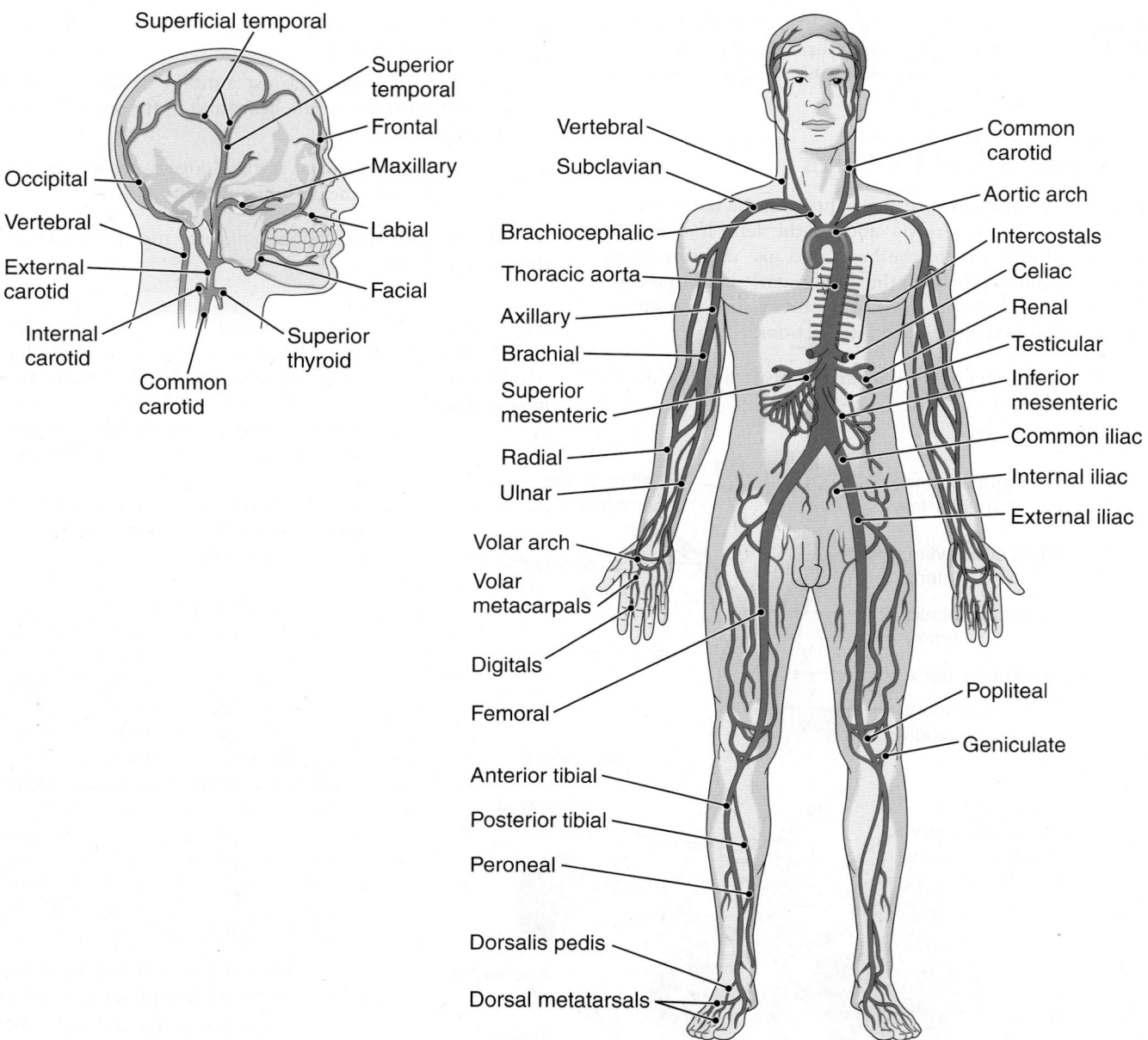

Figure 15-5 **Principal systemic arteries.**

and paired branches extending laterally. The unpaired vessels are large arteries that supply the abdominal viscera. The most important of these visceral branches are as follows:

1. The **celiac** (SE-le-ak) **trunk** is a short artery, about 1.25 cm (1/2 inch) long, that subdivides into three branches: the **left gastric artery** goes to the stomach, the **splenic** (SPLEN-ik) **artery** goes to the spleen, and the **hepatic** (heh-PAT-ik) **artery** carries oxygenated blood to the liver.

2. The **superior mesenteric** (mes-en-TER-ik) **artery**, the largest of these branches, carries blood to most of the small intestine and to the first half of the large intestine.

3. The much smaller **inferior mesenteric artery**, located below the superior mesenteric artery and near the end of the abdominal aorta, supplies the second half of the large intestine.

The abdominal aorta's paired lateral branches include the following right and left vessels:

1. The **phrenic** (FREN-ik) **arteries** supply the diaphragm.

2. The **suprarenal** (su-prah-RE-nal) **arteries** supply the adrenal (suprarenal) glands.

3. The **renal** (RE-nal) **arteries,** the largest in this group, carry blood to the kidneys.

4. The **ovarian arteries** in females and **testicular** (tes-TIK-u-lar) **arteries** in males (formerly called the spermatic arteries) supply the sex glands.

5. Four pairs of **lumbar** (LUM-bar) **arteries** extend into the musculature of the abdominal wall.

CHECKPOINT **15-5** ➤ What are the subdivisions of the aorta, the largest artery?

The Iliac Arteries and Their Subdivisions

The abdominal aorta finally divides into two **common iliac** (IL-e-ak) **arteries**. These vessels, which are about 5 cm (2 inches) long, extend into the pelvis, where each subdivides into an **internal** and an **external iliac artery** (see Fig. 15-5). The internal iliac vessels then send branches to the pelvic organs, including the urinary bladder, the rectum, and some reproductive organs.

Each external iliac artery continues into the thigh as the **femoral** (FEM-or-al) **artery**. This vessel gives rise to branches in the thigh and then becomes the **popliteal** (pop-LIT-e-al) **artery**, which subdivides below the knee. The subdivisions include the posterior and anterior **tibial arteries** and the **dorsalis pedis** (dor-SA-lis PE-dis), which supply the leg and the foot.

Arteries That Branch to the Arm and Head

Each common carotid artery travels along the trachea enclosed in a sheath with the internal jugular vein and the vagus nerve. Just anterior to the angle of the mandible (lower jaw) it branches into the **external** and **internal carotid arteries** (see Fig. 15-5). You can feel the pulse of the carotid artery just anterior to the large sternocleidomastoid muscle in the neck and below the jaw. The internal carotid artery travels into the head and branches to supply the eye, the anterior portion of the brain, and other structures in the cranium. The external carotid artery branches to the thyroid gland and to other structures in the head and upper part of the neck.

The **subclavian** (sub-KLA-ve-an) **artery** supplies blood to the arm and hand. Its first branch, however, is the **vertebral** (VER-the-bral) **artery**, which passes though the transverse processes of the first six cervical vertebrae and supplies blood to the posterior brain. The subclavian artery changes names as it travels through the arm and branches to the arm and hand. It first becomes the **axillary** (AK-sil-ar-e) **artery** in the axilla (armpit). The longest part of this vessel, the **brachial** (BRA-ke-al) **artery**, is in the arm proper. The brachial artery subdivides into two branches near the elbow: the **radial artery**, which continues down the thumb side of the forearm and wrist, and the **ulnar artery**, which extends along the medial or little finger side into the hand.

Just as the larger branches of a tree divide into limbs of varying sizes, so the arterial tree has a multitude of sub-divisions. Hundreds of names might be included. We have mentioned only some of them.

CHECKPOINT **15-6** ➤ What arteries are formed by the final division of the abdominal aorta?

CHECKPOINT **15-7** ➤ What areas are supplied by the brachiocephalic artery?

Anastomoses

A communication between two vessels is called an **anastomosis** (ah-nas-to-MO-sis). By means of arterial anastomoses, blood reaches vital organs by more than one route. Some examples of such end-artery unions are as follows:

- The **circle of Willis** (Fig. 15-6) receives blood from the two internal carotid arteries and from the **basilar** (BAS-il-ar) **artery**, which is formed by the union of the two vertebral arteries. This arterial circle lies just under the brain's center and sends branches to the cerebrum and other parts of the brain.

- The **superficial palmar arch** is formed by the union of the radial and ulnar arteries in the hand. It sends branches to the hand and the fingers.

- The **mesenteric** arches are made of communications between branches of the vessels that supply blood to the intestinal tract.

- **Arterial arches** are formed by the union of tibial artery branches in the foot. There are similar anastomoses in other parts of the body.

Arteriovenous anastomoses are blood shunts found in a few areas, including the external ears, the hands, and the feet. In this type of shunt, a small vessel known as a **metarteriole** (met-ar-TE-re-ole) or *thoroughfare channel*, connects the arterial system directly with the venous system, bypassing the capillaries (Fig. 15-7). This pathway provides a more rapid flow and a greater blood volume to these areas, thus protecting these exposed parts from freezing in cold weather.

CHECKPOINT **15-8** ➤ What is an anastomosis?

Systemic Veins

Whereas most arteries are located in protected and rather deep areas of the body, many of the principal systemic veins are found near the surface (Fig. 15-8). The most important of the **superficial veins** are in the extremities, and include the following:

- The veins on the back of the hand and at the front of the elbow. Those at the elbow are often used for drawing blood for test purposes, as well as for intravenous injections. The largest of this venous group are the **cephalic** (seh-FAL-ik), the **basilic** (bah-SIL-ik), and the **median cubital** (KU-bih-tal) **veins**.

15

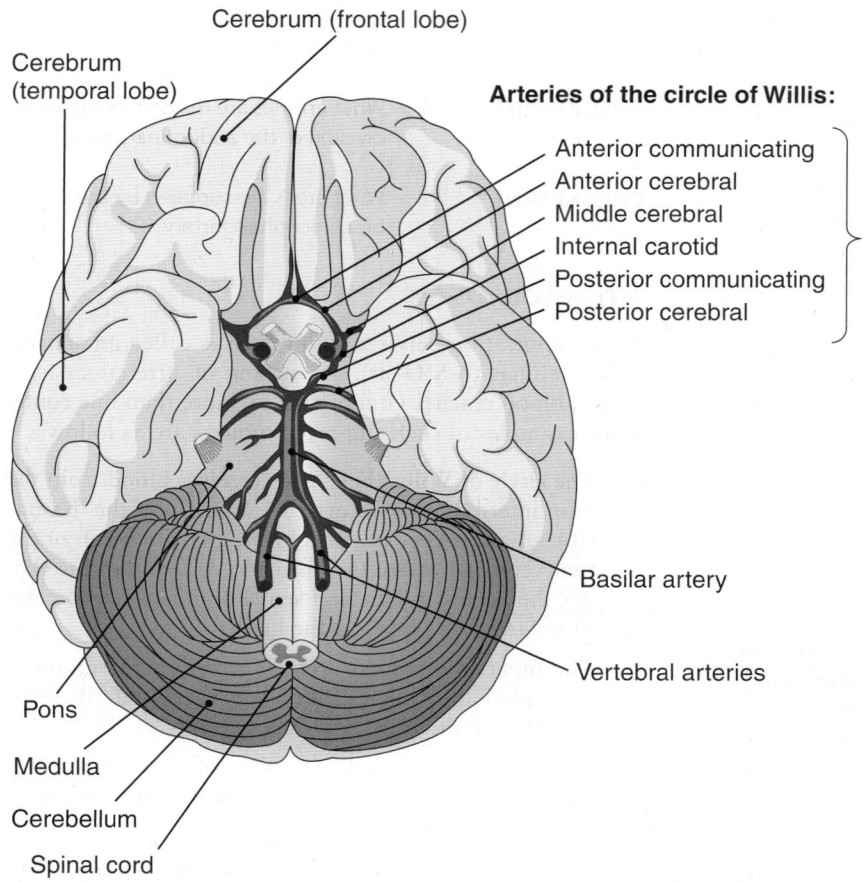

Cerebrum (frontal lobe)

Cerebrum (temporal lobe)

Arteries of the circle of Willis:
Anterior communicating
Anterior cerebral
Middle cerebral
Internal carotid
Posterior communicating
Posterior cerebral

Basilar artery

Vertebral arteries

Pons

Medulla

Cerebellum

Spinal cord

Figure 15-6 **Arteries that supply the brain.** The bracket at right groups the arteries that make up the circle of Willis.

- The **saphenous** (sah-FE-nus) **veins** of the lower extremities, which are the body's longest veins. The great saphenous vein begins in the foot and extends up the medial side of the leg, the knee, and the thigh. It finally empties into the femoral vein near the groin.

The **deep veins** tend to parallel arteries and usually have the same names as the corresponding arteries. Examples of these include the **femoral** and the external and internal **iliac** vessels of the lower body, and the **brachial, axillary,** and **subclavian** vessels of the upper extremities. Exceptions are found in the veins of the head and the neck. The two **jugular** (JUG-u-lar) **veins** on each side of the neck drain the areas supplied by the carotid arteries (*jugular* is from a Latin word meaning "neck"). The larger of the two veins, the internal jugular, receives blood from the large veins (cranial venous sinuses) that drain the head and also from regions of the face and neck. The smaller external jugular drains the areas supplied by the external carotid artery. Both veins empty directly into a subclavian vein. A **brachiocephalic vein** is formed on each side by the union of the subclavian and the jugular veins (see Fig. 15-8). (Remember, there is only *one* brachiocephalic artery.)

The Venae Cavae and Their Tributaries

Two large veins receive blood from the systemic vessels and empty directly into the heart's right atrium. The veins of the head, neck, upper extremities, and chest all drain into the **superior vena cava** (VE-nah KA-vah). This vessel is formed by the union of the right and left brachiocephalic veins, which drain the head, neck, and upper extremities. The unpaired **azygos** (AZ-ih-gos) **vein** drains the veins of the chest wall and empties into the superior vena cava just before the latter empties into the heart (see Fig. 15-8) (*azygous* is from a Greek word meaning "unpaired").

The **inferior vena cava,** which is much longer than the superior vena cava, returns blood from areas below the diaphragm. It begins in the lower abdomen with the union of the two common iliac veins. It then ascends along the abdomen's posterior wall, through a groove in the posterior part of the liver, through the diaphragm, and finally through the lower thorax to empty into the heart's right atrium.

Drainage into the inferior vena cava is more complicated than drainage into the superior vena cava. The large veins below the diaphragm may be divided into two groups:

- The right and left veins that drain paired parts and organs. They include the **iliac** veins from near the groin; four pairs of **lumbar veins** from the dorsal trunk and from the spinal cord; the **testicular veins** from the male testes and the **ovarian veins** from the female ovaries; the **renal** and **suprarenal veins** from the kidneys and adrenal glands near the kidneys; and finally the large **hepatic veins** from the liver. For the most part, these vessels empty directly into the inferior vena cava. The left testicular in the male and the left ovarian in the female empty into the left renal vein, which then takes this blood to the inferior vena cava; these veins thus constitute exceptions to the rule that the paired veins empty directly into the vena cava.

- Unpaired veins that drain the spleen and parts of the digestive tract (stomach and intestine) empty into a vein called the **hepatic portal vein.** Unlike other lower veins, which empty into the inferior vena cava, the hepatic portal vein is part of a special system that enables blood to circulate through the liver before returning to the heart. This system, the hepatic portal system, will be described in more detail later.

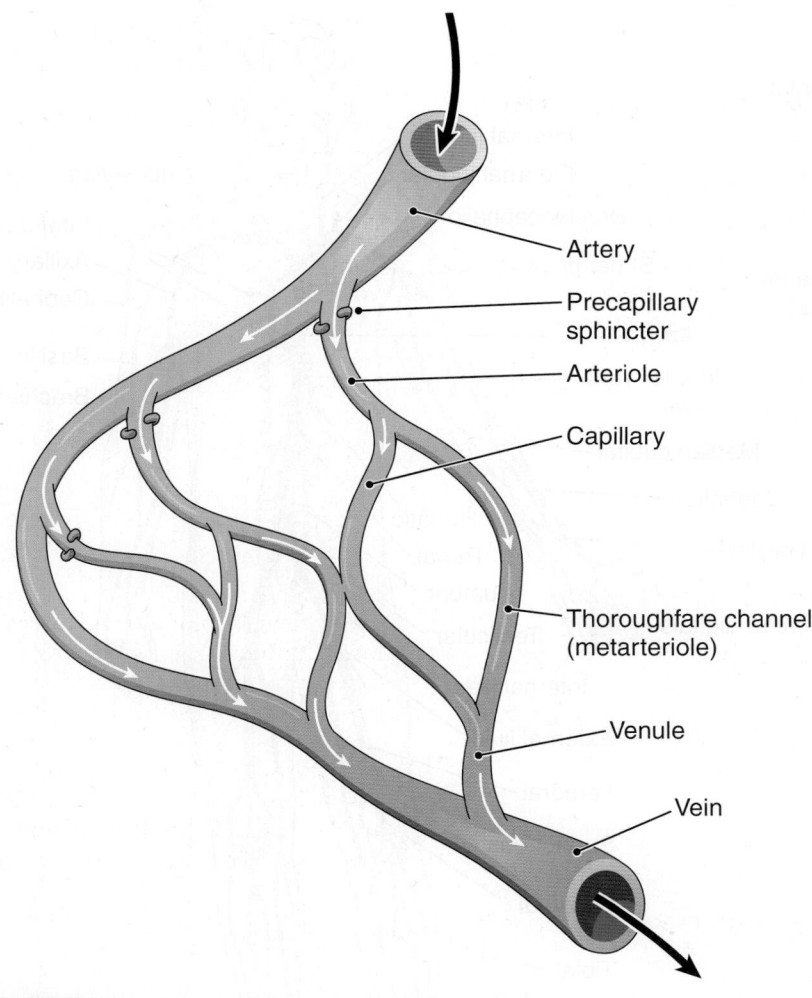

Artery

Precapillary sphincter

Arteriole

Capillary

Thoroughfare channel (metarteriole)

Venule

Vein

Figure 15-7 **Capillary network showing an arteriovenous shunt (anastomosis).** A connecting vessel, known as a thoroughfare channel or metarteriole, carries blood directly from an arteriole to a venule, bypassing the capillaries.

Other important venous sinuses are the **cranial venous sinuses**, which are located inside the skull and drain the veins from all over the brain (Fig. 15-9). The largest of the cranial venous sinuses are the following:

- The two **cavernous sinuses**, situated behind the eyeballs, drain the eyes' **ophthalmic** (of-THAL-mik) **veins**. They give rise to the **petrosal** (peh-TRO-sal) **sinuses**, which drain into the jugular veins.

- The **superior sagittal** (SAJ-ih-tal) **sinus** is a single long space located in the midline above the brain and in the fissure between the two cerebral hemispheres. It ends in an enlargement called the **confluence** (KON-flu-ens) **of sinuses**.

- The two **transverse sinuses**, also called the **lateral sinuses**, are large spaces between the layers of the dura mater (the outermost membrane around the brain). They begin posteriorly from the confluence of sinuses and then extend laterally. As each sinus extends around the skull's interior, it receives additional blood, including blood draining through the inferior sagittal sinus and straight sinus. Nearly all of the blood leaving the brain eventually empties into one of the transverse sinuses. Each sinus extends anteriorly to empty into an internal jugular vein, which then passes through a channel in the skull to continue downward in the neck.

CHECKPOINT 15-9 ➤ Veins are described as superficial or deep. What does superficial mean?

CHECKPOINT 15-10 ➤ What two large veins drain the systemic blood vessels and empty into the right atrium?

Venous Sinuses

The word *sinus* means "space" or "hollow." A **venous sinus** is a large channel that drains deoxygenated blood, but does not have the usual tubular structure of the veins. One example of a venous sinus is the **coronary sinus**, which receives most of the blood from the heart wall (see Fig. 14-8 in Chapter 14). It lies between the left atrium and left ventricle on the heart's posterior surface, and empties directly into the right atrium, along with the two venae cavae.

CHECKPOINT 15-11 ➤ What is a venous sinus?

The Hepatic Portal System

Almost always, when blood leaves a capillary bed, it flows directly back to the heart. In a portal system, however, blood circulates through a second capillary bed, usually in a second organ, before it returns to the heart. A portal system is a kind of detour in the pathway of venous return that transports materials directly from one organ to another. Chapter 12 described the small local portal system that carries secretions from the hypothalamus to the pituitary gland. A much larger portal system is the **hepatic portal system**, which carries blood from the abdominal organs to the liver (Fig. 15-10).

The hepatic portal system includes the veins that drain blood from capillaries in the spleen, stomach, pancreas, and intestine. Instead of emptying their blood di-

15

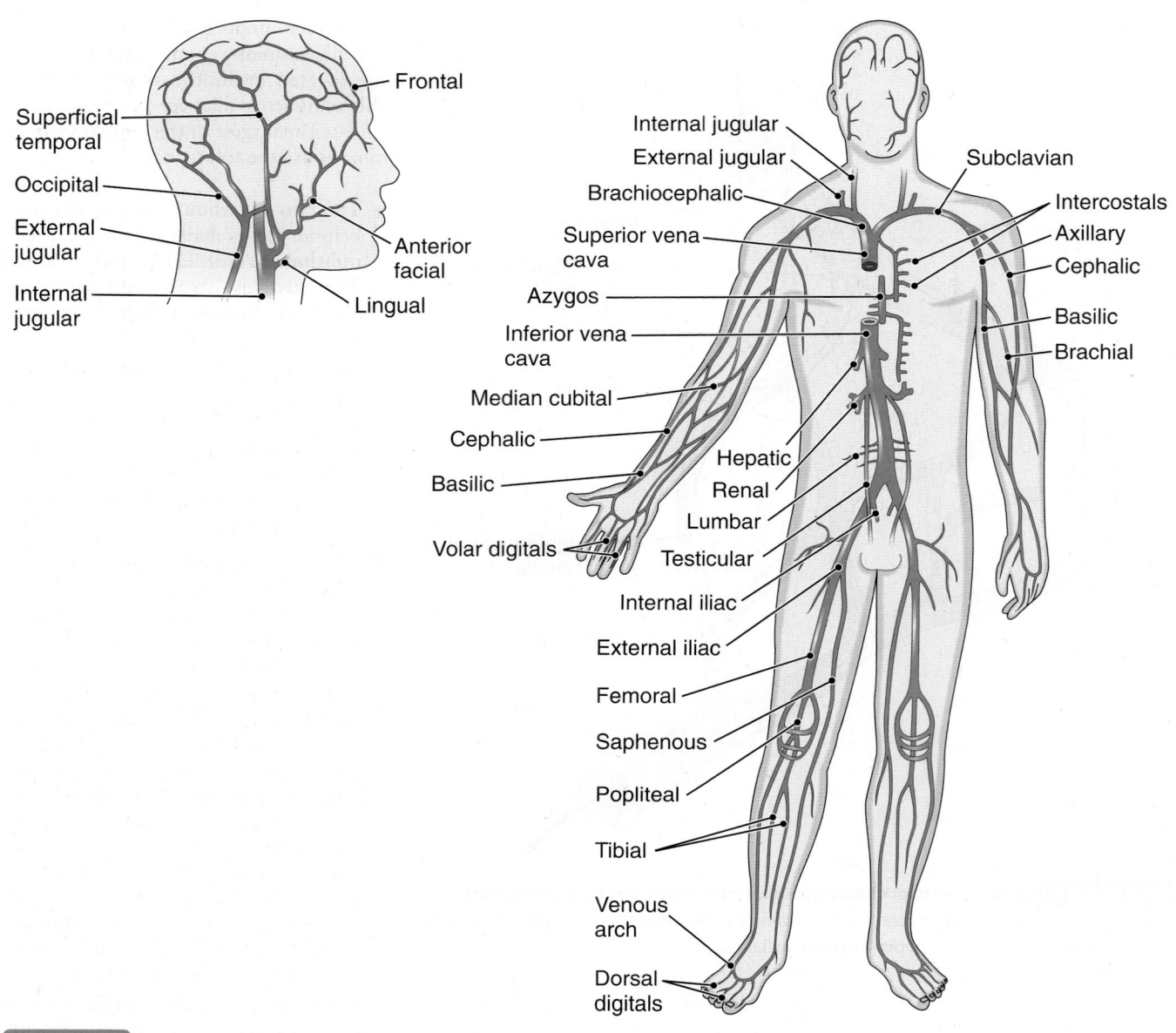

Figure 15-8 Principal systemic veins. [ZOOMING IN ➤ How many brachiocephalic veins are there?]

rectly into the inferior vena cava, they deliver it through the hepatic portal vein to the liver. The portal vein's largest tributary is the **superior mesenteric vein**, which drains blood from the proximal portion of the intestine. It is joined by the **splenic vein** just under the liver. Other tributaries of the portal circulation are the **gastric, pancreatic,** and **inferior mesenteric veins.** As it enters the liver, the portal vein divides and subdivides into ever smaller branches.

Eventually, the portal blood flows into a vast network of sinuslike vessels called **sinusoids** (SI-nus-oyds). These enlarged capillary channels allow liver cells close contact with the blood coming from the abdominal organs. (Similar blood channels are found in the spleen and endocrine glands, including the thyroid and adrenals.)

After leaving the sinusoids, blood is finally collected by the hepatic veins, which empty into the inferior vena cava.

The purpose of the hepatic portal system is to transport blood from the digestive organs and the spleen to the liver sinusoids, so that the liver cells can carry out their functions. For example, when food is digested, most of the end products are absorbed from the small intestine into the bloodstream and transported to the liver by the portal system. In the liver, these nutrients are processed, stored, and released as needed into the general circulation.

CHECKPOINT **15-12** ➤ The hepatic portal system takes blood from the abdominal organs to what organ?

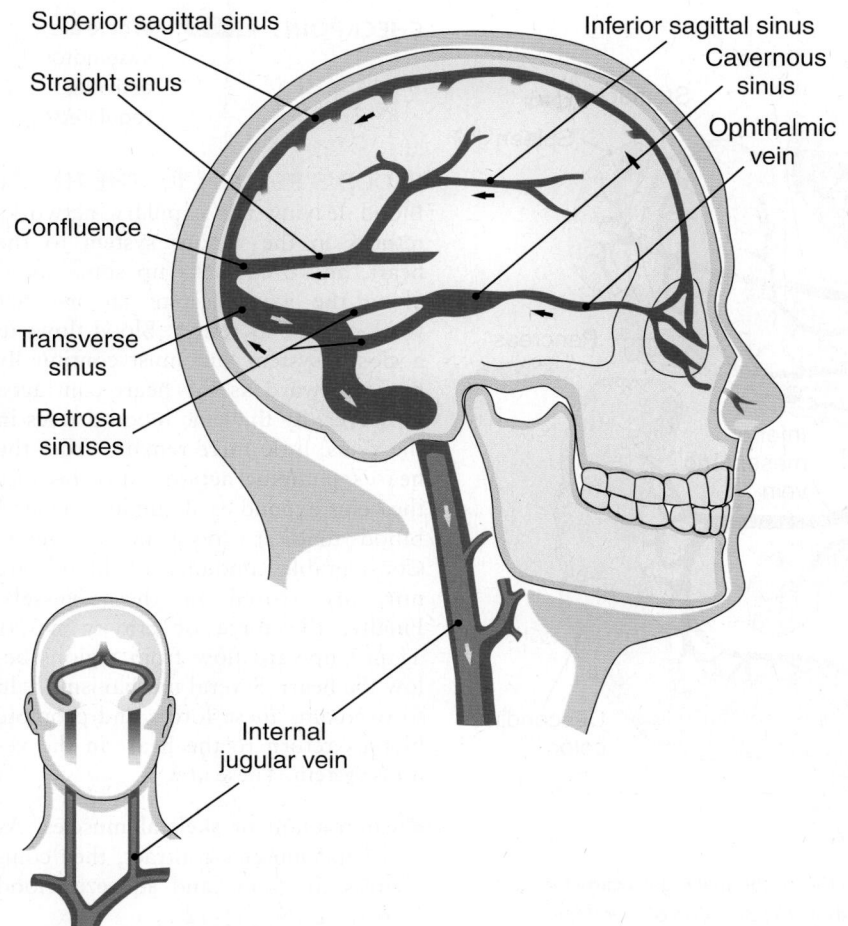

Superior sagittal sinus

Straight sinus

Confluence

Transverse sinus

Petrosal sinuses

Inferior sagittal sinus

Cavernous sinus

Ophthalmic vein

Internal jugular vein

Figure 15-9 **Cranial venous sinuses.** The inset shows the paired transverse sinuses, which carry blood from the brain to the jugular veins.

Circulation Physiology

Circulating blood might be compared to a bus that travels around the city, picking up and delivering passengers at each stop on its route. For example, as blood flows through capillaries surrounding the air sacs in the lungs, it picks up oxygen and unloads carbon dioxide. Later, when this oxygenated blood is pumped to capillaries in other parts of the body, it unloads the oxygen and picks up carbon dioxide and other substances generated by the cells (Fig. 15-11). The microscopic capillaries are of fundamental importance in these activities. It is only through the cells of these thin-walled vessels that the necessary exchanges can occur.

All living cells are immersed in a slightly salty liquid called **tissue fluid,** or **interstitial fluid.** Looking again at Figure 15-11, one can see how this fluid serves as "middleman" between the capillary membrane and the neighboring cells. As water, oxygen, and other necessary cellular materials pass through the capillary walls, they enter the tissue fluid. Then, these substances make their way by diffusion to the cells. At the same time, carbon dioxide and

other metabolic end products leave the cells and move in the opposite direction. These substances enter the capillaries and are carried away in the bloodstream for processing in other organs or elimination from the body.

Capillary Exchange

Diffusion is the main process by which substances move between the cells and the capillary blood. Recall that diffusion is the movement of a substance from an area where it is in higher concentration to an area where it is in lower concentration. Diffusion does not require transporters or cellular energy.

An additional force that moves materials from the blood into the tissues is the pressure of the blood as it flows through the capillaries. Blood pressure is the force that filters, or "pushes," water and dissolved materials out of the capillary into the tissue fluid. Fluid is drawn back into the capillary by osmotic pressure, the "pulling force" of substances dissolved and suspended in the blood. Osmotic pressure is maintained by plasma proteins (mainly albumin), which are too large to go through the capillary wall. These processes result in the constant exchange of fluids across the capillary wall.

The movement of blood through the capillaries is relatively slow, owing to the much larger cross-sectional area of the capillaries compared with that of the vessels from which they branch. This slow progress through the capillaries allows time for exchanges to occur. Note that even when the capillary exchange process is most efficient, some water is left behind in the tissues. Also, some proteins escape from the capillaries into the tissues. The lymphatic system, discussed in Chapter 16, collects this extra fluid and protein and returns them to the circulation (see Fig. 15-11).

CHECKPOINT 15-13 ➤ As materials diffuse back and forth between the blood and tissue fluid across the capillary wall, what force helps to push materials out of the capillary? What force helps to draw materials into the capillary?

The Dynamics of Blood Flow

Blood flow is carefully regulated to supply tissue needs without unnecessary burden on the heart. Some organs, such as the brain, liver, and kidneys, require large quanti-

15

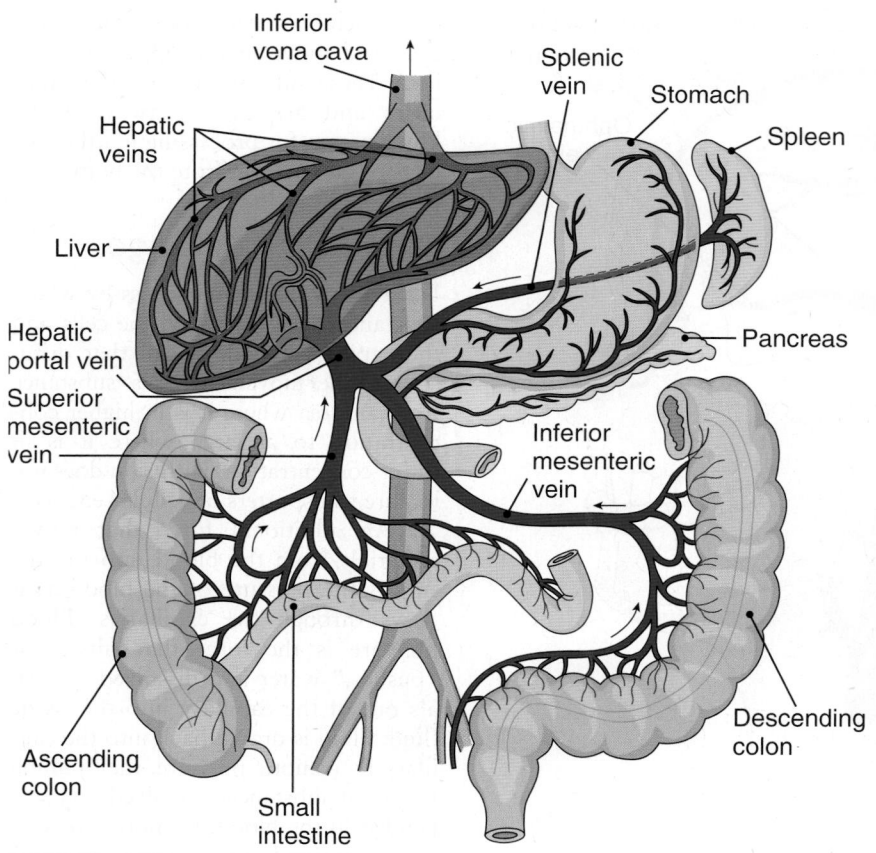

Figure 15-10 **Hepatic portal system.** Veins from the abdominal organs carry blood to the hepatic portal vein leading to the liver. Arrows show the direction of blood flow. [**ZOOMING IN** ➤ What vessel do the hepatic veins drain into?]

ties of blood even at rest. The requirements of some tissues, such as the skeletal muscles and digestive organs, increase greatly during periods of activity. For example, the blood flow in muscle can increase 25 times during exercise. The volume of blood flowing to a particular organ can be regulated by changing the size of the blood vessels supplying that organ.

An increase in a blood vessel's diameter is called **vasodilation**. This change allows for the delivery of more blood to an area. **Vasoconstriction** is a decrease in a blood vessel's diameter, causing a decrease in blood flow. These *vasomotor activities* result from the contraction or relaxation of smooth muscle in the walls of the blood vessels, mainly the arterioles. A **vasomotor center** in the medulla of the brain stem regulates vasomotor activities, sending its messages through the autonomic nervous system.

Blood flow into an individual capillary is regulated by a **precapillary sphincter** of smooth muscle that encircles the entrance to the capillary (see Fig. 15-7). This sphincter widens to allow more blood to enter when tissues need more oxygen.

CHECKPOINT **15-14** ➤ Name the two types of vasomotor changes.

CHECKPOINT **15-15** ➤ Where are vasomotor activities regulated?

BLOOD'S RETURN TO THE HEART

Blood leaving the capillary networks returns in the venous system to the heart, and even picks up some speed along the way, despite factors that work against its return. Blood flows in a closed system and must continually move forward as the heart contracts. However, by the time blood arrives in the veins, little force remains from the heart's pumping action. Also, because the veins expand easily under pressure, blood tends to pool in the veins. Considerable amounts of blood are normally stored in these vessels. Finally, the force of gravity works against upward flow from regions below the heart. Several mechanisms help to overcome these forces and promote blood's return to the heart in the venous system. These are:

- **Contraction of skeletal muscles.** As skeletal muscles contract, they compress the veins and squeeze blood forward (Fig. 15-12).

- **Valves** in the veins prevent back flow and keep blood flowing toward the heart.

- **Breathing.** Pressure changes in the abdominal and thoracic cavities during breathing also promote blood return in the venous system. During inhalation, the diaphragm flattens and puts pressure on the large abdominal veins. At the same time, chest expansion causes pressure to drop in the thorax. Together, these actions serve to both push and pull blood through these cavities and return it to the heart.

As evidence of these effects, if a person stands completely motionless, especially on a hot day when the superficial vessels dilate, enough blood can accumulate in the lower extremities to cause fainting from insufficient oxygen to the brain.

The Pulse

The ventricles regularly pump blood into the arteries about 70 to 80 times a minute. The force of ventricular contraction starts a wave of increased pressure that begins at the heart and travels along the arteries. This wave, called the **pulse**, can be felt in any artery that is relatively close to the surface, particularly if the vessel can be pressed down against a bone. At the wrist, the radial artery passes

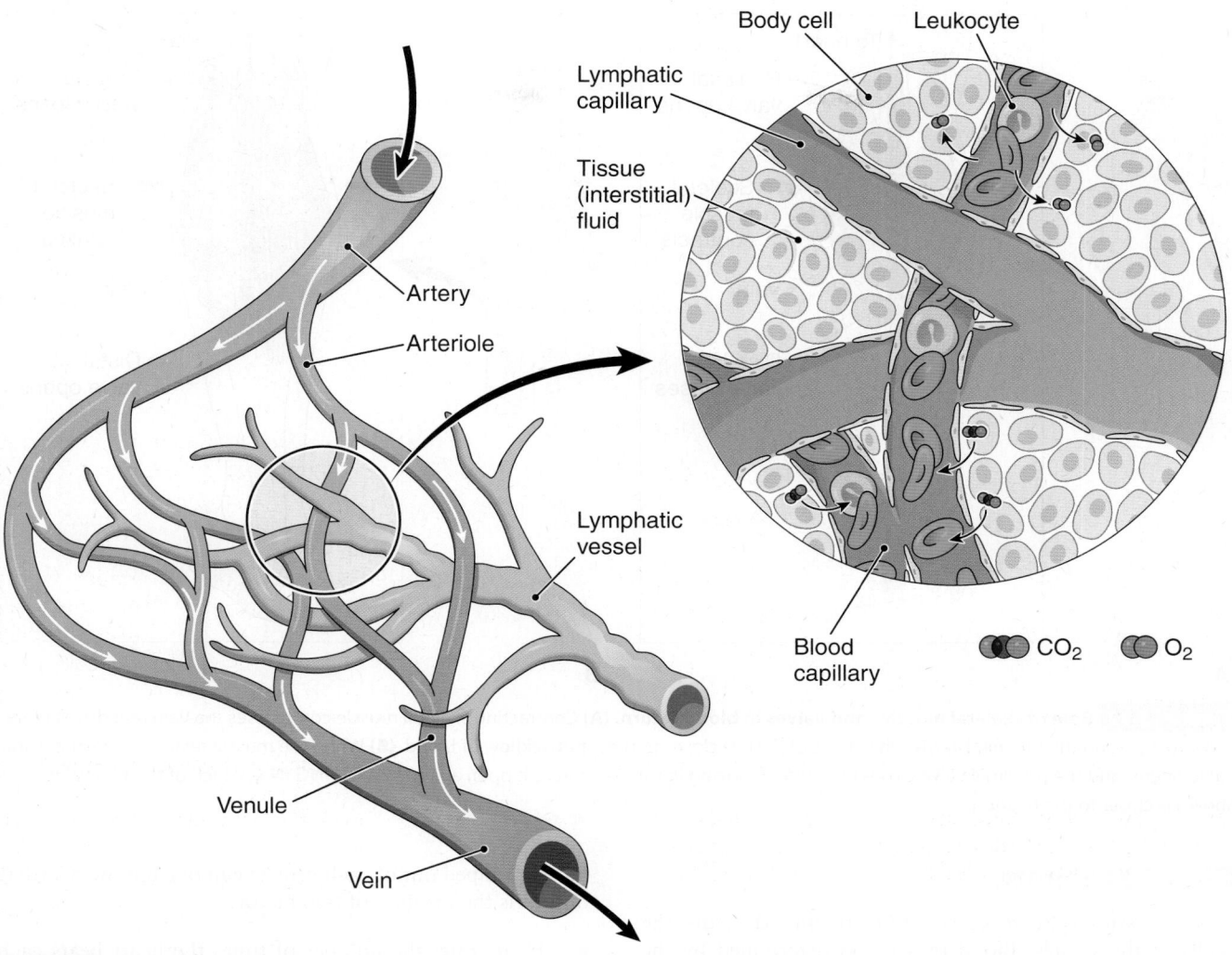

Figure 15-11 Connection between small blood vessels through capillaries. The blood delivers oxygen (O_2) to the tissues and picks up carbon dioxide (CO_2) for transport to the lungs. Note the lymphatic capillaries, which aid in tissue drainage.

15

over the bone on the forearm's thumb side, and the pulse is most commonly obtained here. Other vessels sometimes used for taking the pulse are the carotid artery in the neck and the dorsalis pedis on the top of the foot.

Normally, the pulse rate is the same as the heart rate, but if a heartbeat is abnormally weak, or if the artery is obstructed, the beat may not be detected as a pulse. In checking another person's pulse, it is important to use your second or third finger. If you use your thumb, you may be feeling your own pulse. When taking a pulse, it is important to gauge the strength as well as the regularity and rate.

PULSE RATE Various factors may influence the pulse rate. We describe just a few here:

- The pulse is somewhat faster in small people than in large people and usually is slightly faster in women than in men.

- In a newborn infant, the rate may be from 120 to 140 beats/minute. As the child grows, the rate tends to become slower.

- Muscular activity influences the pulse rate. During sleep, the pulse may slow down to 60 beats/minute, whereas during strenuous exercise, the rate may go up to well over 100 beats/minute. For a person in good condition, the pulse does not go up as rapidly as it does in an inactive person, and it returns to a resting rate more quickly after exercise.

- Emotional disturbances may increase the pulse rate.

- In many infections, the pulse rate increases with the increase in temperature.

- Excessive secretion of thyroid hormone may cause a rapid pulse.

CHECKPOINT 15-16 ➤ What is the definition of *pulse*?

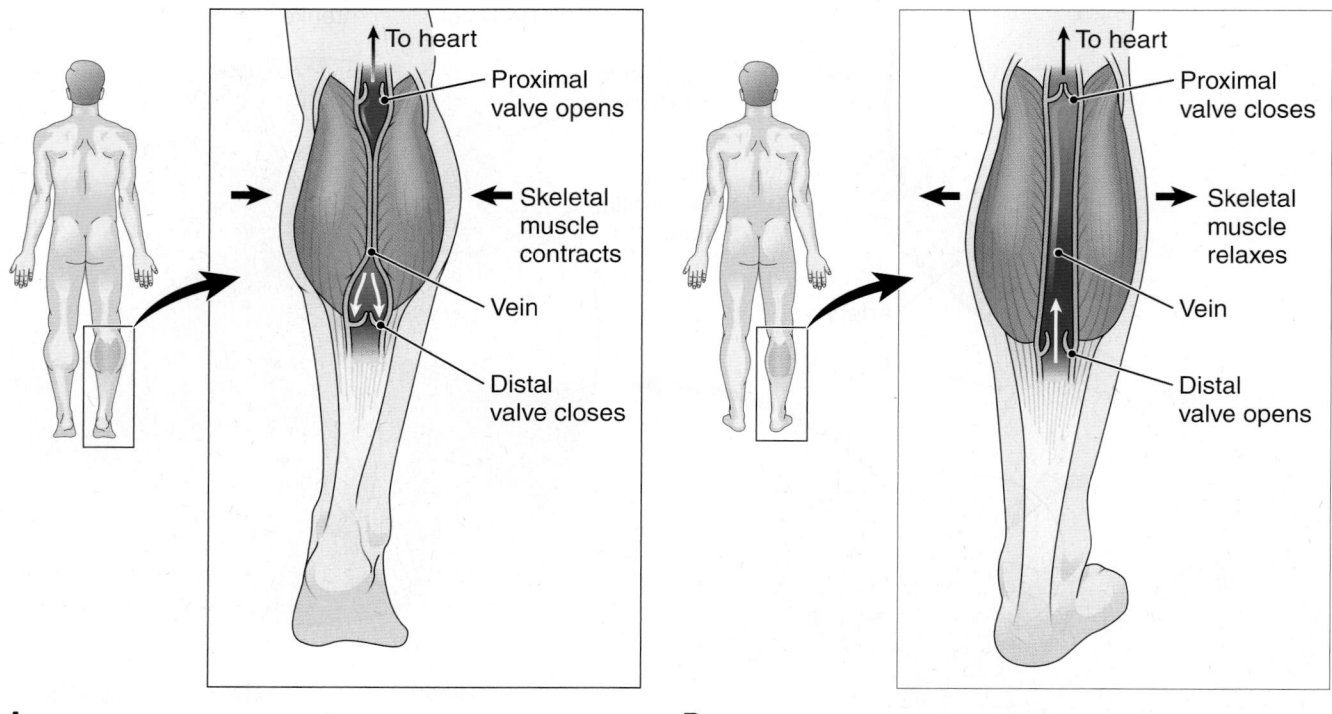

A   **B**

Figure 15-12 **Role of skeletal muscles and valves in blood return. (A)** Contracting skeletal muscle compresses the vein and drives blood forward, opening the proximal valve, while the distal valve closes to prevent backflow of blood. **(B)** When the muscle relaxes again, the distal valve opens, and the proximal valve closes until blood moving in the vein forces it open again. [**ZOOMING IN ➤** Which of the two valves shown is closer to the heart?]

Blood Pressure

Blood pressure is the force exerted by the blood against the walls of the vessels. Blood pressure is determined by the heart's output and resistance to blood flow in the vessels. If either of these factors changes and there are no compensating changes, blood pressure will change (Fig. 15-13).

CARDIAC OUTPUT As described in Chapter 14, the output of the heart, or cardiac output (CO), is the volume of

blood pumped out of each ventricle in one minute. Cardiac output is the product of two factors:

- **Heart rate**, the number of times the heart beats each minute. The basic heart rate is set internally by the SA node, but can be influenced by the autonomic nervous system, hormones, and other substances circulating in the blood, such as ions.

- **Stroke volume**, the volume of blood ejected from the ventricle with each beat. The sympathetic nervous system can stimulate more forceful heart contractions to increase blood ejection. Also, if more blood returns to the heart in the venous system, stretching of the heart muscle will promote more forceful contractions.

RESISTANCE TO BLOOD FLOW
Resistance is opposition to blood flow owing to friction generated as blood slides along the vessel walls. Because the effects of resistance are seen mostly in small arteries and arterioles that are at a distance from the heart and large vessels, this factor is often described as *peripheral resistance*. Resistance in the vessels is affected by the following factors:

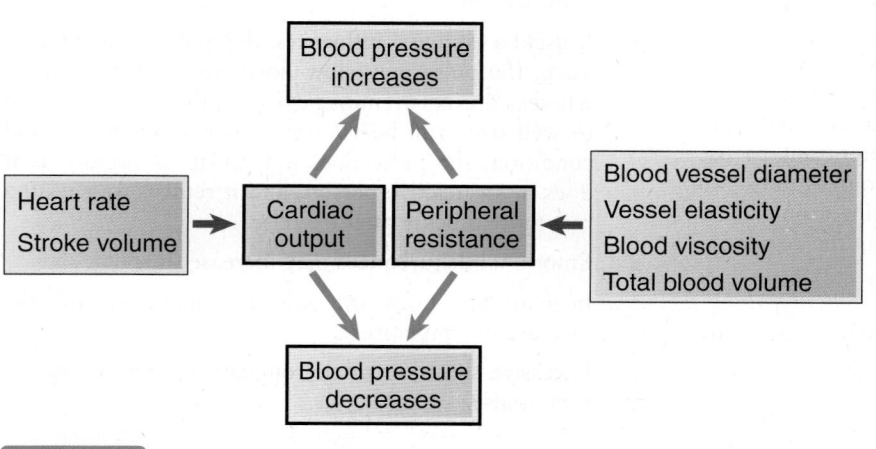

Figure 15-13 **Factors that influence blood pressure.**

- **Vasomotor changes.** A narrow vessel offers more resistance to blood flow than a wider vessel, just as it is harder to draw fluid through a narrow straw than through a wide straw. Thus, vasoconstriction increases resistance to flow and vasodilation lowers resistance.

   The medulla's vasomotor center, which controls vessel diameter, responds mainly to impulses from sensory receptors in the large vessels. The carotid arteries and the aorta have **baroreceptors** (bar-o-re-SEP-torz) in their walls that respond to changes in pressure. When they are stretched by increased blood pressure, they transmit signals that result in vasodilation. At the same time, central controls slow the heart rate to reduce cardiac output. With less stretching, the sympathetic nervous system causes the vessels to constrict and causes the heart rate to increase.

- **Elasticity of blood vessels.** Arteries normally expand to receive blood and then return to their original size. If vessels lose elasticity, as by atherosclerosis, they offer more resistance to blood flow. You've probably experienced this phenomenon if you've tried to blow up a firm, new balloon. More pressure is generated as you blow, and the balloon is a lot harder to inflate than a softer balloon, which expands more easily under pressure. Blood vessels lose elasticity with aging, thus increasing resistance and blood pressure.

- **Viscosity,** or thickness of the blood. Just as a milkshake is harder to suck through a straw than milk is, increased blood viscosity will increase blood pressure. Increased numbers of red blood cells, as in polycythemia, or a loss of plasma volume, as by dehydration, will increase blood viscosity. The hematocrit test described in Chapter 13 is one measure of blood viscosity; it measures the relative percentage of packed cells in whole blood.

- **Total blood volume,** the total amount of blood that is in the vascular system at a given time. A loss of blood volume, as by hemorrhage, will lower blood pressure. An increase in blood volume will generate more pressure within the vessels. It will also increase cardiac output by increasing venous return of blood to the heart.

To summarize, all of these relationships are expressed together by the following equation:

$$\text{Blood pressure} = \text{cardiac output} \times \text{peripheral resistance}$$

MEASUREMENT OF BLOOD PRESSURE The measurement and careful interpretation of blood pressure may prove a valuable guide in the care and evaluation of a person's health. Because blood pressure decreases as the blood flows from arteries into capillaries and finally into veins, healthcare providers ordinarily measure arterial pressure only, most commonly in the brachial artery of the arm. They use an instrument called a **sphygmomanometer** (sfig-mo-mah-NOM-eh-ter) (Fig. 15-14), more simply called a blood pressure cuff or blood pressure apparatus. This instrument measures two variables:

- **Systolic pressure,** which occurs during heart muscle contraction
- **Diastolic pressure,** which occurs during relaxation of the heart muscle

The sphygmomanometer is an inflatable cuff attached to a pressure gauge. Pressure is expressed in millimeters mercury (mm Hg), that is, the height to which the pressure can push a column of mercury in a tube. The examiner

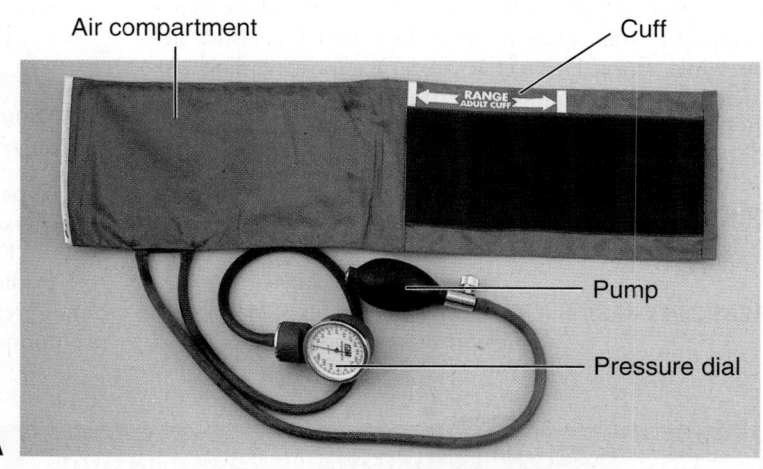

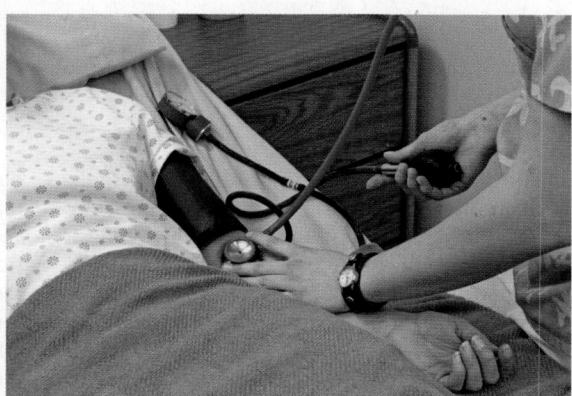

Figure 15-14 **Measurement of blood pressure. (A)** A sphygmomanometer, or blood pressure cuff. **(B)** Once the cuff is inflated, the examiner releases the pressure and listens for sounds in the vessels with a stethoscope. (A, Reprinted with permission from Bickley LS. *Bates' Guide to Physical Examination and History Taking*, 8th ed. Philadelphia: Lippincott Williams & Wilkins, 2003; B, reprinted with permission from Taylor C, Lillis C, LeMone P. *Fundamentals of Nursing*, 5th ed. Philadelphia: Lippincott Williams & Wilkins, 2004.)

wraps the cuff around the patient's upper arm and inflates it with air until the brachial artery is compressed and the blood flow is cut off. Then, listening with a stethoscope, he or she slowly lets air out of the cuff until the first pulsations are heard. At this point, the pressure in the cuff is equal to the systolic pressure, and this pressure is read. Then, more air is let out gradually until a characteristic muffled sound indicates that the vessel is open and the diastolic pressure is read. Original-style sphygmomanometers display readings on a graduated column of mercury, but newer types display them on a dial or measure blood pressure electronically and give a digital reading. A typical normal systolic pressure is 120 mm Hg; a typical normal diastolic pressure is 80 mm Hg. Blood pressure is reported as systolic pressure first, then diastolic pressure, separated by a slash, such as 120/80.

Considerable experience is required to ensure an accurate blood pressure reading. Often it is necessary to repeat measurements. Note also that blood pressure varies throughout the day and under different conditions, so a single reading does not give a complete picture. Some people typically have a higher reading in a doctor's office because of stress. People who experience such "white coat hypertension" may need to take their blood pressure at home while relaxed to get a more accurate reading. A physician might recommend treatment for mild hypertension. Box 15-2 explains how cardiac catheterization is used to measure blood pressure with high accuracy.

CHECKPOINT `15-17` ➤ What is the definition of blood pressure?

CHECKPOINT `15-18` ➤ What two components of blood pressure are measured?

ABNORMAL BLOOD PRESSURE Lower-than-normal blood pressure is called **hypotension** (hi-po-TEN-shun). Because of individual variations in normal pressure levels, however, what would be a low pressure for one person might be normal for someone else. For this reason, hypotension is best evaluated in terms of how well the body tissues are being supplied with blood. A person whose systolic blood pressure drops to below his or her normal range may experience fainting episodes because of inadequate blood flow to the brain. The sudden lowering of blood pressure to below a person's normal level is one sign of shock; it may also occur in certain chronic diseases and in heart block.

Hypertension (hi-per-TEN-shun), or high blood pressure, has received a great deal of attention in medicine. Hypertension normally occurs temporarily as a result of excitement or exertion. However, it may persist in a number of conditions, including the following:

- Kidney disease and uremia (excess nitrogenous waste in the blood) or other toxic conditions

- Endocrine disorders, such as hyperthyroidism and acromegaly

- Arterial disease, including hardening of the arteries (atherosclerosis), which reduces vacular elasticity

- Tumors of the adrenal medulla (central portion) with the release of excess epinephrine

Hypertension that has no apparent medical cause is called **essential hypertension**. Excess of an enzyme called **renin** (RE-nin), produced in the kidney, appears to play a role in the severity of essential hypertension. Renin raises blood pressure by causing blood vessels to constrict and by promoting the kidney's retention of salt and water.

Box 15-2 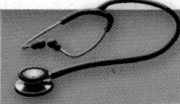 **Clinical Perspectives**

Cardiac Catheterization: Measuring Blood Pressure from Within

Because arterial blood pressure decreases as blood flows farther away from the heart, measurement of blood pressure with a simple inflatable cuff around the arm is only a reflection of the pressure in the heart and pulmonary arteries. Precise measurement of pressure in these parts of the cardiovascular system is useful in diagnosing certain cardiac and pulmonary disorders.

More accurate readings can be obtained using a catheter (thin tube) inserted directly into the heart and large vessels. One type commonly used is the pulmonary artery catheter (also known as the Swan-Ganz catheter), which has an inflatable balloon at the tip. This device is threaded into the right side of the heart through a large vein. Typically, the right internal jugular vein is used because it is the shortest and most

direct route to the heart, but the subclavian and femoral veins may be used instead. The catheter's position in the heart is confirmed by a chest x-ray and, when appropriately positioned, the atrial and ventricular blood pressures are recorded. As the catheter continues into the pulmonary artery, pressure in this vessel can be read. When the balloon is inflated, the catheter becomes wedged in a branch of the pulmonary artery, blocking blood flow. The reading obtained is called the **pulmonary capillary wedge (PCW) pressure**. It gives information on pressure in the heart's left side and on resistance in the lungs. Combined with other tests, cardiac catheterization can be used to diagnose cardiac and pulmonary disorders such as shock, pericarditis, congenital heart disease, and heart failure.

It is important to treat even mild hypertension because this condition can eventually:

- Weaken vessels and lead to saclike bulges (aneurysms) in vessel walls that are likely to rupture. In the brain, vessel rupture is one cause of stroke. Rupture of a vessel in the eye may lead to blindness.

- Stress the heart by causing it to work harder to pump blood into the arterial system. In response to this greater effort, the heart enlarges, but eventually it weakens and becomes less efficient.

- Stress the kidneys and damage renal vessels.

- Damage the lining of vessels, predisposing to atherosclerosis.

> **PASSport to Success**
> Visit **thePoint** or see the Student Resource CD in the back of this book for an animation on hypertension.

Although medical caregivers often place emphasis on the systolic blood pressure, in many cases, the diastolic pressure is even more important. The total fluid volume in the vascular system and the condition of small arteries may have a greater effect on diastolic pressure. Table 15-1 lists degrees of hypertension as compared with normal blood pressure values.

TREATMENT OF HYPERTENSION Even though there is much individual variation in blood pressure, physicians have established guidelines for the diagnosis and treatment of hypertension. The first stage of hypertension begins at 140/90 mm Hg. Treatment at this point should be based on diet, exercise, and weight loss, if necessary. Drug therapy should be added to this regimen for people with pressure readings above 159/99 mm Hg. Drugs used to treat hypertension include the following:

- Diuretics, which promote water loss
- Drugs that limit production of renin
- Drugs that relax blood vessels

CHECKPOINT 15-19 ➤ What is meant by *hypertension* and *hypotension*?

Arterial Degeneration and Other Vascular Disorders

As a result of age or other degenerative changes, materials may be deposited within the arterial walls. These deposits cause an irregular thickening of the wall at the expense of the lumen (space inside the vessel), as well as a loss of elasticity. In some cases, calcium salts and scar tissue may cause this hardening of the arteries, technically called **arteriosclerosis** (ar-te-re-o-skle-RO-sis). The most common form of this disorder is **atherosclerosis** (ath-er-o-skle-RO-sis) (Fig. 15-15), in which areas of yellow, fatlike material, called **plaque** (PLAK), accumulate in the vessels and separate the muscle and elastic tissue. Sometimes, the arterial lining is also damaged, leading to possible blood clot (thrombus) formation and partial or complete obstruction of the vessel, as occurs in coronary thrombosis. Atherosclerosis begins with microscopic damage to the arterial endothelium caused by direct contact with LDL (the "bad" cholesterol), oxidizing chemicals, such as free-radicals, and some proteins. Lipids begin to accumulate in the arterial wall, followed by aggregation of platelets and macrophages, and plaque formation. The arterial wall soon bulges into the lumen and obstructs blood flow. Arteries in the heart, brain, kidneys, and the extremities seem to be especially vulnerable to this process.

Atherosclerosis and its complications (heart disease, stroke, and thrombosis) account for 40% of all deaths in the United States! A diet high in fats, particularly saturated fats, is known to contribute to atherosclerosis. Cigarette smoking also increases the extent and severity of this disorder. Arterial damage may be present for years without causing any noticeable symptoms. As the thickening of the wall continues and the lumen's diameter decreases, limiting blood flow, a variety of symptoms can appear. The nature of these disturbances varies with the area affected and with the extent of the arterial changes. Some examples are as follows:

- Leg cramps, pain, and sudden lameness while walking may be caused by insufficient blood supply to the lower extremities resulting from arterial damage.

- Headaches, dizziness, and mental disorders may be the result of cerebral artery sclerosis.

- Hypertension may result from a decrease in lumen size within many arteries throughout the body. Although hypertension may be present in young people with no apparent arterial damage, and atherosclerosis may be present without causing hypertension, the two are often found together in elderly people.

Table 15-1	Blood Pressure	

Blood Pressure Classification (Adults)*

Category	Systolic (mm Hg)	Diastolic (mm Hg)
Optimal	<120	<80
Normal	<130	<85
High normal	130–139	85–89
Hypertension		
Stage 1 (mild)	140–159	90–99
Stage 2 (moderate)	160–179	100–109
Stage 3 (severe)	≥180	≥110

*When the systolic and diastolic pressures are in different categories, the higher category is used.

15

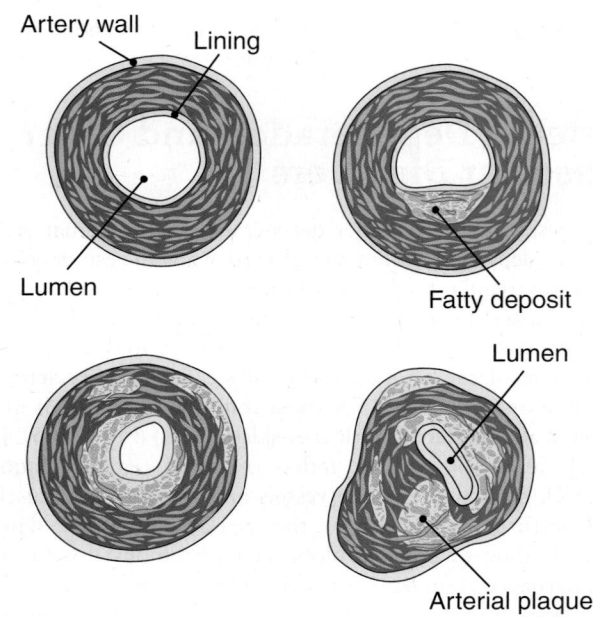

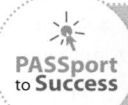

Figure 15-15 Stages in atherosclerosis.

■ Palpitations, dyspnea (difficulty in breathing), paleness, weakness, and other symptoms may be the result of coronary artery arteriosclerosis. The severe pain of

angina pectoris may follow the lack of oxygen and the myocardial damage associated with sclerosis of the vessels that supply the heart.

■ An increase in the amount of urine with the appearance of albumin. Albumin is a normal plasma protein usually found in the urine only if there is kidney damage. Other symptoms referable to the kidneys may be caused by renal artery damage.

■ Ulceration and tissue necrosis (death) as a result of ischemia (lack of blood supply), especially in the extremities. If the dead tissue is invaded by bacteria, the result is **gangrene** (GANG-grene). The arterial damage that is caused by diabetes, for example, often leads to gangrene in the extremities of elderly diabetic patients.

> **PASSport to Success**
> Visit **thePoint** or see the Student Resource CD in the back of this book for illustrations of atherosclerosis development and its clinical effects.

TREATMENT FOR ARTERIAL DEGENERATION Balloon catheterization and bypass grafts used to treat arterial disease were discussed with reference to the heart in Chapter 14. Stents, small tubes inserted to keep vessels open, also discussed in relation to the heart, are used for other vessels as well. An additional treatment approach is **endarterectomy** (end-ar-ter-EK-to-me), removal of a ves-

Disease in Context revisited

▶ Reggie's Pulmonary Embolism

As soon as the blood clot broke free in Reggie's femoral vein, it began its journey to the heart. The clot (now called an embolus) traveled within the right femoral vein, which entered the abdominal cavity and widened, becoming the external iliac vein. The embolus flowed into the large right common iliac vein, mixing with pelvic blood from the internal iliac vein. Then, the embolus was carried toward the even larger inferior vena cava. As the embolus traveled superiorly toward the heart, it joined with blood from the kidneys and intestines. The inferior vena cava carried the embolus through the diaphragm into the thoracic cavity and into the right atrium of the heart. The embolus flowed past the tricuspid valve into the right ventricle, which contracted and propelled the embolus past the pulmonary valve and into the pulmonary trunk. The embolus entered the left pulmonary artery and then traveled through successively

smaller arterial branches until finally it became wedged in one of the small arteries supplying blood to his left lung. Reggie had developed a pulmonary embolism!

Reggie felt a sharp crushing pain in his chest and woke with a start. He knew something was terribly wrong and pressed the panic button clipped to his hospital bed. Reggie's nurse rushed to his bedside and recognized that Reggie was in life-threatening danger. He received immediate treatment of tissue plasminogen activator (tPA) to dissolve the clots in his pulmonary artery and femoral vein and several doses of heparin to prevent more clots from forming. Reggie had survived his second medical emergency!

In this case, we followed an embolus as it traveled from Reggie's femoral vein to his pulmonary artery. Using the diagrams in this chapter, can you trace its pathway?

sel's thickened, atheromatous lining. Common sites for this procedure are the carotid artery or vertebral artery leading to the brain and the common iliac or femoral arteries leading to the lower limbs. Surgeons can remove a blockage by direct incision of a vessel. More commonly, to remove plaque, they use a cutting tool inserted with a catheter through the vessel opening.

ANEURYSM An **aneurysm** (AN-u-rizm) is a bulging sac in a blood vessel's wall caused by a localized weakness in that part of the vessel (Fig. 15-16). The aorta and vessels in the brain are common aneurysm sites. The damage to the wall may be congenital or a result of arteriosclerosis. Whatever the cause, the aneurysm may continue to grow in size. As it swells, it may cause some derangement of other structures, in which case definite symptoms are present. If undiagnosed, the weakened area eventually yields to the pressure, and the aneurysm bursts like a balloon, usually causing death. Surgical replacement of the damaged segment with a synthetic graft may be lifesaving.

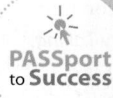
PASSport to Success   Visit *thePoint* or see the Student Resource CD in the back of this book for a photograph of an aortic aneurysm.

Hemorrhage

A profuse escape of blood from the vessels is known as **hemorrhage** (HEM-or-ij), a word that means "a bursting forth of blood." Such bleeding may be external or internal, from vessels of any size, and may involve any part of the body. Capillary oozing usually is stopped by the normal process of clot formation.

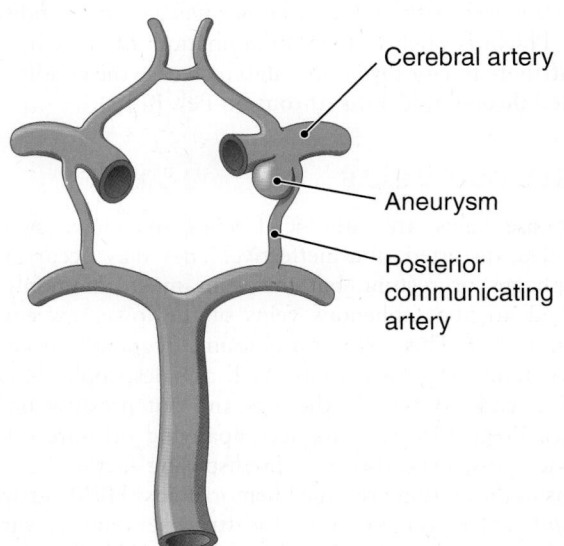

Figure 15-16 **A cerebral aneurysm in the circle of Willis.** (Reprinted with permission from Cohen BJ. *Medical Terminology*, 4th ed. Philadelphia: Lippincott Williams & Wilkins, 2004.)

FIRST AID FOR HEMORRHAGE The loss of a small amount of blood will cause no problem for a healthy adult, but loss of one liter or more of blood is life-threatening. The first step to control bleeding is the application of direct pressure to the wound using a clean cloth. An assisting person should wear gloves to protect from blood-borne diseases. A bleeding extremity should be elevated above the heart level. In cases of severe, persistent bleeding, application of pressure where a local artery can be pressed against a bone slows the bleeding. The most important of these "pressure points" are the following:

- The **facial artery**, which may be pressed against the lower jaw for hemorrhage around the nose, mouth, and cheek. One can feel the pulse of the facial artery in the depression about 1 inch anterior to the lower jaw's angle.

- The **temporal artery**, which may be pressed against the side of the skull just anterior to the ear to stop hemorrhage on the side of the face and around the ear.

- The **common carotid artery** in the neck, which may be pressed back against the spinal column for bleeding in the neck and the head.

- The **subclavian artery**, which may be pressed against the first rib by a downward push with the thumb to stop bleeding from the shoulder or arm.

- The **brachial artery**, which may be pressed against the humerus (arm bone) by a push inward along the natural groove between the arm's two large muscles. This stops hand, wrist, and forearm hemorrhage.

- The **femoral artery** (in the groin), which may be pressed to avoid serious hemorrhage of the lower extremity.

It is important not to leave the pressure on too long, as this may cause damage to tissues supplied by arteries past the pressure point.

Shock

The word **shock** has a number of meanings. In terms of the circulating blood, it refers to a life-threatening condition in which there is inadequate blood flow to the body tissues. A wide range of conditions that reduce effective circulation can cause shock. The exact cause is often not known. However, a widely used classification is based on causative factors, the most important of which include the following:

- **Cardiogenic** (kar-de-o-JEN-ik) **shock**, sometimes called *pump failure*, is often a complication of heart muscle damage, as occurs in myocardial infarction. It is the leading cause of shock death.

- **Septic shock** is second only to cardiogenic shock as a cause of shock death. It is usually the result of an overwhelming bacterial infection.

- **Hypovolemic** (hi-po-vo-LE-mik) **shock** is caused by a decrease in the volume of circulating blood and may follow severe hemorrhage or burns.

- **Anaphylactic** (an-ah-fih-LAK-tik) **shock** is a severe allergic reaction to foreign substances to which the person has been sensitized (see Chapter 17 on Immunity).

When the cause is not known, shock is classified according to its severity.

In **mild shock**, regulatory mechanisms relieve the circulatory deficit. Signs are often subtle changes in heart rate and blood pressure. Constriction of small blood vessels and the detouring of blood away from certain organs increase the effective circulation. Mild shock may develop into a severe, life-threatening circulatory failure.

Severe shock is characterized by poor circulation, which causes further damage and deepening of the shock. Late shock symptoms include clammy skin, anxiety, low blood pressure, rapid pulse, and rapid, shallow breathing. Heart contractions are weakened, owing to the decrease in the heart's blood supply. The vascular walls also are weakened, so that the vessels dilate. The capillaries become more permeable and lose fluid, owing to the accumulation of metabolic wastes.

The victim of shock should first be placed in a horizontal position and covered with a blanket. If there is bleeding, it should be stopped. The patient's head should be kept turned to the side to prevent aspiration (breathing in) of vomited material, an important cause of death in shock cases. Further treatment of shock depends largely on treatment of the causative factors. For example, shock resulting from fluid loss, as in hemorrhage or burns, is best treated with blood products or plasma expanders (intravenous fluids). Shock caused by heart failure should be treated with drugs that improve heart muscle contractions. In any case, all measures are aimed at supporting the circulation and improving the cardiac output. Oxygen is frequently administered to improve oxygen delivery to the tissues.

CHECKPOINT 15-20 ➤ With regard to the circulation, what is meant by shock?

Thrombosis

Formation of a blood clot in a vessel is **thrombosis** (throm-BO-sis). A blood clot in a vein, termed *deep venous thrombosis* (DVT), most commonly develops in the deep veins of the calf muscle, although it may appear elsewhere. Thromboses typically occur in people who are recovering from surgery, injury, or childbirth or those who are bedridden. Clot formation may also be associated with some diseases, with obesity, and with certain drugs, such as hormonal medications. Symptoms are pain and swelling, often with warmth and redness below or around

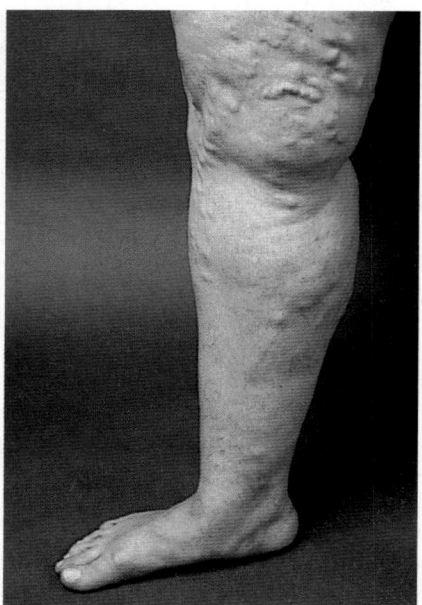

Figure 15-17 **Varicose veins.** (Reprinted with permission from Bickley LS. *Bates' Guide to Physical Examination and History Taking*, 8th ed. Philadelphia: Lippincott Williams & Wilkins, 2003.)

the clot. Thrombosis can be diagnosed with ultrasound or with magnetic resonance imaging (MRI).

A dangerous complication of thrombosis is formation of an **embolus** (EM-bo-lus), a piece of the clot that becomes loose and floats in the blood. An embolus is carried through the circulatory system until it lodges in a vessel. If it reaches the lungs, sudden death from **pulmonary embolism** (EM-bo-lizm) may result. Prevention of infections, early activity to promote circulation after an injury or an operation, and the use of anticoagulant drugs when appropriate have greatly reduced the incidence of this condition.

Phlebitis (fleh-BI-tis), inflammation of a vein, may contribute to clot formation, in which case the condition is called **thrombophlebitis** (throm-bo-fleh-BI-tis).

Varicose Veins

Varicose veins are superficial veins that have become swollen, distorted, and ineffective. They may occur in the esophagus or rectum, but the veins most commonly involved are the saphenous veins of the lower extremities (Fig. 15-17). This condition is found frequently in people who stand for long periods, such as salespeople, because blood tends to pool in the legs and put pressure on the veins. Pregnancy, with its accompanying pressure on the pelvic veins, may also be a predisposing factor. Varicose veins in the rectum are called **hemorrhoids** (HEM-o-royds), or *piles*. The general term for varicose veins is **varices** (VAR-ih-seze); the singular form is **varix** (VAR-iks).

Word Anatomy

Medical terms are built from standardized word parts (prefixes, roots, and suffixes). Learning the meanings of these parts can help you remember words and interpret unfamiliar terms.

WORD PART	MEANING	EXAMPLE
Systemic Arteries		
brachi/o	arm	The *brachiocephalic* artery supplies blood to the arm and head on the right side.
cephal/o	head	See preceding example.
clav/o	clavicle	The *subclavian* artery extends under the clavicle on each side.
cost/o	rib	The *intercostal* arteries are between the ribs.
celi/o	abdomen	The *celiac* trunk branches to supply blood to the abdominal organs.
gastr/o	stomach	The *gastric* artery goes to the stomach.
splen/o	spleen	The *splenic* artery goes to the spleen.
hepat/o	liver	The *hepatic* artery supplies blood to the liver.
enter/o	intestine	The *mesenteric* arteries supply blood to the intestines.
phren/o	diaphragm	The *phrenic* artery supplies blood to the diaphragm.
ped/o	foot	The dorsalis *pedis* artery supplies blood to the foot.
stoma	mouth	An *anastomosis* is a communication between two vessels.
Circulation Physiology		
bar/o	pressure	A *baroreceptor* responds to changes in pressure.
sphygm/o	pulse	A *sphygmomanometer* is used to measure blood pressure.
man/o	pressure	See preceding example.
Arterial Degeneration and Other Vascular Disorders		
-ectomy	surgical removal	*Endarterectomy* is a procedure for removing plaque from the lining of a vessel.
phleb/o	vein	*Phlebitis* is inflammation of a vein.

15

Summary

I. **BLOOD VESSELS**
  A. Categories
    1. Arteries—carry blood away from heart
    2. Arterioles—small arteries
    3. Capillaries—allow for exchanges between blood and tissues, or blood and air in lungs; connect arterioles and venules
    4. Venules—small veins
    5. Veins—carry blood toward heart
  B. Blood circuits
    1. Pulmonary circuit—carries blood to and from lungs
    2. Systemic circuit—carries blood to and from rest of body
  C. Vessel structure
    1. Artery walls—layers (tunics)
      a. Innermost—single layer of flat epithelial cells (endothelium)
      b. Middle—thicker layer of smooth muscle and elastic connective tissue
      c. Outer—connective tissue
    2. Arterioles—thinner walls, less elastic tissue, more smooth muscle
    3. Capillaries—only endothelium; single layer of cells
    4. Venules—wall slightly thicker than capillary wall
    5. Veins—all three layers; thinner walls than arteries, less elastic tissue

II. **SYSTEMIC ARTERIES**
  A. The aorta and its parts
    1. Largest artery
    2. Divisions
      a. Ascending aorta
        (1) Left and right coronary arteries
      b. Aortic arch
        (1) Brachiocephalic artery—branches to arm and head on right
        (2) Left common carotid artery—supplies left side of neck and the head
        (3) Left subclavian artery—supplies left arm
      c. Descending aorta
        (1) Thoracic aorta—branches to chest wall, esophagus, bronchi
        (2) Abdominal aorta—supplies abdominal viscera
  B. Iliac arteries and their subdivisions
    1. Final divisions of aorta

    2. Branch to pelvis and legs
  C. Arteries that branch to the arm and head—common carotid, subclavian, brachial
  D. Anastomoses—communications between vessels

III. **SYSTEMIC VEINS**
  A. Location
    1. Superficial—near surface
    2. Deep—usually parallel to arteries with same names as corresponding arteries
  B. The venae cavae and their tributaries
    1. Superior vena cava—drains upper body
      a. Jugular veins drain head and neck
      b. Brachiocephalic veins empty into superior vena cava
    2. Inferior vena cava—drains lower body
  C. Venous sinuses—enlarged venous channels
  D. Hepatic portal system—carries blood from abdominal organs to liver, where it is processed before returning to heart

IV. **CIRCULATION PHYSIOLOGY**
  A. Capillary exchange
    1. Primary method—diffusion
    2. Medium—tissue fluid
    3. Blood pressure—drives fluid into tissues
    4. Osmotic pressure—pulls fluid into capillary
  B. Dynamics of blood flow
    1. Vasomotor activities
      a. Vasodilation—increase in diameter of blood vessel
      b. Vasoconstriction—decrease in diameter of blood vessel
      c. Vasomotor center—in medulla; controls contraction and relaxation of smooth muscle in vessel wall
    2. Precapillary sphincter—regulates blood flow into capillary
    3. Return of blood to heart
      a. Pumping action of heart
      b. Pressure of skeletal muscles on veins
      c. Valves in veins
      d. Breathing—changes in pressure move blood toward heart
  C. The pulse
    1. Wave of pressure that travels along arteries as ventricles contract
    2. Rate affected by size, age, gender, activity, and other factors
  D. Blood pressure
    1. Force exerted by blood against vessel walls

2. Factors
   a. Cardiac output—stroke volume x heart rate
   b. Resistance to blood flow—vessel diameter, vessel elasticity, blood viscosity, blood volume
      (1) Baroreceptors in large arteries respond to changes in pressure
      (2) Activate vasomotor center in medulla
3. Measured in arm with sphygmomanometer
   a. Systolic pressure
      (1) Occurs during heart contraction
      (2) Averages 120 mm Hg
   b. Diastolic pressure
      (1) Occurs during heart relaxation
      (2) Averages 80 mm Hg
4. Abnormal blood pressure
   a. Hypotension—low blood pressure
   b. Hypertension—high blood pressure
      (1) Essential hypertension—has no apparent medical cause
      (2) May involve renin, enzyme released from kidneys
      (3) May lead to aneurysm, stroke, stress on heart and kidneys, atherosclerosis
5. Treatment of hypertension—diuretics, reduction of renin, relaxation of blood vessels

V. **ARTERIAL DEGENERATION AND OTHER VASCULAR DISORDERS**
   A. Arteriosclerosis—hardening of arteries with scar tissue, calcium salts, or fatty deposits
      1. Atherosclerosis—deposits of fatty material (plaque) in vessels
      2. Possible results—pain, breathing problems, angina pectoris, thrombosis (blood clot), tissue necrosis, gangrene
   B. Aneurysm—weakness and bulging of a vessel; may burst
   C. Hemorrhage
      1. Profuse loss of blood
      2. First aid measures: direct pressure, elevation of limb, pressure on artery
   D. Shock—inadequate blood flow to tissues
   E. Thrombosis—formation of blood clot in a vessel
      1. Embolus—piece of a clot traveling in circulation
         a. Pulmonary embolism—clot lodged in lung
      2. Phlebitis—inflammation of a vein; may lead to thrombophlebitis
         a. Varicose veins—swelling and loss of function in superficial veins, usually in legs and rectum (hemorrhoids)

Questions for Study and Review

BUILDING UNDERSTANDING

Fill in the blanks

1. Capillaries receive blood from vessels called _____.

2. The specific part of the brain that regulates blood pressure is the _____.

3. The flow of blood into an individual capillary is regulated by a(n) _____.

4. Lower-than-normal blood pressure is called _____.

5. Inflammation of a vein is called_____.

Matching > Match each numbered item with the most closely related lettered item.

___ **6.** Lack of blood supply to a tissue or organ

___ **7.** Bulging sac in the wall of a vessel

___ **8.** Loss of blood

___ **9.** An immobile blood clot within a vessel

___ **10.** A mobile blood clot within a vessel

a. embolus

b. thrombus

c. ischemia

d. aneurysm

e. hemorrhage

Multiple choice

___ **11.** The innermost layer of a blood vessel is composed of

    a. smooth muscle
    b. epithelium
    c. connective tissue
    d. nervous tissue

___ **12.** The largest artery in the body is the

    a. aorta
    b. brachiocephalic trunk
    c. splenic artery
    d. superior mesenteric artery

___ **13.** The main process by which substances move between the cells and the capillary blood is

    a. endocytosis
    b. exocytosis
    c. osmosis
    d. diffusion

___ **14.** The stomach, spleen, and liver receive blood via the

    a. hepatic portal system
    b. superior mesenteric artery
    c. inferior mesenteric artery
    d. celiac trunk

___ **15.** The medical term describing the deposition of material within arterial walls is

    a. shock
    b. gangrene
    c. arteriosclerosis
    d. stasis

UNDERSTANDING CONCEPTS

16. Differentiate between the terms in each of the following pairs:

    a. artery and vein
    b. arteriole and venule
    c. anastomosis and venous sinus
    d. vasoconstriction and vasodilation
    e. systolic and diastolic pressure

17. How does the structure of the blood vessels correlate with their function?

18. Trace a drop of blood from the left ventricle to the:

    a. right side of the head and neck
    b. lateral surface of the left hand
    c. right foot
    d. liver
    e. small intestine

19. Trace a drop of blood from capillaries in the wall of the small intestine to the right atrium. What is the purpose of going through the liver on this trip?

20. What physiological factors influence blood pressure?

21. Describe three mechanisms that promote the return of blood to the heart in the venous system.

22. What are some symptoms of arteriosclerosis and how are these produced?

23. What is shock and why is it so dangerous? Name some symptoms of shock and identify the types of shock based on (a) cause and (b) severity.

CONCEPTUAL THINKING

24. Kidney disease usually results in the loss of protein from the blood into the urine. One common sign of kidney disease is edema. Based on this information and your understanding of capillary exchange, explain why edema is often associated with kidney disease.

25. Cliff C., a 49-year-old self-described "couch potato," has a blood pressure of 162/100 mm Hg. What is Cliff's diagnosis? What can this disorder lead to? If you were Cliff's doctor, what treatments might you discuss with him?

26. In Reggie's case, an embolus traveled from his femoral vein to his pulmonary artery. Describe the pathway the embolus would take if it traveled from his femoral vein to the middle cerebral artery supplying blood to his left frontal lobe. What deficits would you suspect to see from this brain stroke? (*Hint*: consult Chapter 10!)

15

CHAPTER 16

The Lymphatic System and Lymphoid Tissue

Learning Outcomes

After careful study of this chapter, you should be able to:

1. List the functions of the lymphatic system
2. Explain how lymphatic capillaries differ from blood capillaries
3. Name the two main lymphatic ducts and describe the area drained by each
4. List the major structures of the lymphatic system and give the locations and functions of each
5. Describe the composition and function of the reticuloendothelial system
6. Describe the major lymphatic system disorders
7. Show how word parts are used to build words related to the lymphatic system (see Word Anatomy at the end of the chapter)

Selected Key Terms

The following terms and other boldface terms in the chapter are defined in the Glossary

adenoids
chyle
lacteal
lymph
lymphadenitis
lymphadenopathy
lymphangitis
lymphatic duct
lymph node
spleen
thymus
tonsil

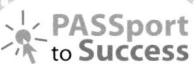

PASSport to Success

Visit *thePoint* or see the Student Resource CD in the back of this book for definitions and pronunciations of key terms as well as a pretest for this chapter.

Disease
in Context

> ## Mike's Second Case: Emergency Splenectomy

Alek, a 4th-year medical student, slumped into a chair in the lounge and closed his eyes. It was only a few hours into his shift, but he was already exhausted. Then, Alek's pager buzzed—*get to the operating room immediately*! Minutes later, he donned a sterile gown and gloves and entered the operating room, which buzzed with activity as the surgical team prepped the patient for emergency abdominal surgery. Alek listened carefully to the surgeon as she explained the case to the team. "Patient's name is Mike. He's 21 years old and was in a car accident about an hour ago. Paramedics noted significant bruising of the left upper quadrant, tachycardia, and hypotension." The surgeon glanced at the medical student and asked, "Alek, what does that suggest to you?"

Alek thought quickly and answered, "The location of the injury and cardiovascular problems suggest a ruptured spleen."

"That's exactly what the emergency team thought," replied the surgeon. "OK folks, let's open Mike up and see if Alek's right." Using a scalpel, the surgeon made a midsagittal incision through Mike's abdominal wall. Then, she made a transverse incision to open the left side of his abdominal cavity and suctioned out the blood that filled it. She located the purple-colored spleen in the left hypochondriac region and noted a large tear in the connective tissue capsule surrounding it. "You're right, Alek. We've got a ruptured spleen here, which we'll have to remove." The surgeon searched for the splenic artery supplying blood to the damaged organ and when she found it, tied it shut, and cut it. Then, she cut the ligaments that suspended the spleen between the stomach and transverse colon. Finally, she tied and cut the splenic vein and removed Mike's spleen. "OK," said the surgeon, "Let's close him up and get him to intensive care. Alek, good job today."

Mike's spleen, a lymphoid organ, was injured during a car accident and had to be removed. In this chapter, you will learn about the spleen and other organs that make up the lymphatic system. Later, we'll check in on Mike and learn about splenectomy's long-term consequences.

The Lymphatic System

The lymphatic system is a widespread system of tissues and vessels. Its organs are not in continuous order, but are scattered throughout the body, and it services almost all regions. Only bone tissue, cartilage, epithelium, and the central nervous system are not in direct communication with this system.

Functions of the Lymphatic System

The lymphatic system's functions are just as varied as its locations. These functions fall into three categories:

- **Fluid balance.** As blood circulates through the capillaries in the tissues, water and dissolved substances are constantly exchanged between the bloodstream and the interstitial (in-ter-STISH-al) fluids that bathe the cells. Ideally, the volume of fluid that leaves the blood should be matched by the amount that returns to the blood. However, there is always a slight excess of fluid left behind in the tissues. In addition, some proteins escape from the blood capillaries and are left behind. This fluid and protein would accumulate in the tissues if not for a second drainage pathway through lymphatic vessels (Fig. 16-1).

In addition to the blood-carrying capillaries, the tissues also contain microscopic lymphatic capillaries. These small vessels pick up excess fluid and protein left behind in the tissues (Fig. 16-2). The capillaries then drain into larger vessels, which eventually return these materials to the venous system near the heart.

The fluid that circulates in the lymphatic system is called **lymph** (limf), a clear fluid similar in composi-

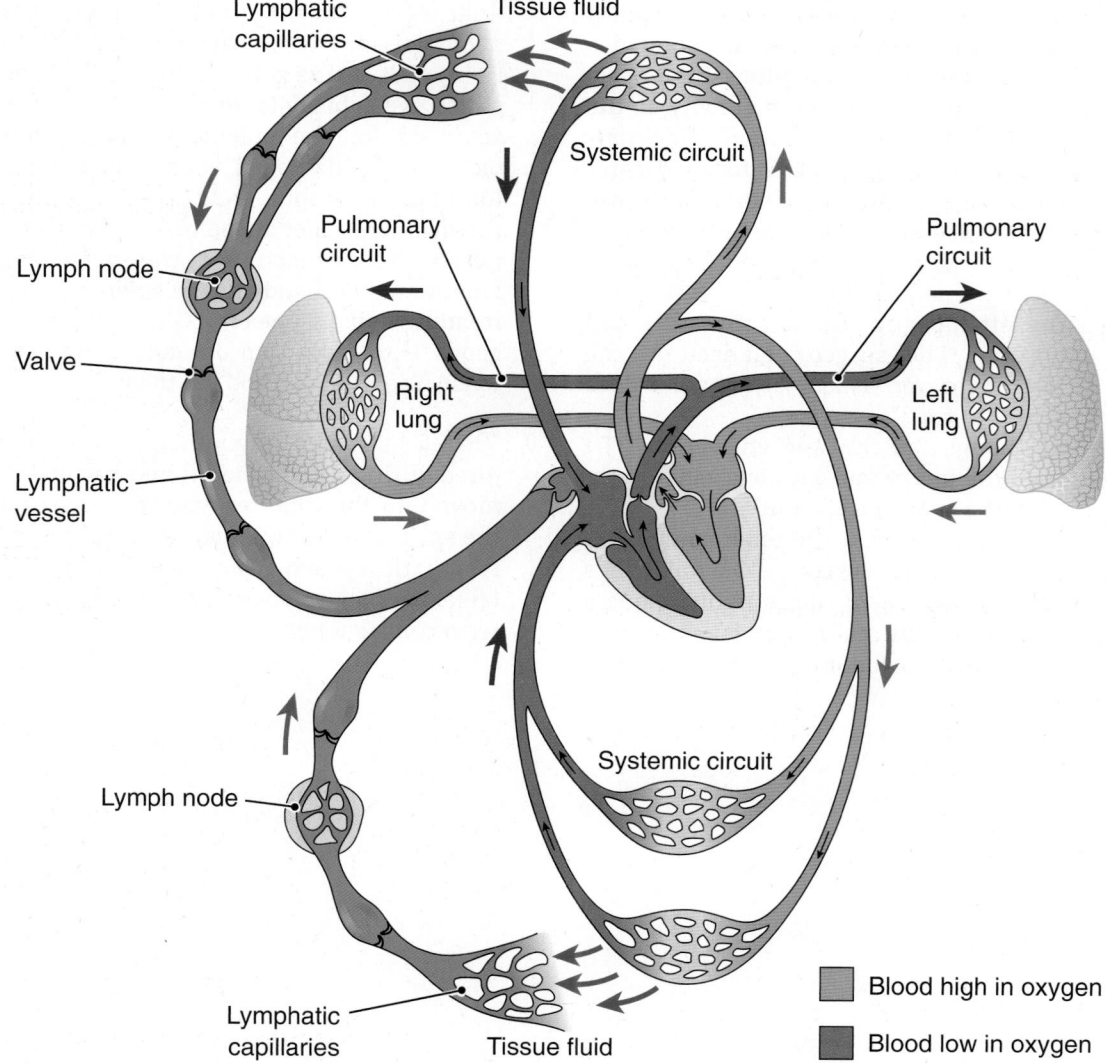

Figure 16-1 **The lymphatic system in relation to the cardiovascular system.** Lymphatic vessels pick up fluid in the tissues and return it to the blood in vessels near the heart. [**ZOOMING IN** ➤ What type of blood vessel receives lymph collected from the body?]

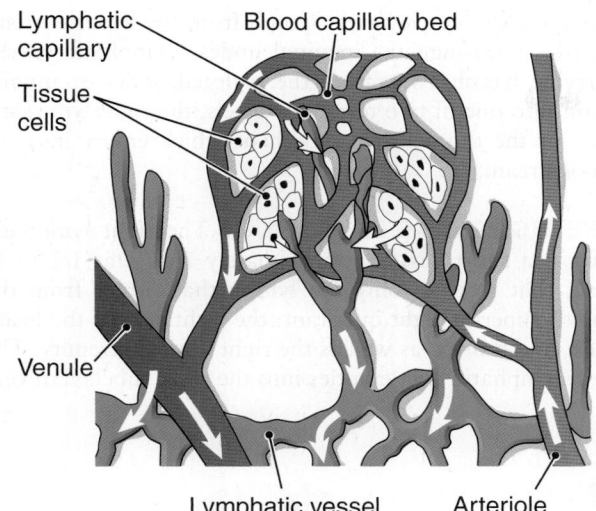

Lymphatic capillary

Blood capillary bed

Tissue cells

Venule

Lymphatic vessel

Arteriole

Figure 16-2 **Pathway of lymphatic drainage in the tissues.**
Lymphatic capillaries are more permeable than blood capillaries
and can pick up fluid and proteins left in the tissues as blood leaves
the capillary bed to travel back toward the heart.

tion to interstitial fluid. Although lymph is formed
from the components of blood plasma, it differs from
the plasma in that it has much less protein.

■ **Protection from infection.** The lymphatic system is an
important component of the immune system, which
fights infection. One group of white blood cells, the
lymphocytes, can live and multiply in the lymphatic
system, where they attack and destroy foreign organisms. Lymphoid tissue scattered throughout the body
filters out pathogens, other foreign matter, and cellular debris in body fluids. More will be said about the
lymphocytes and immunity in Chapter 17.

■ **Absorption of fats.** Following the chemical and mechanical breakdown of food in the digestive tract, most
nutrients are absorbed into the blood through intestinal capillaries. Many digested fats, however, are too
large to enter the blood capillaries and are instead absorbed into lymphatic capillaries. These fats are added
to the blood when lymph joins the bloodstream. The
topic of digestion is covered in Chapter 19.

CHECKPOINT **16-1** ➤ What are three functions of the
lymphatic system?

Lymphatic Circulation

Lymph travels through a network of small and large channels that are in some ways similar to the blood vessels.
However, the system is not a complete circuit. It is a one-way system that begins in the tissues and ends when the
lymph joins the blood (see Fig. 16-1).

Lymphatic Capillaries

The walls of the lymphatic capillaries resemble those of the
blood capillaries in that they are made of one layer of flattened (squamous) epithelial cells. This thin layer, also
called *endothelium*, allows for easy passage of soluble materials and water (Fig. 16-3). The gaps between the endothelial cells in the lymphatic capillaries are larger than
those of the blood capillaries. The lymphatic capillaries are
thus more permeable, allowing for easier entrance of relatively large protein molecules. The proteins do not move
back out of the vessels because the endothelial cells overlap slightly, forming one-way valves to block their return.

Unlike the blood capillaries, the lymphatic capillaries
arise blindly; that is, they are closed at one end and do not
form a bridge between two larger vessels. Instead, one end
simply lies within a lake of tissue fluid, and the other communicates with a larger lymphatic vessel that transports
the lymph toward the heart (see Figs. 16-1 and 16-2).

Some specialized lymphatic capillaries located in the
small intestine's lining absorb digested fats. Fats taken into
these **lacteals** (LAK-te-als) are transported in the lymphatic
vessels until the lymph is added to the blood. More information on the lymphatic system's role in digestion is found
in Chapter 19.

CHECKPOINT **16-2** ➤ What are two differences between
blood capillaries and lymphatic
capillaries?

Lymphatic Vessels

The lymphatic vessels are thin-walled and delicate and have
a beaded appearance because of indentations where valves
are located (see Fig. 16-1). These valves prevent back flow
in the same way as do those found in some veins.

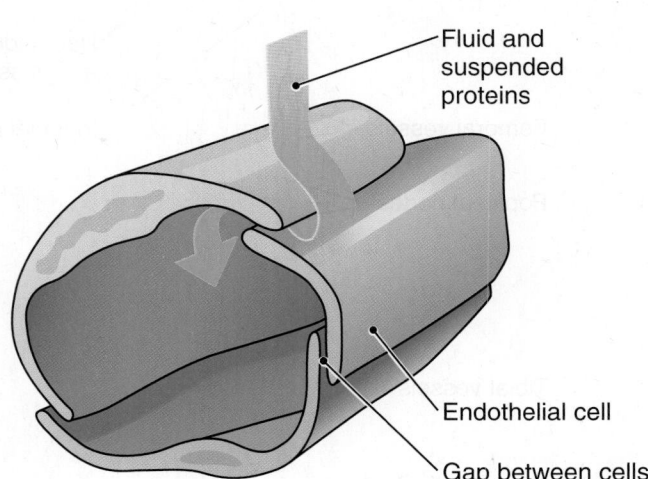

Fluid and suspended proteins

Endothelial cell

Gap between cells

Figure 16-3 **Structure of a lymphatic capillary.** Fluid and
proteins can enter the capillary with ease through gaps between
the endothelial cells. Overlapping cells act as valves to prevent the
material from leaving.

16

Lymphatic vessels (Fig. 16-4) include **superficial** and **deep** sets. The surface lymphatics are immediately below the skin, often lying near the superficial veins. The deep vessels are usually larger and accompany the deep veins.

Lymphatic vessels are named according to location. For example, those in the breast are called **mammary** lymphatic vessels, those in the thigh are called **femoral** lymphatic vessels, and those in the leg are called **tibial** lymphatic vessels. At certain points, the vessels drain through lymph nodes, small masses of lymphatic tissue that filter the lymph. The nodes are in groups that serve a particular region. For example, nearly all the lymph from the upper extremity and the breast passes through the **axil-** **lary lymph nodes**, whereas lymph from the lower extremity passes through the **inguinal nodes**. Lymphatic vessels carrying lymph away from the regional nodes eventually drain into one of two terminal vessels, the right lymphatic duct or the thoracic duct, both of which empty into the bloodstream.

THE RIGHT LYMPHATIC DUCT The **right lymphatic duct** is a short vessel, approximately 1.25 cm (1/2 inch) long, that receives only the lymph that comes from the body's superior right quadrant: the right side of the head, neck, and thorax, as well as the right upper extremity. The right lymphatic duct empties into the right subclavian vein

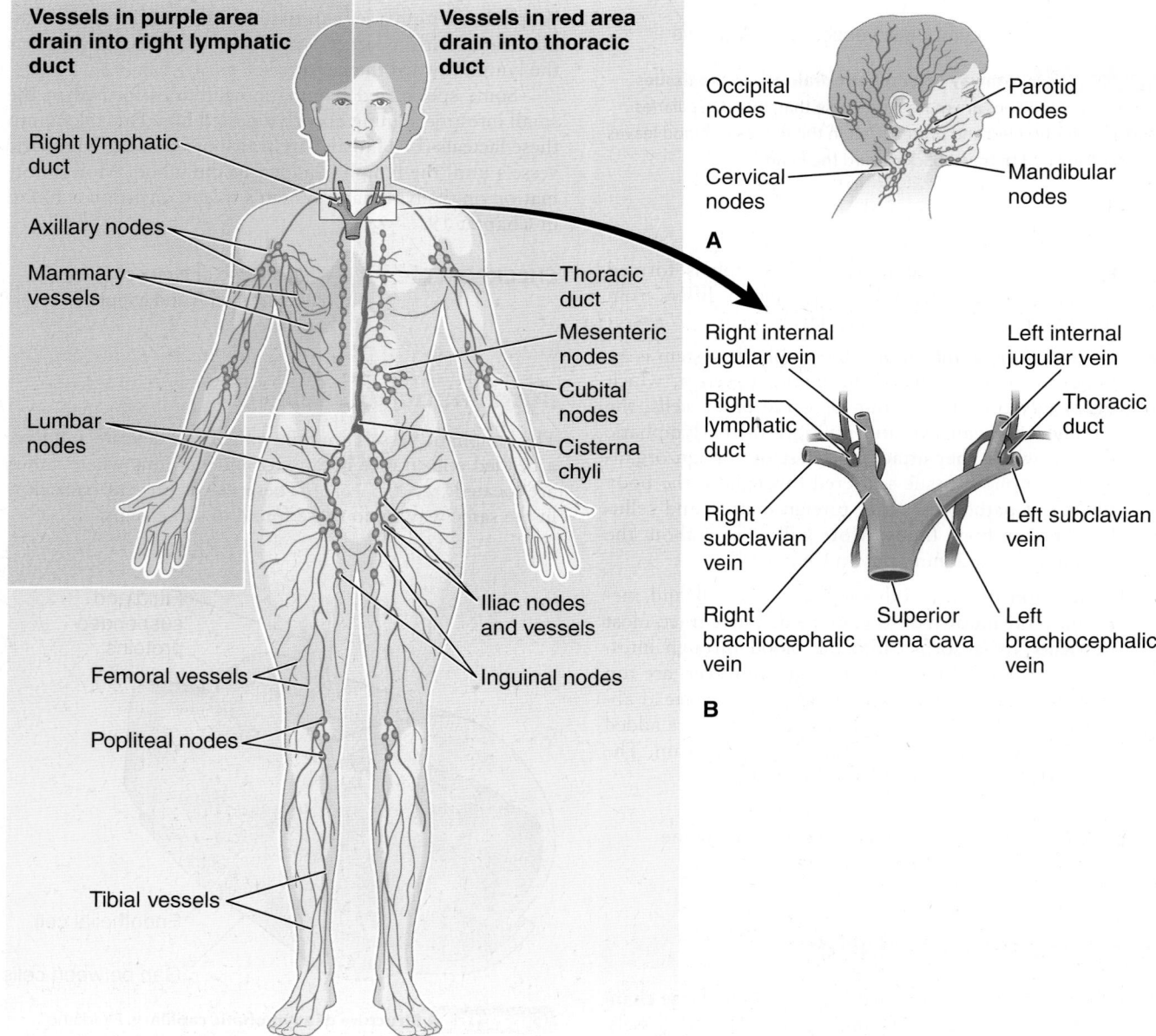

Figure 16-4 **Vessels and nodes of the lymphatic system. (A)** Lymph nodes and vessels of the head. **(B)** Drainage of right lymphatic duct and thoracic duct into subclavian veins.

near the heart (see Fig. 16-4B). Its opening into this vein is guarded by two pocket-like semilunar valves to prevent blood from entering the duct. The rest of the body is drained by the thoracic duct.

THE THORACIC DUCT The **thoracic duct**, or left lymphatic duct, is the larger of the two terminal vessels, measuring approximately 40 cm (16 inches) in length. As shown in Figure 16-4, the thoracic duct receives lymph from all parts of the body except those superior to the diaphragm on the right side. This duct begins in the posterior part of the abdominal cavity, inferior to the attachment of the diaphragm. The duct's first part is enlarged to form a cistern, or temporary storage pouch, called the **cisterna chyli** (sis-TER-nah KI-li). **Chyle** (kile) is the milky fluid that drains from the intestinal lacteals; it is formed by the combination of fat globules and lymph. Chyle passes through the intestinal lymphatic vessels and the lymph nodes of the mesentery (membrane around the intestines), finally entering the cisterna chyli. In addition to chyle, all the lymph from below the diaphragm empties into the cisterna chyli, passing through the various clusters of lymph nodes. The thoracic duct then carries this lymph into the bloodstream.

The thoracic duct extends upward through the diaphragm and along the posterior thoracic wall into the base of the neck on the left side. Here, it receives the left jugular lymphatic vessels from the head and neck, the left subclavian vessels from the left upper extremity, and other lymphatic vessels from the thorax and its parts. In addition to the valves along the duct, there are two valves at its opening into the left subclavian vein to prevent the passage of blood into the duct.

CHECKPOINT 16-3 ➤ What are the two main lymphatic vessels?

Movement of Lymph

The segments of lymphatic vessels located between the valves contract rhythmically, propelling the lymph forward. The contraction rate is related to the fluid volume in the vessel—the more fluid, the more rapid the contractions.

Lymph is also moved by the same mechanisms that promote venous return of blood to the heart. As skeletal muscles contract during movement, they compress the lymphatic vessels and drive lymph forward. Changes in pressures within the abdominal and thoracic cavities caused by breathing aid lymphatic movement during passage through these body cavities. Box 16-1, Lymphedema, describes what happens when lymph does not flow properly.

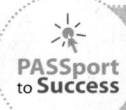

PASSport to Success Massage therapy can improve lymphatic drainage and blood circulation as well as benefit muscles. Visit **thePoint** or see the Student Resource CD in the back of this book for more information about this field.

Lymphoid Tissue

Lymphoid (LIM-foyd) **tissue** is distributed throughout the body and makes up the lymphatic system's specialized organs. The lymph nodes have already been described rela-

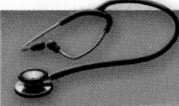

Box 16-1   Clinical Perspectives

16

Lymphedema: When Lymph Stops Flowing

The body's fluid balance requires appropriate fluid distribution among the cardiovascular system, lymphatic system, and the tissues. **Edema** occurs when the balance is tipped toward excess fluid in the tissues. Often, edema is due to heart failure. However, blockage of lymphatic vessels (and the resulting fluid accumulation in the subcutaneous tissues) can cause another form of edema called **lymphedema**. The clinical hallmark of lymphedema is chronic swelling of an arm or leg, whereas heart failure usually causes swelling of both legs.

Lymphedema may be either primary or secondary. Primary lymphedema is a rare congenital condition caused by abnormal development of lymphatic vessels. Secondary lymphedema, or acquired lymphedema, can develop as a result of trauma to a limb, surgery, radiation therapy, or infection of the lymphatic vessels (lymphangitis). One of lymphedema's most common causes is the removal of axillary lymph nodes

during mastectomy (breast removal), which disrupts lymph flow from the adjacent arm. Lymphedema may also occur following prostate surgery.

Therapies that encourage flow through the lymphatic vessels are useful in treating lymphedema. These therapies may include elevation of the affected limb, manual lymphatic drainage through massage, light exercise, and firm wrapping of the limb to apply compression. In addition, changes in daily habits can lessen lymphedema's effects. For example, further blockage of lymph drainage can be prevented by wearing loose-fitting clothing and jewelry, carrying a purse or handbag on the unaffected arm, and sitting with legs uncrossed. Lymphangitis requires the use of appropriate antibiotics. Prompt treatment is necessary because, in addition to swelling, other complications include poor wound healing, skin ulcers, and increased risk of infection.

tive to describing lymphatic circulation, but these tissues and other lymphatic system components are discussed in greater detail in the next section.

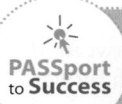

Lymph Nodes

The lymph nodes, as noted, are designed to filter the lymph once it is drained from the tissues (Fig. 16-5). They are also sites where lymphocytes of the immune system multiply and work to combat foreign organisms. The lymph nodes are small, rounded masses varying from pinhead size to as long as 2.5 cm (1 inch). Each has a fibrous connective tissue capsule from which partitions (trabeculae) extend into the node's substance. At various points in the node's surface, afferent lymphatic vessels pierce the capsule to carry lymph into the node. An indented area called the **hilum** (HI-lum) is the exit point for efferent lymphatic vessels carrying lymph out of the node. At this region, other structures, including blood vessels and nerves, connect with the node.

Each node is subdivided into lymph-filled spaces (sinuses) and cords of lymphatic tissue. Pulplike nodules in the outer region, or cortex, have germinal centers where certain immune lymphocytes multiply. The inner region, the medulla, has populations of immune cells, including lymphocytes and macrophages (phagocytes), along open channels that lead into the efferent vessels.

Lymph nodes are seldom isolated. As a rule, they are massed together in groups, varying in number from 2 or 3 to well over 100. Some of these groups are placed deeply, whereas others are superficial. The main groups include the following:

- **Cervical nodes,** located in the neck in deep and superficial groups, drain various parts of the head and neck. They often become enlarged during upper respiratory infections.
- **Axillary nodes,** located in the axillae (armpits), may become en-

larged after infections of the upper extremities and the breasts. Cancer cells from the breasts often metastasize (spread) to the axillary nodes.

- **Tracheobronchial** (tra-ke-o-BRONG-ke-al) **nodes** are found near the trachea and around the larger bronchial tubes. In people living in highly polluted areas, these nodes become filled with air contaminants.

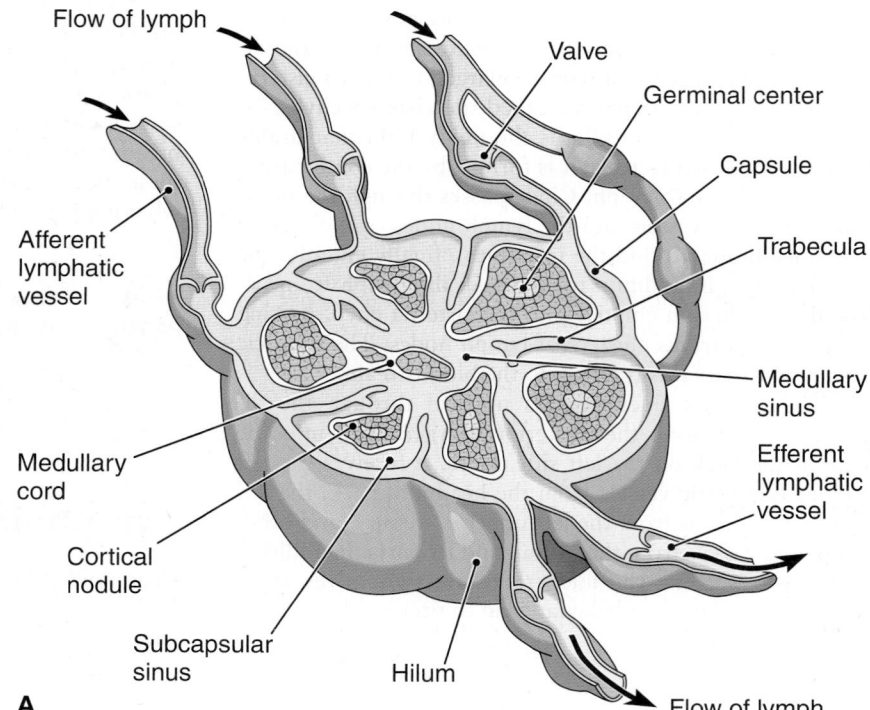

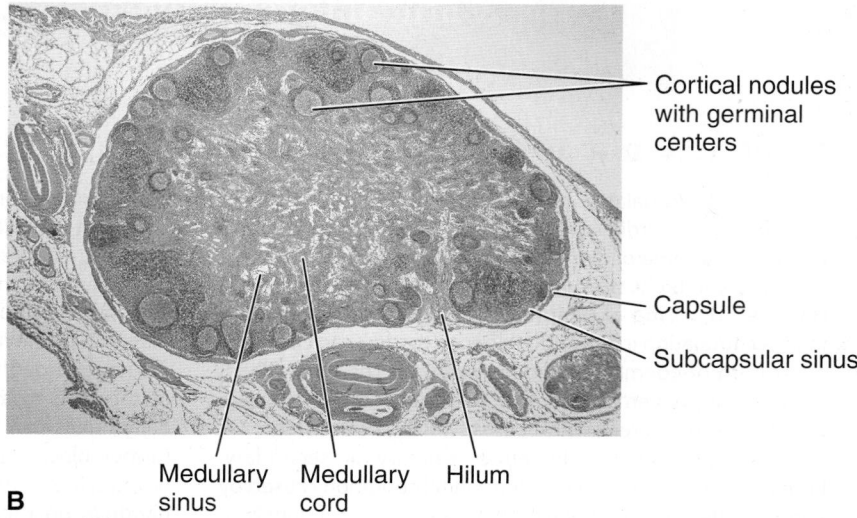

Figure 16-5 **Structure of a lymph node. (A)** Arrows indicate the flow of lymph through the node. **(B)** Section of a lymph node as seen under the microscope (low power). (B, Reprinted with permission from Cormack DH. *Essential Histology*, 2nd ed. Philadelphia: Lippincott Williams & Wilkins, 2001.) [**ZOOMING IN** ➤ What type of lymphatic vessel carries lymph into a node? What type of lymphatic vessel carries lymph out of a node?]

- **Mesenteric** (mes-en-TER-ik) **nodes** are found between the two layers of peritoneum that form the mesentery. There are some 100 to 150 of these nodes.

- **Inguinal nodes,** located in the groin region, receive lymph drainage from the lower extremities and from the external genital organs. When they become enlarged, they are often referred to as **buboes** (BU-bose), from which bubonic plague got its name.

Box 16-2 explains the role of lymph node biopsy in the treatment of cancer.

CHECKPOINT **16-4** ➤ What is the function of the lymph nodes?

The Spleen

The spleen is an organ that contains lymphoid tissue designed to filter blood. It is located in the superior left hypochondriac region of the abdomen, high up under the dome of the diaphragm, and normally is protected by the lower part of the rib cage (Fig. 16-6). The spleen is a soft, purplish, and somewhat flattened organ, measuring approximately 12.5 to 16 cm (5 to 6 inches) long and 5 to 7.5 cm (2 to 3 inches) wide. The spleen's capsule, as well as its framework, is more elastic than that of the lymph nodes. It contains involuntary muscle, which enables the splenic capsule to contract and also to withstand some swelling.

Considering its size, the spleen has an unusually large blood supply. The organ is filled with a soft pulp that filters the blood. It also harbors phagocytes and lympho-

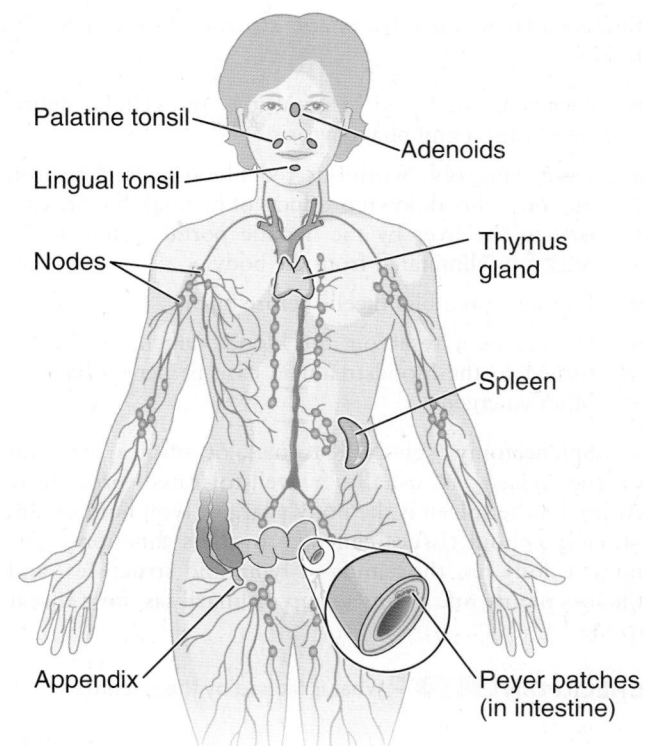

Figure 16-6 **Location of lymphoid tissue.**

Labels: Palatine tonsil, Adenoids, Lingual tonsil, Nodes, Thymus gland, Spleen, Appendix, Peyer patches (in intestine)

cytes, which are active in immunity. The spleen is classified as part of the lymphatic system because it contains prominent masses of lymphoid tissue. However, it has wider

---

Box 16-2   Hot Topics

Sentinel Node Biopsy: Finding Cancer Before It Spreads

Ordinarily, the lymphatic system is one of the body's primary defenses against disease. In cancer, though, it can be a vehicle for the spread (metastasis) of disease. When cancer cells enter the lymphatic vessels, they travel to other parts of the body, where they may establish new tumors. Along the way, some cancer cells become lodged in the lymph nodes.

In breast cancer, the degree of invasion of nearby lymph nodes helps determine what treatments are required after surgical removal of the tumor. Until recently, a mastectomy often included the removal of nearby lymphatic vessels and nodes (a procedure called axillary lymph node dissection). Biopsy of the nodes determined whether or not they contained cancerous cells. If they did, radiation treatment or chemotherapy was required. In many women with early-stage breast cancer, however, the axillary bodies do not contain cancerous cells. In addition, about 20% of the women

whose lymphatic vessels and nodes have been removed suffer impaired lymph flow, resulting in lymphedema, pain, disability, and an increased risk of infection.

Sentinel node biopsy is a diagnostic procedure that may minimize the need to perform axillary lymph node dissection, while still detecting metastasis. Surgeons use radioactive tracers to identify the first nodes that receive lymph from the area of a tumor. Biopsy of only these "sentinel nodes" reveals whether tumor cells are present, providing the earliest indication of metastasis. Research shows that sentinel lymph node biopsy is associated with less pain, fewer complications, and faster recovery than axillary lymph node dissection. However, clinical trials are ongoing to determine whether sentinel node biopsy is as successful as axillary dissection in finding cancer before it spreads.

16

functions than other lymphatic structures, including the following:

- Cleansing the blood of impurities and cellular debris by filtration and phagocytosis.
- Destroying old, worn-out red blood cells. The iron and other breakdown products of hemoglobin are carried to the liver by the hepatic portal system to be reused or eliminated from the body.
- Producing red blood cells before birth.
- Serving as a reservoir for blood, which can be returned to the bloodstream in case of hemorrhage or other emergency.

Splenectomy (sple-NEK-to-me), or surgical removal of the spleen, is usually a well-tolerated procedure. Although the spleen is the body's largest lymphoid organ, other lymphoid tissues can take over its functions. The human body has thousands of lymphoid structures, and the loss of any one or any group ordinarily is not a threat to life.

CHECKPOINT 16-5 ➤ What is filtered by the spleen?

The Thymus

Because of its appearance under a microscope, the **thymus** (THI-mus), located in the superior thorax deep to the sternum, traditionally has been considered part of the lymphoid system (see Fig. 16-6). Recent studies, however, suggest that this structure has a much wider function than other lymphoid tissue. It appears that the thymus plays a key role in immune system development before birth and during the first few months of infancy. Certain lymphocytes must mature in the thymus gland before they can perform their functions in the immune system (see Chapter 17). These T cells (T lymphocytes) develop under the effects of the thymus gland hormone called **thymosin** (THI-mo-sin), which also promotes lymphocyte growth and lymphoid tissue activity throughout the body. Removal of the thymus causes a generalized decrease in the production of T cells, as well as a decrease in the size of the spleen and of lymph nodes throughout the body.

The thymus is most active during early life. After puberty, the tissue undergoes changes; it shrinks in size and is replaced by connective tissue and fat.

CHECKPOINT 16-6 ➤ What kind of immune system cells develop in the thymus?

The Tonsils

The **tonsils** are unencapsulated masses of lymphoid tissue located in the vicinity of the pharynx (throat) where they remove contaminants from materials that are inhaled or swallowed (Fig. 16-7). The tonsils have deep grooves lined with lymphatic nodules. Lymphocytes attack pathogens

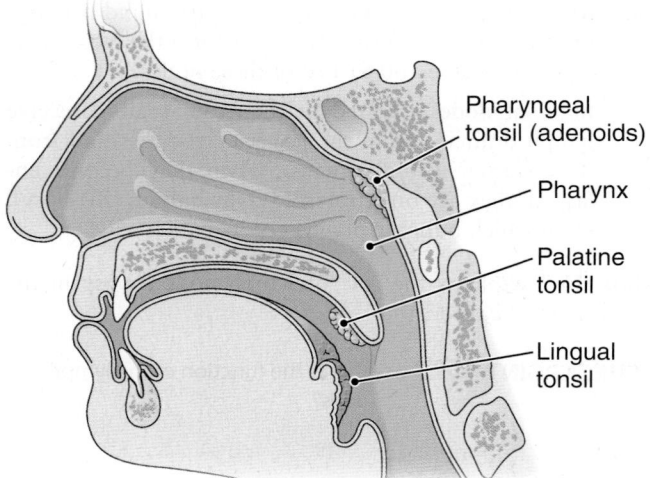

Figure 16-7   Location of the tonsils. All are in the vicinity of the pharynx (throat).

trapped in these grooves. The tonsils are located in three areas:

- The **palatine** (PAL-ah-tine) **tonsils** are oval bodies located at each side of the soft palate. These are generally what is meant when one refers to "the tonsils."
- The single **pharyngeal** (fah-RIN-je-al) **tonsil** is commonly referred to as the **adenoids** (from a general term that means "gland-like"). It is located behind the nose on the posterior wall of the upper pharynx.
- The **lingual** (LING-gwal) **tonsils** are little mounds of lymphoid tissue at the posterior of the tongue.

Any of these tonsils may become so loaded with bacteria that they become reservoirs for repeated infections and their removal is advisable. In children, a slight enlargement of any of them is not an indication for surgery, however, because all lymphoid tissue masses tend to be larger in childhood. A physician must determine whether these masses are abnormally enlarged, taking the patient's age into account, because the tonsils function in immunity during early childhood. Surgery is considered if there is recurrent infection or if the enlarged tonsils make swallowing or breathing difficult. Their removal may also help children suffering from otitis media, because bacteria infecting the tonsils may travel to the middle ear. The surgery to remove the palatine tonsils is a tonsillectomy; an adenoidectomy is removal of the adenoids. Often these two procedures are done together and abbreviated as T & A. Most tonsillectomies are performed by electrocautery, which uses an electric current to burn the tissue away. A newer technique, which allows faster recovery and fewer complications, uses radiowaves to break down the tonsillar tissue.

CHECKPOINT 16-7 ➤ Tonsils filter tissue fluid. What is the general location of the tonsils?

Other Lymphoid Tissue

The **appendix** (ah-PEN-diks) is a fingerlike tube of lymphatic tissue, measuring approximately 8 cm (3 inches) long. It is attached, or "appended" to the first portion of the large intestine (see Fig. 16-6). Like the tonsils, it seems to be noticed only when it becomes infected, causing appendicitis. The appendix may, however, figure in the development of immunity, as do the tonsils.

In the mucous membranes lining portions of the digestive, respiratory, and urogenital tracts, there are areas of lymphatic tissue that help destroy outside contaminants. By means of phagocytosis and production of antibodies, substances that counteract infectious agents, this **m**ucosal-associated lymphatic tissue, or MALT, prevents microorganisms from invading deeper tissues.

Peyer (PI-er) **patches** are part of the MALT system. These clusters of lymphoid nodules are located in the mucous membranes lining the distal small intestine. Peyer patches, along with the tonsils and appendix, are included in the specific network known as GALT, or **g**ut-associated lymphoid tissue. All of these lymphatic tissues associated with mucous membranes are now recognized as an important first barrier against invading microorganisms.

The Reticuloendothelial System

The **reticuloendothelial** (reh-tik-u-lo-en-do-THE-le-al) **system** consists of related cells responsible for the destruction of worn-out blood cells, bacteria, cancer cells, and other foreign substances that are potentially harmful. Included among these cells are monocytes, relatively large white blood cells (see Fig. 13-4E in Chapter 13) that are formed in the bone marrow and then circulate in the bloodstream to various areas. Upon entering the tissues, monocytes develop into **macrophages** (MAK-ro-faj-ez), a term that means "big eaters."

Macrophages in some organs are given special names; **Kupffer** (KOOP-fer) **cells**, for example, are located in the lining of the liver sinusoids (blood channels). Other parts of the reticuloendothelial system are found in the spleen, bone marrow, lymph nodes, and brain. Some macro-phages are located in the lungs, where they are called *dust cells* because they ingest solid particles that enter the lungs; others are found in soft connective tissues all over the body.

This widely distributed protective system has been called by several other names, including tissue macrophage system, mononuclear phagocyte system, and monocyte-macrophage system. These names describe the type of cells found within this system.

Disorders of the Lymphatic System and Lymphoid Tissue

Lymphangitis (lim-fan-JI-tis), which is inflammation of lymphatic vessels, usually begins in the region of an infected and neglected injury and can be seen as red streaks extending along an extremity. Such inflamed vessels are a sign that bacteria have spread into the lymphatic system. If the lymph nodes are not able to stop the infection, pathogens may enter the bloodstream, causing **septicemia** (sep-tih-SE-me-ah), or blood poisoning. Streptococci often are the invading organisms in such cases.

In **lymphadenitis** (lim-fad-en-I-tis), or inflammation of the lymph nodes, the nodes become enlarged and tender. This condition reflects the body's attempt to combat an infection. Cervical lymphadenitis occurs during measles, scarlet fever, septic sore throat, diphtheria, and, frequently, the common cold. Chronic lymphadenitis may be caused by the bacillus that causes tuberculosis. Infections of the upper extremities cause enlarged axillary nodes, as does breast cancer. Infections of the external genitals or the lower extremities may cause enlargement of the inguinal lymph nodes.

Lymphedema

Edema is tissue swelling due to excess fluid. The condition has a variety of causes, but edema due to obstruction of lymph flow is called **lymphedema** (lim-feh-DE-mah). Possible causes of lymphedema include infection of the lymphatic vessels, a malignant growth that obstructs lymph flow, or loss of lymphatic vessels and nodes as a result of injury or surgery. Areas affected by lymphedema are more prone to infection because the lymphatic system's filtering activity is diminished. Mechanical methods to improve drainage and drugs to promote water loss are possible treatments for lymphedema (see Box 16-1, Lymphedema).

As mentioned in Chapter 5, **elephantiasis** is a great enlargement of the lower extremities resulting from lymphatic vessel blockage by small worms called **filariae** (fi-LA-re-e). These tiny parasites, carried by insects such as flies and mosquitoes, invade the tissues as embryos or immature forms. They then grow in the lymph channels and obstruct lymphatic flow. The swelling of the legs or, as sometimes happens in men, the scrotum, may be so great that the victim becomes incapacitated. This disease is especially common in certain parts of Asia and in some of the Pacific islands. No cure is known.

Lymphadenopathy

Lymphadenopathy (lim-fad-en-OP-ah-the) is a term meaning "disease of the lymph nodes." Enlarged lymph nodes are a common symptom in a number of infectious and cancerous diseases. For example, generalized lymphadenopathy is an early sign of infection with HIV (human immunodeficiency virus), the virus that causes AIDS (acquired immunodeficiency syndrome). **Infectious mononucleosis** (mon-o-nu-kle-O-sis) is an acute viral infection, the hallmark of which is a marked enlargement of the cervical lymph nodes. Mononucleosis is fairly common among college students. Enlarged lymph nodes are commonly referred to as glands, as in "swollen glands." However, they do not produce secretions and are not glands.

16

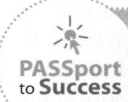

Visit *thePoint* or see the Student Resource CD in the back of this book for a picture of cervical lymphadenopathy.

Splenomegaly

Enlargement of the spleen, known as **splenomegaly** (sple-no-MEG-ah-le), accompanies certain acute infectious diseases, including scarlet fever, typhus fever, typhoid fever, and syphilis. Many tropical parasitic diseases cause splenomegaly. A certain blood fluke (flatworm) that is fairly common among workers in Japan and other parts of Asia causes marked splenic enlargement.

Splenic anemia is characterized by enlargement of the spleen, hemorrhages from the stomach, and fluid accumulation in the abdomen. In this and other similar diseases, splenectomy appears to constitute a cure.

Lymphoma

Lymphoma (lim-FO-mah) is any tumor, benign or malignant, that occurs in lymphoid tissue. Two examples of malignant lymphoma are described next.

Hodgkin disease is a chronic malignant disease of lymphoid tissue, especially the lymph nodes. The incidence of this disease rises in two age groups: in the early 20s among both men and women, and again after age 50, more commonly among men. The cause is unknown, but in some cases may involve a viral infection. Hodgkin disease appears as painless enlargement of a lymph node or close group of nodes, often in the neck, but also in the armpit, thorax, and groin. It may spread throughout the lymphatic system and eventually to other systems if not controlled by treatment. Early signs are weight loss, fever, night sweats, fatigue, anemia, and decline in immune defenses. A clear sign of the disease is the presence of Reed-Sternberg cells in lymph node biopsy tissue (Fig. 16-8). Chemotherapy and radiotherapy, either separately or in

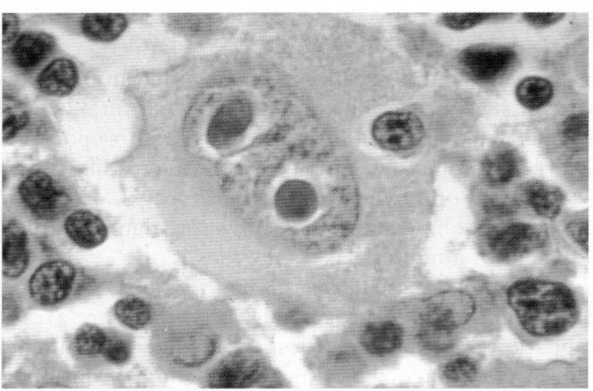

Figure 16-8 Reed-Sternberg cell characteristic of Hodgkin disease. A typical cell has two nuclei with large, dark-staining nucleoli. (Reprinted with permission from Rubin E, Farber JL. *Pathology*, 3rd ed. Philadelphia: Lippincott Williams & Wilkins, 1999.)

combination, have been used with good results, affording patients many years of life.

Non-Hodgkin lymphoma is more common than Hodgkin disease. It appears mostly in older adults and patients with deficient immune systems, such as those with AIDS. Enlargement of the lymph nodes (lymphadenopathy), especially in the cervical region, is an early sign in many cases. It is more widespread through the lymphatic system than Hodgkin disease and spreads more readily to other tissues, such as the liver. Like Hodgkin disease, it may be related to a viral infection. It shares many of the same symptoms as are seen in Hodgkin disease, but there are no Reed-Sternberg cells on biopsy. The current cure rate with chemotherapy and radiation is approximately 50%.

CHECKPOINT 16-8 ➤ What is lymphadenopathy?

CHECKPOINT 16-9 ➤ What is lymphoma and what are two examples of malignant lymphoma?

Disease in Context revisited

➤ Mike's Splenectomy

Mike lay in his hospital bed thinking about the past couple of days. After the surgery, his doctor had explained that removal of his spleen had been necessary because it had ruptured during the car accident. He was still coming to terms with what that meant. In fact, until today, he wasn't even sure what the spleen was!

Earlier in the morning, Mike's physician came by to check in on him. During their conversation, Mike learned that the spleen is a bean-shaped purple organ about the size of a large bar of soap. It is normally located underneath the diaphragm in the upper left part of the abdomen. Given how little he knew about it, Mike was surprised to learn that one of the spleen's functions is to filter foreign substances from the blood and remove worn-out red blood cells. "You mean it's like an oil filter on a car?" asked Mike. "Sort of," replied the doctor. "But don't worry, other parts of your circulatory system will help clean your blood now."

Mike also learned that the spleen acts like a large lymph node, detecting and fighting disease-causing organisms. "So, now that my spleen is gone, am I going to be sick all the time?" asked Mike. "Well," answered the doctor, "As you recover, you'll need to take antibiotics to reduce the risk of infection. In the long term, if you have a fever or any sign of illness, come see me right away. In addition, make sure that you get your yearly flu vaccinations."

During this case, we saw that the spleen filters blood and protects the body from harmful organisms. In Chapter 17, we'll learn more about how certain blood cells and the lymphatic system protect us from disease.

Word Anatomy

Medical terms are built from standardized word parts (prefixes, roots, and suffixes). Learning the meanings of these parts can help you remember words and interpret unfamiliar terms.

WORD PART	MEANING	EXAMPLE
Lymphoid Tissue		
–oid	like, resembling	*Lymphoid* tissue makes up the specialized organs of the lymphatic system.
aden/o	gland	The *adenoids* are gland-like tonsils.
lingu/o	tongue	The *lingual* tonsils are at the back of the tongue.
Disorders of the Lymphatic System and Lymphoid Tissue		
-pathy	any disease	*Lymphadenopathy* is any disease of the lymph nodes.
-megaly	excessive enlargement	*Splenomegaly* is excessive enlargement of the spleen.

Summary

I. **LYMPHATIC SYSTEM**
   A. Functions
      1. Fluid balance—drains excess fluid and proteins from the tissues and returns them to the blood
      2. Protection from infection
         a. Lymphocytes fight foreign organisms
         b. Lymphoid tissue filters body fluids
      3. Absorption of fats—lacteals absorb digested fats from small intestine

II. **LYMPHATIC CIRCULATION**
   A. Lymphatic capillaries
      1. Made of endothelium (simple squamous epithelium)
      2. More permeable than blood capillaries
      3. Overlapping cells form one-way valves
   B. Lymphatic vessels
      1. Superficial and deep sets
      2. Right lymphatic duct
         a. Drains upper right part of body
         b. Empties into right subclavian vein
      3. Thoracic duct
         a. Drains remainder of body
         b. Empties into left subclavian vein
   C. Movement of lymph
      1. Valves in vessels
      2. Contraction of vessels
      3. Skeletal muscle contraction
      4. Breathing

III. **LYMPHOID TISSUE**
   A. Lymph nodes
      1. Along path of lymphatic vessels
      2. Filter lymph
   B. Spleen
      1. Filtration of blood
      2. Destruction of old red cells
      3. Production of red cells before birth
      4. Storage of blood
   C. Thymus
      1. Processing of T lymphocytes (T cells)
      2. Secretion of thymosin—stimulates T lymphocytes in lymphoid tissue

   D. Tonsils
      1. Filter swallowed and inhaled material
      2. Located near pharynx (throat)
         a. Palatine—near soft palate
         b. Pharyngeal (adenoids)—behind nose
         c. Lingual—back of tongue
   E. Other
      1. Appendix—attached to large intestine
      2. Mucosal—associated lymphoid tissue (MALT)
         a. Gut-associated lymphoid tissue (GALT)
            (1) Example—Peyer patches in lining of small intestine

IV. **THE RETICULOENDOTHELIAL SYSTEM**
   A. Cells throughout body that remove impurities
   B. Macrophages
      1. From monocytes
      2. Localize and given special names—e.g., Kuppfer cells, dust cells

V. **DISORDERS OF THE LYMPHATIC SYSTEM AND LYMPHOID TISSUE**
   A. Inflammations
      1. Lymphangitis—inflammation of lymphatic vessels
      2. Lymphadenitis—inflammation of lymph nodes that occurs during infection
   B. Lymphedema—swelling due to obstruction of lymph flow
      1. Removal of lymph nodes and vessels by injury, surgery
      2. Infection—e.g., elephantiasis caused by filariae (parasitic worms)
   C. Lymphadenopathy—disease of lymph nodes
   D. Splenomegaly—enlargement of the spleen
   E. Lymphoma—tumor of lymphoid tissue
      1. Hodgkin disease—chronic malignancy with enlarged lymph nodes
      2. Non-Hodgkin lymphoma—more common in older adults

Questions for Study and Review

BUILDING UNDERSTANDING

Fill in the blanks

1. The fluid that circulates in the lymphatic system is called _____.

2. Digested fats enter the lymphatic circulation through vessels called_____.

3. Fat globules and lymph combine to form a milky fluid called _____.

4. Surgical removal of the spleen is termed _____.

5. When filariae block lymphatic vessels they cause the disease called _____.

Matching > Match each numbered item with the most closely related lettered item.

___ **6.** Inflammation of lymphatic vessels

___ **7.** Inflammation of lymph nodes

___ **8.** Fluid retention due to obstruction of lymph vessels

___ **9.** Tumor that occurs in lymphoid tissue

a. lymphoma

b. lymphangitis

c. lymphedema

d. lymphadenitis

Multiple choice

___ **10.** Compared to plasma, lymph contains much less
   a. fat
   b. protein
   c. carbohydrate
   d. water

___ **11.** Lymph from the lower extremities returns to the cardiovascular system via the
   a. cisterna chyli
   b. right lymphatic duct
   c. thymus
   d. thoracic duct

___ **12.** Macrophages and monocytes found throughout the body make up the
   a. tonsils
   b. Peyer patches
   c. reticuloendothelial system
   d. appendix

___ **13.** The hallmark clinical sign of infectious mononucleosis is:
   a. splenomegaly
   b. lymphadenopathy
   c. lymphangitis
   d. edema

UNDERSTANDING CONCEPTS

14. How does the structure of lymphatic capillaries correlate with their function? List some differences between lymphatic and blood capillaries.

15. Describe three mechanisms that propel lymph through the lymphatic vessels.

16. Trace a globule of fat from a lacteal in the small intestine to the right atrium.

17. Describe the structure of a typical lymph node.

18. State the location of the spleen and list several of its functions.

19. Describe two forms of lymphoma.

CONCEPTUAL THINKING

20. Explain the absence of arteries in the lymphatic circulatory system.

21. In Mike's second case, he presented with hypotension and tachycardia due to a ruptured spleen. Explain how a ruptured spleen can cause these disorders.

22. In the case story, why was Mike treated with antibiotics and vaccinated for influenza following his splenectomy?

16

CHAPTER 17

Body Defenses, Immunity, and Vaccines

Learning Outcomes

After careful study of this chapter, you should be able to:

1. List the factors that determine the occurrence of infection
2. Differentiate between nonspecific and specific body defenses and give examples of each
3. Briefly describe the inflammatory reaction
4. List several types of innate immunity
5. Define *antigen* and *antibody*
6. Compare T cells and B cells with respect to development and type of activity
7. Explain the role of macrophages in immunity
8. Describe some protective effects of an antigen–antibody reaction
9. Differentiate between natural and artificial adaptive immunity
10. Differentiate between active and passive immunity
11. Define the term *vaccine* and give several examples of vaccines
12. Define the term *immune serum* and give several examples of immune sera
13. List several disorders of the immune system
14. Explain the possible role of the immune system in preventing cancer
15. Explain the role of the immune system in tissue transplantation
16. Show how word parts are used to build words related to body defenses, immunity, and vaccines (see Word Anatomy at the end of the chapter)

Selected Key Terms

The following terms and other boldface terms in the chapter are defined in the Glossary

allergy
anaphylaxis
antibody
antigen
antiserum
attenuated
autoimmunity
B cell
complement
gamma globulin
immunity
immunization
immunodeficiency
inflammation
interferon
interleukin
lymphocyte
macrophage
plasma cell
T cell
toxin
toxoid
transplantation
vaccine

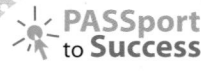

PASSport to Success

Visit *thePoint* or see the Student Resource CD in the back of this book for definitions and pronunciations of key terms as well as a pretest for this chapter.

Disease in Context

➤ Maria's Second Case: Fighting Back Against Disease

"Hi there," the receptionist called out, as Maria Sanchez entered the senior personal care facility where she worked. "You've been out a while."

"Yes," said Maria, "over a week; a run-in with the flu."

"I suppose you're still on antibiotics then," added the receptionist.

"No," Maria replied. "Antibiotics don't work against viruses. It was just the old rest, fluids, and aspirin solution for me." Maria hung up her coat, changed out of her boots, and moved on toward the activities center to resume her duties as coordinator. Her assistant, Anna, was already there.

"So good to have you back, Maria. The residents say that things aren't the same without you," declared Anna. "You look a little pale, though. Are you feeling okay?"

"Pretty good, said Maria, "but I hope I don't have to go through that flu again."

"Well, the staff doctor is coming in this afternoon to give the residents their flu shots. Why don't you ask him about getting one yourself this time?" Anna suggested.

Later that day, the physician agreed that Maria should be included in the group getting immunized against the flu. "I've already had the flu. Aren't I immune now?" Maria asked.

"Not necessarily," replied Dr. Andrews. "Because there are many strains of the influenza virus around, you could still pick up an infection with another variety. You're not allergic to eggs are you?"

"No, but why do you ask?" Maria wanted to know.

"Well," explained Dr. Andrews, "even though newer methods of producing the vaccine are under development, the vaccine we're using now is still made the old-fashioned way by growing the virus in fertilized chicken eggs. There's another form of the vaccine given as a nasal spray, but in the older population, we still use the injectable one."

"Okay," said Maria, "shoot."

In Chapter 5 we followed the path of Maria's influenza virus infection. Later in this chapter, we'll learn how her body responds to the flu vaccine and how well the vaccine will protect her from another bout of the disease.

Chapter 5 presents a rather frightening list of harmful organisms that surround us in our environment. Fortunately, most of us survive contact with these invaders and even become more resistant to disease in the process. The job of protecting us from these harmful agents belongs in part to certain blood cells and to the lymphatic system, which together make up our **immune system**.

The immune system is part of our general body defenses against disease. Some of these defenses are **nonspecific**; that is, they are effective against any harmful agent that enters the body. Other defenses are referred to as **specific**; that is, they act only against a certain agent and no others.

Why Do Infections Occur?

Although the body is constantly exposed to pathogenic invasion, many conditions determine whether an infection will actually occur. Pathogens have a decided preference for certain body tissues and must have access to these tissues. The polio virus, for example, may be inhaled or swallowed in large numbers and at first may come into direct contact with the mucous membranes lining the respiratory and digestive tracts. However, it causes no apparent disorder of these tissues but goes on to attack only nervous tissue. In contrast, the viruses that cause influenza and the common cold do attack the respiratory mucous membranes. HIV, the virus that causes AIDS, attacks a certain type of T cell (T-lymphocyte) which has surface receptors for the virus.

The **portal of entry** is an important condition influencing infection. The respiratory tract is a common entrance route for pathogens. Other important entry points include the digestive system and the tubes that open into the urinary and reproductive systems. Any break in the skin or in a mucous membrane allows organisms such as staphylococci easy access to deeper tissues and may lead to infection, whereas unbroken skin or mucous membranes are usually not affected.

The **virulence** (VIR-u-lens) of an organism, or the organism's power to overcome its host's defenses, is another important factor. Virulence has two aspects: one may be thought of as "aggressiveness," or invasive power; the other is the organism's ability to produce **toxins** (poisons) that damage the body. Different organisms vary in virulence. A specific organism's virulence also can change; variants of the influenza virus, for example, can be more dangerous in some years than in others. Organisms may gain virulence as they pass from one infected host to another.

The **dose** (number) of pathogens that invade the body also is a determining factor in whether or not an infection develops. Even if the virulence of a particular organism happens to be low, infection may occur if a large number enter the body.

Finally, an individual's condition, or **predisposition**, to infection is also important. Disease organisms are around us all the time. Why does a person only occasion-

ally get a cold, flu, or other infection? Part of the answer lies in the person's condition, as influenced by general physical and emotional health, nutrition, living habits, and age.

CHECKPOINT 17-1 ➤ What are some factors that influence the occurrence of infection?

Nonspecific Defenses

The features that protect the body against disease are usually considered as successive "lines of defense," beginning with the relatively simple or outer barriers and proceeding through progressively more complicated responses until the ultimate defense mechanism—immunity—is reached.

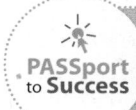 **PASSport to Success** Visit **thePoint** or see the Student Resource CD in the back of this book for illustrations of nonspecific defenses.

Chemical and Mechanical Barriers

The first line of defense against invaders includes:

- The skin serves as a mechanical barrier as long as it remains intact. A serious danger to burn victims, for example, is the risk of infection as a result of skin destruction.

- The mucous membranes that line the passageways leading into the body also act as barriers, trapping foreign material in their sticky secretions. The cilia in membranes in the upper respiratory tract help to sweep impurities out of the body.

- Body secretions, such as tears, perspiration, and saliva, wash away microorganisms and may contain acids, enzymes, or other chemicals that destroy invaders. Digestive juices destroy many ingested bacteria and their toxins.

- Certain reflexes aid in the removal of pathogens. Sneezing and coughing, for instance, tend to remove foreign matter, including microorganisms, from the upper respiratory tract. Vomiting and diarrhea are ways in which toxins and bacteria may be expelled.

CHECKPOINT 17-2 ➤ What tissues constitute the first line of defense against the invasion of pathogens?

Phagocytosis

Phagocytosis is part of the second line of defense against invaders. In the process of phagocytosis, white blood cells take in and destroy waste and foreign material (see Fig. 13-6 in Chapter 13). Neutrophils and macrophages are the main phagocytic white blood cells. Neutrophils are a type of granular leukocyte. Macrophages are derived from monocytes, a type of agranular leukocyte. Both kinds of cells travel in the blood to infection sites. Some of the macrophages remain fixed in the tissues, for example, in the skin, liver, lungs, lymphoid tissue, and bone marrow, to fight infection and remove debris. Macrophages were mentioned in Chapter 16 as part of the reticuloendothelial system.

Natural Killer Cells

The **natural killer (NK) cell** is a type of lymphocyte different from those active in specific immunity, which are described later. NK cells can recognize body cells with abnormal membranes, such as tumor cells and cells infected with virus, and, as their name indicates, can destroy them on contact. NK cells are found in the lymph nodes, spleen, bone marrow, and blood. They destroy abnormal cells by secreting a protein that breaks down the cell membrane, but the way in which they find their targets is not yet completely understood.

Inflammation

Inflammation is a nonspecific defensive response to a tissue-damaging irritant. Any irritant can cause inflammation: friction, x-rays, fire, extreme temperatures, and wounds, as well as caustic chemicals and contact with allergens—all can be classified as irritants. Often, however, inflammation results from irritation caused by infection. With the entrance and multiplication of pathogens, a whole series of defensive processes begins. This **inflammatory reaction** is accompanied by four classic symptoms: heat, redness, swelling, and pain, as described below.

When tissues are injured, damaged cells release **histamine** (HIS-tah-mene) and other substances that cause the small blood vessels to dilate (widen). They also release attractant substances that bring a variety of white blood cells to the area, including granulocytes, macrophages, and **mast cells**, which are similar to basophils but reside in the tissues. These cells also secrete vasodilators and other substances that promote and prolong the inflammatory response. Increased blood flow causes heat, redness, and swelling in the tissues. Some of these substances also irritate pain receptors.

The cellular secretions then cause the epithelial cells in the capillary walls to contract, thus widening the gaps between the cells and increasing permeability. As blood flows through the vessels, leukocytes move through these altered walls and into the tissue, where they can reach the irritant directly. Fluid from the blood plasma also leaks out of the vessels into the tissues and begins to clot, thus limiting the spread of infection to other areas. The mixture of leukocytes and fluid, the **inflammatory exudate**, contributes to swelling and puts pressure on nerve endings, adding to the pain of inflammation.

Phagocytes are destroyed in large numbers as they work, and dead cells gradually accumulate in the area.

The mixture of exudate, living and dead white blood cells, pathogens, and destroyed tissue cells is **pus**.

Meanwhile, the lymphatic vessels begin to drain fluid from the inflamed area and carry it toward the lymph nodes for filtration. The regional lymph nodes become enlarged and tender, a sign that they are performing their protective function by working overtime to produce phagocytic cells that "clean" the lymph flowing through them.

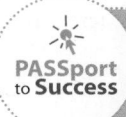 Visit **thePoint** or see the Student Resource CD in the back of this book for a diagram summarizing the events in inflammation and for the animation *Acute Inflammation*.

Fever

An increase in body temperature above the normal range can be a sign that body defenses are active. When phagocytes are exposed to infecting organisms, they release substances that raise body temperature. Fever boosts the immune system in several ways. It stimulates phagocytes, increases metabolism, and decreases certain disease organisms' ability to multiply.

A common misperception is that fever is a dangerous symptom that should always be eliminated. Control of fever in itself does little to alter the course of an illness. Healthcare workers, however, should always be alert to fever development as a possible sign of a serious disorder and should recognize that an increased metabolic rate may have adverse effects on a weak patient's heart.

Interferon

Certain cells infected with a virus release a substance that prevents nearby cells from producing more virus. This substance was first found in cells infected with influenza virus, and it was called **interferon** because it "interferes" with multiplication and spread of the virus. Interferon is now known to be a group of substances. Each is abbreviated IFN with a Greek letter, alpha (α), beta (β), or gamma (γ), to indicate the category of interferon and additional letters or numbers to indicate more specific types, such as α2a or β1b.

Pure interferons are now available in adequate quantities for treatment because they are produced by genetic engineering in microorganisms. They are used to treat certain viral infections, such as hepatitis. Interferons are also of interest because they act nonspecifically on cells of the immune system. They have been used with varying success to boost the immune response in the treatment of malignancies, such as melanoma, leukemia, and Kaposi sarcoma, a cancer associated with AIDS. Interestingly, interferon β is used to treat the autoimmune disorder multiple sclerosis (MS), because it stimulates cells that depress the immune response.

CHECKPOINT 17-3 ➤ What are some nonspecific factors that help to control infection?

17

Immunity

Immunity is the final line of defense against disease. Immunity to disease can be defined as an individual's power to resist or overcome the effects of a *particular* disease agent or its harmful products. In a broader sense, the immune system will recognize *any* foreign material and attempt to get rid of it, as occurs in tissue transplantation from one individual to another. Immunity is a selective process; that is, immunity to one disease does not necessarily cause immunity to another. This selective characteristic is called **specificity** (spes-ih-FIS-ih-te).

There are two main categories of immunity:

- **Innate immunity** is inborn and is inherited along with other characteristics in a person's genes.

- **Adaptive immunity** develops after birth. Adaptive immunity may be acquired by **natural** or **artificial** means; in addition, it may be either **active** or **passive**.

Figure 17-1 summarizes the different types of immunity. Refer to this diagram as we investigate each category in turn.

Innate Immunity

Both humans and animals have what is called a **species immunity** to many of each other's diseases. Although certain diseases found in animals may be transmitted to humans, many infections, such as chicken cholera, hog cholera, distemper, and other animal diseases, do not affect human beings. However, the constitutional differences that make human beings immune to these disorders also make them susceptible to others that do not affect different species. Such infections as measles, scarlet fever, and diphtheria do not appear to affect animals who come in contact with infected humans.

Some members of a given group have a more highly developed **individual immunity** to specific diseases. For example, some people are prone to cold sores (fever blisters) caused by herpes virus, whereas others have never shown signs of this infection. Newspapers and magazines sometimes feature the advice of an elderly person who is asked to give his or her secret for living to a ripe old age. Some elderly people may say that they lived a carefully regulated life with the right amount of rest, exercise, and work, whereas others may boast of drinking alcohol, smoking, not exercising, and other kinds of unhealthy behavior. However, it is possible that the latter group resisted infection and maintained health despite their habits, rather than because of them, thanks to inherited resistance factors.

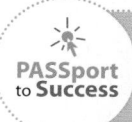 **PASSport to Success** Visit *thePoint* or see the Student Resource CD in the back of this book for the animation *Immune Response*, which illustrates the following reactions.

Adaptive Immunity

Unlike innate immunity, which is due to inherited factors, adaptive immunity develops during a person's lifetime as that person encounters various specific harmful agents.

If the following description of the immune system seems complex, bear in mind that from infancy on, your immune system is able to protect you from millions of foreign substances, even synthetic substances not found in nature. All the while, the system is kept in check, so that it does not usually overreact to produce allergies or mistakenly attack and damage your own body tissues.

CHECKPOINT 17-4 ➤ What is the difference between innate and adaptive immunity?

ANTIGENS An **antigen** (AN-te-jen) (**Ag**) is any foreign substance that enters the body and induces an immune response. (The word is formed from *anti*body + *gen* because an antigen stimulates antibody production.) Most antigens are large protein molecules, but carbohydrates and some lipids may act as antigens. Antigens may be found on the surface of pathogenic organisms,

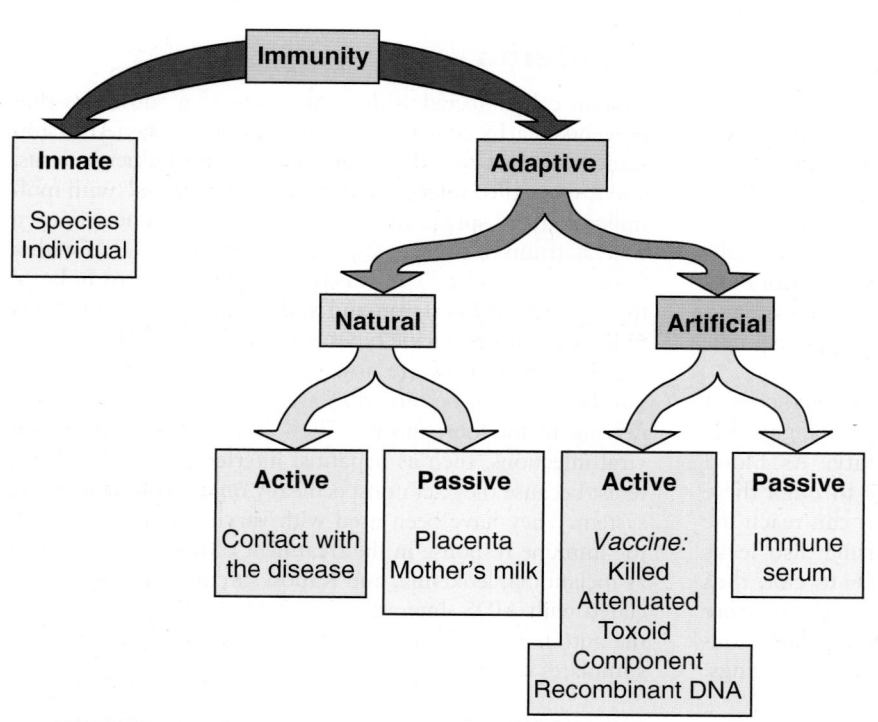

Figure 17-1 **Types of immunity.**

on the surface of red blood cells and tissue cells, on pollens, in toxins, and in foods. The critical feature of any substance described as an antigen is that it stimulates the activity of certain lymphocytes classified as T or B cells.

T CELLS Both T and B cells come from hematopoietic (blood-forming) stem cells in bone marrow, as do all blood cells. The T and B cells differ, however, in their development and their method of action. Some of the immature stem cells migrate to the thymus and become T cells, which constitute about 80% of the lymphocytes in the circulating blood. While in the thymus, these T lymphocytes multiply and become capable of combining with specific foreign antigens, at which time they are described as **sensitized**. These thymus-derived cells produce an immunity that is said to be **cell-mediated** immunity.

There are several types of T cells, each with different functions. The different types and some of their functions are as follows:

- **Cytotoxic T cells** (T_c) destroy foreign cells directly.

- **Helper T cells** (T_h) release substances known as **interleukins** (in-ter-LU-kinz) (IL) that stimulate other lymphocytes and macrophages and thereby assist in the destruction of foreign cells. (These substances are so named because they act between white blood cells). There are several subtypes of these helper T cells, one of which is infected and destroyed by the AIDS virus (HIV). The HIV-targeted T cells have a special surface receptor (CD_4) to which the virus attaches.

- **Regulatory T cells** (T_{reg}) suppress the immune response in order to prevent overactivity. These T cells may inhibit or destroy active lymphocytes.

- **Memory T cells** remember an antigen and start a rapid response if that antigen is contacted again.

The T cell portion of the immune system is generally responsible for defense against cancer cells, certain viruses, and other pathogens that grow within cells (intracellular parasites), as well as for the rejection of tissue transplanted from another person.

The Role of Macrophages Macrophages are phagocytic white blood cells derived from monocytes (their name means "big eater"). They act as processing centers for foreign antigens. They ingest foreign proteins, such as disease organisms, and break them down within phagocytic vesicles (Fig. 17-2). They then insert fragments of the foreign antigen into their plasma membrane. The foreign antigens are displayed on the macrophage's surface in combination with antigens that a T cell can recognize as belonging to the "self." Self-antigens are known as MHC (major histocompatibility complex) antigens because of their importance in cross-matching for tissue transplantation. They are also known as HLAs (human leukocyte antigens), because white blood cells are used in testing tissues for compatibility. Macrophages and other cells that present antigens to T cells are known as APCs (antigen-presenting cells).

For a T cell to react with a foreign antigen, that antigen must be presented to the T cell along with the MHC proteins. A special receptor on the T cell must bind with both the MHC protein and the foreign antigen fragment (see Fig. 17-2). The activated T_h then produces interleukins (ILs), which stimulate other leukocytes, such as B cells. There are many different types of interleukins, and they participate at different points in the immune response. They are produced by white cells and also by fibroblasts (cells in connective tissue that produce fibers) and by epithelial cells. Because ILs stimulate the cells active in immunity, they are used medically to boost the immune system.

CHECKPOINT **17-5** ➤ What is an antigen?

CHECKPOINT **17-6** ➤ List four types of T cells.

B CELLS AND ANTIBODIES An **antibody** (Ab), also known as an **immunoglobulin** (Ig), is a substance produced in response to an antigen. Antibodies are manufactured by **B**

17

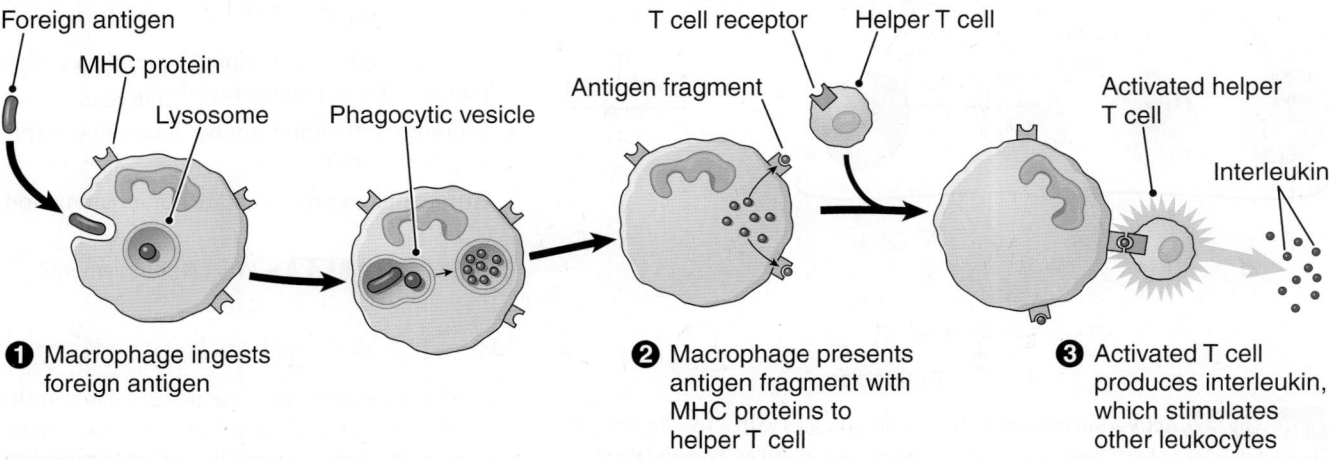

1 Macrophage ingests foreign antigen

2 Macrophage presents antigen fragment with MHC proteins to helper T cell

3 Activated T cell produces interleukin, which stimulates other leukocytes

Foreign antigen
MHC protein
Lysosome
Phagocytic vesicle
Antigen fragment
T cell receptor   Helper T cell
Activated helper T cell
Interleukin

Figure 17-2 **Activation of a helper T cell by a macrophage (antigen-presenting cell).** [ZOOMING IN ➤ What is contained in the lysosome that joins the phagocytic vesicle?]

cells (B lymphocytes), another type of lymphocyte active in the immune system. These cells must mature in the fetal liver or in lymphoid tissue before becoming active in the blood.

B cells have surface receptors that bind with a specific type of antigen (Fig. 17-3). Exposure to the antigen stimulates the cells to multiply rapidly and produce large numbers (clones) of **plasma cells**. These mature cells produce antibodies against the original antigen and release them into the blood, providing the form of immunity described as **humoral immunity** (the term *humoral* refers to body fluids).

Humoral immunity generally protects against circulating antigens and bacteria that grow outside the cells (extracellular pathogens). All antibodies are contained in a portion of the blood plasma called the **gamma globulin** fraction. Box 17-1, Antibodies, provides further information about the different types of antibodies.

Some antibodies produced by B cells remain in the blood to give long-term immunity. In addition, some of the activated B cells do not become plasma cells but, like certain T cells, become memory cells. On repeated contact with an antigen, these cells are ready to produce antibodies immediately. Because of this "immunologic memory," one is usually immune to a childhood disease after having it.

CHECKPOINT **17-7** ➤ What is an antibody?

CHECKPOINT **17-8** ➤ What type of cells produce antibodies?

The Antigen–Antibody Reaction

The antibody that is produced in response to a specific antigen, such as a bacterial cell or a toxin, has a shape that matches some part of that antigen, much in the same way that a key's shape matches the shape of its lock. The antibody can bind specifically to the antigen that caused its production and thereby destroy or inactivate it. Antigen–antibody interactions are illustrated and their protective effects are described in Table 17-1.

COMPLEMENT The destruction of foreign cells sometimes requires the enzymatic activity of a group of nonspecific proteins in the blood, together called **complement**. Complement proteins are always present in the blood, but they must be activated by antigen–antibody complexes or by foreign cell surfaces. Complement is so named because it assists with immune reactions. Some of complement's actions are to:

- Coat foreign cells to help phagocytes recognize and engulf them
- Destroy cells by forming complexes that punch holes in plasma membranes
- Promote inflammation by increasing capillary permeability
- Attract phagocytes to an area of inflammation

CHECKPOINT **17-9** ➤ What is complement?

Natural Adaptive Immunity

Adaptive immunity may be acquired naturally through contact with a specific disease organism, in which case, antibodies manufactured by the infected person's cells act against the infecting agent or its toxins. The infection that trig-

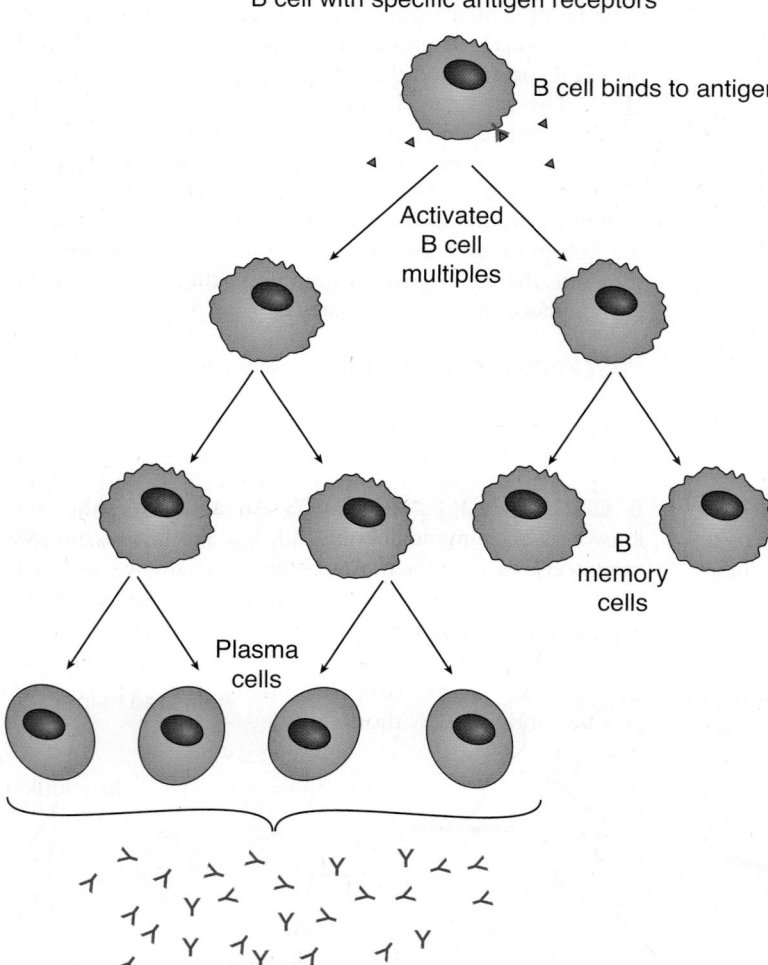

B cell with specific antigen receptors

B cell binds to antigen

Activated B cell multiples

B memory cells

Plasma cells

Antibodies

Figure 17-3 **Activation of B cells.** The B cell combines with a specific antigen. The cell divides to form plasma cells, which produce antibodies. Some of the cells develop into memory cells, which protect against reinfection. [**ZOOMING IN** ➤ What two types of cells develop from activated B cells?]

Box 17-1	A Closer Look

Antibodies: A Protein Army That Fights Disease

Antibodies are proteins secreted by plasma cells (activated B cells) in response to specific antigens. They are all contained in a fraction of the blood plasma known as gamma globulin. Because the plasma contains other globulins as well, antibodies have become known as immunoglobulins (Ig). Immunologic studies have shown that there are several classes of immunoglobulins that vary in molecular size and in function (see below). Studies of these antibody fractions can be helpful in making a diagnosis. For example, high levels of IgM antibodies, because they are the first to be produced in an immune response, indicate a recent infection.

Class	Abundance	Characteristics and Function
IgG	75%	Found in the blood, lymph, and intestines Enhances phagocytosis, neutralizes toxins, and activates complement Crosses the placenta and confers passive immunity from mother to fetus
IgA	15%	Found in glandular secretions such as sweat, tears, saliva, mucus, and digestive juices Provides local protection in mucous membranes against bacteria and viruses Also found in breast milk, providing passive immunity to newborn
IgM	5%–10%	Found in the blood and lymph The first antibody to be secreted after infection Stimulates agglutination and activates complement
IgD	<1%	Located on the surface of B cells
IgE	<0.1%	Located on basophils and mast cells Active in allergic reactions and parasitic infections

gers the immunity may be so mild as to cause no symptoms (is subclinical). Nevertheless, it stimulates the host's cells to produce an active immunity.

Each time a person is invaded by disease organisms, his or her cells manufacture antibodies that provide immunity against the infection. Such immunity may last for years, and in some cases for life. Because the host is actively involved in the production of antibodies, this type of immunity is called **active immunity**. See Box 17-2, Too Much Stress, for information on how stress affects the immune system.

Adaptive immunity also may be acquired naturally by the passage of antibodies from a mother to her fetus through the placenta. Because these antibodies come from an outside source, this type of immunity is called **passive immunity**. The antibodies obtained in this way do not last as long as actively produced antibodies, but they do help protect the infant for about 6 months, at which time the child's own immune system begins to function. Nursing an infant can lengthen this protective period because the mother's specific antibodies are present in her breast milk and colostrum (the first breast secretion). These are the only known examples of naturally acquired passive immunity.

CHECKPOINT 17-10 ➤ What is the difference between the active and passive forms of natural adaptive immunity?

Artificial Adaptive Immunity

A person who has not been exposed to repeated small doses of a particular organism has no antibodies against that organism and may be defenseless against infection. Therefore, medical personnel may use artificial measures to cause a person's immune system to manufacture antibodies. The administration of virulent pathogens obviously would be dangerous. Instead, laboratory workers treat the harmful agent to reduce its virulence before it is administered. In this way, the immune system is made to produce antibodies without causing a serious illness. This protective process is known as **vaccination** (vak-sin-A-shun), or **immunization**, and the solution used is called a **vaccine** (vak-SENE). Ordinarily, the administration of a vaccine is a preventive measure designed to provide protection in anticipation of invasion by a certain disease organism.

Originally, the word *vaccination* meant inoculation against smallpox. (The term even comes from the Latin word for *cow*, referring to cowpox, which is used to vaccinate against smallpox.) According to the World Health Organization, however, smallpox has now been eliminated as a result of widespread immunization programs. Mandatory vaccination has been discontinued because the chance of adverse side effects from the vaccine is thought

Table 17-1	Antigen–Antibody Interactions and Their Effects

Interaction	Effects
Prevention of attachment	A pathogen coated with antibody is prevented from attaching to a cell.
Clumping of antigen	Antibodies can link antigens together, forming a cluster that phagocytes can ingest.
Neutralization of toxins	Antibodies bind to toxin molecules to prevent them from damaging cells.
Help with phagocytosis	Phagocytes can attach more easily to antigens that are coated with antibody.
Activation of complement	When complement attaches to antibody on a cell surface, a series of reactions begins that activates complement to destroy cells.
Activation of NK cells	NK cells respond to antibody adhering to a cell surface and attack the cell.

to be greater than the probability of contracting the disease.

All vaccines carry a risk of adverse side effects and may be contraindicated in some cases. People who are immunosuppressed, for example, should not be given vaccines that contain live virus. Also, pregnant women should not receive live virus vaccine because the virus could cross the placenta and harm the fetus.

TYPES OF VACCINES Vaccines can be made with live organisms or with organisms killed by heat or chemicals. If live organisms are used, they must be nonvirulent for humans, such as the cowpox virus used for smallpox immunization, or they must be treated in the laboratory to

weaken them as human pathogens. An organism weakened for use in vaccines is described as **attenuated**. In some cases, just an antigenic component of the pathogen is used as a vaccine. Another type of vaccine is made from the toxin produced by a disease organism. The toxin is altered with heat or chemicals to reduce its harmfulness, but it can still function as an antigen to induce immunity. Such an altered toxin is called a **toxoid**.

The newest types of vaccines are produced from antigenic components of pathogens or by genetic engineering. By techniques of recombinant DNA, the genes for specific disease antigens are inserted into the genetic material of harmless organisms. The antigens produced by these organisms are extracted and purified and used for

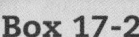 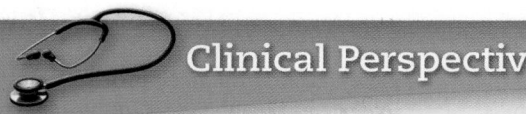

Box 17-2 **Clinical Perspectives**

Too Much Stress Makes the Immune System Sick

The impact of stress on the immune system is the most wide-ranging and significant of its many effects on the body. Stressors such as trauma, infection, debilitating disease, surgery, pain, extreme environmental conditions, and emotional distress all hamper immune function. The mechanisms responsible for these changes are not yet fully understood. Scientists do know that stress causes the hypothalamus to promote the release of ACTH from the anterior pituitary. This hormone stimulates the adrenal cortex to release the hormone cortisol, which influences a person's immediate ability to overcome any challenge, even stress itself. However, the abnormally high levels of cortisol that appear during periods of intense stress can actually be harmful. Such levels can:

- inhibit histamine release from damaged tissues, thereby blocking inflammation and the arrival of phagocytic leukocytes.
- reduce phagocytosis in damaged tissues, thus preventing antigen presentation to (and activation of) both killer T cells and helper T cells.
- inhibit interleukin secretion from helper T cells, thus preventing the immune system from mounting a coordinated response to infection.

---

immunization. The hepatitis B vaccine is produced in this manner.

BOOSTERS In many cases, an active immunity acquired by artificial (or even natural) means does not last a lifetime. Circulating antibodies can decline with time. To help maintain a high titer (level) of antibodies in the blood, repeated inoculations, called *booster shots*, are administered at intervals. The number of booster injections recommended varies with the disease and with an individual's environment or range of exposure. On occasion, epidemics in high schools or colleges may prompt recommendations for specific boosters. Table 17-2 lists the vaccines currently recommended in the United States for childhood immunizations. The number and timing of doses varies with the different vaccines.

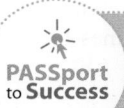

PASSport to **Success**

Nurse practitioners often administer vaccines. Visit **thePoint** or see the Student Resource CD in the back of this book to read about this career, and specifically about pediatric nurse practitioners.

EXAMPLES OF BACTERIAL VACCINES Children are routinely immunized with vaccines against bacteria or their toxins. Because of whooping cough's seriousness in young infants, early inoculation with whooping cough, or **pertussis** (per-TUS-is), vaccine is recommended. A new form of the vaccine containing pertussis toxoid causes fewer adverse reactions than older types that contained heat-killed organisms. This acellular (aP) vaccine usually is given in a mixture with diphtheria toxoid and tetanus tox-

17

Table 17-2	Childhood Immunizations*	
Vaccine	**Disease(s)**	**Schedule**
DTaP	Diphtheria, tetanus, pertussis (whooping cough)	2, 4, 6, and 15–18 months; booster at 4–6 years Diphtheria and tetanus toxoid (Td) at 11–12 years
Hib	*Haemophilus influenza* type b (spinal meningitis)	2 and 4 months or 2, 4, and 6 months depending on type used
PCV	Pneumococcus (pneumonia, meningitis)	2, 4, 6, and 12–15 months
MMR	Measles, mumps, rubella	15 months and 4–6 years
HBV	Hepatitis B	Birth, 1–2 months, 6–18 months
Polio vaccine (IPV)	Poliomyelitis	2 and 4 months, 6–18 months, and 4–6 years
Varicella	Chickenpox	12–15 months and 4–6 years
Rotavirus	Rotavirus gastroenteritis	2, 4, and 6 months

*Recommended by the Advisory Committee on Immunization Practices (www.cdc.gov/vaccines/recs/acip), the American Academy of Pediatrics (www.aap.org), and the American Academy of Family Physicians (www.aafp.org). Information is also available through the National Immunization Program website (www.cdc.gov/vaccines).

oid. The combination, referred to as *DTaP*, may be given as early as 2 months of age and should be followed by additional injections at 4, 6, and 15 months and again when the child enters day care, a school, or any other environment in which he or she might be exposed to one of these contagious diseases. Diphtheria and tetanus toxoid (Td) is given again at 11 to 12 years of age. A tetanus booster is given when there is a disease risk and the last booster was administered more than 10 years prior to exposure.

Routine inoculation against *Haemophilus influenzae* type B (Hib) has nearly eliminated the life-threatening meningitis caused by this organism among preschool children. Hib also causes pneumonia and recurrent ear infections in young children. Depending on the type used, the vaccine is given in either two doses or three doses beginning at 2 months of age.

Pneumococcal vaccine (PCV) protects against infection with pneumococcus, an organism that can cause pneumonia and meningitis. Four doses are given between the ages of 2 and 15 months.

EXAMPLES OF VIRAL VACCINES Intensive research on viruses has resulted in the development of vaccines for an increasing number of viral diseases.

■ The medical community has achieved spectacular results in eliminating poliomyelitis by the use of vaccines. The first of these was an inactivated polio vaccine (IVP) developed by Dr. Jonas Salk and made with killed poliovirus. A more convenient oral vaccine (OPV), made with live attenuated virus, was then developed by Dr. Albert Sabin. Both vaccine types are presently used in worldwide immunization programs, but IPV is preferred for routine childhood immunizations. A series of three doses is given between 2 and 18 months, and a fourth dose is given before entry into school.

■ MMR, made with live attenuated viruses, protects against measles (rubeola), mumps, and rubella (German measles). Rubella is a very mild disease, but it causes birth defects in a developing fetus (see Table 2 in Appendix 5). A first dose of MMR is given at 15 months and a second between 4 and 6 years of age.

■ Infants are now routinely immunized against hepatitis B, receiving the first of three shots just after birth and two more before the age of 18 months. The vaccine is also recommended for people at high risk of hepatitis B infection, including healthcare workers, people on kidney dialysis, people receiving blood clotting factors, injecting drug users, and those with multiple sexual partners. A vaccine against hepatitis A virus is recommended for travelers and others at high risk for infection.

■ A vaccine against chicken pox (varicella) has been available since 1995. Children who have not had the disease by 1 year of age should be vaccinated. Although chicken pox is usually a mild disease, it can cause encephalitis, and infection in a pregnant woman can cause congenital malformation of the fetus. Because varicella is the same virus that causes shingles, vaccination may prevent this late-life sequel. A live virus shingles vaccine is also now available for people 60 years or older.

■ A number of vaccines have been developed against influenza, which is caused by a variety of different viral strains. Laboratories produce a new vaccine each year to combat what they expect will be the most common strains in the population. The elderly, the debilitated, and children, especially those with certain risk factors, including asthma, heart disease, sickle cell disease, HIV infection, and diabetes, should be immunized yearly against influenza.

■ Rotavirus causes a highly contagious gastrointestinal infection among babies and toddlers worldwide. The vomiting and diarrhea that result from infection can lead rapidly to life-threatening dehydration. A new vaccine has been approved to prevent this disease and should be administered at 2, 4, and 6 months of age.

■ The human papilloma virus (HPV) causes sexually transmitted genital warts in both men and women and is associated with almost all cases of cervical cancer in women. Vaccines against the most prevalent HPV strains are now available and immunization is recommended for girls at age 11 to 12 years and those 13 to 26 years of age who have not yet been vaccinated.

■ The rabies vaccine is an exception to the rule that a vaccine should be given before invasion by a disease organism. Rabies is a viral disease transmitted by the bite of wild animals such as raccoons, bats, foxes, and skunks. Mandatory vaccination of domestic animals has practically eliminated this source of rabies in some countries, including the United States, but worldwide, a variety of wild and domestic animals are host to the virus. There is no cure for rabies; it is fatal in nearly all cases. The disease develops so slowly, however, that affected people vaccinated after transmission of the organism still have time to develop an active immunity. The vaccine may be given preventively to people who work with animals.

CHECKPOINT `17-11` ➤ What are some bacterial diseases for which there are vaccines?

CHECKPOINT `17-12` ➤ What are some viral diseases for which there are vaccines?

ARTIFICIAL PASSIVE IMMUNITY It takes several weeks to produce a naturally acquired active immunity and even longer to produce an artificial active immunity through the administration of a vaccine. Therefore, a person who receives a large dose of virulent organisms and has no established immunity to them is in great danger. To prevent illness, the person must quickly receive counteracting antibodies from an outside source. This is accomplished through the administration of an **immune serum,** or **antiserum.** The "ready-made" serum gives short-lived but effective protection against the invaders in the form of an artificially acquired passive immunity. Immune sera are used in emergencies, that is, in situations in which there is no time to wait until an active immunity has developed.

Preparation of Antisera Immune sera often are derived from animals, mainly horses. It has been found that the horse's tissues produce large quantities of antibodies in response to the injection of organisms or their toxins. After repeated injections, the horse is bled according to careful sterile technique; because of the animal's size, it is possible to remove large quantities of blood without causing injury. The blood is allowed to clot, and the serum is removed and packaged in sterile containers.

Injecting humans with serum derived from animals is not without its problems. The foreign proteins in animal sera may cause an often serious sensitivity reaction, called **serum sickness.** To avoid this problem, human antibody in the form of gamma globulin may be used.

CHECKPOINT 17-13 ➤ What is an immune serum and when are immune sera used?

Examples of Antisera Some immune sera contain antibodies, known as **antitoxins,** that neutralize toxins but have no effect on the toxic organisms themselves. Certain antibodies act directly on pathogens, engulfing and destroying them or preventing their continued reproduction. Some antisera are obtained from animal sources, others from human sources. Examples of immune sera are:

■ Diphtheria antitoxin is obtained from immunized horses.

■ Tetanus immune globulin is effective in preventing lockjaw (tetanus), which is often a complication of neglected wounds. Because tetanus immune globulin is of human origin, it carries less risk of adverse reactions than do sera obtained from horses.

■ Immune globulin (human) is given to people exposed to hepatitis A, measles, polio, or chickenpox. It is also given on a regular basis to people with congenital (present at birth) immune deficiencies.

■ Hepatitis B immune globulin, used after hepatitis B exposure, is given principally to infants born to mothers who have hepatitis.

■ The immune globulin Rh_o(D) (trade name RhoGAM), is a concentrated human antibody given to prevent an Rh-negative mother from forming Rh antibodies. It is given during pregnancy if maternal antibodies develop and after the birth of an Rh-positive infant (or even after a miscarriage of a presumably Rh-positive fetus) (see Chapter 13). It is also given when Rh transfusion incompatibilities occur.

■ Anti-snake bite sera, or **antivenins** (an-te-VEN-ins) are used to combat the effects of certain poisonous snake bites.

■ Botulism antitoxin, an antiserum from horses, offers the best hope for botulism victims, although only if given early.

■ Rabies antiserum, from humans or horses, is used with the vaccine to treat victims of rabid animal bites.

Disorders of the Immune System

Immune system disorders may result from overactivity or underactivity. Allergy and autoimmune diseases fall into the first category; hereditary, infectious, and environmental immune deficiency disease fall into the second.

Allergy

Allergy involves antigens and antibodies, and its chemical processes are much like those of immunity. Allergy—a broader term for which is **hypersensitivity**—can be defined informally as a tendency to react unfavorably to certain substances that are normally harmless to most people.

These reaction-producing substances are called **allergens** (AL-er-jens), and like most antigens, they are usually proteins. Examples of typical allergens are pollens, house dust, animal dander (*dander* is the term for the minute scales that are found on hairs and feathers), and certain food proteins. Many drugs can induce allergy, particularly aspirin, barbiturates, and antibiotics (especially penicillin).

When a susceptible person's tissues are repeatedly exposed to an allergen—for example, exposure of the nasal mucosa to pollens—those tissues become **sensitized**; that is, antibodies are produced in them. When the next exposure to the allergen occurs, there is an antigen–antibody reaction. Normally, this type of reaction takes place in the blood without harm, as in immunity. In allergy, however, the antigen–antibody reaction takes place within the cells of the sensitized tissues, with results that are disagreeable and sometimes dangerous. In the case of the nasal mucosa that has become sensitized to pollen, the allergic manifestation is **hay fever,** with symptoms much like those of the common cold.

The antigen–antibody reaction in sensitized individuals promotes the release of excessive histamine. Histamine causes dilation and leaking from capillaries as well as contraction of involuntary muscles (e.g., in the bronchi). Antihistamines are drugs that counteract histamine and may be effective in treating the symptoms of certain allergies. Sometimes, it is possible to desensitize an allergic person by repeated intermittent injections of the offending allergen. Unfortunately, this form of protection does not last long.

Serum sickness is an example of an allergic manifestation that may occur in response to various sera. People who are allergic to the proteins in serum from a horse or some other animal show such symptoms as fever, vomit-

17

ing, joint pain, enlargement of the regional lymph nodes, and **urticaria** (ur-tih-KA-re-ah), also called hives. This type of allergic reaction can be severe but is rarely fatal.

ANAPHYLAXIS Anaphylaxis (an-ah-fih-LAK-sis) is a severe, life-threatening allergic response in a sensitized individual. (The term actually means excess "guarding," in this case, immune protection, from the Greek word *phylaxis*.) Any allergen can provoke an anaphylactic response, but common causes are drugs, insect venom, and foods. Symptoms appear within seconds to minutes after contact and include breathing problems, swelling of the throat and tongue, urticaria, edema, and decreased blood pressure with cardiovascular shock. Anaphylaxis is treated with injectable epinephrine, antihistamine, administration of oxygen, and plasma expanders to increase blood volume. People subject to severe allergic reactions must avoid contact with known allergens. They should be sensitivity tested before administration of a new drug and should also carry injectable epinephrine and wear a medical bracelet identifying their allergy.

Autoimmunity

The term **autoimmunity** refers to an abnormal reactivity to one's own tissues. In autoimmunity, the immune system reacts to the body's own antigens, described as "self," as if they were foreign antigens, or "nonself." Normally, the immune system learns before birth to ignore (tolerate) the body's own tissues by eliminating or inactivating those lymphocytes that will attack them. Some factors that might result in autoimmunity include:

- A change in "self" proteins, as a result of disease, for example.
- Loss of immune system control, as through loss of regulatory T cell activity, for example.
- Cross-reaction of antibodies with "self" antigens. This reaction occurs in rheumatic fever, for example, when antibodies to streptococci damage the heart valves.

Autoimmunity is involved in a long list of diseases, including rheumatoid arthritis, multiple sclerosis, lupus erythematosus, psoriasis, inflammatory bowel diseases, Graves disease, glomerulonephritis, and type I diabetes. All of these diseases probably result to varying degrees from the interaction of individual genetic makeup with environmental factors, including infections. Autoimmune diseases are three times more prevalent in women than in men, perhaps related to hormonal differences.

Autoimmunity is treated with drugs that suppress the immune system and with antibodies to lymphocytes. Pure antibodies, such as these, are prepared in the laboratory and are known as *monoclonal antibodies*. A newer approach uses chemotherapy to destroy immune cells followed by their replacement with healthy stem cells from bone marrow.

Immune Deficiency Diseases

An immune deficiency is some type of failure of the immune system. This failure may involve any part of the system, such as T cells, B cells, or the thymus gland, and it may vary in severity. Such disorders may be congenital (present at birth) or may be acquired as a result of malnutrition, infection, or treatment with x-rays or certain drugs.

The disease **AIDS** (acquired immunodeficiency syndrome) is a devastating example of an infection that attacks the immune system. It is caused by **HIV** (human immunodeficiency virus), which destroys the specific helper T cells that have a receptor (CD_4) for the virus. Its first appearance in the United States in the early 1980s was among homosexual men and injecting drug users. It now occurs worldwide in heterosexual populations of all ages. AIDS is considered to be a pandemic, especially in sub-Saharan Africa and in some parts of Asia. It is spread through unprotected sexual activity and the use of contaminated injection needles. It can also be transmitted from a mother to her fetus. The testing of donated blood has virtually eliminated the spread of AIDS through blood transfusions.

HIV belongs to a group of viruses that is unique in its method of reproduction. The group's name, **retroviruses** (RET-ro-vi-rus-es), which means "backward viruses," refers to the way in which the viruses reverse the typical order of genetic action. Retroviruses have RNA instead of DNA as their genetic material. Unlike other RNA viruses, however, they transcribe (copy) the RNA into DNA to reproduce inside the host. To accomplish this unusual feat, the virus has an enzyme called **reverse transcriptase** (tran-SKRIP-tase). The DNA formed using reverse transcriptase enters the host cell's nucleus and becomes part of its genetic material. There, it may direct the formation of more viruses or lie dormant and undetected for long periods, even years, before being triggered to multiply and cause disease. Some retroviruses can transform the host DNA and produce cancer. These viruses have been associated with leukemia in both humans and animals and with other types of tumors in animals.

Diagnosis of HIV infection is based on the presence of HIV antibodies, the virus, or viral components in the blood. The disease is monitored with CD4+ T cell counts and measurement of HIV RNA in the blood.

Patients with AIDS succumb easily to disease, including rare diseases such as a fungal (*Pneumocystis*) pneumonia and an especially malignant skin cancer, **Kaposi** (*KAP-o-se*) **sarcoma**. Drugs active against HIV stop viral growth at different stages of replication. Some, such as AZT, inhibit reverse transcriptase. These drugs, often used in combination, can slow the progress of HIV replication, but so far, do not prevent infection or cure AIDS. An obstacle to the development of a vaccine against HIV is the tremendous variability of the virus.

Visit *thePoint* or see the Student Resource CD in the back of this book for illustrations on the course of HIV infection and the pathology of AIDS.

Multiple Myeloma

Multiple myeloma is a cancer of the blood-forming cells in bone marrow, mainly the plasma cells that produce antibodies. These cells produce an excess of a particular antibody, but the antibody is not effective. The disease causes loss of resistance to infection, anemia, bone pain, and bone weakening, owing to production of a factor that accelerates loss of bone tissue. High blood levels of calcium and proteins secreted by the plasma cells often lead to kidney failure. Multiple myeloma is treated with chemotherapy. A new approach is high-dose chemotherapy combined with bone marrow transplants. Blood-forming stem cells in the bone marrow replace cells killed by the chemotherapy. This treatment is expensive, and stem cell transplants in themselves are dangerous, but this combined treatment has improved survival rates.

CHECKPOINT 17-14 ➤ What are some disorders of the immune system?

The Immune System and Cancer

Cancer cells differ slightly from normal body cells and therefore the immune system should recognize them as "nonself." The fact that people with AIDS and other immune deficiencies develop cancer at a higher rate than normal suggests that this is true. Cancer cells probably form continuously in the body but normally are destroyed by NK cells and the immune system, a process called **immune surveillance** (sur-VAY-lans). As a person ages, cell-mediated immunity declines and cancer is more likely to develop.

Medical scientists are attempting to treat cancer by stimulating the patient's immune system, a practice called **immunotherapy**. In one approach, T cells are removed from the patient, activated with interleukin, and then reinjected. This method has given some positive results, especially in treatment of melanoma, a highly malignant form of skin cancer. In the future, a vaccine against cancer may become a reality. Vaccines that target specific proteins produced by cancer cells have already been tested in a few forms of cancer.

Transplantation and the Rejection Syndrome

Transplantation is the grafting to a recipient of an organ or tissue from an animal or other human to replace an injured or incompetent body part. Much experimental work preceded transplantation surgery in humans. Tissues that have been transplanted include: bone marrow, lymphoid tissue, skin, corneas, parathyroid glands, ovaries, kidneys, lungs, heart, and liver.

Every organism's natural tendency to destroy foreign substances, including tissues from another person or any other animal, has been the most formidable obstacle to complete success. This normal antigen–antibody reaction has, in this case, been called the **rejection syndrome**.

In all cases of transplantation or grafting, the tissues of the donor, the person donating the part, should be typed in much the same way that blood is typed when a transfusion is given. Blood type antigens are much fewer in number than tissue antigens; thus, the process of obtaining matching blood is much less involved than is the process of obtaining matching tissues. Laboratories do tissue typing in an effort to obtain donors whose tissues contain relatively few antigens that might cause transplant rejection in a recipient, the person receiving the part. (One exception to the need for careful cross-matching is corneal transplantation in the eye. Corneal proteins don't enter the circulation to stimulate an immune response.)

Because it is impossible to match all of a donor's antigens with those of the recipient, physicians give the recipient drugs that will suppress an immune response to the transplanted tissue. These include drugs that suppress synthesis of nucleic acids; drugs or antibodies that inhibit lymphocytes; and adrenal glucocorticoid hormones, such as cortisol, that suppress immunity. These drugs cause a variety of adverse side effects, such as hypertension, kidney damage, and osteoporosis (glucocorticoids). Most importantly, they reduce a patient's ability to fight infection. Because T cells cause much of the reaction against the foreign material in transplants, scientists are trying to use drugs and antibodies to suppress the action of these lymphocytes without damaging the B cells. B cells produce circulating antibodies and are most important in preventing infections. Success with transplantation will increase when methods are found to selectively suppress the immune attack on transplants without destroying the recipient's ability to combat disease.

CHECKPOINT 17-15 ➤ What is the greatest obstacle to tissue transplantation from one individual to another?

17

Disease in Context revisited

➤ Annual Flu Shots for Maria

Maria has taken precautions against contracting the flu again. Once Dr. Andrews gave her the flu shot, her immune system began to respond to the inactivated viral antigens in the vaccine. Many of the components of Maria's immune system are activated, ending with plasma cells, derived from B cells, producing specific antibodies that will grant immunity to the virus.

Several days later, Maria met Dr. Andrews in the hall. "Thanks for the flu shot," she said. "I guess I'm safe against influenza now for life, or at least for a few years. I remember my mom telling me that if I was good when I had to take my childhood shots, I'd never have to get them again."

"Well, not exactly," the doctor replied. "Your immune system will remember the organisms that were in that vaccine, and protect you against them. But, each year new strains arise in humans or develop in animals and can be transmitted to humans." Maria realized that she'd heard over the years about swine influenza, bird influenza, and different types, such as A and B. She also knew about the Asian flu and the big Spanish flu epidemic of the early 1900s. "The vaccine is made from the three viral strains that are expected to cause the greatest problem each year," Dr. Andrews continued. "But if you get the shot annually, you should be relatively safe."

During this case we learned that vaccination stimulates the immune system to manufacture antibodies against disease organisms. Usually, the immune system protects us from infectious disease, but sometimes the system works to our disadvantage. We saw an example of that in Chapter 9, with Susan's case of multiple sclerosis.

Word Anatomy

Medical terms are built from standardized word parts (prefixes, roots, and suffixes). Learning the meanings of these parts can help you remember words and interpret unfamiliar terms.

WORD PART	MEANING	EXAMPLE
Why Do Infections Occur?		
tox	poison	A *toxin* is a substance that is poisonous.
Disorders of the Immune System		
erg	work	In cases of *allergy*, the immune system overworks.
ana-	excessive	*Anaphylaxis* is a life-threatening condition that results from an excessive immune reaction.
myel/o	marrow	Multiple *myeloma* is a cancer (-oma) of blood-forming cells in bone marrow.

Summary

I. **WHY DO INFECTIONS OCCUR?**
   A. Tissue preference of pathogen
   B. Portal of entry of pathogen
   C. Virulence of pathogen
      1. Invasive power
      2. Production of toxins (poisons)
   D. Dose (number) of pathogens
   E. Predisposition of host

II. **NONSPECIFIC DEFENSES**
   A. Chemical and mechanical barriers
      1. Skin
      2. Mucous membranes
      3. Body secretions
      4. Reflexes—coughing, sneezing, vomiting, diarrhea
   B. Phagocytosis—mainly by neutrophils and macrophages
   C. Natural killer (NK) cells—attack tumor cells and virus-infected cells
   D. Inflammation
   E. Fever
   F. Interferon
      1. Substances released from virus-infected cells
      2. Prevent virus production in nearby cells
      3. Stimulate the immune response nonspecifically

III. **IMMUNITY**—specific defense against disease
   A. Innate immunity
      1. Inborn, inherited with genes
      2. Types: species, individual
   B. Adaptive immunity—acquired after birth
      1. Antigens—stimulate immune response by lymphocytes
      2. T cells (T lymphocytes)
         a. Processed in thymus
         b. Types: cytotoxic, helper, regulatory, memory
         c. Involved in cell-mediated immunity
      3. Macrophages
         a. Derived from monocytes
         b. Present antigen to T cells in combination with MHC ("self") proteins
         c. Stimulate the release of interleukins (IL)
      4. B cells (B lymphocytes)
         a. Mature in lymphoid tissue
         b. Develop into plasma cells
            (1) Produce circulating antibodies
            (2) Antibodies counteract antigens
         c. Also develop into memory cells
         d. Involved in humoral immunity
   C. The antigen–antibody reaction
      1. Shape of antibody matches shape of antigen
      2. Results

         a. Prevention of attachment
         b. Clumping of antigen
         c. Neutralization of toxins
         d. Help in phagocytosis
         e. Activation of complement
         f. Activation of NK cells
      3. Complement
         a. Group of proteins in blood
         b. Actions
            (1) Coats foreign cells
            (2) Damages plasma membranes
            (3) Promotes inflammation
            (4) Attracts phagocytes
   D. Natural adaptive immunity
      1. Active—acquired through contact with the disease
      2. Passive—acquired from antibodies obtained through placenta and mother's milk
   E. Artificial adaptive immunity
      1. Active—immunization with vaccines
         a. Types: live (attenuated), killed, toxoid, recombinant DNA
         b. Boosters—keep antibody titers high
         c. Examples of bacterial vaccines
         d. Examples of viral vaccines
      2. Passive—administration of immune serum (antiserum)

IV. **DISORDERS OF THE IMMUNE SYSTEM**
   A. Allergy—hypersensitivity to normally harmless substances (allergens)
      1. Anaphylaxis—severe, life-threatening allergic response
   B. Autoimmunity—abnormal response to body's own tissues
   C. Immune deficiency diseases—failure in the immune system
      1. Congenital (present at birth)
      2. Acquired (e.g., AIDS)
   D. Multiple myeloma—cancer of blood-forming cells in bone marrow

V. **THE IMMUNE SYSTEM AND CANCER**
   A. Immune surveillance—ability of immune system to find and destroy abnormal cells (e.g., cancer cells)
   B. Immunotherapy—stimulating the immune system to treat cancer

VI. **TRANSPLANTATION AND THE REJECTION SYNDROME**
   A. Grafting of an organ or tissue to replace injured or incompetent part
   B. Requirements
      1. Tissue typing
      2. Suppression of immune system

17

Questions for Study and Review

BUILDING UNDERSTANDING

Fill in the blanks

1. The power of the organism to overcome its host's defenses is called _____.

2. Heat, redness, swelling, and pain are classic signs of _____.

3. Any foreign substance that enters the body and induces an immune response is called a(n)_____.

4. All antibodies are contained in a portion of the blood plasma termed the _____.

5. Substances capable of inducing a hypersensitivity reaction are called _____.

Matching > Match each numbered item with the most closely related lettered item.

___ 6. Destroy foreign cells directly.

___ 7. Release interleukins, which stimulate other cells to join the immune response.

___ 8. Suppress the immune response in order to prevent overactivity.

___ 9. Remember an antigen and start a rapid response if the antigen is contacted again.

___ 10. Manufacture antibodies when activated by antigens.

a. regulatory T cells

b. memory T cells

c. cytotoxic T cells

d. B cells

e. helper T cells

Multiple choice

___ 11. All of the following are part of the first line of defense against invaders *except*

   a. tears
   b. saliva
   c. neutrophils
   d. skin

___ 12. Damaged cells release a vasodilator substance called

   a. interleukin
   b. interferon
   c. histamine
   d. complement

___ 13. Which of the following cells mature in the thymus?

   a. T cell
   b. B cell
   c. plasma cell
   d. natural killer cell

___ 14. Sensitivity to animal-derived immune serum may lead to a serious condition called

   a. serum sickness
   b. hay fever
   c. Kaposi sarcoma
   d. rejection syndrome

___ 15. An abnormal reactivity to one's own tissues is called

   a. allergy
   b. autoimmunity
   c. anaphylaxis
   d. rejection

UNDERSTANDING CONCEPTS

16. Describe four factors that influence the occurrence of infection.

17. What causes the symptoms of inflammation?

18. Differentiate between the terms in each of the following pairs:

    a. interferon and interleukin
    b. antibody and complement
    c. innate immunity and adaptive immunity
    d. cell-mediated immunity and humoral immunity
    e. active immunity and passive immunity
    f. toxin and toxoid

19. Describe the events that must occur for a T cell to react with a foreign antigen. Once activated, what do the T cells do?

20. What role do antibodies play in immunity? How are they produced? How do they work?

21. Compare and contrast the four types of adaptive immunity.

22. What is an immune serum? Give examples. Define antitoxin.

23. Define allergy. How is the process of allergy like that of immunity, and how do they differ?

24. What is meant by rejection syndrome, and what is being done to offset this syndrome?

CONCEPTUAL THINKING

25. While in the garden with his father, Alek, a 4-year-old boy was, in his own words, "kicked by a bee." Shortly afterward, Alek developed hives near the affected area, which he began to scratch. About 10 minutes later, Alek's father noticed that his son was wheezing. What is happening to Alek? Describe the inflammatory events that are occurring in his body. How should Alek's father respond?

26. Why is HIV's attack on helper T cells so devastating to the entire immune system?

27. In Maria's case, she received an injectable influenza vaccine made with killed virus. The nasal spray flu vaccine is made with live attenuated virus. What is the difference between these two types of vaccines? In the future, what other types of influenza vaccines might be developed?

17

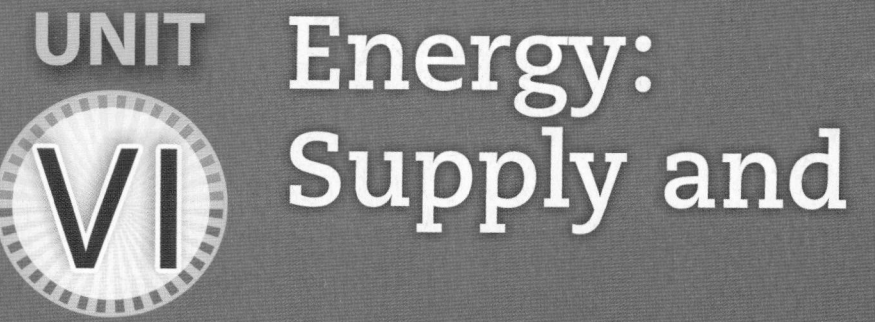

UNIT VI

Energy: Supply and Use

The five chapters in this unit show how oxygen and nutrients are processed, taken up by the body fluids, and used by the cells to yield energy. This unit also describes how the stability of body functions (homeostasis) is maintained and how waste products are eliminated.

CHAPTER 18

The Respiratory System

Learning Outcomes

After careful study of this chapter, you should be able to:

1. Define *respiration* and describe the three phases of respiration
2. Name and describe all the structures of the respiratory system
3. Explain the mechanism for pulmonary ventilation
4. List the ways in which oxygen and carbon dioxide are transported in the blood
5. Describe nervous and chemical controls of respiration
6. Give several examples of altered breathing patterns
7. List and define four conditions that result from inadequate breathing
8. Describe several types of respiratory infection
9. Describe some allergic responses that affect the respiratory system
10. Name the diseases involved in chronic obstructive pulmonary disease (COPD)
11. Describe some disorders that involve the pleura
12. Describe equipment used to treat respiratory disorders
13. Show how word parts are used to build words related to respiration (see Word Anatomy at the end of the chapter)

Selected Key Terms

The following terms and other boldface terms in the chapter are defined in the Glossary

alveolus (pl., alveoli)
asthma
bronchiole
bronchus (pl., bronchi)
chemoreceptor
compliance
diaphragm
emphysema
epiglottis
epistaxis
hemoglobin
hilum
hypercapnia
hypoxia
larynx
lung
mediastinum
pharynx
phrenic nerve
pleura
pneumothorax
respiration
surfactant
trachea
ventilation

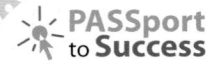

PASSport to Success

Visit *thePoint* or see the Student Resource CD in the back of this book for definitions and pronunciations of key terms as well as a pretest for this chapter.

Disease in Context

➤ Emily's Case: Advances in Asthma Therapy

"Remind me to mention to Dr. Martinez that Emily still has that nagging cough," Nicole told her husband.

"I've been worried about that," he replied. "You know, I had asthma as a kid—I hope she doesn't. I could hardly do any sports without taking a couple puffs of my inhaler."

Later that week, Dr. Martinez listened carefully to 3-year-old Emily's lungs for any sign of inflammation. He knew that the common symptoms of asthma—coughing, wheezing, and shortness of breath—were due to swelling of the airway tissues and spasm of the smooth muscle wrapped around them. "I don't hear any wheezing, but given the family history, we can't rule out asthma. In addition to the genetic component, asthma can have several environmental triggers such as respiratory infections, allergies, cold air, and exercise."

"Well," replied Nicole, "Emily did have a cold right before the coughing began. I haven't noticed any allergies, but now that I think about it, she did have a persistent cough last winter too. And, she is getting lots of exercise at preschool and dance class. So, if Emily does have asthma, what will that mean for her? I know that it limited my husband's activities when he was a kid."

"Asthma is rarely life-threatening," answered the doctor. "And the drug therapies that we now have to control asthma are much better than when your husband was young. But, first, I think we need to figure out if Emily's cough is really due to asthma. I suggest that you monitor Emily for the next few weeks and see if anything exacerbates it. In the event that she does have asthma, we might be able to treat it with a relatively new medication called an antileukotriene. This medication is taken orally every day and prevents the lungs from producing substances called leukotrienes, which cause the smooth muscle in the airways to constrict. Blocking leukotrienes helps prevent narrowing of the airways, and thus, the symptoms of asthma. With this medication, Emily may not even need an inhaler."

Dr. Martinez su.spects that Emily has asthma, the most common chronic respiratory disease of childhood. In this chapter, we'll examine the respiratory system and the components involved in this disease. Later in the chapter, we'll check in on Emily and learn about other medications used to treat asthma.

Phases of Respiration

Most people think of respiration simply as the process by which air moves into and out of the lungs, that is, *breathing*. By scientific definition, respiration is the process by which oxygen is obtained from the environment and delivered to the cells. Carbon dioxide is transported to the outside in a reverse pathway (Fig. 18-1).

Respiration includes three phases:

- **Pulmonary ventilation,** which is the exchange of air between the atmosphere and the air sacs (alveoli) of the lungs. This is normally accomplished by the inhalation and exhalation of breathing.

- **External exchange of gases,** which occurs in the lungs as oxygen (O_2) diffuses from the air sacs into the blood and carbon dioxide (CO_2) diffuses out of the blood to be eliminated.

- **Internal exchange of gases,** which occurs in the tissues as oxygen diffuses from the blood to the cells, whereas carbon dioxide passes from the cells into the blood.

Gas exchange requires close association of the respiratory system with the circulatory system, as the circulating blood is needed to transport oxygen to the cells and transport carbon dioxide back to the lungs.

The term *respiration* is also used to describe a related process that occurs at the cellular level. In **cellular respiration,** oxygen is taken into a cell and used in the breakdown of nutrients with the release of energy. Carbon dioxide is the waste product of cellular respiration (see Chapter 20's discussion of metabolism).

CHECKPOINT 18-1 ➤ What are the three phases of respiration?

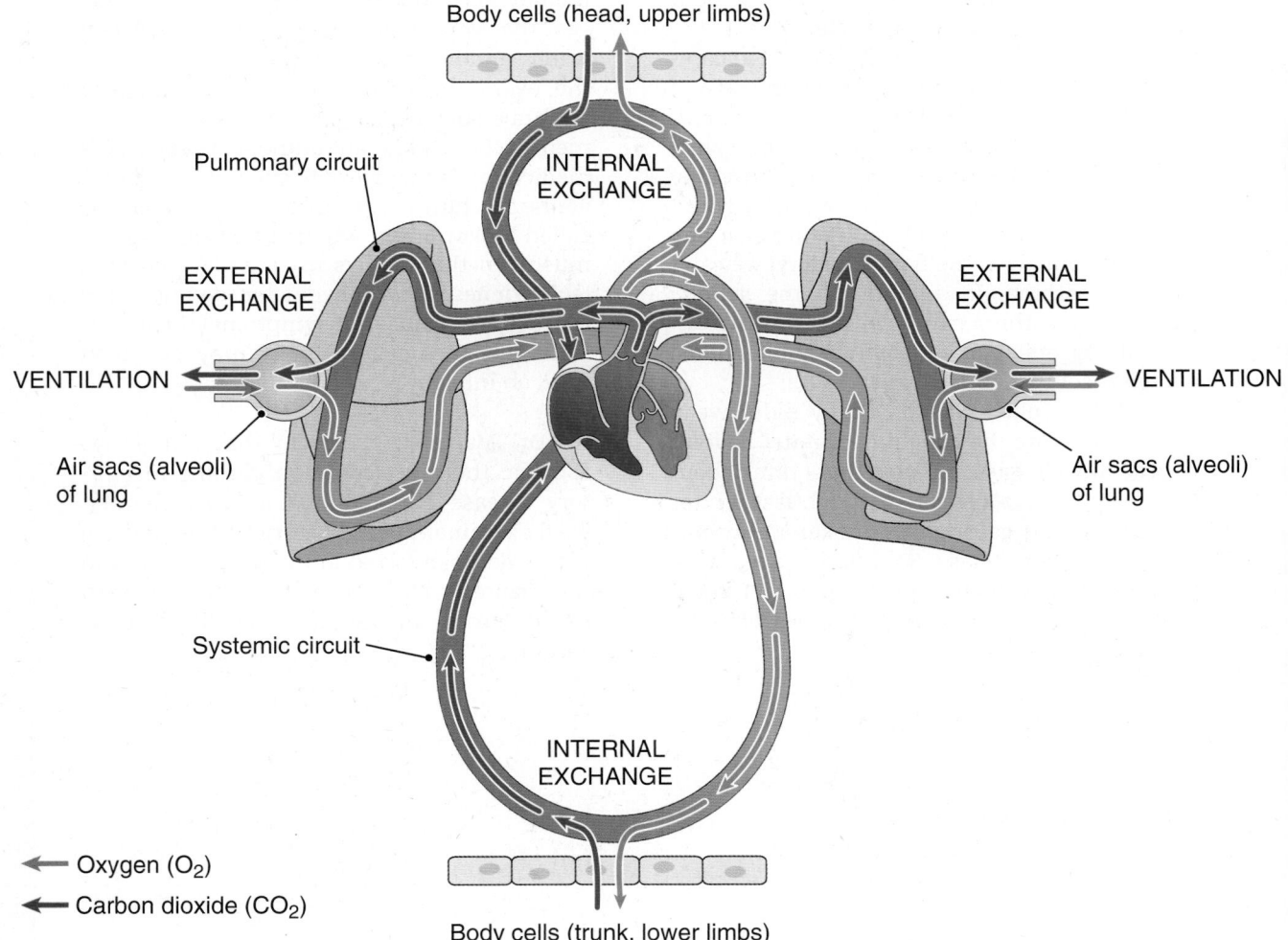

Figure 18-1 **Overview of respiration.** In ventilation, gases are moved into and out of the lungs. In external exchange, gases move between the air sacs (alveoli) of the lungs and the blood. In internal exchange, gases move between the blood and body cells. The circulation transports gases in the blood.

The Respiratory System

The respiratory system is an intricate arrangement of spaces and passageways that conduct air into the lungs (Fig. 18-2). These spaces include the nasal cavities; the pharynx, which is common to the digestive and respiratory systems; the voice box, or larynx; the windpipe, or trachea; and the lungs themselves, with their conducting tubes and air sacs. The entire system might be thought of as a pathway for air between the atmosphere and the blood.

The Nasal Cavities

Air enters the body through the openings in the nose called the **nostrils,** or **nares** (NA-reze) (sing. naris). Immediately inside the nostrils, located between the roof of the mouth and the cranium, are the two spaces known as the **nasal cavities.** These two spaces are separated from each other by a partition, the **nasal septum.** The septum's superior portion is formed by a thin plate of the ethmoid bone that extends downward, and the inferior portion is formed by the vomer (see Fig. 7-5A in Chapter 7). An anterior extension of the septum is made of hyaline cartilage. The sep-

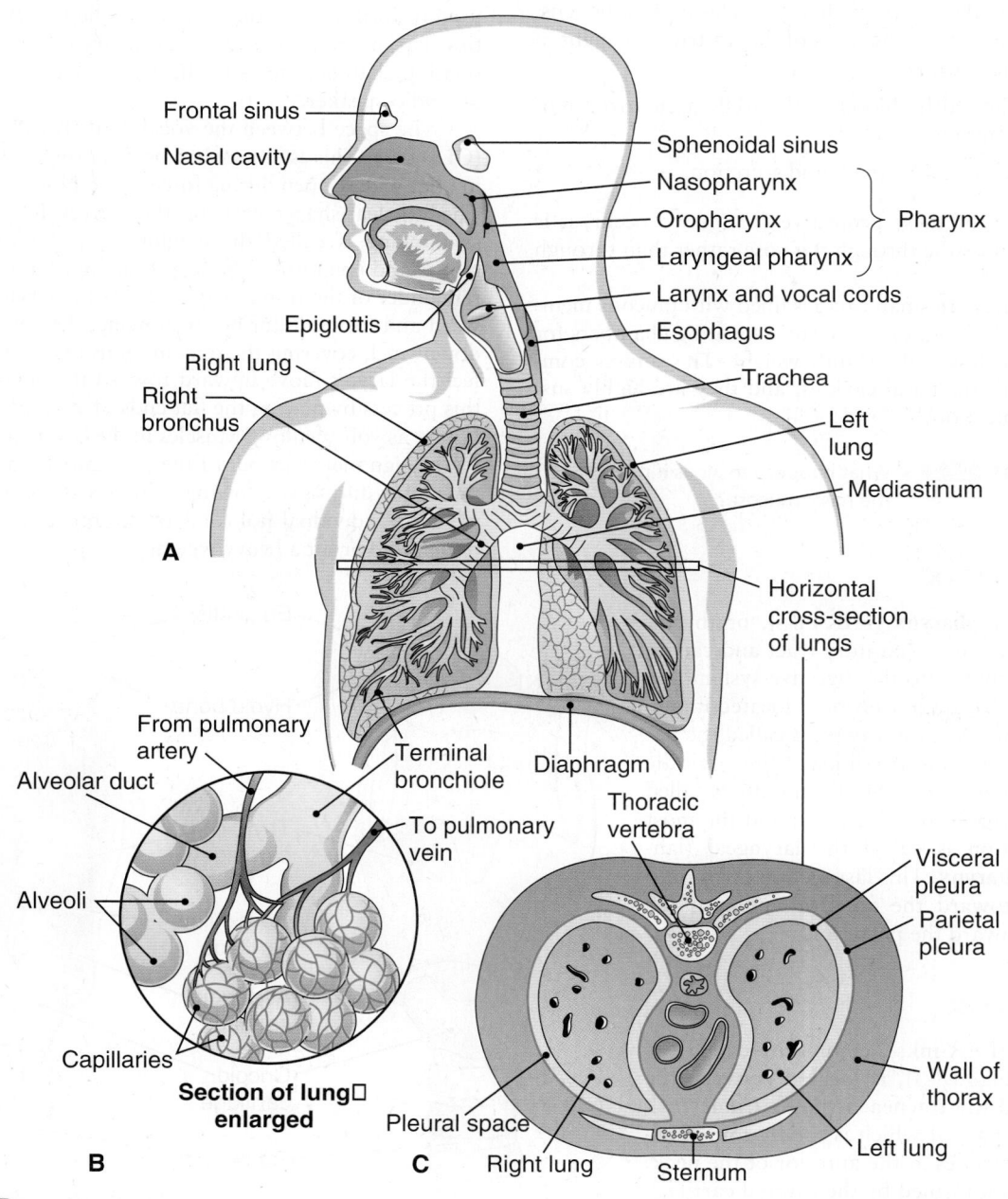

Figure 18-2   **The respiratory system. (A)** Overview. **(B)** Enlarged section of lung tissue showing the relationship between the alveoli (air sacs) of the lungs and the blood capillaries. **(C)** A transverse section through the lungs. [ZOOMING IN ▸ What organ is located in the medial depression of the left lung?]

tum and the walls of the nasal cavity are covered with mucous membrane, consisting of stratified squamous (flat) epithelium, tissue that is resistant to wear.

On the lateral walls of each nasal cavity are three projections called the **conchae** (KONG-ke) (see Figs. 7-5A and 7-8 in Chapter 7). The shell-like conchae greatly increase the surface area of the mucous membrane over which air travels on its way through the nasal cavities. This membrane contains many blood vessels that deliver heat and moisture. The membrane's cells secrete a large amount of fluid—up to 1 quart each day. The following changes occur as air comes in contact with the nasal lining:

■ Foreign bodies, such as dust particles and pathogens, are filtered out by the hairs of the nostrils or caught in the surface mucus.

■ Air is warmed by blood in the well-vascularized mucous membrane.

■ Air is moistened by the liquid secretion.

To allow for these protective changes to occur, it is preferable to breathe through the nose rather than through the mouth.

The **sinuses** are small cavities lined with mucous membrane in the skull bones. They are resonating chambers for the voice and lessen the skull's weight. The sinuses communicate with the nasal cavities, and they are highly susceptible to infection.

CHECKPOINT **18-2** ➤ What happens to air as it passes over the nasal mucosa?

The Pharynx

The muscular **pharynx** (FAR-inks), or throat, carries air into the respiratory tract and carries foods and liquids into the digestive system (see Fig. 18-2). The superior portion, located immediately behind the nasal cavity, is called the **nasopharynx** (na-zo-FAR-inks); the middle section, located posterior to the mouth, is called the **oropharynx** (o-ro-FAR-inks); and the most inferior portion is called the **laryngeal** (lah-RIN-je-al) **pharynx**. This last section opens into the larynx toward the anterior and into the esophagus toward the posterior.

The Larynx

The **larynx** (LAR-inks), commonly called the *voice box* (Fig. 18-3), is located between the pharynx and the trachea. It has a framework of cartilage, part of which is the thyroid cartilage that protrudes at the anterior of the neck. The projection formed by the thyroid cartilage is commonly called the *Adam's apple* because it is considerably larger in men than in women.

Folds of mucous membrane used in producing speech are located on both sides at the superior portion of the larynx. These are the vocal folds, or **vocal cords** (Fig. 18-4), which vibrate as air flows over them from the lungs. Variations in the length and tension of the vocal cords and the distance between them regulate the pitch of sound. The amount of air forced over them regulates volume. A difference in the size of the larynx and the vocal cords is what accounts for the difference between adult male and female voices. In general, a man's larynx is larger than a woman's. His vocal cords are thicker and longer, so they vibrate more slowly, resulting in a lower range of pitch. Muscles of the pharynx, tongue, lips, and face also are used to form clear pronunciations. The mouth, nasal cavities, paranasal sinuses, and the pharynx all serve as resonating chambers for speech, just as does the cabinet for an audio speaker.

The space between the vocal cords is called the **glottis** (GLOT-is). This is somewhat open during normal breathing but widely open during forced breathing (see Fig. 18-4). The little leaf-shaped cartilage that covers the larynx during swallowing is called the **epiglottis** (ep-ih-GLOT-is). The glottis and epiglottis help keep food and liquids out of the remainder of the respiratory tract. As the larynx moves upward and forward during swallowing, the epiglottis moves downward, covering the opening into the larynx. You can feel the larynx move upward toward the epiglottis during this process by placing the flat ends of your fingers on your larynx as you swallow. Muscles in the larynx assist in keeping foreign materials out of the respiratory tract by closing the glottis during swallowing. Muscles also close the glottis when an individual holds his or her breath and strains, as to defecate or lift a heavy weight.

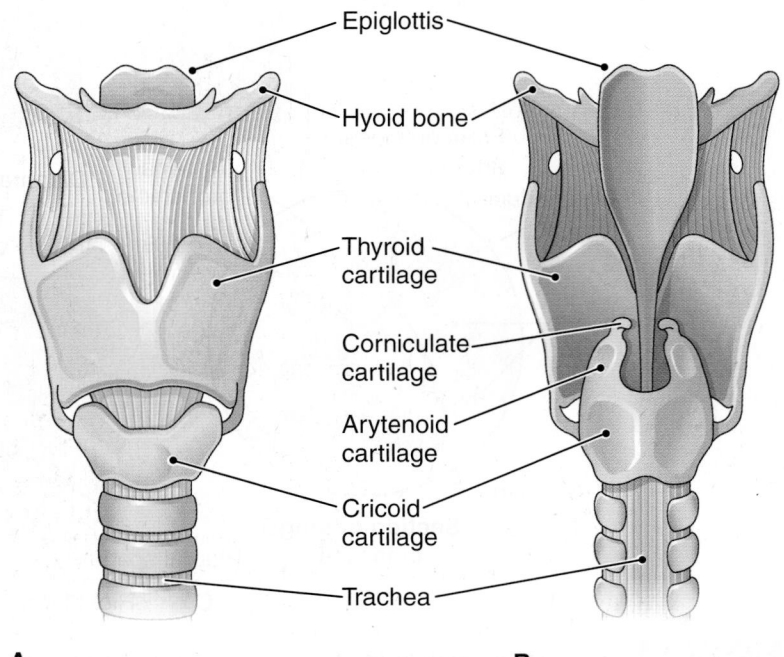

A   **B**

Figure 18-3 **The larynx. (A)** Anterior view. **(B)** Posterior view.

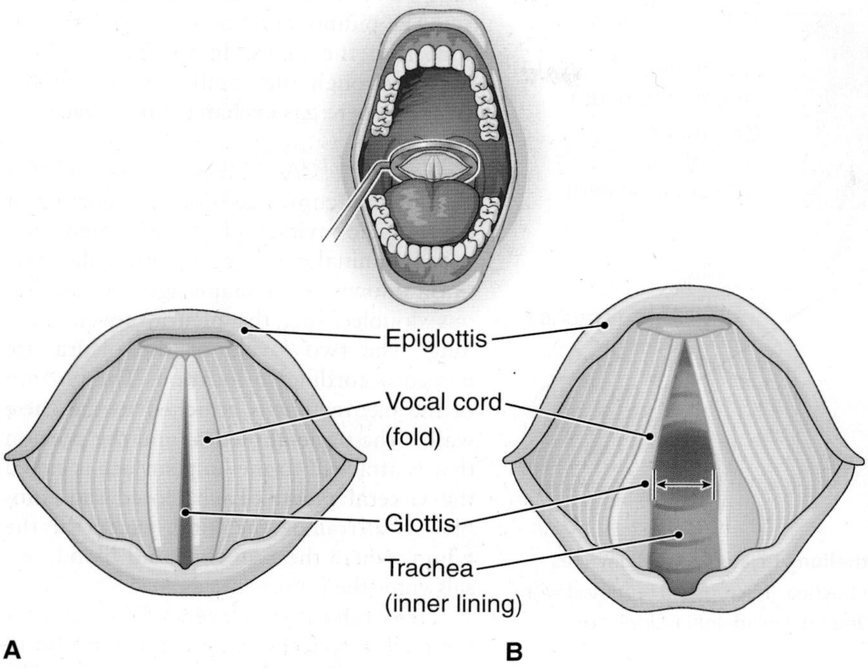

A   **B**

Epiglottis

Vocal cord (fold)

Glottis

Trachea (inner lining)

Figure 18-4 **The vocal cords, superior view. (A)** The glottis in closed position. **(B)** The glottis in open position. [**ZOOMING IN ➤** What cartilage is named for its position above the glottis?]

The Trachea

The **trachea** (TRA-ke-ah), commonly called the *windpipe*, is a tube that extends from the inferior edge of the larynx to the upper part of the chest superior to the heart. The trachea's purpose is to conduct air between the larynx and the lungs.

A framework of separate cartilages reinforces the trachea and keeps it open. These cartilages, each shaped somewhat like a tiny horseshoe or the letter C, are found along the trachea's entire length. The open sections in the cartilages are lined up at their posterior so that the esophagus can expand into this region during swallowing.

CHECKPOINT 18-3 ➤ What are the scientific names for the throat, voice box, and windpipe?

CHECKPOINT 18-4 ➤ What are the three regions of the pharynx?

The Bronchi

At its inferior end, the trachea divides into two primary, or mainstem, **bronchi** (BRONG-ki), which enter the lungs (see Fig. 18-2). The right bronchus is considerably larger in diameter than the left and extends downward in a more vertical direction. Therefore, if a foreign body is inhaled, it is likely to enter the right lung. Each bronchus enters the lung at a notch or depression called the **hilum** (HI-lum). Blood vessels and

nerves also connect with the lung here and, together with the bronchus, make up a region known as the *root* of the lung.

THE LINING OF THE AIR PASSAGEWAYS The trachea, bronchi, and other conducting passageways of the respiratory tract are lined with a special type of epithelium (Fig. 18-5). Basically, it is simple columnar epithelium, but the cells are arranged in such a way that they appear stratified. The tissue is thus described as *pseudostratified*, meaning "falsely stratified." These epithelial cells have cilia to filter out impurities and to create fluid movement within the conducting tubes. The cilia beat to drive impurities toward the throat, where they can be swallowed or eliminated by coughing, sneezing, or blowing the nose.

The Lungs

The **lungs** are the organs in which gas diffusion takes place through the extremely thin and delicate lung tissues (see Fig. 18-2). The two lungs are set side by side in the thoracic (chest) cavity. Between them are the heart, the great blood vessels, and other organs of the **mediastinum** (me-de-as-TI-num), the space between the lungs, including the esophagus, trachea, and lymph nodes. (See Appendix 7 for a dissection photograph showing the lungs in relation to the heart and diaphragm.)

On its medial side, the left lung has an indentation that accommodates the heart. The right lung is subdivided by fissures into three lobes; the left lung is divided into two lobes. Each lobe is then further subdivided into segments and then lobules. These subdivisions correspond to subdivisions of the bronchi as they branch throughout the lungs.

Each primary bronchus enters the lung at the hilum and immediately subdivides. The right bronchus divides into three secondary bronchi, each of which enters one of the right lung's three lobes. The left bronchus gives rise to two secondary bronchi, which enter the left lung's two lobes. Because the bronchial subdivisions resemble the branches of a tree, they have been given the common name *bronchial tree*. The bronchi subdivide again and again, becoming progressively smaller as they branch through lung tissue.

18

CHECKPOINT 18-5 ➤ The cells that line the respiratory passageways help to keep impurities out of the lungs. What feature of these cells enables them to filter impurities and move fluids?

The smallest of these conducting tubes are called

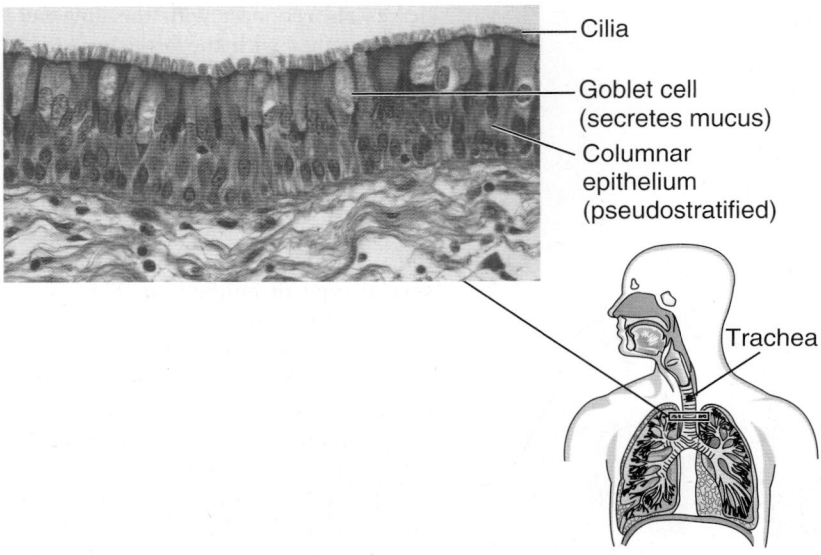

Cilia
Goblet cell (secretes mucus)
Columnar epithelium (pseudostratified)
Trachea

Figure 18-5 **Microscopic view of ciliated epithelium.** Ciliated epithelium lines the respiratory passageways, as shown here in the trachea. (Micrograph reprinted with permission from Cormack DH. *Essential Histology*, 2nd ed. Philadelphia: Lippincott Williams & Wilkins, 2001.)

bronchioles (BRONG-ke-oles). With branching, the histology of the tubes gradually changes. The bronchi contain small bits of cartilage, which give firmness to their walls and hold the passageways open so that air can pass in and out easily. As the bronchi become smaller, however, the cartilage decreases in amount. In the bronchioles, there is no cartilage at all; what remains is mostly smooth muscle, which is under the control of the autonomic (involuntary) nervous system.

THE ALVEOLI At the end of the **terminal bronchioles**, the smallest subdivisions of the bronchial tree, there are clusters of tiny air sacs in which most gas exchange takes place. These sacs are the **alveoli** (al-VE-o-li) (sing. alveolus) (see Fig. 18-2). The wall of each alveolus is made of a single-cell layer of squamous epithelium. This thin wall provides easy passage for the gases entering and leaving the blood as the blood circulates through the millions of tiny capillaries covering the alveoli.

Certain cells in the alveolar wall produce **surfactant** (sur-FAK-tant), a substance that reduces the surface tension ("pull") of the fluids that line the alveoli. This surface action prevents collapse of the alveoli and eases lung expansion.

There are about 300 million alveoli in the human lungs. The resulting surface area in contact with gases approximates 60 square meters (some books say even more). This area is equivalent, as an example, to the floor surface of a classroom that measures about 24 by 24 feet. As with many other body systems, there is great functional reserve; we have about three times as much lung tissue as is minimally necessary to sustain life. Because of the many air spaces, the lung is light in weight; normally, a piece of lung tissue dropped into a glass of water will float. Figure 18-6

shows a microscopic view of lung tissue.

The pulmonary circuit brings blood to and from the lungs. In the lungs, blood passes through the capillaries around the alveoli, where gas exchange takes place.

THE LUNG CAVITIES AND PLEURA
The lungs occupy a considerable portion of the thoracic cavity, which is separated from the abdominal cavity by the muscular partition known as the **diaphragm**. A continuous doubled sac, the **pleura**, covers each lung. The two layers of the pleura are named according to location. The portion of the pleura that is attached to the chest wall is the **parietal pleura**, and the portion that is attached to the lung surface is called the **visceral pleura**. Each closed sac completely surrounds the lung, except at the hilum, where the bronchus and blood vessels enter the lung.

Between the two layers of the pleura is the **pleural space**, containing a thin film of fluid that lubricates the membranes. The effect of this fluid is the same as between two flat pieces of glass joined by a film of water; that is, the surfaces slide easily on each other but strongly resist separation. Thus, the lungs are able to move and enlarge effortlessly in response to changes in the thoracic volume that occur during breathing.

CHECKPOINT 18-6 ➤ In what structures does gas exchange occur in the lung?

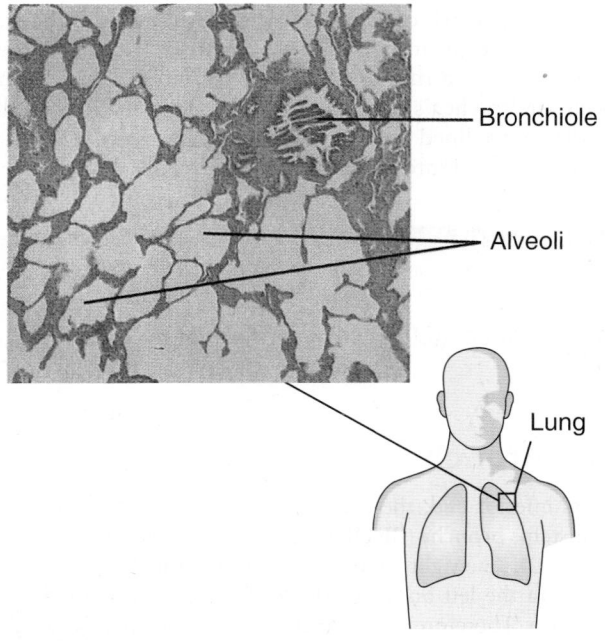

Bronchiole
Alveoli
Lung

Figure 18-6 **Lung tissue viewed through a microscope.** (Micrograph courtesy of Dana Morse Bittus and BJ Cohen.)

CHECKPOINT **18-7** ➤ What is the name of the membrane that encloses the lung?

The Process of Respiration

Respiration involves ventilation of the lungs, exchange of gases, and their transport in the blood. Respiratory needs are met by central and peripheral controls of breathing.

Pulmonary Ventilation

Ventilation is the movement of air into and out of the lungs, normally accomplished by breathing. There are two phases of ventilation (Fig. 18-7):

■ **Inhalation**, or inspiration, is the drawing of air into the lungs.

■ **Exhalation**, or expiration, is the expulsion of air from the lungs.

In **inhalation**, the active phase of breathing, respiratory muscles of the thorax and diaphragm contract to en-large the thoracic cavity. During quiet breathing, the diaphragm's movement accounts for most of the increase in thoracic volume. The diaphragm is a strong, dome-shaped muscle attached to the body wall around the base of the rib cage. The diaphragm's contraction and flattening cause a piston-like downward motion that increases the chest's vertical dimension. Other muscles that participate in breathing are the external and internal intercostal muscles. These muscles run at different angles in two layers between the ribs. As the external intercostals contract for inhalation, they lift the rib cage upward and outward. Put the palms of your hands on either side of the rib cage to feel this action as you inhale. During forceful inhalation, the rib cage is moved further up and out by contraction of muscles in the neck and chest wall.

As the thoracic cavity increases in size, gas pressure within the cavity decreases. This phenomenon follows a law in physics stating that when the volume of a given amount of gas increases, the pressure of the gas decreases. Conversely, when the volume decreases, the pressure increases. If you blow air into a tight balloon that does not expand very much, the gas particles are in close contact and will hit the wall of the balloon frequently, creating greater pressure (Fig. 18-8). If you tap this balloon, it will spring back to its original shape. When you blow into a soft balloon that expands easily under pressure, the gas particles spread out into a larger area and will not hit the balloon's wall as often. If you tap the balloon, your finger will make an indentation. Thus, pressure in the chest cavity drops as the thorax expands. When the pressure drops to slightly below the air pressure outside the lungs, air is drawn into the lungs, as by suction.

The ease with which one can expand the lungs and thorax is called **compliance**. Normal elasticity of the lung tissue, aided by surfactant, allows the lungs to expand under pressure and fill adequately with air during inhalation. Compliance is decreased when the lungs resist expansion. Conditions that can decrease compliance include diseases that damage or scar lung tissue, fluid accumulation in the lungs, deficiency of surfactant, and interference with the action of breathing muscles.

Air enters the respiratory passages and flows through the ever-dividing tubes of the bronchial tree. As the air traverses this route, it moves more and more slowly through the great number of bronchial tubes until there is virtually no forward flow as it reaches the alveoli. The incoming air mixes with the residual air remaining in the respiratory passageways, so that the gases

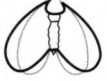

Left lung

External intercostal muscles

Diaphragm

During inhalation the diaphragm presses the abdominal organs downward and forward.

A. Action of rib cage in inhalation

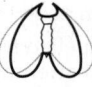

Left lung

Internal intercostal muscles

Diaphragm

During exhalation the diaphragm rises and recoils to the resting position.

B. Action of rib cage in exhalation

Figure 18-7 **Pulmonary ventilation. (A)** Inhalation. **(B)** Exhalation. **[ZOOMING IN ➤** What muscles are located between the ribs? **]**

18

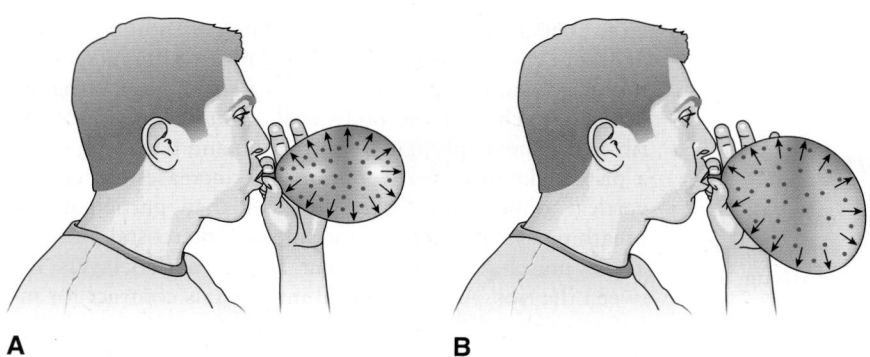

A   **B**

Figure 18-8 **The relationship of gas pressure to volume. (A)** Inflation of a stiff balloon creates strong air pressure against the wall of the balloon. **(B)** The same amount of air in a soft balloon spreads out into the available space, resulting in lower gas pressure. [ZOOMING IN ➤ What happens to gas pressure as the volume of its container increases?]

soon are evenly distributed. Each breath causes relatively little change in the gas composition of the alveoli, but normal continuous breathing ensures the presence of adequate oxygen and the removal of carbon dioxide.

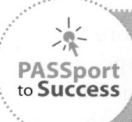 **PASSport to Success** Visit *thePoint* or see the Student Resource CD in the back of this book for illustrations of the breathing muscles and for the animation *Pulmonary Ventilation.*

In **exhalation**, the passive phase of breathing, the respiratory muscles relax, allowing the ribs and diaphragm to return to their original positions. The lung tissues are elastic and recoil to their original size during exhalation. Surface tension within the alveoli aids in this return to resting size. During forced exhalation, the internal intercostal muscles contract, pulling the bottom of the rib cage in and down. The muscles of the abdominal wall contract, pushing the abdominal viscera upward against the relaxed diaphragm.

Table 18-1 gives the definitions and average values for some of the breathing volumes and capacities that are important in evaluating respiratory function. A lung *capacity* is a sum of volumes. These same values are shown on a graph as they might appear on a tracing made by a **spirometer** (spi-ROM-eh-ter), an instrument for recording lung volumes (Fig. 18-9). The tracing is a **spirogram** (SPI-ro-gram).

CHECKPOINT 18-8 ➤ What are the two phases of breathing? Which is active and which is passive?

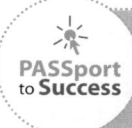 **PASSport to Success** Respiratory therapists evaluate and treat breathing disorders. Visit *thePoint* or see the Student Resource CD in the back of this book for a description of this career.

Gas Exchange

External exchange is the movement of gases between the alveoli and the capillary blood in the lungs (see Fig. 18-1). The barrier that separates alveolar air from the blood is composed of the alveolar wall and the capillary wall, both of which are extremely thin. This respiratory membrane is not only very thin, it is also moist. The moisture is important because the oxygen and carbon dioxide must go into solution before they can diffuse across the membrane. Recall that **diffusion** refers to the movement of molecules from an area in which they are in higher concentration to

Table 18-1	Lung Volumes and Capacities	
Volume	**Definition**	**Average Value (mL)**
Tidal volume	The amount of air moved into or out of the lungs in quiet, relaxed breathing	500
Residual volume	The volume of air that remains in the lungs after maximum exhalation	1,200
Inspiratory reserve volume	The additional amount that can be breathed in by force after a normal inhalation	2,600
Expiratory reserve volume	The additional amount that can be breathed out by force after a normal exhalation	900
Vital capacity	The volume of air that can be expelled from the lungs by maximum exhalation after maximum inhalation	4,000
Functional residual capacity	The amount of air remaining in the lungs after normal exhalation	2,100
Total lung capacity	The total volume of air that can be contained in the lungs after maximum inhalation	5,200

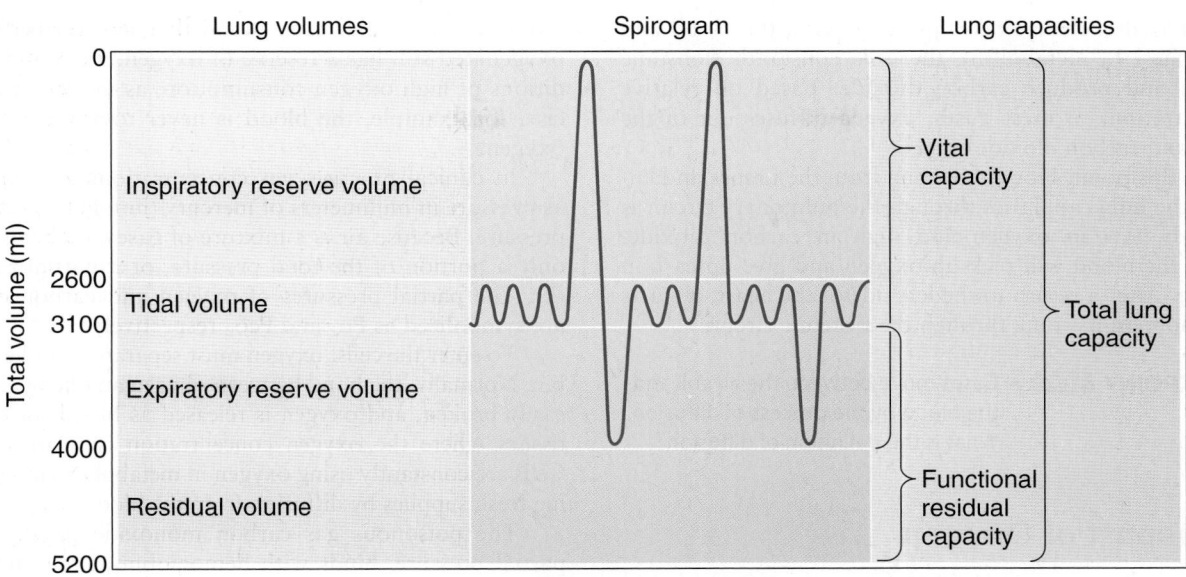

Figure 18-9 **A spirogram.** The tracing of lung volumes is made with a spirometer. [**ZOOMING IN** ➤ What lung volume cannot be measured with a spirometer?]

an area in which they are in lower concentration. Therefore, the relative concentrations of a gas on the two sides of a membrane determine the direction of diffusion. Normally, inspired air contains about 21% oxygen and 0.04%

carbon dioxide; expired air has only 16% oxygen and 3.5% carbon dioxide. These values illustrate that a two-way diffusion takes place through the walls of the alveoli and capillaries (Fig. 18-10).

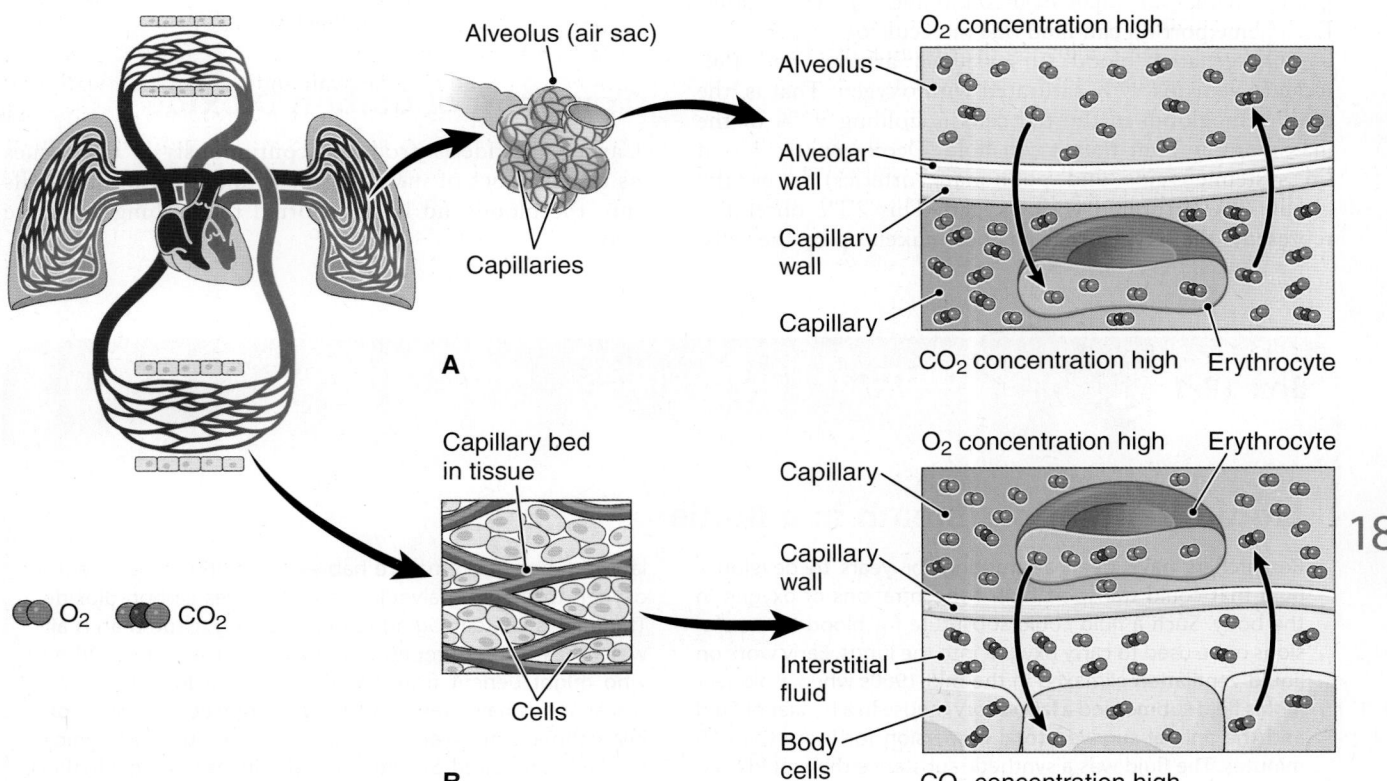

Figure 18-10 **Gas exchange. (A)** External exchange between the alveoli and the blood. Oxygen diffuses into the blood and carbon dioxide diffuses out, based on concentrations of the two gases in the alveoli and in the blood. **(B)** Internal exchange between the blood and the cells. Oxygen diffuses out of the blood and into tissues, while carbon dioxide diffuses from the cells into the blood.

Internal exchange takes place between the blood and the tissues. In metabolism, the cells constantly consume oxygen and produce carbon dioxide. Based on relative concentrations of these gases, oxygen diffuses out of the blood and carbon dioxide enters.

At this point, blood returning from the tissues and entering the lung capillaries through the pulmonary circuit is relatively low in oxygen and high in carbon dioxide. Again, the blood will pick up oxygen and give up carbon dioxide. After a return to the left side of the heart, it starts once more on its route through the systemic circuit.

CHECKPOINT `18-9` ➤ Gases move between the alveoli and the blood by the process of diffusion. What is the definition of diffusion?

Transport of Oxygen

A very small percentage (1.5%) of the oxygen in the blood is carried in solution in the plasma. (Oxygen does dissolve in water, as shown by the fact that aquatic animals get their oxygen from water.) However, almost all (98.5%) of the oxygen that diffuses into the capillary blood in the lungs binds to **hemoglobin** in the red blood cells. If not for hemoglobin and its ability to hold oxygen in the blood, the heart would have to work much harder to supply enough oxygen to the tissues. The hemoglobin molecule is a large protein with four small iron-containing "heme" regions. Each heme portion can bind one molecule of oxygen.

Oxygenated blood (in systemic arteries and pulmonary veins) is 97% saturated with oxygen. That is, the total hemoglobin in the red cells is holding 97% of the maximum amount that it can hold. Deoxygenated blood (in systemic veins and pulmonary arteries) is usually about 70% saturated with oxygen. This 27% difference represents the oxygen that has been taken up by the cells.

Note, however, that even blood that is described as deoxygenated still has a reserve of oxygen. Even under conditions of high oxygen consumption, as in vigorous exercise, for example, the blood is never totally depleted of oxygen.

In clinical practice, gas concentrations are expressed as pressure in millimeters of mercury (mm Hg), as is blood pressure. Because air is a mixture of gases, each gas exerts only a portion of the total pressure, or a **partial pressure** (P). The partial pressures of oxygen and carbon dioxide are symbolized as P_{O_2} and P_{CO_2} respectively.

To enter the cells, oxygen must separate from hemoglobin. Normally, the bond between oxygen and hemoglobin is easily broken, and oxygen is released as blood travels into tissues where the oxygen concentration is relatively low. Cells are constantly using oxygen in metabolism and obtaining fresh supplies by diffusion from the blood.

The poisonous gas carbon monoxide (CO), at low partial pressure, binds with hemoglobin at the same molecular sites as does oxygen. However, it binds more tightly and displaces oxygen. Even a small amount of carbon monoxide causes a serious reduction in the blood's ability to carry oxygen.

For an interesting variation on normal gas transport, see Box 18-1 on liquid ventilation.

CHECKPOINT `18-10` ➤ What substance in red blood cells carries almost all of the oxygen in the blood?

Transport of Carbon Dioxide

Carbon dioxide is produced continuously in the tissues as a byproduct of metabolism. It diffuses from the cells into the blood and is transported to the lungs in three ways:

Box 18-1 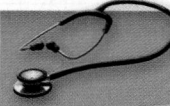 Clinical Perspectives

Liquid Ventilation: Breath in a Bottle

Researchers have been attempting for years to develop a fluid that could transport high concentrations of oxygen in the body. Such a fluid could substitute for blood in transfusions or be used to carry oxygen into the lungs. Early work on liquid ventilation climaxed in the mid-1960s when a pioneer in this field submerged a laboratory mouse in a beaker of fluid and the animal survived total immersion for more than 10 minutes. The fluid was a synthetic substance that could hold as much oxygen as does air.

A newer version of this fluid, a fluorine-containing chemical known as PFC, has been tested to ventilate the collapsed lungs of premature babies. In addition to delivering oxygen to the lung alveoli, it also removes carbon dioxide. The fluid is less damaging to delicate lung tissue than is air, which has to be pumped in under higher pressure. Others who might benefit from liquid ventilation include people whose lungs have been damaged by infection, inhaled toxins, asthma, emphysema, and lung cancer, but more clinical research is required. Scientists are also investigating whether liquid ventilation could be used to deliver drugs directly to lung tissue.

- About 10% is dissolved in the plasma and in the fluid within red blood cells. (Carbonated beverages are examples of water in which CO_2 is dissolved.)

- About 15% is combined with the protein portion of hemoglobin and with plasma proteins.

- About 75% is transported as an ion, known as a **bicarbonate** (bi-KAR-bon-ate) **ion**, which is formed when carbon dioxide undergoes a chemical change after it dissolves in blood fluids. It first combines with water to form **carbonic** (kar-BON-ik) **acid**, which then separates (ionizes) into hydrogen and bicarbonate ions.

The bicarbonate ion is formed slowly in the plasma but much more rapidly inside the red blood cells, where an enzyme called **carbonic anhydrase** (an-HI-drase) increases the speed of the reaction. The bicarbonate formed in the red blood cells moves to the plasma and then is carried to the lungs. In the lungs, the process is reversed as bicarbonate reenters the red blood cells and releases carbon dioxide for diffusion into the alveoli and exhalation. For those with a background in chemistry, the equation for these reactions follows. The arrows going in both directions signify that the reactions are reversible. The upper arrows describe what happens as CO_2 enters the blood; the lower arrows indicate what happens as CO_2 is released from the blood to be exhaled from the lungs.

$$CO_2 \; + \; H_2O \rightleftarrows H_2CO_3 \rightleftarrows \; H^+ \; + \; HCO_3^-$$

carbon   water   carbonic   hydrogen   bicarbonate
dioxide   acid   ion   ion

Carbon dioxide is important in regulating the blood's pH (acid–base balance). As a bicarbonate ion is formed from carbon dioxide in the plasma, a hydrogen ion (H^+) is also produced. Therefore, the blood becomes more acidic as the amount of carbon dioxide in the blood increases to yield more hydrogen and bicarbonate ions. The exhalation of carbon dioxide shifts the blood's pH more toward the alkaline (basic) range. The bicarbonate ion is also an important buffer in the blood, acting chemically to help keep the pH of body fluids within a steady range of 7.35 to 7.45.

CHECKPOINT `18-11` ➤ What is the main form in which carbon dioxide is carried in the blood?

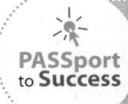 **PASSport to Success**   Visit **thePoint** or see the Student Resource CD in the back of this book to view the animation *Oxygen Transport* and *Carbon Dioxide Exchange*.

Regulation of Respiration

Centers in the central nervous system control the fundamental respiratory pattern. This pattern is modified by special receptors that detect changes in the blood's chemical composition.

NERVOUS CONTROL Regulation of respiration is a complex process that must keep pace with moment-to-moment changes in cellular oxygen requirements and carbon dioxide production. Regulation depends primarily on a respiratory control center located partly in the medulla and partly in the pons of the brain stem. The control center's main part, located in the medulla, sets the basic pattern of respiration. This pattern can be modified by centers in the pons. These areas continuously regulate breathing, so that levels of oxygen, carbon dioxide, and acid are kept within normal limits.

From the respiratory center in the medulla, motor nerve fibers extend into the spinal cord. From the cervical (neck) part of the cord, these nerve fibers continue through the **phrenic** (FREN-ik) **nerve** (a branch of the vagus nerve) to the diaphragm. The diaphragm and the other respiratory muscles are voluntary in the sense that they can be regulated consciously by messages from the higher brain centers, notably the cerebral cortex. It is possible for a person to deliberately breathe more rapidly or more slowly or to hold his or her breath and not breathe at all for a while. In a short time, however, the respiratory center in the brain stem will override the voluntary desire to not breathe, and breathing will resume. Most of the time, we breathe without thinking about it, and the respiratory center is in control.

CHECKPOINT `18-12` ➤ What part of the brain stem sets the basic pattern of respiration?

CHECKPOINT `18-13` ➤ What is the name of the motor nerve that controls the diaphragm?

CHEMICAL CONTROL Of vital importance in the control of respiration are **chemoreceptors** (ke-mo-re-SEP-tors) which, like the receptors for taste and smell, are sensitive to chemicals dissolved in body fluids. The chemoreceptors that regulate respiration are located centrally (near the brain stem) and peripherally (in arteries).

The central chemoreceptors are on either side of the brain stem near the medullary respiratory center. These receptors respond to the CO_2 level in circulating blood, but the gas acts indirectly. CO_2 is capable of diffusing through the capillary blood–brain barrier. It dissolves in CSF (the fluid in and around the brain) and separates into hydrogen ion and bicarbonate ion, as explained previously. It is the presence of hydrogen ion and its effect in lowering pH that actually stimulates the central chemoreceptors. The rise in blood CO_2 level, known as **hypercapnia** (hi-per-KAP-ne-ah), thus triggers ventilation.

The peripheral chemoreceptors that regulate respiration are found in structures called the *carotid* and *aortic bodies*. The carotid bodies are located near the bifurcation (forking) of the common carotid arteries in the neck, whereas the aortic bodies are located in the aortic arch. These bodies contain sensory neurons that respond mainly to a decrease in oxygen supply. They are not usually involved in regulating breathing, because they don't act until oxygen drops to a very low level. Because there is usually an ample reserve of oxygen in the blood, carbon dioxide

18

has the most immediate effect in regulating respiration at the level of the central chemoreceptors. When the carbon dioxide level increases, breathing must be increased to blow off the excess gas. Oxygen only becomes a controlling factor when its level falls considerably below normal.

CHECKPOINT 18-14 ▸ What gas is the main chemical controller of respiration?

Abnormal Ventilation

In **hyperventilation** (hi-per-ven-tih-LA-shun), an increased amount of air enters the alveoli. This condition results from deep and rapid respiration that commonly occurs during anxiety attacks, or when a person is experiencing pain or other forms of stress. Hyperventilation causes an increase in the oxygen level and a decrease in the carbon dioxide level of the blood, a condition called **hypocapnia** (hi-po-KAP-ne-ah). The loss of carbon dioxide increases the blood's pH (alkalosis) by removing acidic products, as shown by the equation cited previously. The change in pH results in dizziness and tingling sensations. Breathing may stop because the respiratory control center is not stimulated. Gradually, the carbon dioxide level returns to normal, and a regular breathing pattern is resumed. In extreme cases, a person may faint, and then breathing will involuntarily return to normal. In assisting a person who is hyperventilating, one should speak calmly, reassure him or her that the situation is not dangerous, and encourage even breathing from the diaphragm.

In **hypoventilation**, an insufficient amount of air enters the alveoli. The many possible causes of this condition include respiratory obstruction, lung disease, injury to the respiratory center, depression of the respiratory center, as by drugs, and chest deformity. Hypoventilation results in an increase in the carbon dioxide concentration in the blood, leading to a decrease in the blood's pH (acidosis), again according to the equation previously mentioned.

Breathing Patterns

Normal breathing rates vary from 12 to 20 breaths per minute for adults. In children, rates may vary from 20 to 40 breaths per minute, depending on age and size. In infants, the respiratory rate may be more than 40 breaths per minute. Changes in respiratory rates are important in various disorders and should be recorded carefully. To determine the respiratory rate, the healthcare worker counts the client's breathing for at least 30 seconds, usually by watching the chest rise and fall with each inhalation and exhalation. The count is then multiplied by 2 to obtain the rate in breaths per minute. It is best if the person does not realize that he or she is being observed because awareness of the measurement may cause a change in the breathing rate.

SOME TERMS FOR ALTERED BREATHING The following is a list of terms designating various respiratory abnormalities. These are symptoms, not diseases. Note that the word ending -*pnea* refers to breathing.

- **Hyperpnea** (hi-PERP-ne-ah) refers to an abnormal increase in the depth and rate of breathing.
- **Hypopnea** (hi-POP-ne-ah) is a decrease in the rate and depth of breathing.
- **Tachypnea** (tak-IP-ne-ah) is an excessive rate of breathing that may be normal, as in exercise.
- **Apnea** (AP-ne-ah) is a temporary cessation of breathing. Short periods of apnea occur normally during deep sleep. More severe sleep apnea can result from obstruction of the respiratory passageways or, less commonly, by failure in the central respiratory center.
- **Dyspnea** (disp-NE-ah) is a subjective feeling of difficult or labored breathing.
- **Orthopnea** (or-THOP-ne-ah) refers to a difficulty in breathing that is relieved by sitting in an upright position, either against two pillows in bed or in a chair.
- **Kussmaul** (KOOS-mowl) **respiration** is deep, rapid respiration characteristic of acidosis (overly acidic body fluids) as seen in uncontrolled diabetes.
- **Cheyne-Stokes** (CHANE-stokes) **respiration** is a rhythmic variation in the depth of respiratory movements alternating with periods of apnea. It is caused by depression of the breathing centers and is seen in certain critically ill patients.

RESULTS OF INADEQUATE BREATHING Conditions that may result from decreased respiration include the following:

- **Cyanosis** (si-ah-NO-sis) is a bluish color of the skin and mucous membranes caused by an insufficient amount of oxygen in the blood (see Fig. 6-6).
- **Hypoxia** (hi-POK-se-ah) means a lower than normal oxygen level in the tissues. The term **anoxia** (ah-NOK-se-ah) is sometimes used instead, but is not as accurate because it means a total lack of oxygen.
- **Hypoxemia** (hi-pok-SE-me-ah) refers to a lower than normal oxygen concentration in arterial blood.
- **Suffocation** is the cessation of respiration, often the result of a mechanical blockage of the respiratory passages.

Box 18-2, Adaptations to High Altitudes, offers information on adjusting to high altitudes and other hypoxic conditions.

Disorders of the Respiratory System

Infection is a major cause of respiratory disorders. These may involve any portion of the system. Allergies and environmental factors also affect respiration, and lung cancer is a major cause of cancer deaths in both men and women.

Box 18-2   A Closer Look

Adaptations to High Altitude: Living with Hypoxia

Our bodies work best at low altitudes where oxygen is plentiful. However, people are able to live at high altitudes where oxygen is scarce and can even survive climbing Mount Everest, the tallest peak on our planet, showing that the human body can adapt to hypoxic conditions. This adaptation process compensates for decreased atmospheric oxygen by increasing the efficiency of the respiratory and cardiovascular systems.

The body's immediate response to high altitude is to increase the rate of ventilation (hyperventilation) and raise the heart rate to increase cardiac output. Hyperventilation makes more oxygen available to the cells and increases blood pH (al-

kalosis), which boosts hemoglobin's capacity to bind oxygen. Over time, the body adapts in additional ways. Hypoxia stimulates the kidneys to secrete erythropoietin, prompting red bone marrow to manufacture more erythrocytes and hemoglobin. Also, capillaries proliferate, increasing blood flow to the tissues. Some people are unable to adapt to high altitudes, and for them, hypoxia and alkalosis lead to potentially fatal **altitude sickness**.

Successful adaptation to high altitude illustrates the principle of homeostasis and also helps to explain how the body adjusts to hypoxia associated with disorders such as chronic obstructive pulmonary disease.

Disorders of the Nasal Cavities and Related Structures

The paranasal sinuses are located in the skull bones in the vicinity of the nasal cavities. Infection may easily travel into these sinuses from the mouth, nose, and throat along their mucous membranes. The resulting inflammation is called **sinusitis**. Chronic (long-standing) sinus infection may cause changes in the epithelial cells, resulting in tumor formation. Some of these growths have a grapelike appearance and cause airway obstruction; such tumors are called polyps (POL-ips).

The partition separating the two nasal cavities is called the *nasal septum*. Because of minor structural defects, the nasal septum is rarely exactly in the midline. If it is markedly to one side, it is described as a **deviated septum**. In this condition, one nasal space may be considerably smaller than the other. If an affected person has an attack of hay fever or develops a cold with accompanying swelling of the mucosa, the smaller nasal cavity may be completely closed. Sometimes, the septum is curved in such a way that both nasal cavities are occluded, forcing the person to breathe through his or her mouth. Such an occlusion may also prevent proper drainage from the sinuses and aggravate a case of sinusitis.

The most common cause of nosebleed, also called **epistaxis** (ep-e-STAK-sis) (from a Greek word meaning "to drip"), is injury to the mucous membranes in the nasal cavity. Causes of injury include infection, drying of the membranes, picking the nose, or other forms of trauma. These simple nosebleeds usually stop on their own, but some measures that help are applying pressure to the upper lip under the nose, pinching the nose together, or applying ice to the forehead. Epistaxis may signal more serious problems, such as blood clotting abnormalities, excessively high blood pressure, or tumors.

Serious injuries that lead to nosebleed, or a nosebleed that will not stop, require professional medical care. Treatment may include packing the nose with gauze or other material, administering vasoconstrictors, or cauterizing the wound.

Infection

The respiratory tract mucosa is one of the most important portals of entry for disease-producing organisms. The transfer of disease organisms from one person's respiratory system to another's occurs most rapidly in crowded places, such as schools, theaters, and institutions. Droplets from one sneeze may be loaded with many billions of disease-producing organisms.

Mucous membranes can resist infection to some degree by producing larger quantities of mucus. The runny nose, an unpleasant symptom of the common cold, is the body's attempt to wash away pathogens and protect deeper tissues from further infection. If the membrane's resistance is reduced, however, the membrane may act as a pathway for the spread of disease. The infection may travel by that route into the nasal sinuses, or middle ear, along the respiratory passageways, or into the lung. Each infection is named according to the part involved, such as pharyngitis (commonly called a *sore throat*), laryngitis, or bronchitis.

Among the infections transmitted through the respiratory passageways are the common cold, diphtheria, chickenpox, measles, influenza, pneumonia, and tuberculosis. Any infection that is confined to the nose and throat is called an **upper respiratory infection** (URI). Very often, an upper respiratory infection is the first evidence of infectious disease in children. Such an infection may precede the onset of a serious disease, such as rheumatic fever, which may follow a streptococcal throat infection.

18

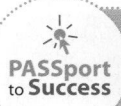

Visit **thePoint** or see the Student Resource CD in the back of this book for a summary diagram of respiratory infections.

THE COMMON COLD The common cold is the most widespread of all respiratory diseases—of all communicable diseases, for that matter. More time is lost from school and work because of the common cold than any other disorder. (See Box 5-2 in Chapter 5.) The causative agents are viruses that probably number more than 200 different types. Medical science has yet to establish the effectiveness of any method for preventing the common cold. Because there are so many organisms involved, the production of an effective vaccine against colds seems unlikely.

The symptoms of the common cold are familiar: first the swollen and inflamed mucosa of the nose and the throat, then the copious discharge of watery fluid from the nose, and finally the thick and ropy discharge that occurs when the cold is subsiding. The scientific name for the common cold is **acute coryza** (ko-RI-zah); the word coryza can also mean simply "a nasal discharge."

RESPIRATORY SYNCYTIAL VIRUS (RSV) RSV is the most common cause of lower respiratory tract infections in infants and young children worldwide. The name comes from the fact that the virus induces fusion of cultured cells (formation of a syncytium) when grown in the laboratory. Infection may result in bronchiolitis or pneumonia, but the virus may affect the upper respiratory tract as well. Most susceptible are premature infants, those with congenital heart disease, and those who are immunodeficient. Exposure to cigarette smoke is a definite risk factor.

The virus usually enters through the eyes and nose following contact with contaminated air, nasal secretions, or objects. The incubation period is 3 to 5 days, and an infected person sheds virus particles during the incubation period and up to 2 weeks thereafter. Thorough handwashing helps to reduce spread of the virus. Infection usually resolves in 5 to 7 days, although some cases require hospitalization and antiviral drug treatments.

CROUP Croup usually affects children under 3 years of age and is associated with a number of different infections that result in upper respiratory inflammation. Airway constriction produces a loud, barking cough, wheezing, difficulty in breathing, and hoarseness. If croup is severe, the child may produce a harsh, squeaking noise (stridor) when breathing in through a narrowed trachea. Viral infections, such as those involving parainfluenza, adenovirus, RSV, influenza, or measles, are usually the cause. Although croup may be frightening to parents and children, recovery is complete in most cases within a week. Home treatments include humidifying room air or having the child breathe in steam. Also, cool air may shrink the respiratory tissues enough to bring relief.

INFLUENZA Influenza (in-flu-EN-zah), or "flu," is an acute contagious disease characterized by an inflammatory condition of the upper respiratory tract accompanied by generalized aches and pains. It is caused by a virus and may spread to the sinuses and downward to the lungs. Inflammation of the trachea and the bronchi causes the characteristic cough of influenza, and the general infection causes an extremely weakened condition. The great danger of influenza is its tendency to develop into a particularly severe form of pneumonia. At intervals in history, there have been tremendous epidemics of influenza in which millions of people have died. Vaccines have been effective, although the protection is of short duration.

PNEUMONIA Pneumonia (nu-MO-ne-ah) is an inflammation of the lungs in which the air spaces become filled with fluid. A variety of organisms, including staphylococci, pneumococci, streptococci, *Legionella pneumophila* (cause of Legionnaires disease), chlamydias, and viruses may be responsible. Many of these pathogens may be carried by a healthy person in the upper respiratory mucosa. If the person remains in good health, they may be carried for a long time with no ill effect. If the patient's resistance to infection is lowered, however, the pathogens may invade the tissues and cause disease.

Susceptibility to pneumonia is increased in patients with chronic, debilitating illness or chronic respiratory disease, in smokers, and in people with alcoholism. It is also increased in cases of exposure to toxic gases, suppression of the immune system, or viral respiratory infections.

There are two main kinds of pneumonia as determined by the extent of lung involvement and other factors:

- **Bronchopneumonia**, in which the disease process is scattered throughout the lung. The cause may be infection with a staphylococcus, gram-negative *Proteus* species, colon bacillus (not normally pathogenic), or a virus. Bronchopneumonia most often is secondary to an infection or to some factor that has lowered the patient's resistance to disease. This is the most common form of pneumonia.

- **Lobar pneumonia**, in which an entire lobe of the lung is infected at one time. The causative organism is usually a pneumococcus, although other pathogens may also cause this disease. *Legionella* is the agent of Legionnaires disease, or legionellosis, severe lobar pneumonia that occurs mostly in localized epidemics.

Most types of pneumonia are characterized by the formation of a fluid, or **exudate** (EKS-u-date), in the infected alveoli; this fluid consists chiefly of serum and pus, products of infection. Some red blood cells may be present, as indicated by red streaks in the sputum. Sometimes, so many air sacs become filled with fluid that the victim finds it hard to absorb enough oxygen to maintain life.

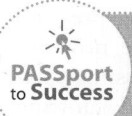

Visit **thePoint** or see the Student Resource CD in the back of this book for an illustration of the two types of pneumonia.

Pneumocystis Pneumonia (PCP) PCP occurs mainly in people with weakened immune systems, such as HIV-positive individuals or transplant recipients on immunosuppressant drugs. The infectious agent was originally called P. carinii and classified as a protozoon. It has now been reclassified as an atypical fungus and renamed P. jiroveci. The organism grows in the fluid that lines the alveoli of the lungs. Laboratories diagnose the disease by microscopic identification of the organism in a sputum sample, bronchoscopy specimen, or lung biopsy specimen. PCP is treated with antimicrobial drugs, although these medications may cause serious side effects in immunocompromised patients.

TUBERCULOSIS Tuberculosis (tu-ber-ku-LO-sis) (**TB**) is an infectious disease caused by the bacillus *Mycobacterium tuberculosis*. Although the tubercle bacillus may invade any body tissue, it usually grows in the lung. Tuberculosis remains a leading cause of death from communicable disease, primarily because of the relatively large numbers of cases among recent immigrants, elderly people, and poor people in metropolitan areas. The spread of AIDS has been linked with a rising incidence of TB because this viral disease weakens host defenses.

The name *tuberculosis* comes from the small lesions, or tubercles, that form where the organisms grow. If unchecked, these lesions degenerate and may even liquefy to cause cavities within an organ. In early stages, the disease may lie dormant, only to flare up at a later time. The tuberculosis organism can readily spread into the lymph nodes or into the blood and be carried to other organs. The lymph nodes in the thorax, especially those surrounding the trachea and bronchi, are frequently involved. Infection of the pleura results in tuberculous pleurisy (inflammation of the pleura). In this case, a collection of fluid, known as an effusion (e-FU-zhun), accumulates in the pleural space.

Drugs can be used successfully in many cases of tuberculosis, although strains of the TB organism that are resistant to multiple antibiotics have appeared recently. The best results have been obtained by use of a combination of several drugs, with prompt, intensive, and uninterrupted treatment once a program is begun. Therapy is usually continued for a minimum of 6 to 18 months; therefore, close supervision by the healthcare practitioner is important. Adverse drug reactions are rather common, necessitating changes in the drug combinations. Drug treatment of patients whose infection has not progressed to active disease is particularly effective.

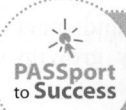 **PASSport to Success** Visit **thePoint** or see the Student Resource CD in the back of this book for a micrograph of the acid-fast TB organism and a diagram of TB infection.

Hay Fever and Asthma

Hypersensitivity to plant pollens, dust, certain foods, and other allergens may lead to **hay fever** or **asthma** (AZ-mah) or both. Hay fever, known medically as *allergic rhinitis*, is characterized by a watery discharge from the eyes and nose. Hay fever often appears in a seasonal pattern due to pollen allergy. The response may be chronic if the allergen is present year round. The symptoms of asthma are caused by reversible changes, which include inflammation of airway tissues and spasm of the involuntary muscle in bronchial tubes. Spasm constricts the tubes, causing resistance to air flow. The person experiences a sense of suffocation and has labored breathing (dyspnea), often with wheezing. Treatment may include inhaled steroids to prevent inflammation and inhaled bronchodilators to open airways during acute episodes.

Patients vary considerably in their responses, and most cases of asthma involve multiple causes. Respiratory infection, noxious fumes, or drug allergy can initiate episodes, but one of the more common triggers for asthma attacks is exercise. The rapid air movement in sensitive airways causes smooth muscle spasm in the breathing passages.

A great difficulty in the treatment of hay fever or asthma is identification of the particular substance to which the patient is allergic. Allergists usually give a number of skin tests, but in most cases, the results are inconclusive. People with allergies may benefit from a series of injections to reduce their sensitivity to specific substances.

Chronic Obstructive Pulmonary Disease (COPD)

Chronic obstructive pulmonary disease (COPD) is the term used to describe several lung disorders, including **chronic bronchitis** and **emphysema** (em-fih-SE-mah). Most affected patients have symptoms and lung damage characteristic of both diseases. In chronic bronchitis, the airway linings are chronically inflamed and produce excessive secretions. Emphysema is characterized by dilation and finally destruction of the alveoli.

In COPD, respiratory function is impaired by obstruction to normal air flow, reducing exchange of oxygen and carbon dioxide. There is air trapping and over-inflation of parts of the lungs. In the early stages of these diseases, the small airways are involved, and several years may pass before symptoms become evident. Later, the affected person develops dyspnea as a result of difficulty in exhaling air through the obstructed air passages.

In certain smokers, COPD may result in serious disability and death within 10 years of the onset of symptoms. Giving up smoking may reverse progression of the disorder, especially when it is diagnosed early and other respiratory irritants also are eliminated. Sometimes, the word *emphysema* is used to mean COPD.

COPD is also called COLD (chronic obstructive lung disease).

18

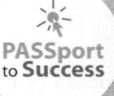 **PASSport to Success** Visit **thePoint** or see the Student Resource CD in the back of this book for a photograph showing emphysema in lung tissue.

Sudden Infant Death Syndrome (SIDS)

SIDS, also called "crib death," is the unexplained death of a seemingly healthy infant under 1 year of age. Death usually occurs during sleep, leaving no signs of its cause. Neither autopsy nor careful investigation of family history and circumstances of death provides any clues. Certain maternal conditions during pregnancy are associated with an increased risk of SIDS, although none is a sure predictor. These include cigarette smoking, age under 20, low weight gain, anemia, illegal drug use, and infections of the reproductive or urinary tracts.

Some guidelines that have reduced the SIDS incidence are:

- Place the baby supine (on its back) for sleep, unless there is some medical reason not to do so. A reminder for parents and other caregivers is the slogan "Back to sleep." A side position is not as effective, as the baby can roll over, and it should never be put to sleep prone (face down). In the prone position, the baby can re-breathe its own CO_2, building up CO_2 and diminishing blood O_2 levels. The position may also cause obstruction in the upper airways or lead to overheating by reducing loss of body heat.

- Keep the baby in a smoke-free environment. Maternal smoking during pregnancy, or smoking in the baby's environment after birth, increases the SIDS risk.

- Use a firm, flat baby mattress, not soft foam, fur, or fiber-filled bedding.

- Avoid overheating the baby with room air, clothing, or bedding, especially when the baby has a cold or other infection.

CHECKPOINT `18-15` ➤ What does COPD mean and what two diseases are commonly involved in COPD?

Respiratory Distress Syndrome (RDS)

RDS covers a range of inflammatory disorders that result from other medical problems or from direct injury to the lungs. **Acute respiratory distress syndrome** (ARDS), or shock lung, usually appears in adults, in contrast to a form of the syndrome that occurs in premature newborns, as described later. Some causes of ARDS are:

- Airway obstruction as from mucus, foreign bodies, emboli, or tumors
- Sepsis (systemic infection)
- Aspiration (inhalation) of stomach contents
- Allergy
- Lung trauma

Inflammation and damage to the alveoli results in pulmonary edema, dyspnea (difficulty in breathing), de-

creased compliance, hypoxemia, and formation of fibrous scar tissue in the lungs. The incomplete expansion of a lung or portion of a lung, such as results from ARDS, is called **atelectasis** (at-e-LEK-tah-sis), or collapsed lung.

In premature newborns, atelectasis may result from insufficient surfactant production by the immature lungs. **Respiratory distress syndrome of the newborn** is now treated by administration of surfactant that is produced in bacteria by genetic engineering. The syndrome was formerly called *hyaline membrane disease* because of the clear membrane formed from lung exudates in the alveoli.

Cancer

Tumors can arise in all portions of the respiratory tract. Two common sites are described as follows.

LUNG CANCER Cancer of the lungs is the most common cause of cancer-related deaths in both men and women. The incidence rate in women continues to increase, whereas the rate in men has been decreasing recently. By far, the most important cause of lung cancer is cigarette smoking. Smokers suffer from lung cancer 10 times as often as do nonsmokers. The risk of getting lung cancer is increased in people who started smoking early in life, smoke large numbers of cigarettes daily, and inhale deeply. Smokers who are exposed to toxic chemicals or particles in the air have an even higher lung cancer rate. Smoking has also been linked with an increase in COPD and cancers of respiratory passages.

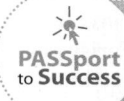 **PASSport to Success** Visit **thePoint** or see the Student Resource CD in the back of this book for an illustration of the effects of smoking.

A common form of lung cancer is **bronchogenic** (brong-ko-JEN-ik) **carcinoma**, so called because the malignancy originates in a bronchus. The tumor may grow until the bronchus is blocked, cutting off the air supply to that lung. The lung then collapses, and the secretions trapped in the lung spaces become infected, with a resulting pneumonia or lung abscess formation. This type of lung cancer can spread, causing secondary growths in the lymph nodes of the chest and neck and in the brain and other parts of the body. A treatment that offers a possibility of cure before secondary growths have had time to form is complete removal of the lung. This operation is called a **pneumonectomy** (nu-mo-NEK-to-me).

Malignant tumors of the stomach, breast, and other organs may spread to the lungs as secondary growths (metastases).

CANCER OF THE LARYNX Cancer of the larynx usually involves squamous cell carcinoma, and its incidence is definitely linked to cigarette smoking and alcohol consumption. Symptoms include sore throat, hoarseness, ear pain, and enlarged cervical lymph nodes. The cure rate is high for small tumors that have not spread when treated with radiation and (sometimes) surgery. Total or partial removal of the larynx is necessary in cases of advanced cancer that do not respond to radiation or chemotherapy. During and after laryngectomy a patient may need a surgically-created opening, or stoma, in the trachea with a tube (tracheostomy tube) for breathing. Patients have to care for the stoma and the "trach" (trake) tube. If the vocal cords are removed, a patient can learn to speak by using air forced out of the esophagus or by using a mechanical device to generate sound.

Disorders Involving the Pleura

Pleurisy (PLUR-ih-se), or inflammation of the pleura, usually accompanies a lung infection—particularly pneumonia or tuberculosis. This condition can be quite painful because the inflammation produces a sticky exudate that roughens the pleura of both the lung and the chest wall; when the two surfaces rub together during ventilation, the roughness causes acute irritation. The sticking together of two surfaces is called an adhesion (ad-HE-zhun). Infection of the pleura also causes an increase in the amount of pleural fluid. This fluid may accumulate in the pleural space in quantities large enough to compress the lung, resulting in an inability to obtain enough air.

Pneumothorax (nu-mo-THOR-aks) is an accumulation of air in the pleural space (Fig. 18-11). The lung on the affected side collapses, causing the patient to have great difficulty breathing. Pneumothorax may be caused by a wound in the chest wall or by rupture of the lung's air spaces. In pneumothorax caused by a penetrating wound in the chest wall, an airtight cover over the opening prevents further air from entering. The remaining lung can then function to provide adequate oxygen.

Blood in the pleural space, a condition called **hemothorax**, is also caused by penetrating chest wounds. In such cases, the first priority is to stop the bleeding.

The abnormal accumulation of fluid or air in the pleural space from any of the above conditions may call for procedures to promote lung expansion. In **thoracentesis** (thor-ah-sen-TE-sis) a large-bore needle is inserted between ribs into the pleural space to remove fluid (Fig. 18-12). The presence of both air and fluid in the pleural space may require insertion of a chest tube, a large tube with several openings along the internal end. The tube is securely connected to a chest drainage system. These procedures restore negative pressure in the pleural space and allow reexpansion of the lung.

Age and the Respiratory Tract

With age, the tissues of the respiratory tract lose elasticity and become more rigid. Similar rigidity in the chest wall, combined with arthritis and loss of strength in the breathing muscles, results in an overall decrease in compliance and in lung capacity. Reduction in protective mechanisms in the lungs, such as phagocytosis, leads to increased susceptibility to infection. The incidence of lung disease increases with age, hastened by cigarette smoking and by exposure to other environmental irritants. Although there is much individual variation, especially related to one's customary level of activity, these changes gradually lead to reduced capacity for exercise.

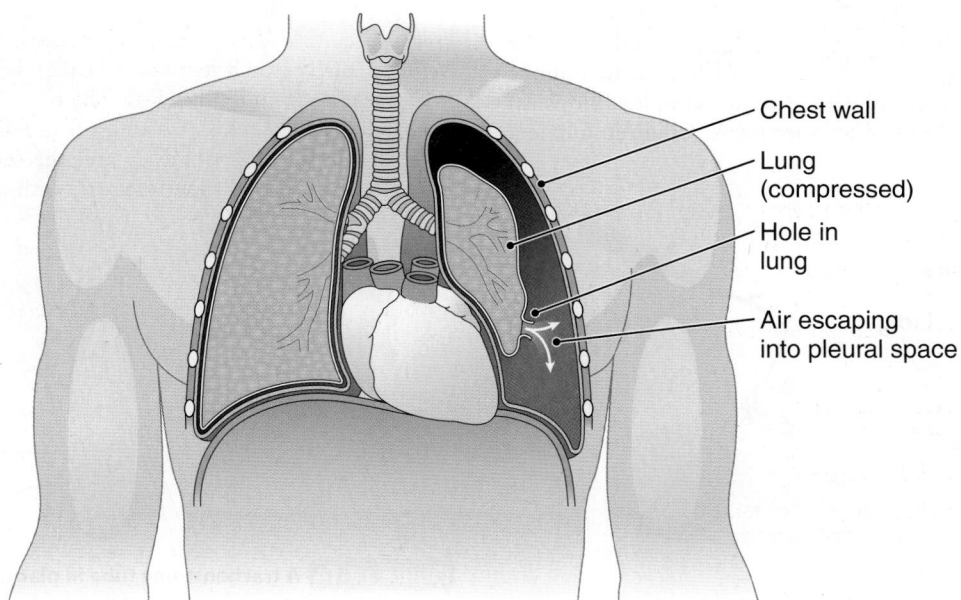

Chest wall

Lung (compressed)

Hole in lung

Air escaping into pleural space

18

Figure 18-11 **Pneumothorax.** Injury to lung tissue allows air to leak into the pleural space and put pressure on the lung. (Reprinted with permission from Cohen BJ. *Medical Terminology*, 5th ed. Philadelphia: Lippincott Williams & Wilkins, 2008.)

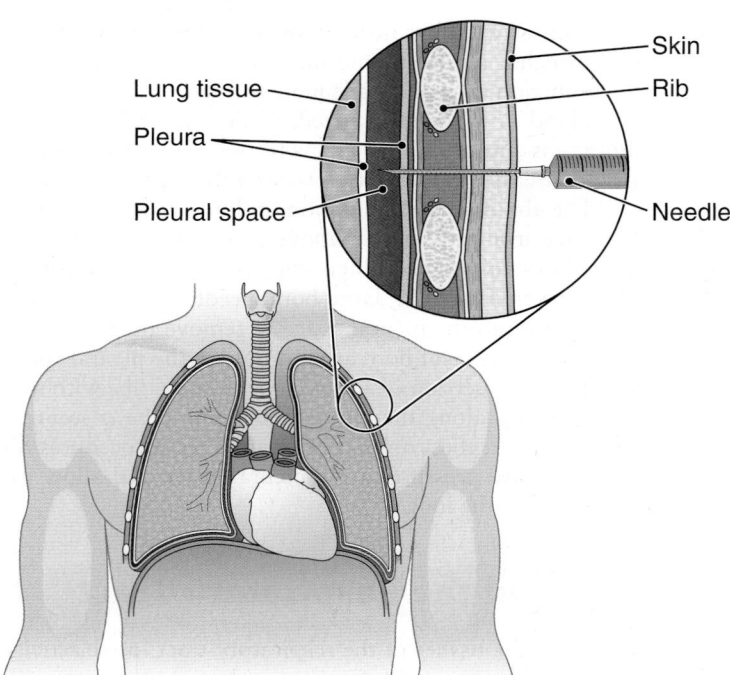

Figure 18-12 **Thoracentesis.** A needle is inserted into the pleural space to withdraw fluid. (Reprinted with permission from Cohen BJ. *Medical Terminology*, 4th ed. Philadelphia: Lippincott Williams & Wilkins, 2004.)

Special Equipment for Respiratory Treatment

The **bronchoscope** (BRONG-ko-skope) is a rigid or flexible fiberoptic tubular instrument used for inspection of the primary bronchi and the larger bronchial tubes (Fig. 18-13). Most bronchoscopes are now attached to video recording equipment. The bronchoscope is passed into the respiratory tract by way of the nose or mouth and the pharynx. Physicians may use a bronchoscope to remove foreign bodies, inspect and take tissue samples (biopsies) from tumors, or collect other specimens. Children inhale a

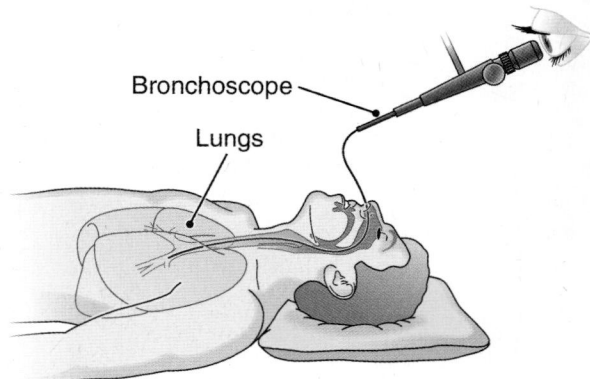

Figure 18-13 **Use of a bronchoscope.** (Reprinted with permission from Cohen BJ. *Medical Terminology,* 4th ed. Philadelphia: Lippincott Williams & Wilkins, 2004.)

variety of objects, such as pins, beans, pieces of nuts, and small coins, all of which a physician may remove with the aid of a bronchoscope. If such items are left in the lung, they may cause an abscess or other serious complication and may even lead to death.

Oxygen therapy is used to sustain life when a condition interferes with adequate oxygen supply to the tissues. The oxygen must first have moisture added by bubbling it through water that is at room temperature or heated. Therapists may deliver oxygen to the patient by mask, catheter, or nasal prongs. Because there is danger of fire when oxygen is being administered, smoking in the room is absolutely prohibited.

A **suction apparatus** is used for removing mucus or other substances from the respiratory tract by means of negative pressure. A container to trap secretions is located between the patient and the machine. The tube leading to the patient has an opening to control the suction. When suction is applied, the drainage flows from the patient's respiratory tract into the collection container.

A **tracheostomy** (tra-ke-OS-to-me) **tube** is used if the pharynx or the larynx is obstructed. It is a small metal or plastic tube that is inserted through a cut made in the trachea, and it acts as an artificial airway for ventilation (Fig. 18-14). The procedure

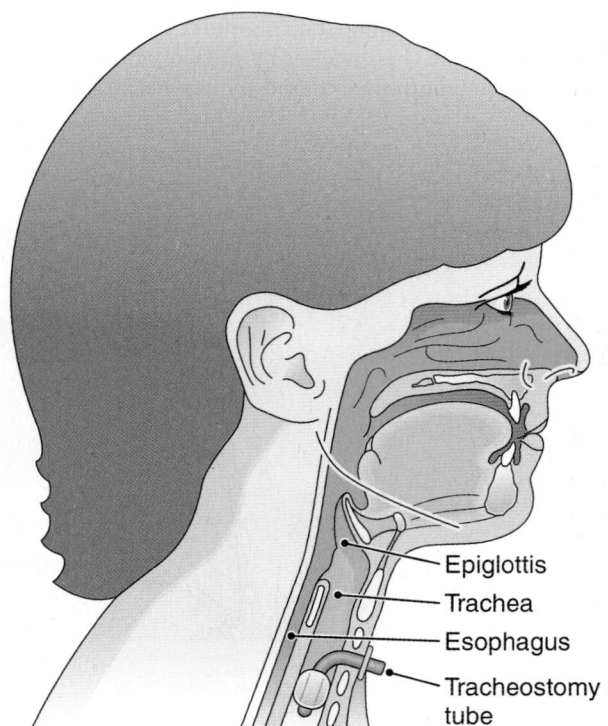

Figure 18-14 **A tracheostomy tube in place.** (Reprinted with permission from Cohen BJ. *Medical Terminology*, 5th ed. Philadelphia: Lippincott Williams & Wilkins, 2008.) [**ZOOMING IN** ➤ What structure is posterior to the trachea?]

for the insertion of such a tube is a *tracheostomy*. The word **tracheotomy** (tra-ke-OT-o-me) refers to the incision in the trachea.

Artificial respiration is used when a patient has temporarily lost the capacity to perform normal ventilation. Such emergencies include cases of gas or smoke inhalation, electric shock, drowning, poisoning, or paralysis of the breathing muscles. A number of different apparatuses are used for artificial respiration in a clinical setting.

There are also some techniques that can be used in an emergency.

Many public agencies offer classes in the techniques of mouth-to-mouth respiration and cardiac massage to revive people experiencing respiratory or cardiac arrest. This technique is known as **cardiopulmonary resuscitation**, or **CPR**. These classes also include instruction in emergency airway clearance using abdominal thrusts (Heimlich maneuver), chest thrusts, or back blows to open obstructed airways.

Disease in Context revisited

➤ Emily's Asthma

It had been about a month since Emily's appointment with Dr. Martinez. During that time, her parents had monitored her breathing very carefully and had noticed patterns in her coughing bouts. "It does seem that Emily gets out of breath sooner than the other kids when she exercises," Emily's mother reported to Dr. Martinez during her follow-up appointment. "And now that the weather has cooled off, I do notice that she coughs more," continued Nicole.

"Let's take a listen to Emily's lungs," replied the doctor as he placed his stethoscope on the little girl's chest. "Yes," he continued, "I hear wheezing today, which suggests that Emily's airways are narrowed. Based on this finding, your observations, and the family history, I think Emily has asthma."

Although Nicole had expected the doctor's diagnosis, it was still a shock to hear him say it. Seeing her look of alarm, Dr. Martinez continued, "Most kids with asthma lead very normal, active lives. The medications available today target asthma right at its source—inflammation. In fact, with proper treatment, many kids maintain near-normal pulmonary function. Let's start with an oral antileukotriene medication that Emily will take daily to control airway inflammation. If, after a few weeks, we don't see any improvement, we'll supplement her treatment with an anti-inflammatory in the form of a low-dose corticosteroid inhaler. I'm also going to prescribe an inhaler to use if Emily has a severe asthma episode. The inhaler contains a medication that relaxes the smooth muscle of her airways, giving her short-term relief of symptoms."

In this case, we learned that Emily's asthma was caused by airway inflammation. Medications that limit the inflammatory response in the respiratory passages can prevent the symptoms of asthma. For a review of the role of inflammation in normal body defense mechanisms, see Chapter 17.

18

Word Anatomy

Medical terms are built from standardized word parts (prefixes, roots, and suffixes). Learning the meanings of these parts can help you remember words and interpret unfamiliar terms.

WORD PART	MEANING	EXAMPLE
The Respiratory System		
nas/o	nose	The *nasopharynx* is behind the nasal cavity.
or/o	mouth	The *oropharynx* is behind the mouth.
laryng/o	larynx	The *laryngeal* pharynx opens into the larynx.
pleur/o	side, rib	The *pleura* covers the lung and lines the chest wall (rib cage).
The Process of Respiration		
spir/o	breathing	A *spirometer* is an instrument used to record breathing volumes.
capn/o	carbon dioxide	*Hypercapnia* is a rise in the blood level of carbon dioxide.
-pnea	breathing	*Hypopnea* is a decrease in the rate and depth of breathing.
orth/o-	straight	*Orthopnea* can be relieved by sitting in an upright position.
Disorders of the Respiratory System		
pneumon/o	lung	*Pneumonia* is inflammation of the lung.
atel/o	incomplete	*Atelectasis* is incomplete expansion of the lung.
pneum/o	air, gas	*Pneumothorax* is accumulation of air in the pleural space.
–centesis	tapping, perforation	In *thoracentesis* a needle is inserted into the pleural space to remove fluid.

Summary

I. **PHASES OF RESPIRATION**
   A. Pulmonary ventilation
   B. External gas exchange
   C. Internal gas exchange

II. **THE RESPIRATORY SYSTEM**
   A. Nasal cavities—filter, warm, and moisten air
   B. Pharynx (throat)—carries air into respiratory tract and food into digestive tract
   C. Larynx (voice box)—contains vocal cords
      1. Glottis—space between the vocal cords
      2. Epiglottis—covers larynx on swallowing to help prevent food from entering
   D. Trachea (windpipe)
   E. Bronchi—branches of trachea that enter lungs and then subdivide
      1. Bronchioles—smallest subdivisions

   F. Lungs
      1. Organs of gas exchange
      2. Lobes—three on right; two on left
      3. Alveoli
         a. Tiny air sacs where gases are exchanged
         b. Surfactant—reduces surface tension in alveoli; eases expansion of lungs
      4. Pleura—membrane that encloses the lung
         a. Visceral pleura—attached to surface of lung
         b. Parietal pleura—attached to chest wall
         c. Pleural space—between layers
      5. Mediastinum—space and organs between lungs

III. **THE PROCESS OF RESPIRATION**
   A. Pulmonary ventilation
      1. Inhalation—drawing of air into lungs

a. Compliance—ease with which lungs and thorax can be expanded

2. Exhalation—expulsion of air from lungs

3. Lung volumes—used to evaluate respiratory function

B. Gas exchange

1. Gases diffuse from area of higher concentration to area of lower concentration

2. In lungs—oxygen enters blood and carbon dioxide leaves (external exchange)

3. In tissues—oxygen leaves blood and carbon dioxide enters (internal exchange)

C. Oxygen transport

1. Almost totally bound to heme portion of hemoglobin in red blood cells

2. Separates from hemoglobin when oxygen concentration is low (in tissues)

a. Carbon monoxide replaces oxygen on hemoglobin

D. Carbon dioxide transport

1. Most carried as bicarbonate ion

2. Regulates pH of blood

E. Regulation of respiration

1. Nervous control—centers in medulla and pons

2. Chemical control

a. Central chemoreceptors respond to CO_2, which decreases pH

b. Peripheral chemorecptors—respond to low levels of O_2

F. Abnormal ventilation

1. Hyperventilation—rapid, deep respiration

2. Hypoventilation—inadequate air in alveoli

G. Breathing patterns

1. Normal—12 to 20 breaths per minute in adult

2. Types of altered breathing

a. Hyperpnea—increase in depth and rate of breathing

b. Tachypnea—excessive rate of breathing

c. Apnea—temporary cessation of breathing

d. Dyspnea—difficulty in breathing

e. Orthopnea—difficulty relieved by upright position

f. Kussmaul—characterizes acidosis

g. Cheyne-Stokes—irregularity found in critically ill

3. Possible results—cyanosis, hypoxia (anoxia), hypoxemia, suffocation

IV. **DISORDERS OF THE RESPIRATORY SYSTEM**

A. Disorders of the nasal cavities and related structures—sinusitis, polyps, deviated septum, nosebleed (epistaxis)

B. Infection—colds, RSV, croup, influenza, pneumonia, tuberculosis

C. Hay fever and asthma—hypersensitivity (allergy)

D. COPD—involves emphysema and bronchitis

E. SIDS—sudden infant death syndrome

F. Respiratory distress syndrome (RDS)

1. Acute (ARDS)—due to other medical problem or direct injury to lung

2. RDS of newborn—due to lack of surfactant

G. Cancer—smoking a major causative factor

H. Disorders involving the pleural space

1. Pleurisy—inflammation of pleura

2. Pneumothorax—air in pleural space

3. Hemothorax—blood in pleural space

V. **AGE AND THE RESPIRATORY TRACT**

VI. **SPECIAL EQUIPMENT FOR RESPIRATORY TREATMENT**

A. Bronchoscope—tube used to examine air passageways and remove foreign bodies

B. Oxygen therapy

C. Suction apparatus—removes mucus and other substances

D. Tracheostomy—artificial airway

a. Tracheotomy—incision into trachea

E. Artificial respiration—cardiopulmonary resuscitation (CPR)

Questions for Study and Review

18

BUILDING UNDERSTANDING

Fill in the blanks

1. The exchange of air between the atmosphere and the lungs is called _____.

2. The space between the vocal cords is the _____.

3. The ease with which the lungs and thorax can be expanded is termed _____.

4. A lower than normal level of oxygen in the tissues is called _____.

5. Inflammation of the pleura is termed _____.

Matching > Match each numbered item with the most closely related lettered item.

___ **6.** A decrease in the rate and depth of breathing

___ **7.** An increase in the rate and depth of breathing

___ **8.** A temporary cessation of breathing

___ **9.** Difficult or labored breathing

___ **10.** Difficult breathing that is relieved by sitting up

a. dyspnea

b. hyperpnea

c. orthopnea

d. hypopnea

e. apnea

Multiple choice

___ **11.** The bony projections in the nasal cavities that increase surface area are called

  a. nares
  b. septae
  c. conchae
  d. sinuses

___ **12.** Which of the following structures produces speech?

  a. pharynx
  b. larynx
  c. trachea
  d. lungs

___ **13.** The leaf-shaped cartilage that covers the larynx during swallowing is the

  a. epiglottis
  b. glottis
  c. conchae
  d. sinus

___ **14.** Respiration is centrally regulated by the

  a. cerebral cortex
  b. diencephalon
  c. brain stem
  d. cerebellum

___ **15.** Incomplete expansion of a lung or portion of a lung is called

  a. effusion
  b. adhesion
  c. epistaxis
  d. atelectasis

UNDERSTANDING CONCEPTS

16. Differentiate between the terms in each of the following pairs:

  a. internal and external gas exchange
  b. pleura and diaphragm
  c. inhalation and exhalation
  d. spirometer and spirogram

17. Trace the path of air from the nostrils to the lung capillaries.

18. What is the function of the cilia on cells that line the respiratory passageways?

19. Compare and contrast the transport of oxygen and carbon dioxide in the blood.

20. Define hyperventilation and hypoventilation. What is the effect of each on blood CO_2 levels and blood pH?

21. What are chemoreceptors and how do they function to regulate breathing?

22. Describe the structural and functional changes that occur in the respiratory system in chronic obstructive pulmonary disease.

23. Compare and contrast the following disease conditions:

  a. Kussmaul and Cheyne-Stokes respiration
  b. acute coryza and influenza
  c. bronchopneumonia and lobar pneumonia
  d. pneumothorax and hemathorax

CONCEPTUAL THINKING

24. Jake, a sometimes exasperating 4-year-old, threatens his mother that he will hold his breath until "he dies." Should his mother be concerned that he might succeed?

25. Why is it important that airplane interiors are pressurized? If the cabin lost pressure, what physiological adaptations to respiration might occur in the passengers?

26. In Emily's case, an anti-inflammatory medication was used to control her asthma symptoms. Explain how this drug works in the respiratory system.

18

CHAPTER 19

The Digestive System

Learning Outcomes

After careful study of this chapter, you should be able to:

1. Name the three main functions of the digestive system
2. Describe the four layers of the digestive tract wall
3. Differentiate between the two layers of the peritoneum
4. Name and locate the different types of teeth
5. Name and describe the functions of the organs of the digestive tract
6. Name and describe the functions of the accessory organs of digestion
7. Describe how bile functions in digestion
8. Name and locate the ducts that carry bile from the liver into the digestive tract
9. Explain the role of enzymes in digestion and give examples of enzymes
10. Name the digestion products of fats, proteins, and carbohydrates
11. Define *absorption*
12. Define *villi* and state how villi function in absorption
13. Explain the use of feedback in regulating digestion and give several examples
14. List several hormones involved in regulating digestion
15. Describe common disorders of the digestive tract and the accessory organs
16. Show how word parts are used to build words related to digestion (see Word Anatomy at the end of the chapter)

Selected Key Terms

The following terms and other boldface terms in the chapter are defined in the Glossary

absorption
bile
chyle
chyme
defecation
deglutition
digestion
duodenum
emulsify
enzyme
esophagus
gallbladder
hydrolysis
intestine
lacteal
liver
mastication
pancreas
peristalsis
peritoneum
saliva
stomach
ulcer
villi

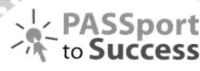

Visit *thePoint* or see the Student Resource CD in the back of this book for definitions and pronunciations of key terms as well as a pretest for this chapter.

Disease in Context

▶ Adam's Case: The Picture of Health

Adam was okay with everything his family doctor had described about his routine physical examination. "We'll draw some blood for testing," Dr. Michaels explained. "You didn't have anything to eat since last night, did you? We'll send your specimen to the lab to get information on your blood cells and blood chemistry, hemoglobin, lipoproteins, and such. You need to leave a urine sample to check for sugar, and then Annette will take your blood pressure and run an ECG. I'll be in to ask you some general questions and do some 'hands-on' examination, including, of course, a check on your prostate. And, Adam, since you are well past your 50th birthday, you need to stop stalling on getting that colonoscopy."

Sending in the stool sample later to test for signs of blood wasn't a problem for Adam, and he could live with the prostate exam, but he wasn't so happy about the colonoscopy! He had heard that the prep to clean out the colon was unpleasant. "You know," Adam protested, "I'm healthy and have no family history of colon cancer or polyps, so why do I need to do this?"

"Actually," replied Dr. Michaels, "most colorectal cancers appear in people with no symptoms and with no family history or genetic predisposition. In that higher risk population, we recommend earlier and more frequent testing. There is a new 'virtual colonoscopy' procedure that uses computerized x-rays instead of an endoscope to generate detailed images of the colon, but for a baseline study, your proctologist might prefer the routine method. Besides, if we have to remove any polyps or other abnormal tissue, we'd have to resort to that anyway. When you're ready to leave the office, ask Jean at the front desk to set up an appointment for you."

As part of Adam's physical, the doctor examined many of Adam's organ systems, including his digestive system. Because of his age, the doctor recommended a closer inspection of Adam's colon. In this chapter, we'll learn about the digestive tract and the accessory organs that contribute to digestion. We'll also visit Adam again and find out how the colonoscopy went!

Function and Design of the Digestive System

Every body cell needs a constant supply of nutrients. The energy contained in these nutrients is used to do cell work. In addition, the cell rearranges the nutrients' chemical building blocks to manufacture cellular materials for metabolism, growth, and repair. Food as we take it in, however, is too large to enter the cells. It must first be broken down into particles small enough to pass through the cells' plasma membrane. This breakdown process is known as **digestion**.

After digestion, the circulation must carry nutrients to the cells in every part of the body. The transfer of nutrients into the circulation is called **absorption**. Finally, undigested waste material must be eliminated. Digestion, absorption, and elimination are the three chief functions of the digestive system.

For our purposes, the digestive system may be divided into two groups of organs:

- The **digestive tract**, a continuous passageway beginning at the mouth, where food is taken in, and terminating at the anus, where the solid waste products of digestion are expelled from the body.

- The **accessory organs**, which are necessary for the digestive process but are not a direct part of the digestive tract. They release substances into the digestive tract through ducts. These organs are the salivary glands, liver, gallbladder, and pancreas.

Before describing the individual organs of the digestive tract, we will pause to discuss the general structure of these organs. We will also describe the large membrane (peritoneum) that lines the abdominopelvic cavity, which contains most of the digestive organs.

CHECKPOINT 19-1 ➤ Why does food have to be digested before cells can use it?

The Wall of the Digestive Tract

Although modified for specific tasks in different organs, the wall of the digestive tract, from the esophagus to the anus, is similar in structure throughout. The general pattern consists of four layers, which are, from innermost to outermost:

1. Mucous membrane
2. Submucosa
3. Smooth muscle
4. Serous membrane

Refer to the diagram of the small intestine in Figure 19-1 as we describe the individual layers of this wall in greater detail.

First is the **mucous membrane**, or **mucosa**, so called because its epithelial layer contains many mucus-secreting cells. From the mouth through the esophagus, and also in the anus, the epithelium consists of multiple layers of squamous (flat) cells, which help to protect deeper tissues.

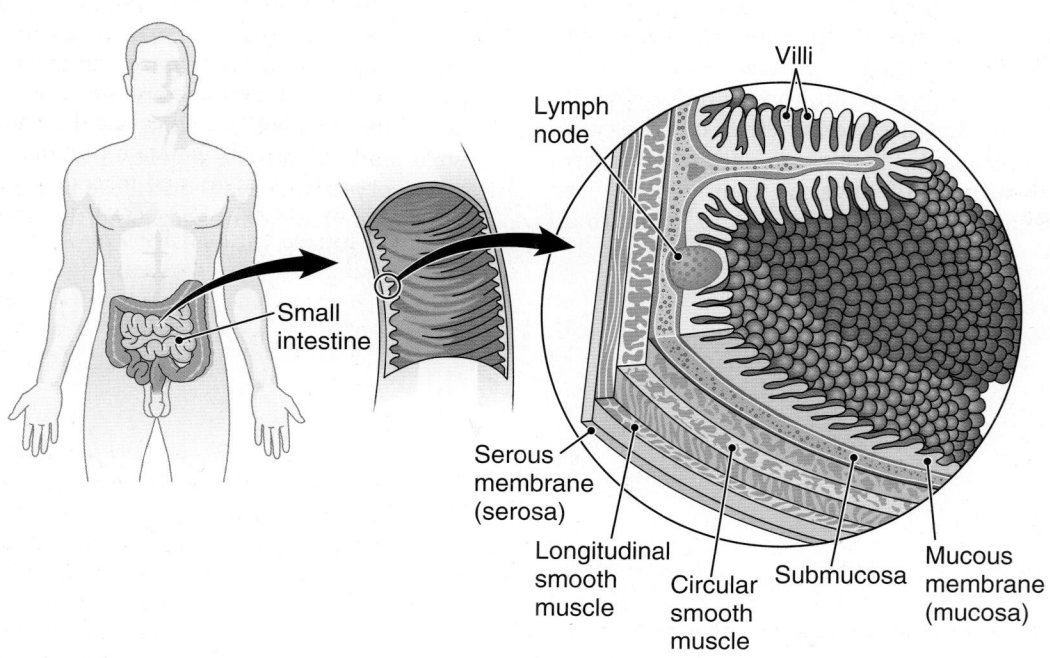

Figure 19-1 **Wall of the digestive tract.** The mucous membrane of the small intestine shown here has numerous projections called villi.
[ZOOMING IN ➤ What type of tissue is between the submucosa and the serous membrane in the digestive tract wall? **]**

Throughout the remainder of the digestive tract, the type of epithelium in the mucosa is simple columnar. Many of the cells that secrete digestive juices are located in the mucosa. Figure 19-2 is a microscopic view of a representative section of the digestive tract taken from the small intestine. Mucus-secreting cells (goblet cells) appear as clear areas between epithelial cells. Note that the small intestine's lining has fingerlike extensions (villi) that aid in the absorption of nutrients, as will be described later.

The layer of connective tissue beneath the mucosa is the **submucosa**, which contains blood vessels and some of the nerves that help regulate digestive activity. In the small intestine, the submucosa has many glands that produce mucus to protect that organ from the highly acidic material it receives from the stomach.

The next layer is composed of **smooth muscle**. Most of the digestive organs have two layers of smooth muscle: an inner layer of circular fibers, and an outer layer of longitudinal fibers. When a section of the circular muscle contracts, the organ's lumen narrows; when the longitudinal muscle contracts, a section of the wall shortens and the lu-

men becomes wider. These alternating muscular contractions create the wavelike movement, called **peristalsis** (per-ih-STAL-sis), that propels food through the digestive tract and mixes it with digestive juices.

The esophagus differs slightly from this pattern in having striated muscle in its upper portion, and the stomach has an additional third layer of smooth muscle in its wall to add strength for churning food.

The digestive organs in the abdominopelvic cavity have an outermost layer of **serous membrane**, or **serosa**, a thin, moist tissue composed of simple squamous epithelium and loose connective tissue. This membrane forms part of the **peritoneum** (per-ih-to-NE-um). The esophagus above the diaphragm has instead an outer layer composed of fibrous connective tissue.

CHECKPOINT 19-2 ➤ The digestive tract has a wall that is basically similar throughout its length and is composed of four layers. What are the typical four layers of this wall?

The Peritoneum

The abdominopelvic cavity is lined with a thin, shiny serous membrane that also folds back to cover most of the organs contained within the cavity (Fig. 19-3). The outer portion of this membrane, the layer that lines the cavity, is called the **parietal** (pah-RI-eh-tal) **peritoneum**; that covering the organs is called the **visceral** (VIS-eh-ral) **peritoneum**. This slippery membrane allows the organs to slide over each other as they function. The peritoneum also carries blood vessels, lymphatic vessels, and nerves. In some places, it supports the organs and binds them to each other. The peritoneal cavity is the potential space between the membrane's two layers and contains serous fluid (peritoneal fluid). The greater peritoneal cavity is the main portion, located in the abdominal cavity and extending into the pelvic cavity (see Fig. 19-3). The lesser peritoneal cavity is formed by a smaller extension of these membranes dorsal to the stomach, extending dorsal to the liver to the posterior attachment of the diaphragm. Subdivisions of the peritoneum around the various organs have special names.

SUBDIVISIONS OF THE PERITONEUM The **mesentery** (MES-en-ter-e) is a double-layered portion of the peritoneum shaped somewhat like a fan. The handle portion is attached to the posterior abdominal wall, and the expanded long edge is attached to the small intestine. Between the two membranous layers of the mesentery are the vessels and nerves that supply the intestine. The section of the peritoneum that extends from the colon to the posterior abdominal wall is the **mesocolon** (mes-o-KO-lon).

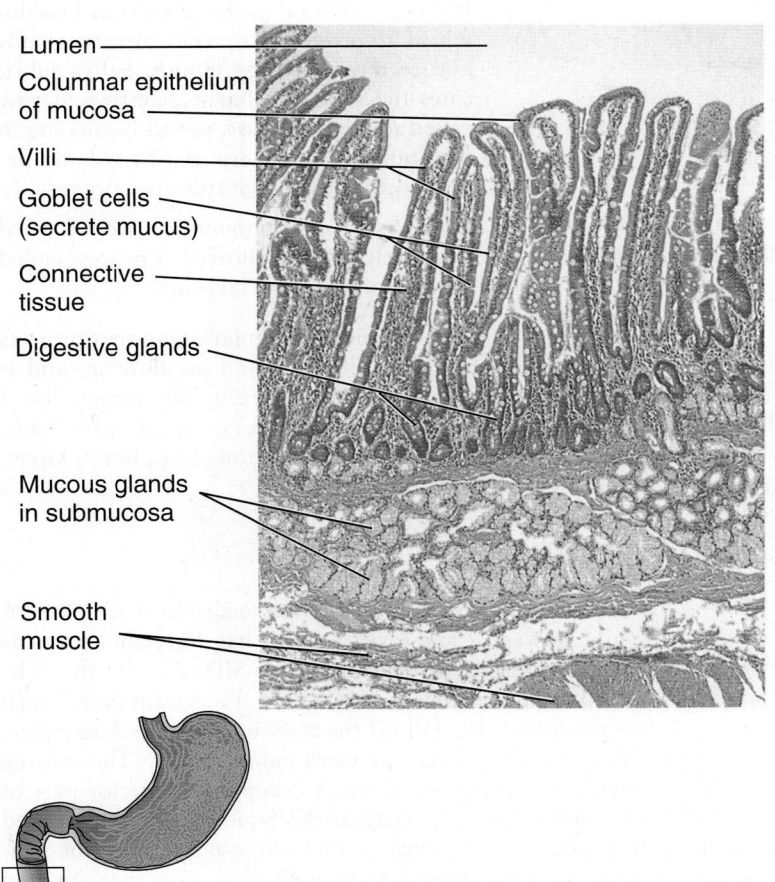

Lumen

Columnar epithelium of mucosa

Villi

Goblet cells (secrete mucus)

Connective tissue

Digestive glands

Mucous glands in submucosa

Smooth muscle

Figure 19-2 **Microscopic view of small intestine.** The layers of the intestinal wall are visible (except for the serous membrane). (Micrograph reprinted with permission from Cormack DH. *Essential Histology*, 2nd ed. Philadelphia: Lippincott Williams & Wilkins, 2001.)

19

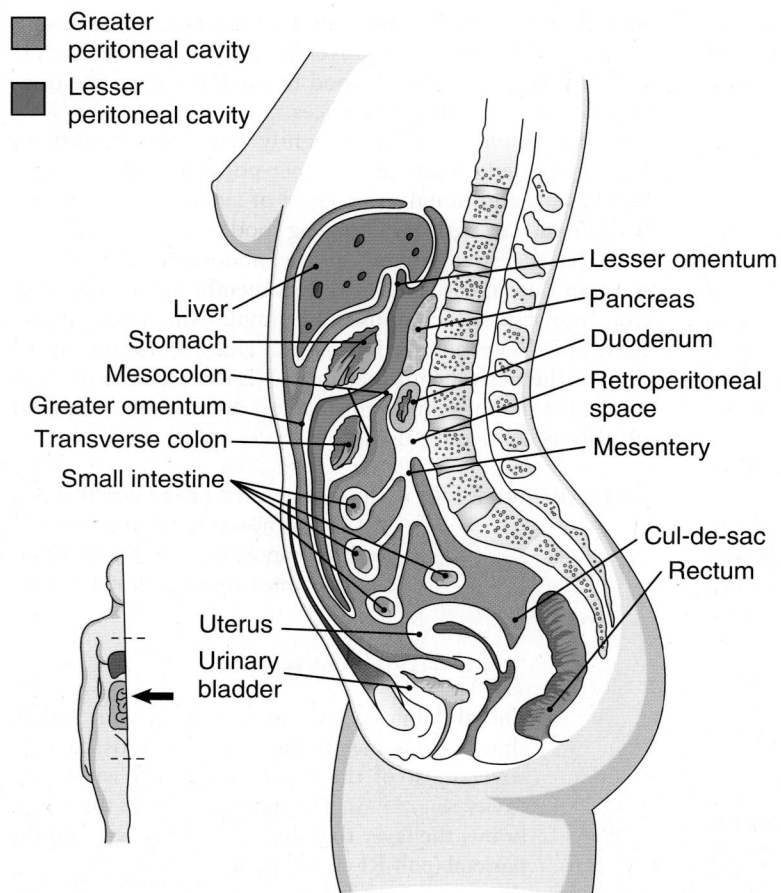

Greater peritoneal cavity

Lesser peritoneal cavity

Liver
Stomach
Mesocolon
Greater omentum
Transverse colon
Small intestine
Uterus
Urinary bladder

Lesser omentum
Pancreas
Duodenum
Retroperitoneal space
Mesentery
Cul-de-sac
Rectum

Figure19-3 **The abdominopelvic cavity.** Subdivisions of the peritoneum fold over, supporting and separating individual organs. **[ZOOMING IN ▶** What part of the peritoneum is around the small intestine? **]**

A large double layer of the peritoneum containing much fat hangs like an apron over the front of the intestine. This **greater omentum** (o-MEN-tum) extends from the lower border of the stomach into the pelvic cavity and then loops back up to the transverse colon. A smaller membrane, called the **lesser omentum**, extends between the stomach and the liver.

CHECKPOINT **19-3** ➤ What is the name of the large serous membrane that lines the abdominopelvic cavity and covers the organs it contains?

Organs of the Digestive Tract

As we study the organs of the digestive system, locate each in Figure 19-4. The digestive tract is a muscular tube extending through the body. It is composed of several parts: the **mouth, pharynx, esophagus, stomach, small intestine,** and **large intestine.** The digestive tract is sometimes called the alimentary tract, from the word *aliment*, meaning "food." It is more commonly referred to as the **gastroin-**

testinal **(GI)** tract because of the major importance of the stomach and intestine in the digestive process.

The next section describes the structure and function of each digestive organ. These descriptions are followed by an overview of how the organs work together in digestion. See Appendix 7 for a dissection photograph showing the digestive organs in place.

The Mouth

The **mouth,** also called the **oral cavity,** is where a substance begins its travels through the digestive tract (Fig. 19-5). The mouth has the following digestive functions:

■ It receives food, a process called **ingestion.**

■ It breaks food into small portions. This is done mainly by the teeth in the process of chewing or **mastication** (mas-tih-KA-shun), but the tongue, cheeks, and lips are also used.

■ It mixes the food with **saliva** (sah-LI-vah), which is produced by the salivary glands and secreted into the mouth. Saliva lubricates the food and has a digestive enzyme called *salivary amylase,* which begins starch digestion. The salivary glands will be described with the other accessory organs.

■ It moves proper amounts of food toward the throat to be swallowed, a process called **deglutition** (deg-lu-TISH-un).

The tongue, a muscular organ that projects into the mouth, aids in chewing and swallowing, and is one of the principal organs of speech. The tongue has a number of special surface receptors, called *taste buds,* which can differentiate taste sensations (e.g., bitter, sweet, sour, or salty) (see Chapter 11).

The Teeth

The oral cavity also contains the teeth (see Fig. 19-5). A child between 2 and 6 years of age has 20 teeth, known as the baby teeth or **deciduous** (de-SID-u-us) teeth. (The word deciduous means "falling off at a certain time," such as the leaves that fall off the trees in autumn.) A complete set of adult permanent teeth numbers 32. The cutting teeth, or **incisors** (in-SI-sors), occupy the anterior part of the oral cavity. The **cuspids** (KUS-pids), commonly called the *canines* (KA-nines) or *eyeteeth,* are lateral to the incisors. They are pointed teeth with deep roots that are used for more forceful gripping and tearing of food. The **molars** (MO-lars), the larger grinding teeth, are posterior. There are two premolars and three molars. In an adult, each quadrant (quarter) of the mouth, moving from anterior to posterior, has two incisors, one cuspid, and five molars.

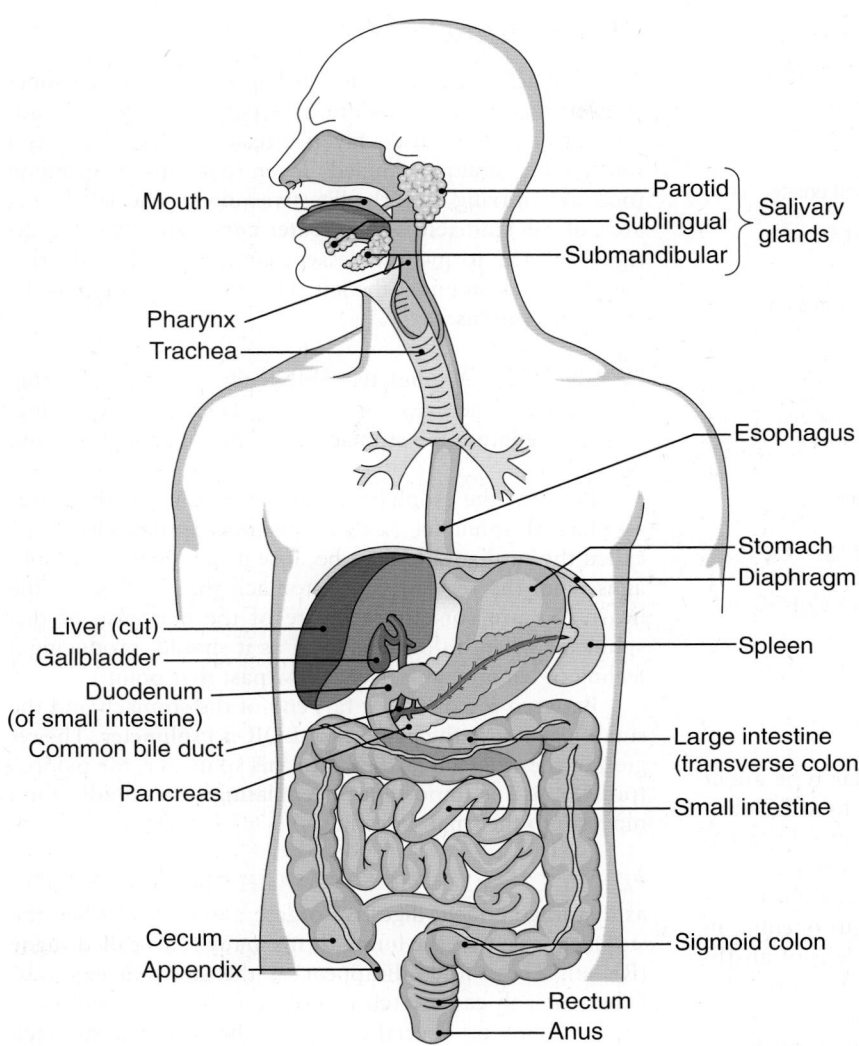

Figure 19-4 **The digestive system.** The figure also shows nearby structures for orientation. [**ZOOMING IN** ➤ What accessory organs of digestion secrete into the mouth?]

so-called *wisdom teeth*, may appear. In some cases, the jaw is not large enough for these teeth, or there are other abnormalities, so that the third molars may not erupt or may have to be removed. Figure 19-6 shows the parts of a molar.

The main substance of the tooth is **dentin**, a calcified substance harder than bone. Within the tooth is a soft pulp containing blood vessels and nerves. The tooth's crown projects above the gum, the **gingiva** (JIN-jih-vah), and is covered with **enamel**, the hardest substance in the body. The roots of the tooth, below the gum line in a bony socket, are covered with a rigid connective tissue (cementum) that helps to hold the tooth in place. Each root has a canal containing extensions of the pulp.

The Pharynx

The **pharynx** (FAR-inks) is commonly referred to as the throat (see Fig. 19-5). The oral part of the pharynx, the oropharynx, is visible when you look into an open mouth and depress the tongue. The palatine tonsils may be seen at either side of the oropharynx. The pharynx also extends upward to the nasal cavity, where it is referred to as the nasopharynx and downward to the larynx, where it is called the laryngeal pharynx. The **soft palate** is tissue that forms the posterior roof of the oral cavity. From it hangs a soft, fleshy, V-shaped mass called the **uvula** (U-vu-lah).

In swallowing, the tongue pushes a **bolus** (BO-lus) of food, a small portion of chewed food mixed with saliva, into the pharynx. Once the food reaches the pharynx, swallowing occurs rapidly by an involuntary reflex action. At the same time, the soft palate and uvula are raised to prevent food and liquid from entering the nasal cavity, and the tongue is raised to seal the back of the oral cavity. The entrance of the trachea is guarded during swallowing by a leaf-shaped cartilage, the **epiglottis**, which covers the opening of the larynx. The swallowed food is then moved into the esophagus.

The first eight deciduous (baby) teeth to appear through the gums are the incisors. Later, the cuspids and molars appear. Usually, the 20 baby teeth all have appeared by the time a child has reached the age of 2 to 3 years. During the first 2 years, the permanent teeth develop within the upper jaw (maxilla) and lower jaw (mandible) from buds that are present at birth. The first permanent teeth to appear are the four 6-year molars, which come in before any baby teeth are lost. Because decay and infection of deciduous molars may spread to new, permanent teeth, deciduous teeth need proper care.

As a child grows, the jawbones grow, making space for additional teeth. After the 6-year molars have appeared, the baby incisors loosen and are replaced by permanent incisors. Next, the baby canines (cuspids) are replaced by permanent canines, and finally, the baby molars are replaced by the permanent bicuspids (premolars).

At this point, the larger jawbones are ready for the appearance of the 12-year, or second, permanent molar teeth. During or after the late teens, the third molars, or

PASSport to Success Visit ***thePoint*** or see the Student Resource CD in the back of this book for information on dental hygienists and their role in maintaining the health of the teeth and gums.

CHECKPOINT 19-4 ➤ How many baby teeth are there and what is the scientific name for the baby teeth?

19

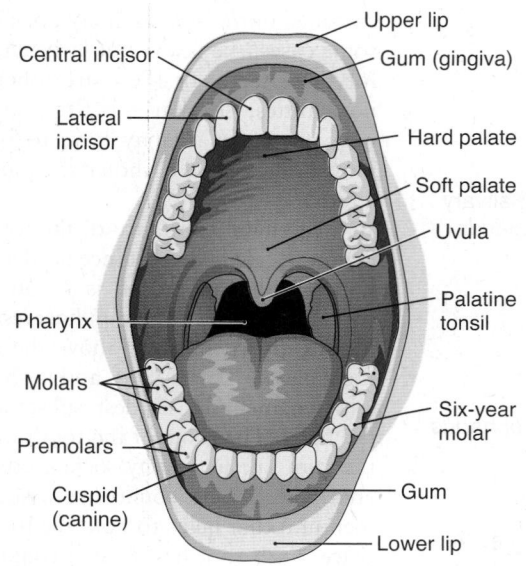

Figure 19-5   **The mouth.** The teeth and tonsils are visible in this view.

The Esophagus

The **esophagus** (eh-SOF-ah-gus) is a muscular tube about 25 cm (10 inches) long. In the esophagus, food is lubricated with mucus and moved by peristalsis into the stomach. No additional digestion occurs in the esophagus.

Before joining the stomach, the esophagus must pass through the diaphragm. It travels through an opening in the diaphragm called the **esophageal hiatus** (eh-sof-ah-JE-al hi-A-tus). If there is a weakness in the diaphragm at this point, a portion of the stomach or other abdominal organ may protrude through the space, a condition called *hiatal hernia.*

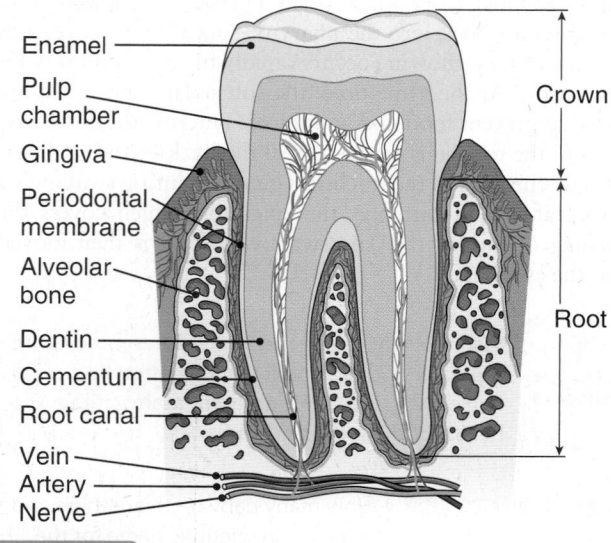

Figure 19-6   **A molar tooth.**

The Stomach

The stomach is an expanded J-shaped organ in the superior left region of the abdominal cavity (Fig. 19-7). In addition to the two muscle layers already described, it has a third, inner oblique (angled) layer that aids in grinding food and mixing it with digestive juices. The left-facing arch of the stomach is the **greater curvature**, whereas the right surface forms the **lesser curvature**. The superior rounded portion under the left side of the diaphragm is the stomach's **fundus.**

SPHINCTERS   A **sphincter** (SFINK-ter) is a muscular ring that regulates the size of an opening. There are two sphincters that separate the stomach from the organs above and below.

Between the esophagus and the stomach is the **lower esophageal sphincter (LES)**. This muscle has also been called the **cardiac sphincter** because it separates the esophagus from the region of the stomach that is close to the heart. We are sometimes aware of the existence of this sphincter when it does not relax as it should, producing a feeling of being unable to swallow past that point.

Between the distal, or far, end of the stomach and the small intestine is the **pyloric** (pi-LOR-ik) **sphincter**. The region of the stomach leading into this sphincter, the **pylorus** (pi-LOR-us), is important in regulating how rapidly food moves into the small intestine.

FUNCTIONS OF THE STOMACH   The stomach serves as a storage pouch, digestive organ, and churn. When the stomach is empty, the lining forms many folds called **rugae** (RU-je). These folds disappear as the stomach expands. (The stomach can stretch to hold one half of a gallon of food and liquid.) Special cells in the lining of the stomach secrete substances that mix together to form gastric juice. Some of the cells secrete a great amount of mucus to protect the stomach lining from digestive secretions. Other cells produce the active components of the gastric juice, which are:

- Hydrochloric acid (HCl), a strong acid that helps break down protein and destroys foreign organisms.

- Pepsin, a protein-digesting enzyme produced in an inactive form and activated only when food enters the stomach and HCl is produced.

Chyme (*kime*), from a Greek word meaning "juice," is the highly acidic, semiliquid mixture of gastric juice and food that leaves the stomach to enter the small intestine.

CHECKPOINT **19-5** ➤ What type of food is digested in the stomach?

The Small Intestine

The small intestine is the longest part of the digestive tract (Fig. 19-8). It is known as the small intestine because, although it is longer than the large intestine, it is smaller in di-

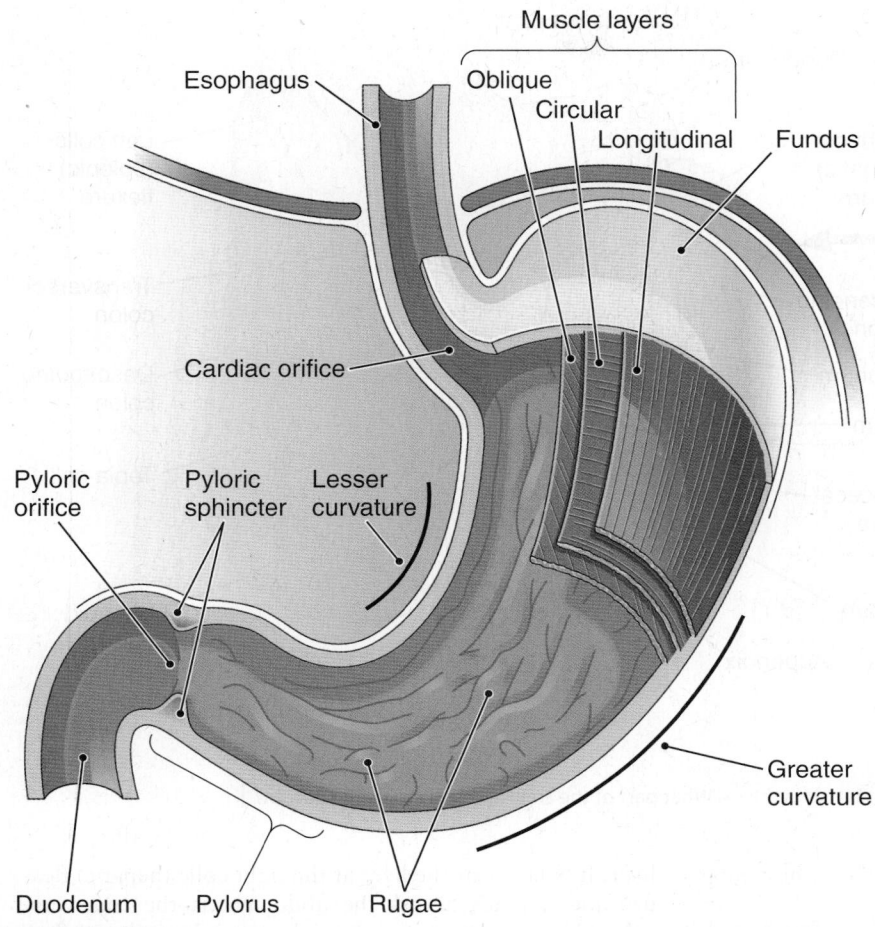

Muscle layers

Esophagus

Oblique
Circular
Longitudinal   Fundus

Cardiac orifice

Pyloric orifice

Pyloric sphincter   Lesser curvature

Greater curvature

Duodenum   Pylorus   Rugae

Figure 19-7 **Longitudinal section of the stomach.** The stomach's interior is visible, along with a portion of the esophagus and the duodenum. [**ZOOMING IN** ➤ What additional muscle layer is in the wall of the stomach that is not found in the rest of the digestive tract?]

ameter, with an average width of approximately 2.5 cm (1 inch). After death, when relaxed to its full length, the small intestine is approximately 6 m (20 feet) long. In life, the small intestine averages 3 m (10 feet) in length. The first 25 cm (10 inches) or so of the small intestine make up the **duodenum** (du-o-DE-num) (named for the Latin word for "twelve," based on its length of twelve finger widths). Beyond the duodenum are two more divisions: the **jejunum** (je-JU-num), which forms the next two-fifths of the small intestine, and the **ileum** (IL-e-um), which constitutes the remaining portion.

FUNCTIONS OF THE SMALL INTESTINE The duodenal mucosa and submucosa contain glands that secrete large amounts of mucus to protect the small intestine from the strongly acidic chyme entering from the stomach. Mucosal cells of the small intestine also secrete enzymes that digest proteins and carbohydrates. In addition, digestive juices from the liver and pancreas enter the small intestine through a small opening in the duodenum. Most digestion takes place in the small intestine under the effects of these juices.

Most absorption of digested food, water, and minerals also occurs through the walls of the small intestine. To increase the organ's surface area for this purpose, the mucosa is formed into millions of tiny, fingerlike projections, called **villi** (VIL-li) (Fig. 19-9), which give the inner surface a velvety appearance (see also Figs. 19-1 and 19-2). The epithelial cells of the villi also have small projecting folds of the plasma membrane known as **microvilli**. These create a remarkable increase in the total surface area available for absorption in the small intestine.

Each villus contains blood vessels through which most digestion products are absorbed into the blood. Each one also contains a specialized lymphatic capillary called a **lacteal** (LAK-tele) through which fats are absorbed into the lymph. Box 19-1, The Folded Intestine, provides more information on the relationship of surface area to absorption.

The Large Intestine

The large intestine is approximately 6.5 cm (2.5 inches) in diameter and approximately 1.5 m (5 feet) long (see Fig. 19-8). It is named for its wide diameter, rather than its length. The outer longitudinal muscle fibers in its wall form three separate surface bands (see Fig. 19-8). These bands, known as **teniae** (TEN-e-e) **coli,** draw up the organ's wall to give it its distinctive puckered appearance. (Spelling is also *taeniae*; the singular is *tenia* or *taenia*).

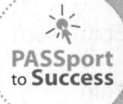 PASSport to Success — Visit **thePoint** or see the Student Resource CD in the back of this book for a photomicrograph of a villus showing a lacteal.

CHECKPOINT **19-6** ➤ What are the three divisions of the small intestine?

CHECKPOINT **19-7** ➤ How does the small intestine function in the digestive process?

SUBDIVISIONS OF THE LARGE INTESTINE The large intestine begins in the lower right region of the abdomen. The first part is a small pouch called the **cecum** (SE-kum). Between the ileum of the small intestine and the cecum is a sphincter, the **ileocecal** (il-e-o-SE-kal) **valve,** that prevents food from traveling backward into the small intestine. Attached to the cecum is a small, blind tube containing lymphoid tissue; its full name is **vermiform** (VER-mih-

19

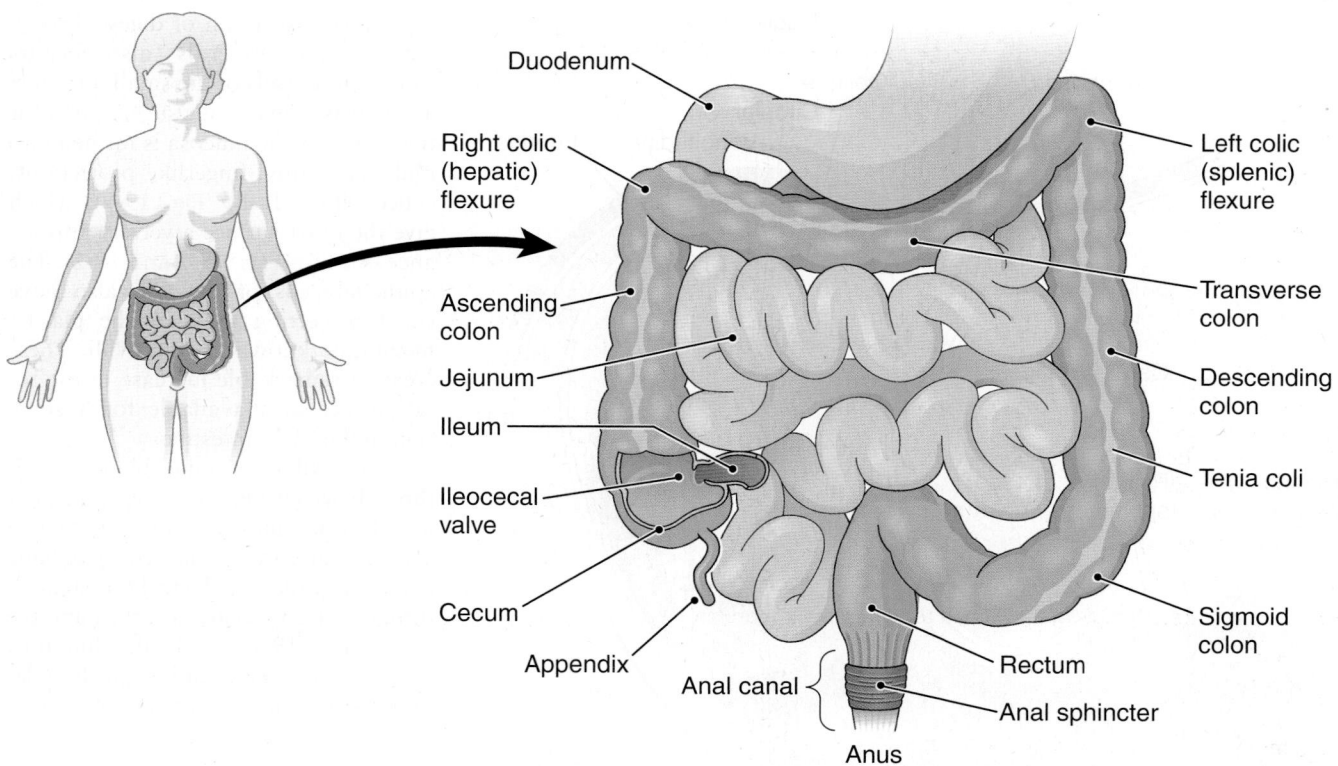

Labels (clockwise): Duodenum, Left colic (splenic) flexure, Transverse colon, Descending colon, Tenia coli, Sigmoid colon, Rectum, Anal sphincter, Anus, Anal canal, Appendix, Cecum, Ileocecal valve, Ileum, Jejunum, Ascending colon, Right colic (hepatic) flexure

Figure 19-8 **The small and large intestines.** [ZOOMING IN ➤ What part of the small intestine joins the cecum?]

form) **appendix** (*vermiform* means "wormlike"), but usually just "appendix" is used.

The second portion, the **ascending colon**, extends superiorly along the right side of the abdomen toward the

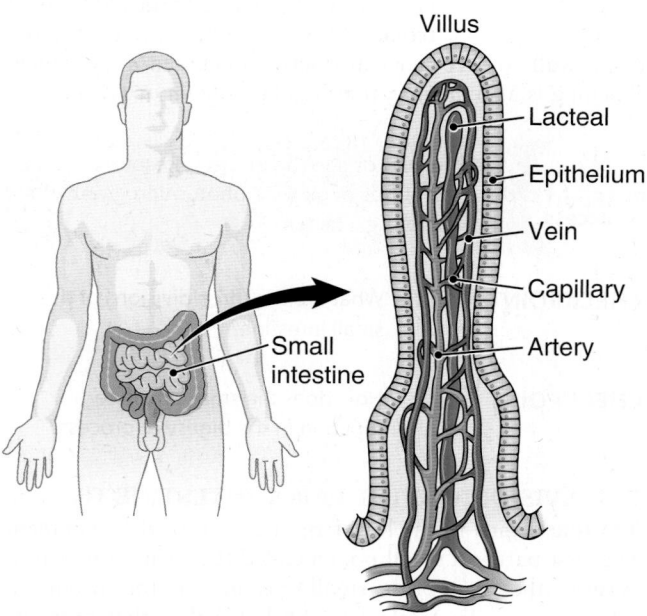

Labels: Villus, Lacteal, Epithelium, Vein, Capillary, Artery, Small intestine

Figure 19-9 **A villus of the small intestine.** Each villus has blood vessels and a lacteal (lymphatic capillary) for absorption of nutrients.

liver. It bends near the liver at the right colic (hepatic) flexure and extends across the abdomen as the **transverse colon**. It bends again sharply at the left colic (splenic) flexure and extends inferiorly on the left side of the abdomen into the pelvis, forming the **descending colon**. The distal colon bends backward into an S shape forming the **sigmoid colon** (named for the Greek letter *sigma*), which continues downward to empty into the **rectum**, a temporary storage area for indigestible or nonabsorbable food residue (see Fig. 19-8). The narrow terminal portion of the large intestine is the **anal canal**, which leads to the outside of the body through an opening called the **anus** (A-nus).

FUNCTIONS OF THE LARGE INTESTINE The large intestine secretes a great quantity of mucus, but no enzymes. Food is not digested in this organ, but some water is reabsorbed, and undigested food is stored, formed into solid waste material, called **feces** (FE-seze) or stool, and then eliminated.

At intervals, usually after meals, the involuntary muscles within the walls of the large intestine propel solid waste toward the rectum. Stretching of the rectum stimulates contraction of smooth muscle in the rectal wall. Aided by voluntary contractions of the diaphragm and the abdominal muscles, the feces are eliminated from the body in a process called **defecation** (def-e-KA-shun). An anal sphincter provides voluntary control over defecation (see Fig. 19-8).

While food residue is stored in the large intestine, bacteria that normally live in the colon act on it to produce

Box 19-1 A Closer Look

The Folded Intestine: More Absorption With Less Length

Whenever materials pass from one system to another, they must travel through a cellular membrane. A major factor in how much transport can occur per unit of time is the total surface area of the membrane; the greater the surface area, the higher the rate of transport. The problem of packing a large amount of surface into a small space is solved in the body by folding the membranes. We do the same thing in everyday life. Imagine trying to store a bed sheet in the closet without folding it!

In the small intestine, where digested food must absorb into the bloodstream, there is folding of membranes down to the level of single cells.

■ The 6-meter-long organ is coiled to fit into the abdominal cavity.

■ The inner wall of the organ is thrown into circular folds called plicae circulares, which not only increase surface area, but aid in mixing.

■ The mucosal villi project into the lumen, providing more surface area than a flat membrane would.

■ The individual cells that line the small intestine have microvilli, tiny fingerlike folds of the plasma membrane that increase surface area tremendously.

Together, these structural features of the small intestine result in an absorptive surface area estimated to be about 250 square meters! Folding is present in other parts of the digestive system and in other areas of the body as well. Can you name other systems that show this folding pattern?

---

vitamin K and some of the B-complex vitamins. As mentioned, systemic antibiotic therapy may destroy these symbiotic (helpful) bacteria living in the large intestine, causing undesirable side effects.

CHECKPOINT 19-8 ➤ What are the divisions of the large intestine?

CHECKPOINT 19-9 ➤ What are the functions of the large intestine?

The Accessory Organs

The accessory organs (Fig. 19-10) release secretions through ducts into the digestive tract. The salivary glands deliver their secretions into the mouth. All of the other accessory organs release secretions into the duodenum.

The Salivary Glands

While food is in the mouth, it is mixed with **saliva** (sah-LI-vah), which moistens the food and facilitates mastication (chewing) and deglutition (swallowing). Saliva helps to keep the teeth and mouth clean. It also contains some antibodies and an enzyme (lysozyme) that help reduce bacterial growth.

This watery mixture contains mucus and an enzyme called **salivary amylase** (AM-ih-laze), which begins the

digestive process by converting starch to sugar. Saliva is manufactured by three pairs of glands (see Fig. 19-4):

■ The **parotid** (pah-ROT-id) **glands,** the largest of the group, are located inferior and anterior to the ear.

■ The **submandibular** (sub-man-DIB-u-lar), or **submaxillary** (sub-MAK-sih-ler-e), **glands** are located near the body of the lower jaw.

■ The **sublingual** (sub-LING-gwal) **glands** are under the tongue.

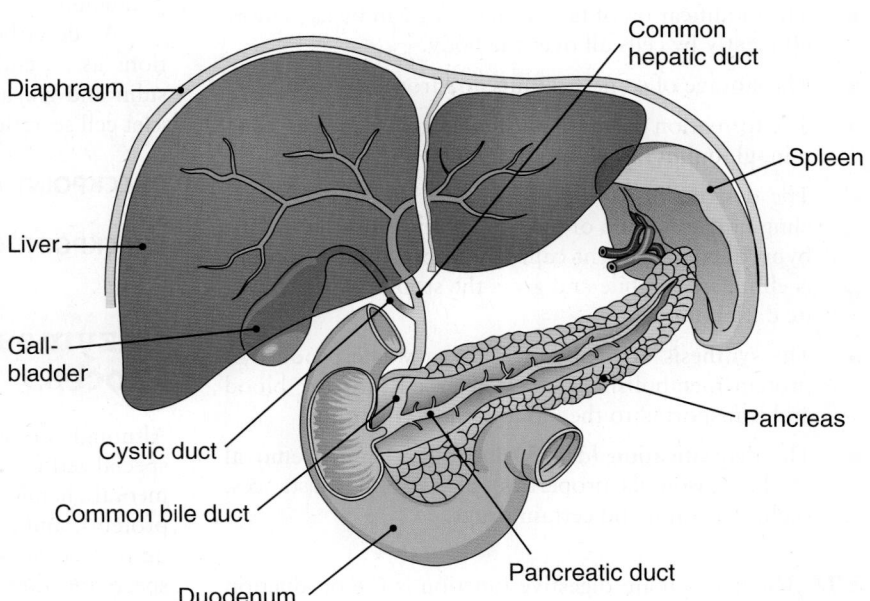

Figure 19-10 Accessory organs of digestion. [**ZOOMING IN** ➤ Into what part of the intestine do these accessory organs secrete?]

19

All these glands empty through ducts into the oral cavity.

CHECKPOINT **19-10** ➤ What are the names of the salivary glands?

The Liver

The **liver** (LIV-er), often referred to by the word root *hepat*, is the body's largest glandular organ (see Fig. 19-10). It is located in the superior right portion of the abdominal cavity under the dome of the diaphragm. The lower edge of a normal-sized liver is level with the lower margin of the ribs. The human liver is the same reddish brown color as animal liver seen in the supermarket. It has a large right lobe and a smaller left lobe; the right lobe includes two inferior smaller lobes. The liver is supplied with blood through two vessels: the portal vein and the hepatic artery (the portal system and blood supply to the liver were described in Chapter 15). These vessels deliver about 1.5 quarts (1.6 L) of blood to the liver every minute. The hepatic artery carries oxygenated blood, whereas the venous portal system carries blood that is rich in digestive end products. This most remarkable organ has many functions that affect digestion, metabolism, blood composition, and elimination of waste. Some of its major activities are:

- The manufacture of **bile**, a substance needed for the digestion of fats.

- The storage of glucose (a simple sugar) in the form of **glycogen**, the animal equivalent of the starch found in plants. When the blood sugar level falls below normal, liver cells convert glycogen to glucose, which is released into the blood to restore the normal blood sugar concentration.

- The modification of fats so that they can be used more efficiently by cells all over the body.

- The storage of some vitamins and iron.

- The formation of blood plasma proteins, such as albumin, globulins, and clotting factors.

- The destruction of old red blood cells and the recycling or elimination of their breakdown products. One byproduct, a pigment called **bilirubin** (BIL-ih-ru-bin), is eliminated in bile and gives the stool its characteristic dark color.

- The synthesis of **urea** (u-RE-ah), a waste product of protein metabolism. Urea is released into the blood and transported to the kidneys for elimination.

- The **detoxification** (de-tok-sih-fih-KA-shun) (removal of the poisonous properties) of harmful substances, such as alcohol and certain drugs.

BILE The liver's main digestive function is the production of bile, a substance needed for the processing of fats. The salts contained in bile act like a detergent to **emulsify** fat, that is, to break up fat into small droplets that can be acted on more effectively by digestive enzymes. Bile also aids in fat absorption from the small intestine.

Bile leaves the lobes of the liver by two ducts that merge to form the **common hepatic duct**. After collecting bile from the gallbladder, this duct, now called the **common bile duct**, delivers bile into the duodenum. These and the other accessory ducts are shown in Figure 19-10.

The Gallbladder

The **gallbladder** (GAWL-blad-er) is a muscular sac on the inferior surface of the liver that stores bile. Although the liver may manufacture bile continuously, the body needs it only a few times a day. Consequently, bile from the liver flows into the hepatic ducts and then up through the **cystic** (SIS-tik) **duct**, connected with the gallbladder (see Fig. 19-10). When chyme enters the duodenum, the gallbladder contracts, squeezing bile through the cystic duct and into the common bile duct, leading to the duodenum.

The Pancreas

The **pancreas** (PAN-kre-as) is a long gland that extends from the duodenum to the spleen (see Fig. 19-10). The pancreas produces enzymes that digest fats, proteins, carbohydrates, and nucleic acids. The protein-digesting enzymes are produced in inactive forms which must be converted to active forms in the small intestine by other enzymes.

The pancreas also releases large amounts of sodium bicarbonate ($NaHCO_3$), an alkaline (basic) fluid that neutralizes the acidic chyme in the small intestine, thus protecting the lining of the digestive tract. These juices collect in a main duct that joins the common bile duct or empties into the duodenum near the common bile duct. Most people have an additional smaller duct that opens into the duodenum.

As described in Chapter 12, the pancreas also functions as an endocrine gland, producing the hormones insulin and glucagon that regulate sugar metabolism. These islet cell secretions are released into the blood.

CHECKPOINT **19-11** ➤ What is the role of the gallbladder?

CHECKPOINT **19-12** ➤ What is the role of bile in digestion?

Enzymes and the Digestive Process

Although the individual organs of the digestive tract are specialized for digesting different types of food, the fundamental chemical process of digestion is the same for fats, proteins, and carbohydrates. In every case, this process requires enzymes. Enzymes are catalysts, substances that speed the rate of chemical reactions, but are not themselves changed or used up in the reaction.

All enzymes are proteins, and they are highly specific in their actions. In digestion, an enzyme acts only in a certain type of reaction involving a certain type of nutrient molecule. For example, the carbohydrate-digesting enzyme amylase only splits starch into the disaccharide (double sugar) maltose. Another enzyme is required to split maltose into two molecules of the monosaccharide (simple sugar) glucose. Other enzymes split fats into their building blocks, glycerol and fatty acids, and still others split proteins into smaller units called *peptides* and into their building blocks, amino acids (see Enzymes in Chapter 2).

The Role of Water

Because water is added to nutrient molecules as they are split by enzymes, the process of digestion is referred to chemically as **hydrolysis** (hi-DROL-ih-sis), which means "splitting by means of water" (see Fig. 2-2). In this chemical process, water's hydroxyl group (OH^-) is added to one fragment and the hydrogen ion (H^+) is added to the other, splitting the molecule. About 7 liters of water are secreted into the digestive tract each day, in addition to the nearly 2 liters taken in with food and drink. You can now understand why so large an amount of water is needed. Water not only is used to produce digestive juices and to dilute food so that it can move more easily through the digestive tract, but also is used in the chemical process of digestion itself.

Digestion, Step-by-Step

Let us see what happens to a mass of food from the time it is taken into the mouth to the moment that it is ready to be absorbed (see Table 19-1).

In the mouth, the food is chewed and mixed with saliva, softening it so that it can be swallowed easily. Salivary amylase initiates the digestive process by changing some of the starches into sugar.

DIGESTION IN THE STOMACH When the food reaches the stomach, it is acted on by gastric juice, with its hydrochloric acid (HCl) and enzymes. The hydrochloric acid has the important function of breaking down proteins and preparing them for digestion. In addition, HCl activates the enzyme pepsin, which is secreted by gastric cells in an inactive form. Once activated by hydrochloric acid, pepsin works to digest protein; this enzyme is the first to digest nearly every type of protein in the diet. The stomach also secretes a fat-digesting enzyme (lipase), but it is of little importance in adults.

The food, gastric juice, and mucus (which is also secreted by cells of the gastric lining) are mixed to form chyme. This semiliquid substance is moved from the stomach to the small intestine for further digestion.

DIGESTION IN THE SMALL INTESTINE In the duodenum, the first part of the small intestine, chyme is mixed with the greenish-yellow bile delivered from the liver and the gallbladder through the common bile duct. Bile does not contain enzymes; instead, it contains salts that emulsify fats to allow the powerful secretions from the pancreas to act on them most efficiently.

Pancreatic juice contains a number of enzymes, including:

- **Lipase.** After bile divides fats into tiny particles, the highly active pancreatic enzyme lipase digests almost all of them. In this process, fats are usually broken down into two simpler compounds, glycerol (glycerin) and fatty acids, which are more readily absorbable. If pancreatic lipase is absent, fats are expelled with the feces in undigested form.

- **Amylase.** This enzyme changes starch to sugar.

Table 19-1	Summary of Digestion		
Organ	**Activity**	**Nutrients Digested**	**Active Secretions**
Mouth	Chews food and mixes it with saliva; forms into bolus for swallowing	Starch	Salivary amylase
Esophagus	Moves food by peristalsis into stomach	—	—
Stomach	Stores food, churns food, and mixes it with digestive juices	Proteins	Hydrochloric acid, pepsin
Small intestine	Secretes enzymes, neutralizes acidity, receives secretions from pancreas and liver, absorbs nutrients and water into the blood or lymph	Fats, proteins, carbohydrates, nucleic acids	Intestinal enzymes, pancreatic enzymes, bile from liver
Large intestine	Reabsorbs some water; forms, stores, and eliminates stool	—	—

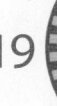

19

- **Trypsin** (TRIP-sin). This enzyme splits proteins into amino acids, which are small enough to be absorbed through the intestine.
- **Nucleases** (NU-kle-ases). These enzymes digest the nucleic acids DNA and RNA.

It is important to note that most digestion occurs in the small intestine under the action of pancreatic juice, which has the ability to break down all types of foods. When pancreatic juice is absent, serious digestive disturbances always occur.

The small intestine also produces a number of enzymes, including three that act on complex sugars to transform them into simpler, absorbable forms. These enzymes are **maltase**, **sucrase**, and **lactase**, which act on the disaccharides maltose, sucrose, and lactose, respectively.

Table 19-2 summarizes the main substances used in digestion. Note that, except for HCl, sodium bicarbonate, and bile salts, all the substances listed are enzymes.

CHECKPOINT **19-13** ➤ What organ produces the most complete digestive secretions?

Absorption

The means by which digested nutrients reach the blood is known as **absorption**. Most absorption takes place through the villi in the mucosa of the small intestine (see Fig. 19-9). Within each villus is an arteriole and a venule bridged with capillaries. Simple sugars, small proteins (peptides), amino acids, some simple fatty acids, and most of the water in the digestive tract are absorbed into the blood through these capillaries. From here, they pass by way of the portal system to the liver, to be processed, stored, or released as needed.

Absorption of Fats

Most fats have an alternative method of reaching the blood. Instead of entering the blood capillaries, they are absorbed by the villi's more permeable lymphatic capillaries, the lacteals. The absorbed fat droplets give the lymph a milky appearance. The mixture of lymph and fat globules that drains from the small intestine after fat has been digested is called **chyle** (kile). Chyle merges with the lymphatic circulation and eventually enters the blood when the lymph drains into veins near the heart. The absorbed fats then circulate to the liver for further processing.

Absorption of Vitamins and Minerals

Minerals and vitamins ingested with food are also absorbed from the small intestine. The minerals and some of the vitamins dissolve in water and are absorbed directly into the blood. Other vitamins are incorporated in fats and are absorbed along with the fats. Vitamin K and some B vitamins are produced by bacterial action in the colon and are absorbed from the large intestine.

CHECKPOINT **19-14** ➤ What is absorption?

Control of Digestion

As food moves through the digestive tract, its rate of movement and the activity of each organ it passes through must be carefully regulated. If food moves too slowly or digestive secretions are inadequate, the body will not get enough nourishment. If food moves too rapidly or excess secretions are produced, digestion may be incomplete or the digestive tract's lining may be damaged. There are two

Table 19-2	**Digestive Juices Produced by Digestive Tract Organs and Accessory Organs**	
Organ	**Main Digestive Juices Secreted**	**Action**
Salivary glands	Salivary amylase	Begins starch digestion
Stomach	Hydrochloric acid (HCl)*	Breaks down proteins
	Pepsin	Begins protein digestion
Small intestine	Peptidases	Digests proteins to amino acids
	Lactase, maltase, sucrase	Digests disaccharides to monosaccharides
Pancreas	Sodium bicarbonate*	Neutralizes HCl
	Amylase	Digests starch
	Trypsin	Digests protein to amino acids
	Lipases	Digests fats to fatty acids and glycerol
	Nucleases	Digests nucleic acids
Liver	Bile salts*	Emulsifies fats

*Not enzymes.

types of control over digestion: nervous and hormonal. Both illustrate the principles of feedback control.

The nerves that control digestive activity are located in the submucosa and between the muscle layers of the organ walls. Instructions for action come from the autonomic (visceral) nervous system. In general, parasympathetic stimulation increases activity, and sympathetic stimulation decreases activity. Excess sympathetic stimulation, as in stress, can block food's movement through the digestive tract and inhibit mucus secretion, which is crucial in protecting the lining of the digestive tract.

The digestive organs themselves produce the hormones involved in the regulation of digestion. The following is a discussion of some of these controls (Table 19-3).

The sight, smell, thought, taste, or feel of food in the mouth stimulates, through the nervous system, the secretion of saliva and the release of gastric juice. Once in the stomach, food stimulates the release into the blood of the hormone **gastrin**, which promotes stomach secretions and motility (movement).

When chyme enters the duodenum, nerve impulses inhibit stomach motility, so that food will not move too rapidly into the small intestine. This action is a good example of negative feedback. At the same time, hormones released from the duodenum not only function in digestion, but also feed back to the stomach to reduce its activity. **Gastric-inhibitory peptide (GIP)** is one such hormone. It acts on the stomach to inhibit the release of gastric juice. Its more important action is to stimulate insulin release from the pancreas when glucose enters the duodenum. Another of these hormones, **secretin** (se-KRE-tin) stimulates the pancreas to release water and bicarbonate to dilute and neutralize chyme. **Cholecystokinin** (ko-le-sis-to-KI-nin) **(CCK)**, stimulates the release of enzymes from the pancreas and causes the gallbladder to release bile.

CHECKPOINT 19-15 ➤ What are the two types of control over the digestive process?

Hunger and Appetite

Hunger is the desire for food, which can be satisfied by the ingestion of a filling meal. Hunger is regulated by hypothalamic centers that respond to the levels of nutrients in the blood. When these levels are low, the hypothalamus stimulates a sensation of hunger. Strong, mildly painful contractions of the empty stomach may stimulate a feeling of hunger. Messages received by the hypothalamus reduce hunger as food is chewed and swallowed and begins to fill the stomach. The short-term regulation of food intake works to keep the amount of food eaten within the limits of what the intestine can process. The long-term regulation of food intake maintains appropriate blood levels of nutrients.

Appetite differs from hunger in that, although it is basically a desire for food, it often has no relationship to the need for food. Even after an adequate meal that has relieved hunger, a person may still have an appetite for additional food. A variety of factors, such as emotional state, cultural influences, habit, and memories of past food intake, can affect appetite. The regulation of appetite is not well understood. Despite day-to-day variations in food intake and physical activity, a healthy individual maintains a constant body weight and energy reserves of fat over long periods. With the discovery of the hormone **leptin** (from the Greek word *leptos*, meaning "thin"), researchers have been able to piece together one long-term mechanism for regulating weight. Leptin is produced by adipocytes in adipose tissue. When fat is stored because of excess food intake, the cells release more leptin. Centers in the hypothalamus respond to the hormone by decreasing food intake and increasing energy expenditure, resulting in weight loss. If this feedback mechanism is disrupted, obesity will result. Early hopes of using leptin to treat human obesity have dimmed, however, because obese people do not have a leptin deficiency. This system's failure in humans appears to be caused by the hypothalamus' inability to respond to leptin rather than our inability to make the hormone.

Table 19-3	Hormones Active in Digestion	19

Hormone	Source	Action
Gastrin	Stomach	Stimulates release of gastric juice
Gastric-inhibitory peptide (GIP)	Duodenum	Stimulates insulin release from pancreas when glucose enters duodenum; inhibits release of gastric juice
Secretin	Duodenum	Stimulates release of water and bicarbonate from pancreas, stimulates release of bile from liver; inhibits the stomach
Cholecystokinin (CCK)	Duodenum	Stimulates release of digestive enzymes from pancreas, stimulates release of bile from gallbladder; inhibits the stomach

CHECKPOINT 19-16 ➤ What is the difference between hunger and appetite?

Eating Disorders

A chronic loss of appetite, called **anorexia** (an-o-REK-se-ah), may be caused by a great variety of physical and mental disorders. Because the hypothalamus and the higher brain centers are involved in the regulation of hunger, it is possible that emotional and social factors contribute to the development of anorexia.

Anorexia nervosa is a psychological disorder that predominantly afflicts young women. In a desire to be excessively thin, affected people literally starve themselves, sometimes to the point of death. A related disorder, **bulimia** (bu-LIM-e-ah), is also called the *binge-purge syndrome*. Affected individuals eat huge quantities of food at one time, and then induce vomiting or take large doses of laxatives to prevent absorption of the food.

These disorders stress all body systems. In women, a lack of estrogen production may cause menstrual periods to cease. Loss of bone mass may lead to osteoporosis. Degeneration of the myocardium can result in heart failure. Mental function is impaired. The reflux of acidic substances in bulimia causes erosion of the esophagus and destruction of tooth enamel.

Disorders of the Digestive System

Infections, ulcers, cancer, and structural abnormalities all affect the digestive system at almost any level. Stones may form in the accessory organs or their ducts. Mechanical, nervous, chemical, and hormonal factors may be at the source of digestive problems.

Peritonitis

Inflammation of the peritoneum, termed **peritonitis** (per-ih-to-NI-tis), is a serious complication that may follow infection of an organ covered by the peritoneum—often, the appendix. The frequency and severity of peritonitis have been greatly reduced by the use of antibiotics. The disorder still occurs, however, and can be dangerous. If the infection is kept in one area, it is said to be *localized peritonitis*. A *generalized peritonitis*, as may be caused by a ruptured appendix, a perforated ulcer, or a penetrating wound, may lead to the growth of so many disease organisms and the release of so much bacterial toxin as to be fatal. Immediate surgery to repair the rupture and medical care are needed.

Diseases of the Mouth and Teeth

Tooth decay is also termed dental **caries** (KA-reze) (from Latin meaning "rottenness"). It has a number of causes, including diet, heredity, mechanical problems, and endocrine disorders. People who ingest a lot of sugar are particularly prone to this disease. Because a baby's teeth begin to develop before birth, a mother's diet during pregnancy is important in ensuring the formation of healthy teeth in her baby.

Any infection of the gum is called **gingivitis** (jin-jih-VI-tis). If such an infection continues untreated, it may lead to a more serious condition, **periodontitis** (per-e-o-don-TI-tis), which involves not only the gum tissue but also the teeth's supporting bone. Tooth loosening and bone destruction follow unless periodontitis is halted by proper treatment and improved dental hygiene. Periodontitis is responsible for nearly 80% of tooth loss in people older than 45 years of age.

Vincent disease, a kind of gingivitis caused by a spirochete or a bacillus, is most prevalent in teenagers and young adults. Characterized by inflammation, ulceration, and infection of the oral mucous membranes, this disorder is highly contagious, particularly by oral contact. Patients on antibiotic therapy are more likely than normal to develop fungal infections of the mouth and tongue because these drugs may destroy the normal bacterial flora and allow other organisms to grow.

Leukoplakia (lu-ko-PLA-ke-ah) is characterized by thickened white patches on the mucous membranes of the mouth. It is common in smokers and is considered precancerous.

CHECKPOINT 19-17 ➤ What are some common diseases of the mouth and teeth?

Disorders of the Esophagus and Stomach

The distal portion of the esophagus is a common site for ulcer development due to acid reflux (backflow) from the stomach. In cases of liver disease, the esophagus is prone to develop varicose veins, which are subject to severe bleeding.

As noted, a weakness in the diaphragm at the point where the esophagus joins the stomach may allow the stomach to protrude upward as a **hiatal** (hi-A-tal) **hernia**. Minor irregularities in this area are common and may cause no problem, but the incidence and severity of hiatal hernia increase with age. A hiatal hernia may cause discomfort after meals, gastritis, or ulceration, and serious cases may need surgical repair.

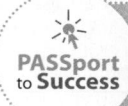 **PASSport to Success** Visit *thePoint* or see the Student Resource CD in the back of this book for an illustration of hiatal hernia.

Weakness in the lower esophageal sphincter (LES) may allow the acidic stomach contents to flow back into the distal esophagus. The result is a burning sensation below or behind the sternum that is described as *heartburn*. The symptom does not involve the heart in any way, but is felt in the vicinity of the heart. Often it is mistaken for a heart attack. More dangerously, a heart attack can be mistaken for heartburn, and people may fail to seek medical attention thinking they have a minor disturbance. Chronic reflux is referred to as **gastroesophageal reflux disease (GERD)**. Overfilling of the stomach and meals high in fat contribute to reflux and GERD by initiating nervous responses that relax the LES. Acid reflux irritates the esophageal mucous membrane, leading to esophagitis. Eventually there may be edema and scar tissue formation that narrows the esophagus and interferes with digestion. GERD also increases the risk of esophageal cancer.

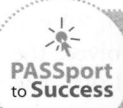 Visit *thePoint* or see the Student Resource CD in the back of this book for an illustration of the causes and effects of GERD.

Acid reflux and GERD are treated with antacids and drugs that inhibit the production of HCl. People with this problem should avoid certain foods and beverages, including fats, caffeine, chocolate, and alcohol, and should not smoke. Other measures that may help are eating in an upright position, not bending down for long periods, not lying down for several hours after eating, and sleeping with the head elevated. Weight loss may also help in cases of obesity.

Nausea is an unpleasant sensation that may follow distention or irritation of the distal esophagus or the stomach as a result of various nervous and mechanical factors. It may be a symptom of interference with normal peristalsis in the stomach and intestine, and thus may be followed by vomiting.

Vomiting, also called **emesis** (EM-eh-sis), is the expulsion of gastric (and sometimes intestinal) contents through the mouth by reverse peristalsis. The contraction of muscles in the abdominal wall forcibly empties the stomach. Vomiting is frequently caused by overeating or by inflammation of the stomach lining, a condition called **gastritis** (gas-TRI-tis). Gastritis results from irritation of the mucosa by certain drugs, food, or drinks. For example, the long-term use of aspirin, highly spiced foods, or alcohol can lead to gastritis. The nicotine in cigarettes can also cause gastritis.

Flatus (FLA-tus) usually refers to excessive amounts of air (gas) in the stomach or intestine. The resulting condition is referred to as **flatulence** (FLAT-u-lens). In some cases, a physician may need to insert a tube into the stomach or rectum to aid the patient in expelling flatus.

STOMACH CANCER Although stomach cancer has become rare in the United States, it is common in many parts of the world, and it is a serious disorder because of its high death rate. Men are more susceptible than women to stomach cancer. The tumor nearly always develops from the stomach's epithelial or mucosal lining, and is often of the type called **adenocarcinoma** (ad-en-o-kar-sih-NO-mah). Sometimes, the victim has suffered from long-standing indigestion (discomfort after meals) but has failed to consult a physician until the cancer has metastasized (spread) to other organs, such as the liver or lymph nodes. Persistent indigestion is one of the important warning signs of stomach cancer.

PEPTIC ULCER An ulcer is an area of the skin or mucous membrane in which the tissues are gradually destroyed. **Peptic ulcers** (named for the enzyme pepsin) occur in the mucous membrane of the esophagus, stomach, or duodenum (the first part of the small intestine) and are most common in people between the ages of 30 and 45 years. Peptic ulcers in the stomach are termed *gastric ulcers*; those in the duodenum are *duodenal* (du-o-DE-nal) *ulcers*.

Smoking cigarettes and taking aspirin or other anti-inflammatory drugs are major causative factors. It also has been found that infection with a bacterium, *Helicobacter pylori*, is a factor in causing peptic ulcers. The organism is associated with inflammation of the stomach and duodenum, and most people with ulcers who have an *H. pylori* infection are cured when the organism is eliminated with antibiotics. Drugs that inhibit the secretion of stomach acids are often effective in treating peptic ulcers.

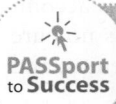 Visit *thePoint* or see the Student Resource CD in the back of this book for common ulcer types and sites.

PYLORIC STENOSIS Normally, the stomach contents are moved through the pyloric sphincter within approximately 2 to 6 hours after eating. Some infants, however, most often boys, are born with an obstruction of the pyloric sphincter, a condition called **pyloric stenosis** (steh-NO-sis). Usually, surgery is required in these cases to modify the muscle, so that food can pass from the stomach into the duodenum.

 Visit *thePoint* or see the Student Resource CD in the back of this book for an illustration of pyloric stenosis.

Intestinal Disorders

Many intestinal disorders involve inflammation. **Appendicitis** (ah-pen-dih-SI-tis) is inflammation of the appendix, which may result from infection or obstruction. The cause of obstruction is usually a **fecalith** (FE-cah-lith), a hardened piece of fecal material. The first sign of acute appendicitis is usually abdominal pain, with loss of appetite and sometimes nausea or vomiting. Pain eventually localizes in the right lower quadrant of the abdomen. Laboratory blood tests show elevated leukocytes. Surgery (appendectomy) is required to remove an inflamed appendix. Untreated, it can rupture to spread infection into the peritoneal cavity.

Two similar diseases are included under the heading of **inflammatory bowel disease** (IBD): **Crohn** (krone) **disease** and **ulcerative colitis**. Both occur mainly in adolescents and young adults and cause similar symptoms of pain, diarrhea, weight loss, and rectal bleeding. Crohn disease usually involves inflammation of the distal small intestine. It is an autoimmune disease, which may in part be

19

hereditary. Ulcerative colitis involves inflammation and ulceration of the colon, and usually the rectum.

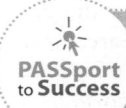

PASSport to Success Visit *thePoint* or see the Student Resource CD in the back of this book for information on the complications of ulcerative colitis.

Irritable bowel syndrome (IBS) is a common gastrointestinal disorder seen typically in young to middle-aged women. Symptoms include pain and constipation or diarrhea, or sometimes both conditions in alternation. In IBS, the intestine is overly sensitive to stimulation, often brought on by stress. Although the condition is chronic and causes much pain, frustration, and anxiety, it is not life-threatening and does not develop into more serious bowel diseases.

Difficulties with digestion or absorption may be due to **enteritis** (en-ter-I-tis), an intestinal inflammation. When both the stomach and the small intestine are involved, the disorder is called **gastroenteritis** (gas-tro-en-ter-I-tis). The symptoms of gastroenteritis include nausea, vomiting, and diarrhea as well as acute abdominal pain (colic). The disorder may be caused by a variety of pathogenic organisms, including viruses, bacteria, and protozoa. Chemical irritants, such as alcohol, certain drugs (e.g., aspirin), and other toxins, have been known to cause this disorder as well.

Diverticula (di-ver-TIK-u-lah) are small pouches in the wall of the intestine, most commonly in the colon. A diet low in fiber contributes to the formation of large numbers of diverticula, a condition called **diverticulosis** (di-ver-tik-u-LO-sis). Collection of waste and bacteria in these sacs leads to **diverticulitis** (di-ver-tik-u-LI-tis), which is accompanied by pain and sometimes bleeding. There is no cure for diverticulitis; it is treated with diet, stool softeners, and drugs to reduce intestinal motility.

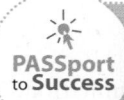

PASSport to Success Visit *thePoint* or see the Student Resource CD in the back of this book for an illustration of diverticulitis.

CHECKPOINT 19-18 ➤ What two diseases fall into the category of inflammatory bowel disease?

DIARRHEA Diarrhea is a symptom characterized by abnormally frequent watery bowel movements. The danger of diarrhea is dehydration and loss of salts, especially in infants. Diarrhea may result from excess activity of the colon, faulty absorption, or infection. Infections resulting in diarrhea include cholera, dysentery, and food poisoning. Tables 1 and 5 in Appendix 5 list some of the organisms causing these diseases. Such infections are often spread by poor sanitation and contaminated food, milk, or water. A stool examination may be required to establish the cause of diarrhea; examination may reveal the presence of pathogenic organisms, worm eggs, or blood.

CONSTIPATION Millions of dollars are spent each year in an effort to remedy a condition called **constipation**. What is constipation? Many people erroneously think they are constipated if they go a day or more without having a bowel movement. Actually, what is normal varies greatly; one person may normally have a bowel movement only once every 2 or 3 days, whereas another may normally have more than one movement daily. The term *constipation* is also used to refer to hard stools or difficulty with defecation.

On the basis of its onset, constipation may be classified as acute or chronic. Acute constipation occurs suddenly and may be due to an intestinal obstruction, such as a tumor or diverticulitis. Extreme constipation is termed **obstipation** (ob-stih-PA-shun). Chronic constipation, in contrast, has a more gradual onset and may be divided into two groups:

- **Spastic constipation,** in which the intestinal musculature is overstimulated so that the canal becomes narrowed and the lumen (space) inside the intestine is not large enough to permit the passage of fecal material.

- **Flaccid** (FLAK-sid) **constipation,** which is characterized by a lazy, or **atonic** (ah-TON-ik), intestinal muscle. Elderly people and those on bed rest are particularly susceptible to this condition. Often, it results from repeated denial of the urge to defecate. Regular bowel habits, moderate exercise, eating more vegetables and other bulky foods, and an increase in fluid may help people who have sluggish intestinal muscles.

People should avoid the chronic use of laxatives and enemas, which interfere with the natural defecation reflex. They may also alter electrolyte balance and result in fluid loss. The streams of fluid used in enemas may injure the intestinal lining by removing the normal protective mucus. In addition, enemas aggravate hemorrhoids. Enemas should be done only on a physician's order, and sparingly.

INTESTINAL OBSTRUCTION **Intussusception** (in-tuh-suh-SEP-shun) is the slipping of a part of the intestine into an adjacent part (Fig. 19-11). It occurs mainly in male infants in the ileocecal region. **Volvulus** (VOL-vu-lus) is a twisting of the intestine, usually the sigmoid colon. It may be a congenital malformation or the result of a foreign body. Both intussusception and volvulus can be fatal if not treated quickly. **Ileus** (IL-e-us) is an intestinal obstruction caused by lack of peristalsis or by muscle contraction. A physician can insert a tube to release intestinal material. **Hemorrhoids** (HEM-o-roydz) are varicose veins in the rectum. These enlarged veins may cause pain and bleeding and may eventually extend out through the rectum.

CANCER OF THE COLON AND RECTUM Tumors of the colon and rectum are among the six most common types of cancer in the United States. These tumors are usually adenocarcinomas that arise from the mucosal lining.

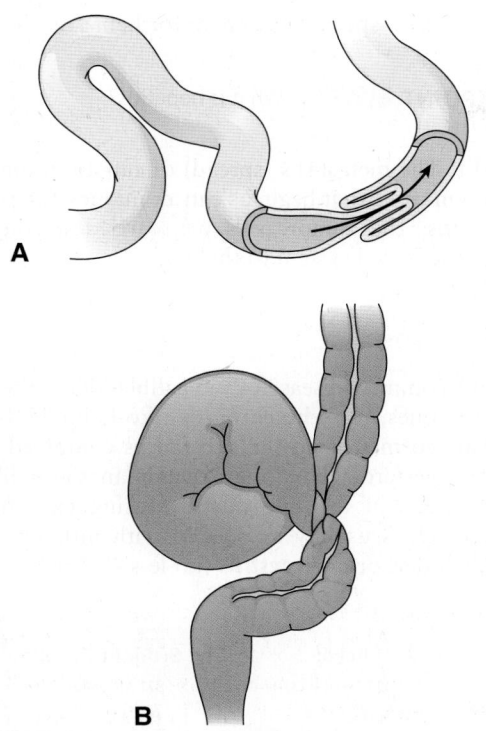

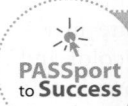

Figure 19-11 **Intestinal obstructions. (A)** Intussusception. A part of the intestine slips into an adjacent part. **(B)** Volvulus. A twisting of the intestine. (Modified with permission from Cohen BJ. *Medical Terminology*, 5th ed. Philadelphia: Lippincott Williams & Wilkins, 2008.)

The occurrence of colon cancer is evenly divided between the sexes, but malignant tumors of the rectum are more common in men than in women.

Tumors may be detected by direct examination of the rectum and lower colon with an instrument called a **sigmoidoscope** (sig-MOY-do-skope) (named for the sigmoid colon). A **colonoscope** (ko-LON-o-skope) is used to examine deeper regions of the colon (see Box 19-2, Endoscopy). The presence of blood in the stool may indicate cancer of the bowel or some other gastrointestinal disturbance. A simple chemical test can detect extremely small quantities of blood in the stool, referred to as *occult* ("hidden") *blood*. Early detection and treatment are the keys to increasing survival rates.

PASSport to Success Visit *thePoint* or see the Student Resource CD in the back of this book for illustrations of colonoscopy and a colonoscopic image.

Infection of the Salivary Glands

The contagious disease commonly called *mumps* is a viral infection of the parotid salivary glands. This type of **parotitis** (par-o-TI-tis), or inflammation of the parotid glands, may lead to inflammation of the testicles by the same virus. Males affected after puberty are at risk for permanent damage to these sex organs, resulting in sterility. Another complication of mumps that occurs in about 10% of cases is meningitis. Mumps now can be prevented by childhood immunization with a vaccine (MMR).

Cirrhosis and Other Liver Diseases

Cirrhosis (sih-RO-sis) of the liver is a chronic disease in which active liver cells are replaced by inactive connective (scar) tissue. The most common type of cirrhosis is alcoholic

---

Box 19-2 Clinical Perspectives

Endoscopy: A View From Within

Modern medicine has made great strides toward looking into the body without resorting to invasive surgery. An instrument that has made this possible in many cases is the **endoscope**, which is inserted into the body through an orifice or small incision and used to examine passageways, hollow organs, and body cavities. The first endoscopes were rigid lighted telescopes that could be inserted only a short distance into the body. Today, physicians are able to navigate the twists and turns of the digestive tract using long **fiberoptic endoscopes** composed of flexible bundles of glass or plastic that transmit light.

In the gastrointestinal tract, endoscopy can detect structural abnormalities, bleeding ulcers, inflammation, and tumors. In addition, endoscopes can be used to remove fluid samples or tissue biopsy specimens. Some surgery can even be done with an endoscope, such as polyp removal from the colon or expansion of a sphincter. Endoscopy can also be used to examine and operate on joints (arthroscopy), the bladder (cystoscopy), respiratory passages (bronchoscopy), and the abdominal cavity (laparoscopy).

Capsular endoscopy, a recent technological advance, has made examination of the gastrointestinal tract even easier. It uses a pill-sized camera that can be swallowed! As the camera moves through the digestive tract, it transmits video images to a data recorder worn on the patient's belt.

19

(portal) cirrhosis. Alcohol has a direct damaging effect on liver cells that is compounded by malnutrition. Hepatic cell destruction hampers the portal circulation, causing blood to accumulate in the spleen and gastrointestinal tract and causing fluid (ascites) to accumulate in the peritoneal cavity.

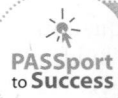

Visit *thePoint* or see the Student Resource CD in the back of this book for a photograph of a cirrhotic liver.

JAUNDICE Damage to the liver or blockage in any of the bile ducts may cause bile pigment to accumulate in the blood. As a result, the stool may become pale in color and the skin and sclera of the eyes may become yellowish; this symptom is called **jaundice** (JAWN-dis) (from French *jaune* for "yellow") (see Fig. 6-6B). Jaundice may also be caused by excess destruction of red blood cells. In addition, it is often seen in newborns, in whom the liver is immature and not yet functioning efficiently.

HEPATITIS Inflammation of the liver, called **hepatitis** (hep-ah-TI-tis), may be caused by drugs, alcohol, or infection (see Table 2 in Appendix 5). The known viruses that cause hepatitis are named A through E. These vary in route (pathway) of infection, severity, and complications. All types of hepatitis are marked by hepatic cell destruction and such symptoms as loss of appetite, jaundice, and liver enlargement. In most patients, the liver cells regenerate with little residual damage. The types of hepatitis virus and their primary routes of transmission are as follows:

Hepatitis A (HAV): commonly transmitted in fecal matter and contaminated food and water. There is a vaccine for hepatitis A, which is recommended for people traveling to areas where this disease is a threat.

Hepatitis B (HBV): transmitted by exposure to the virus in blood or body fluids, although it also can be spread by fecal contamination. This is the most prevalent form of hepatitis. HBV and other blood-borne types of hepatitis virus (C and D) have been linked to long-term development of liver cancer. Also, people with these forms of hepatitis may develop into carriers, able to transmit the disease but not showing any symptoms. HBV is usually transmitted by use of improperly sterilized needles. A vaccine is available that is now recommended for childhood immunization and for people working in healthcare and childcare.

Hepatitis C (HCV): transmitted primarily by exposure to infected blood. There is some evidence of limited sexual transmission. Clinical symptoms of hepatitis C may develop many years after exposure to the virus.

Hepatitis D (HDV): transmitted by direct exchange of blood. It occurs only in those with hepatitis B infection.

Hepatitis E (HEV): transmitted by fecal contamination of water. Most cases have been linked to epidemics in Asia, Africa, and Central America.

An additional related virus has been designated hepatitis G. It is similar in structure to HCV and is found in blood, but does not appear to cause hepatitis.

There is no specific treatment for hepatitis.

CHECKPOINT 19-19 ➤ What is hepatitis?

CANCER The metastasis (spread) of cancer to the liver is common in cases that begin as cancer in one of the abdominal organs; the tumor cells are carried in the blood through the portal system to the liver.

Gallstones

The most common disease of the gallbladder is the formation of stones, or **cholelithiasis** (ko-le-lih-THI-ah-sis). Stones are formed from the substances contained in bile, mainly cholesterol. They may remain in the gallbladder or may lodge in the bile ducts, causing extreme pain. Cholelithiasis is usually associated with inflammation of the gallbladder, or **cholecystitis** (ko-le-sis-TI-tis).

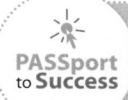

Visit *thePoint* or see the Student Resource CD in the back of this book for an illustration of gallstones.

Pancreatitis

Because they are usually confined to proper channels, pancreatic enzymes do not damage body tissues. If the bile ducts become blocked, however, pancreatic enzymes back up into the pancreas. Also, in some cases of gastric inflammation from excess alcohol consumption or in gallbladder disease, irritation may extend to the pancreas and cause abnormal activation of the pancreatic enzymes. In either circumstance, the pancreas suffers destruction by its own juice, and the outcome can be fatal; this condition is known as **acute pancreatitis**.

Aging and the Digestive System

With age, receptors for taste and smell deteriorate, leading to a loss of appetite and decreased enjoyment of food. A decrease in saliva and poor gag reflex make swallowing more difficult. Tooth loss or poorly fitting dentures may make chewing food more difficult.

Activity of the digestive organs decreases. These changes can be seen in poor absorption of certain vitamins and poor protein digestion. Slowing of peristalsis in the large intestine and increased consumption of easily chewed, refined foods contribute to the common occurrence of constipation.

The tissues of the digestive system require constant replacement. Slowing of this process contributes to a variety of digestive disorders, including gastritis, ulcers, and diverticulosis. As with many body systems, tumors and cancer occur more frequently with age.

Disease in Context revisited

➤ Adam's Colonoscopy

At his scheduled time, Adam reported to the hospital as an outpatient for his colonoscopy. He had stayed on a clear liquid diet for a day and done the required laxative prep to clear his colon. He met with Dr. Clarkson who described the procedure. "We'll give you light sedation, and then use a flexible lighted endoscope with a camera to examine the entire colon. The procedure should take only about half an hour and has a very low risk. You have made arrangements for someone to go home with you, haven't you?" Adam said his brother was coming. After the test Dr. Clarkson reported that everything looked fine and that he would send the results to Dr. Michaels. "The good news, Adam, is that you have 10 years before you have to do this again.

Maybe next time we'll be able to get our pictures with a small camera in a pill that you can swallow. That's already being tested. With the excellent medical care you're getting, you'll probably be alive to see the screening done by genetic study of cells sloughed off in the stool—and that won't require a prep."

Adam's case shows the importance of anatomic studies in the diagnosis and treatment of disease. Box 1-2 has general information on medical imaging, and various methods are mentioned in chapters and cases throughout this book. We'll visit Adam again in Chapter 22 when he finds out that his prostate gland is affecting his urinary system.

Word Anatomy

Medical terms are built from standardized word parts (prefixes, roots, and suffixes). Learning the meanings of these parts can help you remember words and interpret unfamiliar terms.

WORD PART	MEANING	EXAMPLE
Function and Design of the Digestive System		
ab-	away from	In *absorption*, digested materials are taken from the digestive tract into the circulation.
enter/o	intestine	The *mesentery* is the portion of the peritoneum around the intestine.
mes/o-	middle	The *mesocolon*, like the mesentery, comes from the middle layer of cells in the embryo, the mesoderm.
Organs of the Digestive Tract		
gastr/o	stomach	The *gastrointestinal* tract consists mainly of the stomach and intestine.
The Accessory Organs		
amyl/o	starch	The starch-digesting enzyme in saliva is salivary *amylase*.
lingu/o	tongue	The *sublingual* salivary glands are under the tongue.
hepat/o	liver	The *hepatic* portal system carries blood to the liver.
bil/i	bile	*Bilirubin* is a pigment found in bile.
cyst/o	bladder, sac	The *cystic* duct carries bile into and out of the gallbladder.

19

WORD PART	MEANING	EXAMPLE
Control of Digestion		
chole	bile, gall	*Cholecystokinin* is a hormone that activates the gallbladder (cholecyst/o).
Disorders of the Digestive System		
odont/o	tooth	*Periodontitis* is a disease of the gums and the tissue around a tooth.
-lith	stone	A *fecalith* is a hardened piece of fecal material.
-rhea (the r is doubled when added to a word)	flow, discharge	*Diarrhea* is flow of watery bowel movements through (dia-) the digestive tract.

Summary

I. **FUNCTION AND DESIGN OF THE DIGESTIVE SYSTEM**
   A. Functions—digestion, absorption, elimination
   B. Two groups of organs—digestive tract and accessory organs
   C. The wall of the digestive tract—mucous membrane (mucosa), submucosa, smooth muscle, serous membrane (serosa)
   D. The peritoneum
      1. Serous membrane that lines the abdominal cavity and folds over organs
      2. Divisions—mesentery, mesocolon, greater omentum, lesser omentum

II. **ORGANS OF THE DIGESTIVE TRACT**
   A. Mouth
      1. Functions
         a. Ingest food
         b. Begin digestion of starch with salivary amylase
         c. Mastication (chewing)
         d. Deglutition (swallowing)
      2. Tongue—aids mastication and deglutition; has taste buds
   B. Teeth
      1. Deciduous (baby) teeth—20 (incisors, canines, molars)
      2. Permanent teeth—32 (incisors, canines, premolars, molars)
   C. Pharynx (throat)—moves bolus (portion) of food into esophagus by reflex swallowing
   D. Esophagus—long muscular tube that carries food to stomach by peristalsis
   E. Stomach
      1. Functions
         a. Storage of food
         b. Breakdown of food by churning to form chyme
         c. Breakdown of protein with hydrochloric acid (HCl)
         d. Digestion of protein with enzyme pepsin
   F. Small intestine
      1. Functions
         a. Digestion of food
         b. Absorption of nutrients and water through villi (small projections of intestinal lining)
      2. Divisions—duodenum, jejunum, ileum
   G. Large intestine
      1. Functions
         a. Storage and elimination of waste (defecation)
         b. Reabsorption of water
      2. Divisions—cecum; ascending, transverse, descending, and sigmoid colons; rectum; anus

III. **ACCESSORY ORGANS**
   A. Salivary glands—secrete saliva
      1. Functions of saliva
         a. Moistening food—aids chewing and swallowing
         b. Cleaning of mouth and teeth
         c. Digestion of starch with amylase
      2. Three pairs—parotid, submandibular, sublingual
   B. Liver
      1. Functions
         a. Manufacture of bile—emulsifies fats
         b. Storage of glucose
         c. Modification of fats
         d. Storage of vitamins and iron
         e. Formation of blood plasma proteins
         f. Destruction of old red blood cells
         g. Synthesis of urea—waste product of proteins
         h. Detoxification of harmful substances

C. Gallbladder
  1. Stores bile until needed for digestion
D. Pancreas
  1. Secretes powerful digestive juice
  2. Secretes sodium bicarbonate ($NaHCO_3$), an alkali (base) to neutralize chyme
IV. **ENZYMES AND THE DIGESTIVE PROCESS**
  A. Enzymes—catalysts that speed reactions
    1. Products of digestion
      a. Simple sugars (monosaccharides) from carbohydrates
      b. Peptides and amino acids from proteins
      c. Glycerol and fatty acids from fats
  B. The role of water
    1. Used to split foods (hydrolysis)
    2. Lubricates and dilutes food
  C. Digestion, step-by-step
    1. Mouth—starch
    2. Stomach—protein
    3. Small intestine—remainder of food
V. **ABSORPTION**
  A. Movement of nutrients into the circulation
  B. Absorption of fats—most enter lymphatic system
  C. Absorption of vitamins and minerals
VI. **CONTROL OF DIGESTION**
  A. Nervous control
    1. Parasympathetic system—generally increases activity
    2. Sympathetic system—generally decreases activity
  B. Hormonal control
    1. Stimulation of digestive activity
    2. Feedback to inhibit stomach activity
    3. Examples—gastrin, GIP, secretin, CCK
  C. Hunger and appetite

D. Eating disorders—e.g., anorexia, bulimia
VII. **DISORDERS OF THE DIGESTIVE SYSTEM**
  A. Peritonitis
  B. Diseases of the mouth and teeth—caries, gingivitis, periodontitis, Vincent disease, leukoplakia
  C. Disorders involving the esophagus and stomach
    1. Hiatal hernia—protrusion of organ through diaphragm
    2. Gastroesophageal reflux disease (GERD)
    3. Nausea, vomiting (emesis)
    4. Cancer
    5. Ulcer—peptic ulcer in esophagus, stomach, or duodenum
    6. Pyloric stenosis
  D. Intestinal disorders ·
    1. Inflammatory diseases—appendicitis, Crohn disease, ulcerative colitis, irritable bowel syndrome (IBS), diverticulitis
    2. Diarrhea
    3. Constipation
    4. Obstruction—intussusception, volvulus, ileus, hemorrhoids
    5. Cancer
  E. Infection of the salivary glands
    1. Mumps—viral infection of parotid salivary gland
  F. Cirrhosis and other diseases of the liver
    1. Jaundice—yellow color due to bile pigments in blood
    2. Hepatitis—viruses A to E
    3. Cancer
  G. Gallstones—cholelithiasis
  H. Pancreatitis
VIII. **AGING AND THE DIGESTIVE SYSTEM**

Questions for Study and Review

BUILDING UNDERSTANDING

Fill in the blanks

1. The wave-like movement of the digestive tract wall is called _____.

2. The small intestine is connected to the posterior abdominal wall by _____.

3. The liver can store glucose in the form of _____.

4. The parotid glands secrete _____.

5. Inflammation of the gallbladder is termed _____.

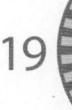

19

Matching > Match each numbered item with the most closely related lettered item.

____ **6.** Digests starch

____ **7.** Begins protein digestion

____ **8.** Digests fats

____ **9.** Digests protein to amino acids

____ **10.** Emulsify fats

a. lipase

b. amylase

c. trypsin

d. pepsin

e. bile salts

Multiple choice

____ **11.** The teeth break up food into small parts by a process called

    a. absorption
    b. deglutition
    c. ingestion
    d. mastication

____ **12.** Hydrochloric acid and pepsin are secreted by the

    a. salivary glands
    b. stomach
    c. pancreas
    d. liver

____ **13.** The double layer of peritoneum that extends from the lower border of the stomach and hangs over the intestine is the

    a. greater omentum
    b. lesser omentum
    c. mesentery
    d. mesocolon

____ **14.** The soft, fleshy V-shaped mass of tissue that hangs from the soft palate is the

    a. epiglottis
    b. esophageal hiatus
    c. uvula
    d. gingiva

____ **15.** Thickened white patches on the oral mucous membranes characterizes the disorder called

    a. periodontitis
    b. cholelithiasis
    c. pancreatitis
    d. leukoplakia

UNDERSTANDING CONCEPTS

16. Differentiate between the terms in each of the following pairs:

    a. digestion and absorption
    b. parietal and visceral peritoneum
    c. gastrin and gastric-inhibitory peptide
    d. secretin and cholecystokinin

17. Name the four layers of the digestive tract. What tissue makes up each layer? What is the function of each layer?

18. Trace the path of a bolus of food through the digestive system.

19. Describe the structure and function of the liver, pancreas, and gallbladder. How are the products of these organs delivered to the digestive tract?

20. Where does absorption occur in the digestive tract, and what structures are needed for absorption? What types of nutrients are absorbed into the blood? Into the lymph?

21. Name several hormones that regulate digestion.

22. Compare and contrast the following disorders:

    a. anorexia and bulimia
    b. inflammatory bowel disease and irritable bowel syndrome
    c. intussusception and volvulus

23. What are the causes and effects of hepatitis?

CONCEPTUAL THINKING

24. Why should a person who suffers from peptic ulcers avoid the use of aspirin (acetylsalicylic acid)?

25. Cholelithiasis can cause pancreatitis. Why?

26. In Adam's case, the proctologist described a future test in which pathologists would look for genetic changes in sloughed off colon cells. What kind of changes might they look for?

27. Colorectal cancer often develops from polyps in the intestinal lining. What is a polyp and why might a polyp become cancerous?

19

CHAPTER 20
Metabolism, Nutrition, and Body Temperature

Learning Outcomes

After careful study of this chapter, you should be able to:

1. Differentiate between catabolism and anabolism
2. Differentiate between the anaerobic and aerobic phases of cellular respiration and give the end products and the relative amount of energy released by each
3. Define *metabolic rate* and name several factors that affect the metabolic rate
4. Explain the roles of glucose and glycogen in metabolism
5. Compare the energy contents of fats, proteins, and carbohydrates
6. Define *essential amino acid*
7. Explain the roles of minerals and vitamins in nutrition and give examples of each
8. List the recommended percentages of carbohydrate, fat, and protein in the diet
9. Distinguish between simple and complex carbohydrates, giving examples of each
10. Compare saturated and unsaturated fats
11. List some adverse effects of alcohol consumption
12. Describe some nutritional disorders
13. Explain how heat is produced and lost in the body
14. Describe the role of the hypothalamus in regulating body temperature
15. Explain the role of fever in disease
16. Describe some adverse effects of excessive heat and cold
17. Show how word parts are used to build words related to metabolism, nutrition, and body temperature (see Word Anatomy at the end of the chapter)

Selected Key Terms

The following terms and other boldface terms in the chapter are defined in the Glossary

anabolism

catabolism

fever

glucose

glycogen

hypothalamus

hypothermia

kilocalorie

malnutrition

metabolic rate

mineral

oxidation

pyrogen

vitamin

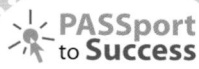

PASSport to Success

Visit *thePoint* or see the Student Resource CD in the back of this book for definitions and pronunciations of key terms as well as a pretest for this chapter.

Disease in Context

> Becky's Second Case: Managing Her Metabolism

"Becky, are you sure you packed everything? Glucose monitor, insulin, needles..." asked Becky's mom as she loaded her daughter's knapsack and sleeping bag into the car. Becky rolled her eyes and said, "Yeah mom, I've got everything. Don't worry; I'll only be at camp for a week!"

Becky's mom sighed. She knew her daughter was right. Besides, *this* summer camp was for children with diabetes mellitus. Not only would she get to do all the fun things that kids normally do at camp, she would also be safe. After all, there was experienced medical staff on site and many of the camp counselors were diabetic themselves. Becky's mom knew that this was a great opportunity for her daughter to learn more about managing her condition and meet other kids with diabetes.

At camp, Becky was having a great time. Her cabin leader, Wanda, was really cool. Today, Wanda was going to teach them how to paddle a canoe! "OK girls," said Wanda, "before we head out to the dock, we need to check our blood glucose levels. Does anyone remember why?"

"Paddling a canoe takes a lot of effort and we have to make sure that we have energy for our muscles to do the work," answered Becky's bunkmate.

"That's right!" replied Wanda. She went on to explain that blood glucose is the main energy source for the body. The pancreas releases the hormone insulin, which signals body cells to absorb glucose from the blood stream. Then, the cells run a series of chemical reactions (called cellular respiration) that convert glucose into carbon dioxide and water. During these catabolic reactions, the cells manufacture adenosine triphosphate (ATP), which they use to run their cellular activities. People with diabetes mellitus don't make enough insulin, so their cells aren't able to absorb glucose from the bloodstream and use it to make ATP. To ensure a constant supply of cellular ATP, diabetics must monitor their blood glucose levels and inject themselves with insulin.

Diabetes mellitus is a disorder that affects glucose metabolism. In this chapter, we'll learn more about metabolism as well as nutrition and body temperature regulation. Later in the chapter, we'll revisit Becky and see what else she's learned at camp.

Metabolism

Nutrients absorbed from the digestive tract are used for all the body's cellular activities, which together make up **metabolism**. These activities fall into two categories:

- **Catabolism**, the breakdown of complex compounds into simpler compounds. Catabolism includes the digestion of food into small molecules and the release of energy from these molecules within the cell.

- **Anabolism**, the building of simple compounds into substances needed for cellular activities and for the growth and repair of tissues.

Through the steps of catabolism and anabolism, there is a constant turnover of body materials as energy is consumed, cells function and grow, and waste products are generated.

CHECKPOINT **20-1** ➤ What are the two phases of metabolism?

Cellular Respiration

Energy is released from nutrients in a series of reactions called **cellular respiration** (Table 20-1 and Fig. 20-1). Early studies on cellular respiration were done with **glucose** as the starting compound. Glucose is a simple sugar that is the body's main energy source.

THE ANAEROBIC PHASE The first steps in the breakdown of glucose do not require oxygen; that is, they are **anaerobic**. This phase of catabolism, known as **glycolysis** (gli-KOL-ih-sis), occurs in the cell's cytoplasm. It yields a small amount of energy, which is used to make ATP (adenosine triphosphate), the cell's energy compound. Each glucose molecule yields enough energy by this process to produce two molecules of ATP.

The anaerobic breakdown of glucose is incomplete and ends with formation of an organic product called **pyruvic** (pi-RU-vik) **acid**. This organic acid is further metabolized in the next phase of cellular respiration, which requires oxygen. In muscle cells operating briefly under anaerobic conditions, pyruvic acid is converted to lactic acid, which accumulates as the cells build up an oxygen debt (described in Chapter 8). Lactic acid induces muscle fatigue, so the body is forced to rest and recover. During the recovery phase immediately after exercise, breathing

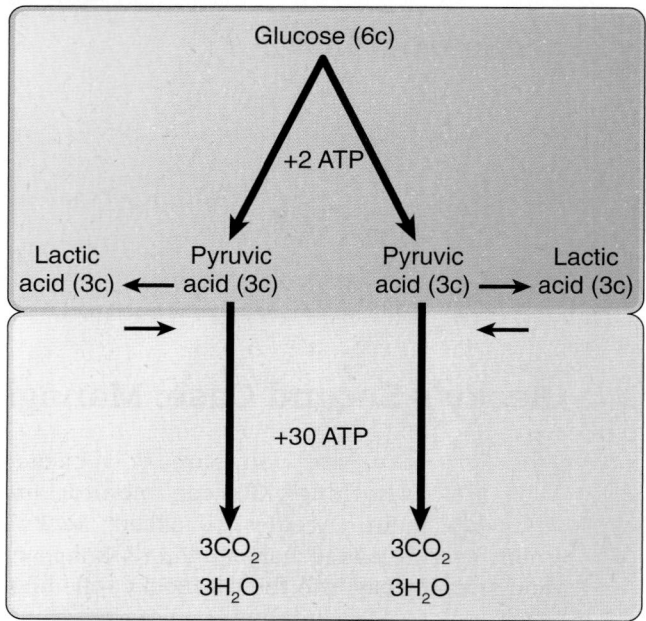

ANAEROBIC

AEROBIC

Figure 20-1 **Cellular respiration.** This diagram shows the catabolism of glucose without oxygen (anaerobic) and with oxygen (aerobic). (c, carbon atoms in one molecule of a substance.) In cellular respiration, glucose first yields two molecules of pyruvic acid, which will convert to lactic acid under anaerobic conditions, as during intense exercise. (Lactic acid must eventually be converted back to pyruvic acid.) Typically, however, pyruvic acid is broken down aerobically (using oxygen) to CO_2 and H_2O. [**ZOOMING IN** ➤ What does pyruvic acid produce in cellular respiration under anaerobic conditions? Under aerobic conditions?]

restores the oxygen needed to convert lactic acid back to pyruvic acid, which is then metabolized further. During this recovery phase, reserves stored in muscles are also replenished. These compounds are myoglobin, which stores oxygen; glycogen, which can be broken down into glucose; and creatine phosphate, which stores energy.

THE AEROBIC PHASE To generate enough energy for survival, the body's cells must break pyruvic acid down more completely in the second phase of cellular respiration, which requires oxygen. These **aerobic** reactions occur within the cell's mitochondria. They result in transfer of most of the energy remaining in the nutrients to ATP. On

Table 20-1	Summary of Cellular Respiration of Glucose		
Phase	**Location in Cell**	**End Product(s)**	**Energy Yield/Glucose**
Anaerobic (glycolysis)	Cytoplasm	Pyruvic acid	2 ATP
Aerobic	Mitochondria	Carbon dioxide and water	30 ATP

average, cells are able to form about 30 molecules of ATP aerobically per glucose molecule. Statements on energy yields may differ slightly, because cells in different tissues vary in their metabolic pathways and in the amount of energy they use to power cellular respiration. In any case, this additional yield is quite an increase over anaerobic metabolism alone, resulting in a total of 32 molecules of ATP per glucose as compared to two.

During the aerobic steps of cellular respiration, the cells form carbon dioxide, which then must be transported to the lungs for elimination. In addition, water is formed by the combination of oxygen with the hydrogen that is removed from nutrient molecules. Because of the type of chemical reactions involved, and because oxygen is used in the final steps, cellular respiration is described as an **oxidation** of nutrients. Note that enzymes are required as catalysts in all these metabolic reactions. Many of the vitamins and minerals described later in this chapter are parts of these enzymes.

Although the oxidation of food is often compared to the burning of fuel, this comparison is inaccurate. Burning fuel results in a sudden and often wasteful release of energy in the form of heat and light. In contrast, metabolic oxidation occurs in small steps, and much of the energy released is stored as ATP for later use by the cells; some of the energy is released as heat, which is used to maintain body temperature, as discussed later in this chapter.

For those who know how to read chemical equations, the net balanced equation for cellular respiration, starting with glucose, is as follows:

$$C_6H_{12}O_6 + 6O_2 \rightarrow 6CO_2 + 6H_2O$$

glucose   oxygen   carbon dioxide   water

CHECKPOINT 20-2 ➤ What name is given to the series of cellular reactions that releases energy from nutrients?

METABOLIC RATE **Metabolic rate** refers to the rate at which energy is released from nutrients in the cells. It is affected by a person's size, body fat, sex, age, activity, and hormones, especially thyroid hormone (thyroxine). Metabolic rate is high in children and adolescents and decreases with age. **Basal metabolism** is the amount of energy needed to maintain life functions while the body is at rest.

The unit used to measure energy is the kilocalorie (kcal), which is the amount of heat needed to raise 1 kilogram of water 1°C. To estimate the daily calories needed taking activity level into account, see Box 20-1, Calorie Counting.

Box 20-1   A Closer Look

Calorie Counting: Estimating Daily Energy Needs

Basal energy requirements for a day can be estimated with a simple formula. An average woman requires 0.9 kcal/kg/hour, and a man, 1.0 kcal/kg/hour. Multiplying 0.9 by body weight in kilograms* by 24 for a woman, or 1.0 by body weight in kilograms by 24 for a man, yields the daily basal energy requirement. For example, if a woman weighed 132 pounds, the equation would be as follows:

132 pounds ÷ 2.2 pounds/kg = 60 kg

0.9 kcal/kg/hour × 60 kg = 54 kcal/hour

54 kcal/hour × 24 hours/day = 1,296 kcal/day

To estimate total energy needs for a day, a percentage based on activity level ("couch potato" to serious athlete) must also be added to the basal requirement. These percentages are shown in the table that follows.

The equation to calculate total energy needs for a day is:

Basal energy requirement + (basal energy requirement × activity level)

Using our previous example, and assuming light activity levels, the following equations apply:

At 40% activity:

**1,296 kcal/day + (1,296 kcal/day × 40%)
= 1,814.4 kcal/day**

At 60% activity:

**1,296 kcal/day + (1,296 kcal/day × 60%)
= 2,073.6 kcal/day**

Therefore, the woman in our example would require between 1,814 and 2,073 kcal/day.

Activity Level	Male	Female
Little activity ("couch potato")	25%–40%	25%–35%
Light activity (e.g., walking to and from class, but little or no intentional exercise)	50%–75%	40%–60%
Moderate activity (e.g., aerobics several times a week)	65%–80%	50%–70%
Heavy activity (serious athlete)	90%–120%	80%–100%

*To convert pounds to kilograms, divide weight in pounds by 2.2.

20

The Use of Nutrients for Energy

As noted, glucose is the body's main energy source. Most of the carbohydrates in the diet are converted to glucose in the course of metabolism. Reserves of glucose are stored in liver and muscle cells as **glycogen** (GLI-ko-jen), a compound built from glucose molecules. When glucose is needed for energy, glycogen is broken down to yield glucose. Glycerol and fatty acids (from fat digestion) and amino acids (from protein digestion) can also be used for energy, but they enter the breakdown process at different points.

Fat in the diet yields more than twice as much energy as do protein and carbohydrate (e.g., it is more "fattening"); fat yields 9 kcal of energy per gram, whereas protein and carbohydrate each yield 4 kcal per gram. Calories that are ingested in excess of need are converted to fat and stored in adipose tissue.

Before they are oxidized for energy, amino acids must have their nitrogen (amine) groups removed. This removal, called **deamination** (de-am-ih-NA-shun), occurs in the liver, where the nitrogen groups are then formed into urea by combination with carbon dioxide. The blood transports urea to the kidneys to be eliminated.

There are no specialized storage forms of proteins, as there are for carbohydrates (glycogen) and fats (adipose tissue). Therefore, when one needs more proteins than are supplied in the diet, they must be obtained from body substance, such as muscle tissue or plasma proteins. Drawing on these resources becomes dangerous when needs are extreme. Fats and carbohydrates are described as "protein sparing," because they are used for energy before proteins are and thus spare proteins for the synthesis of necessary body components.

CHECKPOINT 20-3 ➤ What is the main energy source for the cells?

Anabolism

Nutrient molecules are built into body materials by anabolic steps, all of which are catalyzed by enzymes.

ESSENTIAL AMINO ACIDS Eleven of the 20 amino acids needed to build proteins can be synthesized internally by metabolic reactions. These 11 amino acids are described as *nonessential* because they need not be taken in as food (Table 20-2). The remaining 9 amino acids cannot be made metabolically and therefore must be taken in as part of the diet; these are the **essential amino acids**. Note that some nonessential amino acids may become essential under certain conditions, as during extreme physical stress, or in certain hereditary metabolic diseases.

ESSENTIAL FATTY ACIDS There are also two essential fatty acids, **linoleic** (lin-o-LE-ik) **acid** and **linolenic** (lin-o-LEN-ik) **acid**, that must be taken in as food. These are easily obtained through a healthful, balanced diet.

CHECKPOINT 20-4 ➤ What is meant when an amino acid or a fatty acid is described as essential?

Minerals and Vitamins

In addition to needing fats, proteins, and carbohydrates, the body requires minerals and vitamins.

Table 20-2	**Amino acids**		

Nonessential Amino Acids*		**Essential Amino Acids****	
Name	**Pronunciation**	**Name*****	**Pronunciation**
Alanine	AL-ah-nene	Histidine	HIS-tih-dene
Arginine	AR-jih-nene	Isoleucine	i-so-LU-sene
Asparagine	ah-SPAR-ah-jene	Leucine	LU-sene
Aspartic acid	ah-SPAR-tik AH-sid	Lysine	LI-sene
Cysteine	SIS-teh-ene	Methionine	meh-THI-o-nene
Glutamic acid	glu-TAM-ik AH-sid	Phenylalanine	fen-il-AL-ah-nene
Glutamine	GLU-tah-mene	Threonine	THRE-o-nene
Glycine	GLY-sene	Tryptophan	TRIP-to-fane
Proline	PRO-lene	Valine	VA-lene
Serine	SERE-ene		
Tyrosine	TI-ro-sene		

*Nonessential amino acids can be synthesized by the body.
**Essential amino acids cannot be synthesized by the body; they must be taken in as part of the diet.
***If you are ever called upon to memorize the essential amino acids, the mnemonic (memory device) Pvt. T. M. Hill gives the first letter of each name.

Minerals are chemical elements needed for body structure, fluid balance, and such activities as muscle contraction, nerve impulse conduction, and blood clotting. Some minerals are components of vitamins. A list of the main minerals needed in a proper diet is given in Table 20-3. Some additional minerals not listed are also required for good health. Minerals needed in extremely small amounts are referred to as **trace elements.**

Vitamins are complex organic substances needed in very small quantities. Vitamins are parts of enzymes or other substances essential for metabolism, and vitamin deficiencies lead to a variety of nutritional diseases.

The water-soluble vitamins are the B vitamins and vitamin C. These are not stored and must be taken in regularly with food. The fat-soluble vitamins are A, D, E, and K. These vitamins are kept in reserve in fatty tissue. Excess intake of the fat-soluble vitamins can lead to toxicity. A list of vitamins is given in Table 20-4.

Certain substances are valuable in the diet as **antioxidants.** They defend against the harmful effects of **free radicals,** highly reactive and unstable molecules produced from oxygen in the normal course of metabolism (and also from UV radiation, air pollution, and tobacco smoke). Free radicals contribute to aging and disease. Antioxidants react with free radicals to stabilize them and minimize their harmful effects on cells. Vitamins C and E and beta-carotene, an orange pigment found in plants that is converted to vitamin A, are antioxidants. There are also many compounds found in plants (e.g., soybeans and tomatoes) that are antioxidants.

CHECKPOINT 20-5 ➤ Both vitamins and minerals are needed in metabolism. What is the difference between vitamins and minerals?

Table 20-3   Minerals

Mineral	Functions	Sources	Results of Deficiency
Calcium (Ca)	Formation of bones and teeth, blood clotting, nerve conduction, muscle contraction	Dairy products, eggs, green vegetables, legumes (peas and beans)	Rickets, tetany, osteoporosis
Phosphorus (P)	Formation of bones and teeth; found in ATP, nucleic acids	Meat, fish, poultry, egg yolk, dairy products	Osteoporosis, abnormal metabolism
Sodium (Na)	Fluid balance; nerve impulse conduction, muscle contraction	Most foods, especially processed foods, table salt	Weakness, cramps, diarrhea, dehydration
Potassium (K)	Fluid balance, nerve and muscle activity	Fruits, meats, seafood, milk, vegetables, grains	Muscular and neurologic disorders
Chloride (Cl)	Fluid balance, hydrochloric acid in stomach	Meat, milk, eggs, processed foods, table salt	Rarely occurs
Iron (Fe)	Oxygen carrier (hemoglobin, myoglobin)	Meat, eggs, fortified cereals, legumes, dried fruit	Anemia, dry skin, indigestion
Iodine (I)	Thyroid hormones	Seafood, iodized salt	Hypothyroidism, goiter
Magnesium (Mg)	Catalyst for enzyme reactions, carbohydrate metabolism	Green vegetables, grains, nuts, legumes	Spasticity, arrhythmia, vasodilation
Manganese (Mn)	Catalyst in actions of calcium and phosphorus; facilitator of many cellular processes	Many foods	Possible reproductive disorders
Copper (Cu)	Necessary for absorption and use of iron in formation of hemoglobin; part of some enzymes	Meat, water	Anemia
Chromium (Cr)	Works with insulin to regulate blood glucose levels	Meat, unrefined food, fats and oils	Inability to use glucose
Cobalt (Co)	Part of vitamin B_{12}	Animal products	Pernicious anemia
Zinc (Zn)	Promotes carbon dioxide transport and energy metabolism; found in enzymes	Meat, fish, poultry, grains, vegetables	Alopecia (baldness); possibly related to diabetes
Fluoride (F)	Prevents tooth decay	Fluoridated water, tea, seafood	Dental caries

20

Table 20-4	Vitamins		
Vitamins	**Functions**	**Sources**	**Results of Deficiency**
A (retinol)	Required for healthy epithelial tissue and for eye pigments; involved in reproduction and immunity	Orange fruits and vegetables, liver, eggs, dairy products, dark green vegetables	Night blindness; dry, scaly skin; decreased immunity
B$_1$ (thiamin)	Required for enzymes involved in oxidation of nutrients; nerve function	Pork, cereal, grains, meats, legumes, nuts	Beriberi, a disease of nerves
B$_2$ (riboflavin)	In enzymes required for oxidation of nutrients	Milk, eggs, liver, green leafy vegetables, grains	Skin and tongue disorders
B$_3$ (niacin, nicotinic acid)	Involved in oxidation of nutrients	Yeast, meat, liver, grains, legumes, nuts	Pellagra with dermatitis, diarrhea, mental disorders
B$_6$ (pyridoxine)	Amino acid and fatty acid metabolism; formation of niacin; manufacture of red blood cells	Meat, fish, poultry, fruit, grains, legumes, vegetables	Anemia, irritability, convulsions, muscle twitching, skin disorders
Pantothenic acid	Essential for normal growth; energy metabolism	Yeast, liver, eggs, and many other foods	Sleep disturbances, digestive upset
B$_{12}$ (cyanocobalamin)	Production of cells; maintenance of nerve cells; fatty acid and amino acid metabolism	Animal products	Pernicious anemia
Biotin (a B vitamin)	Involved in fat and glycogen formation, amino acid metabolism	Peanuts, liver, tomatoes, eggs, oatmeal, soy, and many other foods	Lack of coordination, dermatitis, fatigue
Folate (folic acid, a B vitamin)	Required for amino acid metabolism, DNA synthesis, maturation of red blood cells	Vegetables, liver, legumes, seeds	Anemia, digestive disorders, neural tube defects in the embryo
C (ascorbic acid)	Maintains healthy skin and mucous membranes; involved in synthesis of collagen; antioxidant	Citrus fruits, green vegetables, potatoes, orange fruits	Scurvy, poor wound healing, anemia, weak bones
D (calciferol)	Aids in absorption of calcium and phosphorus from intestinal tract	Fatty fish, liver, eggs, fortified milk	Rickets, bone deformities
E (tocopherol)	Protects cell membranes; antioxidant	Seeds, green vegetables, nuts, grains, oils	Anemia, muscle and liver degeneration, pain
K	Synthesis of blood clotting factors, bone formation	Bacteria in digestive tract, liver, cabbage, and leafy green vegetables	Hemorrhage

Nutritional Guidelines

The relative amounts of carbohydrates, fats, and proteins that should be in the daily diet vary somewhat with the individual. Typical recommendations for the number of calories derived each day from the three types of food are as follows:

- Carbohydrate: 55% to 60%.
- Fat: 30% or less.
- Protein: 15% to 20%.

It is important to realize that the type as well as the amount of each nutrient is a factor in good health. A weight loss diet should follow the same proportions as given above, but with a reduction in portion sizes.

Carbohydrates

Carbohydrates in the diet should be mainly complex, naturally occurring carbohydrates, and one should keep simple sugars to a minimum. Simple sugars are monosaccharides, such as glucose and fructose (fruit sugar), and disaccharides, such as sucrose (table sugar) and lactose (milk sugar). Simple sugars are a source of fast energy because they are metabolized rapidly. However, they boost pancreatic insulin output, and as a result, they cause blood glucose levels to rise and fall rapidly. It is healthier to maintain steady glucose levels, which normally range from approximately 85 to 125 mg/dL throughout the day.

The **glycemic effect** is a measure of how rapidly a particular food raises the blood glucose level and stimulates the release of insulin. The effect is generally low for whole grains, fruit, and dairy products and high for sweets and refined ("white") grains. Note, however, that the glycemic effect of a food also depends on when it is eaten during the day, and if or how it is combined with other foods.

Complex carbohydrates are polysaccharides. Examples are:

■ Starches, found in grains, legumes, and potatoes

■ Fibers, such as cellulose, pectins, and gums, which are the structural materials of plants

Fiber adds bulk to the stool and promotes elimination of toxins and waste. It also slows the digestion and absorption of carbohydrates, thus regulating the release of glucose. It helps in weight control by providing a sense of fullness and limiting caloric intake. Adequate fiber in the diet lowers cholesterol and helps to prevent diabetes, colon cancer, hemorrhoids, appendicitis, and diverticulitis. Foods high in fiber, such as whole grains, fruits, and vegetables, are also rich in vitamins and minerals (see Box 20-2).

CHECKPOINT 20-6 ➤ What is the normal range of blood glucose?

Fats

Fats are subdivided into saturated and unsaturated forms based on their chemical structure. The fatty acids in **saturated fats** have more hydrogen atoms in their molecules and fewer double bonds between carbons atoms than do those of unsaturated fats (Fig. 20-2). Most saturated fats are from animal sources and are solid at room temperature, such as butter and lard. Also included in this group are the so-called "tropical oils": coconut oil and palm oil. **Unsaturated fats** are derived from plants. They are liquid at room temperature and are generally referred to as oils, such as corn, peanut, olive, and canola oils.

Saturated fats should make up less than one third of the fat in the diet (less than 10% of total calories). Diets high in saturated fats are associated with a higher than normal incidence of cancer, heart disease, and cardiovascular problems, although the relation between these factors is not fully understood.

Many commercial products contain fats that are artificially saturated to prevent rancidity and provide a more solid consistency. These are listed on food labels as partially hydrogenated (HI-dro-jen-a-ted) vegetable oils and are found in baked goods, processed peanut butter, vegetable shortening, and solid margarine. Evidence shows that components of hydrogenated fats, known as *trans-fatty acids*, may be just as harmful, if not more so, than natural saturated fats and should be avoided.

Proteins

Because proteins, unlike carbohydrates and fats, are not stored in special reserves, protein foods should be taken in on a regular basis, with attention to obtaining the essential amino acids. Most animal proteins supply all of the essential amino acids and are described as complete proteins. Most vegetables are lacking in one or more of the essential amino acids. People on strict vegetarian diets must learn to combine foods, such as legumes (e.g., beans and peas) with

---

Box 20-2 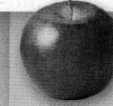 **Health Maintenance**

Dietary Fiber: Bulking Up

Dietary fiber is best known for its ability to improve bowel habits and ease weight loss. But fiber may also help to prevent diabetes, heart disease, and certain digestive disorders such as diverticulitis and gallstones.

Dietary fiber is an indigestible type of carbohydrate found in fruit, vegetables, and whole grains. The amount of fiber recommended for a 2,000-calorie diet is 25 grams per day, but most people in the United States tend to get only half this amount. One should eat fiber-rich foods throughout the day to meet the requirement. It is best to increase fiber in the diet gradually to avoid unpleasant symptoms, such as intestinal bloating and flatulence. If your diet lacks fiber, try adding the following foods over a period of several weeks:

■ Whole grain breads, cereals, pasta, and brown rice. These add 1 to 3 more grams of fiber per serving than the "white" product.
■ Legumes, which include beans, peas, and lentils. These add 4 to 12 grams of fiber per serving.
■ Fruits and vegetables. Whole, raw, unpeeled versions contain the most fiber, and juices, the least. Apple juice has no fiber, whereas a whole apple has 3 grams.
■ Unprocessed bran. This can be sprinkled over almost any food: cereal, soups, and casseroles. One tablespoon adds 2 grams of fiber. Be sure to take adequate fluids with bran.

20

Saturated
fatty acid
(stearic acid)

Unsaturated
fatty acid
(linoleic acid)

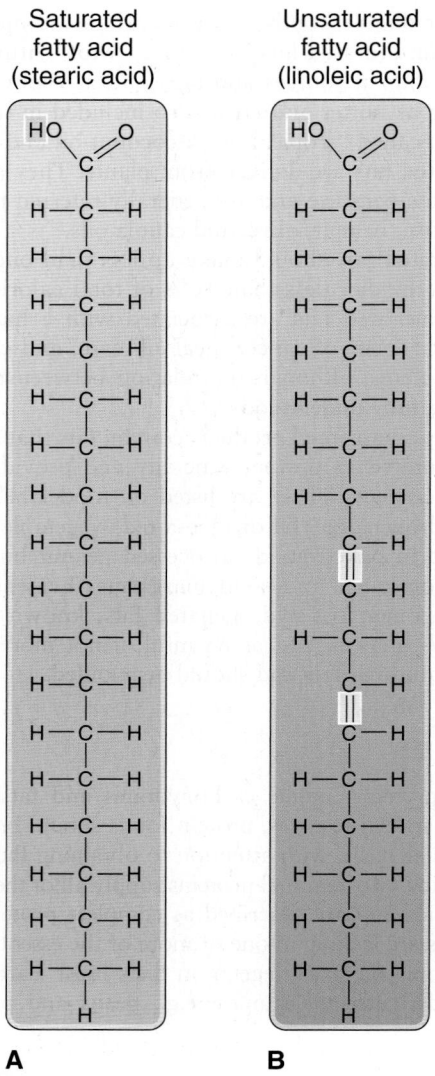

A **B**

Figure 20-2 **Saturated and unsaturated fats.** **(A)** Saturated fatty acids contain the maximum numbers of hydrogen atoms attached to carbons and no double bonds between carbon atoms. **(B)** Unsaturated fatty acids have less than the maximum number of hydrogen atoms attached to carbons and one or more double bonds between carbon atoms (highlighted).

grains (e.g., rice, corn, or wheat), to obtain all the essential amino acids each day. Table 20-5 demonstrates the principles of combining two foods, legumes and grains, to supply essential amino acids that might be missing in one food or the other. Legumes are rich in isoleucine and lysine but poor in methionine and tryptophan, while grains are just the opposite. For illustration purposes, the table includes only the four missing essential amino acids (there are nine total). Traditional ethnic diets reflect these healthy combinations, for example, beans with corn or rice in Mexican dishes or chickpeas and lentils with wheat in Middle Eastern fare.

Vitamin and Mineral Supplements

The need for mineral and vitamin supplements to the diet is a subject of controversy. Some researchers maintain that adequate amounts of these substances can be obtained from a varied, healthful diet. Many commercial foods, including milk, cereal, and bread, are already fortified with minerals and vitamins. Others hold that pollution, depletion of the soils, and the storage, refining, and processing of foods make additional supplementation beneficial. Most agree, however, that children, elderly people, pregnant and lactating women, and teenagers, who often do not get enough of the proper foods, would profit from additional minerals and vitamins.

When required, supplements should be selected by a physician or nutritionist to fit an individual's particular needs. Megavitamin dosages may cause unpleasant reactions and in some cases are hazardous. Vitamins A and D have both been found to cause serious toxic effects when taken in excess.

U.S. Dietary Guidelines

The United States Department of Agriculture (USDA) has published dietary guidelines at regular intervals since 1916. The newest version, incorporating updated nutritional information, is the 2005 guide, MyPyramid (Fig. 20-3). The colored bands in the pyramid show five different categories of foods in widths that indicate relative amounts that should be chosen from each group daily. The narrow yellow band

Table 20-5	Combining Foods for Essential Amino Acids			
	Essential Amino Acids*			
	Isoleucine	Lysine	Methionine	Tryptophan
Legumes	+	+		
Grains			+	+
Legumes and grains combined	+	+	+	+

*There are 9 essential amino acids; the table includes 4 for the purposes of illustration.

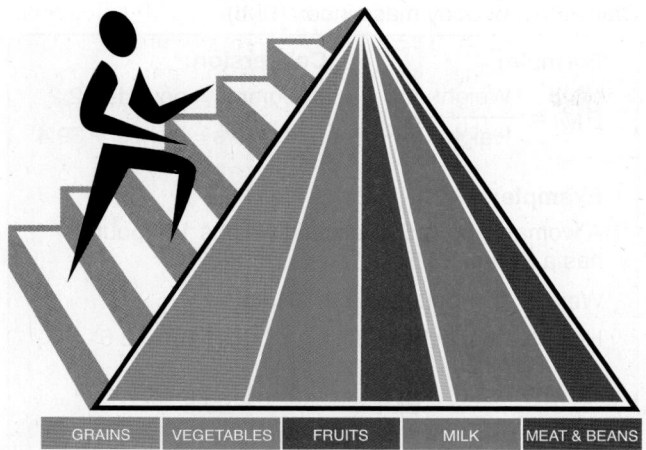

GRAINS | VEGETABLES | FRUITS | MILK | MEAT & BEANS

Figure 20-3 **U.S. Dietary Guidelines.** (MyPyramid, U.S. Department of Agriculture/Center for Nutrition Policy and Promotion.)

between the fruits (red) and milk (blue) represents oils, which should be consumed in moderation.

The pyramid and accompanying guidelines stress:

- Variety in the diet. Foods in all the groups are needed each day for good health.

- Moderation. A single serving or portion is smaller than most people think.

- Eating fruits and vegetables. Most people need more of these in their diets.

- Choice of "nutrient dense" foods that are rich in nutrients compared to their calorie content. This recommendation also includes eating unrefined foods, such as whole grains, and unprocessed foods.

- The importance of exercise, as represented by the climbing figure on the side of the pyramid.

The pyramid graphic does not include sugar, solid fats, or alcohol. The USDA guidelines explain that these are considered "discretionary calories," that is, "extras" that you can eat within your recommended daily energy limit after nutrient needs are met. Of course, you could also select additional foods from among the recommended nutrient-rich groups to satisfy energy needs.

The new guidelines also stress individual variation. On the Internet at http://www.mypyramid.gov/ you can get a personalized estimate of what and how much you should eat based on your height, weight, age, sex, and level of physical activity. You can also assess your diet online with MyPyramid Tracker. Most people will need to make gradual shifts in their diets to reach their healthier eating goals, as suggested by the steps on the side of the pyramid.

Alcohol

Alcohol yields energy in the amount of 7 kcal per gram, but it is not considered a nutrient because it does not yield useful end products. In fact, alcohol interferes with metabolism and contributes to a variety of disorders.

The body can metabolize about one-half ounce of pure alcohol (ethanol) per hour. This amount translates into one glass of wine, one can of beer, or one shot of hard liquor. Consumed at a more rapid rate, alcohol enters the bloodstream and affects many cells, notably in the brain.

Alcohol is rapidly absorbed through the stomach and small intestine and is detoxified by the liver. When delivered in excess to the liver, alcohol can lead to the accumulation of fat as well as inflammation and scarring of liver tissue. It can eventually cause cirrhosis (*sih-RO-sis*), which involves irreversible changes in liver structure. Alcohol metabolism ties up enzymes needed for oxidation of nutrients and also results in byproducts that acidify body fluids. Other effects of alcoholism include obesity, malnutrition, cancer, ulcers, and fetal alcohol syndrome. Health professionals advise pregnant women not to drink any alcohol. In addition, alcohol impairs judgment and leads to increased involvement in accidents.

Although alcohol consumption is compatible with good health and may even have a beneficial effect on the cardiovascular system, alcohol should be consumed only in moderation.

PASSport to Success Visit **thePoint** or see the Student Resource CD in the back of this book for a summary of the effects of alcohol abuse and photographs of its effects on liver and brain tissue.

CHECKPOINT **20-7** ➤ What are typical recommendations for the relative amounts of carbohydrates, fats, and proteins in the diet?

Nutritional Disorders

Diet-related problems may originate from an excess or shortage of necessary nutrients. Another issue in the news today is weight control. Food allergies may also affect some people.

Food Allergies

Some people develop clear allergic (hypersensitive) symptoms if they eat certain foods. Common food allergens are wheat, nuts, milk, shellfish, and eggs, but almost any food might cause an allergic reaction in a given individual. People may also have allergic reactions to food additives, such as flavorings, colorings, or preservatives. Signs of allergic reactions usually involve the skin, respiratory tract, or gastrointestinal tract. Food allergies may provoke potentially fatal anaphylactic shock in extremely sensitive individuals.

20

Malnutrition

If any vital nutrient is missing from the diet, the body will suffer from malnutrition. One commonly thinks of a malnourished person as someone who does not have enough to eat, but malnutrition can also occur from eating too much of the wrong foods. Factors that contribute to malnutrition are poverty, old age, chronic illness, anorexia, poor dental health, and drug or alcohol addiction.

In poor and underdeveloped countries, many children suffer from protein and energy malnutrition (PEM). **Marasmus** (mah-RAZ-mus) is a term used for severe malnutrition in infancy (from Greek meaning "dying away").

Kwashiorkor (kwash-e-OR-kor) typically affects older children when they are weaned because another child is born (and the name means just that). A low protein level in the blood plasma interferes with fluid return to the capillaries, resulting in edema. Often excess fluid accumulates in the abdomen as ascites (ah-SI-teze) fluid, causing the stomach to bulge.

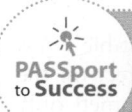 **PASSport to Success** Visit *thePoint* or see the Student Resource CD in the back of this book for the effects of kwashiorkor.

Overweight and Obesity

The causes of obesity are complex, involving social, economic, genetic, psychological, and metabolic factors. It is common knowledge that overweight and obesity have increased in the past several decades in many countries. In the US, 35% of adults are overweight and an additional 30% are obese (see "Body Mass Index" below.) Obesity shortens the life span and is associated with cardiovascular disease, diabetes, some cancers, and other diseases. The incidence of type 2 diabetes, once considered to have an adult onset, has increased greatly among children. Some researchers hold that obesity has a closer correlation to chronic disease than poverty, smoking, or drinking alcohol.

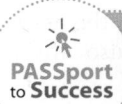 **PASSport to Success** Visit *thePoint* or see the Student Resource CD in the back of this book for a summary of the long-term complications of diabetes.

Scientists are studying the nervous and hormonal controls over weight, but so far they have not found any effective and safe drugs for weight control. For most people, a varied diet eaten in moderation and regular exercise are the surest ways to avoid obesity. At least 30 minutes of moderate to vigorous exercise every day is recommended for health and weight control.

BODY MASS INDEX Body mass index (BMI) is a measurement used to evaluate body size. It is based on the ratio of weight to height (Fig. 20-4). BMI is calculated by

Calculation of body mass index (BMI)

Formula:	**Conversion:**
$BMI = \dfrac{Weight\ (kg)}{Height\ (m)^2}$	Kilograms = pounds ÷ 2.2 Meters = inches ÷ 39.4

Example:
A woman who is 5′4″ tall and weighs 134 pounds has a BMI of 23.5.
Weight: 134 pounds ÷ 2.2 = 61 kg
Height: 64 inches ÷ 39.4 = 1.6 m; $(1.6)^2 = 2.6$

$$BMI = \frac{61\ kg}{2.6\ m} = 23.5$$

Figure 20-4 **Calculation of body mass index (BMI).**
[ZOOMING IN ➤ What is the BMI of a male 5′10″ in height who weighs 170 pounds? (Round off to one decimal place.) **]**

dividing weight in kilograms by height in meters squared. (For those not accustomed to using the metric system, an alternate method is to divide weight in pounds by the square of height in inches and multiply by 703.) A healthy range for this measurement is 19 to 24. Overweight is defined as a BMI of 25 to 30, and obesity as a BMI greater than 30. However, BMI does not take into account the relative amount of muscle and fat in the body. For example, a bodybuilder might be healthy with a higher than typical BMI because muscle has a higher density than fat.

Underweight

People who are underweight have as much difficulty gaining weight as others have losing it. The problem of underweight may result from rapid growth, eating disorders, allergies, illness, or psychological factors. It is associated with low reserves of energy, reproductive disturbances, and nutritional deficiencies. A BMI of less than 18.5 is defined as underweight. To gain weight, people have to increase their intake of calories, but they should also exercise to add muscle tissue and not just fat.

Nutrition and Aging

With age, a person may find it difficult to maintain a balanced diet. Often, the elderly lose interest in buying and preparing food or are unable to do so. Because metabolism generally slows, and less food is required to meet energy needs, nutritional deficiencies may develop. Medications may interfere with appetite and with the absorption and use of specific nutrients.

It is important for older people to seek out foods that are "nutrient dense," that is, foods that have a high proportion of nutrients in comparison with the number of calories they provide. Exercise helps to boost appetite and maintains muscle tissue, which is more active metabolically.

Body Temperature

Heat is an important byproduct of the many chemical activities constantly occurring in body tissues. At the same time, heat is always being lost through a variety of outlets. Under normal conditions, a number of regulatory devices keep body temperature constant within quite narrow limits. Maintenance of a constant temperature despite both internal and external influences is one phase of homeostasis, the tendency of all body processes to maintain a normal state despite forces that tend to alter them.

Heat Production

Heat is a byproduct of the cellular oxidations that generate energy. The amount of heat produced by a given organ varies with the kind of tissue and its activity. While at rest, muscles may produce as little as 25% of total body heat, but when muscles contract, heat production is greatly multiplied, owing to their increased metabolic rate. Under basal conditions (at rest), the liver and other abdominal organs produce about 50% of total body heat. The brain produces only 15% of body heat at rest, and an increase in nervous tissue activity produces little increase in heat production. High heat-generating tissues do not become much warmer than others because the circulating blood distributes the heat fairly evenly.

FACTORS AFFECTING HEAT PRODUCTION The rate at which heat is produced is affected by a number of factors, including exercise, hormone production, food intake, and age. Hormones, such as thyroxine from the thyroid gland and epinephrine (adrenaline) from the adrenal medulla, increase heat production.

The intake of food is also accompanied by increased heat production. The nutrients that enter the blood after digestion are available for increased cellular metabolism. In addition, the glands and muscles of the digestive system generate heat as they set to work. These responses do not account for all the increase, however, nor do they account for the much greater increase in metabolism after a meal containing a large amount of protein.

CHECKPOINT **20-8** ➤ What are some factors that affect heat production in the body?

Heat Loss

Although 15% to 20% of heat loss occurs through the respiratory system and with urine and feces, more than 80% of heat loss occurs through the skin. Networks of blood vessels in the skin's dermis (deeper part) can bring considerable quantities of blood near the surface, so that heat can be dissipated to the outside. This release can occur in several ways.

- Heat can be transferred directly to the surrounding air by means of **conduction**.

- Heat also travels from its source as heat waves or rays, a process termed **radiation**.

- If the air is moving, so that the layer of heated air next to the body is constantly being carried away and replaced with cooler air (as by an electric fan), the process is known as **convection**.

- Finally, heat may be lost by **evaporation**, the process by which liquid changes to the vapor state.

To illustrate evaporation, rub some alcohol on your skin; it evaporates rapidly, using so much heat that your skin feels cold. Perspiration does the same thing, although not as quickly. The rate of heat loss through evaporation depends on the humidity of the surrounding air. When humidity exceeds 60% or so, perspiration does not evaporate so readily, making one feel very uncomfortable unless some other means of heat loss is available, such as convection caused by a fan.

PREVENTION OF HEAT LOSS Factors that play a part in heat loss through the skin include the volume of tissue compared with the amount of skin surface. A child loses heat more rapidly than does an adult. Such parts as fingers and toes are affected most by exposure to cold because they have a great amount of skin compared with total tissue volume.

If the surrounding air temperature is lower than that of the body, excessive heat loss is prevented by both natural and artificial means. Clothing checks heat loss by trapping insulating air in both its material and its layers. An effective natural insulation against cold is the layer of fat under the skin. The degree of insulation depends on the thickness of the subcutaneous layer. Even when skin temperature is low, this fatty tissue prevents the deeper tissues from losing much heat. On the average, this layer is slightly thicker in females than in males.

Temperature Regulation

Body temperature remains almost constant despite wide variations in the rate of heat production or loss, because of internal temperature-regulating mechanisms.

THE ROLE OF THE HYPOTHALAMUS Many body areas take part in heat regulation, but the most important center is the hypothalamus, the area of the brain located just above the pituitary gland. One group of hypothalamic cells controls heat production in body tissues, whereas another group controls heat loss. Regulation is based on the temperature of the blood circulating through the brain and also on input from temperature receptors in the skin.

If these two factors indicate that too much heat is being lost, impulses are sent quickly from the hypothalamus to the autonomic (involuntary) nervous system, which in turn causes constriction of the skin's blood vessels to reduce heat loss. Other impulses are sent to the muscles to

20

cause shivering, a rhythmic contraction that result in increased heat production. Furthermore, epinephrine output may be increased if necessary. Epinephrine increases cellular metabolism for a short period, and this in turn increases heat production.

If there is danger of overheating, the hypothalamus stimulates the sweat glands to increase their activity. Impulses from the hypothalamus also cause cutaneous blood vessels to dilate, so that increased blood flow will promote heat loss. The hypothalamus may also induce muscle relaxation to minimize heat production.

Muscles are especially important in temperature regulation because variations in the activity of these large tissue masses can readily increase or decrease heat generation. Because muscles form roughly one-third of the body, either an involuntary or an intentional increase in their activity can form enough heat to offset a considerable decrease in the temperature of the environment.

CHECKPOINT **20-9** ➤ What part of the brain is responsible for regulating body temperature?

AGE FACTORS Very young and very old people are limited in their ability to regulate body temperature when exposed to environmental extremes. A newborn infant's body temperature decreases if the infant is exposed to a cool environment for a long period. Elderly people also are not able to produce enough heat to maintain body temperature in a cool environment.

With regard to overheating in these age groups, heat loss mechanisms are not fully developed in the newborn. The elderly do not lose as much heat from their skin as do younger people. Both groups should be protected from extreme temperatures.

NORMAL BODY TEMPERATURE The normal temperature range obtained by either a mercury or an electronic thermometer may extend from 36.2°C to 37.6°C (97°F to 100°F). Body temperature varies with the time of day. Usually, it is lowest in the early morning because the muscles have been relaxed and no food has been taken in for several hours. Temperature tends to be higher in the late afternoon and evening because of physical activity and food consumption.

Normal temperature also varies in different parts of the body. Skin temperature obtained in the axilla (armpit) is lower than mouth temperature, and mouth temperature is a degree or so lower than rectal temperature. It is believed that, if it were possible to place a thermometer inside the liver, it would register a degree or more higher than rectal temperature. The temperature within a muscle might be even higher during activity.

Although the Fahrenheit scale is used in the United States, in most parts of the world, temperature is measured with the **Celsius** (SEL-se-us) thermometer. On this scale, the ice point is at 0° and the normal boiling point of water is at 100°, the interval between these two points being divided into 100 equal units. The Celsius scale is also called

the **centigrade scale** (think of 100 cents in a dollar). See Appendix 2 for a comparison of the Celsius and Fahrenheit scales and formulas for converting from one to the other.

CHECKPOINT **20-10** ➤ What is normal body temperature?

Fever

Fever is a condition in which the body temperature is higher than normal. An individual with a fever is described as **febrile** (FEB-ril). Usually, the presence of fever is due to an infection, but there can be many other causes, such as malignancies, brain injuries, toxic reactions, reactions to vaccines, and diseases involving the central nervous system (CNS). Sometimes, emotional upsets can bring on a fever. Whatever the cause, the effect is to reset the body's thermostat in the hypothalamus.

Curiously enough, fever usually is preceded by a chill—that is, a violent attack of shivering and a sensation of cold that blankets and heating pads seem unable to relieve. As a result of these reactions, heat is generated and stored and, when the chill subsides, the body temperature is elevated.

The old adage that a fever should be starved is completely wrong. During a fever, there is an increase in metabolism that is usually proportional to the fever's intensity. The body uses available sugars and fats, and there is an increase in the use of protein. During the first week or so of a fever, there is definite evidence of protein destruction, so a high-calorie diet with plenty of protein is recommended.

When a fever ends, sometimes the drop in temperature to normal occurs very rapidly. This sudden fall in temperature is called the **crisis**, and it is usually accompanied by symptoms indicating rapid heat loss: profuse perspiration, muscular relaxation, and dilation of blood vessels in the skin. A gradual drop in temperature, in contrast, is known as **lysis**. A drug that reduces fever is described as **antipyretic** (an-ti-pi-RET-ik).

The mechanism of fever production is not completely understood, but we might think of the hypothalamus as a thermostat that during fever is set higher than normal. This change in the heat-regulating mechanism often follows the introduction of a foreign protein or the entrance into the bloodstream of bacteria or their toxins. Substances that produce fever are called **pyrogens** (PI-ro-jens).

Up to a point, fever may be beneficial because it steps up phagocytosis (the process by which white blood cells destroy bacteria and other foreign material), inhibits the growth of certain organisms, and increases cellular metabolism, which may help recovery from disease.

Responses to Excessive Heat

The body's heat-regulating devices are efficient, but there is a limit to what they can accomplish. High outside temperature may overcome the body's heat loss mechanisms, in which case body temperature rises and cellular metabolism with accompanying heat production increases. When body temperature rises, the affected person is apt to suffer from a series of disorders: heat cramps are followed by heat exhaustion, which, if untreated, is followed by heat stroke.

In **heat cramps**, there is localized muscle cramping of the extremities and occasionally of the abdomen. The condition abates with rest in a cool environment and adequate fluids.

With further heat retention and more fluid loss, **heat exhaustion** occurs. Symptoms of this disorder include headache, tiredness, vomiting, and a rapid pulse. The victim feels hot, but the skin is cool due to evaporation of sweat. There may be a decrease in circulating blood volume and lowered blood pressure. Heat exhaustion is also treated by rest and fluid replacement.

Heat stroke (also called sunstroke) is a medical emergency. Heat stroke can be recognized by a body temperature of up to 41°C (105°F); hot, dry skin; and CNS symptoms, including confusion, dizziness, and loss of consciousness. The body has responded to the loss of circulating fluid by reducing blood flow to the skin and sweat glands.

It is important to lower the heatstroke victim's body temperature immediately by removing the individual's clothing, placing him or her in a cool environment, and cooling the body with cold water or ice. The patient should be treated with appropriate fluids containing necessary electrolytes, including sodium, potassium, calcium, and chloride. Supportive medical care is also needed to avoid fatal complications.

CHECKPOINT **20-11** ➤ What are some conditions brought on by excessive heat?

Responses to Excessive Cold

The body is no more capable of coping with prolonged exposure to cold than with prolonged exposure to heat. If, for example, the body is immersed in cold water for a time, the water (a better heat conductor than air) removes more heat from the body than can be replaced, and temperature falls. Cold air can produce the same result, particularly when clothing is inadequate. The main effects of an excessively low body temperature, termed **hypothermia** (hi-po-THER-me-ah), are uncontrolled shivering, lack of coordination, and decreased heart and respiratory rates. Speech becomes slurred, and there is overpowering sleepiness, which may lead to coma and death. Outdoor activities in cool, not necessarily cold, weather cause many unrecognized cases of hypothermia. Wind, fatigue, and depletion of water and energy stores all play a part.

When the body is cooled below a certain point, cellular metabolism slows, and heat production is inadequate to maintain a normal temperature. The person must then be warmed gradually by heat from an outside source. The best first aid measure is to remove the person's clothing and put him or her in a warmed sleeping bag with an unclothed companion until shivering stops. Administration of warm, sweetened fluids also helps.

Exposure to cold, particularly to moist cold, may result in **frostbite**, which can cause permanent local tissue damage. The areas most likely to be affected by frostbite are the face, ears, and extremities. Formation of ice crystals and reduction of blood supply to an area leads to necrosis (death) of tissue and possible gangrene. The very young, the very old, and those who suffer from circulatory disorders are particularly susceptible to cold injuries.

A frostbitten area should never be rubbed; rather, it should be thawed by application of warm towels or immersion in circulating lukewarm (not hot) water for 20 to 30 minutes. The affected area should be treated gently; a person with frostbitten feet should not be permitted to walk. People with cold-damaged extremities frequently have some lowering of body temperature. The whole body should be warmed at the same time that the affected part is warmed.

Hypothermia is employed in certain types of surgery. In these circumstances, drugs are used to depress the hypothalamus and reduce the body temperature to as low as 25°C (77°F) before the surgeon begins the operation. In heart surgery, the blood is cooled further to 20°C (68°F) as it goes through the heart-lung machine. This method has been successful even in infants.

CHECKPOINT **20-12** ➤ What is the term for excessively low body temperature?

20

Disease in Context revisited

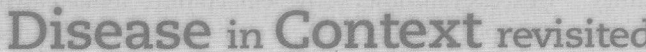

➤ Becky Learns to Manage Her Diabetes

"Hi Mom!" Becky shouted into the camp phone. "No, everything's fine… Actually, I'm calling because I knew you were probably worried! I'm having an awesome time. I've gone canoeing, hiking, and swimming every day. At night, we've been sitting around the campfire telling ghost stories… Yeah, I've made some new friends too—everyone's really great. Wanda, my cabin leader, is so cool. She has diabetes too and she knows a lot about it. We did this neat experiment the other day where we tested our blood glucose levels before and after going on a hike. Did you know that glucose levels drop after exercise because the body uses glucose to make ATP? … And at lunch today we learned that foods are made up of car-bohydrates, fats, and proteins. Did you know that glucose is a carbohydrate? And that some foods can raise your blood sugar really fast. Wanda called it the 'glycemic effect' or something like that. Anyways, that's why it's better to eat brown bread and fruit instead of white bread and candy. We also learned about saturated and unsaturated fats. Tell Dad that when I get home he and I need to talk. If he keeps eating all those fatty foods he likes, he's going to get heart disease!"

In this case, we saw that diabetes mellitus is an endocrine disorder that prevents cells from metabolizing glucose. To review the topic of diabetes mellitus, refer back to Chapter 12.

Word Anatomy

Medical terms are built from standardized word parts (prefixes, roots, and suffixes). Learning the meanings of these parts can help you remember words and interpret unfamiliar terms.

WORD PART	MEANING	EXAMPLE
Metabolism		
glyc/o	sugar, sweet	*Glycogen* yields glucose molecules when it breaks down.
-lysis	separating, dissolving	*Glycolysis* is the breakdown of glucose for energy.
Body Temperature		
pyr/o	fire, fever	An *antipyretic* drug reduces fever.
therm/o	heat	*Hypothermia* is an excessively low body temperature.

Summary

I. **METABOLISM**
    A. Phases
        1. Catabolism—breakdown of complex compounds into simpler compounds
        2. Anabolism—building of simple compounds into substances needed for cellular activities, growth, and repair

    B. Cellular respiration—a series of reactions in which food is oxidized for energy
        1. Anaerobic phase—does not require oxygen
            a. Location—cytoplasm
            b. Yield—2 ATP per glucose
            c. End product—organic (i.e., pyruvic acid)

2. Aerobic phase—requires oxygen
   a. Location—mitochondria
   b. Yield—30 ATP per glucose on average
   c. End products—carbon dioxide and water
3. Metabolic rate—rate at which energy is released from food in the cells
   a. Basal metabolism—amount of energy needed to maintain life functions while at rest
C. Use of nutrients for energy
   1. Glucose—main energy source
   2. Fats—highest energy yield
   3. Proteins—can be used for energy after removal of nitrogen (deamination)
D. Anabolism
   1. Essential amino acids and fatty acids must be taken in as part of diet
E. Minerals and vitamins
   1. Minerals—elements needed for body structure and cell activities
      a. Trace elements—elements needed in extremely small amounts
   2. Vitamins—organic substances needed in small amounts
      a. Antioxidants (e.g., vitamins C and E) protect against free radicals

II. **NUTRITIONAL GUIDELINES**
A. Carbohydrates
   1. 55% to 60% of calories
   2. Should be complex (unrefined) not simple (sugars)
      a. Glycemic effect—how quickly a food raises blood glucose and insulin
      b. Plant fiber important
B. Fats
   1. 30% or less of calories
   2. Unsaturated healthier than saturated
      a. Hydrogenated fats artificially saturated
C. Proteins
   1. 15% to 20% of calories
   2. Complete—all essential amino acids
      a. Need to combine plant foods
D. Vitamin and mineral supplements
E. U.S. dietary guidelines—USDA MyPyramid
F. Alcohol—metabolized in liver

III. **NUTRITIONAL DISORDERS**
A. Food allergies
B. Malnutrition

C. Overweight and obesity
   1. Body mass index (BMI)—weight (kg) ÷ (height [m])^2
D. Underweight

IV. **NUTRITION AND AGING**
V. **BODY TEMPERATURE**
A. Heat production
   1. Most heat produced in muscles and glands
   2. Distributed by the circulation
   3. Affected by exercise, hormones, food, age
B. Heat loss
   1. Avenues—skin, urine, feces, respiratory system
   2. Mechanisms—conduction, radiation, convection, evaporation
   3. Prevention of heat loss—clothing, subcutaneous fat
C. Temperature regulation
   1. Hypothalamus—main temperature-regulating center
      a. Responds to temperature of blood in brain and temperature receptors in skin
   2. Conservation of heat
      a. Constriction of blood vessels in skin
      b. Shivering
      c. Increased release of epinephrine
   3. Release of heat
      a. Dilation of skin vessels
      b. Sweating
      c. Relaxation of muscles
   4. Age factors
   5. Normal body temperature—ranges from 36.2°C to 37.6°C; varies with time of day and location measured
D. Fever—higher than normal body temperature resulting from infection, injury, toxin, damage to CNS, etc.
   1. Pyrogen—substance that produces fever
   2. Antipyretic—drug that reduces fever
E. Response to excessive heat—heat cramps, heat exhaustion, heat stroke
F. Response to excessive cold
   1. Hypothermia—low body temperature
      a. Results—coma and death
      b. Uses—surgery
   2. Frostbite—reduction of blood supply to areas such as face, ears, toes, fingers
      a. Results—necrosis and gangrene

20

Questions for Study and Review

BUILDING UNDERSTANDING

Fill in the blanks

1. Building glycogen from glucose is an example of _____.
2. The amount of energy needed to maintain life functions while at rest is _____.
3. Reserves of glucose are stored in liver and muscle as _____.
4. The most important area of the brain for temperature regulation is the _____.
5. A drug that reduces fever is described as _____.

Matching > Match each numbered item with the most closely related lettered item.

___ **6.** Main energy source for the body

___ **7.** Chemical element required for normal body function

___ **8.** Complex organic substance required for normal body function

___ **9.** Energy storage molecule with only single bonds between carbon atoms

___ **10.** Energy storage molecule with one or more double bonds between carbon atoms

a. saturated fat

b. vitamin

c. mineral

d. unsaturated fat

e. glucose

Multiple choice

___ **11.** During amino acid catabolism, nitrogen is removed by
   a. oxidation
   b. the glycemic effect
   c. lysis
   d. deamination

___ **12.** Which of the following would have the lowest glycemic effect?
   a. glucose
   b. sucrose
   c. lactose
   d. starch

___ **13.** Alcohol is catabolized by the
   a. small intestine
   b. liver
   c. pancreas
   d. spleen

___ **14.** Amino acids that cannot be made by metabolism are said to be
   a. essential
   b. nonessential
   c. antioxidants
   d. free radicals

UNDERSTANDING CONCEPTS

15. In what part of the cell does anaerobic respiration occur and what are its end products? In what part of the cell does aerobic respiration occur? What are its end products?

16. About how many kilocalories are released from a tablespoon of butter (14 grams)? a tablespoon of sugar (12 grams)? a tablespoon of egg white (15 grams)?

17. If you eat 2,000 kcal a day, how many kilocalories should come from carbohydrates? from fats? from protein?

18. How is heat produced in the body? What structures produce the most heat during increased activity?

19. Emily's body temperature increased from 36.2°C to 36.5°C and then decreased to 36.2°C. Describe the feedback mechanism regulating Emily's body temperature.

20. Define *fever*. Name some aspects of the course of fever, and list some of its beneficial and harmful effects.

21. What is hypothermia? Under what circumstances does it usually occur? List some of its effects.

22. Differentiate between the terms in the following pairs:
  a. conduction and convection
  b. radiation and evaporation
  c. marasmus and kwashiorkor
  d. lysis and crisis
  e. heat exhaustion and heat stroke

CONCEPTUAL THINKING

23. The oxidation of glucose to form ATP is often compared to the burning of fuel. Why is this analogy inaccurate?

24. In the case story, Becky learned about the glycemic effect. In order to prevent hyperglycemia, which foods should Becky avoid or eat in moderation?

25. Richard M, a self-described couch potato, is 6 feet tall and weighs 240 pounds. Calculate Richard's body mass index. Is Richard overweight or obese? List some diseases associated with obesity.

20

Body Fluids

Selected Key Terms

The following terms and other boldface terms in the chapter are defined in the Glossary

acidosis
alkalosis
ascites
buffer
dehydration
edema
effusion
electrolyte
extracellular
interstitial
intracellular
pH

Learning Outcomes

After careful study of this chapter, you should be able to:

1. Compare intracellular and extracellular fluids
2. List four types of extracellular fluids
3. Name the systems that are involved in water balance
4. Explain how thirst is regulated
5. Define *electrolytes* and describe some of their functions
6. Describe the role of hormones in electrolyte balance
7. Describe three methods for regulating the pH of body fluids
8. Compare acidosis and alkalosis, including possible causes
9. Describe three disorders involving body fluids
10. Specify some fluids used in therapy
11. Show how word parts are used to build words related to bodily fluids (see Word Anatomy at the end of the chapter)

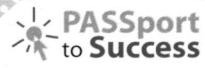

PASSport
to Success

Visit *thePoint* or see the Student Resource CD in the back of this book for definitions and pronunciations of key terms as well as a pretest for this chapter.

Disease
in Context

> ### Margaret's Second Case: A Fluid Balancing Act

Angela, a nurse in the intensive care unit (ICU), sat down at her station to review her patient's chart. During last week's heat wave, Margaret Ringland, 78-years-old, was admitted to the hospital with dehydration (severe water loss). This was evident by her low urine output and high urine concentration. While in emergency, she received intravenous fluids to replace the water she had lost. In the ICU, Margaret was encouraged to drink plenty of fluids so that she would remain hydrated. Over the past several days, the ICU team had kept a 24-hour intake–output record of all the liquid Margaret had ingested and excreted. Today, she was going home. But before Margaret could be discharged, Angela needed to provide her with some information to help prevent this condition from happening again.

Given the current heat wave, Angela wasn't surprised with Margaret's diagnosis. Elderly patients like Margaret are particularly susceptible to dehydration because they often have less water stored in their body fluid compartments than younger adults. In addition, their kidneys tend to be less efficient at reabsorbing water. Margaret also presented with hypernatremia (excess sodium ions in the body fluids). Angela knew this was directly related to Margaret's water loss—as her total body fluid volume dropped, the concentration of sodium in that fluid increased. Sodium is essential for body functions such as nerve impulse transmission. However, too much sodium can cause problems, including hypertension, edema, convulsions, and even coma. Now that Margaret was rehydrated, her sodium ion concentration had dropped to normal levels as well.

While reviewing Margaret's chart, Angela noted that Margaret was also deficient in two other essential electrolytes—potassium and calcium. Like sodium, potassium is required for proper nerve impulse conduction. Calcium is required for bone formation and blood clotting. Margaret's hypokalemia was probably due to the diuretic medication her doctor had prescribed to lower her blood pressure, which caused her to lose potassium as a side effect. Her hypocalcemia was probably associated with her age-related osteoporosis. Angela reminded herself that she would have to give Margaret a list of foods rich in potassium and calcium.

For Margaret, abnormal body water volume and ion concentrations had serious health consequences. In this chapter we'll learn more about body fluid and electrolyte balance. Later, we'll check in on Margaret as Angela prepares her for discharge.

The Importance of Water

Water is important to living cells as a solvent, a transport medium, and a participant in metabolic reactions. The normal proportion of body water varies from 50% to 70% of a person's weight. It is highest in the young and in thin, muscular individuals. As the amount of fat increases, the percentage of water in the body decreases, because adipose tissue holds very little water compared with muscle tissue. In infants, water makes up 75% of the total body mass. That's why infants are in greater danger from dehydration than adults.

Various electrolytes (salts), nutrients, gases, waste, and special substances, such as enzymes and hormones, are dissolved or suspended in body water. The composition of body fluids is an important factor in homeostasis. Whenever the volume or chemical makeup of these fluids deviates even slightly from normal, disease results. (See Appendix 4, Table 3, for normal values.) The constancy of body fluids is maintained in the following ways:

- The thirst mechanism maintains the volume of water at a constant level

- Kidney activity regulates the volume and composition of body fluids (see Chapter 22)

- Hormones serve to regulate fluid volume and electrolytes (see section on electrolytes later in the chapter)

- Regulators of pH (acidity and alkalinity), including buffers, respiration, and kidney function

The maintenance of proper fluid balance involves many of the principles discussed in earlier chapters, such as pH and buffers, the effects of respiration on pH, tonicity of solutions, and forces influencing capillary exchange. Some of these chapters will be referenced in the following sections. Additional information follows in Chapter 22 on the urinary system.

Fluid Compartments

Although body fluids have much in common no matter where they are located, there are some important differences between fluid inside and outside cells. Accordingly, fluids are grouped into two main compartments (Fig. 21-1):

- **Intracellular fluid** (ICF) is contained within the cells. About two-thirds to three-fourths of all body fluids are in this category.

- **Extracellular fluid** (ECF) includes all body fluids outside of cells. In this group are included the following:

    > **Interstitial** (in-ter-STISH-al) **fluid,** or more simply, tissue fluid. This fluid is located in the spaces between the cells in tissues all over the body. It is estimated that tissue fluid constitutes about 15% of body weight.

    > **Blood plasma,** which constitutes about 4% of a person's body weight.

    > **Lymph,** the fluid that drains from the tissues into the lymphatic system. This is about 1% of body weight.

    > **Fluid in special compartments,** such as cerebrospinal fluid, the aqueous and vitreous humors of the eye, serous fluid, and synovial fluid. Together, these make up about 1% to 3% of total body fluids.

Fluids are not locked into one compartment. There is a constant interchange between compartments as fluids are transferred across semipermeable plasma membranes by diffusion and osmosis (see Fig. 21-1). Also, fluids are lost and replaced on a daily basis.

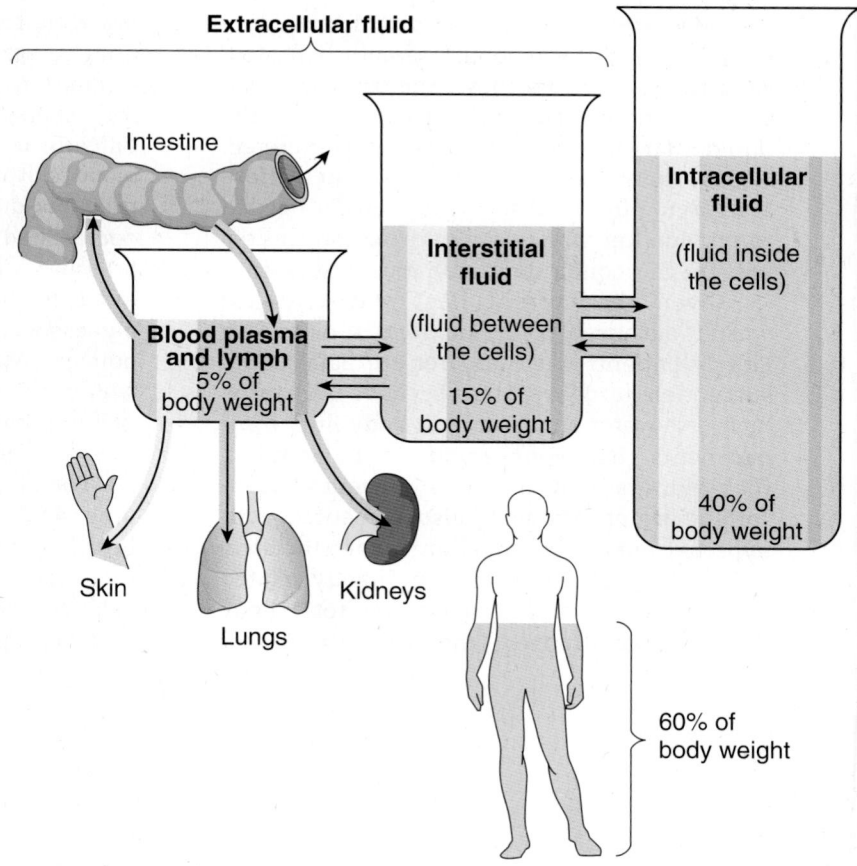

Figure 21-1 **Main fluid compartments showing relative percentage by weight of body fluid.** Fluid percentages vary but total about 60% of body weight. Fluids are constantly exchanged among compartments, and each day fluids are lost and replaced. **[ZOOMING IN ➤** What are some avenues through which water is lost? **]**

CHECKPOINT **21-1** ➤ What are the two main compartments into which body fluids are grouped?

Water Balance

In a healthy person, the quantity of water gained in a day is approximately equal to the quantity lost (output) (Fig. 21-2). The quantity of water consumed in a day (intake) varies considerably. The average adult in a comfortable environment takes in about 2,300 mL of water (about 2 1/2 quarts) daily. About two-thirds of this quantity comes from drinking water and other beverages; about one-third comes from foods—fruits, vegetables, and soups. About 200 mL of water is produced each day as a by-product of cellular respiration. This water, described as *metabolic water*, brings the total average gain to 2,500 mL each day.

The same volume of water is constantly being lost from the body by the following routes:

- The **kidneys** excrete the largest quantity of water lost each day. About 1 to 1.5 liters of water are eliminated daily in the urine. (Note that beverages containing alcohol or caffeine act as diuretics and increase water loss through the kidneys.)

- The **skin**. Although sebum and keratin help prevent dehydration, water is constantly evaporating from the skin's surface. Larger amounts of water are lost from the skin as sweat when it is necessary to cool the body.

- The **lungs** expel water along with carbon dioxide.

- The **intestinal tract** eliminates water along with the feces.

In many disorders, it is important for the healthcare team to know whether a patient's intake and output are equal; in such a case, a 24-hour intake–output record is kept. The intake record includes *all* the liquid the patient has taken in. This means fluids administered intravenously as well as those consumed by mouth. The healthcare worker must account for water, other beverages, and liquid foods, such as soup and ice cream. The output record includes the quantity of urine excreted in the same 24-hour period as well as an estimation of fluid losses due to fever, vomiting, diarrhea, bleeding, wound discharge, or other causes.

CHECKPOINT **21-2** ➤ What are four routes for water loss from the body?

Sense of Thirst

The control center for the sense of thirst is located in the brain's hypothalamus. This center plays a major role in the regulation of total fluid volume. A decrease in fluid volume or an increase in the concentration of body fluids stimulates the thirst center, causing a person to drink water or other fluids containing large amounts of water. Dryness of the mouth also causes a sensation of thirst. Excessive thirst, such as that caused by excessive urine loss in cases of diabetes, is called **polydipsia** (pol-e-DIP-se-ah).

The thirst center should stimulate enough drinking to balance fluids, but this is not always the case. During vigorous exercise, especially in hot weather, the body can dehydrate rapidly. People may not drink enough to replace needed fluids. In addition, if plain water is consumed, the dilution of body fluids may depress the thirst center. Athletes who are exercising very strenuously may need to drink beverages with some carbohydrates for energy and also some electrolytes to keep fluids in balance. (See Box 21-1, Osmoreceptors: Thinking About Thirst, for more about thirst regulation.)

CHECKPOINT **21-3** ➤ Where is the control center for the sense of thirst located?

Electrolytes and Their Functions

Electrolytes are important constituents of body fluids. These compounds separate into positively and negatively charged ions in solution. Positively charged ions are called *cations*; negatively charged ions are called *anions*. Electrolytes are so-named because they conduct an electrical current in solution. A few of the most important ions are reviewed next:

- Positive ions (cations):

  > **Sodium** is chiefly responsible for maintaining osmotic balance and body fluid volume. It is the main positive ion in extracellular fluids. Sodium is

Water gain / Water loss

Water gain 2500 mL/day	Water loss 2500 mL/day
Metabolism 200 mL	Feces 200 mL
Food 700 mL	Lungs 300 mL
	Skin 500 mL
Drink 1600 mL	Urine 1500 mL

Figure 21-2 **Daily gain and loss of water.**

21

Box 21-1   A Closer Look

Osmoreceptors: Thinking About Thirst

Osmoreceptors are specialized neurons that help to maintain water balances by detecting changes in the concentration of extracellular fluid (ECF). They are located in the hypothalamus of the brain in an area adjacent to the third ventricle, where they monitor the osmotic pressure (concentration) of the circulating blood plasma.

Osmoreceptors respond primarily to small increases in sodium, the most common cation in ECF. As the blood becomes more concentrated, sodium draws water out of the cells, initiating nerve impulses. Traveling to different regions of the hypothalamus, these impulses may have two different but related effects:

■ They stimulate the hypothalamus to produce antidiuretic hormone (ADH), which is then released from the posterior pituitary. ADH travels to the kidneys and causes these organs to conserve water.

■ They stimulate the thirst center of the hypothalamus, causing increased consumption of water. Almost as soon as water consumption begins, however, the sensation of thirst disappears. Receptors in the throat and stomach send inhibitory signals to the thirst center, preventing overconsumption of water and allowing time for ADH to affect the kidneys.

Both of these mechanisms serve to dilute the blood and other body fluids. Either mechanism alone can maintain water balance. If both fail, a person soon becomes dehydrated.

---

required for nerve impulse conduction and is important in maintaining acid–base balance.

> **Potassium** is also important in the transmission of nerve impulses and is the major positive ion in intracellular fluids. Potassium is involved in enzymatic activities, and it helps regulate the chemical reactions by which carbohydrate is converted to energy and amino acids are converted to protein.

> **Calcium** is required for bone formation, muscle contraction, nerve impulse transmission, and blood clotting.

■ Negative ions (anions):

> **Phosphate** is essential in carbohydrate metabolism, bone formation, and acid–base balance. Phosphates are found in plasma membranes, nucleic acids (DNA and RNA), and ATP.

> **Chloride** is essential for the formation of hydrochloric acid in the stomach. It also helps to regulate fluid balance and pH. It is the most abundant anion in extracellular fluids.

CHECKPOINT 21-4 ➤ What is the main cation in extracellular fluid? In intracellular fluid?

CHECKPOINT 21-5 ➤ What is the main anion in extracellular fluid?

Electrolyte Balance

The body must keep electrolytes in the proper concentration in both intracellular and extracellular fluids (see Box 21-2, Sodium and Potassium). The maintenance of water

and electrolyte balance is one of the most difficult problems for health workers in caring for patients. Although some electrolytes are lost in the feces and through the skin as sweat, the job of balancing electrolytes is left mainly to the kidneys, as described in Chapter 22 on the urinary system.

THE ROLE OF HORMONES Several hormones are involved in balancing electrolytes (see Chapter 12). Aldosterone, produced by the adrenal cortex, promotes the reabsorption of sodium (and water) and the elimination of potassium. In Addison disease, in which the adrenal cortex does not produce enough aldosterone, there is a loss of sodium and water and an excess of potassium.

When the blood concentration of sodium rises above the normal range, the pituitary secretes more antidiuretic hormone (ADH). This hormone increases water reabsorption in the kidney to dilute the excess sodium.

The most recently discovered hormone active in electrolyte regulation comes from the heart. Atrial natriuretic peptide (ANP) is secreted by specialized atrial myocardial cells when blood pressure rises too high. As its name implies, ANP causes the kidneys to excrete sodium and water, thus decreasing blood volume and lowering blood pressure.

Hormones from the parathyroid and thyroid glands regulate calcium and phosphate levels. Parathyroid hormone increases blood calcium levels by causing the bones to release calcium and the kidneys to reabsorb calcium. The thyroid hormone calcitonin lowers blood calcium by causing calcium to be deposited in the bones.

CHECKPOINT 21-6 ➤ What are some mechanisms for regulating electrolytes in body fluids?

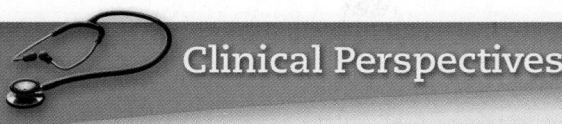

Box 21-2 · Clinical Perspectives

Sodium and Potassium: Causes and Consequences of Imbalance

The concentrations of sodium and potassium in body fluids are important measures of water and electrolyte balance. An excess of sodium in body fluids is termed **hypernatremia**, taken from the Latin name for sodium, *natrium*. This condition accompanies dehydration and severe vomiting and may cause hypertension, edema, convulsions, and coma. **Hyponatremia**, a deficiency of sodium in body fluids, can come from water intoxication, heart failure, kidney failure, cirrhosis of the liver, pH imbalance, or endocrine disorders. It can cause muscle weakness, hypotension, confusion, shock, convulsions, and coma.

The term **hyperkalemia** is taken from the Latin name for potassium, *kalium*. It refers to excess potassium in body fluids, which may result from kidney failure, dehydration, and other causes. Its signs and symptoms include nausea, vomiting, muscular weakness, and severe cardiac arrhythmias. **Hypokalemia**, or low potassium in body fluids, may result from taking diuretics, which cause potassium to be lost along with water. It may also result from pH imbalance or secretion of too much aldosterone from the adrenal cortex, and it causes muscle fatigue, paralysis, confusion, hypoventilation, and cardiac arrhythmias.

PASSport to Success

Visit *thePoint* or see the Student Resource CD in the back of this book for a summary chart of hormones and electrolyte balance.

Acid–Base Balance

The pH scale is a measure of how acidic or basic (alkaline) a solution is. As described in Chapter 2, the pH scale measures the hydrogen ion (H^+) concentration in a solution. Body fluids are slightly alkaline, with a pH range of 7.35 to 7.45. These fluids must be kept within a narrow pH range, or damage, even death, will result. A shift in either direction by three tenths of a point on the pH scale, to 7.0 or 7.7, is fatal.

Regulation of pH

The body constantly produces acids in the course of metabolism. Catabolism of fats yields fatty acids and other acidic byproducts; cellular respiration yields pyruvic acid and, under anaerobic conditions, lactic acid; carbon dioxide dissolves in the blood and yields carbonic acid (see Chapter 18). Conversely, a few abnormal conditions may cause alkaline shifts in pH. Several systems act together to counteract these changes and maintain acid–base balance:

- **Buffer systems.** Buffers are substances that prevent sharp changes in hydrogen ion (H^+) concentration and thus maintain a relatively constant pH. Buffers work by accepting or releasing these ions as needed to keep the pH steady. The main buffer systems in the body are bicarbonate buffers, phosphate buffers, and proteins, such as hemoglobin in red blood cells and plasma proteins.

- **Respiration.** The role of respiration in controlling pH was described in Chapter 18. Recall that carbon dioxide release from the lungs makes the blood more alkaline by reducing the amount of carbonic acid formed. In contrast, carbon dioxide retention makes the blood more acidic. Respiratory rate can adjust pH for short-term regulation.

- **Kidney function.** The kidneys regulate pH by reabsorbing or eliminating hydrogen ions as needed. The kidneys are responsible for long-term pH regulation. The activity of the kidneys is described in Chapter 22.

CHECKPOINT 21-7 ➤ What are three mechanisms for maintaining the acid–base balance of body fluids?

Abnormal pH

If shifts in pH cannot be controlled, either acidosis or alkalosis results (Table 21-1). **Acidosis** (as-ih-DO-sis) is a condition produced by a drop in the pH of body fluids to less than pH 7.35. This condition depresses the nervous system, leading to mental confusion and ultimately coma. Acidosis may result from a respiratory obstruction or any lung disease which prevents the release of CO_2. It may also arise from kidney failure or prolonged diarrhea, which drains the alkaline contents of the intestine. Long-term excessive exercise under anaerobic conditions can produce lactic acidosis.

Acidosis may also result from inadequate carbohydrate metabolism, as occurs in diabetes mellitus, ingestion of a low-carbohydrate diet, or starvation. In these cases, the body metabolizes too much fat and protein from food or body materials, leading to the production of excess acid. When acidosis results from the accumulation of

21

Table 21-1	Causes of Acidosis and Alkalosis	
	Acidosis	**Alkalosis**
Metabolic	Kidney failure; anaerobic metabolism; lack of carbohydrate metabolism, as in diabetes, starvation; prolonged diarrhea	Overuse of antacids; prolonged vomiting
Respiratory	Respiratory obstruction, lung disease such as asthma or emphysema, apnea or decreased ventilation	Hyperventilation (overbreathing due to anxiety or oxygen deficiency)

ketone bodies, as in the case of diabetes, the condition is more accurately described as ketoacidosis.

Alkalosis (al-kah-LO-sis) results from an increase in pH to greater than 7.45. This abnormality excites the nervous system to produce tingling sensations, muscle twitches, and eventually paralysis. The possible causes of alkalosis include hyperventilation (the release of too much carbon dioxide), ingestion of too much antacid, and prolonged vomiting with loss of stomach acids.

It is convenient to categorize acidosis and alkalosis as having either respiratory or metabolic origins. Respiratory acidosis or alkalosis results from either an increase or a decrease in blood CO_2. Metabolic acidosis or alkalosis results from unregulated increases or decreases in any other acids (see Table 21-1).

CHECKPOINT **21-8** ➤ What are the conditions that arise from abnormally low or high pH of body fluids?

Disorders of Body Fluids

Edema is the accumulation of excessive fluid in the intercellular spaces (Fig. 21-3).

Some causes of edema are as follows:

- Interference with normal fluid return to the heart, as caused by congestive heart failure or blockage in the venous or lymphatic systems (see Chapters 14 and 15). A backup of fluid in the lungs, **pulmonary edema**, is a serious potential consequence of congestive heart failure.

- Lack of protein in the blood. This deficiency may result from protein loss or ingestion of too little dietary protein for an extended period. It may also result from failure of the liver to manufacture adequate amounts of the protein albumin, as frequently occurs in liver disease. The decrease in protein lowers the blood's osmotic pressure and reduces fluid return to the circulation. Diminished fluid return results in accumulation of fluid in the tissues.

- Kidney failure, a common clinical cause of edema, resulting from the inability of the kidneys to eliminate adequate amounts of urine.

- Increased loss of fluid through the capillaries, as caused by injury, allergic reaction, or certain infections.

Water intoxication involves dilution of body fluids in both the intracellular and extracellular compartments. Transport of water into the cells results in swelling. In the brain, cellular swelling may lead to convulsions, coma, and finally death. Causes of water intoxication include an excess of ADH and intake of excess fluids by mouth or by intravenous injection.

Effusion (e-FU-zhun) is the escape of fluid into a cavity or a space. An example is pleural effusion, fluid within the pleural space; in this condition fluid compresses the lung, so that normal breathing is not possible. Tuberculosis, cancer, and some infections may give rise to effusion. Effusion into the pericardial sac, which encloses the heart, may occur in autoimmune disorders, such as lupus erythematosus and rheumatoid arthritis. Infection is

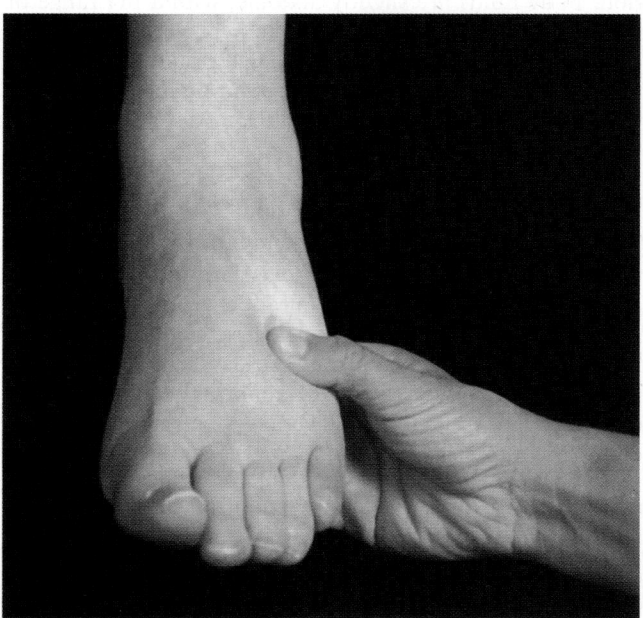

Figure 21-3 **Edema of the foot.** (Reprinted with permission from Bickley LS. *Bates' Guide to Physical Examination and History Taking*, 8th ed. Philadelphia: Lippincott Williams & Wilkins, 2003.)

Disease in Context revisited

➤ Margaret Learns to Avoid Dehydration

"Hello, Margaret. Are you ready to go home today?" Angela asked her patient.

"Oh yes," answered Margaret. "You've made me feel so comfortable, but I'm looking forward to sleeping in my own bed tonight!"

"Well," continued Angela, "before you leave, can we talk a bit about taking care of yourself at home?" With Margaret's permission, Angela explained that Margaret needed to match her fluid intake with her fluid loss to ensure water balance and prevent dehydration. "I know that 2½ quarts of water per day seems like a lot, but don't forget that drinks aren't your only source. You can also get water from foods like fruits, vegetables, and soups," she recommended.

Angela advised Margaret to think about her electrolytes as well. She encouraged Margaret to eat foods low in sodium—not only would it help

her stay hydrated, but it would also help her avoid high blood pressure. Since Margaret's potassium levels were a little low (due to a blood pressure medication she was taking), Angela suggested that she eat potassium-rich foods like cantaloupe, apricots, raisins, and tomatoes. Margaret's calcium levels were also a little low, so Angela suggested that Margaret eat calcium-rich foods like dairy products, fish, and leafy green vegetables such as spinach and broccoli.

During this case, we saw the importance of fluid and electrolyte balance to maintain health. Many of the mechanisms that the body uses to regulate fluid volume and ion concentration occur in the kidneys. In Chapter 22, The Urinary System, we'll examine some of these homeostatic mechanisms.

---

another cause of pericardial effusion. The fluid may interfere with normal heart contractions and can cause death.

Ascites (ah-SI-teze) is effusion with accumulation of fluid within the abdominal cavity. It may occur in disorders of the liver, kidneys, and heart, as well as in cancers, infection, or malnutrition.

Dehydration (de-hi-DRA-shun), a severe deficit of body fluids, will result in death if it is prolonged. The causes include vomiting, diarrhea, drainage from burns or wounds, excessive perspiration, and inadequate fluid intake, as in cases of damage to the thirst mechanism. In such cases, it may be necessary to administer intravenous fluids to correct fluid and electrolyte imbalances.

CHECKPOINT 21-9 ➤ What is edema?

Fluid Therapy

Chapter 3 discussed the rules concerning movement of water into and out of cells when they are placed in different solutions. Recall that an isotonic solution has the same concentration as the cellular fluids and will not cause a net loss or gain of water. A hypertonic solution is more concentrated than cellular fluid and will draw water out of the cells. A hypotonic solution is less concentrated than the cellular fluids and a cell will take in water when placed in this type of solution. These rules must be considered when fluid is administered.

Fluids are administered into a vein under a wide variety of conditions to help maintain normal body functions when natural intake is not possible. Fluids are also administered to correct specific fluid and electrolyte imbalances in cases of losses due to disease or injury.

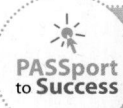 **PASSport to Success** Visit *thePoint* or see the Student Resource CD in the back of this book for information on emergency medical technicians who often must administer fluids in providing health care.

The first fluid administered intravenously in emergencies is normal saline, which contains 0.9% sodium chloride, a concentration equal to that of plasma. Because it is isotonic, this type of solution does not change the ion distribution in the body fluid compartments.

Frequently, a patient receives 5% dextrose (glucose) in 0.45% (1/2 normal) saline. This solution is hypertonic when infused, but becomes hypotonic after the sugar is metabolized. Another common fluid is 5% dextrose in water. This solution is slightly hypotonic when infused. The amount of sugar contained in a liter of this fluid is equal to 170 calories. The sugar is soon used up, resulting in a fluid that is effectively pure water. Use of these hypotonic fluids is not advisable for long-term therapy because of the common occurrence of water intoxication. Both these dextrose solutions increase the

21

plasma fluid volume. Small amounts of potassium chloride are often added to replace electrolytes lost by vomiting or diarrhea.

Ringer lactate solution contains sodium, potassium, calcium, chloride, and lactate. In this formulation, the electrolyte concentrations are equal to normal plasma values. The lactate is metabolized to bicarbonate, which acts as a buffer. This fluid is given when the need is for additional plasma volume with the electrolyte concentration equal to that of the blood.

In 25% serum albumin, the concentration of the plasma protein albumin is five times normal. This hypertonic solution draws fluid from the interstitial spaces into the circulation.

Fluids containing varied concentrations of dextrose, sodium chloride, potassium, and other electrolytes and substances are manufactured. These fluids are used to correct specific imbalances. Nutritional solutions containing concentrated sugar, protein, and fat are available for administration when oral intake is not possible for an extended period.

Word Anatomy

Medical terms are built from standardized word parts (prefixes, roots, and suffixes). Learning the meanings of these parts can help you remember words and interpret unfamiliar terms.

WORD PART	MEANING	EXAMPLE
Fluid Compartments		
intra-	within	*Intracellular* fluid is within a cell.
extra-	outside of, beyond	*Extracellular* fluid is outside the cells.
semi-	partial, half	A *semipermeable* membrane is partially permeable.
Water Balance		
poly-	many	*Polydipsia* is excessive thirst.
osmo-	osmosis	*Osmoreceptors* detect changes in osmotic concentration of fluids.
Acid–Base Balance		
-o/sis	condition, process	*Acidosis* is a condition produced by a drop in the pH of body fluids.
Disorders of Body Fluids		
tox/o	poison	Water *intoxication* is dilution of body fluids by excess water.
hydr/o	water	*Dehydration* is a severe deficit of body fluids.

Summary

I. **THE IMPORTANCE OF WATER**
   A. Functions
      1. Solvent
      2. Transport medium
      3. Participant in metabolic reactions
   B. 50% to 70% of body weight
   C. Contains electrolytes, nutrients, gases, wastes, hormones, and other substances
   D. Important in homeostasis

II. **FLUID COMPARTMENTS**
   A. Intracellular fluid—contained within the cells
   B. Extracellular fluid—outside the cells
      1. Blood plasma
      2. Interstitial (tissue) fluid
      3. Lymph
      4. Fluid in special compartments

III. **WATER BALANCE**
   A. Loss—through kidneys, skin, lungs, intestinal tract

B. Gain—through beverages, food, metabolic water
C. Sense of thirst
   1. Control center in hypothalamus
   2. Responds to fluid volume and concentration of body fluids

IV. **ELECTROLYTES AND THEIR FUNCTIONS**
A. Electrolytes release ions in solution
   1. Positive ions (cations)—e.g., sodium, potassium, calcium
   2. Negative ions (anions)—e.g., phosphate, chloride
B. Electrolyte balance
   1. Kidneys—main regulators
   2. Role of hormones
      a. Aldosterone (from adrenal cortex)
         (1) Promotes reabsorption of sodium
         (2) Promotes excretion of potassium
      b. ADH (from pituitary)
         (1) Causes kidney to retain water
      c. ANP (from heart)
         (1) Causes kidney to excrete sodium and water
      d. Parathyroid hormone (from parathyroid glands)
         (1) Increases blood calcium level
      e. Calcitonin (from thyroid)
         (1) Decreases blood calcium level

V. **ACID–BASE BALANCE**
A. Normal pH range is 7.35 to 7.45
B. Regulation of pH
   1. Buffers—maintain constant pH
   2. Respiration—release of carbon dioxide increases alkalinity; retention of carbon dioxide increases acidity

   3. Kidney—regulates amount of hydrogen ion excreted
C. Abnormal pH
   1. Acidosis—decrease in pH; causes: respiratory obstruction, lung disease, kidney failure, diarrhea, diabetes mellitus, starvation
   2. Alkalosis—increase in pH; causes: hyperventilation, ingestion of antacids, prolonged vomiting

VI. **DISORDERS OF BODY FLUIDS**
A. Edema—accumulation of fluid in tissues
   1. Causes
      a. Interference with fluid return to heart
      b. Lack of proteins in blood
      c. Kidney failure
      d. Fluid loss from capillaries
B. Water intoxication—dilution of body fluids
C. Effusion—escape of fluid into a cavity or space
D. Ascites—accumulation of fluid in abdominal cavity
E. Dehydration—deficiency of fluid

VII. **FLUID THERAPY**
A. Purpose
   1. Correct fluid balance
   2. Correct electrolyte balance
   3. Provide nourishment
B. Commonly used solutions
   1. Normal saline
   2. 5% dextrose (glucose) in 0.45% (1/2 normal) saline
   3. 5% dextrose in water
   4. Ringer lactate
   5. 25% serum albumin

Questions for Study and Review

BUILDING UNDERSTANDING

Fill in the blanks

1. Excessive thirst is termed_____.
2. Loss of sodium and an excess of potassium are classic signs of _____ disease.
3. Substances in the blood that prevent sharp changes in hydrogen ion concentration are called_____.
4. Effusion with accumulation of fluid within the abdominal cavity is termed _____.
5. A severe deficit in body fluid is called _____.

21

Matching > Match each numbered item with the most closely related lettered item.

____ **6.** Essential for maintaining osmotic balance and body fluid volume; this cation is abundant in extracellular fluid

____ **7.** Important in the transmission of nerve impulses and enzyme activities; this cation is abundant in intracellular fluid

____ **8.** Required for bone formation, muscle contraction, and blood clotting

____ **9.** Essential in bone formation and acid–base balance; this anion is found in plasma membranes, ATP, and nucleic acids

____ **10.** Important for gastric acid formation; this anion is abundant in extracellular fluid

a. sodium

b. potassium

c. calcium

d. phosphate

e. chloride

Multiple choice

____ **11.** Body water content is greatest in

    a. infants
    b. children
    c. young adults
    d. elderly adults

____ **12.** Fluid located in the spaces between the cells is called

    a. cytoplasm
    b. plasma
    c. interstitial fluid
    d. lymph

____ **13.** The organ(s) responsible for water loss through evaporation is (are) the

    a. kidneys
    b. skin
    c. lungs
    d. intestinal tract

____ **14.** Which of the following is responsible for long-term regulation of pH?

    a. buffer system
    b. digestive system
    c. respiratory system
    d. urinary system

____ **15.** Increased blood CO_2 causes

    a. respiratory acidosis
    b. respiratory alkalosis
    c. metabolic acidosis
    d. metabolic alkalosis

UNDERSTANDING CONCEPTS

16. Compare the terms in each of the following pairs:

    a. intracellular and extracellular fluid
    b. aldosterone and antidiuretic hormone
    c. calcitonin and parathyroid hormone

17. In a healthy person, what is the ratio of fluid intake to output?

18. Explain the role of the hypothalamus in water balance.

19. How do the respiratory and urinary systems regulate pH?

20. Compare and contrast the following disorders:

    a. acidosis and alkalosis
    b. edema and effusion
    c. water intoxication and dehydration

21. List some causes of edema.

22. List three purposes for administering intravenous fluids.

23. Compare and contrast the following types of intravenous fluids:

    a. normal saline and 5% dextrose saline
    b. Ringer solution and serum albumin

CONCEPTUAL THINKING

24. Patty Grant, 55-years-old, reports severe headaches and excessive thirst and urination. What is the probable cause of Patty's symptoms?

25. Why is emphysema associated with decreased urine pH?

26. In Margaret's case, her dehydration was treated with an isotonic IV solution. What would happen to her intracellular fluid volume if she received a hypertonic IV solution?

21

CHAPTER 22

The Urinary System

Learning Outcomes

After careful study of this chapter, you should be able to:

1. List the systems that eliminate waste and name the substances eliminated by each
2. Describe the parts of the urinary system and give the functions of each
3. List the activities of the kidneys in maintaining homeostasis
4. Trace the path of a drop of blood as it flows through the kidney
5. Describe a nephron
6. Name the four processes involved in urine formation and describe the action of each
7. Identify the role of antidiuretic hormone (ADH) in urine formation
8. Describe the components and functions of the juxtaglomerular (JG) apparatus
9. Describe the process of micturition
10. Name three normal and six abnormal constituents of urine
11. List the common disorders of the urinary system
12. List six signs of chronic renal failure
13. Explain the principle and the purpose of kidney dialysis
14. Show how word parts are used to build words related to the urinary system (see Word Anatomy at the end of the chapter)

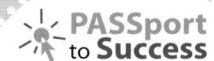

Disease in Context

➤ Adam's Second Case: Urinary Blockade

Adam rolled out of bed and glanced at the clock as he rushed to the bathroom. *Jeez, it's only been a couple of hours since the last time I had to pee*, he thought. *Hopefully this time it won't take as long.* Sure enough, Adam had difficulty voiding. Even once he was able to get started, he only managed to produce a small volume of urine. Lately, this was happening more and more frequently. At first, he chalked it up to getting older, but now he wondered if he had some sort of bladder or kidney infection. As he climbed back into bed, Adam decided that he would make an appointment with his family doctor.

"So let me get this straight," said Dr. Singh. "Over the last several weeks, you've experienced increased frequency and urgency of urination, even at night (nocturia). While urinating, you've had hesitation in starting, decreased volume, and diminished force of the stream. And even after urination, you still feel that your urinary bladder is not completely empty." Based on Adam's symptoms, Dr. Singh suspected that Adam's prostate gland (a male reproductive organ) was causing problems for his urinary system. The prostate gland lies immediately inferior to the urinary bladder, where it surrounds the first part of the urethra. If the gland becomes enlarged, it can obstruct the urethra and prevent the urinary bladder from emptying completely. At 55 years old, Adam was in the right age range for this condition.

Dr. Singh's suspicions were confirmed by the digital rectal exam. Adam's prostate was large and rubbery. The doctor carefully palpated the prostate's surface with his finger—he could not detect any nodules on its smooth surface. "Adam, my initial diagnosis is that you have benign prostatic hypertrophy—your prostate has grown larger and is preventing urine from passing out of your urinary bladder. Your prostate's surface is smooth though, which suggests that the growth is not cancerous, but we'll have to get that ruled out. I'm going to order some blood tests and urinalyses, as well as refer you to a urologist."

Adam's prostate is causing problems for his urinary system. In this chapter, we'll examine the anatomy and physiology of the urinary system. Later, we'll learn how Adam's disorder is resolved.

Excretion

The urinary system is also called the *excretory system* because one of its main functions is **excretion**, removal and elimination of metabolic waste products from the blood. It has many other functions as well, including regulation of the volume, acid–base balance (pH), and electrolyte composition of body fluids.

Although the focus of this chapter is the urinary system, certain aspects of other systems are also discussed, because body systems work interdependently to maintain homeostasis (internal balance). The systems active in excretion and some of the substances they eliminate are the following:

- The **urinary system** excretes water, nitrogen-containing waste products, and salts. These are all constituents of the urine.

- The **digestive system** eliminates water, some salts, and bile, in addition to digestive residue, all of which are contained in the feces. The liver is important in eliminating the products of red blood cell destruction and in breaking down certain drugs and toxins.

- The **respiratory system** eliminates carbon dioxide and water. The latter appears as vapor, as can be demonstrated by breathing on a windowpane or a mirror, where the water condenses.

- The skin, or **integumentary system**, excretes water, salts, and very small quantities of nitrogenous wastes. These all appear in perspiration, although water also evaporates continuously from the skin without our being conscious of it.

CHECKPOINT 22-1 ➤ The main function of the urinary system is to eliminate waste. What are some other systems that eliminate waste?

Organs of the Urinary System

The main parts of the urinary system, shown in Figure 22-1, are as follows:

- Two **kidneys**. These organs extract wastes from the blood, balance body fluids, and form urine.

- Two **ureters** (U-re-ters). These tubes conduct urine from the kidneys to the urinary bladder.

- A single **urinary bladder**. This reservoir receives and stores the urine brought to it by the two ureters.

- A single **urethra** (u-RE-thrah). This tube conducts urine from the bladder to the outside of the body for elimination.

CHECKPOINT 22-2 ➤ What are the organs of the urinary system?

The Kidneys

The kidneys interact with other systems as prime regulators of homeostasis. After a brief overview of the kidney's many activities, we'll describe its structure and specific roles in urine formation and regulation of blood pressure.

Kidney Activities

The kidneys are involved in the following processes:

- Excretion of unwanted substances, such as cellular metabolic waste, excess salts, and toxins. One product of amino acid metabolism is nitrogen-containing waste material, chiefly **urea** (u-RE-ah). After synthesis in the liver, urea is transported in the blood to the kidneys for elimination. The kidneys have a specialized mechanism for the elimination of urea and other nitrogenous (ni-TROJ-en-us) wastes.

- Water balance. Although the amount of water gained and lost in a day can vary tremendously, the kidneys can adapt to these variations, so that the volume of body water remains remarkably stable from day to day.

- Acid–base balance of body fluids. Acids are constantly being produced by cellular metabolism. Certain foods can yield acids or bases, and people may also ingest antacids, such as bicarbonate. However, if the body is to function normally, the pH of body fluids must remain in the range of 7.35 to 7.45 (see Chapter 21).

- Blood pressure regulation. The kidneys depend on blood pressure to filter the blood. If blood pressure falls too low for effective filtration, specialized kidney cells release renin. This enzyme activates a blood protein, angiotensin, that causes blood vessels to constrict, thus raising blood pressure. Angiotensin has additional effects as described later in the chapter.

- Regulation of red blood cell production. When the kidneys do not get enough oxygen, they produce the hormone **erythropoietin** (eh-rith-ro-POY-eh-tin) **(EPO)**, which stimulates red cell production in the bone marrow. EPO made by genetic engineering is now available to treat severe anemia, such as occurs in the end stage of kidney failure.

Kidney Structure

The kidneys lie against the back muscles in the upper abdomen at about the level of the last thoracic and first three lumbar vertebrae. The right kidney is slightly lower than the left to accommodate the liver. Each kidney is firmly enclosed in a membranous **renal capsule** made of fibrous connective tissue. In addition, there is a protective layer of fat called the **adipose capsule** around the organ. An outermost layer of fascia (connective tissue) anchors the kidney to the peritoneum and abdominal wall. The kidneys, as well as the ureters, lie posterior to

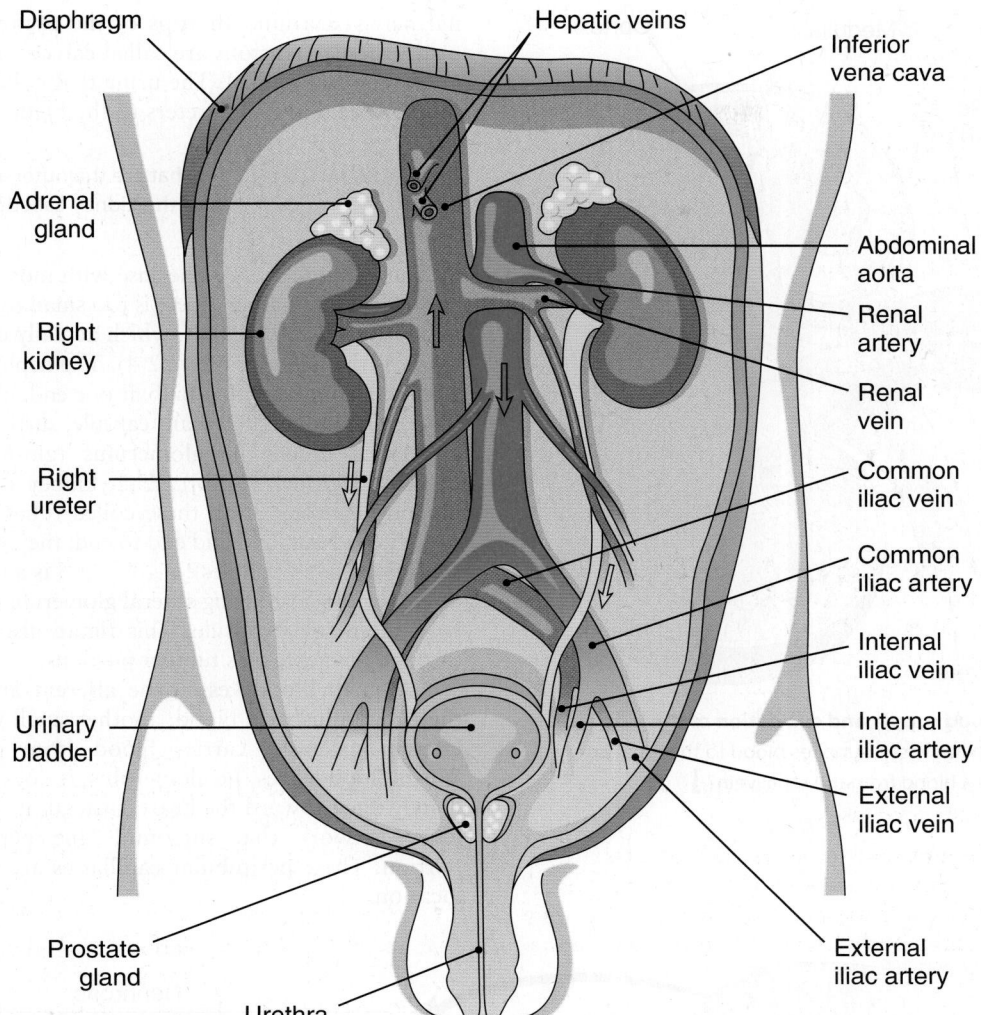

Diaphragm

Hepatic veins

Inferior
vena cava

Adrenal
gland

Abdominal
aorta

Renal
artery

Right
kidney

Renal
vein

Right
ureter

Common
iliac vein

Common
iliac artery

Internal
iliac vein

Urinary
bladder

Internal
iliac artery

External
iliac vein

Prostate
gland

External
iliac artery

Urethra

Figure 22-1 **Male urinary system, showing blood vessels.** [ZOOMING IN ➤ What vessel supplies blood to the kidney? What vessel drains the kidney?]

the peritoneum. Thus, they are not in the peritoneal cavity but rather in an area known as the **retroperitoneal** (ret-ro-per-ih-to-NE-al) **space.** See Appendix 7 for a dissection photograph showing the kidneys and renal vessels in place.

CHECKPOINT 22-3 ➤ The kidneys are located in the retroperitoneal space. Where is this space?

BLOOD SUPPLY The kidney's blood supply is illustrated in Figure 22-2. Blood is brought to the kidney by a short branch of the abdominal aorta called the **renal artery.**

After entering the kidney, the renal artery subdivides into smaller and smaller branches, which eventually make contact with the kidney's functional units, the **nephrons** (NEF-ronz). Blood leaves the kidney by vessels that finally merge to form the **renal vein,** which carries blood into the inferior vena cava for return to the heart.

CHECKPOINT 22-4 ➤ What vessel supplies blood to the kidney and what vessel drains blood from the kidney?

ORGANIZATION The kidney is a somewhat flattened organ approximately 10 cm (4 inches) long, 5 cm (2 inches) wide, and 2.5 cm (1 inch) thick (Fig. 22-3). On the medial border there is a notch called the **hilum,** where the renal artery, the renal vein, and the ureter connect with the kidney. The lateral border is convex (curved outward), giving the entire organ a bean-shaped appearance.

The kidney is divided into two regions: the renal cortex and the renal medulla (Fig. 22-3). The **renal cortex** is the kidney's outer portion. The internal **renal medulla** contains tubes in which urine is formed and collected. These tubes form a number of cone-shaped structures called **renal pyramids.** The tips of the pyramids point toward the **renal pelvis,** a funnel-shaped basin that forms the upper end of the ureter. Cuplike extensions of the re-

22

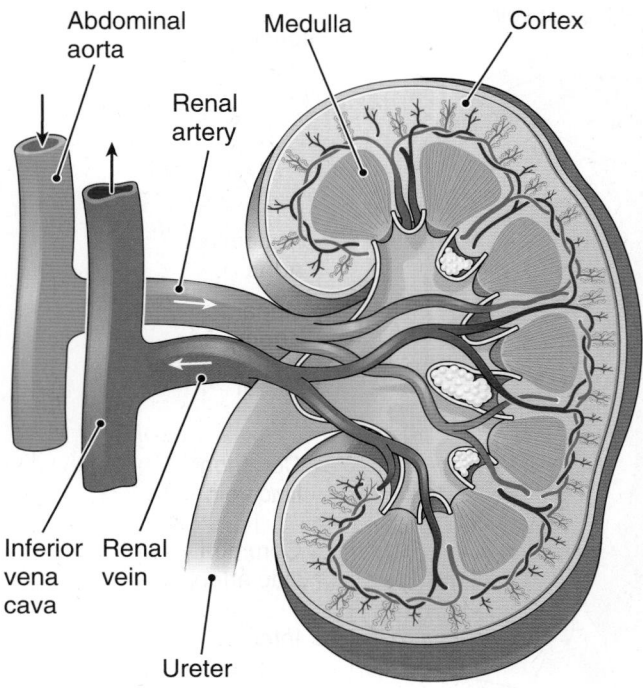

Figure 22-2 **Blood supply and circulation of the kidney.**
[ZOOMING IN ➤ What vessel supplies blood to the renal artery?
What vessel receives blood from the renal vein? **]**

nal pelvis surround the tips of the pyramids and collect urine; these extensions are called **calyces** (KA-lih-seze; singular, **calyx**, KA-liks). The urine that collects in the pelvis then passes down the ureters to the bladder.

CHECKPOINT **22-5** ➤ What are the outer and inner regions of the kidney called?

THE NEPHRON As is the case with most organs, the kidney's most fascinating aspect is too small to be seen with the naked eye. This basic unit, which actually does the kidney's work, is the **nephron** (Fig. 22-4). The nephron is essentially a tiny coiled tube with a bulb at one end. This bulb, known as the **glomerular** (Bowman) **capsule**, surrounds a cluster of capillaries called the **glomerulus** (glo-MER-u-lus) (pl., glomeruli [glo-MER-u-li]). Each kidney contains about 1 million nephrons; if all these coiled tubes were separated, straightened out, and laid end to end, they would span some 120 kilometers (75 miles)! Figure 22-5 is a microscopic view of kidney tissue showing several glomeruli, each surrounded by a glomerular capsule. This figure also shows sections through the nephron's tubular portions.

A small blood vessel, the **afferent arteriole**, supplies the glomerulus with blood; another small vessel, called the **efferent arteriole**, carries blood from the glomerulus. When blood leaves the glomerulus, it does not head immediately back toward the heart. Instead, it flows into a capillary network that surrounds the nephron's tubular portion. These **peritubular capillaries** are named for their location.

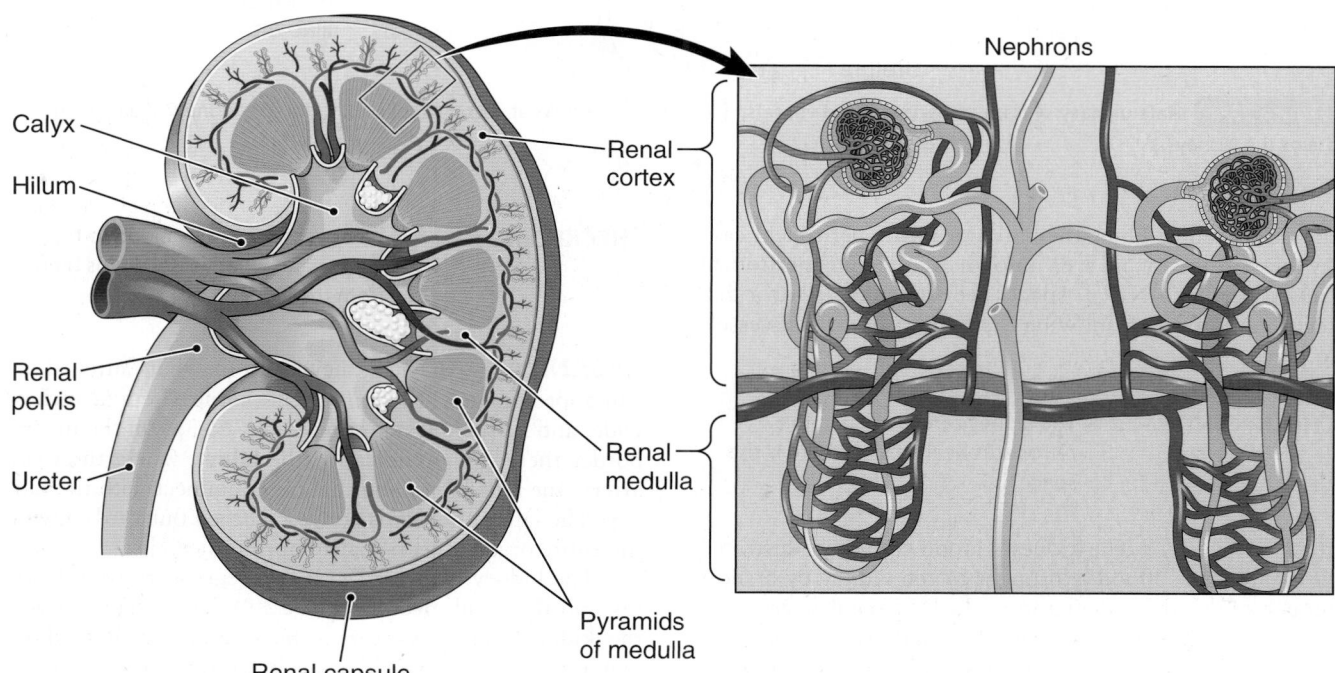

Figure 22-3 **Longitudinal section through the kidney.** Its internal structure is shown *(left)*, along with an enlarged diagram of nephrons *(right)*. Each kidney contains more than 1 million nephrons. **[ZOOMING IN ➤** What is the outer region of the kidney called? What is the inner region of the kidney called? **]**

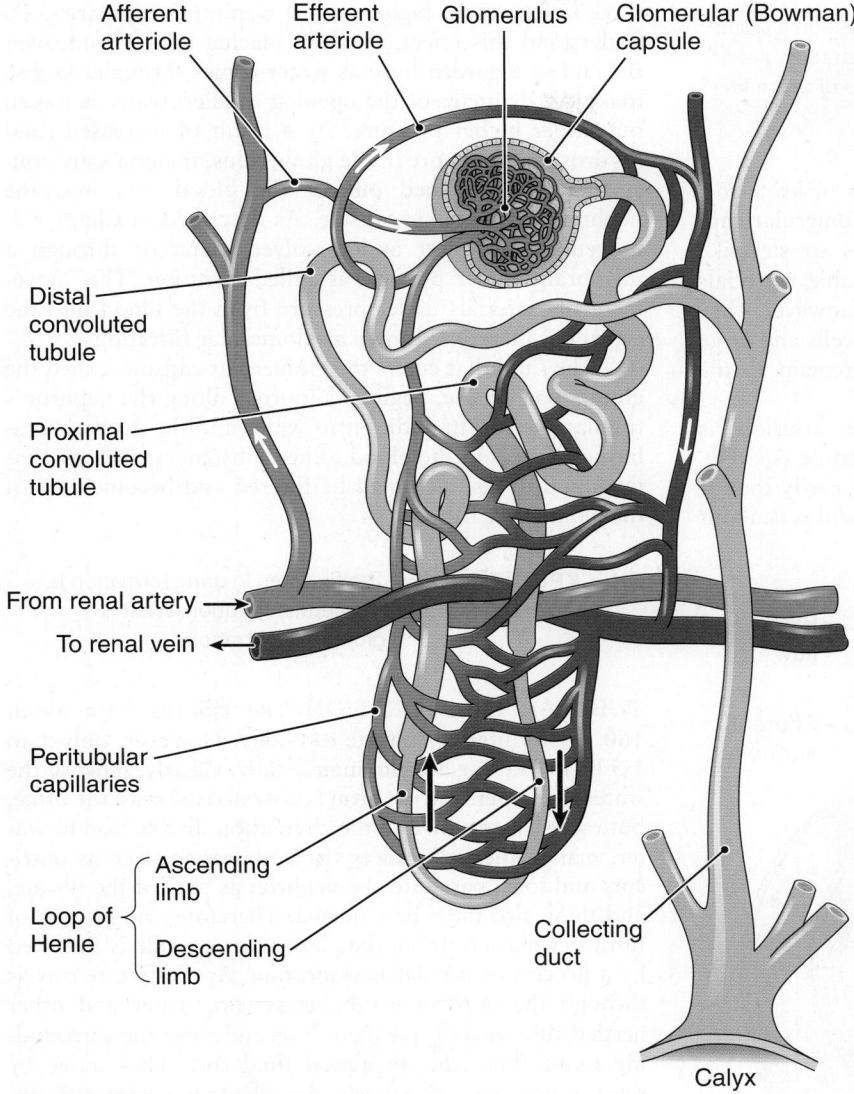

Afferent arteriole

Efferent arteriole

Glomerulus

Glomerular (Bowman) capsule

Distal convoluted tubule

Proximal convoluted tubule

From renal artery

To renal vein

Peritubular capillaries

Ascending limb

Loop of Henle

Descending limb

Collecting duct

Calyx

Figure 22-4 **A nephron and its blood supply.** The nephron regulates the proportions of water, waste, and other materials according to the body's constantly changing needs. Materials that enter the nephron can be returned to the blood through the surrounding capillaries. [**ZOOMING IN** ➤ Which of the two convoluted tubules is closer to the glomerular capsule? Which convoluted tubule is farther away?]

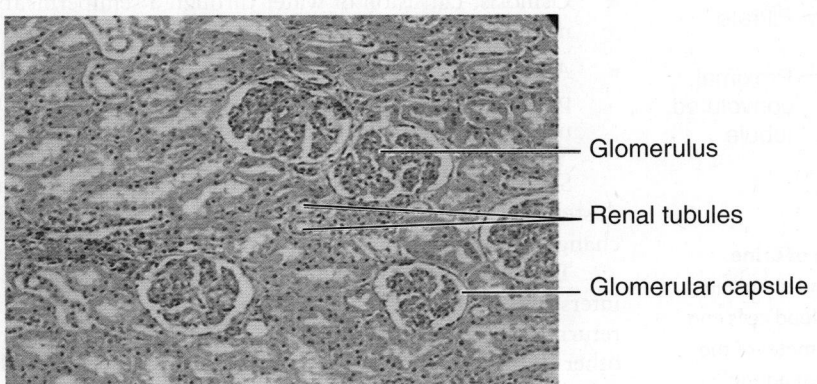

Glomerulus

Renal tubules

Glomerular capsule

Figure 22-5 **Microscopic view of the kidney.** (Courtesy of Dana Morse Bittus and BJ Cohen.)

The nephron's tubular portion consists of several parts. The coiled part leading from the glomerular capsule is called the **proximal convoluted** (KON-vo-lu-ted) **tubule** (PCT, or just proximal tubule). The tubule then uncoils to form a hairpin-shaped segment called the **nephron loop**, or loop of Henle. The first part of the loop, which carries fluid toward the medulla, is the **descending limb** (see Fig. 22-4). The part that continues from the loop's turn and carries fluid away from the medulla, is the **ascending limb**. Continuing from the ascending limb, the tubule coils once again into the **distal convoluted tubule** (DCT, or just distal tubule), so called because it is farther along the tubule from the glomerular capsule than is the PCT. Each tubule empties into a collecting duct, which then continues through the medulla toward the renal pelvis.

The glomerulus, glomerular capsule, and the proximal and distal convoluted tubules of the nephron are within the renal cortex. The nephron loop and collecting duct extend into the medulla (see Fig. 22-3).

CHECKPOINT 22-6 ➤ What is the functional unit of the kidney called?

CHECKPOINT 22-7 ➤ What name is given to the coil of capillaries in the glomerular (Bowman) capsule?

Formation of Urine

The following explanation of urine formation describes a complex process, involving many back-and-forth exchanges between the bloodstream and the kidney tubules. As fluid filtered from the blood travels slowly through the nephron's twists and turns, there is ample time for exchanges to take place. These processes together allow the kidney to "fine tune" body fluids as they adjust the composition of the urine.

22

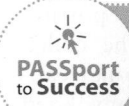

Visit *thePoint* or see the Student Resource CD in the back of this book for the animation Renal Function, which shows the process of urine formation in action.

GLOMERULAR FILTRATION The process of urine formation begins with the glomerulus in the glomerular capsule. The walls of the glomerular capillaries are sievelike and permit the free flow of water and soluble materials through them. Like other capillary walls, however, they are impermeable (im-PER-me-abl) to blood cells and large protein molecules, and these components remain in the blood (Fig. 22-6).

Because the diameter of the afferent arteriole is slightly larger than that of the efferent arteriole (see Fig. 22-6), blood can enter the glomerulus more easily than it can leave. Thus, blood pressure in the glomerulus is about three to four times higher than it is in other capillaries. To understand this effect, think of placing your thumb over the end of a garden hose as water comes through. As you make the diameter of the opening smaller, water is forced out under higher pressure. As a result of increased fluid (hydrostatic) pressure in the glomerulus, materials are constantly being pushed out of the blood and into the nephron's glomerular capsule. As described in Chapter 3, movement of water and dissolved materials through a membrane under pressure is called *filtration*. This movement of materials under pressure from the blood into the capsule is therefore known as **glomerular filtration**.

The fluid that enters the glomerular capsule, called the **glomerular filtrate**, begins its journey along the nephron's tubular system. In addition to water and the normal soluble substances in the blood, other substances, such as vitamins and drugs, also may be filtered and become part of the glomerular filtrate.

CHECKPOINT 22-8 ➤ The first step in urine formation is glomerular filtration. What is glomerular filtration?

TUBULAR REABSORPTION The kidneys form about 160 to 180 liters of filtrate each day. However, only 1 to 1.5 liters of urine are eliminated daily. Clearly, most of the water that enters the nephron is not excreted with the urine, but rather, is returned to the circulation. In addition to water, many other substances the body needs, such as nutrients and ions, pass into the nephron as part of the filtrate, and these also must be returned. Therefore, the process of filtration that occurs in the glomerular capsule is followed by a process of **tubular reabsorption**. As the filtrate travels through the nephron's tubular system, water and other needed substances leave the tubule and enter the surrounding tissue fluid, the interstitial fluid (IF). They move by several processes previously described in Chapter 3, including:

- Diffusion. The movement of substances from an area of higher concentration to an area of lower concentration (following the concentration gradient).

- Osmosis. Diffusion of water through a semipermeable membrane.

- Active transport. Movement of materials through the plasma membrane against the concentration gradient using energy and transporters.

Several hormones noted in Chapter 21, including aldosterone and ANP (atrial natriuretic peptide) affect these changes (Table 22-1).

The substances that leave the nephron and enter the interstitial fluid then enter the peritubular capillaries and return to the circulation. In contrast, most of the urea and other nitrogenous waste materials are kept within the tubule to be eliminated with the urine. Box 22-1, Transport Maximum, presents additional information on tubular reabsorption in the nephron.

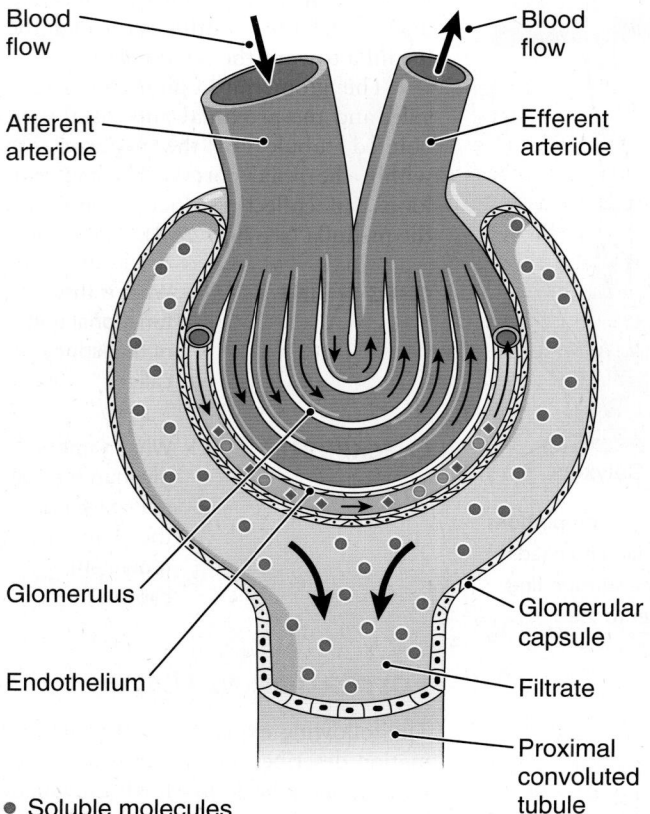

Blood flow

Blood flow

Afferent arteriole

Efferent arteriole

Glomerulus

Glomerular capsule

Endothelium

Filtrate

Proximal convoluted tubule

- Soluble molecules
- Proteins
- Blood cells

Figure 22-6 Filtration process in the formation of urine. Blood pressure inside the glomerulus forces water and dissolved substances into the glomerular (Bowman) capsule. Blood cells and proteins remain behind in the blood. The smaller diameter of the efferent arteriole as compared with that of the afferent arteriole maintains the hydrostatic (fluid) pressure. **[ZOOMING IN ➤** Which arteriole associated with the glomerulus has the wider diameter? **]**

Table 22-1	Substances that Affect Renal Function	
Substance	**Source**	**Action**
Aldosterone (al-DOS-ter-one)	Hormone released from the adrenal cortex under effects of angiotensin	Promotes reabsorption of sodium and water in the kidney to conserve water and increase blood pressure
Atrial natriuretic peptide (na-tre-u-RET-ik) (ANP)	Atrial myocardial cells; released when blood pressure is too high	Causes kidney to excrete sodium and water to decrease blood volume and blood pressure
Antidiuretic hormone (an-te-di-u-RET-ik) (ADH)	Made in the hypothalamus and released from the posterior pituitary; released when blood becomes too concentrated	Promotes reabsorption of water from the distal convoluted tubule and collecting duct to concentrate the urine and conserve water
Renin (RE-nin)	Enzyme produced by renal cells when blood pressure falls too low for effective filtration	Activates angiotensin in the blood
Angiotensin (an-je-o-TEN-sin)	Protein in the blood that is activated by renin	Causes constriction of blood vessels to raise blood pressure; also stimulates release of aldosterone from the adrenal cortex and ADH from the posterior pituitary

TUBULAR SECRETION Before the filtrate leaves the body as urine, the kidney makes final adjustments in composition by means of **tubular secretion**. In this process, some substances are actively moved from the blood into the nephron. Potassium ions are moved into the urine in this manner. Importantly, the kidneys regulate the acid–base (pH) balance of body fluids by the active secretion of hydrogen ions. Some drugs, such as penicillin, also are actively secreted into the nephron for elimination.

CONCENTRATION OF THE URINE The amount of water that is eliminated with the urine is regulated by a complex mechanism within the nephron that is influenced by **antidiuretic hormone (ADH)**, a hormone released from the posterior pituitary gland (see Table 22-1). The process is called the **countercurrent mechanism** because it involves fluid traveling in opposite directions within the ascending and descending limbs of the nephron loop. The countercurrent mechanism is illustrated in Figure 22-7. Its essentials are as follows.

As the filtrate passes through the nephron loop, electrolytes, especially sodium, are actively pumped out by the nephron's cells, resulting in an increased concentration of the interstitial fluid. Because the ascending limb of the loop is not very permeable to water, the filtrate at this point becomes increasingly dilute (see Fig. 22-7). As the filtrate then passes through the more permeable DCT and collecting duct, the concentrated fluids around the nephron draw water out to be returned to the blood. (Remember, according to the laws of osmosis, water fol-

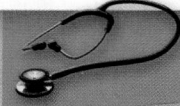

Box 22-1 Clinical Perspectives

Transport Maximum

The kidneys work efficiently to return valuable substances to the blood after glomerular filtration. However, the carriers that are needed for active transport of these substances can become overloaded. Thus, there is a limit to the amount of each substance that can be reabsorbed in a given time period. The limit of this reabsorption rate is called the **transport maximum (Tm)**, or tubular maximum, and it is measured in milligrams (mg) per minute. For example, the Tm for glucose is approximately 375 mg/minute.

If a substance is present in excess in the blood, it may exceed its transport maximum and then, because it cannot be totally reabsorbed, some will be excreted in the urine. Thus, the transport maximum determines the **renal threshold**—the plasma concentration at which a substance will begin to be excreted in the urine, which is measured in mg per deciliter (dL). For example, if the concentration of glucose in the blood exceeds its renal threshold (180 mg/dL), glucose will begin to appear in the urine, a condition called **glycosuria**. The most common cause of glycosuria is uncontrolled diabetes mellitus.

22

KIDNEY CORTEX

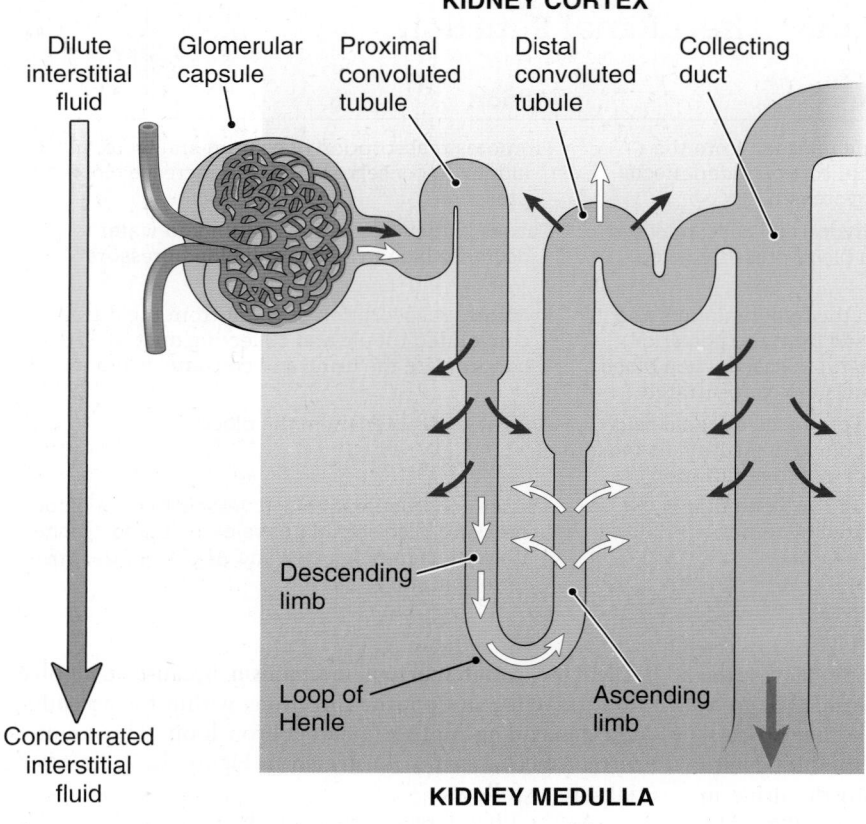

Sodium (Na⁺) Water (H_2O)

Figure 22-7 **Countercurrent mechanism for concentration of urine.** Concentration is regulated by means of intricate exchanges of water and electrolytes, mainly sodium, in the nephron loop, distal convoluted tubule, and collecting duct. The intensity of color shows changing concentrations of the interstitial fluid and filtrate.

lows salt.) In this manner, the urine becomes more concentrated as it leaves the nephron and its volume is reduced.

The hormone ADH makes the walls of the DCT and collecting duct more permeable to water, so that more water will be reabsorbed and less will be excreted with the urine. The release of ADH from the posterior pituitary is regulated by a feedback system. As the blood becomes more concentrated, the hypothalamus triggers more ADH release from the posterior pituitary; as the blood becomes more dilute, less ADH is released. In the disease diabetes insipidus, there is inadequate secretion of ADH from the hypothalamus, which results in the elimination of large amounts of dilute urine accompanied by excessive thirst.

SUMMARY OF URINE FORMATION The processes involved in urine formation are summarized below and illustrated in Figure 22-8.

1. Glomerular filtration allows diffusible materials to pass from the blood into the nephron.

2. Tubular reabsorption moves useful substances back into the blood while keeping waste products in the nephron to be eliminated in the urine.

3. Tubular secretion moves additional substances from the blood into the nephron for elimination. Movement of hydrogen ions is one means by which the pH of body fluids is balanced.

4. The countercurrent mechanism concentrates the urine and reduces the volume excreted. The pituitary hormone ADH allows more water to be reabsorbed from the nephron.

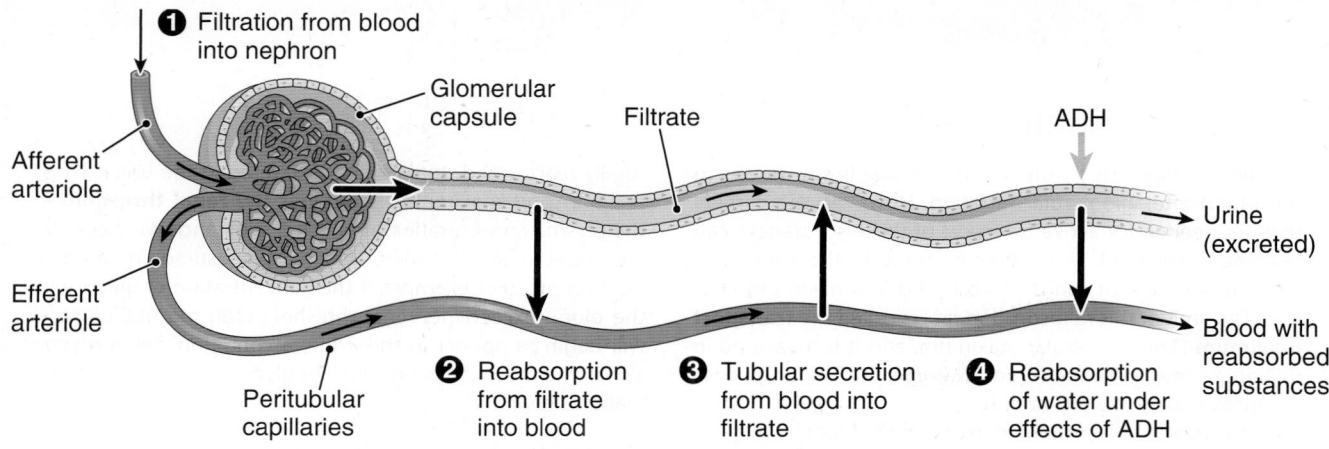

Figure 22-8 **Summary of urine formation in a nephron.**

CHECKPOINT **22-9** ➤ What are the four processes involved in the formation of urine?

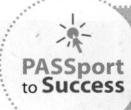

Visit *thePoint* or see the Student Resource CD in the back of this book for a flow chart summarizing kidney regulation of blood pressure.

Control of Blood Pressure

The kidneys have an internal mechanism for maintaining adequate filtration pressure. A specialized portion of the nephron, the **juxtaglomerular (JG) apparatus**, is involved in this control. The JG apparatus includes cells in the DCT, which carries urine from the nephron into the collecting duct, and cells in the afferent arteriole, which carries blood into the glomerulus. As seen in Figure 22-9, the first portion of the DCT curves backward toward the glomerulus to pass between the afferent and efferent arterioles (*juxtaglomerular* means "near the glomerulus"). At the point where the DCT makes contact with the afferent arteriole, there are specialized cells in each that together make up the JG apparatus.

When receptors in the DCT detect low volume or low sodium content in the filtrate leaving the nephron, they trigger cells in the afferent arteriole to secrete the enzyme **renin** (RE-nin) (see Table 22-1). This enzyme initiates the process that activates angiotensin, a protein that elevates blood pressure by several mechanisms. It promotes the release of aldosterone and ADH and stimulates thirst, raising blood pressure by increasing blood volume. It also causes vasoconstriction and stimulates heart activity through the sympathetic nervous system. Box 22-2, The Renin-Angiotensin Pathway, has more details on these events and their clinical applications.

CHECKPOINT **22-10** ➤ What substance is produced by the JG apparatus and under what conditions is it produced?

The Ureters

Each of the two ureters is a long, slender, muscular tube that extends from the kidney down to and through the inferior portion of the urinary bladder (see Fig. 22-1). The ureters, which are located posterior to the peritoneum and distally below the peritoneum, are entirely extraperitoneal. Their length naturally varies with the size of the individual, and they may be anywhere from 25 cm to 32 cm (10 to 13 inches) long. Nearly 2.5 cm (1 inch) of the terminal distal ureter enters the bladder by passing obliquely (at an angle) through the inferior bladder wall. Because of this oblique path through the wall, a full bladder compresses the ureter and prevents the backflow of urine.

The ureteral wall includes a lining of epithelial cells, a relatively thick layer of involuntary muscle, and finally, an outer coat of fibrous connective tissue. The epithelium is the transitional type, which flattens from a cuboidal shape as the tube stretches. This same type of epithelium lines the renal pelvis, the bladder, and the proximal portion of the urethra. The ureteral muscles are capable of the same rhythmic contraction (peristalsis) that occurs in the digestive

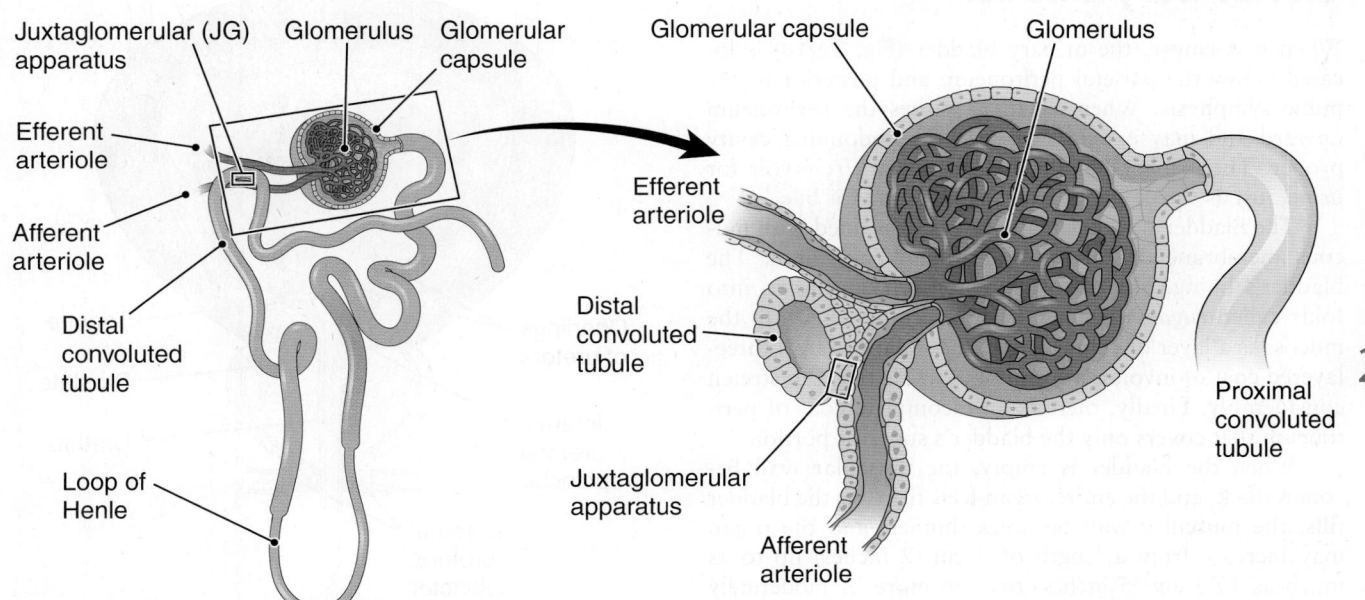

Figure 22-9 **Structure of the juxtaglomerular (JG) apparatus.** Note how the distal convoluted tubule contacts the afferent arteriole *(right)*. Cells in these two structures make up the JG apparatus. [ZOOMING IN ➤ The JG apparatus is made up of cells from which two structures?]

Box 22-2 A Closer Look

The Renin-Angiotensin Pathway: The Renal Route to Blood Pressure Control

In addition to forming urine, the kidneys play an integral role in regulating blood pressure. When blood pressure drops, cells of the juxtaglomerular (JG) apparatus secrete the enzyme renin into the blood. Renin acts on another blood protein, **angiotensinogen**, which is manufactured by the liver. Renin converts angiotensinogen into **angiotensin I** by cleaving off some amino acids from the end of the protein. Angiotensin I is then converted into **angiotensin II** by yet another enzyme called angiotensin-converting enzyme (ACE), which is manufactured by capillary endothelium, especially in the lungs. Angiotensin II increases blood pressure in four ways:

1. It increases cardiac output and stimulates vasoconstriction.

2. It stimulates the release of aldosterone, a hormone that acts on the nephron's distal convoluted tubule to increase sodium reabsorption, and secondarily, water reabsorption.

3. It stimulates the release of antidiuretic hormone (ADH), which acts directly on the distal convoluted tubules to increase water reabsorption.

4. It stimulates thirst centers in the hypothalamus, resulting in increased fluid consumption.

The combined effects of angiotensin II produce a dramatic increase in blood pressure. In fact, angiotensin II is estimated to be four to eight times more powerful than norepinephrine, another potent stimulator of hypertension, and thus is a good target for blood pressure-controlling drugs. One class of drugs used to treat hypertension is the **ACE inhibitors** (angiotensin-converting enzyme inhibitors), which control blood pressure by blocking the production of angiotensin II.

---

system. Urine is moved along the ureter from the kidneys to the bladder by gravity and by peristalsis at frequent intervals.

The Urinary Bladder

When it is empty, the urinary bladder (Fig. 22-10) is located below the parietal peritoneum and posterior to the pubic symphysis. When filled, it pushes the peritoneum upward and may extend well into the abdominal cavity proper. The urinary bladder is a temporary reservoir for urine, just as the gallbladder is a storage sac for bile.

The bladder wall has many layers. It is lined with mucous membrane containing transitional epithelium. The bladder's lining, like that of the stomach, is thrown into folds called *rugae* when the organ is empty. Beneath the mucosa is a layer of connective tissue, followed by a three-layered coat of involuntary smooth muscle that can stretch considerably. Finally, there is an incomplete coat of peritoneum that covers only the bladder's superior portion.

When the bladder is empty, the muscular wall becomes thick, and the entire organ feels firm. As the bladder fills, the muscular wall becomes thinner, and the organ may increase from a length of 5 cm (2 inches) up to as much as 12.5 cm (5 inches) or even more. A moderately full bladder holds about 470 mL (1 pint) of urine.

The **trigone** (TRI-gone) is a triangular-shaped region in the floor of the bladder. It is marked by the openings of the two ureters and the urethra (see Fig. 22-10). As the bladder fills with urine, it expands upward, leaving the

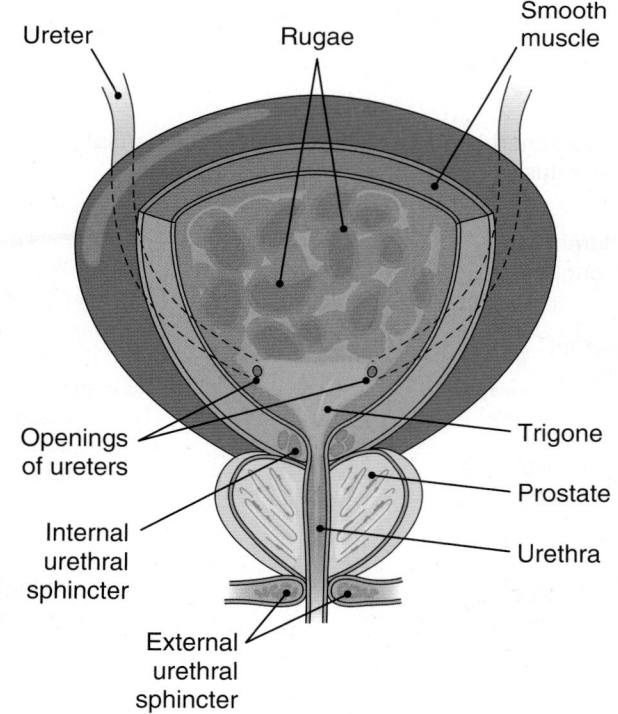

Figure 22-10 **Interior of the male urinary bladder.** The trigone is a triangular region in the floor of the bladder marked by the openings of the ureters and the urethra. [**ZOOMING IN ➤** What gland does the urethra pass through in the male?]

trigone at the base stationary. This stability prevents stretching of the ureteral openings and the possible backflow of urine into the ureters.

The Urethra

The **urethra** is the tube that extends from the bladder to the outside (see Fig. 22-1) and is the means by which the bladder is emptied. The urethra differs in males and females; in the male, it is part of both the reproductive system and the urinary system, and it is much longer than is the female urethra.

The male urethra is approximately 20 cm (8 inches) in length. Proximally, it passes through the prostate gland, where it is joined by two ducts carrying male germ cells (spermatozoa) from the testes and glandular secretions. From here, it leads to the outside through the **penis** (PE-nis), the male organ of copulation. The male urethra serves the dual purpose of conveying semen with the germ cells and draining the bladder.

The urethra in the female is a thin-walled tube about 4 cm (1.5 inches) long. It is posterior to the pubic symphysis and is embedded in the muscle of the anterior vaginal wall. The external opening, called the **urinary meatus** (me-A-tus), is located just anterior to the vaginal opening between the labia minora. The female urethra drains the bladder only and is entirely separate from the reproductive system.

Urination

The process of expelling (voiding) urine from the bladder is called **urination** or **micturition** (mik-tu-RISH-un). This process is controlled both voluntarily and involuntarily with the aid of two rings of muscle (sphincters) that surround the urethra (see Fig. 22-10). Near the bladder's outlet is an involuntary **internal urethral sphincter** formed by a continuation of the bladder's smooth muscle. Below this muscle is a voluntary **external urethral** sphincter formed by the muscles of the pelvic floor. By learning to control the voluntary sphincter, one can gain control over the bladder's emptying.

As the bladder fills with urine, stretch receptors in its wall send impulses to a center in the lower part of the spinal cord. Motor impulses from this center stimulate contraction of the bladder wall, forcing urine outward as both the internal and external sphincters are made to relax. In the infant, this emptying occurs automatically as a simple reflex. Early in life, a person learns to control urination from higher centers in the brain until an appropriate time, a process known as *toilet training*. The impulse to urinate will override conscious controls if the bladder becomes too full.

The bladder can be emptied voluntarily by relaxing the muscles of the pelvic floor and increasing the pressure in the abdomen. The resulting increased pressure in the bladder triggers the spinal reflex that leads to urination.

CHECKPOINT 22-11 ➤ What is the name of the tube that carries urine from the kidney to the bladder?

CHECKPOINT 22-12 ➤ What is the name of the tube that carries urine from the bladder to the outside?

The Urine

Urine is a yellowish liquid that is approximately 95% water and 5% dissolved solids and gases. The pH of freshly collected urine averages 6.0, with a range of 4.5 to 8.0. Diet may cause considerable variation in pH.

The amount of dissolved substances in urine is indicated by its **specific gravity**. The specific gravity of pure water, used as a standard, is 1.000. Because of the dissolved materials it contains, urine has a specific gravity that normally varies from 1.002 (very dilute urine) to 1.040 (very concentrated urine). When the kidneys are diseased, they lose the ability to concentrate urine, and the specific gravity no longer varies as it does when the kidneys function normally.

Normal Constituents

Some of the dissolved substances normally found in the urine are the following:

- **Nitrogenous waste products**, including urea, uric acid, and **creatinine** (kre-AT-ih-nin).

- **Electrolytes**, including sodium chloride (as in common table salt) and different kinds of sulfates and phosphates. Electrolytes are excreted in appropriate amounts to keep their blood concentration constant.

- **Pigment**, mainly yellow pigment derived from certain bile compounds. Pigments from foods and drugs also may appear in the urine.

Abnormal Constituents

Examination of urine, called a **urinalysis** (u-rin-AL-ih-sis) (**UA**), is one of the most important parts of a medical evaluation. A routine urinalysis includes observation of color and turbidity (cloudiness) as well as measurement of pH and specific gravity. Laboratories also test for a variety of abnormal components, including:

- **Glucose** is usually an important indicator of diabetes mellitus, in which the cells do not adequately metabolize blood sugar. The excess glucose, which cannot be reabsorbed, is excreted in the urine. The presence of glucose in the urine is known as **glycosuria** (gli-ko-SU-re-ah) or glucosuria.

- **Albumin.** The presence of this protein, which is normally retained in the blood, may indicate a kidney disorder, such as glomerulonephritis. Albumin in the urine is known as **albuminuria** (al-bu-mih-NU-re-ah).

- **Blood** in the urine is usually an important indicator of urinary system disease, including nephritis. Blood in the urine is known as **hematuria** (hem-ah-TU-re-ah).

22

- **Ketones** (KE-tones) are produced when fats are incompletely oxidized; ketones in the urine are seen in diabetes mellitus and starvation.

- **White blood cells** (pus) are evidence of infection; they can be seen by microscopic examination of a centrifuged specimen. Pus in the urine is known as **pyuria** (pi-U-re-ah).

- **Casts** are solid materials molded within the microscopic kidney tubules. They consist of cells or proteins and, when present in large number, they usually indicate disease of the nephrons.

More extensive tests on urine may include analysis for drugs, enzymes, hormones, and other metabolites, as well as cultures for microorganisms. Normal values for common urine tests are given in Appendix 4, Table 1.

Disorders of the Urinary System

The kidney is more prone to disorders than any other portion of the urinary system.

Kidney Disorders

Kidney disorders may be acute or chronic. Acute conditions usually arise suddenly, most frequently as the result of infection with inflammation of the nephrons. These diseases commonly run a course of a few weeks and are followed by complete recovery. Chronic conditions arise slowly and are often progressive, with gradual loss of kidney function.

Acute glomerulonephritis (glo-mer-u-lo-nef-RI-tis), also known as *acute poststreptococcal glomerulonephritis*, is the most common renal disease. This condition usually occurs in children about 1 to 4 weeks after a streptococcal throat infection. Antibodies formed in response to the streptococci attach to the glomerular membrane and cause injury. These damaged glomeruli allow protein, especially albumin, to filter into the glomerular capsule and ultimately to appear in the urine (albuminuria). They also allow red blood cells to filter into the urine (hematuria). Usually, the patient recovers without permanent kidney damage. In adult patients, the disease is more likely to become chronic, with a gradual decrease in the number of functioning nephrons, leading to chronic renal failure.

Pyelonephritis (pi-el-o-nef-RI-tis), an inflammation of the renal pelvis and the kidney tissue, may be either acute or chronic. In acute pyelonephritis, the inflammation results from a bacterial infection. Bacteria most commonly reach the kidney by ascending along the lining membrane from a distal urinary tract infection (see Fig. 23-14 in Chapter 23). More rarely, the blood carries bacteria to the kidney.

Acute pyelonephritis is often seen in people with partial obstruction of urine flow with stagnation (urinary stasis). It is most likely to occur in pregnant women and in men with an enlarged prostate, because the prostate sur-

rounds the first portion of the urethra in males. Other causes of stasis include neurogenic bladder, which is bladder dysfunction resulting from neurologic lesions, as seen in diabetes mellitus, and structural defects in the area where the ureters enter the bladder. Pyelonephritis usually responds to antibiotic treatment, fluid replacement, rest, and fever control.

Chronic pyelonephritis, a more serious disease, is frequently seen in patients with urinary tract stasis or backflow. It may be caused by persistent or repeated bacterial infections. Progressive kidney damage is evidenced by high blood pressure, continual loss of protein in the urine, and dilute urine.

Hydronephrosis (hi-dro-nef-RO-sis) is the distention of the renal pelvis and calyces with accumulated fluid as a result of urinary tract obstruction. The most common causes of obstruction, in addition to pregnancy or an enlarged prostate, are a kidney stone that has formed in the pelvis and dropped into the ureter, a tumor that presses on a ureter, and scars due to inflammation. Prompt removal of the obstruction may result in complete recovery. If the obstruction is not removed, the kidney will be permanently damaged.

A **polycystic** (pol-e-SIS-tik) **kidney** is one in which many fluid-containing sacs develop in the active tissue and gradually destroy it by pressure. This disorder may run in families, and treatment has not proved very satisfactory, except for the use of dialysis machines or kidney transplantation.

Tumors of the kidneys usually grow rather slowly, but rapidly invading types are occasionally found. Blood in the urine and dull pain in the kidney region are warnings that should be heeded at once. Surgical removal of the kidney offers the best chance of cure because most renal cancers do not respond to chemotherapy or radiation.

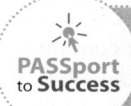 **PASSport to Success** Visit *thePoint* or see the Student Resource CD in the back of this book for illustrations of the kidney disorders discussed here.

KIDNEY STONES Kidney stones, or **calculi** (KAL-ku-li), are made of substances, such as calcium salts or uric acid, that precipitate out of the urine instead of remaining in solution. They usually form in the renal pelvis, but may also form in the bladder.

The causes of stone formation include dehydration, urinary stasis (stagnation), and urinary tract infection. The stones may vary in size from tiny grains resembling bits of gravel up to large masses that fill the renal pelvis and extend into the calyces. The latter are described as **staghorn calculi**.

There is no way of dissolving these stones because substances that could do so would also destroy renal tissue. Sometimes, instruments can be used to crush small stones and thus allow them to be expelled with the urine, but more often, surgical removal is required. A **litho-triptor** (LITH-o-trip-tor), literally a "stone-cracker," is a device that employs external shock waves to shatter kidney stones. The procedure is called **lithotripsy** (LITH-o-trip-se).

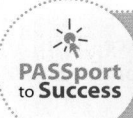

RENAL FAILURE Acute renal failure may result from a medical or surgical emergency or from toxins that damage the tubules. This condition is characterized by a sudden, serious decrease in kidney function accompanied by electrolyte and acid–base imbalances. Acute renal failure occurs as a serious complication of other severe illness and may be fatal.

Chronic renal failure results from a gradual loss of nephrons. As more and more nephrons are destroyed, the kidneys slowly lose the ability to perform their normal functions. As the disease progresses, nitrogenous waste products accumulate to high levels in the blood, causing a condition known as **uremia** (u-RE-me-ah). In many cases, there is a lesser decrease in renal function, known as **renal insufficiency**, that produces fewer symptoms.

A few of the characteristic signs and symptoms of chronic renal failure are the following:

- **Dehydration** (de-hi-DRA-shun). Excessive loss of body fluid may occur early in renal failure, when the kidneys cannot concentrate the urine and large amounts of water are eliminated.

- **Edema** (eh-DE-mah). Accumulation of fluid in the tissue spaces may occur late in chronic renal disease, when the kidneys cannot eliminate water in adequate amounts.

- **Electrolyte imbalance**, including retention of sodium and accumulation of potassium.

- **Hypertension** may occur as the result of fluid overload and increased renin production (see Box 22-2).

- **Anemia** occurs when the kidneys cannot produce the hormone erythropoietin to activate red blood cell production in bone marrow.

- **Uremia** (u-RE-me-ah), an excess of nitrogenous waste products in the blood. When these levels are very high, urea can be changed into ammonia in the stomach and intestine and cause ulcerations and bleeding.

CHECKPOINT 22-13 ➤ What is the difference between acute and chronic kidney disorders?

RENAL DIALYSIS AND KIDNEY TRANSPLANTATION Dialysis (di-AL-ih-sis) means "the separation of dissolved molecules based on their ability to pass through a semipermeable membrane" (Fig. 22-11A). Molecules that can pass through the membrane move from an area of greater concentration to one of lesser concentration. In patients who have defective renal function, the accumulation

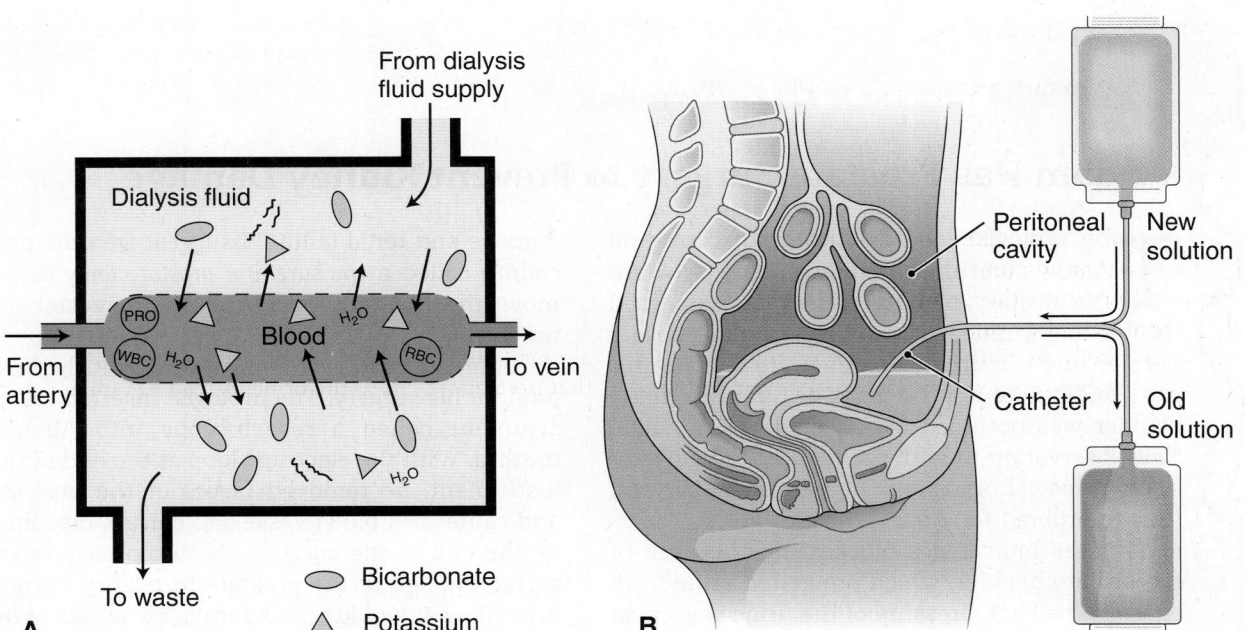

Figure 22-11 **A hemodialysis system and a peritoneal dialysis system. (A)** In hemodialysis, a cellophane membrane separates the blood compartment and dialysis fluid compartment. This membrane is porous enough to allow all of the constituents except the plasma proteins (PRO) and blood cells (WBC, RBC) to diffuse between the two compartments. **(B)** In peritoneal dialysis, a semipermeable membrane richly supplied with blood vessels lines the peritoneal cavity. With dialysate dwelling in the peritoneal cavity, waste products diffuse from the network of blood vessels into the dialysate. (A, Reprinted with permission from Porth CM. *Pathophysiology*, 7th ed. Philadelphia: Lippincott Williams & Wilkins, 2004; B, reprinted with permission from Cohen BJ. *Medical Terminology*, 5th ed. Philadelphia: Lippincott Williams & Wilkins, 2008.)

of urea and other nitrogenous waste products can be reduced by passage of the patient's blood through a dialysis machine. The principle of "molecules leaving the area of greater concentration" thus operates to remove wastes from the blood. The fluid in the dialysis machine, the dialysate, can be adjusted to regulate the flow of substances out of the blood.

There are two methods of dialysis in use: hemodialysis (blood dialysis) and peritoneal dialysis (dialysis in the abdominal cavity). In hemodialysis, the dialysis membrane is made of cellophane or other synthetic material. In peritoneal dialysis, the surface area of the peritoneum acts as the membrane (see Fig. 22-11B). Dialysis fluid is introduced into the peritoneal cavity and then periodically removed along with waste products. This procedure may be done at intervals through the day or during the night.

A 1973 amendment to the Social Security Act provides federal financial assistance for people who have chronic renal disease and require dialysis. Most hemodialysis is performed in freestanding clinics. Treatment time has been reduced; a typical schedule involves 2 to 3 hours, three times a week. Access to the bloodstream has been made safer and easier through surgical establishment of a permanent exchange site (shunt). Peritoneal dialysis also has been improved and simplified, enabling patients to manage treatment at home.

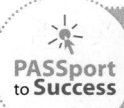

PASSport to Success

Visit *thePoint* or see the Student Resource CD in the back of this book for a description of the career of hemodialysis technician.

The final option for treatment of renal failure is kidney transplantation. Surgeons have successfully performed many of these procedures. Kidneys have so much extra functioning tissue that the loss of one kidney normally poses no problem to the donor. Records show that transplantation success is greatest when surgeons use a kidney from a living donor who is closely related to the patient. Organs from deceased donors have also proved satisfactory in many cases. The problem of tissue rejection (the rejection syndrome) is discussed in Chapter 17.

Disorders of the Ureters

Abnormalities in structure of the ureter include subdivision at the renal pelvis and constricted or abnormally narrow parts, called **strictures** (STRICK-tures). Abnormal pressure from tumors or other outside masses may cause ureteral narrowing. Obstruction also may be caused by stones from the kidneys, or kinking of the tube because of a dropped kidney, a condition known as **renal ptosis** (TO-

Disease in Context revisited

▶ Adam Has Prostate Surgery to Prevent Kidney Damage

The urologist inserted the cystoscope into Adam's urethra, carefully guiding it toward the urinary bladder. When he examined the bladder's mucous membrane lining, he did not see any urinary stones or tumors of the rugae. He did note that the neck of Adam's urinary bladder was occluded by his enlarged prostate. This observation fit with the results of the pyelogram (a special radiograph of the urinary system) he had ordered for Adam a week earlier. The x-ray images indicated a blockage in the neck of the urinary bladder, which prevented urine from exiting. The back-pressure of the urine was causing distention of the ureters (hydroureter) and kidneys (hydronephrosis). The doctor removed the cystoscope and reported his findings to his patient. "Adam, Dr. Singh's diagnosis was correct. The blockage in your urinary system is due to enlargement of your prostate gland. If we don't treat this now, your kidneys are at risk of severe

damage and renal failure. I suggest we do a procedure called a *transurethral prostatectomy* to remove the prostatic overgrowth and reestablish urine flow."

A few days later, Adam was back at the hospital for his surgery. The urologist inserted an instrument called a resectoscope into Adam's urethra. With the electrical loop at the end of the instrument, he removed pieces of the prostate and cauterized blood vessels to control bleeding. By the end of the surgery, the urologist had resected enough of the prostate to restore normal urine flow. It would take Adam a few weeks to recover, but soon he would be back to normal.

During this case, we saw that enlargement of the prostate gland can seriously affect urinary system function. To learn more about the prostate gland and other organs of the male reproductive system, see Chapter 23.

sis). In cases of **ureterocele** (u-RE-ter-o-sele), the end of the ureter bulges into the bladder (Fig. 22-12). The result is urinary obstruction that leads to distention of the ureter (hydroureter) and renal pelvis (hydronephrosis). The usual cause of ureterocele is a congenital (present at birth) narrowing of the ureteral opening.

URETERAL STONES The passage of a small stone along the ureter causes excruciating pain, called *renal colic*. Relief of this pain usually requires morphine or an equally powerful drug. The first "barber surgeons," operating without benefit of anesthesia, were permitted by their patients to cut through the skin and the muscles of the back to remove stones from the ureters. "Cutting for stone" in this way was relatively successful, despite the lack of sterile technique, because the approach through the back avoided the peritoneal cavity and the serious risk of peritonitis.

Modern surgery employs a variety of instruments for removal of stones from the ureter, including endoscopes similar to those described in Chapter 19. The transurethral route through the urethra and urinary bladder and then into the ureter, as well as entrance through the skin and muscles of the back, may be used to remove calculi from the kidney pelvis or from the ureter.

PASSport to Success Visit *thePoint* or see the Student Resource CD in the back of this book for a diagram showing sites of urinary obstruction, reflux, and infection.

CHECKPOINT 22-14 ➤ What is the scientific name for stones, as may occur in the urinary tract?

Bladder Disorders

A full (distended) bladder lies in an unprotected position in the lower abdomen, and a blow may rupture it, necessitating immediate surgical repair. Blood in the urine is a rather common symptom of infection or tumors, which may involve the bladder.

CYSTITIS Inflammation of the bladder, called **cystitis** (sis-TI-tis), is 10 times as common in women as in men. This may be due, at least in part, to the very short urethra of the female compared with that of the male. The usual path of infection is that bacteria ascend from the outside through the urethra into the bladder (see Fig. 23-14 in Chapter 23). The common contaminants are colon bacteria, such as *E. coli*, carried to the urethra from the anus. Urinary stasis and catheterization to remove urine from the bladder are other possible sources of infection. Pain, urgency to urinate, and urinary frequency are common symptoms of cystitis.

Another type of cystitis, called **interstitial cystitis**, may cause pelvic pain with discomfort before and after urination. The tissues below the mucosa are involved. The dis-

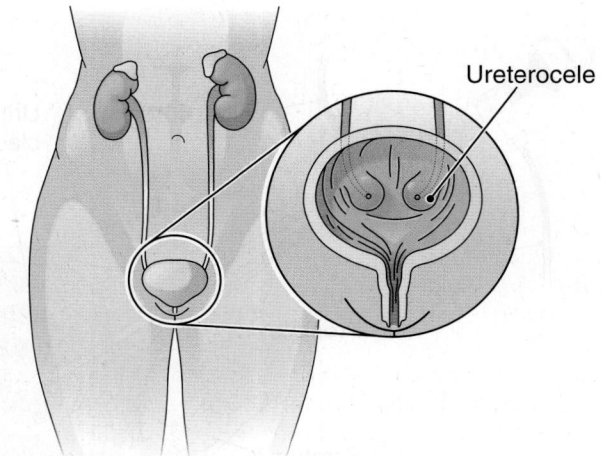

Figure 22-12 Ureterocele. The ureter bulges into the bladder. The resulting obstruction causes urine to back up into the ureter and renal pelvis. (Reprinted with permission from Cohen BJ. *Medical Terminology*, 5th ed. Philadelphia: Lippincott Williams & Wilkins, 2008.)

ease can be diagnosed only with the use of a **cystoscope**, a type of endoscope used to examine the bladder (Fig. 22-13). Because no bacteria are involved, antibiotics are not effective treatment and may even be harmful.

Obstruction by an enlarged prostate gland in a male or from pregnancy may lead to urinary stasis and cystitis. Reduction of a person's general resistance to infection, as in diabetes, may also lead to cystitis. The danger of cystitis is that the infection may ascend to other parts of the urinary tract.

TUMORS Bladder tumors, which are most prevalent in men older than 50 years of age, include benign papillomas and various kinds of cancer. About 90% of these tumors arise from the bladder's epithelial lining. Possible causes include toxins (particularly certain aniline dyes), chronic infestations (e.g., schistosomiasis), heavy cigarette smoking, and the presence of urinary stones, which may develop and increase in size within the bladder.

Blood in the urine (hematuria) and frequent urination, in the absence of pain or fever, are early signs of a bladder tumor. A cystoscopic examination (see Fig. 22-13) and biopsy should be performed as soon as these signs are detected. Treatment includes removal of the tumor, which may be done cystoscopically, and localized chemotherapy. More serious cases may require irradiation. Removal before the tumor invades the muscle wall gives the best prognosis.

If it is necessary to remove the bladder in a **cystectomy** (sis-TEK-to-me), the ureters must be vented elsewhere. They may be diverted to the body surface through a segment of the ileum, a procedure known as an **ileal conduit** (Fig. 22-14), or diverted to some other portion of the intestine. Alternatively, surgeons may create a bladder from a section of the colon.

URINARY INCONTINENCE Urinary incontinence (in-KON-tin-ens) refers to an involuntary loss of urine. The

22

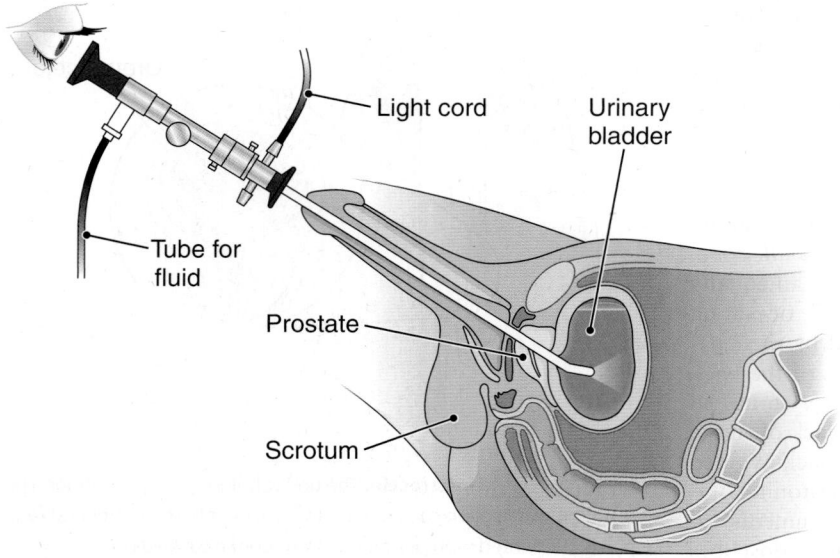

Figure 22-13 **Cystoscopy.** A lighted cystoscope is introduced through the urethra into the bladder of a male subject. Sterile fluid is used to inflate the bladder. The cystoscope is used to examine the bladder, remove specimens for biopsy, and remove tumors. (Reprinted with permission from Cohen BJ. *Medical Terminology,* 5th ed. Philadelphia: Lippincott Williams & Wilkins, 2008.)

condition may originate with a neurologic disorder, trauma to the spinal cord, weakness of the pelvic muscles, impaired bladder function, or medications. Different forms of urinary incontinence have specific names:

- Stress incontinence results from urethral incompetence that allows small amounts of urine to be released when an activity increases pressure in the abdomen. These activities include coughing, sneezing, laughing, lifting, or exercising.

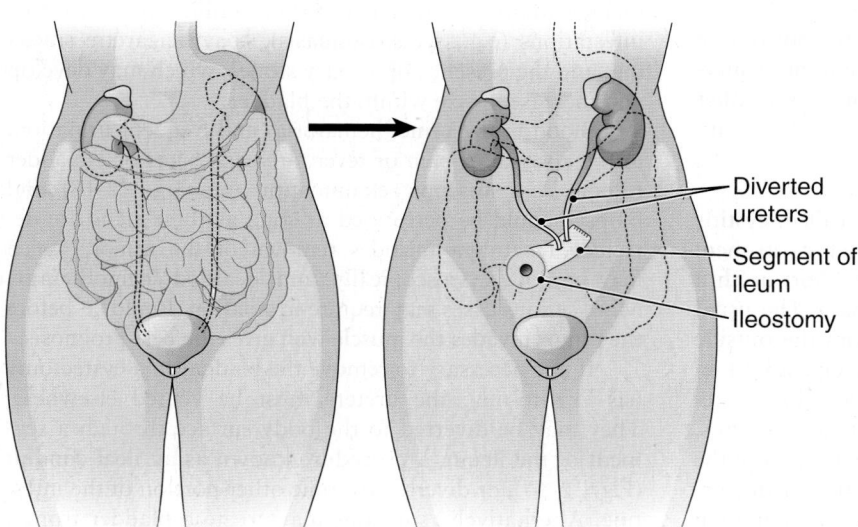

Diverted ureters

Segment of ileum

Ileostomy

Figure 22-14 **Ileal conduit.** The ureters are vented through a segment of the ileum to open at the body surface through an ileostomy. (Reprinted with permission from Cohen BJ. *Medical Terminology,* 5th ed. Philadelphia: Lippincott Williams & Wilkins, 2008.)

- Urge incontinence, also called *overactive bladder*, results from an inability to control bladder contractions once the sensation of bladder fullness is perceived.

- Overflow incontinence arises from neurologic damage or urinary obstruction that causes the bladder to overfill. Excess pressure in the bladder results in involuntary loss of urine.

- **Enuresis** (en-u-RE-sis) is involuntary urination, usually during the night (bed-wetting).

Some treatment approaches to incontinence include muscle exercises, dietary changes, biofeedback, medication, surgery or, in serious cases, self-catheterization.

CHECKPOINT **22-15** ➤ What is the term for inflammation of the bladder?

Disorders of the Urethra

Congenital anomalies may involve the urethra as well as other parts of the urinary tract. The opening of the urethra to the outside may be too small, or the urethra itself may be narrowed. Occasionally, an abnormal valve-like structure is found at the point where the urethra enters the bladder. If it is not removed surgically, it can cause back pressure of the urine, with serious consequences. There is also a condition in the male in which the urethra opens on the undersurface of the penis instead of at the end. This is called **hypospadias** (hi-po-SPA-de-as) (Fig. 22-15).

Urethritis, which is characterized by inflammation of the mucous membrane and the glands of the urethra, is much more common in men than in women. It is often caused by infection with gonococci or chlamydias, although many other bacteria may be involved.

"Straddle" injuries to the urethra are common in men. This type of injury occurs when, for example, a man walking along a raised beam slips and lands with the beam between his legs. Such an accident may catch the urethra between the hard surfaces of the beam and the pubic arch and rupture the urethra. In accidents in which the bones of the pelvis are fractured, rupture of the urethra is fairly common.

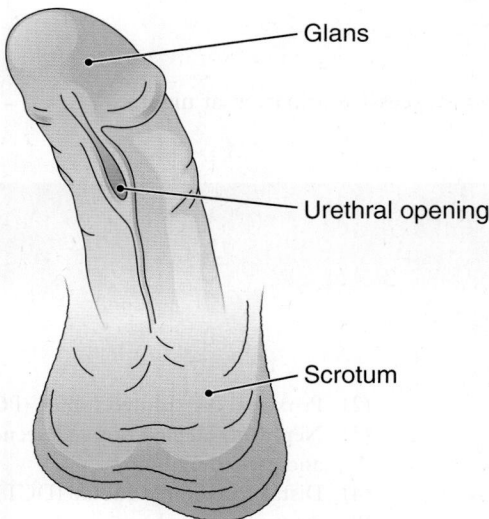

Figure 22-15 **Hypospadias.** A ventral view of the penis is shown here. (Reprinted with permission from Cohen BJ. *Medical Terminology*, 5th ed. Philadelphia: Lippincott Williams & Wilkins, 2008.)

Glans

Urethral opening

Scrotum

The Effects of Aging

Even without renal disease, aging causes the kidneys to lose some of their ability to concentrate urine. With aging, progressively more water is needed to excrete the same amount of waste. Older people find it necessary to drink more water than young people, and they eliminate larger amounts of urine (polyuria), even at night (nocturia).

Beginning at about 40 years of age, there is a decrease in the number and size of the nephrons. Often, more than half of them are lost before the age of 80 years. There may be an increase in blood urea nitrogen (BUN) without serious symptoms. Elderly people are more susceptible than young people to urinary system infections. Childbearing may cause damage to the musculature of the pelvic floor, resulting in urinary tract problems in later years.

Enlargement of the prostate, common in older men, may cause obstruction and back pressure in the ureters and kidneys. If this condition is untreated, it will cause permanent damage to the kidneys. Changes with age, including decreased bladder capacity and decreased muscle tone in the bladder and urinary sphincters, may predispose to incontinence. However, most elderly people (60% in nursing homes, and up to 85% living independently) have no incontinence.

Word Anatomy

Medical terms are built from standardized word parts (prefixes, roots, and suffixes). Learning the meanings of these parts can help you remember words and interpret unfamiliar terms.

WORD PART	MEANING	EXAMPLE
The Kidneys		
retro-	backward, behind	The *retroperitoneal* space is posterior to the peritoneal cavity.
ren/o	kidney	The *renal* artery carries blood to the kidney.
nephr/o	kidney	The *nephron* is the functional unit of the kidney.
juxta-	next to	The *juxtaglomerular* apparatus is next to the glomerulus.
The Ureters		
extra-	beyond, outside of	The ureters are *extraperitoneal*.
Disorders of the Urinary System		
pyel/o	renal pelvis	*Pyelonephritis* is inflammation of the nephrons and renal pelvis.
cyst/o	sac, bladder	A *polycystic* kidney develops many fluid-containing sacs.
dia-	through	*Dialysis* is the separation (-lysis) of molecules based on their ability to pass through a semipermeable membrane.
-cele	swelling, enlarged space	A *uterocele* is formed as the end of the ureter bulges into the bladder.
trans-	across, through	A *transurethral* route is through the urethra.

22

WORD PART	MEANING	EXAMPLE
The Effects of Aging		
noct/i	night	*Nocturia* is excessive urination at night.

Summary

I. **EXCRETION**
  A. Removal and elimination of metabolic waste
  B. Systems that eliminate waste
  1. Urinary—removes waste from blood
    a. Other functions—regulates blood volume, pH, and electrolytes
  2. Digestive system—eliminates water, salts, bile with digestive residue
  3. Respiratory system—eliminates carbon dioxide, water
  4. Skin—eliminates water, salts, nitrogenous waste

II. **ORGANS OF THE URINARY SYSTEM**
  A. Kidneys (2)
  B. Ureters (2)
  C. Urinary bladder (1)
  D. Urethra (1)

III. **KIDNEYS**
  A. Kidney activities
  1. Excretion of waste, excess salts, toxins
  2. Water balance
  3. Acid–base balance (pH)
  4. Blood pressure regulation
  5. Erythropoietin (EPO) secretion—hormone stimulates red blood cell production
  B. Kidney structure
  1. Location
    a. In upper abdomen against the back
    b. In retroperitoneal space (posterior to the peritoneum)
  2. Blood supply
    a. Renal artery—carries blood to kidney from aorta
    b. Renal vein—carries blood from kidney to inferior vena cava
  3. Organization
    a. Cortex—outer portion
    b. Medulla—inner portion
    c. Pelvis
      (1) Upper end of ureter
      (2) Calyces—cuplike extensions that receive urine
  4. Nephron
    a. Functional unit of kidney
    b. Parts
      (1) Glomerular (Bowman) capsule—around glomerulus
      (2) Proximal convoluted tubule (PCT)
      (3) Nephron (Henle) loop—descending and ascending limbs
      (4) Distal convoluted tubule (DCT)
    c. Blood supply to nephron
      (1) Afferent arteriole—enters glomerular capsule
      (2) Glomerulus—coil of capillaries in glomerular capsule
      (3) Efferent arteriole—leaves glomerular capsule
      (4) Peritubular capillaries—surround nephron

  C. Formation of urine
  1. Glomerular filtration—driven by blood pressure in glomerulus
    a. Water and soluble substances forced out of blood and into glomerular capsule
    b. Blood cells and proteins remain in blood
    c. Glomerular filtrate—material that leaves blood and enters the nephron
  2. Tubular reabsorption
    a. Most of filtrate leaves nephron by diffusion, osmosis, and active transport
    b. Influenced by hormones (e.g. aldosterone, ANP)
    c. Returns to blood through peritubular capillaries
  3. Tubular secretion—materials moved from blood into nephron for excretion
  4. Concentration of urine
    a. Countercurrent mechanism—method for concentrating urine based on movement of ions and permeability of tubule
    b. ADH
      (1) Hormone from posterior pituitary
      (2) Promotes reabsorption of water

  D. Regulation of blood pressure
  1. Kidneys need adequate blood pressure to filter blood
  2. Juxtaglomerular apparatus
    a. Consists of cells in afferent arteriole and distal convoluted tubule
    b. Releases renin when blood pressure low

c. Renin activates angiotensin to raise blood pressure
   (1) Stimulates release of aldosterone
   (2) Stimulates release of ADH
   (3) Promotes vasoconstriction
   (4) Stimulates thirst
   (5) Stimulates sympathetic nervous system

IV. **URETERS**
   A. Carry urine from the kidneys to the bladder

V. **URINARY BLADDER**
   A. Stores urine until it is eliminated
   B. Trigone—triangular region in base of bladder; remains stable as bladder fills

VI. **URETHRA**
   A. Carries urine out of body
   B. Male urethra—20 cm long; carries both urine and semen
   C. Female urethra—4 cm long; opening anterior to vagina
   D. Urination (micturition)
      1. Both voluntary and involuntary
      2. Sphincters
         a. Internal urethral sphincter—involuntary (smooth muscle)
         b. External urethral sphincter—voluntary (skeletal muscle)
      3. Stretch receptors in bladder wall signal reflex emptying
      4. Can be controlled through higher brain centers

VII. **URINE**
   A. pH averages 6.0
   B. Specific gravity—measures dissolved substances
   C. Normal constituents—water, nitrogenous waste, electrolytes, pigments
   D. Abnormal constituents—glucose, albumin, blood, ketones, white blood cells, casts

VIII. **DISORDERS OF THE URINARY SYSTEM**
   A. Kidney disorders
      1. Examples
         a. Acute glomerulonephritis—damages glomeruli

b. Pyelonephritis—inflammation of kidney and renal pelvis
c. Hydronephrosis—distention with obstructed fluids
d. Polycystic kidney—fluid-containing sacs develop
e. Tumors
      2. Kidney stones—calculi
      3. Renal failure
         a. Types
            (1) Acute—results from medical emergency or toxins
            (2) Chronic—signs include dehydration, electrolyte imbalance, edema, hypertension, anemia, uremia
         4. Treatment
            a. Renal dialysis—removes unwanted substances from blood when kidneys fail
               (1) Hemodialysis—exchange through synthetic membrane
               (2) Peritoneal dialysis—peritoneum is exchange membrane
            b. Kidney transplantation
   B. Disorders of the ureters
      1. Stricture (narrowing)
      2. Stones (calculi)
   C. Disorders of the bladder
      1. Cystitis—inflammation; most common in females
      2. Tumors
      3. Urinary incontinence
   D. Disorders of the urethra
      1. Hypospadias—urethra opens on underside of penis
      2. Urethritis—inflammation

IX. **EFFECTS OF AGING**
   A. Polyuria—increased elimination of urine
   B. Nocturia—urination at night
   C. Incontinence
   D. Increased blood urea nitrogen (BUN)
   E. Prostate enlargement

Questions for Study and Review

22

BUILDING UNDERSTANDING

Fill in the blanks

1. Each kidney is located outside the abdominal cavity in the _____ space.

2. The renal artery, renal vein, and ureter connect to the kidney at the _____.

3. The part of the bladder marked by the openings of the ureters and urethra is called the _____.

4. The amount of dissolved substances in urine is indicated by its _____.

5. The presence of glucose in the urine is known as _____.

Matching > Match each numbered item with the most closely related lettered item.

___ **6.** Produced by the kidney in response to low blood pressure

___ **7.** Stimulates vasoconstriction

___ **8.** Produced by the kidney in response to hypoxia

___ **9.** Stimulates kidneys to produce concentrated urine

___ **10.** Produced by the liver during protein catabolism

a. urea

b. erythropoietin

c. antidiuretic hormone

d. renin

e. angiotensin

Multiple choice

___ **11.** The functional unit of the renal system is the

    a. renal capsule
    b. kidney
    c. nephron
    d. juxtaglomerular apparatus

___ **12.** The nephron loop is located in the renal

    a. cortex
    b. medulla
    c. pelvis
    d. calyx

___ **13.** Fluid moves out of the glomerulus by

    a. filtration
    b. diffusion
    c. osmosis
    d. active transport

___ **14.** One's ability to delay urination is due to voluntary control of the

    a. trigone
    b. internal urethral sphincter
    c. external urethral sphincter
    d. urinary meatus

___ **15.** Pus in the urine is termed

    a. pyuria
    b. uremia
    c. anemia
    d. enuresis

UNDERSTANDING CONCEPTS

16. List four organ systems active in excretion. What are the products eliminated by each?

17. Compare and contrast the following terms:

    a. glomerular capsule and glomerulus
    b. afferent and efferent arteriole
    c. proximal and distal convoluted tubule
    d. ureter and urethra

18. Trace the pathway of a urea molecule from the afferent arteriole to the urinary meatus.

19. Describe the four processes involved in the formation of urine.

20. Compare the male urethra and female urethra in structure and function. Why is cystitis more common in women than in men?

21. List some of the dissolved substances normally found in the urine.

22. Differentiate between the following disorders:

    a. albuminuria and hematuria
    b. glomerulonephritis and pyelonephritis
    c. hydronephrosis and polycystic kidney
    d. renal ptosis and ureterocele

23. What is meant by the word *dialysis* and how is this principle used for patients with kidney failure? What kinds of membranes are used for hemodialysis? for peritoneal dialysis?

CONCEPTUAL THINKING

24. Christie is 14 years old and suffers from anorexia nervosa. Her parents take her to the hospital after she reports sharp pain in the lumbar region of her back. While there, she is diagnosed with hydronephrosis. What is the relationship between her eating disorder and her renal disorder?

25. A class of antihypertensive drugs called loop diuretics prevents sodium reabsorption in the nephron loop. How could a drug like this lower blood pressure?

26. In Adam's second case, enlargement of the prostate gland led to hydronephrosis. What effect might this have on glomerular filtration?

The final unit includes three chapters on the structures and functions related to reproduction and heredity. The reproductive system is not necessary for the continuation of the life of the individual but rather is needed for the continuation of the human species. The reproductive cells and their genes have been studied intensively during recent years as part of the rapidly advancing science of genetics.

CHAPTER 23

The Male and Female Reproductive Systems

Learning Outcomes

After careful study of this chapter, you should be able to:

1. Name the male and female gonads and describe the function of each
2. State the purpose of meiosis
3. List the accessory organs of the male and female reproductive tracts and cite the function of each
4. Describe the composition and function of semen
5. Draw and label a spermatozoon
6. List in the correct order the hormones produced during the menstrual cycle and cite the source of each
7. Describe the functions of the main male and female sex hormones
8. Explain how negative feedback regulates reproductive function in both males and females
9. Describe the changes that occur during and after menopause
10. Cite the main methods of birth control in use
11. Briefly describe the major disorders of the male and female reproductive tracts
12. Show how word parts are used to build words related to the reproductive systems (see Word Anatomy at the end of the chapter)

Selected Key Terms

The following terms and other boldface terms in the chapter are defined in the Glossary

contraception
corpus luteum
endometrium
estrogen
follicle
follicle-stimulating hormone (FSH)
gamete
infertility
luteinizing hormone (LH)
menopause
menses
menstruation
ovary
ovulation
ovum (pl., ova)
progesterone
semen
spermatozoon (pl., spermatozoa)
testis (pl., testes)
testosterone
uterus

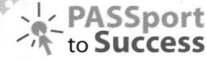

PASSport to Success

Visit *thePoint* or see the Student Resource CD in the back of this book for definitions and pronunciations of key terms as well as a pretest for this chapter.

Disease
in Context

> ## Sylvie's Case: Removal of a Benign Uterine Tumor

"Oooh," Sylvie complained to her husband as she came into the house from gardening. "I know it's unusually hot this summer, but I'm having a hard time gardening this year for some reason. I feel a pull in my hip and groin and some discomfort in my belly. Maybe I've pulled a muscle; I should make an appointment for a massage and maybe talk to the trainers at the gym about getting some exercises to stretch out my hip muscles." "Maybe you should make an extra visit to your gynecologist," Jon suggested. "Remember he said something about a tumor last time you went?" "Right," Sylvie replied, "he said something about a small, benign tumor in my uterus. A fibroid, I think he called it. He didn't think it would cause problems, at least for a while, but maybe I should check it out. I've noticed some irregular bleeding, but chalked that up to my approaching menopause."

When Sylvie later consulted with her gynecologist, Dr. Bernard, she had already had a pelvic ultrasound to check on her uterus. After looking over her results, the doctor told her, "I don't know if this fibroid is the cause of your symptoms, but it has increased in size since your last visit. The ultrasound shows that the myoma, or fibroid, is about 3.5 cm, just about the size of a golf ball. I'm surprised that it has changed so rapidly, but that may be related to hormonal changes. I think because of its interior location we can remove it and repair the uterus through the vagina. We'll schedule you for outpatient surgery at Lincoln Hospital. If all goes well, you should have a very brief recovery period."

Sylvie's case uses some of the terms related to the female reproductive tract. Later, we'll revisit Sylvie to find out the results of her surgery.

Reproduction

The chapters in this unit deal with what is certainly one of the most interesting and mysterious attributes of life: the ability to reproduce. The simplest forms of life, one-celled organisms, usually need no partner to reproduce; they simply divide by themselves. This form of reproduction is known as **asexual** (nonsexual) reproduction.

In most animals, however, reproduction is **sexual**, meaning that there are two kinds of individuals, males and females, each of which has specialized cells designed specifically for the perpetuation of the species. These specialized sex cells are known as **germ cells** or **gametes** (GAM-etes). In the male, they are called **spermatozoa** (sper-mah-to-ZO-ah, sing., **spermatozoon**) or simply sperm cells; in the female, they are called **ova** (O-vah; sing., **ovum**), or egg cells.

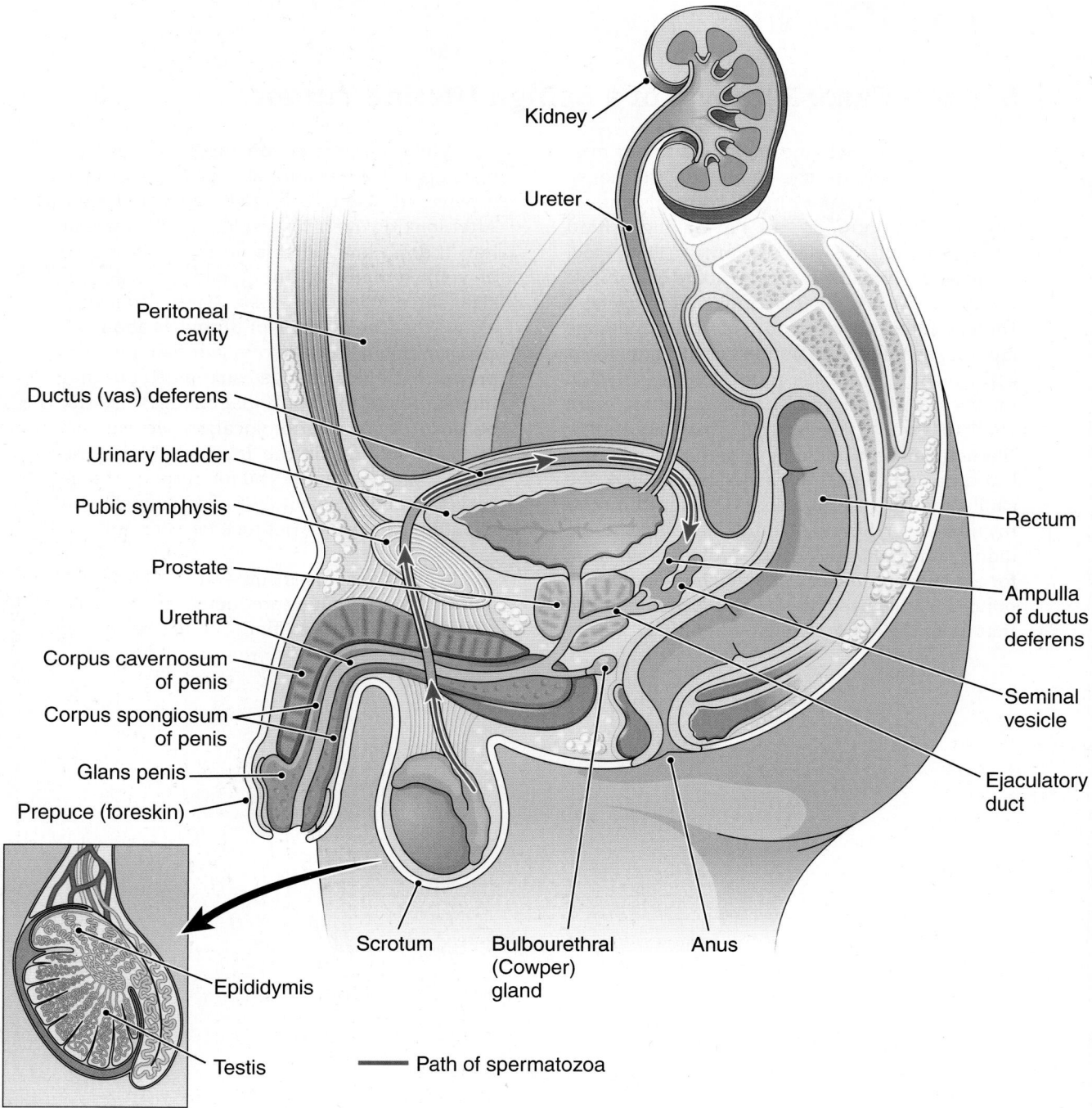

Figure 23-1 **Male reproductive system.** Organs of the urinary system are also shown. **[ZOOMING IN ➤** What four glands empty secretions into the urethra? **]**

Meiosis

Gametes are characterized by having half as many chromosomes as are found in any other body cell. During their formation, they go through a special process of cell division, called **meiosis** (mi-O-sis), which halves the number of chromosomes. In humans, meiosis reduces the chromosome number in a cell from 46 to 23. The role of meiosis in reproduction is explained in more detail in Chapter 25.

CHECKPOINT 23-1 ➤ What is the process of cell division that halves the chromosome number in a cell to produce a gamete?

The Male Reproductive System

The male reproductive system, like that of the female, may be divided into two groups of organs: primary and accessory (see Fig. 23-1).

- The primary organs are the **gonads** (GO-nads), or sex glands; they produce the germ cells and manufacture hormones. The male gonad is the testis. (In comparison, the female gonad is the ovary, as explained below.)

- The **accessory organs** include a series of ducts that transport the germ cells as well as various exocrine glands.

See Appendix 7 for a dissection photograph of the male reproductive system.

The Testes

The male gonads, the paired **testes** (TES-teze) (sing. **testis**), are located outside of the body proper, suspended between the thighs in a sac called the **scrotum** (SKRO-tum). The testes are oval organs measuring approximately 4.0 cm (1.5 inches) in length and approximately 2.5 cm (1 inch) in each of the other two dimensions. During embryonic life, each testis develops from tissue near the kidney.

A month or two before birth, the testis normally descends (moves downward) through the **inguinal** (ING-gwih-nal) **canal** in the abdominal wall into the scrotum. The testis then remains suspended by a **spermatic cord** (Fig. 23-2) that extends through the inguinal canal. This cord contains blood vessels, lymphatic vessels, nerves, and the tube (ductus deferens) that transports spermatozoa away from the testis. The gland must descend completely if it is to function normally; to produce spermatozoa, the testis must be kept at the temperature of the scrotum, which is several degrees lower than that of the abdominal cavity.

> ⚡ **PASSport to Success**
> Visit **thePoint** or see the Student Resource CD in the back of this book for an illustration showing the descent of the testes.

INTERNAL STRUCTURE Most of the specialized tissue of the testis consists of tiny coiled **seminiferous** (seh-mih-

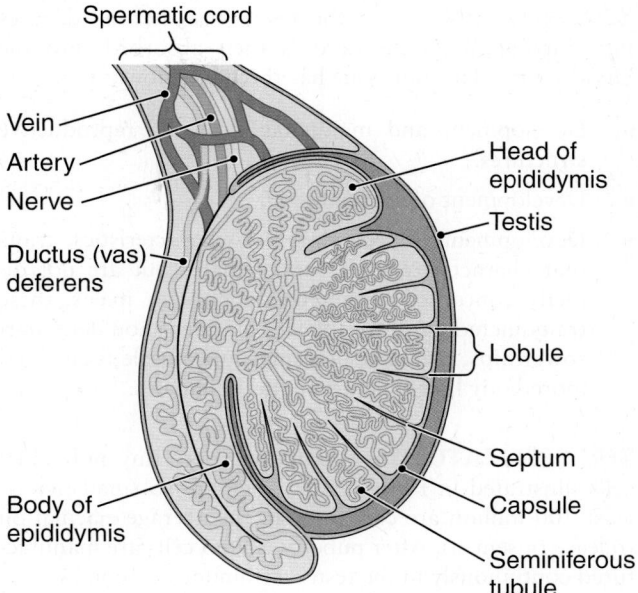

Figure 23-2 **Structure of the testis.** The epididymis and spermatic cord are also shown. [ZOOMING IN ➤ What duct receives secretions from the epididymis?]

NIF-er-us) **tubules.** Primitive cells in the walls of these tubules develop into mature spermatozoa, aided by neighboring cells called **sustentacular** (sus-ten-TAK-u-lar) **(Sertoli) cells.** These so-called "nurse" cells nourish and protect the developing spermatozoa. They also secrete a protein that binds testosterone in the seminiferous tubules.

Specialized **interstitial** (in-ter-STISH-al) **cells** that secrete the male sex hormone **testosterone** (tes-TOS-teh-rone) are located between the seminiferous tubules. Figure 23-3 is a microscopic view of the testis in cross-section, showing the seminiferous tubules, interstitial cells, and developing spermatozoa.

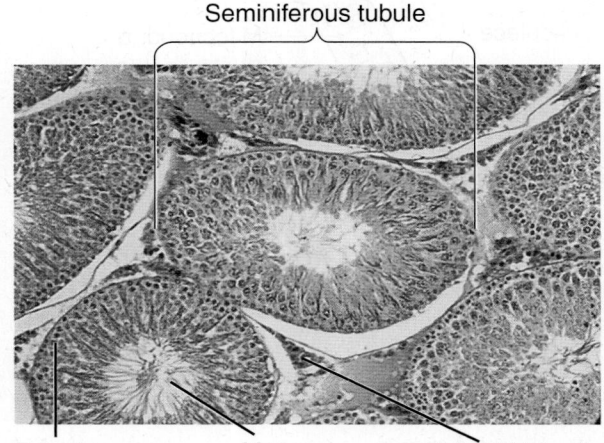

Figure 23-3 **Microscopic view of the testis.** (Courtesy of Dana Morse Bittus and BJ Cohen.)

23

TESTOSTERONE From the testis, testosterone diffuses into surrounding fluids and is then absorbed into the bloodstream. This hormone has three functions:

- Development and maintenance of the reproductive structures.

- Development of spermatozoa.

- Development of **secondary sex characteristics**, traits that characterize males and females but are not directly concerned with reproduction. In males, these traits include a deeper voice, broader shoulders, narrower hips, a greater percentage of muscle tissue, and more body hair than are found in females.

THE SPERMATOZOA Spermatozoa are tiny individual cells illustrated in Figure 23-4. They are so small that at least 200 million are contained in the average ejaculation (release of semen). After puberty, sperm cells are manufactured continuously in the testes' seminiferous tubules.

The spermatozoon has an oval head that is mostly a nucleus containing chromosomes. The **acrosome** (AK-rosome), which covers the head like a cap, contains enzymes that help the sperm cell to penetrate the ovum.

Whiplike movements of the tail (flagellum) propel the sperm through the female reproductive system to the ovum. The cell's middle region (midpiece) contains many mitochondria that provide energy for movement.

CHECKPOINT **23-2** ➤ What is the male gonad? What is the main male sex hormone?

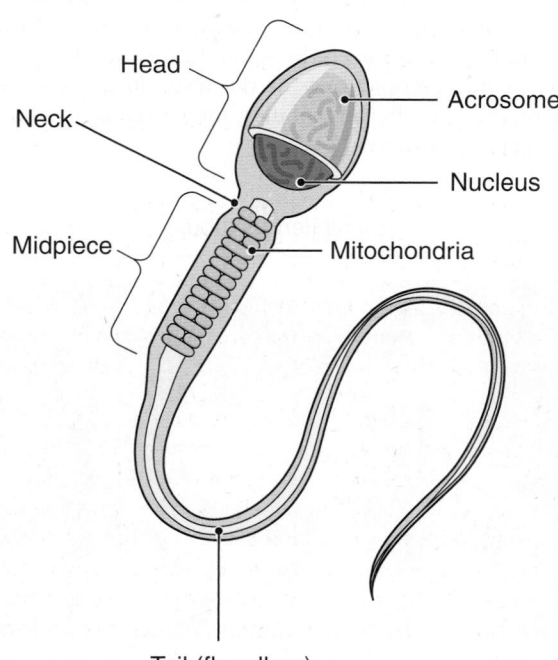

Head
Neck
Acrosome
Nucleus
Midpiece
Mitochondria

Tail (flagellum)

Figure 23-4 **Diagram of a human spermatozoon.** Major structural features are shown. [**ZOOMING IN** ➤ What organelles provide energy for sperm cell motility?]

CHECKPOINT **23-3** ➤ What is the male sex cell (gamete) called?

CHECKPOINT **23-4** ➤ What are the main subdivisions of a spermatozoon?

Accessory Organs

The system of ducts that transports the spermatozoa begins with tubules inside the testis itself. From these tubules, the cells collect in a greatly coiled tube called the **epididymis** (ep-ih-DID-ih-mis), which is 6 meters (20 feet) long and is located on the surface of the testis inside the scrotal sac (see Fig. 23-2). While they are temporarily stored in the epididymis, the sperm cells mature and become motile, able to move or "swim" by themselves.

The epididymis finally extends upward at the **ductus deferens** (DEF-er-enz), also called the **vas deferens**. This tube, contained in the spermatic cord, continues through the inguinal canal into the abdominal cavity. Here, it separates from the remainder of the spermatic cord and curves behind the urinary bladder. The ductus deferens then joins with the duct of the **seminal vesicle** (VES-ih-kl) on the same side to form the **ejaculatory** (e-JAK-u-lah-to-re) **duct**. The right and left ejaculatory ducts travel through the body of the prostate gland and then empty into the urethra.

CHECKPOINT **23-5** ➤ What is the order in which sperm cells travel through the ducts of the male reproductive system?

Semen

Semen (SE-men) (meaning "seed") is the mixture of sperm cells and various secretions that is expelled from the body. It is a sticky fluid with a milky appearance. The pH is in the alkaline range of 7.2 to 7.8. The secretions in semen serve several functions:

- Nourish the spermatozoa

- Transport the spermatozoa

- Neutralize the acidity of the male urethra and the female vaginal tract

- Lubricate the reproductive tract during sexual intercourse

- Prevent infection with antibacterial enzymes and antibodies

The glands discussed next contribute secretions to the semen (see Fig. 23-1).

THE SEMINAL VESICLES The seminal vesicles are twisted muscular tubes with many small outpouchings. They are approximately 7.5 cm (3 inches) long and are attached to the connective tissue at the posterior of the urinary bladder. The glandular lining produces a thick, yellow, alkaline secretion containing large quantities of simple sugar and other substances that provide nourishment for the sperm. The seminal fluid makes up a large part of the semen's volume.

THE PROSTATE GLAND The **prostate gland** lies immediately inferior to the urinary bladder, where it surrounds the first part of the urethra. Ducts from the prostate carry its secretions into the urethra. The thin, alkaline prostatic secretion helps neutralize the acidity of the vaginal tract and enhance the spermatozoa's motility. The prostate gland is also supplied with muscular tissue, which, upon signals from the nervous system, contracts to aid in the expulsion of the semen from the body.

BULBOURETHRAL GLANDS The **bulbourethral** (bulbo-u-RE-thral) **glands**, also called **Cowper glands**, are a pair of pea-sized organs located in the pelvic floor just inferior to the prostate gland. They secrete mucus to lubricate the urethra and tip of the penis during sexual stimulation. The ducts of these glands extend approximately 2.5 cm (1 inch) from each side and empty into the urethra before it extends into the penis.

Other very small glands secrete mucus into the urethra as it passes through the penis.

CHECKPOINT 23-6 ➤ What glands, aside from the testis, contribute secretions to semen?

The Urethra and Penis

The male urethra, as discussed in Chapter 22, serves the dual purpose of conveying urine from the bladder and carrying the reproductive cells with their accompanying secretions to the outside. The ejection of semen is made possible by **erection**, the stiffening and enlargement of the penis, through which the longest part of the urethra extends. The penis is made of spongy tissue containing many blood spaces that are relatively empty when the organ is flaccid but that fill with blood and distend when the penis is erect. This tissue is subdivided into three segments, each called a **corpus** (body) (Fig. 23-5). A single, ventrally located **corpus spongiosum** contains the urethra. On either side is a larger **corpus cavernosum** (pl., corpora cavernosa). At the distal end of the penis, the corpus spongiosum enlarges to form the **glans penis**, which is covered with a loose fold of skin, the **prepuce** (PRE-puse), commonly called the *foreskin*. It is the end of the foreskin that is removed in a **circumcision** (sir-kum-SIZH-un), a surgery frequently performed on male babies for religious or cultural reasons. Experts disagree on the medical value of circumcision with regard to improved cleanliness and disease prevention.

The penis and scrotum together make up the male **external genitalia** (jen-ih-TA-le-ah).

EJACULATION Ejaculation (e-jak-u-LA-shun) is the forceful expulsion of semen through the urethra to the outside. The process is initiated by reflex centers in the spinal cord that stimulate smooth muscle contraction in the prostate.

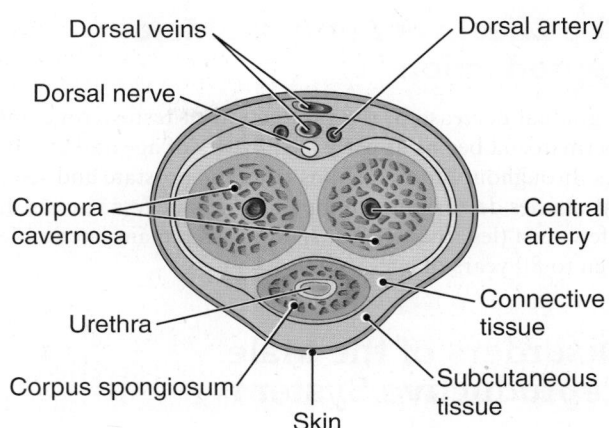

Figure 23-5 **Cross-section of the penis.** [ZOOMING IN ➤ What subdivision of the penis contains the urethra?]

This is followed by contraction of skeletal muscle in the pelvic floor, which provides the force needed for expulsion. During ejaculation, the involuntary sphincter at the base of the bladder closes to prevent the release of urine.

A male typically ejaculates 2 to 5 mL of semen containing 50 to 150 million sperm cells per mL. Out of the millions of spermatozoa in an ejaculation, only one, if any, can fertilize an ovum. The remainder of the cells live from only a few hours up to a maximum of 3 days.

Hormonal Control of Male Reproduction

The activities of the testes are under the control of two hormones produced by the anterior pituitary. These hormones are named for their activity in female reproduction (described later), although they are chemically the same in both males and females.

- **Follicle-stimulating hormone (FSH)** stimulates the sustentacular (Sertoli) cells and promotes the formation of spermatozoa.

- **Luteinizing hormone (LH)** stimulates the interstitial cells between the seminiferous tubules to produce testosterone, which is also needed for sperm cell development.

Starting at puberty, the hypothalamus begins to secrete hormones that trigger the release of FSH and LH. These hormones are secreted continuously in the male.

The activity of the hypothalamus is in turn regulated by a negative feedback mechanism involving testosterone. As the blood level of testosterone increases, the hypothalamus secretes less releasing hormone; as the level of testosterone decreases, the hypothalamus secretes more releasing hormone (see Fig. 12-3 in Chapter 12).

CHECKPOINT 23-7 ➤ What two pituitary hormones regulate both male and female reproduction?

23

The Effects of Aging on Male Reproduction

A gradual decrease in the production of testosterone and spermatozoa begins as early as 20 years of age and continues throughout life. Secretions from the prostate and seminal vesicles decrease in amount and become less viscous. In a few men (less than 10%), sperm cells remain late in life, even to 80 years of age.

Disorders of the Male Reproductive System

A variety of disorders can contribute to **infertility**, a significantly lower than normal ability to reproduce. If the inability is complete, the condition is termed **sterility**. The proportion of infertility in couples that can be attributed to defects involving the male has been estimated from 40% to 50%. (See also Box 23-1, Treating Erectile Dysfunction.)

The tubules of the testes are sensitive to x-rays, infections, toxins, and malnutrition, all of which bring about degenerative changes. Such damage may cause a decrease in the numbers of spermatozoa produced, leading to a condition called **oligospermia** (ol-ih-go-SPER-me-ah). Adequate numbers of sperm are required to disperse the coating around the ovum so that one sperm can fertilize it. Absence of or an inadequate number of sperm cells is a significant cause of infertility.

A male may be intentionally sterilized by an operation called a **vasectomy** (vah-SEK-to-me). In this procedure, a portion of the ductus deferens on each side is removed, and the cut end is closed to keep spermatozoa from reaching the urethra. The tiny sperm cells are simply reabsorbed. A man who has had a vasectomy retains the ability to produce hormones and all other seminal secretions as well as the ability to perform the sex act, but no fertilization can occur.

Structural Disorders

Cryptorchidism (kript-OR-kid-izm) is a failure of the testis to descend into the scrotum. Unless corrected in childhood, this condition results in sterility. Undescended testes are also particularly subject to tumor formation. Most testes that are undescended at birth descend spontaneously by 1 year of age. Surgical correction is the usual remedy in the remaining cases.

Torsion of the testis is a twisting of the spermatic cord that results from rotation of the testis (Fig. 23-6). This turning may occur during descent of the testis or later in life, most commonly between the ages of 8 to 18 years. The condition is accompanied by acute pain, swelling, and shortening of the spermatic cord. It requires emergency surgery to correct the defect, and may involve removal of the testis (orchiectomy). Torsion of the testis is a developmental disorder that often affects both glands, so the other testis must be examined to determine whether or not preventive surgery is needed.

Hernia (HER-ne-ah), or rupture, refers to the abnormal protrusion of an organ or organ part through the wall of the cavity in which it is normally contained (Fig. 23-7).

Box 23-1 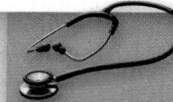 **Clinical Perspectives**

Treating Erectile Dysfunction: When NO Means Yes

Approximately 25 million American men and their partners are affected by **erectile dysfunction** (ED), the inability to achieve an erection. Although ED is more common in men over the age of 65, it can occur at any age and can have many causes. Until recently, ED was believed to be caused by psychological factors, such as stress or depression. It is now known that many cases of ED are caused by physical factors, including cardiovascular disease, diabetes, spinal cord injury, and damage to penile nerves during prostate surgery. Antidepressant and antihypertensive medications also can produce erectile dysfunction.

Erection results from interaction between the autonomic nervous system and penile blood vessels. Sexual arousal stimulates parasympathetic nerves in the penis to release a compound called nitric oxide (NO), which activates the vascular smooth muscle enzyme guanylyl cyclase. This enzyme catalyzes production of cyclic GMP (cGMP), a potent vasodilator that in-

creases blood flow into the penis to cause erection. Physical factors that cause ED prevent these physiologic occurrences.

Until recently, treatment options for ED, such as penile injections, vacuum pumps, and insertion of medications into the penile urethra, were inadequate, inconvenient, and painful. Today, drugs that target the physiologic mechanisms that underlie erection are giving men who suffer from ED new hope. The best known of these is sildenafil (Viagra), which works by inhibiting the enzyme that breaks down cGMP, thus prolonging the effects of NO.

Although effective in about 80% of all ED cases, Viagra can cause some relatively minor side effects, including headache, nasal congestion, stomach upset, and blue-tinged vision. Viagra should never be used by men who are taking nitrate drugs to treat angina. Because nitrate drugs elevate NO levels, taking them with Viagra, a drug that prolongs the effects of NO, can cause life-threatening hypotension.

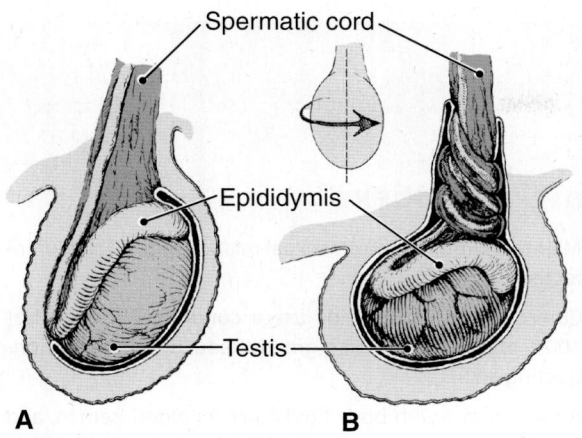

Figure 23-6 **Torsion of the testis. (A)** Normal. **(B)** Torsion. The testis rotates, twisting the spermatic cord. (Reprinted with permission from LifeART Pediatrics 1 [CD-ROM]. Baltimore: Lippincott Williams & Wilkins, 2000.)

Hernias most often occur where there is a weak area in the abdominal wall, at the inguinal canal for example. In this region, during development, the testis pushes its way through the muscles and connective tissues of the abdominal wall, carrying with it the blood vessels and other structures that form the spermatic cord.

Normally, in the adult, the inguinal area is fairly well reinforced with connective tissue, and there is no direct connection between the abdominal cavity and the scrotal sac. As in other regions where an opening permits a structure's passage through the abdominal wall, however, this area constitutes a weak place where a hernia may occur.

Phimosis (fi-MO-sis) is a tightness of the foreskin (prepuce), so that it cannot be drawn back. Phimosis may

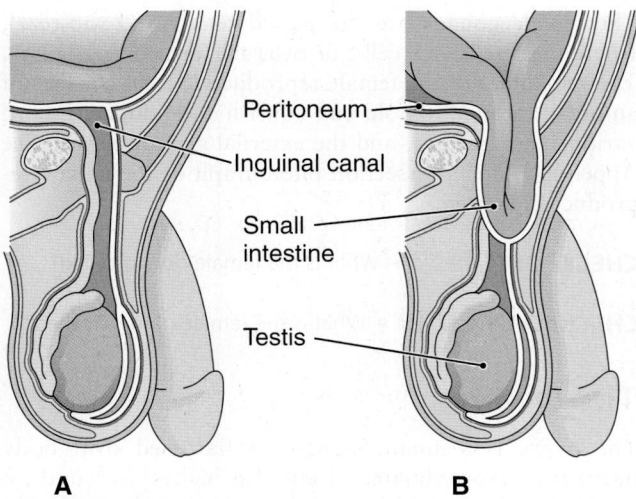

Figure 23-7 **Inguinal hernia. (A)** Normal. **(B)** Hernia. The intestine protrudes through a weakness in the abdominal wall at the inguinal canal. (Reprinted with permission from Cohen BJ. *Medical Terminology*, 4th ed. Philadelphia: Lippincott Williams & Wilkins, 2004.)

be remedied by circumcision, in which part or all of the foreskin is surgically removed.

Infections

Sexually transmitted infections (STI), formerly known as *sexually transmitted diseases* (STD) or *venereal diseases* (VD), are spread through sexual contact in both males and females. They most commonly involve chlamydial infections and gonococcal infections (gonorrhea). In males, these diseases are manifested by a discharge from the urethra, which may be accompanied by burning and pain, especially during urination. The infection may travel along the mucous membrane into the prostate gland and the epididymis; if both sides are affected and enough scar tissue is formed to destroy the tubules, sterility may result.

Another common STI is a persistent infection called **genital herpes**. Caused by a virus, this disorder is characterized by fluid-filled vesicles (blisters) on and around the genital organs.

The sexually transmitted disease **syphilis** is caused by a spirochete (*Treponema pallidum*). Because syphilis spreads quickly in the bloodstream, it is regarded as a systemic disorder (see Appendix 5, Table 1). The genital ulcers caused by syphilis increase the chances of infection with the AIDS virus. HIV itself is considered an STI because of its most common route of spread. (See Box 23-2, Sexually Transmitted Infections.)

EPIDIDYMITIS Organisms from an STI or urinary tract infection (UTI) may travel through the ducts of the reproductive system to the epididymis. A congenital malformation in the urinary tract can predispose to **epididymitis** (ep-ih-did-ih-MI-tis), and infection may also be carried to the organ systemically by blood or lymph. Treatment includes an antibiotic along with bed rest and support of the scrotum to promote lymphatic drainage.

PROSTATITIS The usual cause of prostatic inflammation is bacterial infection secondary to an ascending urinary tract infection. A variety of intestinal organisms and bacteria from other sources may be involved, but *E. coli* is the most common. Treatment with antibiotics usually clears the infection, but tests to diagnose the source of infection may be needed if the condition persists. Other possible causes of **prostatitis** (pros-tah-TI-tis) are bladder-neck obstruction that forces urine into the prostate and autoimmunity.

ORCHITIS Orchitis (or-KI-tis) is inflammation of the testis, which also may follow from infection of the urinary or reproductive tract. Mumps, a viral infection of the parotid salivary gland, may also involve the testes. A mumps infection during or after puberty may result in testicular inflammation, which could lead to sterility.

CHECKPOINT 23-8 ➤ What are some infectious diseases of the reproductive tract?

23

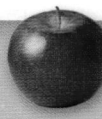

Box 23-2 Health Maintenance

Sexually Transmitted Infections: Lowering Your Risks

Sexually transmitted infections (STIs) such as chlamydia, gonorrhea, genital herpes, HIV, and syphilis are some of the most common infectious diseases in the United States, affecting more than 13 million men and women each year. These diseases are associated with complications such as pelvic inflammatory disease, epididymitis, infertility, liver failure, neurological disorders, cancer, and AIDS. Women are more likely to contract STIs than are men. The same mechanisms that transport sperm cells through the female reproductive tract also move infectious organisms. The surest way to prevent STIs is to avoid sexual contact with others. If you are sexually active, the following techniques can lower your risks:

- Maintain a monogamous sexual relationship with an uninfected partner.

- Correctly and consistently use a condom. Although not 100% effective, condoms greatly reduce the risk of contracting an STI.

- Avoid contact with body fluids such as blood, semen, and vaginal fluids, all of which may harbor infectious organisms.

- Urinate and wash the genitals after sex. This may help remove infectious organisms before they cause disease.

- Have regular checkups for STIs. Most of the time STIs cause no symptoms, particularly in women.

Tumors

Tumors of the prostate may be benign or malignant. Both types cause such pressure on the urethra that urination becomes difficult. Back pressure may destroy kidney tissue and may lead to stasis of urine in the bladder with a resulting susceptibility to infection. Men with benign prostate enlargement, known as benign prostatic hyperplasia (BPH), may respond to medication to shrink the prostate. An herbal remedy that may help to slow progress of BPH is an extract of berries of the saw palmetto, a low-growing palm tree. If urinary function is threatened, however, surgery is needed to reduce the obstruction. Traditionally, this surgery has been performed through the urethra, in a transurethral prostatectomy (TURP). Newer methods include use of laser and ultrasound to destroy excess tissue or placement of a stent to widen the urethra.

Prostatic cancer is the most common cancer of males in the United States, especially among men older than 50 years of age. Other risk factors, in addition to age, are race, family history, and certain environmental agents. A high-fat diet may increase risk by promoting production of male sex hormones. Prostatic cancer is frequently detected as a nodule during rectal examination. Early detection has improved with annual blood tests for prostate-specific antigen (PSA). This protein increases in cases of prostate cancer, although it may increase in other prostatic disorders as well. Depending on the age of the patient and the nature of the cancer, the course of treatment may include surveillance, radiation therapy, surgery, or hormone treatments.

PASSport to Success Visit *thePoint* or see the Student Resource CD in the back of this book for illustrations of prostate surgery procedures.

Testicular cancer affects young to middle-aged adults. Almost all testicular cancers arise in the germ cells, and a tumor can metastasize through the lymphatic system at an early stage of development. Early detection with regular testicular self-examination (TSE), however, improves the chances for effective treatment. The 5-year survival rate for this form of cancer is now greater than 95%. Often fertility can be preserved, although sperm banking is an option for men about to undergo treatment for testicular cancer.

The Female Reproductive System

The female gonads are the paired **ovaries** (O-vah-reze), where the female sex cells, or ova, are formed (Fig. 23-8). The remainder of the female reproductive tract consists of an organ (uterus) to hold and nourish a developing infant, various passageways, and the external genital organs. See Appendix 7 for a dissection photograph of the female reproductive system.

CHECKPOINT 23-9 ➤ What is the female gonad called?

CHECKPOINT 23-10 ➤ What is the female gamete called?

The Ovaries

The ovary is a small, somewhat flattened oval body measuring approximately 4 cm (1.6 inches) in length, 2 cm (0.8 inch) in width, and 1 cm (0.4 inch) in depth. Like the testes, the ovaries descend, but only as far as the pelvic cavity. Here, they are held in place by ligaments, including the broad ligament, the ovarian ligament, and others, that attach them to the uterus and the body wall.

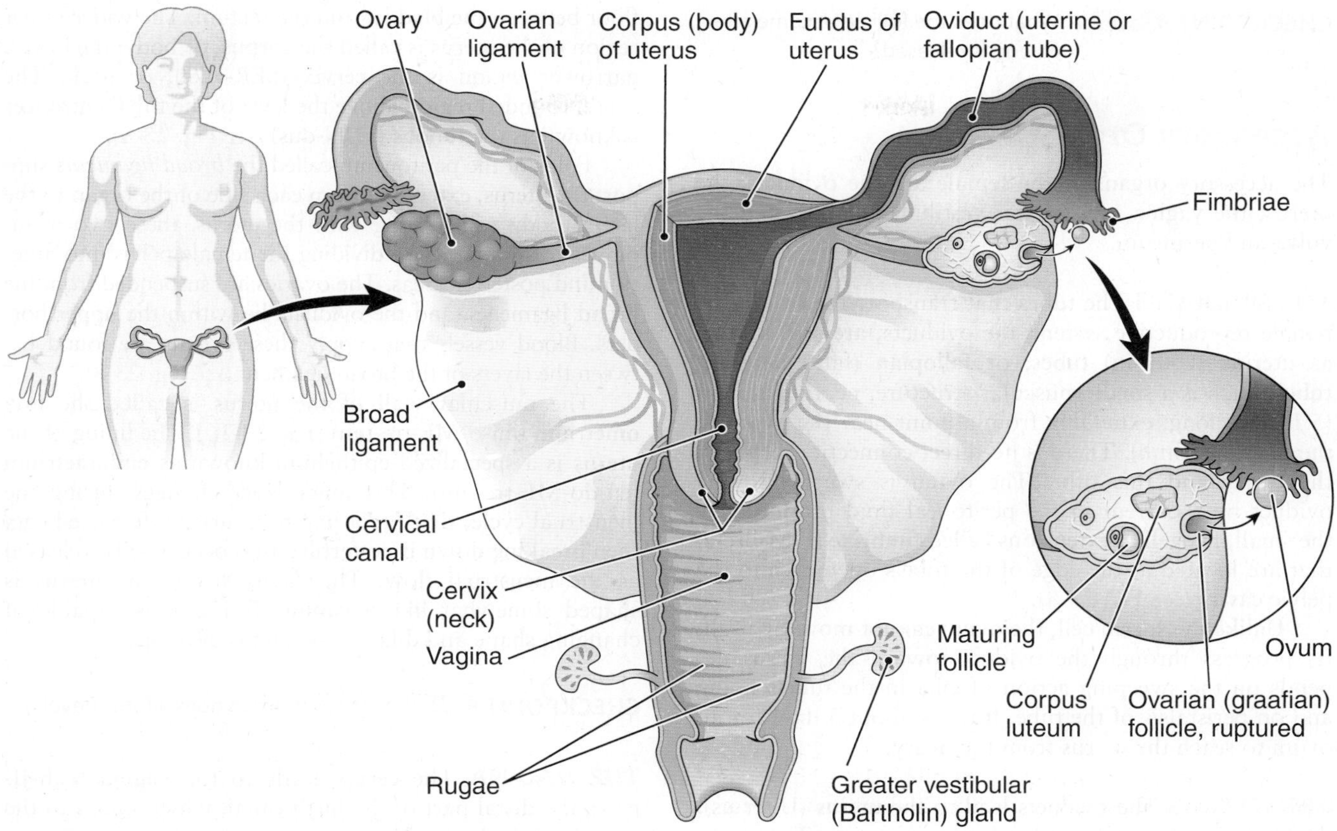

Ovary   Ovarian   Corpus (body)   Fundus of   Oviduct (uterine or
ligament   of uterus   uterus   fallopian tube)

Fimbriae

Broad
ligament

Cervical
canal

Cervix
(neck)

Vagina

Maturing
follicle

Ovum

Corpus
luteum

Ovarian (graafian)
follicle, ruptured

Rugae

Greater vestibular
(Bartholin) gland

Figure 23-8 **Female reproductive system.** The enlargement (*right*) shows ovulation. [ZOOMING IN ➤ What is the deepest part of the uterus called?]

The Ova and Ovulation

The outer layer of the ovary is made of a single layer of epithelium. Beneath this layer, the female gametes, the ova, are produced. The ovaries of a newborn female contain a large number of potential ova. Each month during the reproductive years, several ripen, but usually only one is released.

The complicated process of maturation, or "ripening," of an ovum takes place in a small fluid-filled cluster of cells called the **ovarian follicle** (o-VA-re-an FOL-ih-kl) or **graafian** (GRAF-e-an) **follicle** (Fig. 23-9). As the follicle develops, cells in its wall secrete the hormone estrogen (EStro-jen), which stimulates growth of the uterine lining. When an ovum has ripened, the ovarian follicle may rupture and discharge the egg cell from the ovary's surface. The rupture of a follicle allowing an ovum's escape into the pelvic cavity is called **ovulation** (ov-u-LA-shun). Any developing ova that are not released simply degenerate.

After it is released, the egg cell is swept into the nearest **oviduct** (O-vih-dukt), a tube that arches over the ovary and leads to the uterus (see Fig. 23-8).

CHECKPOINT 23-11 ➤ What is the structure that surrounds the egg as it ripens?

CHECKPOINT 23-12 ➤ What is the process of releasing an egg cell from the ovary called?

THE CORPUS LUTEUM After the ovum has been expelled, the remaining follicle is transformed into a solid glandular mass called the **corpus luteum** (LU-te-um). This structure secretes estrogen and also progesterone (pro-JESter-one), another hormone needed in the reproductive cycle. Commonly, the corpus luteum shrinks and is replaced by scar tissue. When a pregnancy occurs, however, this structure remains active for a while. Sometimes, as a result of normal ovulation, the corpus luteum persists and forms a small ovarian cyst (fluid-filled sac). This condition usually resolves without treatment.

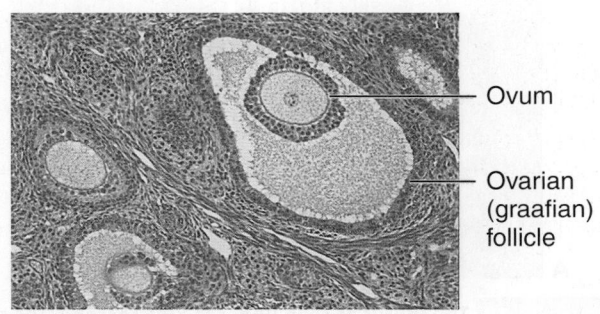

Ovum

Ovarian
(graafian)
follicle

Figure 23-9 **Microscopic view of the ovary.** The photomicrograph shows egg cells (ova) developing within ovarian (graafian) follicles. (Courtesy of Dana Morse Bittus and BJ Cohen.)

23

CHECKPOINT 23-13 ➤ What does the follicle become after its egg is released?

Accessory Organs

The accessory organs in the female are the oviducts, the uterus, the vagina, the greater vestibular glands, and the vulva and perineum.

THE OVIDUCTS The tubes that transport the ova in the female reproductive system, the oviducts, are also known as **uterine** (U-ter-in) **tubes**, or **fallopian** (fah-LO-pe-an) **tubes.** Each is a small, muscular structure, nearly 12.5 cm (5 inches) long, extending from a point near the ovary to the uterus (womb). There is no direct connection between the ovary and this tube. The ovum is swept into the oviduct by a current in the peritoneal fluid produced by the small, fringelike extensions called **fimbriae** (FIM-bre-e) that are located at the edge of the tube's opening into the pelvic cavity (see Fig. 23-8).

Unlike the sperm cell, the ovum cannot move by itself. Its progress through the oviduct toward the uterus depends on the sweeping action of cilia in the tube's lining and on peristalsis of the tube. It takes about 5 days for an ovum to reach the uterus from the ovary.

THE UTERUS The oviducts lead to the **uterus** (U-ter-us), the organ in which a fetus develops to maturity. The uterus is a pear-shaped, muscular organ approximately 7.5 cm (3 inches) long, 5 cm (2 inches) wide, and 2.5 cm (1 inch) deep. (The organ is typically larger in women who have borne children and smaller in postmenopausal women.) The superior portion rests on the upper surface of the urinary bladder; the inferior portion is embedded in the pelvic

floor between the bladder and the rectum. The wider upper region of the uterus is called the **corpus**, or body; the lower, narrower region is the **cervix** (SER-viks), or neck. The small, rounded region above the level of the tubal entrances is known as the **fundus** (FUN-dus) (see Fig. 23-8).

Folds of the peritoneum called the *broad ligaments* support the uterus, extending from each side of the organ to the lateral body wall. Along with the uterus, these two membranes form a partition dividing the female pelvis into anterior and posterior areas. The ovaries are suspended from the broad ligaments, and the oviducts lie within the upper borders. Blood vessels that supply these organs are found between the layers of the broad ligament (see Fig. 23-8).

The muscular wall of the uterus is called the **myometrium** (mi-o-ME-tre-um) (Fig. 23-10). The lining of the uterus is a specialized epithelium known as **endometrium** (en-do-ME-tre-um). This inner layer changes during the menstrual cycle, first preparing to nourish a fertilized egg, then breaking down if no fertilization occurs to be released as the menstrual flow. The cavity inside the uterus is shaped somewhat like a capital T, but it is capable of changing shape and dilating as a fetus develops.

CHECKPOINT 23-14 ➤ In what organ does a fetus develop?

THE VAGINA The cervix leads to the **vagina** (vah-JI-nah), the distal part of the birth canal, which opens to the outside of the body. The vagina is a muscular tube approximately 7.5 cm (3 inches) long. The cervix dips into the superior portion of the vagina forming a circular recess known as the **fornix** (FOR-niks). The deepest area of the fornix, located behind the cervix, is the **posterior fornix** (Fig. 23-11). This recess in the posterior vagina lies adjacent to the most inferior portion of the peritoneal cavity, a

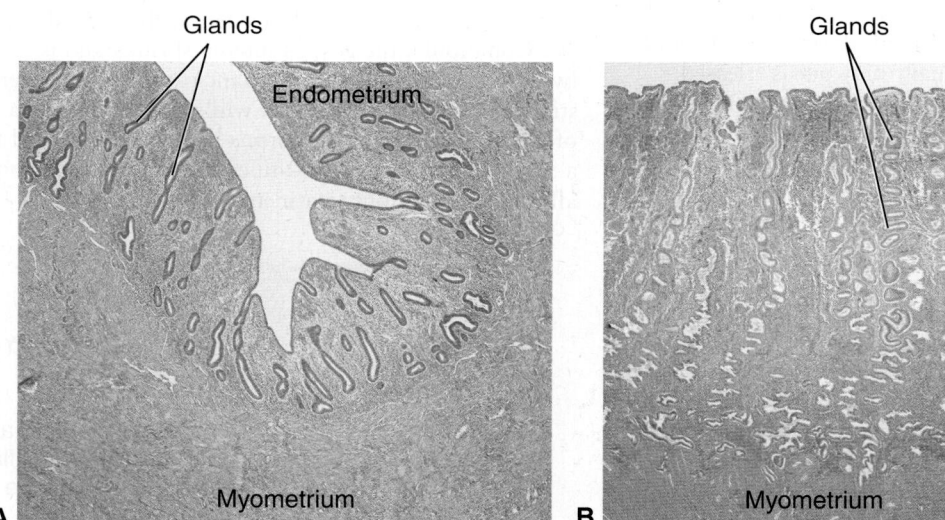

Figure 23-10 **The uterus as seen under the microscope.** The photomicrographs show the myometrium and endometrium and illustrate the changes that occur in the endometrium during the menstrual cycle. **(A)** Proliferative phase (first part of cycle). **(B)** Secretory phase (second part of cycle). (Reprinted with permission from Cormack DH. *Essential Histology*, 2nd ed. Philadelphia: Lippincott Williams & Wilkins, 2001.) [**ZOOMING IN** ➤ In which part of the menstrual cycle is the endometrium most highly developed?]

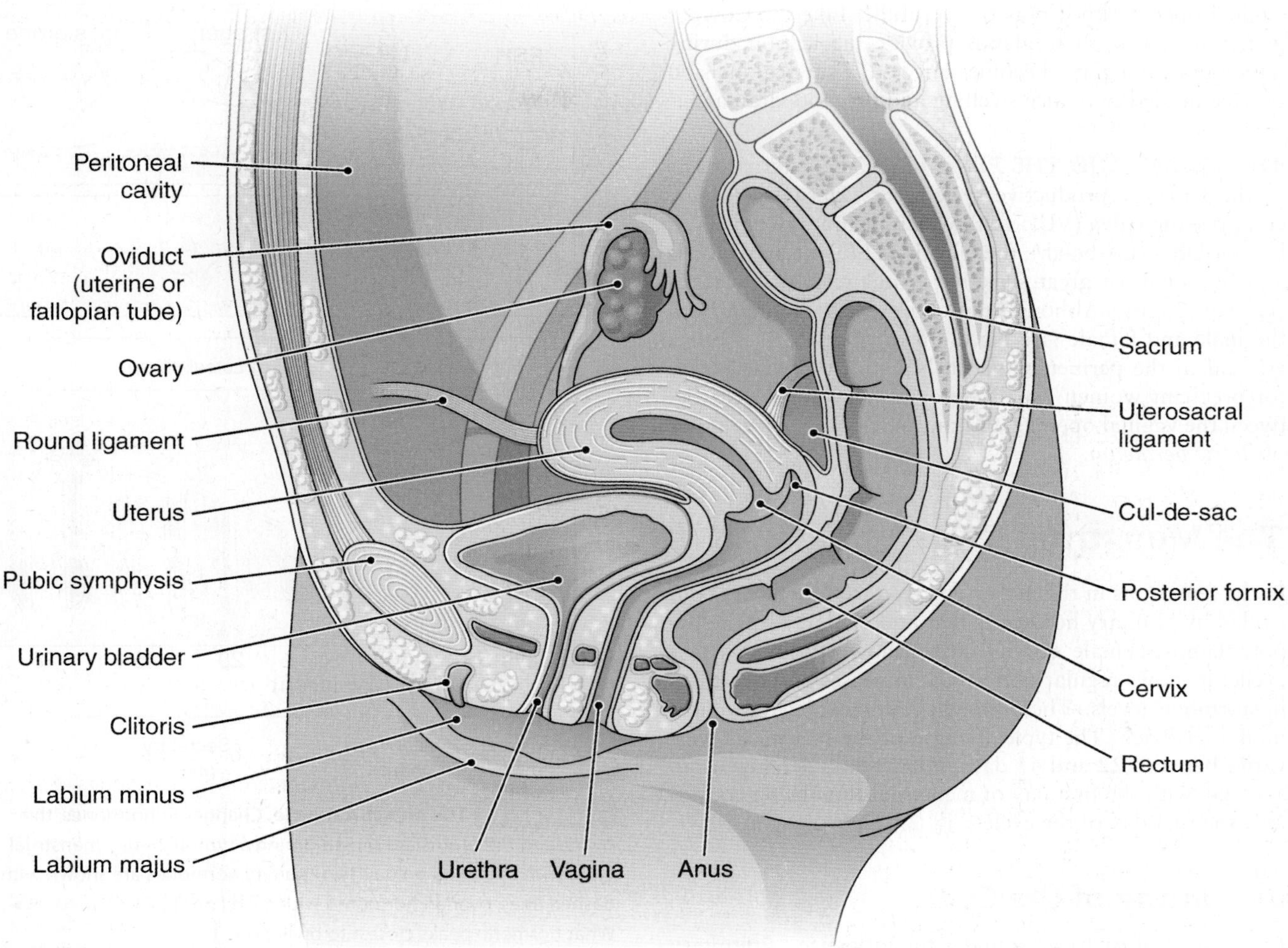

Peritoneal cavity

Oviduct (uterine or fallopian tube)

Ovary

Round ligament

Uterus

Pubic symphysis

Urinary bladder

Clitoris

Labium minus

Labium majus

Sacrum

Uterosacral ligament

Cul-de-sac

Posterior fornix

Cervix

Rectum

Urethra   Vagina   Anus

Figure 23-11 **Female reproductive system (sagittal section).** This view shows the relationship of the reproductive organs to each other and to other structures in the pelvic cavity. [**ZOOMING IN ➤** Which has the more anterior opening, the vagina or the urethra?]

narrow passage between the uterus and the rectum named the **cul-de-sac** (from the French meaning "bottom of the sack"). This area is also known as the *rectouterine pouch* or the *pouch of Douglas*. A rather thin layer of tissue separates the posterior fornix from this region, so that abscesses or tumors in the peritoneal cavity can sometimes be detected by vaginal examination.

The lining of the vagina is a wrinkled mucous membrane similar to that found in the stomach. The folds (rugae) permit enlargement so that childbirth usually does not tear the lining. In addition to being a part of the birth canal, the vagina is the organ that receives the penis during sexual intercourse. A fold of membrane called the **hymen** (HI-men) may sometimes be found at or near the vaginal (VAJ-ih-nal) canal opening (Fig. 23-12).

THE GREATER VESTIBULAR GLANDS Just superior and lateral to the vaginal opening are the two mucus-producing **greater vestibular** (ves-TIB-u-lar) **(Bartholin) glands** (see Fig. 23-8). These glands secrete into an area near the

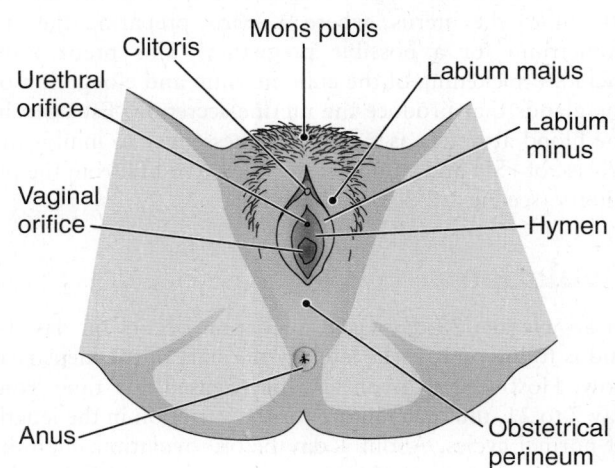

Clitoris

Urethral orifice

Vaginal orifice

Anus

Mons pubis

Labium majus

Labium minus

Hymen

Obstetrical perineum

Figure 23-12 **External parts of the female reproductive system.** Nearby structures are also shown.

23

vaginal opening known as the **vestibule**. Like the Cowper glands in males, these glands provide lubrication during intercourse. If a gland becomes infected, a surgical incision may be needed to reduce swelling and promote drainage.

THE VULVA AND THE PERINEUM The external parts of the female reproductive system, or external genitalia, comprise the **vulva** (VUL-vah), which includes two pairs of lips, or **labia** (LA-be-ah); the **clitoris** (KLIT-o-ris), which is a small organ of great sensitivity; and related structures (see Fig. 23-12). Although the entire pelvic floor in both the male and female (see Fig. 8-15 in Chapter 8) is properly called the **perineum** (per-ih-NE-um), those who care for pregnant women usually refer to the limited area between the vaginal opening and the anus as the *perineum* or *obstetric perineum*.

The Menstrual Cycle

In the female, as in the male, reproductive function is controlled by pituitary hormones that are regulated by the hypothalamus. Female activity differs, however, in that it is cyclic; it shows regular patterns of increases and decreases in hormone levels. These changes are regulated by hormonal feedback. The typical length of the menstrual cycle varies between 22 and 45 days, but 28 days is taken as an average, with the first day of menstrual flow being considered the first day of the cycle (Fig. 23-13).

Beginning of the Cycle

At the start of each cycle, under the influence of pituitary FSH, several follicles, each containing an ovum, begin to develop in the ovary. Usually, only one of these follicles will ultimately release an ovum from the ovary in a single month. The follicle produces increasing amounts of **estrogen** as it matures (see Fig. 23-13). (*Estrogen* is the term used for a group of related hormones, the most active of which is estradiol.) The estrogen is carried in the bloodstream to the uterus, where it starts preparing the endometrium for a possible pregnancy. This preparation includes thickening of the endometrium and elongation of the glands that produce the uterine secretion. Estrogen in the blood also acts as a feedback messenger to inhibit the release of FSH and stimulate the release of LH from the pituitary (see Fig. 12-3 in Chapter 12).

Ovulation

In an average 28-day cycle, ovulation occurs on day 14 and is followed 2 weeks later by the start of the menstrual flow. However, an ovum can be released any time from day 7 to 21, thus accounting for the variation in the length of normal cycles. About 1 day before ovulation, high estrogen levels cause an **LH surge**, a sharp rise of LH in the blood. (Note that there is also a small rise in FSH at this time—shown in Figure 23-13—caused by the increase in

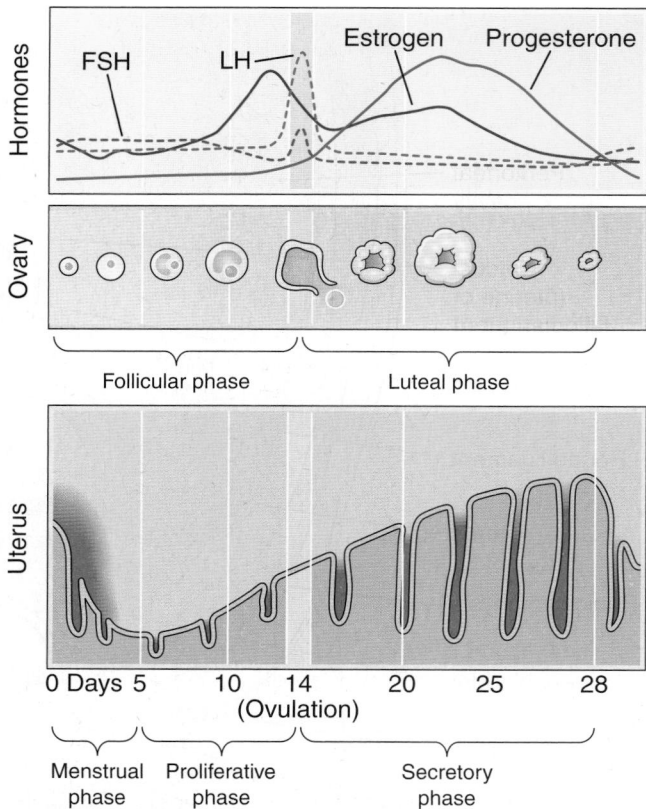

Figure 23-13 **The menstrual cycle.** Changes in hormones, the ovary, and the uterus are shown during a typical 28-day menstrual cycle with ovulation on day 14. (Pituitary hormones are shown with dashed lines, ovarian hormones with solid lines.) [ZOOMING IN ➤ What hormone peaks closest to ovulation?]

gonadotropin-releasing hormone [Gn-RH] from the hypothalamus that promotes the rise in LH.) It is LH that causes ovulation and transforms the ruptured follicle into the corpus luteum, which produces some estrogen and large amounts of **progesterone**. Under the influence of these hormones, the endometrium continues to thicken, and the glands and blood vessels increase in size. The rising levels of estrogen and progesterone feed back to inhibit the release of FSH and LH from the pituitary. During this time, the ovum makes its journey to the uterus by way of the oviduct. If the ovum is not fertilized while passing through the uterine tube, it dies within 2 to 3 days and then disintegrates.

During each menstrual cycle, changes occur in both the ovary and the uterus (see Fig. 23-13). The time before ovulation is described as the follicular phase in the ovary, because it encompasses development of the ovarian follicle. The uterus during this same time is in a proliferative phase, marked by growth of the endometrium. After ovulation, the ovary is in a luteal phase, with conversion of the follicle to the corpus luteum, and the uterus is described as being in a secretory phase, based on activity of the endometrial glands.

CHECKPOINT **23-15** ➤ What are the two hormones produced in the ovaries?

Visit **thePoint** or see the Student Resource CD in the back of this book for a summary chart on reproductive hormones and the animation *Ovulation and Fertilization.*

The Menstrual Phase

If fertilization does not occur, the corpus luteum degenerates, and the levels of estrogen and progesterone decrease. Without the hormones to support growth, the endometrium degenerates. Small hemorrhages appear in this tissue, producing the bloody discharge known as **menstrual flow**, or **menses** (MEN-seze). Bits of endometrium break away and accompany the blood flow during this period of **menstruation** (men-stru-A-shun). The average duration of menstruation is 2 to 6 days.

Even before the menstrual flow ceases, the endometrium begins to repair itself through the growth of new cells. The low levels of estrogen and progesterone allow the release of FSH from the anterior pituitary. FSH causes new follicles to begin to ripen within the ovaries, and the cycle begins anew.

The activity of ovarian hormones as negative feedback messengers is the basis of hormonal methods of contraception (birth control). Estrogen and progesterone inhibit the release of FSH and LH from the pituitary, preventing ovulation. The menstrual period that follows withdrawal of estrogen and progesterone supplementation is anovulatory, that is, it is not preceded by ovulation.

Menopause

Menopause (MEN-o-pawz) is the period during which menstruation ceases altogether. It ordinarily occurs gradually between the ages of 45 and 55 years and is caused by a normal decline in ovarian function. The ovary becomes chiefly scar tissue and no longer produces ripe follicles or appreciable amounts of estrogen. Eventually, the uterus, oviducts, vagina, and vulva all become somewhat atrophied and the vaginal mucosa becomes thinner, dryer, and more sensitive.

Menopause is an entirely normal condition, but its onset sometimes brings about effects that are temporarily disturbing. The decrease in estrogen levels can cause nervous symptoms, such as anxiety and insomnia. Because estrogen also helps maintain the vascular dilation that promotes heat loss, low levels may result in "hot flashes."

Hormone Replacement Therapy

Physicians may prescribe hormone replacement therapy (HRT) to relieve the discomforts associated with menopause. This medication is usually a combination of estrogen with a synthetic progesterone (progestin), which is included to prevent overgrowth of the endometrium and the risk of endometrial cancer. Early assumptions about the role of estrogen in preventing heart attacks have been disproved by carefully controlled studies, at least with regard to the most commonly prescribed form of HRT. The hormone therapy did lower the incidence of colorectal cancer and hip fractures, a sign of osteoporosis. Studies are continuing with estrogen alone, generally prescribed for women who have undergone a hysterectomy and do not have a uterus.

In addition to an increased risk of breast cancer, HRT also carries a risk of thrombosis and embolism, which is highest among women who smoke. All HRT risks increase with the duration of therapy. Therefore, treatment should be given for a short time and at the lowest effective dose. Women with a history or family history of breast cancer or circulatory problems should not take HRT.

CHECKPOINT **23-16** ➤ What is the definition of menopause?

Birth Control

Birth control is most commonly achieved by **contraception**, which is the use of artificial methods to prevent fertilization of the ovum. Birth control measures that prevent implantation of the fertilized ovum are also considered contraceptives, although technically they do not prevent conception and are more accurately called **abortifacients** (ah-bor-tih-FA-shents) (agents that cause abortion). Some of the birth control methods act by both mechanisms. Table 23-1 presents a brief description of the main contraceptive methods currently in use along with some advantages and disadvantages of each. The list is given in rough order of decreasing effectiveness. Unless specifically mentioned as doing so, a given method does *not* prevent the transmission of STIs.

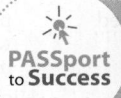

Visit **thePoint** or see the Student Resource CD in the back of this book for an illustration of surgical sterilization.

The various hormonal methods of birth control basically differ in how they administer the hormones. The emergency contraceptive pill (ECP) is a synthetic progesterone (progestin) taken within 72 hours after intercourse, usually in two doses 12 hours apart. It reduces the risk of pregnancy following unprotected intercourse. This so-called "morning after pill" is intended for emergency use and not as a regular birth control method. Birth control hormones can also be implanted as capsules under the skin of the upper arm. This method is highly effective and lasts for 3 to 5 years, but the capsules must be implanted and removed by a health professional, and they have been difficult to remove in some cases.

Researchers have done trials with a male contraceptive pill, but none is on the market as yet. The male version

23

| Table 23-1 | Main Methods of Birth Control Currently in Use |

Method	Description	Advantages	Disadvantages
Surgical			
Vasectomy/tubal ligation	Cutting and tying of tubes carrying gametes	Nearly 100% effective; involves no chemical or mechanical devices	Not usually reversible; rare surgical complications
Hormonal			
Birth control pills	Estrogen and progestin, or progestin alone, taken orally to prevent ovulation	Highly effective; requires no last-minute preparation	Alters physiology; return to fertility may be delayed; risk of cardiovascular disease in older women who smoke or have hypertension
Birth control shot	Injection of synthetic progesterone every 3 months to prevent ovulation	Highly effective; lasts for 3 to 4 months	Alters physiology; same possible side effects as birth control pill; also possible menstrual irregularity, amenorrhea
Birth control patch	Adhesive patch placed on body that administers estrogen and progestin through the skin; left on for 3 weeks and removed for a fourth week	Protects long-term; less chance of incorrect use; no last-minute preparation	Alters physiology; same possible side effects as birth control pill
Birth control ring	Flexible ring inserted into vagina that releases hormones internally; left in place for 3 weeks and removed for a fourth week	Long-lasting; highly effective; no last-minute preparation	Possible infections, irritation; same possible side effects as birth control pill
Barrier			
Male condom	Sheath that fits over erect penis and prevents release of semen	Easily available, does not affect physiology; protects against sexually transmitted infection (STI)	Must be applied just before intercourse; may slip or tear
Diaphragm (with spermicide)	Rubber cap that fits over cervix and prevents entrance of sperm	Does not affect physiology; some protection against STI; no side effects	Must be inserted before intercourse and left in place for 6 hours; requires fitting by physician
Contraceptive sponge (with spermicide)	Soft, disposable foam disk containing spermicide, which is moistened with water and inserted into the vagina	Protects against pregnancy for 24 hours; non-hormonal; some STI protection; available without prescription; inexpensive	85%–90% effective depending on proper use; possible skin irritation
Intrauterine device (IUD)	Metal or plastic device inserted into uterus through vagina; prevents fertilization and implantation by release of copper or birth control hormones	Highly effective for 5–10 years depending on type; reversible; no last-minute preparation	Must be introduced and removed by health professional; heavy menstrual bleeding
Other			
Spermicide	Chemicals used to kill sperm; best when used in combination with a barrier method	Available without prescription; inexpensive; does not affect physiology; some protection against STI	May cause local irritation; must be used just before intercourse
Fertility awareness	Abstinence during fertile part of cycle as determined by menstrual history, basal body temperature, or quality of cervical mucus	Does not affect physiology; accepted by certain religions	High failure rate; requires careful record-keeping

of "the pill" also works by suppressing GnRH to inhibit release of FSH and LH, which are important in spermatogenesis. Use of testosterone as a negative feedback messenger requires regular injections and has some undesirable side effects at the doses needed. Administration of the female hormone progesterone prevents spermatogenesis, but also inhibits normal testosterone production. Studies are ongoing to find the best way to deliver the right male contraceptive hormones at safe and effective doses.

The female condom is a sheath that fits into the vagina. It does protect against STIs, but is not very convenient to use. Mifepristone (RU 486) is a drug taken after conception to terminate an early pregnancy. It blocks the action of progesterone, causing the uterus to shed its lining and release the fertilized egg. It must be combined with administration of prostaglandins to expel the uterine tissue. Mifepristone is not in widespread use in the United States, but it has been used in other countries.

CHECKPOINT **23-17** ➤ What is the definition of contraception?

Disorders of the Female Reproductive System

Female reproductive disorders include menstrual disturbances, various forms of tumors, and infections, any of which can contribute to infertility.

Menstrual Disorders

Absence of menstrual flow is known as **amenorrhea** (ah-men-o-RE-ah). This condition can be symptomatic of insufficient hormone secretion or congenital abnormality of the reproductive organs. Stress and other psychological factors often play a part in cessation of the menstrual flow. For example, any significant change in a woman's general state of health or change in her living habits, such as a shift in working hours, can interfere with menstruation. Very low body weight with a low percentage of body fat can lead to amenorrhea by reducing estrogen synthesis, as may occur in athletes who overtrain without eating enough and in women who are starving or have eating disorders.

Dysmenorrhea (dis-men-o-RE-ah) means painful or difficult menstruation. In young women, this may be due to immaturity of the uterus. Often, the pain can be relieved by drugs that block prostaglandins, because some prostaglandins are known to cause painful uterine contractions.

In many cases, women have been completely relieved of menstrual cramps by their first pregnancies. Apparently, enlargement of the cervical opening remedies the condition. Artificial dilation of the cervical opening may alleviate dysmenorrhea for several months. Often, such health measures as sufficient rest, a well-balanced diet, and appropriate exercise remedy the disorder. In cases of dysmenorrhea, the application of heat over the abdomen may relieve the pain, just as it may ease other types of muscular cramps.

Another possible cause of menstrual disorders is **endometriosis** (en-do-me-tre-O-sis). This is growth of endometrial tissue outside the uterus, commonly on the ovaries, oviducts, peritoneum, or other pelvic organs. Endometriosis results in inflammation and other complications and may require surgical removal.

Abnormal uterine bleeding includes excessive menstrual flow, too-frequent menstruation, and nonmenstrual bleeding. Any of these may cause serious anemias and deserve careful medical attention. Nonmenstrual bleeding may be an indication of a tumor, possibly cancer.

Premenstrual syndrome (PMS), also called **premenstrual tension**, is a condition in which nervousness, irritability, and depression precede the menstrual period. It is thought to be caused by fluid retention in various tissues, including the brain. Sometimes, a low-salt diet and appropriate medication for 2 weeks before the menses prevent this disorder. This treatment may also avert dysmenorrhea.

Benign and Malignant Tumors

Fibroids, which are more correctly called *myomas*, are common tumors of the uterus. Studies indicate that about 50% of women who reach the age of 50 have one or more of these growths in the uterine wall. Often, these tumors are small; they usually remain benign and produce no symptoms. They develop between puberty and menopause and ordinarily stop growing after a woman has reached the age of 50. In some cases, these growths interfere with pregnancy. In a patient younger than 40 years of age, a surgeon may simply remove the tumor and leave the uterus fairly intact. Normal pregnancies have occurred after such surgery.

Fibroids may become so large that pressure on adjacent structures causes problems. Sometimes, invasion of blood vessels near the uterine cavity causes serious hemorrhages. Treatment may be suppression of hormones that stimulate fibroid development, blocking blood supply to the fibroid, or surgical removal of the growth. In some cases, surgeons may need to remove the entire uterus or a large part of it, a procedure called a **hysterectomy** (his-ter-EK-to-me).

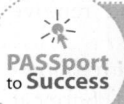 **PASSport to Success** Visit **thePoint** or see the Student Resource CD in the back of this book for an illustration of possible fibroid formation sites.

BREAST CANCER Cancer of the breast is the most commonly occurring malignant disease in women. The risk factors in breast cancer are age past 40, family history of breast cancer, and factors that increase exposure to estrogen, such as early onset of menstruation, late menopause, late or no pregnancies, long-term HRT, and obesity (fat cells produce estrogen). Mutations in two genes (BRCA1 and BRCA2) are responsible for hereditary forms of breast cancer, which make up only about 8% of all cases. These

23

Disease in Context revisited

▶ Sylvie's Myomectomy

Dr. Bernard visited Sylvie in the outpatient recovery room to discuss the results of her myomectomy. "The procedure was successful," he reported. "We were able to remove the fibroid completely and repair the uterus with a hysteroscope, a type of endoscope. There are several methods available now to avoid hysterectomy in cases of myomas, and many people believe you should preserve the uterus if possible, even after child-bearing years. If fibroids are larger, or more numerous, or in certain other locations in the uterus, we sometimes need to use a laparoscope or do an abdominal incision. But you're fine for now. Take it easy for the rest of the week, and don't drive for a couple of days. Call my office if you have any pain or bleeding. You should schedule a check-up in 6 months to see how you are doing."

"Thanks Doctor," Sylvie said. "I feel pretty good right now, so I assume I'll be fine. I'll be sure to let you know if I'm not."

Sylvie's case contains medical terms that can be divided into standardized parts. Each chapter in this book contains a section on "word anatomy" that gives the meanings of the prefixes, roots, and suffixes used in the chapter. Knowledge of these word elements helps you to remember scientific terms and to make guesses about the meaning of new terms. You can find the definitions of many scientific word parts in a good dictionary.

---

same genetic mutations are associated with an increased risk of ovarian cancer.

A breast tumor is usually a painless, movable mass that is often noticed by a woman and all too frequently ignored. In recent years, however, there has been increasing emphasis on the importance of regular breast self-examination (BSE). (Most breast lumps are discovered by women themselves.) Any lump, no matter how small, should be reported to a physician immediately. The **mammogram**, a radiographic study of the breast, has improved the detection of early breast cancer. Guidelines recommend regular mammograms after the age of 40 years, and earlier if there is a family history of breast cancer. Some physicians now recommend adding MRI scans for high-risk patients. Suspicious areas require further study by ultrasonography or biopsy (either a needle aspiration, removal of a core of tissue, or excision of the lump). In a stereotactic biopsy, a physician uses a computer-guided imaging system to locate suspicious tissue and remove samples with a needle.

Breast cancer treatment consists of surgery with follow-up therapy of radiation, chemotherapy, or both. Surgical treatment by removal of the lump ("lumpectomy") or a segment of the breast is most common. Removal of the entire breast and dissection of the lymph nodes in the axilla (armpit) is called **modified radical mastectomy** (mas-TEK-to-me). The extent of tumor spread through the lymph nodes is an important factor in prognosis. In a sentinel lymph node biopsy, the first (sentinel) lymph nodes to receive lymph from the tumor are identified and tested for cancerous cells. Treatment is based on how much spread has occurred (see Box 16-2). Treatment of breast cancer is often followed by administration of drugs that inhibit estrogen production or block estrogen receptors in breast tissue (if the tumor responds to that hormone), or drugs that inhibit tumor growth factors.

Note that the incidence of the various types of cancer should not be confused with the death rates for each type. Owing to education of the public and increasingly better methods of diagnosis and treatment, some forms of cancer have a higher cure rate than others. For example, breast cancer appears much more often in women than does lung cancer, but more women now die each year from lung cancer than from breast cancer.

ENDOMETRIAL CANCER The most common cancer of the female reproductive tract is cancer of the endometrium (the lining of the uterus). This type of cancer usually affects women during or after menopause. It is seen most frequently in women who have been exposed to high levels of estrogen, which causes overgrowth of the endometrium. This group includes those who have received estrogen therapy unopposed by progesterone, those who have had few or no pregnancies, and the obese. Symptoms include an abnormal discharge or irregular bleeding; later, there is cramping and pelvic pain. This type of cancer is diagnosed by endometrial biopsy. The usual methods of treatment include surgery and irradiation. Endometrial cancer grows slowly in its beginning stages, so early, aggressive treatment usually saves a patient's life.

OVARIAN CANCER Ovarian cancer is the second most common reproductive tract cancer in the female, usually occurring in women between the ages of 40 and 65 years. It is a leading cause of cancer deaths in women. Although most ovarian cysts are not malignant, they should always be investigated for possible malignant change. Ovarian cancer is highly curable if treated before it has spread to other organs. However, these malignancies tend to progress rapidly, and they are difficult to detect because symptoms are vague, there are few recognized risk factors, and at present there is no reliable screening test.

CERVICAL CANCER Cancer of the cervix is linked to infection with human papilloma virus (HPV), which causes genital warts and is spread through sexual contact. Thus, cervical cancer can be considered a sexually transmitted disease. Risk factors for the disease are related to exposure to HPV, such as early age of sexual activity and multiple sex partners. Certain strains of the virus are found in cervical carcinomas and precancerous cervical cells.

Early detection is often possible because the cancer develops slowly from atypical cervical cells. The decline in the death rate from cervical cancer is directly related to use of the **Papanicolaou** (pap-ah-nik-o-LAH-o) **test**, also known as the *Pap test* or *Pap smear*. The Pap smear is a microscopic examination of cells obtained from cervical scrapings and swabs of the cervical canal. All women should be encouraged to have this test every year. Even girls younger than 18 years of age should be tested if they are sexually active. Guidelines now recommend less frequent testing after normal results are obtained in three annual tests.

A vaccine against the most prevalent HPV strains is recommended for females from 11 to 12 years of age.

Infections

Infections that affect the male reproductive system also infect the female genital organs (Fig. 23-14), although these diseases may be less apparent in women. The most common STIs in women are chlamydial infections, gonorrhea, HIV, and genital herpes, caused by herpes simplex virus (HSV). Syphilis also occurs in women and can be passed through the placenta from mother to fetus, causing stillbirth or birth of an infected infant.

The incidence of **genital warts**, caused by human papillomavirus (HPV), has increased in recent years. These infections have been linked to cancer of the reproductive tract, especially, as noted, cancer of the uterine cervix.

Salpingitis (sal-pin-JI-tis) means inflammation of any tube, but usually refers to disease of the uterine tubes (oviducts). Most uterine tube infections are caused by gonococci or by the bacterium *Chlamydia trachomatis*, but other bacteria may be the cause. Salpingitis may lead to sterility by obstructing the tubes, thus preventing the passage of ova.

Pelvic inflammatory disease (PID) results from extension of infections from the reproductive organs into the pelvic cavity, and it often involves the peritoneum. (See the purple arrow pathway in Fig. 23-14.) Gonococcus or chlamydia is usually the initial cause of infection, but most cases of PID involve multiple organisms.

Infertility

Infertility is much more difficult to diagnose and evaluate in women than in men. Whereas a microscopic examination of properly collected semen may be enough to determine the presence of abnormal or too few sperm cells in the male, no such simple study can be made in the female. Infertility in women, as in men, may be relative or absolute. Causes of female infertility include infections, endocrine disorders, psychogenic factors, and abnormalities in the structure and function of the reproductive organs themselves. In all cases of apparent infertility, the male partner should be investigated first because the procedures for determining lack of fertility in the male are much simpler and less costly than those in the female, as well as being essential for the evaluation.

PASSport to Success

Clinics and medical offices may employ physician assistants. Visit **thePoint** or see the Student Resource CD in the back of this book for a description of this career.

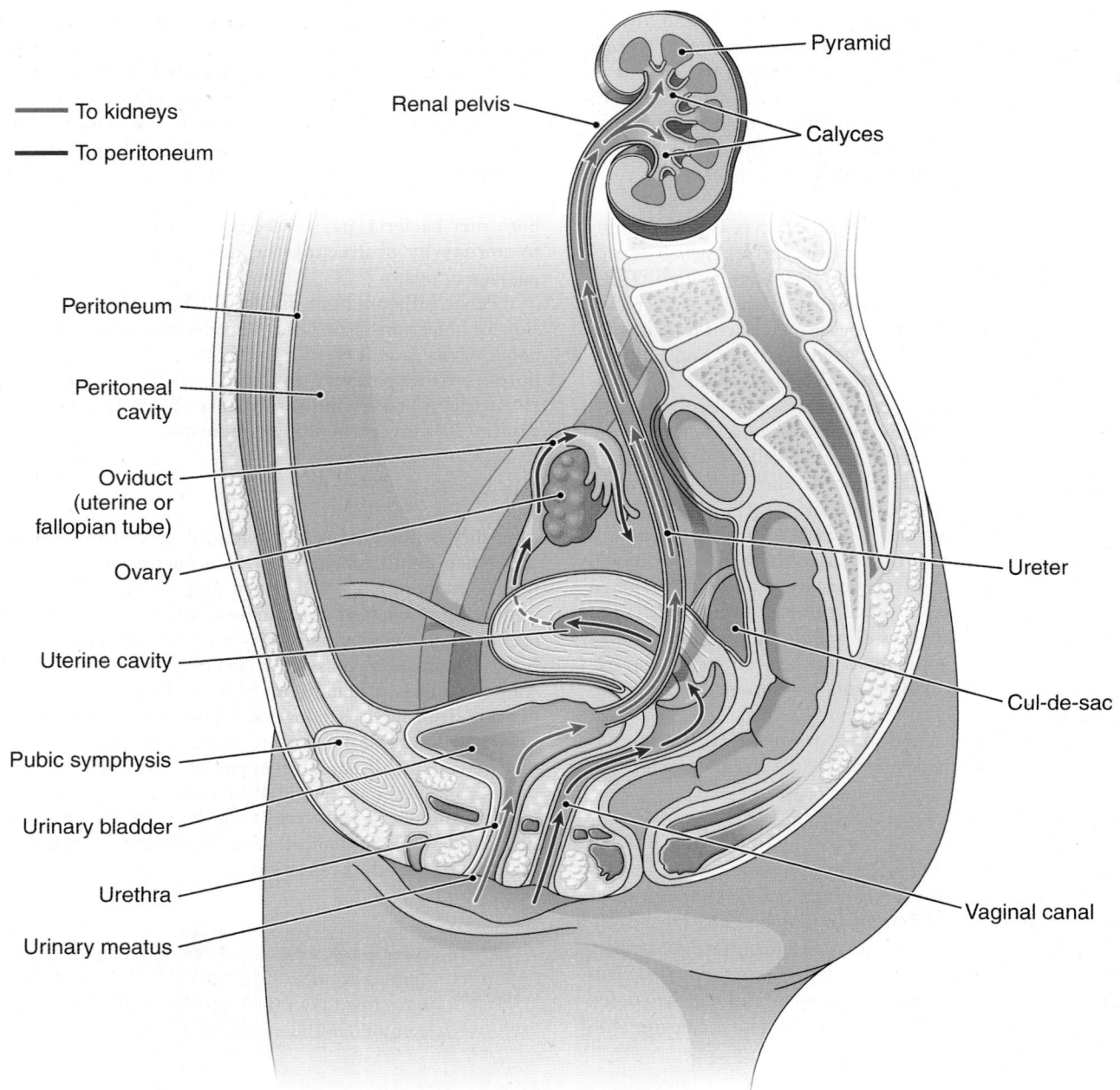

— To kidneys
— To peritoneum

Pyramid

Renal pelvis

Calyces

Peritoneum

Peritoneal cavity

Oviduct (uterine or fallopian tube)

Ovary

Uterine cavity

Pubic symphysis

Urinary bladder

Urethra

Urinary meatus

Ureter

Cul-de-sac

Vaginal canal

Figure 23-14 **Pathway of infection.** Disease organisms can travel from outside to the peritoneum and into the urinary system.

Word Anatomy

Medical terms are built from standardized word parts (prefixes, roots, and suffixes). Learning the meanings of these parts can help you remember words and interpret unfamiliar terms.

WORD PART	MEANING	EXAMPLE
The Male Reproductive System		
semin/o	semen, seed	Sperm cells are produced in the *seminiferous* tubules.
test/o	testis	The hormone *testosterone* is produced in the testis.
acr/o	extremity, end	The *acrosome* covers the head of a sperm cell.
fer	to carry	The ductus *deferens* carries spermatozoa away from (de-) the testis.
circum-	around	A cut is made around the glans to remove part of the foreskin in a *circumcision*.
Disorders of the Male Reproductive System		
oligo/o-	few, deficiency	*Oligospermia* is a deficiency in the numbers of spermatozoa produced.
crypto/o-	hidden	*Cryptorchidism* refers to an undescended testis (orchid/o).
orchid/o, orchi/o	testis	*Orchiectomy* is removal of the testis.
The Female Reproductive System		
ov/o, ov/i	egg	An *ovum* is an egg cell.
ovar, ovari/o	ovary	The *ovarian* follicle encloses a maturing ovum.
metr/o	uterus	The *myometrium* is the muscular (my/o) layer of the uterus.
rect/o	rectum	The *rectouterine* pouch is between the uterus and rectum.
Disorders of the Female Reproductive System		
men/o	uterine bleeding; menses	*Amenorrhea* is absence of menstrual flow.
hyster/o	uterus	*Hysterectomy* is surgical removal of the uterus.
mamm/o	breast, mammary gland	A *mammogram* is radiographic study of the breast.
mast/o	breast	A *mastectomy* is surgical removal of the breast.
salping/o	tube	*Salpingitis* is inflammation of a tube, such as the oviduct.

Summary

I. **REPRODUCTION**
   A. Meiosis—reduces chromosome number from 46 to 23
      1. Gametes (sex cells)
         a. Spermatozoa (sperm cells)—male
         b. Ova (egg cells)—female

II. **MALE REPRODUCTIVE SYSTEM**
   A. Primary organs—gonads
   B. Accessory organs—ducts and exocrine glands

C. Testes
   1. Scrotum—sac that holds the testes
   2. Inguinal canal—channel through which testis descends
   3. Internal structure
      a. Seminiferous tubules—tubes in which sperm cells are produced
         (1) Sustentacular (Sertoli) cells—aid in development of spermatozoa

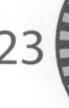
23

b. Interstitial cells (between tubules)—secrete hormones

4. Testosterone—main male hormone
   a. Maintains reproductive structures
   b. Aids development of secondary sex characteristics

5. Spermatozoa
   a. Head—contains chromosomes
   b. Acrosome—covers head; has enzymes to help penetration of ovum
   c. Midpiece—contains mitochondria
   d. Tail (flagellum)—propels sperm

D. Accessory organs
   1. Epididymis—stores spermatozoa until ejaculation
   2. Ductus (vas) deferens—conducts sperm cells through spermatic cord
   3. Ejaculatory duct—empties into urethra

E. Semen
   1. Functions
      a. Nourish spermatozoa
      b. Transport spermatozoa
      c. Neutralize male urethra and vaginal tract
      d. Lubricate reproductive tract during intercourse
      e. Prevent infection
   2. Glands
      a. Seminal vesicles
      b. Prostate—around first portion of urethra
      c. Bulbourethral (Cowper) glands

F. Urethra and penis
   1. Urethra
      a. Conveys urine and semen through penis
   2. Penis
      a. Structure
         (1) Corpus spongiosum—central; contains urethra
         (2) Corpora cavernosa—lateral
         (3) Glands—distal enlargement of corpus spongiosum
         (4) Prepuce—foreskin
      b. Erection—stiffening and enlargement of penis
   3. Ejaculation—forceful expulsion of semen

III. **HORMONAL CONTROL OF MALE REPRODUCTION**
   A. Pituitary hormones
      1. FSH (follicle stimulating hormone)
         a. Stimulates Sertoli cells
         b. Promotes formation of spermatozoa
      2. LH (luteinizing hormone)
         a. Stimulates interstitial cells to produce testosterone
   B. Effects of aging on male reproduction
      1. Decline in testosterone, spermatozoa, and semen

IV. **DISORDERS OF THE MALE REPRODUCTIVE SYSTEM**
   A. Infertility—lower than normal ability to reproduce
   B. Structural disorders
      1. Cryptorchidism—failure of testis to descend

2. Torsion of the testis—twisting of spermatic cord
3. Inguinal hernia
4. Phimosis—tightness of the foreskin

C. Infections
   1. Sexually transmitted infections (STI)
   2. Epididymitis—inflammation of the epididymis
   3. Prostatitis—inflammation of the prostate
   4. Orchitis—inflammation of the testis

D. Tumors
   1. Tumors of the prostate
      a. Benign prostatic hyperplasia (BPH)
   2. Cancer of the testis

V. **FEMALE REPRODUCTIVE SYSTEM**
   A. Ovaries—gonads in which ova form
   B. Ova and ovulation
      1. Egg ripens in graafian follicle
      2. Ovulation—release of ovum from ovary
      3. Corpus luteum
         a. Remainder of follicle in ovary
         b. Continues to function if egg fertilized
         c. Disintegrates if egg not fertilized
   C. Accessory organs
      1. Oviducts (uterine tubes, fallopian tubes)
         a. Fimbriae—fringelike extensions that sweep egg into oviduct
      2. Uterus
         a. Holds developing fetus
         b. Supported by broad ligament
         c. Endometrium—lining of uterus
         d. Myometrium—muscle layer
         e. Cervix—narrow, lower part
      3. Vagina
         a. Tube connecting uterus to outside
         b. Hymen—fold of membrane over vaginal opening
         c. Greater vestibular (Bartholin) glands—secrete mucus
      4. Vulva and perineum
         a. Vulva—external genitalia
            (1) Labia—two sets of folds (majora, minora)
            (2) Clitoris—organ of great sensitivity
         b. Perineum—pelvic floor
            (1) In obstetrics—area between vagina and anus

VI. **MENSTRUAL CYCLE**
   A. Average 28 days
   B. Beginning of the cycle
      1. FSH stimulates follicle—follicular phase
      2. Follicle secretes estrogen
      3. Estrogen thickens lining of uterus—proliferative phase
   C. Ovulation
      1. LH surge 1 day before
      2. Corpus luteum produces progesterone—luteal phase

3. Progesterone continues growth of endometrium—secretory phase
4. Ovum disintegrates if not fertilized

D. Menstrual phase (menstruation)
1. If egg not fertilized, corpus luteum degenerates
2. Lining of uterus breaks down releasing menses

VII. **MENOPAUSE**
   A. Period during which menstuation stops
   B. Hormone replacement therapy (HRT)
   1. Reduces adverse symptoms of menopause
   2. Risks of HRT—cardiovascular disorders, breast cancer

VIII. **BIRTH CONTROL**
   A. Contraception—use of artificial methods to prevent fertilization or implantation of fertilized egg
   B. Methods—surgery, hormonal, barrier, IUD, spermicides, fertility awareness

IX. **DISORDERS OF THE FEMALE REPRODUCTIVE SYSTEM**
   A. Menstrual disorders
   1. Amenorrhea—absence of menstrual flow
   2. Dysmenorrhea—painful or difficult menstruation

3. Abnormal uterine bleeding
4. Premenstrual syndrome

B. Benign and malignant tumors
1. Fibroids (myomas)—common tumors of uterus
2. Breast cancer
   a. Mammogram—radiographic study of the breast
   b. Mastectomy—removal of breast or breast tissue
3. Endometrial cancer—cancer of uterine lining
4. Ovarian cancer
5. Cervical cancer—due to human papilloma virus (HPV) infection
   a. Pap test (smear) for cervical cancer

D. Infections
1. Sexually transmitted infections
2. Genital warts—caused by HPV
3. Salpingitis—inflammation of uterine tubes
4. Pelvic inflammatory disease (PID)

E. Infertility

Review

BUILDING UNDERSTANDING

Fill in the blanks

1. Gametes go through a special process of cell division called _____.

2. Spermatozoa begin their development in tiny coiled _____.

3. An ovum matures in a small fluid-filled cluster of cells called the _____.

4. Failure of the testis to descend into the scrotum results in the disorder _____.

5. Surgical removal of the uterus is called a(n) _____.

Matching > Match each numbered item with the most closely related lettered item.

___ **6.** A hormone released by the pituitary that promotes follicular development in the ovary

___ **7.** A hormone released by developing follicles that promotes thickening of the endometrium

___ **8.** A hormone released by the pituitary that stimulates ovulation

___ **9.** A hormone released by the corpus luteum that promotes thickening of the endometrium

a. follicle stimulating hormone

b. estrogen

c. luteinizing hormone

d. progesterone

23

Multiple choice

___ **10.** A month or two before birth, the testis travels from the abdominal cavity to the scrotum through the

    a. spermatic cord
    b. inguinal canal
    c. seminiferous tubule
    d. vas deferens

___ **11.** Enzymes that help the sperm cell to penetrate the ovum are found in the

    a. acrosome
    b. head
    c. midpiece
    d. flagellum

___ **12.** Inflammation of the testis is called

    a. phimosis
    b. epididymitis
    c. prostatitis
    d. orchitis

___ **13.** The uterus and ovaries are supported by the

    a. uterine tubes
    b. broad ligaments
    c. fimbriae
    d. fornix

___ **14.** The area between the vaginal opening and the anus is referred to as the

    a. vestibule
    b. vulva
    c. hymen
    d. perineum

___ **15.** The most common site of cancer in the female reproductive tract is the

    a. endometrium
    b. myometrium
    c. ovaries
    d. cervix

UNDERSTANDING CONCEPTS

16. Compare and contrast the following terms:

    a. asexual reproduction and sexual reproduction
    b. spermatozoa and ova
    c. sustentacular cell and interstitial cell
    d. ovarian follicle and corpus luteum
    e. myometrium and endometrium

17. Trace the pathway of sperm from the site of production to the urethra.

18. Describe the components of semen, their sites of production, and their functions.

19. List the hormones that control male reproduction and state their functions.

20. Trace the pathway of an ovum from the site of production to the site of implantation.

21. Beginning with the first day of the menstrual flow, describe the events of one complete cycle, including the role of the hormones involved.

22. Define *contraception*. Describe methods of contraception that involve (1) barriers; (2) chemicals; (3) hormones; (4) prevention of implantation.

23. Compare and contrast the following disorders:

    a. epididymitis and prostatitis
    b. benign prostatic hyperplasia and prostatic cancer
    c. amenorrhea and dysmenorrhea
    d. fibroids and endometrial cancer
    e. ovarian cancer and cervical cancer

CONCEPTUAL THINKING

24. Theoretically, it is possible for a brain-dead man to ejaculate. What anatomical and physiological feature makes this possible?

25. Nicole, a middle-aged mother of three, is considering a tubal ligation, a contraceptive procedure that involves cutting the uterine tubes. Nicole is worried that this might cause her to enter early menopause. Should she be worried?

26. Sylvie's case involves a myoma. Define a myoma. Identify the two word parts in the term *myoma* and give the meaning of each. Identify and define the word parts in other terms used in the case history and the remainder of the chapter, including fibroid, myomectomy, hysteroscope, and laparoscope.

23

CHAPTER 24

Development and Birth

Learning Outcomes

After careful study of this chapter, you should be able to:

1. Describe fertilization and the early development of the fertilized egg
2. Describe the structure and function of the placenta
3. Describe how fetal circulation differs from adult circulation
4. Briefly describe changes that occur in the fetus and the mother during pregnancy
5. Briefly describe the four stages of labor
6. Compare fraternal and identical twins
7. Cite the advantages of breastfeeding
8. Describe several disorders associated with pregnancy, childbirth, and lactation
9. Show how word parts are used to build words related to development and birth (see Word Anatomy at the end of the chapter)

Selected Key Terms

The following terms and other boldface terms in the chapter are defined in the Glossary

abortion
amniotic sac
embryo
fertilization
fetus
gestation
human chorionic gonadotropin (hCG)
implantation
lactation
oxytocin
parturition
placenta
prolactin
umbilical cord
zygote

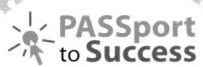

PASSport to Success

Visit *thePoint* or see the Student Resource CD in the back of this book for definitions and pronunciations of key terms as well as a pretest for this chapter.

Disease in Context

> Sue's Third Case: Emma's Arrival

"Your reflexes are fine," said Sue's neurologist. "Have you had any unusual symptoms since your last appointment?"

"No," replied Sue. "I feel really good. My MS hasn't been a problem lately."

"That's excellent," replied the neurologist. "I'll write a refill for your medications—is there anything else for you today?"

"Actually, there is," replied Sue. She told her doctor that she and her husband were thinking about starting a family, but were concerned about the potential negative effects of multiple sclerosis on fetal development. Sue also worried that pregnancy might aggravate the neurological disorder.

"There's no evidence that multiple sclerosis negatively affects pregnancy, labor, or delivery, nor does it pose significant risks to the fetus," replied the neurologist. "Pregnancy doesn't seem to have a negative effect on MS either. In fact, many women with MS find that their symptoms actually lessen during pregnancy, especially in the second and third trimesters. We think this is because a pregnant woman's ovaries produce hormones, like progesterone, that act as natural immunosuppressants, preventing her body from rejecting her fetus. Most women do report an in increase in the frequency and severity of their MS symptoms in the first 6 months postpartum. And as you already know, future flare-ups may cause increased fatigue, and pose physical limitations. It will be important for you and your husband to look ahead and make sure you have the resources and people you can rely on for support."

"When you and your husband feel ready to conceive," the doctor continued, "You'll need to come and see me so we can adjust your medications. Unfortunately, corticosteroids and interferon can cross the placenta and have adverse effects on fetal development. Like any other woman in childbearing years, you should also start taking a folic acid supplement. This has been shown to lower the risk of embryonic neural tube defects like spina bifida."

Sue is relieved that her MS will not impact on her desire to start a family. In this chapter, you will learn about pregnancy, labor, and delivery. Later, we will return to Sue as she prepares to deliver her baby.

Pregnancy

Pregnancy begins with fertilization of an ovum and ends with delivery of the fetus and afterbirth. During this approximately 38-week period of development, known as **gestation** (jes-TA-shun), all fetal tissues differentiate from a single fertilized egg. Along the way, many changes occur in both the mother and the developing infant.

Fertilization and the Start of Pregnancy

When semen is deposited in the vagina, the many spermatozoa immediately wriggle about in all directions, some traveling into the uterus and oviducts (Fig. 24-1). If an egg cell is present in the oviduct, many spermatozoa cluster around it. Using enzymes, they dissolve the coating around the ovum, so that eventually one sperm cell can penetrate its plasma membrane. The nuclei of the sperm and egg then combine. (See Box 24-1, Assisted Reproductive Technology.)

The result of this union is a single cell, called a **zygote** (ZI-gote), with the full human chromosome number of 46. The zygote divides rapidly into two cells and then four

cells and soon forms a ball of cells. During this time, the cell cluster is traveling toward the uterine cavity, pushed along by cilia lining the oviduct and by peristalsis (contractions) of the tube. After reaching the uterus, the little ball of cells burrows into the greatly thickened uterine lining and is soon implanted and completely covered. After **implantation** in the uterus, a group of cells within the dividing cluster becomes an **embryo** (EM-bre-o), the term used for the growing offspring in the early stage of gestation. The other cells within the cluster will differentiate into tissue that will support the developing offspring throughout gestation.

CHECKPOINT **24-1** ➤ What structure is formed by the union of an ovum and a spermatozoon?

The Placenta

For a few days after implantation, the embryo gets nourishment from the endometrium. By the end of the second week, however, the outer cells of the embryonic cluster form villi (projections) that invade the uterine wall and maternal blood channels (venous sinuses). Gradually, tissue in the outer embryonic layer and in the uterine lining

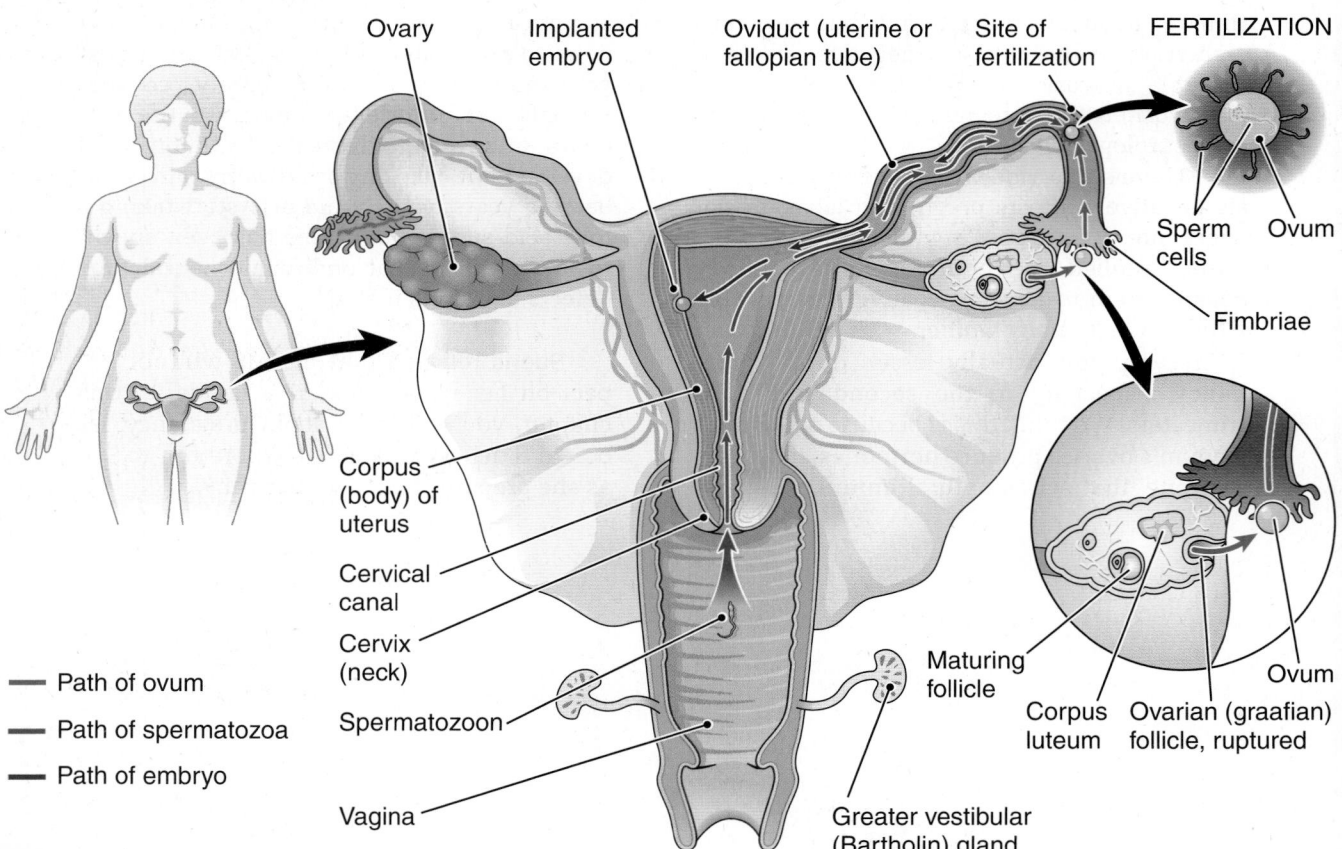

— Path of ovum

— Path of spermatozoa

— Path of embryo

Labels: Ovary, Implanted embryo, Oviduct (uterine or fallopian tube), Site of fertilization, FERTILIZATION, Sperm cells, Ovum, Fimbriae, Corpus (body) of uterus, Cervical canal, Cervix (neck), Spermatozoon, Vagina, Greater vestibular (Bartholin) gland, Maturing follicle, Corpus luteum, Ovarian (graafian) follicle, ruptured, Ovum

Figure 24-1 **The female reproductive system.** Arrows show the pathway of the spermatozoa and ovum and also of the fertilization and implantation of the fertilized ovum. [ZOOMING IN ➤ Where is the ovum fertilized?]

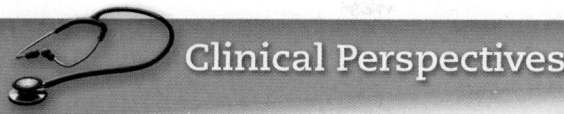

Box 24-1   **Clinical Perspectives**

Assisted Reproductive Technology: The "Art" of Conception

At least one in ten American couples is affected by infertility. Assisted reproductive technologies such as in vitro fertilization (IVF), gamete intrafallopian transfer (GIFT), and zygote intrafallopian transfer (ZIFT) can help these couples become pregnant.

In vitro fertilization refers to fertilization of an ovum outside the mother's body in a laboratory dish. It is often used when a woman's oviducts are blocked or when a man has a low sperm count. The woman participating in IVF is given hormones to cause ovulation of several ova. These are then withdrawn with a needle and fertilized with the father's sperm. After a few divisions, some of the fertilized ova are placed in the uterus, thus bypassing the oviducts. Additional fertilized ova can be frozen to repeat the procedure in case of failure or for later pregnancies.

GIFT can be used when the woman has at least one normal oviduct and the man has an adequate sperm count. As in

IVF, the woman is given hormones to cause ovulation of several ova, which are collected. Then, the ova and the father's sperm are placed into the oviduct using a catheter. Thus, in GIFT, fertilization occurs inside the woman, not in a laboratory dish.

ZIFT is a combination of both IVF and GIFT. Fertilization takes place in a laboratory dish, and then the zygote is placed into the oviduct.

Because of a lack of guidelines or restrictions in the United States in the field of assisted reproductive technology, some problems have arisen. These issues concern the use of stored embryos and gametes, use of embryos without consent, and improper screening for disease among donors. In addition, the implantation of more than one fertilized ovum has resulted in a high incidence of multiple births, even up to seven or eight offspring in a single pregnancy, a situation that imperils the survival and health of the babies.

---

together form the **placenta** (plah-SEN-tah), a flat, circular organ that consists of a spongy network of blood-filled channels and capillary-containing villi (Fig. 24-2). (*Placenta* is from a Latin word meaning "pancake.") The placenta is the organ of nutrition, respiration, and excretion for the developing offspring throughout gestation. Although the blood of the mother and her offspring do not mix—each has its own blood and cardiovascular system—exchanges take place through the capillaries of the placental villi. In this manner, gases (CO_2 and O_2) are exchanged, nutrients are provided to the developing infant, and waste products are released into the maternal blood to be eliminated.

THE UMBILICAL CORD The embryo is connected to the developing placenta by a stalk of tissue that eventually becomes the **umbilical** (um-BIL-ih-kal) **cord**. This structure carries blood to and from the embryo, later called the **fetus** (FE-tus). The cord encloses two arteries that carry deoxygenated blood from the fetus to the placenta, and one vein that carries oxygenated blood from the placenta to the fetus (see Fig. 24-2). (Note that, like the pulmonary vessels, these arteries carry blood low in oxygen and this vein carries blood high in oxygen.)

FETAL CIRCULATION The fetus has special circulatory adaptations to carry blood to and from the umbilical cord and to bypass the non-functional lungs. A small amount of the oxygenated blood traveling toward the fetus in the **umbilical vein** is delivered directly to the liver. However, most of the blood is added to the deoxygenated blood in the inferior vena cava through a small vessel, the **ductus venosus**.

Although mixed, this blood still contains enough oxygen to nourish fetal tissues. Once in the right atrium, some of the blood flows directly into the left atrium through a small hole in the atrial septum, the **foramen ovale** (o-VA-le). This blood bypasses the right ventricle and the pulmonary circuit. Blood that does enter the right ventricle is pumped into the pulmonary artery. Although a small amount of this blood goes to the lungs, most of it shunts directly into the systemic circuit through a small vessel, the **ductus arteriosus**, which connects the pulmonary artery to the descending aorta (see Fig. 24-2). Blood returns to the placenta to be oxygenated through the two **umbilical arteries**. See Appendix 7 for a dissection photograph showing fetal circulation.

After birth, when the baby's lungs are functioning, these adaptations begin to close. The foramen ovale gradually seals and the various vessels constrict into fibrous cords, usually within minutes after birth (only the proximal parts of the umbilical arteries persist as arteries to the urinary bladder). Failure to close results in congenital heart defects, as shown in Figure 14-13B and C.

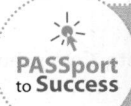

PASSport to Success   Visit ***thePoint*** or see the Student Resource CD in the back of this book to view the animation *Fetal Circulation.*

PLACENTAL HORMONES In addition to maintaining the fetus, the placenta is an endocrine organ. Beginning soon after implantation, some embryonic cells produce the hormone **human chorionic gonadotropin** (ko-re-ON-ik gon-ah-do-TRO-pin) (**hCG**). This hormone stimulates the

24

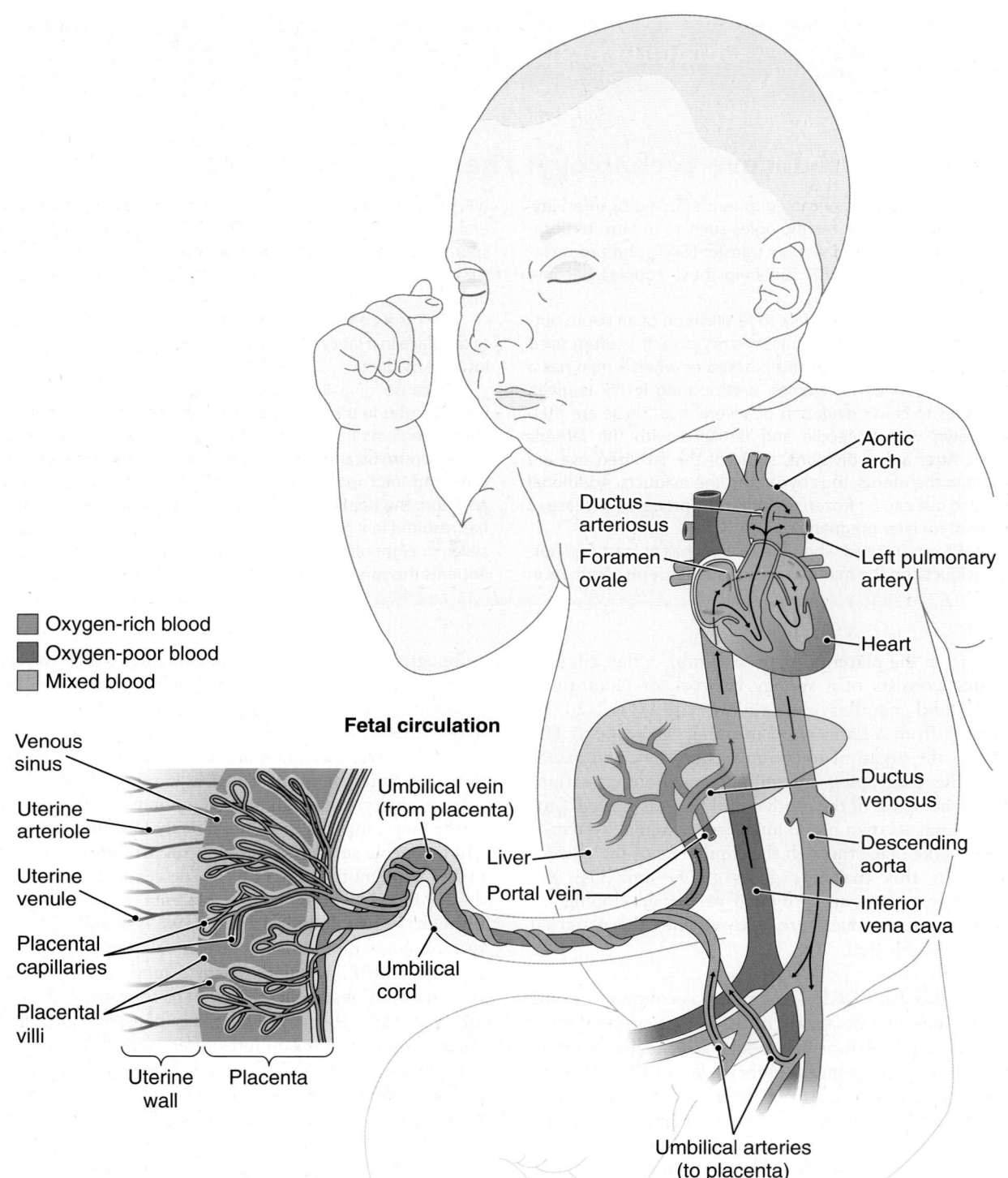

Oxygen-rich blood
Oxygen-poor blood
Mixed blood

Fetal circulation

Venous sinus

Uterine arteriole

Uterine venule

Placental capillaries

Placental villi

Uterine wall   Placenta

Umbilical vein (from placenta)

Liver

Portal vein

Umbilical cord

Umbilical arteries (to placenta)

Aortic arch

Ductus arteriosus

Foramen ovale

Left pulmonary artery

Heart

Ductus venosus

Descending aorta

Inferior vena cava

Figure 24-2 **Fetal circulation and section of placenta.** Colors show relative oxygen content of blood. [ZOOMING IN ➤ What is signified by the purple color in this illustration?]

ovarian corpus luteum, prolonging its life-span to 11 or 12 weeks and causing it to secrete increasing amounts of progesterone and estrogen. It is hCG that is used in tests as an indicator of pregnancy.

Progesterone is essential for the maintenance of preg-

nancy. It promotes endometrial secretion to nourish the embryo, maintains the endometrium, and decreases the uterine muscle's ability to contract, thus preventing the embryo from being expelled from the body. During pregnancy, progesterone also helps prepare the breasts for milk secretion. Estrogen promotes enlargement of the uterus and breasts. By the 11th or 12th week of pregnancy, the corpus luteum is no longer needed; by this time, the placenta itself can secrete adequate amounts of progesterone and estrogen, and the corpus luteum disintegrates. Miscarriages (loss of an embryo or fetus) are most likely to occur during this critical time when hormone secretion is shifting from the corpus luteum to the placenta.

Human placental lactogen (hPL) is a hormone secreted by the placenta during pregnancy, reaching a peak at term, the normal conclusion of pregnancy. hPL stimulates growth of the breasts to prepare the mother for production of milk, or **lactation** (lak-TA-shun). More importantly, it regulates the levels of nutrients in the mother's blood to keep them available for the fetus. This second function leads to an alternate name for this hormone: human chorionic somatomammotropin.

Relaxin is a placental hormone that softens the cervix and relaxes the sacral joints and the pubic symphysis. These changes help to widen the birth canal and aid in delivery.

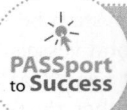

PASSport to Success — Visit *thePoint* or see the Student Resource CD in the back of this book for a summary chart on placental hormones.

CHECKPOINT 24-2 ➤ What organ nourishes the developing fetus?

CHECKPOINT 24-3 ➤ What is the function of the umbilical cord?

CHECKPOINT 24-4 ➤ Fetal circulation is adapted to bypass what organs?

Development of the Embryo

The developing offspring is referred to as an embryo for the first 8 weeks of life (Fig. 24-3), and the study of growth during this period is called **embryology** (em-bre-OL-o-je). The beginnings of all body systems are established during this time. The heart and the brain are among

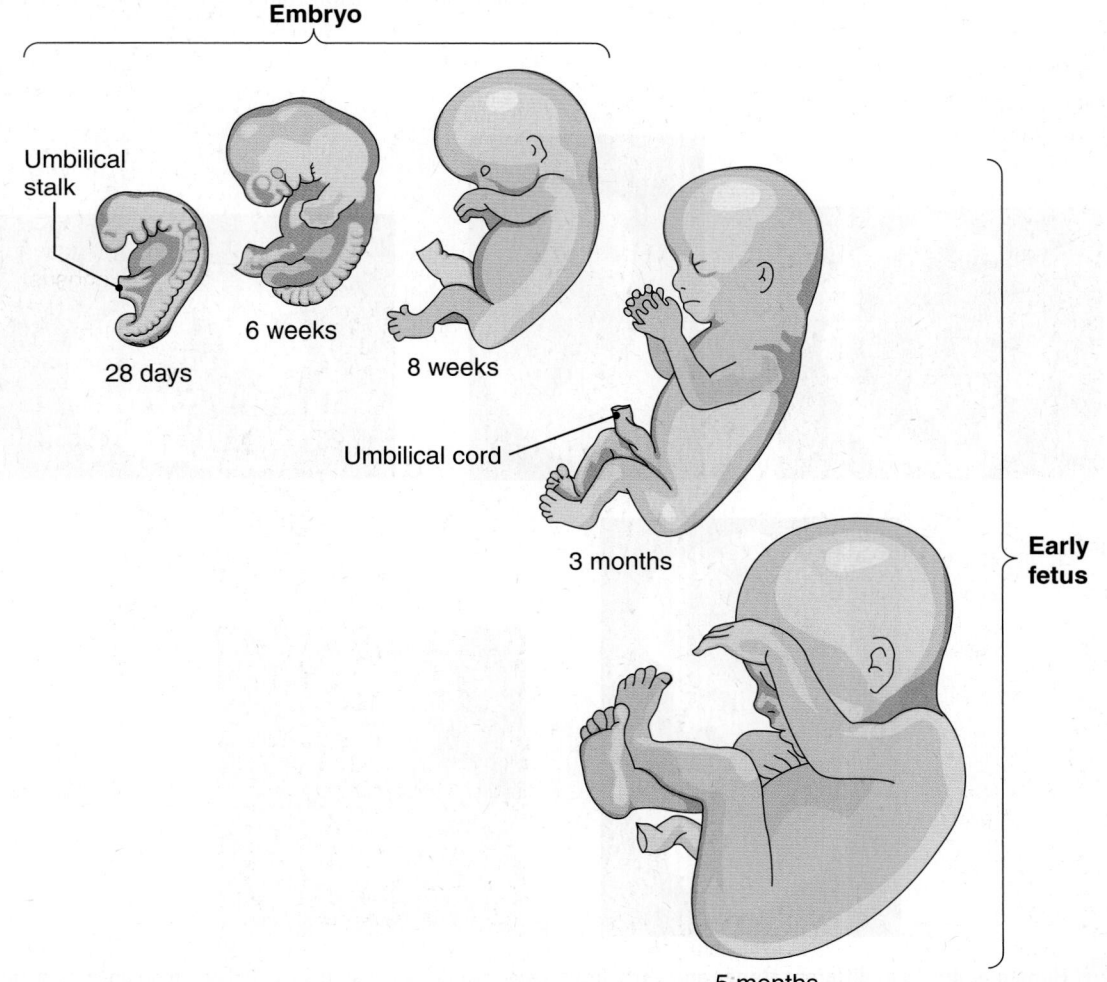

Figure 24-3 Development of an embryo and early fetus.

the first organs to develop. A primitive nervous system begins to form in the third week. The heart and blood vessels originate during the second week, and the first heartbeat appears during week 4, at the same time that other muscles begin to develop.

By the end of the first month, the embryo is approximately 0.62 cm (0.25 inches) long, with four small swellings at the sides called **limb buds**, which will develop into the four extremities. At this time, the heart produces a prominent bulge at the anterior of the embryo.

By the end of the second month, the embryo takes on an appearance that is recognizably human. In male embryos, the primitive testes have formed and have begun to secrete testosterone, which will direct formation of the male reproductive organs as gestation continues. Figure 24-4 shows photographs of embryonic and early fetal development.

CHECKPOINT 24-5 ➤ All body systems originate during the early development of the embryo. At about what time in gestation does the heartbeat first appear?

The Fetus

The term *fetus* is used for the developing offspring from the beginning of the third month until birth. During this period, the organ systems continue to grow and mature. The ovaries form in the female early in this fetal period, and at this stage they contain all the primitive cells (oocytes) that can later develop into mature ova (egg cells).

For study, the entire gestation period may be divided into three equal segments or **trimesters**. The fetus's most rapid growth occurs during the second trimester (months 4 to 6). By the end of the fourth month, the fetus is almost 15 cm (6 inches) long, and its external genitalia are sufficiently developed to reveal its sex. By the seventh month, the fetus is usually approximately 35 cm (14 inches) long and weighs approximately 1.1 kg (2.4 pounds). At the end of pregnancy, the normal length of the fetus is 45 to 56 cm (18 to 22.5 inches), and the weight varies from 2.7 to 4.5 kg (6 to 10 pounds).

The **amniotic** (am-ne-OT-ik) **sac**, which is filled with a clear liquid known as **amniotic fluid**, surrounds the fetus and serves as a protective cushion for it (Fig. 24-5). The amniotic sac ruptures at birth, an event marked by the common expression that the mother's "water broke."

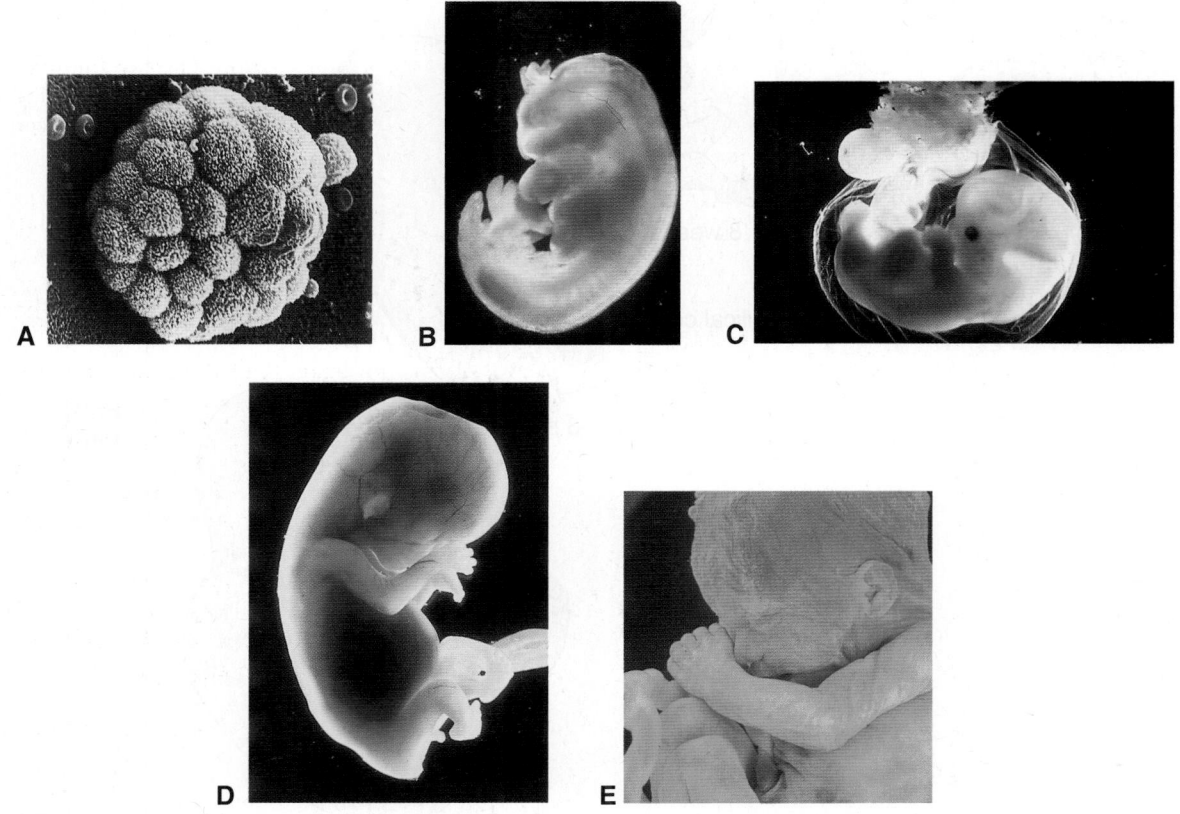

Figure 24-4 **Human embryos at different stages and early fetus. (A)** Implantation in uterus 7 to 8 days after conception. **(B)** Embryo at 32 days. **(C)** At 37 days. **(D)** At 41 days. **(E)** Fetus between 12 and 15 weeks. (Reprinted with permission from Pillitteri A. *Maternal and Child Health Nursing*, 4th ed. Philadelphia: Lippincott Williams & Wilkins, 2003.)

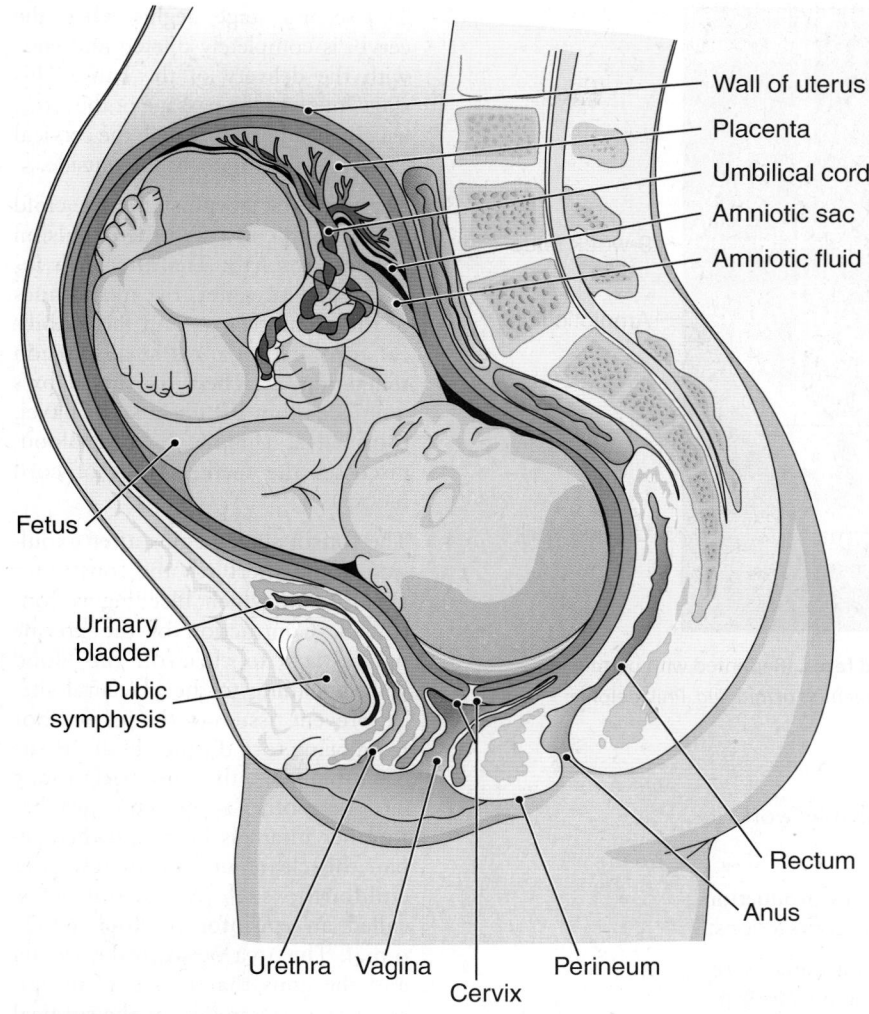

Wall of uterus
Placenta
Umbilical cord
Amniotic sac
Amniotic fluid

Fetus

Urinary
bladder
Pubic
symphysis

Rectum

Anus

Urethra   Vagina   Perineum
              Cervix

Figure 24-5 **Midsagittal section of a pregnant uterus with intact fetus.** [ZOOMING IN ➤ What structure connects the fetus to the placenta?]

■ The lungs provide more oxygen by increasing the rate and depth of respiration.

■ The kidneys excrete nitrogenous wastes from both the fetus and the mother.

■ The digestive system supplies additional nutrients for the growth of maternal organs (uterus and breasts) and fetal growth, as well as for subsequent labor and milk secretion.

Nausea and vomiting are common discomforts in early pregnancy. These most often occur upon arising or during periods of fatigue, and are more common in women who smoke cigarettes. The specific cause of these symptoms is not known, but they may be a result of the great changes in hormone levels that occur at this time. The nausea and vomiting usually last for only a few weeks to several months.

Urinary frequency and constipation are often present during the early stages of pregnancy and then usually disappear. They may reappear late in pregnancy as the head of the fetus drops from the abdominal region down into the pelvis, pressing on the rectum and the urinary bladder.

During development, the fetal skin is protected by a layer of cheeselike material called the **vernix caseosa** (VER-niks ka-se-O-sah) (literally, "cheesy varnish").

CHECKPOINT 24-6 ➤ What is the name of the fluid-filled sac that holds the fetus?

The Mother

The total period of pregnancy, from fertilization of the ovum to birth, is approximately 266 days, also given as 280 days or 40 weeks from the last menstrual period (LMP). During this time, the mother must supply all the food and oxygen for the fetus and eliminate its waste materials. To support the additional demands of the growing fetus, the mother's metabolism changes markedly, and several organ systems increase their output:

■ The heart pumps more blood to supply the needs of the uterus and the fetus.

THE USE OF ULTRASOUND IN OBSTETRICS Ultrasonography (ul-trah-son-OG-rah-fe) is a safe, painless, and noninvasive method for studying soft tissue. It has proved extremely valuable for monitoring pregnancies and deliveries.

An ultrasound image, called a *sonogram*, is made by sending high-frequency sound waves into the body (Fig. 24-6). Each time a wave meets an interface between two tissues of different densities, an echo is produced. An instrument called a *transducer* converts the reflected sound waves into electrical energy, and a computer is used to generate an image on a viewing screen.

Ultrasound scans can be used in obstetrics to diagnose pregnancy, judge fetal age, and determine the location of the placenta. The technique can also show the presence of excess amniotic fluid and fetal abnormalities.

CHECKPOINT 24-7 ➤ What is the approximate duration of pregnancy in days?

Childbirth

The exact mechanisms that trigger the beginning of uterine contractions for childbirth are still not completely known.

24

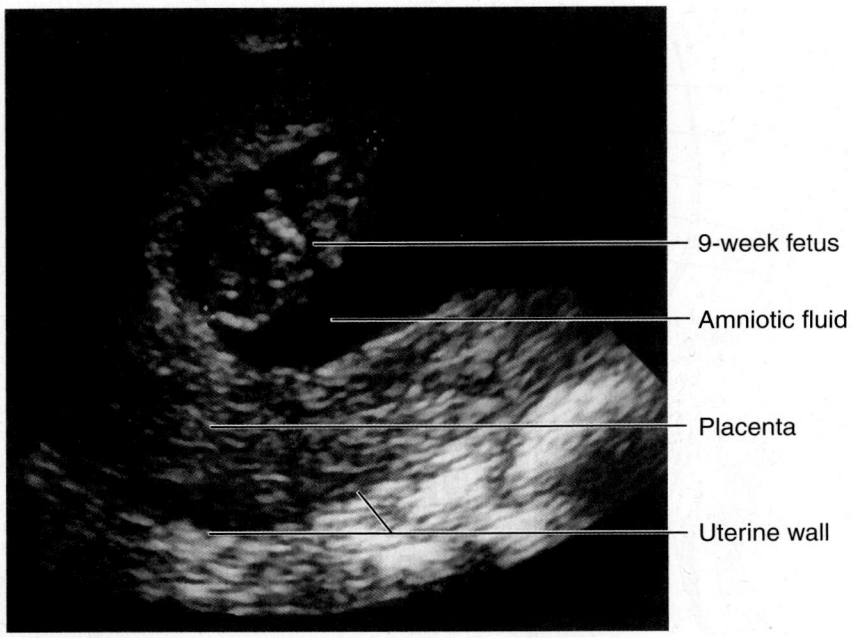

9-week fetus

Amniotic fluid

Placenta

Uterine wall

Figure 24-6 **Sonogram showing a 9-week-old fetus.** (Reprinted with permission from Erkonen WE. *Radiology 101: Basics and Fundamentals of Imaging*. Philadelphia: Lippincott Williams & Wilkins, 1998.)

Some fetal and maternal factors that probably work in combination to start labor are:

- Stretching of the uterine muscle stimulates production of prostaglandin, which promotes uterine contractions.

- Pressure on the cervix from the baby stimulates release of **oxytocin** (ok-se-TO-sin) from the posterior pituitary. The uterine muscle becomes increasingly sensitive to this hormone late in pregnancy.

- Changes in the placenta that occur with time may contribute to the start of labor.

- Cortisol from the fetal adrenal cortex inhibits the mother's progesterone. Increase in the relative amount of estrogen as compared to progesterone stimulates uterine contractions.

After labor begins, stimuli from the cervix and vagina produce reflex secretion of oxytocin, which in turn increases the uterine contractions (an example of positive feedback).

The Four Stages of Labor

The process by which the fetus is expelled from the uterus is known as **labor** and **delivery**; it also may be called **parturition** (par-tu-RISH-un). It is divided into four stages:

1. The **first stage** begins with the onset of regular uterine contractions. With each contraction, the cervix becomes thinner and the opening larger. Rupture of the amniotic sac may occur at any time, with a gush of fluid from the vagina.

2. The **second stage** begins when the cervix is completely dilated and ends with the delivery of the baby. This stage involves the passage of the fetus, usually head first, through the cervical canal and the vagina to the outside.

3. The **third stage** begins after the child is born and ends with the expulsion of the afterbirth. The afterbirth includes the placenta, the membranes of the amniotic sac, and the umbilical cord, except for a small portion remaining attached to the baby's umbilicus (um-BIL-ih-kus), or navel. (Box 24-2, Umbilical Cord Blood, discusses the medical uses of cord blood.)

4. The **fourth stage** begins after expulsion of the afterbirth and constitutes a period in which bleeding is controlled. Contraction of the uterine muscle acts to close off the blood vessels leading to the placental site. To prevent tissues of the pelvic floor from being torn during childbirth, as often happens, the obstetrician may cut the mother's perineum just before her infant is born and then repair this clean cut immediately after childbirth; such an operation is called an **episiotomy** (eh-piz-e-OT-o-me). The area between the vagina and the anus that is cut in an episiotomy is referred to as the surgical or obstetrical perineum (see Fig. 23-12 in Chapter 23).

CHECKPOINT 24-8 ➤ What is parturition?

Cesarean Section

A **cesarean** (se-ZAR-re-an) **section** (C section) is an incision made in the abdominal wall and uterine wall for delivery of a fetus. A cesarean section may be required for a variety of reasons, including placental abnormalities, abnormal fetal position, disproportion between the head of the fetus and the mother's pelvis that makes vaginal delivery difficult or dangerous, and other problems that may arise during pregnancy and delivery.

CHECKPOINT 24-9 ➤ What is a cesarean section?

Multiple Births

Until recently, statistics indicated that twins occurred in about 1 of every 80 to 90 births, varying somewhat in different countries. Triplets occurred much less frequently, usually once in several thousand births, whereas quadru-

Disease in Context revisited

▶ Sue Experiences the Four Stages of Labor

"Ooh, I think it's time," gasped Sue as another wave of uterine contractions began.

"I'll call Dr. Philips and let her know we're on our way," replied Sue's husband, and went to get Sue's overnight bag.

"Hurry, Shawn! I think my water just broke!"

Dr. Philips examined Sue in the labor and delivery room. Sue's cervix was dilating, signaling that she was in the first stage of labor. At Sue's request, the anesthetist gave her an epidural block to help control pain. He inserted a needle between Sue's lumbar vertebrae into the epidural space. Through the needle, he threaded a catheter, which would remain in Sue's back for her entire labor. He removed the needle and administered the pain medication via the catheter.

About an hour later, Sue's labor progressed into the second stage. Her cervix was completely dilated and she was encouraged to push with each contraction. After the baby's head was de-

livered, the obstetrician cleared its airway and checked to make sure that the umbilical cord was free. Shortly after, Sue gave a final push and her baby girl, Emma, was born. The nurse wrapped her in a warm blanket and placed her on Sue's chest. While Sue and Shawn admired their new daughter, Dr. Philips delivered Sue's placenta. This marked the end of the third stage of labor. A couple of hours later, Sue and Emma were in their hospital room resting comfortably. As Sue breastfed Emma, her uterus contracted and began to shrink to its original size. Although Sue was too enamored with her baby daughter to notice, she had just completed the fourth stage of labor.

In this case, Sue learned that multiple sclerosis would not affect her ability to have a baby. Following a normal pregnancy, she successfully delivered a healthy baby girl. To review some of the reproductive anatomy discussed in this case, see Chapter 23.

Box 24-2 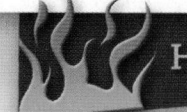 Hot Topics

Umbilical Cord Blood: Giving Life After Birth

Following childbirth, the umbilical cord and placenta are usually discarded. However, research suggests that blood harvested from these structures could save lives. Like bone marrow, umbilical cord blood contains stem cells capable of differentiating into all blood cell types. Cancer patients whose bone marrow is destroyed by chemotherapy often require stem cell transplants, as do those with leukemia, anemia, or certain immune disorders.

Stem cells obtained from umbilical cord blood offer some important advantages over those acquired from bone marrow. These advantages include:

- Greater ease of collection and storage. Whereas bone marrow collection is a surgical procedure, cord blood can be collected immediately after the umbilical cord is cut. The blood can then be stored frozen in a blood bank.

- No risk to the donor. Because cord blood is collected after the cord is cut, the procedure is not dangerous to the donor.

- Lower risk to the recipient. Since cord blood is immature, it does not have to match the recipient's tissues as closely as bone marrow does, so there is less chance of transplant rejection and graft-versus-host disease than with bone marrow. In addition, umbilical cord blood is less likely to contain infectious organisms than is bone marrow.

- Higher chance of finding a donor. Since umbilical cord blood need not closely match a recipient's tissues, the likelihood of finding a match between donor and recipient is higher.

Although umbilical cord blood is a promising stem cell source, only enough cells to treat a child or small adult can be harvested from a single donor. Scientists hope that improved collection techniques and advances in cell culture will increase the number of stem cells available from a single donor, enabling all patients in need to benefit from this treatment.

24

plets occurred very rarely. The birth of quintuplets represented a historic event unless the mother had taken fertility drugs. Now these fertility drugs, usually gonadotropins, are given more commonly, and the number of multiple births has increased significantly. Multiple fetuses tend to be born prematurely and therefore have a high death rate. However, better care of infants and newer treatments have resulted in more living multiple births than ever.

Twins originate in two different ways, and on this basis are divided into two types:

- **Fraternal twins** result from the fertilization of two different ova by two spermatozoa. Two completely different individuals, as distinct from each other as brothers and sisters of different ages, are produced. Each fetus has its own placenta and surrounding sac.

- **Identical twins** develop from a single zygote formed from a single ovum fertilized by a single spermatozoon. Sometime during the early stages of development, the embryonic cells separate into two units. Usually, there is a single placenta, although there must be a separate umbilical cord for each fetus. Identical twins are always the same sex and carry the same inherited traits.

Other multiple births may be fraternal, identical, or combinations of these. The tendency to multiple births seems to be hereditary.

Termination of Pregnancy

A pregnancy may end before its full term has been completed. The term **live birth** is used if the baby breathes or shows any evidence of life such as heartbeat, pulsation of the umbilical cord, or movement of voluntary muscles. An **immature** or **premature** infant is one born before the organ systems are mature. Infants born before the 37th week of gestation or weighing less than 2,500 grams (5.5 pounds) are considered **preterm**.

Loss of the fetus is classified according to the duration of the pregnancy:

- The term **abortion** refers to loss of the embryo or fetus before the 20th week or weight of about 500 grams (1.1 pound). This loss can be either spontaneous or induced.

  > **Spontaneous abortion** occurs naturally with no interference. The most common causes are related to an abnormality of the embryo or fetus. Other causes include abnormality of the mother's reproductive organs, infections, or chronic disorders, such as kidney disease or hypertension. **Miscarriage** is the lay term for spontaneous abortion.

  > **Induced abortion** occurs as a result of artificial or mechanical interruption of pregnancy. A **therapeutic abortion** is an abortion performed by a physician as a treatment for a variety of reasons. More liberal access to this type of abortion has dramatically reduced the incidence of death related to illegal abortion.

- The term **fetal death** refers to loss of the fetus after the eighth week of pregnancy. **Stillbirth** refers to the delivery of an infant who is lifeless.

Immaturity is a leading cause of death in the newborn. After the 20th week of pregnancy, the fetus is considered **viable**, that is, able to live outside the uterus. A fetus expelled before the 24th week or before reaching a weight of 1,000 grams (2.2 pounds) has little more than a 50% chance of survival; one born at a point closer to the full 40 weeks stands a much better chance of living. However, increasing numbers of immature infants are being saved because of advances in neonatal intensive care.

Hospitals use the Apgar score to assess a newborn's health and predict survival. Five features are rated as 0, 1, or 2 at 1 minute and 5 minutes after delivery. The maximum possible score on each test is 10. Infants with low scores require medical attention and have lower survival rates.

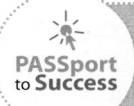

PASSport to Success — Visit **thePoint** or see the Student Resource CD in the back of this book for the Apgar scoring system.

CHECKPOINT **24-10** ➤ What does the term *viable* mean with reference to a fetus?

The Mammary Glands and Lactation

The **mammary glands**, or breasts, of the female are accessories of the reproductive system. They provide nourishment for the baby after its birth. The mammary glands are similar in construction to the sweat glands. Each gland is divided into a number of lobes composed of glandular tissue and fat, and each lobe is further subdivided. Secretions from the lobes are conveyed through **lactiferous** (lak-TIF-er-us) **ducts**, all of which converge at the papilla (nipple) (Fig. 24-7).

The mammary glands begin developing during puberty, but they do not become functional until the end of a pregnancy. Placental lactogen (hPL) helps to prepare the breasts for lactation, and the hormone **prolactin (PRL)**, produced by the anterior pituitary gland, stimulates the mammary glands' secretory cells. The first mammary gland secretion is a thin liquid called **colostrum** (ko-LOS-trum). It is nutritious but has a somewhat different composition from milk. Milk secretion begins within a few days following birth and can continue for several years as long as milk is frequently removed by the suckling baby or by pumping. Stimulation of the breast by the suckling infant causes oxytocin release from the posterior pituitary. This hormone causes the milk ducts to contract, resulting in the ejection, or *letdown*, of milk.

The newborn baby's digestive tract is not ready for the usual adult mixed diet. Mother's milk is more desirable for the young infant than milk from other animals for several reasons, some of which are listed below:

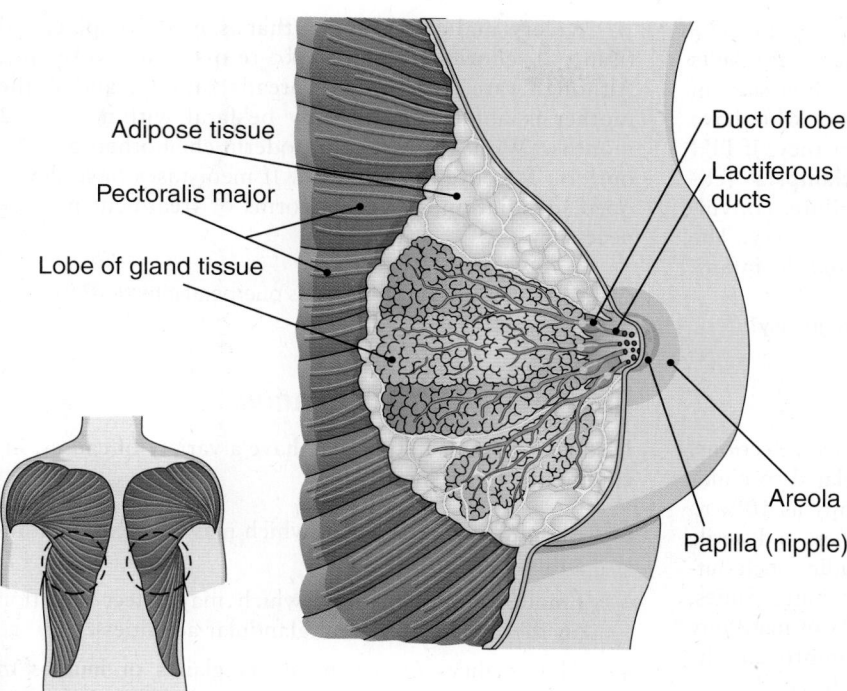

Figure 24-7 **Section of the breast (mammary gland).** [ZOOMING IN ➤ What muscle underlies the breast?]

- Infections that may be transmitted by foods exposed to the outside air are avoided by nursing.
- Both breast milk and colostrum contain maternal antibodies that help protect the baby against pathogens.
- The proportions of various nutrients and other substances in human milk are perfectly suited to the human infant. Substitutes are not exact imitations of human milk. Nutrients are present in more desirable amounts if the mother's diet is well balanced.
- The psychological and emotional benefits of nursing are of infinite value to both the mother and the infant.

CHECKPOINT 24-11 ➤ What is lactation?

Disorders of Pregnancy, Childbirth, and Lactation

A pregnancy that develops in a location outside the uterine cavity is said to be an **ectopic** (ek-TOP-ik) **pregnancy** (Fig. 24-8). The most common type is the tubal ectopic pregnancy, in which the embryo begins to grow in the oviduct. This structure cannot expand to contain the growing embryo and may rupture. Ectopic pregnancy may threaten the mother's life if it does not receive prompt surgical treatment.

In **placenta previa** (PRE-ve-ah) the placenta, which is usually attached to the superior part of the uterus, instead becomes attached at or near the internal opening of the cervix. The normal cervical softening and dilation that occur in later pregnancy separate part of the placenta from

its attachment. The result is painless bleeding and interference with the fetal oxygen supply.

Sometimes the placenta separates from the uterine wall prematurely, often after the 20th week of pregnancy, causing hemorrhage. This disorder, known as **abruptio placentae** (ab-RUP-she-o plah-SEN-te), or *placental abruption*, occurs most often in multigravidas (mul-te-GRAV-ih-dahz), meaning women who have had more than one pregnancy or are older than 35 years of age. Placental abruption is a common cause of bleeding during the second half of pregnancy and may require termination of pregnancy to save the mother's life.

Pregnancy-Induced Hypertension

A serious disorder that can develop in the latter part of pregnancy is **pregnancy-induced hypertension (PIH)**, also called *preeclampsia* (pre-eh-KLAMP-se-ah) or *toxemia of pregnancy*. Signs include hypertension, protein in the urine (pro-

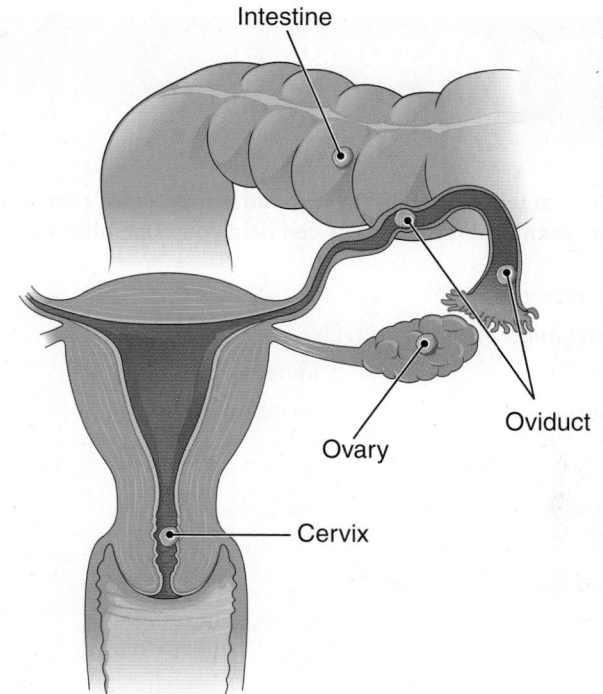

Figure 24-8 **Ectopic pregnancy sites.** The most common site is the oviduct, in which case it is a tubal ectopic pregnancy. (Reprinted with permission from Cohen BJ. *Medical Terminology*, 5th ed. Philadelphia: Lippincott Williams & Wilkins, 2008.)

24

teinuria), general edema, and sudden weight gain. The cause of this disorder is a hormone imbalance that results in constriction of blood vessels. It is most often seen in women whose nutritional state is poor and who have received little or no health care during pregnancy. If PIH remains untreated, it may lead to **eclampsia** (eh-KLAMP-se-ah) with the onset of kidney failure, convulsions, and coma during pregnancy or after delivery. The result may be the death of both the mother and the infant.

CHECKPOINT `24-12` ➤ What is an ectopic pregnancy?

Postpartum Disorders

Childbirth-related deaths are often due to infections. **Puerperal** (pu-ER-per-al) **infections**, those related to childbirth, were once the cause of death in as many as 10% to 12% of women going through labor. Cleanliness and sterile techniques have improved the chances of avoiding such outcomes of pregnancies. Nevertheless, in the United States, puerperal infection still develops in about 6% of maternity patients. Antibiotics have dramatically improved the chances of recovery for both the mother and the child.

A **hydatidiform** (hi-dah-TID-ih-form) **mole**, or hydatid mole, is a benign overgrowth of placental tissue. The placenta dilates and resembles grapelike cysts. The growth may invade the uterine wall, causing it to rupture.

A very malignant tumor that is made of placental tissue is **choriocarcinoma** (ko-re-o-kar-sih-NO-mah). Although rare, this tumor spreads rapidly, and if the mother is not treated, it may be fatal within 3 to 12 months. With the use of modern chemotherapy, the outlook for cure is very good. If metastases have developed, irradiation and other forms of treatment may be necessary.

CHECKPOINT `24-13` ➤ What is puerperal infection?

Lactation Disturbances

Disturbances in lactation may have a variety of causes, including the following:

- Malnutrition or anemia, which may prevent lactation entirely.

- Emotional disturbances, which may affect lactation (as they may affect other glandular activities).

- Abnormalities of the mammary glands or injuries to these organs, which may interfere with their functioning.

- **Mastitis** (mas-TI-tis), or "inflammation of the breast," which is caused by infection. Antibiotic treatment usually allows for the continuation of nursing.

Word Anatomy

Medical terms are built from standardized word parts (prefixes, roots, and suffixes). Learning the meanings of these parts can help you remember words and interpret unfamiliar terms.

WORD PART	MEANING	EXAMPLE
Pregnancy		
zyg/o	joined	An ovum and spermatozoon join to form a *zygote*.
chori/o	membrane, chorion	Human *chorionic* gonadotropin is produced by the outermost cells (chorion) of the embryo and acts on the corpus luteum in the ovary.
somat/o	body	Human chorionic *somatomammotropin* controls nutrients for the body and acts on the mammary glands (mamm/o).
Childbirth		
ox/y	sharp, acute	*Oxytocin* is a hormone that stimulates labor.
toc/o	labor	See preceding example.
Disorders of Pregnancy, Childbirth, and Lactation		
ecto-	outside, external	An *ectopic* pregnancy occurs outside of the uterine cavity.

Summary

I. **PREGNANCY (GESTATION)—LASTS ABOUT 38 WEEKS**
   A. Fertilization and the start of pregnancy
      1. Fertilization occurs in oviduct
      2. Zygote (fertilized egg)—formed by fusion of egg and sperm nuclei
         a. Divides rapidly
         b. Travels to uterus
         c. Implants in lining and becomes embryo
   B. The placenta
      1. Formed by tissue around embryo and in lining of uterus
      2. Functions
         a. Nourishment
         b. Gas exchange
         c. Removal of waste
         d. Production of hormones
      3. Umbilical cord—connects fetus to placenta
         a. Umbilical vein—carries blood high in oxygen
         b. Umbilical arteries (2)—carry blood low in oxygen
      4. Fetal circulation—bypasses lungs
         a. Ductus venosus—carries blood from umbilical vein to inferior vena cava
         b. Foramen ovale—hole in atrial septum that allows blood to flow from right to left atrium
         c. Ductus arteriosus—connects pulmonary artery to descending aorta
      5. Placental hormones
         a. Human chorionic gonadotropin (hCG)—maintains corpus luteum for 11 to 12 weeks
         b. Progesterone—maintains endometrium; limits uterine contractions; prepares breasts for lactation
         c. Estrogen—enlarges uterus and breasts
         d. Human placental lactogen (hPL)—stimulates lactation; regulates nutrients
         e. Relaxin—relaxes birth canal
   C. Development of the embryo
      1. First 8 weeks
      2. All body systems begin to develop
   D. The fetus
      1. Third month to birth
      2. Amniotic sac
         a. Surrounds fetus
         b. Contains fluid to cushion and protect fetus
   E. The mother
      1. Increased demands on heart, lungs, kidneys
      2. Increased nutritional needs
      3. Ultrasound used to monitor pregnancy and delivery

II. **CHILDBIRTH**
   A. Initiated by changes in uterus, placenta, fetus
   B. Four stages of labor
      1. Contractions
      2. Delivery of baby
      3. Expulsion of afterbirth
      4. Contraction of uterus
   C. Cesarean section
      1. Incision to remove fetus
   D. Multiple births
      1. Fraternal twins formed from two different ova
      2. Identical twins develop from a single zygote
      3. Larger multiples follow either pattern or a combination
      4. Increased by fertility drugs
   E. Termination of pregnancy
      1. Immature (premature) infant—born before organ systems mature
      2. Preterm—born before 37th week or weighing less than 2,500 grams
      3. Abortion—loss of fetus before 20th week or weighing less than 500 grams; spontaneous or induced
      4. Fetal death—loss of fetus after 8 weeks of pregnancy

III. **MAMMARY GLANDS AND LACTATION**
   A. Lactation—secretion of milk
      1. Colostrum—first mammary secretion
   B. Hormones
      1. hPL—prepares breasts for lactation
      2. Prolactin—stimulates secretory cells
      3. Oxytocin—promotes letdown (ejection) of milk
   C. Advantages of breastfeeding
      1. Reduces infections
      2. Transfers antibodies
      3. Provides best form of nutrition
      4. Emotional satisfaction

IV. **DISORDERS OF PREGNANCY, CHILDBIRTH, AND LACTATION**
   A. Pregnancy disorders
      1. Ectopic pregnancy—pregnancy outside of uterus; commonly in oviduct
      2. Placenta previa—improper attachment of placenta to uterus
      3. Placental abruption—separation of placenta from uterus
      4. Pregnancy-induced hypertension (PIH)
         a. Also called preeclampsia, toxemia of pregnancy
         b. Eclampsia—results from untreated PIH

24

B. Postpartum disorders
1. Puerperal infection
2. Hydatidiform mole—benign overgrowth of placenta
3. Choriocarcinoma—malignant tumor of placental tissue

C. Lactation disturbances
1. Possible causes
a. Malnutrition
b. Emotional disturbances
c. Abnormalities of mammary glands
d. Mastitis—inflammation of the breast

Questions for Study and Review

BUILDING UNDERSTANDING

Fill in the blanks

1. Fetal skin is protected by a cheeselike material called_____.

2. The first mammary secretion is called _____.

3. Sound waves can be used to safely monitor pregnancy with a technique called _____.

4. A pregnancy that develops in a location outside the uterine cavity is said to be a(n) _____ pregnancy.

5. Inflammation of the breast as a result of infection is named_____.

Matching > Match each numbered item with the most closely related lettered item.

___ 6. A placental hormone that stimulates the ovaries to secrete progesterone and estrogen

___ 7. A placental hormone that regulates maternal blood nutrient levels

___ 8. A placental hormone that softens the cervix, which widens the birth canal

___ 9. A pituitary hormone that stimulates uterine contractions

___ 10. A pituitary hormone that stimulates maternal milk production

a. human placental lactogen

b. prolactin

c. oxytocin

d. relaxin

e. human chorionic gonadotropin

Multiple choice

___ 11. For a few days after implantation, the embryo is nourished by the
a. endometrium
b. placenta
c. yolk sac
d. umbilical cord

___ 12. By what month can the sex of the fetus be accurately determined?
a. second
b. third
c. fourth
d. fifth

___ 13. The total period of pregnancy, from fertilization to birth, is about
a. 37 weeks
b. 38 weeks
c. 39 weeks
d. 40 weeks

___ 14. With regard to identical twins, which of the following statements is incorrect?
a. they develop from a single zygote
b. they each have their own placenta
c. they are always the same sex
d. they carry the same inherited traits

___ 15. The earliest that a fetus could survive outside of the uterus is after the
a. 20th week
b. 24th week
c. 28th week
d. 30th week

UNDERSTANDING CONCEPTS

16. Distinguish among the following: zygote, embryo, and fetus.

17. Explain the role of the placenta in fetal development.

18. Is blood in the umbilical arteries relatively high or low in oxygen? In the umbilical vein?

19. Describe some of the changes that take place in the mother's body during pregnancy.

20. What is the major event of each of the four stages of parturition?

21. List several reasons why breast milk is best for baby.

22. What is a cesarean section? List several reasons why it may be required.

23. Compare and contrast the following disease-related terms:
a. fetal death and still birth
b. spontaneous abortion and induced abortion
c. placenta previa and abruptio placentae
d. pregnancy-induced hypertension and eclampsia
e. hydatidiform mole and choriocarcinoma

CONCEPTUAL THINKING

24. Why is the risk of miscarriage highest at week 12 of pregnancy?

25. Although it is strongly suggested that a woman not drink alcohol during her entire pregnancy, why is this advice particularly important during the first trimester?

26. In Sue's case, breast feeding helped Sue complete the fourth stage of labor. Explain the physiological mechanism responsible for this.

24

CHAPTER 25

Heredity and Hereditary Diseases

Learning Outcomes

After careful study of this chapter, you should be able to:

1. Briefly describe the mechanism of gene function
2. Explain the difference between dominant and recessive genes
3. Compare *phenotype* and *genotype* and give examples of each
4. Describe what is meant by a *carrier* of a genetic trait
5. Define *meiosis* and explain its function in reproduction
6. Explain how sex is determined in humans
7. Describe what is meant by the term *sex-linked* and list several sex-linked traits
8. List several factors that may influence the expression of a gene
9. Define *mutation*
10. Differentiate among congenital, genetic, and hereditary disorders and give several examples of each
11. List several factors that may cause genetic disorders
12. Define *karyotype* and explain how karyotypes are used in genetic counseling
13. Briefly describe several methods used to treat genetic disorders
14. Show how word parts are used to build words related to heredity (see Word Anatomy at the end of the chapter)

Selected Key Terms

The following terms and other boldface terms in the chapter are defined in the Glossary

allele
amniocentesis
autosome
carrier
chromosome
congenital
dominant
gene
genetic
genotype
heredity
heterozygous
homozygous
karyotype
meiosis
mutagen
mutation
pedigree
phenotype
progeny
recessive
sex-linked
trait

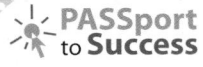

PASSport to Success

Visit *thePoint* or see the Student Resource CD in the back of this book for definitions and pronunciations of key terms as well as a pretest for this chapter.

Disease in Context

► Ben's Second Case: The Genetics of Cystic Fibrosis

When 2-year-old Ben was diagnosed with cystic fibrosis (CF), his parents, Alison and David, were shocked to discover that he had inherited the genetic disease from them. At first, their attention was focused only on Ben and the treatment he would need. Later, they also began to wonder how they had given him the disease and whether or not other children they might have would be at risk. So they made an appointment with a genetic counselor.

Ms. Clarkson explained, "All of a person's traits are inherited from his or her parents in the form of genes, discrete units of DNA carried on chromosomes in the egg and sperm cells. CF is caused by a change, or mutation, in a gene located on chromosome number 7. This gene codes for a chloride ion channel that is important in manufacturing sweat, digestive fluids, and mucus." "But how come Ben has cystic fibrosis, and he inherited it from us, but we don't have any signs of the disease?" Alison asked, perplexed.

"Well," Ms. Clarkson continued, "a genetic disease can arise from a spontaneous mutation, but more likely, you and David are carriers of the CF gene."

"Meaning...?" said David.

"Meaning," replied the counselor, "that all genetic traits are determined by pairs of genes, called alleles. If even one of these alleles is a so-called dominant gene, it will always be expressed. A person with a dominant disease gene will show the disease and you know it's there. However, most genetic diseases, including CF, are caused by recessive genes. These can be masked by a dominant allele, so you need two copies of the gene to show the disease. You and Alison are disease free, but you each carry one CF gene that was passed on to Ben."

"Does this mean all of our children will be sick with CF?" Alison wondered. "Should we stop here with our family?"

"Not necessarily" answered Ms. Clarkson. "We could do a family study to look for evidence of CF in your relatives, and there is a lab test done on blood or saliva to identify carriers, but we can assume at this point that both you and David carry the CF gene. That said, there's a one in four chance that any of your children will have CF. The 25% risk is constant with each birth, whether you've had a child with CF or not. There is a prenatal test that can identify CF in a fetus, and you can choose to make family decisions based on those results. But that's a subject for future discussions. Right now, you have to concentrate on Ben and his care."

In this chapter, we will learn more about heredity and hereditary diseases. Later, we'll see what treatment options are available for Ben.

We are often struck by the resemblance of a baby to one or both of its parents, yet rarely do we stop to consider *how* various traits are transmitted from parents to offspring. This subject—heredity—has fascinated humans for thousands of years. The *Old Testament* contains numerous references to heredity (although, of course, the word was unknown in biblical times). It was not until the 19th century, however, that methodical investigation into heredity was begun. At that time, an Austrian monk, Gregor Mendel, discovered through his experiments with garden peas that there was a precise pattern in the appearance of differences among parents and their **progeny** (PROJ-eh-ne), their offspring or descendents. Mendel's most important contribution to the understanding of heredity was the demonstration that there are independent units of heredity in the cells. Later, these independent units were given the name **genes**.

Genes and Chromosomes

Genes are actually segments of DNA (deoxyribonucleic acid) contained in the threadlike chromosomes within the nucleus of each cell. Genes govern the cell by controlling the manufacture of proteins, especially enzymes, which are necessary for all the chemical reactions that occur within the cell. Other proteins regulated by genes are those used for structural materials, hormones, and growth factors.

When body cells divide by the process of mitosis, the DNA that makes up the chromosomes is replicated and distributed to the daughter cells, so that each daughter cell gets exactly the same kind and number of chromosomes as were in the original cell. Each chromosome (aside from the Y chromosome, which determines male sex) may carry thousands of genes, and each gene carries the code for a specific trait (characteristic). These traits constitute the physical, biochemical, and physiologic make-up of every cell in the body. (See Box 25-1 to learn about the Human Genome Project.)

In humans, every cell except the gametes (sex cells) contains 46 chromosomes. The chromosomes exist in pairs. One member of each pair was received at the time of fertilization from the offspring's father, and one was received from the mother. The paired chromosomes, except for the pair that determines sex, are alike in size and appearance. Thus, each body cell has one pair of sex chromosomes and 22 pairs (44 chromosomes) that are not involved in sex determination and are known as **autosomes** (AW-to-somes).

The paired autosomes carry genes for the same traits at exactly the same sites on each. Any form of a gene that appears at a specific site on a chromosome is called an **allele** (al-LELE). In humans and other organisms with two sets of chromosomes (diploid organisms), the alleles for each trait exist in pairs.

CHECKPOINT `25-1` ➤ What is a gene? What is a gene made of?

Dominant and Recessive Genes

Another of Mendel's discoveries was that genes can be either dominant or recessive. A **dominant** gene is one that expresses its effect in the cell regardless of whether its allele on the matching chromosome is the same as or different from the dominant gene. The gene need be received

---

Box 25-1   Hot Topics

The Human Genome Project: Reading the Book of Life

Packed tightly in nearly every one of your body cells (except the red blood cells) is a complete copy of your genome—the genetic instructions that direct all of your cellular activities. Written in the language of DNA, these instructions consist of genes parceled into 46 chromosomes that code for proteins. In 1990, a consortium of scientists from around the world set out to crack the genetic code and read the human genome, our "book of life." This monumental task, called the Human Genome Project, was completed in 2003 and succeeded in mapping the entire human genome—3 billion DNA base pairs arranged into about 30,000 genes. Now, scientists can pinpoint the exact location and chemical code of every gene in the body.

The human genome was decoded using a technique called sequencing. Samples of human DNA were fragmented into smaller pieces and then inserted into bacteria. As the bacteria multiplied, they produced more and more copies of the human DNA fragments, which the scientists extracted. The DNA copies were loaded into a sequencing machine capable of "reading" the string of DNA nucleotides that composed each fragment. Then, using computers, the scientists put all of the sequences from the fragments back together to get the entire human genome.

Now, scientists hope to use all these pages of the book of life to revolutionize the treatment of human disease. The information obtained from the Human Genome Project may lead to improved disease diagnosis, new drug treatments, and even gene therapy.

from only one parent to be expressed in the offspring. When the matching genes for a trait are different, the alleles are described as **heterozygous** (het-er-o-ZI-gus), or hybrid.

The effect of a **recessive** gene is not evident unless its paired allele on the matching chromosome is also recessive. Thus, a recessive trait appears only if the recessive genes for that trait are received from both parents. For example, the gene for brown eyes is dominant over the gene for blue eyes, which is recessive. Blue eyes appear in the offspring only if genes for blue eyes are received from both parents. When both the genes for a trait are the same, that is, both dominant or both recessive, the alleles are said to be **homozygous** (ho-mo-ZI-gus), or purebred. A recessive trait only appears if a person's genes are homozygous for that trait.

Any characteristic that can be observed or can be tested for is part of a person's **phenotype** (FE-no-tipe). Eye color, for example, can be seen when looking at a person. Blood type is not visible but can be determined by testing and is also a part of a person's phenotype. When someone has the recessive phenotype, his or her genetic make-up, or **genotype** (JEN-o-tipe), is obviously homozygous recessive. When a dominant phenotype appears, the person's genotype can be either homozygous dominant or heterozygous. Only genetic studies or family studies can reveal which it is.

A recessive gene is not expressed if it is present in the cell together with a dominant allele. However, the recessive gene can be passed on to offspring and may thus appear in future generations. An individual who shows no evidence of a trait but has a recessive gene for that trait is described as a **carrier** of the gene. Using genetic terminology, that person shows the dominant phenotype but has a heterozygous genotype for that trait.

CHECKPOINT 25-2 ➤ What is the difference between a dominant and a recessive gene?

Distribution of Chromosomes to Offspring

The reproductive cells (ova and spermatozoa) are produced by a special process of cell division called **meiosis** (mi-O-sis). This process divides the chromosome number in half, so that each reproductive cell has 23 chromosomes. Moreover, the division occurs in such a way that each cell receives one member of each chromosome pair that was present in the original cell. The separation occurs at random, meaning that either member of the original pair may be included in a given germ cell. Thus, the maternal and paternal sets of chromosomes get mixed up and redistributed at this time, leading to increased variety within the population. Children in a family resemble each other, but no two look exactly alike (unless they are identical twins), because they receive different combinations of maternal and paternal chromosomes.

Geneticists use a grid called a **Punnett square** to show all the combinations of genes that can result from a given

parental cross (Fig. 25-1). In these calculations, a capital letter is used for the dominant gene and the recessive gene is represented by the lower case of the same letter. For example, if *B* is the gene for the dominant trait brown eyes, then *b* would be the recessive gene for blue eyes. In the offspring, the genotype BB is homozygous dominant and the genotype Bb is heterozygous, both of which will show the dominant phenotype brown eyes. The homozygous recessive genotype bb will show the recessive phenotype blue eyes.

A Punnett square shows all the possible gene combinations of a given cross and the theoretical ratios of all the genotypes produced. Actual ratios may differ if the number of offspring is small. For example, the chances of having a male or female baby are 50-50 with each birth, but a family might have several girls before having a boy, and vice versa. The chances of seeing the theoretical ratios improve as the number of offspring increases.

CHECKPOINT 25-3 ➤ What is the process of cell division that forms the gametes?

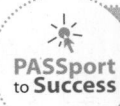 **PASSport to Success** Visit *thePoint* or see the Student Resource CD in the back of this book for a diagram of meiosis in male and female gamete formation.

Sex Determination

The two chromosomes that determine the offspring's sex, unlike the autosomes (the other 22 pairs of chromosomes), are not matched in size and appearance. The female X chromosome is larger than most other chromosomes and carries genes for other characteristics in addition to that

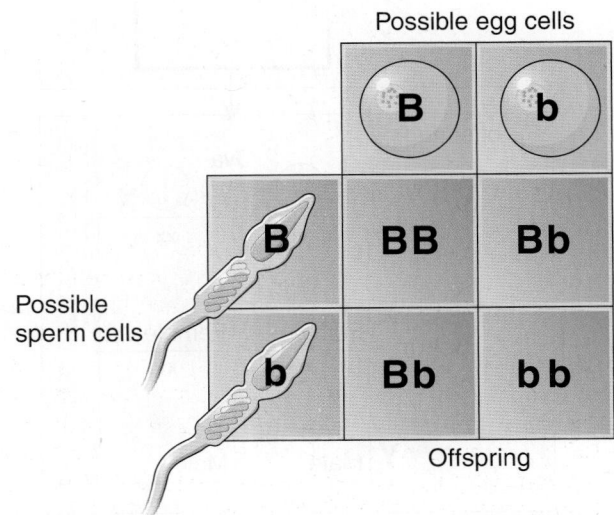

Figure 25-1 **A Punnett square.** Geneticists use this grid to show all the possible combinations of a given cross, in this case, Bb ×Bb. [**ZOOMING IN** ➤ What percentage of children will show the recessive phenotype blond hair?]

25

for sex. The male Y chromosome is smaller than other chromosomes and mainly determines sex. A female has two X chromosomes in each body cell; a male has one X and one Y.

By the process of meiosis, each male sperm cell receives either an X or a Y chromosome, whereas every egg cell receives only an X chromosome (Fig. 25-2). If a sperm cell with an X chromosome fertilizes an ovum, the resulting infant will be female; if a sperm with a Y chromosome fertilizes an ovum, the resulting infant will be male (see Fig. 25-2).

Sex-Linked Traits

Any trait that is carried on a sex chromosome is said to be **sex-linked**. Because the Y chromosome carries few traits aside from sex determination, most sex-linked traits are carried on the X chromosome and are best described as *X-linked*. Examples are hemophilia, certain forms of baldness, and red-green color blindness.

Sex-linked traits appear almost exclusively in males. The reason for this is that most of these traits are recessive, and if a recessive gene is located on the X chromosome in a male it cannot be masked by a matching dominant gene. (Remember that the Y chromosome with which the X chromosome pairs is very small and carries few genes.) Thus, a male who has only one recessive gene for a trait will exhibit that characteristic, whereas a female must have two recessive genes to show the trait. The female must inherit a recessive gene for that trait from each parent and be homozygous recessive in order for the trait to appear.

CHECKPOINT `25-4` ➤ What sex chromosome combination determines a female? A male?

CHECKPOINT `25-5` ➤ What term is used to describe a trait carried on a sex chromosome?

Hereditary Traits

Some observable hereditary traits are skin, eye, and hair color and facial features. Also influenced by genetics are less clearly defined traits, such as weight, body build, life span, and susceptibility to disease.

Some human traits, including the traits involved in many genetic diseases, are determined by a single pair of genes; most, however, are the result of two or more gene pairs acting together in what is termed **multifactorial inheritance**. This type of inheritance accounts for the wide range of variations within populations in such characteristics as coloration, height, and weight, all of which are determined by more than one pair of genes.

Gene Expression

The effect of a gene on a person's phenotype may be influenced by a variety of factors, including the individual's sex and the presence of other genes. For example, the genes for certain types of baldness and certain types of color blindness may be inherited by either males or females, but the traits appear mostly in males under the effects of male sex hormone.

Environment also plays a part in gene expression. One inherits a potential for a given size, for example, but one's actual size is additionally influenced by such factors as nutrition, development, and general state of health. The same is true of life span and susceptibility to diseases.

Genetic Mutation

As a rule, chromosomes replicate exactly during cell division. Occasionally, however, for reasons not yet totally understood, the genes or chromosomes change. This change may involve a single gene or whole chromosomes.

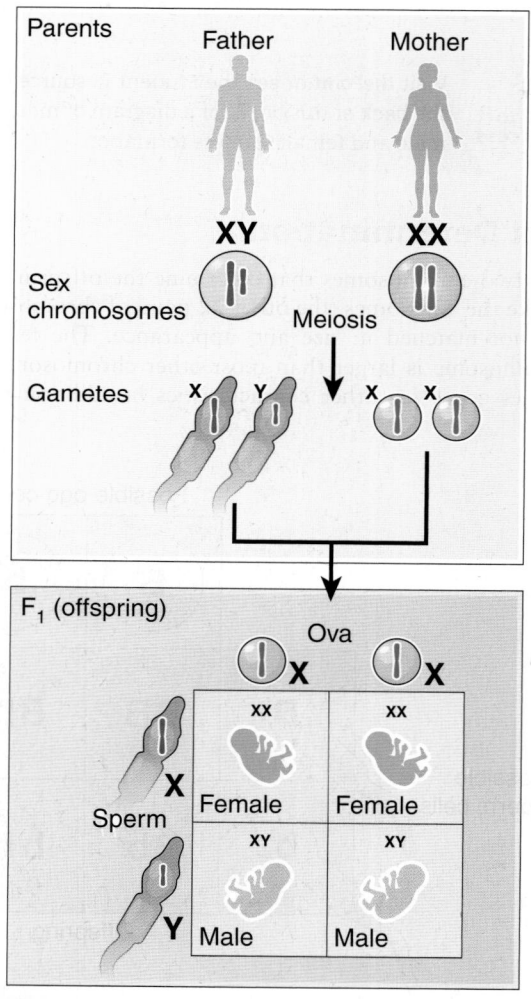

Figure 25-2 **Sex determination.** If an X chromosome from a male unites with an X chromosome from a female, the child is female (XX); if a Y chromosome from a male unites with an X chromosome from a female, the child is male (XY).

Alternatively, it may consist of chromosomal breakage, in which there is loss or rearrangement of gene fragments. Often these changes occur during cell division (mitosis or meiosis) as chromosomes come together, re-assort, and get distributed to two new cells. Such a change is termed a genetic **mutation**. Mutations may occur spontaneously or may be induced by some agent, such as ionizing radiation or chemicals, described as a **mutagen** (MU-tah-jen) or mutagenic agent.

If a mutation occurs in an ovum or a sperm cell, the altered trait will be inherited by the offspring. The vast majority of harmful mutations never are expressed because the affected fetus dies and is spontaneously aborted. Most remaining mutations are so inconsequential that they have no visible effect. Beneficial mutations, on the other hand, tend to survive and increase as a population evolves.

CHECKPOINT 25-6 ➤ What is a mutation?

Genetic Diseases

Any disorders that involve the genes may be said to be genetic, but they are not always hereditary, that is, passed from parent to offspring in the reproductive cells.

Noninherited genetic disorders may begin during maturation of the sex cells or even during development of the embryo.

Advances in genetic research have made it possible to identify the causes of many hereditary disorders and to develop genetic screening methods. In people who are "at risk" for having a child with a genetic disorder, as well as fetuses and newborns with a suspected abnormality, tests can often confirm or rule out the presence of a genetic defect.

Congenital Versus Hereditary Diseases

Before we discuss hereditary diseases, we need to distinguish them from other congenital diseases. To illustrate, let us assume that two infants are born within seconds in adjoining delivery rooms of the same hospital. It is noted that one infant has a clubfoot, a condition called **talipes** (TAL-ih-pes); the second infant has a rudimentary extra finger attached to the fifth finger of each hand, a condition called **polydactyly** (pol-e-DAK-til-e). Are both conditions hereditary? Both congenital? Is either hereditary? We can answer these questions by defining the key terms, *congenital* and *hereditary*. **Congenital** means present at the time of

Disease in Context revisited

➤ Managing Ben's Cystic Fibrosis

After learning Ben's diagnosis, his parents met with his pediatrician to discuss the treatment Ben would require to manage his cystic fibrosis. Although the doctor told them that there was no cure for cystic fibrosis yet, they were relieved to hear that there had been vast improvements in treatment in recent years. He explained that the goals of CF treatment were to minimize respiratory and digestive problems.

Therapies for respiratory problems in people with CF center on keeping the lungs clear of mucus that can block the respiratory passageways and provide an excellent growth medium for infectious organisms. Chest physical therapy, which involves pounding the chest and back with either one's hands or a machine, is the main method of removing mucus from the lungs and is repeated three to four times daily. Anti-inflammatory and mucolytic (mucus-dissolving) drugs are also useful in loosening mucus from the lungs. Unfortunately, it is difficult to remove all of the mucus, so most people with CF have persistent lung infections, which require antibiotic treatment.

Management of digestive problems also centers on clearing the digestive tract of mucus, as well as ensuring adequate nutrition. Enemas and mucolytic medications are used to treat intestinal mucoid blockages. A high-calorie diet (low in fat and high in protein) improves growth and development and helps the immune system to resist lung infections. Oral pancreatic enzymes are taken before every meal to help the small intestine digest fats and proteins and absorb more vitamins.

In this case, Ben's parents learned about the genetic causes of and treatments for cystic fibrosis. It would take them some time to absorb all of this information, but they were confident that they could minimize Ben's respiratory and digestive problems. To review the respiratory system, see Chapter 18. For a review of the digestive system, see Chapter 19.

25

birth; **hereditary** means genetically transmitted or transmissible. Thus, one condition may be both congenital and hereditary; another, congenital yet not hereditary.

Hereditary conditions are usually evident at birth or soon thereafter. However, certain inherited disorders, such as adult polycystic kidney disease and Huntington disease, a nervous disorder, do not manifest themselves until about midlife (40 to 50 years of age). People with these genetic defects may pass them on to their children before they are aware of them unless genetic testing reveals their presence. In the case of our earlier examples, the clubfoot is congenital, but not hereditary, having resulted from severe distortion of the developing extremities during intrauterine growth; the extra fingers are hereditary, a familial trait that appears in another relative, a grandparent perhaps, or a parent, and that is evident at the time of birth.

CAUSES OF CONGENITAL DISORDERS Although causes of congenital deformities and birth defects often are not known, in some cases, they are known and can be avoided. For example, certain infections and toxins may be transmitted from the mother's blood by way of the placenta to the fetal circulation. Some of these cause serious developmental disorders in affected babies.

German measles (rubella) is a contagious viral infection that is ordinarily a mild disease, but if maternal infection occurs during the first 3 or 4 months of pregnancy, the fetus has a 40% chance of developing defects of the eye (cataracts), ear (deafness), brain, and heart. Infection can be prevented by appropriate immunizations.

Ionizing radiation and various toxins may damage the genes, and the disorders they produce are sometimes transmissible. Environmental agents, such as mercury and some chemicals used in industry (e.g., certain phenols and PCB), as well as some drugs, notably LSD, are known to disrupt genetic organization. (See Box 25-2, Preventing Genetic Damage.)

Intake of alcohol and cigarette smoking by a pregnant woman often cause growth retardation and low birthweight in her infant. Smaller than normal infants do not do as well as average weight babies. Some congenital brain and heart defects have been associated with a condition called **fetal alcohol syndrome**. Healthcare professionals strongly recommend total abstinence from alcohol and cigarettes during pregnancy.

Spina bifida (SPI-nah BIF-ih-dah) is incomplete closure of the spine, through which the spinal cord and its membranes may project (Fig. 25-3). The defect usually occurs in the lumbar region. If the meninges protrude (herniate), the defect is termed a meningocele (meh-NIN-go-sele); if both the spinal cord and meninges protrude, it is a myelomeningocele (mi-eh-lo-meh-NIN-go-sele). In the latter case, the spinal cord ends at the point of the defect, which affects function below that point. Folic acid, a B vitamin, reduces the risk of spina bifida and other CNS defects in the fetus. Women of childbearing age should eat foods high in folic acid (green leafy vegetables, fruits, and legumes) and should take folic acid supplements even before pregnancy, as the nervous system develops early. In the United States, folic acid is added to grain products, such as bread, pasta, rice, and cereals.

CHECKPOINT 25-7 ➤ Can a disorder be congenital but not hereditary? Explain.

Box 25-2 🍎 **Health Maintenance**

Preventing Genetic Damage

It is sometimes difficult to determine whether a genetic defect is the result of a spontaneous random mutation or is related to exposure of a germ cell to an environmental toxin. Male and female sex cells are present at birth but do not become active until the reproductive years. This leaves a long time span during which toxic exposure can occur. Most of what we know about chemicals that cause mutations has been learned from environmental accidents. For example, mercury compounds have found their way into the food chain, causing neural damage to the children of parents who consumed foods containing mercury. Lead, which is toxic when ingested, as from air or water pollution, has been implicated in sperm cell abnormalities and in reduced sperm counts. Radiation accidents have been linked to increased susceptibility to certain cancers in children born after these accidents.

Meiosis is the step most prone to genetic errors. This process can be studied in males with specimens obtained from testicular biopsy. Also, samples of sperm cells, which are produced continuously in males, can be obtained easily and studied for visible defects. Advancing age in both the mother and the father is known to increase errors in meiosis. Males between 20 and 45 years of age carry the least risk of transmitting a genetic error. For females, the least risk is between ages 15 to 35 years. Because new sperm cells are produced on a 64-day cycle, men are advised to avoid conception for a few months after exposure to x-rays, cancer chemotherapy, or other chemicals capable of causing mutations.

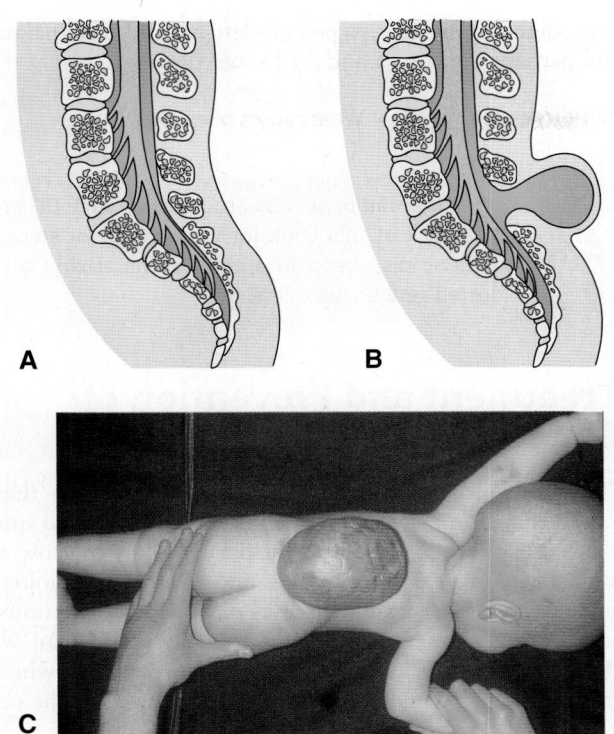

Figure 25-3 **Spina bifida, incomplete closure of the spinal cord. (A)** Normal spinal cord. **(B)** Spina bifida with protrusion of the meninges (meningocele). **(C)** Protrusion of the spinal cord and meninges (myelomeningocele). (Reprinted with permission from Pillitteri A. *Maternal and Child Health Nursing*, 4th ed. Philadelphia: Lippincott Williams & Wilkins, 2003.)

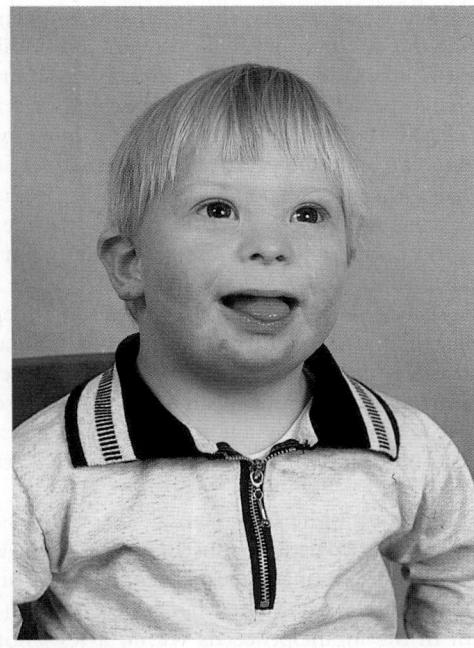

Figure 25-4 **Child with Down syndrome (trisomy 21).** The typical facial features are visible in this photo. (Reprinted with permission from Pillitteri A. *Maternal and Child Health Nursing*, 4th ed. Philadelphia: Lippincott Williams & Wilkins, 2003.)

Examples of Genetic Diseases

The best known example of a genetic disorder that is not hereditary is the most common form of **Down syndrome**, also known as **trisomy 21** because it results from an extra chromosome number 21 in each cell. This abnormality arises during formation of a sex cell. The disorder is usually recognizable at birth by the child's distinctive facial features (Fig. 25-4). Children with Down syndrome have poor muscle tone. They have lowered immunity and are also prone to heart disease, leukemia, and Alzheimer disease. Their intellectual function is impaired. However, the amount of skill they can gain depends on the severity of the disease and their family and school environments. Down syndrome is usually not inherited, although there is a hereditary form of the disorder. In most cases, both parents are normal, as are the child's siblings. The likelihood of having a baby with Down syndrome increases dramatically in women past the age of 35 years and may result from defects in either the male or female germ cells owing to age.

Most genetic diseases are **familial** or **hereditary**; that is, they are passed on from parent to child in the egg or sperm. In the case of a disorder carried by a dominant gene, only one parent needs to carry the abnormal gene to give rise to the disease. Any child who receives the defec-

tive gene will have the disease. Any children who do not show the disease do not have the defective gene nor are they carriers. One example is **Huntington disease**, a progressive degenerative disorder associated with rapid, involuntary muscle activity and mental deterioration. The disease does not appear until about age 40 and leads to death within 15 years. There is no cure for Huntington disease, but people with the defective gene can be identified by genetic testing. Another example is **Marfan syndrome**, a connective tissue disease. People with Marfan syndrome are tall, thin, and have heart defects.

If the disease trait is carried by a recessive gene, as is the case in most inheritable disorders, a defective gene must come from each parent. Some recessively inherited diseases are described next.

In **phenylketonuria** (fen-il-ke-to-NU-re-ah) **(PKU)**, the lack of a certain enzyme prevents the proper metabolism of **phenylalanine** (fen-il-AL-ah-nin), one of the common amino acids. As a result, phenylalanine accumulates in the infant's blood and appears in the urine. If the condition remains untreated, it leads to mental retardation before the age of 2 years. Newborn infants are routinely screened for PKU.

Sickle cell disease is described in Chapter 13, where it is stated that the disease is found almost exclusively among black patients. By contrast, **cystic fibrosis** is most common in white populations; in fact, it is the most frequently inherited disease among this group. Cystic fibrosis is characterized by excessively thickened secretions in the bronchi, the intestine, and the pancreatic ducts, resulting in obstruction of these vital organs. It is associated with fre-

25

quent respiratory infections, intestinal losses, particularly of fats and fat-soluble vitamins, as well as massive salt loss. Treatment includes oral administration of pancreatic enzymes and special pulmonary exercises. Cystic fibrosis was once fatal by the time of adolescence, but now, with appropriate care, life expectancies are extending into the third decade. The gene responsible for the disease has been identified, raising hope of better diagnosis, treatment, and perhaps even correction of the defective gene that causes the disorder.

In **Tay-Sachs disease**, a certain type of fat is deposited in neurons of the CNS and retina because cellular lysosomes lack an enzyme that breaks it down. The disease occurs mainly in eastern European (Ashkenazi) Jews and generally leads to death by age four. There is no cure for Tay-Sachs, but a blood test can identify genetic carriers of the disease.

Another group of heritable muscle disorders is known collectively as the **progressive muscular atrophies**. Atrophy (AT-ro-fe) means wasting due to decrease in the size of a normally developed part. The absence of normal muscle movement in the infant proceeds within a few months to extreme weakness of the respiratory muscles, until ultimately the infant is unable to breathe adequately. Most afflicted babies die within several months. The name *floppy baby syndrome*, as the disease is commonly called, provides a vivid description of its effects.

Albinism is another recessively inherited disorder that affects the cells (melanocytes) that produce the pigment melanin. The skin and hair color are strikingly white and do not darken with age. The skin is abnormally sensitive to sunlight and may appear wrinkled. People with albinism are especially susceptible to skin cancer and to some severe visual disturbances, such as myopia (nearsightedness) and abnormal sensitivity to light (photophobia).

Fragile X syndrome is the most common cause of inherited mental retardation in both males and females. It is an X-linked recessive disorder associated with a fragile site on an arm of the X chromosome. In males, it also causes enlarged testes, hyperactivity, mitral valve malfunction, high forehead, and enlarged jaw and ears.

Other inherited disorders include **osteogenesis** (os-te-o-JEN-eh-sis) **imperfecta**, or *brittle bone disease*, in which multiple fractures may occur during and shortly after fetal life, and a disorder of skin, muscles, and bones called **neurofibromatosis** (nu-ro-fi-bro-mah-TO-sis). In the latter condition, multiple masses, often on stalks (pedunculated), grow along nerves all over the body.

More than 20 different cancers have been linked to specific gene mutations. These include cancers of the breast, ovary, and colon as well as some forms of leukemia. Note, however, that hereditary forms of cancer account for only about 1% of all cancers and that the development of cancer is complex, involving not only specific genes but also gene interactions and environmental factors.

Genetic components have been suggested in some other diseases as well, including certain forms of heart disease, diabetes mellitus, types of cleft lip and cleft palate, and perhaps Parkinson and Alzheimer disease.

CHECKPOINT 25-8 ➤ What causes phenylketonuria?

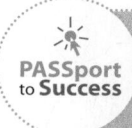

Visit **thePoint** or see the Student Resource CD in the back of this book for illustrations of some genetic diseases and a chart summarizing selected genetic disorders.

Treatment and Prevention of Genetic Diseases

The number of genetic diseases is so great (more than 4,000) that many pages of this book would be needed simply to list them all. Moreover, the list continues to grow as sophisticated research techniques and advances in biology make it clear that various diseases of previously unknown origin are genetic—some hereditary, others not. Can we identify which are inherited genetic disorders and which are due to environmental factors? Can we prevent the occurrence of any of them?

Genetic Counseling

It is possible to prevent genetic disorders in many cases and even to treat some of them. The most effective method of preventing genetic disease is through genetic counseling, a specialized field of health care. Genetic counseling centers use a team approach of medical, nursing, laboratory, and social service professionals to advise and care for clients. People who might consider genetic counseling include prospective parents over the age of 35, those who have a family history of genetic disorders, and those who are considering some form of fertility treatment.

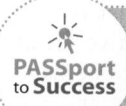

Visit **thePoint** or see the Student Resource CD in the back of this book for a description of careers in genetic counseling.

THE FAMILY HISTORY An accurate and complete family history of both prospective parents is necessary for genetic counseling. This history should include information about relatives with respect to age, onset of a specific disease, health status, and cause of death. The families' ethnic origins may be relevant because some genetic diseases predominate in certain ethnic groups. Hospital and physician records are studied, as are photographs of family members. The ages of the prospective parents are considered as factors, as is parental or ancestral relationship (e.g., marriage between first cousins). The complete, detailed family history, or tree, is called a pedigree. Pedigrees are used to determine the pattern of inheritance of a genetic disease within a family (Fig. 25-5). They may also indicate whether

The recessive trait c is cystic fibrosis.
The dominant normal gene is C.

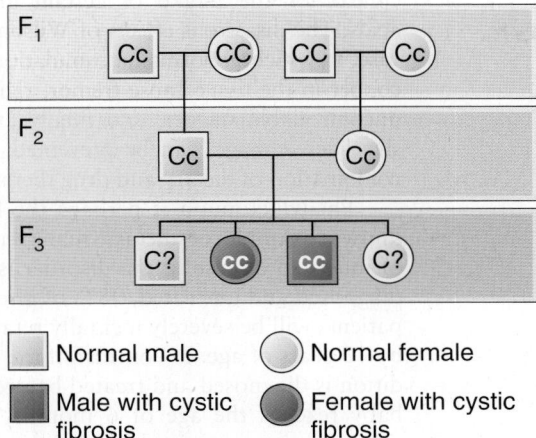

Normal male

Normal female

Male with cystic fibrosis

Female with cystic fibrosis

Figure 25-5 **A pedigree (family history) showing three generations (F₁–F₃).** The pedigree is a tool used in genetic studies and genetic counseling. In this example, one parent in each F₁ cross and both parents in the F₂ cross are normal but carry the recessive gene (c) for cystic fibrosis. For the normal children in F₃, only one gene (the dominant normal gene) is known. Note that the F₃ generation does not show strict predicted genetic ratios. Theoretically, only one in four children should be homozygous recessive (have two recessive genes. [**ZOOMING IN** ➤ What are the possible genotypes of the two normal children in the F₃ generation?]

a given family member is a carrier of the disease. Note that in some cases, there is not enough family data to determine the genotype of all members with regard to a given trait. Also, small numbers of offspring may not show the strict genetic ratios expected from a given cross (see Fig. 25-5).

LABORATORY STUDIES One technique that enables the geneticist to study an unborn fetus is **amniocentesis** (am-ne-o-sen-TE-sis). During this procedure, a small amount of the amniotic fluid that surrounds the fetus is withdrawn (Fig. 25-6). Fetal skin cells in the amniotic fluid are removed, grown (cultured), and separated for study. The chromosomes are examined, and the amniotic fluid is analyzed for biochemical abnormalities. With these methods, almost 200 genetic diseases can be detected before birth.

Another method for obtaining fetal cells for study involves sampling of the chorionic villi through the cervix. The chorionic villi are hairlike projections

of the membrane that surrounds the embryo in early pregnancy. The method is called **chorionic villus sampling (CVS)**. Samples may be taken between 8 and 10 weeks of pregnancy, and the cells obtained may be analyzed immediately. In contrast, amniocentesis cannot be done before the 14th to 16th week of pregnancy, and test results are not available for about 2 weeks.

Abnormalities in the chromosome number and some abnormalities within the chromosomes can be detected by **karyotype** (KAR-e-o-tipe) analysis. A karyotype is produced by growing cells obtained by amniocentesis or CVS in a special medium and arresting cell division at the metaphase stage. A technician uses special stains to reveal certain changes in fine structure within the chromosomes. The chromosomes, visible under the microscope, are then photographed, and the photographs are cut out and arranged in groups according to their size and form (Fig. 25-7). Abnormalities in the number or structure of the chromosomes can thereby be detected.

COUNSELING PROSPECTIVE PARENTS Armed with all the available pertinent facts, and with knowledge of genetic inheritance patterns, the counselor is equipped to inform the prospective parents of the possibility of their having genetically abnormal offspring. The couple may then use this information to make decisions about family planning. Depending on the individuals and their situation, a couple might elect to have no children, have an adoptive family, use a donor gamete, terminate a pregnancy, or accept the risk.

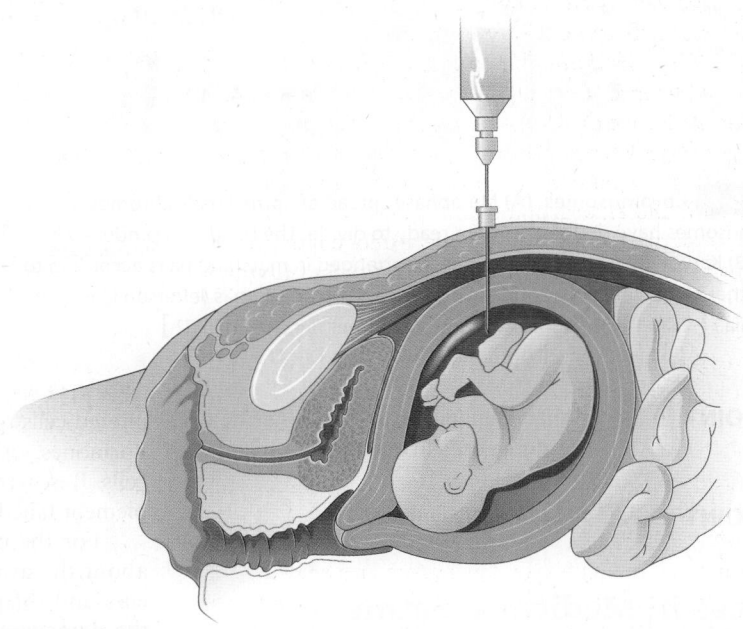

Figure 25-6 **Amniocentesis.** A sample of amniotic fluid is removed from the amniotic sac. Cells and fluid are tested for fetal abnormalities. (Reprinted with permission from Cohen BJ. *Medical Terminology*, 5th ed. Philadelphia: Lippincott Williams & Wilkins, 2008.)

25

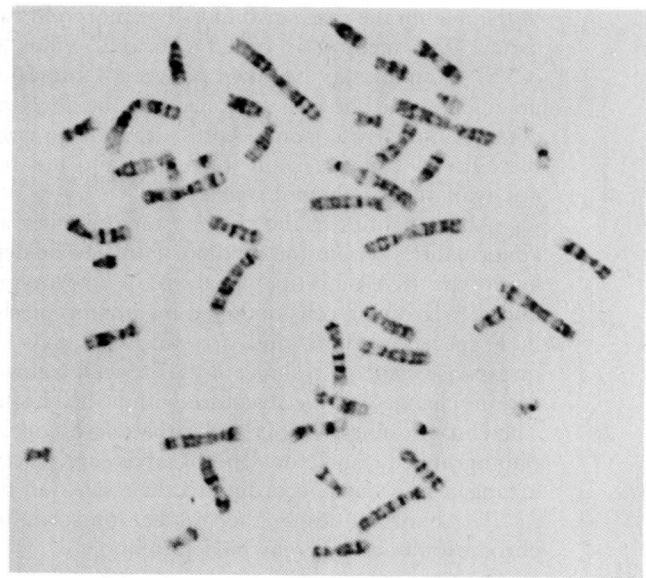

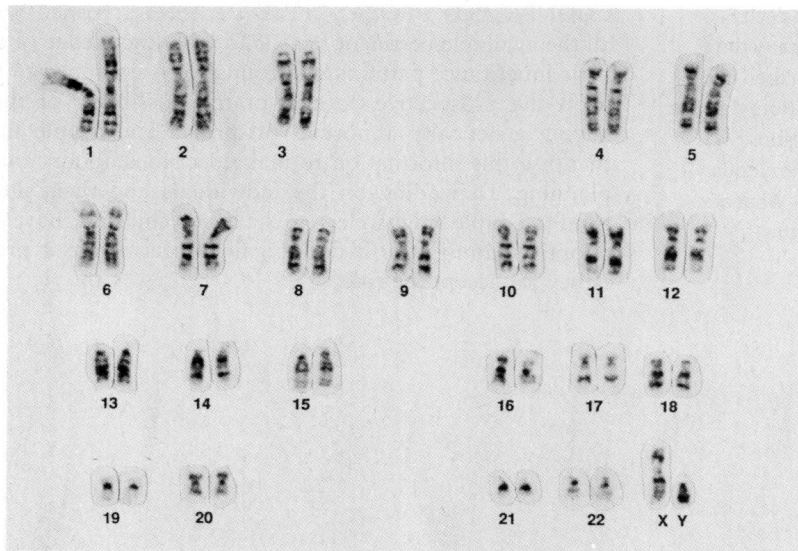

CHECKPOINT **25-9** ➤ What is a pedigree and how is a pedigree used in genetic counseling?

CHECKPOINT **25-10** ➤ What is a karyotype?

Progress in Medical Treatment

The mental and physical ravages of many genetic diseases are largely preventable, provided the diseases are diagnosed and treated early in the individual's life. Some of these diseases respond well to dietary control. One such disease,

called **maple syrup urine disease**, responds to very large doses of thiamin along with control of the intake of certain amino acids. The disastrous effects of **Wilson disease**, in which abnormal accumulations of copper in the tissue cause tremor, rigidity, uncontrollable stagger, and finally extensive liver damage, can be prevented by a combination of dietary and drug therapies.

Phenylketonuria is perhaps the best-known example of dietary management of inherited disease. If the disorder is undiagnosed and untreated, 98% of affected patients will be severely mentally retarded by 10 years of age. In contrast, if the condition is diagnosed and treated before the baby reaches the age of 6 months, and treatment is maintained until the age of 10 years, mental deficiency will be prevented, or at least minimized. A simple blood test for PKU is now done routinely in hospitals throughout the United States. Infants are usually screened immediately after birth, but they should be retested 24 to 48 hours after taking in protein.

Klinefelter (KLINE-fel-ter) **syndrome**, which occurs in about 1 in 600 males, is a common cause of underdevelopment of the gonads with resulting infertility. Inheritors of this disorder have abnormal sex chromosome patterns, usually an extra X chromosome. Instead of the typical male XY pattern, the cells contain an XXY combination owing to failure of the sex chromosomes to separate during cell division. Treatment of this disorder includes the use of hormones and psychotherapy.

In the future, we can anticipate greatly improved methods of screening, diagnosis, and treatment of genetic diseases. There have been reports of fetuses being treated with vitamins or hormones after prenatal diagnosis of a genetic disorder. Ahead lies the possibility of treating or correcting genetic disorders through genetic engineering—introducing genetically altered cells to produce missing factors, such as enzymes or hormones, or even correcting faulty genes in the patient's cells. Researchers have already made some attempts to supplement failed genes with healthy ones.

For the present, it is important to educate the public about the availability of screening methods for both parents and offspring. People should also be made aware of the damaging effects of radiation, drugs, and other toxic substances on the genes. Because so many congenital disorders are associated with environmental factors, public education and better health habits will probably yield greater overall benefits than genetic manipulations.

Word Anatomy

Medical terms are built from standardized word parts (prefixes, roots, and suffixes). Learning the meanings of these parts can help you remember words and interpret unfamiliar terms.

WORD PART	MEANING	EXAMPLE
Genes and Chromosomes		
chrom/o	color	*Chromosomes* color darkly with stains.
aut/o-	self	*Autosomes* are all the chromosomes aside from the two that determine sex.
heter/o	other, different	*Heterozygous* paired genes (alleles) are different from each other.
homo-	same	*Homozygous* paired genes (alleles) are the same.
phen/o	to show	Traits that can be observed or tested for make up a person's *phenotype*.
Hereditary Traits		
multi-	many	*Multifactorial* traits are determined by multiple pairs of genes.
Genetic Diseases		
dactyl/o	digit (finger or toe)	In *polydactyly* there is an extra finger on each hand.
con-	with	A *congenital* defect is present at the time of birth.
-cele	swelling	In spina bifida, the meninges can protrude through the spine as a *meningocele*.
Treatment and Prevention of Genetic Diseases		
-centesis	tapping, perforation	*Amniocentesis* is a tap of the amniotic fluid.
kary/o	nucleus	A *karyotype* is an analysis of the chromosomes contained in the nucleus of a cell.

Summary

I. **GENES AND CHROMOSOMES**
   A. Genes
      1. Hereditary units
      2. Segments of DNA
      3. Control manufacture of proteins (e.g., enzymes, hormones)
   B. Chromosomes
      1. Threadlike bodies in nucleus; 46 in humans
      2. Composed of genes
      3. 22 pairs autosomes (non-sex chromosomes)
      4. 1 pair sex chromosomes
   C. Dominant and recessive genes
      1. Dominant gene—always expressed
         a. May be heterozygous (two genes different)
         b. May be homozygous dominant (two genes the same)
      2. Recessive gene—expressed only if homozygous recessive (received from both parents)
         a. Carrier—person with recessive gene that is not apparent but can be passed to offspring
         b. Phenotype—characteristic that can be seen or tested for
         c. Genotype—genetic make-up
   D. Distribution of chromosomes to offspring
      1. Meiosis
         a. Cell division that forms sex cells with 23 chromosomes

25

b.   Each cell receives one of each chromosome pair
c.   Punnett square shows results of crosses
E.   Sex determination
1.   X chromosome larger and carries other traits
2.   Y smaller and carries mainly gene for sex determination
3.   Female cells have XX; male cells have XY
F.   Sex-linked traits
1.   Traits carried on sex chromosome (usually X)
2.   Sex-linked traits appear mostly in males
a.   Passed from mother to son on X chromosome
b.   If recessive, not masked by dominant gene on Y
c.   Examples—hemophilia, baldness, red-green color blindness

II.   **HEREDITARY TRAITS**
A.   Genes determine physical, biochemical, and physiologic characteristics of every cell
1.   Some traits determined by single gene pairs
2.   Most determined by multifactorial inheritance
a.   Involves multiple gene pairs
b.   Produces a range of variations in a population
c.   Examples—height, weight, coloration, susceptibility to disease
B.   Gene expression
1.   Factors
a.   Sex
b.   Presence of other genes
c.   Environment
C.   Genetic mutation
1.   Change in genes or chromosomes
2.   May be passed to offspring if occurs in germ cells
3.   Mutagenic agents
a.   Factors causing mutation
b.   Examples—ionizing radiation, chemicals

III.   **GENETIC DISEASES**—disorders involving genes
A.   Congenital versus hereditary diseases
1.   Congenital disorders
a.   Present at birth
b.   May or may not be hereditary
2.   Hereditary (familial) disorders
a.   Passed from parent to offspring in sex cells
3.   Causes—infections, toxins, ionizing radiation, alcohol, smoking
a.   Examples—defects caused by rubella, fetal alcohol syndrome, spina bifida
B.   Examples of genetic diseases
1.   Down syndrome—results from extra chromosome 21 (trisomy 21)
2.   Dominant inheritance—Huntington disease, Marfan sundrome
3.   Recessive inheritance—PKU (phenylketonuria), cystic fibrosis, sickle cell anemia, Tay-Sachs disease, progressive muscular atrophies, albinism, osteogenesis imperfecta, neurofibromatosis

IV.   **TREATMENT AND PREVENTION OF GENETIC DISEASES**
A.   Genetic counseling
1.   Pedigree—family history
2.   Laboratory studies
a.   Amniocentesis—withdrawal of amniotic fluid for study at 14 to 16 weeks of pregnancy
b.   Chorionic villus sampling—done at 8 to 10 weeks of pregnancy
c.   Karyotype—analysis of chromosomes
3.   Counseling the prospective parents
B.   Progress in medical treatment
1.   Dietary control—maple syrup urine disease, Wilson disease, PKU
2.   Hormone therapy—Klinefelter disease
3.   Fetal therapy
4.   Correction of faulty genes—experimental

Questions for Study and Review

BUILDING UNDERSTANDING

Fill in the blanks

1.   The basic unit of heredity is a(n) _____.

2.   Chromosomes not involved in sex determination are known as _____.

3.   Any trait that is carried on a sex chromosome is said to be _____.

4.   Change in a gene or chromosome is called _____.

5.   Incomplete closure of the spine results in a disorder called _____.

Matching > Match each numbered item with the most closely related lettered item.

___ **6.** A gene that is always expressed if present

___ **7.** A gene that is not always expressed if present

___ **8.** Term for paired genes for a trait that are the same

___ **9.** Term for paired genes for a trait that are different

a. dominant

b. recessive

c. homozygous

d. heterozygous

Multiple choice

___ **10.** The genetic code is composed of
   a. deoxyribonucleic acid
   b. ribonucleic acid
   c. protein
   d. nuclear membrane

___ **11.** Genes govern the cell by controlling the manufacture of
   a. carbohydrates
   b. lipids
   c. proteins
   d. electrolytes

___ **12.** Paired genes for a given trait are known as
   a. chromosomes
   b. ribosomes
   c. nucleotides
   d. alleles

___ **13.** A condition characterized by extra fingers or toes is called
   a. talipes
   b. polydactyly
   c. osteogenesis imperfecta
   d. neurofibromatosis

___ **14.** A complete detailed family history can be obtained by doing
   a. chorionic villus sampling
   b. amniocentesis
   c. a karyotype
   d. a pedigree

UNDERSTANDING CONCEPTS

15. How many chromosomes are there in a human body cell? In a human gamete?

16. Dana has one dominant allele for brown eyes (*B*) and one recessive allele for blue eyes. What is Dana's genotype? What is her phenotype?

17. Describe the process of meiosis and explain how it results in genetic variation.

18. Explain the great variation in the color of skin and hair in humans.

19. Describe how a mutagenic agent can produce genetic variation.

20. What is the difference between a congenital disease and a hereditary disease? List some congenital and hereditary diseases.

21. What is PKU and how should this disease be treated?

22. Compare and contrast amniocentesis and chorionic villus sampling. List some diseases that can be diagnosed using these techniques.

23. What is the most common inheritable disease among black people? Among white people? What are the symptoms of these two diseases?

CONCEPTUAL THINKING

24. If mitosis were used to produce gametes, what consequences would this have on the offspring's genotype, phenotype, and chromosome number?

25. Jason and Nicole are expecting their first child and are wondering what their child's eye color might be. Jason has blue eyes (a recessive trait) and Nicole has brown eyes (a dominant trait). Both of Jason's parents have blue eyes. One of Nicole's parents has brown eyes, the other has blue eyes. What are Jason's and Nicole's genotype and phenotype? What are the possible genotypes and phenotypes of their children?

26. In the case story, Ben's parents were both carriers of the cystic fibrosis trait. Using a Punnett square, calculate the possible genotypic and phenotypic combinations for their offspring.

25

Glossary

A

abdominopelvic (ab-dom-ih-no-PEL-vik) Pertaining to the abdomen and pelvis.

abduction (ab-DUK-shun) Movement away from the midline.

abortifacient (ah-bor-tih-FA-shent) Agent that induces an abortion.

abortion (ah-BOR-shun) Loss of an embryo or fetus before the 20th week of pregnancy.

abscess (AB-ses) Area of tissue breakdown; a localized space in the body containing pus and liquefied tissue.

absorption (ab-SORP-shun) Transfer of digested nutrients from the digestive tract into the circulation.

accommodation (ah-kom-o-DA-shun) Coordinated changes in the lens of the eye that enable one to focus on near and far objects.

acetylcholine (as-e-til-KO-lene) (**ACh**) Neurotransmitter; released at synapses within the nervous system and at the neuromuscular junction.

acid (AH-sid) Substance that can donate a hydrogen ion to another substance.

acid-fast stain Procedure used to color cells for viewing under the microscope.

acidosis (as-ih-DO-sis) Condition that results from a decrease in the pH of body fluids.

acne (AK-ne) Disease of the sebaceous glands.

acquired immunodeficiency syndrome (**AIDS**) Viral disease that attacks the immune system, specifically the T-helper lymphocytes with CD4 receptors.

acromegaly (ak-ro-MEG-ah-le) Condition caused by oversecretion of growth hormone in adults; there is overgrowth of some bones and involvement of multiple body systems.

acrosome (AK-ro-some) Caplike structure over the head of the sperm cell that helps the sperm to penetrate the ovum.

ACTH See adrenocorticotropic hormone.

actin (AK-tin) One of the two contractile proteins in muscle cells, the other being myosin.

action potential Sudden change in the electrical charge on a cell membrane, which then spreads along the membrane; nerve impulse.

active transport Movement of a substance into or out of a cell in an opposite direction to the way in which it would normally flow by diffusion; active transport requires energy and transporters.

acupuncture (AK-u-punk-chur) Ancient Chinese method of inserting thin needles into the body at specific points to relieve pain or promote healing.

acute (ah-KUTE) Referring to a severe but short-lived disease or condition.

Addison disease Condition caused by hypofunction of the adrenal cortex.

adduction (ad-DUK-shun) Movement toward the midline.

adenoids (Ad-eh-noyds) Popular name for pharygeal tonsil located in the nasopharynx.

adenosine triphosphate (ah-DEN-o-sene tri-FOS-fate) (**ATP**) Energy-storing compound found in all cells.

ADH See antidiuretic hormone.

adhesion (ad-HE-zhun) Holding together of two surfaces or parts; band of connective tissue between parts that are normally separate; molecular attraction between contacting bodies.

adipose (AD-ih-pose) Referring to fats or a type of connective tissue that stores fat.

adrenal (ah-DRE-nal) **gland** Endocrine gland located above the kidney; suprarenal gland.

adrenaline (ah-DREN-ah-lin) See epinephrine.

adrenergic (ad-ren-ER-jik) An activity or structure that responds to epinephrine (adrenaline).

adrenocorticotropic (ah-dre-no-kor-tih-ko-TRO-pik) **hormone** (**ACTH**) Hormone produced by the pituitary that stimulates the adrenal cortex.

aerobic (air-O-bik) Requiring oxygen.

afferent (AF-fer-ent) Carrying toward a given point, such as a sensory neuron that carries nerve impulses toward the central nervous system.

agglutination (ah-glu-tih-NA-shun) Clumping of cells due to an antigen–antibody reaction.

agranulocyte (a-GRAN-u-lo-site) Leukocyte without visible granules in the cytoplasm when stained; lymphocyte or monocyte.

AIDS See acquired immunodeficiency syndrome.

albinism (AL-bih-nizm) A hereditary disorder that affects melanin production.

albumin (al-BU-min) Protein in blood plasma and other body fluids; helps maintain the osmotic pressure of the blood.

albuminuria (al-bu-mih-NU-re-ah) Presence of albumin in the urine, usually as a result of a kidney disorder.

aldosterone (al-DOS-ter-one) Hormone released by the adrenal cortex that promotes sodium and water reabsorption in the kidneys.

alkali (AL-kah-li) Substance that can accept a hydrogen ion (H^+); substance that donates a hydroxide ion (OH^-); a base.

alkalosis (al-kah-LO-sis) Condition that results from an increase in the pH of body fluids.

allele (al-LELE) One member of the gene pair that controls a given trait.

allergen (AL-er-jen) Substance that causes hypersensitivity; substance that induces allergy.

allergy (AL-er-je) Tendency to react unfavorably to a certain substance that is normally harmless to most people; hypersensitivity.

alopecia (al-o-PE-she-ah) Baldness.

alveolus (al-VE-o-lus) Small sac or pouch; usually a tiny air sac in the lungs through which gases are exchanged between the outside air and the blood; tooth socket; pl., alveoli.

Alzheimer (ALZ-hi-mer) **disease** Unexplained degeneration of the cerebral cortex and hippocampus with intellectual impairment, mood changes, and confusion.

amblyopia (am-ble-O-pe-ah) Vision loss in a healthy eye because it cannot work properly with the other eye.

amino (ah-ME-no) **acid** Building block of protein.

amniocentesis (am-ne-o-sen-TE-sis) Removal of fluid and cells from the amniotic sac for prenatal diagnostic tests.

amniotic (am-ne-OT-ik) Pertaining to the sac that surrounds and cushions the developing fetus or to the fluid that fills that sac.

amniotic (am-ne-OT-ik) **sac** Fluid-filled sac that surrounds and cushions the developing fetus.

amphiarthrosis (am-fe-ar-THRO-sis) Slightly movable joint.

amyotrophic (ah-mi-o-TROF-ik) **lateral sclerosis** (**ALS**) Disorder of the nervous system in which motor neurons are destroyed.

anabolism (ah-NAB-o-lizm) Metabolic building of simple compounds into more complex substances needed by the body.

anaerobic (an-air-O-bik) Not requiring oxygen.

analgesic (an-al-JE-zik) Relieving pain; a pain-relieving agent that does not cause loss of consciousness.

anaphase (AN-ah-faze) The third stage of mitosis in which chromosomes separate to opposite sides of the cell.

anaphylaxis (an-ah-fih-LAK-sis) Severe, life-threatening allergic response.

anastomosis (ah-nas-to-MO-sis) Communication between two structures, such as blood vessels.

anatomy (ah-NAT-o-me) Study of body structure.

anemia (ah-NE-me-ah) Abnormally low level of hemoglobin or red cells in the blood, resulting in inadequate delivery of oxygen to the tissues.

androgen (AN-dro-jen) Any male sex hormone.

anesthesia (an-es-THE-ze-ah) Loss of sensation, particularly of pain; drug with this effect is an anesthetic.

aneurysm (AN-u-rizm) Bulging sac in the wall of a vessel.

angiotensin (an-je-o-TEN-sin) Substance formed in the blood by the action of the renal enzyme renin; it increases blood pressure by causing vascular constriction and stimulating the release of aldosterone from the adrenal cortex.

angina (an-JI-nah) Severe choking pain; disease or condition producing such pain. Angina pectoris is suffocating pain in the chest, usually caused by lack of oxygen supply to the heart muscle.

angioplasty (AN-je-o-plas-te) Use of a balloon inserted with a catheter to open a blocked vessel.

anion (AN-i-on) Negatively charged particle (ion).

anorexia (an-o-REK-se-ah) Chronic loss of appetite. Anorexia nervosa is a psychological condition in which a person may become seriously, even fatally, weakened from lack of food.

anoxia (ah-NOK-se-ah) See hypoxia.

ANP See atrial natriuretic peptide.

ANS See autonomic nervous system.

antagonist (an-TAG-o-nist) Muscle that has an action opposite that of a given movement; substance that opposes the action of another substance.

anterior (an-TE-re-or) Toward the front or belly surface; ventral.

anthelmintic (ant-hel-MIN-tik) Agent that acts against worms; vermicide; vermifuge.

antibiotic (an-te-bi-OT-ik) Substance produced by living cells that kills or arrests the growth of bacteria.

antibody (AN-te-bod-e) **(Ab)** Substance produced in response to a specific antigen; immunoglobulin.

antidiuretic (an-ti-di-u-RET-ik) **hormone (ADH)** Hormone released from the posterior pituitary gland that increases water reabsorption in the kidneys, thus decreasing the urinary output.

antigen (AN-te-jen) **(Ag)** Foreign substance that produces an immune response.

antineoplastic (an-ti-ne-o-PLAS-tik) Acting against a neoplasm (tumor).

antioxidant (an-te-OX-ih-dant) Substances in the diet that protect against harmful free radicals.

antipyretic (an-ti-pi-RET-ik) Drug that reduces fever.

antiseptic (an-tih-SEP-tik) Substance that prevents pathogens from multiplying but does not necessarily kill them.

antiserum (an-te-SE-rum) Serum containing antibodies that may be given to provide passive immunity; immune serum.

antitoxin (an-te-TOKS-in) Antibody that neutralizes a toxin.

antivenin (an-te-VEN-in) Antibody that neutralizes a snake venom.

anus (A-nus) Inferior opening of the digestive tract.

aorta (a-OR-tah) The largest artery; carries blood out of the heart's left ventricle.

apex (A-peks) Pointed region of a cone-shaped structure.

aphasia (ah-FA-ze-ah) Loss or defect in language communication; loss of the ability to speak or write is expressive aphasia; loss of understanding of written or spoken language is receptive aphasia.

apnea (AP-ne-ah) Temporary cessation of breathing.

apocrine (AP-o-krin) Referring to a gland that releases some cellular material along with its secretions.

aponeurosis (ap-o-nu-RO-sis) Broad sheet of fibrous connective tissue that attaches muscle to bone or to other muscle.

appendicular (ap-en-DIK-u-lar) **skeleton** Part of the skeleton that includes the bones of the upper extremities, lower extremities, shoulder girdle, and hips.

appendix (ah-PEN-diks) Fingerlike tube of lymphatic tissue attached to the first portion of the large intestine; vermiform (wormlike) appendix.

aqueous (A-kwe-us) Pertaining to water; an aqueous solution is one in which water is the solvent.

aqueous (A-kwe-us) **humor** Watery fluid that fills much of the eyeball anterior to the lens.

arachnoid (ah-RAK-noyd) Middle layer of the meninges.

areolar (ah-RE-o-lar) Referring to loose connective tissue, any small space, or to an areola, a circular area of marked color.

arrector pili (ah-REK-tor PI-li) Muscle attached to a hair follicle that raises the hair.

arrhythmia (ah-RITH-me-ah) Abnormal rhythm of the heartbeat; dysrhythmia.

arteriole (ar-TE-re-ole) Vessel between a small artery and a capillary.

arteriosclerosis (ar-te-re-o-skle-RO-sis) Hardening of the arteries.

artery (AR-ter-e) Vessel that carries blood away from the heart.

arthritis (arth-RI-tis) Inflammation of the joints.

arthrocentesis (ar-thro-sen-TE-sis) Puncture of a joint to withdraw fluid.

arthroscope (AR-thro-skope) Instrument for examining the interior of the knee and surgically repairing the knee.

articular (ar-TIK-u-lar) Pertaining to a joint.

ascites (ah-SI-teze) Abnormal collection of fluid in the abdominal cavity.

asepsis (a-SEP-sis) Condition in which no pathogens are present; adj., aseptic.

asthma (AZ-mah) Allergy-induced inflammation and constriction of the air passageways.

astigmatism (ah-STIG-mah-tizm) Visual defect due to an irregularity in the curvature of the cornea or the lens.

ataxia (ah-TAK-se-ah) Lack of muscular coordination; irregular muscular action.

atelectasis (at-e-LEK-tah-sis) Incomplete lung expansion; collapsed lung.

atherosclerosis (ath-er-o-skleh-RO-sis) Hardening of the arteries due to the deposit of yellowish, fatlike material in the lining of these vessels.

atom (AT-om) Smallest subunit of a chemical element.

atomic number The number of protons in the nucleus of an element's atoms; a number characteristic of each element.

atopic dermatitis (ah-TOP-ik der-mah-TI-tis) Skin condition that may involve redness, blisters, pimples, scaling, and crusting; eczema.

ATP See adenosine triphosphate.

atrial natriuretic (na-tre-u-RET-ik) **peptide (ANP)** Hormone produced by the atria of the heart that lowers blood pressure.

atrioventricular (a-tre-o-ven-TRIK-u-lar) **(AV) node** Part of the heart's conduction system.

atrium (A-tre-um) One of the heart's two upper chambers; adj., atrial.

atrophy (AT-ro-fe) Wasting or decrease in size of a part.

attenuated (ah-TEN-u-a-ted) Weakened.

autoclave Instrument used to sterilize material with steam under pressure.

autoimmunity (aw-to-ih-MU-nih-te) Abnormal reactivity to one's own tissues.

autologous (aw-TOL-o-gus) Related to self, such as blood or tissue taken from one's own body.

autonomic (aw-to-NOM-ik) **nervous system (ANS)** The part of the nervous system that controls smooth muscle, cardiac muscle, and glands; the visceral or involuntary nervous system.

autosome (AW-to-some) A chromosome not involved in sex determination. There are 44 autosomes (22 pairs) in humans.

AV node See atrioventricular node.

axial (AK-se-al) **skeleton** The part of the skeleton that includes the skull, spinal column, ribs, and sternum.

axilla (ak-SIL-ah) Hollow beneath the arm where it joins the body; armpit.

axon (AK-son) Fiber of a neuron that conducts impulses away from the cell body.

B

bacillus (bah-SIL-us) Rod-shaped bacterium; pl., bacilli (bah-SIL-i).

bacterium (bak-TE-re-um) Type of microorganism; pl., bacteria (bak-TE-re-ah).

bacteriostasis (bak-te-re-o-STA-sis) Condition in which bacterial growth is inhibited but the organisms are not killed.

band cell Immature neutrophil.

baroreceptor (bar-o-re-SEP-ter) Receptor that responds to pressure, such as those in vessel walls that respond to stretching and help regulate blood pressure; a type of mechanoreceptor.

basal ganglia (BA-sal GANG-le-ah) Gray masses in the lower part of the forebrain that aid in muscle coordination.

base Substance that can accept a hydrogen ion (H^+); substance that donates a hydroxide ion (OH^-); an alkali.

basophil (BA-so-fil) Granular white blood cell that shows large, dark blue cytoplasmic granules when stained with basic stain.

B cell Agranular white blood cell that gives rise to antibody-producing plasma cells in response to an antigen; B lymphocyte.

Bell palsy Facial paralysis caused by damage to the facial nerve (VII), usually on one side of the face.

benign (be-NINE) Denoting a mild condition, favorable for recovery, or a tumor that does not metastasize (spread).

bicarbonate ion (bi-KAR-bon-ate I-on) Ion formed from carbonic acid along with hydrogen ion.

bile Substance produced in the liver that emulsifies fats.

bilirubin (BIL-ih-ru-bin) Pigment derived from the breakdown of hemoglobin and found in bile.

biofeedback (bi-o-FEED-bak) A method for controlling involuntary responses by means of electronic devices that monitor changes and feed information back to a person.

biopsy (BI-op-se) Removal of tissue or other material from the living body for examination, usually under the microscope.

blood urea nitrogen (BUN) Amount of nitrogen from urea in the blood; test to evaluate kidney function.

bolus (BO-lus) A concentrated mass; the portion of food that is moved to the back of the mouth and swallowed.

Bowman capsule Enlarged portion of the nephron that contains the glomerulus; glomerular capsule.

bone Hard connective tissue that makes up most of the skeleton, or any structure composed of this type of tissue.

bradycardia (brad-e-KAR-de-ah) Heart rate of less than 60 beats per minute.

brain The central controlling area of the central nervous system (CNS).

brain stem Portion of the brain that connects the cerebrum with the spinal cord; contains the midbrain, pons, and medulla oblongata.

Broca (bro-KAH) **area** Area of the cerebral cortex concerned with motor control of speech.

bronchiole (BRONG-ke-ole) Microscopic branch of a bronchus.

bronchoscope (BRONG-ko-skope) Endoscope for examination of the bronchi and removal of small objects from the bronchi.

bronchus (BRONG-kus) Large air passageway in the lung; pl., bronchi (BRONG-ki).

buffer (BUF-er) Substance that prevents sharp changes in the pH of a solution.

bulbourethral (bul-bo-u-RE-thral) **gland** Gland that secretes mucus to lubricate the urethra and tip of penis during sexual stimulation; Cowper gland.

bulimia (bu-LIM-e-ah) Eating disorder also known as binge–purge syndrome.

bulk transport Movement of large amounts of material through a cell's plasma membrane.

bulla (BUL-ah) Vesicle.

BUN See blood urea nitrogen.

bursa (BER-sah) Small, fluid-filled sac found in an area subject to stress around bones and joints; pl., bursae (BER-se).

bursitis (ber-SI-tis) Inflammation of a bursa.

C

calcitonin (kal-sih-TO-nin) Hormone from the thyroid gland that lowers blood calcium levels and promotes deposit of calcium in bones; thyrocalcitonin.

calcitriol (kal-sih-TRI-ol) The active form of vitamin D; dihydroxycholecalciferol (di-hi-drok-se-ko-le-kal-SIF-eh-rol).

calculus (KAL-ku-lus) Stone, such as a urinary stone; pl., calculi (KAL-ku-li).

calyx (KA-liks) Cuplike extension of the renal pelvis that collects urine; pl., calyces (KA-lih-seze).

cancellous (KAN-sel-us) Referring to spongy bone tissue.

cancer (KAN-ser) Tumor that spreads to other tissues; a malignant neoplasm.

capillary (CAP-ih-lar-e) Microscopic vessel through which exchanges take place between the blood and the tissues.

carbohydrate (kar-bo-HI-drate) Simple sugar or compound made from simple sugars linked together, such as starch or glycogen.

carbon Element that is the basis of organic chemistry.

carbon dioxide (di-OX-ide) (CO2) Gaseous waste product of cellular metabolism.

carbonic acid (kar-BON-ik) Acid formed when carbon dioxide dissolves in water; carbonic acid then separates into hydrogen ion and bicarbonate ion.

carbonic anhydrase (an-HI-drase) Enzyme that catalyzes the interconversion of carbon dioxide with bicarbonate ion and hydrogen ion.

carcinogen (kar-SIN-o-jen) Cancer-causing substance.

carcinoma (kar-sih-NO-mah) Malignant growth of epithelial cells; a form of cancer.

cardiac (KAR-de-ak) Pertaining to the heart.

cardiopulmonary resuscitation (CPR) Method to restore heartbeat and breathing by mouth-to-mouth resuscitation and closed chest cardiac massage.

cardiovascular system (kar-dE-o-VAS-ku-lar) System consisting of the heart and blood vessels that transports blood throughout the body.

caries (KA-reze) Tooth decay.

carotenemia (kar-o-te-NE-me-ah) Yellowish skin color caused by eating excessive amounts of carrots and other deeply colored vegetables.

carrier Individual who has a gene that is not expressed but that can be passed to offspring.

cartilage (KAR-tih-lij) Type of hard connective tissue found at the ends of bones, the tip of the nose, larynx, trachea, and the embryonic skeleton.

CAT See computed tomography.

catabolism (kah-TAB-o-lizm) Metabolic breakdown of substances into simpler substances; includes the digestion of food and the oxidation of nutrient molecules for energy.

catalyst (KAT-ah-list) Substance that speeds the rate of a chemical reaction.

cataract (KAT-ah-rakt) Opacity of the eye's lens or lens capsule.

catheter (KATH-eh-ter) Tube that can be inserted into a vessel or cavity; may be used to remove fluid, such as urine or blood; v., catheterize.

cation (KAT-i-on) Positively charged particle (ion).

caudal (KAWD-al) Toward or nearer to the sacral region of the spinal column.

CCK See cholecystokinin.

cecum (SE-kum) Small pouch at the beginning of the large intestine.

cell Basic unit of life.

cell membrane Outer covering of a cell; regulates what enters and leaves cell; plasma membrane.

cellular respiration Series of reactions by which nutrients are oxidized for energy within the cell.

central nervous system (CNS) Part of the nervous system that includes the brain and spinal cord.

centrifuge (SEN-trih-fuje) An instrument that separates materials in a mixture based on density.

centriole (SEN-tre-ole) Rod-shaped body near the nucleus of a cell; functions in cell division.

cerebellum (ser-eh-BEL-um) Small section of the brain located under the cerebral hemispheres; functions in coordination, balance, and muscle tone.

cerebral (SER-e-bral) **cortex** Very thin outer layer of gray matter on the surface of the cerebral hemispheres.

cerebral palsy (PAWL-ze) Disorder caused by brain damage occurring before or during the birth process.

cerebrospinal (ser-e-bro-SPI-nal) **fluid (CSF)** Fluid that circulates in and around the brain and spinal cord.

cerebrovascular (ser-e-bro-VAS-ku-lar) **accident (CVA)** Condition involving obstruction of blood flow to brain tissue or bleeding into brain tissue, usually as a result of hypertension or atherosclerosis; stroke.

cerebrum (SER-e-brum) Largest part of the brain; composed of two cerebral hemispheres.

cerumen (seh-RU-men) Earwax; adj., ceruminous (seh-RU-min-us).

cervix (SER-vix) Constricted portion of an organ or part, such as the lower portion of the uterus; neck; adj., cervical.

chemistry (KEM-is-tre) Study of the composition and properties of matter.

chemoreceptor (ke-mo-re-SEP-tor) Receptor that responds to chemicals in body fluids.

chemotherapy (ke-mo-THER-ah-pe) Treatment of a disease by administration of a chemical agent.

Cheyne-Stokes (CHANE-stokes) **respiration** Rhythmic variation in the depth of respiratory movements alternating with periods of apnea due to depression of the breathing centers.

chlamydia (klah-MID-e-ah) Type of very small bacterium that can exist only within a living cell; members of this group cause inclusion conjunctivitis, trachoma, sexually transmitted infections, and respiratory diseases.

cholecystokinin (ko-le-sis-to-KI-nin) **(CCK)** Duodenal hormone that stimulates release of pancreatic enzymes and bile from the gallbladder.

cholelithiasis (ko-le-lih-THI-ah-sis) Gallstones.

cholesterol (ko-LES-ter-ol) Organic fatlike compound found in animal fat, bile, blood, myelin, liver, and other parts of the body.

cholinergic (ko-lin-ER-jik) Activity or structure that responds to acetylcholine.

chondrocyte (KON-dro-site) Cell that produces cartilage.

chordae tendineae (KOR-de ten-DIN-e-e) Fibrous threads that stabilize the heart's AV valve flaps.

choriocarcinoma (ko-re-o-kar-sih-NO-mah) Very malignant tumor made of placental tissue.

choroid (KO-royd) Pigmented middle layer of the eye.

choroid plexus (KO-royd PLEKS-us) Vascular network in the brain's ventricles that forms cerebrospinal fluid.

chromosome (KRO-mo-some) Dark-staining, threadlike body in a cell's nucleus; contains genes that determine hereditary traits.

chronic (KRON-ik) Referring to a disease that develops slowly, persists over a long time, or is recurring.

chyle (kile) Milky-appearing fluid absorbed into the lymphatic system from the small intestine. It consists of lymph and droplets of digested fat.

chyme (kime) Mixture of partially digested food, water, and digestive juices that forms in the stomach.

cicatrix (SIK-ah-trix) Scar.

cilia (SIL-e-ah) Hairs or hairlike processes, such as eyelashes or microscopic extensions from a cell's surface; sing., cilium.

ciliary (SIL-e-ar-e) **muscle** Eye muscle that controls the shape of the lens.

circumduction (ser-kum-DUK-shun) Circular movement at a joint.

circumcision (sir-kum-SIJ-un) Surgery to remove the foreskin of the penis.

cirrhosis (sih-RO-sis) Chronic disease, usually of the liver, in which active cells are replaced by inactive scar tissue.

cisterna chyli (sis-TER-nah KI-li) First part of the thoracic lymph duct, which is enlarged to form a temporary storage area.

CK See creatine kinase.

clitoris (KLIT-o-ris) Small organ of great sensitivity in the external genitalia of the female.

CNS See central nervous system.

coagulation (ko-ag-u-LA-shun) Clotting, as of blood.

coccus (KOK-us) Round bacterium; pl., cocci (KOK-si).

cochlea (KOK-le-ah) Coiled portion of the inner ear that contains the organ of hearing.

colic (KOL-ik) Spasm of visceral muscle.

collagen (KOL-ah-jen) Flexible white protein that gives strength and resilience to connective tissue, such as bone and cartilage.

colloid (kol-OYD) Mixture in which suspended particles do not dissolve but remain distributed in the solvent because of their small size (e.g., cytoplasm); colloidal suspension.

colon (KO-lon) Main portion of the large intestine.

colostrum (ko-LOS-trum) Secretion of the mammary glands released prior to secretion of milk.

communicable (kom-MU-nih-kabl) Capable of being transmitted from one person to another, such as disease; contagious.

complement (KOM-ple-ment) Group of blood proteins that helps antibodies to destroy foreign cells.

compliance (kom-PLI-ans) The ease with which the lungs and thorax can be expanded.

compound Substance composed of two or more chemical elements.

computed tomography (to-MOG-rah-fe) **(CT)** Imaging method in which multiple radiographic views taken from different angles are analyzed by computer to show an area cross-section; used to detect tumors and other abnormalities; also called computed axial tomography (CAT).

concha (KON-ka) Shell-like bone in the nasal cavity; pl., conchae (KON-ke).

concussion (kon-CUSH-on) Injury resulting from a violent blow or shock.

condyle (KON-dile) Rounded projection, as on a bone.

cone Receptor cell in the eye's retina; used for vision in bright light.

congenital (con-JEN-ih-tal) Present at birth.

conjunctiva (kon-junk-TI-vah) Membrane that lines the eyelid and covers the anterior part of the sclera (white of the eye).

constipation (kon-stih-PA-shun) Infrequency of or difficulty with defecation.

contraception (con-trah-SEP-shun) Prevention of an ovum's fertilization or implantation of a fertilized ovum; birth control.

convergence (kon-VER-jens) The centering of both eyes on the same visual field.

convulsion (kon-VUL-shun) Series of muscle spasms; seizure.

Cooley anemia Severe form of β thalassemia, a hereditary blood disorder that impairs hemoglobin formation.

cornea (KOR-ne-ah) Clear portion of the sclera that covers the anterior of the eye.

coronary (KOR-on-ar-e) Referring to the heart or to the arteries supplying blood to the heart.

coronary thrombosis (throm-BO-sis) Formation of a blood clot in a vessel of the heart.

corpus callosum (kal-O-sum) Thick bundle of myelinated nerve cell fibers, deep within the brain, that carries nerve impulses from one cerebral hemisphere to the other.

corpus luteum (LU-te-um) Yellow body formed from ovarian follicle after ovulation; produces progesterone.

cortex (KOR-tex) Outer layer of an organ, such as the brain, kidney, or adrenal gland.

coryza (ko-RI-zah) Nasal discharge; acute coryza is the common cold.

countercurrent mechanism Mechanism for concentrating urine as it flows through the distal nephron.

covalent (KO-va-lent) **bond** Chemical bond formed by the sharing of electrons between atoms.

CPR See cardiopulmonary resuscitation.

cranial (KRA-ne-al) Pertaining to the cranium, the part of the skull that encloses the brain; toward the head or nearer to the head.

creatine (KRE-ah-tin) **phosphate** Compound in muscle tissue that stores energy in high energy bonds.

creatinine (kre-AT-ih-nin) Nitrogenous waste product eliminated in urine.

creatine kinase (CK) (KRE-ah-tin KI-nase) Enzyme in muscle cells that is released in increased amounts when muscle tissue is damaged; the form specific to cardiac muscle cells is creatine kinase MB (CK-MB).

crenation (kre-NA-shun) Shrinking of a cell, as when placed in a hypertonic solution.

crista (KRIS-tah) Receptor for the sense of dynamic equilibrium; pl., cristae.

croup (krupe) Loud barking cough associated with upper respiratory infection in children.

cryoprecipitate (kri-o-pre-SIP-ih-tate) Precipitate formed when plasma is frozen and then thawed.

cryptorchidism (kript-OR-kid-izm) Failure of the testis to descend into the scrotum; undescended testicle.

CSF See cerebrospinal fluid.

CT See computed tomography.

Cushing syndrome Condition caused by overactivity of the adrenal cortex.

cutaneous (ku-TA-ne-us) Referring to the skin.

cuticle (KU-tih-kl) Extension of the stratum corneum that seals the space between the nail plate and the skin above the nail root.

cyanosis (si-ah-NO-sis) Bluish discoloration of the skin and mucous membranes resulting from insufficient oxygen in the blood.

cystic (SIS-tik) **duct** Duct that carries bile into and out of the gallbladder.

cystic fibrosis (SIS-tik fi-BRO-sis) Hereditary disease involving thickened secretions and electrolyte imbalances.

cystitis (sis-TI-tis) Inflammation of the urinary bladder.

cytology (si-TOL-o-je) Study of cells.

cytoplasm (SI-to-plazm) Substance that fills the cell, consisting of a liquid cytosol and organelles.

cytosol (SI-to-sol) Liquid portion of the cytoplasm, consisting of nutrients, minerals, enzymes and other materials in water.

D

deamination (de-am-ih-NA-shun) Removal of amino groups from proteins in metabolism.

decubitus (de-KU-bih-tus) Lying down.

defecation (def-eh-KA-shun) Act of eliminating undigested waste from the digestive tract.

degeneration (de-jen-er-A-shun) Breakdown, as from age, injury, or disease.

deglutition (deg-lu-TISH-un) Act of swallowing.

dehydration (de-hi-DRA-shun) Excessive loss of body fluid.

dementia (de-MEN-she-ah) Gradual and usually irreversible loss of intellectual function.

denaturation (de-nah-tu-RA-shun) Change in structure of a protein, such as an enzyme, so that it can no longer function.

dendrite (DEN-drite) Neuron fiber that conducts impulses toward the cell body.

deoxyribonucleic (de-OK-se-ri-bo-nu-kle-ik) **acid (DNA)** Genetic material of the cell; makes up the chromosomes in the cell's nucleus.

depolarization (de-po-lar-ih-ZA-shun) Sudden reversal of the charge on a cell membrane.

dermal papillae (pah-PIL-le) Extensions of the dermis that project up into the epidermis; they contain blood vessels that supply the epidermis.

dermatitis (der-mah-TI-tis) Inflammation of the skin.

dermatome (DER-mah-tome) A region of the skin supplied by a single spinal nerve.

dermatosis (der-mah-to-sis) Any skin disease.

dermis (DER-mis) True skin; deeper part of the skin.

dextrose (DEK-strose) Glucose, a simple sugar.

diabetes insipidus (in-SIP-ih-dus) Condition due to insufficient ADH secretion by the posterior pituitary; there is excessive water loss.

diabetes mellitus (di-ah-BE-teze mel-LI-tus) Disease of insufficient insulin in which excess glucose is found in blood and urine; characterized by abnormal metabolism of glucose, protein, and fat.

diagnosis (di-ag-NO-sis) Identification of an illness.

dialysis (di-AL-ih-sis) Method for separating molecules in solution based on differences in their ability to pass through a semipermeable membrane; method for removing nitrogenous waste products from the body, as by hemodialysis or peritoneal dialysis.

diaphragm (DI-ah-fram) Dome-shaped muscle under the lungs that flattens during inhalation; separating membrane or structure.

diaphysis (di-AF-ih-sis) Shaft of a long bone.

diarrhea (di-ah-RE-ah) Abnormally frequent watery bowel movements.

diarthrosis (di-ar-THRO-sis) Freely movable joint; synovial joint.

diastole (di-AS-to-le) Relaxation phase of the cardiac cycle; adj., diastolic (di-as-TOL-ik).

diencephalon (di-en-SEF-ah-lon) Region of the brain between the cerebral hemispheres and the midbrain; contains the thalamus, hypothalamus, and pituitary gland.

diffusion (dih-FU-zhun) Movement of molecules from a region where they are in higher concentration to a region where they are in lower concentration.

digestion (di-JEST-yun) Process of breaking down food into absorbable particles.

digestive system (di-JES-tiv) The system involved in taking in nutrients, converting them to a form the body can use, and absorbing them into the circulation.

dihydroxycholecalciferol (di-hi-drok-se-ko-le-kal-SIF-eh-rol) The active form of vitamin D.

dilation (di-LA-shun) Widening of a part, such as the pupil of the eye, a blood vessel, or the uterine cervix; dilatation.

disaccharide (di-SAK-ah-ride) Compound formed of two simple sugars linked together, such as sucrose and lactose.

disease Illness; abnormal state in which part or all of the body does not function properly.

disinfection (dis-in-FEK-shun) Killing of pathogens but not necessarily harmless microbes.

dissect (dis-sekt) To cut apart or separate tissues for study.

distal (DIS-tal) Farther from a structure's origin or from a given reference point.

diverticulosis (di-ver-tik-u-LO-sis) Presence of diverticuli (small pouches) in the intestinal wall.

DNA See deoxyribonucleic acid.

dominant (DOM-ih-nant) Referring to a gene that is always expressed if present.

dopamine (DO-pah-mene) A neurotranmitter.

dorsal (DOR-sal) Toward the back; posterior.

dorsiflexion (dor-sih-FLEK-shun) Bending the foot upward at the ankle.

Down syndrome A congenital disorder usually due to an extra chromosome 21; trisomy 21.

duct Tube or vessel.

ductus arteriosus (DUK-tus ar-te-re-O-sus) Small vessel in the fetus that carries blood from the pulmonary artery to the descending aorta.

ductus deferens (DEF-er-enz) Tube that carries sperm cells from the testis to the urethra; vas deferens.

ductus venosus (ve-NO-sus) Small vessel in the fetus that carries blood from the umbilical vein to the inferior vena cava.

duodenum (du-o-DE-num) First portion of the small intestine.

dura mater (DU-rah MA-ter) Outermost layer of the meninges.

dysmenorrhea (dis-men-o-RE-ah) Painful or difficult menstruation.

dyspnea (disp-NE-ah) Difficult or labored breathing.

E

eccrine (EK-rin) Referring to sweat glands that regulate body temperature and vent directly to the surface of the skin through a pore.

ECG See electrocardiograph.

echocardiograph (ek-o-KAR-de-o-graf) Instrument to study the heart by means of ultrasound; the record produced is an echocardiogram.

eclampsia (eh-KLAMP-se-ah) Serious and sometimes fatal condition involving convulsions, liver damage, and kidney failure that can develop from pregnancy-induced hypertension.

ectopic (ek-TOP-ik) Out of a normal place, as a pregnancy or heartbeat.

eczema (EK-ze-mah) See atopic dermatitis.

edema (eh-DE-mah) Accumulation of fluid in the tissue spaces.

EEG See electroencephalograph.

effector (ef-FEK-tor) Muscle or gland that responds to a stimulus; effector organ.

efferent (EF-fer-ent) Carrying away from a given point, such as a motor neuron that carries nerve impulses away from the central nervous system.

effusion (eh-FU-zhun) Escape of fluid into a cavity or space; the fluid itself.

ejaculation (e-jak-u-LA-shun) Expulsion of semen through the urethra.

EKG See electrocardiograph.

electrocardiograph (e-lek-tro-KAR-de-o-graf) **(ECG, EKG)** Instrument to study the heart's electrical activity; record made is an electrocardiogram.

electroencephalograph (e-lek-tro-en-SEF-ah-lo-graf) **(EEG)** Instrument used to study the brain's electrical activity; record made is an electroencephalogram.

electrolyte (e-LEK-tro-lite) Compound that separates into ions in solution; substance that conducts an electrical current in solution.

electron (e-LEK-tron) Negatively charged particle located in an energy level outside an atom's nucleus.

electrophoresis (e-lek-tro-fo-RE-sis) Separation of components in a mixture by passing an electrical current through it; components separate on the basis of their charge.

element (EL-eh-ment) One of the substances from which all matter is made; substance that cannot be decomposed into a simpler substance.

elephantiasis (el-eh-fan-TI-ah-sis) Enlargement of the extremities due to blockage of lymph flow by small filariae (fi-LA-re-e) worms.

embolism (EM-bo-lizm) The condition of having an embolus (obstruction in the circulation).

embolus (EM-bo-lus) Blood clot or other obstruction in the circulation.

embryo (EM-bre-o) Developing offspring during the first 2 months of pregnancy.

emesis (EM-eh-sis) Vomiting.

emphysema (em-fih-SE-mah) Pulmonary disease characterized by dilation and destruction of the alveoli.

emulsify (e-MUL-sih-fi) To break up fats into small particles; n., emulsification.

endarterectomy (end-ar-ter-EK-to-me) Procedure to remove plaque associated with atherosclerosis from a vessel's lining.

endocardium (en-do-KAR-de-um) Membrane that lines the heart chambers and covers the valves.

endocrine (EN-do-krin) Referring to a gland that secretes directly into the bloodstream.

endocrine system The system composed of glands that secrete hormones.

endocytosis (en-do-si-TO-sis) Movement of large amounts of material into a cell (e.g., phagocytosis and pinocytosis).

endolymph (EN-do-limf) Fluid that fills the membranous labyrinth of the inner ear.

endomysium (en-do-MIS-e-um) Connective tissue around an individual muscle fiber.

endometrium (en-do-ME-tre-um) Lining of the uterus.

endoplasmic reticulum (en-do-PLAS-mik re-TIK-u-lum) **(ER)** Network of membranes in the cellular cytoplasm; may be smooth or rough based on absence or presence of ribosomes.

end-organ Modified ending on a dendrite that functions as a sensory receptor.

endorphin (en-DOR-fin) Pain-relieving substance released naturally from the brain.

endosteum (en-DOS-te-um) Thin membrane that lines a bone's marrow cavity.

endothelium (en-do-THE-le-um) Epithelium that lines the heart, blood vessels, and lymphatic vessels.

enucleation (e-nu-kle-A-shun) Removal of the eyeball.

enzyme (EN-zime) Organic catalyst; speeds the rate of a reaction but is not changed in the reaction.

eosinophil (e-o-SIN-o-fil) Granular white blood cell that shows bead-like, bright pink cytoplasmic granules when stained with acid stain; acidophil.

epicardium (ep-ih-KAR-de-um) Membrane that forms the heart wall's outermost layer and is continuous with the lining of the fibrous pericardium; visceral pericardium.

epicondyle (ep-ih-KON-dile) Small projection on a bone above a condyle.

epidemic (ep-ih-DEM-ik) Occurrence of a disease among many people in a given region at the same time.

epidermis (ep-ih-DER-mis) Outermost layer of the skin.

epididymis (ep-ih-DID-ih-mis) Coiled tube on the surface of the testis in which sperm cells are stored and in which they mature.

epigastric (ep-ih-GAS-trik) Pertaining to the region just inferior to the sternum (breastbone).

epiglottis (ep-e-GLOT-is) Leaf-shaped cartilage that covers the larynx during swallowing.

epilepsy (EP-ih-lep-se) Chronic neurologic disorder involving abnormal electrical activity of the brain; characterized by seizures of varying severity.

epimysium (ep-ih-MIS-e-um) Sheath of fibrous connective tissue that encloses a muscle.

epinephrine (ep-ih-NEF-rin) Neurotransmitter and hormone; released from neurons of the sympathetic nervous system and from the adrenal medulla; adrenaline.

epiphysis (eh-PIF-ih-sis) End of a long bone; adj., epiphyseal (ep-ih-FIZ-e-al).

episiotomy (eh-piz-e-OT-o-me) Cutting of the perineum between the vaginal opening and the anus to reduce tissue tearing in childbirth.

epistaxis (ep-e-STAK-sis) Nosebleed.

epithelium (ep-ih-THE-le-um) One of the four main types of tissue; forms glands, covers surfaces, and lines cavities; adj., epithelial.

EPO See erythropoietin.

equilibrium (e-kwih-LIB-re-um) Sense of balance.

ER See endoplasmic reticulum.

eruption (e-RUP-shun) Raised skin lesion; rash.

erythema (er-eh-THE-mah) Redness of the skin.

erythrocyte (eh-RITH-ro-site) Red blood cell.

erythropoietin (EPO) (eh-rith-ro-POY-eh-tin) Hormone released from the kidney that stimulates red blood cell production in the red bone marrow.

esophagus (eh-SOF-ah-gus) Muscular tube that carries food from the throat to the stomach.

estrogen (ES-tro-jen) Group of female sex hormones that promotes development of the uterine lining and maintains secondary sex characteristics.

etiology (e-te-OL-o-je) Study of a disease's cause or the theory of its origin.

eustachian (u-STA-shun) **tube** Tube that connects the middle ear cavity to the throat; auditory tube.

eversion (e-VER-zhun) Turning outward, with reference to movement of the foot.

excitability In cells, the ability to transmit an electrical current along the plasma membrane.

excoriation (eks-ko-re-A-shun) Scratch into the skin.

excretion (eks-KRE-shun) Removal and elimination of metabolic waste products from the blood.

exfoliation (eks-fo-le-A-shun) Loss of cells from the surface of tissue, such as the skin.

exhalation (eks-hah-LA-shun) Expulsion of air from the lungs; expiration.

exocrine (EK-so-krin) Referring to a gland that secretes through a duct.

exocytosis (eks-o-si-TO-sis) Movement of large amounts of material out of the cell using vesicles.

exophthalmos (ek-sof-THAL-mos) Protrusion (bulging) of the eyes, commonly seen in Graves disease.

extension (eks-TEN-shun) Motion that increases the angle at a joint.

extracellular (EK-strah-sel-u-lar) Outside the cell.

extremity (ek-STREM-ih-te) Limb; an arm or leg.

exudate (EKS-u-date) Any fluid or semisolid that oozes out of tissue, particularly as a result of injury or inflammation.

F

facilitated diffusion Movement of material across the plasma membrane as it would normally flow by diffusion but using transporters to speed movement.

fallopian (fah-LO-pe-an) **tube** See oviduct.

fascia (FASH-e-ah) Band or sheet of fibrous connective tissue.

fascicle (FAS-ih-kl) Small bundle, as of muscle cells or nerve cell fibers.

fat Type of lipid composed of glycerol and fatty acids; triglyceride.

febrile (FEB-ril) Pertaining to fever.

fecalith (FE-kah-lith) Hardened piece of fecal material that may cause obstruction.

feces (FE-seze) Waste material discharged from the large intestine; excrement; stool.

feedback Return of information into a system, so that it can be used to regulate that system.

fertilization (fer-til-ih-ZA-shun) Union of an ovum and a spermatozoon.

fetus (FE-tus) Developing offspring from the third month of pregnancy until birth.

fever (FE-ver) Abnormally high body temperature.

fibrillation (fih-brih-LA-shun) Very rapid, uncoordinated beating of the heart.

fibrin (FI-brin) Blood protein that forms a blood clot.

fibrinogen (fi-BRIN-o-jen) Plasma protein that is converted to fibrin in blood clotting.

filtration (fil-TRA-shun) Movement of material through a semipermeable membrane under mechanical force.

fimbriae (FIM-bre-e) Fringelike extensions of the oviduct that sweep a released ovum into the oviduct.

fissure (FISH-ure) Deep groove.

flaccid (FLAK-sid) Flabby, limp, soft.

flagellum (flah-JEL-lum) Long whiplike extension from a cell used for locomotion; pl., flagella.

flatus (FLA-tus) Gas in the digestive tract; condition of having gas is flatulence (FLAT-u-lens).

flexion (FLEK-shun) Bending motion that decreases the angle between bones at a joint.

follicle (FOL-ih-kl) Sac or cavity, such as the ovarian follicle or hair follicle.

follicle-stimulating hormone (FSH) Hormone produced by the anterior pituitary that stimulates development of ova in the ovary and spermatozoa in the testes.

fontanel (fon-tah-NEL) Membranous area in the infant skull where bone has not yet formed; also spelled fontanelle; "soft spot."

foramen (fo-RA-men) Opening or passageway, as into or through a bone; pl., foramina (fo-RAM-in-ah).

foramen magnum Large opening in the skull's occipital bone through which the spinal cord passes to join the brain.

foramen ovale (o-VA-le) Small hole in the fetal atrial septum that allows blood to pass directly from the right atrium to the left atrium.

formed elements Cells and cell fragments in the blood.

fornix (FOR-niks) A recess or archlike structure.

fossa (FOS-sah) Hollow or depression, as in a bone; pl., fossae (FOS-se).

fovea (FO-ve-ah) Small pit or cup-shaped depression in a surface; the fovea centralis near the center of the retina is the point of sharpest vision.

fragile (FRAH-jil) **X syndrome** Hereditary form of mental retardation; x-linked recessive disorder that appears in both males and females.

frontal (FRONT-al) Describing a plane that divides a structure into anterior and posterior parts.

FSH See follicle-stimulating hormone.

fulcrum (FUL-krum) Pivot point in a lever system; joint in the skeletal system.

fundus (FUN-dus) The deepest portion of an organ, such as the eye or the uterus.

fungus (FUN-gus) Type of plantlike microorganism; yeast or mold; pl., fungi (FUN-ji).

G

gallbladder (GAWL-blad-er) Muscular sac on the inferior surface of the liver that stores bile.

gamete (GAM-ete) Reproductive cell; ovum or spermatozoon.

gamma globulin (GLOB-u-lin) Protein fraction in the blood plasma that contains antibodies.

ganglion (GANG-le-on) Collection of nerve cell bodies located outside the central nervous system.

gangrene (GANG-grene) Death of tissue accompanied by bacterial invasion and putrefaction.

gastric-inhibitory peptide (GIP) Duodenal hormone that inhibits release of gastric juice and stimulates insulin release from the pancreas.

gastrin (GAS-trin) Hormone released from the stomach that stimulates stomach activity.

gastrointestinal (gas-tro-in-TES-tih-nal) **(GI)** Pertaining to the stomach and intestine or the digestive tract as a whole.

gene Hereditary factor; portion of the DNA on a chromosome.

genetic (jeh-NET-ik) Pertaining to the genes or heredity.

genitalia (jen-ih-TA-le-ah) Reproductive organs, both external and internal.

genotype (JEN-o-tipe) Genetic make-up of an organism.

gestation (jes-TA-shun) Period of development from conception to birth.

GH See growth hormone.

GI See gastrointestinal.

gigantism (ji-GAN-tizm) Excessive growth due to oversecretion of growth hormone in childhood.

gingiva (JIN-jih-vah) Tissue around the teeth; gum.

glans Enlarged distal portion of the penis.

glaucoma (glaw-KO-mah) Disorder involving increased fluid pressure within the eye.

glial cells (GLI-al) Cells that support and protect the nervous system; neuroglia.

glioma (gli-O-mah) Tumor of neuroglial tissue.

glomerular (glo-MER-u-lar) **filtrate** Fluid and dissolved materials that leave the blood and enter the kidney nephron through the glomerular (Bowman) capsule.

glomerulonephritis (glo-mer-u-lo-nef-RI-tis) Kidney disease often resulting from antibodies to a streptococcal infection.

glomerulus (glo-MER-u-lus) Cluster of capillaries in the nephron's glomerular (Bowman) capsule.

glottis (GLOT-is) Space between the vocal cords.

glucagon (GLU-kah-gon) Hormone from the pancreatic islets that raises blood glucose level.

glucocorticoid (glu-ko-KOR-tih-koyd) Steroid hormone from the adrenal cortex that raises nutrients in the blood during times of stress, e.g., cortisol.

glucose (GLU-kose) Simple sugar; main energy source for the cells; dextrose.

glycemic (gli-SE-mik) **effect** Measure of how rapidly a food raises the blood glucose level and stimulates release of insulin.

glycogen (GLI-ko-jen) Compound built from glucose molecules that is stored for energy in liver and muscles.

glycolysis (gli-KOL-ih-sis) First, anaerobic phase of the metabolic breakdown of glucose for energy.

glycosuria (gli-ko-SU-re-ah) Presence of glucose in the urine.

goblet cell Single-celled gland that secretes mucus.

goiter (GOY-ter) Enlargement of the thyroid gland.

Golgi (GOL-je) **apparatus** System of cellular membranes that formulates special substances; also called Golgi complex.

gonad (GO-nad) Sex gland; ovary or testis.

gonadotropin (gon-ah-do-TRO-pin) Hormone that acts on a reproductive gland (ovary or testis) e.g., FSH, LH.

gout Type of arthritis caused by a metabolic disturbance.

Graafian (GRAF-e-an) **follicle** See ovarian follicle.

gram (g) Basic unit of weight in the metric system.

gram stain Procedure used to color microorganisms for viewing under the microscope.

granulocyte (GRAN-u-lo-site) Leukocyte with visible granules in the cytoplasm when stained.

Graves disease Common form of hyperthyroidism.

gray matter Nervous tissue composed of unmyelinated fibers and cell bodies.

greater vestibular (ves-TIB-u-lar) **gland** Gland that secretes mucus into the vagina; Bartholin gland.

growth hormone (GH) Hormone produced by anterior pituitary that promotes tissue growth; somatotropin.

gustation (gus-TA-shun) Sense of taste; adj., gustatory.

gyrus (JI-rus) Raised area of the cerebral cortex; pl., gyri (JI-ri).

H

Haversian (ha-VER-shan) **canal** Channel in the center of an osteon (Haversian system), a subunit of compact bone.

Haversian system See osteon.

hay fever Seasonal allergy often due to pollen.

heart (hart) Organ that pumps blood through the cardiovascular system.

helminth (HEL-minth) Worm.

hemapheresis (hem-ah-fer-E-sis) Return of blood components to a donor following separation and removal of desired components.

hematocrit (he-MAT-o-krit) **(Hct)** Volume percentage of red blood cells in whole blood; packed cell volume.

hematoma (he-mah-TO-mah) Tumor or swelling filled with blood.

hematuria (hem-ah-TU-re-ah) Blood in the urine.

hemocytometer (he-mo-si-TOM-eh-ter) Device used to count blood cells under the microscope.

hemodialysis (he-mo-di-AL-ih-sis) Removal of impurities from the blood by their passage through a semipermeable membrane in a fluid bath.

hemoglobin (he-mo-GLO-bin) **(Hb)** Iron-containing protein in red blood cells that binds oxygen.

hemolysis (he-MOL-ih-sis) Rupture of red blood cells; v., hemolyze (HE-mo-lize).

hemolytic (he-mo-LIT-ik) **disease of the newborn (HDN)** Condition that results from Rh incompatibility between a mother and her fetus; erythroblastosis fetalis.

hemophilia (he-mo-FIL-e-ah) Hereditary bleeding disorder associated with a lack of clotting factors in the blood.

hemopoiesis (he-mo-poy-E-sis) Production of blood cells; hematopoiesis.

hemorrhage (HEM-eh-rij) Loss of blood.

hemorrhoids (HEM-o-royds) Varicose veins in the rectum.

hemostasis (he-mo-STA-sis) Stoppage of bleeding.

hemothorax (he-mo-THOR-aks) Accumulation of blood in the pleural space.

heparin (HEP-ah-rin) Substance that prevents blood clotting; anticoagulant.

hepatitis (hep-ah-TI-tis) Inflammation of the liver.

heredity (he-RED-ih-te) Transmission of characteristics from parent to offspring by means of the genes; the genetic makeup of the individual.

hereditary (he-RED-ih-tar-e) Transmitted or transmissible through the genes; familial.

hernia (HER-ne-ah) Protrusion of an organ or tissue through the wall of the cavity in which it is normally enclosed.

heterozygous (het-er-o-ZI-gus) Having unmatched alleles for a given trait; hybrid.

hilum (HI-lum) Indented region of an organ where vessels and nerves enter or leave.

hippocampus (hip-o-KAM-pus) Sea horse–shaped region of the limbic system that functions in learning and formation of long-term memory.

histamine (HIS-tah-mene) Substance released from tissues during an antigen–antibody reaction.

histology (his-TOL-o-je) Study of tissues.

HIV See human immunodeficiency virus.

Hodgkin disease Chronic malignant disease of lymphoid tissue.

homeostasis (ho-me-o-STA-sis) State of balance within the body; maintenance of body conditions within set limits.

homozygous (ho-mo-ZI-gus) Having identical alleles for a given trait; purebred.

hormone Secretion of an endocrine gland; chemical messenger that has specific regulatory effects on certain other cells.

host An organism in or on which a parasite lives.

human chorionic gonadotropin (ko-re-ON-ik gon-ah-do-TRO-pin) **(hCG)** Hormone produced by embryonic cells soon after implantation that maintains the corpus luteum.

human immunodeficiency virus (HIV) Virus that causes AIDS.

human placental lactogen (hPL) Hormone produced by the placenta that prepares the breasts for lactation and maintains nutrient levels in maternal blood.

humoral (HU-mor-al) Pertaining to body fluids, such as immunity based on antibodies circulating in the blood.

Huntington disease Progressive degenerative disorder carried by a dominant gene.

hyaline (HI-ah-lin) Clear, glasslike; referring to a type of cartilage.

hydatidiform (hi-dah-TID-ih-form) **mole** Benign overgrowth of placental tissue.

hydrocephalus (hi-dro-SEF-ah-lus) Abnormal accumulation of CSF within the brain.

hydrolysis (hi-DROL-ih-sis) Splitting of large molecules by the addition of water, as in digestion.

hydrophilic (hi-dro-FIL-ik) Mixing with or dissolving in water, such as salts; literally "water-loving."

hydrophobic (hi-dro-FO-bik) Repelling and not dissolving in water, such as fats; literally "water-fearing."

hymen Fold of membrane near the opening of the vaginal canal.

hypercapnia (hi-per-KAP-ne-ah) Increased level of carbon dioxide in the blood.

hyperglycemia (hi-per-gli-SE-me-ah) Abnormal increase in the amount of glucose in the blood.

hyperopia (hi-per-O-pe-ah) Farsightedness.

hyperpnea (hi-PERP-ne-ah) Abnormal increase in the depth and rate of breathing.

hypersensitivity (hi-per-SEN-sih-tiv-ih-te) Exaggerated reaction of the immune system to a substance that is normally harmless to most people; allergy.

hypertension (hi-per-TEN-shun) High blood pressure.

hypertonic (hi-per-TON-ik) Describing a solution that is more concentrated than the fluids within a cell.

hypertrophy (hy-PER-tro-fe) Enlargement or overgrowth of an organ or part.

hyperventilation (hi-per-ven-tih-LA-shun) Increased amount of air entering the alveoli of the lungs due to deep and rapid respiration.

hypocapnia (hi-po-KAP-ne-ah) Decreased level of carbon dioxide in the blood.

hypochondriac (hi-po-KON-dre-ak) Pertaining to a region just inferior to the ribs.

hypogastric (hi-po-GAS-trik) Pertaining to an area inferior to the stomach or the most inferior midline region of the abdomen.

hypoglycemia (hi-po-gli-SE-me-ah) Abnormal decrease in the amount of glucose in the blood.

hypophysis (hi-POF-ih-sis) Pituitary gland.

hypopnea (hi-POP-ne-ah) Decrease in the rate and depth of breathing.

hypospadias (hi-po-SPA-de-as) Opening of the urethra on the undersurface of the penis.

hypotension (hi-po-TEN-shun) Low blood pressure.

hypothalamus (hi-po-THAL-ah-mus) Region of the brain that controls the pituitary and maintains homeostasis.

hypothermia (hi-po-THER-me-ah) Abnormally low body temperature.

hypotonic (hi-po-TON-ik) Describing a solution that is less concentrated than the fluids within a cell.

hypoventilation (hi-po-ven-tih-LA-shun) Insufficient amount of air entering the alveoli.

hypoxemia (hi-pok-SE-me-ah) Lower than normal concentration of oxygen in arterial blood.

hypoxia (hi-POK-se-ah) Lower than normal level of oxygen in the tissues.

hysterectomy (his-ter-EK-to-me) Surgical removal of the uterus.

I

iatrogenic (i-at-ro-JEN-ik) Resulting from the adverse effects of treatment.

idiopathic (id-e-o-PATH-ik) Describing a disease without known cause.

ileum (IL-e-um) Third portion of the small intestine.

ileus (IL-e-us) Intestinal obstruction caused by lack of peristalsis or by muscle contraction.

iliac (IL-e-ak) Pertaining to the ilium, the upper portion of the hipbone.

immunity (ih-MU-nih-te) Power of an individual to resist or overcome the effects of a particular disease or other harmful agent.

immunization (ih-mu-nih-ZA-shun) Use of a vaccine to produce immunity; vaccination.

immunodeficiency (im-u-no-de-FISH-en-se) Any failure of the immune system.

immunoglobulin (im-mu-no-GLOB-u-lin) **(Ig)** See antibody.

immunotherapy (im-mu-no-THER-a-pe) Stimulation of the immune system to fight disease, such as cancer.

impetigo (im-peh-TI-go) Acute, contagious staphylococcal or streptococcal skin infection.

implantation (im-plan-TA-shun) Embedding of a fertilized ovum into the uterine lining.

incidence (IN-sih-dense) In epidemiology, the number of new disease cases appearing in a particular population during a specific time period.

infarct (IN-farkt) Area of tissue damaged from lack of blood supply caused by a vessel blockage.

infection (in-FEK-shun) Invasion by pathogens.

infectious mononucleosis (mon-o-nu-kle-O-sis) Acute viral infection associated with enlargement of the lymph nodes.

inferior (in-FE-re-or) Below or lower.

inferior vena cava (VE-nah KA-vah) Large vein that drains the lower body and empties into the heart's right atrium.

infertility (in-fer-TIL-ih-te) Decreased ability to reproduce.

inflammation (in-flah-MA-shun) Response of tissues to injury; characterized by heat, redness, swelling, and pain.

influenza (in-flu-EN-zah) Acute contagious viral disease of the upper respiratory tract.

infundibulum (in-fun-DIB-u-lum) Stalk that connects the pituitary gland to the brain's hypothalamus.

ingestion (in-JES-chun) The intake of food.

inguinal (IN-gwih-nal) Pertaining to the groin region or the region of the inguinal canal.

inhalation (in-hah-LA-shun) Drawing of air into the lungs; inspiration.

insertion (in-SER-shun) Muscle attachment connected to a movable part.

insulin (IN-su-lin) Hormone from the pancreatic islets that lowers blood glucose level.

integument (in-TEG-u-ment) Skin; adj., integumentary.

integumentary system The skin and all its associated structures.

intercalated (in-TER-cah-la-ted) **disk** A modified plasma membrane in cardiac tissue that allows rapid transfer of electrical impulses between cells.

intercellular (in-ter-SEL-u-lar) Between cells.

intercostal (in-ter-KOS-tal) Between the ribs.

interferon (in-ter-FERE-on) **(IFN)** Group of substances released from virus-infected cells that prevent spread of infection to other cells; also nonspecifically boost the immune system.

interleukin (in-ter-LU-kin) Substance released by a T cell or macrophage that stimulates other cells of the immune system.

interneuron (in-ter-NU-ron) Nerve cell that transmits impulses within the central nervous system.

interphase (IN-ter-faze) Stage in a cell's life between one mitosis and the next when the cell is not dividing.

interstitial (in-ter-STISH-al) Between; pertaining to an organ's spaces or structures between active tissues.

intestine (in-TES-tin) Organ of the digestive tract between the stomach and the anus, consisting of the small and large intestine.

intracellular (in-trah-SEL-u-lar) Within a cell.

intussusception (in-tuh-suh-SEP-shun) Slipping of a part of the intestine into a part below it.

inversion (in-VER-zhun) Turning inward, with reference to movement of the foot.

ion (I-on) Charged particle formed when an electrolyte goes into solution.

ionic bond Chemical bond formed by the exchange of electrons between atoms.

iris (I-ris) Circular colored region of the eye around the pupil.

ischemia (is-KE-me-ah) Lack of blood supply to an area.

islets (I-lets) Groups of cells in the pancreas that produce hormones; islets of Langerhans (LAHNG-er-hanz).

isometric (i-so-MET-rik) **contraction** Muscle contraction in which there is no change in muscle length but an increase in muscle tension, as in pushing against an immovable force.

isotonic (i-so-TON-ik) Describing a solution that has the same concentration as the fluid within a cell.

isotonic contraction Muscle contraction in which the tone within the muscle remains the same but the muscle shortens to produce movement.

isotope (I-so-tope) Form of an element that has the same atomic number as another form of that element but a different atomic weight; isotopes differ in their numbers of neutrons.

isthmus (IS-mus) Narrow band, such as the band that connects the two lobes of the thyroid gland.

J

jaundice (JAWN-dis) Yellowish skin discoloration that is usually due to the presence of bile in the blood.

jejunum (je-JU-num) Second portion of the small intestine.

joint Area of junction between two or more bones; articulation.

juxtaglomerular (juks-tah-glo-MER-u-lar) **(JG) apparatus** Structure in the kidney composed of cells of the afferent arteriole and distal convoluted tubule that secretes the enzyme renin when blood pressure decreases below a certain level.

K

karyotype (KAR-e-o-tipe) Picture of the chromosomes arranged according to size and form.

keloid (KE-loyd) Mass or raised area that results from excess production of scar tissue.

keratin (KER-ah-tin) Protein that thickens and protects the skin; makes up hair and nails.

ketoacidosis (ke-to-as-ih-DO-sis) Acidosis that results from accumulation of ketone bodies in the blood.

kidney (KID-ne) Organ of excretion.

kilocalorie (kil-o-KAL-o-re) Measure of the energy content of food; technically, the amount of heat needed to raise 1 kg of water 1° centigrade.

kinesthesia (kin-es-THE-ze-ah) Sense of body movement.

Klinefelter (KLINE-fel-ter) **syndrome** Genetic disorder involving abnormal sex chromosomes, usually an extra X chromosome.

Kupffer (KOOP-fer) **cells** Macrophages in the liver that help to fight infection.

Kussmaul (KOOS-mowl) **respiration** Deep, rapid respiration characteristic of acidosis (overly acidic body fluids) as seen in uncontrolled diabetes.

kwashiorkor (kwash-e-OR-kor) Severe protein and energy malnutrition seen in children after weaning.

kyphosis (ki-FO-sis) Exaggerated lumbar curve of the spine.

L

labium (LA-be-um) Lip; pl., labia (LA-be-ah).

labyrinth (LAB-ih-rinth) Inner ear, named for its complex shape.

laceration (las-er-A-shun) Rough, jagged skin wound.

lacrimal (LAK-rih-mal) Referring to tears or the tear glands.

lacrimal apparatus lacrimal (tear) gland and its associated ducts.

lactation (lak-TA-shun) Secretion of milk.

lacteal (LAK-te-al) Lymphatic capillary that drains digested fats from the villi of the small intestine.

lactic (LAK-tik) **acid** Organic acid that accumulates in muscle cells functioning without oxygen.

laryngeal (lah-RIN-je-al) **pharynx** Lowest portion of the pharynx, opening into the larynx and esophpagus.

larynx (LAR-inks) Structure between the pharynx and trachea that contains the vocal cords; voice box.

laser (LA-zer) Device that produces a very intense light beam.

lateral (LAT-er-al) Farther from the midline; toward the side.

lens Biconvex structure of the eye that changes in thickness to accommodate for near and far vision; crystalline lens.

leptin (LEP-tin) Hormone produced by adipocytes that aids in weight control by decreasing food intake and increasing energy expenditure.

lesion (LE-zhun) Wound or local injury.

leukemia (lu-KE-me-ah) Malignant blood disease characterized by abnormal development of white blood cells.

leukocyte (LU-ko-site) White blood cell.

leukocytosis (lu-ko-si-TO-sis) Increase in the number of white cells in the blood, such as during infection.

leukopenia (lu-ko-PE-ne-ah) Deficiency of leukocytes in the blood.

leukoplakia (lu-ko-PLA-ke-ah) Thickened white patches on the oral mucous membranes, often due to smoking.

LH See luteinizing hormone.

ligament (LIG-ah-ment) Band of connective tissue that connects a bone to another bone; thickened portion or fold of the peritoneum that supports an organ or attaches it to another organ.

limbic (LIM- bik) **system** Area between the brain's cerebrum and diencephalon that is involved in emotional states and behavior.

lipid (LIP-id) Type of organic compound, one example of which is a fat.

liter (LE-ter) **(L)** Basic unit of volume in the metric system; 1,000 mL; 1.06 qt.

lithotripsy (LITH-o-trip-se) Use of external shock waves to shatter stones (calculi).

liver (LIV-er) Large gland inferior to the diaphragm in the superior right abdomen; has many functions, including bile secretion, detoxification, storage, and interconversion of nutrients.

loop of Henle (HEN-le) Hairpin shaped segment of the renal tubule between the proximal and distal convoluted tubules; nephron loop.

lordosis (lor-DO-sis) Exaggerated lumbar curve of the spine.

lumbar (LUM-bar) Pertaining to the region of the spine between the thoracic vertebrae and the sacrum.

lumen (LU-men) Central opening of an organ or vessel.

lung Organ of respiration.

lunula (LU-nu-la) Pale half-moon shaped area at the proximal end of the nail.

lupus erythematosus (LU-pus er-ih-the-mah-TO-sis) Chronic inflammatory autoimmune disease that involves the skin and sometimes other organs.

luteinizing (LU-te-in-i-zing) **hormone (LH)** Hormone produced by the anterior pituitary that induces ovulation and formation of the corpus luteum in females; in males, it stimulates cells in the testes to produce testosterone.

lymph (limf) Fluid in the lymphatic system.

lymph node Mass of lymphoid tissue along the path of a lymphatic vessel that filters lymph and harbors white blood cells active in immunity.

lymphadenitis (lim-fad-en-I-tis) Inflammation of lymph nodes.

lymphadenopathy (lim-fad-en-OP-ah-the) Any disorder of lymph nodes.

lymphangitis (lim-fan-JI-tis) Inflammation of lymphatic vessels.

lymphatic duct (lim-FAH-tic) Vessel of the lymphatic system.

lymphatic system System consisting of the lymphatic vessels and lymphoid tissue; involved in immunity, digestion, and fluid balance.

lymphedema (lim-feh-DE-mah) Edema due to obstruction of lymph flow.

lymphocyte (LIM-fo-site) Agranular white blood cell that functions in immunity.

lymphoma (lim-FO-mah) Any tumor, benign or malignant, that occurs in lymphoid tissue.

lysosome (LI-so-some) Cell organelle that contains digestive enzymes.

M

macrophage (MAK-ro-faj) Large phagocytic cell that develops from a monocyte; presents antigen to lymphocytes in immune response.

macula (MAK-u-lah) Spot; flat, discolored spot on the skin, such as a freckle or measles lesion; also called macule; small yellow spot in the eye's retina that contains the fovea, the point of sharpest vision; receptor for the sense of static equilibrium.

magnetic resonance imaging (MRI) Method for studying tissue based on nuclear movement after exposure to radio waves in a powerful magnetic field.

major histocompatibility complex (MHC) Group of genes that codes for specific proteins (antigens) on cellular surfaces; these antigens are important in cross-matching for tissue transplantation; they are also important in immune reactions.

malignant (mah-LIG-nant) Describing a tumor that spreads; describing a disorder that tends to become worse and cause death.

malnutrition (mal-nu-TRISH-un) State resulting from lack of food, lack of an essential dietary component, or faulty use of food in the diet.

MALT Mucosal-associated lymphoid tissue; tissue in the mucous membranes that helps fight infection.

mammary (MAM-er-e) **gland** Breast.

mammogram (MAM-o-gram) Radiographic study of the breast.

maple syrup urine disease Recessive hereditary disease that affects amino acid metabolism and, among other symptoms, produces the smell of maple syrup in urine and on the body.

marasmus (mah-RAZ-mus) Severe malnutrition in infants.

mast cell White blood cell related to a basophil that is present in tissues; active in inflammatory and allergic reactions.

mastectomy (mas-TEK-to-me) Removal of the breast; mammectomy.

mastication (mas-tih-KA-shun) Act of chewing.

mastitis (mas-TI-tis) Inflammation of the breast.

matrix (MA-triks) The nonliving background material in a tissue; the intercellular material.

meatus (me-A-tus) Short channel or passageway, as in a bone.

medial (ME-de-al) Nearer the midline of the body.

mediastinum (me-de-as-TI-num) Region between the lungs and the organs and vessels it contains.

medulla (meh-DUL-lah) Inner region of an organ; marrow.

medullary (MED-u-lar-e) **cavity** Channel at the center of a long bone that contains bone marrow.

medulla oblongata (ob-long-GAH-tah) Part of the brain stem that connects the brain to the spinal cord.

megakaryocyte (meg-ah-KAR-e-o-site) Very large cell that gives rise to blood platelets.

meibomian (mi-BO-me-an) **gland** Gland that produces a secretion that lubricates the eyelashes.

meiosis (mi-O-sis) Process of cell division that halves the chromosome number in the formation of the reproductive cells.

melanin (MEL-ah-nin) Dark pigment found in skin, hair, parts of the eye, and certain parts of the brain.

melanocyte (MEL-ah-no-site) Cell that produces melanin.

melanoma (mel-ah-NO-mah) Malignant tumor of melanocytes.

melatonin (mel-ah-TO-nin) Hormone produced by the pineal gland.

membrane Thin sheet of tissue.

Mendelian (men-DE-le-en) **laws** Principles of heredity discovered by an Austrian monk named Gregor Mendel.

meninges (men-IN-jeze) Three layers of fibrous membranes that cover the brain and spinal cord.

menopause (MEN-o-pawz) Time during which menstruation ceases.

menses (MEN-seze) Monthly flow of blood from the female reproductive tract.

menstruation (men-stru-A-shun) The period of menstrual flow.

mesentery (MES-en-ter-e) Membranous peritoneal ligament that attaches the small intestine to the dorsal abdominal wall.

mesocolon (mes-o-KO-lon) Peritoneal ligament that attaches the colon to the dorsal abdominal wall.

mesothelium (mes-o-THE-le-um) Epithelial tissue found in serous membranes.

metabolic rate Rate at which energy is released from nutrients in the cells.

metabolic syndrome Condition related to type 2 diabetes mellitus with insulin resistance, obesity, hyperglycemia, high blood pressure, and metabolic disturbances; also called syndrome X.

metabolism (meh-TAB-o-lizm) All the physical and chemical processes by which an organism is maintained.

metaphase (MET-ah-faze) Second stage of mitosis, during which the chromosomes line up across the equator of the cell.

metarteriole (met-ar-TE-re-ole) Small vessel that connects the arterial system directly with the venous system in a blood shunt; thoroughfare channel.

metastasis (meh-TAS-tah-sis) Spread of tumor cells; pl., metastases (meh-TAS-tah-seze).

meter (ME-ter) (**m**) Basic unit of length in the metric system; 1.1 yards.

MHC See Major histocompatibility complex.

microbiology (mi-kro-bi-OL-o-je) Study of microscopic organisms.

micrometer (MI-kro-me-ter) (**μm**) 1/1,000th of a millimeter; micron; an instrument for measuring through a microscope (pronounced mi-KROM-eh-ter).

microorganism (mi-kro-OR-gan-izm) Microscopic organism.

microscope (MI-kro-skope) Magnifying instrument used to examine cells and other structures not visible with the naked eye; exam-

ples are the compound light microscope, transmission electron microscope (TEM) and scanning electron microscope (SEM).

microvilli (mi-kro-VIL-li) Small projections of the plasma membrane that increase surface area; sing., microvillus.

micturition (mik-tu-RISH-un) Act of urination; voiding of the urinary bladder.

midbrain Upper portion of the brainstem.

mineral (MIN-er-al) Inorganic substance; in the diet, an element needed in small amounts for health.

mineralocorticoid (min-er-al-o-KOR-tih-koyd) Steroid hormone from the adrenal cortex that regulates electrolyte balance, e.g. aldosterone.

mitochondria (mi-to-KON-dre-ah) Cell organelles that manufacture ATP with the energy released from the oxidation of nutrients; sing., mitochondrion.

mitosis (mi-TO-sis) Type of cell division that produces two daughter cells exactly like the parent cell.

mitral (MI-tral) **valve** Valve between the heart's left atrium and left ventricle; left AV valve; bicuspid valve.

mixture Blend of two or more substances.

molecule (MOL-eh-kule) Particle formed by chemical bonding of two or more atoms; smallest subunit of a compound.

monocyte (MON-o-site) Phagocytic agranular white blood cell.

monosaccharide (mon-o-SAK-ah-ride) Simple sugar; basic unit of carbohydrates.

mortality (mor-TAL-ih-te) **rate** Percentage of a population that dies from a given disease within a given time period.

motor (MO-tor) Describing structures or activities involved in transmitting impulses away from the central nervous system; efferent.

motor end plate Region of a muscle cell membrane that receives nervous stimulation.

motor unit Group consisting of a single neuron and all the muscle fibers it stimulates.

mouth Proximal opening of the digestive tract where food is ingested, chewed, mixed with saliva, and swallowed.

MRI See magnetic resonance imaging.

mucosa (mu-KO-sah) Lining membrane that produces mucus; mucous membrane.

mucus (MU-kus) Thick protective fluid secreted by mucous membranes and glands; adj., mucous.

multiple (SKLE-ro-SIS) **sclerosis** Disease that affects the myelin sheath around axons leading to neuron degeneration.

murmur Abnormal heart sound.

muscle (MUS-l) Tissue that contracts to produce movement; includes skeletal, smooth, and cardiac types; adj., muscular.

muscular (MUS-ku-lar) **system** The system of skeletal muscles that moves the skeleton, supports and protects the organs, and maintains posture.

mutagen (MU-tah-jen) Agent that causes mutation; adj., mutagenic (mu-tah-JEN-ik).

mutation (mu-TA-shun) Change in a gene or a chromosome.

myalgia (mi-AL-je-ah) Muscular pain.

mycology (mi-KOL-o-je) Study of fungi (yeasts and molds).

myelin (MI-el-in) Fatty material that covers and insulates the axons of some neurons.

myocardium (mi-o-KAR-de-um) Middle layer of the heart wall; heart muscle.

myoglobin (MI-o-glo-bin) Compound that stores oxygen in muscle cells.

myoma (mi-O-mah) Usually benign tumor of the uterus; fibroma; fibroid.

myometrium (mi-o-ME-tre-um) Muscular layer of the uterus.

myopia (mi-O-pe-ah) Nearsightedness.

myosin (MI-o-sin) One of the two contractile proteins in muscle cells, the other being actin.

myxedema (mik-seh-DE-mah) Condition that results from hypothyroidism in adults.

N

narcotic (nar-KOT-ik) Drug that acts on the CNS to alter perception and response to pain.

nasopharynx (na-zo-FAR-inks) Upper portion of the pharynx located posterior to the nasal cavity.

natural killer (**NK**) **cell** Type of lymphocyte that can nonspecifically destroy abnormal cells.

naturopathy (na-chur-OP-a-the) Philosophy of helping people to heal themselves by developing healthy lifestyles.

nausea (NAW-ze-ah) Unpleasant sensation due to disturbance in the upper GI tract that may precede vomiting.

necrosis (neh-KRO-sis) Tissue death.

negative feedback Self-regulating system in which the result of an action is the control over that action; a method for keeping body conditions within a normal range and maintaining homeostasis.

neoplasm (NE-o-plazm) Abnormal growth of cells; tumor; adj., neoplastic.

nephron (NEF-ron) Microscopic functional unit of the kidney.

nephron loop Hairpin shaped segment of the renal tubule between the proximal and distal convoluted tubules; loop of Henle.

nerve Bundle of neuron fibers outside the central nervous system.

nerve impulse Electrical charge that spreads along the membrane of a neuron; action potential.

nervous system (NER-vus) The system that transports information in the body by means of electrical impulses.

neuralgia (nu-RAL-je-ah) Pain in a nerve.

neurilemma (nu-rih-LEM-mah) Thin sheath that covers certain peripheral axons; aids in axon regeneration.

neuritis (nu-RI-tis) Inflammation of a nerve, with pain, tenderness, and loss of sensation.

neuroglia (nu-ROG-le-ah) Supporting and protective cells of the nervous system; glial cells.

neuromuscular junction Point at which a nerve fiber contacts a muscle cell.

neuron (NU-ron) Conducting cell of the nervous system.

neurotransmitter (nu-ro-TRANS-mit-er) Chemical released from the ending of an axon that enables a nerve impulse to cross a synapse.

neutron (NU-tron) Noncharged particle in an atom's nucleus.

neutrophil (NU-tro-fil) Phagocytic granular white blood cell; polymorph; poly; PMN; seg.

nevus (NE-vus) Mole or birthmark.

nitrogen (NI-tro-jen) Chemical element found in all proteins.

node Small mass of tissue, such as a lymph node; space between cells in the myelin sheath.

norepinephrine (nor-epi-ih-NEF-rin) Neurotransmitter similar to epinephrine; noradrenaline.

normal saline Isotonic or physiologic salt solution.

nosocomial (nos-o-KO-me-al) Acquired in a hospital, as an infection.

nucleic acid (nu-KLE-ik) Complex organic substance composed of nucleotides that makes up DNA and RNA.

nucleolus (nu-KLE-o-lus) Small unit within the nucleus that assembles ribosomes.

nucleotide (NU-kle-o-tide) Building block of DNA and RNA.

nucleus (NU-kle-us) Largest cellular organelle, containing the DNA, which directs all cell activities; group of neurons in the central nervous system; in chemistry, the central part of an atom.

O

obstipation (ob-stih-PA-shun) Extreme constipation.

occlusion (ok-LU-zhun) Closing, as of a vessel.

olfaction (ol-FAK-shun) Sense of smell; adj., olfactory.

omentum (o-MEN-tum) Portion of the peritoneum; greater omentum extends over the anterior abdomen; lesser omentum extends between the stomach and liver.

oncology (on-KOL-o-je) Study of tumors.

ophthalmic (of-THAL-mik) Pertaining to the eye.

ophthalmoscope (of-THAL-mo-skope) Instrument for examining the posterior (fundus) of the eye.

opportunistic (op-por-tu-NIS-tik) Describing an infection that takes hold because a host has been compromised (weakened) by disease.

organ (OR-gan) Body part containing two or more tissues functioning together for specific purposes.

organelle (or-gan-EL) Specialized subdivision within a cell.

organic (or-GAN-ik) Referring to the complex compounds found in living things that contain carbon, and usually hydrogen, and oxygen.

organism (OR-gan-izm) Individual plant or animal; any organized living thing.

organ of Corti (KOR-te) Receptor for hearing located in the cochlea of the internal ear.

origin (OR-ih-jin) Source; beginning; muscle attachment connected to a nonmoving part.

oropharynx (o-ro-FAR-inks) Middle portion of the pharynx, located behind the mouth.

orthopnea (or-THOP-ne-ah) Difficulty in breathing that is relieved by sitting in an upright position.

osmosis (os-MO-sis) Diffusion of water through a semipermeable membrane.

osmotic (os-MOT-ik) **pressure** Tendency of a solution to draw water into it; directly related to a solution's concentration.

osseus (OS-e-us) Pertaining to bone tissue.

ossicle (OS-ih-kl) One of three small bones of the middle ear: malleus, incus, or stapes.

ossification (os-ih-fih-KA-shun) Process of bone formation.

osteoblast (OS-te-o-blast) Bone-forming cell.

osteoclast (OS-te-o-clast) Cell that breaks down bone.

osteocyte (OS-te-o-site) Mature bone cell; maintains bone but does not produce new bone tissue.

osteon (OS-te-on) Subunit of compact bone, consisting of concentric rings of bone tissue around a central channel; haversian system.

osteopenia (os-te-o-PE-ne-ah) Reduction in bone density to below average levels.

osteoporosis (os-te-o-po-RO-sis) Abnormal loss of bone tissue with tendency to fracture.

otoliths (O-to-liths) Crystals that add weight to fluids in the inner ear and function in the sense of static equilibrium.

ovarian follicle (o-VA-re-an FOL-ih-kl) Cluster of cells in which the ovum develops within the ovary; Graafian follicle.

ovary (O-vah-re) Female reproductive gland.

oviduct (O-vih-dukt) Tube that carries ova from the ovaries to the uterus; fallopian tube, uterine tube.

ovulation (ov-u-LA-shun) Release of a mature ovum from an ovarian follicle.

ovum (O-vum) Female reproductive cell or gamete; pl., ova.

oxidation (ok-sih-DA-shun) Chemical breakdown of nutrients for energy.

oxygen (OK-sih-jen) (O_2) The gas needed to break down nutrients completely for energy within the cell.

oxygen debt Amount of oxygen needed to reverse the effects produced in muscles functioning without oxygen.

oxytocin (ok-se-TO-sin) Hormone from the posterior pituitary that causes uterine contraction and milk ejection ("letdown") from the breasts.

P

pacemaker Sinoatrial (SA) node of the heart; group of cells or artificial device that sets the rate of heart contractions.

palate (PAL-at) Roof of the oral cavity; anterior portion is hard palate, posterior portion is soft palate.

pallor (PAL-or) Paleness of the skin.

pancreas (PAN-kre-as) Large, elongated gland behind the stomach; produces digestive enzymes and hormones (e.g., insulin).

pandemic (pan-DEM-ik) Disease that is prevalent throughout an entire country, continent, or the world.

Papanicolaou (pap-ah-nik-o-LAH-o) **test** Histologic test for cervical cancer; Pap test or smear.

papilla (pah-PIL-ah) Small nipplelike projection or elevation.

papillary muscles (PAP-ih-lar-e) Columnar muscles in the heart's ventricular walls that anchor and pull on the chordae tendineae to prevent the valve flaps from everting when the ventricles contract.

papule (PAP-ule) Firm, raised lesion of the skin.

paracentesis (par-eh-sen-TE-sis) Puncture of the abdominal cavity, usually to remove a fluid accumulation, such as ascites; abdominocentesis.

parasite (PAR-ah-site) Organism that lives on or within another (the host) at the other's expense.

parasympathetic nervous system Craniosacral division of the autonomic nervous system; generally reverses the fight-or-flight (stress) response.

parathyroid (par-ah-THI-royd) **gland** Any of four to six small glands embedded in the capsule enclosing the thyroid gland; produces parathyroid hormone, which raises the blood calcium level by causing calcium release from bones.

parietal (pah-RI-eh-tal) Pertaining to the wall of a space or cavity.

Parkinson disease Progressive neurologic condition characterized by tremors, rigidity of limbs and joints, slow movement, and impaired balance.

parturition (par-tu-RISH-un) Childbirth; labor.

pathogen (PATH-o-jen) Disease-causing organism; adj., pathogenic (path-o-JEN-ik).

pathology (pah-THOL-o-je) Study of disease.

pathophysiology (path-o-fiz-e-OL-o-je) Study of the physiologic basis of disease.

pedigree (PED-ih-gre) Family history; used in the study of heredity; family tree.

pelvic inflammatory disease (PID) Ascending infection that involves the pelvic organs; common causes are gonorrhea and chlamydia.

pelvis (PEL-vis) Basinlike structure, such as the lower portion of the abdomen or the upper flared portion of the ureter (renal pelvis).

pemphigus (PEM-fih-gus) An autoimmune skin disease with blistering of the skin.

penis (PE-nis) Male organ of urination and sexual intercourse.

perforating canal Channel across a long bone that contains blood vessels and nerves; Volkmann canal.

pericardium (per-ih-KAR-de-um) Fibrous sac lined with serous membrane that encloses the heart.

perichondrium (per-ih-KON-dre-um) Layer of connective tissue that covers cartilage.

perilymph (PER-e-limf) Fluid that fills the inner ear's bony labyrinth.

perimysium (per-ih-MIS-e-um) Connective tissue around a fascicle of muscle tissue.

perineum (per-ih-NE-um) Pelvic floor; external region between the anus and genital organs.

periosteum (per-e-OS-te-um) Connective tissue membrane covering a bone.

peripheral (peh-RIF-er-al) Located away from a center or central structure.

peripheral nervous system (PNS) All the nerves and nervous tissue outside the central nervous system.

peripheral neuritis (peh-RIF-er-al nu-RI-tis) Degeneration of nerves supplying the distal extremities; polyneuritis.

peristalsis (per-ih-STAL-sis) Wavelike movements in the wall of an organ or duct that propel its contents forward.

peritoneum (per-ih-to-NE-um) Serous membrane that lines the abdominal cavity and forms outer layer of abdominal organs; forms supporting ligaments for some organs.

peritonitis (per-ih-to-NI-tis) Inflammation of the peritoneum.

peroxisome (per-OK-sih-some) Cell organelle that enzymatically destroys harmful substances produced in metabolism.

Peyer (PI-er) **patches** Clusters of lymphatic nodules in the mucous membranes lining the distal portion of the small intestine.

pH Symbol indicating hydrogen ion (H$^+$) concentration; scale that measures the relative acidity and alkalinity (basicity) of a solution.

phagocyte (FAG-o-site) Cell capable of engulfing large particles, such as foreign matter or cellular debris, through the plasma membrane.

phagocytosis (fag-o-si-TO-sis) Engulfing of large particles through the plasma membrane.

pharynx (FAR-inks) Throat; passageway between the mouth and esophagus.

phenotype (FE-no-tipe) All the characteristics of an organism that can be seen or tested for.

phenylketonuria (fen-il-ke-to-NU-re-ah) **(PKU)** Hereditary metabolic disorder involving inability to metabolize the amino acid phenylalanine.

phimosis (fi-MO-sis) Tightness of the foreskin.

phlebitis (fleh-BI-tis) Inflammation of a vein.

phospholipid (fos-fo-LIP-id) Complex lipid containing phosphorus.

phrenic (FREN-ik) Pertaining to the diaphragm.

phrenic nerve Nerve that activates the diaphragm.

physiology (fiz-e-OL-o-je) Study of the function of living organisms.

pia mater (PI-ah MA-ter) Innermost layer of the meninges.

PID See pelvic inflammatory disease.

pineal (PIN-e-al) **gland** Gland in the brain that is regulated by light; involved in sleep–wake cycles.

pinna (PIN-nah) Outer projecting portion of the ear; auricle.

pinocytosis (pi-no-si-TO-sis) Intake of small particles and droplets by the plasma membrane of a cell.

pituitary (pih-TU-ih-tar-e) **gland** Endocrine gland located under and controlled by the hypothalamus; releases hormones that control

other glands; hypophysis.

placenta (plah-SEN-tah) Structure that nourishes and maintains the developing fetus during pregnancy.

plaque (PLAK) A patch or flat area; fatty material that deposits in vessel linings in atherosclerosis.

plasma (PLAZ-mah) Liquid portion of the blood.

plasma cell Cell derived from a B cell that produces antibodies.

plasma membrane Outer covering of a cell; regulates what enters and leaves cell; cell membrane.

plasmapheresis (plas-mah-fer-E-sis) Separation and removal of plasma from a blood donation and return of the formed elements to the donor.

platelet (PLATE-let) Cell fragment that forms a plug to stop bleeding and acts in blood clotting; thrombocyte.

pleura (PLU-rah) Serous membrane that lines the chest cavity and covers the lungs.

pleurisy (PLUR-ih-se) Inflammation of the pleura; pleuritis.

plexus (PLEK-sus) Network of vessels or nerves.

pneumonia (nu-MO-ne-ah) Inflammation of the lungs, commonly due to infection; pneumonitis.

pneumothorax (nu-mo-THO-raks) Accumulation of air in the pleural space.

PNS See peripheral nervous system.

poliomyelitis (po-le-o-mi-eh-LI-tis) (polio) Viral disease of the nervous system that occurs most commonly in children.

polycythemia (pol-e-si-THE-me-ah) Increase in the number of red cells in the blood.

polydipsia (pol-e-DIP-se-ah) Excessive thirst.

polyp (POL-ip) Protruding growth, often grapelike, from a mucous membrane.

polysaccharide (pol-e-SAK-ah-ride) Compound formed from many simple sugars linked together, such as starch and glycogen.

pons (ponz) Area of the brain between the midbrain and medulla; connects the cerebellum with the rest of the central nervous system.

portal system Venous system that carries blood to a second capillary bed through which it circulates before returning to the heart.

positive feedback A substance or condition that acts within a system to promote more of the same activity.

positron emission tomography (to-MOG-rah-fe) **(PET)** Imaging method that uses a radioactive substance to show activity in an organ.

posterior (pos-TE-re-or) Toward the back; dorsal.

potential (po-TEN-shal) An electrical charge, as on the neuron plasma membrane.

precipitation (pre-sip-ih-TA-shun) Clumping of small particles as a result of an antigen–antibody reaction; seen as a cloudiness.

preeclampsia (pre-eh-KLAMP-se-ah) See pregnancy induced hypertension.

pregnancy (PREG-nan-se) Period during which an embryo or fetus is developing in the body.

pregnancy-induced hypertension (PIH) Hypertension, proteinuria, and edema associated with a hormone imbalance in the latter part of pregnancy; if untreated, may lead to eclampsia; preeclampsia, toxemia of pregnancy.

prepuce (PRE-puse) Loose fold of skin that covers the glans penis; foreskin.

presbycusis (pres-be-KU-sis) Slowly progressive hearing loss that often accompanies aging.

presbyopia (pres-be-O-pe-ah) Loss of visual accommodation that occurs with age, leading to farsightedness.

prevalence (PREV-ah-lens) In epidemiology, the overall frequency of a disease in a given group.

prime mover Muscle that performs a given movement; agonist.

prion (PRI-on) An infectious protein particle that causes progressive neurodegenerative disease.

PRL see prolactin.

progeny (PROJ-eh-ne) Offspring, descendent.

progesterone (pro-JES-ter-one) Hormone produced by the corpus luteum and placenta; maintains the uterine lining for pregnancy.

prognosis (prog-NO-sis) Prediction of the probable outcome of a disease based on the condition of the patient and knowledge about the disease.

prolactin (pro-LAK-tin) Hormone from the anterior pituitary that stimulates milk production in the breasts; PRL.

prone Face down or palm down.

prophase (PRO-faze) First stage of mitosis, during which the chromosomes become visible and the organelles disappear.

prophylaxis (pro-fih-LAK-sis) Prevention of disease.

proprioceptor (pro-pre-o-SEP-tor) Sensory receptor that aids in judging body position and changes in position; located in muscles, tendons, and joints.

prostaglandin (pros-tah-GLAN-din) Any of a group of hormones produced by many cells; these hormones have a variety of effects.

prostate (PROS-tate) **gland** Gland that surrounds the urethra below the bladder and contributes secretions to the semen.

protein (PRO-tene) Organic compound made of amino acids; contains nitrogen in addition to carbon, hydrogen, and oxygen (some contain sulfur or phosphorus).

prothrombin (pro-THROM-bin) Clotting factor; converted to thrombin during blood clotting.

prothrombinase (pro-THROM-bih-nase) Blood clotting factor that converts prothrombin to thrombin.

proton (PRO-ton) Positively charged particle in an atom's nucleus.

protozoon (pro-to-ZO-on) Animal-like microorganism; pl., protozoa.

proximal (PROK-sih-mal) Nearer to point of origin or to a reference point.

pruritis (pru-RI-tis) Intense itching of the skin.

psoriasis (so-RI-ah-sis) Chronic skin disease with red, flat areas covered with silvery scales.

ptosis (TO-sis) Dropping down of a part.

puerperal (pu-ER-per-al) Related to childbirth.

pulmonary circuit Pathway that carries blood from the heart to the lungs for oxygenation and then returns the blood to the heart.

pulse Wave of increased pressure in the vessels produced by heart contraction.

pupil (PU-pil) Opening in the center of the eye through which light enters.

Purkinje (pur-KIN-je) **fibers** Part of the heart's conduction system; conduction myofibers.

pus Mixture of bacteria and leukocytes formed in response to infection.

pustule (PUS-tule) Vesicle filled with pus.

pyelonephritis (pi-eh-lo-neh-FRI-tis) Inflammation of the liver, calyces, and renal pelvis, often due to bacterial infection.

pylorus (pi-LOR-us) Distal region of the stomach that leads to the pyloric sphincter.

pyrogen (PI-ro-jen) Substance that produces fever.

pyruvic (pi-RU-vik) **acid** Intermediate product in the breakdown of glucose for energy.

R

radioactivity (ra-de-o-ak-TIV-ih-te) Emission of atomic particles from an element.

radiography (ra-de-og-rah-fe) Production of an image by passage of x-rays through the body onto sensitized film; record produced is a radiograph.

rash Surface skin lesion.

receptor (re-SEP-tor) Specialized cell or ending of a sensory neuron that can be excited by a stimulus. A site in the cell membrane to which a special substance (e.g., hormone, antibody) may attach.

recessive (re-SES-iv) Referring to a gene that is not expressed if a dominant gene for the same trait is present.

reflex (RE-fleks) Simple, rapid, automatic response involving few neurons.

reflex arc (ark) Pathway through the nervous system from stimulus to response; commonly involves a receptor, sensory neuron, central neuron(s), motor neuron, and effector.

refraction (re-FRAK-shun) Bending of light rays as they pass from one medium to another of a different density.

relaxin (re-LAKS-in) Placental hormone that softens the cervix and relaxes the pelvic joints.

renin (RE-nin) Enzyme released from the kidney's juxtaglomerular apparatus that indirectly increases blood pressure by activating angiotensin.

repolarization (re-po-lar-ih-ZA-shun) Sudden return to the original charge on a cell membrane following depolarization.

resorption (re-SORP-shun) Loss of substance, such as that of bone or a tooth.

respiration (res-pih-RA-shun) Process by which oxygen is obtained from the environment and delivered to the cells.

respiratory system System consisting of the lungs and breathing passages involved in exchange of oxygen and carbon dioxide between the outside air and the blood.

reticular (reh-TIK-u-lar) **formation** Network in the limbic system that governs wakefulness and sleep.

reticuloendothelial (reh-tik-u-lo-en-do-THE-le-al) **system** Protective system consisting of highly phagocytic cells in body fluids and tissues, such as the spleen, lymph nodes, bone marrow, and liver.

retina (RET-ih-nah) Innermost layer of the eye; contains light-sensitive cells (rods and cones).

retroperitoneal (ret-ro-per-ih-to-NE-al) Behind the peritoneum, as are the kidneys, pancreas, and abdominal aorta.

retrovirus (RET-ro-vi-rus) Virus that has RNA as the genetic material and copies the RNA into DNA to replicate in the host cells (e.g., HIV).

reverse transcriptase (tran-SKRIP-tase) Enzyme needed for transcribing RNA into DNA in a retrovirus.

Rh factor A red cell antigen; D antigen.

rheumatoid (RU-mah-toyd) **arthritis** Disease of connective tissue that affects the joints.

rhodopsin (ro-DOP-sin) Light-sensitive pigment in the rods of the eye; visual purple.

rib One of the slender curved bones that make up most of the thorax; costa; adj., costal.

ribonucleic (RI-bo-nu-kle-ik) **acid** (**RNA**) Substance needed for protein manufacture in the cell.

ribosome (RI-bo-some) Small body in the cell's cytoplasm that is a site of protein manufacture.

rickets (RIK-ets) Softening of bone (osteomalacia) in children, usually caused by a deficiency of vitamin D.

Rickettsia (rih-KET-se-ah) Extremely small oval to rod-shaped bacterium that can grow only within a living cell.

RNA See ribonucleic acid.

rod Receptor cell in the retina of the eye; used for vision in dim light.

roentgenogram (rent-GEN-o-gram) Image produced by means of x-rays; radiograph.

rotation (ro-TA-shun) Twisting or turning of a bone on its own axis.

rugae (RU-je) Folds in the lining of an organ, such as the stomach or urinary bladder; sing., ruga (RU-gah).

rule of nines Method for estimating the extent of a burn based on multiples of nine.

S

SA node See sinoatrial node.

saliva (sah-LI-vah) Secretion of the salivary glands; moistens food and contains an enzyme that digests starch.

salt Compound formed by reaction between an acid and a base (e.g. NaCl, table salt).

saltatory (SAL-tah-to-re) **conduction** Transmission of an electrical impulse from node to node along a myelinated fiber; faster than continuous conduction along the entire membrane.

sagittal (SAJ-ih-tal) Describing a plane that divides a structure into right and left portions.

sarcoma (sar-KO-mah) Malignant tumor of connective tissue; a form of cancer.

sarcoplasmic reticulum (sar-ko-PLAS-mik re-TIK-u-lum) (**SR**) Intracellular membrane in muscle cells that is equivalent to the endoplasmic reticulum (ER) in other cells; stores calcium needed for muscle contraction.

saturated fat Fat that has more hydrogen atoms and fewer double bonds between carbons than do unsaturated fats.

scar Fibrous connective tissue that replaces normal tissues destroyed by injury or disease; cicatrix.

Schwann (shvahn) **cell** Cell in the nervous system that produces the myelin sheath around peripheral axons.

sclera (SKLE-rah) Outermost layer of the eye; made of tough connective tissue; "white" of the eye.

scleroderma (skle-ro-DER-mah) An autoimmune disease associated with overproduction of collagen.

scoliosis (sko-le-O-sis) Lateral curvature of the spine.

scrotum (SKRO-tum) Sac in which testes are suspended.

sebaceous (seh-BA-chus) Pertaining to sebum; an oily substance secreted by skin glands.

sebum (SE-bum) Oily secretion that lubricates the skin; adj., sebaceous (se-BA-shus).

secretin (se-KRE-tin) Hormone from the duodenum that stimulates pancreatic release of water and bicarbonate.

seizure (SE-zhur) Series of muscle spasms; convulsion.

selectively permeable Describing a membrane that regulates what can pass through (e.g., a cell's plasma membrane).

sella turcica (SEL-ah TUR-sih-ka) Saddlelike depression in the floor of the skull that holds the pituitary gland.

semen (SE-men) Mixture of sperm cells and secretions from several glands of the male reproductive tract.

semicircular canal Bony canal in the internal ear that contains receptors for the sense of dynamic equilibrium; there are three semicircular canals in each ear.

semilunar (sem-e-LU-nar) Shaped like a half-moon, such as the flaps of the pulmonary and aortic valves.

seminal vesicle (VES-ih-kl) Gland that contributes secretions to the semen.

seminiferous (seh-mih-NIF-er-us) **tubules** Tubules in which sperm cells develop in the testis.

semipermeable (sem-e-PER-me-ah-bl) Capable of being penetrated by some substances and not others.

sensory (SEN-so-re) Describing cells or activities involved in transmitting impulses toward the central nervous system; afferent.

sensory adaptation Gradual loss of sensation when sensory receptors are exposed to continuous stimulation.

sensory receptor Part of the nervous system that detects a stimulus.

sepsis (SEP-sis) Presence of pathogenic microorganisms or their toxins in the bloodstream or other tissues; adj., septic.

septicemia (sep-tih-SE-me-ah) Presence of pathogenic organisms or their toxins in the bloodstream; blood poisoning.

septum (SEP-tum) Dividing wall, as between the chambers of the heart or the nasal cavities.

serosa (se-RO-sah) Serous membrane; epithelial membrane that secretes a thin, watery fluid.

Sertoli cells See sustentacular cells.

serum (SE-rum) Liquid portion of blood without clotting factors; thin, watery fluid; adj., serous (SE-rus).

sex-linked Referring to a gene carried on a sex chromosome, usually the X chromosome.

sexually transmitted infection (STI) Communicable disease acquired through sexual relations; sexually transmitted disease (STD); venereal disease (VD).

shingles Viral infection that follows the nerve pathways; caused by the same virus that causes chicken pox; herpes zoster.

shock Pertaining to the circulation: a life-threatening condition in which there is inadequate blood flow to the tissues.

sickle cell disease Hereditary disease in which abnormal hemoglobin causes red blood cells to change shape (sickle) when they release oxygen.

sign Manifestation of a disease as noted by an observer.

sinoatrial (si-no-A-tre-al) **(SA) node** Tissue in the right atrium's upper wall that sets the rate of heart contractions; the heart's pacemaker.

sinus (SI-nus) Cavity or channel, such as the paranasal sinuses in the skull bones.

sinus rhythm Normal heart rhythm originating at the SA node.

sinusoid (SI-nus-oyd) Enlarged capillary that serves as a blood channel.

skeletal (SKEL-eh-tal) **system** The body system that includes the bones and joints.

skeleton (SKEL-eh-ton) Bony framework of the body; adj., skeletal.

skull Bony framework of the head.

solute (SOL-ute) Substance that is dissolved in another substance (the solvent).

solution (so-LU-shun) Homogeneous mixture of one substance dissolved in another; the components in a mixture are evenly distributed and cannot be distinguished from each other.

solvent (SOL-vent) Substance in which another substance (the solute) is dissolved.

somatic (so-MAT-ik) **nervous system** Division of the nervous system that controls voluntary activities and stimulates skeletal muscle.

somatotropin (so-mah-to-TRO-pin) Growth hormone.

spasm Sudden and involuntary muscular contraction.

specific gravity The weight of a substance as compared to the weight of an equal volume of pure water.

spermatic (sper-MAT-ik) **cord** Cord that extends through the inguinal canal and suspends the testis; contains blood vessels, nerves, and ductus deferens.

spermatozoon (sper-mah-to-ZO-on) Male reproductive cell or gamete; pl., spermatozoa; sperm cell.

sphincter (SFINK-ter) Muscular ring that regulates the size of an opening.

sphygmomanometer (sfig-mo-mah-NOM-eh-ter) Device used to measure blood pressure; blood pressure apparatus or cuff.

spina bifida (SPI-nah BIF-ih-dah) Incomplete closure of the spine.

spinal cord Nervous tissue contained in the spinal column; major relay area between the brain and the peripheral nervous system.

spirillum (spi-RIL-um) Corkscrew or spiral-shaped bacterium; pl., spirilla.

spirochete (SPI-ro-kete) Spiral-shaped microorganism that moves in a waving and twisting motion.

spirometer (spi-ROM-eh-ter) Instrument for recording lung volumes; tracing is a spirogram.

spleen Lymphoid organ in the upper left region of the abdomen.

spore Resistant form of bacterium; reproductive cell in lower plants.

squamous (SKWA-mus) Flat and irregular, as in squamous epithelium.

SR See sarcoplasmic reticulum.

staging A procedure for evaluating the extent of tumor spread.

stain (stane) Dye that aids in viewing structures under the microscope.

staphylococcus (staf-ih-lo-KOK-us) Round bacterium found in a cluster resembling a bunch of grapes; pl., staphylococci (staf-ih-lo-KOK-si).

stasis (STA-sis) Stoppage in the normal flow of fluids, such as blood, lymph, urine, or contents of the digestive tract.

stem cell Cell that has the potential to develop into different types of cells.

stenosis (sten-O-sis) Narrowing of a duct or canal.

stent Small tube inserted into a vessel to keep it open.

sterility Complete inability to reproduce.

sterilization (ster-ih-li-ZA-shun) Process of killing every living microorganism on or in an object; procedure that makes an individual incapable of reproduction.

steroid (STE-royd) Category of lipids that includes the hormones of the sex glands and the adrenal cortex.

stethoscope (STETH-o-skope) Instrument for conveying sounds from the patient's body to the examiner's ears.

STI See sexually transmitted infection.

stimulus (STIM-u-lus) Change in the external or internal environment that produces a response.

stomach (STUM-ak) Organ of the digestive tract that stores food, mixes it with digestive juices, and moves it into the small intestine.

strabismus (strah-BIZ-mus) Deviation of the eye resulting from lack of eyeball muscle coordination.

stratified In multiple layers (strata).

stratum (STRA-tum) A layer; pl., strata.

stratum basale (bas-A-le) Deepest layer of the epidermis; layer that produces new epidermal cells; stratum germinativum.

stratum corneum (KOR-ne-um) The thick uppermost layer of the epidermis.

striations (stri-A-shuns) Stripes or bands, as seen in skeletal muscle and cardiac muscle.

stricture (STRICK-ture) Narrowing of a part.

stroke Damage to the brain due to lack of oxygen; usually caused by a blood clot in a vessel (thrombus) or rupture of a vessel; cerebrovascular accident (CVA).

subacute (sub-a-KUTE) Not as severe as an acute infection nor as long-lasting as a chronic disorder.

subcutaneous (sub-ku-TA-ne-us) Under the skin.

submucosa (sub-mu-KO-sah) Layer of connective tissue beneath the mucosa.

substrate Substance on which an enzyme works.

sudoriferous (su-do-RIF-er-us) Producing sweat; referring to the sweat glands.

sulcus (SUL-kus) Shallow groove, as between convolutions of the cerebral cortex; pl., sulci (SUL-si).

superior (su-PE-re-or) Above; in a higher position.

superior vena cava (VE-nah KA-vah) Large vein that drains the upper part of the body and empties into the heart's right atrium.

supine (SU-pine) Face up or palm up.

surfactant (sur-FAK-tant) Substance in the alveoli that prevents their collapse by reducing surface tension of the contained fluids.

suspension (sus-PEN-shun) Heterogeneous mixture that will separate unless shaken.

suspensory ligaments Filaments attached to the ciliary muscle of the eye that hold the lens in place.

sustentacular (sus-ten-TAK-u-lar) **cells** Cells in the seminiferous tubules that aid in development of spermatozoa; Sertoli cells.

suture (SU-chur) Type of joint in which bone surfaces are closely united, as in the skull; stitch used in surgery to bring parts together or to stitch parts together in surgery.

sympathetic nervous system Thoracolumbar division of the autonomic nervous system; stimulates a fight-or-flight (stress) response.

symptom (SIMP-tom) Evidence of disease noted by the patient; such evidence noted by an examiner is called a sign or an objective symptom.

synapse (SIN-aps) Junction between two neurons or between a neuron and an effector.

synarthrosis (sin-ar-THRO-sis) Immovable joint.

syndrome (SIN-drome) Group of symptoms characteristic of a disorder.

synergist (SIN-er-jist) Substance or structure that enhances the work of another. A muscle that works with a prime mover to produce a given movement.

synovial (sin-O-ve-al) Pertaining to a thick lubricating fluid found in joints, bursae, and tendon sheaths; pertaining to a freely movable (diarthrotic) joint.

system (SIS-tem) Group of organs functioning together for the same general purposes.

systemic (sis-TEM-ik) Referring to a generalized infection or condition.

systemic circuit Pathway that carries blood to all tissues of the body except the lungs.

systole (SIS-to-le) Contraction phase of the cardiac cycle; adj., systolic (sis-TOL-ik).

T

tachycardia (tak-e-KAR-de-ah) Heart rate more than 100 beats per minute.

tachypnea (tak-IP-ne-ah) Excessive rate of respiration.

tactile (TAK-til) Pertaining to the sense of touch.

target tissue Tissue that is capable of responding to a specific hormone.

Tay-Sachs disease Hereditary disease affecting fat metabolism.

T cell Lymphocyte active in immunity that matures in the thymus gland; destroys foreign cells directly; T lymphocyte.

tectorial (tek-TO-re-al) **membrane** Part of the hearing apparatus; generates nerve impulses as cilia move against it in response to sound waves.

telophase (TEL-o-faze) Final stage of mitosis, during which new nuclei form and the cell contents usually divide.

tendinitis (ten-din-I-tis) Inflammation of a tendon.

tendon (TEN-don) Cord of fibrous connective tissue that attaches a muscle to a bone.

teniae (TEN-e-e) **coli** Bands of smooth muscle in the wall of the large intestine.

testis (TES-tis) Male reproductive gland; pl., testes (TES-teze).

testosterone (tes-TOS-ter-one) Male sex hormone produced in the testes; promotes sperm cell development and maintains secondary sex characteristics.

tetanus (TET-an-us) Constant contraction of a muscle; infectious disease caused by a bacterium (*Clostridium tetani*); lockjaw.

tetany (TET-an-e) Muscle spasms due to low blood calcium, as in parathyroid deficiency.

thalassemia (thal-ah-SE-me-ah) Hereditary blood disorder that impairs hemoglobin production; the two forms are alpha (α) and beta (β).

thalamus (THAL-ah-mus) Region of the brain located in the diencephalon; chief relay center for sensory impulses traveling to the cerebral cortex.

therapy (THER-ah-pe) Treatment.

thoracentesis (thor-a-sen-TE-sis) Puncture of the chest for aspiration of fluid in the pleural space.

thorax (THO-raks) Chest; adj., thoracic (tho-RAS-ik).

thrombocyte (THROM-bo-site) Blood platelet; cell fragment that participates in clotting.

thrombocytopenia (throm-bo-si-to-PE-ne-ah) Deficiency of platelets in the blood.

thrombolytic (throm-bo-LIT-ik) Dissolving blood clots.

thrombosis (throm-BO-sis) Condition of having a thrombus (blood clot in a vessel).

thrombus (THROM-bus) Blood clot within a vessel.

thymosin (THI-mo-sin) Hormone produced by the thymus gland.

thymus (THI-mus) Endocrine gland in the upper portion of the chest; stimulates development of T cells.

thyroid (THI-royd) Endocrine gland in the neck.

thyroiditis (thi-royd-I-tis) Inflammation of the thyroid gland.

thyroid-stimulating hormone (TSH) Hormone produced by the anterior pituitary that stimulates the thyroid gland; thyrotropin.

thyroxine (thi-ROK-sin) Hormone produced by the thyroid gland; increases metabolic rate and needed for normal growth; T_4.

tinea (TIN-e-ah) Common term for fungal skin infection.

tissue Group of similar cells that performs a specialized function.

tonicity (to-NIS-ih-te) The osmotic concentration or osmotic pressure of a solution. The effect that a solution will have on osmosis.

tonsil (TON-sil) Mass of lymphoid tissue in the region of the pharynx.

tonus (TO-nus) Partially contracted state of muscle; also, tone.

toxemia (tok-SE-me-ah) General toxic condition in which poisonous bacterial substances are absorbed into the bloodstream; presence of harmful substances in the blood as a result of abnormal metabolism.

toxin (TOK-sin) Poison.

toxoid (TOK-soyd) Altered toxin used to produce active immunity.

trachea (TRA-ke-ah) Tube that extends from the larynx to the bronchi; windpipe.

tracheostomy (tra-ke-OS-to-me) Surgical opening into the trachea for the introduction of a tube through which a person may breathe.

trachoma (trah-KO-mah) Acute eye infection caused by chlamydia.

tract Bundle of neuron fibers within the central nervous system.

trait Characteristic.

transfusion (trans-FU-zhun) Introduction of blood or blood components directly into the bloodstream.

transplantation (trans-plan-TA-shun) The grafting to a recipient of an organ or tissue from an animal or other human to replace an injured or incompetent body part.

transverse Describing a plane that divides a structure into superior and inferior parts.

trauma (TRAW-mah) Injury or wound.

tricuspid (tri-KUS-pid) **valve** Valve between the heart's right atrium and right ventricle.

trigeminal neuralgia (tri-JEM-ih-nal nu-RAL-je-ah) Severe spasmodic pain affecting the fifth cranial nerve; tic douloureux (tik du-lu-RU).

triglyceride (tri-GLIS-er-ide) Simple fat composed of glycerol and three fatty acids.

trigone (TRI-gone) Triangular-shaped region in the floor of the bladder that remains stable as the bladder fills.

triiodothyronine (tri-i-o-do-THI-ro-nin) Thyroid hormone that functions with thyroxine to raise cellular metabolism; T_3.

tropomyosin (tro-po-MI-o-sin) Protein that works with troponin to regulate contraction in skeletal muscle.

troponin (tro-PO-nin) Protein that works with tropomyosin to regulate contraction in skeletal muscle.

TSH See thyroid-stimulating hormone.

tuberculosis (tu-ber-ku-LO-sis) (TB) Infectious disease, often of the lung, caused by the bacillus *Mycobacterium tuberculosis*.

tumor (TU-mor) Abnormal growth or neoplasm.

tympanic (tim-PAN-ik) **membrane** Membrane between the external and middle ear that transmits sound waves to the bones of the middle ear; eardrum.

U

ulcer (UL-ser) Sore or lesion associated with death and disintegration of tissue.

ultrasound (UL-trah-sound) Very high frequency sound waves.

umbilical (um-BIL-ih-kal) **cord** Structure that connects the fetus with the placenta; contains vessels that carry blood between the fetus and placenta.

umbilicus (um-BIL-ih-kus) Small scar on the abdomen that marks the former attachment of the umbilical cord to the fetus; navel.

universal solvent Term used for water because it dissolves more substances than any other solvent.

unsaturated fat Fat that has fewer hydrogen atoms and more double bonds between carbons than do saturated fats.

urea (u-RE-ah) Nitrogenous waste product excreted in the urine; end product of protein metabolism.

uremia (u-RE-me-ah) Accumulation of nitrogenous waste products in the blood.

ureter (U-re-ter) Tube that carries urine from the kidney to the urinary bladder.

urethra (u-RE-thrah) Tube that carries urine from the urinary bladder to the outside of the body.

urinalysis (u-rin-AL-ih-sis) Laboratory examination of urine's physical and chemical properties.

urinary bladder Hollow organ that stores urine until it is eliminated.

urinary (U-rin-ar-e) **system** The system involved in elimination of soluble waste, water balance, and regulation of body fluids.

urination (u-rin-A-shun) Voiding of urine; micturition.

urine (U-rin) Liquid waste excreted by the kidneys.

urticaria (ur-tih-KA-re-ah) Hives; allergic skin reaction with elevated red patches (wheals).

uterus (U-ter-us) Muscular, pear-shaped organ in the female pelvis within which the fetus develops during pregnancy; adj., uterine.

uvea (U-ve-ah) Middle coat of the eye, including the choroid, iris, and ciliary body; vascular and pigmented structures of the eye.

uvula (U-vu-lah) Soft, fleshy, V-shaped mass that hangs from the soft palate.

V

vaccination (vak-sin-A-shun) Administration of a vaccine to protect against a specific disease; immunization.

vaccine (vak-SENE) Substance used to produce active immunity; usually, a suspension of attenuated or killed pathogens or some component of a pathogen given by inoculation to prevent a specific disease.

vagina (vah-JI-nah) Distal part of the birth canal that opens to the outside of the body; female organ of sexual intercourse.

valence (VA-lens) The combining power of an atom; the number of electrons lost or gained by atoms of an element in chemical reactions.

valve Structure that prevents fluid from flowing backward, as in the heart, veins, and lymphatic vessels.

varicose (VAR-ih-kose) Pertaining to an enlarged and twisted vessel, as in varicose vein.

vas deferens (DEF-er-enz) Tube that carries sperm cells from the testis to the urethra; ductus deferens.

vascular (VAS-ku-lar) Pertaining to blood vessels.

vasectomy (vah-SEK-to-me) Surgical removal of part or all of the ductus (vas) deferens; usually done on both sides to produce sterility.

vasoconstriction (vas-o-kon-STRIK-shun) Decrease in a blood vessel's diameter.

vasodilation (vas-o-di-LA-shun) Increase in a blood vessel's diameter.

VD Venereal disease; see sexually transmitted infection.

vector (VEK-tor) An insect or other animal that transmits a disease-causing organism from one host to another.

vein (vane) Vessel that carries blood toward the heart.

vena cava (VE-nah KA-vah) Large vein that carries blood into the heart's right atrium; superior vena cava or inferior vena cava.

venereal (ve-NE-re-al) **disease** (VD) Infectious disease acquired through sexual activity; sexually transmitted infection (STI).

venous sinus (VE-nus SI-nus) Large channel that drains deoxygenated blood.

ventilation (ven-tih-LA-shun) Movement of air into and out of the lungs.

ventral (VEN-tral) Toward the front or belly surface; anterior.

ventricle (VEN-trih-kl) Cavity or chamber; one of the heart's two lower chambers; one of the brain's four chambers in which cerebrospinal fluid is produced; adj., ventricular (ven-TRIK-u-lar).

venule (VEN-ule) Vessel between a capillary and a vein.

vernix caseosa (VEr-niks ka-se-O-sah) Cheeselike sebaceous secretion that covers a newborn.

vertebra (VER-teh-brah) A bone of the spinal column; pl., vertebrae (VER-teh-bre).

verruca (veh-RU-kah) Wart.

vesicle (VES-ih-kl) Small sac or blister filled with fluid.

vesicular transport Use of vesicles to move large amounts of material through the plasma membrane of a cell.

vestibular apparatus (ves-TIB-u-lar) Part of the inner ear concerned with equilibrium; consists of the semicircular canals and vestibule.

vestibule (VES-tih-bule) Part of the internal ear that contains receptors for the sense of static equilibrium; any space at the entrance to a canal or organ.

vibrio (VIB-re-o) Slight curved or comma-shaped bacterium; pl., vibrios.

villi (VIL-li) Small fingerlike projections from the surface of a membrane; projections in the lining of the small intestine through which digested food is absorbed; sing., villus.

viroid (VI-royd) Infectious agent composed of RNA with no protein. Viroids are intracellular parasites linked so far only to diseases in plants.

virulence (VIR-u-lens) Power of an organism to overcome a host's defenses.

virus (VI-rus) Extremely small infectious agent that can reproduce only within a living cell.

viscera (VIS-er-ah) Organs in the ventral body cavities, especially the abdominal organs; adj., visceral.

viscosity (vis-KOS-ih-te) Thickness, as of the blood or other fluid.

vitamin (VI-tah-min) Organic compound needed in small amounts for health.

vitreous (VIT-re-us) **body** Soft, jellylike substance that fills the eyeball and holds the shape of the eye; vitreous humor.

vocal cords Folds of mucous membrane in the larynx used in producing speech.

Volkmann canal See perforating canal.

volvulus (VOL-vu-lus) Twisting of the intestine.

von Willebrand disease Hereditary blood clotting disorder in which there is a shortage of von Willebrand factor.

W

Wernicke (VER-nih-ke) **area** Portion of the cerebral cortex concerned with speech recognition and the meaning of words.

white matter Nervous tissue composed of myelinated fibers.

Wilson disease Recessive hereditary disease associated with a defect in copper metabolism and accumulation of copper in the liver, brain, or other tissues.

X

x-ray Ray or radiation of extremely short wavelength that can penetrate opaque substances and affect photographic plates and fluorescent screens.

Z

zygote (ZI-gote) Fertilized ovum; cell formed by the union of a sperm and an egg.

Glossary of Word Parts

Use of Word Parts in Medical Terminology

Medical terminology, the special language of the health occupations, is based on an understanding of a few relatively basic elements. These elements—roots, prefixes, and suffixes—form the foundation of almost all medical terms. A useful way to familiarize yourself with each term is to learn to pronounce it correctly and say it aloud several times. Soon it will become an integral part of your vocabulary.

The foundation of a word is the word root. Examples of word roots are *abdomin*, referring to the belly region; and *aden*, pertaining to a gland. A word root is often followed by a vowel to facilitate pronunciation, as in *abdomino* and *adeno*. We then refer to it as a "combining form."

A prefix is a part of a word that precedes the word root and changes its meaning. For example, the prefix *mal-* in malnutrition means "abnormal." A suffix, or word ending, is a part that follows the word root and adds to or changes its meaning. The suffix *-rhea* means "profuse flow" or "discharge," as in diarrhea, a condition characterized by excessive discharge of liquid stools.

Many medical words are compound words; that is, they are made up of more than one root or combining form. Examples of such compound words are *erythrocyte* (red blood cell) and *hydrocele* (fluid-containing sac), and many more difficult words, such as *sternoclavicular* (indicating relations to both the sternum and the clavicle).

A general knowledge of language structure and spelling rules is also helpful in mastering medical terminology. For example, adjectives include words that end in *-al*, as in sternal (the noun is sternum), and words that end in *-ous*, as in mucous (the noun is mucus).

The following list includes some of the most commonly used word roots, prefixes, and suffixes, as well as examples of their use. Prefixes are followed by a hyphen; suffixes are preceded by a hyphen; and word roots have no hyphen. Commonly used combining vowels are added following a slash.

Word Parts

a-, an- absent, deficient, lack of: *aphasia, atrophy, anemia, anuria*
ab- away from: *abduction, aboral*
abdomin/o belly or abdominal area: *abdominocentesis, abdominoscopy*
acous, acus hearing, sound: *acoustic, presbyacusis*
acr/o end, extremity: *acromegaly, acromion*
actin/o, actin/i relation to raylike structures or, more commonly, to light or roentgen (x-) rays, or some other type of radiation: *actiniform, actinodermatitis*
ad- (sometimes converted to *ac-, af-, ag-, ap-, as-, at-,*) toward, added to, near: *adrenal, accretion, agglomerated, afferent*
aden/o gland: *adenectomy, adenitis, adenocarcinoma*
aer/o air, gas: *aerobic, aerate*
-agogue inducing, leading, stimulating: *cholagogue, galactagogue*
-al pertaining to, resembling: *skeletal, surgical, ileal*
alb/i- white: *albinism, albiduria*
alge, alg/o, alges/i pain: *algetic, algophobia, analgesic*
-algia pain, painful condition: *myalgia, neuralgia*
amb/i- both, on two sides: *ambidexterity, ambivalent*
ambly- dimness, dullness: *amblyopia*
amphi on both sides, around, double: *amphiarthrosis, amphibian*
amyl/o starch: *amylase, amyloid*
an- absent, deficient, lack of: *anaerobic, anoxia, anemic*
ana- upward, back, again, excessive: *anatomy, anastomosis, anabolism*
andr/o male: *androgen, androgenous*
angi/o vessel: *angiogram, angiotensin*
ant/i- against; to prevent, suppress, or destroy: *antarthritic, antibiotic, anticoagulant*
ante- before, ahead of: *antenatal, antepartum*
anter/o- position ahead of or in front of (i.e., anterior to) another part: *anterolateral, anteroventral*
-apheresis take away, withdraw: *hemapheresis, plasmapheresis*
ap/o- separation, derivation from: *apocrine, apoptosis, apophysis*
aqu/e water: *aqueous, aquatic, aqueduct*
-ar pertaining to, resembling: *muscular, nuclear*

arthr/o joint or articulation: *arthrolysis, arthrostomy, arthritis*
-ary pertaining to, resembling: *salivary, dietary, urinary*
-ase enzyme: *lipase, protease*
-asis *See –sis*
atel/o- imperfect: *atelectasis*
ather/o gruel: *athersclerosis, atheroma*
audi/o sound, hearing: *audiogenic, audiometry, audiovisual*
aut/o- self: *autistic, autodigestion, autoimmune*

bar/o pressure: *baroreceptor, barometer*
bas/o- alkaline: *basic, basophilic*
bi- two, twice: *bifurcate, bisexual*
bil/i bile: *biliary, bilirubin*
bio- life, living organism: *biopsy, antibiotic*
blast/o, -blast early stage of a cell, immature cell: *blastula, blastophore, erythroblast*
bleph, blephar/o eyelid, eyelash: *blepharism, blepharitis, blepharospasm*
brachi, brachi/o arm: *brachial, brachiocephalic, brachiotomy*
brachy- short: *brachydactylia, brachyesophagus*
brady- slow: *bradycardia*
bronch/o-, bronch/i bronchus: *bronchiectasis, bronchoscope*
bucc cheek: *buccal*

capn/o carbon dioxide: *hypocapnia, hypercapnia*
carcin/o cancer: *carcinogenic, carcinoma*
cardi/o, cardi/a heart: *carditis, cardiac, cardiologist*
cata- down: *catabolism, catalyst*
-cele swelling; enlarged space or cavity: *cystocele, meningocele, rectocele*
celi/o abdomen: *celiac, celiocentesis*
centi- relating to 100 (used in naming units of measurements): *centigrade, centimeter*
-centesis perforation, tapping: *aminocentesis, paracentesis*
cephal/o head: *cephalalgia, cephalopelvic*

cerebr/o brain: *cerobrospinal, cerebrum*
cervi neck: *cervical, cervix*
cheil/o lips; brim or edge: *cheilitis, cheilosis*
chem/o, chem/i chemistry, chemical: *chemotherapy, chemocautery, chemoreceptor*
chir/o, cheir/o hand: *cheiralgia, cheiromegaly, chiropractic*
chol/e, chol/o bile, gall: *chologogue, cholecyst, cholelith*
cholecyst/o gallbladder: *cholecystitis, cholecystokinin*
chondr/o, chondri/o cartilage: *chondric, chondrocyte, chondroma*
chori/o membrane: *chorion, choroid, choriocarcinoma*
chrom/o, chromat/o color: *chromosome, chromatin, chromophilic*
-cid, -cide to cut, kill or destroy: *bactericidal, germicide, suicide*
circum- around, surrounding: *circumorbital, circumrenal, circumduction*
-clast break: *osteoclast*
clav/o, cleid/o clavicle: *cleidomastoid, subclavian*
co- with, together: *cofactor, cohesion, coinfection*
colp/o vagina: *colpectasia, colposcope, colpotomy*
con- with: *concentric, concentrate, conduct*
contra- opposed, against: *contraindication, contralateral*
corne/o horny: *corneum, cornified, cornea*
cortic/o cortex: *cortical, corticotropic, cortisone*
cost/a, cost/o- ribs: *intercostal, costosternal*
counter- against, opposite to: *counteract, counterirritation, countertraction*
crani/o skull: *cranium, craniotomy*
cry/o- cold: *cryalgesia, cryogenic, cryotherapy*
crypt/o- hidden, concealed: *cryptic, cryptogenic, cryptorchidism*
-cusis hearing: *acusis, presbyacusis*
cut- skin: *subcutaneous*
cyan/o- blue: *cyanosis, cyanogen*
cyst/i, cyst/o sac, bladder: *cystitis, cystoscope*
cyt/o, -cyte cell: *cytology, cytoplasm, osteocyte*

dactyl/o digits (usually fingers, but sometimes toes): *dactylitis, polydactyly*
de- remove: *detoxify, dehydration*
dendr tree: *dendrite*
dent/o, dent/i tooth: *dentition, dentin, dentifrice*
derm/o, dermat/o skin: *dermatitis, dermatology, dermatosis*
di- twice, double: *dimorphism, dibasic, dihybrid*
dipl/o- double: *diplopia, diplococcus*
dia- through, between, across, apart: *diaphragm, diaphysis*
dis- apart, away from: *disarticulation, distal*
dors/i, dors/o- back (in the human, this combining form is the same as poster/o-): *dorsal, dorsiflexion, dorso-nuchal*
dys- disordered, difficult, painful: *dysentery, dysphagia, dyspnea*

e- out: *enucleation, evisceration, ejection*
-ectasis expansion, dilation, stretching: *angiectasis, bronchiectasis*
ecto- outside, external: *ectoderm, ectogenous*
-ectomy surgical removal or destruction by other means: *appendectomy, thyroidectomy*
edem swelling: *edema*
-emia condition of blood: *glycemia, hyperemia*
encephal/o brain: *encephalitis, encephalogram*
end/o- in, within, innermost: *endarterial, endocardium, endothelium*
enter/o intestine: *enteritis, enterocolitis*
epi- on, upon: *epicardium, epidermis*
equi- equal: *equidistant, equivalent, equilibrium*
erg/o work: *ergonomic, energy, synergy*
eryth-, erythr/o red: *erythema, erythrocyte*
-esthesia sensation: *anesthesia, paresthesia*
eu- well, normal, good: *euphoria, eupnea*
ex/o- outside, out of, away from: *excretion, exocrine, exophthalmic*
extra- beyond, outside of, in addition to: *extracellular, extrasystole, extravasation*

fasci fibrous connective tissue layers: *fascia, fascitis, fascicle*
fer, -ferent to bear, to carry: *afferent, efferent, transfer*
fibr/o threadlike structures, fibers: *fibrillation, fibroblast, fibrositis*

gastr/o stomach: *gastritis, gastroenterostomy*
-gen an agent that produces or originates: *allergen, pathogen, fibrinogen*
-genic produced from, producing: *neurogenic, pyogenic, psychogenic*

genit/o organs of reproduction: *genitoplasty, genitourinary*
gen/o- a relationship to reproduction or sex: *genealogy, generate, genetic, genotype*
-geny manner of origin, development or production: *ontogeny, progeny*
gest/o gestation, pregnancy: *progesterone, gestagen*
glio, -glia gluey material; specifically, the support tissue of the central nervous system: *glioma, neuroglia*
gloss/o tongue: *glossitis, glossopharyngeal*
glyc/o- relating to sugar, glucose, sweet: *glycemia, glycosuria*
gnath/o related to the jaw: *prognathic, gnathoplasty*
gnos to perceive, recognize: *agnostic, prognosis, diagnosis*
gon seed, knee: *gonad, gonarthritis*
-gram record, that which is recorded: *electrocardiogram, electroencephalogram*
graph/o, -graph instrument for recording, record, writing: *electrocardiograph, electroencephalograph, micrograph*
-graphy process of recording data: *photography, radiography*
gyn/o, gyne, gynec/o female, woman: *gynecology, gynecomastia, gynoplasty*
gyr/o circle: *gyroscope, gyrus, gyration*

hema, hemo, hemat/o blood: *hematoma, hematuria, hemorrhage*
hemi- one half: *hemisphere, heminephrectomy, hemiplegia*
hepat/o liver: *hepatitis, hepatogenous*
heter/o- other, different: *heterogenous, heterosexual, heterochromia*
hist/o, histi/o tissue: *histology, histiocyte*
homeo-, homo- unchanging, the same: *homeostasis, homosexual*
hydr/o water: *hydrolysis, hydrocephalus*
hyper- above, over, excessive: *hyperesthesia, hyperglycemia, hypertrophy*
hypo- deficient, below, beneath: *hypochondrium, hypodermic, hypogastrium*
hyster/o uterus: *hysterectomy*

-ia state of, condition of: *myopia, hypochondria, ischemia*
-iatrics, -trics medical specialty: *pediatrics, obstetrics*
iatr/o physician, medicine: *iatrogenic*
-ic pertaining to, resembling: *metric, psychiatric, geriatric*
idio- self, one's own, separate, distinct: *idiopathic, idiosyncrasy*
-ile pertaining to, resembling: *febrile, virile*
im-, in- in, into, lacking: *implantation, infiltration, inanimate*
infra- below, inferior: *infraspinous, infracortical*
insul/o pancreatic islet, island: *insulin, insulation, insulinoma*
inter- between: *intercostal, interstitial*
intra- within a part or structure: *intracranial, intracellular, intraocular*
isch suppression: *ischemia*
-ism state of: *alcoholism, hyperthyroidism*
iso- same, equal: *isotonic, isometric*
-ist one who specializes in a field of study: *cardiologist, gastroenterologist*
-itis inflammation: *dermatitis, keratitis, neuritis*

juxta- next to: *juxtaglomerular, juxtaposition*

kary/o nucleus: *karyotype, karyoplasm*
kerat/o cornea of the eye, certain horny tissues: *keratin, keratitis, keratoplasty*
kine movement: *kinetic, kinesiology, kinesthesia*

lacri- tear: *lacrimal*
lact/o milk: *lactation, lactogenic*
laryng/o larynx: *laryngeal, laryngectomy, laryngitis*
later/o side: *lateral*
-lemma sheath: *neurilemma, sarcolemma*
leuk/o- (also written as *leuc-, leuco-*) white, colorless: *leukocyte, leukoplakia*
lip/o lipid, fat: *lipase, lipoma*
lig- bind: *ligament, ligature*
lingu/o tongue: *lingual, linguadental*
lith/o stone (calculus): *lithiasis, lithotripsy*
-logy study of: *physiology, gynecology*
lute/o yellow: *macula lutea, corpus luteum*
lymph/o lymph, lymphatic system, lymphocyte: *lymphoid, lymphedema*
lyso-, -lysis, -lytic: loosening, dissolving, separating: *hemolysis, paralysis, lysosome*

macr/o- large, abnormal length: *macrophage, macroblast*. **See also** -mega, mega/o-

mal- bad, diseased, disordered, abnormal: *malnutrition, malocclusion, malunion*

malac/o, -malacia softening: *malacoma, osteomalacia*

mamm/o breast, mammary gland: *mammogram, mammoplasty, mammal*

man/o pressure: *manometer, sphygmomanometer*

mast/o breast: *mastectomy, mastitis*

meg/a-, megal/o, -megaly unusually or excessively large: *megacolon, megaloblast, splenomegaly, megakaryocyte*

melan/o dark, black: *melanin, melanocyte, melanoma*

men/o physiologic uterine bleeding, menses: *menstrual, menorrhagia, menopause*

mening/o membranes covering the brain and spinal cord: *meningitis, meningocele*

mes/a, mes/o- middle, midline: *mesencephalon, mesoderm*

meta- change, beyond, after, over, near: *metabolism, metacarpal, metaplasia*

-meter, metr/o measure: *hemocytometer, sphygmomanometer, spirometer, isometric*

metr/o uterus: *endometrium, metroptosis, metrorrhagia*

micro- very small: *microscope, microbiology, microsurgery, micrometer*

mon/o- single, one: *monocyte, mononucleosis*

morph/o shape, form: *morphogenesis, morphology*

multi- many: *multiple, multifactorial, multipara*

my/o muscle: *myenteron, myocardium, myometrium*

myc/o, mycet fungus: *mycid, mycete, mycology, mycosis, mycelium*

myel/o marrow (often used in reference to the spinal cord): *myeloid, myeloblast, osteomyelitis, poliomyelitis*

myring/o tympanic membrane: *myringotomy, myringitis*

myx/o mucus: *myxoma, myxovirus*

narc/o stupor: *narcosis, narcolepsy, narcotic*

nas/o nose: *nasopharynx, paranasal*

natri sodium: *hyponatremia, natriuretic*

necr/o death, corpse: *necrosis*

neo- new: *neoplasm, neonatal*

neph, nephr/o kidney: *nephrectomy, nephron*

neur/o, neur/i nerve, nervous tissue: *neuron, neuralgia, neuroma*

neutr/o neutral: *neutrophil, neutropenia*

noct/i night: *noctambulation, nocturia, noctiphobia*

ocul/o eye: *oculist, oculomotor, oculomycosis*

odont/o tooth, teeth: *odontalgia, orthodontics*

-odynia pain, tenderness: *myodynia, neurodynia*

-oid like, resembling: *lymphoid, myeloid*

olig/o- few, a deficiency: *oligospermia, oliguria*

-oma tumor, swelling: *hematoma, sarcoma*

-one ending for steroid hormone: *testosterone, progesterone*

onych/o nails: *paronychia, onychoma*

oo, ovum, egg: *oocyte, oogenesis*, (do not confuse with oophor-)

oophor/o ovary: *oophorectomy, oophoritis, oophorocystectomy*. **See also** ovar-

ophthalm/o eye: *ophthalmia, ophthalmologist, ophthalmoscope*

-opia disorder of the eye or vision: *heterotropia, myopia, hyperopia*

or/o mouth: *oropharynx, oral*

orchi/o, orchid/o testis: *orchitis, cryptorchidism*

orth/o- straight, normal: *orthopedics, orthopnea, orthosis*

-ory pertaining to, resembling: *respiratory, circulatory*

oscill/o to swing to and fro: *oscilloscope*

osmo- osmosis: *osmoreceptor; osmotic*

oss/i, osse/o, oste/o bone, bone tissue: *osseous, ossicle, osteocyte, osteomyelitis*

ot/o ear: *otalgia, otitis, otomycosis*

-ous pertaining to, resembling: *fibrous, venous, androgynous*

ov/o egg, ovum: *oviduct, ovulation*

ovar, ovari/o ovary: *ovariectomy*. **See also** oophor

ox-, -oxia pertaining to oxygen: *hypoxemia, hypoxia, anoxia*

oxy sharp, acute: *oxygen, oxytocia*

pan- all: *pandemic, panacea*

papill/o nipple: *papilloma, papillary*

para- near, beyond, apart from, beside: *paramedical, parametrium, parathyroid, parasagittal*

pariet/o wall: *parietal*

path/o, -pathy disease, abnormal condition: *pathogen, pathology, neuropathy*

ped/o, pedia child, foot: *pedophobia, pediatrician, pedialgia*

-penia lack of: *leukopenia, thrombocytopenia*

per- through, excessively: *percutaneous, perfusion*

peri- around: *pericardium, perichondrium*

-pexy fixation: *nephropexy, proctopexy*

phag/o to eat, to ingest: *phagocyte, phagosome*

-phagia, -phagy eating, swallowing: *aphagia, dysphagia*

-phasia speech, ability to talk: *aphasia, dysphasia*

phen/o to show: *phenotype*

-phil, -philic to like, have an affinity for: *eosinophilia, hemophilia, hydrophilic*

phleb/o vein: *phlebitis, phlebotomy*

-phobia fear, dread, abnormal aversion: *phobic, acrophobia, hydrophobia*

phot/o light: *photoreceptor, photophobia*

phren/o diaphragm: *phrenic, phrenicotomy*

physi/o natural, physical: *physiology, physician*

pil/e, pil/i, pil/o hair, resembling hair: *pileous, piliation, pilonidal*

pin/o to drink: *pinocytosis*

-plasty molding, surgical formation: *cystoplasty, gastroplasty, kineplasty*

-plegia stroke, paralysis: *paraplegia, hemiplegia*

pleur/o side, rib, pleura: *pleurisy, pleurotomy*

-pnea air, breathing: *dyspnea, eupnea*

pneum/o, pneumat/o air, gas, respiration: *pneumothorax, pneumograph, pneumatocele*

pneumon/o lung: *pneumonia, pneumonectomy*

pod/o foot: *podiatry, pododynia*

-poiesis making, forming: *erythropoiesis, hematopoiesis*

polio- gray: *polioencephalitis, poliomyelitis*

poly- many: *polyarthritis, polycystic, polycythemia*

post- behind, after, following: *postnatal, postocular, postpartum*

pre- before, ahead of: *precancerous, preclinical, prenatal*

presby- old age: *presbycusis, presbyopia*

pro- before, in front of, in favor of: *prodromal, prosencephalon, prolapse, prothrombin*

proct/o rectum: *proctitis, proctocele, proctologist*

propri/o own: *proprioception*

pseud/o false: *pseudoarthrosis, pseudostratified, pseudopod*

psych/o mind: *psychosomatic, psychotherapy*

-ptosis downward displacement, falling, prolapse: *blepharoptosis, enteroptosis, nephroptosis*

pulm/o, pulmon/o lung: *pulmonic, pulmonology*

py/o pus: *pyuria, pyogenic, pyorrhea*

pyel/o renal pelvis: *pyelitis, pyelogram, pyelonephrosis*

pyr/o fire, fever: *pyrogen, antipyretic, pyromania*

quadr/i- four: *quadriceps, quadriplegic*

rachi/o spine: *rachicentesis, rachischisis*

radio- emission of rays or radiation: *radioactive, radiography, radiology*

re- again, back: *reabsorption, reaction, regenerate*

rect/o rectum: *rectal, rectouterine*

ren/o kidney: *renal, renopathy*

reticul/o network: *reticulum, reticular*

retro- backward, located behind: *retrocecal, retroperitoneal*

rhin/o nose: *rhinitis, rhinoplasty*

-rhage, -rhagia* bursting forth, excessive flow: *hemorrhage, menorrhagia*

-rhaphy* suturing or sewing up a gap or defect in a part: *herniorrhaphy, gastrorrhaphy, cystorrhaphy*

-rhea* flow, discharge: *diarrhea, gonorrhea, seborrhea*

sacchar/o sugar: *monosaccharide, polysaccharide*

salping/o tube: *salpingitis, salpingoscopy*

sarc/o flesh: *sarcolemma, sarcoplasm, sarcomere*

scler/o hard, hardness; *scleroderma, sclerosis*

scoli/o- twisted, crooked: *scoliosis, scoliosometer*

* When a suffix beginning with *rh* is added to a word root, the *r* is doubled.

-scope instrument used to look into or examine a part: *bronchoscope, endoscope, arthroscope*

semi- partial, half: *semipermeable, semicoma*

semin/o semen, seed: *seminiferous, seminal*

sep, septic poison, rot, decay: *sepsis, septicemia*

sin/o sinus: *sinusitis, sinusoid, sinoatrial*

-sis condition or process, usually abnormal: *dermatosis, osteoporosis*

soma-, somat/o, -some body: *somatic, somatotype, somatotropin*

son/o sound: *sonogram, sonography*

sphygm/o pulse: *sphygmomanometer*

spir/o breathing: *spirometer, inspiration, expiration*

splanchn/o- internal organs: *splanchnic, splanchnoptosis*

splen/o spleen: *splenectomy, splenic*

staphyl/o grapelike cluster: *staphylococcus*

stat, -stasis stand, stoppage, remain at rest: *hemostasis, static, homeostasis*

sten/o- contracted, narrowed: *stenosis*

sthen/o, -sthenia, -sthenic strength: *asthenic, calisthenics, neurasthenia*

steth/o chest: *stethoscope*

stoma, stomat/o mouth: *stomatitis*

-stomy surgical creation of an opening into a hollow organ or an opening between two organs: *colostomy, tracheostomy, gastroenterostomy*

strept/o chain: *streptococcus, streptobacillus*

sub- under, below, near, almost: *subclavian, subcutaneous, subluxation*

super- over, above, excessive: *superego, supernatant, superficial*

supra- above, over, superior: *supranasal, suprarenal*

sym-, syn- with, together: *symphysis, synapse*

syring/o fistula, tube, cavity: *syringectomy, syringomyelia*

tach/o-, tachy- rapid: *tachycardia, tachypnea*

tars/o eyelid, foot: *tarsitis, tarsoplasty, tarsoptosis*

-taxia, -taxis order, arrangement: *ataxia, chemotaxis, thermotaxis*

tel/o end: *telophase, telomere*

tens- stretch, pull: *extension, tensor*

test/o testis: *testosterone, testicular*

tetr/a four: *tetralogy, tetraplegia*

therm/o-, -thermy heat: *thermalgesia, thermocautery, diathermy, thermometer*

thromb/o blood clot: *thrombosis, thrombocyte*

toc/o labor: *eutocia, dystocia, oxytocin*

tom/o, -tomy incision of, cutting: *anatomy, phlebotomy, laparotomy*

ton/o tone, tension: *tonicity, tonic*

tox, toxic/o poison: *toxin, cytotoxic, toxemia, toxicology*

trache/o trachea, windpipe: *tracheal, tracheitis, tracheotomy*

trans- across, through, beyond: *transorbital, transpiration, transplant, transport*

tri- three: *triad, triceps*

trich/o hair: *trichiasis, trichosis, trichology*

troph/o, -trophic, -trophy nutrition, nurture: *atrophic, hypertrophy*

trop/o, -tropin, -tropic turning toward, acting on, influencing, changing: *thyrotropin, adrenocorticotropic, gonadotropic*

tympan/o drum: *tympanic, tympanum*

ultra- beyond or excessive: *ultrasound, ultraviolent, ultrastructure*

uni- one: *unilateral, uniovular, unicellular*

-uria urine: *glycosuria, hematuria, pyuria*

ur/o urine, urinary tract: *urology, urogenital*

vas/o vessel, duct: *vascular, vasectomy, vasodilation*

viscer/o internal organs, viscera: *visceral, visceroptosis*

vitre/o glasslike: *vitreous*

xer/o dryness: *xeroderma, xerophthalmia, xerosis*

-y condition of: *tetany, atony, dysentery*

zyg/o joined: *zygote, heterozygous, monozygotic*

Appendices

Metric Measurements

Appendix 1-1	**Metric Measurements**

Unit	Abbreviation	Metric Equivalent	U.S. Equivalent
Units of length			
Kilometer	km	1,000 meters	0.62 miles; 1.6 km/mile
Meter*	m	100 cm; 1,000 mm	39.4 inches; 1.1 yards
Centimeter	cm	1/100 m; 0.01 m	0.39 inches; 2.5 cm/inch
Millimeter	mm	1/1,000 m; 0.001 m	0.039 inches; 25 mm/inch
Micrometer	μm	1/1,000 mm; 0.001 mm	
Units of Weight			
Kilogram	kg	1,000 g	2.2 lb
Gram*	g	1,000 mg	0.035 oz.; 28.5 g/oz
Milligram	mg	1/1,000 g; 0.001 g	
Microgram	μg	1/1,000 mg; 0.001 mg	
Units of volume			
Liter*	L	1,000 mL	1.06 qt
Deciliter	dL	1/10 L; 0.1 L	
Milliliter	mL	1/1,000 L; 0.001 L	0.034 oz.; 29.4 mL/oz
Microliter	μL, mcL	1/1,000 mL; 0.001 mL	

* Basic unit.

Celsius–Fahrenheit Temperature Conversion Scale

Celsius to Fahrenheit

Use the following formula to convert Celsius readings to Fahrenheit readings:

$$°F = 9/5°C + 32$$

For example, if the Celsius reading is 37°

$$°F = (9/5 \times 37) + 32$$

$$= 66.6 + 32$$

98.6°F (normal body temperature)

Fahrenheit to Celsius

Use the following formula to convert Fahrenheit readings to Celsius readings:

$$°C = 5/9 (°F - 32)$$

For example, if the Fahrenheit reading is 68°

$$°C = 5/9 (68 - 32)$$

$$= 5/9 \times 36$$

20°C (a nice spring day)

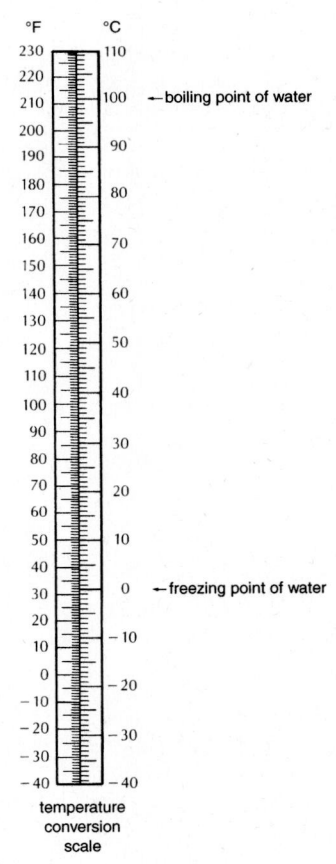

temperature
conversion
scale

Periodic Table of the Elements

The periodic table lists the chemical elements according to their atomic numbers. The boxes in the table have information about the elements, as shown by the example at the top of the chart. The upper number in each box is the atomic number, which represents the number of protons in the nucleus of the atom. Under the name of the element is its chemical symbol, an abbreviation of its modern or Latin name. The Latin names of four common elements are shown below the chart. The bottom number in each box gives the atomic weight (mass) of that element's atoms compared with the weight of carbon atoms. Atomic weight is the sum of the weights of the protons and neutrons in the nucleus.

All the elements in a column share similar chemical properties based on the number of electrons in their outermost energy levels. Those in column VIII are non-reactive (inert) and are referred to as the noble gases. The 26 elements found in the body are color coded according to quantity (see totals above the chart). Carbon, hydrogen, oxygen, and nitrogen make up 96% of body weight. The first three of these are present in all carbohydrates, lipids, proteins, and nucleic acids. Nitrogen is an additional component of all proteins. Nine other elements make up almost all the rest of body weight. The remaining 13 elements are present in very small amounts and are referred to as trace elements. Although needed in very small quantities, they are essential for good health, as they are parts of enzymes and other compounds used in metabolism.

PERIODIC TABLE OF THE ELEMENTS

Notation:

6	Atomic number
Carbon	Name
C	Symbol
12.01	Atomic weight

- 96% of body weight
- 3.9% of body weight
- 0.1% of body weight

I	II												III	IV	V	VI	VII	VIII
1 Hydrogen **H** 1.01																		2 Helium **He** 4.00
3 Lithium **Li** 6.94	4 Beryllium **Be** 9.01												5 Boron **B** 10.81	6 Carbon **C** 12.01	7 Nitrogen **N** 14.01	8 Oxygen **O** 16.00	9 Fluorine **F** 19.00	10 Neon **Ne** 20.18
11 Sodium **Na** 22.99	12 Magnesium **Mg** 24.31												13 Aluminum **Al** 26.98	14 Silicon **Si** 28.09	15 Phosphorus **P** 30.97	16 Sulfur **S** 32.07	17 Chlorine **Cl** 35.45	18 Argon **Ar** 39.95
19 Potassium **K** 39.10	20 Calcium **Ca** 40.08	21 Scandium **Sc** 44.96	22 Titanium **Ti** 47.88	23 Vanadium **V** 50.94	24 Chromium **Cr** 52.00	25 Manganese **Mn** 54.94	26 Iron **Fe** 55.85	27 Cobalt **Co** 58.93	28 Nickel **Ni** 58.69	29 Copper **Cu** 63.55	30 Zinc **Zn** 65.39		31 Gallium **Ga** 69.72	32 Germanium **Ge** 72.59	33 Arsenic **As** 74.92	34 Selenium **Se** 78.96	35 Bromine **Br** 79.90	36 Krypton **Kr** 83.80
37 Rubidium **Rb** 85.47	38 Strontium **Sr** 87.62	39 Yttrium **Y** 88.91	40 Zirconium **Zr** 91.22	41 Niobium **Nb** 92.91	42 Molybdenum **Mo** 95.94	43 Technetium **Tc** (98)	44 Ruthenium **Ru** 101.1	45 Rhodium **Rh** 102.9	46 Palladium **Pd** 106.4	47 Silver **Ag** 107.9	48 Cadmium **Cd** 112.4		49 Indium **In** 114.8	50 Tin **Sn** 118.7	51 Antimony **Sb** 121.8	52 Tellurium **Te** 127.6	53 Iodine **I** 126.9	54 Xenon **Xe** 131.3
55 Cesium **Cs** 132.91	56 Barium **Ba** 137.34		72 Hafnium **Hf** 178.5	73 Tantalum **Ta** 180.9	74 Tungsten **W** 183.9	75 Rhenium **Re** 186.2	76 Osmium **Os** 190.2	77 Iridium **Ir** 192.2	78 Platinum **Pt** 195.1	79 Gold **Au** 196.9	80 Mercury **Hg** 200.6		81 Thallium **Tl** 204.4	82 Lead **Pb** 207.2	83 Bismuth **Bi** 209.0	84 Polonium **Po** (210)	85 Astatine **At** (210)	86 Radon **Rn** (222)
87 Francium **Fr** (223)	88 Radium **Ra** (226)		104 Rutherfordium **Rf** (257)	105 Dubnium **Db** (260)	106 Seaborgium **Sg** (263)	107 Bohrium **Bh** (262)	108 Hassium **Hs** (265)	109 Meitnerium **Mt** (267)	110 Darmstadtium **Ds** (271)	111 Unnamed (272)	112 Unnamed (277)							

57-71 Lanthanides

57 Lanthanum **La** 138.9	58 Cerium **Ce** 140.1	59 Praseodymium **Pr** 140.9	60 Neodymium **Nd** 144.2	61 Promethium **Pm** (145)	62 Samarium **Sm** (150.4)	63 Europium **Eu** 152.0	64 Gadolinium **Gd** 157.3	65 Terbium **Tb** 158.9	66 Dysprosium **Dy** 162.5	67 Holmium **Ho** 164.9	68 Erbium **Er** 167.3	69 Thulium **Tm** 168.9	70 Ytterbium **Yb** 173.0	71 Lutetium **Lu** 175.0

89-103 Actinides

89 Actinium **Ac** (227)	90 Thorium **Th** 232.0	91 Protactinium **Pa** (231)	92 Uranium **U** (238)	93 Neptunium **Np** (237)	94 Plutonium **Pu** (244)	95 Americium **Am** (243)	96 Curium **Cm** (247)	97 Berkelium **Bk** (247)	98 Californium **Cf** (251)	99 Einsteinium **Es** (254)	100 Fermium **Fm** (257)	101 Mendelevium **Md** (256)	102 Nobelium **No** (259)	103 Lawrencium **Lr** (257)

Name	Latin name	Symbol
Copper	*cuprium*	Cu
Iron	*ferrum*	Fe
Potassium	*kalium*	K
Sodium	*natrium*	Na

Tests

Appendix 4-1 Routine Urinalysis

Test	Normal Value	Clinical Significance
General characteristics and measurements		
Color	Pale yellow to amber	Color change can be due to concentration or dilution, drugs, metabolic or inflammatory disorders
Odor	Slightly aromatic	Foul odor typical of urinary tract infection, fruity odor in uncontrolled diabetes mellitus
Appearance (clarity)	Clear to slightly hazy	Cloudy urine occurs with infection or after refrigeration; may indicate presence of bacteria, cells, mucus, or crystals
Specific gravity	1.003–1.030 (first morning catch; routine is random)	Decreased in diabetes insipidus, acute renal failure, water intoxication; increased in liver disorders, heart failure, dehydration
pH	4.5–8.0	Acid urine accompanies acidosis, fever, high protein diet; alkaline urine in urinary tract infection, metabolic alkalosis, vegetarian diet
Chemical determinations		
Glucose	Negative	Glucose present in uncontrolled diabetes mellitus, steroid excess
Ketones	Negative	Present in diabetes mellitus and in starvation
Protein	Negative	Present in kidney disorders, such as glomerulonephritis, acute kidney failure
Bilirubin	Negative	Breakdown product of hemoglobin; present in liver disease or in bile blockage
Urobilinogen	0.2–1.0 Ehrlich units /dL	Breakdown product of bilirubin; increased in hemolytic anemias and in liver disease; remains negative in bile obstruction
Blood (occult)	Negative	Detects small amounts of blood cells, hemoglobin, or myoglobin; present in severe trauma, metabolic disorders, bladder infections
Nitrite	Negative	Product of bacterial breakdown of urine; positive result suggests urinary tract infection and needs to be followed up with a culture of the urine
Microscopic		
Red blood cells	0–3 per high-power field	Increased because of bleeding within the urinary tract from trauma, tumors, inflammation, or damage within the kidney
White blood cells	0–4 per high-power field	Increased by kidney or bladder infection
Renal epithelial cells	Occasional	Increased number indicates damage to kidney tubules
Casts	None	Hyaline casts normal; large number of abnormal casts indicates inflammation or a systemic disorder
Crystals	Present	Most are normal; may be acid or alkaline
Bacteria	Few	Increased in urinary tract infection or contamination from infected genitalia
Others		Any yeasts, parasites, mucus, spermatozoa, or other microscopic findings would be reported here

Appendix 4-2   Complete Blood Count

Test	Normal Value*	Clinical Significance
Red blood cell (RBC) count	Men: 4.2–5.4 million/μL Women: 3.6–5.0 million/μL	Decreased in anemia; increased in dehydration, polycythemia
Hemoglobin (Hb)	Men: 13.5–17.5 g/dL Women: 12–16 g/dL	Decreased in anemia, hemorrhage, and hemolytic reactions; increased in dehydration, heart and lung disease
Hematocrit (Hct) or packed cell volume (PCV)	Men: 40%–50% Women: 37%–47%	Decreased in anemia; increased in polycythemia, dehydration These values, calculated from the RBC count, Hb, and Hct, give information valuable in the diagnosis and classification of anemia
Red blood cell (RBC) indices (examples)		
Mean corpuscular volume (MCV)	87–103 μL/red cell	Measures the average size or volume of each RBC: small size (microcytic) in iron-deficiency anemia; large size (macrocytic) typical of pernicious anemia
Mean corpuscular hemoglobin (MCH)	26–34 pg/red cell	Measures the weight of hemoglobin per RBC; useful in differentiating types of anemia in a severely anemic patient
Mean corpuscular hemoglobin concentration (MCHC)	31–37 g/dL	Defines the volume of hemoglobin per RBC; used to determine the color or concentration of hemoglobin per RBC
White blood cell (WBC) count	5,000–10,000μL	Increased in leukemia and in response to infection, inflammation, and dehydration; decreased in bone marrow suppression
Platelets	150,000–350,000/μL	Increased in many malignant disorders; decreased in disseminated intravascular coagulation (DIC) or toxic drug effects; spontaneous bleeding may occur at platelet counts below 20,000 μL
Differential (Peripheral blood smear)		A stained slide of the blood is needed to perform the differential. The percentages of the different WBCs are estimated, and the slide is microscopically checked for abnormal characteristics in WBCs, RBCs, and platelets
WBCs		
Segmented neutrophils (SEGs, POLYs)	40%–74%	Increased in bacterial infections; low numbers leave person very susceptible to infection
Immature neutrophils (BANDs)	0%–3%	Increased when neutrophil count increases
Lymphocytes (LYMPHs)	20%–40%	Increased in viral infections; low numbers leave person dangerously susceptible to infection
Monocytes (MONOs)	2%–6%	Increased in specific infections
Eosinophils (EOs)	1%–4%	Increased in allergic disorders
Basophils (BASOs)	0.5%–1%	Increased in allergic disorders

* *Values vary depending on instrumentation and type of test.*

Appendix 4-3 Blood Chemistry Tests

Test	Normal Value	Clinical Significance
Basic panel: An overview of electrolytes, waste product management, and metabolism		
Blood urea nitrogen (BUN)	7–18 mg/dL	Increased in renal disease and dehydration; decreased in liver damage and malnutrition
Carbon dioxide (CO_2) (includes bicarbonate)	23–30 mmol/L	Useful to evaluate acid-base balance by measuring total carbon dioxide in the blood: Elevated in vomiting and pulmonary disease; decreased in diabetic acidosis, acute renal failure, and hyperventilation
Chloride (Cl)	98–106 mEq/L	Increased in dehydration, hyperventilation, and congestive heart failure; decreased in vomiting, diarrhea, and fever
Creatinine	0.6–1.2 mg/dL	Produced at a constant rate and excreted by the kidney; increased in kidney disease
Glucose	Fasting: 70–110 mg/dL Random: 85–125 mg/dL	Increased in diabetes and severe illness; decreased in insulin overdose or hypoglycemia
Potassium (K)	3.5–5 mEq/L	Increased in renal failure, extensive cell damage, and acidosis; decreased in vomiting, diarrhea, and excess administration of diuretics or IV fluids
Sodium (Na)	101–111 mEq/L or 135–148 mEq/L (depending on test)	Increased in dehydration and diabetes insipidus; decreased in overload of IV fluids, burns, diarrhea, or vomiting
Additional blood chemistry tests		
Alanine amino-transferase (ALT)	10–40 U/L	Used to diagnose and monitor treatment of liver disease and to monitor the effects of drugs on the liver; increased in myocardial infarction
Albumin	3.8–5.0 g/dL	Albumin holds water in blood; decreased in liver disease and kidney disease
Albumin-globulin ratio (A/G ratio)	Greater than 1	Low A/G ratio signifies a tendency for edema because globulin is less effective than albumin at holding water in the blood
Alkaline phosphatase (ALP)	20–70 U/L (varies by method)	Enzyme of bone metabolism; increased in liver disease and metastatic bone disease
Amylase	21–160 U/L	Used to diagnose and monitor treatment of acute pancreatitis and to detect salivary gland inflammation
Aspartate amino-transferase (AST)	0–41 U/L (varies)	Enzyme present in tissues with high metabolic activity; increased in myocardial infarction and liver disease
Bilirubin, total	0.2–1.0 mg/dL	Breakdown product of hemoglobin from red blood cells; increased when excessive red blood cells are being destroyed or in liver disease
Calcium (Ca)	8.8–10.0 mg/dL	Increased in excess parathyroid hormone production and in cancer; decreased in alkalosis, elevated phosphate in renal failure, and excess IV fluids
Cholesterol	120–220 mg/dL desirable range	Screening test used to evaluate risk of heart disease; levels of 200 mg/dL or above indicate increased risk of heart disease and warrant further investigation
Creatine kinase (CK)	Men: 38–174 U/L Women: 96–140 U/L	Elevated enzyme level indicates myocardial infarction or damage to skeletal muscle. When elevated, specific fractions (isoenzymes) are tested for
Gamma-glutamyl transferase (GGT)	Men: 6–26 U/L Women: 4–18 U/L	Used to diagnose liver disease and to test for chronic alcoholism
Globulins	2.3–3.5 g/dL	Proteins active in immunity; help albumin keep water in blood
Iron, serum (Fe)	Men: 75–175 µg/dL Women: 65–165 µg/dL	Decreased in iron deficiency and anemia; increased in hemolytic conditions
High-density lipoproteins (HDLs)	Men: 30–70 mg/dL Women: 30–85 mg/dL	Used to evaluate the risk of heart disease

(continued)

Appendix 4-3	Blood Chemistry Tests (*continued*)	

Test	Normal Value	Clinical Significance
Lactic dehydrogenase (LDH or LD)	95–200 U/L (Normal ranges vary greatly)	Enzyme released in many kinds of tissue damage, including myocardial infarction, pulmonary infarction, and liver disease
Lipase	4–24 U/L (varies with test)	Enzyme used to diagnose pancreatitis
Low-density lipoproteins (LDLs)	80–140 mg/dL	Used to evaluate the risk of heart disease
Magnesium (Mg)	1.3–2.1 mEq/L	Vital in neuromuscular function; decreased levels may occur in malnutrition, alcoholism, pancreatitis, diarrhea
Phosphorus (P) (inorganic)	2.7–4.5 mg/dL	Evaluated in response to calcium; main store is in bone: elevated in kidney disease; decreased in excess parathyroid hormone
Protein, total	6–8 g/dL	Increased in dehydration, multiple myeloma; decreased in kidney disease, liver disease, poor nutrition, severe burns, excessive bleeding
Serum glutamic oxalacetic transaminase (SGOT)		See Aspartate aminotransferase (AST)
Serum glutamic pyruvic transaminase (SGPT)		See Alanine aminotransferase (ALT)
Thyroxin (T_4)	5–12.5 µg/dL (varies)	Screening test of thyroid function; increased in hyperthyroidism; decreased in myxedema and hypothyroidism
Thyroid-stimulating hormone (TSH)	0.5–6 mIU/L	Produced by pituitary to promote thyroid gland function; elevated when thyroid gland is not functioning
Triiodothyronine (T_3)	120–195 mg/dL	Elevated in specific types of hyperthyroidism
Triglycerides	Men: 40–160 mg/dL Women: 35–135 mg/dL	An indication of ability to metabolize fats; increased triglycerides and cholesterol indicate high risk of atherosclerosis
Uric acid	Men: 3.5–7.2 mg/dL Women: 2.6–6.0 mg/dL	Produced by breakdown of ingested purines in food and nucleic acids; elevated in kidney disease, gout, and leukemia

Appendix 5-1	**Bacterial Diseases**

Organism	Disease and Description
Cocci	
Neisseria gonorrhoeae (gonococcus)	Gonorrhea. Acute inflammation of mucous membranes of the reproductive and urinary tracts (with possible spread to the peritoneum in the female). Systemic infection may cause gonococcal arthritis and endocarditis. Organism also causes ophthalmia neonatorum, an eye inflammation of the newborn.
Neisseria meningitidis (meningococcus)	Epidemic meningitis. Inflammation of the membranes covering brain and spinal cord. A vaccine is available for use in high-risk populations.
Staphylococcus aureus and other staphylococci	Boils, carbuncles, impetigo, osteomyelitis, staphylococcal pneumonia, cystitis, pyelonephritis, empyema, septicemia, toxic shock, and food poisoning. Strains resistant to antibiotics are a cause of infections originating in hospitals, such as wound infections.
Streptococcus pneumoniae	Pneumonia; inflammation of the alveoli, bronchioles, and bronchi; middle ear infections; meningitis. May be prevented by use of polyvalent pneumococcal vaccine.
Streptococcus pyogenes, Streptococcus hemolyticus, and other streptococci	Septicemia, septic sore throat, scarlet fever, puerperal sepsis, erysipelas, streptococcal pneumonia, rheumatic fever, subacute bacterial endocarditis, acute glomerulonephritis.
Bacilli	
Bordetella pertussis	Pertussis (whooping cough). Severe infection of the trachea and bronchi. The "whoop" is caused by the effort to recover breath after coughing. All children should be immunized against pertussis.
Brucella abortus (and others)	Brucellosis, or undulant fever. Disease of animals such as cattle and goats transmitted to humans through unpasteurized dairy products or undercooked meat. Acute phase of fever and weight loss; chronic disease with abscess formation and depression.
Clostridium botulinum	Botulism. Very severe poisoning caused by eating food in which the organism has been allowed to grow and excrete its toxin. Causes muscle paralysis and may result in death from asphyxiation. Infant botulism results from ingestion of spores. It causes respiratory problems and flaccid paralysis, which usually respond to treatment.
Clostridium perfringens	Gas gangrene. Acute wound infection. Organisms cause death of tissues accompanied by the generation of gas within them.
Clostridium tetani	Tetanus. Acute, often fatal poisoning caused by introduction of the organism into deep wounds. Characterized by severe muscular spasms. Also called *lockjaw*.
Corynebacterium diphtheriae	Diphtheria. Acute throat inflammation with the formation of a leathery membranelike growth (pseudomembrane) that can obstruct air passages and cause death by asphyxiation. Toxin produced by this organism can damage heart, nerves, kidneys, and other organs. Disease preventable by appropriate vaccination.
Escherichia coli, Proteus spp., and other colon bacilli	Normal inhabitants of the colon, and usually harmless there. Cause of local and systemic infections, food poisoning, diarrhea (especially in children), septicemia, and septic shock. E. coli is a common hospital-acquired infection.

(continued)

Appendix 5-1   Bacterial Diseases (continued)

Organism	Disease and Description
Francisella tularensis	Tularemia, or deer fly fever. Transmitted by contact with an infected animal or by a tick or fly bite. Symptoms are fever, ulceration of the skin, and enlarged lymph nodes.
Haemophilus influenzae type b (Hib)	Severe infections in children under 3 years of age. Causes meningitis, also epiglottitis, septicemia, pneumonia, pericarditis, and septic arthritis. Preschool vaccinations are routine.
Helicobacter pylori	Acute inflammation of the stomach (gastritis), ulcers of the stomach's pyloric area and the duodenum.
Legionella pneumophila	Legionnaires disease (pneumonia). Seen in localized epidemics; may be transmitted by air conditioning towers and by contaminated soil at excavation sites. Not spread person to person. Characterized by high fever, vomiting, diarrhea, cough, and bradycardia. Mild form of the disease called Pontiac fever.
Mycobacterium leprae (Hansen bacillus)	Leprosy. Chronic illness in which hard swellings occur under the skin, particularly of the face, causing a distorted appearance. In one form of leprosy, the nerves are affected, resulting in loss of sensation in the extremities.
Mycobacterium tuberculosis (tubercle bacillus)	Tuberculosis. Infectious disease in which the organism causes primary lesions called *tubercles*. These break down into cheeselike masses of tissue, a process known as *caseation*. Any body organ can be infected, but in adults, the usual site is the lungs. Still one of the most widespread diseases in the world, tuberculosis is treated with chemotherapy; strains of the bacillus have developed resistance to drugs.
Pseudomonas aeruginosa	Common organism is a frequent cause of wound and urinary infections in debilitated hospitalized patients. Often found in solutions that have been standing for long periods.
Salmonella typhi (and others)	Salmonellosis occurs as enterocolitis, bacteremia, localized infection, or typhoid. Depending on type, presenting symptoms may be fever, diarrhea, or abscesses; complications include intestinal perforation and endocarditis. Carried in water, milk, meat, and other food.
Shigella dysenteriae (and others)	Serious bacillary dysentery. Acute intestinal infection with diarrhea (sometimes bloody); may cause dehydration with electrolyte imbalance or septicemia. Transmitted through fecal-oral route or other poor sanitation.
Yersinia pestis	Plague, the "black death" of the Middle Ages. Transmitted to humans by fleas from infected rodents. Symptoms of the most common form are swollen, infected lymph nodes, or *buboes*. Another form may cause pneumonia. All forms may lead to a rapidly fatal septicemia.

Curved rods

Vibrio

Vibrio cholerae	Cholera. Acute intestinal infection characterized by prolonged vomiting and diarrhea, leading to severe dehydration, electrolyte imbalance, and in some cases, death.

Spirochetes

Borrelia burgdorferi	Lyme disease, transmitted by the extremely small deer tick. Usually starts with a bulls-eye rash followed by flulike symptoms, at which time antibiotics are effective. May progress to neurologic problems and joint inflammation.
Borrelia recurrentis (and others)	Relapsing fever. Generalized infection in which attacks of fever alternate with periods of apparent recovery. Organisms spread by lice, ticks, and other insects.
Treponema pallidum	Syphilis. Infectious disease transmitted mainly by sexual intercourse. Untreated syphilis is seen in the following three stages: primary—formation of primary lesion (chancre); secondary—skin eruptions and infectious patches on mucous membranes; tertiary—development of generalized lesions (gummas) and destruction of tissues resulting in aneurysm, heart disease, and degenerative changes in brain, spinal cord, ganglia, and meninges. Also a cause of intrauterine fetal death or stillbirth.
Treponema vincentii	Vincent disease (trench mouth). Infection of the mouth and throat accompanied by formation of a pseudomembrane, with ulceration.

(continued)

Appendix 5-1 Bacterial Diseases (continued)

Organism	Disease and Description
Other bacteria	
(*Note:* The following organisms are smaller than other bacteria and vary in shape. Like viruses, they grow within cells, but they differ from viruses in that they are affected by antibiotics.)	
Chlamydia oculogenitalis	Inclusion conjunctivitis, acute eye infection. Carried in genital organs; transmitted during birth or through water in inadequately chlorinated swimming pools.
Chlamydia psittaci	Psittacosis, also called ornithosis. Disease transmitted by various birds, including parrots, ducks, geese, and turkeys. Primary symptoms are chills, headache, and fever, more severe in older people. The duration may be from 2 to 3 weeks, often with a long convalescence. Antibiotic drugs are effective remedies.
Chlamydia trachomatis	Sexually transmitted infection causing pelvic inflammatory disease and other reproductive tract infections. Also causes inclusion conjunctivitis, an acute eye infection, and trachoma, a chronic infection that is a common cause of blindness in underdeveloped areas of the world. Infection of the conjunctiva and cornea characterized by redness, pain, and lacrimation. Antibiotic therapy is effective if begun before there is scarring. The same organism causes lymphogranuloma venereum (LGV), a sexually transmitted infection characterized by swelling of inguinal lymph nodes and accompanied by signs of general infection
Coxiella burnetti	Q fever. Infection transmitted from cattle, sheep, and goats to humans by contaminated dust and also carried by arthropods. Symptoms are fever, headache, chills, and pneumonitis. This disorder is almost never fatal.
Rickettsia prowazekii	Epidemic typhus. Transmitted to humans by lice; associated with poor hygiene and war. Main symptoms are headache, hypotension, delirium, and a red rash. Frequently fatal in older people.
Rickettsia rickettsii	Rocky Mountain spotted fever. Tick-borne disease occurring throughout the United States. Symptoms are fever, muscle aches, and a rash that may progress to gangrene over bony prominences. The disease is rarely fatal.
Rickettsia typhi	Endemic or murine typhus. A milder disease transmitted to humans from rats by fleas. Symptoms are fever, rash, headache, and cough. The disease is rarely fatal.

Appendix 5-2 Viral Diseases

Organism	Disease and Description
Common cold viruses	Common cold (coryza), viral infection of the upper respiratory tract. A wide variety of organisms may be involved. May lead to complications, such as pneumonia and influenza.
Cytomegalovirus (CMV)	Common mild salivary gland infection. In an immunosuppressed person may cause infection of the retina, lung, and liver, GI tract ulceration, and brain inflammation. Causes severe fetal or neonatal damage.
Encephalitis viruses	Encephalitis, which usually refers to any brain inflammation accompanied by degenerative tissue changes. Encephalitis has many causes besides viruses. Viral forms of encephalitis include Western and Eastern epidemic, equine, St. Louis, Japanese B, and others. Some are known to be transmitted from birds and other animals to humans by insects, principally mosquitoes.
Epstein-Barr virus (EBV)	Mononucleosis, a highly infectious disease spread by saliva. Common among teenagers and young adults. There is fever, sore throat, marked fatigue, and enlargement of the spleen and lymph nodes. Infects B lymphocytes (mononuclear leukocytes) causing them to multiply. Virus remains latent for life after infection. EBV also causes Burkitt lymphoma, a malignant B lymphocyte tumor common in parts of Africa.
Hantavirus	Hantavirus pulmonary syndrome (HPS) with high mortality rate. Spread through inhalation of virus from dried urine of infected rodents.

(continued)

Appendix 5-2   Viral Diseases *(continued)*

Organism	Disease and Description
Hepatitis viruses	Liver inflammation. Varieties A through E are recognized.
Hepatitis A virus (HAV)	Transmitted by fecal contamination. Does not become chronic or produce carrier state. Infection provides lifelong immunity. Vaccine is available.
Hepatitis B virus (HBV)	Transmitted by direct exchange of blood and body fluids. Can cause rapidly fatal disease or develop into chronic disease and carrier state. Risk of progress to liver cancer. Vaccine is available.
Hepatitis C virus (HCV)	Spread through blood exchange (usually transfusions before 1992 when screening began) or shared needles. May become chronic and lead to cirrhosis, liver failure, liver cancer. Antiviral drugs may limit infection.
Hepatitis D virus (HDV)	Spread by blood exchange and occurs as coinfection with hepatitis B. Responsible for half of rapidly fatal liver failure cases and also a high rate of chronic disease that progresses to death.
Hepatitis E virus (HEV)	Transmitted by fecal contamination and occurs in epidemics in Middle East and Asia. Resembles hepatitis A. Can be fatal in pregnant women.
Herpes simplex virus type 1	Cold sores or fever blisters that appear around the mouth and nose of people with colds or other illnesses accompanied by fever.
Herpes simplex virus type 2	Genital herpes. Acute inflammatory disease of the genitalia, often recurring. A very common sexually transmitted infection.
Human immunodeficiency virus (HIV)	Acquired immunodeficiency syndrome (AIDS). Disease that infects T cells of the immune system and is usually fatal if untreatd. Diagnosed by antibody tests, decline in specific (CD4) cells, and presenting disease, including *Candida albicans* infection, *Pneumocystis jirovici* pneumonia (PCP), Kaposi sarcoma, persistent swelling of lymph nodes (lymphadenopathy), chronic diarrhea, and wasting. Spread by contact with contaminated body fluids and by transplacental route.
Human papillomavirus (HPV)	Genital warts (condylomata acuminata). Sexually transmitted warts of the genital and perianal area in men and women. Associated with cervical dysplasia and cancer. A vaccine against the most prevalent strains is available.
Influenza virus	Epidemic viral infection, marked by chills, fever, muscular pains, and prostration. The most serious complication is bronchopneumonia caused by *Haemophilus influenzae* (a bacillus) or streptococci.
Mumps virus	Epidemic parotitis. Acute inflammation with swelling of the parotid salivary glands. Mumps can have many complications, such as orchitis (inflammation of the testes) in young men and meningitis in young children.
Pneumonia viruses	Lung infections caused by a number of different viruses, such as the influenza and parainfluenza viruses, adenoviruses, and varicella viruses.
Poliovirus	Poliomyelitis (polio). Acute viral infection that may attack the anterior horns of the spinal cord, resulting in paralysis of certain voluntary muscles. Most countries have eliminated polio through vaccination programs.
Rhabdovirus	Rabies. An acute, fatal disease transmitted to humans through the saliva of an infected animal. Rabies is characterized by violent muscular spasms induced by the slightest sensations. Because the swallowing of water causes throat spasms, the disease is also call hydrophobia ("fear of water"). The final stage of paralysis ends in death. Rabies vaccines are available for humans and animals.
Rotavirus	Attacks lining of small intestine causing severe diarrhea in children. A new vaccine was approved in 2006.
Rubella virus	Rubella or German measles. A less severe form of measles, but especially dangerous during the first 3 months of pregnancy because the disease organism can cause heart defects, deafness, mental deficiency, and other permanent damage in the fetus.
Rubeola virus	Measles. An acute respiratory inflammation followed by fever and a generalized skin rash. Patients are prone to the development of dangerous complications, such as bronchopneumonia and other secondary infections caused by staphylococci and streptococci.
SARS virus	Highly infectious respiratory disease called severe acute respiratory syndrome (SARS). Emerged in China early in 2003 and spread to other countries before it was isolated and identified as a viral infection. Believed to have spread from small mammals to humans.

(continued)

Appendix 5-2 Viral Diseases (continued)

Organism	Disease and Description
Varicella zoster	Chickenpox (varicella). A usually mild infection, almost completely confined to children, characterized by blisterlike skin eruptions. Vaccine now available.
	Shingles (herpes zoster). A very painful eruption of skin blisters that follows the course of certain peripheral nerves. These blisters eventually dry up and form scabs that resemble shingles. Vaccine now available for people 60 years and older.

Appendix 5-3 Prion Diseases

Agent	Disease
(Note: Prions are infectious agents that contain protein but no nucleic acid. They cause slow, spongy degeneration of brain tissue, known as spongiform encephalitis, in humans and animals.)	
Chronic wasting disease agent	Chronic wasting disease in deer and elk.
Creutzfeldt-Jakob agent	Creutzfeldt-Jacob disease (CJD), a spongiform encephalopathy in humans.
Kuru agent	Kuru spongiform encephalopathy in humans.
Mad cow agent	Mad cow spongiform encephalopathy, or bovine spongiform encephalopathy (BSE) in cows and humans.
Scrapie agent	Scrapie spongiform encephalopathy in sheep.

Appendix 5-4 Fungal Diseases

Disease/Organism	Description
Actinomycosis	"Lumpy jaw" in cattle and humans. The organisms cause the formation of large tissue masses, which are often accompanied by abscesses. The lungs and liver may be involved.
Blastomycosis (*Blastomyces dermatitidis*)	General term for any infection caused by a yeastlike organism. There may be skin tumors and lesions in the lungs, bones, liver, spleen, and kidneys.
Candidiasis (*Candida albicans*)	Infection that can involve the skin and mucous membranes. May cause diaper rash, infection of the nail beds, and infection of the mucous membranes of the mouth (thrush), throat, and vagina.
Coccidioidomycosis (*Coccidioides immitis*)	Systemic fungal disease also called *San Joaquin Valley fever*. Because it often attacks the lungs, it may be mistaken for tuberculosis.
Histoplasmosis (*Histoplasma capsulatum*)	Variety of disorders, ranging from mild respiratory symptoms or enlargement of liver, spleen, and lymph nodes to cavities in the lungs with symptoms similar to those of tuberculosis.
Pneumocystis jiroveci (formerly carinii)	Pneumonia (PCP). Opportunistic infection in people with a depressed immune system. Invades lungs and causes a foamy exudate to collect in alveoli.
Ringworm Tinea capitis Tinea corporis Tinea pedis	Common fungal skin infections, many of which cause blisters and scaling with discoloration of the affected areas. All are caused by similar organisms from a group of fungi called *dermatophytes*. They are easily transmitted by person to person contact or by contaminated articles.

Appendix 5-5   Protozoal Diseases

Organism	Disease And Description
Amebae	
Entamoeba histolytica	Amebic dysentery. Severe ulceration of the wall of the large intestine caused by amebae. Acute diarrhea may be an important symptom. This organism also may cause liver abscesses.
Ciliates	
Balantidium coli	Gastrointestinal disturbances and ulcers of the colon.
Flagellates	
Giardia lamblia	Gastrointestinal disturbances.
Leishmania donovani (and others)	Kala-azar. In this disease, there is enlargement of the liver and spleen as well as skin lesions.
Trichomonas vaginalis	Inflammation and discharge from the vagina. In males, it involves the urethra and causes painful urination.
Trypanosoma	African sleeping sickness. Disease begins with a high fever, followed by invasion of the brain and spinal cord by the organisms. Usually, the disease ends with continued drowsiness, coma, and death.
Sporozoa (apicomplexans)	
Cryptosporidium	Cramps and diarrhea that can be long term and severe in people with a weakened immune system, such as those with AIDS. Spread in water and by personal contact in close quarters.
Plasmodium; varieties include *vivax, falciparum, malariae*	Malaria. Characterized by recurrent attacks of chills followed by high fever. Severe malarial attacks can be fatal because of kidney failure, cerebral disorders, and other complications.
Toxoplasma gondii	Toxoplasmosis. Common infectious disease transmitted by cats and raw meat. Mild forms cause fever and lymph node enlargement. May cause fatal encephalitis in immunosuppressed patients. Infection of a pregnant woman is a cause of fetal stillbirth or congenital damage.

APPENDIX 6
Answers to Chapter Checkpoint and Zooming In Questions

Chapter 1

Answers to Checkpoint Questions

1-1 Study of body structure is anatomy; study of body function is physiology.

1-2 The breakdown phase of metabolism is catabolism; the building phase of metabolism is anabolism.

1-3 Negative feedback systems are primarily used to maintain homeostasis.

1-4 The three planes in which the body can be cut are sagittal, frontal (coronal), and transverse (horizontal). The midsagittal plane divides the body into two equal halves.

1-5 The posterior cavity is the dorsal cavity; the anterior cavity is the ventral cavity.

1-6 The three central regions of the abdomen are the epigastric, umbilical, and hypogastric regions; the three left and right lateral regions of the abdomen are the hypochondriac, lumbar, and iliac (inguinal) regions.

1-7 The basic unit of length in the metric system is the meter; of weight, the gram; of volume, the liter.

Answers to Zooming In Questions

1-7 The figures are standing in the anatomic position.

1-8 The transverse (horizontal) plane divides the body into superior and inferior parts. The frontal (coronal) plane divides the body into anterior and posterior parts.

1-11 The ventral cavity contains the diaphragm.

Chapter 2

Answers to Checkpoint Questions

2-1 Atoms are subunits of elements.

2-2 Three types of particles found in atoms are protons, neutrons, and electrons.

2-3 Molecules are units composed of two or more atoms. They are the subunits of compounds.

2-4 Water is the most abundant compound in the body.

2-5 In a solution, the components dissolve and remain evenly distributed (the mixture is homogeneous); in a suspension, the particles settle out unless the mixture is shaken (the mixture is heterogeneous).

2-6 When an electrolyte goes into solution, it separates into charged particles called ions (cations and anions).

2-7 A covalent bond is formed by the sharing of electrons.

2-8 A value of 7.0 is neutral on the pH scale. An acid measures lower than 7.0; a base measures higher than 7.0.

2-9 A buffer is a substance that maintains a steady pH of a solution.

2-10 Isotopes that break down to give off radiation are termed radioactive.

2-11 Organic compounds are found in living things.

2-12 The element carbon is the basis of organic chemistry.

2-13 The three main categories of organic compounds are carbohydrates, lipids, and proteins.

2-14 A catalyst is a compound that speeds up the rate of a chemical reaction.

Answers to Zooming In Questions

2-1 The number of protons is equal to the number of electrons. There are eight protons and eight electrons.

2-2 Two hydrogen atoms bond with an oxygen atom to form water.

2-4 Two electrons are needed to complete the energy level of each hydrogen atom.

2-5 The amount of hydroxide ion (OH^-) in a solution decreases when the amount of hydrogen ion (H^+) increases.

2-7 Monosaccharides are the building blocks of disaccharides and polysaccharides.

2-8 There are three carbon atoms in glycerol.

2-9 The amino group of an amino acid contains nitrogen.

2-10 The shape of the enzyme after the reaction is the same as it was before the reaction.

Chapter 3

Answers to Checkpoint Questions

3-1 The cell shows organization, metabolism, responsiveness, homeostasis, growth, and reproduction.

3-2 Three types of microscopes are the compound light microscope, transmission electron microscope (TEM), and scanning electron microscope (SEM).

3-3 The main substance of the plasma membrane is a bilayer of phospholipids. Three types of materials found within the membrane are cholesterol, proteins, and carbohydrates (glycoproteins and glycolipids).

3-4 The cell organelles are specialized structures that perform different tasks.

3-5 The nucleus is called the control center of the cell because it contains the chromosomes, hereditary units that control all cellular activities.

3-6 The two types of organelles used for movement are the cilia, which are small and hairlike, and the flagellum, which is long and whiplike.

3-7 Nucleotides are the building blocks of nucleic acids.

3-8 DNA codes for proteins in the cell.

3-9 The three main types of RNA active in protein synthesis are messenger RNA (mRNA), ribosomal RNA (rRNA) and transfer RNA (tRNA).

3-10 Before mitosis can occur, the DNA must replicate (double). The replication occurs during interphase.

3-11 The four stages of mitosis are prophase, metaphase, anaphase, and telophase.

3-12 Diffusion, osmosis, filtration, and facilitated diffusion do not require cellular energy; active transport, endocytosis (phagocytosis and pinocytosis), and exocytosis require cellular energy.

3-13 An isotonic solution is the same concentration as the fluid within the cell; a hypotonic solution is less concentrated; a hypertonic solution is more concentrated.

Answers to Zooming In Questions

3-1 The transmission electron microscope (TEM) shows the most internal structure (B). The scanning electron microscope (SEM) shows the cilia in three dimensions (C).

3-2 Ribosomes attached to the ER make it look rough. Cytosol is the liquid part of the cytoplasm.

3-3 Two layers make up the main substance of the plasma membrane.

3-4 Epithelial cells (B) would best cover a large surface area because they are flat.

3-6 The nucleotides pair up so that there is one large nucleotide and one smaller nucleotide in each pair.

3-9 If the original cell has 46 chromosomes, each daughter cell will have 46 chromosomes after mitosis.

3-11 If diffusion were occurring in the body, the net would be the plasma membrane.

3-12 If the solute could pass through the membrane, the solute and solvent molecules would equalize on the two sides of the membrane, and the fluid level would be the same on both sides.

3-13 If the concentration of solute was increased on side B of this system, the osmotic pressure would increase.

3-15 An increase in the number of transporters would increase the rate of facilitated diffusion. A decrease in the number of transporters would decrease the rate of facilitated diffusion.

3-16 A lysosome would likely help to destroy a particle taken in by phagocytosis.

3-18 If lost blood were replaced with pure water, red blood cells would swell because the blood would become hypotonic to the cells.

Chapter 4

Answers to Checkpoint Questions

4-1 The three basic shapes of epithelium are squamous (flat and irregular), cuboidal (square), and columnar (long and narrow).

4-2 Exocrine glands secrete through ducts; endocrine glands do not have ducts and secrete directly into surrounding tissue and the bloodstream.

4-3 The intercellular material in connective tissue is the matrix.

4-4 The main type of fiber in connective tissue is composed of collagen.

4-5 Circulating connective tissues are blood and lymph. Generalized connective tissues are loose (areolar, adipose) and dense, as found in membranes, capsules, ligaments, and tendons. Structural connective tissues are cartilage and bone.

4-6 The three types of muscle tissue are skeletal (voluntary), cardiac, and smooth (visceral) muscle.

4-7 The basic cellular unit of the nervous system is the neuron and it carries nerve impulses.

4-8 The nonconducting support cells of the nervous system are neuroglia (glial cells).

4-9 The three types of epithelial membranes are the cutaneous membrane (skin), serous membranes, and mucous membranes.

4-10 A benign tumor does not spread; a malignant tumor spreads (metastasizes) to other tissues.

4-11 The three standard approaches to treatment of cancer are surgery, radiation, and chemotherapy.

Answers to Zooming In Questions

4-1 The epithelial cells are in a single layer.

4-5 Areolar connective tissue has the most fibers; adipose tissue is modified for storage.

Chapter 5

Answers to Checkpoint Questions

5-1 Disease is an abnormality of the structure or function of a part, organ, or system.

5-2 A predisposing cause of disease is a factor that may not in itself give rise to a disease but that increases the probability of a person's becoming ill.

5-3 The two medical sciences that are involved in study of disease are pathology (study of disease) and physiology (study of function).

5-4 A communicable disease is one that can be transmitted from one person to another.

5-5 A diagnosis is the identification of an illness based on signs and symptoms.

5-6 A parasite is an organism that lives on or within a host and at the host's expense.

5-7 A pathogen is any disease-causing organism.

5-8 The skin, respiratory tract, digestive, urinary and reproductive systems are portals of entry and exit for microorganisms.

5-9 Microbiology includes the study of bacteria, viruses, fungi, protozoa, and algae.

5-10 The term normal flora refers to the microorganisms that normally live in or on the body.

5-11 Resistant forms of bacteria are called endospores.

5-12 The three basic shapes of bacteria are cocci (round), bacilli (rod-shaped), and curved rods, including vibrios, spirilla, and spirochetes.

5-13 Viruses are smaller than bacteria, are not cellular, and have no enzyme system. They contain only DNA or RNA, not both.

5-14 The protozoa are most animal-like.

5-15 Helminthology is the study of worms.

5-16 Three levels of asepsis are sterilization, disinfection, and antisepsis.

5-17 Handwashing is the single most important measure for preventing the spread of infection.

5-18 An antibiotic is a substance produced by living cells that has the power to kill or arrest the growth of bacteria.

5-19 Stains are used to color cells so that they can be examined under the microscope.

Answers to Zooming In Questions

5-3 Streptococci are the cells shown in Figure 5-3D.

5-5 Flagella indicate that the cells in A are capable of movement.

5-9 The term intracellular means that the parasites are inside cells. Vectors transmit disease organisms from one host to another.

5-10 Skeletal (striated) muscle tissue is shown in B.

Chapter 6
Answers to Checkpoint Questions

6-1 The skin and all its associated structures make up the integumentary system.

6-2 The superficial layer of the skin is the epidermis; the deeper layer is the dermis.

6-3 The subcutaneous layer is composed of loose connective tissue and adipose (fat) tissue.

6-4 The sebaceous glands produce an oily secretion called sebum.

6-5 The sweat glands are the sudoriferous glands.

6-6 Each hair develops within a sheath called the hair follicle.

6-7 Temperature is regulated through the skin by dilation (widening) and constriction (narrowing) of blood vessels and by evaporation of perspiration from the body surface.

6-8 Melanin, hemoglobin, and carotene impart color to the skin.

6-9 A lesion is any wound or local damage to tissue.

6-10 Epithelial and connective tissues repair themselves most easily.

6-11 Dermatosis is any skin disease; dermatitis is inflammation of the skin.

6-12 Melanoma is a cancer of the skin's pigment-producing cells.

6-13 Some viruses that affect the skin are herpes simplex virus, herpes zoster virus, and papillomavirus.

6-14 A fungus causes a tinea or ringworm infection.

6-15 Some autoimmune disorders that involve the skin are pemphigus, lupus erythematosus, and scleroderma.

Answers to Zooming In Questions

6-4 The sebaceous glands and apocrine sweat glands secrete to the outside through the hair follicles. The sweat glands are made of simple cuboidal epithelium.

6-6 Blue color is associated with cyanosis. Yellow color is associated with jaundice.

Chapter 7
Answers to Checkpoint Questions

7-1 The shaft of the long bone is the diaphysis; the end of a long bone is the epiphysis.

7-2 Compact bone makes up the main shaft of long bones and the outer layer of other bones; spongy (cancellous) bone makes up the ends of the long bones and the center of other bones.

7-3 The cells found in bone are osteoblasts, which build bone tissue, osteocytes, which maintain bone, and osteoclasts, which break down (resorb) bone.

7-4 Calcium compounds are deposited in the matrix of bone to harden it.

7-5 The epiphyseal plates are the secondary growth centers of a long bone.

7-6 The markings on bones help to form joints, serve as points for muscle attachments, and allow passage of nerves and blood vessels.

7-7 The skeleton of the trunk consists of the vertebral column and the bones of the thorax, which are the ribs and the sternum.

7-8 The five regions of the vertebral column are the cervical vertebrae, thoracic vertebrae, lumbar vertebrae, sacrum, and coccyx.

7-9 The appendicular skeleton consists of bones of the shoulder girdle, hip, and extremities.

7-10 The three types of joints classified according to the material between the adjoining bones are fibrous, cartilaginous, and synovial.

7-11 A synovial joint or diarthrosis is the most freely movable type of joint.

7-12 Arthritis is the most common type of joint disorder.

Answers to Zooming In Questions

7-5 A suture is the type of joint between bones of the skull.

7-6 The maxilla and palatine bones make up each side of the hard palate.

7-7 A foramen is a hole.

7-9 The anterior fontanel is the largest fontanel.

7-10 The cervical and lumbar vertebrae form a convex curve; the thoracic and sacral vertebrae form a concave curve.

7-14 The costal cartilages attach to the ribs.

7-15 The prefix *supra* means above; the prefix *infra* means below.

7-17 The radius is the lateral bone of the forearm.

7-19 The olecranon of the ulna forms the bony prominence of the elbow.

7-21 The ischium is nicknamed the "sit bone."

7-24 The tibia is the medial bone of the leg.

7-25 The calcaneus is the heel bone.

Chapter 8
Answers to Checkpoint Questions

8-1 The three types of muscle are smooth muscle, cardiac muscle, and skeletal muscle.

8-2 The three main functions of skeletal muscle are movement of the skeleton, maintenance of posture, and generation of heat.

8-3 The neuromuscular junction is the special synapse where a nerve cell makes contact with a muscle cell.

8-4 Acetylcholine (ACh) is the neurotransmitter involved in the stimulation of skeletal muscle cells.

8-5 Excitability and contractility are the two properties of muscle cells that are needed for response to a stimulus.

8-6 Actin and myosin are the filaments that interact to produce muscle contraction.

8-7 Calcium is needed to allow actin and myosin to interact.

8-8 ATP is the compound produced by the oxidation of nutrients that supplies the energy for muscle cell contraction.

8-9 Lactic acid is produced when muscles work without oxygen, causing muscle fatigue.

8-10 A muscle's attachment to a less movable part of the skeleton is the origin; a muscle's attachment to a movable part of the skeleton is the insertion.

8-11 The muscle that produces a movement is called the prime mover; the muscle that produces an opposite movement is the antagonist.

8-12 The action of most muscles is represented by a third-class lever in which the fulcrum is behind the point of effort and the weight.

8-13 The diaphragm is the muscle most important in breathing.

8-14 The muscles of the abdominal wall are strengthened by having the muscle fibers run in different directions.

Answers to Zooming In Questions

8-1 The endomysium is the innermost layer of connective tissue in a skeletal muscle. Perimysium surrounds a fascicle of muscle fibers.

8-5 The actin and myosin filaments do not change in length as muscle contracts, they simply overlap more.

8-7 Contraction of the biceps brachii produces flexion at the elbow.

8-11 The frontalis, temporalis, nasalis, and zygomaticus are named for the bones they are near.

Chapter 9
Answers to Checkpoint Questions

9-1 Structurally, the nervous system can be divided into a central and a peripheral nervous system.

9-2 The somatic nervous system is voluntary and controls skeletal muscle; the autonomic (visceral) nervous system is involuntary and controls involuntary muscles and glands.

9-3 The fiber of the neuron that carries impulses toward the cell body is the dendrite; the fiber that carries impulses away from the cell body is the axon.

9-4 Myelinated fibers are white, and unmyelinated tissues are gray.

9-5 Sensory (afferent) nerves convey impulses toward the CNS; motor (efferent) nerves convey impulses away from the CNS.

9-6 Neuroglia (glial cells) are the nonconducting cells of the nervous system that protect, nourish, and support the neurons.

9-7 In an action potential, depolarization is the stage when the charge on the membrane reverses; repolarization is when the charge returns to the resting state.

9-8 Sodium ion (Na^+) and potassium ion (K^+) are the two ions involved in the generation of an action potential.

9-9 Neurotransmitters are the chemicals used to carry information across the synaptic cleft.

9-10 In the spinal cord, an H-shaped section of gray matter is located internally, and the white matter is located around it. The gray matter extends in two pairs of columns called dorsal and ventral horns.

9-11 The tracts in the white matter of the spinal cord carry impulses to and from the brain. Ascending tracts conduct toward the brain; descending tracts conduct away from the brain.

9-12 A reflex arc is a pathway through the nervous system from a stimulus to an effector.

9-13 There are 31 pairs of spinal nerves.

9-14 There are two neurons in each motor pathway of the autonomic nervous system.

9-15 The sympathetic system stimulates a stress response, and the parasympathetic system reverses it.

Answers to Zooming In Questions

9-2 The neuron shown is a motor neuron.

9-11 No. The spinal cord is not as long as the spinal column. There are seven cervical vertebrae and eight cervical spinal nerves.

9-13 The reflex arc shown is a somatic reflex arc. An interneuron is located between the sensory and motor neurons in the CNS.

9-14 There are two neurons in this spinal reflex. Acetylcholine is the neurotransmitter released at the synapse shown by number 5, as this is a somatic reflex arc involving skeletal muscle.

9-15 The sacral spinal nerves (S1) carry impulses from the skin of the toes. The cervical spinal nerves (C6,7,8) carry impulses from the skin of the anterior hand and fingers.

9-16 The parasympathetic division of the autonomic nervous system has ganglia closer to the effector organ than does the sympathetic system.

Chapter 10

Answers to Checkpoint Questions

10-1 The main divisions of the brain are the cerebrum, diencephalon, brain stem, and cerebellum.

10-2 The three layers of the meninges are the dura mater, arachnoid, and pia mater.

10-3 CSF is produced in the ventricles of the brain. The two lateral ventricles are in the cerebral hemispheres, the third ventricle is in the diencephalon, and the fourth is between the brain stem and the cerebellum.

10-4 The frontal, parietal, temporal and occipital are the four surface lobes of each cerebral hemisphere.

10-5 The cerebral cortex is the outer layer of gray matter of the cerebral hemispheres where higher functions occur.

10-6 The thalamus of the diencephalon directs sensory input to the cerebral cortex; the hypothalamus helps to maintain homeostasis.

10-7 The three subdivisions of the brain stem are the midbrain, pons, and medulla oblongata.

10-8 The cerebellum aids in coordination of voluntary muscles, maintenance of balance, and maintenance of muscle tone.

10-9 Stroke is the common term for cerebrovascular accident.

10-10 Neuroglia are commonly involved in brain tumors.

10-11 There are 12 pairs of cranial nerves.

10-12 A mixed nerve has both sensory and motor fibers.

Answers to Zooming In Questions

10-3 Dural (venous) sinuses are located in the space where the dura mater divides into two layers.

10-4 The fourth ventricle is continuous with the central canal of the spinal cord.

10-5 The lateral ventricles are the largest ventricles.

10-6 The central sulcus separates the frontal from the parietal lobe.

10-7 Folding provides the cortex with increased surface area.

10-8 The primary sensory area (cortex) is posterior to the central sulcus. The primary motor area (cortex) is anterior to the central sulcus.

10-10 The pituitary gland is attached to the hypothalamus of the brain.

Chapter 11

Answers to Checkpoint Questions

11-1 Structures that protect the eye include the skull bones, eyelid, eyelash, eyebrow, conjunctiva, and lacrimal gland.

11-2 The sclera, choroid, and retina are the tunics (coats) of the eyeball.

11-3 The structures that refract light as it passes through the eye are the cornea, aqueous humor, lens, and vitreous body.

11-4 The rods and cones are the receptor cells of the retina.

11-5 The extrinsic eye muscles pull on the eyeball so that both eyes center on one visual field, a process known as convergence.

11-6 The iris adjusts the size of the pupil to regulate the amount of light that enters the eye.

11-7 The ciliary muscle adjusts the thickness of the lens to accommodate for near vision.

11-8 Cranial nerve II is the optic nerve. It carries impulses from the retinal rods and cones to the brain.

11-9 Hyperopia, myopia, and astigmatism are some errors of refraction.

11-10 The ossicles of the middle ear are three small bones, the malleus, incus, and stapes, that transmit sound waves from the tympanic membrane to the inner ear.

11-11 The organ of hearing is the organ of Corti located in the cochlear duct within the cochlea.

11-12 The receptors for equilibrium are located in the vestibule and semicircular canals.

11-13 Static equilibrium and dynamic equilibrium are the two forms of equilibrium.

11-14 The senses of taste and smell are the special senses that respond to chemical stimuli.

11-15 The general senses are touch, pressure, temperature, position (proprioception), and pain.

11-16 Proprioceptors are the receptors that respond to change in position. They are located in muscles, tendons, and joints.

Answers to Zooming In Questions

11-6 Location and direction of fibers are characteristics used in naming the extrinsic eye muscles.

11-7 The circular muscles of the iris contract to make the pupil smaller; the radial muscles contract to make the pupil larger.

11-8 The suspensory ligaments of the ciliary muscle hold the lens in place.

11-10 The oculomotor nerve (III) moves the eye.

11-16 The cilia on the receptor cells bend when the fluid around them moves.

Chapter 12
Answers to Checkpoint Questions

12-1 Hormones are chemicals that have specific regulatory effects on certain cells or organs in the body. Some of their effects are to regulate growth, metabolism, reproduction, and behavior.

12-2 Negative feedback is the main method used to regulate the secretion of hormones.

12-3 The hypothalamus controls the pituitary.

12-4 The anterior pituitary produces growth hormone (GH), thyroid-stimulating hormone (TSH), adrenocorticotropic hormone (ACTH), prolactin (PRL) follicle stimulating hormone (FSH) and luteinizing hormone (LH).

12-5 The posterior pituitary releases antidiuretic hormone (ADH) and oxytocin.

12-6 Thyroid hormones increase the metabolic rate in cells.

12-7 The mineral calcium is regulated by calcitonin and parathyroid hormone (PTH).

12-8 Epinephrine (adrenaline) is the main hormone from the adrenal medulla.

12-9 Glucocorticoids, mineralocorticoids, and sex hormones are released by the adrenal cortex.

12-10 Cortisol raises glucose levels in the blood.

12-11 Insulin and glucagon are the two hormones produced by the pancreatic islets to regulate glucose levels.

12-12 Insulin is low or ineffective in cases of diabetes mellitus.

12-13 Secondary sex characteristics are features associated with gender other than reproductive activity.

12-14 The stomach, small intestine, kidney, brain, heart and placenta are some organs other than endocrine glands that produce hormones.

12-15 Epinephrine, norepinephrine, ACTH, cortisol, growth hormone, thyroid hormones, sex hormones, and insulin are some hormones released in time of stress.

Answers to Zooming In Questions

12-3 The infundibulum connects the hypothalamus and the pituitary gland.

12-4 The larynx is superior to the thyroid; the trachea is inferior to the thyroid.

12-7 The outer region of the adrenal is the cortex; the inner region is the medulla.

Chapter 13
Answers to Checkpoint Questions

13-1 Some substances transported in blood are oxygen, carbon dioxide, nutrients, electrolytes, vitamins, hormones, urea, and toxins.

13-2 7.35 to 7.45 is the pH range of the blood.

13-3 The two main components of the blood are the liquid portion or plasma, and the formed elements, which include the cells and cell fragments.

13-4 Protein is the most abundant type of substance in plasma aside from water.

13-5 Blood cells form in the red bone marrow.

13-6 Hematopoietic stem cells give rise to all blood cells.

13-7 The main function of hemoglobin is to carry oxygen in the blood.

13-8 Neutrophils, eosinophils, and basophils are the granular leukocytes. Lymphocytes and monocytes are the agranular leukocytes.

13-9 The main function of leukocytes is to destroy pathogens.

13-10 The blood platelets are essential to blood coagulation (clotting).

13-11 When fibrinogen converts to fibrin a blood clot forms.

13-12 A, B, AB and O are the four ABO blood type groups.

13-13 The blood antigens most often involved in incompatibility reactions are the A antigen, B antigen, and Rh antigen.

13-14 Blood is commonly separated into its component parts by a centrifuge.

13-15 Anemia is an abnormally low level of red cells or hemoglobin in the blood.

13-16 Leukemia is a cancer of the tissues that produce white cells, resulting in an excess number of white cells in the blood.

13-17 Platelets are low in cases of thrombocytopenia.

13-18 The hematocrit is the percentage of red cell volume in whole blood.

Answers to Zooming In Questions

13-2 Erythrocytes (red blood cells) are the most numerous cells in the blood.

13-3 Erythrocytes are described as biconcave because they have an inward depression on both sides.

13-4 The granulocytes have segmented nuclei. Monocytes are the largest in size. Lymphocytes are the smallest in size.

13-6 Simple squamous epithelium makes up the capillary wall.

13-8 Fibrin in the blood forms a clot.

13-9 No. To test for Rh antigen, you have to use anti-Rh serum. The two types of antigens are independent.

13-10 A neutrophil is in the upper left corner of the picture. Platelets are the small dark bodies between the cells.

Chapter 14
Answers to Checkpoint Questions

14-1 The innermost layer of the heart is the endocardium, the middle is the myocardium, and the outermost is the epicardium.

14-2 The pericardium is the sac that encloses the heart.

14-3 The upper chamber on each side of the heart is the atrium; each lower chamber is the ventricle.

14-4 Valves direct the flow of blood through the heart.

14-5 The coronary circulation is the blood supply to the myocardium.

14-6 The contraction phase of the cardiac cycle is systole; the relaxation phase is diastole.

14-7 Cardiac output is determined by the stroke volume, the volume of blood ejected from the ventricle with each beat, and by the heart rate, the number of times the heart beats per minute.

14-8 The small mass of tissue that starts the heartbeat is the sinoatrial (SA) node.

14-9 The autonomic nervous system is the main influence on the rate and strength of heart contractions.

14-10 A heart murmur is an abnormal heart sound.

14-11 Congenital heart disease is a defect present at birth.

14-12 Rheumatic fever is caused by certain streptococci.

14-13 Atherosclerosis commonly causes narrowing of the coronary vessels.

14-14 ECG and EKG stand for electrocardiography.

14-15 Coronary angioplasty is the technique used to open a restricted coronary artery with a balloon catheter.

Answers to Zooming In Questions

14-1 The left lung is smaller than the right lung because the heart is located more toward the left of the thorax.

14-2 The left ventricle has the thickest wall.

14-4 The aorta carries blood into the systemic circuit.

14-5 The myocardium is the thickest layer of the heart wall.

14-6 The right AV valve has three cusps; the left AV valve has two.

14-10 The AV (tricuspid and mitral) valves close when the ventricles contract, and the semilunar (pulmonary and aortic) valves open.

14-11 The internodal pathways connect the SA and AV nodes.

14-12 The SA and AV nodes are affected by the autonomic nervous system.

14-16 The cardiac cycle shown in the diagram is 0.8 seconds.

Chapter 15
Answers to Checkpoint Questions

15-1 The five types of blood vessels are arteries, arterioles, capillaries, venules, and veins

15-2 The pulmonary circuit carries blood from the heart to the lungs and back to the heart; the systemic circuit carries blood to and from all remaining tissues in the body.

15-3 Smooth muscle makes up the middle layer of arteries and veins. Smooth muscle is involuntary muscle controlled by the autonomic nervous system.

15-4 There is one cell layer in the wall of a capillary.

15-5 The aorta is divided into the ascending aorta, aortic arch, thoracic aorta, and abdominal aorta.

15-6 The common iliac arteries are formed by the final division of the abdominal aorta.

15-7 The brachiocephalic artery supplies the arm and head on the right side.

15-8 An anastomosis is a communication between two vessels.

15-9 Superficial means near the surface.

15-10 The superior vena cava and inferior vena cava drain the systemic circuit and empty into the right atrium.

15-11 A venous sinus is a large channel that drains deoxygenated blood.

15-12 The hepatic portal system takes blood from the abdominal organs to the liver.

15-13 As materials diffuse across the capillary wall, blood pressure helps to push materials out of the capillaries, and the blood osmotic pressure helps to draw materials into the capillaries.

15-14 Vasodilation and vasoconstriction are the two type of vasomotor changes.

15-15 Vasomotor activities are regulated in the medulla of the brain stem.

15-16 The pulse is the wave of pressure that begins at the heart and travels along the arteries.

15-17 Blood pressure is the force exerted by blood against the walls of the vessels.

15-18 Systolic and diastolic blood pressure are measured.

15-19 Hypertension is high blood pressure, and hypotension is low blood pressure.

15-20 Circulatory shock is inadequate blood flow to the tissues.

Answers to Zooming In Questions

15-1 Pulmonary capillaries pick up oxygen. Systemic capillaries release oxygen.

15-2 Veins have valves to control blood flow.

15-3 The artery has a thicker wall than the vein.

15-4 There is one brachiocephalic artery.

15-8 There are two brachiocephalic veins.

15-10 The hepatic veins drain into the inferior vena cava.

15-12 The proximal valve is closer to the heart.

Chapter 16

Answers to Checkpoint Questions

16-1 The lymphatic system drains excess fluid and proteins from the tissues, protects against pathogens, and absorbs fats from the small intestine.

16-2 The lymphatic capillaries are more permeable than blood capillaries and begin blindly. They are closed at one end and do not bridge two vessels.

16-3 The two main lymphatic vessels are the right lymphatic duct and the thoracic duct.

16-4 The lymph nodes filter lymph. They also have lymphocytes and monocytes to fight infection.

16-5 The spleen filters blood.

16-6 T cells of the immune system develop in the thymus.

16-7 Tonsils are located in the vicinity of the pharynx (throat).

16-8 Lymphadenopathy is any disease of the lymph nodes.

16-9 Lymphoma is any tumor of lymphoid tissue. Two examples of malignant lymphoma are Hodgkin disease and nonHodgkin lymphoma.

Answers to Zooming In Questions

16-1 A vein receives lymph collected from the body.

16-5 An afferent vessel carries lymph into a node. An efferent vessel carries lymph out of a node.

Chapter 17

Answers to Checkpoint Questions

17-1 Factors that influence the occurrence of infection include access to preferred body tissues, the portal of entry, virulence, dose, and the individual's predisposition to infection.

17-2 The unbroken skin and mucous membranes constitute the first line of defense against the invasion of pathogens.

17-3 Some nonspecific factors that help to control infection are chemical and mechanical barriers, phagocytosis, natural killer cells, inflammation, fever, and interferon.

17-4 Innate immunity is inherited in a person's genetic material; adaptive immunity is acquired during an individual's lifetime.

17-5 An antigen is any foreign substance, usually a protein, that induces an immune response.

17-6 Four types of T cells are cytotoxic, helper, regulatory, and memory.

17-7 An antibody is a substance produced in response to an antigen.

17-8 Plasma cells, derived from B cells, produce antibodies.

17-9 Complement is a group of proteins in the blood that sometimes is required for the destruction of foreign cells.

17-10 The active form of natural adaptive immunity comes from contact with a disease organism; the passive form comes from the passage of antibodies from a mother to her fetus through the placenta, colostrum, or breast milk.

17-11 Bacterial diseases for which there are vaccines include smallpox, whooping cough (pertussis), diphtheria, tetanus, *Haemophilus influenzae* type b (Hib), and pneumococcus.

17-12 Viral diseases for which there are vaccines include poliomyelitis, measles (rubeola), mumps, rubella (German measles), hepatitis A and B, chicken pox (varicella), influenza, rotavirus, human papilloma virus (HPV), and rabies.

17-13 An immune serum is an antiserum prepared in an animal; immune sera can be used in emergencies to provide passive immunization.

17-14 Disorders of the immune system include allergy, autoimmunity, and immune deficiency diseases.

17-15 The tendency of every organism to destroy foreign substances is the greatest obstacle to transplantation of tissues from one individual to another.

Answers to Zooming In Questions

17-2 Digestive enzymes are contained in the lysosome that joins the phagocytic vesicle.

17-3 Plasma cells and memory cells develop from activated B cells.

Chapter 18

Answers to Checkpoint Questions

18-1 The three phases of respiration are pulmonary ventilation, external exchange of gases, and internal exchange of gases.

18-2 As air passes over the nasal mucosa, it is filtered, warmed, and moistened.

18-3 The scientific name for the throat is pharynx, for the voice box is larynx, and for the windpipe is trachea.

18-4 The three regions of the pharynx are the nasopharynx, oropharynx, and laryngeal pharynx.

18-5 The cells that line the respiratory passageways have cilia to filter impurities and to move fluids.

18-6 Gas exchange in the lungs occurs in the alveoli.

18-7 The pleura is the membrane that encloses the lung.

18-8 The two phases of breathing are inhalation, which is active, and exhalation, which is passive.

18-9 Diffusion is the movement of molecules from an area in which they are in higher concentration to an area where they are in lower concentration.

18-10 Hemoglobin is the substance in red blood cells that carries almost all of the oxygen in the blood.

18-11 The main form in which carbon dioxide is carried in the blood is as bicarbonate ion.

18-12 The medulla of the brain stem sets the basic pattern of respiration.

18-13 The phrenic nerve is the motor nerve that controls the diaphragm.

18-14 Carbon dioxide is the main chemical controller of respiration.

18-15 COPD is chronic obstructive pulmonary disease. Chronic bronchitis and emphysema are commonly involved in COPD.

Answers to Zooming In Questions

18-2 The heart is located in the medial depression of the left lung.

18-4 The epiglottis is named for its position above the glottis.

18-7 The external and internal intercostals are the muscles between the ribs.

18-8 Gas pressure decreases as the volume of its container increases.

18-9 Residual volume can not be measured with a spirometer.

18-14 The esophagus is posterior to the trachea.

Chapter 19

Answers to Checkpoint Questions

19-1 Food must be broken down by digestion into particles small enough to pass through the plasma membrane.

19-2 The digestive tract has a wall composed of a mucous membrane (mucosa), a submucosa, smooth muscle, and a serous membrane (serosa).

19-3 The peritoneum is the large serous membrane that lines the abdominopelvic cavity and covers the organs it contains.

19-4 There are 20 baby teeth, which are also called deciduous teeth.

19-5 Proteins are digested in the stomach.

19-6 The three divisions of the small intestine are the duodenum, jejunum, and ileum.

19-7 Most digestion takes place in the small intestine under the effects of digestive juices from the small intestine and the accessory organs. Most absorption of digested food and water also occurs in the small intestine.

19-8 The divisions of the large intestine are the cecum, ascending colon, transverse colon, descending colon, sigmoid colon, and rectum.

19-9 The large intestine reabsorbs some water and stores, forms, and eliminates the stool. It also houses bacteria that provide some vitamins.

19-10 The salivary glands are the parotid, submandibular (submaxillary), and sublingual.

19-11 The gallbladder stores bile.

19-12 Bile emulsifies fats.

19-13 The pancreas produces the most complete digestive secretions.

19-14 Absorption is the movement of digested nutrients into the circulation.

19-15 The two types of control over the digestive process are nervous control and hormonal control.

19-16 Hunger is the desire for food that can be satisfied by the ingestion of a filling meal. Appetite is a desire for food that is unrelated to a need for food.

19-17 Caries, gingivitis, and periodontitis are common diseases of the mouth and teeth.

19-18 Crohn disease and ulcerative colitis are inflammatory bowel diseases.

19-19 Hepatitis is inflammation of the liver.

Answers to Zooming In Questions

19-1 Smooth muscle (circular and longitudinal) is between the submucosa and the serous membrane in the digestive tract wall.

19-3 The mesentery is the part of the peritoneum around the small intestine.

19-4 The salivary glands are the accessory organs that secrete into the mouth.

19-7 The oblique muscle layer is an additional muscle layer in the stomach as compared to the rest of the digestive tract.

19-8 The ileum of the small intestine joins the cecum.

19-10 The accessory organs shown secrete into the duodenum.

Chapter 20

Answers to Checkpoint Questions

20-1 The two phases of metabolism are catabolism, the breakdown phase of metabolism, and anabolism, the building phase of metabolism.

20-2 Cellular respiration is the series of reactions that releases energy from nutrients in the cell.

20-3 Glucose is the main energy source for the cells.

20-4 An essential amino acid or fatty acid cannot be made metabolically and must be taken in as part of the diet.

20-5 Minerals are chemical elements, and vitamins are complex organic substances.

20-6 The normal range of blood glucose is 85 to 125 mg/dL

20-7 Typical recommendations are 55% to 60% carbohydrate; 30% or less fat; 15% to 20% protein.

20-8 Some factors that affect heat production are exercise, hormone production, food intake, and age.

20-9 The hypothalamus of the brain is responsible for regulating body temperature.

20-10 Normal body temperature is 36.2°C to 37.6°C (97°F to 100°F).

20-11 Heat cramps, heat exhaustion, and heat stroke are brought on by excessive heat.

20-12 Hypothermia is excessively low body temperature.

Answers to Zooming In Questions

20-1 Pyruvic acid produces lactic acid under anaerobic conditions; it produces CO_2 and H_2O under aerobic conditions.

20-4 The BMI is 24 (77 ÷ 3.2 = 24).

Chapter 21

Answers to Checkpoint Questions

21-1 Body fluids are grouped into intracellular fluid and extracellular fluid.

21-2 Water is lost from the body through the kidneys, the skin, the lungs, and the intestinal tract.

21-3 The control center for the sense of thirst is located in the hypothalamus of the brain.

21-4 Sodium is the main cation in extracellular fluid. Potassium is the main cation in intracellular fluid.

21-5 Chloride is the main anion in extracellular fluid.

21-6 Some electrolytes are lost through the feces and sweat. The kidneys have the main job of balancing electrolytes. Several hormones, such as aldosterone, parathyroid hormone, and calcitonin, are also involved.

21-7 The acid–base balance of body fluids is maintained by buffer systems, respiration, and kidney function.

21-8 Abnormally low pH of body fluids results in acidosis; abnormally high pH of body fluids results in alkalosis.

21-9 Edema is the accumulation of excessive fluid in the intercellular spaces.

Answers to Zooming In Questions

21-1 Water is lost through the skin, lungs, kidneys, and intestine.

Chapter 22

Answers to Checkpoint Questions

22-1 Systems other than the urinary system that eliminate waste include the digestive, respiratory, and integumentary systems.

22-2 The urinary system consists of two kidneys, two ureters, the bladder, and the urethra.

22-3 The retroperitoneal space is posterior to the peritoneum.

22-4 The renal artery supplies blood to the kidney, and the renal vein drains blood from the kidney.

22-5 The outer region of the kidney is the renal cortex; the inner region is the renal medulla.

22-6 The nephron is the functional unit of the kidney.

22-7 The glomerulus is the coil of capillaries in the glomerular (Bowman) capsule.

22-8 Glomerular filtration is the movement of materials under pressure from the blood into the glomerular capsule of the nephron.

22-9 The four processes involved in the formation of urine are glomerular filtration, tubular reabsorption, tubular secretion, and the countercurrent mechanism for concentrating the urine.

22-10 The JG apparatus produces renin when blood pressure falls too low for the kidneys to function effectively. The signal for renin production is low volume or low sodium in the filtrate leaving the nephron.

22-11 The ureter carries urine from the kidney to the bladder.

22-12 The urethra carries urine from the bladder to the outside.

22-13 Acute kidney disorders arise suddenly, usually as a result of infection. Chronic conditions arise slowly and are often progressive, with gradual loss of kidney functions.

22-14 The scientific name for stones is calculi.

22-15 Inflammation of the bladder is cystitis.

Answers to Zooming In Questions

22-1 The renal artery supplies blood to the kidney. The renal vein drains blood from the kidney.

22-2 The aorta supplies blood to the renal artery. The inferior vena cava receives blood from the renal vein.

22-3 The outer region of the kidney is the renal cortex. The inner region of the kidney is the renal medulla.

22-4 The proximal convoluted tubule is closer to the glomerular capsule. The distal convoluted tubule is farther away from the glomerular capsule.

22-6 The afferent arteriole has a wider diameter than the efferent arteriole.

22-9 The juxtaglomerular apparatus is made up of cells from the afferent arteriole and the distal convoluted tubule.

22-10 The urethra passes through the prostate gland in the male.

Chapter 23

Answers to Checkpoint Questions

23-1   Meiosis is the process of cell division that halves the chromosome number in a cell to produce a gamete.

23-2   The testis is the male gonad. Testosterone is the main male sex hormone.

23-3   The spermatozoon, or sperm cell, is the male sex cell (gamete).

23-4   The main subdivisions of the sperm cell are the head, midpiece, and tail (flagellum).

23-5   Sperm cells leave the seminiferous tubules within the testis and then travel through the epididymis, ductus (vas) deferens, ejaculatory duct, and urethra.

23-6   Glands that contribute secretions to the semen, aside from the testes, are the seminal vesicles, prostate, and bulbourethral glands.

23-7   Follicle-stimulating hormone (FSH) and luteinizing hormone (LH) are the pituitary hormones that regulate male and female reproduction.

23-8   Infectious diseases of the reproductive tract include chlamydial and gonococcal infections, genital herpes, syphilis, *E. coli* infections, mumps.

23-9   The ovary is the female gonad.

23-10 The ovum (egg cell) is the female gamete.

23-11 The ovarian (graafian) follicle surrounds the egg as it ripens.

23-12 Ovulation is the process of releasing an egg cell from the ovary.

23-13 The follicle becomes the corpus luteum after ovulation

23-14 The fetus develops in the uterus.

23-15 The two hormones produced in the ovaries are estrogen and progesterone.

23-16 Menopause is the period during which menstruation ceases.

23-17 Contraception is the use of artificial methods to prevent fertilization of the ovum or implantation of the fertilized ovum.

Answers to Zooming In Questions

23-1   The four glands that empty secretions into the urethra are the testes, seminal vesicles, prostate, and bulbourethral glands.

23-2   The ductus (vas) deferens receives secretions from the epididymis.

23-4   Mitochondria are the organelles that provide energy for sperm cell motility.

23-5   The corpus spongiosum of the penis contains the urethra.

23-8   The fundus of the uterus is the deepest part.

23-10 The endometrium is most highly developed in the second part of the menstrual cycle.

23-11 The opening of the urethra is anterior to the opening of the vagina.

23-13 LH shows the greatest increase at the time of ovulation.

Chapter 24

Answers to Checkpoint Questions

24-1   A zygote is formed by the union of an ovum and a spermatozoon.

24-2   The placenta nourishes the developing fetus.

24-3   The umbilical cord carries blood between the fetus and the placenta.

24-4   Fetal circulation is adapted to bypass the lungs

24-5   The heartbeat first appears during the fourth week of embryonic development.

24-6   The amniotic sac is the fluid-filled sac that holds the fetus.

24-7   The approximate length of pregnancy in days is 266.

24-8   Parturition is the process of labor and delivery.

24-9   A cesarean section is an incision made in the abdominal wall and the uterine wall for delivery of a fetus.

24-10 The term viable with reference to a fetus means able to live outside the uterus.

24-11 Lactation is the secretion of milk from the mammary glands.

24-12 An ectopic pregnancy is one that develops in a location outside the uterine cavity.

24-13 Puerperal infection is an infection that is related to childbirth.

Answers to Zooming In Questions

24-1   The ovum is fertilized in the oviduct (fallopian, uterine) tube.

24-2   The purple color signifies a mixture of oxygenated and unoxygenated blood.

24-5   The umbilical cord connects the fetus to the placenta.

24-7   The pectoralis major underlies the breast.

Chapter 25

Answers to Checkpoint Questions

25-1   A gene is an independent unit of heredity. Each is a segment of DNA contained in a chromosome.

25-2   A dominant gene is always expressed, regardless of the gene on the matching chromosome. A recessive gene is only expressed if the gene on the matching chromosome is also recessive.

25-3 Meiosis is the process of cell division that forms the gametes.

25-4 The sex chromosome combination that determines a female is XX; a male is XY.

25-5 A trait carried on a sex chromosome is described as sex-linked.

25-6 A mutation is a change in a cell's genetic material (a gene or chromosome).

25-7 A congenital disease is present at birth. A hereditary disease is genetically transmitted or transmissible. A disorder may occur during development and be present at birth but not be inherited through the genes.

25-8 Phenylketonuria is caused by a hereditary lack of an enzyme needed for phenylalanine metabolism.

25-9 A pedigree is a complete, detailed family history. It is used to determine the inheritance pattern of a genetic disease within a family.

25-10 A karyotype is a picture of the chromosomes cut out and arranged in groups according to size and form.

Answers to Zooming In Questions

25-1 25% of children will show the recessive phenotype blond hair. 50% of children will be heterozygous.

25-5 The possible genotypes of the two normal children in the F3 generation are CC or Cc.

25-7 There are 44 autosomes shown in B.

Dissection Atlas

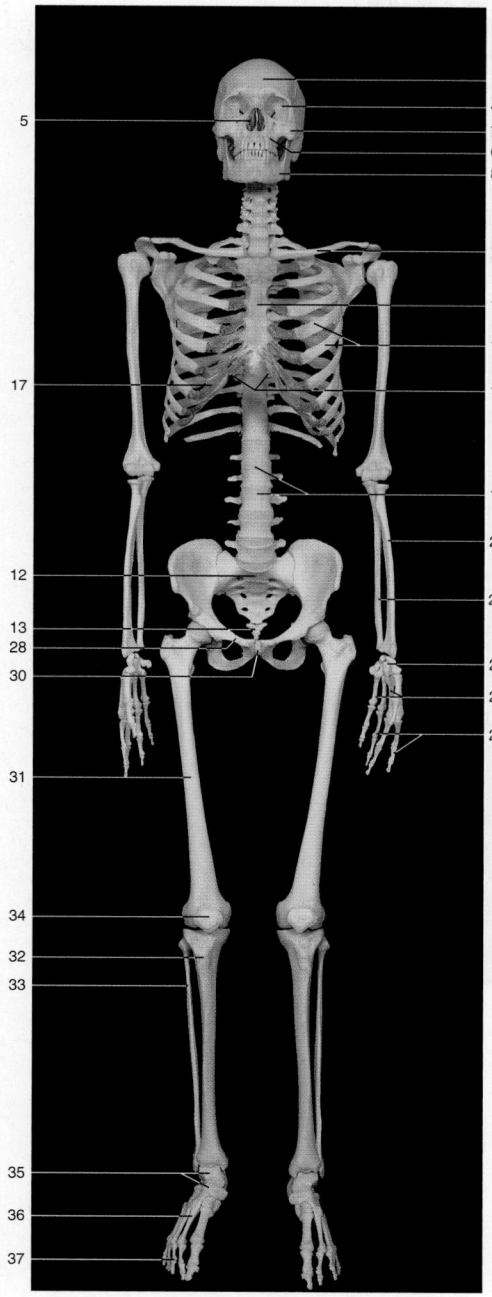

Axial skeleton
Head

1	Frontal bone
4	Orbit
5	Nasal cavity
6	Maxilla
7	Zygomatic bone
8	Mandible

Trunk and thorax
Vertebral column

12	Sacrum
13	Coccyx
14	Intervertebral discs

Thorax

15	Sternum
16	Ribs
17	Coastal cartilate
18	Infrasternal angle

Appendicular skeleton
Upper limb and shoulder girdle

19	Clavicle
22	Radius
23	Ulna
24	Carpal bones
25	Metacarpal bones
26	Phalanges of the hand

Lower limb and pelvis

28	Pubix
30	Symphysis pubix
31	Femur
32	Tibia
33	Fibula
34	Patella
35	Tarsal bones
36	Metatarsal bones
37	Phalanges of the foot

Figure A7-1 **Skeleton of a female adult (anterior aspect).** (Reprinted with permission from Rohen JW, Yokochi C, Lütjen-Drecoll E. *Color Atlas of Anatomy*, 6th ed. Stuttgart, New York: Schattauer, 2006.)

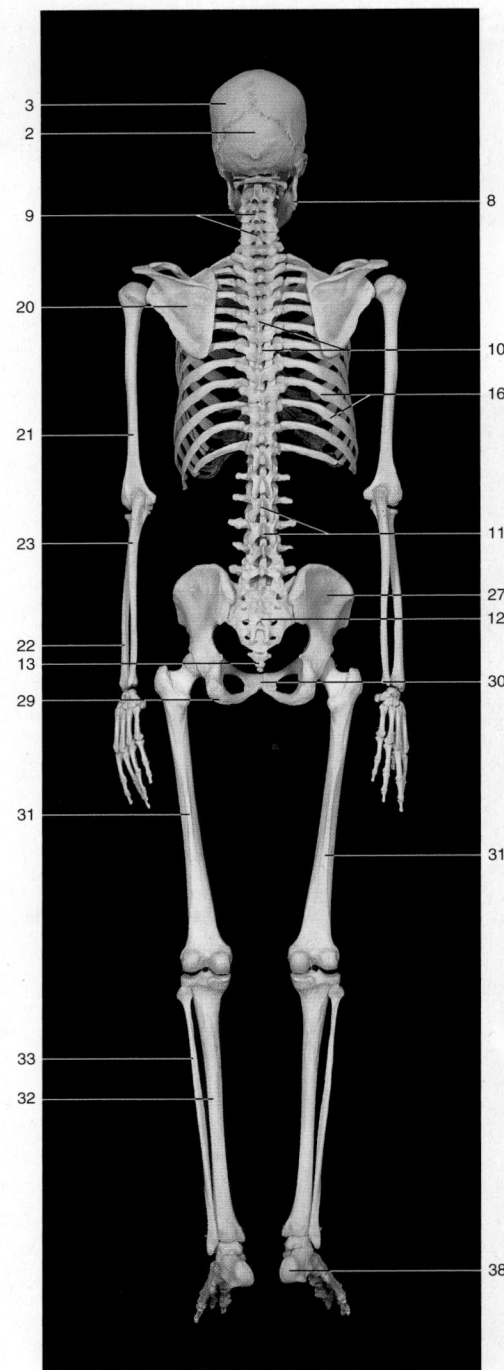

Axial skeleton
Head

2 Occipital bone
3 Parietal bone
8 Mandible

Trunk and thorax
Vertebral column

9   Cervical vertebrae
10 Thoracic vertebrae
11 Lumbar vertebrae
12 Sacrum
13 Coccyx

Thorax

16 Ribs

Appendicular skeleton
Upper limb and shoulder girdle

20 Scapula
21 Humerus
22 Radius
23 Ulna

Lower limb and pelvis

27 Ilium
29 Ischium
30 Symphysis pubix
31 Femur
32 Tibia
33 Fibula
38 Calcaneus

Figure A7-2 **Skeleton of a female adult (posterior aspect).** (Reprinted with permission from Rohen JW, Yokochi C, Lütjen-Drecoll E. *Color Atlas of Anatomy,* 6th ed. Stuttgart, New York: Schattauer, 2006.)

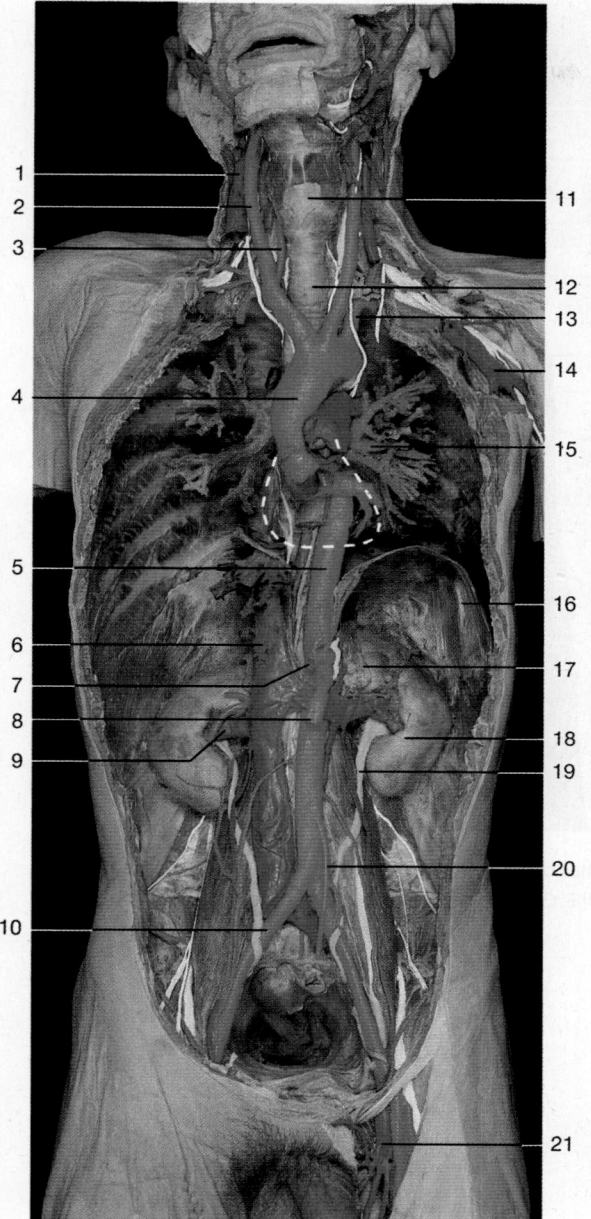

1	Internal jugular vein
2	Common carotid artery
3	Vertebral artery
4	Ascending aorta
5	Descending aorta
6	Inferior vena cava
7	Celiac trunk
8	Superior mesenteric artery
9	Renal vein
10	Common iliac artery
11	Larynx
12	Trachea
13	Left subclavian artery
14	Left axillary vein
15	Pulmonary veins
16	Diaphragm
17	Suprarenal gland
18	Kidney
19	Ureter
20	Inferior mesenteric artery
21	Femoral vein

Figure A7-3 **Major vessels of the trunk.** The position of the heart is indicated by the dotted line. (Reprinted with permission from Rohen JW, Yokochi C, Lütjen-Drecoll E. *Color Atlas of Anatomy*, 6th ed. Stuttgart, New York: Schattauer, 2006.)

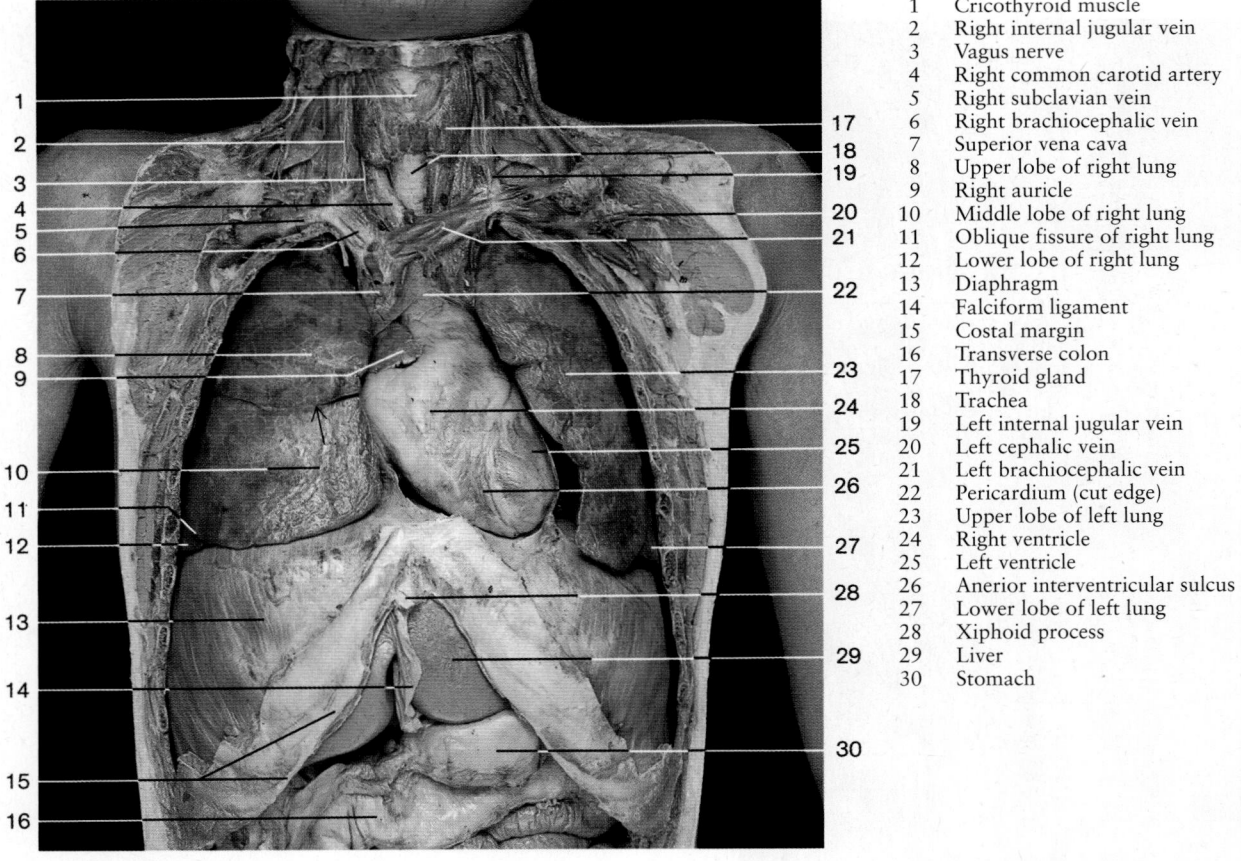

1   Cricothyroid muscle
2   Right internal jugular vein
3   Vagus nerve
4   Right common carotid artery
5   Right subclavian vein
6   Right brachiocephalic vein
7   Superior vena cava
8   Upper lobe of right lung
9   Right auricle
10 Middle lobe of right lung
11 Oblique fissure of right lung
12 Lower lobe of right lung
13 Diaphragm
14 Falciform ligament
15 Costal margin
16 Transverse colon
17 Thyroid gland
18 Trachea
19 Left internal jugular vein
20 Left cephalic vein
21 Left brachiocephalic vein
22 Pericardium (cut edge)
23 Upper lobe of left lung
24 Right ventricle
25 Left ventricle
26 Anerior interventricular sulcus
27 Lower lobe of left lung
28 Xiphoid process
29 Liver
30 Stomach

Figure A7-4 **Positions of thoracic organs.** The anterior thoracic wall has been removed. Arrow: horizontal fissure of the right lung. (Reprinted with permission from Rohen JW, Yokochi C, Lütjen-Drecoll E. *Color Atlas of Anatomy*, 6th ed. Stuttgart, New York: Schattauer, 2006.)

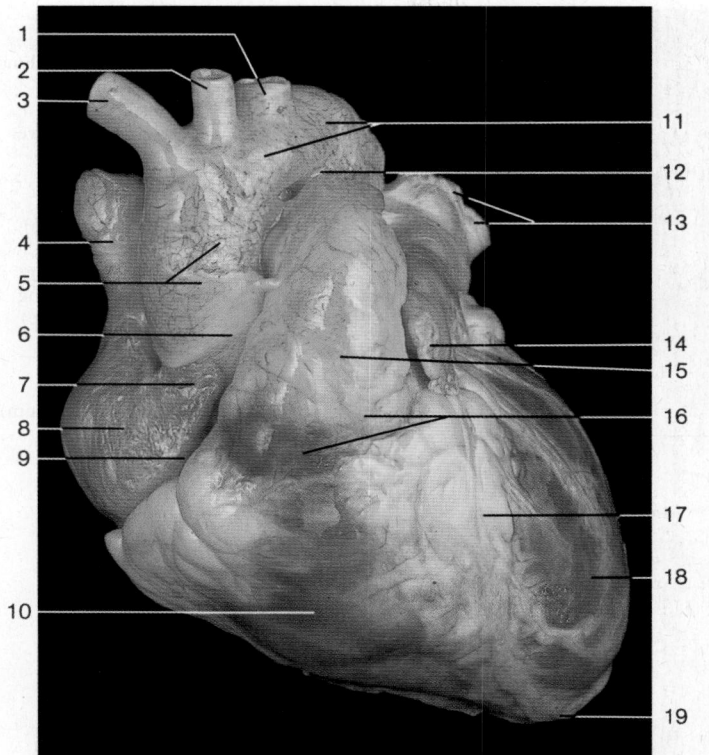

1   Left subclavian artery
2   Left common carotic artery
3   Brachiocephalic trunk
4   Superior vena cava
5   Ascending aorta
6   Bulb of the aorta
7   Right auricle
8   Right atrium
9   Coronary sulcus
10 Right ventricle
11 Aortic arch
12 Ligamentum arteriosum
13 Left pulmonary veins
14 Left auricle
15 Pulmonary trunk
16 Sinus of pulmonary trunk
17 Anterior interventricular sulcus
18 Left ventricle
19 Apex of the heart

Figure A7-5 **Heart of a 30-year-old woman (anterior aspect).** (Reprinted with permission from Rohen JW, Yokochi C, Lütjen-Drecoll E. *Color Atlas of Anatomy*, 6th ed. Stuttgart, New York: Schattauer, 2006.)

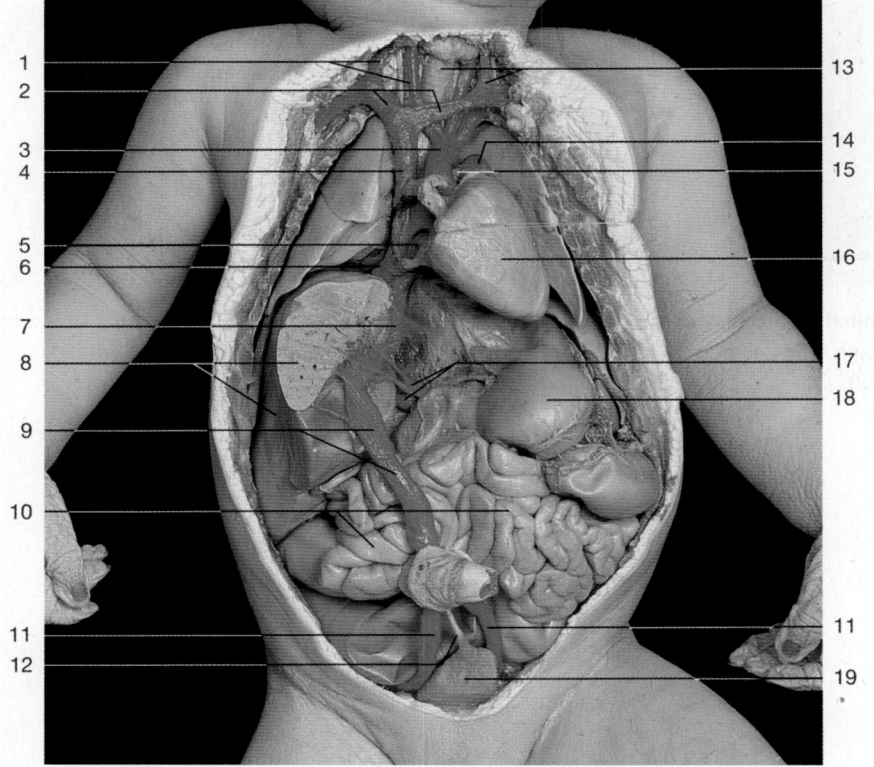

1   Internal jugular vein and right common carotid artery
2   Right and left brachiocephalic vein
3   Aortic arch
4   Superior vena cava
5   Foramen ovale
6   Inferior vena cava
7   Ductus venosus
8   Liver
9   Umbilical vein
10 Small intestine
11 Umbilical artery
12 Urachus
13 Trachea and left internal jugular vein
14 Left pulmonary artery
15 Ductus arteriosus (Botalli)
16 Right ventricle
17 Hepatic arteries (red) and portal vein (blue)
18 Stomach
19 Urinary bladder

Figure A7-6 **Thoracic and abdominal regions in the newborn (anterior aspect).** The right atrium has been opened to show the foramen ovale. The left lobe of the liver has been removed. (Reprinted with permission from Rohen JW, Yokochi C, Lütjen-Drecoll E. *Color Atlas of Anatomy*, 6th ed. Stuttgart, New York: Schattauer, 2006.)

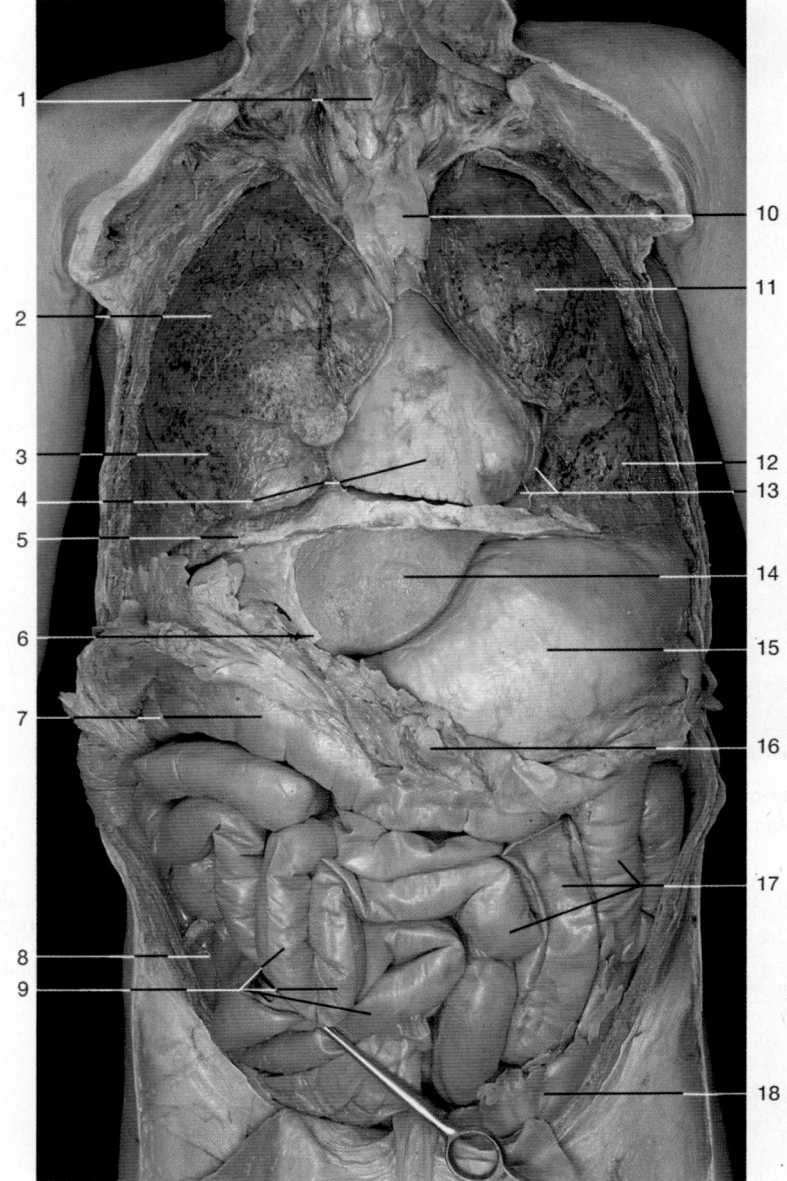

1   Thyroid gland
2   Upper lobe of right lung
3   Middle lobe of right lung
4   Heart
5   Diaphragm
6   Round ligament of liver
      (ligamentum teres)
7   Transverse colon
8   Cecum
9   Small intestine (ileum)
10   Thymus
11   Upper lobe of left lung
12   Lower lobe of left lung
13   Pericardium (cut edge)
14   Liver (left lobe)
15   Stomach
16   Greater omentum
17   Small intestine (jejunum)
18   Sigmoid colon

Figure A7-7 **Abdominal organs in situ.** The greater omentum has been partly removed or reflected. (Reprinted with permission from Rohen JW, Yokochi C, Lütjen-Drecoll E. *Color Atlas of Anatomy*, 6th ed. Stuttgart, New York: Schattauer, 2006.)

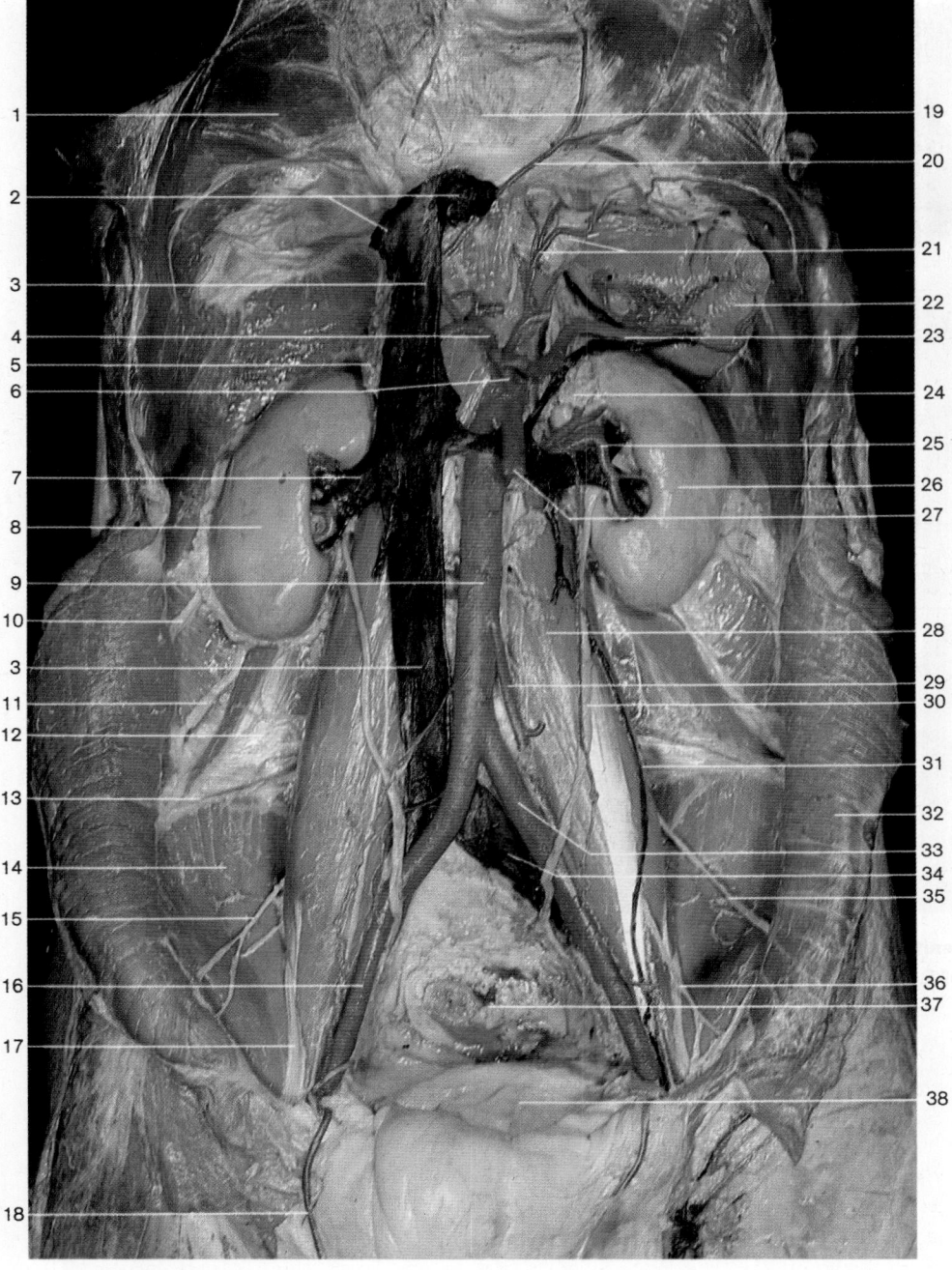

1   Diaphragm
2   Hepatic veins
3   Inferior vena cava
4   Common hepatic artery
5   Suprarenal gland
6   Celiac trunk
7   Right renal vein
8   Kidney
9   Abdominal aorta
10 Subcostal nerve
11 Iliohypogastric nerve
12 Central tendon of di-
    aphragm
13 Inferior phrenic artery
14 Cardiac part of stomach
15 Spleen
16 Splenic artery
17 Superior renal artery
18 Superior mesenteric artery
19 Psoas major muscle
20 Inferior mesenteric artery
21 Ureter

Figure A7-8 **Retroperitoneal organs, kidneys, and suprarenal glands in situ (anterior aspect).** Red, arteries; blue, veins. (Reprinted with permission from Rohen JW, Yokochi C, Lütjen-Drecoll E. *Color Atlas of Anatomy*, 6th ed. Stuttgart, New York: Schattauer, 2006.)

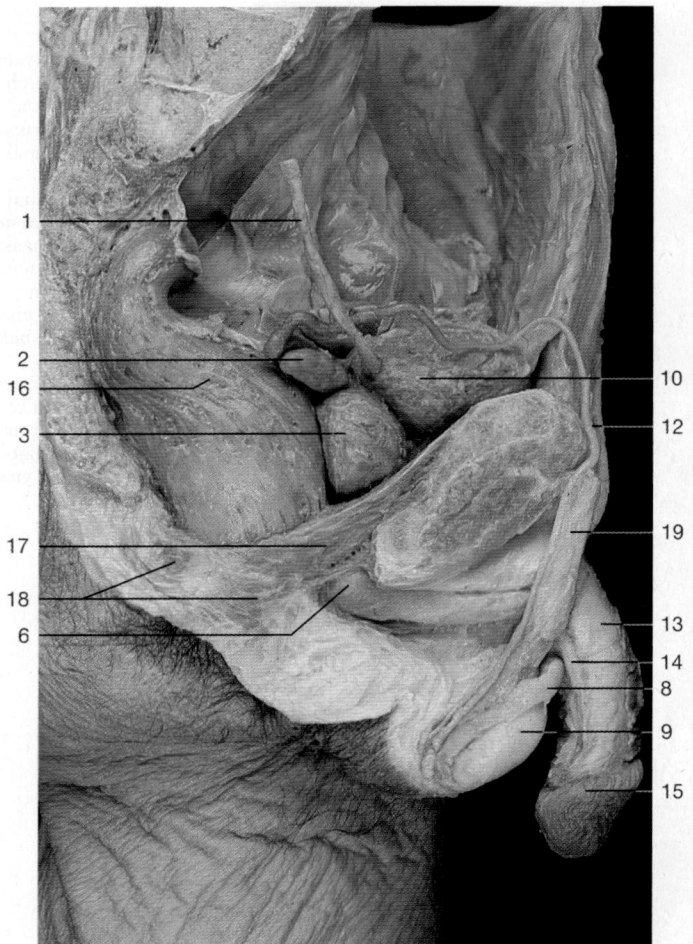

1   Ureter
2   Seminal vesicle
3   Prostate gland
6   Bulb of penis
8   Epididymis
9   Testis
10 Urinary bladder
12 Ductus deferens
13 Corpus cavernosum of penis
14 Corpus spongiosum of penis
15 Glans penis
16 Ampulla of rectum
17 Levator ani muscle
18 Anal canal and external anal
    sphincter muscle
19 Spermatic cord (cut)

Figure A7-9 **Male genital organs in situ (right lateral aspect).** (Reprinted with permission from Rohen JW, Yokochi C, Lütjen-Drecoll E. *Color Atlas of Anatomy*, 6th ed. Stuttgart, New York: Schattauer, 2006.)

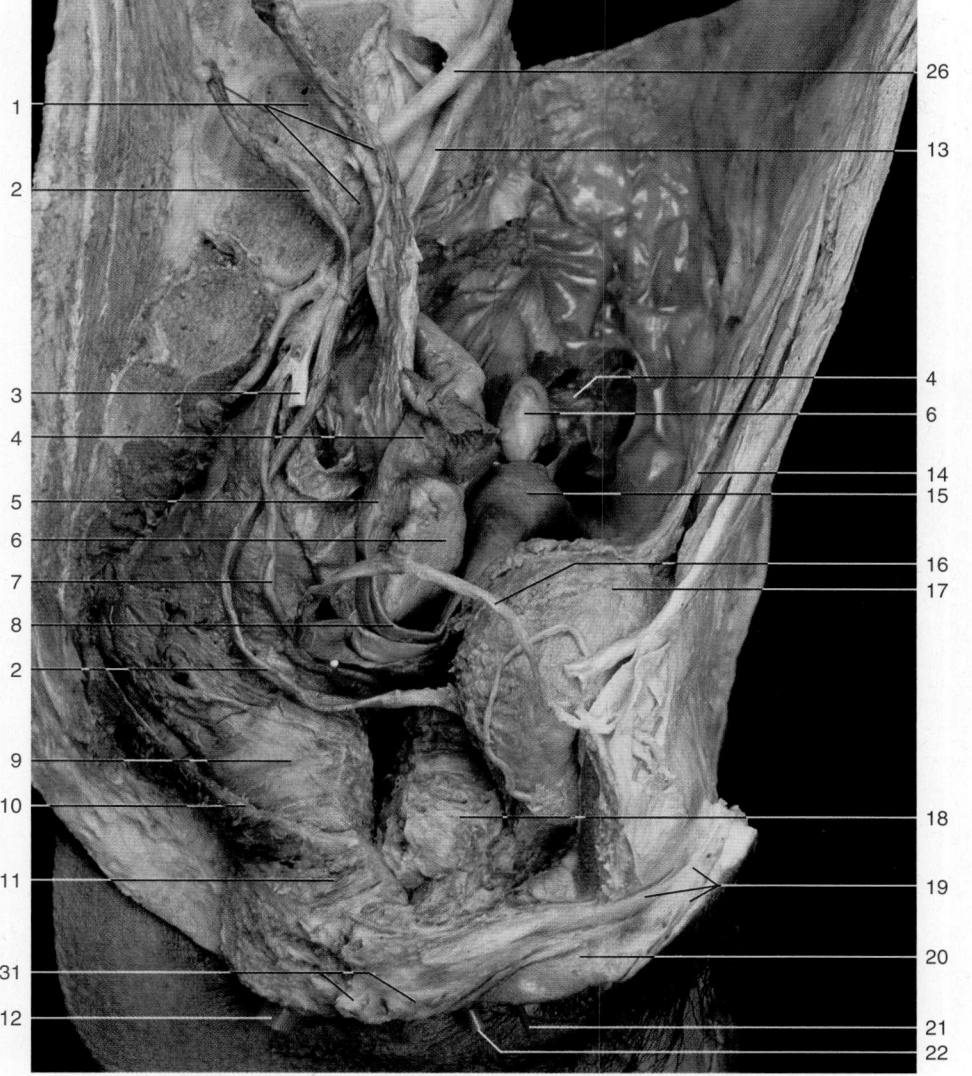

1   Body of fifth lumbar vertebra, suspensory ligament of ovary, and sacral promontory
2   Ureter
3   Medial umbilical ligament (remnant of umbilical artery) (cut)
4   Infundibulum of uterine tube
5   Ampulla of uterine tube
6   Ovary
7   Uterine artery
8   Uterine tube
9   Rectum
10   Levator ani muscle (pelvic diaphragm – cut edge)
11   External anal sphincter muscle
12   Anus (probe)
13   Internal iliac artery
14   Remnant of urachus (median umbilical ligament)
15   Uterus
16   Round ligament of uterus
17   Urinary bladder
18   Vagina
19   Clitoris
20   Labium minus
21   External orifice of urethra (red probe)
22   Vaginal orifice (green probe)
26   External iliac artery
31   Greater vestibular gland and bulb of the vestibule

Figure A7-10 **Female internal genital organs in situ.** Right half of the pelvis and sacrum have been removed. (Reprinted with permission from Rohen JW, Yokochi C, Lütjen-Drecoll E. *Color Atlas of Anatomy*, 6th ed. Stuttgart, New York: Schattauer, 2006.)

Index

Page numbers in *italics* denote figures; page numbers followed by *t* denote tables; and page numbers followed by *B* denote boxes.

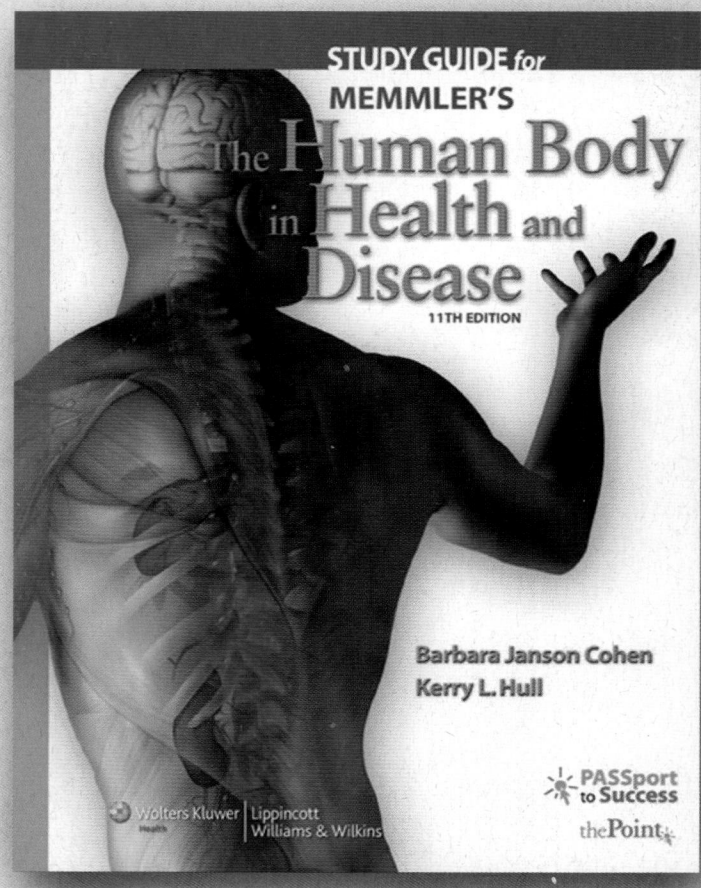